OH'S INT[illegible] RE MANUAL

SEVENTH EDITION

Content Strategist: Michael Houston
Content Development Specialist: Nani Clansey
Content Coordinator: Sam Crowe, Humayra Rahman
Project Manager: Umarani Natarajan
Design: Miles Hitchen
Illustration Manager: Jennifer Rose
Illustrator: Kinesis Illustration
Marketing Manager: Abigail Swartz

Seventh Edition

OH'S INTENSIVE CARE MANUAL

Edited by

Andrew D Bersten
MB BS MD FCICM

Director, Intensive Care Unit, Flinders Medical Centre
Professor and Head, Department of Critical Care Medicine
Flinders University
Adelaide, SA, Australia

Neil Soni
MB ChB MD FANZCA FRCA FCICM FFICM

Consultant in Intensive Care
Chelsea and Westminster Hospital
Honorary Senior Lecturer
Imperial College Medical School
London, United Kingdom

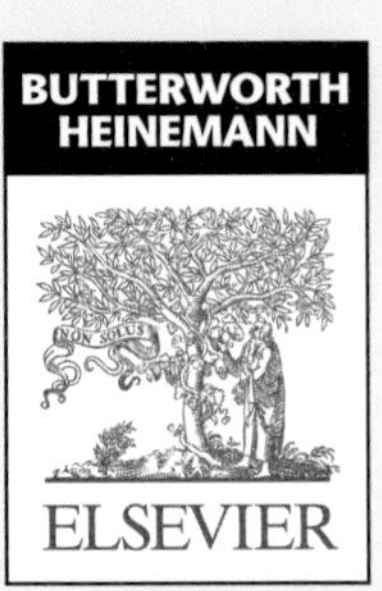

For additional online content visit expertconsult.com

Expert CONSULT

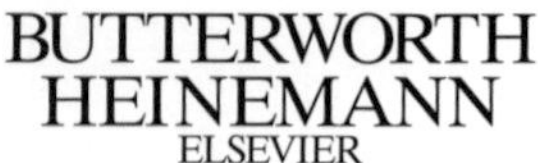

First edition 1979
Second edition 1985
Third edition 1990
Fourth edition 1997
Fifth edition 2003
Sixth edition 2009
Seventh edition 2014
Reprinted 2014

ISBN: 978-0-7020-4762-6
Ebook ISBN: 978-1-4557-5013-9

British Library Cataloguing in Publication Data
A catalogue record for this book is available from the British Library

Library of Congress Cataloging in Publication Data
A catalog record for this book is available from the Library of Congress

Notices
Knowledge and best practice in this field are constantly changing. As new research and experience broaden our understanding, changes in research methods, professional practices, or medical treatment may become necessary.

Practitioners and researchers must always rely on their own experience and knowledge in evaluating and using any information, methods, compounds, or experiments described herein. In using such information or methods they should be mindful of their own safety and the safety of others, including parties for whom they have a professional responsibility.

With respect to any drug or pharmaceutical products identified, readers are advised to check the most current information provided (i) on procedures featured or (ii) by the manufacturer of each product to be administered, to verify the recommended dose or formula, the method and duration of administration, and contraindications. It is the responsibility of practitioners, relying on their own experience and knowledge of their patients, to make diagnoses, to determine dosages and the best treatment for each individual patient, and to take all appropriate safety precautions.

To the fullest extent of the law, neither the Publisher nor the authors, contributors, or editors, assume any liability for any injury and/or damage to persons or property as a matter of products liability, negligence or otherwise, or from any use or operation of any methods, products, instructions, or ideas contained in the material herein.

Printed in China
Last digit is the print number: 9 8 7 6 5 4 3 2

Contents

List of Contributors

Timothy M Alce BSc MB BS PhD
Clinical Research Fellow, Department of Anaesthesia, Chelsea and Westminster Hospital, London, UK

Sumesh Arora MD EDIC FCICM
Staff Specialist, Intensive Care Medicine, Prince of Wales Hospital; Conjoint Lecturer, University of New South Wales, Sydney, NSW, Australia

Thearina de Beer MBchB FRCA DICM FFICM
Consultant AICU, Neuro-ICU and Anaesthetics, Department of Critical Care, Nottingham University Hospitals NHS Trust, Nottingham, UK

Rinaldo Bellomo MB BS FRACP MD FCICM
Professor, The University of Melbourne, Honorary Professor, Monash University, Melbourne; Honorary Professor, Sydney University, Sydney, NSW, Australia; Concurrent Professor, University of Nanjing, Nanjing, China

Andrew D Bersten MB BS MD FCICM
Director, Intensive Care Unit, Flinders Medical Centre; Professor and Head, Department of Critical Care Medicine, Flinders University, Adelaide, SA, Australia

Tim Bowles BSc (Hons) MB BS FRCA
Senior Registrar, Intensive Care Unit, Royal Perth Hospital, Perth, WA, Australia

Jeremy P Campbell MB ChB (Hons) MRCS FRCA
Consultant Anaesthetist, Queen Charlotte's and Chelsea Hospital, Imperial College Healthcare NHS Trust, London, UK

Alastair C Carr MB ChB MSc DA FRCA DICM FFICM MBA
Consultant in Intensive Care Medicine, The Royal Marsden Hospital, London, UK

Marianne J Chapman BM BS PhD FCICM
Associate Professor, Discipline of Acute Care Medicine, University of Adelaide; Director of Research and Senior Staff Specialist, Intensive Care Unit, Royal Adelaide Hospital, Adelaide, SA, Australia

Kai Man Chan MBChB FHKCA (IC) FHKCA FHKAM FCICM
Associate Consultant, Department of Anaesthesia and Intensive Care, Prince of Wales Hospital, Shatin, NT, Hong Kong

Gordon YS Choi BSc MB BS FHKCA (IC) CICM
Consultant, Intensive Care Unit, Prince of Wales Hospital, Shatin, NT, Hong Kong

Christine Chung BPharm MSc
Lead Directorate Pharmacist, Imaging and Anaesthetics, Department of Pharmacy, Chelsea and Westminster NHS Foundation Trust, London, UK

Jeremy Cohen FRCA MRCP FCICM PhD
Department of Intensive Care, Royal Brisbane and Ipswich Hospitals, University of Queensland, Brisbane, QLD, Australia

David Collins BSc (Hons) MN MAppMgt (Nursing) Grad Dip Haem Nursing
Clinical Nurse Consultant – Apheresis, Northern Sydney Cancer Centre, Royal North Shore Hospital, Sydney, NSW, Australia

D James Cooper BM BS MD FRACP FCICM
Professor of Intensive Care Medicine, Director, Australian and New Zealand Intensive Care Research Centre, Monash University and Alfred Hospital, Melbourne, VIC, Australia

Evelyn Corner BSc (Hons) MRes MCSP
Clinical Lead Respiratory Physiotherapist, Chelsea and Westminster NHS Foundation Trust; Research Fellow, Imperial College Medical School, London, UK

Simon Cottam MB ChB FRCA
Consultant Anaesthetist, King's College Hospital, London, UK

Sarah Cox BSc MB BS FRCP
Consultant in Palliative Medicine, Chelsea and Westminster NHS Foundation Trust and Trinity Hospice; Honorary Senior Lecturer, Imperial College School of Medicine, London, UK

Lester AH Critchley MD FFARCSI FHKAM
Professor, Honorary Consultant, Specialist Anaesthetist, Department of Anaesthesia and Intensive Care, The Chinese University of Hong Kong, Shatin, NT, Hong Kong

Andrew R Davies MB BS FRACP FCICM
Intensive Care Specialist, Melbourne, VIC, Australia

Anthony Delaney MB BS MSc FACEM FCICM
Staff Specialist in Intensive Care, Royal North Shore Hospital; Senior Lecturer, Northern Clinical School, Sydney Medical School, University of Sydney, Sydney, NSW, Australia

Rishi H-P Dhillon MB ChB FRCPath MRCP DTM&H
Consultant in Microbiology, Public Health Wales Microbiology, University Hospital of Wales, Cardiff, Wales, UK

Tavey Dorofaeff MB ChB FRACP (NZ) CICM
Senior Lecturer, University of Queensland; Specialist Paediatric Intensivist, PICU Royal Children's Hospital, Brisbane, QLD, Australia

Graeme J Duke MB BS MD FCICM FANZCA
Senior Staff Specialist, Intensive Care Department, Box Hill Hospital, Box Hill, VIC, Australia

Cyrus Edibam MB BS (UWA) FANZCA FCICM DDU
Director, Intensive Care Medicine, Royal Perth Hospital, Perth, WA, Australia

Evan R Everest BSc MB ChB FRACP FCICM
Senior Consultant Intensive and Critical Care Unit, Flinders Medical Centre; Retrieval Consultant, MedSTAR Emergency Retrieval Service; Operations Manager, SA State Rescue Helicopter Service; Senior Lecturer, Department of Intensive Care School of Medicine, Flinders University, Adelaide, SA, Australia

Simon Finfer MB BS FRCP FRCA FCICM MD
Professor, Sydney Medical School, University of Sydney; Senior Staff Specialist in Intensive Care, Intensive Care Unit, Royal North Shore Hospital, Pacific Highway, St Leonards, NSW, Australia

Malcolm M Fisher AO MB ChB MD FCICM FRCA
Clinical Professor, Departments of Medicine and Anaesthesia, University of Sydney, Sydney, NSW, Australia

Oliver J Flower BMedSci MB BS FCICM
Staff Specialist, Royal North Shore Hospital, Clinical Lecturer, University of Sydney, Sydney, NSW, Australia

Carole Foot MB BS (Hons) MSc FACEM FCICM
Intensive Care Specialist, Royal North Shore Hospital; Clinical Associate Professor, University of Sydney, Sydney, NSW, Australia

David Fraenkel BM BS FRACP FCICM
Senior Staff Specialist, Department of Intensive Care, Princess Alexandra Hospital, Brisbane, QLD, Australia

Steven T Galluccio MB BS FCICM FRACP PGDipClinUS
Consultant, Department of Intensive and Critical Medicine, Flinders Medical Centre, Adelaide, SA, Australia

A Raffaele De Gaudio MD
Professor of Anesthesiology and Intensive Care, Department of Health Sciences, University of Florence, Florence, Italy

Tony Gin MB ChB FRCA FANZCA FHKAM MD
Chairman, Department of Anaesthesia and Intensive Care, The Chinese University of Hong Kong, Hong Kong; COS and Head of Department, Department of Anaesthesia and Intensive Care, Prince of Wales Hospital, Shatin, NT, Hong Kong

Charles D Gomersall BSc MB BS FRCA EDIC FCICM FHKCA (IC) FHKAM FRCP (Glasg)
Professor, Department of Anaesthesia and Intensive Care, The Chinese University of Hong Kong, Shatin, NT, Hong Kong

Anthony C Gordon MB BS MD FRCA FFICM
Clinical Senior Lecturer, Section of Anaesthetics, Pain Medicine and Intensive Care, Faculty of Medicine, Imperial College, London, UK

Munita Grover BSc (Hons) MB BS FRCA MD FFICM
Consultant Intensivist, North West London Hospitals NHS Trust, Northwick Park Hospital, Watford, UK

Pascale Gruber MB BS MRCP FRCA EDIC FFICM
Consultant in Intensive Care Medicine and Anaesthesia, The Royal Marsden NHS Foundation Trust, London, UK

Anish Gupta BSc MB BS FRCA
Consultant Anaesthetist, King's College Hospital, London, UK

Jonathan M Handy BSc MB BS FRCA EDIC FFICM
Consultant, Magill Department of Anaesthetics, Intensive Care and Pain Management, Chelsea and Westminster Hospital; Honorary Senior Lecturer, Imperial College School of Medicine, London, UK

Sara Hanna MB B Chir MRCPCH
Consultant, Intensive Care, Evelina Children's Hospital, Guy's and St Thomas' Foundation Trust, London, UK

James Hatcher MBChB DTM&H MRCP
Specialty Registrar in Infectious Diseases and Medical Microbiology, Chelsea and Westminster NHS Foundation Trust, London, UK

Felicity H Hawker MB BS FCICM
Intensive Care Specialist, Cabrini Hospital, Melbourne, VIC, Australia

Michelle Hayes MD FRCA FFICM
Consultant in Anaesthetics and Intensive Care, Magill Department of Anaesthetics, Chelsea and Westminster Hospital, London, UK

Victoria Heaviside MB BS FRCA FFICM
Consultant in Intensive Care Medicine and Anaesthesia, St Bartholomew's Hospital, Barts and The London NHS Trust, London, UK

Liz Hickson MB ChB (Hons) MMedSci MRCP (UK) FCICM
Intensive Care Specialist, Royal North Shore Hospital; Clinical Senior Lecturer, University of Sydney, Sydney, NSW, Australia

Alisa Higgins MPH BPhysio (Hons)
Research Fellow, Australian and New Zealand Intensive Care Research Centre, Department of Epidemiology and Preventive Medicine, Monash University, Melbourne, VIC, Australia

Pierre Hoffmeyer MD
Professor and Head, Division of Orthopaedics and Traumatology; Chair, Department of Surgery, Geneva University Hospital, Geneva, Switzerland

Andrew Holt MB BS FCICM
Critical Care Specialist, Department of Critical Care Medicine, Flinders Medical Center, Bedford Park, SA, Australia

Matthew R Hooper MB BS DipIMC RCS (Ed) FACEM FCICM PGCertClinUS
Associate Professor, Anton Breinl Centre, James Cook University, Townsville; Senior Consultant, MedSTAR Emergency Medical Retrieval Service; Senior Staff Specialist, Intensive and Critical Care Unit, Flinders Medical Centre; Squadron Leader, Royal Australian Air Force Specialist Reserve, Adelaide, SA, Australia

Li C Hsee BSc MB BCh BAO LRCP LRCS (I) FRACS
Consultant Trauma and Acute Care Surgeon, Trauma Service, Auckland City Hospital, Auckland, New Zealand

Nicholas Ioannou BA MB BS MA MRCP FRCA FFICM
Consultant Intensivist and Anaesthetist, Guy's and St Thomas' NHS Foundation Trust, London, UK

James P Isbister BSc (Med) MB BS FRACP FRCPA
Consultant in Haematology and Transfusion Medicine, Clinical Professor of Medicine, Sydney Medical School, Royal North Shore Hospital of Sydney; Adjunct Professor, University of Technology, Sydney; Adjunct Professor of Medicine, Monash University, Melbourne, VIC, Australia

Matthias Jacob MD PhD
Associate Professor, Department of Anaesthesiology, University Hospital Munich, Munich, Germany

Paul James BSc MBBCh FRCA
Consultant in Paediatric Intensive Care and Anaesthesia, Evelina Children's Hospital, Guys and St Thomas NHS Trust, London, UK

Paul Cassius Jansz MB BS FRACS PhD
Senior Cardiothoracic Surgeon, Heart and Lung Transplant Unit, St Vincent's Hospital, Sydney, NSW, Australia

Mandy O Jones MSc PhD MCSP SRP
Course Director Physiotherapy, School of Health Science and Social Care, Brunel University, London, UK

Gavin M Joynt MB BCh FFA (SA)(CritCare) FHKCA (IC) CICM
Professor, Department of Anaesthesia and Intensive Care, The Chinese University of Hong Kong; Head, Intensive Care Unit, Prince of Wales Hospital, Shatin, NT, Hong Kong

James A Judson MNZM MB ChB FFARACS FCICM
Honorary Specialist Intensivist, Department of Critical Care Medicine, Auckland City Hospital, Auckland, New Zealand

Richard Keays MB BS MD FRCP FRCA FFICM
Director of Intensive Care, Magill Department of Anaesthetics and Intensive Care, Chelsea and Westminster Hospital, London, UK

Angus M Kennedy MB BS MRCP MD
Consultant Neurologist, Department of Neurology, Chelsea and Westminster Hospital, London, UK

Ian Kerridge BA BMed (Hons) MPhil (Cantab) FRACP FRCPA
Associate Professor, Haematology Department, Royal North Shore Hospital, St Leonards, Sydney, NSW, Australia

Geoff Knight MMBS FRACP FCICM
Director, Paediatric Intensive Care, Princess Margaret Hospital for Children, Perth, WA, Australia

Stephen W Lam MB BS (Hons) FRACP FCICM
Consultant, Department of Critical Care Medicine, Flinders Medical Centre, Adelaide, SA, Australia

Richard Leonard MB BChir FRCP FRCA FANZCA FCICM FFICM
Consultant, Adult Intensive Care Unit, St Mary's Hospital, Imperial College Healthcare NHS Trust, London, UK

Daniel Lew MD
Director, Infectious Diseases Service, Department of Internal Medicine, Geneva Hospitals and Faculty of Medicine, Geneva, Switzerland

Alexander M Man Ying Li MA (Cantab) MB BChir MRCP FRCA EDIC FCICM FICM
Consultant, Magill Department of Anaesthetics, Intensive Care and Pain Management, Chelsea and Westminster Hospital, London, UK

Jeffrey Lipman MB BCh DA FFA(Crit Care) FCICM MD
Head of Anaesthesiology and Critical Care, University of Queensland; Director ICU, Royal Brisbane and Women's Hospital, Brisbane, QLD, Australia

Pieter HW Lubbert MD PhD
Fellow, Trauma Service, Department of Surgery, Auckland City Hospital, Auckland, New Zealand

Peter S Macdonald MB BS MD PHD FRACP
Professor of Medicine, University of New South Wales; Head, Transplantation Research Laboratory, Victor Chang Cardiac Research Institute; Senior Staff Cardiologist, Heart and Lung Transplant Unit, St Vincent's Hospital, Sydney, NSW, Australia

David P Mackie MB ChB FRCA
Anesthesiologist/Intensivist, Department of Intensive Care, Red Cross Hospital, Beverwijk, The Netherlands

Matthew Maiden BSc BM BS FCICM FACEM
Intensive Care Physician, Royal Adelaide Hospital, Adelaide, SA, Australia; Emergency Physician, Barwon Health, Geelong, VIC, Australia

Colin McArthur MB ChB FANZCA FCICM
Clinical Director, Department of Critical Care Medicine, Auckland City Hospital, Auckland, New Zealand

Kevin McCaffery MB ChB MRCP (UK) FCICM
Senior Staff Specialist in Paediatric Intensive Care Medicine, Royal Hospital for Sick Children and Mater Children's Hospital, Brisbane, Australia; Honorary Senior Lecturer, University of Queensland, Brisbane, QLD, Australia

Steve McGloughlin BMed FRACP FCICM
Intensive Care Physician, The Alfred Hospital, Melbourne, VIC, Australia

Johnny Millar MB ChB PhD MRCP FRACP FCICM
Head of Cardiac Intensive Care, Royal Children's Hospital, Melbourne, VIC, Australia

Wai Ka Ming MB ChB FHKCA (IC)
Resident Specialist, Department of Anaesthesia and Intensive Care, Prince of Wales Hospital, Shatin, NT, Hong Kong

Fiona H Moffatt BSc (Hons) MSc MCSP SRP
Lecturer University of Nottingham, School of Nursing, Midwifery and Physiotherapy, Nottingham, UK

Thomas J Morgan FCICM
Senior Lecturer, School of Medicine, Anaesthesiology and Critical Care, University of Queensland; Senior Critical Care Physician, Mater Adult Hospital, Brisbane, QLD, Australia

Peter T Morley MB BS FRACP FANZCA FCICM
Associate Professor, Department of Medicine, Director of Medical Education, Senior Specialist, Intensive Care, Royal Melbourne Hospital and Royal Melbourne Hospital Clinical School, University of Melbourne, Melbourne, VIC, Australia

John A Myburgh MB BCh FCICM PhD
Professor of Critical Care Medicine, University of New South Wales, Department of Intensive Care Medicine, St George Hospital; Director, Division of Critical Care and Trauma, The George Institute for Global Health, Sydney, NSW, Australia

Michael MG Mythen MB BS FRCA MD FFICM
Smiths Medical Professor of Anaesthesia and Critical Care, University College London (UCL), London, UK

Matthew T Naughton MD FRACP
Head, General Respiratory and Sleep Medicine Service, Department of Allergy, Immunology and Respiratory Medicine, The Alfred Hospital; Adjunct Professor of Medicine, Monash University, Melbourne, VIC, Australia

Alistair D Nichol MB BCh BAO BA PhD FCICM FJFICMI FCARCSI
Professor of Critical Care Medicine, School of Medicine and Medical Sciences, University College Dublin, Ireland; Associate Professor, Department of Epidemiology and Preventive Medicine, Monash University, Australia; Consultant Intensivist/Anaesthetist, St Vincent's University Hospital Dublin, Ireland; Honorary Intensivist, Alfred Hospital, Melbourne, VIC, Australia

Gerry O'Callaghan MB FCARCSI FCICM
Senior Consultant in Intensive Care Medicine, Flinders Medical Centre; Senior Lecturer Faculty of Health Sciences, Flinders University of South Australia, Adelaide, SA, Australia

Helen I Opdam MB BS FRACP FCICM
Intensive Care Specialist, Austin Hospital, Heidelberg, VIC, Australia

Aaisha Opel BSc MB BS MRCP PhD
Specialist Registrar in Cardiology, University College London, London, UK

Alexander A Padiglione MB BS FRACP PhD
Infectious Diseases Physician, Department of Infectious Diseases, The Alfred Hospital and Monash Medical Centre, Melbourne, VIC, Australia

Simon PG Padley BSc MB BS MRCP FRCR
Consultant Radiologist, Chelsea and Westminster Hospital and Royal Brompton Hospital; Reader in Radiology, Imperial College School of Medicine, London, UK

Valerie Page MB BCh FRCA FFICM
Consultant in Anaesthesia and Critical Care, Department of Anaesthesia, West Hertfordshire Hospitals NHS Trust, Watford General Hospital, Watford, UK

Mark Palazzo MB ChB FRCA FRCP FFICM MD
Consultant Critical Care Medicine, Department of Critical Care Medicine, Imperial College Healthcare NHS Trust, London, UK

Sandra L Peake BSc (Hons) BM BS FCICM PhD
Associate Professor, School of Medicine, University of Adelaide; Adjunct Associate Professor, School of Epidemiology and Preventive Medicine, Monash University, Victoria; Senior Staff Specialist, Department of Intensive Care Medicine, The Queen Elizabeth Hospital, Adelaide, SA, Australia

Vincent Pellegrino MB BS FRACP FCICM
Senior Intensivist, Alfred Hospital, Melbourne, VIC, Australia

Michael E Pelly MSc (Clin Trop Med) FRCP DTM&H
Consultant Physician, Chelsea and Westminster Hospital, London, UK

David Pilcher MB BS FCICM
Associate Professor, Department of Intensive Care Medicine, The Alfred Hospital, Melbourne, VIC, Australia

Didier Pittet MD MS
Director, Infection Control Program, WHO Collaborating Centre on Patient Safety, University of Geneva Hospitals and Faculty of Medicine, Geneva, Switzerland

Kevin Plumpton MB ChB FRACP FCICM
Senior Staff Specialist, Paediatric Intensive Care, Royal Children's Hospital and Mater Children's Hospital; Honorary Senior Lecturer, University of Queensland, Brisbane, QLD, Australia

Brad Power MB BS FRACP FCICM
Intensive Care Specialist, Department of Intensive Care, Sir Charles Gairdner Hospital, Perth, WA, Australia

Susanna Price BSc MB BS MRCP PhD EDICM FFICM FESC
Consultant Cardiologist and Intensivist, Royal Brompton Hospital; Honorary Senior Lecturer, Imperial College, London, UK

Raymond F Raper AM MB BS BA MD FRACP FCICM
Head, Department of Intensive Care Medicine, Royal North Shore Hospital, Sydney, NSW, Australia

Michael C Reade MB BS MPH DPhil DIMCRCSEd DMCC FANZCA FCICM
Lieutenant Colonel, Joint Health Command, Australian Defence Force; Professor of Military Medicine and Surgery, University of Queensland; Consultant Intensivist, Royal Brisbane and Women's Hospital, Brisbane, QLD, Australia

Bernard Riley BSc MBE FRCA FFICM
Consultant in Adult Critical Care, Queen's Medical Centre, Nottingham University Hospitals NHS Trust, Nottingham, UK

Shelley D Riphagen MBChB Dip Obs (SA) FCP (Paeds) SA
Consultant, Paediatric Intensive Care, Evelina Children's Hospital, London, UK

Hayley Robinson BMedSci (Hons) MB BS (Hons)
Intensive Care Registrar, Intensive Care Unit, Royal Perth Hospital, Perth, WA, Australia

Vineet V Sarode MB BS MD IDCCM FCICM PGCertCU (Melb)
Specialist Intensive Care Physician, Cabrini Hospital, Melbourne, VIC, Australia

Hugo Sax MD
Private Docent, Division of Infectious Diseases and Hospital Epidemiology, University Hospital of Zurich, Zurich, Switzerland

Manoj K Saxena BSc MB BChir MRCP (UK) FRACP (AUS) FCICM
Intensive Care Physician, St George Hospital, Kogarah; Conjoint Lecturer, University of New South Wales; Honorary Fellow, The George Institute for Global Health, Kogarah, NSW, Australia

Oliver R Segal MD FRCP FHRS
Consultant Electrophysiologist, The Heart Hospital, University College London Hospitals, London, UK

Frank Shann AM MB BS MD FRACP FCICM
Professor of Critical Care Medicine, Department of Paediatrics, University of Melbourne; Staff Specialist in Intensive Care, Royal Children's Hospital, Melbourne, VIC, Australia

Pratik Sinha BSc (Hons) MB ChB MCEM PhD
Specialist Registrar, Intensive Care and Emergency Medicine, Guy's and St Thomas' NHS Foundation Trust, London, UK

Ramachandran Sivakumar MD FRCP
Consultant Physician, Colchester Hospital University NHS Foundation Trust, Colchester, UK

George Skowronski MB BS (Hons) FRCP FRACP FCICM
Director, ICU, St George Private Hospital, Sydney; Senior Specialist, ICU, St George (Public) Hospital, Sydney; Conjoint Associate Professor, Critical Care, University of New South Wales, Sydney, NSW, Australia

Anthony J Slater FRACP FCICM
Director, Paediatric Intensive Care Unit, Royal Children's Hospital, Herston, QLD, Australia

Martin Smith MB BS FRCA FFICM
Consultant and Honorary Professor, Department of Neurocritical Care, The National Hospital for Neurology and Neurosurgery, University College London Hospitals, London, UK

Neil Soni MB ChB MD FANZCA FRCA FCICM FFICM
Consultant in Intensive Care, Chelsea and Westminster Hospital; Honorary Senior Lecturer, Imperial College Medical School, London, UK

Stephen J Streat MB ChB FRACP
Intensivist, Department of Critical Care Medicine; Clinical Director, Organ Donation New Zealand, Auckland District Health Board, Auckland, New Zealand

Richard Strickland FACEM FCICM DDU
Consultant, Critical Care, Royal Adelaide Hospital, Adelaide, SA, Australia

David J Sturgess MB BS PhD PGDipCU FRACGP FANZCA FCICM
Senior Lecturer, Discipline of Anaesthesiology and Critical Care, School of Medicine, The University of Queensland; Specialist Anaesthetist and Intensive Care Physician, Mater Health Services, Raymond Terrace; Program Leader, Improving Acute Care Program, Mater Medical Research Institute, Brisbane, QLD, Australia

Christian P Subbe DM MRCP
Senior Clinical Lecturer, Consultant Acute, Respiratory and Critical Care Medicine, School of Medical Sciences, Bangor University, Bangor, Wales, UK

Joseph JY Sung MD PhD
Mok Hing Yiu Professor of Medicine, The Chinese University of Hong Kong, Shatin, NT, Hong Kong

Chee Wee Tan MB BS (Hons) FRACP FRCPA
Consultant Haematologist, Department of Haematology, Royal Adelaide Hospital / Institute of Medical and Veterinary Science, Adelaide, SA, Australia

Guido Tavazzi MD
University of Pavia, Department of Anaesthesia and Intensive Care I, Foundation Policlinico San Matteo IRCCS, Pavia, Italy; Echocardiography Fellow, Royal Brompton Hospital, London, UK

Peter D (Toby) Thomas MB BS FRACP FANZCA FCICM
Colonel, 3rd Health Support Battalion, Royal Australian Army Medical Corps; Director, Intensive Care Unit, Lyell McEwin Hospital, Elizabeth Vale, SA, Australia

James Tibballs BMedSc (Hons) MB BS MEd MD MBA MHlth&MedLaw PGDipArts (Fr) DALF FANZCA FCICM FACLM
Deputy Director, Paediatric Intensive Care Unit, The Royal Children's Hospital; Associate Professor, Departments of Paediatrics and Pharmacology, The University of Melbourne, Melbourne, VIC, Australia

Luke E Torre MB BS (Hons) FCICM FANZCA
Associate Professor, School of Medicine, Notre Dame University, Fremantle; Intensivist, Sir Charles Gairdner Hospital, Nedlands; Anaesthetist, Joondalup Health Campus, Joondalup, WA, Australia

David Treacher MA FRCP
Consultant Physician, Intensive Care and Respiratory Medicine, Guy's and St Thomas' NHS Foundation Trust, London, UK

David V Tuxen MB BS MD FRACP DipDHM FJFICM
Senior Intensivist, Intensive Care, The Alfred Hospital, Melbourne, VIC, Australia

Ilker Uçkay MD
Senior Attending, Infection Control Program, Service of Infectious Diseases, Orthopaedic Surgery Service, University of Geneva Hospitals, Geneva, Switzerland

Balasubramanian Venkatesh MB BS MD (IntMed) FRCA (UK) FFARCSI MD(UK) FCICM (ANZ)
Professor in Intensive Care, Princess Alexandra and Wesley Hospitals, University of Queensland, Brisbane, QLD; Honorary Professor, University of Sydney, Sydney, NSW, Australia

Jacqueline EHM Vet MD
Anaesthesiologist-intensivist, Department of Intensive Care, Red Cross Hospital, Beverwijk, The Netherlands

Marcela P Vizcaychipi MD PhD FRCA EDIC FFICM
Consultant in Anaesthesia and Intensive Care, Honorary Clinical Senior Lecturer, Chelsea and Westminster Hospital, Imperial College, London, UK

Adrian J Wagstaff BSc MB BS MD FFICM
Consultant in Anaesthesia and Intensive Care, Humphrey Davy Department of Anaesthesia, University Hospitals, Bristol, UK

Carl S Waldmann MA MB BChir FRCA EDIC FFICM
Consultant in Intensive Care and Anaesthesia, Royal Berkshire Hospital, Reading, UK

Christopher M Ward MB ChB PhD
Associate Professor, Sydney Medical School, Sydney, Australia; Head and Director of Research, Department of Haematology and Transfusion Medicine, Royal North Shore Hospital, Sydney, NSW, Australia

John R Welch BSc (Hons) MSc RGN ENB 100
Consultant Nurse, Critical Care, University College London Hospitals NHS Foundation Trust; Honorary Senior Lecturer, City University, London, UK

Julia Wendon MB ChB FRCP
Professor of Hepatolgy and Consultant in Intensive Care, Liver Intensive Care Unit, King's College Hospital, London, UK

Mary White MB BAO BCh MSc FCAI PhD
Consultant Intensivist and Anaesthetist, Royal Brompton Hospital, London, UK

Ubbo F Wiersema MB BS FRACP FCICM
Intensive Care Consultant, Intensive and Critical Care Unit, Flinders Medical Centre, Adelaide, SA, Australia

Timothy Wigmore MA FRCA FCICM FFICM
Consultant Anaesthetist and Intensivist, Critical Care Department, Royal Marsden Foundation Trust, London, UK

Christopher Willars MB BS FRCA FFICM
Consultant Intensivist, Liver Intensive Care Unit, King's College Hospital, London, UK

Wan Tsz Pan Winnie MB ChB FHKCA (IC) FHKAM FCICM
Resident Specialist, Department and Anaesthesia and Intensive Care, Prince of Wales Hospital, Shatin, NT, Hong Kong

David M Wood MD FACMT FBPharmacolS FRCP
Consultant Physician and Clinical Toxicologist, Guy's and St Thomas' NHS Foundation Trust and King's Health Partners; Senior Lecturer, King's College London, London, UK

Duncan LA Wyncoll MB BS FRCA EDIC DipICM FFICM
Consultant Intensivist, Guy's and St Thomas' NHS Trust, London, UK

Steve M Yentis BSc MB BS FRCA MD MA
Consultant Anaesthetist, Chelsea and Westminster Hospital, Honorary Reader, Imperial College, London, UK

Preface

The first edition of *Oh's Intensive Care Manual* was published in 1979, when intensive care may not have been in its infancy but it certainly wasn't far beyond. Teik Oh, with tremendous foresight, brought together the fundamental elements of managing the critically ill in a particularly pragmatic manner, which could be considered a guideline for the development of the specialty. Thirty-four years on, the seventh edition reflects both the maturation of that specialty and the phenomenal progress medically, technically, scientifically, ethically and educationally in all areas of management of the critically ill.

As with previous editions, each and every chapter has been updated, and there are many areas where new sections reflect the changing nature of the specialty and the subtle shifts in emphasis in the workplace. These include the growing interest in critical care both before and after the intensive care unit, including the role of palliative care. There is increasing focus on the ethical dilemmas, which cannot be separated from legal considerations that beset critical care in all age groups. Team working is fundamental to delivering intensive care and this is formally addressed, as is education and examination. As bedside ultrasound has been incorporated into clinical examination and many procedures, this is now recognised in addition to the chapter on echocardiography. Extracorporeal membrane oxygenation (ECMO) is increasingly being used for both respiratory and circulatory support, with a unique double chapter dedicated to this area. Almost every chapter has new developments while in some, such as liver failure, there are new sections to address the increasing complexity of the field as it impacts on intensive care. Malignant disease is a common co-morbidity or cause for admission postoperatively so this has been included, as has delirium, which is a common problem.

There has been discussion about the relevance of the paediatric section in this era of specialisation. It is the editors' contention that populations outside of hospital include paediatrics and so a working knowledge of paediatric intensive care should be an integral part of any intensivist's knowledge. With this in mind, this section has been significantly, and in our opinion impressively, updated.

We sincerely hope that this edition will achieve several goals. It will update the previous edition in terms of the changing knowledge base, it will address emerging issues in intensive care, it will be of use to both medical and paramedical staff, but most importantly it will adhere to the pragmatic and clinically useful style so effectively promulgated by Teik Oh when it was originally published 34 years ago. If clinicians can reach for it in the early hours of the morning, easily locate the information they require and feel either guided or reassured, it will have served its purpose. If those passing examinations can say it helped, that would be gilding the lily.

ADB
NS

ACKNOWLEDGEMENTS

It is a fitting time to use this opportunity to acknowledge the tremendous achievement of Teik Oh in the creation of this book back in 1979 and for many editions following. It has been a massive asset in the development of the specialty, especially in the early days, and there are hundreds, indeed thousands, of intensivists across much of the world, including both of us, who have been the benefactors of the enthusiasm, energy and sheer work that Teik put into this book. The real beneficiaries have been the countless patients over all those years whose management was enhanced by access to this book either during training or when it has been reached for on the intensive care unit.

ADB
NS

Part One

Organisation Aspects

1

Design and organisation of intensive care units

Vineet V Sarode and Felicity H Hawker

The intensive care unit (ICU) is a distinct organisational and geographic entity for clinical activity and care, operating in cooperation with other departments integrated in a hospital. The ICU is used to monitor and support threatened or failing vital functions in critically ill patients, who have illnesses with the potential to endanger life, so that adequate diagnostic measures and medical or surgical therapies can be performed to improve outcome.[1] Hence intensive care patients may be:

1. Patients requiring monitoring and treatment because one or more vital functions are threatened by an acute (or an acute-on-chronic) disease (e.g. sepsis, myocardial infarction, gastrointestinal haemorrhage), or by the sequelae of surgical or other intensive treatment (e.g. percutaneous interventions) with the potential for developing life-threatening conditions
2. Patients already having failure of one or more vital functions such as cardiovascular, respiratory, renal, metabolic, or cerebral function but with a reasonable chance of a meaningful functional recovery. In principle, patients in known end-stages of untreatable terminal diseases are not admitted.

ICUs developed from the postoperative recovery rooms and respiratory units of the mid twentieth century when it became clear that concentrating the sickest patients in one area was beneficial. Intermittent positive-pressure ventilation (IPPV) was pioneered in the treatment of respiratory failure in the 1948–9 poliomyelitis epidemics, and particularly in the 1952 Copenhagen poliomyelitis epidemic when IPPV was delivered using an endotracheal tube and a manual bag, before the development of manual ventilators.

As outlined below, the ICU is a department with dedicated medical, nursing and allied health staff that operates with defined policies and procedures and has its own quality improvement, continuing education and research programmes. Through its care of critically ill patients in the ICU and its outreach activities (see Ch. 2), the intensive care department provides an integrated service to the hospital, without which many programmes (e.g. cardiac surgery, trauma and transplantation) could not function.

CLASSIFICATION AND ROLE DELINEATION OF AN ICU

The delineation of roles of hospitals in a region or area is necessary to rationalise services and optimise resources. Each ICU should similarly have its role in the region defined, and should support the defined duties of its hospital. In general, small hospitals require ICUs that provide basic intensive care services. Critically ill patients who need complex management and sophisticated investigative back-up should be managed in an ICU located in a large tertiary referral hospital. Three levels of adult ICUs are classified as follows by the College of Intensive Care Medicine (Australia and New Zealand).[2] The European Society of Intensive Care Medicine has a similar classification. The American College of Critical Care Medicine also has a similar classification but uses a reversed-numbering system.[3] It should be noted that full-time directors and directors with qualifications in intensive care medicine are less common in the USA,[4] as are the requirements for a dedicated doctor for the ICU around the clock, and referral to the attending ICU specialist for management.[5] Nurse staffing should be in line with accepted standards that are outlined in Chapter 6, Critical Care Nursing.

1. *Level I ICU*: a Level I ICU has a role in small district hospitals. It should be able to provide resuscitation and short-term cardiorespiratory support of critically ill patients. It will have a major role in monitoring and preventing complications in 'at-risk' medical and surgical patients. It must be capable of providing mechanical ventilation and simple invasive cardiovascular monitoring for a period of several hours. A Level I ICU should have an established relationship with a Level II or a Level III unit that should include mutual transfer and back transfer policies and an established joint review process. The medical director should be a certified intensive care specialist.
2. *Level II ICU*: a Level II ICU is located in larger general hospitals. It should be capable of providing a high standard of general intensive care, including multisystem life support, in accordance with the role of its hospital (e.g. regional centre for acute medicine,

general surgery, trauma). It should have a medical officer on site and access to pharmacy, pathology and radiology facilities at all times, but it may not have all forms of complex therapy and investigations (e.g. interventional radiology, cardiac surgical service). The medical director and at least one other specialist should be certified intensive care specialists. Patients admitted must be referred to the attending intensive care specialists for management. Referral and transport policies should be in place with a Level III unit to enable escalation of care.
3. *Level III ICU*: a Level III ICU is located in a major tertiary referral hospital. It should provide all aspects of intensive care management required by its referral role for indefinite periods. These units should have a demonstrated commitment to education and research. Large ICUs should be divided into smaller 'pods' of 8–15 patients for the purpose of clinical management. The unit should be staffed by intensive care specialists with trainees, critical care nurses, allied health professionals and clerical and scientific staff. Complex investigations and imaging and support by specialists of all disciplines required by the referral role of the hospital must be available at all times. All patients admitted to the unit must be referred to the attending intensive care specialist for management.

The classification of types of ICU must not be confused with the description of intensive care beds within a hospital, as with the UK classification of intensive care beds.

TYPE AND SIZE OF AN ICU[2]

An institution may organise its intensive care beds into multiple units under separate management by single-discipline specialists (e.g. medical ICU, surgical ICU, burns ICU). Although this may be functional in some hospitals, the experience in Australia and New Zealand has favoured the development of general multidisciplinary ICUs. Thus, with the exception of dialysis units, coronary care units and neonatal ICUs, critically ill patients are admitted to the hospital's multidisciplinary ICU and are managed by intensive care specialists (or paediatric intensive care specialists in paediatric hospitals).

There are good economic and operational arguments for a multidisciplinary ICU as against separate, single-discipline ICUs. Duplication of equipment and services is avoided. Critically ill patients develop the same pathophysiological processes no matter whether they are classified as medical or surgical and they require the same approaches to support of vital organs.

The ICU may constitute up to 10% of total hospital beds. The number of beds required depends on the role and type of ICU. Multidisciplinary ICUs require more beds than single-specialty ICUs, especially if high-dependency beds are integrated into the unit. ICUs with fewer than four beds are considered not to be cost-effective and are too small to provide adequate clinical experience for skills maintenance for medical and nursing staff. On the other hand, the emerging trend of very large ICUs[6] can create major management problems. There is a suggestion that efficiency deteriorates once the number of critically ill patients per medical team exceeds 12.[7] Consequently as detailed above these unit should be divided into 'pods'. Cohorting of patients in these subunits may be based on specific processes of care or the underlying clinical problem.

HIGH-DEPENDENCY UNIT (HDU)[8–10]

An HDU is a specially staffed and equipped area of a hospital that provides a level of care intermediate between intensive care and the general ward care. Although HDUs may be located in or near specialty wards, increasingly they are located within or immediately adjacent to an ICU complex and are often staffed by the ICU.

The HDU provides invasive monitoring and support for patients with or at risk of developing acute (or acute-on-chronic) single-organ failure, particularly where the predicted risk of clinical deterioration is high or unknown. It may act as a 'step-up' or 'step-down' unit between the level of care delivered on a general ward and that in an ICU. Equipment should be available to manage short-term emergencies (e.g. need for mechanical ventilation). Earlier studies have shown conflicting results about benefits to outcome associated with the introduction of HDUs,[8] whereas a more recent survey where HDU care was based on a 'single-organ failure and support model' has shown that HDUs play a crucial role in management.[10]

DESIGN OF AN ICU[1,2,11]

The goal of design is to create a healing environment – a design that produces a measurable improvement in the physical or psychological states of patients, staff and visitors. Optimal ICU design helps to reduce medical errors, improve patient outcomes, reduce length of stay, increase social support for patients and can play a role in reducing costs.[11]

The layout of the ICU should allow rapid access to relevant acute areas including operating theatres and postoperative areas, the emergency department, functional testing departments (e.g. cardiac catheterisation laboratory, endoscopy) and the medical imaging department. Lines of communication must be available around the clock. Safe transport of critically ill patients to and from the ICU should be facilitated by centrally located, keyed, oversized lifts and doors, and corridors should allow easy passage of beds and equipment. There should be a single entry and exit point, attended by the unit receptionist. Through traffic of goods or people to other hospital areas must never be allowed. An ICU should have areas and rooms for public reception, patient management and support services. The total area of the unit should be 2.5–3 times the area devoted to patient care.

PATIENT CARE ZONE

An ideal patient room should incorporate three zones: a patient zone, a family zone and a caregiver zone.[11] Each patient bed area in an adult ICU requires a minimum floor space of 20 m^2 with single rooms being larger (at least 25 m^2), to accommodate patient, staff and equipment. There should be at least 2.5 m traffic area beyond the bed area. Single rooms should have an optimal clearance of not less than 1.2 m at the head and the foot of the bed, and not less than 1.8 m on each side. The ratio of single-room beds to open-ward beds will depend on the role and type of the ICU. Single rooms are essential for isolation; with the emergence of resistant bacterial strains in ICUs around the world, single rooms are recommended. They have been shown to decrease acquisition of resistant bacteria and antibiotic use.[12] Isolation rooms should be equipped with an anteroom of at least 3 m^2 for hand washing, gowning and storage of isolation material. Some isolation rooms should be negative-pressure ventilated for contagious respiratory infections. A non-splash hand wash basin with elbow- or foot-operated taps and a hand disinfection facility should be available for each bed.

Bedside service outlets should conform to local standards and requirements (including electrical safety and emergency supply, such as to the Australian Standard, Cardiac Protected Status AS3003).

Utilities per bed space as recommended for a Level III ICU are:

- 4 oxygen
- 3 air outlets
- 3 suction inlets
- 16–20 power outlets
- a bedside light
- 4 data outlets.

Adequate and appropriate lighting for clinical observation must be available. Patients should be able to be seen at all the times to allow detection of changes in status. All patient rooms should have access to natural light. Patients exposed to sunlight have been shown to experience less stress, require fewer analgesics and have improved sleep quality and quantity.[13] Lack of natural light or outside view increases the incidence of disorientation in patients and stress levels in staff.[14,15]

Efforts should be made to reduce sound transmission and therefore noise levels (e.g. walls and ceilings should be constructed of materials with high sound-absorbing capability). Suitable and safe air quality should be maintained at all times. Air conditioning and heating should be provided with an emphasis on patient comfort. A clock and a calendar at each bed space are useful for patient orientation. It is widely held that transporting long-stay ICU patients outdoors is good for their morale, and access to an outside area should be considered in the design process.

The medical utility distribution systems configuration (e.g. floor column, wall mounted, or ceiling pendant) depends on individual preference. There should be room to place or attach additional portable monitoring equipment and, as far as possible, equipment should be kept off the floor. Space for charts, syringes, sampling tubes, pillows, suction catheters and patient personal belongings should be available, often in one or more moveable bedside trolleys.

CLINICAL SUPPORT ZONE

Since critical care nursing is primarily at the bedside, staffing of a central nurse station is less important and emphasis should be on 'decentralised' stations just inside the room or outside the room - often paired to permit observation of two adjacent rooms. Nevertheless, the central station and other work areas should have adequate space for staff to allow centralised clinical management, staff interaction, mentoring and socialisation. This central station usually houses a central monitor, satellite pharmacy and drug preparation area, satellite storage of sterile and non-sterile items, telephones, computers with internet connections, patient records, reference books and policy and procedure manuals. A dedicated computer for the picture archive and communication system (PACS) or a multi-display X-ray viewer should be located within the patient care area.

UNIT SUPPORT ZONE

Storage areas should take up a total floor space of at least 10 m^2 per bed.[11] They should have separate access remote from the patient area for deliveries, and be no farther than 30 m from the patient area. Frequently used items (e.g. intravenous fluids and giving sets, sheets and dressing trays) should be located closer to patients than infrequently used or non-patient items. There should be an area for storing emergency and transport equipment within the patient area with easy access to all beds.

Two separate spaces for clean (15 m^2) and dirty (25 m^2) utility rooms with separate access are necessary. Facilities for estimating blood gases, glucose, electrolytes, haemoglobin, lactate and sometimes clotting status are usually sufficient for the unit's laboratory. There should be a pneumatic tube or equivalent system to transfer specimens to pathology. Adequate arrangements for offices (receptionist, medical and nursing), doctor-on-call rooms (15 m^2), staff lounge (with food/drinks facilities) (40 m^2 per eight beds), wash rooms and seminar room (40 m^2) should be available and an interview room should be taken into consideration.

EQUIPMENT

The type and quantity of equipment will vary with the type, size and function of the ICU and must be appropriate to the workload of the unit. There must be a regular programme in place for checking its safety. Protocols and in-service training for medical and nursing staff must be available for the use of all equipment, including steps to be taken in the event of malfunction. There should also be a system in place for regular maintenance and service. The intensive care budget should include provision to replace old or obsolete equipment at appropriate times. A system of stock control should be in place to ensure consumables are always in adequate supply. The ICU director should have a major role in the purchase of new equipment to ensure it is appropriate for the activities of the unit. Level II and III ICUs should have an equipment officer to coordinate these activities.

FAMILY SUPPORT ZONE

For relatives, there should be a separate area of at least 10 m^2 per eight beds (two chairs per bed), and an additional facility with bed and shower as sleep or rest cubicles can be considered. There should be facilities for tea/coffee making and a water dispenser, and toilets should be located close by. Television and/or music should be provided. It is desirable to have separate entrances to the ICU for visitors and health care professionals. One or more separate areas for distressed relatives should be available.

ICU ORGANISATION

STAFFING[1,2,5,6,11,12,15]

The level of staffing depends on the type of hospital, and tertiary hospital ICUs require large teams. Whatever the size of the team, it is crucial that there is clear and proper communication and collaboration among team members and a true multidisciplinary approach. Knaus et al in a classic study[16] first showed the importance of the relationship between the degree of coordination in an ICU and the effectiveness of its care. Other studies have shown relationships between collaboration and teamwork and better outcomes for patients and staff.[17,18] Inadequate communication is the most frequent root cause of sentinel events.[19]

MEDICAL STAFF[20]

An intensive care department should have a medical director who is qualified in intensive care medicine and who coordinates the clinical, administrative and educational activities of the department. The duties of the director should involve patient care, supervision of trainees/other junior doctors, the drafting of diagnostic and therapeutic protocols, responsibility for the quality, safety and appropriateness of care provided and education, training and research. It is recommended that the director be full time in the department.

The director should be supported by a group of other specialists trained in intensive care medicine who provide patient care and contribute to non-clinical activities. In an ICU of Level II or III there must be at least one specialist exclusively rostered to the unit at all times. Specialists should have a significant or full-time commitment to the ICU ahead of clinical commitments elsewhere. There should be sufficient numbers to allow reasonable working hours, protected non-clinical time and leave of all types. Participation in ICU outreach activities (rapid response calls, outpatient review; see Ch. 2) has increased the workload of intensive care specialists as well as junior staff in many hospitals, resulting in the need to increase the size of the medical team.

There should also be at least one junior doctor with an appropriate level of experience rostered exclusively to Level II and III units at all times. Junior medical staff in the ICU may be intensive care trainees, but should ideally also include trainees of other acute disciplines (e.g. anaesthesia, medicine, surgery and emergency medicine). It is imperative that junior doctors are adequately supervised, with specialists being readily available at all times.

Medical work patterns are important for quality of treatment and should be supervised by the director. These patterns include rosters, structure of handover and daily rounds. Appropriate rostering influences satisfaction and avoids burnout syndrome in staff. It reduces tiredness after night shifts or long shifts and consequently improves attention and reduces errors. It also improves the quality of information transfer during handovers and daily rounds.[21]

This physician-staffing model has been used in Australia and New Zealand for many years, but has not been common in the USA. A systematic review[22] has shown that when there has been mandatory intensive care specialist consultation (or closed ICU), compared with no or elective intensive care specialist consultation or open ICU, both ICU and hospital survival were improved and there was a reduced length of stay in ICU and in hospital.

NURSING STAFF

Critical care nursing is covered in Chapter 6. The bedside nurse conducts the majority of patient assessment, evaluation and care in an ICU. When leave of all kinds is factored in, long-term 24-hour cover of a single bed requires a staff complement of six nurses. Nurse shortages have been shown to be associated with increased patient mortality and nurse burnout, and adversely affect outcome and job satisfaction in the ICU.[23,24]

There should be a nurse manager who is appointed with authority and responsibility for the appropriateness of nursing care and who has extensive experience in intensive care nursing as well as managerial experience. In tertiary units the nurse manager should participate in teaching, continuing education and research. Ideally, all nurses working in an ICU should have training and certification in critical care nursing.

ALLIED HEALTH

Access to physiotherapists, dietitians, social workers and other therapists should also be available. A dedicated ward clinical pharmacist is invaluable and participation of a pharmacist on ward rounds has been associated with a reduction in adverse drug events.[25] Respiratory therapists are allied health personnel trained in and responsible for the equipment and clinical aspects of respiratory therapy, a concept well established in North America, but not the UK, continental Europe and Australasia. Technical support staff, either members of the ICU staff or seconded from biomedical departments, is necessary to service, repair and develop equipment.

OTHER STAFF

Provision should be made for adequate secretarial support.[15] Transport and 'lifting' orderly teams will reduce physical stress and possible injuries to nurses and doctors. If no mechanical system is available to transport specimens to the laboratories (e.g. air-pressurised chutes), sufficient and reliable couriers must be provided to do this day and night. The cleaning personnel should be familiar with the ICU environment and infection control protocols. There should also be a point of contact for local interpreters, chaplains, priests or officials of all religions when there is need for their services.

CLINICAL ACTIVITIES

OPERATIONAL POLICIES[2]

Clear-cut administrative policies are vital to the functioning of an ICU. An *open* ICU has unrestricted access to multiple doctors who are allowed to admit and manage their patients. A *closed* ICU has admission, discharge and referral policies under the control of intensive care specialists. Improved cost benefits are likely with a closed ICU and patient outcomes are better, especially if the intensive care specialists have full clinical responsibilities.[22,26] Consequently ICUs should be *closed* under the charge of a medical specialist director. All patients admitted to the ICU are referred to the director and his/her specialist staff for management, although it is important for the ICU team to communicate regularly with the parent unit and to make referrals to other specialty units when appropriate.

There must be clearly defined policies for admission, discharge, management and referral of patients. Lines of responsibilities must be delineated for all staff members and their job descriptions defined. The director must have final overall authority for all staff and their actions, although in other respects each group may be responsible to respective hospital heads (e.g. the Director of Nursing).

Policies for the care of patients should be formulated and standardised. They should be unambiguous, periodically reviewed and familiarised by all staff. Examples include infection control and isolation policies, policies for intra- and inter-facility transport, end-of-life policies (e.g. do not resuscitate (DNR) procedure) and sedation and restraint protocols. A rigorous fire safety and evacuation plan should be in place. It should be noted, however, that when protocols involve complex issues (such as weaning from mechanical ventilation) they might be less efficient than the judgement of experienced clinicians.[27] Clinical management protocols (e.g. for feeding and bowel care) can be laminated and placed in a folder at each bed or loaded on to the intranet.

PATIENT CARE

ICU patient management should be multidisciplinary, with medical, nursing and other staff working together to provide the best care for each patient. The critical care nurse is the primary carer at the bedside and monitors, manages and supports the critically ill patient (see Ch. 6). The medical team consists of one or more registrars, residents or fellows who direct medical care with an intensive care specialist. The patient should be assessed by a formal ward round of the multidisciplinary team twice daily, usually at a time when the junior medical staff members are handing over. The nurse coordinating the floor, pharmacists and dietitians should also take part in daily rounds. Each patient should be assessed clinically (examination, observations and pathology, radiological and other investigation results), the medication chart reviewed, progress determined and a management plan developed for the immediate and longer term. The ward round is also an opportunity to assess compliance with checklists such as Fast Hug (Feeding Analgesia Sedation Thromboembolic prophylaxis Head of bed elevation stress Ulcer prophylaxis Glyceamic control).[28] Clearly, unstable patients will require much more frequent assessment and intervention.

It is crucial that all observations, examination findings, investigations, medical orders, management plans (including treatment limitations) and important communications with other medical teams and patients' families are clearly documented in the appropriate chart or part of the medical record either electronically or in writing.

Wherever possible clinical management should be evidence based and derived through consensus of the members of the ICU team, accepting, however, that evidence-based medicine has limitations when applied to intensive care medicine.[29]

Well-structured collaboration among physicians, nurses and the other professionals is essential for best possible patient care, which includes presence of inter-professional clinical rounds, standardised and structured processes of handover of inter-disciplinary and inter-professional information and use of clinical information systems.[1]

CARE OF FAMILIES[30]

ICU care includes sensitive handling of relatives. It is important that there are early and repeated discussions with patients' families to reduce family stress and improve consistency in communication. Ideally one senior doctor should be identified as the ICU representative to liaise with a particular family. Discussions should be interactive and honest and an attempt made to predict the likely course, especially with respect to outcome, potential complications and the duration of intensive care management required. The time, date and discussion of each interview should be recorded. Cultural factors should be acknowledged and spiritual support available, especially before, during and after a death. Open visiting hours allow families maximum contact with their loved one and promote an atmosphere of openness and transparency.

OUTREACH

ICU outreach activities are described in Chapter 2.

NON-CLINICAL ACTIVITIES[2]

Non-clinical activities are very important in the ICU, as they enhance the safety, quality and currency of patient care. The College of Intensive Care Medicine recommends that full-time intensive care specialists should have as protected non-clinical time three sessions per fortnight.[20] Nursing and allied health staff should also seek protected time for these activities.

QUALITY IMPROVEMENT[31,32]

It is essential that staff members promote a culture of quality improvement (QI) within the ICU, whatever its size and role. Every ICU should maintain a database that is sufficiently well structured to allow easy extraction of benchmarking, quality control and research data. All ICUs should have demonstrable and documented formal audit and review of its processes and outcomes in a regular multidisciplinary forum. Staff members who collect and process the data should have dedicated QI time.

There are three types of quality indicators:

1. *Structure:* structural indicators assess whether the ICU functions according to its operational guidelines and conforms to the policies of training and specialist bodies (e.g. clinical work load and case mix, staffing establishment and levels of supervision).
2. *Clinical processes*: clinical process indicators assess the way care is delivered. Examples include whether deep-vein thrombosis prophylaxis is given, time to administration of antibiotics and glycaemic control.
3. *Outcomes*: examples of outcome measures include survival rate, quality of life of survivors and patient satisfaction.

The QI process involves *identification* of the indicator to be improved (e.g. high ventilator-associated pneumonia (VAP) rate), *development* of a method to improve it (e.g. checklist such as Fast Hug[28]), *implementation* of the method to improve it (e.g. requirement to tick off the checklist on the morning ward round), and re-evaluation of the indicator (e.g. VAP rate) to ensure the intervention has improved the outcome and finally to *ensure sustainability* (e.g. print checklist on ICU chart).

Activities that assess processes include clinical audit, compliance with protocols, guidelines and checklists and critical incident reporting. Activities that assess outcomes are calculating risk-adjusted mortality using a scoring system such as the Acute Physiology and Chronic Health Evaluation III (APACHE III) and calculation of standardised mortality ratios (see Ch. 3), measurement of rates of adverse events, and surveys.

Risk management is a closely related field. In the ICU, risks can be identified from critical incident reports, morbidity and mortality reviews and complaints from staff, patients or family members. Using similar methodology to the QI process, risks must be identified, assessed and analysed, managed and re-evaluated. A major patient safety incident should result in a root cause analysis.

EDUCATION

All ICUs should have a documented orientation programme for new staff. There should be educational programmes for medical staff and a formal nursing education programme. Educational activities for intensive care trainees include lectures, tutorials, bedside teaching and trial examinations. Clinical reviews and meetings to review journals and new developments should be held regularly. Regular assessments for advanced life support and sometimes other assessments (e.g. medication safety) are often required. Increasingly, simulation centres are used to teach and assess skills and teamwork in crisis scenarios.[33] A number of ICUs are also involved in undergraduate medical teaching. All staff should also participate in continuing education activities outside the hospital (e.g. local, national or international meetings) and specialists should be involved in College CPD.

RESEARCH

Level III ICUs should have an active research programme, preferably with dedicated research staff, but all units should attempt to undertake some research projects whether these are unit-based or contributions to multicentre trials.

THE FUTURE

In the USA critical care medicine is thought to account for 1–2% of the gross domestic product[34] and has become increasingly used and prominent in the delivery of health care. Although the total number of hospitals, hospital beds and inpatient days has decreased, there has been shown to be a large increase in the number of intensive care beds and bed days.[35] There is every reason to expect that other developed countries will follow this trend. As ICUs become larger and ICU staff numbers become larger still, it is crucial that the basic principles outlined in this chapter are followed and that standards of ICU design, staffing and clinical and non-clinical activities are maintained.

Access the complete references list online at http://www.expertconsult.com

9. College of Intensive Care Medicine of Australia and New Zealand. IC-13 Recommendations on standards for high dependency units for training in intensive care medicine 2010. Online. Available: http://www.cicm.org.au.
10. Scala R, Corrado A, Confalonieri M, et al. Increased number and expertise of Italian respiratory high-dependency care units: the second national survey. Resp Care 2011;56:1100–7.
11. Thompson DR, Hamilton DK, Cadenhead CD, et al. Guidelines for intensive care unit design. Crit Care Med 2012;40:1586–600. Epub 2012/04/19.
12. Levin PD, Golovanevski M, Moses AE, et al. Improved ICU design reduces acquisition of antibiotic-resistant bacteria: a quasi-experimental observational study. Crit Care 2011;15:R211.
15. College of Intensive Care Medicine of Australia and New Zealand. IC-07 Administrative Services to Intensive Care Units. 2010. Online. Available: http://www.cicm.org.au.
20. College of Intensive Care Medicine of Australia and New Zealand. IC-02 Intensive care specialist practice in hospitals accredited for training in intensive care medicine 2011. Online. Available: http://www.cicm.org.au.
21. Dierk A. Vagts K KaCWM. Organisation and management of intensive care. Berlin: Medizinisch Wissenschaftliche Verlagsgesellschaft; 2010. p. 197–204.
31. College of Intensive Care Medicine of Australia and New Zealand. IC-08 Quality Improvement 2010. Online. Available: http://www.cicm.org.au.

2

Critical care outreach and rapid response systems

John R Welch and Christian P Subbe

Hospitals around the world are increasingly deploying dedicated outreach, medical emergency or rapid response teams to provide 'critical care without walls'.[1] The objective is to 'ensure equity of care for all critically ill patients irrespective of their location',[2] particularly focusing on those with potential or actual critical illness in general wards.

Outreach and similar services are key components of what are known as rapid response systems. These are based on multidisciplinary 'collaboration and partnership between critical care and other departments to ensure a continuum of care for patients, and [on enhancing] the skills and understanding of all staff in the delivery of critical care'.[3] However, such services are not a replacement for insufficient critical care beds or under-resourced wards.

BACKGROUND

Critical care units contain a small proportion of all hospital beds and have high rates of occupancy. Hospital admission criteria have become more stringent and lengths of stay have decreased in recent years. The result is that many ward patients have serious medical problems but only the most unstable gain admission to a critical care unit. Hence many at-risk patients remain in areas with staff inexperienced in managing critical illness. The problem has been compounded by changes in nursing education that have reduced training time in acute and critical care areas. Key tasks such as measuring physiological signs are often delegated to untrained staff who may not understand the significance of abnormal values; added to this many hospitals use temporary staff less likely to provide the continuity and team working essential for effective care. Medical education is also problematic;[4] training is shorter and more specialised than before, and even senior doctors may be relatively inexperienced.[5]

Comparisons of outcomes of patients admitted to a critical care unit from either the emergency department, operating theatre/recovery area or the wards show that those coming from wards have the highest mortality.[6] Suboptimal treatment is common before transfer to critical care, and is associated with worse outcomes.[7,8] Crucially, differences in mortality have been shown to be due to variations in care rather than differences between the patients themselves and the longer patients are in hospital before admission to critical care, the higher is their mortality.[7,9] Management is often performed by junior teams that fail to appreciate clinical urgency and the importance of senior advice. Inadequate supervision, poor organisation, gaps in communication and continuity of care are also factors.[7,8,10]

Patients who experience lengthy periods of instability before there is an effective medical response are said to have suffered 'failure to rescue'. Such failures are common.[7,8,10–12] In a national review of medical patients subsequently transferred to a critical care unit, many had sustained up to 72 hours of physiological instability.[8] Analysis of 1000 deaths in 10 hospitals concluded that 52 deaths would have had a 50% or greater chance of being prevented; although it is noteworthy that most of these preventable deaths were in elderly, frail patients judged to have had a life expectancy of less than 12 months.[13]

Other groups of patients at risk are those recently discharged from the critical care unit or from the operating theatre after major surgery: about one-quarter of all 'critical care deaths' occur after discharge back to the ward. In particular, patients discharged prematurely suffer increased mortality.[14,15]

OUTREACH, MEDICAL EMERGENCY AND RAPID RESPONSE TEAMS

Medical emergency teams (METs) were introduced in Australia in the 1990s, usually comprising critical care residents and medical registrars. These teams could be directly activated by any member of staff bypassing traditional hospital hierarchies. METs expanded the role of the cardiac arrest team to include the pre-arrest period, generally using call-out criteria based on deranged physiological values or staff concern.[16] In the UK, a review of critical care services in 2000[17] led to increased funding for critical care beds and also the creation of critical care outreach teams, largely staffed by critical care nurses. Similar services have emerged in the USA, driven by the Institute for Healthcare Improvement[18] with more consideration of a whole 'rapid response system' (RRS). This highlights the principle that it is necessary to develop complete, coordinated systems to avoid failures to rescue reliably and consistently.

The RRS can be divided into:

- an afferent component designed to ensure timely escalation of the deteriorating patient, usually using agreed physiological values as a trigger
- an efferent component comprising an individual or team of clinicians who can promptly respond to deterioration
- governance and administrative structures to oversee and organise the service and its ways of working
- mechanisms to improve hospital processes.[19]

Another approach is to think of the RRS as being built on development of a 'chain of prevention' made up of education, monitoring, recognition, call and response.[20]

There are now many models and terms used.[19,21] METs are usually physician led. Critical care outreach (CCO) and rapid response teams (RRTs) are typically nurse led, but may also include physiotherapists and other allied health professionals as well as doctors. Most teams respond to defined physiological triggers, although some also work proactively with known at-risk patients such as those discharged from the critical care unit.

The aim is to prevent unnecessary critical care admissions, to ensure timely transfer to the critical care unit when needed, to facilitate safe return to the ward, to share critical care skills,[17] and to improve care throughout the hospital. There may also be a role in support for patients and their families after hospital discharge (**Box 2.1**).

Box 2.1 Functions of critical care outreach

- Identification of at-risk patients
- Support for ward staff caring for at-risk patients and those recovering from critical illness
- Referral pathways for obtaining timely, effective critical care treatments
- Immediate availability of expert critical care and resuscitation skills when required
- Facilitation of timely transfer to a critical care facility when needed
- Education for ward staff in recognition of fundamental signs of deterioration, and in understanding how to obtain appropriate help promptly
- Outpatient support to patients and their families following discharge from hospital
- Development of systems of coordinated, collaborative, continuous care of critically ill and recovering patients across the hospital and also in the community
- Audit and improvement of basic standards of acute and critical care – and of the outreach team itself – to minimise risk and optimise treatment of the critically ill throughout the hospital

Together, these elements comprise a system to deliver safe, quality care with proactive management of risk and timely treatment of critical illness.

RECOGNISING CRITICAL ILLNESS

Patients with potential or actual critical illness can be identified by review of the history, by examination and by investigations. Higher risks are associated with extremes of age, with significant co-morbidities or with serious presenting conditions.

The timeliness of response depends largely on the quality of monitoring. Patients at risk of deterioration require either very frequent or continuous monitoring to optimise the effect of a rapid response intervention. A conference on the afferent limb of the RRS found that: '(1) vital sign aberrations predict risk, (2) monitoring patients more effectively may improve outcome, although some risk is random, (3) the workload implications of monitoring on the clinical workforce have not been explored, but … should be investigated, (4) the characteristics of an ideal monitoring system are identifiable, and it is possible to categorize monitoring modalities. It may also be possible to describe monitoring levels, and a system'.[22] Currently, measuring and recording of vital signs on general wards are often inadequate.[8,10]

For early recognition of deterioration to be effective:

- the physiological values, laboratory results or other data used for patient monitoring should enable timely identification of deterioration
- there must be enough time to identify at-risk patients and then obtain expert assistance before irreversible deterioration has occurred.

ABNORMAL PHYSIOLOGY AND ADVERSE OUTCOME

There is a known association between abnormal physiology and adverse outcomes,[23,24] and critical care severity scoring systems such as APACHE II[25] are based upon this relationship. Patients who suffer cardiopulmonary arrest or who die in hospital generally have abnormal physiological values recorded in the preceding period, as do patients requiring transfer to the critical care unit.[8,10–12,23,24]

The finding that abnormal physiology precedes adverse events has led to key signs being incorporated into various early warning scoring (EWS) systems. These systems use different combinations of parameters including respiratory rate, oxygen saturation, heart rate, blood pressure, temperature and level of consciousness as well as other indicators such as urine output and pain.[26] The patient's measured vital signs are compared with a set of reference values, with measurements above or below designated points used as triggers for escalation. Formats vary but generally use similar approaches, awarding points for varying degrees of derangement of different functions. Improvement or further deterioration can then be tracked by changes in EWS recorded over time, so that an EWS used in this way can be described as a 'track and trigger system'. Track and trigger systems are broadly categorised as single or multiple parameter systems, aggregate weighted scoring systems or combinations[2] (**Box 2.2**).

Many different systems with variable trigger thresholds have been developed.[27–29] This variance has led to calls for standardised systems to improve training and reliability of response, with the UK National Early Warning Score (NEWS) published in 2012[30] (**Table 2.1**) and now adopted in Wales, Ireland and England. It is based on the analysis of a large database of patients' vital signs recorded in different acute hospitals.[31]

A different approach has been taken by Australian METs, where the calling-out criteria are usually based upon single, markedly deranged physiological values, although ward staff concern is also a trigger[32] (**Box 2.3**).

As well as EWS systems based simply on acute physiology, there are also published methods using other data to risk stratify patients at hospital admission. These systems aim to differentiate patients who need to stay in hospital for further monitoring or treatment and those who need only minimal monitoring or may even be discharged home. Systems based on laboratory parameters alone,[33] laboratory parameters in conjunction with vital sign observations,[34] or indicators of acute physiology, chronic illness and functional status[35] have all been validated against hospital mortality.

Another possible method of activating the RRS is for patients themselves – or their relatives – to call. This method was first used in paediatric settings but may also be useful for adults.[36]

MEASURING OUTCOME

The use of critical care outreach and other RRSs is based on the premise that early detection and treatment of critical illness should improve patient outcomes. The quality of these services may be evaluated against such outcomes but also other indicators including process measures (e.g. numbers of trained staff, completeness of bedside observations, timeliness of escalation and speed of response). The time from patient trigger to transfer to a critical care unit – or initiation of critical care treatments on the ward – may be a useful indicator too (i.e. the 'Score-to-Door time'[37]).

Table 2.2 shows one system that can be used to evaluate outcomes of RRS interventions 24 hours after the initial event, with outcomes classified as being either positive or negative. The proportion of positive interventions provides a measure of the quality of the service.

Box 2.2 Classification of track and trigger warning systems[2]

Single-parameter systems
- Tracking: periodic observation of selected basic signs
- Trigger: one or more extreme observational values

Multiple parameter systems
- Tracking: periodic observation of selected basic vital signs
- Trigger: two or more extreme observational values

Aggregate weighted scoring systems
- Tracking: periodic observation of selected basic vital signs and the assignment of weighted scores to physiological values with calculation of a total score
- Trigger: achieving a previously agreed trigger threshold with the total score
- Combination systems
- Elements of single- or multiple-parameter systems in combination with aggregate weighted scoring

Box 2.3 Medical emergency team calling-out criteria as used in the 23-site MERIT study[32]

Airway	Threatened
Breathing	Respiratory rate <5 or >36 per min Respiratory arrest
Circulation	Systolic blood pressure <90 mmHg (11.97 kPa) Pulse rate <40 or >140 per min
Neurology	Sudden fall in level of consciousness (fall in GCS of >2 points) Repeated or extended seizures
Other	Any patient you are seriously worried about

Table 2.1 National early warning score (NEWS)[31]

PHYSIOLOGICAL PARAMETERS	3	2	1	0	1	2	3
Respiration rate	≤8		9–11	12–20		21–24	≥25
Oxygen saturations	≤91	92–93	94–95	≥96			
Any supplemental oxygen?		Yes		No			
Temperature	≤35.0		35.1–36.0	36.1–38.0	38.1–39.0	≥39.1	
Systolic BP	≤90	91–100	101–110	111–219			≥220
Heart rate	≤40		41–50	51–90	91–110	111–130	≥131
Level of consciousness (AVPU (Alert, Voice, Pain, Unresponsive) scale)				A	V	P	U

Table 2.2 Matrix of possible outcomes of RRS intervention: the '**M**ulti-disciplinary **A**udit **E**va**L**uating **O**utcomes of **R**apid response' (MAELOR) tool

OUTCOMES	POSITIVE	NEGATIVE
Transfer to critical care unit, high-dependency area or operating theatre	1. Timely transfer, e.g. <4 hours after the first trigger	2. Delayed transfer, e.g. >4 hours after the first trigger
Alive on ward	3. No longer triggering	4. Still triggering
Deceased	5. On terminal care pathway/with DNAR order	6. Following cardiopulmonary arrest
Others	7. Alive with documented treatment limitations and DNAR order in place 8. a. Trigger from new pathology unrelated to previous call-out b. Chronic condition leading to continuous trigger (e.g. tachypnoea in advanced pulmonary fibrosis) c. Discharged from hospital	9. Outcome not known/lost to follow-up

Data from Morris A, Owen HM, Jones K, et al. Objective patient-related outcomes of rapid-response systems – a pilot study to demonstrate feasibility in two hospitals. Crit Care Resusc. 2013;15(1):33–9.

RRSs have highlighted shortcomings in the care of ward patients, and contributed to a significant change in attitude to at-risk patients. They have been instrumental in improving ward monitoring, and in disseminating critical care skills. There are anecdotal reports of benefit to individuals,[38] and published evidence that these services improve recognition of at-risk patients, reduce length of stay, cardiac arrest rates, unplanned admissions to critical care, and morbidity and mortality.[39–43] However, some reports do not show significant effects. There are in fact few good quality studies, with just two randomised controlled trials published to date.[32,43]

Positive studies include a UK randomised trial of phased introduction of a 24-hour outreach service to 16 wards in a general acute hospital.[43,44] The outreach team routinely followed up patients discharged from critical care to wards and also saw referrals generated by ward staff concern or use of an EWS system. There was a statistically significant reduction in mortality in wards where the service was operational. In contrast, a large prospective randomised trial of METs in Australia found no improvements in cardiac arrests, unplanned admissions to critical care or unexpected deaths in comparison to the control hospitals in the primary analysis.[32] A secondary analysis was able to show improved outcomes in most hospitals in both the intervention and control groups, with dramatic improvements in those with the weakest baseline performance.[45] This study revealed many shortcomings in identification and care of critically ill patients, with one possible conclusion being that it is essential to take a whole systems approach to early recognition of deterioration and achievement of an effective response.

Several studies have shown an inverse relation between the number of calls to the MET and the rates of cardiac arrest.[46] The explanation for this is not completely clear. It may be that reductions in cardiac arrests are linked to increased proportions of patients surviving to discharge, but it is as likely that decreased cardiac arrest calls are a reflection of better patient assessment and more timely implementation of Do-Not-Attempt-Resuscitation orders and involvement of palliative care specialists in patients with terminal illness. This is not a negative: delivery of good palliative care might be one of the positive outcomes supported by a RRS.[47]

There has been less investigation of the follow-up of patients discharged from critical care units, although this group is known to remain at significant risk. A matched-cohort analysis of 5924 patients found follow-up by an outreach team reduced length of stay and mortality when compared with historical controls and matched patients from hospitals with no outreach.[48]

SETTING UP AN OUTREACH SERVICE

Patients with potential or actual critical care illness are found in every area of the hospital, so systems to identify and treat those patients need to be planned at an organisational level. Involvement of managerial and clinical staff is essential, especially from the wards. It is particularly important that there is agreement and clarity about how the outreach team or equivalent interacts with the parent/primary medical team.

KEY STEPS IN PLANNING AN RRS

- Appoint senior clinical and managerial leads to develop the service.
- Institute organisational needs analysis, audit and evaluation, asking:
  - which patients are at risk of critical illness and where are they located?

- where do cardiopulmonary arrests and unexpected deaths occur?
- what is the source of unplanned admissions to the critical care unit?
- what is the pattern of adverse events where harm can be attributed to the process of care?
- what are the other relevant clinical governance/risk management issues (e.g. complaints), or morbidity and mortality data?

- A point prevalence study can give a snapshot view of the location of patients with physiological derangement.
- Review of unplanned admissions to the critical care unit can identify systems failings including quality of patient management and appropriateness and timeliness of escalation. Key practices can be assessed against specific, measurable standards.
- Such analyses should also highlight staff education and training needs.

Other factors to consider include:

- the patient case-mix
- existing skills of ward staff
- proposed hours of service
- size of hospital – and likely demand
- existing services such as pain teams, nutrition teams, tracheostomy specialist practitioners respiratory specialists, renal specialists, night teams, etc.
- training facilities
- outreach service location and equipment needs including information technology
- funding.

Various bodies in the UK, Australia and USA have published useful guides to setting up and developing a RRS; all are available online.[2,3,49,50]

THE OUTREACH TEAM

The composition and skills of the team should be designed to meet the specific needs identified by individual organisations. At a minimum, the team should be capable of assessment, diagnosis, initiation of resuscitation, and rapid triage of the critically ill patient to a higher level of care with authority to so act. Such clinical competencies as airway management techniques, venepuncture and cannulation are essential, and so are skills in education and training, research and audit. A multiprofessional team is required for this range of skills to be available, and to enable communication with other staff across the hospital. The UK Department of Health has detailed the competencies required for care of at-risk and deteriorating patients, specifying what should be expected of junior, middle-grade and senior staff.[51]

A pragmatic, staged implementation could include:

1. Establishing an education programme in care of the critically ill for ward staff so that they can recognise signs of deterioration and understand the necessity and means of obtaining timely help. Staff should update their skills annually.
2. Introducing a physiological track and trigger warning system and defined referral/response protocols.
3. Developing clinical bedside support – incrementally if necessary – increasing the number of clinical areas covered by the team, and the hours of work. This might include follow-up of patients discharged from critical care and responding to patients identified through the track and trigger system or other means.[2]

It is essential that robust data are collected and used for audit and evaluation – and for feedback to ward managers and clinical staff. Successes should be highlighted and areas for improvement identified. Data may include:

- numbers of referrals and patient follow-ups
- date and time of each episode
- patient details (e.g. age, sex, date of hospital admission, location, emergency/elective admission, medical/surgical, resuscitation status)
- trigger event (e.g. early warning score, cardiac arrest call)
- significant problems identified
- interventions performed
- patient outcomes.

THE FUTURE: TECHNOLOGY TO MITIGATE HUMAN FACTORS

In an increasingly safety conscious society, 'failure to rescue' becomes less and less acceptable. It is clear that many of the errors that lead to 'failure to rescue' are caused by human factors and flaws in the design of hospital systems.[52-54] This was shown by the MERIT study finding that of patients needing escalation to the critical care unit – with signs that should have been referred to the MET – only 30% were actually referred.[32] Hierarchical thinking, inflexible mental modelling, highly variable performance and uncoordinated, inefficient hospital organisation are all factors.[52-54] Even relatively simple matters such as the documentation for vital sign recording have a role: research from Australia has shown that attention to the layout of charts is likely to promote more reliable detection of deterioration.[55]

Automation has the potential to improve reliability of some key processes. Technological aids that automate calculation of early warning scores and communication of abnormal trigger scores are available. These systems are able to perform calculations of EWS with fewer errors and have been shown to improve outcomes.[56] The development of increasingly sophisticated expert systems will enable analysis of patterns of abnormal vital signs that can produce specific alerts as well as prompts and advice about individual patients, with due consideration of their particular pathophysiology.

CONCLUSION

There is no doubt that there are significant numbers of patients on hospital wards with potential or actual critical illness whose care should and could be improved. The RRS represents one method of addressing these issues. In the future, it may turn out to be that the most useful contribution of RRSs is the highlighting of defects in current ways of working, and the application of what has been learned from RRS initiatives to the whole hospital.

Key features include:

- Deteriorating patients can be identified by careful monitoring of physiological signs.
- Timely escalation of appropriate patients to critical care should improve outcomes.
- Effective response to acute deterioration depends on complex human interactions that are prone to error.
- Rapid response systems standardise the response to at-risk and deteriorating patients, and improve process and clinical outcomes for critically ill patients presenting outside the critical care unit.
- Successful systems are based upon multiprofessional working, and effective communication education, data collection/audit, learning from errors, and planned improvement of whole systems of care.

Access the complete references list online at http://www.expertconsult.com

8. Cullinane M, Findlay G, Hargraves C, et al. An Acute Problem? London: National Confidential Enquiry into Patient Outcome and Death; 2005.
13. Hogan H, Healey F, Neale G, et al. Preventable deaths due to problems in care in English acute hospitals: a retrospective case record review study. BMJ Qual Saf 2012;21(9):737–45.
31. Prytherch DR, Smith GB, Schmidt PE, et al. ViEWS - towards a national early warning score for detecting adult inpatient deterioration. Resuscitation 2010;81(8):932–7.
32. Hillman K, Chen J, Cretikos M, et al. Introduction of the medical emergency team (MET) system: a cluster-randomised controlled trial. Lancet 2005;365(9477):2091–7.
37. Oglesby KJ, Durham L, Welch J, et al. 'Score to Door Time', a benchmarking tool for rapid response systems: a pilot multi-centre service evaluation. Crit Care 2011;15(4):R180.
43. Priestley G, Watson W, Rashidian A, et al. Introducing Critical Care Outreach: a ward-randomised trial of phased introduction in a general hospital. Intensive Care Med 2004;30(7):1398–1404.
48. Harrison DA, Gao H, Welch CA, et al. The effects of critical care outreach services before and after critical care: a matched-cohort analysis. J Crit Care 2010;25(2):196–204.
50. 5 Million Lives Campaign. Getting started kit: rapid response teams. Cambridge, MA: Institute for Healthcare Improvement; 2008. Online. Available: www.ihi.org (accessed 1st October 2012).
52. Shearer B, Marshall S, Buist MD, et al. What stops hospital clinical staff from following protocols? An analysis of the incidence and factors behind the failure of bedside clinical staff to activate the rapid response system in a multi-campus Australian metropolitan healthcare service. BMJ Qual Saf 2012;21(7):569–755.
56. Bellomo R, Ackerman M, Bailey M, et al. A controlled trial of electronic automated advisory vital signs monitoring in general hospital wards. Crit Care Med 2012;40(8):2349–61.

FURTHER READING

Morris A, Owen HM, Jones K, et al. Objective patient-related outcomes of rapid-response systems – a pilot study to demonstrate feasibility in two hospitals. Crit Care Resusc 2013;15(1):33–9.

National Institute for Health and Clinical Excellence. Acutely ill patients in hospital: recognition of and response to acute illness in adults in hospital. NICE clinical guideline 50. London: National Institute for Health and Clinical Excellence; 2007. Online. Available: www.nice.org.uk (accessed 1st October 2012).

National Institute for Health and Clinical Excellence. Critical illness rehabilitation. NICE clinical guideline 83. London: National Institute for Health and Clinical Excellence; 2009. Online. Available: www.nice.org.uk (accessed 1st October 2012).

Shekelle PG, Pronovost PJ, Wachter RM, et al. Advancing the science of patient safety. Ann Intern Med 2011;154(10):693–6.

Winters BD, Weaver SJ, Pfoh ER, et al. Rapid-response systems as a patient safety strategy: a systematic review. Ann Intern Med 2013;158(5 Pt 2):417–25.

3

Severity of illness and likely outcome from critical illness

Mark Palazzo

It is intuitive that severity of illness might be related to eventual outcome. It is also not unreasonable to assume that outcome might also be related to whether a condition is reversible or to the presence of co-morbidities that might modify resilience. However, although acuity may be related to outcome, the speed of delivery of care, its organisation and avoidance of iatrogenicity can also be expected to play their part. Many patients also acquire conditions and complications that they were not admitted with whilst in the intensive care unit (ICU).

In many conditions there has been a long history of attempting to relate acuity to outcome. For example, the New York Heart Association first classified patients with cardiac disease based on clinical severity and prognosis in 1928 and this has subsequently been updated seven times, the last in 1994. Similarly the Glasgow Coma Scale described the changes in coma following head injury and its association with prognosis.[1-3] The Ranson score related outcome to severity of acute pancreatitis,[4] while the Pugh modification of Child–Turcotte classification for patients undergoing porto-systemic shunt surgery is widely used for classification of end-stage liver disease.[5] More recently the Euroscore has been used to calculate likely mortality following cardiac surgery.[6]

The earliest attempt to quantify severity of illness in a heterogeneous critically ill population was by Cullen, who devised a score in which therapeutic intervention was used as a surrogate for illness.[7] This was followed in 1981 with the introduction of the Acute Physiology, Age and Chronic Health Evaluation (APACHE) scoring system and shortly after by the Simplified Acute Physiology Score (SAPS) and Mortality Prediction Model (MPM).[8-10] These scores have since been updated for international use while others have been introduced and calibrated to meet a specific population – such as the ICNARC model for the UK.[11]

The advantages of quantifying critical illness with scores and relating this to outcome include:

- a common language for discussion of severity of illness
- a method by which critical care practice and processes can be compared both within and between units
- provision of risk-adjusted mortality predictions facilitating acuity comparisons for clinical trials
- indication of likely post-ICU morbidity and survival.

Limitations of quantifying critical illness with scores are:

- they cannot provide individual patient prognosis
- they cannot be meaningfully used for treatment decisions.

Although mortality prediction is the focus of scoring systems, the numerically greater burden of critical illness is continuing physical and social disablement; indeed the survivors of critical care have a higher mortality than the normal population. There is an inherent temptation to use scoring systems to indicate an individual patient's prognosis, but this would be statistically incorrect. The scores were derived from very large cohorts of heterogeneous patients and the prognostic output is a mortality probability estimate for a similar cohort not an individual.

Less controversial has been the common use of scoring systems to demonstrate there is balance in the acuity of patients admitted into the arms of a clinical trial, but even there the use of the score rather than the calculated risk of death can be misleading in heterogeneous patient groups.[12] Despite the known controversy in using individual patient scores for predicting outcome, studies have used APACHE II scores as a guide to enrolment for treatment.[13]

It is of interest that, although the critical care community widely accepts acuity scores to demonstrate balance between groups in clinical trials, it is less enthusiastic to accept the same systems as comparators for between unit and between country performances, citing calibration and case mix as confounders.[14] That is unless, of course, the same said individuals' unit performances compare favourably!

Poor calibration (model under or over estimates mortality rate for the cohort under study) can be due to numerous reasons. The patient population may be from a different health system to the one where the model was developed, or there may be a systematic error in documenting the raw data, or the case-mix is very different to the original model, or indeed the model fails to include an important prognostic variable that is present in the cohort. For example, it has become clearer that prognosis is as much affected by local organisation, patient pathways, patient's pre-admission condition or their location prior to admission as it is by acute physiological disturbances.[15,16]

Scoring systems would be better calibrated if the models were used only on patient populations similar to those from which the models were constructed, but this would limit their international usefulness. An alternative approach would be to develop the model from a wider international cohort, but then such a model could calibrate poorly when used in an individual country. SAPS III (developed internationally) provided a solution to this with customised formulae so that the risk-adjusted expected mortality could be related to geographical location.[16]

Inevitably, as medical services progress and new treatments become available, risk-adjusted mortality predictions become outdated and trend towards overestimated expected mortality.[17,18] Consequently the designers of the scoring systems have reviewed their models every few years. **Table 3.1** outlines some of the upgraded systems.

FACTORS INDICATING SEVERITY OF ILLNESS AND RISKS THAT MIGHT CONTRIBUTE TO OUTCOME

- Acute physiological disturbance
- Primary pathological process causing physiological disturbance
- Age, co-morbid states and 'physiological reserve'
- Location prior to admission and emergency status
- Unit organisation and processes.

ACUTE PHYSIOLOGICAL DISTURBANCE

It is a reasonable assumption that the degree of physiological disturbance may bear some relationship to severity of illness. This is based on the observation that an untreated pathological insult is followed by increasing compensatory activity in order to retain vital organ function. Most compensatory mechanisms are mediated through neuroendocrine responses directed to maintaining tissue oxygenation ensuring mitochondrial and ultimately organ function. Compensatory signs such as hyperventilation, tachycardia and oliguria associated with cerebral dysfunction are hallmarks of early, untreated critical illness and if decompensation ensues hypotension, metabolic acidosis and stupor develop. Regardless of the insult, organs have limited ways in which they manifest dysfunction and decompensation. Quantifying these common responses is a logical starting point for the basis of a generic scoring system. It is notable that some scoring systems such as SAPS are based solely on the acute physiological disturbance with little or no reference to the driving pathology.

However, acute physiological measurements present some challenges if they are to be translated to scores. The relationship between acute response and insult is non-linear; furthermore anatomical organ damage may not be reflected by measured function until quite extensive. For example, the liver and kidney manifest biochemical abnormality only when a significant proportion of organ mass is malfunctioning. Equally we

Table 3.1 Revision dates for the most common internationally recognised risk-adjusted models for mortality prediction

SEVERITY OF ILLNESS MODEL	YEAR	TIMING OF SCORE	COHORT SIZE	ICU UNITS	WORLD REGIONS OF ICUS PARTICIPATING IN DEVELOPMENT OF MODEL
SAPS	1984	1st 24 h	679	8	France
SAPS II	1993	1st 24 h	13,152	137	Europe/USA
SAPS III	2005	Admission	16,784	303	Europe, Australia, South and Central America
MPM I	1987	Admission	1997	1	USA
MPM II_0	1993	Admission	19,124	137	USA/Europe
MPM_0III	2007	Admission	124,855	135	USA/Canada Brazil
APACHE I	1981	1st 24 h	805	2	USA
APACHE II	1985	1st 24 h	5815	13	USA
APACHE III	1991	1st 24 h	17,440	40	USA
APACHE IV	2006	1st 24 h	110,558	104	USA
ICNARC	2007	1st 24 h	216,626	163	UK
ICNARC revised coefficients for APACHE II and ICNARC	2011 model	1st 24 h			UK

have a poor understanding of the equivalency of malfunction between organs (e.g. what degree of acidosis is equivalent to a given tachycardia or hypotension).

A further consideration for severity of illness estimation is its timing. Ideally a true estimate of physiological disturbance would be in an untreated state. Logistically this may be quite difficult, and indeed most scores arbitrarily took the first 24 hours after admission to intensive care as the period to estimate severity of illness. However, logic would dictate that estimates would be more appropriate in the hours prior to admission when fluid resuscitation, early antibiotic treatment, ventilation or inotropes have not had time to modify the acute response or extent of decompensation. Such support for the seriously ill can diminish the difference between such patients and, for example, elective surgical admissions who have for convenience been kept ventilated until reaching the ICU. The risk of underestimating physiological disturbance has been mitigated either by taking account of the organ support on admission or by including estimates of physiological disturbance before support has been commenced. For example, SAPS III makes an adjustment for patients on inotropes, whereas MPM II allows measurements for the hour on either side of admission.[15,16,19]

PRIMARY PATHOLOGICAL PROCESS

It would be expected that, for a given degree of acute physiological disturbance, the most serious primary pathologies are likely to have the worst predicted outcomes. For example, for a given degree of acute respiratory disturbance at admission a patient with community-acquired pneumonia is likely to have a better outcome than an immunosuppressed patient with an unknown opportunist pneumonia. Furthermore, the potential reversibility of a primary pathological process with specific therapies also greatly influences outcome. For example, patients with diabetic ketoacidosis can be extremely unwell, but specific therapy with insulin and volume therapy can rapidly reverse the physiological disturbance. Conversely failure to identify organisms or sources of sepsis delays specific therapy and adversely affects outcome.

Both APACHE and the most recent SAPS systems include diagnostic categories with the acute physiological data to estimate risk of hospital death.

AGE, CO-MORBID STATES AND PHYSIOLOGICAL RESERVE

Increasing age is normally associated with diminishing capacity to respond to an insult and decompensation occurs earlier. However, this capacity is only broadly predictable. 'Biological' age is a vague term used to imply physiological reserve below that expected for a patient's chronological age. Biological age greater than chronological age is commonly perceived in heavy smokers or abusers of alcohol. These patients may or may not have diminished organ function, but are generally expected to more readily reach a decompensated state. Physiological reserve is a term that hints at the likely ability to cope with an insult and its physiological demands, it is often inferred from age and co-morbidity. Conditions such as diabetes and chronic pulmonary disease are generally considered to have some bearing on physiological reserve, but not always as much as might be expected. On the other hand, co-morbid states such as immunosuppression, cirrhosis and haematological malignancies do result in significant diminution of resistance to infection. These co-morbidities are commonly included in critical illness severity scoring systems, unlike diabetes.

LOCATION PRIOR TO ADMISSION AND EMERGENCY STATUS

The location of a patient prior to admission to ICU is a factor recognised by the more recent scoring systems as having an influence on outcome.[11,15] This might in part be because location influences the lead time to definitive treatment, or is a health care environment where the likelihood of carrying resistant organisms is higher.

The emergency status of a patient has equally been recognised by all scoring systems to influence outcome. Acute medical and emergency surgery admissions are associated with poorer outcomes than those following elective surgery.

UNIT ORGANISATION AND PROCESSES

Soon after the introduction of APACHE II it was recognised that units with effective nursing and medical leadership, good communications and dedicated intensive care specialists had better outcomes than those without such characteristics.[20–25] Additionally, factors such as genetic variables, socioeconomic status, access to investigations and normal medical care are likely to have a quantifiable but as yet indeterminate bearing on the widest aspects of outcome.

RISK-ADJUSTED EXPECTED OUTCOME

Prior to the advent of scoring systems, expected outcome from critical illness was not calculated and it was difficult to have confidence that control groups in clinical trials were representative or internationally relevant. The common outcome measures are ICU, 28-day and hospital mortalities. Scoring systems provide calculations which can demonstrate that active and control groups have similar risks of death and, importantly, that the control group had observed outcomes similar to those expected. Similarly risk-adjusted expected outcome is a standard tool for monitoring the performance of an ICU and offers some indication of comparative performance particularly when patient case-mix is similar.

However, whereas hospital death and risk of death is a clear-cut outcome measure, morbidity in the guise of serious psychological or physical functional impairment is far more common.[26-29] Indeed there is a case that risk-adjusted outcome should be extended to consider time to return to normal function or work as well as survival at 1 year.[30,31] Longer-term outcome is confounded by premorbid chronic health status.

PRINCIPLES OF SCORING SYSTEM DESIGN

CHOICE OF INDEPENDENT PHYSIOLOGICAL VARIABLES AND THEIR TIMING

The designers of the APACHE and SAPS systems originally chose physiological variables that they felt would represent measures of acute illness. The variables chosen by experts were weighted equally on a linear scale with the highest value given to the worst physiological deviation from normal.[9,32] In these early models diagnostic details, premorbid conditions, age and emergency status were also included to create a score that was then used in an equation to provide risk of death. Later upgrades to these systems, SAPS, APACHE and MPM, used logistic regression analysis to determine which variables should be included to explain the observed hospital mortality.[33] Variables were no longer given equal importance nor their weightings linearly related to the physiological disturbance. Furthermore this statistical approach to developing a scoring system confirmed that factors suspected of influencing outcome such as location prior to admission, cardiopulmonary resuscitation (CPR) or dependence on inotropes prior to admission indeed had discriminatory power and were included in the logistic regression equation from which risk of death could be calculated.[11,16]

DEVELOPING A SCORING METHODOLOGY AND ITS VALIDATION

All the commonly used acuity scoring systems have been based on large databases derived from several ICUs (see Table 3.1). Typically more than 50% of the database is used to provide a cohort of patients to act as a developmental group. A number of independent categorical or continuous variables that could feasibly influence outcome are collected. These variables are used in a logistic regression equation to achieve the best fit to explain the dichotomous dependent variables survival or hospital death. The starting point is to include all variables that by univariate analysis are moderately related to outcome, perhaps at the $p<0.15$ level. The logistic equation is then modified through multiple iterations during which variables are either removed or combined in order to improve the fit to explaining outcome. Each variable is weighted with a coefficient to provide the best fit that distinguishes survival from non-survival. The best fit is assessed by the Hosmer–Lemeshow test for goodness of fit.[34] The model is initially tested on the developmental cohort. This is done by exploring the model's ability to discriminate between survivors and non-survivors by plotting positive predictions of death against false-positive predictions in a receiver operator curve (see below). The area under the curve (AUC) sometimes referred to as the c-statistic (or concordance index), is a value that varies from 0.5 (discriminating power not better than chance) to 1.0 (perfect discriminating power). Clearly when tested on the developmental cohort the discriminatory power would be expected to be high. This is done through statistical techniques such as 'jack-knifing' or 'boot-strapping' that take numerous small samples of the developmental cohort to demonstrate stability of the chosen variables. The next step is to test the model against a new set of patients, the validation dataset (the other 50% of patients from the database who were not in the developmental set). The aim of validation is to demonstrate that the model can be used to predict likely hospital outcome, which is again measured with the concordance index.

Once a satisfactory equation has been developed it can be used to calculate the overall probability of death for a group of patients.

A perfect model should ideally be able to predict which patients will survive and which will die (discrimination) and correctly predict the overall observed mortality (calibration). Discriminating power is assessed by construction of a receiver operator curve (ROC).

ROC CONSTRUCTION

The area under a ROC is constructed by using the logistic regression model to indicate the number of patients predicted to die and comparing this with the observed numbers who died. This is undertaken at different thresholds of predictions of death. So, for example, if the threshold is set at 50% the assumption is that any patient at or above that calculated risk counts as a prediction to die. This in turn is compared with what actually happened. Clearly many patients predicted to die do die, but a not-insignificant number predicted to die at the 50% threshold will survive. One can determine just how unreliable that threshold is as a predictor by determining the true-positive predictions (sensitivity) – that is, the observed deaths among those who were predicted to die – and compare these with the false-positive predictions – that is, the survivors among all those predicted to die. This exercise can be repeated using different thresholds such as 60, 70, 80, 90% where again it is assumed that those with calculated risks at the threshold value or above would all be predicted to die. At each threshold point the sensitivity and false-positive rates are calculated. The false-positive predictions of death can be reduced only if the model also has high specificity, in other words it correctly predicts survivors. It is therefore common for the false-positive rate to be expressed as 1 – specificity or 100 – specificity if expressed as percentages. The ROC convention is to plot sensitivity on the y-axis against 1 - specificity on the x-axis, with each x and y value representing sensitivity and false-positive rates at each threshold point (**Fig. 3.1**).

A perfect model would be 100% sensitive and 100% specific and would therefore follow the y-axis with a sensitivity value of 1 and a false-positive value of 0.

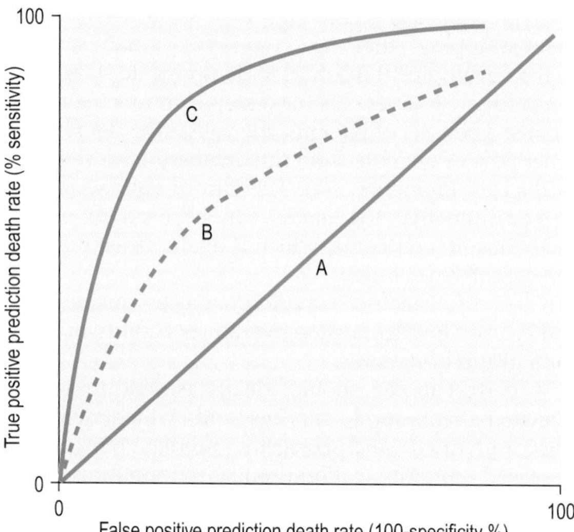

Figure 3.1 A receiver operator curve (ROC) plots true-positive against false-positive rates for a series of cut-off points for risk of death. As sensitivity or true positives increase there is a tendency for more false-positive results. There is a trade-off in making a test or predictor tool very sensitive because it loses specificity. The best curve is one that is above the line of no discrimination (A) and tends towards the y-axis. Therefore the model represented by line C is better than model B. The curve is made up of a series of sensitivity and false-positive estimates based on changing the threshold decision cut-offs. Typically the thresholds would be between 10 and 90% (i.e. when set at 10% the model predicts that every patient above a 10% risk of death will die). This level of cut-off will find every single death, but unfortunately there will be many false positives. This would provide a point towards the right-hand corner of the graph. When the cut-off point is made very high, such as 90%, the model will find only some of the true deaths, but there is less likelihood of a false positive and this will provide a point towards the origin of the graph closely applied to the y-axis.

The curve can be quantified by the area under the curve with higher values indicating more discriminatory power. For binary outcomes such as death and survival the area under the curve expressed as a fraction is the same as the concordance statistic, which varies between 0.5 and 1.

Conversely a curve that demonstrated no ability to discriminate between survivors and non-survivors would be represented by a line at 45 degrees going through the origin (non-discriminator line). The further the ROC is above the non-discriminator line and towards the y-axis the greater is the model's power of discrimination. This can be quantified by the c-statistic, which is a rank order statistic, or quantified by the area under the curve. The two measures are synonymous when the discrimination is between two mutually exclusive outcomes such as survival and non-survival. Prediction models that have AUC 0.7–0.8 are considered fair, those with AUC 0.8–0.9 are good, while those above 0.9 are considered excellent.

It is also possible to calculate the misclassification rate (patients predicted to die who survived and those predicted to survive who died). For example, in the APACHE II system the misclassification rates were 14.5, 15.2, 16.7 and 18.5% respectively at 50, 70, 80 and 90% predicted risk of death cut-off points, indicating that the best trade-off point between sensitivity and specificity with this model was when it was assumed that any patient with a risk of death greater than 50% would be a non-survivor. The calculations of sensitivity, specificity and misclassification rates are outlined in the (**Box 3.1**). **Table 3.2** indicates the AUC for the commonly used scoring systems.

CALIBRATION

A model with good calibration is one that for a given cohort predicts a similar overall percentage mortality to that observed. The extent to which this is achieved can be explored with the Hosmer–Lemeshow goodness-of-fit c-statistic. This compares the model's prediction of death and the actual outcome. The model is deemed to fit well and be well calibrated when there is no statistical difference between the two (i.e. the p value is larger than 0.05).[34]

Observations with many models have revealed that, unless the case-mix of the test patients is similar to those that were used to develop the model, the models may underperform owing to poor calibration. This is particularly true when the testing is done for patients in different countries.[16,35–37]

COMMONLY USED SCORING SYSTEMS

ACUTE PHYSIOLOGY AGE AND CHRONIC HEALTH EVALUATION (APACHE) SYSTEMS I, II, III, IV

In 1981 Knaus described APACHE, a physiologically based classification system for measuring severity of illness in groups of critically ill patients.[32] They suggested that it could be used to control for case-mix, compare outcomes, evaluate new therapies, and study the utilisation of ICUs. APACHE II, a simplified version,

Box 3.1 Calculations of sensitivity and specificity for a prediction model for mortality

When a model is tested against a cohort of patients its ability to correctly discriminate between predicted survivors and non-survivors is a measure of its power and ultimate usefulness.

Based on the data below a number of measures can be determined.

	OBSERVED DEATHS	OBSERVED SURVIVORS	TOTAL
Predicted deaths	450	100	550
Predicted survivors	40	410	450
Total	490	510	1000

Sensitivity: the proportion of observed deaths correctly predicted to die (true positive).
Sensitivity = 450/490 = 0.92.
Specificity: the proportion of survivors correctly predicted to survive (true negative).
Specificity = 410/510 = 0.80.
1 – specificity is the proportion of survivors that were predicted to be dead (false positive).
Positive predictive value: observed predicted deaths as a proportion of the total predicted deaths = 450/550 = 0.82.
Negative predictive value: observed predicted survivors as a proportion of the total predicted to survive = 410/450 = 0.91.
Misclassification rate is the proportion of patients wrongly predicted: (100+40)/1000 = 14%.
Correct classification rate is the proportion of patients correctly predicted: (450+410)/1000 = 86%.
False-positive rate = 100%–positive predictive value=18%.
False-negative rate = 100%–negative predictive value=9%.
Prevalence of death = 490/1000 =49%.

Table 3.2 AUCs for commonly used scoring systems

SCORE	AREA UNDER ROC CURVE
APACHE II	0.85
APACHE III	0.90
SAPS II	0.86
MPM II_0	0.82
$MPMII_{24}$	0.84
SAPS III	0.84
APACHE IV	0.88
ICNARC 2007	0.87
MPM_0III	0.82

In effect these models are only powerful enough to discriminate between likely survivors and non-survivors between 80 and 90% of the time.

was introduced in 1985, which was superseded in 1991 by a proprietary version, APACHE III.[32,38] APACHE IV was introduced in 2006, but remains a proprietary system.[18] APACHE II rather than the later versions has become the most widely studied and used system worldwide for reporting severity of illness.

APACHE II was developed and validated on 5030 ICU patients (excluding coronary bypass patients). The score is the sum of three components:

- an acute physiology score (APS)
- a chronic health score based on defined premorbid states
- a score based on the patient's age.

The 12 variables of the APS and their relative weights were decided by expert opinion. These variables are collected in the first 24 hours after admission to ICU and should represent the worst physiological values. The APACHE II score can be included in a logistic regression equation with a coefficient for one of 50 diagnostic categories representing the reason for admission and a coefficient for admission following emergency surgery. The equation will calculate a probability of death. The probability of death, although calculated for each single individual, will only approximate the model's claimed calibration when a large cohort of patients with the same diagnostic grouping is examined (groups of at least 50). Furthermore, as in all prediction models, although the number of deaths might be predicted correctly, discriminating those who will die from those who will survive will be fraught by misclassification errors and therefore the prediction remains a probability with a defined error and cannot be used for decision making.

APACHE II has functioned best when the ICU patient cohort under test is similar to the original North American development database. The system is now old and overestimates mortality predictions, mainly because critical care management and organisation have improved significantly over the last 30 years. However, simply modifying an old scoring system does not readily correct the calibration problems, hence the need to upgrade the system using recent databases.

APACHE III was introduced in 1991 and was designed to:

- improve prognostic estimates by re-evaluating the selection and weighting of physiological variables with an expanded reference database
- examine how outcome is related to patient selection for ICU admission and its timing
- attempt individual estimates of mortality.

APACHE III was based on a large database (17 440 patients) from 40 US hospitals that was equally divided between developmental and validation groups.

Patients who were admitted for less than 4 hours, with burn injuries or with chest pain were excluded. Coronary artery bypass patients were considered as a separate group.

A total of 17 physiological variables, including a revised version of the Glasgow Coma Scale, were identified through statistical analysis and the diagnostic categories were increased from 50 to 78. The patient location immediately prior to ICU admission was included and only those co-morbidities that affected a patient's immune status were considered. Chronic disease states and age contributed 15% of the calculated mortality risk, the rest being based on the acute physiology disturbance.

APACHE III represented an advance over APACHE II with improved discriminatory power (ROC 0.9 vs 0.85), and better calibration.[38] In an early comparative study, Castella et al reported that, although APACHE II proved better calibrated than SAPS and MPM I in a 14745 mixed patient cohort from European and American ICUs, APACHE III was better calibrated and more discriminating.[39]

A new characteristic introduced in the APACHE system was not only a calculated risk of death based on the first day values, but also serial calculations on subsequent days to provide an updated risk of death calculation for an individual. The coefficients for the regression equations are not in the public domain, and this has made independent assessment of the predictive aspect of the scoring system difficult.

APACHE IV

It was failure of customisation techniques with APACHE III to account for observations in subgroups that led to development of a new model. The authors of APACHE IV revealed that when APACHE III in its modified form was applied to patients collected between 2002 and 2003 calibration was poor.[18]

APACHE IV was based on a new database of 131618 admissions from 104 US ICU in 45 hospitals. The selected hospitals had the APACHE III computerised data collection and analysis system already installed. Of the admissions, 110558 patients had completed datasets and 60% were randomly selected to make up the developmental dataset. The exclusions included patients who were in hospital for more than a year or admitted from another ICU. Only first admissions were counted. The diagnostic groups were increased to 116 and not only was the location prior to admission included but also the hospital length of stay prior to ICU. The statistical and modelling techniques included cubic regression splines, which allow for a non-linear relationship between variables and outcome.

The AUC ROC derived from the model used on a validation dataset was 0.88, indicating very good discrimination. The relative contribution of the predictor variables for estimating hospital mortality is shown in **Table 3.3**.

The APACHE IV system has not been tested outside the US and therefore how it calibrates in the rest of the world is unknown. Indeed this might also be the case in the US given the selected units used for the database.[40]

Table 3.3 The relative contribution of the predictor variables for estimating hospital mortality in APACHE IV

Acute physiology	65.5%
Diagnosis	16.5%
Age	9.4%
Chronic health	5.0%
Admission source and previous length of stay	2.9%
Mechanical ventilation	0.6%

SIMPLIFIED ACUTE PHYSIOLOGY SCORE (SAPS I–III)

The Simplified Acute Physiology Score (SAPS) was originally based on data derived from French ICU, and based almost entirely on acute physiological variables.[9] The chosen 14 physiological variables were selected by experts and arbitrary scores were based on the degree of deviation from normal. Initially the score was not related to an equation for predicting probability of death, although later this was possible. Unlike APACHE II this system included neither diagnostic categories nor chronic health status as part of the severity of illness estimate.

In 1993 SAPS II was introduced and this was based on European and North American patients.[41] The database contained 13152 patients, divided 65% and 35% between developmental and validation cohorts. Excluded patients included those under 18 years, with burns, receiving coronary care or post cardiac surgery.

The weightings given to physiological derangements were derived from logistic regression analysis. The variables included 12 physiological measurements and specific chronic health conditions such as the presence of AIDS, haematological malignancies, cirrhosis and metastasis. Like the original SAPS there was no requirement for inclusion of diagnostic groups. The probability for hospital death could be readily calculated from a logistic regression equation. In the validation sample the area under the ROC was 0.86 with equivalent calibration and discrimination to APACHE III and MPM II. It is the most commonly used scoring system in continental Europe.

SAPS III

SAPS III was introduced in 2005 and developed from a database of 16784 patients from 303 ICU from around the world including South and Central America.[15,16] The model used multilevel logistic regression equations based on 20 variables.

The authors separated variables into those related to the period prior to admission, those concerning the admission itself and those of the acute physiological derangement (**Table 3.4**).

The SAPS III score can be used to derive a risk of death from a logistic regression equation. Discrimination was

Table 3.4 Factors considered in SAPS III

PATIENT CHARACTERISTICS BEFORE ADMISSION	CIRCUMSTANCES SURROUNDING ADMISSION	ACUTE PHYSIOLOGICAL CHANGES WITHIN 1 HOUR BEFORE AND AFTER ADMISSION
Age	Planned or unplanned	GCS
Comorbidities	Reason for admission (diagnostic group)	Bilirubin
Length of stay before ICU admission	Medical or surgical	Temperature
Hospital location before admission	Anatomical site of surgery	Creatinine
Vasoactive agents before admission	Acute infection at time surgery	Leucocytes pH Systolic BP Oxygenation and mechanical ventilation

good, with ROC AUC 0.848. The calibration varied, however, depending on the geographical area tested. The best fits for the general SAPS III risk adjustment model were for Northern European patients while the worst was for Central and South America. This simply reflected the lower number of patients from those areas in the developmental dataset. However, the model can be customised with alternative equations to improve calibration for different regions of the world.

The authors found that 50% of the model's explanatory power for predicting hospital mortality was from patient characteristics prior to admission, while circumstances surrounding admission and acute physiology parameters accounted for 22.5 and 27.5% respectively. The lower explanatory power compared with APACHE IV is notable and may be due to the absence of diagnostic weights in SAPS III.

MORTALITY PREDICTION MODELS (MPM I–III)

MPM was introduced in 1985 to provide an evidence-based approach to constructing a scoring system.[42] The data were derived from a single US institution and included observations at the time of admission to ICU and within the first 24 hours. MPM I_0 was based on the absence or presence of some physiological and diagnostic features at the time of admission, while a further prediction model MPM I_{24} was based on variables reflecting the effects of treatment at the end of the first ICU day. Unlike APACHE and SAPS systems it does not calculate a score based on the extent of physiological derangement, but computes the hospital risk of death from a logistic regression equation from coefficients based on the presence or absence of 15 factors such as coma, chronic renal failure, cirrhosis, heart rate over 150, systolic blood pressure below 90 mmHg (≈12 kPa) and several others.

MPM II is based on the same dataset as SAPS II.[33] The system is a series of four models which provide an outcome prediction estimate for ICU patients at admission and at 24, 48 and 72 hours. In common with the early APACHE and SAPS systems, the models excluded burns, coronary care and cardiac surgery patients. The models were derived by using logistic regression techniques to choose and weight the variables with an additional criterion that variables had to be 'clinically plausible'.

MPM_0 and $MPMII_{24}$ have similar discriminatory power to SAPS II, with ROC AUCs of 0.82 and 0.84 respectively.

In a comparison between MPM II, SAPS II and APACHE III and the earlier versions of these systems, all the newer systems performed better than their respective older versions; however, no system stood out as being superior to the others.[39]

In 2007 MPM_0III was introduced because it was noted that MPM II had lost its calibration against patients who were being recruited into the ongoing Project IMPACT.[43] This was probably due to changes in practice rather than case-mix. MPM_0III was based on retrospective data from 135 ICUs and 124 855 patients collected between 2001 and 2004. The patients were randomly divided into development (60%) and validation (40%) sets. The same variables as MPM II were collected, but included whether the patient was 'do not attempt resuscitation' at the time of admission (1 hour before or after admission). The resulting statistical analysis revealed that not only were the same variables retained but also there was a need to include interactions between age and each of the variables of systolic pressure, cirrhosis, metastatic neoplasms, cardiac dysrhythmia, intracranial mass effect and CPR prior to admission in order to correct overprediction of mortality. The authors achieved better calibration with MPM_0III than with their earlier model. The strengths of the MPM systems are that the burdens of data collection are low and the variables are boolean. The data are collected at the time of admission. This simplicity of collecting fewer variables at admission unfortunately has a trade-off in that discriminatory power is lost compared with other models. However, discriminatory power with ROC AUC at 0.82 remains acceptable.

ICNARC MODELS

ICNARC (Intensive Care National Audit and Research Centre) is a UK organisation dedicated to the collection and analysis of critical care data derived from over 160 ICU on a regular basis. It initially collected data for SAPS, APACHE II and MPM, and in the APACHE II model replaced the original diagnostic categories with its own to improve calibration for the UK. Its success has been based on a consistent methodology for data collection and therefore year-on-year data can be used to update diagnostic coefficients for APACHE II to ensure contemporary calibration. Furthermore, confidence in the data has allowed development of its own ICNARC mortality prediction model. The current ICNARC model was introduced in 2007 and upgraded with new coefficients in 2011. The model was originally based on 163 general ICUs using data collected between 1995 and 2003.[11] The model ultimately included data from 216626 patients. Re-admissions during the same hospital spell were not included. This model was also based on logistic regression analysis and isolated 12 physiological variables, which if all at their worst added up to a score of 100. The model also included age, diagnostic categories, source of admission and whether a patient had received CPR prior to admission. The model showed a high degree of discrimination (0.874) and calibration when applied to a validation set. Interestingly the impact of chronic health was found to be less than expected. Its weakness like the APACHE system is that it is entirely based on a national cohort and may not be suitable outside the UK.

ORGAN FAILURE SCORES

It is intuitive that as more organs fail the likelihood of death increases. As part of his work with APACHE, Knaus devised a simple predictive table in which, depending on age, the number of organs failed and the duration of failure he could estimate the likely risk of death. The organ system failures (OSFs) were defined for 5 organs.[44]

The notable observations were that:

- a single OSF lasting more than 1 day resulted in a hospital mortality rate of 40%
- two OSFs for more than 1 day increased rates to 60%
- three or more OSFs lasting more than 3 days were associated with a mortality of 98%.

Advanced chronological age increased both the probability of developing OSF and the probability of death once OSF occurred. These figures probably overestimate the risk of death in most parts of the world today.

Scores have been described that take account of grades of dysfunction and the supportive therapy required. One of these is the Multiple Organ Dysfunction Score (MODS), which was based on specific descriptors in six organ systems (respiratory, renal, neurological, haematological, cardiovascular and hepatic). Progressive organ dysfunction was measured on a scale of 0 to 4; the intervals were statistically determined for each organ based on associated mortality. The summed score (maximum 24) on the first day score was correlated with mortality in a graduated fashion.[45]

In this organ failure system the ICU mortality was approximately:

- 25% at 9–12 points
- 50% at 13–16 points
- 75% at 17–20 points
- 100% at levels of >20 points.

The score demonstrated good discrimination with areas under the ROC of 0.936 in the development set and 0.928 in the validation set.

Another organ failure score that is commonly used is the Sequential Organ Failure Assessment (SOFA). This score was originally constructed to provide a simple score for daily organ dysfunction in sepsis trials. Subsequently the 'sepsis' in SOFA was renamed 'sequential' to broaden its use. It takes into account six organs (brain, cardiovascular, coagulation, renal, hepatic, respiratory) and scores function from 0 (normal) to 4 (extremely abnormal). Experts defined the parameter intervals.[46] It has the merit of including supportive therapy and, although increasing scores can be shown to be associated with increasing mortality, it was not designed for estimation of outcome probability.

Around the same time as the introduction of SOFA the more scientifically based LODS (Logistic Organ Dysfunction Score) was also described. LODS is an organ failure score that could be used for hospital outcome prediction.[47] It was based on the first-day data of patients who made up the SAPS II and MPM II developmental cohort. The LODS system identified up to three levels of organ dysfunction for six organ systems. Between 1 and 5 LODS points were assigned to the levels of dysfunction. The resulting total LODS scores ranged from 0 to 22 points. Calibration and discrimination were good. It demonstrated that neurological, cardiovascular and renal dysfunction carried the most weight for predictive purposes whereas pulmonary, haematological and hepatic dysfunction carried the least. Unlike SOFA it weights the severity of illness between organs and the degree of severity within an organ system.

SCORES FOR INJURY AND TRAUMA

Patients who suffer physical injury are a relatively homogeneous group, which facilitates categorisation of their illness severity on anatomical damage (Injury Severity Score, ISS) and/or disturbance of vital physiology (Revised Trauma Score, RTS).

ISS is based on the Abbreviated Injury Scale (AIS), which is a consensus-derived anatomically based method for ranking injury for six body regions (head and neck, abdomen, pelvis contents, face, chest and body surface). Unlike the physiologically based general severity of illness scores, which use data at the height of acuity, ISS is anatomical and therefore any injury no matter when detected is relevant; hence data obtained from post-mortem evidence are included.

The first AIS was published in 1969 by the Society of Automotive Engineers.[48] The original reason was to provide standardisation for degree of injury for motor vehicle crash investigators to inform vehicle design. Subsequently other organisations became interested, namely the American Medical Association, and Association for the Advancement of Automotive Medicine. The latter has since taken the lead in updating AIS with major changes in 1976, 1980, 1985, 1990, 1998, 2005 and 2008. The changes have been recoding and alteration of the values for injury.[49,50] AIS values range from 1 (minor) to 6 (untreatable).[49,50] ISS is calculated from the sum of the squares of the highest AIS score (1–5 excluding 6 the non-survivable score) in the three most severely injured body regions. Baker noted that an injury in a second and third region, even if minor, significantly increased mortality; additionally it was observed that the sum of the squares of each score was more linearly related to mortality than the sum of individual scores.[51] The highest score in each body region is 5 and consequently the highest ISS is 75. However, the sum of squares means that certain scores such as 7 and 15 will never be obtained, whereas numbers such as 9 and 16 will be common. This means that statistical analysis should avoid parametric tests on the scores.

Major trauma is defined as an ISS greater than 15 and is associated with a greater than 10% risk of mortality. However, ISS is a purely anatomical system and ignores physiological derangements or chronic health status, this reduces its usefulness for predicting the outcome of cohorts. Care should also be taken when using ISS to compare data year on year if the ISS calculation has been based on different versions of AIS.[52]

A modification of the ISS, the New Injury Severity Score (NISS) has been suggested and considered a better model relating AIS to outcome.[53,54] NISS, unlike ISS, uses the three highest AIS scores even if they are in the same anatomical region, because it was felt that ISS would underestimate the effect on outcome of two very severe injuries in one body region. NISS has been adopted as the standard by the EuroTarn (Trauma audit and research network) project, which aims to establish a consistent dataset and registry for data collection and outcome comparisons in Europe.

The Trauma Score (TS) was introduced as a physiologically based triage tool for use in the field, based on systolic blood pressure, capillary refill, respiratory rate, chest expansion and the Glasgow Coma Scale (GCS). It was suggested along with age to compliment the anatomical scores derived from AIS.[55] However, incorporation of the TS was later reviewed owing to the difficulties of assessing capillary refill and chest expansion in the field and modified to the Revised Trauma Score (RTS).[56]

RTS is based on disturbances in three variables, each coded between 1 and 4:

- GCS
- systolic blood pressure (BP)
- respiratory rate.

Individually, both ISS and RTS had flaws as predictors of outcome from trauma. Boyd imaginatively combined these physiological and anatomical measures with coefficients to provide the Trauma Injury Severity Score (TRISS) methodology for outcome prediction.[57] TRISS, which was developed from the data of 30 000 injured patients, included the presence of penetrating injury and age in its methodology for outcome prediction.[51,56,57] Like other scoring systems it facilitates comparisons between trauma centres and year on year within centres by using expected and observed outcomes. However, because it uses the standard ISS rather than NISS, TRISS is exposed to the same tendency to underestimate the impact of more than one severe injury in the same anatomical region and risks poor calibration.[58–61] TRISS was found to be no better than APACHE II for the patients requiring ICU admission.[62] Also, as might be expected with improvements in trauma care, the TRISS coefficients have become progressively misaligned so that the original model has become less well calibrated.[63,64]

ASCOT (A Severity Characterization Of Trauma) was introduced to rectify perceived problems with TRISS.[65] There are more details on injuries in the same body region, more age subdivisions and the use of emergency room acute physiology details rather than field values. ASCOT predicted survival better than TRISS, particularly for blunt injury. However, there has been reluctance to use ASCOT owing to its increased complexity for only a modest gain in predictive value.

APPLICATION OF SCORING SYSTEMS

Since their introduction, scoring systems for general ICU patients have acquired a more defined role. Having originally been considered a method for quantifying risk of death and potentially managing ICU resources, they have found a more comfortable niche as the accepted tool for benchmarking research trials where case-mix is often similar in the control and active treatment groups. For an individual ICU the Standardized Mortality Ratio (SMR), which compares the observed hospital outcome with the expected one, is a useful measure. It is particularly helpful when used year on year to follow progress in quality of care. Even if a unit is poorly calibrated nationally, longitudinal within-unit performance comparisons remain valid assuming a wonder drug or treatment has not intervened and the case-mix has remained unchanged.

Traditionally SMR values of 1 indicate expected performance, whereas values below 1 and above 1 indicate respectively better and worse performances than expected.

SMR values, which are surrogates for quality of care, have to be used with caution when comparisons are made between intensive care units. A case-mix that deviates from the original developmental case-mix can cause anomalies and variance in calibration from one unit to another.[37]

When calibration is not a cause for concern it still remains difficult to quantify whether a SMR of 1 is significantly worse than one of 0.8. This assessment would have to take account of the standard deviations around the logistic regression equations. As a rule it is wise to avoid comparisons unless samples are very large and with a similar distribution of similar case-mix.

Scoring systems have also been used to explore the association between nursing resource needs and acuity at presentation, however assessing nurse:patient ratios might be more simply based on organ support requirements. Scoring systems have also been used to predict length of stay and therefore estimate bed requirements.[66]

Decision making for an individual patient based on the predictions of scoring systems is universally considered inappropriate because these systems are unable to discriminate with certainty and have misclassification rates in excess of 15%.[14,32,67,68] The logistic regression equations derived from large cohorts of mixed populations provide a probability for the dichotomous events of death or survival and therefore they have no potential use as a guide to further treatment or limitation orders for an individual.

While there are always attempts to correct for calibration and discrimination through new coefficients or new databases, the closest one can get to providing a system for individual prediction is through on-going recalibration with neural networks. Simplistically these systems use patient data feeding back to continually modify predictor equations. This approach theoretically gets closer and closer to predicting outcome, but it never reaches certainty.

Although it is important to recognise the hopelessly ill patient as early as possible, it is likely that management decisions will remain firmly based on clinical judgement rather than scores for the foreseeable future.

Access the complete references list online at http://www.expertconsult.com

10. Teres D, Lemeshow S, Avrunin JS, et al. Validation of the mortality prediction model for ICU patients. Crit Care Med 1987;15(3):208–13.
11. Harrison DA, Parry GJ, Carpenter JR, et al. A new risk prediction model for critical care: the Intensive Care National Audit & Research Centre (ICNARC) model. Crit Care Med 2007;35(4):1091–8. Epub 2007/03/06.
15. Metnitz PG, Moreno RP, Almeida E, et al. SAPS 3 – from evaluation of the patient to evaluation of the intensive care unit. Part 1: Objectives, methods and cohort description. Intensive Care Med 2005;31(10):1336–44.
16. Moreno RP, Metnitz PG, Almeida E, et al. SAPS 3 – from evaluation of the patient to evaluation of the intensive care unit. Part 2: Development of a prognostic model for hospital mortality at ICU admission. Intensive Care Med 2005;31(10):1345–55.
18. Zimmerman JE, Kramer AA, McNair DS, et al. Acute Physiology and Chronic Health Evaluation (APACHE) IV: hospital mortality assessment for today's critically ill patients. Crit Care Med 2006;34(5):1297–310.
32. Knaus WA, Draper EA, Wagner DP, et al. APACHE II: a severity of disease classification system. Crit Care Med 1985;13(10):818–29.
33. Lemeshow S, Teres D, Klar J, et al. Mortality Probability Models (MPM II) based on an international cohort of intensive care unit patients. Journal of the American Medical Association 1993;270(20):2478–86.
41. Le Gall JR, Lemeshow S, Saulnier F. A new Simplified Acute Physiology Score (SAPS II) based on a European/North American multicenter study. JAMA 1993;270(24):2957–63.
45. Marshall JC, Cook DJ, Christou NV, et al. Multiple organ dysfunction score: a reliable descriptor of a complex clinical outcome. Crit Care Med 1995;23(10):1638–52.
47. Le Gall JR, Klar J, Lemeshow S, et al. The Logistic Organ Dysfunction system. A new way to assess organ dysfunction in the intensive care unit. ICU Scoring Group. JAMA 1996;276(10):802–10.
57. Boyd CR, Tolson MA, Copes WS. Evaluating trauma care: the TRISS method. Trauma Score and the Injury Severity Score. J Trauma 1987;27(4):370–8.
66. Zimmerman JE, Kramer AA, McNair DS, et al. Intensive care unit length of stay: Benchmarking based on Acute Physiology and Chronic Health Evaluation (APACHE) IV. Crit Care Med 2006;34(10):2517–29.
67. Metnitz PG, Lang T, Vesely H, et al. Ratios of observed to expected mortality are affected by differences in case mix and quality of care. Intens Care Med 2000;26(10):1466–72.

4

Transport of critically ill patients

Evan R Everest and Matthew R Hooper

Critical illness and injury are not necessarily defined by patient location. In addition, patients may overwhelm the level of care at their current location or require specific investigations or treatments not immediately available to them. For this reason, transport of critically ill and injured patients occurs frequently.

Critical care patient transport has traditionally been divided into two groups; patient movement within a hospital (intra-hospital) or movement between hospitals (inter-hospital or inter-facility). In addition, a select group of critically ill or injured patients not located in a hospital facility may be managed by physician-based medical teams prior to retrieval to a medical facility. Therefore, a third division (primary response or pre-hospital care) is well recognised.

The internationally widespread deployment of medical teams for critically ill patient management and retrieval from both health care facilities and pre-hospital locations has resulted in the developing recognition of pre-hospital and retrieval medicine as a distinct subspecialty.[1]

INTRA-HOSPITAL TRANSPORT

Transports are usually required to facilitate critical investigations and interventions or to move the patient from one critical care area to another. Critically ill or injured patients with limited or no physiological reserve undergoing such transports are at risk of clinical deterioration and adverse events are well reported.[2,3] In order to reduce the mortality and morbidity associated with patient movement, a structured approach utilising high-level clinical personnel who have the correct equipment, training and sufficient planning time is required.

Moving the patient should be associated with little or no compromise in their condition. Unfortunately this is not the case with an adverse event occurring in up to 70% of transports. One-third of these events are equipment related,[4] whereas deterioration in gas exchange[5] and increased rates of ventilator-associated pneumonia are common.[6] However, management is changed in 40–50% of patients, thus justifying the risk.

Patients with unstable physiology should not be transported for non-urgent interventions or investigations. However, where the intervention or investigation is deemed critical to achieving patient stability or providing definitive management, the benefits in patient outcome will outweigh the inherent risks of transport. The transport can therefore be seen as part of the patient's therapeutic requirement and stabilisation process. On occasions when the patient's need is so acute and/or the likelihood of irreversible deterioration in transit is so high consideration should be given to facilitating such interventions or investigations in the ICU rather than the locality where these procedures would normally occur.

When preparing for intra-hospital transport, the following structured approach is recommended:

- Clinical reassessment should occur swiftly, systematically and, whenever possible, with the patient already supported on the equipment that will be used during transport.
- The airway should be checked and secured, endotracheal suction performed, ventilation and oxygenation optimised, adequate and patent vascular access secured and drainage devices measured and emptied.
- Sedation and analgesic requirements should be addressed and any drugs required for transport (including additional infused agents) pre-drawn and labelled for immediate use.
- Ensure that the patient clinical record remains with the team caring for the patient.

COMPUTED TOMORAPHY AND MAGNETIC RESONANCE IMAGING SCANNING

CT scanning is the most common ICU diagnostic intervention requiring patient movement. Head injury patients and those requiring previous administration of oral contrast with decreased gut motility (and thus increasing risk of aspiration) require extra attention. The administration of i.v. contrast through standard multi-lumen central lines is not possible and a large-bore intravenous cannula needs to be inserted and well secured prior to leaving the ICU. Single-lumen large-bore central catheters are an alternative but should be used only as a last resort.

Repeated CT scanning of head-injured patients is common. In these patients with decreased cerebral compliance, movement or changes in body position or Pa_{CO_2} can result in significant elevations in intracranial pressure. Although movement-induced changes in ICP can be reduced with sedation, very little can be done about body position. Changes in Pa_{CO_2} are usually due to variation between ICU and transport ventilators. Most transport ventilators are less precise at setting tidal volume, respiratory rate and PEEP compared with standard ICU ventilators. These changes can have significant effects on minute volume and lung compliance. If time permits, Et_{CO_2} should be established using the transport monitor for 10–15 minutes. This sets the baseline Et_{CO_2} that must be maintained when the patient is connected to the transport ventilator. Respiratory rate or tidal volume is adjusted to maintain the Et_{CO_2}. Ideally the ICP should also be measured but at times this may not be possible.

Radiation exposure for both the patient and staff needs to be considered. A stable patient who is adequately monitored with alarms activated can be observed by staff outside the room. The patient should be moved back to the ICU as soon as scanning is completed.

The use of MRI for ICU is increasing as a diagnostic and prognostic tool for a wide range of ICU patients. The major problems with MRI are the effect that the magnetic field may have on ventilators, monitors and infusion pumps and the potential for these items to become effectively a missile by being attracted to the magnet. The last 5–10 years have seen the development of monitoring and ventilators that are MRI compatible and the acceptance of standards for equipment in the MRI. These magnetic resonance standards are: MR safe, conditional or unsafe. Safe and unsafe are self-explanatory, while conditional relates to equipment that is safe when kept at a predetermined distance from the magnet. Although a lot of equipment has been developed as MR safe, it has been developed from anaesthetic practice for the provision of general anaesthesia during the MRI examination for some patients. This equipment is 'foreign' to most ICU staff and often is not used owing to lack of familiarity. As a result there has been a blending of practice: using some of the 'anaesthesia' equipment but also continuing to use ICU infusions and ventilators at some distance from the magnet. Distance from the magnet is achieved by the insertion of extension tubing but this must be balanced with the risk of disconnection.

Thermal dilution pulmonary artery catheters are probably safe, although opinion varies. Absolute contraindications for MRI scanning include pacemakers, internal defibrillators and cerebral aneurysm clips, whereas other clips may require a period of time, up to 6 weeks, to allow stabilisation within the tissues before scanning can occur. Prior discussion with the MRI unit must occur before the patient is moved from the ICU. Most MRI units will require an MRI checklist to be completed prior to scanning.

STAFFING

A team consisting of at least one ICU medical officer and nurse should be free from other duties. Both team members should be thoroughly familiar with the transport process, equipment and environment. The team should possess the requisite skills and knowledge to independently manage critically ill patients in transit and to deal with anticipated emergencies. The more complex and unstable the patient is, the more capable the team must be. For very unstable patients an additional nurse and more senior doctors may be required. Assistance with safe patient, trolley and equipment movement will also be needed. Non-clinical hospital support staff are therefore part of the team and should be included in all briefs and contingency planning.

EQUIPMENT

Transport equipment should be regularly checked and serviceable. Powered devices should be fully charged, with power cords accessible to facilitate use of mains power in the event of delay. Where possible, equipment should be lightweight, robust and standardised throughout the ICU and hospital. In transit, equipment should be secured (not resting on the patient) but readily accessible. Dedicated transport bridges or gantries are commonly used. Dedicated transport packs or boxes ensure safe carriage of consumable items, resuscitation equipment and drugs. Equipment required for emergency airway management (e.g. bag valve mask, laryngoscope, airway devices and endotracheal tubes) should be immediately available.

MONITORING

As a minimum, intubated and ventilated patients requiring intra-hospital transport should have the following monitoring instituted:[7]

- continuous Et_{CO_2}
- continuous Sa_{O_2}
- continuous invasive or intermittent non-invasive BP
- continuous three-lead ECG.

Ideally, a cardiac monitoring device should also provide cardiac defibrillation and external cardiac-pacing capacity. Patients requiring transport with more advanced monitoring in situ should be considered on a case-by-case basis. For example, ongoing ICP monitoring is critical to ensure avoidance of profound unmonitored falls in cerebral perfusion pressure in an ICU patient with a severe head injury, whereas pulmonary artery pressure monitoring may be excluded from the transport requirements in the haemodynamically stable patient.

INTER-HOSPITAL TRANSPORT

Historical models of inter-hospital patient transfer utilising junior medical staff as 'patient escorts' have much higher rates of hypotension, acidosis and death.[8] Thankfully this type of transport has become increasingly rare with the introduction of specialist retrieval services.

The general principles of patient transport, irrespective of the physical location of the patient, regarding equipment, patient monitoring and clinical requirements remain the same. Standards for transportation of the critically ill have been widely promulgated and must be followed whether it is a complex unstable patient being moved long distances or a semi-elective CT in a stable ICU patient.

With rising expectations for high-level care by the community in both metropolitan and rural locations and with the care for critically ill and injured patients becoming increasingly centralised in large, tertiary, metropolitan ICUs, the need to transfer patients between health care facilities has also increased. Such a demand has seen the development of dedicated specialist retrieval teams. These teams are trained to manage patients in the inter-hospital environment and have varied professional backgrounds. Although these teams can deal with most inter-hospital transfers there are a number where the patient complexity may be beyond the standard retrieval team and additional clinical personnel need to be added for the patient transfer. Inter-hospital transfer of a patient on ECMO (see below) is an example where a complex patient is being managed by a highly specialised team with little or no experience of moving patients in the inter-hospital environment. In these relatively rare cases the role of the retrieval team is to assist by providing the logistical and inter-hospital expertise to allow the ECMO team to concentrate on caring for the patient.

RETRIEVAL CLINICAL COORDINATION AND ADVICE

Retrieval clinical coordination describes the process whereby specialist medical, nursing, paramedic and ambulance service staff are involved in direct supervision of the primary and inter-hospital transport or retrieval of patients. This is to ensure the:

- safe and efficient use of expensive transport and retrieval services
- high-level clinical advice is available prior to and during transport
- the patient is delivered in a timely manner to the most appropriate receiving hospital

safe and efficient use of expensive transport and retrieval services, that high-level clinical advice is available prior to and during transport, and that the patient is directed in a timely manner to the most appropriate receiving facility.

Not all patients who are referred for retrieval will require transport. Of those who do, not all will require emergency retrieval and not all will require a retrieval team. To ensure that this is addressed, an integrated systems approach is required. In general a retrieval service will be used when the complexity of the patient exceeds the ambulance service's ability to transport the patient. Patients requiring a retrieval response may be identified by:

- a diagnosis with the potential to deteriorate
- a clinical requirement for invasive physiological monitoring or acute intervention
- to facilitate continuity of already instituted critical care supports.

Tele-medicine is playing an important and increasing role in this process – not only in assisting decision making regarding retrieval activities (resulting in potential cost savings), but also in supporting remote and regional medical practitioners faced with acutely ill or injured patients and in supporting a retrieval team before and during patient transport.

When there is a requirement for a rapid medical response to a time-critical pre-hospital or retrieval incident, a retrieval service must be able to be activated swiftly and in a coordinated approach with other emergency services. For this reason, many retrieval coordination centres are co-located with ambulance service communication centres. In this way, clinical and logistic expertise is integrated.

Retrieval coordination centres should ideally be accessed by a single number and provide early teleconferencing of the referral agency, a senior critical care clinician (such as a receiving intensive care specialist, relevant specialist clinician or medical retrieval specialist), and occasionally the retrieval team.

Knowing where key assets (transport platforms such as road ambulances, helicopters and fixed wing aircraft) and retrieval teams are at any one time is crucial to effective retrieval clinical coordination. Real-time asset tracking or mapping systems and advanced radio or phone communication networks assist in this regard.

RETRIEVAL TEAM STAFFING

The aim of the team is to at least maintain, but ideally to increase the level of care during transport. This requires a team of sufficient size and skill to provide the full complement of care for the majority of patients being transported.

The minimum team should comprise two people; occasionally a very-low-acuity stable patient may be escorted by a single person. If multiple patients are to be transported a recommended staffing level is $n+1$ where n equals the number of patients.[10]

Who makes up the team continues to be debated. In most cases a doctor will be one member while the other can be a person with either acute care nursing or ambulance background. For a primary pre-hospital response, the combination of a doctor and paramedic is the best mix; the paramedic is familiar with the pre-hospital scene environment and can often guide and support a doctor, especially one early in their retrieval career, while a doctor/nurse combination may be appropriate for complex inter-hospital transfers. The future second person will potentially be someone who has both an acute care nursing and paramedic background and will feel comfortable operating in both environments. Other requirements include the ability to work and communicate as a team, have reasonable body habitus and physical fitness and have no visual or auditory impairment or a susceptibility to motion sickness. In aviation transport the weight of the teams and their equipment is important as there is a maximum weight available. High team weights can limit the amount of fuel able to be carried, which may compromise some missions.

As discussed above there will be some highly complex cases that may be outside of the team's capability and supplementation of the retrieval team by additional specialist personnel may be required. An example of obstetricians or neurosurgeons[11] depending on the type of mission may be added. It is mandatory that the specialist is added to a standard team because of the latter's familiarity with working in the retrieval environment.

TRAINING

Training should cover the following:

- standard operating procedures for the service
- the use of scenarios to teach common procedures and also principles
- familiarity in the various transport platforms to be used; this would include safety briefings on aerial assets and may include helicopter underwater escape training (HUET) and crew (cockpit) resource management (CRM)
- communication procedures
- understanding of the effects of altitude and flight on patient (and team) physiology.

EQUIPMENT

GENERAL CONSIDERATIONS

Minimum equipment standards for supplies, equipment and monitoring have been published.[7] The equipment carried is often a compromise between providing for every conceivable situation and lightweight and mobile. In some cases it is appropriate to have additional or procedure packs that are taken only when warranted by the clinical situation; for example, a Sengstaken–Blakemore tube or temporary transvenous pacing wire is taken only when a GI haemorrhage occurs in a patient who might have varices or the patient has symptomatic complete heart block. This requires a good communication and coordination process.

A suggested list of equipment is given in **Box 4.1**.

Transport monitors, infusion pumps and ventilators must work out of the transport vehicle. They must be battery powered whilst ideally allowing for utilisation of ambulance or aircraft power during transport. Batteries in most modern systems are either sealed lead acid or lithium. There is no place for the older-style Nicad battery, which needs to be totally discharged prior to recharging to overcome memory effect. Battery life is quoted for new batteries and with time this value decreases. Planning on a battery life of 50% of that quoted is prudent. Spare batteries can be carried but changing them usually result in temporary interruption of monitoring. With the newer, smaller defibrillators at least one spare battery is essential. During transport the equipment must be securely stowed. There are international standards in the 'G force' that securing systems must withstand in the event of a crash. In some modern road vehicles or helicopters the requirement is 20 G. The use of a suitability engineered 'stretcher bridge' attached to the patient's stretcher and to which the equipment can be secured provides the most safety.[12]

MONITORING

Clinical observation by experienced clinicians remains an important facet of monitoring.[13] However, there are significant limitations to this approach. It is difficult to auscultate adequately in a moving vehicle and impossible in a helicopter. As a minimum, ECG, pulse oximetry and non-invasive blood pressure (BP) measurement must be provided with the addition of end-tidal CO_2 (Et_{CO_2}) for any intubated patient. Non-invasive BP measurements are often subject to interference, and for critically ill patients invasive arterial access is essential, especially if the length of the transport is long.[14] Newer defibrillators combine defibrillation and the monitoring aspects as outlined above may be an advantage. However, non-invasive BP and defibrillation uses a lot of battery power and spare batteries are essential or must be carried. The use of portable biochemical analysers provides additional management information in long transports.

VENTILATORS

A mechanical ventilator must be used on all intubated patients as manual ventilation cannot reliably deliver constant tidal volumes and a stable Et_{CO_2}.[15] However, a manual system must be available in the rare event of a ventilator failure. Transport ventilators are a compromise between portability and features. Over the last 5 years the desired features as listed in **Box 4.2** have almost been met apart from the ability to ventilate neonates to large adults. Small neonates still require a specific ventilator.

The provision of non-invasive ventilation (NIV) such as continuous positive airway pressure (CPAP) or BiPAP now possible on most modern transport ventilators. An improvement with inspiratory valve-triggering technology has resulted in substantial reductions in

Box 4.1 Suggested equipment schedule for inter-hospital critical care transport

Respiratory equipment

Intubation kit:

- Endotracheal tubes and connectors – adult and paediatric sizes
- Introducers, bougies, Magill forceps
- Laryngoscopes, blades, spare globes and batteries
- Ancillaries: cuff syringe and manometer, clip forceps, 'gooseneck' tubing, HME/filter(s), securing ties, lubricant

Alternative airways:

- Simple: Geudel and nasopharyngeal
- Supraglottic: laryngeal masks and/or Combitube
- Infraglottic: cricothyrotomy kit and tubes

Oxygen masks (including high $F_{I_{O_2}}$ type), tubing, nebulisers

Suction equipment:

- Main suction system – usually vehicle mounted
- Spare (portable) suction – hand-, O_2-, or battery-powered
- Suction tubing, handles, catheters and spare reservoir.

Self-inflating hand ventilator, with masks and PEEP valve

Portable ventilator with disconnect and overpressure alarms

Ventilator circuit and spares

Spirometer and cuff manometer

Capnometer/capnograph

Pleural drainage equipment:

- Intercostal catheters and cannulae
- Surgical insertion kit and sutures (see below)
- Heimlich-type valves and drainage bags

Main oxygen system (usually vehicle-mounted) of adequate capacity with flowmeters and standard wall outlets

Portable/reserve oxygen system with flowmeter and std outlet

Circulatory equipment

Defibrillator/monitor/external pacemaker, with leads, electrodes and pads

IV fluid administration equipment:

- Range of fluids: isotonic crystalloid, dextrose, colloids
- High-flow and metered flow-giving sets
- IV cannulae in range of sizes: peripheral and central/long lines
- IV extension sets, 3-way taps and needle-free injection system
- Syringes, needles and drawing-up cannulae
- Skin preparation wipes, IV dressings and Band-Aid
- Pressure infusion bags (for arterial line also).

Blood pressure monitoring equipment:

- Arterial cannulae with arterial tubing and transducers
- Invasive and non-invasive (automated) BP pressure monitors
- Aneroid (non-mercury) sphygmomanometer and range of cuffs (preferably compatible with NIBP also)

Pulse oximeter, with finger and multi-site probes

Syringe/infusion pumps (minimum two) and appropriate tubing

Miscellaneous equipment

Urinary catheters and drainage/measurement bag

Gastric tubes and drainage bag.

Minor surgical kit (for ICC, CV lines, cricothyrotomy, etc.):

- Sterile instruments: scalpels, scissors, forceps, needle holders
- Suture material and needles
- Antiseptics, skin preparation packs and dressings
- Sterile gloves (various sizes); drapes +/– gowns

Cervical collars, spinal immobilisation kit, splints

Pneumatic anti-shock garment (MAST suit)

Thermometer (non-mercury) and/or temperature probe/monitor

Reflective (space) blanket and thermal insulation drapes

Bandages, tapes, heavy-duty scissors (shears)

Gloves and eye protection

Sharps and contaminated waste receptacles

Pen and folder for paperwork

Torch +/– head light

Drug/additive labels and marker pen

Nasal decongestant (for barotitis prophylaxis)

Pharmacological agents

CNS drugs:

- Narcotics +/– non-narcotic analgesics
- Anxiolytics/sedatives
- Major tranquillisers
- Anticonvulsants
- IV hypnotics/anaesthetic agents
- Antiemetics
- Local anaesthetics

Cardiovascular drugs:

- Antiarrhythmics
- Anticholinergics
- Inotropes/vasoconstrictors
- Nitrates
- Alpha and beta blockers, other hypotensives

Electrolytes and renal agents:

- Sodium bicarbonate
- Calcium (chloride)
- Magnesium
- Potassium
- Loop diuretics
- Osmotic diuretics

Endocrine and metabolic agents:

- Glucose (concentrate) +/– glucagon
- Insulin
- Steroids

Other agents:

- Neuromuscular blockers: depolarising and non-depolarising
- Anticholinesterases (neuromuscular block reversal)
- Narcotic and benzodiazepine antagonists
- Bronchodilators
- Antihistamines
- H_2 blockers/proton pump inhibitors
- Anticoagulants
- Thrombolytics
- Vitamin K
- Antibiotics
- Oxytocics
- Tocolytics
- Diluents (saline and sterile water)

Additional/optional equipment

- Portable ultrasound machine
- Transvenous temporary pacing kit and pacemaker
- Blood (usually O negative) and/or blood products
- Additional infusion pumps and associated IV sets
- Obstetrics kit
- Additional paediatric equipment (depending on capability of basic kit)
- Antivenin (polyvalent or specific)
- Specific drugs or antagonists

Box 4.2 Features of an ideal transport ventilator

- Small, light, robust, and cheap
- Not dependent on external power source
- Easy to use and clean, with foolproof assembly
- Economical on gas consumption
- Suitable for patients from neonates through to large adults
- F_{IO_2} continuously variable from ambient air to 100% oxygen
- Able to deliver PEEP, CPAP, SIMV and pressure support
- Variable I:E ratios
- Flow or pressure generator modes
- Integrated monitoring and alarm functions with audio and visual signals
- Altitude compensated

circuit work with concurrent reduction in the work of breathing. Although clapperboard CPAP systems provide the least circuit work and are optimal for patients with high work of breathing, the new transport ventilators are close enough to ideal to be used. Most patients will tolerate NIV with the modern ventilators, but it does require a different approach by retrieval teams. There needs to be a period of observation prior to transport as the ability to provide advanced airway support in transit is limited.

In most cases heat moisture exchangers (HME) will provide adequate humidification for intubated patients.

A suction system and reserve are required. In most transport vehicles this can be provided by electrically powered devices and a back up such as a gas powered venturi system as a back-up.

INFUSIONS

Critically ill patients often need multiple infusions to be continued during transport. Some drugs that ideally should be given as infusions can be consolidated by combining sedation drugs, or the infusion stopped and given instead by frequent boluses. The older-style volumetric and drop-counting pumps have been superseded by lightweight syringe drivers, which should be the only method used for drug infusions in contemporary retrieval practice.

INTRA-AORTIC BALLOON PUMP (IABP) AND EXTRACORPOREAL MEMBRANE OXYGENATION (ECMO)

Retrieval of patients with IABP in situ has been occurring for many years and, in general, a team with some experience in trouble shooting any pump alarms can manage these patients. The IABP machines are reasonably bulky and heavy with an internal battery life of 1–2 hours. The type of transport vehicle has to be considered to ensure that the pump can be safely secured and can be connected to an external power source

Box 4.3 Essential features of transport vehicles

- Readily available
- Adequate operational safety
- Capable of carrying (at least one) stretcher and mobile intensive care equipment set
- Safe seating for full medical team, including at head and side of patient
- Adequate space and patient access for observation and procedures
- Equipped with adequate supply of oxygen/other gases for duration of transports
- Fitted with medical power supply of appropriate voltage and current capacity
- Appropriate speed (coupled with) comfortable ride, without undue exposure to accelerations in any axis
- Acceptable noise and vibration levels
- Adequate cabin lighting, ventilation and climate control
- Fitted with overhead IV hooks, and sharps/biohazard waste receptacles
- Straightforward embarkation and disembarkation of patient and team
- Fitted with appropriate radios and mobile telephone

either 12–28 V or mains power equivalent. Although the pump will run on external 12–28 V, most pumps require connection to mains power to recharge the battery, so it is essential to limit the time on internal batteries. Insertion of an IABP catheter requires some experience and some pre-departure consideration of the team's capabilities must be made. The addition of an extra doctor experienced in IABP insertion to the standard retrieval team should be considered.

The 'swine flu' epidemic in 2010 saw the rapid emergence of ECMO as a valid treatment for severe viral-induced respiratory failure.[16] It was recognised that ECMO should be provided in a relatively small number of institutions and that ideally patients likely to need ECMO should be transferred early. However, significant numbers of patients deteriorated rapidly and rescue ECMO was instituted in many non-ECMO centres, hence requiring the patient to be transported on ECMO. Most ECMO centre staff will not be familiar with the retrieval environment. The principles of retrieval therefore need to be understood by the ECMO teams with the ideal solution being to combine the ECMO team with a standard retrieval team.

MODE OF TRANSPORT

There are three common types of transport vehicle used: road vehicles, aeroplanes (fixed wing) and helicopters (rotary wing). The basic requirements are listed in **Box 4.3** and their features and limitations are summarised in **Table 4.1**.

Ideally, dedicated vehicles should be used. Often the workload is insufficient to justify this and non dedicated

Table 4.1 Properties of transport vehicles

	ROAD	HELICOPTER	FIXED WING
Launch time	3–5 min	5–10 min (more if IFR)	30–60 min
Speed	10–120 km/h dependent on roads and traffic	120–150 knots (220–290 km/h), straight line	140–180 knots (piston) 230–270 knots (turboprop) 375–460 knots (jet)
Secondary transport	Not applicable	Sometimes	Inevitable
Effective range	0–100 km (longer if required)	50–300 km (longer or shorter in special cases)	200–2000 km
Noise	Low, except at high speed	Moderate to high (headsets required)	Low to moderate (cruise); higher on takeoff/landing
Vibrations	Variable with speed and road surface	Moderate in most phases (varies with rotor type)	Low in cruise; moderate or high on takeoff/landing
Accelerations	Variable and sometimes unpredictable in all axes	Minimal, and usually vertical only	Significant (fore/aft) on takeoff and landing
Special features	Base vehicles readily available	Versatility; point to point capability	Cabin pressurisation and all-weather capability (most)
Acquisition cost	Lowest	High (US$1–4.5 million new, depending on capabilities)	Moderate (piston) to very high (jet)
Operating costs (per km)	Intermediate	Intermediate to high	Low to intermediate

vehicles needing to be reconfigured are used. The mode of transport is based on a number of criteria:

- the availability of the transport vehicle
- the weather, especially if flying
- the distance to be travelled
- location and capability of the retrieval team
- the urgency of the case
- the clinical capability of the referring hospital.

The coordination and tasking centre takes all these into consideration. All things being equal, road is used for distances up to 40–80 km, rotary wing for 60–200 km and fixed wing for over 200 km.

ROAD AMBULANCE

This remains the most common form of transport and for some patients the safest even for long distances.

FIXED WING

Both propeller-driven and jet aircraft are used. Compared with helicopters, their faster speed needs to be offset with the need for a road leg at each end of the transfer. In comparison to helicopters lower noise and cabin pressurisation, often to sea level, and ability to fly in 'icing' conditions increase there utility. Most aeromedical fixed-wing aircraft are specifically configured with stretcher loading devices to assist in loading. Jets tend to be reserved for longer distance, greater than 800–1000 km.

HELICOPTERS

These remain the most high-profile and expensive vehicles used for patient transport. Most will require significant adaption to provide a reasonable working space. The lack of space makes procedures such as intubation almost impossible. They are very noisy to work in, with conversation only possible via intercom systems. This makes communication with patients difficult. It is only recently that the benefits of using a helicopter have been mainly for longer distances. Whereas a mix of single-engine and twin-engine aircraft have been used in the past, changes by regulatory authorities in Europe and Australia mean that most helicopter transports are now being performed in more suitable, larger twin-engine aircraft. The optimal range for use is a 'donut' of 40–300 km and their main advantage is the ability to land on hospital helipads, removing an additional road leg. This, of course, requires the hospital to have a helipad. Helicopter also have a role in the delivery of retrieval teams to trauma cases in high traffic density areas such as London.

SAFETY

Any mode of transport involves some risk to patients and staff. In the aeromedical environment unfamiliar personnel perform clinical tasks poorly,[17] so teams must be appropriately trained and equipped to function effectively and safely in each mode of transport. A senior member of the professional group concerned should train and mentor new personnel on their first few trips.

A safety brief encompassing the use of safety equipment carried on the aircraft, emergency egress and actions to take during an emergency is essential. Daily meetings with helicopter flight crews is essential to improve effective communication between members of the team. This leads to an enhancing the safety of missions understanding between individual team members.

Dangerous activities such as unsafe driving and flying below safe minima are unacceptable. For aviation missions the decision whether a mission proceeds rests entirely with the aircraft pilot, and the attempt to coerce pilots to take risks has been recognised as a contributor to air ambulance accidents.[18] The pilot should be provided with only the details of where the team needs to go. Clinical details should generally not be given as this may influence the decision to proceed with the mission.

ALTITUDE AND TRANSPORT PHYSIOLOGY

Teams need to be aware of altitude-related changes in gas, volume, temperature and partial pressures of oxygen (**Table 4.2**).

Patients already dependent on oxygen will be further compromised by even modest increases in height requiring further oxygen supplementation. It is the partial pressure not the percentage of oxygen

Table 4.2 Changes with altitude

ALTITUDE (FEET/M)	PRESSURE (MMHG/KPA)	ALVEOLAR P_{O_2} (ON AIR)	(100% O_2)	GAS SPACE EXPANSION (%)	STD TEMP (°CELSIUS)	NOTES
Sea level	760 (≈100)	103	663	–	15	15°C is 'reference' average temp – actual obviously varies
1000 (300)	733 (≈97)	98	636	+3.6	13	Minimum altitude above ground level for helicopter transports
2000 (600)	706 (≈94)	94	609	+8	11	Likely altitude for most (VFR) helicopter flights over sea-level terrain
3000 (900) 4000 (1200)	681 (≈91) 656 (≈87)	89 85	584 559	+12 +16	9 7	Likely range of cabin altitude for standard flights in most turboprop air ambulance craft (e.g. Raytheon–Beech King Air series)
7000 (2000)	586 (≈78)	73	489	+29	1	Standard cabin altitude for airliners and most jet air ambulances (e.g. Lear 35)
10000 (3000)	523 (≈70)	61	426	+45	–5	Likely ceiling of helicopter ops and hypoxic threshold in normal individuals
15000 (4500)	429 (≈57)	45	332	+77	–14.5	Threshold for hypoxic decompensation in non-acclimatised individuals
20000 (6000) 25000 (7500)	349 (≈50) 282 (≈37.5)	34 30	252 185	+117 +170	–24.5 –34	Likely upper range of cruise altitude for turboprop aircraft Decompression at these altitudes causes rapid loss of consciousness and death without O_2
40000 (12000)	141 (≈19)	<10	61	+439	–56	Cruise ceiling for airliners and jets Limit for survivable decompression, even with 100% O_2 for flight crew

that is critical. Monitoring of Sa_{O_2} during ascent is essential.

GAS EXPANSION

Expansion of trapped gas in accordance with Boyle's law occurs in physiological and pathological air spaces and air-containing equipment such as endotracheal or tracheostomy tube cuffs, Sengstaken–Blakemore tubes and pulmonary artery balloons. Endotracheal tube cuff pressures will need to be adjusted during flight. Delivered tidal volumes may increase spontaneously in some ventilators, necessitating setting adjustments.

Physiological air spaces include the middle ear, nasal sinuses and GI tract. They can affect both patients and staff; consequently staff with upper respiratory tract infections or gastrointestinal disturbances should not fly.

Pathological air spaces include pneumothoraces, emphysematous lung bullae or cysts, intraocular and intracranial open injuries, bowel obstructions and gas emboli. These patients need to be transported at the lowest altitude possible. Most modern fixed-wing aircraft are capable of cabin pressurization, which decreases hypoxia and gas expansion. The pressurisation effectively replicates flying at a lower altitude – the so-called 'cabin altitude'. The difference between actual altitude and cabin altitude varies, with most air ambulances providing about 350 mmHg (≈50 kPa) differential. This equates to a cabin pressure of 3000 ft (≈900 m) while flying at 20 000 feet (≈6000 m). Most commercial airliners fly with a cabin altitude of around 7–9000 ft (≈2000–2700 m). Once the maximum differential is reached a lower cabin pressure can only be achieved by flying lower, which is often associated with more turbulence and increased fuel consumption. The medical team should only request a lower cabin height if clinically indicated.

Temperature falls 2°C for every 1000 ft (≈300 m) increase in height, as does the partial pressure of water, which is not corrected by cabin pressurisation. This can lead to dehydration especially on long trips.

PREPARATION FOR TRANSPORT

The preparation phase for transport will depend on the patient's clinical condition. The ideal is to spend sufficient time, including any urgent surgery, stabilising the patient so that the transport phase is uneventful. As with intra-hospital transport, this ideal may not be achievable, especially when the patient requires a time-critical intervention available only at the receiving destination. These missions are higher risk but are likely to be less futile than trying to stabilise an inevitably deteriorating patient. Prior to transport all patients must have a secure airway, either self-maintained or intubated and ventilated, and well-secured intravenous access. External bleeding should be controlled and investigations that may impact on the transport performed, if they can be performed in a short time frame. Heimlich-type valves may be attached to any chest drains rather than bulky UWSD (underwater seal drain) devices. The patient is transferred to the stretcher and secured with the patient harness. Any equipment is also attached securely to the stretcher bridge. Any documentation and copies of investigations need also to be taken. A checklist for departure and transport is recommended and provided in **Box 4.4**.

During the early stages of movement, special vigilance must be employed as this is the stage when equipment disconnections or physiological decompensation is likely to occur. During transport the patient is vulnerable to hypothermia and heating in the vehicle should be used.

Box 4.4 Suggested pre-departure checklists

A. Before leaving hospital:	
• Patient identity and next of kin	Recorded
• Consent for transport	Obtained and documented
• Paperwork and X-rays	Collected
• Drugs for transport	Present and sufficient
• Emergency drugs/equipment	Available
• Medical equipment	Collected and repacked
• Monitors, ventilator and infusions	Connected and on
• Tubes, lines, drains and catheters	Secured
• Altitude request (if applicable)	Passed to pilot
• Receiving unit	Contacted and updated
B. In vehicle and pre-departure	
• Stretcher and patient restraints	Secured and checked
• Oxygen supply	On and sufficient
• Monitors, ventilator and infusions	Working and secure
• Emergency drugs/equipment	Stowed and accessible
• Other medical packs	Stowed
• Intravenous fluids	Hung and running
• Intravenous injection port	Accessible
• Medical power	On and connected
• Communications	Checked as applicable
• Seatbelts	On and checked
• Staff/patient headsets	On/checked (if applicable)

HANDOVER

Handover to the receiving hospital is critical. Unless the patient needs immediate resuscitation there should be an opportunity for the retrieval team to have the exclusive attention of the receiving hospital. Various handover tools such as MIST (Mechanism of injury, Injuries suspected or found, Signs (vital signs) and Treatment given) are useful for trauma cases. ISOBAR has a wider application to all patient groups and is being promoted as the standard handover tool in many areas:

- I – introduction
- S – situation
- O – observations
- B – background
- A – assessment
- R – recommendations.

Retrieval teams should use which handover tool is used in local practice. If one is not commonly used then ISOBAR will cover all the essential elements.

PRE-HOSPITAL CARE

Pre-hospital care of the acutely injured and critically ill is a complex and challenging field of medical practice. Ideally, patients should receive the most advanced required level of care at the earliest possible time, integrated with expedient transfer to the most appropriate definitive care facility. The ability to achieve this is both resource and system dependent with unique modifiers including transport platform logistics, environmental concerns and the need to integrate with other responding emergency services.

The benefits of adding a skilled critical care physician to the pre-hospital team are well recognised. Service models across Australasia and Europe reflect this belief.[19] The potential care delivered by such a team approaches or matches that only usually available in a tertiary hospital environment and may represent a 'definitive' requirement for the patient. However, the benefit of a physician and the safety and effectiveness of the team are maximised only if staff involved in such activities have the requisite skills and knowledge and are familiar with the pre-hospital and retrieval environment.

APPROACH TO THE SCENE AND SCENE SAFETY

During the approach to a trauma scene an opportunity exists to:

- identify potential hazards
- briefly 'read' the likely mechanism
- identify patient numbers, distribution and acuity of injury
- commence formulating a pre-hospital plan.

Scene assessment is critical to ensuring team, scene and, ultimately, patient safety.

It begins as soon as details of the task become available. The tasking agency may have access to further information that may be forwarded to the team en route.

In any pre-hospital emergency situation, scene safety is the primary concern and, as detailed above, plans for approaching the scene should be made on or prior to arriving.

The pre-hospital retrieval (PHR) team should adopt the 'safe self, safe team, safe scene, safe patient' approach.

PRE-HOSPITAL PLAN

A pre-hospital plan is a continuously evolving mental plan of action that the team will make as soon as it is activated, using the information given by the tasking agency. In many cases, this initial information is vague or incomplete, which reflects the problems experienced when receiving early phone calls about an incident. Although making a plan prior to arrival with limited information has drawbacks, there are clear benefits in arriving at the incident with a strategy for scene and patient management already in place. The plan often develops as the team travels to the scene and therefore valuable time en route should not be wasted.

When at the scene, the PHR team must have the skill to listen to all members of the emergency services and weigh up their suggestions as part of the overall plan. The ambulance service is the primary provider of pre-hospital care and paramedics are likely to be very experienced. It is worthwhile remembering that the physician-based pre-hospital teams are an extension of the ambulance service and not a replacement for them.

A generic pre-hospital plan could be:

- *the scene:*
  - a safe approach (self, team, scene and others)
- *the patient:*
  - likely requirements, need for extrication, assessment and stabilisation
- *the destination:*
  - triage options
  - transport platform options.

By having a pre-hospital plan, the team can add structure to their actions and, in doing so, develop a shared mental model inherent in teams that function in such high-acuity, high-consequence environments.

ENTRAPMENT AND EXTRICATION

Relative entrapment is a situation in which patients are trapped because of their injuries (e.g. a broken leg with disabling pain), location (e.g. a cave) or the ambient environment (e.g. a blizzard). If it were not for these factors, they would not require help in extricating themselves.

Actual entrapment occurs when patients are physically held in a location by the structure itself – for example, a major vehicle deformation with cabin intrusion, or a building collapse.

The aim is to remove the patient from an entrapped situation as safely and as quickly as possible. The key determinant in this plan (apart from safety) is the condition of the patient. The PHR team must decide on how to compromise between the slower, methodical extrication with total spinal control and the quicker extrication of the less stable patient. Clearly, unstable patients will need rapid extrication but the ability to predict which patients are unsuitable for prolonged extrication due to the anticipated clinical course is more challenging. It may be better to compromise a degree of spinal protection earlier rather than have an emergency ('crash') extrication situation develop 30 minutes later.

The fire and rescue services will have access to the specialised equipment required. Without good teamwork between the services, the extrication will be significantly hindered.

ULTRASOUND IN THE FIELD

The availability of robust portable ultrasound machines has resulted in increased use in the pre-hospital or retrieval environment with good success; however, their use must be limited to people accredited in its use and must not result in undue delays in the patient management.

Access the complete references list online at http://www.expertconsult.com

1. Laird C. Prehospital and retrieval medicine. Emerg Med J 2005;22(4):236.
3. Ridley S, Carter R. The effects of secondary transport on critically ill patients. Anaesthesia 1989;44:822–7.
5. Marx G, Vangerow B, Hecker H, et al. Predictors of respiratory function deterioration after transfer of critically ill patients. Intensive Care Med 1998;24:1157–62.
7. College of Intensive Care Medicine of Australia and New Zealand. Minimum standards for inter-hospital transport of critically ill patients. Joint Faculty of Intensive Care Medicine Policy Document IC10. Melbourne: College of Intensive Care Medicine of Australia and New Zealand; 2010.
8. Bellingan G, Olivier T, Batson S, et al. Comparison of a specialist retrieval team with current United Kingdom practice for the transport of critically ill patients. Intensive Care Med 2000;26:740–4.
16. Burns BJ, Habig K, Reid C, et al. Logistics and safety of extracorporeal membrane oxygenation in medical retrieval. Prehosp Emerg Care 2011;15(2):246–53. Epub 2011 Feb.
19. Garner A, Rashford S, Lee A, et al. Addition of physicians to paramedic helicopter services decreases blunt trauma mortality. Aust NZ J Surg 1999;69:697–700.

5

Physiotherapy in intensive care

Fiona H Moffatt and Mandy O Jones

Historically, physiotherapy in the ICU was confined to the treatment of respiratory problems performed routinely on all patients. Evidence-based practice has demonstrated that there is no longer a place for routine physiotherapy treatment in the ICU.[1] Physiotherapeutic intervention is based on clinical reasoning following the identification of physiotherapy-amenable problems, which are elucidated from a thorough systematic assessment.

There is still some debate about the precise role of the physiotherapist within the ICU, which may vary,[2] but the main features include:

- optimisation of cardiopulmonary function
- assistance in the weaning process utilising ventilatory support and oxygen therapy
- instigation of an early rehabilitation/mobilisation program to assist in preventing the consequences of enforced immobility
- advise on positioning to protect joints and to minimise potential muscle, soft tissue shortening and nerve damage
- optimisation of body position to effect muscle tone in the brain-injured patient
- optimisation of voluntary movement to promote functional independence and improve exercise tolerance
- management of presenting musculoskeletal pathology
- advise and education of family and carers
- liaison with medical and nursing staff on the continuation and monitoring of ongoing physiotherapy-devised care plans.

CARDIOPULMONARY PHYSIOTHERAPY

TREATMENT MODALITIES TO OPTIMISE CARDIOPULMONARY FUNCTION

Patients who are critically ill may present with impaired cardiopulmonary physiology secondary to both the underlying pathology and the therapeutic interventions employed to treat them. In their approach to any individual patient, the physiotherapist may use specific treatment techniques targeted at improving ventilation/perfusion (V/Q) disturbances, increasing lung volumes, reducing the work of breathing and removing pulmonary secretions. Physiotherapy treatment modalities may differ depending on the presence of an endotracheal tube, although patient participation with treatment is encouraged and promoted at the earliest point during intubation. Each intervention is rarely used in isolation, but rather as part of an effective treatment plan. Some physiotherapeutic techniques may have short-lived beneficial effects on pulmonary function, and some have no clear evidence to validate their effectiveness **(Table 5.1).**

LUNG HYPERINFLATION

Therapeutic lung hyperinflation has been used for many years by physiotherapists in the management of patients in the ICU.[3–7] Lung hyperinflation can be achieved through two techniques: manual hyperinflation (MHI) or ventilator hyperinflation (VHI).

Manual hyperinflation uses a self-inflating circuit to deliver a volume of gas 50% greater than tidal volume (V_T), to airway pressures up to 40 cmH_2O, via an endotracheal or tracheostomy tube. An augmented V_T may improve pulmonary compliance and aid recruitment of atelectatic lung, secondary to reduced air-flow resistance and enhanced interdependence via the collateral channels of ventilation.[8] Bronchial secretions may be mobilised by the increased expiratory flow rate and/or stimulation of a cough following a quick release of pressure from the bag on expiration.[9] The net effect can result in improved oxygenation.[8] However, MHI may be contraindicated in some ICU patients; therefore the use of ventilator hyperinflation offers an alternative method to augment lung volume whilst potentially avoiding cardiopulmonary instability associated with ventilator disconnection and loss of positive end-expiratory pressure (PEEP). The delivery of an augmented V_T via the ventilator (200 mL increments until a peak airway pressure of 40 cmH_2O is reached) has been shown to be as effective as conventional MHI in the removal of secretions and maintenance of static lung compliance.[10,11] In an emergency situation an Ambu-bag and facemask can be used to perform MHI in the self-ventilating patient. However, an alternative technique such as IPPB should be considered when an augmented V_T is required during a therapeutic intervention (**Box 5.1**).

Table 5.1 Treatment modalities to optimise cardiopulmonary function

INVASIVELY VENTILATED PATIENTS	NON-INVASIVE/SELF-VENTILATING PATIENTS
Manual hyperinflation (MHI) ventilator hyperinflation (VHI)	Active cycle of breathing technique (ACBT)
Suction	Manual techniques
Inspiratory muscle training	Positioning
Manual techniques	Intermittent positive-pressure breathing (IPPB)
Positioning	Continuous positive airways pressure (CPAP)
Mobilisation/ rehabilitation	Non-invasive ventilation (NIV) Nasopharyngeal/oral suction PEP mask, flutter valve, acapella Mobilisation/rehabilitation

Box 5.1 Potential advantages and complications of MHI

Potential advantages

Reversal of acute lobar atelectasis[8]

Alveolar recruitment via channels of collateral ventilation[8]

Improvement in arterial oxygenation

Mobilisation of secretions and contents of aspiration[11]

Improved static lung compliance[11]

Effectiveness may be increased when combined with appropriate positioning and manual techniques[1]

Potential complications

Absolute contraindications include undrained pneumothorax and unexplained haemoptysis

Cardiovascular and haemodynamic instability[6]

Loss of PEEP, inducing hypoxia and potential lung damage. This can be minimised by incorporating a PEEP valve into the circuit of a 'PEEP-dependent' patient

Risk of volutrauma, barotrauma and pneumothorax, which can be reduced by including a manometer in the circuit

Risk of increased intracranial pressure

Increased patient stress and anxiety

RECRUITMENT MANOEUVRES

Recruitment manoeuvres may be employed to reverse hypoxaemia in patients with ALI/ARDS. A recruitment manoeuvre involves a transient increase in transpulmonary pressure in an attempt to re-inflate and maintain atelectatic lung units.[12] No standard approach exists; however, common options include: the application of incremental levels of continuous positive airways pressure (CPAP) with no tidal excursion, incremental increases in positive end-expiratory pressure (PEEP) with additional V_T, and the application of intermittent larger 'sigh' breaths. In randomised studies, although recruitment manoeuvres may transiently improve oxygenation, there is as yet no proven outcome benefit.[13]

Box 5.2 Potential advantages and complications of suction

Potential advantages

Stimulation of a cough when reflex is impaired by mechanical stimulation of the larynx, trachea or large bronchi

Removal of secretions from central airways when cough is ineffective or absent

Potential complications

Tracheal suction is an invasive procedure and should be undertaken only when there is a clear indication

Absolute contraindications to suctioning are unexplained haemoptysis, severe coagulopathies, severe bronchospasm, laryngeal stridor, base of skull fracture and a compromised cardiovascular system

Hypoxaemia can be induced secondary to suctioning. This can be limited by pre- and post-oxygenation

Cardiac arrhythmias may be more common in the presence of hypoxia

Tracheal stimulation may produce increased sympathetic nervous system activity or a vasovagal reflex producing cardiac arrhythmias and hypotension

SUCTION

Suction is used to clear secretions from central airways when a cough reflex is impaired or absent. A suction catheter is passed via an endotracheal or tracheostomy tube or via a nasal/oral airway to the carina, which may stimulate a cough in a non-paralysed patient (**Box 5.2**). The catheter is pulled back 1 cm before suction is applied on withdrawal. The suction catheter diameter should not be greater than 50% of the diameter of the airway through which it is inserted as large negative pressure can be generated intrathoracically without air entrainment. The use of suction following effective MHI optimises removal of secretions.[14] Instillation of normal saline prior to suctioning remains controversial; however, it may stimulate a cough, maximising secretion mobilisation and clearance.

INSPIRATORY MUSCLE TRAINING

It is recognised that mechanical ventilation and prolonged immobility may result in widespread deconditioning; this can include weakness or fatigue of the diaphragm and inspiratory muscles, plus poor respiratory muscle endurance,[15] resulting in slow or failed weaning from ventilatory support.[16] It has been suggested that mechanical ventilation per se may adversely alter diaphragmatic myofibril length and function, leading to rapid atrophy.[15] A recent systematic review evaluating the effect of inspiratory muscle training on muscle strength in adults weaning from mechanical ventilation reported a significant increase in inspiratory muscle strength following muscle training.[17] However, it remains unclear whether this increased strength is associated with a shorter duration of mechanical ventilation, improved weaning or patient survival.

MANUAL TECHNIQUES

CHEST SHAKING AND VIBRATIONS

Shaking and vibrations are oscillatory movements of large and small amplitude performed during expiration, which are thought to increase expiratory flow rate, aiding mucociliary clearance.[18] The application of chest wall shaking and vibrations is not standardised, but their effectiveness is thought to be influenced by the timing of their application within the breath cycle. Shaking and vibrations applied early in the expiratory cycle have been shown to generate high peak inspiratory pressures, whereas shaking and vibrations applied late in the expiratory cycle are not effective at increasing peak expiratory flow.[19]

CHEST WALL COMPRESSION

Compression of the chest wall can be used to augment an expiratory manoeuvre such as a 'huff' (see section on ACBT) or a cough by providing tactile stimulation or wound support.

CHEST CLAPPING/PERCUSSION

Chest clapping is a rhythmical percussion applied over specific areas of the chest, which may mobilise secretions secondary to the transmission of mechanical oscillations through the chest wall. However, there is little evidence to support this claim.

NEUROPHYSIOLOGICAL FACILITATION (NPF) OF RESPIRATION

NPF of respiration is a set of techniques designed for the treatment of the neurologically impaired adult. Manual externally applied stimuli to the thorax, abdomen and mouth can be used to stimulate increased V_T, a cough reflex, augmented contraction of the abdominal muscles, or an increased conscious level.[20,21]

POSITIONING

A simple change of position can have a profound effect on cardiopulmonary physiology (**Fig. 5.1**).[22,23] As such, positioning is commonly utilised to achieve several different goals: drainage of secretions using gravity-assisted positioning (GAP), reduction of the work of breathing/breathlessness or to optimise ventilation/perfusion (V/Q) matching.

GRAVITY-ASSISTED POSITIONING (GAP)

GAP facilitates the removal of excess bronchial secretions by positioning a specific bronchopulmonary segment perpendicular to gravity (**Box 5.3**). This technique is not used in isolation but in conjunction with augmented VT, either via the ventilator, MHI or the active cycle of breathing techniques (ACBT) in a spontaneously breathing patient. An individual position exists for each bronchopulmonary segment based on the anatomy of the bronchial tree;[24] however, these may need modification in the ICU setting.

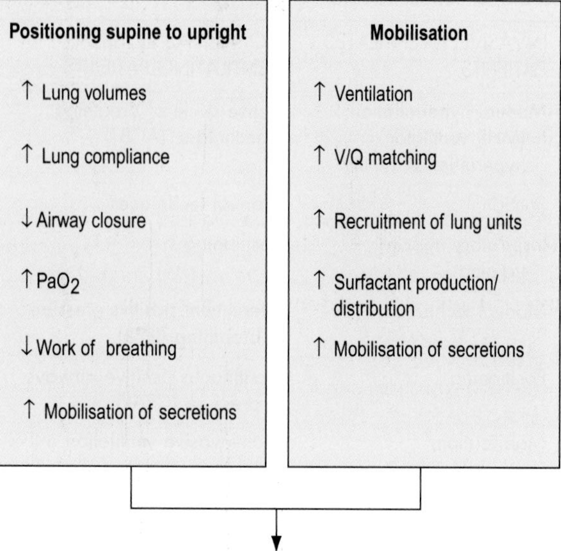

Figure 5.1 Potential advantages and complications of mobilisation. *(Adapted from Dean 1998,[22] with permission.)*

Box 5.3 Potential advantages and complications of GAP

Potential advantages

- Maximises removal of excess bronchial secretions when combined with ACBT
- Allows accurate treatment of specific bronchopulmonary segments
- Self treatment can be included in a home programme on discharge

Potential complications

- Positions need modification when used in the presence of cardiovascular/neurological instability, haemoptysis or gastric reflux

REDUCTION OF THE WORK OF BREATHING

A reduction in the work of breathing/breathlessness can be achieved by putting a patient in a position that optimises the length–tension relationship of the diaphragm, promotes relaxation of the shoulder girdle and upper chest and facilitates the use of breathing control.[25] This approach to positioning is particularly effective when used in conjunction with non-invasive ventilation (NIV). Adequately supported high-side lying is a useful position to promote relaxation of the breathless patient. In addition, it can discourage the overuse of accessory muscles of respiration, which may reduce energy expenditure. Some patients prefer forward lean sitting with their arms placed in front of them on a high table. In this position the length–tension relationship of the diaphragm is optimised secondary to forward displacement of the abdominal contents.

VENTILATION/PERFUSION

Appropriate positioning of a patient can maximise V/Q.[26] In the self-ventilating adult, V/Q matching increases from non-dependent to dependent areas of lung.[27] However, in adults receiving positive-pressure ventilation lung mechanics are altered producing V/Q inequality. In this situation non-dependent areas of lung are preferentially ventilated while dependent regions are optimally perfused; as such a regular change of position is recommended.

In an extreme form prone positioning has been used to improve refractory hypoxaemia in patients with acute lung injury (ALI)/acute respiratory distress syndrome (ARDS). The mechanisms behind these improvements are complex, but probably centre around a combination of a redistribution of some pulmonary perfusion together with a more homogeneous distribution of ventilation leading to improved V/Q matching. Although prone positioning improves oxygenation in up to 70% of those with ALI/ARDS, its role in improving outcome remains controversial.[28]

ACTIVE CYCLE OF BREATHING TECHNIQUE

The ACBT is a cycle of breathing exercises used to remove excess bronchial secretions (**Box 5.4**).[5] The cycle can be adapted for each patient according to existing underlying pathology and presenting clinical signs. It consists of:

- breathing control × 4–6 breaths
- normal tidal breathing using the lower chest
- minimising the use of accessory muscles of respiration
- promoting relaxation
- lower thoracic expansion × 4–6 breaths
- can be used with/without an inspiratory hold
- forced expiration technique
- expiration with an open glottis ('huff'), combined with breathing control.

Although mainly used in the self-ventilating patient, alert, cooperative, ventilated patients can participate with this technique. The ACBT can be delivered via MHI in sedated and ventilated patients requiring mobilisation of secretions and airway clearance.

Box 5.4 Potential advantages and complications of ACBT

Potential advantages

- Mobilises and clears excess bronchial secretions[28]
- Improves lung function[28]
- Minimises the work of breathing
- Individual components of the cycle can be utilised/emphasised to target specific problems
- Can be used in combination with other manual techniques, GAP, V/Q matching, positioning to reduce breathlessness, and during activities such as walking
- Self treatment can be included in a home programme

Potential complications

- Without adequate periods of breathing control, bronchospasm and desaturation can occur
- Poor technique can lead to ineffective treatment and unnecessary energy expenditure

MECHANICAL ADJUNCTS

INTERMITTENT POSITIVE-PRESSURE BREATHING

IPPB is a patient-triggered, pressure-cycled mechanical device mainly used in self-ventilating patients to increase ventilation, mobilise bronchial secretions and re-expand lung tissue by augmenting V_T (**Table 5.2**).[29] Positive airway pressure is maintained throughout inspiration. Expiration is passive. IPPB requires constant adjustment of pressure and flow rates and careful patient monitoring to maintain effectiveness and cooperation. Effectiveness is increased when used in conjunction with positioning, ACBT and manual techniques (**Box 5.5**).

Table 5.2 Site and action of IPPB, CPAP and NIV

	IPPB	CPAP	NIV
Lung volume affected	↑ V_T	↑ FRC	↑ V_T and FRC
Action	Assists removal of excess bronchial secretions	Reverses atelectasis	Ventilatory support

CONTINUOUS POSITIVE AIRWAYS PRESSURE

CPAP maintains a positive airway pressure throughout inspiration and expiration. It is used in both intubated and self-ventilating patients to increase/normalise functional residual capacity (FRC) via recruitment of atelectatic lung. Clinically increased FRC is associated with improved lung compliance, improved oxygenation and reduced work of breathing.[29] Effectiveness is increased when used in conjunction with appropriate positioning. The self-ventilating patient must be able to generate an adequate V_T as this volume is not augmented with CPAP (see Table 5.2).

NON-INVASIVE VENTILATION

In recent years there has been an expansion in the role of NIV in the ICU. This includes the prevention of invasive ventilation in patients with COPD,[30] pulmonary oedema and immunocompromise; early weaning from mechanical ventilation and potentially the prevention

Box 5.5 Potential advantages and complications of IPPB, CPAP and NIV

Potential advantages
Improves lung volumes
Improves gaseous exchange
Decreases the work of breathing
IPPB and NIV can mobilise excess bronchial secretions by improving V_T
IPPB and NIV can improve lung and chest wall compliance
CPAP reduces left ventricular afterload by reducing the transmural pressure gradient
Patients can be mobilised while on CPAP and some modes of NIV; alteration of ventilator settings might be indicated to maximise patient potential/exercise tolerance during treatment
Settings can be adjusted to augment physiotherapy intervention, e.g. increased IPAP to assist removal of secretions

Potential complications
Absolute contraindications include severe bronchospasm, undrained pneumothorax, pneumomediastinum, unexplained haemoptysis and facial fractures; use with care in pre-existing bullous lung disease
Haemodynamic/neurological instability
Risk of decreased urine output with CPAP and NIV
Risk of carbon dioxide retention with CPAP
Risk of aspiration

of re-intubation in those who suffer extubation failure. In addition, V_T may be augmented during physiotherapy treatment to remove secretions, or when mobilising the patient (see Table 5.2). Improved oxygenation may be achieved using NIV when the patient is positioning to optimise V/Q (see Box 5.5).

TREATMENT ADJUNCTS AND TECHNIQUES

PEP mask and oscillating PEP devices such as the Flutter and acapella® are specialised mucociliary clearance devices used by some patients with chronic lung disease. These devices are rarely introduced in the ICU setting.

CRITICAL CARE REHABILITATION

The effects of deconditioning on the cardiovascular (**Box 5.6**), respiratory (**Box 5.7**) and neuromusculoskeletal (**Box 5.8**) systems are well documented.[31–33] This phenomenon occurs as a result of restricted physical activity, and reduces the ability to perform work. Such physical dysfunction can occur with even relatively short periods of immobility, and is significantly influenced by age, pre-morbid condition, nature of the illness/injury, and biochemical/pharmacological factors.[34,35] The consequences of physical dysfunction are significant in terms of patient outcome, length of hospital stay, duration of rehabilitation and subsequent ability to function independently in the community.[34–38] Consequently, there has been a paradigm shift

Box 5.6 Deconditioning and the cardiovascular system[31,33]

↓ stroke volume – ventricular remodeling and reduced preload (see ↓ plasma volume)
↑ heart rate (resting and exercising) – ↓ vagal tone, ↑ sympathetic catecholamine secretion and ↑ cardiac β-receptor activity
↓ cardiac output and systemic oxygen delivery
↓ V_{O_2}max – magnitude highly correlated to duration, static exercise effective in preventing some of decrease. Related to changes centrally (cardiac output) and peripherally (oxygen delivery and utilisation)
↓ plasma volume – secondary to fluid shift and altered renin–antiotensin–aldosterone activity. Contributes to ↓ orthostatic tolerance
Orthostatic intolerance develops more rapidly in the elderly or those with cardiovascular pathology; often slow to resolve
Increased blood viscosity and vascular stasis – predisposition to thromboembolism
Altered cardiovascular reflexes – proposed attenuated baroreflex-mediated sympathoexcitation and enhanced cardiopulmonary receptor-mediated sympathoinhibition; contributes to orthostatic intolerance
Altered arterial/venous vascular function

Box 5.7 Deconditioning and the respiratory system

Adverse effects on:
- FRC
- Compliance (lung and chest wall)
- Resistance
- Closing volume
- Respiratory muscle function – impaired strength and endurance, reduced performance of ventilatory pump, ↑ days of mechanical ventilation, complex weaning issues
- Concept of ventilator-induced diaphragmatic dysfunction proposed (atrophy, fibre remodelling, oxidative stress, and structural injury); time-dependent reduction in force-generating capacity, secondary to disuse and passive shortening
- Respiratory muscle weakness may be limited by judicious choice of ventilation mode; role of inspiratory muscle training unclear

in critical care management to reduce confounding iatrogenic factors and minimise immobility. Care bundles such as the ABCDE (Awakening and Breathing coordination, Choice of sedative or analgesic exposure, Delirium monitoring and management, Early mobility and Exercise) approach have been advocated in order to optimise patient recovery and outcome.[38,39]

The role of early mobility and exercise in attenuating the deleterious effects of immobility during critical illness is now widely reported.[40] Early mobilisation and/or exercise of critically ill patients via selected rehabilitation strategies has been demonstrated to be

Box 5.8 Deconditioning and the neuromusculoskeletal system

Muscle atrophy – protein degradation (loss of contractile protein, increased non-contractile tissue, e.g. collagen) and cytokine activity. Reduction in strength, especially lower-limb antigravity muscles (i.e. those involved with transferring and ambulation). Inactivity amplifies the catabolic response of skeletal muscle to cortisol, therefore more marked atrophy following trauma or illness. Particularly significant in patient groups with low relative muscle mass, e.g. the elderly. Nutritional countermeasures should be considered and carefully titrated to best meet demands

↓ Muscle endurance (cf. Box 5.7 Respiratory system) – reduced muscle blood flow/red cell volume/capillarisation/oxidative enzymes, and biochemical changes. Generally longer to rehabilitate compared with reduction in muscle strength

Muscle shortening or changes in peri/intra-articular connective tissue (including chest wall and thoracic spine) → contractures, ↓ joint range of motion, pain. Positioning and stretching maintain range and delay invasion of non-contractile protein

Decreased bone mineral density (particularly trabecular bone) – may be attenuated by standing or resistance exercise. Rate of recovery tends to lag behind that of muscle strength. Increased risk of fracture on remobilisation, especially in elderly

Microvascular and biochemical changes in peripheral nerves impair neuromuscular function. Adversely affects maximal voluntary contraction, and balance/proprioceptive activity

Critical illness neuropathy and myopathy frequently develop in patients hospitalised in an ICU for >1 week. Risk factors include sepsis, SIRS and severe MOF. Associated with higher mortality rate, prolonged ventilation and rehabilitation, disability and reduced quality of life

safe, feasible, reduce length of stay, decrease the incidence of delirium and improve physical function.[40–43] Based on growing evidence, the European Respiratory Society, the European Society of Intensive Care Medicine, and the National Institute For Health and Clinical Excellence[44] have promoted early instigation of individualised rehabilitation programmes to prevent avoidable physical dysfunction.[44,45] Early mobilisation programmes may, however, face cultural and technological barriers[34,46] and proponents advocate a shift from multidisciplinary 'silos' to collaborative interdisciplinary care.[38,47] The physiotherapist, possessing expertise in rehabilitation and exercise physiology, should play a key coordination role in these programmes by evaluating individual patients, devising a shared therapeutic strategy, and referring to other rehabilitative specialties (e.g. speech and language therapy, occupational therapy) as required.[45]

Careful assessment both before (and during) implementation of an early mobilisation/exercise programme must be undertaken by a suitably experienced physiotherapist. A number of authors have suggested algorithms or criteria for this process,[40,42,48,49] which are summarised in **Box 5.9**.

Box 5.9 Criteria to consider before mobilising a critically ill patient[40,41,46,48]

Past history
Premorbid physiological reserve
Premorbid functional ability
Current cardiovascular reserve
Resting HR <50% of age-predicted maximum
BP <20% variability recently
No new MI or arrhythmias
No orthostatic intolerance
No new antiarrhythmics or vasopressors (or escalating doses of vasopressors)
Other significant cardiovascular concerns excluded
Current respiratory reserve
$Pa_{O_2}:Fi_{O_2}$ >40 kPa
Sa_{O_2} >90% and <4% recent drop
Satisfactory respiratory pattern
PEEP <10, Fi_{O_2} <60%
Concern for airway integrity
Patient–ventilator synchrony
Other factors
Risk assessment undertaken (including environment, staffing, expertise, equipment)
Patient consent
No neurological contraindications
No orthopaedic contraindications
No undue pain, fatigue, anxiety or dyspnoea
Adequate nutritional status
Liaison with interdisciplinary team, patient and/or family
Consideration of objectives and outcome measures

Traditionally, exercise rehabilitation has progressed linearly from activity in bed, then sitting, and finally to standing/walking. The model demonstrated in **Figure 5.2** represents a three-stage functional rehabilitation programme. It is supported by evidence that suggests a multimodal training regimen is required to maintain/restore both physiological and psychological performance after a period of immobility and illness.[50] The use of interlinking circles is intended to reflect the non-linear pattern of exercise progression more commonly utilised in patients with critical illness (e.g. patients may be able to stand using a tilt-table before they are able to tolerate sitting out of bed). The central shaded area represents the core components that should be addressed at every stage in the patient's recovery. The areas bordered by the broken lines represent the progression or regression from one stage to the next. During all stages, the patient's cardiopulmonary response must be closely monitored and exercise titrated accordingly. Modifications (e.g. temporarily increasing the Fi_{O_2} and/or level of ventilatory assistance) during exercise and in the early post-exercise period may be necessary. Such modifications are

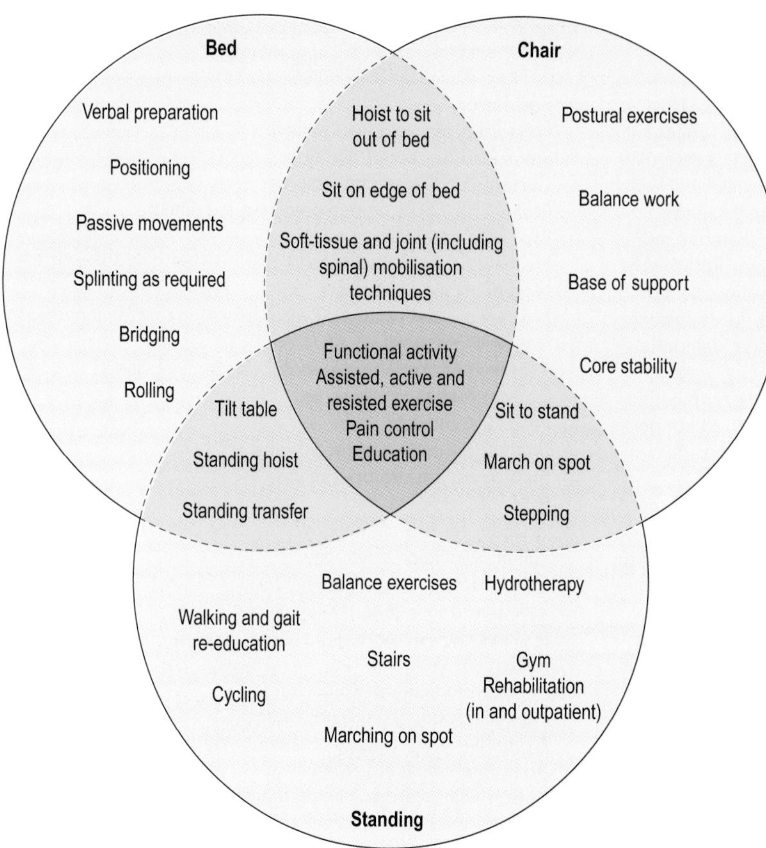

Figure 5.2 Schemata representing three-stage functional rehabilitation programme (the Nottingham Critical Care Rehabilitation Model). *(Douglas E. The Nottingham Critical Care Rehabilitation Model, University of Nottingham Division of Physiotherapy, Personal Communication, 2006, with permission.)*

commonly required as increasing physical activity often coincides with weaning from ventilatory support – both significant challenges to the physiological reserve. All aspects of progressive exercise therapy should be considered including positioning, passive and active mobilisation, aerobic training and muscle strengthening.[45] Adjuncts such as continuous passive motion, splinting or neuromuscular electrical stimulation may also be warranted.

The wealth of evidence regarding deconditioning should play a central role in planning treatment, both preventative and rehabilitative. For example, those muscle groups known to be most adversely affected by disuse should be the first to be targeted with a gradual, progressive regimen. During the remobilisation period, the interdisciplinary team must be particularly mindful of those elements with delayed recovery – for example, orthostatic tolerance and bone mass (predisposition to falls and fractures), and muscle endurance (diminished exercise tolerance).

It has been suggested that, in order to improve long-term outcomes for survivors of ICU (e.g. late mortality, ongoing morbidity, neurocognitive defects, functional disability, quality of life, economic burden), critical illness and its management should be viewed on a continuum and not merely the time spent in a critical care facility.[36] As such, rehabilitation should reflect this, continuing into the community, outpatient or follow-up clinic setting (Douglas, personal communication, 2006). Although the psychological, cardiopulmonary and functional sequelae of critical care survival may be profound (**Table 5.3**) to date, the optimal strategies for delivering post-critical care rehabilitation services remain unclear.[51,52]

PHYSIOTHERAPY ROLE EXPANSION

The nature of the critical care environment offers diverse opportunities for role expansion. The lead physiotherapist for the service must possess specialist cardiopulmonary and rehabilitative skills, as well as an expert knowledge of exercise physiology in health and disease. Furthermore, as a member of a dynamic interdisciplinary team, it may be appropriate to extend diagnostic or clinical skills beyond the remit of conventional physiotherapy (e.g. developing weaning strategies, advanced tracheostomy management, bronchoscopy, prescription, arterial blood gas sampling, managing non-invasive ventilation services, etc.).

As an educator, the clinician must ensure that all professionals who provide physiotherapy input are competent in their assessment, clinical reasoning and

Table 5.3 Psychological, cardiopulmonary and functional problems often encountered after ICU discharge

PSYCHOLOGICAL	CARDIOPULMONARY	FUNCTIONAL
Depression	Compromised cardiopulmonary system	Back pain
Fear	Difficulty clearing retained secretions (trache tube, mini-trach in situ)	Shoulder pain
Anxiety	Decreased lung volumes	Muscle atrophy/decreased strength
Confusion	Oxygen dependency	Inability to carry out activities of daily living independently
Disorientation		Limited mobility
Flashbacks		Poor exercise tolerance
Lack of motivation		Poor gait pattern
Functional dependence		

skill execution. A commitment to audit and research is essential in order to ensure evidence-based service provision, clinical governance and best possible patient outcome.

PHYSIOTHERAPY AND CRITICAL CARE OUTREACH TEAMS

The development of specialist physiotherapist posts within critical care outreach teams (CCOT) constitutes a prime example of role expansion. Following the publication of 'Comprehensive critical care',[53] CCOT services were developed to meet the actual or potential needs of patients through critical care provision 'without walls':

- avert critical care admission where possible
- facilitate timely critical care admission when appropriate
- empower all health care staff by disseminating ward-based critical care skills
- optimise patient management and make best use of critical care resources via effective clinical decision making.

The introduction of CCOT has been associated with a varied approach to team configuration; however, it has been suggested that those following a multiprofessional model are most likely to affect clinical and organisational improvements.[54] Consequently, many teams have elected to employ a designated specialist physiotherapist who can bring physiotherapeutic expertise to the service whilst also developing generic outreach practitioner skills (e.g. advanced tracheostomy management, cannulation, venipuncture, prescription via patient group directions, arterial blood gas sampling, drug administration, advanced life support, management of central/peripheral lines, 12-lead ECG interpretation, ordering/interpreting blood results, non-invasive ventilation, intravenous fluid management and chest X-rays).

SUMMARY

The physiotherapist has an important and varied role within the ICU/HDU setting working as part of the interdisciplinary team to optimise cardiopulmonary function and functional ability. The physiotherapist is often uniquely placed to follow and treat a patient from the acute stages at ICU admission, through the rehabilitation process to subsequent discharge from hospital and, if necessary, treatment can be continued in the outpatient setting.

There is no longer a place for routine physiotherapy treatment. Regular systematic assessment will identify physiotherapy-amenable problems that contribute to an interdisciplinary care plan. Implementation of any physiotherapy treatment should always utilise continuous analytical reassessment.

Acknowledgement

The authors wish to acknowledge the contributions made by Eleanor Douglas and Bronwen Jenkinson.

Access the complete references list online at http://www.expertconsult.com

1. Stiller, K. Physiotherapy in intensive care. Towards an evidence-based practice. Chest 2000;118:1801–13.
10. Dennis D, Jacob W, Budgeon C. Ventilator versus manual hyperinflation in clearing sputum in ventilated intensive care patients. Anaesth Intensive Care 2012;40(1):142–9.
17. Moodie L, Reeve J, Elkin M. Inspiratory muscle training increases inspiratory muscle strength in patients weaning from mechanical ventilation: a systematic review. J Physiother 2011;57:213–21.

19. Shannon H, Stiger R, Gregson RS, et al. Effect of chest wall vibration timing on peak expiratory flow and inspiratory pressure in a ventilator lung model. Physiotherapy 2010;96(4):344–9.
40. Adler J, Malone D. Early mobilization in the Intensive Care Unit: a systematic review. Cardiopulm Phys Ther J 2012;23(1):5–13.
45. Gosselink R, Bott J, Johnson M, et al. Physiotherapy for adult patients with critical illness: recommendations of the European Respiratory Society and European Society of Intensive Care Medicine Task Force on Physiotherapy for Critically Ill Patients. Intensive Care Med 2008;34(7):1188–99.
52. Connolly B, Denehy L, Brett S, et al. Exercise rehabilitation following hospital discharge in survivors of critical illness: An integrative review. Crit Care 2012;16(3):226.

6

Critical care nursing

John R Welch

NATURE AND FUNCTION OF CRITICAL CARE NURSING

Nurses are the round-the-clock constant for critically ill patients and their families, providing continuity and acting as the 'glue' that holds the service together. Nurses fine-tune, coordinate and communicate the many aspects of treatment and care needed by the patient, with:

- continuous, close monitoring of the patient and attached apparatus
- dynamic analysis and synthesis of complex data
- anticipation of complications
- complex decision making, execution and evaluation of interventions so as to minimise adverse effects
- enhancement of the speed and quality of recovery
- emotional support of the patient and family, including support through the end-of-life.[1]

Nursing in critical care is influenced by the essential nature of nursing as well as the specific requirements of the speciality. Key concepts for all nurses are said to include an appreciation of holism and the whole range of influences on all areas of life, and the pursuit of health rather than treatment of illness.[2]

There is inevitably an emphasis on technology in the intensive care unit (ICU): nurses must be technically competent. It is all too easy to neglect the human aspects of care. Expert nurses connect with patients both physically and psychologically,[3] but patient-centred care and emotional support can be lost when the nursing resource is reduced.[4] One ICU patient described his treatment as 'rooted in the minute analysis of charts and the balancing of chemicals, not so much in the warmth of human contact'.[5] Others reported feelings of helplessness, desertion and powerlessness.[6] ICU patients are less heavily sedated and therefore more aware than previously, but can rarely control what happens to them during critical illness, especially in the acute phase. They usually wish to reassert their autonomy as they recover (e.g. during weaning from ventilation or when moving to a lower level of care). Nurses can enable patients to have a say in the management of these processes while still ensuring a safe progression. Essential personal care is invariably undertaken or supervised by nurses; and although important functions such as chest physiotherapy, mobilisation and administration of nutrition may be prescribed by other specialists, they will still be integrated and delivered by nurses.

A SYSTEMATIC APPROACH TO CARE

Nursing the critically ill patient is complex. The clinical review should be structured in order to clarify and prioritise patient needs so that all possible problems are addressed. In acute situations, assessment in turn of the fundamental A–B–C–D–E aspects of care is a useful method:

A. *airway:* with establishment and maintenance of airway patency (using artificial devices when necessary, removal of pulmonary secretions, etc.)

B. *breathing:* ensuring adequacy of oxygenation and ventilation, etc.

C. *circulation:* assessing blood volume and pressures; perfusion of brain, heart, lungs, kidneys, gut and other organs; control of bleeding, haematology, etc.

D. *disability:* checking level of consciousness/reduced consciousness, and the factors that affect it; systemic and localised neurology

E. *exposure:* hands-on, head to toe, front and back examination, and review of everything else; with consideration of wounds and drains; electrolytes and biochemistry, renal function, etc.

Treatment strategies can be prioritised using this schema, which has the additional benefit that it will be familiar to colleagues trained in advanced life support and similar systems.

Further detail may be gained from review of:

F. *fluid* and electrolyte balance, fluid input, urine output

G. *gastrointestinal function:* nutritional needs; elimination

H. *history* and holistic overview of the patient as a person and their socio-cultural context

I. *infection* and infection control; microbiology

L. *lines:* utility and risks

M. *medications*

N. *nursing* and interdisciplinary teamwork: ensuring resources are sufficient for the patient's severity of illness and the physical demands of care

P. *psychology*: and the plan of care and prognosis in the short, medium and longer term.[7]

More sophisticated models can be used to frame a wider impression of the patient or to reflect a particular philosophy or approach to care.[8] There is a great benefit in developing a shared vision within the department, and in articulating how agreed values will be demonstrated in practice.[9] These might include emphasising the primary importance of patient safety and well-being, ensuring that the kindness an individual would want for their own loved ones is always offered, effective teamworking, and having systems in place to achieve continuous improvement.[10] Whichever method is used, there must be explicit definitions of the patient's problems and a clear statement of measurable therapeutic goals.

NURSING AND PATIENT SAFETY

Many patients suffer iatrogenic harm, but bedside nurses have the opportunity to prevent such incidents by intercepting and mitigating errors made by others.[11] No particular system of critical care nursing has been shown to be definitively superior to others,[12] but nursing surveillance is key to patient safety.[13] Insufficient staffing has been linked to increased adverse events, morbidity and mortality.[14] At the minimum, 5.6 nurses need to be employed for each patient requiring 1:1 care 24 hours a day.

EVOLVING ROLES OF CRITICAL CARE NURSES

Critical care nurses' range of practice has widened with progress in technology and changes in the working of other professionals, although the benefits of developing new skills must be balanced against ensuring the maintenance of fundamental care. There is great variation in the array of tasks undertaken by nurses in critical care in different institutions, with invasive procedures and drug prescriptions still usually performed by doctors. Since 2006 qualified nurse prescribers in the UK have been enabled – in theory at least – to prescribe licensed medicines for the whole range of medical conditions. As yet, nurse prescribing is not a widespread phenomenon in critical care but is likely to become a routine part of practice in the future.

Critical care nurses have a rapidly developing role in decision making regarding the adjustment, titration and troubleshooting of such key therapies as ventilation, fluid and inotrope administration, and renal replacement therapy. The use of less-invasive techniques (e.g. transoesophageal Doppler ultrasonography for cardiac output estimation) mean it is possible for nurses to institute sophisticated monitoring and administer appropriate treatments. There is evidence that nurses can achieve good outcomes in these areas, especially with the use of clinical guidelines and protocols (e.g. by reducing the time to wean respiratory support[15]). It is clear that further development of protocols, guidelines and care pathways can be used to enhance the nursing contribution to critical care.

NEW NURSING ROLES IN CRITICAL CARE

Maintaining adequate numbers of staff with the experience and skills to meet the increasing needs of critically ill patients is a challenge. Nurses constitute the largest part of the workforce and represent a significant cost. Changes in training arrangements and the demographics of nurses in general have meant that there are relatively fewer applicants for ICU posts. This has necessitated the development of various new ways of working to deliver both fundamental and more sophisticated aspects of care. New nursing roles include some that substitute for medical roles, as well as those that retain a nursing focus and aim to fill gaps in health care with nursing practice rather than medical care. The UK has designated a number of senior 'nurse consultant' posts in all areas of health, but with the largest proportion in critical care, particularly in outreach roles.[16] These are advanced practitioners focusing primarily on clinical practice but also required to demonstrate professional leadership and consultancy, development of practical education and training, macro-level practice, and service development, research and evaluation.

Other staff – such as 'nursing' or 'health care assistants' – are increasingly and successfully employed to deliver what has previously been seen as core nursing care, in order to support trained nurses and free them to concentrate on more advanced practice.[17] Reductions in health care funding and shortages of trained staff are likely to make such developments more common, but it is imperative that this is a managed process so as to ensure the best outcomes for patients, with proper arrangements for training, support and systems of work.

CRITICAL CARE NURSING BEYOND THE ICU: CRITICAL CARE OUTREACH (SEE CH. 2)

Around the world, general ward staff are required to manage an increasing throughput of patients who are, on average, older than before, with more chronic diseases, and more acute and critical illness. A national review of critically ill ward patients showed that the majority experienced substandard care before transfer to the ICU.[18] Various factors are implicated, including knowledge deficits and failure to appreciate clinical urgency or seek advice, compounded by poor organisation. It is nurses who record or supervise the recording of vital signs, but there is often poor understanding of the importance of such indicators, ineffective communication with senior staff, and difficulties ensuring that appropriate treatments are prescribed and administered. Nurse-led critical care outreach teams support ward staff caring for at-risk and deteriorating patients, and facilitate transfer to ICU when appropriate.[19] They can also support the care of patients on wards after discharge from ICU,[20] and after discharge from the hospital too. Potential problems with these approaches include a loss of specialist critical care staff from the ICU, and being sure that outreach teams have the necessary skills to manage high-risk patients in less well-equipped areas, particularly when there are limitations placed on nurses prescribing and administering treatments.

NURSING IN THE INTERDISCIPLINARY TEAM

High-quality critical care requires genuine interdisciplinary teamwork, with:

- 'clear individual roles
- members who share knowledge, skills, best practice and learning
- systems that enable shared clinical governance, individual and team accountability, risk analysis and management'.[21]

ICUs where team performance is not so well developed are likely to have less effective processes and worse outcomes. Aspects of team leadership, coordination, communication and decision making can be measured against defined criteria, as can outcome indicators relating to patients and staff.[22] Indicators of team performance include:

- compliance with protocols
- adverse events/critical incidents
- patient length of stay
- mortality
- staff satisfaction
- staff retention.[22]

Identified deficiencies in teamworking can then be addressed, although some investment may be needed. A recent study focused on nurses as the main drivers of improvement in the ICU. Units engaged in a structured improvement programme entailing analysis of the prevailing culture in the department, followed by tailored training in teamworking, ways of achieving safer practice, and performance measurement.[23] ICUs that completed this programme had significantly better outcomes than those that did not, even though both groups were required to use the same clinical protocols.[23]

QUALITY OF CARE

Robust audit is the foundation of quality care. Potential indicators include pressure ulcer prevalence, nosocomial infection rates, errors in drug administration, and patient satisfaction.[24] Nurses must measure the quality and take responsibility for the care that they deliver, although it should be appreciated that nursing care cannot be considered entirely separately from other variables that influence patient outcomes. The interdependence of different critical care personnel was illustrated in a multicentre investigation where interaction and communication between team members were more significant predictors of patient mortality than the therapies used or the status of the institution.[25] Quality care depends on a collective interdisciplinary commitment to continuous improvement.[26]

CRITICAL CARE NURSING MANAGEMENT

The nurse manager role is crucial to service performance. The most important priority is the challenge of attracting and retaining a flexible, effective and progressive nursing team that works well with other health care professionals in order to meet patient needs, but within a limited budget.

STAFFING THE CRITICAL CARE UNIT

The starting point for calculations of staffing requirements is the detailing of patient needs – and of the knowledge and skills that will be required to meet those needs – with an appreciation that there will be unpredictable variations over time (**Box 6.1**).

Patient need has many components, including:

- the severity and complexity of acute illness and chronic disease
- other physical characteristics (e.g. mobility, body weight, skin integrity, continence)
- consciousness and cognition
- mood and emotionality (e.g. anxiety, depression, motivation to engage in rehabilitation)
- the frequency and complexity of observation/monitoring and interventions
- the needs of relatives.

The staff resource includes members of the clinical team, the whole range of ancillary staff, and support services. Collectively, these personnel must be adequate to meet patient needs. This requires evaluation of:

- nursing numbers and skill mix
- interdisciplinary team skill mix, with consideration of variations in the availability of team members (e.g. doctors, respiratory/physiotherapists, equipment technicians out of hours).

The context of care is also significant, that is:

- the physical environment (e.g. the ease with which patients can be observed, whether cohorted in groups or in separate rooms)
- workload variations – peaks, troughs and overall activity in the department (e.g. admissions, discharges, transport to other areas (e.g. imaging), transfers).

Box 6.1 Standards for nurse staffing in critical care[27]

1. Critical care patients must have immediate access to a registered nurse with a post-registration qualification in the speciality.
2. Ventilated patients should have a minimum of one nurse to one patient.
3. The nurse–patient ratio should not go below 1 : 2.
4. Patients' care needs should equate to the skills and knowledge of nurses delivering and/or supervising that care.
5. Units should employ flexible working patterns as determined by unit size, activity, case-mix and the fluctuating levels of care for each patient.
6. Supernumerary clinical coordinators who are senior critical care qualified nurses will be required for larger/geographically diverse units of more than six beds. Their role is to ensure effective, safe and appropriate care, by managing and supporting staff and patients, and acting as communicator and liaison between team members.
7. The layout of beds and use of side wards must be taken into account when setting staffing levels.
8. Ongoing education for all staff is of principal importance to ensure knowledgeable and competent staff care for patients. Clinical educator posts should be utilised to support this practice.
9. Health care assistants have a key role in assisting registered nurses deliver direct care and in maintaining patient safety. These roles should be developed to meet the demands of patients and of the unit. However, the registered nurse remains responsible for the assessment, planning, delivery and evaluation of care.
10. Assistant practitioners can provide direct care under the indirect supervision of a registered nurse, who will remain responsible for the assessment, planning and evaluation of patient care. The role of assistant practitioners requires further evaluation.
11. Administrative staff should be employed to ensure nurses are free to give direct care, and to support essential data collection.

OTHER RESPONSIBILITIES

The manager is also responsible for:

- coordinated operational management of the area
- quality of nursing care
- management of nursing pay and non-pay budgets
- personnel management
- dealing with complaints and investigating adverse incidents.

There are always dynamic political, social and economic forces bearing on the organisational objectives and resources of the hospital and the ICU. The nurse manager needs to understand these factors and how they influence the delivery of patient care and the maintenance of a healthy environment for individual and team development. The manager must be able to communicate the key issues to the whole team in the form of an agreed strategy and a clear, regularly updated operational plan for the department. There needs to be a working system that addresses and integrates the views and needs of all users of the service, including patients and their families. Such a system should enable a shared understanding of exactly what needs to be done in practice, and where each team member fits into the plan.

Externally, the manager represents the service and ensures that other disciplines and the bigger organisation are informed about critical care issues.

Teams perform most effectively when individuals believe that they are working toward some common and worthwhile goals. The principles of shared governance can be usefully applied in this perspective, whereby staff collectively review and learn from their own practices. This has to be in the context of:

- the strategic agendas of the unit and the hospital
- the development of the service
- financial issues, budgets and budgetary restraints
- an appreciation of day-to-day working issues.

STRESS MANAGEMENT AND MOTIVATION

The ICU can be extremely stressful, demanding considerable cognitive, affective and psychomotor effort from staff. Supervisory and feedback arrangements should be in place to alleviate such demands, and to enable identification of staff members who are having difficulties at work. Studies of human resource practices in hospitals have found an association between the quantity and quality of staff appraisal and patient mortality, with organisations that emphasise training and teamworking having better outcomes.[28] Regular individual performance reviews and formulation of development plans provide positive assurance and encouragement, and can identify specific personal requirements such as educational needs.

Providing staff at all levels with opportunities to feel that they can influence and perhaps modify the working environment tends to decrease stress and increase motivation. Flexibility to work in different ways at different times while still meeting the overall demands of the department is important. It is the manager's job to balance and meet the needs of staff, patients and the organisation. One method is to give staff choice regarding rostering, partly to help with work–life balance, but also so that the nurse can opt to work with particular patients for a period so as to practise certain skills, and to promote continuity of care. This can have real benefits for patients.

NURSE EDUCATION

There are well-established educational programmes for critical care nurses, although the content and quality vary. There is a role for study of relevant

Box 6.2 Critical care competency framework[29]

Key competencies for critical care nurses education
- Respiratory system, e.g. safe, effective, appropriate nursing management of patient requiring invasive ventilation, using a range of suitable ventilatory modes, pulmonary recruitment manoeuvres (e.g. prone positioning), strategies for weaning, consideration of patient comfort (sedation, etc.)
- Cardiovascular system, e.g. safe, effective, appropriate nursing management of patients suffering from cardiovascular instability, including acute coronary syndromes, cardiac dysrhythmia, haemodynamic instability secondary to other factors, circulatory failure, peri-arrest situations, cardiopulmonary arrest
- Renal system, e.g. safe, effective, appropriate nursing management of patients with acute kidney injury, including fluid and drug therapies, urinary drainage devices, renal replacement techniques
- Gastrointestinal (including liver and biliary) system
- Neurological system
- Integumentary system

Other essential areas
- Medicines management
- Admission and discharge
- End-of-life care
- Rehabilitation
- Psychosocial well-being
- Communication and teamwork
- Infection prevention and control
- Inter- and intra-hospital transfer
- Evidenced-based practice
- Professionalism
- Defensible documentation
- Leadership

philosophy, nursing theory and research methods, but the fundamental requirement is for learning that focuses on clinical practice and practical problem solving (**Box 6.2**).

A competency framework can be used to structure descriptors of the skills, knowledge and attitudes needed to achieve specific patient outcomes. There needs to be consideration of both how individual actions are integrated into holistic care, and the role of independent clinical judgement. Developing nurses' critical thinking and decision-making skills are also important. Appraisal of learners' performance requires assessors to observe and question the nurse in practice; although this places significant demands on hard-pressed clinical areas. It may be that high-fidelity simulators can be used to test performance away from the practice setting in future.

Frameworks to identify different levels of performance have been developed – for example, based on Benner's novice-to-expert hierarchy (**Table 6.1**). UK critical care nursing organisations have described a three-stage version of the model; novice critical care nurses should spend up to 12 months acquiring the core competencies under supervision, then undertake a formal course of training (stage 2), and finally progressing to practice without direct supervision (stage 3).[29]

CRITICAL CARE NURSING RESEARCH

Critical care services treat small numbers of patients at high cost. Critical care has great physical and psychological impact, but often uses somewhat untested methods. Patient outcomes are influenced by different organisational approaches, staff characteristics, varied working practices and treatment methods, as well as differences between patients themselves. Therefore, a range of quantitative and qualitative investigative procedures is needed to gain an understanding of the issues. The approach chosen depends on the nature of the research question, and also the objectives of the researcher and the resources available.

REVIEWING RESEARCH

The methods used to appraise research depend partly on the type of work under review. The following questions may help clarification:

- *Justification for the research:* are the background and rationale of the study clearly established?
- *Scientific content:* is there a specific question/hypothesis?
- *Originality:* is it a new idea, or re-examining an old problem differently or better?
- *Methodology and study design:* are the methods appropriate and are they likely to produce an answer to the question? For example:
  - comparisons of different treatments generally require quantitative measurements of particular end-points (e.g. the dose of a drug needed to achieve a target physiological variable)
  - understanding how an individual thinks or feels usually involves analysis of qualitative material (e.g. data from interviews with patients and families).
- Is the research method described in a way that can be readily understood, and replicated?
- Are the relevant results shown? Are data given that provide details of the individuals under investigation and details of how representative these might be of a larger population?
- Is the analysis appropriate and is the power of the study adequate? (This is determined by the numbers involved and the size of the difference being examined.)
- Interpretation and discussion: are the conclusions and comments reasonable in the light of the results? Do the conclusions follow from the analysis?
- Are any references to background literature comprehensive and appropriate?

Table 6.1 Assessment of critical care nurses' performance (*after* Benner[3])

RATING	DEFINITION	OBSERVED BEHAVIOUR	PROMPTS
Novice	Limited skill and/or knowledge, inconsistent practice, variable interpersonal skill Limited understanding of wider context, inflexible rule-governed behaviour	Lacks coordination and confidence Potential for omissions or inaccuracies Unable to demonstrate accurate and safe performance despite repeated attempts	Requires frequent directive prompts, supervision and advice
Advanced beginner	Some skill and knowledge, generally consistent practice and interpersonal skill; variable ethical thought Some appreciation of situational influences	Coordinated and confident in fundamental tasks Easily distracted or unable to integrate other aspects of patient care	Requires occasional directive prompts and some supervision
Competent	Consistent safe, accurate and effective practice, interpersonal skill and ethical thought Conscious and deliberate planning with consideration of immediate context	Skilful, confident and coordinated patient-focused practice, with evident integration of other aspects of care Prioritisation of workload	Self-directing without supervision
Proficient	Consistent safe, accurate and effective practice, higher-level interpersonal skill and ethical reasoning Conscious and deliberate planning with consideration of longer-term goals Adapts care in response to changing situations	Skilled and accomplished practice, proactive and flexible approach to care Problem solving and decision making through reflection Role model	Capable of supporting and demonstrating skills to others

- What can be taken from the study – that is, what value does the study have in terms of supporting or developing clinical practice?
- What is the overall impression of the work? Is it credible? Is the presentation clear and informative?
- If evaluating a paper, has the work undergone proper peer review?

UNDERTAKING A RESEARCH PROJECT

STAGE 1: IDENTIFY AND CLARIFY THE TOPIC TO BE EXAMINED

Research is most valued when it is relevant to practice. The researcher is more likely to gain support for investigation of high-risk and high-cost processes. Many everyday methods and treatments warrant examination too, particularly when there are significant variations in practice. The researcher should determine how the topic of interest might be described in a measurable way, and formulate the investigation as a question, with consideration of how answers can be obtained.

STAGE 2: GATHER RELEVANT BACKGROUND INFORMATION

It is important to collect information that enables an understanding of the issues under investigation, and helps justify performing the study. Hospital libraries are useful, not least because there may be staff members who can give advice about the project. Indexes for journals and books are in print- and computer-based formats, with databases and texts also available through the internet. A good starting point is Google Scholar (http://scholar.google.co.uk//). This uses a broad approach to locating articles across many disciplines and sources. Specific medical/nursing websites include:

- PubMed, from the US National Library of Medicine (www.nlm.nih.gov/), with access to the MEDLINE (Medical Literature, Analysis, and Retrieval System Online) biomedical database
- the Cumulative Index to Nursing and Allied Health (CINAHL) at www.ebscohost.com/biomedical-libraries/the-cinahl-database
- the Cochrane Collaboration of systematic reviews of health care interventions (www.cochrane.org)
- EMBASE (www.embase.com/), which is particularly good for pharmacological information.

The researcher must also evaluate the quality of the information gathered. Different types of research are traditionally held to have different weights (e.g. results obtained from randomised controlled trials are considered to be high-grade evidence, whereas observational studies are deemed less useful). This hierarchy is not always applicable and may devalue some valuable work, but it does emphasise the need to critically examine the credibility of research.

Box 6.3 Issues for consideration in the review of research proposals

Particular to the patient/research subject
- The possibility of risk of harm
- The degree of inconvenience to the patient/research subject (or associated persons, e.g. patients' relatives)
- The duration of the study period (for the patient/subject)
- Whether the individual patient or research subject may obtain a direct or indirect benefit from participating
- The characteristics of the population to be studied
- Inclusion and exclusion criteria, and the rationale for inclusion and exclusion
- Whether any of the patients/research subjects are enrolled into other research projects that could influence the new study

Particular to study design/integrity
- The credentials of the researchers
- Whether the researchers are subject to any conflicts of interest
- The benefits of the research balanced against its detriments
- What is needed to fund and resource the study
- Whether there is an effective mechanism for managing adverse events
- Whether there is an effective mechanism for terminating the study
- The frequency of occurrence of the phenomenon to be studied
- The duration of the study
- The feasibility of recruiting sufficient patients or research subjects to meet statistical power requirements
- Where, when and how patients or research subjects are to be recruited, and who will be doing the recruiting
- How long the patient or research subject will be given to decide whether or not to take part
- What happens if the patient agrees to take part but subsequently wishes to withdraw
- How data will be collected, scrutinised, stored – and subsequently disposed of – in order to protect patient confidentiality
- Whether the research is analysing an established procedure or a novel method

STAGE 3: DESIGN A METHOD THAT:

- will provide data that will answer the question
- is adequate to answer the question (e.g. studies that use statistics require consideration of the numbers of data items needed to demonstrate differences between different groups or categories)
- is feasible to do in practice
- is ethical.

STAGE 4: COLLECT THE DATA

This is relatively simple provided that the data items to be collected are clearly defined. A common pitfall is to collect lots of unnecessary data and lose the focus of the original question. Data should be collected in a manageable format/database.

STAGE 5: ORGANISE THE DATA

By this stage, a large amount of material may have been gathered. It is important that:

- a system of categorisation and analysis is used that meets the objectives of the investigation
- the analysis addresses the original question
- appropriate statistical methods are used (specialist advice may be required).

STAGE 6: PRESENT AND EXPLAIN THE DATA

Presentation can take many forms, but it is always necessary to:

- set out the question asked
- describe the research method so that it is clear what was done
- illustrate the results and their analysis and
- present the key findings and conclusions.

The conclusions should follow from the analysis without inappropriate extrapolations. Any applications to clinical practice should be highlighted. The report must be presented succinctly and in a constructive manner, but with any shortcomings or problems in the study acknowledged. The goal is that the reader can understand the methodology and how the results were interpreted, as well as any limitations of the work. The main point of research is to share what has been learnt.

STAGE 7: EVALUATE THE PROJECT

The final phase is reflective. Conducting research is a process that can always be improved. Constructive feedback from colleagues should be sought. The researcher should review what has been learnt from the process as well as from the results of the study, and consider how the work might be further developed in the future.

RESEARCH ETHICS

The practitioner must always consider the ethical issues associated with conducting research. It may be necessary to submit an application for approval to an ethics committee. There are local differences in the process of obtaining ethical approval for research on humans, but most systems incorporate the principles of the Declaration of Helsinki (see the World Medical Association website at www.wma.net/en/30publications/10policies/b3/index.html). The ethics committee looks beyond the stated necessity and significance of the proposed research to evaluate a range of matters particular to the patients who may be involved, and to aspects of the study design. Some of these issues are summarised in **Box 6.3**.

Access the complete references list online at http://www.expertconsult.com

1. British Association of Critical Care Nurses, Critical Care Networks National Nurse Leads, Royal College of Nursing Critical Care and In-flight Forum. Standards for nurse staffing in critical care units. Newcastle upon Tyne: British Association of Critical Care Nurses; 2009 (rev. 2010). Online. Available: www.ics.ac.uk/professional/standards_safety_quality/standards_and_guidelines/nurse_staffing_in_critical_care_2009 (accessed 12 January 2013).
3. Benner P. From Novice to Expert: Excellence and Power in Clinical Nursing Practice (commemorative edn). Upper Saddle River, NJ: Prentice-Hall; 2001.
4. Ball C, McElligot M. "Realising the potential of critical care nurses": an exploratory study of the factors that affect and comprise the nursing contribution to the recovery of critically ill patients. Intensive Crit Care Nurs 2003;19(4):226–38.
14. Penoyer DA. Nurse staffing and patient outcomes in critical care: a concise review. Crit Care Med 2010;38(7):1521–8.
22. Reader TW, Flin R, Mearns K, et al. Developing a team performance framework for the intensive care unit. Crit Care Med 2009;37(5):1787–93.
26. Curtis JR, Cook DJ, Wall RJ, et al. Intensive care unit quality improvement: a 'how-to' guide for the interdisciplinary team. Crit Care Med 2006;34(1):211–18.
29. The National Competency Working Group. National Competency Framework for Critical Care Nurses. Critical Care Networks National Nurse Leads; 2013. Online. Available: www.baccn.org.uk/news/121105.asp (accessed 12 January 2013).

7

Ethics in intensive care

Raymond F Raper and Malcolm M Fisher

DEFINITION

Ethics is the study of how one ought to behave. In contrast, the law defines how one must behave to avoid punishment. Ethics is concerned with differentiating right from wrong behaviour. For most people, a sense of ethics is innate. Medical ethics particularly relates to the relationships between health care practitioners and patients and is not limited to doctors even if it is particularly applicable to doctors. Ethical conflict almost always involves a clash of values and appropriate resolution depends on recognition of the conflicting interests and values.

ETHICAL FRAMEWORK

Medical ethics are usually discussed in the context of principles. These principles inform ethical behaviour and can be summarised as:

1. *Autonomy*: the principle of individual self-determination in respect of medical care
2. *Beneficence*: the principle of 'doing good', an obligation always to act in the best interests of patients with respect to saving lives, curing illness and alleviating pain and suffering
3. *Non-maleficence*: the principle of doing no harm
4. *Fidelity*: faithfulness to duties and obligations, a principle underlying confidentiality, telling the truth, keeping up with medical knowledge (i.e. continuing professional development) and not neglecting patient care
5. *Social justice*: the principle of equitable access of all citizens to medical care according to medical need
6. *Utility*: the principle of doing most good for the most number of people – that is, achieving maximum benefits for society without wasting health resources.

Utility is a consequentialist concept, where the right or wrong of an action is determined by the outcome rather than by an a priori principle. The 'correct' action may thus vary with the particular circumstances. This is sometimes seen as an entirely different framework from the rights or principles-based system. The utility principle is more applicable to systems development in medical practice and may create conflict with responsibility for individual patients. It is important that intensivists participate in the public debate that determines how much of society's goods are to be allocated to medicine and how much of the health budget is to be allocated to intensive care without, at the same time, surrendering responsibility for the interests of individual patients. Moving between these collective and individual spheres of functioning can be challenging, but is essential to good medical practice.

Ethical conflict is most often encountered where there is a clash of values. Rationing, for instance, involves a clash between the values of individual rights and collective rights. Euthanasia usually involves a clash between the values of sanctity of life and autonomy. Resolution of ethical conflict depends on recognition both of the values that are in dispute and of the principles that are operative. Absolutist terms such as 'futility' tend to mask the values-in-clash and are thus unhelpful in resolution of ethical conflict. Consideration of the various interests involved is also helpful in foregrounding the real issues behind an ethical conflict.

ICU ETHICAL PROBLEMS

END-OF-LIFE MANAGEMENT

During its relatively brief history, intensive care has seen a dramatic increase in both capacity and capability. Practice has become codified and at least partly standardised and intensive care is more generally accessible. Greater emphasis on individual rights has seen an increased demand for medical resources in general and this has flowed on to intensive care. The great challenge for intensive care lies in the reality that prolonged life support is often quite easily achieved without there being either inevitable recovery or intractable demise. Of the sickest patients in the intensive care unit (ICU), only a proportion ultimately recovers and can be returned to a reasonable quality of life. Even this would not be a problem were it possible to predict survival with any degree of certainty and a great deal of effort has been expended in an attempt to achieve this. Unfortunately, this has met with only limited success and consideration of the appropriateness of ongoing intensive care is necessarily conducted against a background of prognostic uncertainty.[1]

In consequence of this, death in ICU usually involves some limitation or withholding of life-sustaining treatment.[2,3] This has now been well documented in many studies from around the world and the driving factors are now reasonably well understood.[2–9] The ethical principles underpinning this practice are those described above. Intensive care is inevitably burdensome and requires a commensurate benefit to conform to beneficence and non-maleficence. Although life itself has a value, this is considerably offset if it is brief, painful and non-interactive. As death becomes increasingly imminent, its deferment at any cost becomes less appropriate. Considerations of justice should rarely intrude at the bedside. However, prolongation of life by artificial means in a patient with little or no chance of survival may challenge the rights of survivable patients to limited intensive care resources.[10] Where resources are publicly owned, offering to one patient treatment that cannot be made available to all patients in similar circumstances is fundamentally unethical. The collective has the ethical right to regulate access to even beneficial therapy provided it does so in a non-discriminatory fashion. The intensive care specialist does not have a right to unilaterally apply or withhold resources against the will of the collective. Unfortunately, the will of the collective is rarely known.

End-of-life management in the intensive care setting has been subjected to a considerable research endeavour over the past several years.[2,4,11–13] Insights that can be gleaned from published studies include:

- Patients not infrequently die in some discomfort in ICU receiving unwanted therapy.
- Considerable dissatisfaction has been reported by both patients and families with management at the end of life.
- Patients' wishes with respect to end-of-life treatment are commonly unknown.
- Patients and families may be quite ignorant of the nature and prognosis of end-of-life initiatives such as cardiopulmonary resuscitation.[14]
- Active interventions including obligatory, outside consultations have not been particularly effective in improving the quality of end-of-life management.
- There is a good deal of practice variability across countries and communities with respect to attitudes to death, dying and the withholding and withdrawing of active treatment.[2,8]
- The reported variability in practice relates to attitudes of doctors and nurses, decision-making processes and to actual practices once a treatment-limiting decision has been made.
- Although some form of treatment limitation is common, withdrawal of treatment is not practised and is even illegal in some communities, whereas active foreshortening and active euthanasia are reported in others.
- Some confusion remains over the distinction between active foreshortening of life and administration of drugs that both relieve unwanted symptoms and shorten the dying process. The nature and doses of agents used to shorten life actively are not necessarily different from those used to relieve symptoms without the intention of accelerating death, and the time to death may also not be affected.[2]
- Most patients and families report a preference for some form of collaboration in end-of-life decision making.[15–17]
- Involvement in decision making is burdensome for families and can be associated with long-term sequelae.
- Clinicians are now frequently involved in the delivery of care they consider inappropriate. This poses a risk of moral distress and consequent burnout. Inappropriateness involves a very subjective assessment and better reflects the organisational culture of the ICU than patient characteristics.[18]

PRACTICAL CONSIDERATIONS

- Decisions to limit treatment in ICU depend on a careful consideration of the burdens and benefits of treatment.
- Prognostication in ICU practice is imperfect so that decision making is often based on probability rather than certainty. This has led to formulation of concepts such as 'practical certainty'.[19]
- Decision making is usually an evolving process, commonly involving several discussions of therapeutic possibilities, quality of life and patient preferences.[9,11]
- Competent patients should always be involved in discussions, and inclusion of family members should be encouraged and fostered.
- Given the common desire for collaborative decision making, seeking patient preferences and consensus in a proposed management plan is more appropriate than either surrendering decision-making responsibility to patients or surrogates or systematically excluding patients and/or carers.
- The important role of nurses and allied health practitioners in the management of critically ill patients warrants respect by inclusion in discussions. Failure to do so has resulted in nurses inappropriately taking unilateral, surreptitious action justified as patient advocacy. Legal action for unlawful termination of life has also resulted.

ADVANCE DIRECTIVES AND POWER OF ATTORNEY

Patients may formally signal their preferences for end-of-life care in a written document or may nominate a surrogate decision maker in the event of future incompetence. The legal standing of such documents is highly variable. Nevertheless, as expressions of self-determination they have considerable ethical validity and warrant respect. Unfortunately, advance directives are often insufficiently specific and it is not always possible to be sure that decisions included in such documents were fully informed and rational. Given the frequent reticence of patients to consider end-of-life matters,[14] advance directives are unlikely to become widely pervasive.

EUTHANASIA

This term is strictly applicable only to situations of active termination of life with the knowledge of and usually at the request of a patient suffering a terminal and/or debilitating, incurable illness. Physician-assisted suicide is a variation of this practice. This is a subject of considerable debate and is now legal in a small number of jurisdictions though probably practised surreptitiously in many more. Ethicists, largely on consequentialist grounds, maintain no distinction between this and the terminal withdrawal or withholding of treatment[20] (sometimes inappropriately termed 'passive euthanasia'). For intensive care practice, however, the distinction seems obvious and essential. The distinction is most often argued on the basis of intent. Although there may well be a difference in intent between active euthanasia and withdrawal of treatment, relief of pain and suffering may be at the heart of both activities. Even if this is the case, active euthanasia in the ICU context is generally a disproportionate means to the end. Treatment limitation is, arguably, an essential component of intensive care practice whereas euthanasia is not and there is usually a clear and obvious difference in the acts themselves. Thus although it may be true that in some instances there is no moral distinction between euthanasia and withdrawal of treatment, this does not mean that there is never such a distinction.

TREATMENT WITHDRAWAL

- Once a decision has been made to withdraw or withhold treatment, the decision, the participants, the rationale and the details of the treatment limitation should be clearly documented in the patient records. Surreptitious treatment limitation is difficult to justify and potentially hazardous.
- There is no moral hierarchy of treatments, but ventilator withdrawal is more obviously terminal than, say, withdrawal of renal replacement therapy or antibiotics.
- Although treatment may sometimes be withdrawn or withheld in ICU, care must never be withdrawn. An alternative, palliative management plan focusing on symptom relief and patient dignity should be documented and instituted.
- From a practical perspective, progressive treatment withdrawal enables progressive management of any resultant discomfort. It also helps foster an appreciation that death is a consequence of disease or organ system failure rather than of the withdrawal of treatment.
- Symptom relief, especially with sedatives and narcotics, may sometimes appear to hasten death. This is often justified on the 'double effect' principle, as the acceleration of death though foreseen was not intended. More relevantly, however, this can be seen simply as a trade-off of two aims where the relief of unwanted symptoms assumes a higher priority than avoidance of the foreshortening of life. Certainly, it is difficult to justify unnecessary pain and suffering at the end of life on ethical grounds. Finally, clinical experience suggests that, rather than shortening life, narcotics and sedatives commonly prolong the dying process by reducing cardiovascular stress.

CONSENT

Informed consent lies at the heart of the doctor–patient relationship and has both ethical and legal implications. Consent relates both to treatment (especially to invasive procedures) and to participation in research. General principles relating to consent can be listed:

- Patient consent is a fundamental tenet of medical practice. Routine or minor procedures may be included in the general consent to treatment.
- Consent may be waived in an emergency for treatment that is immediately necessary to save life or avoid significant physical deterioration. This applies whether or not the patient is technically competent.
- Valid consent is dependent on the provision of adequate information, including benefits and risks, and must be voluntary and free from coercion.
- Written consent provides evidence of the consent process, but consent itself need not be in writing, unless specifically required by a local authority.
- Competent patients are entitled to refuse consent to treatment even when doing so may result in harm or death.
- Surrogate consent for more elective procedures relies for ethical justification on the principle of autonomy. Patients' interests must thus be paramount. Legal requirements relating to surrogate consent are highly variable and 'surrogate' is often formally defined and limited by local statute.
- Autonomy also provides the ethical justification for advance directives, the legal status of which is also highly variable.
- An enduring power of attorney generally applies to financial affairs rather than to consent to treatment. Again, self-determination constitutes the ethical basis.
- Competent minors may or may not have a legal right to consent, but age does not affect ethical considerations independently of insight and understanding. Even incompetent minors have some entitlement to confidentiality and all are entitled to protection from harm, even if that harm devolves from parental or

guardian decisions based on well-meaning conviction or prejudice.
- Consent is especially required to involve a patient in research, where the importance of full disclosure is even greater. Medical research imposes some particular ethical issues, to be discussed below.
- Consent is also required for teaching purposes, such as video recording and photographing patients and teaching practical procedures.
- There may be a legal requirement for consent for testing for diseases such as human immunodeficiency virus (HIV)/acquired immunodeficiency syndrome (AIDS) and hepatitis. These diseases are not especially unique from an ethical perspective, however, and patients' rights to privacy are not absolute.

Because intensive care patients are often unable to provide formal consent and because critical illness itself may negate the preconditions for consent, this issue is commonly neglected. Consent to 'routine' or everyday procedures in critically ill patients is often presumed or rather subsumed under the general consent to treatment. Near-universal consent is possible, however.[21] The precise role for consent in the intensive care context has not been fully defined, but deviations from the general requirement for consent require some justification. The legal requirement for consent varies with different interpretations and jurisdictions. If taken to extreme, such as enabling surrogate refusal for 'routine' procedures such as central venous access, consent-related autonomy may become incompatible with the beneficence and non-maleficence principles and may largely become untenable.

RATIONING AND SOCIETAL ROLE

Intensive care is, by nature, expensive. This creates a tension and a potential ethical conflict for intensive care practitioners. It is essential to find a balance between responsibilities to individual patients and those to the collective. In theory, this is achieved by removing all rationing decisions from the bedside. Established norms rather than temporal availability or personal influence should determine access to ICU. Treatment is withheld or withdrawn not because there is a 'more deserving' patient at the door but because it would always be withheld or withdrawn under the particular clinical circumstances. Wide variations in access to medical care for similar patients across a single society cannot be ethically justified. More challenging is the definition of society. If a sufficiently broad perspective is adopted, most intensive care is difficult to justify. The ethically responsible intensive care practitioner will both advocate for individual patients and participate in the mostly unstructured social debate that determines what proportion of community resources is expended on medicine and on intensive care in particular.

PROFESSIONALISM

Medical practitioners occupy a unique and, usually, a privileged position in society. With this come a number of responsibilities. These are generally well covered in codes of conduct issued from time to time by professional societies and institutions of learning. The oldest and perhaps best known is the hippocratic oath. Professional, ethical responsibilities may be sorely tested where the well-being of the practitioner is at risk from medical practice, as with infectious disease epidemics and acts of terrorism. Resolution of this potential conflict has not been satisfactorily determined to date.

Among the ethical responsibilities of medical practitioners are:

- maintenance of professional standards by continuing education and professional development
- maintenance of appropriate professional relationships with patients
- appropriate documentation of medical interactions
- participation in quality and safety initiatives and practices
- respect for patient and staff confidentiality
- respect for the tenets of the law.

INDUSTRY AND CONFLICT OF INTEREST

Relationships among doctors and the medical technology and pharmaceutical companies are complex.[22] Doctors and industry are somewhat interdependent. Medical advances do not occur in a vacuum and the invention, assessment, development and marketing of new drugs and technologies necessitate close relationships between doctors and industry. Although doctors are entitled to fair consideration for their skills and effort, the relationships must be overt and openly scrutinised if conflicts of interests are not to occur. The nature of the rewards offered by companies for medical involvement in product development is diverse but includes both direct and indirect payments. The economic justification for all these payments depends on their effects on subsequent product marketing. The propriety of travel and related support is questionable unless it is directly and attributably related to openly contracted services. Involvement of companies with vested interests in pseudoeducational initiatives and even guideline development may be little more than covert marketing.[23] Some open labelled research initiatives with large, practitioner reward programmes are similarly worrisome. Initiatives designed to limit these conflicts of interest include open disclosure of all financial relationships and voluntary and involuntary codes of conduct on both sides of the relationship. Financial inducements can be easily concealed, however, and specific financial relationships can be obscured by their volume and pervasiveness. Although this potential for ethical conflict exists in many other commercial relationships, the nature of medicine and the associated expenditure of, often, public funds dictate that this is not an entirely private consideration.

RESEARCH

Critically ill patients can rarely consent themselves to participation in research projects and yet they are able to benefit from the results of earlier studies with similarly problematic consent issues. Locating surrogate decision makers within a timeframe appropriate for some types of research can also be impossible. This has been recognised and enacted in a consent waiver for even randomised clinical trials. The potential ethical conflict in this situation lies in the use of a patient as an instrument to achieve another's end without express consent. There is a potential 'slippery slope' in valuing the rights of the collective over those of the individual, and yet the individual can be seen to have an interest in the resolution of some of these important clinical questions. The conduct of such research must be carefully scrutinised by outside agents and careful consideration must be given to the balance between risk and benefit. A potentially greater benefit might help justify a potentially greater risk even if the benefit might not be directly applicable to the subject. Studies of, for example, disease mechanisms involving little or no potential direct patient benefit would need to involve no material risk. In general, the principles of consent detailed above are applicable. When a waiver is applied, patients and/or surrogates should be afforded an opportunity to withdraw from the study at the earliest opportunity.

ORGAN DONATION

Concern has been raised over possible or apparent conflict of interest with ICU practitioner involvement in organ donation. This has become especially at issue with the worldwide drive to increase donation for transplantation and the re-emergence of donation after death established on circulatory criteria. The ethical problem, as for research, lies in the use of one patient for the benefit of another or of society in general. The ethical justification for donation depends, again, on autonomy as most citizens when asked express a willingness to be involved in posthumous donation for transplantation. Provided that the focus remains on the patient's interests (including the fulfillment of the known or projected wishes of the patient and the sensitive care of their family), there is no real ethical conflict intrinsic to the involvement of ICU practitioners in the donation process. More and more, donation is being enacted as part of appropriate end-of-life management and is thus easily justified.

RESOLVING ETHICAL CONFLICT

Ethical conflict most commonly arises where there is a clash of values or interests. Resolution is often difficult because of entrenched positions and convictions. The innate sense of right and wrong lends itself to strong convictions in a way not seen in other human activities. The fundamental basis of resolution is discussion, enabling exposure of the values or interests that are in conflict. This may require a third party or mediator. Absolutist convictions such as 'sanctity of life' and absolutist terminology such as 'futility' impede conflict resolution and have to be unravelled.

Actual and potential conflict can frequently be resolved during end-of-life discussions. When this is not possible, outside mediation may be beneficial. The precise utility of this is difficult to establish but it is likely to be most beneficial if initiated early. Ethics committees have an important role in establishing frameworks for ethical practice. There is some evidence that formal ethics consultations facilitate end-of-life management, but the principles utilised are those of open discussion and full disclosure and these should characterise all bedside communication.

Recourse to legal processes may be essential, especially where an impasse has developed and families insist on continuing management felt inappropriate by care givers. There has been a small number of cases where the legal system has been able to respond swiftly and to cope quite well with the complexity of medical decision making, although this is not always the case. It is likely that conflict over end-of-life decision making will increase, particularly in multicultural democracies, and that court intervention will become mere routine rather than a last resort in the face of communication failure.

There are several useful guidelines informing practice, particularly in relation to end-of-life decision making. Individual practitioners should be aware of these and adapt them to local circumstances. Institution-based guidelines that conform to more overarching documents are probably most useful. Most learned colleges and professional societies now promulgate such practice guidelines in various forms.

Access the complete references list online at http://www.expertconsult.com

3. Prendergast TJ, Luce JM. Increasing incidence of withholding and withdrawing of life support from the critically ill. Am J Respir Crit Care Med 1997; 155:15–20.

8. Fisher M. An international perspective on dying in the ICU. In: Curtis JR, Rubenfeld GD, editors. Managing Death in the ICU. New York: Oxford University Press; 2001. p. 273–88.

10. Fisher M, Raper RF. Delay in stopping treatment can become unreasonable and unfair. BMJ 2000;320: 1268–9.
12. The SUPPORT investigators. A controlled trial to improve care for seriously ill, hospitalized patients. The Study to Understand Prognoses and Preferences for Outcomes and Risks of Treatment (SUPPORT). JAMA 1995;274:1591–8.
13. Angus DC, Barnato AE, Linde-Zwirble WT, et al. Use of intensive care at the end of life in the United States: an epidemiologic study. Crit Care Med 2004; 32:638–43.
19. Fisher M, Ridley S. Uncertainty in end-of-life care and shared decision making. Crit Care Resusc 2012;14:1–7.
21. Davis N, Pohlman A, Gehlbach B, et al. Improving the process of informed consent in the critically ill. JAMA 2003;289:1963–8.
22. Gale EAM. Between two cultures: the expert clinician and the pharmaceutical industry. Clin Med 2003; 3:538–41.

8

Common problems after ICU

Carl S Waldmann and Evelyn Corner

Until recently, an intensive care unit (ICU) stay was deemed successful if a patient survived to go to the ward. No consideration was taken of the patient dying on the ward or soon after leaving hospital, or indeed if the patient went home with an appalling quality of life.

Mortality figures for patients leaving our own ICU recently are shown in **Figure 8.1**.

A Kings Fund report in 1989 concluded that it was necessary to look at the morbidity following critical illness as well as mortality: 'There is more to life than measuring death'.[1]

Publications such as that of the Audit Commission (Critical to Success)[2] and that of the National Expert Group[3] (Comprehensive Critical Care) have supported the development of follow-up for patients following a stay in intensive care. In 2009 the National Institute for Health and Clinical Excellence published its guidance and recommendations to facilitate the introduction of rehabilitation programmes in all hospitals looking after critically ill patients.

In Reading, a follow-up programme has been ongoing since 1993. Until recently the rehabilitation of patients after a critical illness has fallen between too many stools. Following multi-organ dysfunction, it is difficult to categorise a patient to an individual specialty such as cardiac, respiratory or the stroke rehabilitation teams. Family doctors often have difficulty taking on the complexity of these patients, with the result that they are denied vital advice and assistance and lack an advocate with 'teeth' to ensure timely help.

SETTING UP A FOLLOW-UP SERVICE

Funding such a follow-up programme has posed local problems in many trusts. The service in Reading was initially approved and funded by local, then regional, audit committees.

The service is staffed by a follow-up sister who spends most of her time in this role helped by a staff nurse and an ICU consultant for the clinics held as a formal outpatient clinic 2–3 times monthly.

Invitations to patients who were in ICU were initially extended to all patients that had been in the ICU for more than 4 days; they were and are seen in clinic at 2 months, 6 months and 1 year after discharge and occasionally, but with time the invitation was extended to patients who have been in ICU for a shorter time period. Referrals are also sent from other hospitals where follow-up wasn't happening. It is important to identify clerical and IT support, and to achieve good collaboration with other hospital departments and general practitioners (GPs) to ensure patients do not make unnecessary journeys to the hospital, by trying to coordinate the patients' visits and ensuring that transport is organised where necessary. Very often, patients will voluntarily come from long distances if they had initially been admitted from other geographical locations – out-of-area transfers.

The logistics of running the service include arranging specific tests that may be required for the visit, such as pulmonary function tests and blood/urine for creatinine clearance. There may be special tests such as magnetic resonance imaging (MRI)[4] for patients who had a tracheostomy during their stay in ICU.

The service in Reading costs £30 000 annually, which, in the context of the bigger picture (£4.5 million budget for our ICU), is a small price to pay (**Table 8.1**). An unexpected bonus is that the clinic is often seen by the patients as a convenient place to make donations to the ICU.

Recently the clinic visits have been funded exactly the same as any other outpatient appointment attracting about £160 for the first visit and £80 for subsequent visits.

SPECIFIC PROBLEMS POST-ICU

The range of problems seen after intensive care is vast and ranges from nightmares and sleep disturbance through to ill-fitting clothes. Many of the problems are very specific to the individual but there are also recurrent themes. Flashbacks are common, as are taste loss, poor appetite, nail and hair disorders and sexual dysfunction.

There are several quality-of-life tools used in follow-up studies (**Box 8.1**).[5–9] Objective measurements may be inappropriate because they look at aspects such as return to work; often, patients in their 50s may not return to work after a traumatic episode, including ICU, and subjective measures would be more applicable, such as Perceived Quality Of Life (PQOL).

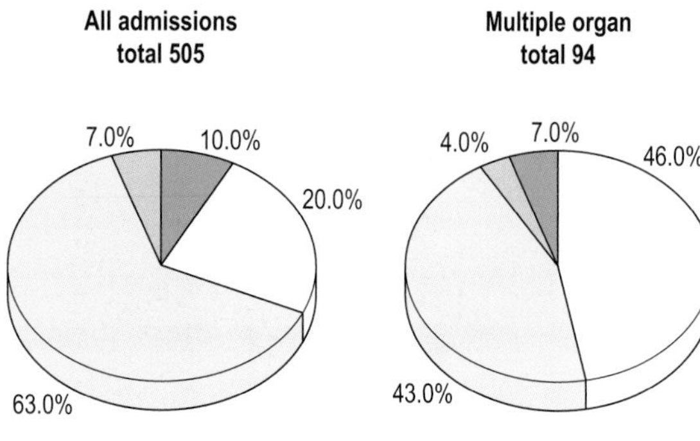

Figure 8.1 Mortality rates for leaving the intensive care unit (ICU).

Table 8.1 Costs of running a service

FOLLOW-UP CLINIC	COST (£)
Nursing	18000
Medical	6000
Administration	4000
Laboratory tests and X-rays	2000
Total	30000

Box 8.1 Quality-of-life tool examples

Objective
QALY Quality of Life tool[5]
Subjective
HAD Hospital Anxiety and Depression[6]
PQOL Perceived Quality of Life[7]
EuroQol 'European' tool[8]
SF 36 36-item short-form survey[9]

TRACHEOSTOMY

Since percutaneous techniques performed by intensivists started to replace surgical tracheostomy in 1991, we have seen an increasing number of patients tracheostomised earlier in their ICU stay.

The long-term sequelae have been assessed by lung function tests, nasoendoscopy and MRI screening (**Fig. 8.2**). There are minor cosmetic problems, such as tethering (**Fig. 8.3**). Tethering is easily dealt with in ear, nose and throat outpatients under local anaesthetic.

More difficult to manage is tracheal stenosis, defined as a 15% reduction in tracheal diameter. However, there have only been two cases to date. These were seen in the first series of 30 cases.[4]

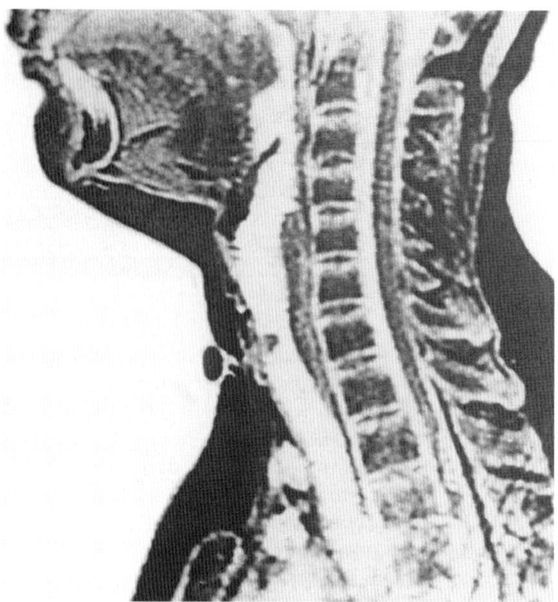

Figure 8.2 Assessment of long-term sequelae.

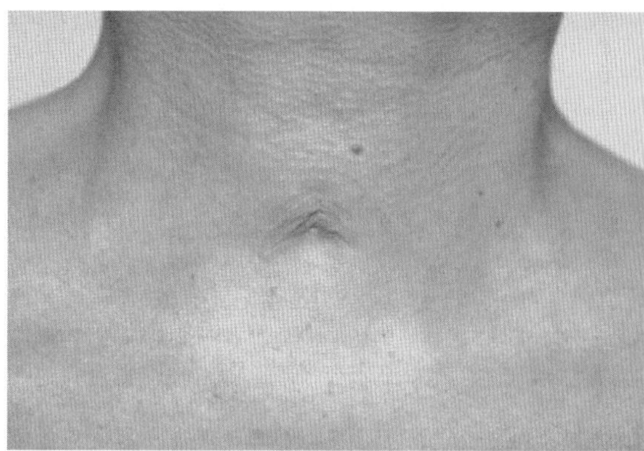

Figure 8.3 Tethering.

MOBILITY

Even in the absence of trauma, patients can expect to need 9 months to 1 year to regain full mobility. This is usually due to a mixture of joint pain, stiffness and muscle weakness. In one study[10] the duration of ICU stay was associated with mobility problems probably associated with loss of muscle mass. If questioned, patients will often report climbing stairs on all fours and descending on their bottoms (**Fig. 8.4**). Muscle wasting can present as a severe localised problem.

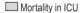

This may be associated with critical illness polyneuropathy (CIP),[11] which not only prolongs ventilatory weaning but also frequently both complicates and

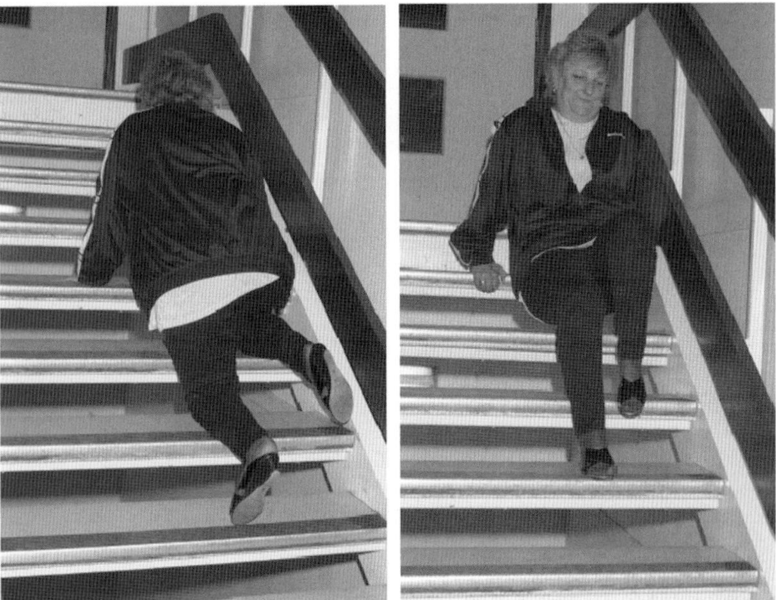

Figure 8.4 Climbing and descending stairs.

delays rehabilitation. Muscle relaxants have been implicated in the development of CIP[12] but have not been shown to cause statistically significant increases in time to wean from ventilation and duration of stay in ICU.[13]

Until recently, there have been no specific rehabilitation programmes for patients recovering from critical illness, although rehabilitation programmes for heart attack, stroke and respiratory disease are well established. A three-centre study has shown that a self-help physiotherapy-guided rehabilitation exercise programme will speed up physical recovery after intensive care.[14]

It is important occasionally for a member of the team to try to spend time with patients at their homes to assess their special needs and liaise with the GPs, district nurses, community physiotherapists and occupational therapists.

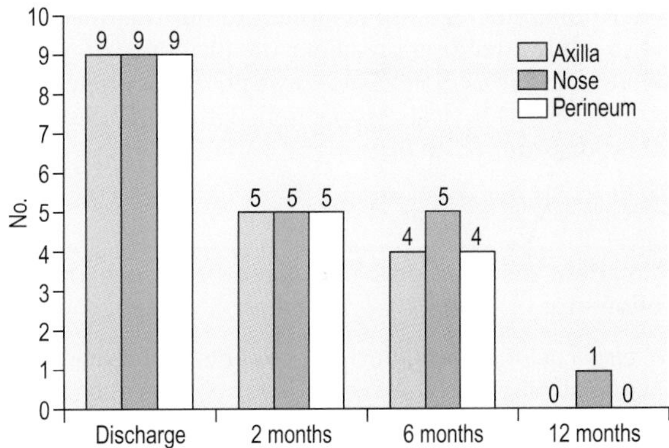

Figure 8.5 Colonisation with meticillin-resistant *Staphylococcus aureus* (MRSA).

SKIN

Patients complain of a variety of non-specific disorders, including hair loss and nail ridging. Severe pruritus used to be common and not amenable to treatment and was traced back to the use of high-molecular-weight starch solutions in ICU. Described in 2000,[15] in 85 cardiac surgical patients, pruritus was absent in the 26 patients who did not receive starch, but there was a 22% incidence in the 59 patients who did receive starch. This is now supposedly less of a problem with the newer starches.

Colonisation with MRSA used to be common after intensive care and often persisted for up to 9 months or longer (**Fig. 8.5**). It was common to hear that patients were being treated as 'lepers' by their own family.

SEXUAL DYSFUNCTION

Any patients who estimate their sex-life activity to be less active than before ICU admission are deemed to have sexual dysfunction.

In a group of 57 patients in one study[16] there was a 39% incidence of sexual dysfunction, although 4 patients' sex life had improved. Sexual dysfunction improves with time, from a frequency of about 26% at 2 months post-ICU down to 16% at 1 year.[17] Sexual dysfunction is often thought to be a psychological problem but, interestingly, following severe burns it has been reported that there is no correlation between the incidence of post-traumatic stress syndrome and sexual dysfunction.[18] Nevertheless, withdrawing sexual intimacy because of fear of failure can damage relationships. Often sexual dysfunction may go untreated because people are too embarrassed to mention the problem when they have recovered from a life-threatening illness.

Sexual dysfunction affects both men and women. In men it usually manifests itself as impotence or inability to maintain an erection sufficient for satisfactory sexual activity. For management guidelines for erectile dysfunction, see Ralph & McNicholas.[19]

In investigating sexual dysfunction, it is important to eliminate causes such as the use of drugs (e.g.L-dopa and H_2-blockers) and certain types of surgery (aortic aneurysm) or trauma/radiotherapy to the pelvic region. The patients may be diabetic.

Treatments available include intracavernous or transureteral alprostadil or oral Viagra. Patients with cardiovascular dysfunction have to be carefully assessed before being given Viagra. Non-pharmacological therapies include the use of vacuum devices and inflatable penile prostheses.

In females, sexual dysfunction may occur due to surgery or trauma to the pelvis. More commonly, there is a reduction in desire. Various lubricating gels can be used. As yet, the role of Viagra for women has to be determined. In 127 patients asked to fill in a questionnaire while attending the clinic, the incidence of sexual dysfunction was 45%.[20] There was no link with gender, but there was a close association with post-traumatic stress disorder (PTSD).

OTHER PHYSICAL PROBLEMS

A variety of other problems have been seen during follow-up:

- *visual acuity:* particularly in patients who have been profoundly hypotensive, visual problems may occur. Occasionally ischaemic changes may be seen on fundoscopy (**Fig. 8.6a**), which may be amenable to laser therapy (**Fig. 8.6b**)
- *facial scarring:* where the tape securing the endotracheal tube has been too tight; this scarring can affect the whole thickness of the cheek
- *unneccessary medication:* frequently medication started in ICU as a temporary measure may have been continued (e.g. amiodarone started for sepsis-related arrhythmias).

PSYCHOLOGICAL PROBLEMS

Most patients admitted to ICU have no warning of their admission (emergency admission) and these are the patients who are very much at risk of psychological sequelae post-ICU.

The majority of patients do not have a structured memory of their ICU stay. Those who do may have upsetting memories, which may be relatively innocuous, such as being thirsty and hearing a can of Coke being opened, or of a far more profound nature.

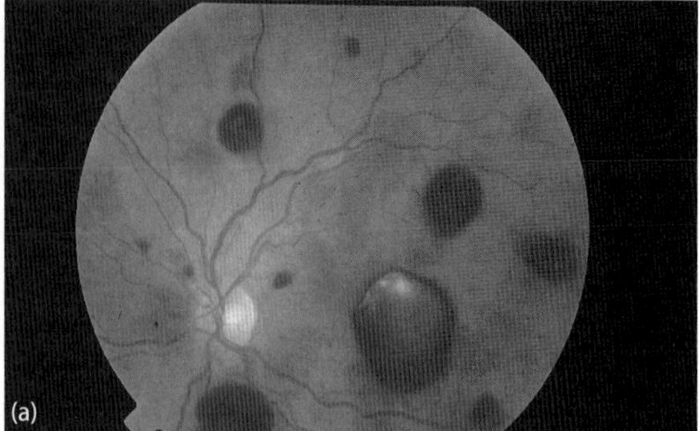

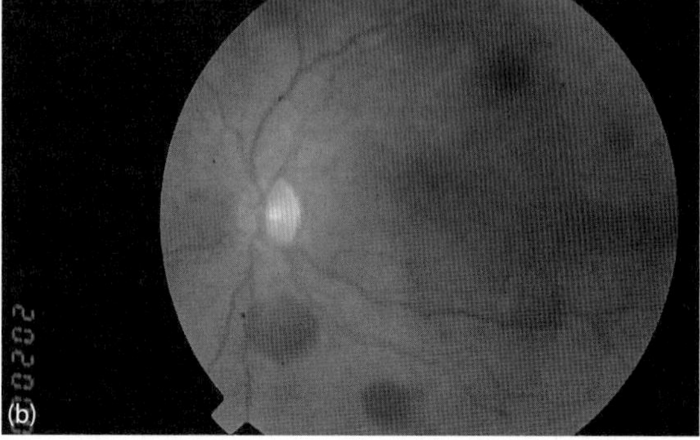

Figure 8.6 (a, b) Ischaemic changes in fundoscopy.

The story of 'torture' experiences is not unusual when you talk to an ex-ICU patient. The psychological impact of the experience may be formidable and may be resented by the patient. The memory of hearing that a patient is about to be 'bagged' was interpreted as being put into a body bag rather than a physiotherapy manoeuvre and the use of a tape measure was interpreted as being measured for a coffin and not as part of the cardiac output measurements. Previous studies demonstrate a high incidence of anxiety, depression and post-traumatic stress.[21] It is common for patients to have memories of being trapped, of being unable to move easily, of being unable to see what is happening and of feeling intensely vulnerable. The anxiety of impending death is also reported.

Below is a typical nightmare of one of our patients:

> *I was in a tunnel knee-deep in mud. It was pitch black, but I could see light at the end. I felt a cold chill on my neck as if someone was breathing down my neck. I thought it was the grim reaper, I knew I had to get to the light.*

There may be several reasons for these experiences (**Box 8.2**). There is a common belief that, when on ICU, it is better that a patient does not remember anything. However, it is increasingly realised that false memories or delusions during an ICU stay can have a significant impact on psychological recovery after ICU[22] whereas factual memories of ICU may reduce anxiety.[23]

Box 8.2 Psychological problems

Illness
Sedation technique
Withdrawal
No communication aids
Lack of clear night/day
Continuous noise of alarms
Sleep disturbance – lack of rapid-eye-movement sleep

It now seems likely that delusional memories of ICU and nightmares are associated with post-traumatic stress disorder (PTSD). PTSD is a normal reaction to severe stress and is similar to a grief reaction to bereavement. It occurs in about 1% of the population and increases to 10% in victims of road traffic accidents and 65% in prisoners of war. About 15% of patients have the typical disorder post-ICU. In those with adult respiratory distress syndrome, the incidence increases to 27.5%.

PTSD is the development of characteristic symptoms after being subjected to a traumatic event. PTSD can be triggered by any memory or mention of something to do with the traumatic event and is characterised by intrusive recollections, avoidance behaviour and hyperarousal symptoms.[24]

There is no doubt that a graded exercise programme is of benefit to aid physical recovery in such ICU patients.[14] Drugs such as fluoxetime (Prozac) do not seem to benefit such patients, even though there is a great temptation to use antidepressants in these patients.[25]

Various strategies to deal with the psychological sequelae of ICU stay have been tried.

- *During ICU stay:* There is no doubt that continuous intravenous sedation has been identified as an independent predictor of a longer duration of mechanical ventilation, ICU stay and total hospital stay.[26] Kreiss et al[27] demonstrated that, in 128 adults, ICU stay was reduced from an average of 7.3 to 4.9 days by the daily interruption of the sedative regimen. This regimen may have had an impact by reducing PTSD as the patients are more likely to have some recollection of their ICU stay, thus helping them to understand the reasons for the need for their prolonged rehabilitation period. However, a recent article[28] demonstrated no difference in length of stay with protocolised sedation with or without daily interruption of sedation. Concerns have been raised as to the type of sedative agent used in ICU. It is well known that etomidate may cause an excess in mortality in trauma patients in ICU[29] and propofol may do the same in head-injured patients at doses greater than 5 mg/kg per hour.[30] The decision to use benzodiazepines such as midazolam increasingly may be associated with dependence. This has been studied; 21 out of 148 ICU patients were discharged home on oral benzodiazepine, of whom 10 were still taking them at 6 months post-discharge having not been on them pre-ICU.[31] Lorazepam has been promoted as the benzodiazepine of choice for sedation in ICU[32] and was preferred by a task force in the USA for adult patients in ICU.[33] More recently, however, Panharipande et al have found a dose-dependent increase in delirium with the use of lorazepam.[34]

  The whole concept of delirium in patients including those who are critically ill has now been reviewed and monitoring and management of delirium is now published as a NICE guidance document.[35]
- *When building or modifying ICUs:* remember that windows and 24-hour clocks visible to patients may help re-establish circadian rhythms and the use of curtains to ensure patient dignity should not be forgotten. There has been some interest in appropriate colours that should be used in ICU décor, avoiding colours that cause alarm in the animal kingdom, such as red, yellow and black.

POST-ICU DISCHARGE

Visiting patients on the ward post ICU discharge and giving them an information booklet helps to prepare them better for the long rehabilitation process ahead.

As well as three ICU follow-up clinic appointments in the year after their discharge, patients with PTSD are encouraged to visit the ICU and, with the help of a diary, reconstruct the lost period of time in the patient's life. We are considering the use of photos of patients whilst they are on ICU to help them understand how ill they actually were.

CONCLUSION

It is important to assess patient satisfaction or dissatisfaction with their follow-up. This may be audited by questionnaire during their third visit to the follow-up clinic at 1-year post ICU discharge.[36]

In the UK, follow-up clinics were recommended by the Audit Commission in 1999 (Criticial to Success)[2] and in the Comprehensive Critical Care document in 2000,[3] yet only a small number of hospitals have been able to fund such a service. Griffiths et al[37] demonstrated that clinics are not widely established and show marked heterogeneity. Of those established, only two-thirds are funded and most do not have a prenegotiated access to other outpatient services. The PRaCTICaL study is, to date, the only evaluation of follow-up clinics that were nurse-led and did not demonstrate a cost-benefit analysis.[38] A similar study measuring the impact of a multidisciplinary clinic might come up with a different conclusion. The NICE 083 Guideline[39] has now been around for 3 years and has yet to be widely implemented. It requires a rehabilitation coordinator. Effective follow-up of patients after their critical illness may

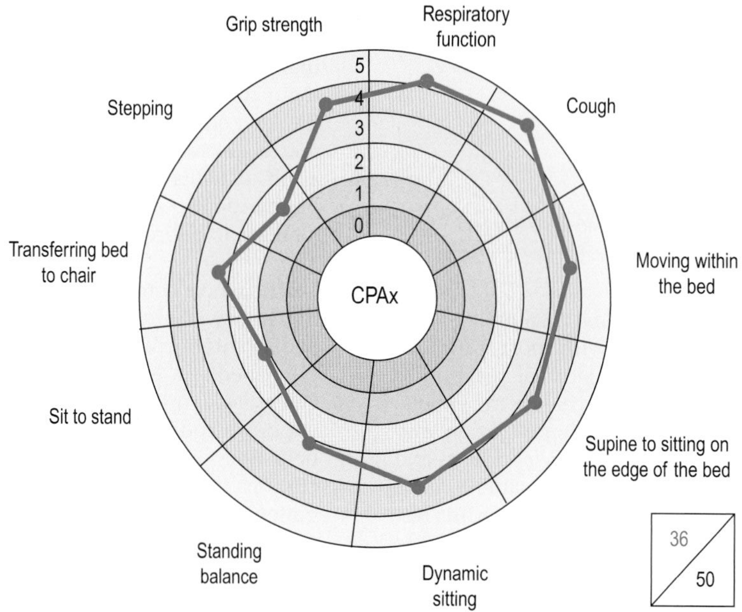

Figure 8.7 This radar chart is plotted to represent a patient's CPAx score. The image demonstrates that his respiratory function, cough and bed mobility are strong, but we can clearly see that his rehabilitation should be tailored to work on gait re-education, transferring from bed to chair and sit to stand. *(From Chelsea and Westminster NHS Foundation Trust (01/03/2010), with permission.)*

well be a future quality indicator of a hospital's critical care service. Meanwhile there is a massive increase in literature related to outcome following critical illness as health economists and intensivists try to make some sense out of the cost-effectiveness of intensive care.[40–43] Further studies are under way. The DiPEx study seeks to obtain a variety of patient and relative experiences of critical care (www.dipex.org). I-CANUK is a website that is being set up to provide a forum and voice for those involved in patient care following intensive care discharge and to support research into potential therapies following critical illness.

There have been few validated tools for the assessment of intensive-care-associated weakness, but recently the Chelsea Critical Care Physical Assessment tool (CPAx) has been developed.[44] The CPAx is a numerical and pictorial scoring system, based on a composite of ten commonly assessed components of physical function, as well as grip strength, measured as a percentage of those predicted for age and gender (**Table 8.2** and **Fig. 8.7**). Each component is graded on a six-point Guttman scale from complete dependence to independence, giving an overall score out of 50. The CPAx is completed daily by the physiotherapist and the score is plotted on a radar chart at the patient's bedside. Progress can be monitored as a daily trend, which lends itself well to the fluctuating status of the critically ill patient.

Preliminary work suggests that the CPAx is a valid measure that can be administered consistently between therapists. In an ongoing project, unpublished data of 314 patients also suggest predictive validity for hospital discharge location. Empirically, it appears to be a useful tool for motivating patients in rehabilitation and for communication with patients and relatives. It is hopeful that following full evaluation of the CPAx, it could be implemented as a universal method for monitoring progress during and after critical illness. Further results of this project will be published in 2013.

Lastly, much work needs to be done to provide an evidence base for the impact of critical care on carers and relatives. The King's College London and the King's Fund have tested the use of patient experience interviews using experience-based co-design (EBCD).[45] In EBCD, trained interviewers interview local patients and staff over several months, and then use edited films of the patient interviews to stimulate work between patients and staff to redesign services.

In a recent modification of the EBCD known as AEBCD (accelerated experience-based co-design) edited films are being produced not from local interviews but from an existing archive of patient interviews held by the University of Oxford, potentially saving several months of work and staff time. Films of patients talking about their experiences of two different conditions (intensive care and lung cancer) are being used in close partnership with patients, relatives and staff in two different hospital trusts (Royal Brompton and Harefield and Royal Berkshire) to help them together plan and implement improvements in care. The approach is being tested in a National Institute for Health Research study (HS&DR 10/1009/14); results of this project should be available in 2013.[46]

Table 8.2 The Chelsea Critical Care Physical Assessment tool (CPAx)

ASPECT OF PHYSICALITY	LEVEL 0	LEVEL 1	LEVEL 2	LEVEL 3	LEVEL 4	LEVEL 5
Respiratory function	Complete ventilator dependence Mandatory breaths only May be fully sedated/paralysed	Ventilator dependence Mandatory breaths with some spontaneous effort	Spontaneously breathing with continuous invasive or non-invasive ventilatory support	Spontaneously breathing with intermittent invasive or non-invasive ventilatory support Or continuous high-flow oxygen (>15 L)	Receiving standard oxygen therapy (<15 L)	Self-ventilating with no oxygen therapy
Cough	Absent cough, may be fully sedated or paralysed	Cough stimulated on deep suctioning only	Weak ineffective voluntary cough, unable to clear independently (e.g. requires deep suction)	Weak, partially effective voluntary cough, sometimes able to clear secretions (e.g. requires yanker suctioning)	Effective cough, clearing secretions with airways clearance techniques	Consistent effective voluntary cough, clearing secretions independently
Moving within the bed (e.g. rolling)	Unable, maybe fully sedated/paralysed	Initiates movement Requires assistance ≥2 people (maximal)	Initiates movement Requires assistance ≥1 person (moderate)	Initiates movement Requires assistance 1 person (minimal)	Independent in ≥3 seconds	Independent in <3 seconds
Supine to sitting on the edge of the bed	Unable/unstable	Initiates movement. Requires assistance ≥2 people (maximal)	Initiates movement. Requires assistance ≥1 person (moderate)	Initiates movement. Requires assistance 1 person (minimal)	Independent in ≥3 seconds	Independent in <3 seconds
Dynamic sitting (i.e. when sitting on the edge of the bed/unsupported sitting)	Unable/unstable	Requires assistance ≥2 people (maximal)	Requires assistance ≥1 person (moderate)	Requires assistance 1 person (minimal)	Independent with some dynamic sitting balance (i.e. able to alter trunk position within base of support)	Independent with full dynamic sitting balance (i.e. able to reach out of base of support)
Standing balance	Unable/unstable/bedbound	Tilt table or similar	Standing hoist or similar	Dependent on frame, crutches or similar	Independent without aides	Independent without aids and full dynamic standing balance (i.e. able to reach out of base of support)
Sit to stand (starting position: ≤90° hip flexion)	Unable/unstable	Sit to stand with maximal assistance (e.g. standing hoist or similar)	Sit to stand with moderate assistance (e.g. 1–2 people)	Sit to stand with minimal assistance (e.g. 1 person)	Sit to stand independently pushing through arms of the chair	Sit to stand independently without upper limb involvement
Transferring from bed to chair	Unable/unstable	Full hoist	Standing hoist or similar	Pivot transfer (no stepping) with mobility aid or physical assistance	Stand and step transfer with mobility aid *or* physical assistance	Independent transfer without equipment
Stepping	Unable/unstable	Using a standing hoist, or similar	Using mobility aids *and* assistance >1 person (moderate)	Using mobility aid *and* assistance 1 person (minimal)	Using mobility aid *or* assistance 1 person (minimal)	Independent without aid
Grip strength (predicted mean for age and gender on the strongest hand)	Unable to assess	<20%	<40%	<60%	<80%	≥80%

Access the complete references list online at http://www.expertconsult.com

14. Jones C, Skirrow P, Griffith RD. Rehabilitation after critical illness, a randomised controlled trial. Crit Care Med 2003;31:2456–61.
34. Panharipande P, Shintani A, Peterson J, et al. Lorazepam is an independent risk factor for transitioning to delirium in intensive care unit patients. Anesthesiology 2006;104(1):21–6.
35. NICE Delirium guidelines. 2010. Online. Available: http://guidance.nice.org.uk/CG103.
37. Griffiths JA, Barber VS, Cuthbertson BH, et al. A national survey of intensive care follow up clinics. Anaesthesia 2006;61:950–5.
38. Cuthbertson BH, Rattray J, Campbell MF, et al. The PRaCTICaL study of a nurse led, intensive care follow-up programme for improving long term outcomes from critical illness: a pragmatic randomised controlled trial. BMJ 2009;339:b3723.
39. NICE 083 Rehabilitation after critical illness. 2009. Online. Available: http://www.nice.org.uk/nicemedia/pdf/CG083NICEGuideline.pdf.
44. Corner EJ, Wood H, Englebretsen C, et al. The Chelsea Critical Care Physical Assessment Tool (CPAx): validation of an innovative new tool to measure physical morbidity in the general adult critical care population; an observational proof-of-concept pilot study. Physiotherapy 2013;99(1):33–41.

9 Clinical information systems

David Fraenkel

Clinical record keeping requires an integrated system to manage the information, including its acquisition during clinical care, and archiving and availability for future clinical, business and research uses.

The term 'clinical information systems' (CIS) refers to computerised systems for managing the clinical record, often within specialised areas of a hospital, such as intensive care, emergency medicine, operating theatres or cardiology. CIS for intensive care units (ICUs) have been developing since the late 1980s; however, their implementation has been limited by cost, functionality and clinician acceptance.[1–9]

The electronic medical record (EMR) and electronic health care records (EHR) embrace respective hospital and community-wide electronic systems for managing patient records, which may be integrated with the more specialised CIS. Over the next decade we can expect to see EHR implementation throughout the health systems of the more developed nations. The driving incentive is community concern for safety and quality in health care and the EHR is the single most powerful measure to produce a safer, more effective and efficient health care system.[1,2,9]

In 2002 the National Health Service (NHS) in the UK embarked on an ambitious National Programme for Information Technology (NPfIT) featuring a national summary care record (SCR) or 'spine' to hold limited essential information on each consenting patient. Additional features included picture archiving and communication systems (PACS), more detailed data held on integrated local computer systems, electronic prescribing and computerised physician order entry (CPOE).[4] NPfIT was described as the largest ever IT project and organisational change in the largest global organisation. Not surprisingly it has encountered major difficulties and deficiencies, with some suggesting it was the largest ever civil IT project disaster, leading towards a more localised and modest set of objectives.[5]

The US government has placed a high priority on electronic health records.[1,2,9] The US implementation rate of EMR and CIS is one of the highest in the world as a result of these quality, governance and financial incentives. However, as would be expected from the heterogeneous nature of the health care system, the capacity for transferring patient records and data sharing is restricted by the lack of common standards.[8,9] Some of the European nations have the most complete roll-out of EMR and CIS, although variations in systems and standards also produce similar challenges.

In Australia, the HealthConnect strategy has been largely focused on broadband connections for primary health care providers and establishing data dictionaries and standards, with limited strategies or funding for actual implementation of EHRs. Efforts to establish EHRs and EMRs have been hindered by the difficulties of establishing a national unique patient identifier. Meanwhile there has been a slow increase in ICU-CIS with some attempts at a regional approach.

The current best examples of effective national strategies are provided by Canada and New Zealand. They have worked to establish common minimal standards, rather than being overly inclusive, and required vendors to comply. Implementation has been focused on incremental and iterative change on a more regional basis, with smaller projects and clinical inclusiveness.

FUNCTIONS AND ADVANTAGES OF CIS

CIS seek to deliver several key benefits (**Box 9.1**).[1] These include the automation of repetitive manual tasks, improved accuracy through reductions in human error, attributable records simultaneously available from multiple points of care and integration with other bedside equipment and information systems. The built-in error checking and knowledge-based systems should also provide a safer and higher-quality clinical process. The CIS electronically capture the data and make this information potentially available to a multitude of systems. This obviates the need for repetitive manual data entry or transcription, while making the data accessible for a range of purposes that may include clinical, business and research reporting.

The ICU is already a technology-rich environment, where bedside devices process and provide data elements in electronic format. Similarly, many clinical measurements are available on monitors, ventilators and pumps. Traditionally, these electronically derived values are transcribed onto observation charts and paper-based clinical records, as are repetitive clinical observations and arithmetic calculations, which are often performed manually or with the aid of a

Box 9.1 Clinical information systems (CIS) benefits

1. Recording of bedside observations
   a. Automation of physiological data collection
   b. Reduction in transcription and arithmetic errors
   c. Downloading from bedside therapeutic devices (e.g. pumps, ventilators)
2. Clinical documentation
   a. Legible and attributable clinical record
   b. Structures and cues encourage comprehensive documentation
   c. Electronic record of drug prescription and administration
   d. Attributable record simultaneously available from multiple points of care
3. Access to additional clinical information at the bedside
   a. Pathology results
   b. Digitised medical imaging and reports
   c. Digital clinical photographs
   d. Other hospital systems (e.g. admission/discharge/transfer (ADT), CIS)
4. Bedside decision support systems
   a. Passive
      (i) Improved and accessible clinical record
      (ii) Online clinical policies and procedures
      (iii) Online knowledge bases
      (iv) Online literature searches
   b. Active
      (i) Investigative and therapeutic management algorithms
      (ii) Clinical pathways
      (iii) Drug allergy and interaction alerts
      (iv) Drug dosing and monitoring support
      (v) Antibiotic selection and prescribing
      (vi) Ventilation and haemodynamic management systems
5. Medicolegal archiving
   a. Audit trail for all changes during episode of care
   b. No ability to change once archived
   c. Secure long-term storage and ensured availability
6. Clinical database
   a. Long-term accessible storage of relevant clinical data
   b. Industry-standard database format
   c. Efficient and flexible query and reporting solutions
   d. Scheduled and ad hoc reports
   e. Clinical, research and management requirements

calculator. The voluminous observation charts present a challenge for both storage and access, and transcription errors and arithmetic errors are prolific in these paper systems.

The CIS automates the process of electronic data collection from monitors, ventilators, infusion pumps, dialysis/filtration equipment, cardiac assist devices and other bedside devices and provides a real-time spreadsheet with arithmetic accuracy. Incorporation of clinical documentation and progress notes provides a legible and attributable record of events.

The patient record can then be accessed from geographically distant workstations in the ICU, the hospital, and even from other more remote sites. As long as the system is running, the record is easy to locate and always available.

A major contribution of CIS to clinical safety and quality is through the provision of an electronic prescribing and administration record for drugs and fluids. Errors in prescription and administration are a leading cause of adverse events with associated morbidity.[1,2] CIS ensure legibility, attribution and completeness of administration and prescribing. However, more active forms of decision support such as dose modification for organ failure, preventing prescription in allergy and identifying important drug–drug interactions are not standardised and require further development.[6–9]

ARCHITECTURE AND COMPONENTS OF CIS

BASIC CIS ARCHITECTURE

All CIS share certain basic components consisting of workstations, a network and central servers (**Fig. 9.1**). The user interface is presented at the workstation, which is usually at each bedside but may also be in nearby central and administrative areas, such as the nurses' station, or more distant in the offices of clinical or administrative staff. Workstations commonly consist of relatively standard personal computer (PC) hardware being desk, pendant or trolley mounted, but may include laptops or personal digital assistants (PDAs) with wireless systems where technical challenges related to speed and reliability of data transmission can be overcome.

Most CIS allow other applications, such as PACS, word processing or email, to be run on the same PC, but this is potentially a rich source of system conflicts and requires careful administration.

Workstations are linked to each other and a centralised set of servers through a network of communication cables. Hubs, switches and routers control network traffic. A dedicated network, either actual or virtual, enhances system performance, but it is important to ensure built-in redundancy in network loops and power sources to minimise potential interruptions from physical disruption or component failure.

The configuration of computer servers varies widely and the best solutions may depend upon organisational IT architecture. Locally installed servers are becoming less common, whereas centralised and physically remote servers still offer technical challenges but some advantages in support.

CIS usually require a separate workstation or server to manage the interfaces with other systems. These include hospital demographics (ADT systems for admission/discharge/transfer), pathology laboratory, pharmacy, radiology and hospital finance. Interfacing requires a software platform known as an interface

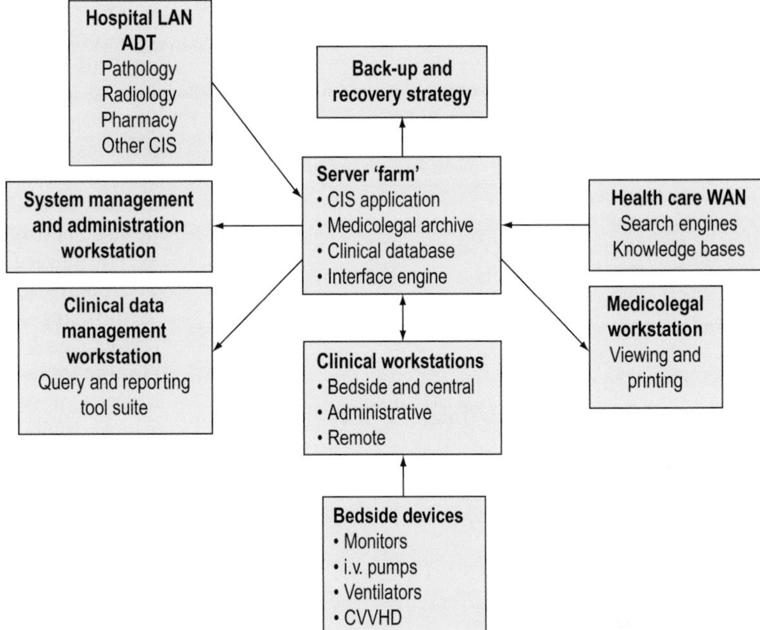

Figure 9.1 Clinical information systems (CIS) architecture. LAN, local area network; WAN, wide area network; ADT, admission/discharge/transfer; CVVHD, continuous venovenous haemodialysis.

engine. Additional software identifies the relevant data and directs and processes these data to the correct field in the appropriate format. Due to the huge variety of current and legacy systems, this process almost always requires custom-written code and programming, representing one of the major risks and expenses of systems integration.[4,5]

Bedside monitoring systems usually include a central station or server that can be linked with the CIS servers to transfer their downloaded information back to the bedside. Transferring data from other bedside devices is usually achieved by a cable connection from the device to a bedside concentrator in the patient bay. The connection requires an electronic decoder, which is specific to the manufacturer and model of the device. The decoder must then communicate with the central servers via a subsidiary server that provides the software translator to complete the interface. A selection of established interfaces to commonly utilised equipment exists, but often additional customised interfaces must be written.

MEDICOLEGAL STORAGE

Electronic data capture does not necessarily result in long-term electronic data storage. Many CIS sites have continued to require the printing out of all reports from the patient episode to store in the paper-based hospital medical record, although this is increasingly because of local politicolegal requirements rather than technical limitations. Modern servers have extensive and expandable storage capacity, albeit this can be rapidly consumed by the equally enormous amount of data being collected from every patient. When the choice of storage solution is made, it is equally important to be aware that the format of data storage is determined by the anticipated use of the data and to ensure that future software upgrades do not render the stored data unreadable.

Data archiving for medicolegal purposes requires that the clinical information be readily accessible and preferably presented in exactly the same format as it was recorded and reviewed by the clinicians during the episode of patient care. Any changes to the clinical record during the patient episode must be clearly displayed and attributable – this is known as an audit trail or change history. An audit trail is a standard feature of most CIS and actually offers improved accountability over paper-based systems. It may be desirable to make it impossible to alter the record after the patient episode, which requires specialised storage formats or strict access restrictions to the data archive.

Once the record is stored, by whatever method, it must be protected from accidental loss. This usually requires a carefully engineered and documented management plan with regular scheduled back-ups, off-site storage of duplicates and robust recovery strategies. When these requirements are fulfilled, the electronic medicolegal archive can readily exceed the performance of a paper-based record through its assured availability and authenticity.

CLINICAL DATABASE STORAGE

A major objective of CIS is to provide a comprehensive clinical database that will accumulate data in real time

Box 9.2 Clinical information systems (CIS) implementation

1. Professional project management
   a. Structured multidisciplinary team
      (i) Sponsor, director, manager, representatives
      (ii) Medical, nursing, allied health, managerial
   b. Comprehensive documentation
   c. Consultative approach
      (i) Medical records department
      (ii) IT/IM department
      (iii) Hospital and business managers
2. Project framework
   a. Needs analysis
   b. Definition of scope
   c. Management of expectation and scope creep
3. Tender evaluation (see Box 9.3)
4. Implementation process
   a. Implementation plan and schedule
   b. Training
   c. Installation
   d. Schedule of payments
   e. Quality monitoring of process
5. Postimplementation review
   a. Actual outcomes of plan
   b. Unresolved issues
   c. Process improvement
6. System management plan
   a. Identification of system components
   b. Departmental and individual roles and responsibilities
   c. Identification of vendor responsibilities
   d. Back-up schedules and recovery plans
7. Support contracts
   a. Scope and level of support
   b. Pricing
8. Future issues
   a. Ongoing management of 'special projects'
   b. Continued development and innovation
   c. System upgrades
   d. Scheduled hardware replacement
   e. System obsolescence and replacement

that can be stored and queried for a wide range of reports for a variety of purposes. The relevant data need to be held in an accessible and readily searchable database that will allow a variety of sophisticated reports to be prepared on both a scheduled and an ad hoc basis. These requirements are quite different from those of medicolegal storage and usually require a separate form of data storage, commonly known as a clinical database, data repository, data warehouse or data management solution.

There may be a requirement to adopt a significantly different database structure from the core CIS database, which may have been designed with prospective user configurability in mind, rather than allowing easy location of data fields in a structure designed for rapidly processing queries. The design of the clinical database is a compromise between saving effectively the large amount of data collected while maintaining speed and ease of use in running queries. Even when the vendor has utilised an industry-standard database application, such as Oracle or SQL, in the core CIS application designing and running queries may still present a challenging specialist task because of the complexity of the table structure or the huge amount of aggregated data.

The clinical data management solutions currently offered are quite diverse. One solution simply provides an industry-standard data transfer protocol (e.g. 'ODBC driver') as a means of accessing the data. The local circumstances of each hospital then dictate customised queries or secondary database designs for local use. Alternatively, an industry-standard query tool is used to generate reports from the core CIS database, but the number of queries that can be designed and preconfigured in this fashion is often limited, particularly as the user configurations of the CIS vary widely. There is inevitably a compromise between standardisation and flexibility. Data fields must be standardised in the configuration of the CIS to allow standard queries to be performed. Some CIS solutions offer a proprietary subsidiary database containing selected clinical data with a wider range of reports preconfigured into the query tool.

EVALUATION AND IMPLEMENTATION OF CIS

Clinicians always underestimate the managerial requirements, human resource demands and opportunity costs of CIS implementation.[1-5] The process should be viewed as a major project requiring advanced planning and management skills (**Box 9.2**). A single site project may take 1–2 years, and a multisite or regional project 2–5 years. The project team must be multidisciplinary, consult widely and consider workplace flows and processes, or else a suboptimal result is guaranteed.[4-8] The CIS will impact on medical, nursing, allied health, managerial and technical staff within the ICU, together with those from other clinical disciplines. Involvement of hospital information management staff is essential. Extensive documentation and continued scheduled reviews are required throughout the process.

Business case development to secure funding is always problematic and may be assisted by the quality benefits of CIS implementation.[3] The most basic system can be expected to cost in the order of AUD $25 000–50 000 per bed, while more advanced systems may be two to three times that cost. Annual recurrent costs are significant and usually exceed 20% of the capital cost of the system.

The CIS industry is subject to the same vagaries as other parts of the IT industry, including high turnover of personnel and frequent inability to deliver on promised functionality and timelines. CIS selection is best conducted as a formal tender process, and the

Box 9.3 Clinical information systems (CIS) evaluation

1. Vendor characteristics
   a. Monitoring of software experience
   b. Niche specialty products, cf. health care-wide
   c. Development base by specialty and geography
2. Preliminary evaluation
   a. Evaluate tender documents
   b. Product demonstration
   c. Prepared and impromptu scenario testing of product
   d. Ensure all required components identified, e.g. database, interfaces, etc.
   e. Comparative levels of best fit for needs and specifications
3. Site visits to installed customer base
   a. Reference sites and 'sites like us'
   b. Demonstrations with vendor
   c. Candid visits without vendor
   d. Observe functionality
   e. Examine interfaces
   f. Explore support issues
4. Interfaces
   a. Identify requirements
   b. Assess vendor capabilities
   c. Inspect working interfaces
   d. Customisation scope and cost
5. Technical issues
   a. Industry-standard hardware and software
   b. Local acceptability
   c. Integration with existing systems
   d. Upgrade paths
   e. Network specifications
   f. Network costs and management
6. Support issues
   a. Location and availability
   b. Product support specialists
   c. Technical engineers
   d. Level of risk sharing
   e. Whole-of-life costing

evaluation of submissions is a complex task (**Box 9.3**). Availability and expense of on-site support during and following implementation are also critical factors.

Implementation planning should be detailed and requires a full-time project officer on site. A standard implementation for a single site needs 4–6 months prior to the 'go live' date with hospital-wide consultation, issue management and carefully scheduled staff training. Multisite and regional implementations may shorten individual implementation times, but require sophisticated management that still allows for site-specific issues. It is desirable to have as many as possible of the interfaces and bedside devices linked to the CIS at the implementation date. This will maximise perceived benefits early and thereby encourage acceptance of the system. It should be implemented through the whole ICU as partial implementations are rarely successful.

Post-implementation review is essential to progress outstanding issues, which are usually prolific, and help establish the arrangements for the support and continued development of the system. A system management plan identifies the responsibility centres for management of the CIS components and clarifies requirements and expectations. A permanent on-site system management position is required for system maintenance, progressing outstanding issues and managing future upgrades and developments.

BENEFITS OF CIS: THE STATE OF THE ART

Basic CIS requirements are fulfilled by the majority of systems currently available:

- Charting, including tabulation of bedside observations and measurements such as fluid balance – the flow sheets are usually more than adequately flexible and configurable to meet local requirements.
- Bedside device interfaces – new devices may not have the necessary decoders and software. The expense of developing new interfaces can be considerable when calculated on a per-bed basis.
- Clinical progress notes – these are adequate but the free text may not be 'searchable', and structured text may be only marginally better.
- Keyboard skills are increasingly widespread, but may still be an issue with some clinicians.
- Drug and fluid prescription and administration are good, but not always incorporated in some systems, necessitating a separate system.

Decision support systems have previously been disappointing but their further development offers substantial benefits.[3,6–9] A legible and available record of previous and ongoing care does offer an improved level of decision support, albeit one that the general community would already expect and see as mandatory. Passive decision support with access to knowledge-based systems through CIS and hospital intranets, as well as resources such as pharmacopoeia, literature search engines and online texts and journals, is widely available. It is intuitive that these resources would improve the quality of clinical outcomes; but there is little evidence to support this.

Active decision support has not been generally available, including the flagging of drug allergies and interactions and the integration of relevant information, such as baseline renal function, recent urine output, last-measured creatinine and required dose of aminoglycoside.[3,6–9] Decision support systems to recommend antimicrobial prescribing, ventilatory therapy or haemodynamic measurement have been developed in dedicated centres of excellence, but are also not generally available, nor are they necessarily able to be migrated successfully across boundaries of international practice. The provision of prompts has been shown to be effective for routine prophylaxis and care processes, supported by clinical pathways and guidelines.

Computerised physician order entry (CPOE) is exemplified in electronic prescribing, but its benefits extend to other areas such as pathology and radiology orders and results viewing. There is good evidence that a reduction in ordering occurs through reduced duplication and timeliness and access to results. The availability of CPOE varies with the level of systems integration and compatibility with other legacy and proprietary computer systems.[3,4,6–9] Standardised communications protocols (e.g. HL-7) are helpful but provide only similarities of electronic language. High-level interfaces require continued maintenance and development and therefore expenditure. Clinical databases remain a significant challenge, whether at a local departmental, hospital, regional or national level. Although many products are purported to include data management and query solutions, those that are available 'off the shelf' may be quite rudimentary and their development may require additional expenditure and a major commitment from the clinical staff. Part of the problem is the need for clinicians to define prospectively what is expected of the system. This requires exhaustive definition of the questions that the system should be able to answer and therefore also specification of the detailed nature of the data and queries that will be required.

Accurate analysis of diagnoses and procedures requires that key information is entered correctly and consistently and that reliable and high-quality data capture is achieved. Data entry should be 'once-only', simple and robust, and should be easily performed as the clinical scenario unfolds. There is very limited agreement and standardisation between clinicians with respect to mandatory data fields, diagnostic criteria and classifications. Standardised reports are therefore difficult to develop in different clinical environments, let alone regions or countries. The eventual adoption of common international standards and classifications (e.g. SNOMED for diagnoses, National Library of Medicines for pharmaceuticals) would greatly facilitate solution design and querying.[4] Other issues, including the speed of data access in huge data repositories, the development of unique patient/episode identifiers and privacy considerations, are still significant.[4–9]

FUTURE DEVELOPMENTS

Over the next decade CIS and the EHR should provide the most significant and comprehensive improvement in the delivery of health care in developed nations. It is difficult to justify continuing with archaic methods of record keeping, which are no longer adequate in almost all other professional, commercial, regulatory and day-to-day activities. Although financial obstacles may seem significant, the human resources and project management required for successful CIS planning and implementation are the most difficult to achieve. Clinical involvement throughout is mandatory. Prospective and cohesive clinician agreement on the identity and method of capture of data elements, together with configuration and reporting requirements, is essential. CIS implementation is not merely a technical process. Changes in work processes and cultural practices will be required, and offer some of the greatest challenges and opportunities to achieve the expected benefits.

Access the complete references list online at http://www.expertconsult.com

1. Bates DW, Gawande AA. Improving safety with information technology. N Engl J Med 2003;348: 2526–34.
2. Leape LL, Berwick DM. Five years after To Err Is Human: what have we learned? JAMA 2005;293: 2384–90.
3. Frisse ME. Comments on return on investment (ROI) as it applies to clinical systems. J Am Med Inform Assoc 2006;13:365–7.
4. Tackley R. Integrating anaesthesia and intensive care into the national care record. Br J Anaesth 2006;97: 69–76.
5. Cross M. There IT goes again. BMJ 2011;343:d5317.
6. Gross PA, Bates DW. A pragmatic approach to implementing best practices for clinical decision support systems in computerized provider order entry systems. J Am Med Inform Assoc 2007;14: 25–8.
7. Mack EH, Wheeler DS, Embi PJ. Clinical decision support systems in the paediatric intensive care unit. Paediatr Crit Care Med 2009;10:23–8.
8. Maslove DM, Rizk N, Lowe HJ. Computerised physician order entry in the critical care environment: A review of the current literature. J Intensive Care Med 2011;26:165–71.
9. Classen D, Bates DW, Denham CR. Meaningful use of computerised prescriber order entry. J Patient Saf 2010;6:15–23.

10

Clinical trials in critical care

Simon Finfer and Anthony Delaney

> *Evidence based medicine is the conscientious, explicit, and judicious use of current best evidence in making decisions about the care of individual patients. The practice of evidence based medicine means integrating individual clinical expertise with the best available external clinical evidence from systematic research.*[1]

The most reliable evidence, and thus the best evidence for guiding clinical practice will generally come from adequately powered and properly conducted randomised clinical trials (RCTs). It is commonly the case, however, that there are no individual RCTs that adequately address a particular question, and so clinicians may have to assess the ability of other studies such as cohort studies, case–control studies and systematic reviews to supplement their clinical expertise. It is important that clinicians are familiar with the underlying principles and potential sources of bias in each of these study designs, so that they can incorporate evidence from reliable trials into their clinical practice and treat with appropriate caution those studies whose design makes it likely that they will produce unreliable results.

RANDOMISED CLINICAL TRIALS

The result of any clinical trial may be due to three factors: a true treatment effect, the effects of bias or confounding, or the play of chance. Randomised clinical trials, when properly designed, conducted and analysed, offer the optimal conditions to minimise bias and confounding, and to define the role that chance may have played in the results. As such, they represent the best study design to delineate true treatment effects under most circumstances. However, it is imperative that RCTs are designed, conducted, analysed and reported correctly. Studies that have not adhered to the principles outlined below may produce results that do not reflect a true estimate of treatment effects.

THE QUESTION TO BE ADDRESSED

Every trial should seek to answer a focused clinical question that can be clearly articulated at the outset. For example, 'we sought to assess the influence of different volume replacement fluids on outcomes of intensive care patients', is better expressed as the focused clinical question; 'we sought to address the hypothesis that when 4% albumin is compared with 0.9% sodium chloride (normal saline) for intravascular fluid resuscitation in adult patients in the ICU, there is no difference in the rate of death from any cause at 28 days'.[2] The focused clinical question defines the interventions to be compared, the population to be studied and the primary outcome to be considered. This approach can be formalised using the PICO system: PICO stands for Patient, Intervention, Comparison, and Outcome. In the example above:

- Patient=adult ICU patient
- Intervention=albumin
- Comparison=saline
- Outcome=28-day all-cause mortality.

The question that a trial is designed to address will vary somewhat depending on the stage of development of the proposed treatment. After development and testing in animal models, the testing of pharmaceutical agents in humans is generally conducted in three phases. Sometimes a fourth phase is added:

1. Phase I trial: testing in healthy volunteers
2. Phase II trial: first testing in population of patients with disease to be modified, usually small trials focused on establishing safety and evidence of efficacy using surrogate outcome measures. Phase II trials provide an estimate of treatment effect and baseline outcomes which can be used to calculate the sample size for phase III trials
3. Phase III: large-scale trial in patients that has sufficient statistical power to determine the effect of the treatment on the primary outcome
4. Phase IV: post-marketing open-label trials to confirm efficacy and safety once the agent is introduced into clinical practice.

Trials may be designed to answer two quite different questions about the same treatment and the design will be quite different depending on the questions to be answered. An 'efficacy trial' seeks to determine whether a treatment will work under optimal conditions, whereas an 'effectiveness' trial seeks to determine the effects of the intervention when applied in normal clinical practice. A comparison of the features of efficacy and effectiveness trials is given in **Table 10.1** from Hébert et al.[3]

Table 10.1 Comparison of study characteristics using either an efficacy or an effectiveness approach when designing a study

STUDY CHARACTERISTICS	EFFICACY TRIAL	EFFECTIVENESS TRIAL
Research question	Will the intervention work under ideal conditions?	Will the intervention result in more good than harm under usual practice conditions?
Setting	Restricted to specialised centres	Open to all institutions
Patient selection	Selected, well-defined patients	A wide range of patients identified using broad eligibility criteria
Study design	Smaller RCT using parallel group or factorial or other approaches (crossover design)	Large multicentre RCT using parallel groups, or factorial cluster
Baseline assessment	Elaborate and detailed	Simple and clinician-friendly
Study intervention	Tightly protocolised. Optimal therapy under optimal conditions	Less tightly protocolised. Implemented in usual clinical practice
Co-interventions	Tightly controlled protocols for many aspects of care	All therapy based on local practice/ experience/minimal control
Compliance	Compliance essential	Non-compliance expected and considered in sample size/analysis
End-points	Disease-related. Related to biological effect 'Surrogate' end-points	Patient-related such as all-cause mortality or quality of life
Analysis	By treatment received	Intention to treat
Sample size	Generally <1000 and often <100 patients	Several thousand patients
DATA MANAGEMENT		
Data collection	Elaborate	Minimal and simple
Data monitoring*	Detailed and rigorous	Minimal
Study management	Significant interventions and support from research staff	Minimal support and interventions from research team

Adapted from Hébert et al.[3]
*Data monitoring refers to the review of source documents and adjudication/verification of outcomes.

POPULATION AND SAMPLE SIZE

The population to be studied will be defined by the study question. Efficacy trials may have a very narrowly defined population, with strict eligibility criteria and many exclusion criteria. Effectiveness trials are likely to have more broad inclusion criteria and few exclusion criteria. Regardless of the design, the population to be studied should be well described. This will allow readers to assess the scientific merit of the study and allows clinicians to judge whether the results of the study could apply to their patients, to assess the 'generalisability' of the results. Trials that include only a very narrowly defined population may also face difficulties in recruiting sufficient participants to reach a definitive conclusion.

How large do trials need to be to reach a definitive conclusion? In a parallel group trial, with a dichotomous outcome (for example, alive or dead), the number of patients required to answer a question depends on four factors:

1. The percentage of patients expected to have the outcome in the control group – the control group outcome rate
2. The expected change (usually reduction) that may result from the treatment being tested – the treatment effect
3. The level of probability to be accepted to indicate that the difference did not occur by chance (i.e. the probability level at which a treatment effect will be deemed to be real) – significance level or α (alpha)
4. The desired percentage chance of detecting a clinically important treatment effect if one truly exists (power).

In the past, trials addressing issues of importance in intensive care medicine were commonly too small to detect clinically important treatment effects,[4] but fortunately this is now changing.[2,5] The conduct of underpowered trials has almost certainly given rise to a significant number of false-negative results (type II errors) leading to potentially beneficial treatments being

Table 10.2 Examples of sample size calculations

CONTROL GROUP OUTCOME RATE (%)	TREATMENT GROUP OUTCOME RATE (%)	ARR	POWER (β)	TOTAL SAMPLE SIZE
50	30	20	80	206
50	30	20	90	268
30	15	15	90	348
30	20	10	90	824
30	25	5	90	3428
15	10	5	90	1914
15	12	3	90	5582
10	8	2	80	6626
10	8	2	90	8802

ARR = absolute risk reduction.
All calculations performed with STATA 8.2, assuming a two-sided $\alpha = 0.05$.

discarded. In order to avoid these errors, clinical trials have to include a surprisingly large number of participants. Examples of sample size calculations based on different baseline incidences, different treatment effects and different statistical power are given in **Table 10.2.**

RANDOMISATION AND ALLOCATION CONCEALMENT

Two components of the randomisation procedure are critically important. The first is the generation of a truly random allocation sequence; modern computer programs make this relatively straightforward. The second is the concealment of this allocation sequence from the investigators, so that the investigators and participants are unaware of the treatment allocation (group) prior to each participant entering the study.

There are a number of benefits to using a random process to determine treatment allocation. Firstly, it eliminates the possibility of bias in treatment assignment (selection bias). In order for this to be ensured, both a truly random sequence of allocation must be produced and this sequence must not be known to the investigators prior to each participant entering the trial. Secondly, it reduces the chance that the trial results are affected by confounding. It is important that, prior to the intervention in a RCT being delivered, both groups have an equal chance of developing the outcome of interest. A clinical characteristic (such as advanced age, gender or disease severity as measured by APACHE or SOFA scores) that is associated with the outcome is known as a confounding factor. Randomisation of a sufficient number of participants ensures that both known and unknown confounding factors (e.g. genetic polymorphisms) are evenly distributed between the two treatment groups. The play of chance may result in uneven distribution of known confounding factors between the groups and this is particularly likely in trials with fewer than 200 participants.[6] The third benefit of randomisation is that it allows the use of probability theory to quantify the role that chance could have played when differences are found between groups.[7] Finally, randomisation with allocation concealment facilitates blinding, another important component in the minimisation of bias in clinical trials.[8]

The generation of the allocation sequence must be truly random. There are a number of approaches to generating a truly random allocation sequence, most commonly using a computer-generated sequence of random numbers. More complicated processes where randomisation is performed in blocks, or is stratified to ensure that patients from each hospital in a multi-centred trial or those with certain baseline characteristics are equally distributed between treatment groups, can also be used. Allocation methods based upon predictable sequences, such as those based on medical record numbers or days of the week, do not constitute true randomisation and should be avoided. These methods allow researchers to predict to which group a participant will be allocated prior to them entering the trial, which introduces the possibility of selection bias.

Whatever method is used to produce a random allocation sequence, it is important that allocation concealment is maintained. Methods to ensure the concealment of allocation may be as simple as using sealed opaque envelopes,[9] or as complex as the centralised automated telephone-based or web-based systems commonly used in large multi-centred trials. In recent years web-based randomisation has become the predominant method of assigning trial participants to treatment groups. Appropriate attention to this aspect of a clinical trial is essential as trials with poor allocation concealment produce estimates of treatment effects that may be exaggerated by up to 40%.[10]

THE INTERVENTIONS

The intervention being evaluated in any clinical trial should be described in sufficient detail that clinicians could implement the therapy if they so desired, or researchers could replicate the study to confirm the results. This may be a simple task if the intervention is a single drug given once at the beginning of an illness, or may be complex if the intervention being tested is the introduction of a process of care, such as the introduction of a medical emergency team.[11] There are two additional areas with regards to the interventions delivered in clinical trials that require some thought by those conducting the trial and by clinicians evaluating the results, namely blinding and the control of concomitant interventions.

BLINDING

Blinding, also known as masking, is the practice of keeping trial participants (and, in the case of critically ill patients, their relatives or other legal surrogate decision makers), caregivers, data collectors, those adjudicating outcomes and sometimes those analysing the data and writing the study reports, unaware of which treatment is being given to individual participants. Blinding serves to reduce bias by preventing clinicians from consciously or subconsciously treating patients differently on the basis of their treatment assignment within the trial. It prevents data collectors from introducing bias when recording parameters that require a subjective assessment (e.g. pain scores, sedation scores or the Glasgow Coma Score). Although many ICU trials cannot be blinded (e.g. trials of intensive insulin therapy cannot blind treating staff who are responsible for monitoring blood glucose and adjusting insulin infusion rates), the successful blinding of the Saline versus Albumin Fluid Evaluation trial demonstrated the possibility of blinding even large complex trials if investigators are sufficiently committed and innovative.[2] Blinded outcome assessment is also necessary when the chosen outcome measure requires a subjective judgement. In such cases the outcome measure is said to be subject to the potential for ascertainment bias. For example, a blinded outcome assessment committee should adjudicate the diagnosis of ventilator-associated pneumonia (VAP) and blinded assessors should be used when assessing functional neurological recovery using the extended Glasgow outcome scale; both the diagnosis of VAP and assessment of the Glasgow outcome scale require a degree of subjective assessment and are therefore said to be prone to ascertainment bias.

It has been traditional to describe trials as single blinded, double blinded or even triple blinded. These terms, however, can be interpreted by clinicians to mean different things, and the terminology may be confusing.[12] It is recommended that reports of RCTs include a description of who was blinded and how this was achieved, rather than a simple statement that the trial was 'single blind' or 'double blind'.[13] Blinding is an important safeguard against bias in RCTs and, although not thought to be as essential as maintenance of allocation concealment, empirical studies have shown that unblinded studies may produce results that are biased by as much as 17%.[10]

CONCOMITANT TREATMENTS

Concomitant treatments are all treatments that are administered to patients during the course of a trial other than the study treatment. With the exception of the study treatment, patients assigned to the different treatment groups should be treated equally. When one group is treated in a way that is dependent on the treatment assignment but not directly related to the treatment, there is the possibility that this third factor will influence the outcome. An example might be a trial of pulmonary artery catheters (PAC) compared with management without a PAC. If the group assigned to receive management based on the data from a PAC received an additional daily chest X-ray to confirm the position of the PAC, they could conceivably have other important complications noted earlier, such as pneumonia, pulmonary oedema or pneumothoraces, and this may affect outcome in a fashion unrelated to the data available from the PAC. Maintenance of balance in concomitant treatments is facilitated by blinding. When trials cannot be blinded, use of concomitant treatments that may alter outcome should be recorded and reported, so that the potential impact of different concomitant treatments can be assessed.

ADAPTIVE TRIAL DESIGNS

Traditional clinical trials have followed a fixed design from the start of participant recruitment until trial completion. This approach has many advantages including simplicity and transparency, which should make the trial results more compelling. In recent years, interest in the use of adaptive trial designs has increased. An adaptive trial is one in which the trial design is changed while the trial is being conducted. The change may be quite simple and easy to understand, such as changing the sample size, and in practice most trials have an adaptive design as they allow early stopping for either efficacy or futility in response to recommendations from an independent data-monitoring committee. A less well-established but equally simple adaptive design is increasing the sample size due to a lower than expected event rate; an example of this is the PROWESS-SHOCK study where a predetermined increase in the sample size occurred in response to a lower than expected mortality rate in patients with septic shock.[14] More complex adaptive designs are used in other fields of medicine such as oncology,[15] where design changes may include changing drug doses or dropping or adding trial arms or drug doses, changing the proportion of patients assigned to each arm of a trial or seamlessly moving from phase II to phase III within a single trial.[15] Although such designs have been rare in critical care research, the failure of clinical trials in areas such as industry-sponsored sepsis research may see adaptive designs becoming more accepted in future years.

OUTCOME MEASUREMENT

All clinical trials should be designed to detect a difference in a single outcome. In general there are two types of outcomes, clinically meaningful outcomes and surrogate outcomes.

A clinically meaningful outcome is a measure of how patients feel, function or survive.[16] Clinically meaningful outcomes are the most credible end-points for clinical trials that seek to change clinical practice. Phase III trials should always use clinically meaningful outcomes as the primary outcome. Examples of clinically meaningful outcomes include mortality and measures of health-related quality of life. In contrast, a surrogate outcome is a substitute for a clinically meaningful outcome; a reasonable surrogate outcome would be expected to predict clinical benefits based upon epidemiological, therapeutic, pathophysiological or other scientific evidence.[16] Examples of surrogate end-points would include cytokine levels in sepsis trials, changes in oxygenation in ventilation trials, or blood pressure and urine output in a fluid resuscitation trial.

Unless a surrogate outcome has been validated, it is unwise to rely on changes in surrogate outcomes to guide clinical practice. For example, it seemed intuitively sensible that after myocardial infarction the suppression of ventricular premature beats (a surrogate outcome), which were known to be linked to mortality (the clinically meaningful outcome), would be beneficial; unfortunately the CAST trial found increased mortality in participants assigned to receive antiarrhythmic therapy.[17] The process for determining whether a surrogate outcome is a reliable indicator of clinically meaningful outcomes has been described.[18]

ANALYSIS

Even when trials are well designed and conducted, inappropriate statistical analyses may result in uncertain or erroneous conclusions. A detailed discussion of the statistical analysis of large-scale trials is well beyond the scope of this chapter but certain guiding principles can be articulated:

- All trials should adhere to a predetermined statistical analysis plan as otherwise the temptation to perform multiple analyses and report only those that support the preconceived ideas of the investigators may prove irresistible. A predetermined analysis plan protects the investigators from such temptation and allows readers to give appropriate weighting to the results.
- The convention of accepting a p value of <0.05 to indicate 'statistical significance' is based on assessment of a single outcome. Assessing multiple outcomes increases the likelihood of finding a p value of <0.05 purely due to the play of chance. Each trial should have a single predefined primary outcome measure. If more than one primary outcome measure is used then the p value used to indicate statistical significance should be reduced. The simplest method is to perform a Bonferoni correction, which divides 0.05 by the number of outcomes examined to determine the new level of statistical significance. Thus for two outcomes the p value must be below 0.025, and for three it must be below 0.017. The p value may also have to be reduced further if the trial employs interim analyses.

Clinicians should pay close attention to the analysis to make certain that a true intention-to-treat analysis is presented, and that any subgroup analysis is viewed with an appropriate amount of caution.

INTENTION-TO-TREAT ANALYSIS

Trials should be analysed using the 'intention-to-treat' principle. This means that all participants are analysed in the group to which they were randomised regardless of whether they received all or any of the treatment to which they were assigned. To some readers the intention-to-treat principle may appear intuitively incorrect; it is reasonable to ask why patients who did not receive the intended treatment should be included in the analysis. Use of intention-to-treat analysis prevents bias arising from the selective exclusion of patients – termed attrition bias. In an appropriately sized trial, loss of patients at random should occur equally in both groups and inclusion of those patients will not alter the result. If loss of patients is occurring as a non-random event (e.g. because of protocol violations or intolerance of the treatment in one arm of the trial) then the trial result will be different if the lost patients are excluded. Consider a trial of a 5-day course of L-NMMA for the treatment of patients with septic shock; in the trial a number of patients who receive L-NMMA die in the first 24–48 hours and are excluded from the analysis as they have received only a little of the study treatment. A trial report based on the remaining patients who completed the treatment protocol (per-protocol analysis) will not give a true estimate of the effect of using L-NMMA in clinical practice. Although this is an extreme example, once a patient is included in a trial his/her outcome should always be accounted for in the study report.

SUBGROUP ANALYSIS

Particular difficulties arise from the selection, analysis and reporting of subgroups. Subgroups should be predefined and kept to the minimum number possible. When many subgroups are examined, the likelihood of finding a subgroup where the treatment effect is different from that seen in the overall population increases. A well-known example of this was the analysis of the treatment effect of aspirin in patients with myocardial infarction in the large Second International Study of Infarct Survival (ISIS-2) trial. Overall the trial indicated that aspirin reduced the relative risk of death at 1 month by 23%. To illustrate the unreliability of subgroup analyses, the participants were divided into subgroups according to their astrological birth signs; the analysis showed that patients born under Libra or Gemini did not benefit from treatment with aspirin.[19] Although it is easy to identify this as a chance subgroup finding, this may be much harder when the choice of the subgroup appears rational and a theoretical explanation for the findings can be advanced. For example in the Gruppo Italiano per lo Studio della Streptochinasi nell'infarto miocardico (GISSI) trial, subgroup analysis suggested that fibrinolytic therapy did not reduce mortality in patients who had suffered a previous myocardial infarct.[20] Although this finding appears biologically plausible, subsequent trials have shown quite clearly that fibrinolytic therapy is just as effective in patients with prior infarction as in those without.[21]

Separation of patients into subgroups should be on the basis of characteristics that are apparent at the time of randomisation. Selection of subgroups using features identified after randomisation risks introducing bias as the patients have already been subjected to the different study treatments and the subgroup analysis will therefore not be comparing like with like.

TESTS OF INTERACTION VERSUS WITHIN-SUBGROUP COMPARISONS

Even when subgroups are selected appropriately, many readers will be tempted to draw inappropriate conclusions from the results. As the trial will have been designed to examine the effect of the treatment on the primary outcome in the whole study population, the best assessment of the treatment effect in any subgroup will be the effect seen in the trial as a whole. When analysing a subgroup result, the investigators should seek to answer the following question: 'Is the treatment effect in the subgroup different from the treatment effect seen in the remaining participants?' This is a test of interaction or of heterogeneity. Often the investigators err and perform within-subgroup comparisons, which instead answer the question: 'What was the effect of treatment A versus treatment B in this subgroup?' Within-subgroup comparisons are more likely to lead to unreliable results. Journals such as the New England Journal of Medicine provide guidelines for the analysis and reporting of subgroup effects.[22]

REPORTING

The reporting of randomised controlled trials has been greatly improved by the work of the CONSORT (Consolidated standards of Reporting Trials) group.[13,23] The consort statement provides a framework and checklist (**Table 10.3**) that can be followed by investigators and authors to provide a standardised high-quality report.[23] An increasing number of journals require authors to follow the CONSORT recommendations when reporting the results of a randomised controlled trial. The group also recommends the publication of a structured diagram that documents the flow of patients through four stages of the trial – namely enrolment, allocation, follow-up and analysis (**Fig. 10.1**). It is likely that the use of the CONSORT statement to guide the reporting of RCTs does lead to improvements, at least in the quality of reporting of randomised controlled trials.[24]

Trials may report results using a number of values that, taken together, will give readers a full understanding of the trial results. These may include a

Table 10.3 The Consort 2010 checklist[23] of information to include when reporting a randomised trial*

SECTION/TOPIC	ITEM NO.	CHECKLIST ITEM
TIME AND ABSTRACT		
	1a	Identification as a randomised trial in the title
	1b	Structured summary of trial design, methods, results, and conclusions (for specific guidance see CONSORT for abstracts)
INTRODUCTION		
Background and objectives	2a	Scientific background and explanation of rationale
	2b	Specific objectives or hypothesis
METHODS		
Trial design	3a	Description of trial design (such as parallel, factorial) including allocation ratio
	3b	Important changes to methods after trial commencement (such as eligibility criteria), with reasons
Participants	4a	Eligibility criteria for participants
	4b	Settings and locations where the data were collected
Interventions	5	The interventions for each group were sufficient
Outcomes	6a	Completely defined pre-specified primary and secondary outcome measures, including how and when they were assessed
	6b	Any changes to trial outcomes after the trial commenced, with reasons
Sample size	7a	How sample size was determined
	7b	When applicable, explanation of any interim analyses
RANDOMISATION		
Sequence generation	8a	Method used to generate the random allocation sequence
	8b	Type of randomisation; details of any restriction (such as blocking and block size)

Table 10.3 The Consort 2010 checklist of information to include when reporting a randomised trial—cont'd

SECTION/TOPIC	ITEM NO.	CHECKLIST ITEM
Allocation concealment mechanism	9	Mechanism used to implement the random allocation sequence (such as sequentially numbered containers), describing any steps take to conceal the sequence until interventions were assigned
Implementation	10	Who generated the random allocation sequence, who enrolled participants, and who assigned participants to interventions
Blinding	11a	If done, who was blinded after assignment to interventions (for example, participants, care providers, those assessing outcomes and how)
	11b	If relevant, description of the similarity of interventions
Statistical methods	12a	Statistical methods used to compare groups for primary and secondary outcomes
	12b	Methods for additional analyses, such as subgroup analyses and adjusted analyses
RESULTS		
Participant flow (a diagram is strongly recommended)	13a	For each group, the numbers of participants who were randomly assigned, received intended treatment, and were analysed for the primary outcome
	13b	For each group, losses and exclusions after randomisation, together with reasons
Recruitment	14a	Dates defining the periods of recruitment and follow-up
	14b	Why the trial ended or was stopped
Baseline data	15	A table showing baseline demographic and clinical characteristics for each group
Numbers analysed	16	For each group, number of participants (denominator) included in each analysis and whether the analysis was by original assigned groups
Outcomes and estimation	17a	For each primary and secondary outcome, results for each group, and the estimated effect size and its precision (such as 95% confidence interval)
	17b	For binary outcomes, presentation of both absolute and relative effect sizes is recommended
Ancillary analyses	18	Results of any other analyses performed, including subgroup analyses and adjusted analyses, distinguishing pre-specified from exploratory
Harms	19	All important harms or unintended effects in each group for (specific guidance see CONSORT for harms)
DISCUSSION		
Limitations	20	Trial limitations, addressing sources of potential bias, imprecision, and, if relevant, multiplicity of analyses
Generalisability	21	Generalisability (external validity, applicability) of the trial findings
Interpretation	22	Interpretation consistent with results, balancing benefits and harms, and considering other relevant evidence
OTHER INFORMATION		
Registration	23	Registration number and name of trial registry
Protocol	24	Where the full trial protocol can be accessed, if available
Funding	25	Sources of funding and other support (such as supply of drugs), role of funders

Reproduced with permission from Schulz KF, Altman DG, Moher D, CONSORT Group. CONSORT 2010 statement: updated guidelines for reporting parallel group randomised trials. BMJ 2010;340:c332.

*We strongly recommend reading this statement in conjunction with the CONSORT 2010 Explanation and Elaboration for important clarifications on all the items. If relevant, we also recommend reading CONSORT extensions for cluster randomised trials, non-inferiority and equivalence trials, non-pharmacological treatments, herbal interventions, and pragmatic trials. Additional extensions are forthcoming: for this and for up-to-date references relevant to this checklist see www.consort-statement.org.

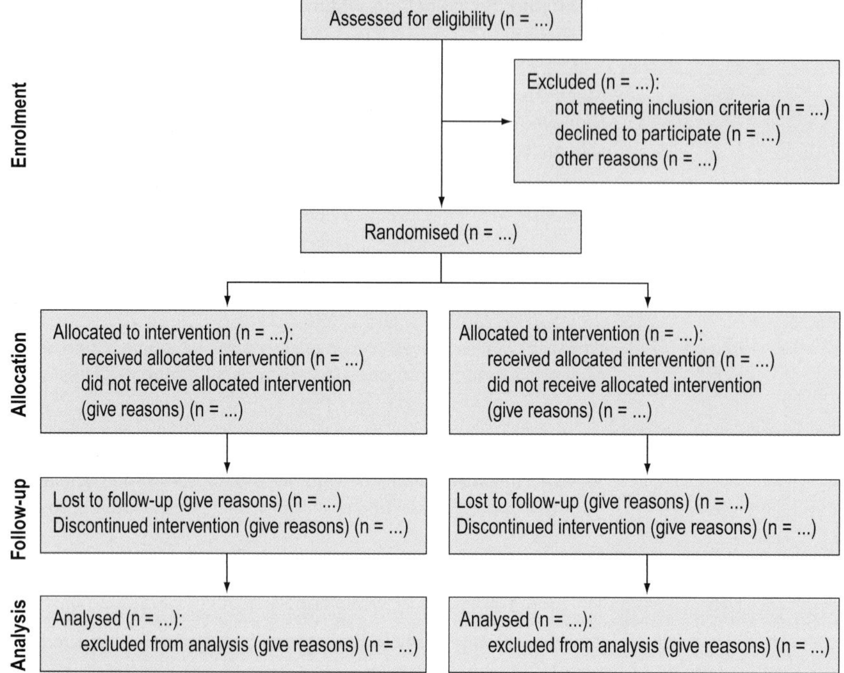

Figure 10.1 Flow diagram of the progress through the phases of a randomised trial.[23] *(From Schulz KF, Altman DG, Moher D, CONSORT Group. CONSORT 2010 statement: updated guidelines for reporting parallel group randomised trials. BMJ 2010;340:c332, with permission.)*

p value, confidence intervals and number needed to treat (or harm).

- *Probabilities:* the *p* value represents the probability that a difference has arisen by chance. In very large trials, small and clinically insignificant differences may give rise to *p* value of less than 0.05 and, conversely, a moderately sized trial may report a clinically important difference with a *p* value that is close to or greater than 0.05; *p* values should not be viewed in isolation but assessed in combination with other measures such as confidence intervals and the number needed to treat (or harm).
- *Confidence intervals:* give an indication of the precision of the result. Whenever a trial reports a difference it is reporting a difference found in a finite sample of the population of interest. If the same trial is repeated it is highly likely a slightly or very different result will be reported. If the trial is reporting a relatively small number of patients with the outcome of interest (small number of events) then the difference between the results may be large, if the trial reports a large number of events then it is likely the two results will be quite close to each other. Confidence intervals give a range of values within which it is likely the 'true' result lies – they give an indication of the precision of the result. The most commonly quoted are the 95% confidence intervals; these are the limits within which we would expect 95% of study results to lie if the study were repeated an infinite number of times, though they are often interpreted to mean that we can be 95% confident that the 'true' result lies within these limits.
- *Number needed to treat (or harm):* a useful concept for clinicians is the number needed to treat (or harm). This is the reciprocal of the absolute difference in outcomes arising from two treatments. For example in the ISIS-2 trial, patients randomised to intravenous streptokinase had an absolute reduction in mortality of 2.8%. Thus the number needed to treat to prevent one death is 100/2.8 or 35.7 patients. As the trial was very large with a large number of events (17187 participants and 1820 deaths), this relatively small absolute reduction in mortality (2.8%) yielded a *p* value of less than 0.000001. The same calculation can be performed to calculate the number needed to harm. For example, in the CRASH trial, patients with traumatic brain injury treated with high-dose steroids had a 3.4% increase in the absolute risk of death. The number needed to harm is calculated as 100/3.4, or one extra death for every 29.4 patients treated with high-dose corticosteroids. Again, as this was a large trial (10008 participants and 1945 deaths) the *p* value is small ($p = 0.00001$).

ETHICAL ISSUES SPECIFIC TO CLINICAL TRIALS IN CRITICAL CARE

The ethical principles guiding the conduct of research in critical care are outlined in the International Ethical

Guidelines for Biomedical Research Involving Human Subjects,[25] in addition country-specific guidelines are provided by various national bodies. The ethical principles of integrity, respect for persons, beneficence and justice, should be considered whenever research is conducted and an appropriately convened human research ethics committee or the equivalent should assess all research to ensure adherence to these principles. As the potential participants in critical care research are particularly vulnerable, owing to the nature of the conditions and the limitations to communication that exist, special consideration needs to be given to a number of areas including informed consent.

INFORMED CONSENT

That all mentally competent participants in clinical research should give informed consent prior to entering a study is an important ethical principle. This is rarely possible for people suffering critical illness, where the disease process (e.g. traumatic brain injury, encephalitis, severe hypoxaemia) or the required treatment (e.g. intubation, use of sedative medications) may make it impossible to obtain informed consent. Even awake, alert patients may not be able to give fully informed consent when they are facing stressful and potentially life-threatening situations.[26] This applies equally to surrogate decision makers. However, the treatment of critically ill patients can be improved only through the conduct of research and in many jurisdictions this has been recognised by making special provisions for consent in emergency research including research in the critically ill. In some circumstances, it may be ethical to allow a waiver of consent for research involving treatments that must be given in a time-dependent fashion (e.g. in the setting of cardiac arrest). A waiver of consent may well improve recruitment into clinical trials; it is unclear whether this approach is universally acceptable. Another approach has been to allow delayed consent, where patients are included in the study and consent from the patient or the relevant surrogate decision maker is sought as soon as practical. Neither approach is without problems.[27]

CRITICAL APPRAISAL

Clinicians reading reports of randomised controlled trials should use a structured framework to assess the methodological quality of the trial and the adequacy of the trial report. They should also address the magnitude and precision of reported treatment effects and ask themselves whether the results of the trial can be applied to their own clinical practice. There are a number of resources available to assist clinicians in this task, notably the Users' Guides to the Medical Literature, originally published in JAMA and the Critical Appraisal Skills Program from Oxford, UK, both of which are freely available on the internet.[28,29] These resources provide a structured framework that allows any reader to perform a systematic critical appraisal of

Box 10.1 Critical appraisal checklist for randomised controlled trials[28]

I. Are the results of the study valid?

Primary guides: Was the assignment of patients to treatments randomised?

1. Were all patients who entered the trial properly accounted for and attributed at its conclusion?
2. Was follow-up complete?
3. Were patients analysed in the groups to which they were randomised?

Secondary guides: Were patients, health workers, and study personnel 'blind' to treatment?

1. Were the groups similar at the start of the trial?
2. Aside from the experimental intervention, were the groups treated equally?

II. What were the results?

How large was the treatment effect?

1. How precise was the estimate of the treatment effect?

III. Will the results help me in caring for my patients?

Can the results be applied to my patient care?

1. Were all clinically important outcomes considered?
2. Are the likely treatment benefits worth the potential harms and costs?

almost any piece of medical literature. A checklist is provided for the appraisal of randomised controlled trials (**Box 10.1**).

OBSERVATIONAL STUDIES

Although RCTs are the optimal study design for deciding whether or not a treatment 'works', not all research questions can be addressed with this type of study. When the disease is rare, the outcome is rare or the treatment may be associated with harm, other study designs may be more appropriate. In these circumstances a cohort study or case–control study may be used to explore potential associations between exposure to a treatment and the occurrence of outcomes.

DESCRIPTIVE STUDIES

Case reports, case series and cross-sectional studies are all examples of descriptive studies. These types of studies may be important in the initial identification of new diseases such as HIV/AIDS[30–33] and SARS.[34] The purpose of these studies will be to describe the 'who, when, where, what and why' of the condition, and so further the understanding of the epidemiology of the disease. It is important that clear and standardised definitions of cases are used, so that clinicians and researchers can identify similar cases from the information provided. Although there are some famous examples where data from simple observational studies has been used to solve particular problems,[35]in general only very limited inferences can be drawn from descriptive data. In particular, it is dangerous to draw conclusions about 'cause and effect' using data from descriptive studies alone.[36]

ANALYTICAL OBSERVATIONAL STUDIES

There are two main types of analytical observational studies: case–control studies and cohort studies.

Case–control studies are performed by identifying patients with a particular condition (the 'cases'), and a group of people who do not have the condition (the 'controls'). The researchers then look back in time to ascertain the exposure of the members of each group to the variables of interest.[37] A case–control design may be appropriate when the disease has a long latency period and is rare. Cohort studies are performed by identifying a group of people who have been exposed to a certain risk factor and a group of people who are similar in most respects apart from their exposure to the risk factor. Both groups are then followed to ascertain whether they develop the outcome of interest. Cohort studies may be the appropriate design to determine the effects of a rare exposure, and have the advantage of being able to detect multiple outcomes that are associated with the same exposure.[38]

Both types of observational studies are prone to bias. In particular, although it is possible to correct for known confounding factors using multivariate statistical techniques, it is not possible to control for unknown or unmeasured confounding factors. There are a number of other biases that may distort the results of observational studies; these include selection bias, information bias and differential loss to follow-up.[38,39] Critical appraisal guides for observational studies are available to help readers assess the validity of these studies.[40] These limitations and inherent biases mean that observational studies may not always provide reliable evidence to guide clinical practice, although it has been argued that this is not always the case.[41,42]

SYSTEMATIC REVIEWS AND META-ANALYSIS

Systematic reviews have been proposed as a solution to the problem of the ever expanding medical literature.[43] A systematic review utilises specific methods to identify and critically appraise all the RCTs that address a particular clinical question and, if appropriate, statistically combine the results of the primary RCTs in order to arrive at an overall estimate of the effect of the treatment. By systematically assembling all RCTs that address one specific topic, methodologically sound systematic reviews can provide a valuable overview for the busy clinician. They play an important role in providing an objective appraisal of all available evidence and may reduce the possibility that treatments with moderate effects will be discarded owing to false-negative results from small or underpowered studies.[44] The use of meta-analysis could have resulted in the earlier introduction of life-saving therapies such as thrombolysis.[45] By using systematic methods, meta-analyses can provide more accurate and unbiased overviews, drawing conclusions that are often at odds with those of 'experts' and narrative reviews.[46,47]

In spite of these advantages and benefits, there are still problems with interpretation of meta-analyses. Like all clinical trials, they need to be performed with attention to methodological detail. There are guidelines for performing and reporting systematic reviews.[48,49] It is clear that in the critical care literature these guidelines are not always followed.[50] Clinicians should critically appraise the reports of all systematic reviews and meta-analyses regardless of the source of the review, using an appropriate guide.[51,52] Problems with interpretation can arise when the results of meta-analysis are at odds with the results of large RCTs that address the same issue;[53,54] this is not uncommon and clinicians will have to compare the methodological quality of the meta-analysis and the RCTs included in it with the validity of the large RCT in order to decide which provides the most reliable evidence.[55,2]

Access the complete references list online at http://www.expertconsult.com

3. Hébert PC, Cook DJ, Wells G, et al. The design of randomized clinical trials in critically ill patients. Chest 2002;121(4):1290–300.
13. Altman DG, Schulz KF, Moher D, et al. The revised CONSORT statement for reporting randomized trials: explanation and elaboration. Ann Intern Med 2001;134(8):663–94.
22. Wang R, Lagakos SW, Ware JH, et al. Statistics in medicine – Reporting of subgroup analyses in clinical trials. N Engl J Med 2007;357(21):2189–94.
23. Schulz KF, Altman DG, Moher D, CONSORT Group. CONSORT 2010 statement: updated guidelines for reporting parallel group randomised trials. BMJ 2010;340:c332.
39. MacMahon S, Collins R. Reliable assessment of the effects of treatment on mortality and major morbidity, II: observational studies. Lancet 2001;357(9254): 455–62.
49. Moher D, Cook DJ, Eastwood S, et al. Improving the quality of reports of meta-analyses of randomised controlled trials: the QUOROM statement. Quality of Reporting of Meta-analyses. Lancet 1999;354(9193): 1896–900.

11

Palliative care

Sarah Cox and Neil Soni

The World Health Organisation defines palliative care as an approach that improves the quality of life of patients and their families facing the problems associated with life-threatening illness, through the prevention and relief of suffering by means of early identification and impeccable assessment and treatment of pain and other problems, physical, psychosocial and spiritual (**Box 11.1**).[1]

Palliative care should be part of the care of patients identified as dying on ICU. In addition, the principles of palliative care may be appropriate for patients with life-limiting disease admitted to ICU for treatment of reversible causes such as neutropenic sepsis as a consequence of palliative chemotherapy. The palliative care team may also have a role in the care-of-patients with long-term conditions being considered for ICU admission. This chapter reviews the issues around identification and management of palliative and end-of-life care for ICU patients. It will also address the practical, ethical and emotional issues that arise.

PRE-ADMISSION TO ICU

Admission to ICU requires a judgement about the likelihood of benefit for the individual patient. Whilst this is often a discussion between the ICU or critical care outreach team, the usual medical team and the patient and family, the palliative care team may have an important role to play. Firstly, they can be part of a discussion about appropriateness of aggressive treatment. Secondly, it may be helpful to underline that if ICU care is not the chosen course of action, there is another specialist team who will be involved to ensure good symptom control and emotional support. Their expertise in communication can be useful in clarifying goals according to the patient's wishes, if known, including access to pre-existing advance care plans from community health care teams. They can support family and ward staff with alternative care plans. They may become the point of contact for the family providing continuity and reassurance in what is often an emotionally fraught situation.

PATIENTS ON ICU WHO ARE DYING

Around 5% of deaths in the UK and 20% of deaths in the USA occur on the intensive care unit.[2–4] Not all of these deaths could or should be predicted, but the proportion that follows a period of treatment withdrawal is increasing in both North America and Europe. This suggests an identifiable end-of-life phase, which could be managed with palliative care principles in mind, or as shared care with a specialist palliative care team.

There is great variability between services and cultures in identification of an end-of-life phase. Up to 90% of deaths in North American ICUs happen after decisions to limit life-sustaining treatment.[2] In northern Europe the figure is lower at around 50%, and 20% in southern Europe.[3,4] While these differences might be explained by the greater availability of ICU beds in America or less selective admission criteria, it is likely that they reflect, at least in part, cultural differences of expectations of treatment.

Scales such as APACHE III have been developed to help predict outcomes of ICU intervention,[5] but they are not sufficiently precise to be helpful in end-of-life decision making for an individual.[4] Frequently ICU admission represents a therapeutic trial with both clinicians and family sustaining hope until it is clear the trial has failed. Only then, which may be very late in the acute illness, will a transition to the goals of palliative care be considered appropriate. There may be an opportunity therefore to communicate uncertainty earlier on in the ICU stay so that active and palliative care can occur together.

What constitutes a good death depends on the views of the individual; however, there are some common themes from the literature including freedom from pain and other symptoms, and the ability to retain some degree of control, autonomy and independence.[6] For patients dying on ICU the last three are difficult to achieve. However, they suggest delivering treatment that supports patients' values and beliefs, including appropriate limitation of the use of aggressive treatments. Surveys of patients and ICU nurses suggest a clear overlap between them in the priority of avoiding prolongation of dying (**Box 11.2**).[6,7]

For relatives of patients dying on ICU, a good death requires attention to comfort, and more particularly to pain management. Families rate whole-person concerns highly, including feeling that their relative was at peace and retained dignity and self-respect.[8] Increased satisfaction of families is also related to clarity around the

Box 11.1 World Health Organization definition of palliative care[1]

- Provides relief from pain and other distressing symptoms
- Affirms life and regards dying as a normal process
- Intends neither to hasten nor postpone death
- Integrates the psychological and spiritual aspects of patient care
- Offers a support system to help patients live as actively as possible until death
- Offers a support system to help family members cope during the patient's illness and in their own bereavement
- Uses a team approach to address the needs of patients and their families, including bereavement counselling if indicated
- Will enhance quality of life, and may also positively influence the course of illness
- Is applicable early in the course of illness, in conjunction with other therapies that are intended to prolong life, such as chemotherapy or radiation therapy, and includes those investigations needed to better

Based on Sepúlveda C, Marlin A, Yoshida T, Ullrich A. Palliative Care: The World Health Organization's Global Perspective. J Pain Sympt Manage 2002;24(2):91–6.

Box 11.2 Patients' and ICU nurses' priorities for a good death

Patients[6]	*ICU nurses*[7]
Adequate pain and symptom management	Managing pain and other symptoms
Avoiding inappropriate prolongation of dying	Promoting earlier cessation of treatment or not initiating aggressive treatment at all
Achieving a sense of control	Knowing and following patients' wishes for end-of-life care
Relieving burden on others	Communicating effectively as a health care team
Strengthening relationship with loved ones	

processes of limiting treatment, with trials of treatment being explained and withdrawal or withholding of treatment occurring as expected.[9]

DECISION MAKING FOR PATIENTS AT THE END OF LIFE

INVOLVEMENT OF PATIENTS

In the 1990s the SUPPORT study team reported their prospective observation of over 9000 seriously ill hospitalised patients.[10] The authors identified overaggressive management, inadequate pain control and poor communication amongst a significant number of those who went on to die. There was evidence that physicians were often not aware of patients' wishes around medical care.

Patients' preferences for treatment may be accessed directly in only a small minority of cases admitted to ICU. Occasionally, a valid and applicable advance directive exists, or patients have a statement of wishes or have discussed their preferences for treatment with close family. The majority (up to 95%) of patients requiring admission to ITU will be unable to engage in discussions about treatment choices, and most will not have discussed their wishes with relatives or recorded them in writing.[11] Offering advance care planning to individuals with chronic progressive diseases is being encouraged, but as yet has only been taken up by a small minority. Ideally, in the future, advance care planning in patients with progressive medical conditions may be helpful in respecting patient wishes around ICU care.

Where patients are able to discuss options for treatment, it should be considered that they may have a variable understanding of medical interventions. In essence they tend to overestimate the likelihood of their success, with optimism on the part of the patient, and a reluctance to be pessimistic on the part of the clinicians.[12] However, discussions about treatment that include details of the likely outcome, and potential burden, can significantly reduce patient preferences for those treatments where the medical benefit is uncertain.[13]

INVOLVEMENT OF FAMILIES IN DECISION MAKING

The realisation that active treatment is no longer in the patient's best interests comes to health professionals, patients and families at different times. Partly this is due to experience and training and partly a sometimes-unrealistic belief in what ICU treatment can achieve. Managing the different expectations is challenging. Families want to be involved in decision making, especially around value-laden decisions such as withdrawal of life support,[14] but they will need to have clear explanations of their relative's condition and the purpose and limitations of treatment. Their role, and the role of the health care team, should be to advocate for the patient, making the decision that patient would have made had they been able.[15] Relatives are able to identify patient preferences with agreement of 80% or greater in situations where the impact of the physical insult is either mild or devastating.[16] However, there is a dramatic drop in agreement (down to around 60%) for more ambiguous scenarios associated with long-term physical or cognitive morbidity. In these situations, relatives are more likely than patients to identify the clinical outcome as acceptable.

Effective, frequent and timely communication with relatives increases satisfaction with care and reduces anxiety in bereavement.[17] Insufficient time spent communicating with families results in poor understanding of the diagnosis, prognosis and plan of care and increased conflict.[18] Time spent is not, in itself, enough and far more important is the clinicians' ability to elicit and respond to families' views and concerns. Simply, families judge the quality of the discussion, at least in part, by how much time they are allowed to speak rather than encouraged to listen.[19] Although the communication skills of ICU staff may be excellent, the additional resource of the palliative care team can also be useful in these situations.

INVOLVEMENT OF OTHER HEALTH PROFESSIONALS IN DECISION MAKING

ICU nurses often feel frustrated by the medical plan especially when, in their view, conflicting or over-optimistic messages are given to patients or family members.[20] In contrast, physicians are reported to feel the burden of making decisions about limiting treatment and that 'it's a lot easier to say it than to do it'.[21]

Collaboration between these professionals has the potential to produce better-informed decisions, which can lead to greater satisfaction with care for patients, families and the professionals involved.[22,23] Not surprisingly inconsistent messages and non-collaborative inter-professional behaviours result in family dissatisfaction.[24] Shared decision making will reduce the burden of decision making on senior ICU physicians, but it still usually remains their ultimate responsibility. Three studies of collaborative decision making involving at least nurses, physicians and family have demonstrated the additional benefits of reduced length of ICU stay and lower costs with no increase in mortality.[22,23,25]

There is much published on the involvement of other professionals in end-of-life decision making. Lilly et al included a social worker and a chaplain in their model of family meetings;[22] others have suggested the importance of considering other specialists such as physiotherapists (respiratory therapists)[26] or palliative care clinicians.[27] Involvement of clinical ethicists has been demonstrated to improve satisfaction of both health care professionals and families and to reduce length of ICU stay and costs for patients who died.[28]

WITHDRAWAL OF AND WITHHOLDING TREATMENT

Patients identify the avoidance of inappropriate prolongation of dying in their definition of what a 'good death' might look like.[6] There is agreement in the USA and northern Europe that where treatment is not going to succeed it should be withheld or withdrawn.[4,29,30] However, there is wide variation in withholding and withdrawing treatment across countries.[4] Differences have also been measured in what ICU physicians believe they should do and what actually happens, with physicians identifying a significantly greater need for withholding or withdrawing treatment than their practice demonstrates.[5]

The ethical basis for withholding treatment is the same as that for withdrawal; however, the practice of withdrawal is often emotionally more difficult for all concerned. This may be a result of the more active nature of withdrawal.[29] It is also possible that some ICU treatments, when withdrawn, result in rapid decline and death with a greater requirement for symptomatic medication and this temporal association presents an uncomfortable comparison with the act of euthanasia. However, allowing inevitable death and euthanasia are ethically and, in most countries, legally distinct. It is the intention behind each decision to withhold or withdraw that is critical.

Decisions to limit treatment include discontinuing monitoring vital signs, withholding cardiopulmonary resuscitation, vasopressors, antibiotics and artificial hydration, and removal of mechanical ventilation. All decisions should be considered individually in terms of the benefit and burden to the patient and in the context of the goals of care. In the large, prospective study of end-of-life practices in European ICUs, the Ethicus study group identified wide variation in withdrawal (5–69%) and withholding (16–70%) of therapy.[5]

Decisions to remove or reduce mechanical ventilation at the end of life present particularly difficult ethical and practical issues. Differing practices of weaning ventilation from rapid to prolonged are described. Proponents of the former suggest that prolonged weaning prolongs dying and therefore unnecessary suffering.[31] Those in support of prolonged weaning argue that a rapid reduction in ventilation may be associated with more dyspnoea.[29] Extubation is practised by some ICU physicians who argue that there is discomfort associated with the endotracheal tube itself and that there is no ethical justification in leaving the tube in place once a decision has been made to discontinue life-sustaining treatment.[32,29] However, there is a significant incidence of stridor and laboured breathing in extubated patients, which suggests this approach may induce more symptoms than it relieves.[32]

There has been concern about the doses of opioids and benzodiazepines required to control dyspnoea and agitation, especially in rapid weaning or extubation, and whether in fact these medications themselves bring about the patient's death. The principle of double effect holds that the unintended consequence (death) is ethically acceptable because of the intended effect (symptom control). This is a controversial position with which some are uncomfortable. In fact the principle of double effect may not be relevant as small studies in ICU show

Box 11.3 Recommendations for managing the transition from active to palliative care on the ICU

- Inclusive and collaborative decision making
- Consistent communication with family that begins early
- Identification of trials of therapy with timed reassessment against clinical milestones
- Concurrent attention to symptom control, spiritual and psychological support of patient and family
- Clarity about withholding and withdrawing treatment
- Guidance for 'stepping-down' to general hospital wards
- Inclusion of organ donation in consideration
- Assessment of bereavement risk for onward referral if appropriate
- Support of staff

that the doses of opioids and sedatives required for symptom control are relatively modest[33,34] and in dying palliative care patients these drugs do not appear to hasten death.[35,36]

Given such variations in practice and potential for different interpretations of intentions in withdrawing or withholding life-sustaining treatment, excellent communication between the multiprofessional team and the family, and clear documentation of the intent and decision-making process leading to it are paramount (**Box 11.3**).

SYMPTOM CONTROL

Symptom assessment usually involves taking a detailed history from the patient to understand the cause and severity of the symptom. In many ICU patients at the end of life this is not possible and so physiological variables and behavioural observations are used as surrogate markers, such as heart rate and respiratory rate. The use of validated pain scales such as the Behaviour Pain Scale[37] or Pain Assessment Behaviour Scale[38] may provide more objective records of pain to direct changes in dose of symptomatic medication. Involvement of the specialist palliative care team may be useful when the situation is unclear or symptoms prove difficult to control.

Dyspnoea correlates most strongly with tachycardia and tachypnoea[39] and may be treated symptomatically with opioids with the addition of benzodiazepines to reduce anxiety if necessary. Treatments such as oxygen, corticosteroids and diuretics may be appropriate if they are contributing to symptomatic control of breathlessness. Signs of agitation, anxiety, or behavioural markers of pain that do not respond to opioids and may be caused by general distress can be treated with benzodiazepines. Specialist palliative care input may be helpful if symptoms fail to respond to usual measures.

Choice of opioid and benzodiazepine varies; it is important for units to use the particular drug they are familiar with. Morphine is cheap but should not be used in patients with moderate to severe renal impairment as accumulation can result in additional symptoms. Fentanyl or alfentanil are common alternatives in this situation. Drug doses should be titrated against symptoms and escalated in response to documented markers of distress.

SUPPORT FOR FAMILIES AND STAFF

Patients and families will need support in the form of effective communication and they may also need psychological support. This is often provided by ICU staff, particularly the nursing staff, with whom they may have spent significant time. Offers of additional psychological support should be made to patients and family members and accessed from the specialist palliative care team and from chaplaincy.

Palliative care continues as bereavement care after the patient dies. In practice most bereavement support from ICU is offered immediately after death or by external agencies. Needless to say, relatives need to be informed of the death in a sensitive manner; they also need to understand the cause of death. Identification of family members who may be at risk of complicated bereavement may be guided by features of the illness and death, features of the bereaved person such as psychological morbidity, their relationship with the deceased, and their social supports. Referral to a local bereavement service or requesting permission to call the family doctor and arrange an appointment may be appropriate.

Bereavement surveys suggest ways we could improve the impact of relatives' deaths on ICU including skilled communication during the critical illness and after death. Post-traumatic stress-related symptoms are more common among family members who felt information giving was incomplete.[40] These symptoms can translate subsequently to increased rates of anxiety and depression.

ICU staff have emotional responses to the death of their patients, which need to be addressed to avoid burnout or other negative long-term sequelae.[41,42] Support might include debriefing around deaths, a supportive environment, and access to psychosocial resources. Collaborative decision making would be expected to reduce staff stress about dying patients.

ORGAN DONATION

The topic of organ donation and the ICU is more fully discussed in Chapter 100. Involvement of the palliative care team may be helpful to provide additional emotional support to the family. There may also be an important role in managing signs of distress, especially during withdrawal of treatment in donation by cardiac death (DCD). In DCD the family may wish to be with the patient whilst treatment is withdrawn. This process is an opportunity for them to say goodbye and they may have specific wishes around prayer or cultural rituals that should be elicited and honoured as far as possible. Provision should be made for appropriate symptomatic drugs to be with the patient during DCD to treat signs of distress, as these will be unpleasant for the family, although they may not be experienced as discomfort by the patient. In some units, the palliative care team takes over care of patients if they do not die within the timeframe for DCD, moving them to another ward or palliative care unit within the hospital.[43]

CARE PATHWAYS TO SUPPORT END-OF-LIFE CARE ON ICU

Pathways and protocols have been developed to improve the care of dying patients on the ICU.[44,45] The care of the dying pathway developed by the Marie Curie Centre in Liverpool, UK prompts appropriate assessment of symptoms, communication with family and patient if possible, psychological and spiritual support and support with practical issues such as open visiting and free car parking.[44] It acts as a reminder to consider the appropriateness of each treatment in terms of the burden and benefit and supports the nursing staff in monitoring and maintaining comfort on an ongoing basis.

STEPPING DOWN FROM ICU

Some patients are able to transfer out of ICU for their last days but this transition needs to be managed carefully to avoid additional family distress. The initial suggestion of stepping down from ICU is another opportunity to utilise the palliative care team's expertise.

This transition is both a physical and emotional one for patients and families who may feel that this step away from critical care in some way seals the fate of the patient. They will be concerned about losing the skilled staff and environment they know. Their anxiety may be compounded by the knowledge that there is not the same ratio of staff to patients outside ICU.[46] Clear information about changes in ward and treatments may help to reduce the anxiety.

A member of the palliative care team can be helpful in providing continuity around this transition. If invited to meet the patient and family before transfer, they can begin to understand the specific needs of patient and family members including symptom control, emotional and spiritual issues.

The move should take place in a planned way with the family given as much forewarning as possible. Ideally, the patient should not be transferred at night or weekends if this means there is less support available. Treatments and monitoring should not be discontinued immediately before transfer, although some changes may be necessary if the 'step-down' ward does not usually care for patients with arterial lines or intravenous opioid infusions. The palliative care team can help to advise about practicalities of continuing symptomatic medications after the move, and managing this transition seamlessly.

CONCLUSION

With advances in technology, there is likely to be an increase in trials of ICU treatment, and a corresponding increase in transition to palliative care on the ICU. How this is managed will depend on local access to specialist palliative care resources and the focus of the ICU staff. Limitation of treatment, in whatever guise, is a difficult area and constitutes a significant part of clinical practice on the ICU. It is immensely important to patients, their relatives and clinicians and deserves to be more openly discussed. Review of ICU deaths at mortality and morbidity meetings could include consideration of the quality of the patient's end-of-life care and family support to promote learning and improve care for subsequent patients.

Access the complete references list online at http://www.expertconsult.com

3. Sprung C, Cohen S, Sjokvist P, et al. Ethicus Study Group. End of life practices in European intensive care units – the Ethicus study. JAMA 2003;290(6): 790–7.
4. Carlet J, Thijs L, Antonelli M, et al. Statement of the 5th International Consensus Conference in Critical Care: Brussels, Belgium. Challenges in end-of-life care in the ICU. Intensive Care Med 2004;30(5):770–84.
6. Singer P, Martin D, Kelner M. Quality end-of-life care – patients' perspectives. JAMA 1999;281(2):163–8.
29. Truog R, Campbell M, Curtis R, et al. Recommendations for end-of-life care in the intensive care unit: A consensus statement by the American College of Critical Care Medicine. Crit Care Med 2008;36(3): 953–63.
44. The Marie Curie Palliative Care Institute Liverpool. Intensive Care Unit and the Liverpool Care Pathway for the Dying Patient (LCP). 2011. Online. Available: http://www.mcpcil.org.uk/liverpool-care-pathway/lcp-specialist-icu.htm (accessed 01/06/12).

12

ICU and the elderly

Richard Keays

The proportion of the population that is elderly is increasing in all developed and developing nations. Medical innovation and a belief that old age and disease can be defeated by a combination of personal choice and greater resources has led to rising, often unrealistic, expectations. Increasingly intensive care medicine is becoming a specialty largely focused on care of the elderly and the age-acquired co-morbidities of this patient group complicate their management. The consequence of this demographic shift in the critical care unit population has remained largely unstudied. This chapter seeks to bring together the current information on management of the elderly presenting to critical care.

DEFINITIONS

There is no agreed definition of 'elderly'. It has been defined by chronology, social role, physical capacity, threshold life expectancy and when 'active contribution is no longer possible'. Most commonly it is taken as the pension age – though this is an inherently fluid endpoint. In 1875 over-50s were defined as elderly whereas now it seems around the pension age of 65, although the over-80s are also becoming an 'identifiable' group. These chronological niceties are rarely relevant from a medical perspective as clinicians understand the poor correlation between chronological and physiological age. The medical literature has no common definition and uses a wide range of arbitrary values from 67 to 70, over-70s and, more recently, over-80s to describe population groups.[1]

DEMOGRAPHICS

More people are living longer and this trend has shown little sign of stopping. In the UK, 5 years ago 16% of the population was over 65 and 1.2 million, of a total population of just over 60 million, were over 85 years of age.[2] Current United Nations projections predict the population of over 80s will double by 2050, representing 10% of the total population in developed countries. There are some signs this inexorable rise in life expectancy may have peaked. For the first time in 50 years Spain reported a fall in life expectancy,[3] a finding repeated in some parts of the US.[4] These recent declines have been attributed to familiar factors accounting for poor health: obesity, tobacco and other preventable risks.

Nevertheless, the post-war increase in longevity means many more elderly people present to critical care than previously. This greater longevity may be attributable to improved diet and better lifestyle decisions, but is also explained by improved disease management; however, the resultant gain in survival is at the price of living with morbidity. Not only are there more elderly patients but also they have more significant co-morbidity and thus a greater likelihood of developing a critical illness.

These societal changes are reflected in the ICU demographics. In Australia and New Zealand 13% of ICU admissions were over 80 years old and the numbers had been increasing by about 5% per annum between 2000 and 2005.[5] Unsurprisingly, the chances of being admitted to ICU are somewhat related to resource availability. In 2005 the number of ICU beds per 100 000 population was 3.3 for the UK, 7.8 in Australia, 24 in Germany and 20 in the USA.[6] A study comparing the USA with the UK in terms of hospitalisation and the elderly found that 47% of British over-85s died in hospital, whereas this figure was only 31% in the US; however, only 1.3% of these patients received intensive care in the UK compared with 11% in the USA.[7] Of all hospital discharges, only 2.2% of patients had received intensive care in the UK compared with 19.3% in the USA.

Approaching the problem from a different direction is to consider what happens to a whole cohort of elderly people. One such longitudinal study from America following over 1 million elderly patients over a 5-year follow-up period found that over half were admitted to some higher dependency care unit at some point.[8]

THE AGEING PROCESS

Individuals accumulate co-morbidities with pathophysiological consequences as they age – but these physiological changes are both unpredictable and extremely variable across any population. Ageing is the combination of physiological change and accumulated pathophysiology (**Fig. 12.1**). Examples of physiological

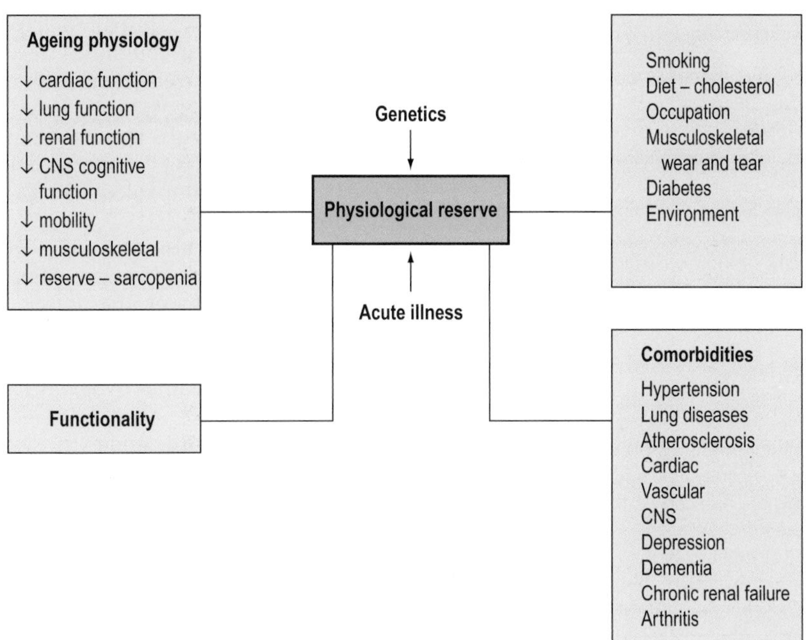

Figure 12.1 Factors affecting physiological reserve.

changes associated with ageing include maximal oxygen uptake, cardiovascular function, muscle mass, tissue elasticity, memory and reaction time, but there are many more.[9]

THE ORGAN SYSTEMS

Each organ system undergoes age-related declines but, in addition, there are specific disease-related organ alterations leading to a net impairment of organ function. A brief overview of changes associated with age and the impact of commoner co-morbidities follows.

CARDIOVASCULAR CHANGES

The heart has reduced contractility and overall mechanical efficiency.[10] This is caused by:

- altered connective tissue compliance due to interstitial collagen being laid down
- reduction in myocyte numbers
- valve hardening and sclerosis, which can affect function
- fibrosis and cell loss in conduction pathways impairing conduction
- deterioration in the sinoatrial node
- ventricular hypertrophy with slower myocardial relaxation.

The result of these changes is a reduction in arterial compliance with an earlier return of the reflected wave in systole. Normally, cardiac pulsatile energy is absorbed at arteriolar segmental level in the young but not in the elderly. Aortic impedance increases and higher blood flow organs show familiar signs of microvasculopathy. This, coupled with the tendency for pulse pressure to rise with age, means that ventricles hypertrophy and cardiac work increases. The resultant increasing oxygen demand occurs against a background fall in diastolic coronary blood flow with ventricular hypertrophy.

Both contraction and relaxation phases are slower. Diastolic filling time is reduced placing an extra emphasis on the atrial component to maintain this filling resulting in a reversal of the *E*/*A* ratio (early to late diastolic-filling velocity). Subsequent atrial dilatation is more likely to lead to atrial fibrillation, significantly compromising ventricular filling. The smaller end-diastolic volume is poorly tolerated and impaired cardiac performance ensues.

In addition to these changes, coronary flow reserve is limited, blood vessels are less easily dilated and there is a chronically elevated basal sympathetic tone. Baroreceptor reflexes are impaired and there is decreased sodium conservation.

In summary, the main ageing changes are myocardial and vascular stiffening, with impaired cardiac and vascular compliance. The blunted sympathetic responses produce the 'hyposympathetic heart' with a tendency to increased end-diastolic volume. Additionally there is an age-related reduction in cardiac contractility. Overall cardiac reserve and flexibility of response are reduced, but are usually more than able to deal with

Box 12.1 Cardiovascular ageing

- Cellular changes: reduced excitation contraction coupling, calcium homeostasis, myocyte function and increased atrial natriuretic peptide
- Decrease in myocytes, altered connective tissues, increased ventricular wall size
- Reduction in conductive tissues and numbers of sinus node cells
- Decreased contractility, reduced ventricular compliance, increased ventricular filling pressure, blunting of β-adrenoceptor responsiveness, reduced coronary flow reserve
- Stiffer arteries, reduced elasticity
- Thicker media and intima
- Alterations in autonomic tone with reduced β-adrenoreceptor-mediated vasodilatation; reduced NO activity
- Reduced heart rate, increased end-diastolic volume, increased stroke volume, reduced peak values for ejection fraction, cardiac output
- Impaired conduction, atrial fibrillation
- Clinical effects: more arrhythmias, hypertension, reduced exercise tolerance, dyspnoea and heart failure

the normal physical requirements of the elderly – though not with more excessive demands (**Box 12.1**).[10,11]

ACQUIRED CARDIOVASCULAR DISEASE

Atherosclerosis is detectable much earlier in life and starts to become relevant around 40 years of age in males and after menopause in females. Forty per cent of deaths over the age of 65 are cardiovascular and this increases with age. Diabetes, smoking, poor blood pressure control and high cholesterol all increase the risk of death from cardiovascular disease and most become more common with age.[12] Myocardial infarction carries a higher mortality in the elderly and the risk associated with interventional treatments is also higher.[10,11] The Framingham study showed that 40% of myocardial infarctions in those over 75 were silent.[13] In addition, arrhythmias such as atrial fibrillation are more common as a chronic feature in the elderly but most particularly affect the postoperative patient. In one study, 22% of over-70-year-olds developed postoperative atrial fibrillation.[14] When it does occur patients may be more at risk from hypotension, cardiac failure and myocardial infarction. The commonest cause of death amongst the over-85s in the postoperative period is myocardial infarction.[15]

RESPIRATORY

Lung function decline starts at around the age of 35 years. Muscle function is impaired by a combination of reduced fast twitch fibres and muscle atrophy such that between the ages of 65 and 85 there is a decrease in maximum inspiratory pressure, maximum voluntary ventilation and FEV1. Impaired diaphragmatic strength impacts on force of coughing. Degeneration of elastic fibres in the lung parenchyma leads to air space enlargement. Chest wall compliance is reduced and a rise in closing volume results in increasing *V/Q* mismatching. This whole effect has been termed 'senile emphysema' and is often accompanied by age-related β-receptor dysfunction.

Gas transfer is also affected – DLCO declines with some impairment of oxygenation (about 0.5 kPa/decade) but no discernible effect on carbon dioxide clearance. Both the hypoxic and hypercapnic respiratory control responses are blunted. Exercise capacity, as shown by V_{max}, declines by about 1% per year after the age of 30.[15–17]

Less direct intrinsic and extrinsic changes also occur that will impair respiratory function. Diminished antioxidant defences have been observed and bronchial lavage sampling shows changes in both immunoglobulin and CD4/CD8 ratios implying chronic antigenic stimulation. There is also an increasing age-related burden of problems such as nocturnal gastroesophageal reflux, kyphosis, vertebral collapse and sleep apnoea. The likelihood of environmental exposure to agents with the potential to cause lung damage, most particularly tobacco smoke, increases with age.

Hence it is predictable not only that more elderly patients will require respiratory support, but also that ventilatory weaning is going to be more challenging in this group. Mortality is also likely to be higher as compared with younger populations. An American study confirms that the likelihood of requiring ventilation does increase with age, with an estimated 10% chance in the over-75s.[18] Amongst those who are ventilated mortality in the over-70s is nearly double that in the under-40s,[19] and there is a high 3-year mortality in those discharged from ICU with 57% of deaths occurring early after discharge.[20] This bleaker picture is offset to some extent in those with chronic obstructive airways disease; patients with acute exacerbations have a lower mortality at 28% as compared with other causes of respiratory failure. Nevertheless, even amongst ICU survivors in this group, the extent of premorbid problems and the need for ongoing care at discharge dictates outcome; if they were not fit to go directly home then mortality is higher[21] and a high proportion will still need help with at least one activity of daily living, and the quality of life scores are low – though not necessarily lower than they were premorbidly.

RENAL

Kidney size becomes smaller with age due to a reduction in the number of nephrons; 20–30% of glomeruli become sclerotic and glomerular filtration rate may diminish by 50% by 80 years of age. However, this is neither consistent nor predictable.[22] Not only does creatinine clearance start to decline from the fourth decade of life but renal blood flow also decreases by about 10% per decade. Tubular exchange of sodium and hydrogen ions is also reduced, with impaired ability to handle fluid loads and academia. Rarely is this ever seen as a clinical or biochemical entity, but it does represent a reduction in reserve capacity and manifests only when acute stressors are applied. In the elderly, the competing needs of the kidney versus the heart make the treatment of incipient failure of either organ problematic, and failure of one organ can cause failure of the other – this has been termed 'cardiorenal syndrome'.[23]

The risk of developing acute renal failure increases with age and is especially associated with co-morbidities such as cardiac failure and renovascular disease and acquired preconditions such as known nephrotoxic drugs, surgical interventions and sepsis. Obstructive uropathy may be a consequence of the increasing prevalence of prostatic disease. Many drugs have been implicated, but non-steroidal analgesics and ACE inhibitors stand out. Surgery involves acute changes to blood pressure and volume status, but carries the additional risk of abdominal hypertension.

There is an attributable mortality associated with acute kidney injury, though it is difficult to tease out. It appears that this may be similar between the young and the old[24] and has been variously quoted at between 15 and 40%. The outcome from acute renal failure is determined by cause and prior functional status, with drug-related renal failure doing better than most other causes. The mean survival of octogenarians after an episode of acute renal failure was 19 months, but complete recovery of renal function occurs in just over half the survivors.[25] In one study, only 3 out of 23 biopsies of acute kidney injury showed evidence of acute tubular necrosis.[26] Those with pre-existing chronic renal failure are seven times more likely to progress to long-term dialysis.[27]

A secondary but important effect in the elderly is that there is often a reduced ability to excrete drugs. The consequence may be prolonged half-life (by a factor of 1.4), altered volumes of distribution (+24%) and reduced clearance.[28] This is probably a source of excess morbidity in the elderly.

LIVER

This is relatively unaffected and has huge intrinsic reserve so that a reduced mass of up to 30% at 80 years probably has little effect, other than loss of reserve. There is a tendency to reduced liver blood flow by up to 40% at 80 years and also reduced metabolic function, in particular demethylation and the production of cholinesterase. It may have some effect on drug handling, but is rarely of clinical relevance.

It is acquired liver disease (most commonly cirrhosis) that is the potent predictor of mortality and this has a peak age of presentation in the sixth or seventh decades of life. Nevertheless, age itself is not a poor prognostic indicator in the context of patients with cirrhosis requiring intensive care.[29]

CENTRAL NERVOUS SYSTEM

There is often some decline in cognitive performance with age, though this is contentious. Memory loss is apparent in 10% of those over 70 years of age and about half of these are due to some variant of Alzheimer's disease. This incidence doubles with each decade.[9] The neurocognitive decline is multifactorial but is associated with cerebral vasculopathy, decline in sex steroids, neurochemical alterations such as melatonin and sleep disorders, which are common in the elderly. Dementia has strong associations with cerebral vascular pathology and strokes, but previous head injury is also important. A new era of dementia treatment is imminent and may alter the ICU perspective about the irreversibility of this condition.

Unsurprisingly, patients with neurocognitive decline are much more likely to experience delirium, which is defined as 'an acute confusional state that occurs in the face of an underlying organic aetiology'. It is distinguished from dementia both by the speed of onset and by changes in the level of consciousness. Up to two-thirds of patients aged over 65 years experience delirium in hospital and, in the ICU, one-third of patients are admitted with it and one-third develop it following admission.[30] Clinically, it has a broad spectrum of presentation from inattention, disorientation and agitation through to apathy, immobility and depression. Coma, sedatives and infection are risk factors but other pharmacological agents, noise, light and other sleep-disturbing factors may all be important.[31] It is common after major surgery and trauma, occurring in up to 60% of patients after hip fracture. Many ICU patients develop delirium and in some it will persist as cognitive dysfunction for years. It lengthens hospital stay and is an independent predictor of 6-monthly mortality.[32]

Age is a risk factor for persistent psychological issues and part of this may be related to post-traumatic stress disorder.

Psychological assessment of the elderly post intensive care is in its infancy. Delirium is common and often persistent. The existing tools for assessing delirium are the Confusion Assessment Method for ICU (CAM-ICU) and Intensive Care Delirium Screening Checklist (ICDSC). An ICDSC score of more than 4 correlates with both increased mortality and, in survivors, persistent cognitive dysfunction. More recently the 10-risk-factor assessment tool PREdiction of DELIRium in ICu patients (PRE-DELIRIC) has been validated for ICU.[33] Awareness of the problem should lower the threshold for diagnosis and then these scores, which have been hard to implement, may be used more widely. Anecdotally, the families of elderly patients discharged home often report behavioural and other changes that imply long-lasting sequelae.

METABOLIC

Over the age of 70 there is a tendency for weight loss with a general change in body composition, leading to increased fat and reduced muscle mass. This sarcopenia is manifested by a 30% reduction in main muscle group strength by the 7th decade of life.[34] With less musculoskeletal activity, there is less energy use, less heat production and a reduced calorie requirement with a 2% decrease in basal metabolic rate (BMR) per decade. Protein requirements stay broadly the same.

Malnutrition is common and calorific intake is often inadequate. This 'anorexia of ageing' is multifactorial and is not just psychosocial – there are some fundamental physiological changes: early satiation is common and gastric emptying is delayed with the feeling of fullness suppressing ghrelin thereby reducing appetite, as do raised cholecystokinin levels, which are also common. Dehydration and micronutrient deficiencies are also frequent; loss of water-soluble vitamins such as thiamine with diuretic therapy, folate and vitamins A, C and E deficiency and vitamin B12 deficiency due to atrophic gastritis and reduced intrinsic factor secretion.[35]

Weight loss, frailty and reduced functional capacity will predispose to morbidity, complications, survival and in survivors reduce the ability to regain independence.

SPECIAL CONSIDERATIONS

In many ways the elderly have the same requirements as any other intensive care unit patient. The lack of functional reserve has been described above under the relevant organ or physiological system headings, but there are some other areas that require special consideration.

PHARMACOLOGY

There are marked changes in pharmacokinetics and pharmacodynamics in the elderly. The impaired ability of the kidneys to excrete drugs influences drug half-lives, which may be prolonged. The volume of distribution may also either increase or decrease depending on the drug and changes in body composition.[28] For example, the aminoglycosides may not only achieve higher concentrations than predicted through distribution changes, but also remain higher for longer due to impaired excretion. NSAIDs may have profound and potentially toxic effects by the potent combination of a relatively smaller volume of distribution and the possibility of relative dehydration producing high drug levels; the associated drug-related inhibition of the prostaglandins would promote renal vasoconstriction, reducing renal blood flow and resulting in renal toxicity.

There may be changes in sensitivity to drugs, partly through altered pharmacokinetics as described, or through interaction with physiology such as the decline in sensitivity to beta-adrenergic agonists and antagonists with age. By a similar mechanism the incidence of orthostatic hypotension with antihypertensive drugs increases. The central nervous system, however, becomes more sensitive to centrally acting drugs.

Fluid management must incorporate some general considerations. These include the potential presence of both cardiovascular and renal impairment (cardiorenal syndrome), a reduced flexibility in cardiac output and an increasing dependence on alterations in systemic vascular resistance. This, along with changes in body composition, may alter fluid distribution. However, it is unpredictable across the population and so should be assessed in the individual.

The biggest single problem in the pharmacology of the elderly is poly-pharmacy. Elderly patients will often be on a panoply of medications depending on their chronic health problems. Most drugs have side-effects and interactions and, as the number of medications increases, so too does the likelihood of complications from their use – especially when the patient is ill. The classic example is antihypertensive drugs in the elderly causing postural hypotension. There is a literature relating to the role of poly-pharmacy in hospital and ICU admission with two very different mechanisms: firstly, the drugs being the source of the problem and, secondly, the impact of inadvertent discontinuation of important medications.[36] It is not a minor issue and an important part of the assessment of the elderly should be rationalisation of medication.

SURGICAL OUTCOME

Increasing numbers of elderly patients are having increasingly complex surgery performed upon them. Both operative mortality and postoperative complications are higher in the elderly and again relate to existence of co-morbid disease and lack of physiological reserve. The fitter the patient, the less likely he/she is to experience complications and this is true for both cardiac and non-cardiac surgery.[37, 38] One study in the over-80s showed that 6-month mortality rates after ICU discharge were 30% for planned surgical patients compared with 76% for emergency surgical patients.[39] Elderly patients presenting as emergencies have been eloquently described as 'a heterogeneous cohort of both potentially treatable patients and those who are dying'.[40] Distinguishing the treatable from the futile is difficult across all age groups but particularly so in the elderly where limited life expectancy is usual and severe but unrecognised co-morbidity may exist. Committing patients and their families to emotional and physical hardship is clearly justifiable with a good outcome, but

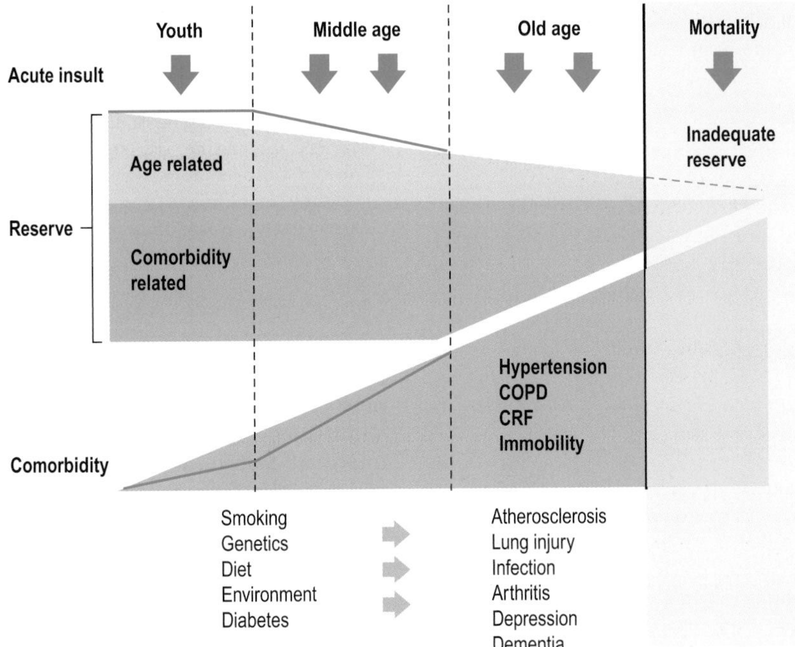

Figure 12.2 Factors affecting ICU outcome. COPD, chronic obstructive pulmonary disease; CRF, chronic renal failure.

far harder to defend if the outcome was never likely to be good. The patient's wishes or preferences should ideally be taken into account, but frequently that is not possible. This is an area of practice that has not been studied but anecdotally is very poorly managed.

ICU OUTCOME

How the interaction between age itself, the severity of the acute illness, or the accumulated co-morbidities and declining functional status due to ageing affects ICU outcome is uncertain (**Fig. 12.2**). APACHE scoring attributes only 7% of the outcome predictive power to age alone. Nevertheless, in some studies of ICU admissions, increasing age does appear to be independently associated with higher 30-day hospital mortality.[41] One study suggests that, for the over-80s, half will not survive ICU but half the survivors will be alive 2 years later.[42] Intuitively, the pre-morbid functional status and presence of co-morbidities should significantly affect ICU outcome. Even supposedly soft indicators such as coming from a care home was associated with higher in-hospital mortality and the medium-term mortality at 6 months is also increased if the patient is discharged to care facilities.[20] In a study of over 15 000 elderly patients compared with non-elderly ICU admissions, the elderly were more likely to have greater co-morbid illnesses and higher illness severity scores, which led to a higher ICU mortality and these patients were more likely to be discharged to either rehabilitation or long-term care.[43] Conversely, other studies have failed to find an association between outcome and pre-existing co-morbidities or functional status.[44]

Age itself is not a useful prognostic indicator and its use as a surrogate for general status is unpredictable. Nevertheless, it is possible to conclude that the outcome for elderly patients admitted to ICU is poorer than for younger patients, but that outcome relates to the pre-morbid state, the severity of the acute illness and the presence of an underlying fatal illness, as in other populations.[42]

Quality of life is probably a more relevant factor than survival. Most patients will have significant functional disability on ICU discharge, which may improve although the evidence is difficult to interpret. In general, those experiencing major acute events with little pre-existing co-morbidities report a substantially lower quality of life afterwards compared with those with significant pre-existing co-morbidities and this is most probably due to relatively lower expectations in the latter group. It is a contentious area with some studies showing no real impairment in quality of life whereas others show significant decline in quality of life.[45]

Probably the best indicators of real outcome for the elderly are measures such as returning home, which has rarely been assessed but is often a very important consideration for the individual. Conti and colleagues assessed this with the results seen in **Box 12.2**; this approach is probably more relevant than mortality figures.[46]

In the future there needs to be more focus on both physical and mental functionality as an outcome

Box 12.2 Factors that influence elderly patients getting home from ICU[46]

Important factors
Over 75 years of age
Neoplasia
Chronic heart failure
Neurological or neurosurgical cause for admission
Trauma
Respiratory failure
Cardiology
Neurological complication
Cardiological complication
Haematological complication
Surgical complication
Less important factors
Planned surgery
Visceral surgery
Chronic renal disease
Living alone

From Conti M, Friolet R, Eckert P, Merlani P. Home return 6 months after an intensive care unit admission for elderly patients. Acta Anaesthesiol Scand 2011;55:387–93, with permission.

measure. Patients need to be not only alive but also have reasonable functional status and ideally be able to return home.

ASSESSMENT FOR ADMISSION

Premorbid functionality and the severity of co-morbid illnesses is of paramount importance when deciding on suitability for admission. This must be put in the context of the acute insult and an analysis of whether the disease process is reversible and if the patient is salvageable. If not then the application of intensive care is likely to impose a physical and mental burden on the patient and their family that cannot be justified by the likely negative outcome. Objective decision making is problematic and it is worth noting that physicians may overestimate the mental and functional status of patients accepted for admission and underestimate it for those whose admission is rejected.[47] Age has little role to play in this decision other than its association with physiological decline and the acquisition of co-morbidity. It is also worth remembering that many elderly patients will have one form or another of advanced directive.

HISTORY

This should involve speaking to the patient or, if impossible, to their relatives to make an assessment of their previous functionality physically and mentally. Establish whether co-morbidities are present and if so how severe. Determine whether the patient is living at home or in a home and how independent he/she is. Living in a nursing home may sometimes, but not always, be a surrogate for significant functional impairment.[43] In the elderly nursing home population anaemia, cancer, heart failure, renal failure and COPD are all related to poor 1-year outcome. For those with previous hospital admissions a history of ventilation is also a potentially important feature. There is a need to know the physical and mental trajectory over the last few months or years, which may indicate significant functional decline. Details relating to level of activity (house, room, chair or bed bound) are powerful indicators (**Box 12.3**).

Box 12.3 History

Where do they live – at home or in care
Independence – how much support
Mobility – shopping, walking
Memory – confusion, sleeping pattern
Previous hospital admissions – in particular ventilation or chronic renal failure
Co-morbidity – respiratory, cardiology and neurology, but also arthritis and mobility
Drugs
Patient's preferences if known

CLINICAL SIGNS

The general habitus is revealing. Posture, muscle bulk, or more often wasting, and the condition of the skin all help indicate long-term physical well-being or otherwise. Ill-health is a potent cause of self-neglect and so the state of the teeth, the lower legs and the feet are very important indicators. Peripheral oedema and infection indicate potential co-morbidities, while chest wall shape may suggest chronic airways disease. Movement and agility are less easily evaluated in acute conditions, but again some impression can be gained by the factors above. Likewise, mental acuity may be difficult to assess in the acute situation.

All of these come together to provide a picture of the level of normal functionality and the degree of co-morbid illnesses, and how they may be contributing to the acute presentation. Then the acute nature of the presentation needs to be evaluated and its reversibility taken in the context of the other problems. The patient's preferences, either declared or previously informed, are a very important part of this assessment. Most importantly no individual part of this should overwhelm all other considerations and age itself is the least relevant factor.

TREATMENT INTENSITY

Elderly patients now present more frequently, have fewer co-morbidities and are more acutely unwell than in the past. They are also more likely to undergo more intensive treatment and are more likely to survive, although the intensity of their treatment may not match that offered to younger patients.[48,49] The conclusion is that high-intensity treatment is appropriate and can produce good results but careful patient selection is key. In a study that followed more than 1 million elderly patients after a diagnosis of serious illness, half were admitted to ICU at some point and, of these, two-thirds were still alive 6 months later.[8]

However, 3% of this cohort accounted for 23% of ICU usage.

EXPECTATIONS AND PREFERENCES

Paradoxically the aim of treating the elderly in the ICU may be more attainable than with younger patients as they may already have adapted to a burden of co-morbid disease and disability and have limited expectations when compared with young previously fit patients. End of life increasingly occurs in a hospital setting, despite the fact that 86% of patients would prefer to die at home, and therefore the level of medical intervention that elderly patients would want is relevant. Only 16% would take life-prolonging drugs if they made them feel worse and most would want palliation even if it shortened life. Most would not want to be put on a ventilator to gain a week of life and the numbers were similar if it were for a month of extra life.[50] Of those octogenarians who survive ICU, half declared they would not want ICU treatment again if it were required.[51] However, one must be careful about making assumptions in this group of patients. The SUPPORT study showed a poor understanding by physicians of patients' preferences[52] and further declared that, despite the fact that more than half of over-70-year-olds would want CPR most physicians substantially underestimated this.[53]

In 1999, Singer and colleagues identified the following as being most important to patients:

- receiving adequate pain and symptom management
- avoiding inappropriate prolongation of dying
- achieving a sense of control
- relieving burden on others
- strengthening their relationship with loved ones.[54]

END OF LIFE

Death in ICU is usually through some form of withdrawal. Only 10% of patients dying in ICU die through failed CPR. Limitation of life support is very common, as is either withdrawing or withholding treatment. There is huge variation in practice between countries, not only in the decision process but also in the issuing of 'Do Not Resuscitate' orders, and the modes of withdrawal and withholding treatment.[55]

Patient preferences are very important, as is physician recognition of medical futility. Key to this area of management is a clear view of what ICU is intended to provide, an understanding of whether the goals are achievable and acceptance that subjecting a patient and their family to the unpleasant rigours of ICU in the sure knowledge that it will achieve no useful outcome is unacceptable. These determinations must be made objectively.

CONCLUSION

The APACHE score demonstrates that most predictive power for outcome is derived from the acute physiological condition; a much smaller component was the admission disease, 13.6%, and age only constituted about 7%.[41] The nature of the acute condition and the severity of co-morbid disease play a far greater part than the known physiological changes that accompany ageing, and thus absolute age itself. The reversibility of these factors should guide management, and this approach is the same for any patient of any age. It is more likely that an older patient will have advance directives and so will have already voiced their personal preferences.

A simplistic view is that intensive care entails reversing an acute episode with the intention of returning the patient to the position they were in before that episode, or close to it. The majority of treatment is supportive and provides the physiological reserve they have lost until it can be regained. Those with less reserve will need more support. The patient will invariably need a certain amount of physical reserve to meet the challenges of the treatment and the recovery. The decision to use ICU requires acknowledgement that ICU has negative as well as positive aspects and that it can be a very unpleasant experience with far-reaching sequelae, both physical and mental, for patients and relatives. Justification is provided by a good outcome so it is implicit that the opinion at the time of admission is that full recovery is possible or indeed probable. As in every other population, appropriate use of intensive care can produce impressive results but inappropriate use can be disastrous for the patient and their family. Age itself is not a contraindication.

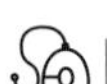
Access the complete references list online at http://www.expertconsult.com

2. Martin JE, Sheaff MT. The pathology of ageing: concepts and mechanisms. J Pathol 2007;211:111–13.
5. Bagshaw SM, Webb SA, Delaney A, et al. Very old patients admitted to intensive care in Australia and New Zealand: a multi-centre cohort analysis. Crit Care 2009;13:R45.
6. Wunsch H, Angus DC, Harrison DA, et al. Variation in critical care services across North America and Western Europe. Crit Care Med 2008;36:2787–93.
16. Marik PE. Management of the critically ill geriatric patient. Crit Care Med 2006;34:S176–182.
42. Roch A, Wiramus S, Pauly V, et al. Long-term outcome in medical patients aged 80 or over following admission to an intensive care unit. Crit Care 2011;15:R36.

13

Health care team in intensive care medicine

Gerry O'Callaghan

The concept of health professionals working in collaboration as part of multidisciplinary teams focused on the requirements of individual patients is a well-established historical tradition.[1] This chapter outlines the benefits and effects of team participation, the characteristics of successful teams and the organisations that foster them in the context of acute health care delivery.

The specific interventions that have been applied to the intensive care setting, the composition of intensive care teams, their function and effect on patient outcome are explored. This overview is not a managerial perspective on the utility of team work in delivering improvements in productivity and quality but seeks to provide practitioners of intensive care medicine with an opportunity to reflect on the variety of ways we work in teams as part of our professional activities and responsibilities.

WHAT IS A TEAM?

Men wanted: for hazardous journey, small wages, bitter cold, long months of complete darkness, constant danger, safe return doubtful. Honour and recognition in case of success.

Sir Ernest Shackleton

The recruitment notice that Sir Ernest Shackleton is purported to have placed in the press in 1914 prior to his Endurance expedition to Antarctica is of interest not solely for its relevance to intensive care medicine, which is undoubtedly also a challenge of endurance, but as an example of the extraordinary power of shared purpose. This is particularly the case when such energy is focused by capable leadership; shared purpose is the foundation of team behaviours and success.

A team is defined as a group of people with clearly defined roles and responsibilities committed to a common purpose or task. The individuals who participate in a team share common values and commit to shared behaviours, for example low-tidal-volume ventilation for ARDS or a full-barrier technique for central venous access. The result of their collective effort is expected to produce more than they could produce working separately. The identity of the team is visible from both within and outside (**Box 13.1**).

It is of value to understand the fundamentals of team dynamics as the heterogeneity and complexity of team composition increase with the increasing array of investigations and treatments for critical illness, emerging roles for non-physician providers and participation by intensive care personnel in roles that extend beyond the traditional physical boundaries of the intensive care unit.

Figure 13.1 illustrates the diversity of individuals and skills involved in caring for critically ill patients. ICU personnel include the medical and nursing staff, allied health including physiotherapists, dieticians, pharmacists and many more. Support personnel include clerks, cleaners and others. External ICU is almost limitless including physicians, surgeons, infectious disease physicians, radiologists and more. Although local factors influence the composition and profile of these categories, the variety and complexity are constant.

The composition of critical care teams has wide regional, national and international variability. Non-physician providers are more common in North America than in the United Kingdom, Europe or Australia where advanced nurse practitioner roles are becoming more common. Such roles are well established in paediatric and neonatal medicine and are often an adjunct rather than an alternative to physicians in training resulting in improved staffing levels and continuity of patient care.[2] More than a quarter of adult academic ICUs in the United States have physician assistants and more than half have nurse practitioners as physician extenders.[3] They have a precisely defined scope of practice, and may order tests, prescribe medications and perform diagnostic and therapeutic procedures under the supervision or on behalf of a nominated responsible physician or surgeon. In a recent review of the impact of non-physician providers on patient outcomes in critical care, there were the following observations.[4]

- Inadequate numbers of qualified intensive care physicians mean that such roles are currently necessary.
- Workforce planning indicates this is likely to remain the case for the foreseeable future.
- There is no evidence that non-physician providers are less safe or effective.
- Non-physician providers contribute important increased capacity in additional areas of intensive care activity such as quality improvement.

The increasing diversity of clinical roles and complexity of therapies (e.g. extracorporeal membrane oxygenation) require that frameworks for improved communication and coordination as well as role delineation have become essential. This view has been endorsed for over a decade by a wide range of professional, academic and government bodies such as The Institute of Medicine, which recommended in To Err is Human, Building a Safer Health System that those who work in teams should train in teams.[5] There is an emerging literature that demonstrates improved outcomes across a range of parameters following implementation of various team-based interventions predominantly using simulation as a platform for improved communication. These innovations are examined later in this chapter.

An explicit team-based approach facilitates continuity of care and effective transfer of information between teams contributing to patient care during the patient's hospital journey. The Australian Commission for Safety and Quality in Health Care describes this transfer of information, accountability and professional responsibility for some or all aspects of care for a patient to another person or professional group on a temporary or permanent basis as clinical handover.[6]

Figure 13.2 illustrates the varying and often asynchronous frequencies of shift changes between nursing, resident and intensive care consultant staff challenging safe and effective continuity of patient care.

The OSSIE Guide to Clinical Handover Improvement summarises the risks to patient safety posed by this high-volume activity as well as providing tools for clinical practice improvement and a comprehensive literature review.[6] Clinical handover is a common cause of adverse events and malpractice claims. It is often of poor quality, infrequently written and generally perceived to be inadequate or unhelpful. A team-based structured approach to handover called the SBAR (situation–background–assessment–recommendation) technique can address these issues effectively.[7]

Much of the language and methodology informing the development of effective teamwork is from a corporate culture that is now being implemented in large health care organisations around the world. The driver for developing effective team-based behaviours is patient safety with strong advocacy and resource allocation from such organisations as the Institute for

Box 13.1 Characteristics of a team

- Common goals
- Shared behaviours and values
- Visible identity
- Clear understanding of roles and responsibilities
- Greater collective than individual effectiveness or potential
- Understanding of shared tools and artefacts such as vocabulary, skills, knowledge
- Mutual trust and respect: solidarity

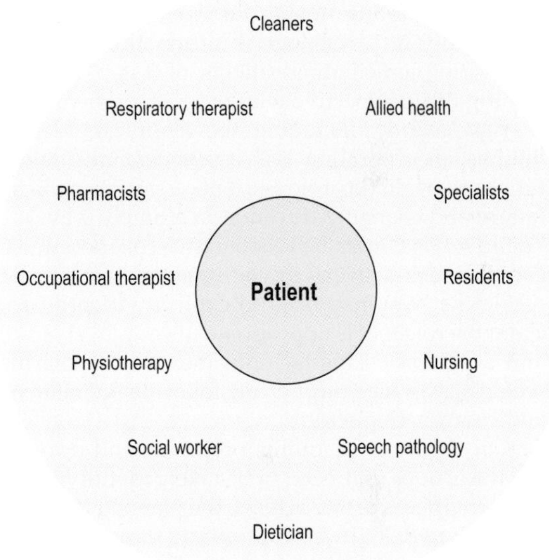

Figure 13.1 The clinical and ancillary care of patients in intensive care is provided by large diverse teams of health care workers. The size, diversity, variability and complexity of these teams make common training in non-technical skills highly desirable.

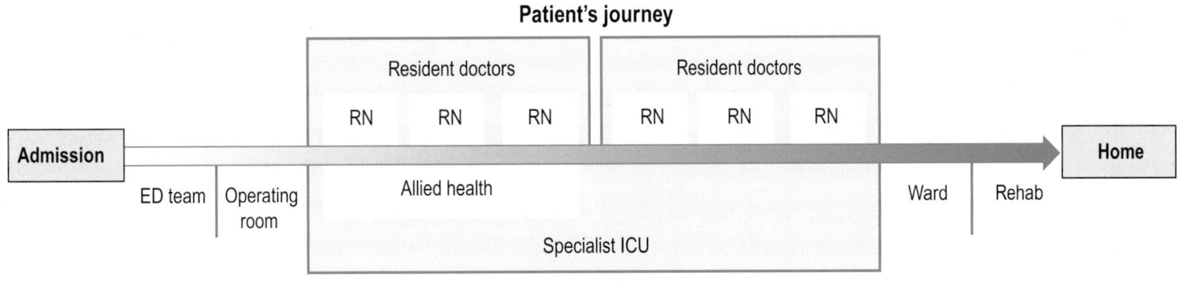

Figure 13.2 Continuity of patient care is the seamless provision of care, transfer of information and communication with relevant stakeholders over time and across multiple locations during a patient's hospitalisation or illness. ED=emergency department; RN=registered nurse.

Health Improvement, the National Health System in the UK, and the Australian Commission for Safety and Quality in Health Care. This derives from the improvements in safety and efficacy demonstrated by team training in the airline industry, the crew resource management (CRM). This is a simulation-based programme that teaches and assesses individual performance of the 'non-technical skills' necessary for effective delivery of complex technical tasks, particularly in high-stress situations. These can be defined as 'the cognitive, social, and personal resource skills that complement technical skills, and contribute to safe and efficient task performance'.[8] The teaching framework has four elements:

- *Situation awareness:* understanding and anticipating the impact of the specific situation on the performance of workers and patient outcome. Examples include requesting further information, confirming the validity of physiological information, checking monitoring, anticipating patients' next steps and confirming this perspective with other team members.
- *Decision making:* including the ability to identify options, incorporating risk assessment and taking time to re-evaluate progress, if necessary recognising failure and changing direction in a timely way.
- *Team work and leadership:* cooperative collaboration in complex task delivery in your assigned role, recognising that you may need to explicitly identify and claim the role that is appropriate to your level of skill and experience. This includes information sharing, seeking assistance, supporting fellow team members and coordinating efforts.
- *Task management:* planning, preparing and prioritising the actions that need to be taken, identifying the resources necessary to achieve the planned tasks and performing them to an appropriate standard.

Tactical thinking is thinking focused on particular tasks. Strategic thinking is a broader consideration of the needs of the patient, team members and organisational requirements and is the responsibility of the team leader.

A training programme based on this approach has been developed for anaesthetists called Anesthetists' Non-Technical Skills (ANTS). Extensive task analysis describing the language and behaviours specific to situations encountered by anaesthetists formed the basis for identifying markers of good or bad performance that could used for assessment.[8] (For details see the website address www.abdn.ac.uk/iprc/ants.)

Rolling out a promising innovation is challenging:

1. It is essential to have a critical mass of course providers who have a sound understanding of the psychology of human performance, the methodology and language of non-technical skills, and the teaching and assessment of colleagues and trainees. Where this is not the case there are unacceptable levels of inter-rater reliability and accuracy.[9]
2. Sustainability of benefit has been shown where training is provided in a similar manner to the CRM programmes in the aviation industry.[10] The authors' recommendation is for a minimum ANTS course length of 2 days to acquire sufficient knowledge and the techniques required. This is an indicator of the organisational support necessary.
3. It provides an insight as to why it is difficult to demonstrate benefit on patient outcomes when few health care providers have the skills or experience necessary to plan and measure the quantum of team building required to address the relevant clinical issue (**Box 13.2**).

Organisational psychology can be used to analyse and assess team dynamics. In one study the communication interactions between 2500 team members for periods of time were reviewed measuring tone of voice, body position relative to other team members, and how much gesturing, talking, listening and interrupting took place.[11] Team communication was categorised in three ways:

- *energy:* how members contribute to a team as a whole
- *engagement:* how members communicate with one another
- *exploration:* how teams communicate with one another.

Team behaviour and patterns of communication were consistent across different contexts and compositions (i.e. different industries including health care workers and a variety of different team sizes). The quantity and quality of interactions can be measured, face-to-face interactions being the most valuable and email or texting the least. Individual talent and reasoning are

Box 13.2 Characteristics of high-performing teams

Leadership that encourages participation from other team members
Effective decision making, clear, transparent, timely and consultative
Open and clear communication
Valuing diversity, welcoming diversity of experience, culture and knowledge
Mutual trust, committing to shared actions and strategies
Managing conflict – dealing with conflict openly and transparently, avoiding the gradual build-up of internal tensions and grudges
Clear goals that have personal meaning and relevance, supported by sharing data and resources
Defined roles and responsibilities – team members understand what they must do and must not
Coordinative relationship, strong bonds between team members supporting frequent interactions
Positive atmosphere, team culture that is open, transparent and positive and believes in the reality of success

Source: www.en.wikipedia.org/wiki/High-Performance.

less important than adopting successful communication patterns.

Successful teams share several defining characteristics:

1. Everyone on the team talks and listens in roughly equal measure, keeping contributions short.
2. Members face one another and their conversations and gestures are energetic.
3. Members connect directly with one another and not just with the team leader.
4. Members carry on back channel or side conversations within the team.
5. Members periodically break, go outside the team and bring information back.

Successful team participation can be learned, and advantage can be taken of the multiple opportunities that present themselves for team working. Critical care physicians are generally expected to take on leadership roles, but few physicians receive any formal training in this area.

A simple checklist can be used for assessing team interactions with colleagues:

- Are my co-workers contributing to ward rounds and patient-centred discussions?
- Do they speak generally or just to one other person?
- Are individuals removing themselves from the group or not facing other team members when they are speaking or listening?
- Am I or the other leadership figures too dominant, speaking too much or too loudly?
- Does everyone get to finish sentences or are people interrupted and cut off?
- Am I (we) happy for any individual team member to speak on behalf of the team?

This final question is a test of mutual trust and respect because it involves accepting reputational risk on behalf of co-workers.

Organisations' attempts to create a high-performance team culture may fail because of:

- insufficient appreciation of the resolve, expertise and resources required to achieve cultural change
- advocacy for team-based training being promotional rather than a full commitment
- provision of insufficient time, opportunity, resources or executive support.

Similar issues have been demonstrated in the implementation of clinical therapeutic guidelines.

NECESSARY OR DESIRABLE ORGANISATIONAL CHARACTERISTICS THAT SUPPORT EFFECTIVE IMPROVEMENT IN CLINICAL PRACTICE AND PATIENT OUTCOMES

Bohmer characterised the four habits of high-value health care organisations[12] (defined as organisations that achieve value in terms of the ratio of long-term outcomes to costs):

1. *Specify and plan in advance:* with decisions based on predetermined explicit criteria
2. *Deliberate design of infrastructure:* including clinical microsystems that align physical environment, business process and clinical pathways in well-defined patient populations
3. *Measurement and oversight targeting:* by predefined metrics, quality and safety goals, which inculcates both accountability and performance
4. *Self-study:* using measurement so that knowledge, data and clinical information can be used not only for assurance of best evidence-based practices but also to identify deviations. Information is shared and not considered to be the property of individuals or departments.

Organisational readiness is a prerequisite to building high-performance critical care teams.

TYPES OF TEAM

A *clinical microsystem* is the most fundamental unit of health care delivery that addresses the needs of a population of patients. It is the dynamic integration of personnel, clinical and support staff, technology, information, care and business processes.[13] Implicit is the participation of all those who have direct patient care responsibilities (**Fig. 13.3**). Participation is compulsory and is the baseline of team participation in the unit, but most participants will also be involved in other team types within this structure. The choice/volition of the

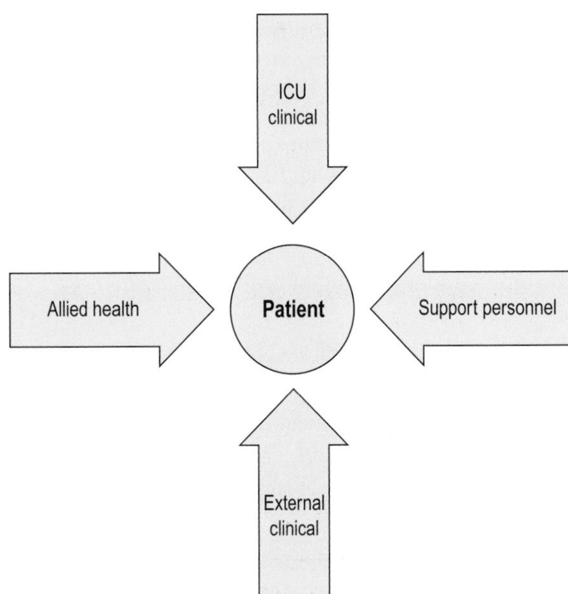

Figure 13.3 Clinical microsystems are the most fundamental units of health care delivery that address the needs of a specific population of patients. This system includes personnel, procedures, business processes and infrastructure.

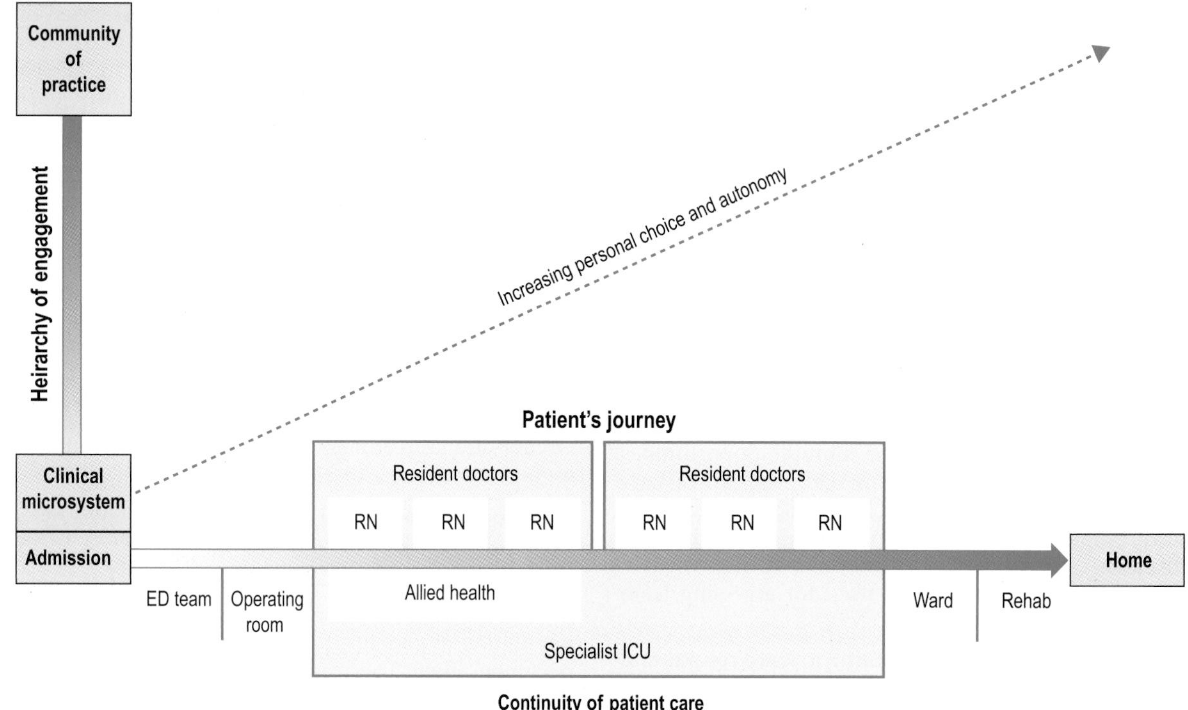

Figure 13.4 The hierarchy of individual integration of team participation represents the relationship between the interests and skills of an individual and the necessary activities that support a clinical microsystem such as an intensive care unit. Activities that are not directly related to patient care provide an opportunity for personnel to choose those activities that are of greatest professional interest. ED=emergency department; RN=registered nurse.

individual within teams is variable. The greater the clinical focus of the team or activity the less choice individuals have in terms of choosing to participate. Resuscitation, diagnosis and treatment are core team activities, while research, safety and quality, administration provide opportunity for choices that align with the interests and expertise of the individual. Collaborations beyond the immediate clinical microsystem in the hospital, professional, interdisciplinary and academic worlds have the greatest degree of choice. Team contexts are relevant to the broad understanding of health care teams.

CRITICAL INCIDENT RESPONSE TEAMS

Medical emergency teams, code and trauma teams need skills designed to meet the crisis, such as airway management, insertion of central venous lines and trauma management. Teams may be nurse or physician led, are highly focused on a single task and often include individuals who interact infrequently owing to the rarity of certain events or the rostering practice. The membership of such teams is highly dynamic, opportunities for training limited and the level of familiarity with local procedures, policies and organisational characteristics varies with the individual team member (**Fig. 13.4**).

Leadership by an easily identifiable authority figure, who has both accountability and responsibility for the outcome, enables the application of well-defined clinical pathways or protocols. This leadership is variously described as top-down, autocratic or transactional[14] and has been demonstrated to improve both process metrics and patient outcomes (**Fig. 13.5**).

ACTIVITY- OR CONTEXT-RELATED TEAMS

These may be described as committees, working groups or parties with variable degrees of formality and stability. These range from ad hoc conversations or correspondence between senior clinicians to formalised adverse event reporting to a committee. The latter has defined terms of reference, meets regularly, keeps records and may be multidisciplinary from both within and outside the ICU and involves clinical governance. They may be temporary, such as implementing a new treatment, or consist of well-established groups responsible for monitoring and communicating clinical outcomes to their peers on a range of clinical indicators. **Figure 13.6** illustrates examples of such clinical contexts.

Critical incident and context teams (see Fig. 13.6) require and benefit from different styles of leadership. Leadership characteristics include inclusiveness, proactive mentorship of less experienced or confident team members, providing a personal example of ethical behaviour and maintaining focus of team members on

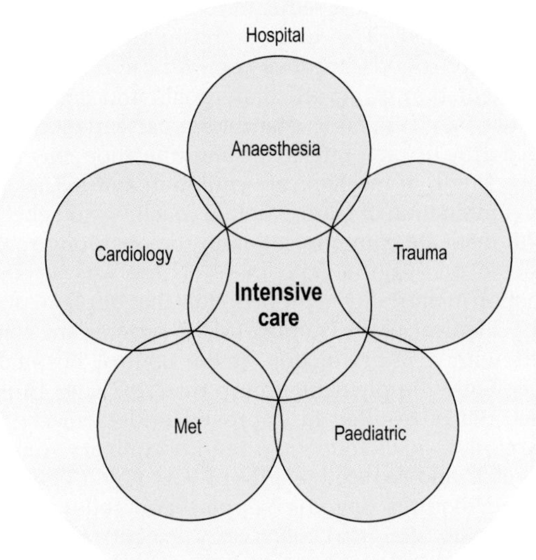

Figure 13.5 Critical incident teams are ad hoc teams of individuals from a range of clinical and professional backgrounds that assemble to meet the clinical needs of a patient experiencing acute physiological deterioration in an acute hospital setting.

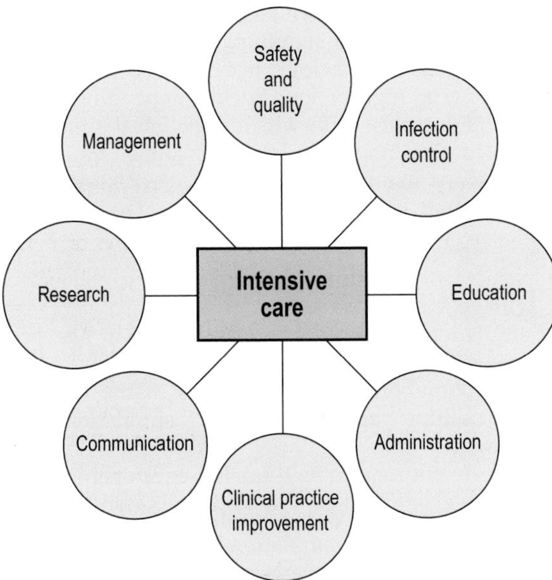

Figure 13.6 Context- or activity-based teams are comprised of individuals from a range of clinical and professional backgrounds who are collectively engaged in administrative, educational and professional activities that support clinical care.

the shared goal. This type of leadership is variously described[12] as democratic, consensus driven, empowering or transformative and is associated with improved staff commitment and participation in safety initiatives. The challenge is adequate flexibility to choose the most appropriate leadership style for each situation, adaptive leadership.

Long-term project outcomes with strong external connections require a different type of team. As such teams are informal and self-organising, often created by the commonality of learning behaviours and activities, consolidated through social interactions, they may not recognise themselves as team members. Examples include research collaboration between clinicians working with laboratory-based scientists and other experts, often from disparate geographical locations. The Community of Practice model first described by Wenger[15] can be used to examine this group. The driving characteristics of working collaborations are a shared knowledge or practice domain, workplace-based context of learning and fluctuating levels of participation. Professional development activities combined with social interaction form an ongoing mechanism that supports professional collaborations and exchange of information such as best practice tools, etc. This formal facilitation of social cohesion in professional groups is part of the community of practice model. Increasing participation and avoiding marginalisation are both important in realising and maximising colleagues' potential.

It is useful to reflect on the numerous types of teams to which intensive care practitioners may belong in order to:

- select the most suitable model for the assigned goal
- measure the overall impact on patient outcomes, staff satisfaction or other parameters
- assess and prioritise workload, taking into account the combination of team-based activities occurring in the intensive care unit.

Effective team-based practices are most commonly described in terms of organisational characteristics or leadership responsibilities, but this fails to emphasise the benefits to team members, which are summarised in **Box 13.3**. These benefits result in improved job satisfaction, which translates into improved staff retention, less sick leave, increased productivity and reduced costs.

SPECIFIC TEAM-BASED INTERVENTIONS AND INNOVATIONS

Broadly there are four categories of intervention that have been applied in critical care areas. These overlap considerably depending on the programme methodology and content.

1. Leadership
2. Team building
3. Simulation
4. Organisational change.

Box 13.3 How team members benefit from team participation

Opportunity to be heard and for effort to be acknowledged
Psychological safety
Clarity of purpose resulting in clear action plans, relevant tools and strategies
Mechanism to resolve conflict and address underperforming co-workers
More positive work environments
Support for professional development
Improved performance in time-critical stressful situations
Situational awareness

Leaders are 'visibly responsible and accountable for achieving the goals of an organisation', and are the people on whom patients and colleagues depend to get things done. The style (autocratic versus democratic) depends on the situation and may change as the situation demands (adaptive leadership). Leadership is the conglomeration of effective behaviours (see Box 13.2) enabling the team in achieving its goal.

In summary, leaders refine and define the team goal, they create a vision and subsequently they include the team in the design of the tools and mechanisms to achieve this vision. They do not avoid hard discussions and difficult decisions; they are honest about the effort and commitment necessary. They create an environment where team members feel secure and are willing to contribute. The culture they create is one of psychological safety, which is important because within teams are hierarchies. Hierarchical discrimination is very variable and has a definite cultural association, so that where there is a high level of respect or fear of authority individuals are extremely unlikely to either challenge or contribute without a specific request or mechanism to do so.

Explicit leadership behaviours such as task assignment, directing co-workers and check-backs of vital signs are associated with fewer task failures and faster instigation of therapies such as intubation and defibrillation in emergency situations. Any group implementation of training or practice improvement processes by definition creates leadership obligations and opportunities. There is no widespread leadership training intervention applied in the intensive care setting, although several studies demonstrate improved outcomes associated with intensive care specialist-led care.[16]

For example, when the impact of multidisciplinary teams on the 30-day mortality of over 100 000 intensive care patients was assessed, intensive care specialist care combined with multidisciplinary teams was associated with a 16% reduction in mortality, which was consistent across patient cohorts and greater severity of illness.[17] This benefit was similar between intensivist-led care or mandatory consult and multidisciplinary care team input, but the greatest reduction was seen when these were combined. The authors postulate that multidisciplinary rounds improve communication, enhance implementation of agreed daily goals and encourage evidence-based care (e.g. pharmacist participation may reduce drug errors). Effective communication may also reduce length of mechanical ventilation and ICU stay.

A combination of team training, coaching and checklists to instigate communication in the operating room impacted on surgical outcomes.[18] There was an 18% reduction in mortality at the hospitals that implemented the US Medical Team Training (MTT) programme compared with a 7% reduction at the control hospitals; subsequently, implementation in over 187 sites in the United States resulted in improved understanding of daily clinical goals following multidisciplinary rounds in the ICU and reduced lengths of ICU stay.[19] The programme requires ongoing support and follow-up at participating sites and mandatory executive support from site administration.

TRAINING

The TeamSTEPPS® training tool is focused on improving patient safety by implementing an evidence-based teamwork system to improve communication and teamwork skills among health care professionals.[20] It has been used in paediatric, medical and surgical ICUs to train acute care teams, reducing times to placing patients on ECMO, and decreasing the nosocomial infection rate.[21] Other team-based initiatives have reduced rates of ventilator-associated pneumonia (VAP)[22] and reduced resuscitation time in trauma situations.[23]

Simulated scenarios can be used to explore, practise and refine the tools of communication, leadership and other team-based behaviours in a clinical context. Simulation may be high or low fidelity depending on the degree of accuracy with which the clinical scenario is replicated. Training may be stand alone, specifically designed and maintained by full-time professional educators or part of a clinical workplace. The important points are:

- participation requires an active choice to collaborate with colleagues
- simulation is an educational tool that has both strengths and limitations
- many common clinical situations in the intensive care setting are suitable for simulation-based training
- most do not require high-fidelity equipment, but do require expert and experienced facilitators.[24]

Using case-based or simulation-based learning, there were significant improvements in leadership, team coordination and verbalising situational information in the intervention group and improved scores for clinical management.[25] Similar results were seen in the paediatric intensive care setting, where most found participation to be of benefit and with a highly effective impact.[26] The authors indicated that there is not only a 6- to 12-month learning curve in programme implementation but repeated exposure is necessary to achieve meaningful benefit.

ORGANISATIONAL CHANGE

This is the final area of intervention. It includes teamwork, simulation and leadership training but the context in which the team model operates is important.[27] The Integrated Team Effectiveness Model (ITEM) illustrates how organisational contexts, such as processes, goals, structure have a direct effect on team effectiveness. The Breakthrough Collaborative Model uses organisational engagement and team alignment to a particular goal to achieve significant changes in clinical outcomes.[28] Such an intervention resulted in a significant increase in the rate of organ donation as measured by both donor identification and consent for donation. Teams use plan-do-study-act (PDSA) cycles to implement change in local practices supported by a senior clinical leader. Each team is provided with strategies and tools for change and participates in educational conferences, which allows the more successful strategies to be shared and adopted more broadly. These educational opportunities foster team development and identify clinical leaders. Although effective in accelerating clinical change these large-scale interventions are expensive and require widespread government, professional and health care organisation support (**Box 13.4**).

SUMMARY

Team-based innovation in the specific context of high-acuity environments such as the intensive care unit is increasing around the world (**Fig. 13.7**). There is an

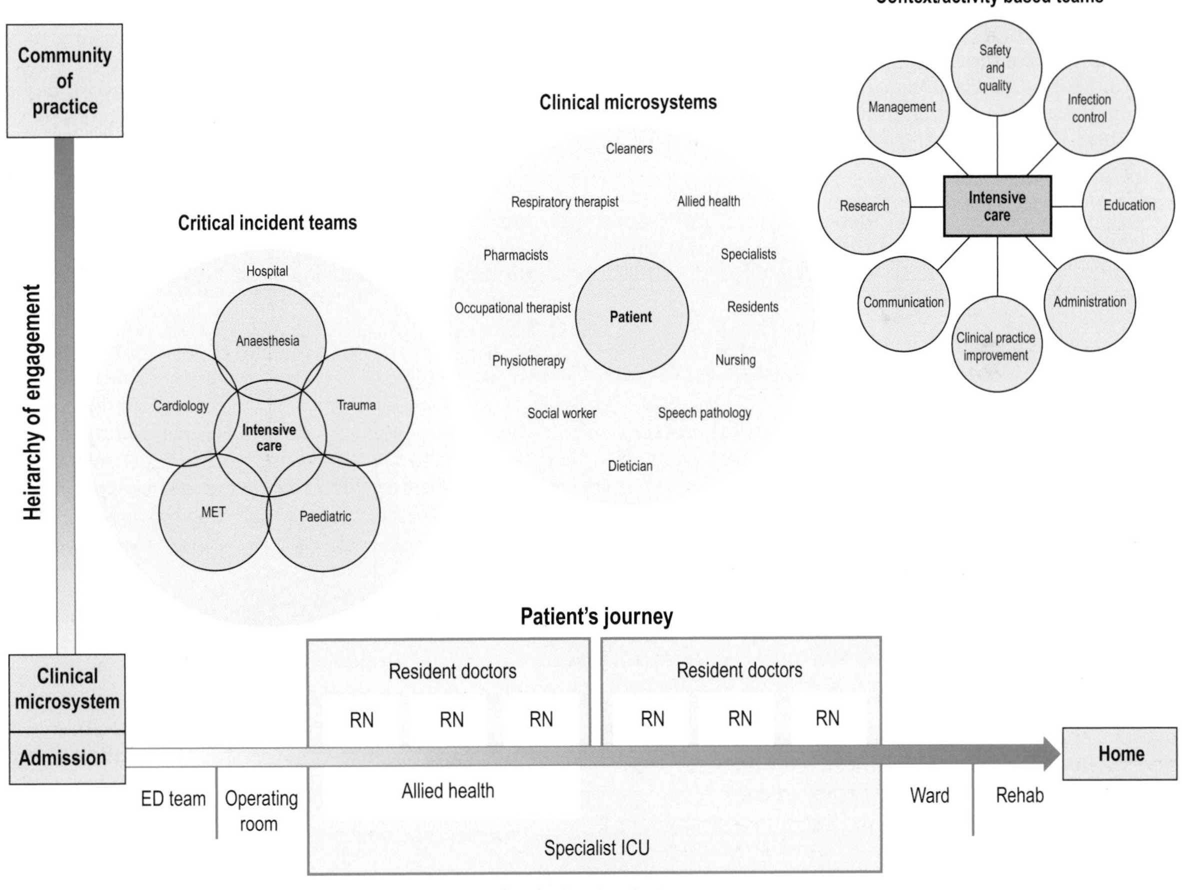

Figure 13.7 Participation in teams which provide specific aspects of clinical care, support professional development and improve quality of care are important articulations of personal preference and autonomy. Such choices are likely to represent important opportunities to increase staff satisfaction and retention and increase system capacity by matching skills and experience with personal interests. ED=emergency department; RN=registered nurse.

Box 13.4 How patients may benefit from team-based health care delivery

Improved continuity of care
Fewer adverse events
Shorter lengths of hospitalisation and mechanical ventilation
Better task delivery in emergency situations
Decreased mortality
Improved family outcomes through better communication

emerging evidence base that supports the following conclusions:

- Team-based interventions result in improved objective and subjective outcomes for patients, health care professionals and provider organisations.
- Well-developed tools, mechanisms and policies are available for the implementation and assessment of such interventions.
- Significant expertise, experience, commitment and resources are necessary to achieve potential benefits.
- The innovation or intervention should be specifically prepared or adapted for the individual circumstances in which it is to be applied.
- Sustainment of improvements in performance requires ongoing maintenance programmes.
- Research to identify the most effective strategies and tools is an appropriate priority for the academic intensive care community.
- Multidisciplinary teams of intensive care health professionals are valuable assets that need to be acknowledged and supported by the organisations in which they work.

Access the complete references list online at http://www.expertconsult.com

4. Gershengorn H, Johnson M, Factor P. The use of nonphysician providers in adult intensive care units. Am J Resp Crit Care Med 2012;185(6):600–5.
8. Flin R, Patey R, Glavin R. Anaesthetists' non-technical skills. British Journal of Anaesthesia 2010;105(1):38–44.
12. Bohmer R. The four habits of high-value health care organisations. New Eng J Med 2011;365(22):2045–7.
14. Manthous C, Hollinghead A. Team science and critical care. Am J Resp Crit Care Med 2011;184:17–25.
15. Wenger E. Communities of practice. Learning as a social system. Systems Thinker 1998;9(5):1–12.
24. Brattebo G. Education and training teamwork using simulation. In: Flatten H, Mureno R, Putensen C, et al, editors. Organisation and Management of Intensive Care. Berlin: Medizinisch Wissenschaftliche Verlagsgesellschaft; 2010:323–34.
25. Frengley R, Weller J, Torrie J. The effect of a simulation-based training intervention on the performance of established critical care unit teams. Crit Care Med 2011;39:2605–11.

14

Preparing for examinations in intensive care medicine

Carole Foot and Liz Hickson

INTRODUCTION

High-stakes postgraduate examinations in intensive care medicine (ICM) are constantly evolving; as diverse in scope as they are in structure; they have paralleled and fuelled the development of what is now a highly respected independent specialty.

For many specialist doctors, the most difficult challenge of their professional career to that point is their fellowship examination. It is viewed by many as a daunting obstacle that grants a right of passage into a fraternity of consultants who share a common commitment to excellence in managing critically ill patients.

This chapter outlines the rationale for these examination processes and their structure. It also reviews various different strategies that may be of benefit to candidates and also of relevance to their supervisors and mentors.

EXAMINATION STRUCTURE AND PROCESS

At the simplest level, professional examinations aim to differentiate candidates who are ready to progress to a higher level of recognition and responsibility. For example, in Australasia since 1979 a fellowship examination in ICM has served as part of an exit criterion to enable recognition as an Intensive Care Specialist.[1]

The challenge of such examinations is to provide a process with content that assesses multiple domains of a candidate's ability to function as a future specialist. Committees of experts in the field have traditionally worked together to devise examinations that test core specialty knowledge and skills. More recently, the importance of assessing competencies that are of more general relevance to a senior health care professional have warranted specific attention.

The CanMEDS initiative of the Royal College of Physicians and Surgeons of Canada has had a significant impact in some regions, with consideration of how to assess the seven roles of a physician: Medical expert, Communicator, Collaborator, Manager, Health Advocate, Scholar and Professional.[2] These have necessitated the inclusion of questions that test beyond pure science, such as the inclusion of role-plays to assess communication with families and other members of the multidisciplinary intensive care unit team.

An evidence-based approach to examinations is now also recognised to be important. Those responsible for credentialing specialists have the challenge of determining how to consistently provide examinations that have high levels of reliability and validity whilst remaining feasible. Issues such as examiner training, standard setting and calibrating, quarantining of candidates on the day of exams, ensuring sufficient exposure to different components of an exam to ensure adequate depth and breadth of testing and transparency of information about the structure and expectations of candidates during examinations are all important.[1, 3] Logistic considerations are of increasing importance, as the numbers of candidates pursuing specialty certification in ICM get bigger and the potential to compromise the quality of the examination process due to feasibility issues is significant. How to optimally examine clinical skills so that the best representation of workplace performance is determined is the subject of ongoing research. For example, when testing a procedural skill (management of a blocked tracheostomy tube) using a simulation as compared with a written format, it was identified that a significant number of critical errors were revealed with simulation that were not detected in a written answer.[4]

Multimodal assessment is now common in ICM examinations. The College of Intensive Care Medicine of Australia and New Zealand fellowship examination utilises a combination of written short-answer questions, vivas that include a communication station with an actor and a procedural skill station, as well as a clinical examination with 'hot cases' involving live ICU patients. The European Diploma in Intensive Care (EDIC) examination process consists of multiple-choice questions, vivas and clinical cases, although this will change to OSCEs shortly. The British Diploma consists of multiple choice questions, structured orals and OSCEs.

DIVERSITY IN ICM TRAINING AND EXAMINATION PROGRAMMES

At a global level there remains great variation in the evolution, practitioner certification and the practice of the specialty. In Europe alone, it was recently concluded that there is 'considerable diversity in pedagogic structure, processes and quality assurance of ICM' and there is 'no harmonisation among European countries'.[5]

The CoBaTrICE (Competency-Based Training in Intensive Care medicine) collaboration is committed to developing an internationally relevant curriculum.[5] The Educational Committee of the WFSICCM (World Federation of Intensive and Critical Care Medicine) supports the development of a common competency-based approach that 'permits diversity of training methods while creating a common outcome: doctors with a universal set of knowledge, skills and attitudes essential for a specialist in ICM'.[6] Although this remains a logical and worthwhile goal that could facilitate and help maintain a high standard of ICM practice, there remains a multitude of political, cultural and financial barriers to achieving this.

A lack of internationally relevant standards is also an obstacle for trainees and specialists wishing to gain experience in different countries or to relocate. It is well described that international medical graduates are at increased risk of experiencing difficulties in passing specialty examinations.[7] The reasons for this are not well described, but are likely to include language barriers, variations in practice standards between countries, isolation from training environments and a lack of knowledge and preparation regarding local examination processes.

GLOBALLY RELEVANT ISSUES REGARDING PREPARATION

Candidates approaching postgraduate examinations spent significant amounts of time preparing for these examinations and universally find the process stressful and for many there is a detrimental impact on their personal lives.[8] Never before has there been such a variety and awareness of strategies to assist the process of exam preparation. There is a paucity of literature regarding which of these many approaches trainees find of greatest utility. A recent survey of emergency medicine specialist trainees found that the most highly valued resources were: attempting practice questions, private study, small group work, a mock examination and access to a local trainer involved in exam preparation. Training courses/workshops are also well received.[9]

PREPARING ALONE

PUBLICATIONS

Training bodies commonly publish a list of recommended books and journals that may be of highest yield to candidates. Books such as this one are highly valued as they distil a vast body of literature into a highly condensed format with identification of relevant evidence underpinning critical care medicine.

Books now exist that focus more specifically on examination processes, providing advice on how to prepare for individual components and some also on how to approach the process in general (e.g. Examination Intensive Care Medicine[10] targets all of the clinical components of the Australasian CICM, EDIC and traditional UK diploma examinations).

Other books, on subjects such as critical care radiology, ECG interpretation, echocardiography and evidence-based medicine/statistics, were written to assist a wider audience but serve as great resources for exam candidates.

PRACTICE QUESTIONS

Training bodies may release past papers and repetition of questions is not uncommon. Some trainers recommend *question mapping*, whereby past papers are analysed to try to detect patterns in topic and style that may assist in predicting future questions. Questions that are answered poorly in an individual exam may be followed by retesting in subsequent ones.

Practising questions under testing conditions, with strict attention to time, may develop candidates' technique, identify gaps in knowledge and serve as variety in study methods. Specific strategies have been suggested for tackling multiple-choice papers that vary with the question type and include encouragement for intuitive guessing when negative marking penalties for incorrect answers are not used. Accessing banks of past questions is helpful (e.g. Multiple Choice Questions in Intensive Care Medicine[11]).

ONLINE RESOURCES

There are a myriad of websites that provide a wealth of material that may assist knowledge acquisition as well as focus on specific regions' exam processes. One of the major difficulties for trainees is to filter through the vast offering and identify reliable information most relevant to their context. It is important to appraise website content, but also authorship validity and the organisation of material when making an evaluation on the potential utility of a source. A considered approach analogous to critically evaluating other forms of medical literature is helpful. See **Box 14.1** for an example of one of the most comprehensive member-only websites currently on offer.

PREPARING WITH OTHERS

LOCAL/REGIONAL TRAINING PROGRAMMES

Coaching for examinations is typically part of a well-structured training programme. The degree of organisation and format of such initiatives varies widely from single institution to regional approaches. In countries where ICM training is well established such processes are well developed, whilst in others the situation is nascent. The situation is rapidly changing in some areas (**Box 14.2**).

Study groups formed from candidates working together in local areas or within large departments are

Box 14.1 Crit-IQ

Todd Fraser, Neil Orford and Kevin Murphy established this in 2008. It began as a training tool for intensive care trainees who were in the process of taking the Joint Faculty of Intensive Care Medicine fellowship exam. It aims to provide a high-quality, interactive, independent medical educational resource to help individuals learn, pass exams and stay up to date. Crit-IQ continues to support and assist organisations and individuals, particularly in developing countries. It is a comprehensive, up-to-date, interactive web-based learning platform for critical care doctors of all levels. It comprises learning modules, podcasts and vodcasts, a journal club, echocardiography and ultrasound learning components, a data interpretation database as well as exam support for trainees at various levels. It has developed into a useful resource for all practitioners of critical care, from anaesthetists to emergency physicians to general physicians at all levels of experience.

About Crit-IQ. Online. Available: http://www.crit-iq.com.au/about.cfm.

Box 14.2 TEaM ICM[12] (Trent and East Midlands ICM training programme)

The move by the new Faculty of Intensive Care Medicine (FICM UK) to approve dual and stand-alone training posts in ICM, allows for ICM trainees to be identified early, guaranteeing a minimum of 5 years of training opportunities. Not all of this training will be in direct ICM posts and suggests that there is an opportunity to model formal ICM education on a long-term commitment to the ICM trainee, rather than to concentrate education into ICM training periods only. A prolonged programme can encourage the sharing of ideas and experiences, and allows the development of a peer group, important for the formation of a cohesive and cooperative group of future colleagues.

The Trent and East Midlands ICM training programme, currently into its seventh year, operates a 5-year rolling syllabus that includes all regional ICM trainees, regardless of which specialty or hospital they are attached to, ensuring that a trainee is regularly exposed to ICM educational initiatives include learning days with lectures, quizzes, debates and field trips (e.g. visits to different units and to the coroner), online discussions and a website with various resources.

Courtesy of Dr Dale Gardiner – Implementing a regional training programme in intensive care medicine. The Royal College of Anaesthetists: Bulletin 2010;61:46–8.

of benefit to some individuals. Benefits may include mutual support, sharing of resources, division of labour in preparing study notes including answers to previous questions, as well as practising exam components together.

COURSES

Opportunities for trainees to attend courses offering concentrated exam preparation exist in various

Box 14.3 Australasian Fellowship examination courses

Australian Short Course on Intensive Care Medicine (also known as 'Tub's Course' after Lindsay (Tub) Worthley who developed the initiative)*
Numbers are limited and it is specifically aimed at trainees sitting their CICM Fellowship examination within the same calendar year. Prospective candidates must have their supervisors of training attest to their suitability as significant pre-course preparation is expected. It consists of tutorials on the written component, vivas and clinical ('hot') cases, simulating the entire exam process. The 28th 3-day course was held in Adelaide this year (2012).
Brisbane Intensive Care Medicine Course**
Courses have been evolving for over a decade and three components are currently offered:
Data Interpretation in Acute Medicine – also open to trainees from diverse backgrounds, this course is in its 8th year
Procedure and Communication Course in Intensive care – a new component with simulations and role plays
Australasian ICM Clinical Refresher Course – now in its 15th year, with over 500 attendees over this time.

*Edwards, N. Royal Adelaide Hospital Intensive Care Unit. Online. Available: http://www.icuadelaide.com.au/course_fellowship.html.
**Venkatesh, B. The Brisbane Course – BICMC 3-day course flyer. Online. Available: http://www.cicm.org.au/courseaus.php.

countries. For over a decade, candidates approaching their fellowship examinations in Australia have commonly attended at least one of the well-known courses that offer mock examination experiences with feedback (**Box 14.3**). More recently, additional courses have targeted those in earlier stages of their preparation.

USEFUL CONCEPTS FROM OTHER DISCIPLINES

EDUCATIONAL THEORY

Much has been written about adult learning theories. Arguably, the best known is from David Kolb. In the early 1970s he concluded that the way people learn is linked to how they *perceive an experience*. The Kolb learning cycle differentiates steps in learning including experiencing, reflecting, thinking and doing. The Kolb Learning Style Inventory has been available for many years and has been used by all disciplines, including health care.[13]

The lesser-known VARK learning style classification is based on systematic differences in how learners prefer to take in and put out information during learning experiences. VARK is an acronym for Visual, Aural, Read/Write and Kinesthetic (concrete experiences).[14]

Such classification tools may offer exam candidates insights into their own most- and least-preferred styles and assist personal preparation. For example, visual

Box 14.4 Mind maps™

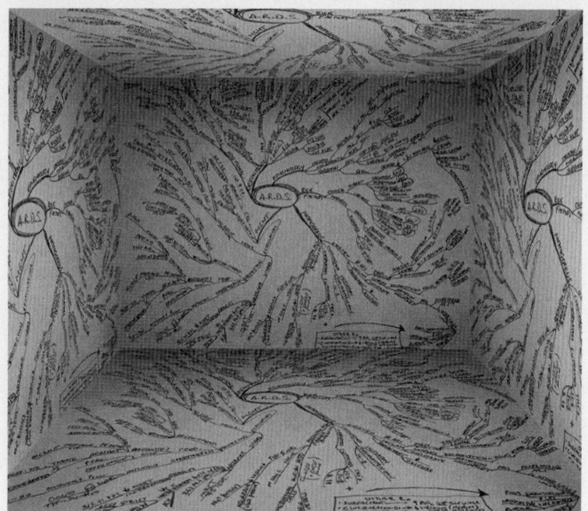

Figure 14.1 'Original mind map'. *(ARDS by Dr Niall Kennedy, Intensive Care Senior Registrar, Sydney. Image courtesy of Matt Tinker photography www.matthewtinker.com.au.)*

Tony Buzan is arguably the modern father of this technique and the term *mind map* is a trademark of his company.

They are used to summarise and link concepts and key terms diagrammatically to facilitate understanding and recall.

Buzan centres. Online. Available: http://www.buzan.com.au/learning/mind_mapping.html.

learners may benefit from utilising techniques such as mind-maps™ (**Box 14.4**) to prepare study notes compared with read/write learners who prefer to make lists and summaries on cards. Non-kinesthetic individuals who prefer reflection and thinking may find learning through simulations difficult and similarly may anticipate the need to work harder to establish comfort with examinations utilising role-plays and manikin-based simulations. Although these assumptions are rational, there are, however, no data supporting the theory that trainees would benefit from formally profiling their learning styles.

SPORTS PSYCHOLOGY

Some trainees, particularly those who have significant performance anxiety or have experienced failure, may benefit from methods used by high-performance athletes. Sports psychology techniques including cognitive behavioural therapy may aid successful performance and hence success. Some critical care trainees have been effectively coached by a performance psychologist (**Box 14.5**) as a major component of their exam preparation.

Box 14.5 Performance psychology for doctors in action

I have been working for many years with hospital registrars to assist with exam preparation, particularly after experiencing failure. This involves looking closely at their lifestyle, family commitments, specific exam requirements, work rosters, overtraining issues, specifics of previous failures and study patterns. It is enormously rewarding.

For the trainee who has failed previously, the immediate reaction is to work harder rather than smarter. Restructuring the study process can break the cycle of frustration and stress after failure. For example, the most opportune time to do creative and productive work is up to midday, as the body reaches maximum activation levels then.[15] So it is suggested that much of the reading and memorizing of material take place on mornings of work-free days. Also important is the daily self-testing on work under timed exam conditions to provide written and oral feedback to the trainee.

Trainees who monitor their study and receive regular feedback are more likely to remain focused on their study goals.[16]

ICM exams are structured in a manner that tests the accuracy of responses under tight time, pressured conditions. It is suggested that sample questions are practised under less than the permitted time per question, in order for the trainee to become accustomed to writing and thinking under pressure. Through overlearning and practice this repetitious behaviour becomes habitual. Compared with non-habitual behaviours, these habits require less conscious attention and effort, and can be performed faster.[17,18]

Issues such as poor oral delivery, low self-esteem, high anxiety, poor motivation, lack of confidence and/or assertiveness can be addressed through the use of goal setting, cognitive restructuring, arousal regulation and imagery. For instance, arousal can mediate attentional focus so that activities that are easy to perform in a stress-free environment become substantially more difficult in a pressure-packed situation.[19] A centring breath can yield physical balance and allow a trainee to mentally focus before attempting a task.[20] Bringing a trainee's focus to the present and enhancing body awareness is a foundation of mindfulness training.[21] Rather than reacting to perceived stressors as if on autopilot, the trainee focuses on breathing and bringing awareness to the inhalation and exhalation of the breath. This is especially useful before oral responses.

Through daily self-monitoring with regular use of a digital voice recorder, a timer, and a diary to record scores for imagery, arousal regulation, effectiveness of study focus, and oral or written feedback, there is a likelihood of better exam results. Trainees report that they feel more in control before exams and they are more likely to experience success.

Dr Patsy Tremayne, Adjunct Associate Professor at the University of Western Sydney, and foundation member of the Australian Psychological Society's College of Sport and Exercise Psychologists (CoSEP).

CONCLUSION

The challenge of examination processes is to help ensure trainees are prepared for the *real world* of specialist practice. It is overly simplistic to think that single examinations will achieve this alone. Comprehensive, quality, patient-centred training programmes, with regulatory bodies with clear governance structures that employ a combination of summative and formative assessment, are likely to achieve closer to the mark.

Access the complete references list online at http://www.expertconsult.com

1. Lee R, Venkatesh B, Morley P. Evidence-based evolution of the high stakes postgraduate intensive care examination in Australia and New Zealand. Br J Hosp Med (Lond) 2007;68:554–6.
2. Frank JR, editor. The CanMEDS 2005 physician competency framework. Better standards. Better physicians. Better care. Ottawa: The Royal College of Physicians and Surgeons of Canada; 2005. Online. Available: http://rcpsc.medical.org/canmeds/index.php.
4. Nunnink L, Venkatesh B, Krishnan A, et al. A prospective comparison between written examination and either simulation-based or oral viva examination of intensive care trainees' procedural skills. Emerg Med Australas 2005;17:263–5.
5. CoBaTrICE Collaboration. The educational environment for training in intensive care medicine: structures, processes, outcomes and challenges in the European region. Intensive Care Med 2009;35: 1575–83.
6. Besso J, Bhagwanjee S, Takezawa J, et al. A global view of eduction and training in critical care medicine. Crit Care Clin 2006;22:539–46.
10. Foot C, Steel L, Vidhani K, et al. Examination Intensive Care Medicine. Chatswood NSW: Elsevier Australasia; 2011.
11. Bennington S, Nightingale P, Shelly M. Multiple Choice Questions in Intensive Care Medicine. Harley Shrewsbury, UK: TFM Publishing; 2009.

Part Two

Shock

15

Overview of shock

Matthew J Maiden and Sandra L Peake

DEFINITION

The answer commonly provided to the question 'what is shock?' is often a vague 'patient with a low blood pressure', followed by some threshold blood pressure below which 'shock' is said to be occurring.

The reason for the uncertainty about what should be a simple concept relates to the fact that the term 'shock' is used in a multitude of contexts (e.g. septic, haemorrhagic, distributive, hypovolaemic, cytotoxic, cardiogenic, anaphylactic, toxic, spinal, neurogenic, cervical and, even electrical shock). However, the unifying feature of shock, irrespective of the initiating disease or clinical features, is *a failure to deliver and/or utilise adequate amounts of oxygen.*[1]

A thorough understanding of what constitutes shock is essential for all critical care practitioners. This chapter will outline the pathophysiology of shock, a classification of diseases that lead to shock and an approach to management.

CIRCULATORY PHYSIOLOGY

OXYGEN DELIVERY

Each day the heart pumps 8000 litres of blood deliver O_2 and nutrients to an estimated 100 trillion cells. This circulatory supply of O_2 and nutrients is tightly regulated by the cardiovascular system. Oxygen delivery (D_{O_2}) is the product of cardiac output (CO) and the oxygen content of arterial blood. D_{O_2} (mL/min) can be summarised by the following equation:

$$D_{O_2} = CO \times ([1.39 \times Hb \times Sa_{O_2}] + [Pa_{O_2} \times 0.003]) \quad (15.1)$$

where Hb is the haemoglobin concentration (g/L), Sa_{O_2} is the arterial Hb saturation and Pa_{O_2} is the arterial oxygen partial pressure. The exact value of the haemoglobin O_2-carrying capacity constant is variably listed as either 1.34 mL O_2/g Hb (directly measured) or 1.39 mL O_2/g Hb (theoretical maximum O_2-carrying capacity).

Assuming adequate arterial oxygen content, CO is the main determinant of D_{O_2}. CO, in turn, is the product of heart rate (HR) and stroke volume (SV) with preload, afterload and myocardial contractility determining SV. Thus:

$$CO = HR \times SV \text{ (preload, afterload, contractility)} \quad (15.2)$$

Alterations in any of these determinants of CO will eventually lead to the development of different 'types' of circulatory shock (e.g. hypovolaemic, distributive, cardiogenic).

D_{O_2}–V_{O_2} RELATIONSHIP

Global D_{O_2} in the adult at rest is approximately 1000 mL/min and oxygen consumption (V_{O_2}) is about 250 mL/min. Under normal circumstances, the extra O_2 being supplied is not required to meet metabolic demand and can conceptually be thought of as a reserve supply (O_2 supply independency). In healthy volunteers at rest, D_{O_2} can be decreased from 14 mL/kg/min to 7 mL/kg/min without signs of inadequate oxygenation.[2]

If D_{O_2} decreases, V_{O_2} initially remains unchanged as the reserve O_2 is utilised. If D_{O_2} falls further, oxygen extraction from Hb is increased to maintain adequate oxygen supply to the tissues. Once O_2 is maximally extracted from Hb, any further reduction of D_{O_2} will limit O_2 supply (O_2 supply dependency). (**Fig. 15.1**).

DYSOXIA

Dysoxia occurs beyond the critical point of supply dependency (critical D_{O_2}). Inadequate O_2 supply leads to anaerobic cellular metabolism, less efficient adenosine triphosphate (ATP) production and consequent cellular and organ dysfunction. Clinically, the expression of dysoxia-induced cellular dysfunction is manifested by features of impaired end-organ perfusion such as drowsiness, delayed capillary refill, oliguria and hyperlactataemia. If the process leading to shock is identified and managed early and appropriately, cellular dysfunction is limited. However if dysoxia persists, the ongoing limitation of O_2 supply affects cell membrane ion channels, leading to an influx of sodium and water, cellular oedema, breaching of cell membrane integrity, cell injury and eventually, cell death.

The ability to withstand limited O_2 supply varies between organs. The heart and brain have high metabolic requirements with a relatively high oxygen extraction, and hence are more vulnerable to reduced O_2 supply. In contrast, the kidney and skin have relatively lower metabolic requirements and lower O_2 extraction and, therefore, are more tolerant of decreased D_{O_2}. The critical D_{O_2} also varies between individuals and is affected by metabolic demand, age, gender, co-morbid diseases, underlying organ function and medications.

Importantly, dysoxia may also occur despite adequate D_{O_2}. In conditions such as sepsis and multi-organ dysfunction syndrome, global D_{O_2} can appear to be adequate and may even be supranormal as a result of increased CO. However, arteriolar shunting around the microvascular beds prevents O_2 delivery to the cells and inflammatory mediators can induce mitochondrial dysfunction, preventing cells from utilising available O_2 (cytotoxic shock).[3-5] Hence *hypotension is not required to define 'shock'.*

'TYPES' OF SHOCK

Clinically, the impairment of circulatory supply of O_2 to the cells is commonly classified according to which component of the circulation is primarily disturbed – that is, hypovolaemic shock (inadequate preload), cardiogenic shock ('pump' failure), obstructive shock (obstructed pump outflow), and distributive or vasodilatory shock (altered vascular capacitance). The classification of shock into various types is clinically useful as it has therapeutic implications; albeit this distinction is sometimes too simplistic. For example, in septic shock, hypovolaemia (decreased preload secondary to increased vascular permeability), vasodilation and myocardial dysfunction may all coexist.

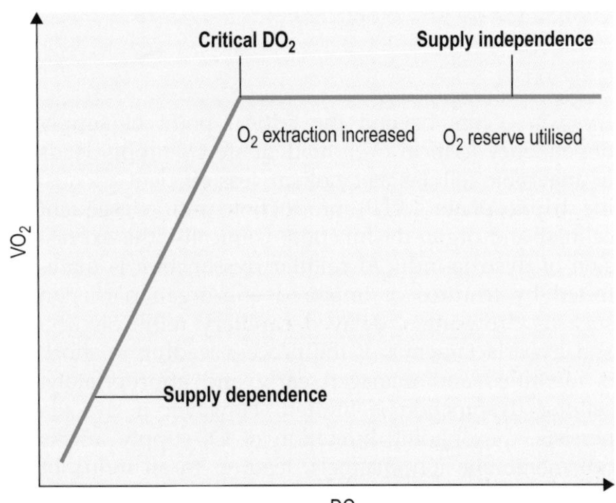

Figure 15.1 Oxygen supply and demand relationship.

HYPOVOLAEMIC SHOCK

Total blood volume is 70 mL/kg and comprises blood cells and serum. Hypovolaemic shock occurs when acute blood loss or excessive fluid losses (e.g. gastrointestinal, urinary tract, burns) lead to decreased circulating blood volume (**Box 15.1**).

Loss of circulatory volume will reduce preload and SV. About 10% of circulating volume loss can be restored by the movement of interstitial fluid into the circulation. Blood loss beyond this invokes cardiovascular compensatory mechanisms in order to restore preload and maintain CO and systemic blood pressure. These mechanisms include:

- *Increasing venous tone:* venoconstriction is an early compensatory response to hypovolaemic shock. The venous system holds about 80% of blood volume and acts as a blood reservoir. The sympathetic nervous system controls venous tone and capacitance of the venous system. Reducing capacitance favours venous return to the heart in an attempt to maintain SV.
- *Increasing arteriolar tone:* sympathetic stimulation of arteriolar resistance vessels increases perfusion pressure to the organs. However, this does not necessarily equate with increased blood flow. The extent of change of arteriolar tone varies between organs in order to ensure adequate blood flow to the vital organs.
- *Increasing HR:* to compensate for the reduction in SV, HR is increased in an attempt to maintain CO.

Box 15.1 Causes of hypovolaemic shock

Blood loss
Vascular injury (e.g. trauma, surgery)
Gastrointestinal bleeding (e.g. peptic ulcer, diverticular, angio-dysplasia, varices)
Obstetric bleeding (e.g. placenta praevia, post-partum haemorrhage)
Intra-abdominal haemorrhage (e.g. splenic laceration, liver injury)
Retroperitoneal (e.g. aortic aneurysm, ectopic rupture, femoral artery bleeding, pelvic fracture)
Long-bone fracture
Pulmonary haemorrhage, haemothorax

Fluid loss
Vomiting
Diarrhoea
Ileostomy losses
Sweating
Polyuria (e.g. glucosuria, diabetes insipidus)
Burns
Pancreatitis
Ascites

Inadequate fluid intake

- *Increasing contractility:* the heart will contract more vigorously in order to increase SV and maintain CO.

The American College of Surgeons classified the severity of haemorrhagic shock according to the presence of certain clinical signs (**Box 15.2**).[6] However, these 'classes' are arbitrary and depend on the rate of blood loss and factors that modulate the critical D_{O_2} (e.g. co-morbidities, medications).

Priorities in the management of hypovolaemic shock are: (1) controlling the source of blood and/or volume loss, and (2) restoring the circulating volume.

CARDIOGENIC SHOCK

The heart is central to the circulatory supply of O_2 and if the pump fails then there are few compensatory mechanisms available. Hence, cardiogenic shock has a very high in-hospital mortality rate ranging from 45–100%, depending on the aetiology.[7] Myocardial ischaemia is the most common cause of cardiogenic shock, but other aetiologies must be considered (**Box 15.3**).

Treatment priorities in cardiogenic shock involve urgent correction of the underlying acute cardiac disease and consideration of afterload reduction while ensuring adequate organ perfusion.

OBSTRUCTIVE SHOCK

Mechanical obstruction to the flow of blood through the cardiac chambers will lead to reduced cardiac output. The limitation of flow may be due to obstruction within the heart (e.g. valve thrombosis, myxoma) or extrinsic compression (e.g. tension pneumothorax, cardiac tamponade). Treatment is directed at urgent removal of the obstruction (e.g. drainage of pericardial effusion, lysis of thromboembolism).

DISTRIBUTIVE SHOCK

Blood distribution around the vascular network is controlled by vascular autoregulation, the autonomic nervous system and hormones. Distributive shock results from the failure of these mechanisms, leading to inappropriate distribution of blood (**Box 15.4**). Unlike other forms of shock, CO may initially be increased as the heart endeavours to compensate for maldistribution of blood.

Management priorities are to identify and treat the precipitating cause and to improve organ perfusion with resuscitation fluids and vasoactive drugs. Sepsis is the most common cause of distributive shock in the ICU and prompt resuscitation of the circulation is essential for improved survival.

CLINICAL SIGNS

The clinical features of shock relate to a critically inadequate circulation and insufficient O_2 delivery and/or utilisation. However, these features are non-specific and will depend on a number of factors including:

- process leading to shock
- severity of precipitating disease or injury
- physiological reserve of the patient
- effects of medications.

The compensatory mechanisms to shock and subsequent clinical manifestations are affected by advancing

Box 15.2 Classes of haemorrhagic shock (American College of Surgeons 2004)

Class 1
<15% blood volume loss
Compensated by shift of interstitial fluid
Minimal clinical changes

Class 2
15–30% blood volume loss
Compensated hypovolaemia
Features include orthostatic hypotension and tachycardia

Class 3
30–40% blood volume loss
Decompensated hypovolaemia
Hypotension, tachypnoea, altered mental state

Modified from American College of Surgeons. Committee on Trauma. ATLS, advanced trauma life support program for doctors. 7th ed. Chicago, IL: American College of Surgeons; 2004.

Box 15.3 Causes of cardiogenic shock

Myocardial ischaemia
Acute valve dysfunction (e.g. chordae rupture, prosthetic valve thrombus)
Myocarditis
Contusion
Septal/ventricular rupture
Drugs (e.g. Ca^{2+} channel blocker overdose, beta blocker overdose)
Bradyarrhythmias (e.g. complete heart block)
Tachyarrhythmias (e.g. atrial or ventricular tachycardias)

Box 15.4 Causes of distributive shock

Septic shock
Toxic shock
Anaphylactic shock
Neurogenic shock
Adrenal/thyroid insufficiency
Toxicity (e.g. drugs)
As a component of multi-organ dysfunction syndrome

age, cardiovascular disease, autonomic disease and medications. For example, patients on beta antagonists will not mount the same tachycardic response to fluid loss and patients with pre-existing cardiac disease are less capable of circulatory compensation and so develop features of shock earlier.

Due to the non-specific and varied clinical signs of shock, repeated assessment with frequent monitoring of vital signs is essential.

Hypotension is a sentinel feature of shock and signifies circulatory failure. However, hypotension develops late as systemic blood pressure is initially maintained by compensatory mechanisms (i.e. vasoconstriction, tachycardia, increased myocardial contractility).

A decline in mean arterial pressure (MAP) below the lower limit of autoregulation results in reduced perfusion to the vital organs. In a healthy adult, tissue perfusion is typically impaired with a MAP of ≤50 mmHg (6.65 kPa). In contrast, elderly patients with pre-existing hypertension or vascular disease generally require a higher MAP to ensure adequate regional blood flow.

If systemic blood pressure cannot be accurately determined by the usual auscultatory techniques, then the patient is likely to be markedly hypotensive. Establish the presence of a central (carotid, femoral) or peripheral (radial, posterior tibial) pulse, followed by palpation of the systolic blood pressure using a blood pressure cuff.

Tachycardia is an early compensatory sign of shock. However, in some conditions bradycardia is the cause of shock (e.g. complete heart block, increased vagal tone in cervical shock, unopposed vagal tone in neurogenic shock).

Tachypnoea steadily increases with worsening shock but falls in the pre-terminal phase of shock.

Oliguria is secondary to reduced glomerular filtration and increased filtrate reabsorption. In shock states, the rate of urine production is a useful guide to adequacy of the circulation.

Altered mental status is a common feature of shock as cerebral function is very sensitive to altered O_2 delivery. During shock, mental state progressively changes from anxiety, agitation, confusion and delirium, toward drowsiness and coma.

Impaired peripheral perfusion provides a clinically useful clue regarding the likely mechanism of shock. Cool, clammy peripheries with pale or mottled skin are suggestive of hypovolaemic or cardiogenic shock, whereas warm peripheries are suggestive of distributive shock.

MANAGEMENT

Resuscitation of shock is a medical emergency. The aim of therapy is to rapidly and effectively restore systemic D_{O_2} and improve tissue perfusion. History, examination and investigation (**Box 15.5**) must occur concurrently with resuscitation. The usual resuscitation principles of airway, breathing, circulation apply.

The principles of management of shock are:

1. Supply O_2
2. Vascular access
3. Volume resuscitation
4. Vasoactive agents
5. Manage precipitating illness or injury
6. Monitoring.

1. Supply oxygen

Ensure any causes of hypoxia are urgently corrected including providing adequate F_{IO_2}, ensuring ventilation is adequate and that any reversible cause of pulmonary shunt is corrected (e.g. pleural collection, bronchus obstruction).

2. Vascular access

Insertion of intravenous cannulae is essential for administration of fluids and medications. Cannula size is an important consideration as it has major implications for the rate of laminar fluid flow. Poiseuille's law describes the variables contributing to laminar flow rates:

$$Q \propto (\Delta P \times \pi r^4) / (8 \times \text{viscosity} \times \text{length}) \qquad (15.3)$$

This emphasises the dramatic effect of radius on flow and that flow is inversely proportional to cannula length. Hence for rapid intravenous fluid administration, venous cannulation using short wide-bore catheters is essential.

Flow rates achieved through different diameter intravenous cannulae are stated to range from 44 mL/

Box 15.5 Investigations for shock (as clinically indicated)

Bedside
Haemoglobin
Arterial blood gas
Lactate
ECG
Ultrasound (e.g. FAST scan, AAA scan)
Echocardiogram

Laboratory
Full blood count, coagulation studies, D-dimer
Electrolytes, creatinine, urea, liver function tests
Cardiac enzymes, lipase
Cultures – urine, blood, sputum, pus
Toxicology assays

Radiology
Chest, abdominal X-ray
Trauma series radiology (chest, pelvis, C-spine)
CT
Angiography (e.g. coronary, visceral, pulmonary)

min (22 G; 0.9 mm diameter) through to 286 mL/min (14 G; 2.1 mm diameter). However, as flow through cannulae is turbulent rather than laminar, flow rates are lower than those quoted.[8]

3. Fluid resuscitation

Fluid resuscitation is usually the first therapeutic strategy in the management of shock, particularly in hypovolaemic or distributive shock. However, it is important to note that not all patients will respond to fluid loading with a significant increase in CO. If the heart is working on the terminal (flat) portion of the Frank–Starling curve, increased preload may not result in a significant increase in SV. Nevertheless, even patients with cardiogenic shock may benefit from a judicious fluid challenge and dynamic assessment of volume responsiveness (i.e. the ability to increase CO with fluid loading or straight leg raise) is preferred to static measurements of volume state (e.g. central venous pressure).

Trendelenburg A quick method to increase venous return is to tilt the patient's pelvis above horizontal (i.e. head down). This will 'auto-transfuse' blood from leg and pelvic veins and increases venous filling pressures and MAP. Increases in CO are minimal if venous capacitance remains high and the extra blood volume is accommodated.

Crystalloids Crystalloid solutions comprise electrolytes (with or without dextrose) and water. These fluids cross semipermeable membranes easily and are rapidly distributed through the intravascular and extravascular spaces. The time for fluid equilibration across the body compartments depends on: (1) osmolality of the fluid, (2) solute clearance and (3) integrity of the vascular endothelium.

Although the choice of fluid should reflect the composition of the fluid lost, 0.9% saline is commonly used for initial volume replacement. 0.9% saline is slightly hyperosmolar (300 mOsm/L) and hyperchloraemic (150 mEq/L) relative to plasma. When large volumes are used for resuscitation, hyperchloraemia can contribute to bicarbonate loss and a normal anion gap metabolic acidosis. Lactated Ringer's solution (Hartmann's) is isotonic and contains lactate (29 mEq/L) and electrolytes in a ratio similar to plasma. However, the calcium in Hartmann's (4 mEq/L) is incompatible with certain drugs and lactate levels may rise if hepatic function is markedly impaired or a lot of fluid is administered. Other crystalloid solutions are available that contain different buffer anions and slightly different composition of electrolytes. These have not been shown to alter clinical outcomes following fluid resuscitation.

Concentrated saline is theoretically a useful resuscitation fluid since a small volume can increase circulating volume (e.g. 250 mL 7.5% saline can increase circulating volume by 500 mL). However, the sodium also passes into interstitial space leading to increased interstitial fluid volume, at the expense of intracellular volume. Volume resuscitation with hypertonic saline may prevent cerebral oedema, but a recent clinical trial of its use in head-injured patients did not show improved outcomes.[9]

Colloids Colloids are solutions containing large molecules that do not pass through a semipermeable membrane. These solutions remain in the circulation for longer, have a smaller volume of distribution and hence are more effective at increasing intravascular volume than the same volume of crystalloid. There are a number of colloid solutions available, which differ based on their type and concentration of colloidal molecules.

Albumin Four per cent normal serum albumin (NSA 40g/L; 260 mOsm/L) is iso-oncotic and infusion rapidly increases circulating volume. NSA is a by-product of whole blood separation; however, it is provided in glass bottles that limit the speed of infusion and the increment in plasma volume lasts only a few hours.[10] Concentrated (20%) albumin is available in smaller volumes (100 mL). It increases circulating fluid volume by drawing fluid from the interstitium. This process takes time and concentrated albumin is not a useful resuscitation fluid.

Whether crystalloid or colloid solution is the better resuscitation fluid is a matter of much debate. Crystalloids are cheap, easy to administer and replete intravascular and extravascular fluid. Their tendency to interstitial oedema and electrolyte alteration is thought to be a problem. Colloids can restore circulating volume more quickly, persist for longer (at least initially) and seem less likely to lead to interstitial oedema. However colloids are more expensive, have a greater risk of side-effects and in critically ill patients can accumulate in the interstitium, contributing to persistent interstitial oedema.

In 1998, a Cochrane review suggested albumin use was associated with increased mortality,[11] but other reviews drew different conclusions.[12–14] To determine the safety of albumin as a resuscitation fluid, the Saline versus Albumin Fluid Evaluation (SAFE) study randomised 7000 patients to receive albumin or crystalloid as their resuscitation fluid.[15] This landmark study revealed that patients receiving albumin required less intravenous fluid, but clinical outcomes were no different to patients who received saline resuscitation. Subgroup analyses suggested that septic patients fared better with 4% NSA, while head-injured patients given saline had better outcomes.

Starch Solutions Starch solutions contain a carbohydrate polymer (starch) as their oncotic molecule and differ according to the type and molecular size of the starch used (high starch 450 000 D, medium starch 200 000 D, low starch 70 000 D). The starch polymers undergo degradation by serum amylase with the fragments cleared by the kidney. The duration of oncotic effect is related to the size of the starch molecule and clearance rates. Whereas starch solutions provide effective intravascular volume replacement and are convenient to administer, their use in patients with septic shock has been associated with increased risk of death, renal impairment and bleeding risk.[16,17] A recent clinical trial of 7000 ICU patients randomised to receive 6% hydroxyethyl starch (HES; 130/0.4) or 0.9% saline as resuscitation fluid found no difference in mortality, but patients who received 6% HES had an increased need for renal replacement therapy and a greater incidence of skin reactions.[18]

Blood The use of blood is essentially limited to shock from acute blood loss or for correcting anaemia that may be contributing to impaired O_2 delivery.

4. Vasoactive agents

When fluid administration alone fails to restore adequate oxygen delivery and organ perfusion, vasoactive agents should be initiated. In extreme shock, it may be necessary to commence fluid resuscitation and vasoactive therapy concurrently.

Vasoactive agents are commonly referred to as 'inotropes' as many of them increase cardiac contractility (i.e. inotropy). However, many agents have their primary effect on vascular tone rather than directly altering contractility. The choice of agent will depend on which aspect of the cardiovascular physiology is deranged and the goals of therapy.

For cardiogenic shock, medications may be required to increase contractility (e.g. dobutamine, milrinone, levosimendan), reduce afterload, maintain adequate systemic and coronary perfusion pressure, increase diastolic relaxation and increase or decrease heart rate. In distributive shock, medications that produce venoconstriction and increased systemic pressures are required. There is little role for cardiovascular medications in hypovolaemic shock; however, the effect of vasopressin is currently being investigated in a prehospital clinical trial.[19]

The choice of which catecholamine to use in shock (i.e. norepinephrine (noradrenaline) vs epinephrine (adrenaline) vs dopamine) has been the subject of considerable debate and opinion. Different catecholamines exhibit different pharmacological properties (e.g. β_1- vs β_2 adrenergic receptor stimulation); however, the superiority of one catecholamine over another has not been demonstrated in any large-scale clinical trials. A large randomised trial of patients with shock reported no difference in 28-day mortality between norepinephrine and dopamine,[20] while an Australian trial found no difference between norepinephrine and epinephrine in patients with shock from any cause.[21] Similarly in septic shock, there is no mortality difference if using epinephrine or norepinephrine with dobutamine.[22] It is not surprising that there is no one 'ideal' vasoactive agent for every patient or for all causes of circulatory shock. Instead these drugs should be chosen based on the desired therapeutic effects on the cardiovascular system.

Although blood pressure is a universal measure of circulation adequacy and often a therapeutic target when using vasoactive agents, there are no randomised controlled trials evaluating the ideal MAP. Choice of ideal MAP remains empirical and is based on the clinician's assessment of the minimum pressure thought to represent adequate blood flow taking into consideration pre-existing comorbidities such as hypertension or vascular disease.

Augmenting the circulation with vasoactive agents to provide 'supranormal' D_{O_2} was previously thought to be a therapeutic option for critically ill patients. However, several clinical trials have repeatedly illustrated that efforts to drive D_{O_2} beyond normal do not improve survival.[23-25]

5. Manage precipitating illness or injury

As the circulation is being resuscitated, the cause of the circulatory disturbance needs to be identified and corrected. Unless this occurs, shock will continue to worsen and death will ensue. Time to definitive treatment of the cause of shock is related to survival. This has been clearly illustrated in cardiogenic shock (time to reperfusion),[26] haemorrhagic shock (time to haemorrhage control)[27] and septic shock (time to appropriate antibiotics).[28]

6. Monitoring

All causes of shock have improved outcomes when managed in an environment that closely monitors clinical signs and physiological parameters (i.e. an ICU).

Clinical monitoring involves frequent assessment of heart rate, blood pressure, respiratory rate, conscious state, urine output, peripheral perfusion and temperature.

An arterial cannula provides beat-to-beat measurement of systemic pressure and is particularly useful for measuring blood pressure when clinical techniques become difficult and unreliable. Arterial cannulae also allow ready sampling for blood gas and lactate measurement.

A central venous cannula allows measurement of central venous pressure (CVP), which is often used as an estimate of venous volume, and hence preload. However, CVP bears a variable relationship to venous volume, as it is dependent on location of the catheter to the right atrium, intrathoracic pressures, venous compliance, position of the patient and tricuspid valve competence. Thus CVP is a guide to the *pressure* status of the venous system rather than a measure of intravascular volume and preload. CVP correlates poorly with fluid response to shock.[29]

Echocardiographic assessment of end-diastolic ventricle volume may better a predictor of preload than invasive pressure measurement, but the technique is operator- and patient-dependent.

As there is no 'gold standard' measure of preload, any monitored variable assessing volume state should be interpreted in conjunction with clinical findings. Repeated assessment and dynamic measures such as systolic pressure variation (in ventilated patients) and response to fluid challenge (e.g. fluid bolus or straight leg raise) are a more useful guide to preload adequacy than static measurements.[30,31]

Some CVCs contain an oximeter in the tip that measures O_2–Hb saturation of central venous blood (Scv_{O_2}). This can be used as a guide to determine O_2 demand and adequacy of D_{O_2}, and to help direct further resuscitation. An $Scv_{O_2} \geq 70\%$ has been proposed as a resuscitation goal.[32] However, Scv_{O_2} is a general measure of global O_2 demand, does not measure the impact of coronary venous blood (from the coronary sinus) and inadequate D_{O_2} may still occur despite a normal or high Scv_{O_2} (viz. anatomical shunts, microcirculation shunting).

Measuring CO in patients with shock is not required routinely. In most patients, clinical assessment provides adequate information regarding CO. There is no evidence that targeting therapy to a specific CO improves outcomes. However, measurement and monitoring may be necessary if a patient's circulatory disturbance does not improve following initial treatment. There is an ever-increasing number of techniques available for estimating CO, all with inherent strengths and limitations. Further discussion of haemodynamic monitoring is found in Chapter 16.

Blood gas, pH and lactate monitoring provide some guidance to the adequacy of cellular resuscitation.[32,33] Inadequate oxygen delivery and/or utilisation is the most common cause of elevated serum lactate (generally defined as >2 mmol/L) in ICU patients. Blood lactate levels, lactate clearance rates and falling base deficit are associated with poor outcomes[34-37] and are a better predictor of mortality than is D_{O_2} or V_{O_2}.[38] However, lactate is not specific for shock, as elevated levels may also occur with liver failure (reduced lactate metabolism), thiamine deficiency (inhibits pyruvate dehydrogenase), lactate administration (e.g. in dialysis fluids), catecholamine administration (beta agonists) and prolonged exercise. Elevated blood lactate levels may also reflect regional dysoxia of an isolated anatomical organ or tissue (e.g. limb or bowel ischaemia) that may not necessarily be associated with a global circulatory disturbance. The role of targeting therapies to lactate clearance or base excess also remains uncertain.

Standard ICU monitoring techniques focus on assessment of the macrocirculation. However, there is growing interest in how the microcirculation can be monitored. Microscopic analysis of the circulation with orthogonal polarisation spectral (OPS) imaging or near infra-red spectroscopy (NIRS) provide fascinating insights into the microcirculatory status, but their use remains experimental.

Access the complete references list online at http://www.expertconsult.com

1. Antonelli M, Levy M, Andrews PJ, et al. Hemodynamic monitoring in shock and implications for management. International Consensus Conference, Paris, France, 27–28 April 2006. Intensive Care Med 2007; 33(4):575–90.
4. Fink MP. Cytopathic hypoxia. Mitochondrial dysfunction as mechanism contributing to organ dysfunction in sepsis. Crit Care Clin 2001;17(1): 219–37.
15. Finfer S, Bellomo R, Boyce N, et al. A comparison of albumin and saline for fluid resuscitation in the intensive care unit. N Engl J Med 2004;350(22): 2247–56.
21. Myburgh JA, Higgins A, Jovanovska A, et al. A comparison of epinephrine and norepinephrine in critically ill patients. Intensive Care Med 2008;34(12): 2226–34.
29. Michard F, Teboul JL. Predicting fluid responsiveness in ICU patients: a critical analysis of the evidence. Chest 2002;121(6):2000–8.

FURTHER READING

Reddi BA, Carpenter RH. Venous excess: a new approach to cardiovascular control and its teaching. J Appl Physiol 2005;98(1):356–64.

16

Haemodynamic monitoring

David J Sturgess

INTRODUCTION

Haemodynamics is the study of blood flow. Haemodynamic monitoring therefore refers to the monitoring of blood flow through the cardiovascular system. In critical care, including the intensive care unit (ICU), haemodynamic monitoring is used to detect cardiovascular insufficiency, differentiate contributing factors, and guide therapy.

There has been debate over the risks and benefits of invasive haemodynamic monitoring in critically ill patients. In the presence of scant data demonstrating an association between invasive monitoring and improved survival, there has been a steady trend toward less invasive monitoring in the ICU.

At the bedside the clinician must work with inexact surrogates of preload, contractility and afterload, measured or derived from arterial blood pressure (systemic or pulmonary), volume or pressure indices of cardiac filling, stroke volume or cardiac output, and various markers of tissue well-being. As a rough guide to the layout of this chapter, clinical observation and evaluation will be considered briefly before progressing to monitoring that is primarily concerned with the measurement of pressures (including catheterisation, equipment and techniques) then flow (cardiac output). The concept of functional haemodynamic monitoring, including the prediction of fluid responsiveness, will be introduced, along with perioperative optimisation. Finally, monitoring of perfusion in the microcirculation will be briefly mentioned.

CLINICAL OBSERVATION AND EVALUATION

The diagnosis of haemodynamic disturbance requires combination and integration of available data.[1] This should include physical examination and review of observations such as pulse, peripheral perfusion (capillary refill and temperature), oedema, urine output, oxygen saturation and end-tidal carbon dioxide.

Electrocardiographic (ECG) monitoring is almost universally indicated in the intensive care unit. Generally a system requiring a reduced number (<10) of electrodes is used. This has benefits in terms of patient comfort and convenience for caregivers. However, it must be kept in mind that when compared to the recorded 12-lead ECG, reconstructed 12-lead ECG data appear to retain specificity but can be significantly less sensitive across a range of rhythmic and morphological abnormalities.[2]

PRESSURE-BASED CARDIOVASCULAR MONITORING

This section will discuss monitoring that is primarily employed for monitoring pressure-based cardiovascular variables. Equipment, techniques and supplementary variables will also be discussed under the most applicable headings.

ARTERIAL BLOOD PRESSURE

The systemic pulse wave propagates from the aortic valve at 6–10 m/s. During its passage into the peripheral vasculature there is a progressive increase in systolic (SBP) and reduction in diastolic blood pressures (DBP), as standing and reflected waves become incorporated into the waveform, a process known as distal pulse amplification. Consequently, systemic arterial pressure measurements vary according to the site of measurement.

Mean arterial pressure (MAP) is arguably a more relevant index to monitor than either SBP or DBP for three reasons:

- MAP is least dependent on measurement site or technique (invasive versus non-invasive).
- MAP is least altered by measurement damping.
- MAP determines tissue blood flow via autoregulation (apart from the left ventricle, which autoregulates from diastolic pressure).

NON-INVASIVE ARTERIAL BLOOD PRESSURE MEASUREMENT

In critical care, most standard non-invasive arterial blood pressure (NIBP) instruments are automated intermittent oscillometric devices. Finger plethysmography and arterial tonometry can monitor both arterial pressure and waveforms continuously, but concerns exist regarding accuracy.

Oscillometric NIBP is often used to check the reliability of invasive measurements, or can be used alone when beat-to-beat monitoring is not required. Contraindications to NIBP are relative, and influence the site of cuff placement. For instance, it is preferable to avoid extremities with severe peripheral vascular disease, venous cannulation, arteriovenous fistula or a predisposition to lymphoedema, as may occur after lymph node clearance.

To make an oscillometric blood pressure measurement, a pneumatic cuff is inflated around a proximal limb until all oscillations in cuff pressure are extinguished. The occluding pressure is then lowered stepwise, so that oscillations reappear over a discrete interval. Proprietary algorithms compute mean, systolic and diastolic pressures from the alterations in oscillatory amplitude during deflation.

Oscillometry overestimates low pressures and underestimates high pressures, but for the normotensive range the 95% confidence limits are ±15 mmHg (2 kPa). Dysrhythmia increases the error. Cuff width should be 40% of the mid-circumference of the limb. Narrower cuffs overestimate and wider cuffs underestimate blood pressures.

Complications are unusual. Repeated cuff inflations can cause skin ulceration, oedema and bruising, more so when the consciousness is impaired by illness and sedation. Ulnar nerve injury is also possible, especially with low cuff placement.

INVASIVE BLOOD PRESSURE MEASUREMENT[3,4]

Invasive blood pressure measurement is desirable in the presence of haemodynamic instability, end-organ disease requiring beat-to-beat blood pressure monitoring, during therapeutic manipulation of the cardiovascular system or if non-invasive methods fail. Cannulation of a systemic artery allows continuous monitoring of the arterial pressure waveform, heart rate and blood pressure, and also facilitates frequent arterial blood gas analysis. Relative contraindications include coagulopathy and vascular abnormality or disease.

The radial artery is the most common site for cannulation; this preference has resulted from ease of cannulation, relatively consistent anatomy and low complication rates (incidence of permanent ischaemic complications ~ 0.09%). Nothing larger than a 20-gauge cannula is advisable, and either a modified Seldinger technique or direct cannulation can be used. Even though anatomical variation is common, adequate collateral flow exists in most patients. The modified Allen's test is sometimes employed prior to cannulation. Evidence is lacking regarding its ability to predict ischaemic complications during radial artery occlusion. Ultrasound (Doppler) might be a more reliable way of confirming collateral perfusion, as well as potentially improving cannulation rates with fewer attempts.

Once inserted, the cannula is usually infused with normal or heparinised saline at 3 mL/h, with a snap flush rate of 30–60 mL/h. The potential use of heparinised saline to prolong catheter patency must be balanced against the potential contamination of blood samples drawn through the cannula (especially APTT) and concerns regarding sensitisation and development of heparin-induced thrombosis thrombocytopenia syndrome (HITTS).

Caution must be used when using a functional end artery (e.g. brachial artery), as complications may manifest as a vascular emergency. In severe circulatory compromise, gaining peripheral arterial access may be difficult and time consuming. Rapid femoral cannulation by the Seldinger percutaneous technique usually remains feasible, with the added advantage that femoral arterial monitoring more accurately reflects aortic pressure in low-output states. This may be relevant in stroke volume estimates based upon arterial waveform characteristics.

No specific recommendations are made regarding planned resiting of cannulae.[5] In practice, cannulae are removed when no longer required, or resited when malfunctioning. This should be expedited if a complication is suspected. Distal perfusion should be checked at least 8-hourly, and the cannula removed if there is persistent blanching, coolness with sluggish capillary refill, loss of pulses, or evidence of raised muscle compartment pressures. Complications associated with arterial cannulation are presented in **Table 16.1**.

Physical properties of clinical pressure measurement systems[6]

In the standard setup, the arterial cannula is connected to a linearly responsive pressure transducer via fluid-filled non-compliant tubing <1 m in length. Modern disposable transducers are precalibrated using electrical signals, and are not normally calibrated further against known pressures. The system is zeroed to the level of the phlebostatic axis, normally the mid-axillary line at the fourth intercostal space. Subsequent lowering of the transducer relative to this axis will cause pressure overestimation, while raising it will cause underestimation.

The *natural resonant frequency* of the system should exceed 36 Hz (>10 harmonics with allowance for optimal damping which allows measurement of up to 67% of resonant frequency) for heart rates up to 180 beats/min (3 Hz), to prevent distortion of the biological signal by sine wave system oscillations. *Damping* refers to any property of an oscillatory system that reduces the amplitude of oscillations. Factors that increase oscillation in the system, such as increased tubing length, diameter or compliance, cause underdamping. Overdamping tends to smooth the waveform, causing underestimation of SBP and overestimation of DBP, while MAP tends to be preserved. Contributing factors include clots, air bubbles and loose connections.

Damping can be assessed clinically by the fast flush test. The fast flush or square wave test is performed by

Table 16.1 Complications of arterial cannulation, with suggested preventative and treatment option

COMPLICATION	PREVENTION	TREATMENT
Vascular thrombosis (ranges from 7–30% following radial artery cannulation). Risk factors for digital ischaemia include: shock, sepsis, embolus of air or clot, hyperlipoproteinaemia, vasculitis, female sex, prothrombotic states, accidental intra-arterial injection of drugs	Risks reduced by smaller catheter, larger artery, decreased duration of cannulation, avoiding traumatic insertion and multiple attempts. Allen's test (including modifications such as Doppler, plethysmography and digital blood pressure) is probably unhelpful	Remove cannula. Arterial thrombosis is usually self-limiting. Severe ischaemic damage estimated at <0.01%. Anticoagulation and/or vascular surgery/intervention may be necessary
Distal embolisation	Diligent catheter care and observation	As for thrombosis
Proximal embolisation of clot or air (can result in stroke)	Diligent catheter care and observation. Exclude air from pressurised system. Avoid axillary, subclavian, or carotid access	Tailored to sequelae
Vascular spasm	Smaller catheter, larger artery, Avoid traumatic insertion and multiple attempts	Remove cannula. Resite if necessary
Skin necrosis at catheter site	Diligent catheter care and observation	Surgical debridement and skin grafting may be necessary
Line disconnection and bleeding/ exsanguination	Minimise connections. Diligent catheter care and observation	Control bleeding. Transfusion may be necessary
Accidental drug injection	Clearly label arterial line near ports	Leave cannula in situ to facilitate treatment if required. Depends on drug injected. May require papaverine or procaine, analgesia, sympathetic block of limb and anticoagulation
Infection – local or systemic	Diligent catheter care and observation	Remove cannula and send tip for culture. Resite if necessary. Immobilise and elevate affected upper limb. Start empiric antibiotics if sepsis or septic shock is present
Damage to nearby structures such as nerves, directly or due to haematoma (e.g. compartment syndrome or carpal tunnel syndrome). Arteriovenous fistula. Femoral approach can be associated with bowel damage	Careful insertion technique. Seek assistance from experienced operator	Haematomas can develop into pseudoaneurysms requiring surgery

Source: Based on information contained in text of reference;[62] Durbin Jr CG. Radial arterial lines and sticks: what are the risks? Respir Care 2001;46(3):229–31.

opening the valve, thus transmitting the pressure from the pressure bag, of the continuous flush apparatus. This is then released/closed abruptly, inducing oscillation. With appropriate damping, the measured pressure should come to reflect the biologic signal within one or two oscillations.

Upstream resistance or turbulence can result in a flow-dependent pressure reduction at the cannula site that differs from damping in that the mean, systolic and diastolic pressures are all reduced. This is described as *attenuation* and is often observed in 'positional' arterial lines.

Estimation of stroke volume and cardiac output

Estimation of stroke volume by analysis of the arterial pressure waveform has been studied for many years. An array of algorithms has resulted, some of which have been incorporated into commercially available monitors. The underlying concepts are discussed further in the cardiac output monitoring section of this chapter.

CENTRAL VENOUS CATHETERISATION

Central venous catheterisation (CVC) is indicated for monitoring of central venous pressure (CVP). It may also be required for administration of certain drugs and parenteral nutrition. In addition, it may be used as a component transpulmonary indicator dilution system for cardiac output monitoring. Modified catheters are also available which continuously monitor central venous oxygen saturation (Scv_{O_2}).

Contraindications to central venous catheterisation are relative and reflect potential complications of the procedure (**Table 16.2**). These should be considered in selecting the site for catheter insertion. The subclavian is preferred to internal jugular or femoral approaches with regarded to minimizing the

Table 16.2 Complications of central venous catheterisation, with preventative and treatment options

COMPLICATION	PREVENTION	TREATMENT
Intravascular loss of guidewire	Ensure guidewire is always secured. Avoid retracting guidewire into insertion needle. Seek assistance from experienced operator	Interventional radiology or surgery may be required for retrieval
Air embolism	Proper patient positioning, including Trendelenburg (head down tilt) for jugular or subclavian insertion. Consider alternative insertion sites. Ensure connections are tight	Left lateral Trendelenburg position. Administer 100% oxygen and ventilatory support. If catheter in place tighten all connections and attempt to aspirate air. Basic/advanced life support if necessary
Dysrhythmias and conduction defects such as right bundle branch block	Continuous electrocardiographic monitoring during insertion. Correct placement of catheter tip	Withdraw or remove guidewire or catheter
Damage to nearby structures: Pneumothorax/haemothorax/chylothorax/hydrothorax, particularly with approaches to subclavian vein. Nerve injury such as phrenic, recurrent laryngeal, Horner's syndrome. Arterial puncture – including injury to carotid, subclavian, aorta or pulmonary artery. Haematoma, pseudoaneurysm, arteriovenous fistula can result. Stroke may result from carotid artery injury. Tracheal injury. Femoral approach can be associated with bowel damage.	Identify risk factors such as previous surgery, skeletal deformity or scarring at site of insertion. Seek assistance from experienced operator. Select insertion site depending on impact of potential complications. Consider ultrasound guidance. Scheduled, routine replacement of catheter increases risk of mechanical complications	Depends on specific complication
Line disconnection and bleeding	Minimise connections. Proper catheter care and observation	Control bleeding. Transfusion may be necessary
Infection – local or systemic (including endocarditis)	Aseptic insertion technique. Lower risk with subclavian compared to internal jugular or femoral insertion. Antimicrobial impregnated catheters. Disinfect catheter hubs. Routine scheduled resiting appears not to reduce systemic infection rates. Remove catheter when no longer required	Remove catheter, resite if necessary. Culture blood and catheter tip. Start empiric antibiotics if sepsis or septic shock is present
Superior vena caval erosion can result in haemothorax or cardiac tamponade	Remove catheter when no longer required	Early detection and surgical intervention
Thrombosis	Remove catheter when no longer required. Subclavian insertion is lower risk than internal jugular or femoral	Anticoagulation, vascular or endovascular intervention may be required

Source: based on information contained in text of reference:[63] McGee DC, Gould MK. Preventing complications of central venous catheterization. N Engl J Med 2003;348(12):1123–33.

risk of central-line-associated bloodstream infections (CLABSI).[7] However, routine replacement of central lines does not appear to reduce CLABSI. Attention should also be given to the coagulation profile and factors that affect coagulation such as thrombolytic therapy.

Traditionally, puncture of the central vein is performed by passing a needle along the anticipated line of the vein with reference to surface anatomical landmarks (landmark method). Catheterisation is usually achieved via the subclavian, internal jugular or external jugular veins into the superior vena cava.[8] Access to the subclavian vein is usually via the infraclavicular approach, but the supraclavicular approach is safe and reliable in experienced hands. Peripherally inserted central catheters (PICC) are inserted via a peripheral vein, such as the cephalic or basilic vein and advanced until the tip lies in a central position.

In the United Kingdom, the National Institute for Health and Clinical Excellence (NICE) has issued guidelines recommending the use of ultrasound for elective catheterisation of the internal jugular vein, and consideration of ultrasound guidance in most clinical situations (formulated 2002, reviewed 2005).[9]

Ultrasound can be used to assist central line placement in a number of ways. Two-dimensional imaging with ultrasound can be used to localise the vein and define anatomy prior to placement of a CVC by standard landmark techniques. Ultrasound can also provide real-time, two-dimensional guidance during CVC insertion. Audio-guided Doppler ultrasound can also aid localisation of the vein and differentiate it from its companion artery during CVC insertion.

For catheters inserted via veins draining to the superior vena cava, the right tracheobronchial angle and carina are common radiological markers of insertion depth. In an attempt to further reduce the incidence of venous erosion (which is rare but potentially catastrophic), some practitioners place the catheter tip lower in the superior vena cava or even in the upper right atrium, ensuring that the catheter is parallel to the long axis of the vein so that the tip does not abut the vein or heart wall end-on.[10]

Many patients with chronic illness, such as malignancy, require long-term central venous catheterization (including PICC). Complications such as central line-associated bloodstream infection and thrombosis (concomitant risk of catheter infection, pulmonary embolus and post-thrombotic syndrome) may require ICU admission and management. Management of such complications is described in **Table 16.2**. In the setting of thrombosis, immediate removal is not necessarily advised.[11]

CENTRAL VENOUS PRESSURE

Jugular venous pressure, CVP and right atrial pressure (RAP) are often used interchangeably. However, in situations associated with increased central venous resistance, such as central vein sclerosis, these pressures may not be the same.

CVP is usually monitored using a fluid-filled pressure transduction system similar to that employed to measure invasive arterial pressures. Waveform analysis is also possible (**Table 16.3**). The normal CVP in the spontaneously breathing supine patient is 0–5 mmHg (0–0.65 kPa), while 10 mmHg (1.3 kPa) is generally accepted as the upper limit during mechanical ventilation. In health there is a good correlation between CVP and pulmonary artery occlusion pressures (PAOP), but this is lost in many types of critical illness such as pulmonary hypertension, pulmonary embolism, right ventricular infarction, left ventricular hypertrophy and myocardial ischaemia. The relationship between CVP and right ventricular end-diastolic volume (preload) is altered in critical illness by changes in right ventricular diastolic compliance and juxta-cardiac pressures.[12]

Except at extreme values, static measures of CVP do not differentiate patients likely to respond to fluid therapy from non-responders (see Functional Haemodynamic Monitoring section). However, dynamic changes in CVP either in response to volume loading or related to respiration can assist in evaluating volume status.[13] For instance, a steep increase in CVP following volume challenge suggests the heart is functioning on the plateau portion of the Frank-Starling curve. Severe hypotension with a low or normal CVP is unlikely to

Table 16.3 Analysis of central venous pressure waveform

CONDITION	PRESSURE CHANGES	WAVEFORM CHANGES
Tricuspid regurgitation	Increased RA pressure	Prominent *v* wave, *x* descent obliterated, *y* descent steep
Right ventricular infarction	RA and RV pressure elevated. RAP does not fall and may rise in inspiration	Prominent *x* and *y* descents
Constrictive pericarditis	RA, RV diastolic, PA diastolic and occlusion pressures elevated and equalised. RAP may rise in inspiration	Prominent *x* and *y* descents
Pericardial tamponade	RA, RV diastolic, PA diastolic and occlusion pressures elevated and equalised. RAP usually falls in inspiration	Y descent damped or absent

RA = right atrial: RV = right ventricular: RAP = right atrial pressure: PA = pulmonary artery.

be due to acute pulmonary embolism, cardiac tamponade or tension pneumothorax.

CENTRAL VENOUS OXYGEN SATURATION

Central venous oxygen saturation (Scv_{O_2}) is an additional variable that may be monitored with a central venous catheter (continuously or via blood gas analysis of samples). It has been proposed as a marker of tissue wellbeing (oxygenation) and will be discussed in a separate chapter. Having been incorporated into a prospective randomised study of patients with severe sepsis and septic shock (Early Goal Directed Therapy),[14] it is mentioned here only as an example of the scant data relating haemodynamic monitoring to improved survival. Results of multicentre evaluation, including the Australasian Resuscitation in Sepsis Evaluation (ARISE Trial, ANZICS Clinical Trials Group) and Protocolized Care for Early Septic Shock (ProCESS Study, NIH funded), are awaited.

PULMONARY ARTERY CATHETER

Right heart catheterisation using a flow-directed balloon-tipped catheter was introduced by Swan et al in 1970.[15] The ability to monitor sophisticated haemodynamic and gas exchange variables at the bedside appealed to clinicians, and the pulmonary artery catheter (PAC) was rapidly accepted into routine critical care. However, this device is potentially associated with a number of risks (**Table 16.4**).

In 1996 a non-randomised cohort study of PAC use in American teaching hospitals appeared to show that PAC in the first 24 hours increased 30-day mortality (odds ratio 1.24, 95% CI 1.03–1.49), mean length of stay and mean cost per hospital stay.[16] An associated editorial called for a moratorium on PAC use, and for a prospective multicentre trial.[17] Prior to this, pulmonary artery catheterisation was regarded by many as the standard of care. Although a moratorium did not eventuate, the debate contributed to clinical equipoise and paved the way for a number of randomised trials.

A recently edited Cochrane database systematic review of PAC monitoring in adult ICU patients incorporated data from 12 randomised controlled trials in adults, comparing management with and without a PAC.[18] The pooled odds ratio for mortality (28-day, 30-day, ICU, hospital) for the eight studies of high-risk surgery patients 0.99 (95% CI 0.73–1.24) and for the four studies of general intensive care patients was 1.05 (95% confidence interval (CI) 0.87–1.26). A subsequent multicentre trial incorporated protocolised haemodynamic management of patients with acute lung injury compared PAC-guided with CVC-guided therapy.[19] There were no significant differences in 60-day mortality or organ function between groups. Overall, these data suggest that PAC monitoring in critically ill patients is neither associated with increased mortality nor with survival benefit.

On the other hand, data do exist that suggest a differential association between PAC use and mortality

Table 16.4 Complications potentially encountered with pulmonary artery catheterisation with proposed measures for prevention and treatment

COMPLICATIONS	PREVENTION	TREATMENT
DURING INSERTION		
Damage to adjacent structures	As for central venous cannulation.	As for central venous cannulation.
Perforation of pulmonary artery	Ensure balloon inflated throughout insertion. Continuously monitor pulmonary artery waveform. Avoid distal PAC tip position.	As for pulmonary artery rupture below.
Air embolism	Raise venous pressure prior to insertion. Always occlude open ends during insertion. Use sheaths with pneumatic valve. Periodically check and tighten all connections. Remove air from fluid bag and tubing. Dress site with occlusive dressing after removal.	Left lateral Trendelenburg position. Administer 100% oxygen and ventilatory support. If PAC in place tighten all connections and attempt to aspirate air from right atrium or right ventricle. Basic/advanced life support if necessary.
Dysrhythmia (12.5–70%)	Keep balloon inflated during passage from RA to PA. Minimise insertion time.	For sustained ventricular tachycardia, remove PAC from right ventricle. For ventricular fibrillation, remove PAC. Advance life support for persistent dysrhythmia.
Right bundle branch block/ Complete heart block	Avoid PAC insertion in patients with left bundle branch block (LBBB) if possible. Insert PAC with pacing electrodes in patients with LBBB.	Use pacing equipment as required.

Table 16.4 Complications potentially encountered with pulmonary artery catheterisation with proposed measures for prevention and treatment—cont'd

COMPLICATIONS	PREVENTION	TREATMENT
Catheter knotting/kinking/ entanglement	Minimise insertion time. Do not advance catheter against resistance. Check for waveform change from RA to RV or RV to PA after advancing 15 cm; if not withdraw catheter. Limit intravascular PAC insertion depth <60 cm. Use of fluoroscopy.	Check chest X-ray. Pull knot back then remove the sheath and catheter. If no sheath used, a cut-down to vein under local anaesthesia may be required. Exploration by a vascular surgeon is indicated if unsuccessful (5% of occasions).
Valve/chordae damage (~0.9%)	Ensure balloon is inflated during forward passage through the heart and deflated prior to any retraction.	Cardiothoracic consultation.
DURING MAINTENANCE		
Dysrhythmia (37%)	Remove PAC when no longer required.	See above.
Thrombosis	As for central venous cannulation.	As for central venous cannulation.
Pulmonary artery rupture (0.2%)	Risk factors include pulmonary hypertension, anticoagulation and *in situ* duration >3 days. Maintain high level of suspicion. Avoid distal PAC tip position. Minimise wedge procedures. Continuously monitor pulmonary artery waveform – withdraw PAC if spontaneous wedging occurs, inflate with only enough air to change PA to PAOP waveform. Withdraw PAC if PAOP obtained with <1.25 mL air.	Check PAC position on CXR, deflate and pull back. If applicable, stop anticoagulation therapy. Lateral position, affected side down. Selective bronchial intubation. PEEP. Surgical repair.
Pulmonary infarction	As for pulmonary artery rupture.	Check PAC position on CXR, deflate and pull back. Observe.
Infection – including blood stream infection/ bacteraemia (1.3–2.3%) and endocarditis (2.2–7.1%)	As for central venous cannulation.	As for central venous cannulation.
Air embolism	High suspicion of balloon rupture. Avoid repeating failed attempts to inflate.	See above.
Misinterpretation/misuse of data	Anticipation and management of common pitfalls related to: Errors of equipment and data acquisition. Factors affecting data interpretation.	Patient selection, individualisation of therapy, an understanding of potentially useful haemodynamic data, as well as an appreciation of alternative monitoring strategies are suggested.

Source: Based upon information contained in text of reference[64]: Evans DC, Doraiswamy VA, Prosciak MP, et al. Complications associated with pulmonary artery catheters: a comprehensive clinical review. Scand J Surg 2009;98:199–208.

dependent upon severity of illness. Multivariate logistic regression analyses of data from a tertiary care university teaching hospital[20] and from the National Trauma Data Bank (American College of Surgeons)[21] suggest that PAC use may be associated with survival benefit in the most severely ill/injured patients.

Overall, the PAC still finds application in anaesthesia and critical care. It potentially offers unique insights into the right heart and pulmonary circulation. However, its role is under increasing scrutiny, and use continues to decline in favour of less invasive alternatives. It is argued that further studies to determine optimal management protocols and appropriate patient groups are required.[18]

Traditional indications for PAC monitoring have been to:

- characterise haemodynamic perturbation (e.g. distributive, cardiogenic, obstructive and hypovolaemic shock or combinations)
- differentiate cardiogenic from non-cardiogenic pulmonary oedema

- guide use of fluids, vasoactive drugs, fluids (including renal replacement therapy) and diuretics, especially when haemodynamic disturbances are coupled with increased lung water, RV or LV dysfunction, pulmonary hypertension and organ dysfunction.

Contraindications for insertion build upon those for central venous catheterisation. If known in advance, atypical cardiac or vascular anatomy, either congenital or secondary to trauma or surgery, should also be considered. Less invasive monitoring might provide the data that are sought. Also, PAC monitoring does not exclude simultaneous recourse to other monitoring techniques.

MEASURED VARIABLES

The PAC remains unique in its ability to measure right ventricular and pulmonary arterial pressures directly at the bedside. While echocardiography might be considered as a less invasive alternative, it is largely confined to intermittent 'snap-shot' evaluation, and can be technically challenging. Normal pressures are given in **Table 16.5**.

Pulmonary artery occlusion pressure

Measurements of pulmonary artery occlusion pressure (PAOP) should be performed by slow injection of air into the balloon while watching the pulmonary artery waveform. Over-wedging can lead to falsely high occlusion pressures or pulmonary arterial rupture. Less than 1.5 mL air (balloon volume) may be required. Deflation after PAOP measurement should re-establish the normal pulmonary arterial waveform. If not, distal migration has occurred and the catheter should be withdrawn until the waveform is re-established.

PAOP should be measured during end expiration and ideally in end diastole, using the ECG p-wave as a marker. When the catheter wedges in a branch of the pulmonary artery it creates a static column of blood which equilibrates with downstream pressure at the site where it rejoins the flowing pulmonary venous system (the j point).[22] Here the blood is very near the left atrium. PAOP therefore closely approximates left atrial pressure (LAP), which approximates left ventricular end-diastolic pressure (LVEDP). The validity of PAOP as a surrogate of preload depends on a number of assumptions (**Fig. 16.1**); these are often incorrect in critically ill patients and the use of PAOP to reflect preload has been questioned.[23]

Table 16.5 Reference range of measured and derived variables from pulmonary artery catheter

SITE	mmHg	(kPa)
Right atrium mean	−1–7	(0.13–0.93)
Right ventricle: systolic	15–25	(2.0–3.3)
Right ventricle: diastolic	0–8	(0–1.1)
Pulmonary artery: systolic	15–25	(2.0–3.3)
Pulmonary artery: diastolic	8–15	(1.1–2.0)
Pulmonary artery: mean	10–20	(1.3–2.6)
Pulmonary artery occlusion pressure	6–15	(0.8–2.0)

Potential substitutes for pulmonary artery occlusion pressure

Measurement of PAOP requires wedging, which is associated with a number of risks (see Table 16.4). The normal pulmonary artery diastolic pressure (PADP) to PAOP gradient is <5 mmHg (0.65 kPa), so that PADP may normally be used as a close approximation for PAOP. However, tachycardia (>120/min) and conditions that increase pulmonary vascular resistance (such as ARDS, chronic obstructive pulmonary disease and pulmonary embolism) variably increase this gradient, invalidating direct substitution of PADP for PAOP. The relationship between PADP and PAOP tends to be stable over hours. Once this is determined, PADP can be used to track PAOP in the short term without repeated wedge manoeuvres.

Echocardiographic measurements, such as transmitral flow and pulmonary venous flow, can provide evidence of elevated left ventricular filling pressure (the hallmark of diastolic dysfunction).[24] Evidence

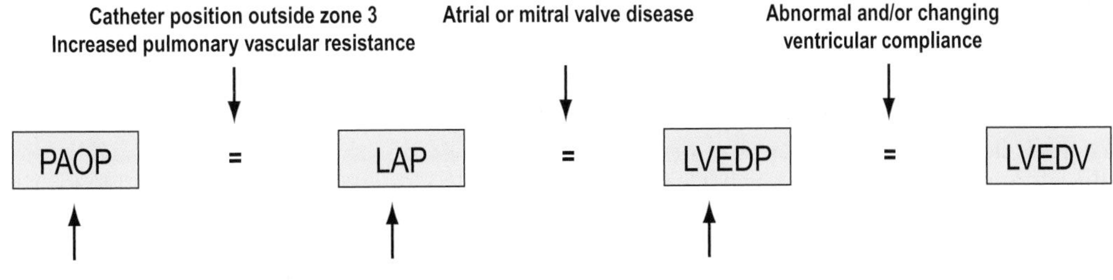

Figure 16.1 Factors affecting the accuracy of PAOP as a measure of preload in critically ill patients. Clinically, LVEDV is usually accepted as a surrogate of preload. PAOP = pulmonary artery occlusion pressure; LAP = left atrial pressure; LVEDP = left ventricular end diastolic pressure; LVEDV = left ventricular end diastolic volume.

Table 16.6 Derived haemodynamic variables

PARAMETER	ABBREVIATION	FORMULA	NORMAL RANGE	UNITS
Mean arterial pressure	MAP	DBP + 0.33 × (SBP – DBP)*	70–105	mmHg
Mean pulmonary artery pressure	MPAP	PADP + 0.33 × (PASP – PADP)*	9–16	mmHg
Mean right ventricular pressure	MRVP	CVP + 0.33 × (PASP – CVP)		mmHg
LV coronary perfusion pressure	LVCCP	DBP – PAOP		mmHg
RV coronary perfusion pressure	RVCCP	MAP – MRVP		mmHg
Cardiac index	CI	CO/BSA	2.8–4.2	$L/min/m^2$
Stroke volume index	SVI	CI/HR	35–70	$mL/beat/m^2$
Systemic vascular resistance index	SVRI	(MAP – CVP)/CI × 79.92	1760–2600	$dyn\ s/cm^5/m^2$
Pulmonary vascular resistance index	PVRI	(PAP – PAOP)/CI × 79.92	44–225	$dyn\ s/cm^5/m^2$
Left ventricular stroke work index	LVSWI	SVI × MAP × 0.0144	44–68	$g\ m/m^2/beat$
Right ventricular stroke work index	RVSWI	SVI × PAP × 0.0144	4–8	$g\ m/m^2/beat$
Body surface area	BSA	Weight $(kg)^{0.425}$ × height $(cm)^{0.725}$ × 0.007184		m^2

* Modern monitors use a more accurate technique; they average the area under the pressure–time curve to estimate mean pressure.
HR = heart rate; CVP = central venous pressure; PAOP = pulmonary artery occlusion pressure; SBP = systolic blood pressure; DBP = diastolic blood pressure; PADP = pulmonary artery diastolic pressure; PASP = pulmonary artery systolic pressure.

increasingly supports the application of such techniques to intensive care patients.[25]

B-type natriuretic peptide (BNP) assay may reflect left ventricular filling pressure, and has demonstrated usefulness in diagnosing cardiac failure in patients presenting to the emergency department with dyspnea. However, preliminary data suggest that BNP is not suitable for evaluating haemodynamic status in critically ill patients.[26]

DERIVED VARIABLES

A number of variables can be derived from the measurements obtained with a standard PAC (see Table 16.5 and **Table 16.6**).

MIXED VENOUS OXYGEN TENSION AND SATURATION

These variables are discussed in Chapter 18 Monitoring oxygenation.

COMPLICATIONS OF PULMONARY ARTERY CATHETERISATION

These are listed in Table 16.4. A catheter may not actually be knotted, despite a chest X-ray appearance to suggest this. If knotting is suspected, other catheters should be removed in reverse order to which they were inserted, and the chest X-ray repeated.

CARDIAC OUTPUT MONITORING

Clinical estimation of cardiac output has been shown to be unreliable until extreme hypotension occurs.[27]

Table 16.7 Classification of methods for evaluating cardiac output in critical care: a variety of techniques primarily estimate stroke volume, multiplication by heart rate calculates cardiac output

CARDIAC OUTPUT	STROKE VOLUME
Fick method (O_2)	Ultrasound • 2D echocardiography (Simpson's method) • Doppler (continuous or pulsed wave)
Indirect Fick method (CO_2) • Partial rebreathing technique	Arterial pressure waveform analysis
Indicator dilution • Thermodilution • Lithium • Indocyanine green • Ultrasound indicator dilution (saline)	Thoracic electrical bioimpedance

A multitude of commercially available devices are approved for cardiac output estimation in critical care. Most devices employ proprietary algorithms. Marketing strategies, patented/trademarked terminology and inconsistencies in nomenclature potentially contribute to confusion. The following discussion of cardiac monitoring techniques attempts to offer the reader an appreciation of fundamental concepts. A classification of techniques is presented in **Table 16.7**.

APPLICATION OF THE FICK PRINCIPLE

The Fick principle is an extension of the law of conservation of mass and states that the amount of a substance taken up by an organ (or the whole body) per unit time is the product of the arteriovenous concentration difference by the blood flow to the organ (or body).

A wide variety of techniques used to measure cardiac output are based upon the Fick principle. The substance measured can include oxygen (Fick method), carbon dioxide (indirect Fick method), or employ an indicator dilution method. Common indicators include thermal energy (thermodilution), lithium and indocyanine green.

THE FICK METHOD

Historically the Fick principle has been applied to determine cardiac output by analysing oxygen uptake from the lungs (direct Fick method). This method requires pulmonary artery catheterisation to sample mixed venous blood. Traditionally, it has been considered the 'gold standard', but in most ICU patients the stringent preconditions for accuracy are not met. Further error is introduced by the elevated oxygen consumption of inflamed lungs. Use is therefore mainly confined to cardiac laboratories.

THE INDIRECT FICK METHOD

The Indirect Fick method employs carbon dioxide (CO_2) as an alternative to oxygen. The use of a partial rebreathing technique, incorporating several assumptions, can be used to eliminate the need to directly measure Cv_{CO_2} with a pulmonary artery catheter.[28,29] The rebreathing values are obtained by introducing an additional 150 mL of dead space into the ventilator circuit (disposable rebreathing loop) and taking measurements once a new equilibrium has been established. Cardiac output can be measured at 3-minute intervals. Assuming that the Cv_{CO_2} concentration does not change significantly throughout the rebreathing period, the terms associated with Cv_{CO2} cancel each other out and are not needed to calculate cardiac output.

Potential issues with the partial rebreathing of CO_2 method include:

- It is unsuitable for non-intubated patients (who have variable tidal volumes and leakage around face-masks).
- Changes in mechanical ventilator settings that alter dead space or ventilation/perfusion relationships may result in an artefactual change in cardiac output measurements. The accuracy of the technique also appears to be challenged by spontaneous mechanically assisted ventilation.
- et_{CO_2} may not accurately reflect change in pulmonary end-capillary and Pa_{CO_2}, especially in chronic lung disease.
- Mathematical models rely upon a series of assumptions that may not be true under certain conditions relevant to critical care.
- There is overall lack of validation in chronic lung disease.

BOLUS THERMODILUTION CARDIAC OUTPUT

This describes the technique utilising a pulmonary artery catheter. It is generally accepted as the de facto clinical gold standard. This reflects applicability at the bedside, clinician familiarity and acceptance of reasonable accuracy.

A bolus injection into the right atrium of cold injectate transiently decreases blood temperature in the pulmonary artery (monitored by a thermistor proximal to the balloon). The mean decrease in temperature (calculated by integrating temperature over time) is inversely proportional to the cardiac output, which can be determined by a modification of the Stewart–Hamilton equation:

$$Q = \frac{V \times (Tb - Ti) K1 \times K2}{Tb(t)\mathrm{d}t} \tag{16.1}$$

where Q = cardiac output; V = volume injected; Tb = blood temperature; Ti = injectate temperature; $K1$ and $K2$ = corrections for specific heat and density of injectate and for blood and dead space volumes; $Tb(t)\mathrm{d}t$ = change in blood temperature as a function of time.

This is an indicator dilution method, using thermal energy (temperature) as the indicator. Advantages of using thermal energy as an indicator are that it is non-toxic (temperature of injectate used does not cause thermal injury) and it does not recirculate. Repeat measurements are limited only by volume constraints and the time to regain temperature stability between injections. A clinically significant change in cardiac output cannot be diagnosed with certainty unless there is a difference of approximately 15% between the mean of three cardiac output determinations and the previous mean.[30]

Too much or too little injectate will respectively under-estimate and over-estimate cardiac output. Cold injectate (preferably 0–4°C but up to 12°C is usually accepted) improves the signal to noise ratio, but causes a brief decrease in heart rate, reducing cardiac output while it is being measured (an example of *biological reactance*). Room temperature injectate introduces a small decrement in bias and precision, but has acceptable accuracy. However, the accuracy using room temperature injectate is further degraded at extremes of cardiac index, high ambient temperatures (and thus injectate temperature) or in patient hypothermia.[31]

Respiration causes fluctuations in cardiac output and PA temperature. Reproducibility is improved by taking measurements in expiration, though this may not reflect cardiac output throughout the respiratory cycle. Timing can be difficult and in practice an average

Box 16.1 Causes of inaccurate bolus thermodilution cardiac output measurements

Catheter malposition
- Wedge position
- Thermistor impinging on vessel wall

Abnormal respiratory pattern
Intracardiac shunts
Tricuspid regurgitation (common in mechanically ventilated patients)
Cardiac dysrhythmias
Incorrect recording of injectate temperature (minimised by siting an additional thermistor on injection port)
Rapid intravenous infusions, especially if administered via the introducer sheath
Injectate port close to or within introducer sheath
Abnormal haematocrit values (affecting *K2* value)
Extremes of cardiac output (room temperature injectate)
Poor technique
- Slow injection (>4 seconds)
- Incorrect injectate volume

of three evenly spaced measurements is taken. Causes of inaccurate measurements are listed in **Box 16.1**.

SEMI-CONTINUOUS THERMODILUTION CARDIAC OUTPUT[32]

This method uses the same principles as bolus thermodilution, but allows semi-continuous measurement by employing a thermal filament wrapped around the right ventricular segment of the catheter. This transmits low-power pulses of heat. 'On–off' heat pulses in pseudo-random binary code are delivered in cycles. The downstream thermistor detects the heat pulses, which are then cross-correlated with the input sequence and power (to allow differentiation of thermal signal from noise).

Potential drawbacks of the technique include:

- inaccuracy during thermal disequilibrium,[33] such as rapid infusions of cool fluids or after cardiac bypass
- delay in detecting sudden changes in cardiac output[33]
- magnetic resonance imaging is contraindicated (it can melt the thermal filament)
- electro-cautery can interfere with measurements.

Additional volumetric data

As well as allowing semicontinuous assessment of cardiac output, incorporation of a rapid response thermistor into the PAC allows estimation of right ventricular ejection fraction (RVEF) and right ventricular end-diastolic volume (RVEDV).[34] Thermodilution techniques appear to overestimate RVEDV and underestimate RVEF.[35] However, right ventricular geometry is complex and there are limited options for bedside volumetric evaluation.

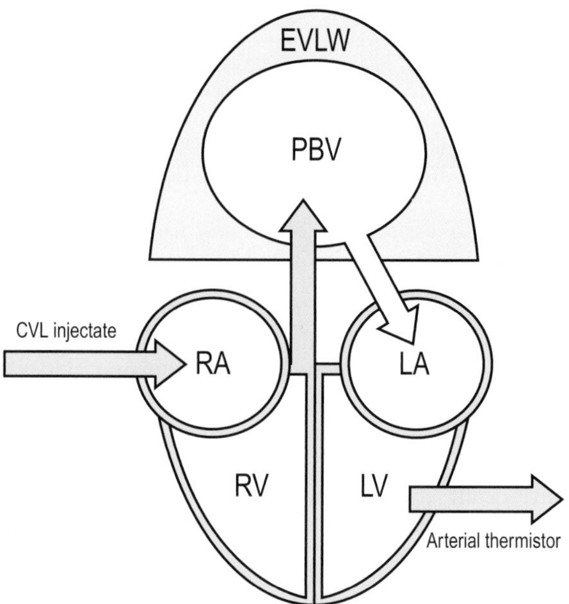

Figure 16.2 Conceptualisation of the transpulmonary mixing chambers of the cardiopulmonary system. Cardiac thermal volumes are proposed to approximate blood volumes at end diastole. CVL = central venous line; EVLW = extravascular lung water; LA = left atrial thermal volume; LV = left ventricular thermal volume; PBV = pulmonary blood volume; RA = right atrial thermal volume; RV = right ventricular thermal volume. Intrathoracic thermal volume (ITTV) is the estimated total thermal volume between the points of central venous injection and peripheral arterial detection, including the EVLW. Pulmonary thermal volume (PTV) is the sum of PBV + EVLW. Intrathoracic blood volume (ITBV) is the sum of RA + RV + PBV + LA + LV, taken to be at end diastole. EVLW = ITTV – ITBV. Global end-diastolic volume (GEDV) is the sum of RAEDV + RVEDV + LAEDV + LVEDV. *(With permission from PULSION Medical Systems SE, www.PULSION.com.)*

TRANSPULMONARY INDICATOR DILUTION

With this technique, thermal and other indicators injected into a central vein are detected in a systemic artery. Because the indicators pass through all chambers of the heart as well as the entire pulmonary circulation, information additional to cardiac output can be gained. In particular, central blood volumes and indices of extravascular lung water can be quantified (**Fig. 16.2**).

Transpulmonary thermodilution[36,37]

A fibreoptic thermistor is usually positioned in the femoral artery at the tip of a modified arterial catheter. Cardiac output is measured by administering a central venous bolus of cold injectate, constructing an arterial thermodilution curve and applying the Stewart-Hamilton equation. The axillary artery can also be used, but placing the sensor in more peripheral arteries such as the radial causes overestimation of cardiac output. Curves are longer and flatter than PAC curves due to thermal equilibration with intrathoracic blood and extravascular lung water, but are unaffected by the respiratory phase of injection. Measurements are in good agreement with pulmonary thermodilution and direct Fick methods. There is a positive bias of about 5%, perhaps because of indicator loss or because transpulmonary measurements are less affected by the transient decrease in heart rate induced by cold thermodilution.

Mathematical models based upon single- or double-indicator techniques allow estimation of intrathoracic blood volume (ITBV), global end-diastolic volume (GEDV) and extravascular lung water (EVLW).[36]

Unlike CVP and PAOP, ITBV is a volumetric preload index. Interpretation is thus independent of alterations in juxta-cardiac pressures or myocardial compliance, and should be superior to conventional pressure indices. There is experimental and clinical evidence that this is so.[38]

EVLW is a marker of the severity of illness. Following EVLW as a therapeutic end-point may reduce positive fluid balances and ventilator and ICU days.[39] EVLW also appears to offer prognostic information in sepsis and acute lung injury.

GEDV is said to represent the volume of blood in all chambers of the heart at end diastole. Like ITBV, GEDV has been shown to be a more reliable measure of cardiac preload than conventional pressure-based surrogates.[40]

LITHIUM DILUTION CARDIAC OUTPUT[41]

Lithium can also serve as a transpulmonary indicator. The small doses of lithium required are non-toxic and easily measured with an ion-selective electrode. Following injection, there is no significant first-pass loss from the circulation. Blood is sampled from an arterial line via a three-way tap. A peristaltic pump limits sampling to 4 mL/min. After passing through the sensor, blood is discarded.

The main advantage over thermodilution is that more peripheral arteries such as the radial can be used without loss of accuracy. Also, injection can be performed peripherally if central venous access is unavailable. The technique shows good agreement with bolus thermodilution (PAC). It is able to safely and accurately measure cardiac output in adult and paediatric populations.

Potential limitations include:

- It cannot be used in patients receiving lithium therapy (background lithium concentration contributes to overestimation of cardiac output).
- Electrode drift can occur in the presence of high-peak doses of muscle relaxants.
- Abnormal shunts can result in erroneous cardiac output measurements (true for all indicator dilution methods).
- Ex vivo analysis requires disposal of sampled blood.

TRANSPULMONARY DYE DILUTION

Transpulmonary indicator dilution can also be performed using injectable dye, usually indocyanine green. Dye dilution (arterial blood analysis) and pulse dye densitometry (transcutaneous optical analysis, comparable to pulse oximetry) have been applied to cardiac output measurement. Concerns exist regarding the accuracy of the transcutaneous method.[42]

ULTRASOUND INDICATOR DILUTION

Whereas transpulmonary thermodilution relies upon changes in temperature induced by injecting saline (other than body temperature), ultrasound indicator dilution relies upon resultant changes in the velocity of sound transmission. Body temperature isotonic saline is injected into a low-volume arteriovenous loop between existing arterial and central venous catheters. The measured change in ultrasound velocity (blood 1560–1585; saline 1533 m/s) allows formulation of an indicator dilution curve with calculation of cardiac output.[43]

ARTERIAL PRESSURE WAVEFORM ANALYSIS[37]

Estimation of stroke volume by analysis of the arterial pressure waveform, in particular various properties of the pulse pressure (pressure above diastolic) component, has been studied for many years. Devices employ different proprietary algorithms (e.g. pulse contour analysis)[44] to calculate flow (cardiac output) from transduced pressure signals. Generic terminology such as arterial pressure waveform analysis is more broadly applicable.

A number of devices require calibration against another method, after which stroke volume can be trended continuously. Accuracy in the presence of arrhythmia has not been established.

Transpulmonary indicator dilution is the usual method of calibration. Devices that use thermodilution or lithium ion calibration are commercially available.[1]

Disadvantages of such techniques can include:

- Recalibration every few hours is advisable to allow for changes in systemic vascular resistance. This is especially important if there is haemodynamic instability or during the administration of vasoactive drugs.
- Alterations in abdominal pressure or changes in body position, particularly in the obese, can alter aortic compliance, necessitating recalibration.
- Dependence on arterial site – clinical validation studies usually document femoral cannulation.
- Aortic aneurysms and significant aortic regurgitation are both difficult to model and invalidate the technique.

Proprietary algorithms for estimating stroke volume and cardiac output (flow) from pressure-based signals without the need for calibration have been incorporated into a number of devices. The principal advantages of these techniques are ease of use and non-invasiveness. However, accuracy is impaired in the presence of major changes in vascular compliance, cardiac dysrhythmia, aortic regurgitation, or poor-quality arterial waveform transduction (under- or overdamping, attenuation).[1]

Although only limited published validation data exist, cardiac output can also be estimated from pulse pressure information acquired completely non-invasively using photoelectric plethysmography in combination with a volume-clamp technique (inflatable finger cuff).[45]

ULTRASOUND

Clinical ultrasound and echocardiographic techniques are becoming indispensible in critical care. Echocardiography is increasingly used in the evaluation of haemodynamically unstable patients. Focused haemodynamic protocols are becoming popular for this purpose and complement other monitoring techniques.

Two approaches are available to measure stroke volume (and thereby cardiac output) using sound waves. The first involves the use of echocardiography to measure systolic and diastolic left-ventricular volumes using Simpson's method (summation of discs). Stroke volume is then calculated. Geometric assumptions, user dependence and access to expensive echocardiographic equipment limit the usefulness of this technique for haemodynamic monitoring. The second method uses Doppler techniques to measure stroke volume (**Fig. 16.3**).[46] This methodology forms the basis of numerous monitoring devices. Doppler is less dependent on image quality, shows better agreement with thermodilution and demonstrates good reproducibility.

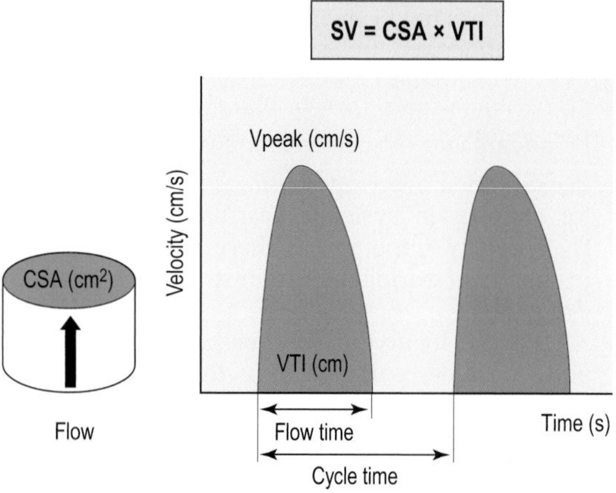

Figure 16.3 Doppler stroke volume calculation. The cross-sectional area of flow (CSA) is calculated as a circle from echocardiographic measurements or nomogram-based estimations. Velocity–time integral (VTI) is the integral of Doppler velocity with regard to time. Stroke volume (SV) is calculated as the product of CSA and VTI (mL/s in this example). Cardiac output is calculated from the product and SV and heart rate. Peak velocity of flow (V_{peak}) is also indicated.

The Doppler principle states that the frequency of reflected sound is altered by a moving target, such as red blood cells. Continuous and pulsed wave Doppler are the main techniques employed to measure flow. Physical principles for the two techniques are similar. Pulsed wave Doppler allows the site of sampling to be specified by transmitting a pulse of sound energy and then 'listening' for a period of time appropriate to catch the signal returning after reflection at the selected depth. With continuous wave Doppler, a piezoelectric crystal transmits the ultrasound beam continuously, while another measures the frequency of reflected waves. The velocities of all the red blood cells moving along the path of the ultrasound beam are recorded. As a result, a continuous wave Doppler recording consists of a full spectral envelope with the outer border corresponding to the fastest moving blood cells. The flow velocity (*V*) of red cells can be determined from the Doppler shift in the frequency of reflected waves:

$$V = (2F_0 \times \cos\theta)^{-1} \times C\Delta F \qquad (16.2)$$

where C is the speed of ultrasound in tissue (1540 m/s), ΔF is the frequency shift, F_0 is the emitted ultrasound frequency, and θ is the angle of incidence. The most accurate results are obtained when the ultrasound beam is parallel to flow ($\theta = 0°$, $\cos\theta = 1$; $\theta = 180°$, $\cos\theta = -1$). However, angles up to 20° still yield acceptable results ($\theta = 20°$, $\cos\theta = 0.94$).

In addition to measuring stroke volume, Doppler assessment of aortic blood flow can provide additional haemodynamic information. For instance, a low duration of aortic velocity signal corrected for heart rate (corrected flow time; FTc) may prompt intravenous fluid challenge.[26,47] The peak velocity of aortic blood flow (V_{peak}) has been proposed as an index of contractility. Also, respiratory variation in V_{peak} (ΔV_{peak}) has been described as a predictor of increased cardiac output in response to fluid challenge.[48]

OESOPHAGEAL DOPPLER MONITORING[37,49]

Oesophageal Doppler measures blood flow velocity in the descending aorta with a Doppler probe (usually 4 MHz continuous wave or 5 MHz pulsed wave depending upon device) incorporated in the tip of a flexible probe. The probe is positioned in the oesophagus about 30–40 cm from the teeth. At this point, the aorta runs parallel to the oesophagus and the systolic cross-sectional area varies least. The probe is rotated to obtain a characteristic aortic signal. The aortic cross-sectional area is either determined from nomograms of age, weight and height, or calculated from a measured diameter (M-mode ultrasound). Calibration against other cardiac output methods is also possible.

Advantages of the technique include:

- Only a short period of training is required. Nurses at the bedside can follow volume challenge protocols guided by Doppler indices.

- The probes (6 mm in diameter) are minimally invasive, and can be inserted nasally or orally.
- Contraindications are few. They include severe agitation, pharyngo-oesophageal pathology, aortic balloon counterpulsation, aortic dissection and severe aortic coarctation.
- Insertion is simple, allowing reduced time to data acquisition and treatment.
- Probes are relatively stable once placed. If displaced they can be repositioned quickly, and can be left in place for days in a sedated, ventilated patient.

Potential disadvantages include:

- Assumptions that descending aortic flow is 70% of total cardiac output and that nomograms accurately determine aortic cross-section can be incorrect. This limits usefulness when there is aortic pathology or compression, or abnormal upper/lower body blood flow distributions.
- Flow in the aorta is not always laminar. Conditions such as tachycardia, anaemia, and aortic valve disease can cause turbulent aortic blood flow and alter velocity measurements.
- Assumptions that the aorta is cylindrical with a fixed systolic cross-section are not always valid. The cross-sectional area of the aorta is actually dynamic and is dependent on the pulse pressure and aortic compliance. This may be particularly relevant in children, where aortic cross-section fluctuates in systole.
- Finding and maintaining optimal probe positioning are important for consistency in trend measurements.
- The probe may be poorly tolerated in non-sedated patients. Oral insertion is usually reserved for intubated patients receiving sedation. Trends toward minimal sedation and shorter duration of endotracheal intubation might decrease the practicality of this technique in many patients.

TRANSCUTANEOUS DOPPLER MONITORING

Externally applied continuous wave Doppler can be used to monitor haemodynamics via transpulmonary (parasternal) and transaortic (suprasternal) windows. If not known or previously measured, flow diameters may be estimated by a proprietary algorithm based upon the linear association between height and cardiovascular dimensions.[50]

Like oesophageal Doppler, this method appears to offer a clinically useful alternative to thermodilution techniques for monitoring cardiac output and its variation.[51] The technique can be used in all age groups and can be comfortably performed in non-sedated patients.

THORACIC ELECTRICAL BIOIMPEDANCE AND BIOREACTANCE[37,52]

An alternating electrical current (high frequency, very low magnitude) is passed through the thorax. Thoracic electrical bioimpedance requires the current to be kept constant while fluctuations in electrical impedance are measured. Six electrodes are usually attached (two in the upper thorax/neck region and four in the lower thorax). These electrodes detect changes in bioimpedance and monitor cardiac electrical signals. The technique is very sensitive to any alteration in position or contact of the electrodes to the patient.

The change in aortic blood flow due to myocardial contraction (stroke volume) is measured from the changes in thoracic bioimpedance through the cardiac cycle. Other factors that contribute to a change in overall thoracic bioimpedance include changes in tissue fluid volume and changes in venous and pulmonary blood volume induced by respiration. Respiratory artefact is eliminated by averaging values over several cardiac cycles using the R–R interval (ECG) as a synchronising signal.

Measuring whole body, rather than truncal, impedance by placing electrodes on wrists and ankles also appears successful.

Inaccuracies can arise from numerous sources that are prevalent in critical care. These include motion artefact, electrical interference, dysrhythmias (including frequent premature atrial contractions and atrial fibrillation) and acute change in tissue water content (such as pulmonary oedema, pleural effusions, or expansion of interstitial fluid). Despite these limitations, it is clinically appealing due to its non-invasive nature.

Bioreactance has built upon the concepts of bioimpedance but, rather than changes in impedance, it measures changes in the frequency of the electrical currents traversing the chest. This potentially improves signal to noise ratio.[1]

FLOW PROBES

In the laboratory, flow probes may be employed to calculate blood flow (including stroke volume and cardiac output). Commercially available systems are ultrasonic or electromagnetic.[53] Though such high-fidelity devices are not readily applied to clinical settings, they are mentioned as the reference or 'gold' standard against which many clinical devices are evaluated experimentally.

STATISTICAL COMPARISON OF CARDIAC OUTPUT MONITORS

Correlation is not an appropriate statistical method for comparing a new measurement device with a reference standard. This is because the new techniques may show high correlation despite being highly inaccurate; for example, the new technique might consistently report cardiac output as double that measured by the reference standard.

A more robust comparison was offered by Bland & Altmann.[54] The Bland–Altmann technique calculates the bias (mean difference between paired measurements), precision (1 standard deviation of the difference

Table 16.8 Variables described as indices of cardiac preload or fluid responsiveness in critically ill patients*

STATIC	DYNAMIC
INTRACARDIAC PRESSURES Central venous pressure (CVP)/right atrial pressure (RAP) Pulmonary artery occlusion pressure (PAOP)	RESPONSE TO FLUID CHALLENGE
CARDIOVASCULAR VOLUMES Thermodilution right ventricular end-diastolic volume (RVEDV) Echocardiographic RVEDV Echocardiographic left ventricular end-diastolic area (LVEDA)/ volume (LVEDV) Transpulmonary thermodilution global end-diastolic volume (GEDV) Transpulmonary thermodilution intrathoracic blood volume (ITBV)	PASSIVE LEG RAISING Change in aortic blood flow Change in pulse pressure SPONTANEOUS RESPIRATORY EFFORT Inspiratory decrease in right atrial pressure (ΔRAP) MANDATORY MECHANICAL VENTILATION Systolic pressure variation (SPV) Decrease in systolic pressure (Δ_{down}) Pulse pressure variation (PPV)
DOPPLER Duration of the aortic velocity signal corrected for heart rate (FTc) Respiratory variation in peak velocity of aortic blood flow (ΔV_{peak})	Pulse contour analysis stroke volume variation (SVV) Respiratory variation in peak aortic blood velocity (ΔV_{peak}) Respiratory change in the pre-ejection period (ΔPEP) Respiratory systolic variation test (RSVT)

* Variables have been divided into static and dynamic categories. Static variables are estimates of ventricular preload at a point in time, usually end-expiration. Dynamic variables are characterised by measurement of variation in haemodynamic measurements in response to changes in cardiac loading conditions.

Source: Based on information contained in text of reference: Sturgess DJ, Joyce C, Marwick TH, Venkatesh B. A clinician's guide to predicting fluid responsiveness in critical illness: applied physiology and research methodology. Anaesth Intensive Care 2007;35(5):669–78. Epub 2007/10/16.

between paired measurements) and limits of agreement (2 standard deviations; describes the range for 95% of comparison points). Based on meta-analysis, Critchley & Critchley proposed that the new technique was interchangeable with the reference technique if the limits of agreement were within ±30%.[55] A recent meta-analysis of minimally invasive techniques challenges this arbitrary threshold, suggesting that limits of agreement of up to 45% may be acceptable in clinical practice.[56]

Given that many new monitors now provide continuous measurements, the ability to trend changes in cardiac output has become an important consideration. This information is not provided by the methods discussed so far. This level of statistical analysis is complex and appropriate methodology is still being determined.[57]

FUNCTIONAL HAEMODYNAMIC MONITORING

Functional haemodynamic monitoring builds upon the observation that functional or 'dynamic' haemodynamic variables are better predictors of haemodynamic response to fluid challenge than 'static' variables (**Table 16.8**).[58] The prediction of fluid responsiveness is an attribute of haemodynamic monitoring technology that would allow rational fluid resuscitation with avoidance of the consequences of excess and unhelpful fluid challenge; these consequences may include excess tissue and pulmonary oedema with deleterious impact upon respiratory function, wound healing and abdominal compartment syndrome.[59]

The potential value of fluid responsiveness hinges upon the ability to predict whether a patient's left ventricle is operating on the plateau (preload independent) portion of the Frank–Starling curve at the time of considering fluid challenge. Thus fluid challenge could be avoided, as it will be ineffective and potentially deleterious. Inotropic support should be considered in preference. It is crucial to appreciate that under normal physiological conditions the left ventricle demonstrates recruitable stroke volume (ascending or 'preload dependent' portion of the Frank–Starling curve). Thus prediction of a fluid responsive state does not mandate fluid challenge.

It must also be appreciated that the majority of 'dynamic' variables posed as predictors of fluid responsiveness have been studied in small samples of highly selected patients under restrictive preconditions (including mandatory mechanical ventilation). In particular techniques, such as pulse pressure variation, have been validated only under a number of caveats including the absence of spontaneous respiratory effort, moderate tidal volumes and normal myocardial contractility. Assessing response to fluid challenge or passive leg raising is more generalisable and is more commonly recommended.[60]

PERIOPERATIVE HAEMODYNAMIC OPTIMISATION

The concept of perioperative haemodynamic optimisation (including 'goal-directed therapy') is not novel. However, evidence increasingly supports a role for haemodynamic monitoring and pre-emptive intervention in high-risk surgical groups, in terms of both reduced morbidity and mortality. The benefit spans monitoring technologies, with potential benefits in terms of reducing mortality as well as surgical complications.[47] Positive results have predominantly followed from protocols incorporating pre- and intraoperative interventions.

MONITORING THE MICROCIRCULATION[60]

Many techniques used to monitor the microcirculation are yet to make the transition to mainstream clinical care. However, there is growing appreciation that perfusion of the microcirculation is adversely affected by many disease states directly relevant to critical care.

Many potential techniques have been studied with varying degrees of success.[61] For reference, a number of techniques for evaluation of perfusion (rather than tissue oxygenation, which is discussed elsewhere) are briefly mentioned here. Clinically, mottled skin, acrocyanosis, delayed capillary refill and increased central to peripheral temperature gradients might disclose an impaired microcirculation. Biomarkers such as lactate and raised plasma hyaluronan (experimental) might also indicate impairment. Laser Doppler flowmetry can be applied to a range of tissues. Microvideoscopic techniques (nailfold videocapillaroscopy; orthogonal polarisation spectral (OPS) and sidestream darkfield (SDF) imaging techniques) can be applied to superficial capillary beds. Except at high levels, blood flow is the major determinant of venous to arterial CO_2 gradient (CO_2 gap). Alternatively, tissue CO_2 can be measured by tissue electrodes, probes or tonometry. Microdialysis and equilibrium analysis allow measurement of molecules from the extracellular environment. These techniques are well suited to quantification of lactate/pyruvate ratio.

Although optimisation of perfusion and oxygenation at a cellular level offers an appealing therapeutic target, a number of practicalities stand in the way. Evaluation of microvascular function at the bedside of critically ill patients remains challenging.[61] Furthermore, many microvascular pathologies may be localised or heterogeneous, in which case the microcirculation being monitored might not offer generalisable data.

Access the complete references list online at http://www.expertconsult.com

1. Vincent JL, Rhodes A, Perel A, et al. Clinical review: update on hemodynamic monitoring – a consensus of 16. Crit Care 2011;15(4):229. Epub 2011/09/03.
5. O'Grady NP, Alexander M, Dellinger EP, et al. Guidelines for the prevention of intravascular catheter-related infections. Centers for Disease Control and Prevention. MMWR Recomm Rep 2002; 51(RR-10):1–29. Epub 2002/09/18.
29. Hofer CK, Ganter MT, Zollinger A. What technique should I use to measure cardiac output? Curr Opin Crit Care 2007;13(3):308–17. Epub 2007/05/01.
36. Hudson E, Beale R. Lung water and blood volume measurements in the critically ill. Curr Opin Crit Care 2000;6(3):222–6.
47. Hamilton MA, Cecconi M, Rhodes A. A systematic review and meta-analysis on the use of preemptive hemodynamic intervention to improve postoperative outcomes in moderate and high-risk surgical patients. Anesth Analg 2011;112(6):1392–402. Epub 2010/10/23.

17

Multiple organ dysfunction syndrome

Matthew J Maiden and Marianne J Chapman

Multi-organ dysfunction syndrome (MODS) is a complex process whereby an acute disease precipitates deranged function of a number of organ systems. MODS is encountered commonly in the intensive care unit (ICU) and accounts for 40–50% of deaths.[1,2] Hence, critical care clinicians require a sound understanding of the pathophysiology and management priorities for MODS.

HISTORY

The development of critical care has improved the survival of severely ill and injured patients but with this has come the recognition that organ failure can develop after the initial injury/illness. This was first described during World War II, where soldiers with severe non-thoracic injuries developed respiratory failure and subsequent renal failure. The incidence of this appeared to be related to the severity and duration of pre-hospital hypotension and the term 'shock lung' was used to describe the subsequent respiratory failure. Although hypoperfusion of the organs may have initiated functional impairment, other factors including blood products, microemboli, fat emboli, endotoxin and excessive oxygen were postulated to contribute.

In the 1970s, similar patterns of 'distant' organ failure were reported in critically ill patients following trauma, surgical haemorrhage, abdominal sepsis, pneumonia and pancreatitis. At autopsy, these patients had similar pathological findings (e.g. microvascular thrombi, tracheobronchial casts, pulmonary congestion, hepatic necrosis, gastric ulcers) irrespective of their admission diagnosis.[3] It was therefore proposed that a common pathogenic process may cause multiple organ failure independent of the precipitating event. If this process could be identified and characterised, it may provide a therapeutic target. Although many pathophysiological processes underlying MODS have been described, it is still not clear what the driving force is and why only some patients develop MODS after a precipitating event.

DEFINITION

In 1973, the term 'sequential organ failure' was used to describe the pattern of multiple organ impairment following resuscitation from aortic aneurysm rupture. Over the next two decades, 40 different names were ascribed to this phenomenon of 'organ disease remote from the site of illness/injury'. The terms 'multiple system failure' or 'multiple organ failure' were commonly used; however, each description and definition differed.

A consensus conference in 1992 proposed the term 'multiple organ dysfunction syndrome' (MODS).[4] This term reflects a distinction between 'dysfunction' and 'failure'. 'Failure' implies a dichotomous outcome that is often irreversible whereas 'dysfunction' describes a spectrum of organ impairment that may change over time. The term 'syndrome' was added to describe a pattern of multiple physiological changes that may have a similar pathogenesis. However, this definition does not characterise or quantify the associated organ dysfunction. Over 20 definitions, classifications and scoring systems of multiple organ dysfunction have been described.[5] These have varied according to which organ systems are assessed, which parameters are measured, and the thresholds of these parameters for the organs to be considered dysfunctional.

The MODS and SOFA (Sepsis-related Organ Failure Assessment) scores (**Tables 17.1** and **17.2**; note the similarity between the scores) were independently developed after the consensus definition of MODS and are commonly used to clinically define the syndrome. Rather than predicting mortality, they were primarily established to describe the severity of MODS and the changes in organ function over time.[6,7] The scores use an equally weighted variable for each of six organ systems that were chosen because they had a strong relationship with mortality and were least influenced by treatment. The score at ICU admission and the change in score over the course of ICU stay strongly correlates with mortality rate with both the MODS and SOFA scores performing similarly.[8] However, these scoring systems use only one parameter for each organ system and thus may underscore patients displaying other features of organ dysfunction. These scores continue to be used to standardise reporting of MODS and provide a quantitative measure of severity that can be followed over time.

AETIOLOGY OF MODS

MODS occurs most commonly as a consequence of the inflammatory response to infection (i.e. sepsis).

Table 17.1 MODS score

MODS SCORE	0	1	2	3	4
Respiratory[a] *(P_{O_2}/Fi_{O_2})*	>300	226–300	151–225	76–150	≤75
Renal[b] *(serum creatinine μmol/L)*	≤100	101–200	201–350	351–500	>500
Hepatic *(serum bilirubin μmol/L)*	≤20	21–60	61–120	121–240	>240
Cardiovascular[c] *(PAR)*	≤10.1	10.1–15.0	15.1–20.0	20.1–30.0	>30.0
Haematologic *(platelet count × 10^3/ml)*	>120	81–120	51–80	21–50	≤20
Neurologic[d] *(Glasgow Coma Score)*	15	13–14	10–12	7–9	≤6

[a]P/F ratio is calculated without reference to the use or mode of mechanical ventilation, and without reference to the use or level of positive end-expiratory pressure;
[b]serum creatinine measured without reference to the use of dialysis;
[c]Pressure-adjusted heart rate (PAR) is calculated as the product of heart rate (HR) multiplied by the ratio of the right atrial (central venous) pressure (RAP) to the mean arterial pressure (MAP): PAR = HR × RAP/MAP;
[d]The Glasgow Coma Score is preferably calculated by the patient's nurse, and is scored conservatively (for the patient receiving sedation or muscle relaxants, normal function is assumed, unless there is evidence of intrinsically altered mentation).

Table 17.2 SOFA score

SOFA SCORE	1	2	3	4
Respiratory *(P_{O_2}/Fi_{O_2})*	<400	<300	<200 With respiratory support	<100
Renal *(serum creatinine μmol/L or urine output)*	110–170	171–299	300–440 or <500 ml/day	>440 or <200 ml/day
Hepatic *(serum bilirubin μmol/L)*	20–32	33–101	102–204	>204
Cardiovascular[a]	MAP < 70mmHg	Dopamine ≤ 5 or Dobutamine (any dose)	Dopamine > 5 or Epinephrine ≤ 0.1 or Norepinephrine ≤ 0.1	Dopamine > 15 or Epinephrine > 0.1 or Norepinephrine > 0.1
Hematologic *(platelet count × 10^3/ml)*	<150	<100	<50	<20
Neurologic *(Glasgow Coma Score)*	13–14	10–12	6–9	<6

[a]Adrenergic agents administered for at least 1h (doses given are in μg/kg/min).

However, almost any disease that invokes tissue injury may progress to MODS (**Box 17.1**).

PATHOGENESIS

MODS is a systemic process with complex pathophysiology. Although inflammation appears to be central to the development of MODS, the extent to which other processes contribute varies according to the precipitating disease, the stage of disease/recovery, the functional reserve of the organs, and the type and timing of the treatments provided. The pathogenesis of MODS is best conceptualised as a complex dynamic non-linear system involving a large number of variables that are highly interdependent (**Fig. 17.1**).[9]

Box 17.1 Diseases that can progress to MODS

Sepsis

Non-sepsis
- Major trauma
- Burns
- Pancreatitis
- Aspiration syndromes
- Extracorporeal circulation (e.g. cardiac bypass)
- Multiple blood transfusion
- Ischaemia–reperfusion injury
- Autoimmune disease
- Heat-induced illness
- Eclampsia
- Poisoning/toxicity

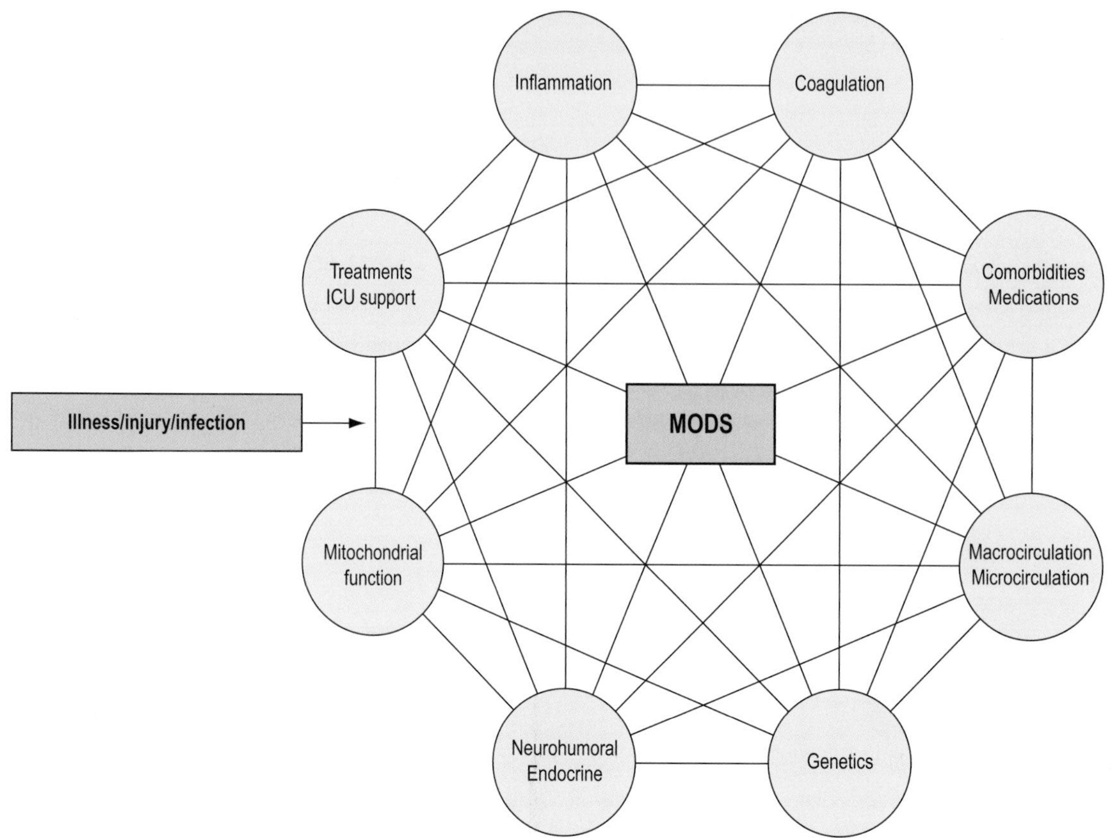

Figure 17.1 MODS results from a complex interaction of a number of different pathogenic processes.

INFLAMMATION

Inflammation is essential to contain infection and for tissue repair. However, the inflammatory response to injury/illness/infection may become 'dys-regulated' during critical illness.[10] Increased levels of pro-inflammatory mediators are associated with worsening organ dysfunction and MODS can be reproduced experimentally by infusion of inflammatory cytokines. As a systemic inflammatory response appears to be central to the development of MODS, the term 'systemic inflammatory response syndrome' (SIRS) was defined in conjunction with the definition of MODS (**Box 17.2**).[4] However, SIRS is non-specific and provides little information about what is provoking the inflammation or the likelihood of progression to MODS.

Many inflammatory mediators have been characterised over the last 50 years (**Box 17.3**). They are released from a variety of inflammatory cells and interact with the immune, endocrine and nervous systems to mediate host defence and tissue repair.

The complex interaction between these mediators has led to the search for common pathways in inflammation that may become therapeutic targets. Intracellular cell signalling molecules that modulate production of cytokines have been the focus of recent research.

Nuclear factor-κB (NF-κB) is a co-factor involved in the transcription of genes that encode inflammatory proteins, apoptotic signalling pathways and nitric oxide production. NF-κB is preformed in the cytoplasm and is activated when the inhibitory subunit (IκBα) is cleaved off, allowing NF-κB to translocate to the nucleus. NF-κB levels are increased in sepsis in proportion to severity.[11]

Box 17.2 Systemic inflammatory response syndrome (SIRS)

Systemic inflammatory response syndrome (SIRS) is defined by the presence of two or more of the following:

1. Temperature >38°C or <36°C
2. Heart rate >90 beats/min
3. Respiratory rate >20 breaths/min or hyperventilation with Pa_{CO_2} <32 mmHg (4.2 kPa)
4. White cell count >12 000 or <4000 cells /μL or >10% immature forms.

Box 17.3 Inflammatory mediators associated with MODS

Interleukin-1β
Interleukin-6
Interleukin-8
Tissue necrosis factor-α
Interferon-γ
Colony stimulating factors
Eicosanoids/platelet-aggregating factor
Soluble adhesion molecules
Complement activation
Heat shock proteins
Free radicals
Pro-calcitonin

Toll-like receptors (e.g. TLR2, TLR4) are activated by bacterial products and necrotic cells and they in turn activate NF-κB and other factors that transcribe inflammatory mediators. The process of TLR activation differs between microbial and non-microbial precipitants.[12] Preclinical studies targeting the non-microbial activation pathways have yielded less organ dysfunction while maintaining anti-microbial efficacy.

High mobility group box protein 1 (HMGB-1) is an evolutionary conserved protein that potentiates binding of inflammatory mediators to inflammatory cells. It also acts as a nuclear co-factor that enhances DNA transcription of inflammatory mediators. Plasma levels of HMGB-1 increase in sepsis and trauma in proportion to the severity of the illness or injury. In experimental studies, anti-HMGB-1 attenuates the inflammatory response to infection, autoimmunity, ischaemia and trauma.[13]

COMPENSATORY ANTI-INFLAMMATORY RESPONSE SYNDROME (CARS)

To ensure a controlled inflammatory response, inflammatory cells also release mediators with anti-inflammatory effects (e.g. IL-4, IL-10). Just as pro-inflammatory mediators may become excessive, the anti-inflammatory response may become predominant, resulting in a state of immunosuppression and anergy.[14] This anti-inflammatory response has been termed the 'compensatory anti-inflammatory response syndrome' (CARS) and is typically encountered some time after the initial inflammatory response.[15] Immunological changes include apoptosis of lymphocytes, release of IL-10, which suppresses TNF-α, decreased cytokine production and down-regulated HLA receptors on monocytes.[16] This relative immunosuppression is often a feature of MODS and is thought to account for why many patients develop iatrogenic infections with organisms that are usually commensal or of low virulence (e.g. *Candida, Pseudomonas, Stenotrophomonas, Enterococcus*).

COAGULATION

The clotting system can be triggered by tissue factor, endotoxin, bacterial antigens and cytokines. Thrombin is produced at the site of infection/injury to isolate infectious sources and initiate tissue repair. However, products of the clotting cascade are pro-inflammatory and the clotting system is central in the inflammatory response. For example, activation of the thrombin receptor induces transcription of NF-κB and stimulation of pro-inflammatory sequelae.

Coagulation is normally controlled by the endogenous anti-coagulant factors anti-thrombin III (AT-III binds to thrombin and endothelium to release endothelial prostacyclin and inhibit platelet aggregation) and protein C (which complexes with protein S to inhibit Va and VIIIa). Levels of these anti-coagulants fall during critical illness and their reduction is proportional to the severity of MODS.[17]

NEUROHUMORAL CHANGES

The autonomic system is closely intertwined with the inflammatory response. The sympathetic and parasympathetic nervous systems innervate lymphoid organs and most immune cells have neurotransmitter receptors. Neural stimulation of the immune cells inhibits cytokine release and suppresses the immune response. Some immune mediators also act as neurohormones providing neural feedback regarding the inflammatory state (**Fig. 17.2**).[18,19]

The 'stress response' to critical illness involves release of the adrenal hormones. This is controlled by hypothalamic secretion of corticotropin-releasing hormone (CRH) under direct neural control and modulated by circulating cytokines. Inadequate hypothalamic–pituitary–adrenal response to critical illness or glucocorticoid resistance may contribute to MODS.

Changes to thyroid metabolism occur during MODS. In health, thyroxine (T_4) is metabolised to the metabolically active tri-iodothyronine (T_3), whereas during critical illness changes to the de-iodination pathways favour production of the biologically inactive reverse-T_3. The consequential fall of plasma T_3 levels is proportional to the severity of MODS and is predictive of mortality.[20]

MACROCIRCULATORY CHANGES

Inadequate circulation of blood resulting in reduced cellular oxygen delivery (DO_2) can lead to anaerobic metabolism and impaired function. This state of circulatory shock contributes to MODS.

Vascular tone is often reduced in MODS with excessive nitric oxide being a well-characterised culprit. Endothelial nitric oxide synthase (iNOS) is induced by many different inflammatory mediators. The nitric oxide (NO) produced is toxic to micro-organisms, acts as an inflammatory signal, produces vascular smooth

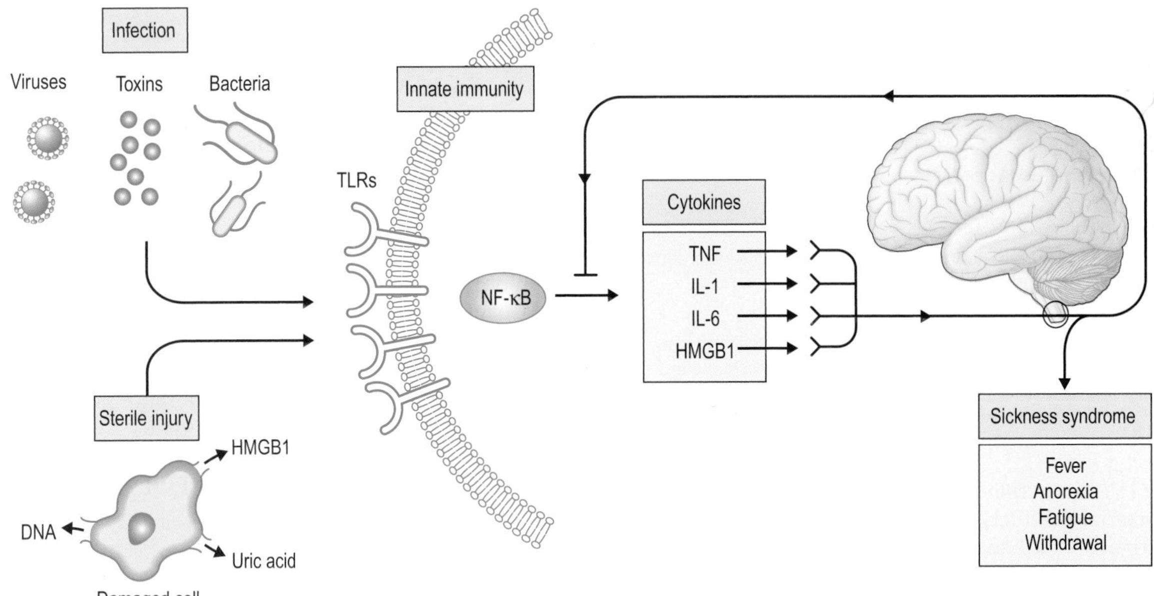

Figure 17.2 Neurohumoral factors influence the response to illness/injury. *(Adapted from Tracey KJ. Understanding immunity requires more than immunology. Nat Immunol 2010;11(7):561–4.)*

muscle relaxation and maintains patency of the microcirculation. However, excessive NO also leads to 'vasoplegia' with low systemic arterial pressures, venodilation and altered blood flow into the organs.

Maintaining sufficient blood circulation is essential for normal organ function. However, attempts to prevent MODS by providing supranormal DO_2 by transfusing red cells or increasing cardiac output with dobutamine have not improved outcomes.[21] Furthermore, clinical studies of agents that inhibit iNOS or antagonise NO have shown haemodynamic benefit but have increased mortality.[22]

MICROCIRCULATORY CHANGES

Using spectral imaging techniques, it has been observed that reduced blood flow through the microcirculation is associated with organ failure and death (**Fig. 17.3**).[23] Microvascular thrombi, reduced red blood cell deformability and increased blood viscosity contribute to reduced microvascular flow.[24] Excessive NO leads to mismatched microvascular flow and shunting.[25] Vascular endothelial disruption increases microvascular permeability favouring formation of interstitial oedema, which further restricts diffusion between the cell and the microcirculation.

APOPTOSIS

Apoptosis is controlled cellular death without provoking inflammation. It is an essential process for normal coordinated function of populations of cells and is involved in cell ageing, immune regulation, epithelial cell turnover and resolution of inflammation. During critical illness, apoptosis is increased in lymphocytes and in cells that typically have a barrier function (e.g. gut epithelium, vascular endothelium).[26] This increases susceptibility to further insults. In contrast, apoptosis of neutrophils is delayed and may lead to an exaggerated inflammatory response.[27] Caspases are central in the regulation of apoptosis and may provide a therapeutic target.

MITOCHONDRIAL DYSFUNCTION

Cell necrosis is an uncommon finding in post-mortem examination of organs that have failed due to MODS. This suggests that processes leading to MODS are primarily a functional disorder rather than structural. Cells may enter a state of 'hibernation' where metabolic activity is reduced. Changes in mitochondrial respiration seen in MODS may be induced by alterations in humoral factors that have metabolic effects (e.g. thyroid hormone, glucocorticoids, catecholamines and cytokines).[28] The cell subsequently fails to utilise available O_2, leading to cellular dysoxia and cellular dysfunction contributing to organ dysfunction.[29,30]

CO-MORBIDITIES

An important consideration in the development of MODS is the patient's premorbid organ function. Patients with pre-existing organ disease are more likely to have further deterioration of organ function as the

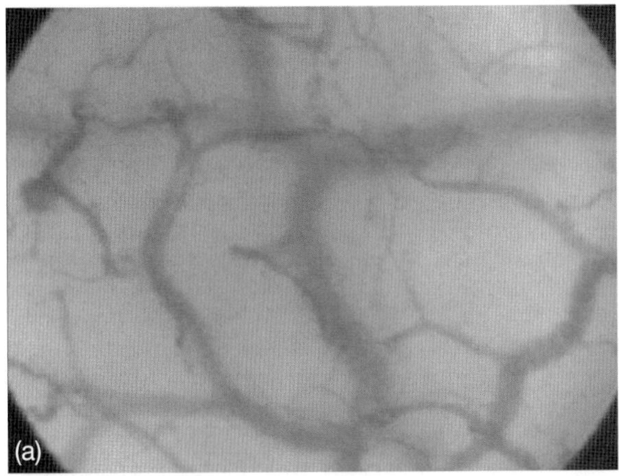

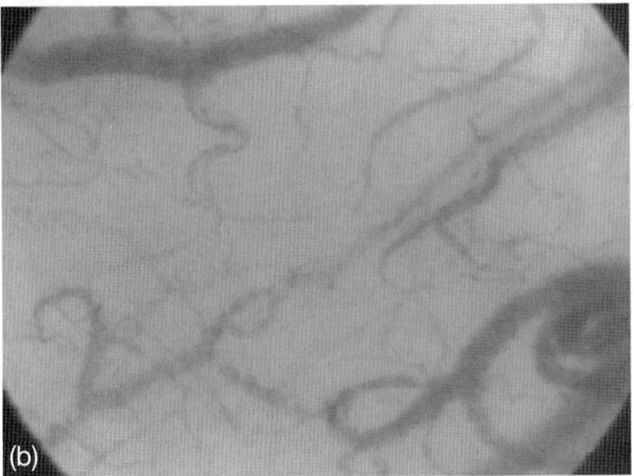

Figure 17.3 Sublingual microcirculatory changes seen in sepsis-induced MODS. (a) Healthy volunteer, and (b) a patient with septic shock. Note the rich density of large and small vessels in the healthy volunteer and the decrease in density of small vessels in sepsis. *(Reprinted with permission of the American Thoracic Society. Copyright ©2012 American Thoracic Society. From: DeBacker et al. Microvascular blood flow is altered in patients with sepsis. American Journal of Respiratory and Critical Care Medicine, 2002;166:98–104. Official journal of the American Thoracic Society.)*

result of acute critical illness (e.g. compromised respiratory reserve in fibrotic lung disease, limited renal function in diabetic nephropathy, reduced marrow response in chronic leukaemia, impaired hepatic function in alcoholic liver disease). These patients will have a lower threshold for developing MODS.

IATROGENESIS

The recognition of MODS corresponded with the development of intensive care supports. It may be that some ICU interventions actually increase the risk of developing MODS or continue to drive the process once it is initiated. For example, the ARDSnet study revealed that 'large tidal-volume ventilation' stimulates the release of pulmonary cytokines leading to worsening lung injury and increased risk of death.[31] ICU patients are now ventilated with smaller tidal volumes. Other ICU interventions such as type of parenteral fluids, immobility, artificial cooling, extracorporeal circulatory support, inotropes, medications, nutrition supplements and blood products may contribute. Providing evidence-based supportive care is a vital aspect of preventing MODS.

GENETICS

For similar disease precipitants and patient baseline characteristics, the phenotypic presentation of MODS differs. Why some patients develop mild organ dysfunction whereas others progress to fulminant MODS may be accounted for by a patient's genotype. For example, differences in genes coding for TNF, TLR, NF-κB, interleukin-1 receptor kinase and caspase-12 have been related to severity of organ dysfunction and extent of ICU supports required following sepsis.[32] Similarly, in patients undergoing elective abdominal aortic aneurysm repair, analysis of preoperative leucocyte genes predicted which patients subsequently developed MODS.[33] Differences in gene expression and proteomic responses may help identify which patients are at risk of MODS and may guide future treatment.

THE GUT IN MODS

The gut and its enteric micro-organisms have been proposed to provide an inflammatory focus during critical illness. Normally these organisms remain commensal due to bowel wall integrity and maintenance of the normal microflora ecosystem. However, when normal conditions are disturbed (e.g. bowel mucosal changes, altered gastric pH, antimicrobial use, overwhelmed reticuloendothelial macrophages), the enteric organisms can invade and perpetuate an inflammatory response. The gut has been described as the 'motor' of MODS and conceptualised as an 'undrained abscess'.[34] However, decontamination of the gut in critical illness remains controversial.

CLINICAL FEATURES OF MODS

The hallmark of MODS is the presence of SIRS with progressive physiological dysfunction in two or more organs.[4] However, there is no one typical constellation or timecourse of organ dysfunction that describes MODS. Some patients may develop only mild organ dysfunction that, with supportive treatment, resolves in days, whereas others can develop fulminant MODS progressing rapidly to death. Which organs become dysfunctional and the timing of their dysfunction depend on the patient's age and phenotype, the inciting injury/illness, premorbid organ function, extent and duration of physiological derangement and the treatments provided.

Identification of MODS as a discrete clinical syndrome has been difficult due to lack of agreement about what characterises an organ dysfunction. There are many ways of measuring organ dysfunction: clinical features, monitored physiological derangement and altered biochemical markers. Each organ system can manifest dysfunction in many different ways. For example, the respiratory system can be considered dysfunctional based on hypoxia (e.g. $Pa_{O_2}:Fi_{O_2}$ ratio), hypercarbia, reduced compliance, radiological change, extent of ventilatory supports or lavage fluid content. The processes that lead to changes in these parameters can be quite different and defining an organ dysfunction based on one variable alone is inadequate to describe the full spectrum of disease.

THERAPIES FOR MODS

The risk of MODS is related to the severity of the precipitating illness/injury, the extent of presenting physiological disturbance, degree of premorbid organ dysfunction and time to definitive care.[35,36] Hence the priorities in the treatment of MODS are:

1. Early recognition of illness
2. Early resuscitation
3. Early definitive treatment
4. Intensive organ support
5. Consideration of premorbid disease
6. Prevention of secondary insults.

The focus of management must be on the immediate treatment of the inflammatory focus (e.g. remove source of sepsis, repair injured tissue, control blood loss, debride burns, stabilise long-bone fractures). Aspects relating to early recognition of the deteriorating patient, resuscitation, specific disease treatments and the methods of organ support are covered in other chapters.

Specific therapies that target the pathogenesis of MODS continue to be extensively studied. Each of the pathophysiological processes described earlier has been targeted in preclinical and clinical trials. However, despite early promise in preclinical studies, no therapy has proven clinical efficacy in the treatment of MODS. The lack of a 'magic bullet' for treatment of MODS is not surprising given the complexity and variability of the pathophysiology, the lack of standardised treatments for some diseases and uncertainty regarding optimal timing of adjunctive therapy.

INFLAMMATION-MODULATING THERAPIES

The pro-inflammatory mediators associated with MODS have been an attractive therapeutic target. In preclinical studies many of these agents have provided physiological benefit, reduced severity of organ dysfunction and improved mortality. However, when these therapies progressed to clinical trials, none have provided benefit and some have worsened outcomes. For example, TNF-α was one of the first cytokines studied as it is released early in the inflammatory process and reducing its effect may attenuate the inflammatory process. Preclinical studies of TNF-α antibodies and soluble TNF-receptors in bacteraemic primates suggested that neutralising TNF-α improved organ function and reduced mortality. However, not only did clinical trials fail to show a benefit but higher doses increased mortality.[37] Similarly, the following agents have shown encouraging results in preclinical trials but no efficacy or adverse outcomes in subsequent clinical studies: endotoxin antibodies, non-steroidal anti-inflammatory drugs, IL-1 receptor antagonists, PAF antagonists, bradykinin antagonists, interferon-γ, nitric oxide synthase inhibition, NO antagonists, AT-III concentrate and activated protein C.[38,39]

The lack of clinical efficacy of immunomodulating therapies for MODS may reflect an inappropriate focus on the harmful effects of cytokines rather than their beneficial role. While inflammatory mediators are associated with MODS, they are also vital for control of infection, tissue repair and healing. Furthermore, the pro-inflammatory mediators also have downstream effects that eventually attenuate inflammation. Although elevated concentrations of pro-inflammatory cytokines are clearly associated with MODS, reduced levels are also associated with increased mortality.[40,41] The inflammatory response involves a very complex interplay of pro- and anti-inflammatory mediators and it is not surprising that targeting one pro-inflammatory mediator has not proven effective.

Future therapies to assist with recovery from MODS may aim to control excess inflammation without interfering with the essential components of the inflammatory process. Agents that modulate the inflammatory process without diminishing anti-microbial mechanisms are currently being investigated.

HUMORAL THERAPY

The role of endocrine manipulation during MODS remains uncertain. 'Tight' blood glucose control with intensive insulin therapy was efficacious in a single centre study of predominantly surgical patients.[42] However, when these blood glucose targets were applied in medical patients in the same centre and in subsequent multicentre studies, no benefit was found and some revealed greater mortality.[43,44]

Glucocorticoids have been a popular experimental therapy. 'High-dose' steroid treatment is known to suppress the inflammatory response but when trialled in critically ill patients with MODS proved to be harmful.[45] As MODS may be associated with relative adrenal insufficiency and/or glucocorticoid resistance, lower-dose steroid treatment has been investigated. Initial studies suggested that septic patients with limited response to ACTH administration had mortality benefit from steroid replacement.[46] However, in the CORTICUS trial, which studied a broader group of septic patients, hydrocortisone did not provide mortality benefit.[47] Whether or not steroid administration is beneficial in sepsis/MODS continues to be debated.

In contrast to steroids, thyroid hormone replacement during MODS has received little attention despite markedly reduced T_3 concentrations. Clinical trials in cardiothoracic ICU patients with low T_3 suggested replacement improves cardiovascular function.[48] This is an area that merits further investigation.

NUTRITION

MODS is a hypercatabolic state and nutritional support is required to ensure adequate energy, protein, fatty acids and trace elements. Nutrition is most safely provided via the gut and delivery by this route may improve intestinal mucosa function.[49] However, the ideal energy delivery and macronutrient composition of nutrition remain unclear. Furthermore the efficacy of supplementing feeds with amino acids (e.g. arginine, glutamine), nucleotides, fatty acids (e.g. omega-3, γ-linoleic acid) and antioxidants (e.g. selenium) is unproven.

OUTCOMES

Despite an increasing prevalence of ICU admissions due to sepsis, outcomes from MODS appear to have improved over time.[50,51] Similarly, patients admitted to ICU with major trauma are now older and have increased injury severity scores but a lower incidence and severity of MODS.[52] As no specific therapies have been developed that 'treat' MODS, the improved outcomes are likely to reflect a greater awareness of the diseases that can progress to MODS, the importance of timely resuscitation and treatment and the application of evidence-based supportive care.

Many questions remain regarding the definition, pathogenesis, diagnosis and treatment of MODS. There has not been a consensus conference on this topic since 1992.[4] Improved clarity in this area is a priority for the ICU community.

Access the complete references list online at http://www.expertconsult.com

9. Seely AJ, Christou NV. Multiple organ dysfunction syndrome: exploring the paradigm of complex nonlinear systems. Crit Care Med 2000;28:2193–200.
14. Boomer JS, To K, Chang KC, et al. Immunosuppression in patients who die of sepsis and multiple organ failure. JAMA 2011;306:2594–605.
19. Tracey KJ. Understanding immunity requires more than immunology. Nat Immunol 2010;11:561–4.
23. Sakr Y, Dubois MJ, De Backer D, et al. Persistent microcirculatory alterations are associated with organ failure and death in patients with septic shock. Crit Care Med 2004;32:1825–31.
28. Singer M, De Santis V, Vitale D, et al. Multiorgan failure is an adaptive, endocrine-mediated, metabolic response to overwhelming systemic inflammation. Lancet 2004;364:545–8.

18

Monitoring oxygenation

Thomas J Morgan and Balasubramanian Venkatesh

THE ROLES OF OXYGEN IN AEROBIC ORGANISMS

Oxygen has several physiological roles:

1. *Bioenergetics:* aerobic mitochondrial respiration accounts for 90% of oxygen consumption, generating adenosine triphosphate (ATP) by oxidative phosphorylation. Mitochondrial electron transfer oxidase systems provide the fundamental machinery, in particular the cytochrome oxidase of complex IV. Oxygen acts as a terminal electron acceptor, combining with two protons to produce water.
2. *Biosynthetics:* oxygen transferase systems incorporate oxygen into substrates, such as prostanoids, catecholamines and some neurotransmitters.
3. *Biodegradation and detoxification reactions:* these mixed function oxidase reactions require oxygen and a co-substrate (e.g. NADPH). The cytochrome P-450 hydroxylases are examples.
4. *Generation of reactive oxygen species:* these are essential anti-microbial defences deployed by neutrophils and macrophages.[1]

'HYPOXIA' AND 'DYSOXIA'

The term 'hypoxia' connotes tissue oxygen deficiency, and has largely superseded the older term 'anoxia'. In 1977 'dysoxia' was introduced as a broader term signifying any form of oxygen-limited cytochrome turnover causing progressive ATP depletion.[2] By this definition dysoxia can occur as a result of hypoxia, but can also be present in states of normal or supranormal oxygen tissue availability.

THE SPECTRUM OF DYSOXIA

1. 'Stagnant' hypoxia, where the primary abnormality is reduced tissue blood flow
2. Oxygen transport block at capillary, interstitial or intracellular levels
3. 'Hypoxaemic' hypoxia, where the primary abnormality is a low arterial oxygen tension
4. 'Anaemic' hypoxia, where the primary abnormality is a low haemoglobin concentration
5. 'Cytopathic' dysoxia, a phenomenon often attributed to sepsis and defined as abnormal cellular oxygen utilisation despite adequate oxygen delivery[3]
6. Oxygen toxicity, defined as abnormal cell function due to high oxygen tensions.

CONSEQUENCES OF TISSUE HYPOXIA

As tissue P_{O_2} falls, biosynthetic and biodegradation systems fail first. Aerobic ATP production initially adjusts to match ATP consumption by several adaptive metabolic mechanisms including increased glycolysis.[4] Cell signalling by reactive oxygen species, released at mitochondrial complex III, activates hypoxia-inducible factor-1, a transcription factor up-regulating genes important in hypoxic cell survival.[5] Oxidative phosphorylation itself begins to fail when intracellular P_{O_2} < 0.1–1 mmHg (0.013–0.13 kPa), equivalent to an extracellular P_{O_2} < 3–5 mmHg (0.39–0.65 kPa). Stopgap ATP production continues by anaerobic glycolysis, but without correction of dysoxia there is progressive lactic acidosis and eventual cell death by apoptosis and necrosis. On reoxygenation, a further release of reactive oxygen species causes oxidant stress, often overshadowing the hypoxic insult.[1]

THE OXYGEN CASCADE

In unicellular organisms, oxygen reaches the mitochondria across a short diffusion path with a steep partial pressure gradient. In multicellular animals the much longer diffusion path traverses a series of stepped partial pressure reductions known as the oxygen cascade. As a result, oxygen tensions in intracellular organelles remain above the anaerobic threshold.

Important steps in the oxygen cascade include:

1. Inspired gas
2. Alveolar gas
3. Arterial blood
4. Microcirculation
5. Interstitium
6. Mitochondria and other intracellular organelles.

The cascade can be jeopardised at any step. If more than one step is involved there is oxygen deprivation amplified downstream in mitochondria and other intracellular organelles. In this chapter we will consider how oxygenation can be monitored at strategic points along the cascade.

INSPIRED GAS

Monitoring the fraction of inspired oxygen (Fi_{O_2}) is necessary to prevent the adverse effects of both hypoxaemia and excess oxygen. The inspired oxygen tension (Pi_{O_2}) of humidified gas is determined by the Fi_{O_2}, the barometric pressure (BP) and the saturated vapour pressure of water (47 mmHg (6.11 kPa)):

$$Pi_{O_2} = Fi_{O_2} \times (\mathrm{BP} - 47) \qquad (18.1)$$

Gas supply pressures are monitored continuously. Ventilators incorporate input pressure alarms and oxygen analysers within the inspiratory module to identify oxygen source failure. Direct measurement of circuit oxygen concentration can be added.

TRANSFER OF INSPIRED GAS TO ALVEOLI

Communication is open between oxygen delivery system and pulmonary alveoli if:

1. There are no signs of upper airway obstruction (Ch. 29)
2. Expired tidal and minute volumes and airway pressures for the ventilated patient are within correctly set alarm limits (Ch. 31)
3. There is an appropriate end-tidal CO_2 waveform (Ch. 38).

ALVEOLAR GAS

In a patient receiving 100% oxygen, alveolar P_{O_2} in individual lung units can range from <40 mmHg to >600 mmHg (<5.2 – >78 kPa). Consequently, end-tidal P_{O_2} monitoring is of little value.

DISTRIBUTION OF ALVEOLAR VENTILATION

Clinicians routinely track chest movement, auscultate air entry, and examine plain chest radiographs. Intermittent CT scanning can reveal occult overdistension,[6] but has logistic disadvantages and is a significant radiation hazard. Electrical impedance tomography shows promise as a real-time non-invasive monitor of recruitment, overdistension and regional lung mechanics. With contrast injections of hypertonic saline it has additional potential for assessment of regional lung perfusion.[7,8]

MATCHING OF VENTILATION AND PERFUSION

For efficient gas exchange, the majority of lung units must receive well-matched alveolar ventilation and perfusion with most V/Q ratios close to unity, but even in health there is some spread to lower and higher ratios. When lungs are diseased, the proportion of lung units with high and low V/Q ratios increases. The adult lung contains at least 100 000 individual gas-exchanging units[9] whose V/Q ratios potentially range from zero to infinity. Such complexity resists simple bedside quantification. The gold standard is the multiple inert gas technique (MIGET), which describes a 50-compartment lung model. By measuring the retention and elimination of six inert gases of varying solubility infused in pre-equilibrated saline, MIGET quantifies the distribution of ventilation and perfusion to 50 lung units spanning a range of V/Q ratios from zero to infinity.[9,10] However, lung models with fewer compartments may suffice for clinical quantification of lung pathophysiology, with the advantage that they can be more easily applied at the bedside. Instead of inert gas infusions, stepped Fi_{O_2} changes can serve as a forcing function while blood gas values and end-tidal gas concentrations are tracked (or pulse oximetry in the least invasive versions).[11–13]

THE 'IDEAL' ALVEOLUS AND THE THREE-COMPARTMENT LUNG MODEL

Meanwhile a three-compartment model devised in the mid twentieth century[14] is still in use, with no need for Fi_{O_2} switching or inert gas infusions. The trade-off is that because the model is overly simplistic it has poor predictive capacity in many respiratory disorders. The three compartments are:

1. The ideal compartment, consisting of alveoli with perfectly matched perfusion and ventilation ($V/Q=1$)
2. The venous admixture or shunt compartment, containing perfused non-ventilated alveoli ($V/Q=0$)
3. The alveolar dead space compartment, consisting of ventilated non-perfused alveoli ($V/Q=\infty$).

The alveolar P_{O_2} in the ideal compartment (PA_{O_2}) is calculated from the alveolar gas equation:

$$PA_{O_2} = -(1 - Fi_{O_2} \times (1 - R)) \times Pa_{CO_2}/R \qquad (18.2)$$

where R is the respiratory exchange ratio, either measured by indirect calorimetry or assumed to be 0.8. Pi_{O_2} is calculated as in Equation 18.1. Pa_{CO_2} is arterial P_{CO_2}.

Most clinicians use the following approximation:

$$PA_{O_2} = Pi_{O_2} - Pa_{CO_2}/0.8$$

It is important to remember that PA_{O_2} is derived from a non-physiological three-compartment lung model. Parameters such as the A–a gradient and venous admixture that are also based on the model (see below) must be regarded in the same light.

TRANSFER FROM ALVEOLI TO ARTERIAL BLOOD (PULMONARY OXYGEN TRANSFER)

The MIGET technique has identified V/Q mismatch and intrapulmonary right-to-left shunt as the two main causes of reduced pulmonary oxygen transfer in critical illness.[15] Intrapulmonary shunt predominates in the acute respiratory distress syndrome (ARDS), lobar pneumonia and after cardiopulmonary bypass, whereas V/Q mismatch without shunt is more prominent in chronic lung disease.[16]

BEDSIDE INDICES OF PULMONARY OXYGEN TRANSFER

These are either tension based or content based.

TENSION-BASED INDICES

A–a gradient

The A–a gradient is calculated as $PA_{O_2} - Pa_{O_2}$, where PA_{O_2} is the 'ideal' compartment alveolar P_{O_2} determined from the alveolar gas equation (Equation 18.2). Hypoxaemia can then be classified under two headings:

Normal A–a gradient

1. Alveolar hypoventilation (elevated PA_{CO_2})
2. Low Pi_{O_2} ($Fi_{O_2} < 0.21$, or barometric pressure <760 mmHg (99 kPa)).

Raised A–a gradient

1. Diffusion defect (rare)
2. V/Q mismatch
3. Right-to-left shunt (intrapulmonary or cardiac)
4. Increased oxygen extraction ($Ca_{O_2} - Cv_{O_2}$).

Although the A–a gradient is a component of the APACHE II, III and IV scoring systems,[17,18] several drawbacks limit its clinical usefulness. They include:

1. Normal values that vary with Fi_{O_2} and age. The normal A–a gradient breathing air is 7 mmHg (0.91 kPa) in young adults and 14 mmHg (1.82 kPa) in the elderly. On 100% oxygen, these values become 31 mmHg (4 kPa) and 56 mmHg (7.3 kPa) respectively.
2. An exaggerated Fi_{O_2} dependence in intrapulmonary shunt (**Fig. 18.1**) and even more so in V/Q mismatch (**Fig. 18. 2**).[19,20]

Pa_{O_2}/Fi_{O_2} ratio

The Pa_{O_2}/Fi_{O_2} ratio is used to define acute lung injury and ARDS,[21] and is an input variable in SAPS II and III,[22] SOFA,[23] APACHE IV[18] and lung injury scoring systems.[24] At sea level its normal value is ≥500 mmHg (65 kPa). In acute lung injury, $Pa_{O_2}/Fi_{O_2} < 300$ mmHg (39 kPa), whilst in ARDS the ratio is <200 mmHg (26 kPa).

Its main advantage is simplicity. There are several disadvantages:

1. Barometric pressure alters the normal Pa_{O_2}/Fi_{O_2} ratio. For a young adult breathing air, a ratio of

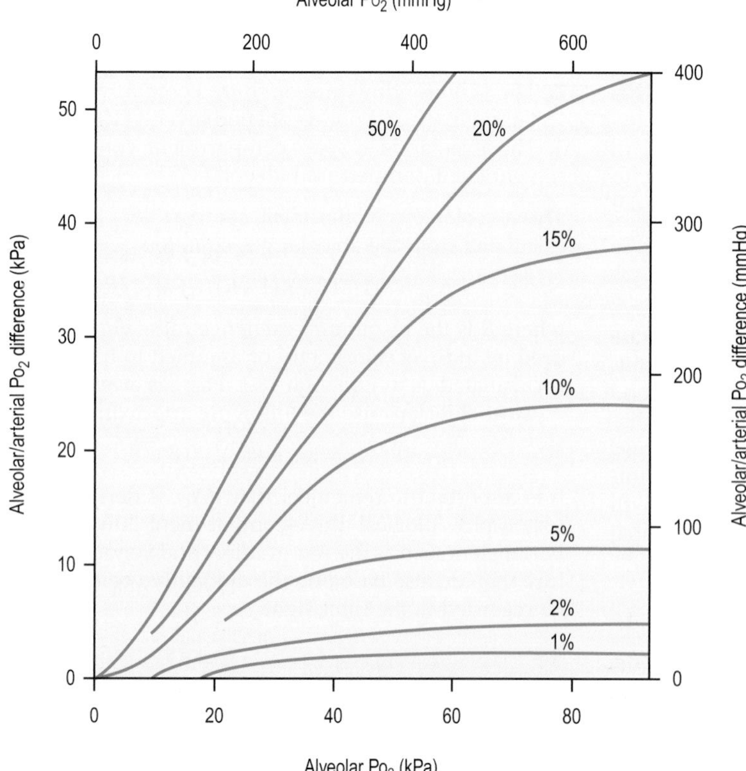

Figure 18.1 Effect of varying Fi_{O_2} (PA_{O_2}) on A–a gradient with different degrees of intrapulmonary shunt. *(Reproduced with permission from Nunn JF. Oxygen. In: Nunn JF, editor. Applied Respiratory Physiology. 4th edn. Oxford, UK: Butterworth-Heinemann; 1993. p. 264.)*

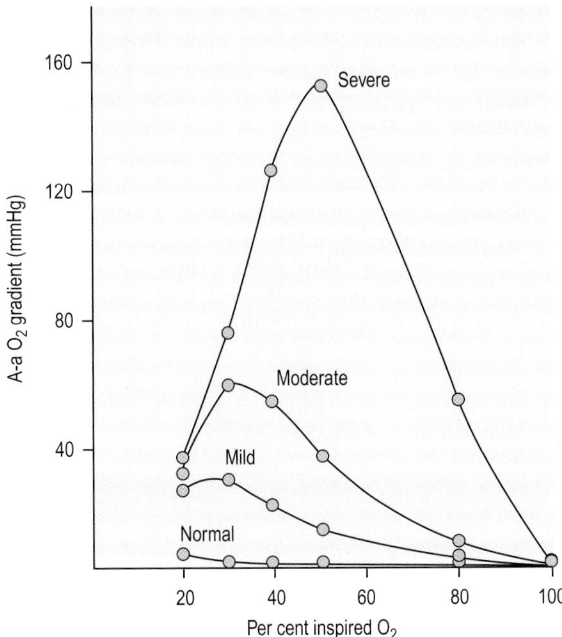

Figure 18.2 Effect of varying Fi_{O_2} on A–a gradient with mild, moderate and severe V/Q mismatch. No allowance is made for absorption atelectasis or alterations in hypoxic pulmonary vasoconstriction. *(Reproduced with permission from D'Alonzo GE, Dantzker DR. Respiratory failure, mechanisms of abnormal gas exchange, and oxygen delivery. Med Clin North Am 1983;67:557–71.)*

380 mmHg (49.4 kPa) is unremarkable at 1600 metres elevation, but not at sea level.

2. Unlike the A–a gradient, the Pa_{O_2}/Fi_{O_2} ratio cannot distinguish hypoxaemia due to alveolar hypoventilation from other causes.
3. The ratio is markedly Fi_{O_2} dependent, both in right-to-left shunt (the predominant ARDS abnormality) and in lungs with a wide V/Q scatter (COPD).[19,20]
4. The ratio is also highly dependent on $Ca_{O_2} - Cv_{O_2}$,[20] which tends to fluctuate markedly in sepsis.

CONTENT-BASED INDICES

Venous admixture (Qs/Qt)

Venous admixture is another construct based on the three-compartment lung model (see above). It represents the proportion of mixed venous blood flowing through the shunt ($V/Q=0$) compartment. It is determined according to the formula:

$$\frac{\dot{Q}_S}{\dot{Q}_T} = \frac{Cc'O_2 - Ca_{O_2}}{Cc'O_2 - C\bar{v}_{O_2}} \qquad (18.3)$$

where Cc_{O_2}, Ca_{O_2} and Cv_{O_2} are the oxygen contents of pulmonary end-capillary, arterial and mixed venous blood respectively. Ca_{O_2} and Cv_{O_2} are calculated using data from arterial and mixed venous blood gas analysis and CO-oximetry (**Table 18.1**). Cc_{O_2} must be derived differently, since pulmonary end-capillary blood cannot be sampled. Pc_{O_2} is assumed to equal PA_{O_2} as derived from the alveolar gas equation (Equation 18.2). Sc_{O_2}

Table 18.1 Oxygen dynamics – measured and derived indices

PARAMETER	ABBREVIATION	FORMULA	NORMAL RANGE	UNITS
Functional haemoglobin concentration	$[Hb_{funct}]$	$[Hb_{O_2}]+[Hb]$	12.0–18.0	g/dL
Arterial oxygen tension	Pa_{O_2}	Measured	95±5 12.5±0,65	mmHg kPa
Mixed venous oxygen tension	Pv_{O_2}	Measured	40±5 5.2±0.65	mmHg kPa
Functional saturation	S_{O_2}	$[Hb_{O_2}]/([Hb_{O_2}]+[Hb])$		
Fractional saturation	FHb_{O_2}	$[Hb_{O_2}]/([Hb_{O_2}]+[Hb]+[COHb]+[MetHb])$		
Arterial functional saturation	Sa_{O_2}		0.97±0.02	
Mixed venous functional saturation	Sv_{O_2}		0.75±0.05	
Blood oxygen content	C_{O_2}	$1.39\times[Hb_{funct}]\times S_{O_2}+0.0031\times P_{O_2}$		mL/dL
Arterial oxygen content	Ca_{O_2}		16–22	mL/dL
Mixed venous oxygen content	Cv_{O_2}		12–17	mL/dL
Cardiac index	CI	CO/BSA	2.5–4.2	L/min/m^2
Oxygen delivery index	$D_{O_2}I$	$CI\times Ca_{O_2}\times 10$	460–650	mL/min/m^2
Oxygen consumption index	$V_{O_2}I$	$CI\times(Ca_{O_2}-Cv_{O_2})\times 10$	96–170	mL/min/m^2
Oxygen extraction ratio	O_2ER	$(Ca_{O_2}-Cv_{O_2})/Ca_{O_2}$ or V_{O_2}/D_{O_2}	0.23–0.32	

Hb_{O_2}=oxyhaemoglobin; Hb=reduced haemoglobin; COHb=carboxyhaemoglobin; MetHb=methaemoglobin, BSA=body surface area.

(normally close to 1) can then be computed from an algorithm for the Hb_{O_2} dissociation curve.[25]

Advantages of venous admixture:

1. Unaffected by barometric pressure
2. Unaffected by alveolar hypoventilation
3. Provided intrapulmonary right-to-left shunt is the dominant pathology (e.g. ARDS), venous admixture is stable across the entire Fi_{O_2} range, despite variations in $Ca_{O_2}-Cv_{O_2}$.[19,26]

Disadvantages of venous admixture:

1. Sampling mixed venous blood requires a PA catheter.
2. In *V/Q* mismatch without right-to-left shunt, venous admixture varies markedly with Fi_{O_2} and virtually disappears at $Fi_{O_2}>0.5$ (**Fig. 18.3**). Venous admixture is thus of little use in conditions where the dominant gas exchange abnormality is not intrapulmonary right-to-left shunt, such as COPD.

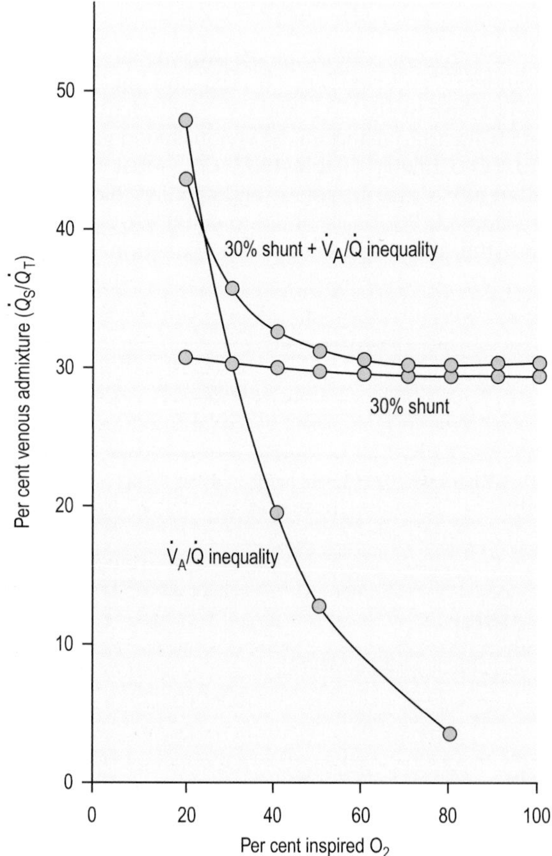

Figure 18.3 Effect of varying Fi_{O_2} on venous admixture in various combinations of *V/Q* mismatch and shunt. No allowance has been made for absorption atelectasis or alterations in hypoxic pulmonary vasoconstriction. *(Reproduced with permission from D'Alonzo GE, Dantzker DR. Respiratory failure, mechanisms of abnormal gas exchange, and oxygen delivery. Med Clin North Am 1983;67:557–71.)*

When determined at $Fi_{O_2}=1$, venous admixture is an accurate measure of right-to-left shunt. However, exposure to 100% oxygen causes absorption atelectasis of unstable low V/Q units, which increases intrapulmonary shunt.

Estimated shunt fraction

If a fixed $Ca_{O_2}-Cv_{O_2}$ is assigned, no PA catheter is necessary. However, in critical illness $Ca_{O_2}-Cv_{O_2}$ can range from 1.3 mL/dL to 7.4 mL/dL. Hence the inaccuracy from assigning a fixed value is such that even the direction of change of estimated shunt can be wrong.[26]

Non-invasive estimates of V/Q mismatch and shunt

Simpler lung models using varying Fi_{O_2} as a forcing function are discussed above.[11-13]

ARTERIAL BLOOD

Indices of arterial oxygenation are Pa_{O_2} and Sa_{O_2}. They are linked by the Hb_{O_2} dissociation curve (**Fig. 18.4**).

Hypoxaemia is defined as $Pa_{O_2}<60$ mmHg (7.8 kPa) or $Sa_{O_2}<0.9$. These values lie near the descending portion of the Hb_{O_2} dissociation curve, so that a further drop in Pa_{O_2} leads to a marked fall in Sa_{O_2} and thus Ca_{O_2}.

BLOOD GAS ANALYSIS AND CO-OXIMETRY

Arterial blood is collected in a purpose-designed syringe containing lyophilised heparin to a final concentration of 20–50 U/mL. Pa_{O_2} measurements are made by a Clark electrode, and Sa_{O_2} by CO-oximetry. The Clark electrode works on polarographic principles,

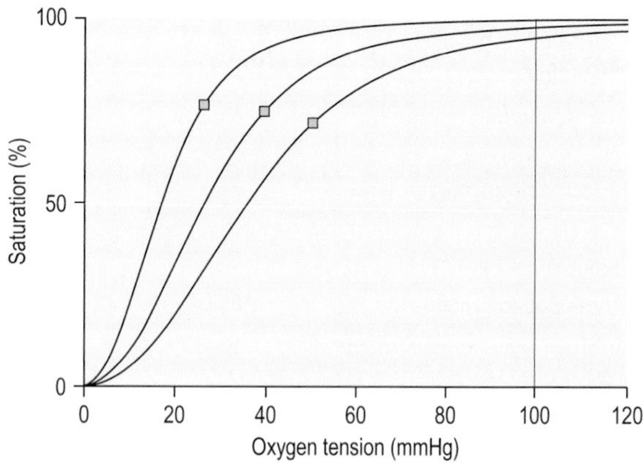

Figure 18.4 Three Hb_{O_2} dissociation curves: normal (P50=26.7 mmHg (3.47 kPa)), left-shifted (P50=17 mmHg (2.21 kPa)) and right-shifted (P50=36 mmHg (4.68 kPa)). The vertical line represents the normal oxygen loading tension (P_{O_2}=100 mmHg (13 kPa)). The filled squares represent an oxygen extraction of 5 mL/dL blood, assuming a haemoglobin concentration of 150 g/L. *(Reproduced with permission from Morgan TJ. The Hb_{O_2} dissociation curve in critical illness. Crit Care Resusc 1999;1:93–100.)*

Table 18.2 Pre-analytic and analytic errors in P_{O_2} measurement

PRE-ANALYTIC	ANALYTIC
Oxygen diffusing into or out of air bubbles along tension gradients	Inter-analyser variability. There is 7–8% measurement variation on the same sample
Contamination with flush solution. Discard volume should be 2–3 times the internal volume of cannula and tubing	Inadequate anticoagulation, allowing protein deposits on electrodes
Pseudohypoxaemia. Oxygen consumption in vitro from extreme leucocytosis	Non-linearity at high P_{O_2} (>150 mmHg (19.5 kPa))
Artefactual Pa_{O_2} elevations. With syringes stored on ice, the semipermeable polypropylene allows oxygen ingress, facilitated by the cold-induced increase in oxygen solubility	Maintenance of electrode temperature within narrow limits (37+/− 0.1°C) is critical. P_{O_2} changes by 7% for every degree Celsius temperature change
	Minimal interference by nitrous oxide and volatile anaesthetic agents unless the polarising voltage of the electrode exceeds 600 mV
	Tonometry is the primary reference method. Quality control materials such as aqueous, perfluorocarbon and bovine haemoglobin solutions are used for convenience
	Arterial blood gas tensions fluctuate breath to breath.[75] Intermittent analysis is a snapshot

and a CO-oximeter computes the concentrations of each of the four main haemoglobin species (Hb_{O_2}, Hb, COHb, MetHb) from light absorbances of haemolysed blood at several wavelengths. Sa_{O_2} is functional saturation, determined from concentrations of Hb_{O_2} and Hb (see Table 18.1). Interference to CO-oximetry arises from substances with competing absorbance spectra, such as bilirubin, HbF, lipid emulsions and intravenous dyes. Increasing the number of wavelengths, for example to 128, can reduce or eliminate interference.

ERRORS

Pre-analytic and analytic errors in P_{O_2} measurement are set out in **Table 18.2**.

TEMPERATURE CORRECTION

All measurements are at 37°C. Temperature-corrected values can be calculated if the core temperature of the patient is entered into the device software. Most clinicians interpret blood gas data at 37°C, except when evaluating the A–a gradient (see Ch. 92, Acid–base balance and disorders).

CONTINUOUS INTRA-ARTERIAL BLOOD GAS MONITORING (Table 18.3)[27]

Multiparameter fibreoptic sensors can be placed in the arterial stream. Fibreoptic sensors are called 'optodes', and those measuring P_{O_2} normally operate by fluorescence quenching. They require calibration with precision gases or solutions before use. Typical sensors are 0.5 mm in diameter, and can be inserted through 20 G arterial cannulae. The 90% in vitro response time to a change in P_{O_2} is 78 seconds. P_{O_2} drift in vivo is 0.03 mmHg/h (0.0039 kPa/h). Recalibration in vivo can be performed against conventional blood gas analysis. Accuracy on in vitro and animal testing is good.

Clinical trials evaluating the accuracy of these monitoring systems have revealed varying degrees of bias and imprecision. Evidence demonstrating an improved outcome when therapeutic decisions are based on data from these devices is lacking. These factors combined with the costs of these devices have limited their bedside application.

Problems encountered with intra-arterial sensors, particularly artefactual due to flow and position, have prompted the development of extracorporeal monitors that can be placed in line but ex vivo. These devices do not provide continuous real-time data. When a measurement is desired, a sample is drawn into the externally located cassette then returned. Results are available in two minutes. In preterm neonates this method can reduce red cell transfusion requirements.[28]

TRANSCUTANEOUS P_{O_2} AND P_{CO_2} MONITORING

Continuous non-invasive assessment of blood gas tensions is possible with transcutaneous P_{O_2} and P_{CO_2} monitoring. Available systems incorporate O_2 and CO_2 electrodes with integral thermistors and servo-controlled heaters. P_{O_2} measurement utilises the principle of the Clark electrode, while the P_{CO_2} device is a pH-sensitive glass electrode. The skin is warmed to

Table 18.3 Continuous intra-arterial Pa_{O_2} monitoring – advantages and disadvantages

ADVANTAGES	DISADVANTAGES
Eliminates pre-analytic errors of intermittent blood gas analysis	The 'wall' effect – a sudden decrease in measured Pa_{O_2} due to contact with the arterial wall, with averaging of arterial and wall oxygen tensions. The problem is reduced in larger arteries such as the femoral artery
More sensitive than pulse oximetry to changes in arterial oxygenation when Pa_{O_2}>70 mmHg (the flat part of the Hb_{O_2} dissociation curve)	The 'flush' effect. Unless the sensor is inserted a sufficient distance beyond the cannula tip, measured Pa_{O_2} can be altered by contamination with the continuous flush solution
Free from the sources of error of pulse oximetry (see Table 18.2)	Damping of the arterial waveform
Near-real-time Pa_{O_2} allows prompt tracking of responses to changed ventilator settings	Large footprint of the free-standing monitor
Reduced exposure of personnel to potentially infected blood	
Reduced blood loss for diagnostic purposes	

42–44°C to achieve good correlation with arterial values. Transcutaneous monitors generate reliable P_{CO_2} values provided perfusion is unimpaired, but P_{O_2} measurements are more for trend analysis. Skin warming necessitates frequent site changes to prevent burns, and there is a need for regular recalibration. Monitoring is not recommended in haemodynamically unstable patients.

Transcutaneous monitors have a role in the prevention of neonatal hyperoxia, which is not reliably detected by pulse oximetry.[29] They may also have a role in the detection of sleep apnoea and hypoventilation syndromes, and for monitoring during nocturnal non-invasive ventilation.[30]

PULSE OXIMETRY[31,32]

Pulse oximetry determines Sp_{O_2} from the absorbance of light at wavelengths 660 nm (red) and 940 nm (infrared) by tissue capillary beds such as fingers, forehead, earlobes and the nasal septum. Two light-emitting diodes cycle on and off at multiples of the mains frequency. A single photodiode detects the transmitted light, and applies a correction for background ambient light. The emergent signal is pulsatile due to arterial volume fluctuations. Subtraction of the background signal (tissue, capillary blood and venous blood) isolates the arterial component.

For both wavelengths, absorbance (A) is determined as follows:

$$A = \log_{10}(I_0 / I)$$

where I_0=incident light intensity and I=emergent light intensity. For a given chromophore, A is proportional to its concentration (Beer's law) and to the path length (Lambert's law). From the pulsatile (AC) and background (DC) absorbance signals at both wavelengths, a ratio (R) is derived:

$$R = (AC_{660} / DC_{660}) / (AC_{940} / DC_{940})$$

Sp_{O_2} is then computed from R, using software 'look-up' tables of empirically derived relationships between R values and either Sa_{O_2} or FHb_{O_2} measured in the arterial blood of volunteers breathing hypoxic gas mixtures.

Sp_{O_2} is usually displayed as a percentage. Since the signal is derived from two wavelengths there is an inherent incorrect assumption that Hb_{O_2} and Hb are the only haemoglobin species in the light path. However, with normal dyshaemoglobin concentrations the error is trivial. Some manufacturers calibrate R against FHb_{O_2} (fractional saturation) rather than Sa_{O_2} (functional saturation). Provided volunteers generating the data have normal dyshaemoglobin concentrations, differences between the two calibrations are small.

SPEED OF RESPONSE

Sp_{O_2} is averaged over 3–6 seconds, and updated every 0.5–1 second. With forehead probes a sudden reduction in Fi_{O_2} produces a response within 10–15 seconds, whereas with finger probes and peripheral vasoconstriction the delay can exceed 1 minute.

ACCURACY

In the 90–97% saturation range, Sp_{O_2} has a mean absolute bias of <1%, and a precision (SD of bias) of <3%. At Sa_{O_2}<0.8 there is significant imprecision and a tendency towards negative bias. This is because very low Sa_{O_2} values are unsafe in volunteers, necessitating extrapolation from Sp_{O_2}/R relationships at higher saturations.

ERROR

Causes of error are set out in **Table 18.4**. A falsely high Sp_{O_2} is of greatest concern.

Unlike CO-oximetry, pulse oximetry is not subject to interference from bilirubin, lipid emulsions and HbF.

Table 18.4 Causes of error in Sp_{O_2} readings

FACTOR	COMMENT
COHb	Measured as $Hb_{O_2}-Sp_{O_2}$ may be falsely high – see text
MetHb	Absorbs both wavelengths – see text
Low saturations	Progressive inaccuracy below 70–80%, usually falsely low Sp_{O_2}
Prominent venous signal	Dependent limb, tricuspid regurgitation (venous pulsations) – falsely low Sp_{O_2}
Non-pulsatile flow	Cardiopulmonary bypass – poor signal
Vasoconstriction, limb ischaemia, shock states	Low pulsatile signal
Motion artefact	Tremor, voluntary movement – falsely low Sp_{O_2}
Ambient light	Strong sunlight, fluorescent and xenon lamps, flickering light– falsely low Sp_{O_2}
Anaemia	No effect
Dyes	Methylene blue, indocyanine green, indigo carmine – falsely low Sp_{O_2}
Black skin pigmentation	Variable precision and bias. May require separate calibration
Nail polish	Especially blue. Falsely low Sp_{O_2}. Acrylic nails do not interfere
Optical shunting	Due to inadequate probe contact – falsely low Sp_{O_2}
Radio-frequency interference	Reported with MRI scanners – falsely high Sp_{O_2}

Dyshaemoglobins and pulse oximetry

Pulse oximeters cannot distinguish COHb from Hb_{O_2}. When [COHb] is elevated, Sp_{O_2} tends to overestimate Sa_{O_2}. Sp_{O_2} can thus provide false reassurance when hypoxaemia is combined with a high [COHb], for example after an inhalational burn injury.

MetHb has more complex effects, since it absorbs both wavelengths. At normal saturations, increased [MetHb] causes underestimation of Sa_{O_2}, but at very low oxygen tensions overestimation is possible. At [MetHb]≥35%, the R value becomes unity, which translates to Sp_{O_2}=85%.

IMPORTANCE OF PULSE OXIMETRY

Pulse oximeters generate accurate real-time information without calibration, within moments of sensor placement. They are mandatory in patient transport, and in high-acuity areas such as operating rooms, recovery rooms and intensive care units. They are also useful screening tools. On the down side, pulse oximeters are insensitive to changes in arterial oxygenation at higher Pa_{O_2} values (>70–100 mmHg (9.1–13 kPa)). They are also the most common source of false alarms in intensive care.

PULSE CO-OXIMETRY[33,34]

Additional continuous real-time non-invasive monitoring of absolute total haemoglobin concentrations and trends becomes possible with these multiwavelength devices. Accuracy remains acceptable in low perfusion states and in patients requiring vasopressor support.

MONITORING HAEMOGLOBIN–OXYGEN AFFINITY

Haemoglobin–oxygen affinity is the relationship between the oxygen tension of blood and its oxygen content, described by the sigmoid-shaped Hb_{O_2} dissociation curve (see Fig. 18.4). The P50 is the oxygen tension at S_{O_2}=0.5. The normal value in humans is 26.7 mmHg (3.47 kPa). Factors that decrease haemoglobin–oxygen affinity increase the P50. They include acidaemia (the Bohr effect), hypercarbia, increased erythrocytic 2,3-DPG and fever, whereas P50 is decreased (increased affinity) by alkalaemia, hypocarbia, low 2,3-DPG concentrations, hypothermia, COHb, MetHb and FHb.

In the intensive care unit, it is possible to calculate accurate P50 values from a single measurement of blood gases and Sa_{O_2} up to Sa_{O_2}=0.97. However, the impact of haemoglobin–oxygen affinity on tissue oxygenation in critical illness appears to be small,[35,36] making routine monitoring unnecessary.

OXYGEN DYNAMICS

Common indices of oxygen dynamics are set out in Table 18.1.

D_{O_2}/V_{O_2} RELATIONSHIPS

Nearly 40 years ago an association was reported between hyperdynamic oxygen flow patterns and survival after high-risk non-cardiac surgery.[37] This led to the concept that maintaining an induced perioperative hyperdynamic state to prevent an acquired oxygen debt might be protective. Although supported at a single-centre level, this hypothesis was not validated by large multicentre studies.[38,39] In fact, aggressive pursuit of hyperdynamic goals seemed counterproductive for the broad ICU population.[40]

Common therapeutic goals were CI>4.5 L/min/m^2, $D_{O_2}I$>600 mL/min/m^2, $V_{O_2}I$>170 mL/min/m^2. However the $V_{O_2}I$ target was especially difficult to achieve. The focus subsequently narrowed to the $D_{O_2}I$ target alone, which removed the need for PA catheterisation. On this basis there is better emerging evidence of benefit in high-risk surgery,[41–43] although definitive multicentre confirmation is awaited.

MEASURING $D_{O_2}I$

Although $D_{O_2}I$ determinations require accurate measurements of CI and Ca_{O_2}, a PA catheter is not essential (see Ch.16). Normal ranges can be quoted (see Table 18.1), but oxygen demand in critical illness is so variable that isolated $D_{O_2}I$ measurements are difficult to interpret.

MEASURING $V_{O_2}I$

The two methods of measuring $V_{O_2}I$ are the reverse Fick method (see Table 18.1), and indirect calorimetry.

Reverse Fick method

The reverse Fick method requires a PA catheter, and has large random errors ranging from 17% overestimation to 13% underestimation. Changes cannot be detected reliably unless they exceed 20%. The error is increased by lung inflammation, when up to 20% of $V_{O_2}I$ can arise from the lungs alone.

Indirect calorimetry

Indirect calorimetry has better accuracy. $V_{O_2}I$ is determined from the volumes and oxygen concentrations of inspired and expired gas. However, high Fi_{O_2} settings introduce error. Newer devices retain accuracy up to Fi_{O_2}=0.8, with relative errors of <5%.

MIXED VENOUS BLOOD

Mixed venous sampling is by gentle aspiration of blood from the distal port of an unwedged PA catheter to ensure complete admixture of blood from superior and inferior venae cavae and coronary sinus. Mixed venous O_2 and CO_2 tensions and content are flow-weighted averages of the venous effluents of multiple tissues. As such they can fail to detect pockets of hypoxia and hypercarbia.

MIXED VENOUS P_{O_2} (Pv_{O_2})

Venous gas tensions reflect post-capillary and tissue gas tensions. A Pv_{O_2} below 26 mmHg (3.38 kPa) is suggestive of cellular hypoxia.[44] Paradoxically, a normal or high Pv_{O_2} does not exclude regional tissue hypoxia, whether cytopathic[45] or as a result of tissue shunting.[46]

MIXED VENOUS OXYGEN SATURATION (Sv_{O_2})[47]

Sv_{O_2} is measured either intermittently by CO-oximetry on mixed venous samples or continuously by fibreoptic reflectance oximetry using a modified PA catheter. Sv_{O_2} measurements have a number of potential uses:

1. To calculate Cv_{O_2} (see Table 18.1). Cv_{O_2} can then be used to determine Qs/Qt, $V_{O_2}I$ by the reverse Fick method, the oxygen extraction ratio (Table 18.1), and cardiac output by the Fick method.
2. As an indirect index of tissue hypoxia. A Sv_{O_2} value of 0.5 corresponds to the theoretical critical Pv_{O_2} of 26 mmHg (3.38 kPa). Values between 0.7 and 0.8 represent a desirable balance between global oxygen supply and demand (see Table 18.1), with lactic acidosis appearing between 0.3 and 0.5.[47] Values exceeding 0.8 can be seen in high-flow states such as sepsis, hyperthyroidism and severe liver disease.

Sv_{O_2} as a therapeutic target (≥0.7) failed to improve survival in a multicentre trial.[48] Only two-thirds of the treatment group achieved the target. Like Pv_{O_2}, Sv_{O_2} is insensitive to cytopathic hypoxia and tissue shunting. In chronic heart failure, low values are surprisingly well tolerated.

CENTRAL VENOUS SATURATION (Scv_{O_2})[47]

As with Sv_{O_2}, Scv_{O_2} can be measured either continuously using a central venous catheter modified for reflectance oximetry, or by intermittent sampling and CO-oximetry. Scv_{O_2} is normally 2–3% lower than Sv_{O_2}. However, in shock this difference can be reversed. Trends in Sv_{O_2} and Scv_{O_2} in response to management usually run in parallel.

In the Rivers single-centre study of early intervention in the hypodynamic phase of severe sepsis and septic shock,[49] resuscitation was directed at a Scv_{O_2} target of >0.7, along with specific central venous pressure and mean arterial pressure goals and an aggressive transfusion policy. There were reductions in 28- and 60-day mortality and in the duration of hospitalisation compared with standard treatment. A target of Scv_{O_2}≥0.7 now has equal billing with Sv_{O_2}≥0.65 in the management guidelines of the Surviving Sepsis Campaign.[50] It is unclear whether intermittent sampling can be substituted with equivalent benefit.

In a subsequent multicentre study with a protocol similar to that of the Rivers study, 10% venous lactate clearance was at least equivalent (non-inferior) to Scv_{O_2} as a therapeutic target in severe sepsis and septic shock.[51] Furthermore, judging by the low take-up in Australia and New Zealand[52] clinicians still question whether the Rivers findings can be generalised to the wider emergency and critical care septic population.[53] This is the subject of a multicentre trial (Australasian Resuscitation in Sepsis Evaluation Randomised

Controlled Trial; ARISE-RCT; ClinicalTrials.gov Identifier: NCT 00975793).

MIXED VENOUS–ARTERIAL P_{CO_2} GRADIENT (ΔP_{CO_2})
ΔP_{CO_2} (normally about 6 mmHg (0.78 kPa)) is markedly increased during cardiac arrest and in experimental low-output states, but lacks sensitivity and specificity as a global index of tissue hypoxia. A sudden increase in the respiratory quotient (V_{CO_2}/V_{O_2}), or in the venoarterial CO_2 tension difference/arteriovenous O_2 content difference to >1.4[54] may be more reliable markers of the onset of anaerobic metabolism. The central venous-arterial P_{CO_2} gradient appears to behave similarly to ΔP_{CO_2} as an index of reduced tissue perfusion.[55]

PLASMA LACTATE AND REDOX INDICES

See Chapter 19.

REGIONAL OXYGENATION INDICES

REGIONAL P_{CO_2}[56]

Regional P_{CO_2} reflects the balance between arterial blood CO_2 content, tissue blood flow and tissue CO_2 production. The CO_2 gap, which is regional $P_{CO_2} - Pa_{CO_2}$, was devised to correct regional P_{CO_2} for varying arterial CO_2 content. As tissue blood flow falls, reduced CO_2 clearance causes the CO_2 gap to increase. With the onset of anaerobic metabolism, tissue CO_2 production steadily decreases, although regional metabolic acidosis generates some CO_2 by proton titration of tissue and capillary HCO_3^-. A rising CO_2 gap signals falling tissue blood flow. It cannot identify the onset of anaerobic metabolism.[57]

GASTRIC TONOMETRY
Gastric tonometry was developed in the knowledge that splanchnic hypoperfusion occurs early in circulatory shock, tends to persist as 'covert shock', and is manifested by intramucosal hypercarbia and acidosis. A gastric tonometer was developed as a modified nasogastric tube with a silicone balloon 11.4 cm from the tip. Gastric mucosal CO_2 equilibrates with luminal CO_2, which equilibrates with (and is measured in) fluid filling the balloon. Early on, this fluid was saline. Subsequently air was found to have more rapid equilibration characteristics.

The original method involved calculation of intramucosal pH (pHi) by substituting gastric luminal P_{CO_2} and arterial [HCO_3^-] in the Henderson–Hasselbalch equation. Intramucosal acidosis was defined as pHi<7.3 and taken to indicate inadequate splanchnic perfusion. However, although pHi can reflect shock severity, it has been difficult to demonstrate its value as a therapeutic target.[58] Changing the monitoring end-point from pHi to the mucosal–arterial CO_2 gap (normally 8–10 mmHg (1.04–1.3 kPa)) has removed the most fundamental flaw: the use of arterial [HCO_3^-] as a surrogate for mucosal [HCO_3^-]. The gastric CO_2 gap derived from air tonometry is an independent prognostic factor in critical illness.[59] Simultaneous end-tidal CO_2 measurement allows the regular calculation of a gastric to end-tidal CO_2 gap, a parameter linked to outcome in high-risk surgery.[60]

Despite these improvements, the technique has not found widespread application. There have been several barriers:

1. The need for a nasogastric tube
2. Signal degradation by luminal contents, including feeds and blood; feeds must be stopped 2 hours prior to measurements, jeopardising nutritional support
3. Inability to identify a clear hypoxic threshold; empirical recommendations have been to target a CO_2 gap <25 mmHg (3.25 kPa)
4. A need to suppress gastric acidity to prevent luminal CO_2 generation by HCl titration of duodenal bicarbonate
5. A lack of convincing evidence that tonometry-guided therapy improves outcome.[58,61]

SUBLINGUAL CAPNOMETRY[56]
Measurement of the sublingual interstitial CO_2 tension has the advantage of accessibility with minimal invasion. Optode sensors provide the most rapid response. As with all tissues, sublingual P_{CO_2} is best combined with Pa_{CO_2} to generate the sublingual CO_2 gap, which tracks sublingual microcirculatory blood flow.[62] The sublingual CO_2 gap has predicted outcome better than lactate or Sv_{O_2} in a limited number of shocked patients. It remains to be seen whether the technique can be used to guide therapy.

More recently earlobe P_{CO_2} has shown similar potential.[63]

CEREBROVENOUS OXYGEN SATURATION MONITORING

See Chapter 75.

DIRECT TISSUE P_{O_2} MEASUREMENT

Measurements have been recorded primarily in animal models in the brain, subcutaneous tissue, muscle and renal beds under a variety of perfusion insults. Tensions are commonly around 30–45 mmHg (3.9–5.85 kPa), but can range from <10 mmHg (1.3 kPa) in the renal medulla to >70 mmHg (9.1 kPa) in subcutaneous tissue. In patients this is largely impractical, although in vivo magnetic resonance imaging is one possible future approach.[64]

OTHER REGIONAL TECHNIQUES

DYNAMIC MICROCIRCULATORY IMAGING
Orthogonal polarisation spectroscopy (OPS) and side-stream dark field (SDF) imaging allow real-time

quantification of microvascular flow via derived indices such as the 'functional capillary density' and 'mean flow index'.[65] The tissue bed most commonly evaluated in intensive care has been the sublingual circulation, but rectal, oral, ileal (via stoma) and other microcirculations can be visualised. The rationale is an extension of the covert or compensated shock concept as originally applied to gastric tonometry, in which multiple organ dysfunction is driven by subtle microcirculatory compromise causing an ongoing tissue oxygen deficit despite acceptable macrocirculatory parameters.[66] Of some concern, the relationship between sublingual and intestinal microcirculations may not be reliably consistent, for example in early abdominal sepsis.[67]

NEAR-INFRARED SPECTROSCOPY (NIRS) WITH FUNCTIONAL OCCLUSION TEST[68]

NIRS uses the differential absorbance properties of Hb_{O_2} and Hb in muscle vessels with diameter <1 mm (arterioles, venules and capillaries) subjected to light of wavelengths 680–800 nm. Light at these wavelengths penetrates >1 cm below the skin, but 95% of the detected signal is from tissue <2.4 mm in depth. The thenar eminence is normally selected for its reliable low subcutaneous thickness at any body mass index and its amenability to induced proximal vascular occlusion via a blood pressure cuff. Device software calculates three main parameters; tissue haemoglobin saturation (St_{O_2}), total tissue haemoglobin (TTH) and absolute tissue haemoglobin index (THI). Preliminary data from patients with septic shock suggest that the thenar eminence and knee area tissue oxygen saturation may be predictive of mortality; however, these variables were not superior to arterial lactate in their predictive ability.[69,70]

The functional occlusion test is designed to detect subtle microcirculatory dysfunction, which may be present in covert shock despite unremarkable resting St_{O_2} values. The sphygmomanometer cuff is inflated >30 mmHg (3.9 kPa) above systolic pressure either for 3 minutes or until St_{O_2} stabilises at 40%,[71] then released. The St_{O_2} desaturation slope ($RdecSt_{O_2}$) during occlusion is an indirect index of muscle V_{O_2} (reduced in sepsis and shock states). On cuff release the resaturation slope ($RincSt_{O_2}$) coupled with the degree of St_{O_2} overshoot (ΔSt_{O_2}) and the THI increment due to the associated reactive hyperaemia quantify reperfusion dynamics and vascular recruitment. These are also decreased in sepsis and shock states (**Fig. 18.5**).

Other regional techniques showing some promise include use of the pulse oximeter plethysmographic curve as a means of monitoring the microcirculation (as well as macrocirculatory fluid responsiveness)[72] and optical spectroscopy.[73]

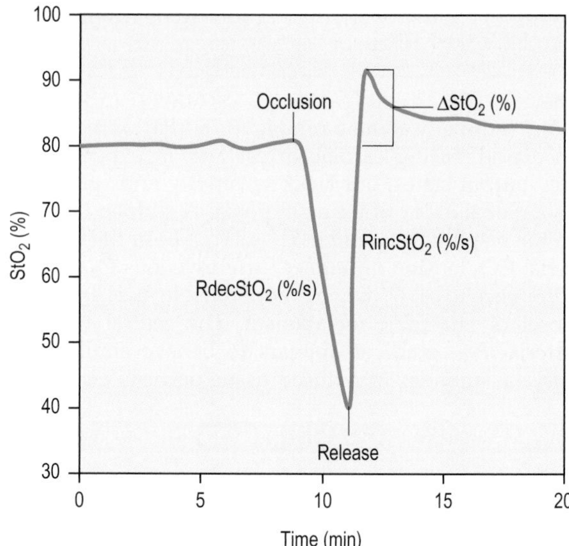

Figure 18.5 Schematic representation of a St_{O_2} curve measured at the thenar eminence during a functional occlusion test. At the point marked 'occlusion' the sphygmomanometer cuff is inflated >30 mmHg (3.9 kPa) above systolic pressure and released when $St_{O_2} \leq 40\%$. The desaturation slope (*Rdec* St_{O_2}) reflects muscle V_{O_2}, and the resaturation slope ($RincSt_{O_2}$) and saturation overshoot (ΔSt_{O_2}) quantify reperfusion dynamics and vascular recruitment. All tend to decrease in sepsis and shock states.

THE PROBLEM OF TISSUE HETEROGENEITY

Despite the emerging human data concerning tissue oxygenation, several areas of uncertainty remain due to the microcirculatory heterogeneity of different tissue beds. There are important differences in both the magnitude and direction of response to a hypoxic or a hypotensive insult.[74] Consequently, identification of a dysoxic threshold in individual tissues remains difficult. More precise knowledge of these variables should eventually provide clinicians with practical resuscitation end-points in hypoxia and shock and may facilitate the practice of 'permissive hypoxia', but at present titration of therapy based on monitoring of tissue oxygenation remains an elusive goal.

Access the complete references list online at http://www.expertconsult.com

4. Loiacono LA, Shapiro DS. Detection of hypoxia at the cellular level. Crit Care Clin 2010;26(2):409–21. Epub 2010/04/13.

7. Muders T, Luepschen H, Putensen C. Impedance tomography as a new monitoring technique. Curr Opin Crit Care 2010;16(3):269–75. Epub 2010/05/07.

19. Kathirgamanathan A, McCahon RA, Hardman JG. Indices of pulmonary oxygenation in pathological lung states: an investigation using high-fidelity, computational modelling. Br J Anaesth 2009;103(2):291–7. Epub 2009/06/23.
31. McMorrow RC, Mythen MG. Pulse oximetry. Curr Opin Crit Care 2006;12(3):269–71. Epub 2006/05/05.
41. Hamilton MA, Cecconi M, Rhodes A. A systematic review and meta-analysis on the use of preemptive hemodynamic intervention to improve postoperative outcomes in moderate and high-risk surgical patients. Anesth Analg 2011;112(6):1392–402. Epub 2010/10/23.
45. Fink MP. Bench-to-bedside review: Cytopathic hypoxia. Crit Care 2002;6(6):491–9. Epub 2002/12/21.
47. Marx G, Reinhart K. Venous oximetry. Curr Opin Crit Care 2006;12(3):263–8. Epub 2006/05/05.
51. Jones AE, Shapiro NI, Trzeciak S, et al. Lactate clearance vs central venous oxygen saturation as goals of early sepsis therapy: a randomized clinical trial. JAMA 2010;303(8):739–46. Epub 2010/02/25.
56. Marik PE. Regional carbon dioxide monitoring to assess the adequacy of tissue perfusion. Curr Opin Crit Care 2005;11(3):245–51. Epub 2005/06/02.
68. Creteur J. Muscle St_{O_2} in critically ill patients. Curr Opin Crit Care 2008;14(3):361–6. Epub 2008/05/10.

19

Lactic acidosis

D James Cooper, Alisa M Higgins and Alistair D Nichol

Lactic acidosis is a metabolic disorder commonly observed in critically ill patients, although the precise prevalence is unknown. The definition of lactic acidosis varies in the literature, although conventionally it is defined as the combination of a blood lactate concentration greater than 5 mmol/L and an arterial blood pH of less than 7.35.[1,2] It has been recognised, however, that the presence of hypoalbuminaemia may mask an anion gap and further that concomitant metabolic or respiratory alkalosis may raise the pH. Lactic acidosis is caused by overproduction of lactate, decreased lactate metabolism, or a combination of the two.

Lactic acidosis in critically ill patients is associated with a high mortality rate,[3] as high as 83%.[1] Lactic acidosis has been associated with higher mortality than other types of acidosis,[3] and increasing blood lactate concentrations have been shown to be associated with increased mortality.[1,4,5] In over 1000 patients with a primary or secondary diagnosis of infection an initial lactate of ≥4 mmol/L was associated with sixfold higher odds of acute-phase death, and acute-phase and in-hospital deaths increased linearly with lactate.[4] However, in 126 patients with severe sepsis or septic shock, lactic acidosis but not hyperlactaemia alone was found to predict in-hospital mortality more exactly.[6] Lactate clearance is also associated with mortality. In 111 patients with severe sepsis, a higher lactate clearance at 6 hours was associated with a decreased mortality rate.[7] Similarly, surgical ICU patients had an increased mortality when the time to normalise lactate levels was greater than 48 hours, with a significantly greater mortality (67% and 100%) when lactate levels failed to normalise.[8,9] In an individual patient, however, prognosis is always dependent on the underlying condition, the initial degree of lactic acidosis being a clinically useful indicator of shock severity, and serial assessment allowing evaluation of overall response to therapy. Recently, blood lactate concentration has been identified as one marker of the degree of shock triggering treatment in septic patients who may benefit from early goal-directed therapy.[10]

Understanding the clinical significance of lactic acidosis is assisted by the knowledge that in healthy athletes very severe but short-lived lactic acidosis during exercise is harmless and insignificant.

PATHOPHYSIOLOGY

There is a continuous cycle of lactate production and metabolism. Lactate is a metabolic end-product of anaerobic glycolysis and is produced by the reduction of pyruvate in a reaction catalysed by lactate dehydrogenase (LDH):

$$\text{pyruvate} + \text{NADH} + \text{H}^+ \xleftrightarrow{\text{LDH}} \text{lactate} + \text{NAD}^+$$

Lactate is produced at about 0.8 mmol/kg per hour, mainly in skeletal muscle, skin, brain, intestine and red blood cells.[11] In critically ill patients, lactate production occurs in many other tissues including lung and liver. Lactate clearance occurs primarily in the liver, with an important contribution from the kidneys, but it can occur to a lesser extent in other organs such as skeletal muscle.[12] Blood lactate levels are normally less than 2 mmol/L and lactic acidosis occurs when lactate production exceeds metabolic capacity, or when the latter is decreased by organ dysfunction. The liver has a key role in lactate homeostasis and many patients who develop lactic acidosis have decreased metabolic capacity due to liver disease.[13]

Lactate formation is dependent upon pyruvate that is produced primarily from the metabolism of glucose by glycolysis, the rate of which is controlled by three unidirectional enzymes and the activity of one of these is increased by increasing intracellular pH. Acidosis therefore decreases (and alkalosis increases) glycolysis and pyruvate, and consequently also lactate production. When oxygen is available, pyruvate enters the mitochondria and is oxidised and lactate does not accumulate. During this process, 36 molecules of adenosine triphosphate (ATP) are produced. Under conditions of hypoxia, pyruvate is unable to enter the mitochondria and is converted to lactate instead. This process generates 2 molecules of ATP; therefore, energy production continues (at a reduced rate) under anaerobic conditions.

In critically ill patients, lactic acidosis is often due to shock. In cardiogenic and hypovolaemic shock, hypoperfusion and tissue hypoxia increase lactic acid production, whereas decreased hepatic perfusion decreases lactic acid metabolism. In septic shock, lactic acidosis is multifactorial and hypoperfusion contributes to it, by microvascular disruption causing regional hypoperfusion and by impaired mitochondrial cellular oxygen utilisation.

CLASSIFICATION OF LACTIC ACIDOSIS

The Cohen & Woods classification of lactic acidosis defines two subgroups of lactic acidosis depending on the presence (type A) or absence (type B) of tissue hypoxia (**Table 19.1**).[14] Type A due to tissue hypoxia is common in critically ill patients, although clinically most patients have features of both type A and type B lactic acidosis, with increased lactate formation from tissue hypoxia and decreased lactate clearance occurring together. Tissue hypoxia is most commonly due to hypoperfusion occurring due to shock (septic, cardiogenic or hypovolaemic), hypotension, cardiac arrest, acute heart failure, or regional hypoperfusion (in particular, mesenteric ischaemia), although it may also be due to reduced tissue oxygen delivery or utilisation due to very severe hypoxaemia, very severe anaemia or carbon monoxide poisoning. Type B lactic acidosis is subdivided into B1 (lactic acidosis occurring in association with an underlying disease), B2 (lactic acidosis due to drugs or toxins), and B3 (lactic acidosis due to inborn errors of metabolism).

Table 19.1 Classification of lactic acidosis

Type A	Shock Very severe hypoxaemia Very severe anaemia Carbon monoxide poisoning
Type B1 (underlying disease)	Sepsis Liver failure Thiamine deficiency Malignancy Phaeochromocytoma Diabetes
Type B2 (drug or toxin)	Epinephrine (adrenaline) Salbutamol Propofol Nucleoside analogue reverse transcriptase inhibitor Ethanol Methanol Paracetamol Nitroprusside Salicylates Ethylene (and propylene) glycol Biguanides Fructose Sorbitol Xylitol Cyanide Isoniazid
Type B3 (rare inborn errors of metabolism)	Glucose-6-phosphatase deficiency Fructose-1,6 diphosphatase deficiency Pyruvate carboxylase deficiency Deficiency of enzymes of oxidative phosphorylation

SEPSIS

There has been much debate[15] whether the hyperlactaemia of sepsis results from net increased cellular production[16] or reduced net clearance.[17] It is likely that, in such patients, the cause of lactic acidosis is multifactorial. As these patients are often haemodynamically unstable, lactate production can increase as a result of inadequate oxygen delivery from hypoperfusion. Other mechanisms thought to contribute to development of lactic acidosis in sepsis include increased pyruvate production,[18] release of lactate from lung parenchyma,[19,20] decreased pyruvate dehydrogenase (PDH) activity,[21,22] and reduced clearance of lactate.[23,24]

Tissue hypoxia may not be a major mechanism for regional lactate production during sepsis: hyperlactaemia is thought to be linked to the severity of the septic cellular inflammatory response and hypermetabolic state.[15,25] Net lactate production from the hepatosplanchnic bed is uncommon in septic patients[26] and nuclear magnetic resonance spectroscopy suggests that hyperlactaemia may occur without tissue hypoxia.[27]

LUNG INJURY

The lung is a primary source of lactate production in patients with ARDS, pulmonary release of lactate being directly related to the severity of lung injury,[20,28] supporting the view that the primary contributors are the tissues with the most inflammation or injury. The increased lactate production by the injured lung is not only secondary to anaerobic metabolism in the hypoxic regions of the lung but also may be due to altered glucose metabolism and a direct effect of cytokines on pulmonary cells.[28]

Laboratory studies suggest that both metabolic and respiratory acidosis protect the lung against injury, whereas correction of acidosis compounds the injury.[29,30] Two ventilator trials[31,32] demonstrating a positive impact on mortality in acute respiratory distress syndrome (ARDS) by limiting tidal volume and airway pressures differed widely on how they regarded the resultant hypercapnic acidosis. Whereas Amato et al[31] allowed elevation of the Pa_{CO_2} (permissive hypercapnia) and resultant acidosis, the ARDSnet group[32] aggressively corrected the hypercapnic acidosis by increasing the respiratory rate and allowing administration of sodium bicarbonate. There is growing evidence that not only may hypercapnic acidosis be beneficial in lung injury,[29,33] but also the ARDSnet intervention aimed at correcting the acidosis may be deleterious.[30,34] These findings have not only promoted a greater tolerance of acidosis in ARDS but also increased reluctance to buffer the acidosis exogenously towards 'normal' values.

ASTHMA

Lactic acidosis often occurs in patients with acute severe asthma, and is often attributed to fatiguing respiratory muscles,[35] inadequate oxygen delivery to the respiratory muscles to meet the elevated oxygen demand[36] and liver ischaemia. However, severe lactic acidosis also occurs in sedated, paralysed mechanically ventilated patients who have no endogenous respiratory muscle activity.[37] Stimulation of beta-adrenergic receptors by beta agonists, including salbutamol and epinephrine, leads to a variety of metabolic effects including an increase in glycogenolysis, gluconeogenesis and lipolysis[38] thus contributing to lactic acidosis. Decrease of intravenous salbutamol infusions to less than 10 μg/min is usually associated with resolution of the acidosis. In asthma, lactic acidosis does not have specific prognostic implications.

MESENTERIC ISCHAEMIA

The diagnosis of mesenteric ischaemia can be challenging to make in the critically ill due to lack of clinical and diagnostic signs, difficulty transferring unstable patients for diagnostic imaging and concern about the deleterious effects of inappropriately administering contrast agents. An ischaemic bowel can produce large amounts of lactate, and the presence of lactic acidosis in the setting of acute abdominal disease has been proposed as an indicator of mesenteric ischaemia. Animal models have shown that lactate increases within 1 hour of induced intestinal ischaemia. In addition, elevated lactate at the time of diagnosis of mesenteric ischaemia is a predictor of mortality.[39] However, although plasma lactate is a very sensitive marker (100%) for detecting acute mesenteric ischaemia, the low specificity of this marker (42%) is a particular problem in the critically ill, who frequently have many plausible alternative diagnoses.

D-lactate is the isomer of lactate produced by intestinal bacterial metabolism and is not produced by humans. Experimental work suggests that ischaemic bowel allows its translocation into the systemic circulation; as D-lactate is not eliminated by the liver, plasma levels may be more specific markers of mesenteric ischaemia. However, many issues need to be clarified, including the effect of antibiotic therapy on the intestinal bacteria, before D-lactate could be considered as a bedside diagnostic test.[40] It is necessary to have a high index of suspicion for mesenteric ischaemia[41] in a deteriorating patient with an elevated lactate in the absence of a convincing alternative diagnosis, as identification of mesenteric ischaemia is frequently made first at laparotomy in the critically ill.

CARDIAC SURGICAL PATIENTS

Hyperlactaemia during cardiopulmonary bypass is relatively frequent and is associated with an increased postoperative morbidity.[42] Recent work has suggested that this 'on pump' hyperlactaemia is secondary to inadequate peripheral oxygen delivery (D_{O_2}), which creates a condition similar to cardiogenic shock leading to both direct lactate formation by dysoxic tissues and to catecholamine release, insulin resistance and hyperglycemia-induced lactate production.

The use of epinephrine after cardiopulmonary bypass precipitates lactic acidosis in some patients.[43] This phenomenon is probably beta agonist mediated, is associated with increased whole body blood flow and resolves after substitution of norepinephrine. However, there is emerging evidence that the severity of lactic acidosis following cardiac surgery is related to certain genetic polymorphisms in tumour necrosis factor and interleukin-10 genes.[44] Similar to asthma, lactic acidosis associated with the administration of epinephrine in this setting does not have the adverse implications of lactic acidosis associated with shock.

OTHER UNDERLYING DISEASES

In patients with cancer, anaerobic glycolysis may be increased whereas hepatic lactate metabolism is impaired by tumour replacement. Diabetic patients may present with shock, but in non-insulin-dependent diabetes there may also be a defect in pyruvate oxidation, and in diabetic ketoacidosis ketones may also inhibit hepatic lactate uptake. Thiamine and biotin are essential co-factors for pyruvate dehydrogenase activity and for conversion of pyruvate to oxaloacetate. Malnutrition (beri-beri) and inadequate parenteral nutrition have therefore been associated with lactic acidosis due to deficiencies of these cofactors. In these cases, pyruvate accumulation increases lactate production.

METFORMIN-ASSOCIATED LACTIC ACIDOSIS (MALA)

Metformin is an oral biguanide used widely in type 2 diabetes mellitus, as it has been shown to decrease cardiovascular morbidity and mortality.[45,46] Metformin-associated lactic acidosis is a rare, but very serious, complication of its use. Two years after its introduction into the US market, an incidence of MALA of 2–9 cases per 100 000 patients treated with metformin each year together with a mortality of up to 50% was reported.[47] A recent study in an Australian tertiary intensive care unit found an incidence of MALA of 6 per 1000 ICU admissions, and a mortality of 29%.[48] A European study found that MALA accounted for 0.84% of all ICU admissions and was associated with a mortality of 30%.[49] In most cases, MALA occurs when the contraindications of metformin have been overlooked or, more commonly, when acute renal failure develops and leads to metformin accumulation.[45,50] Risk factors for developing lactic acidosis while on biguanide treatment include age >60 years, decreased cardiac, hepatic or renal function, diabetic ketoacidosis, surgery, respiratory failure, ethanol intoxication and fasting.[51]

The pathophysiology of MALA remains unclear, and there continues to be controversy about the exact role of metformin in the development of lactic acidosis. A recent Cochrane analysis analysed pooled data from all prospective comparative trials and observational cohorts studies up to 2009 and concluded that there was no current evidence that metformin is associated with an increased risk of lactic acidosis compared with other antihyperglycaemic treatments.[50] However, MALA continues to be reported, frequently in ICU patients,[48,49,52,53] including the Australian cohort described above in which other causes of lactic acidosis were excluded before a diagnosis of MALA was made.[48]

Although the mechanism of MALA is not fully understood, it is thought that biguanides may inhibit oxidative metabolism, and increase the concentration of NADH, reduce gluconeogenesis and suppress gastrointestinal absorption of glucose.[51] A recent retrospective study comparing 10 MALA patients with 187 patients with lactic acidosis of other origin (LAOO) found that the prognosis of MALA was significantly better compared with similarly severe LAOO.[53] Survival of patients with an arterial pH<7.00 was significantly better (50% versus 0%) if MALA was the underlying condition compared with LAOO.[53]

OTHER DRUGS AND TOXINS

The list of potential drugs and toxins that may contribute to the development of lactic acidosis continues to grow. Nucleoside reverse transcriptase inhibitors (NRTIs) used in the treatment of HIV-positive patients cause injury to the mitochondria, which can lead to lactic acidosis. However, NRTI-induced lactic acidosis is rare and is often associated with hepatic steatosis.[54] Acute ethanol intoxication can precipitate lactic acidosis, as ethanol oxidation increases the conversion of pyruvate to lactate and inhibits other pathways of pyruvate accumulation. Underlying alcoholic liver disease and thiamine deficiency may exacerbate the lactic acidosis. Propylene glycol has also been associated with lactic acidosis as it is oxidised by alcohol dehydrogenase in the liver to lactate and pyruvate.[55] It is used as a diluent in many medications such as phenytoin, phenobarbital, lorazepam, diazepam, digoxin and nitroglycerin and, as such, is the most common alcohol intoxication in ICUs.[56]

D-LACTIC ACIDOSIS

D-lactic acidosis is a unique form of lactic acidosis that occurs in patients with short-bowel syndrome, a history of jejuno-ileal bypass surgery or chronic pancreatic insufficiency. Since it was originally described in 1979,[57] there have been numerous reports. Patients typically present with a high-anion-gap metabolic acidosis and neurological manifestations including slurred speech and confusion, triggered by ingestion of large amounts of carbohydrate.

D-lactate is an end-product of the anaerobic metabolism of organic acids produced in the gastrointestinal tract from bacterial metabolism of undigested fibre, sugar and starch.[58] In the setting of carbohydrate malabsorption, the higher concentration of organic acids leads to a decrease in intraluminal pH favouring overpopulation of bacteria such as *Lactobacillus*, one of the main D-lactate-producing bacteria. As D-lactate is metabolised slowly, it can accumulate following a large carbohydrate load. D-lactic acidosis is characterised by a normal lactate level as the assay for lactate measures only L-lactate; a D-lactate level must be specifically requested if D-lactic acidosis is suspected.

CLINICAL PRESENTATION

Patients present with clinical signs appropriate to their primary disorder. Their lactic acidosis is usually evident only after laboratory testing. In critically ill patients with shock, however, the severity of lactic acidosis can be a valuable monitor of the efficacy of resuscitation. Repeated measures of arterial blood gases and blood lactate concentrations are required. In hypovolaemic shock, resolving lactic acidosis along with the clinical signs of improving perfusion is one of several indicators of successful resuscitation. Conversely, failure of lactic acidosis to resolve in hypovolaemic shock suggests inadequate resuscitation or another undetected or unresolved clinical problem. In patients with severe lactic acidosis,[1] a blood lactate concentration of 5 mmol/L indicated a mortality approaching 80%; survival was best in patients whose hyperlactaemia resolved. In septic shock there are many contributors to lactic acidosis, so the time course of acidosis resolution in this setting is a less reliable indicator of the adequacy of shock resuscitation.

Lactic acidosis may also occur in critically ill patients in the absence of shock. Examples include hypermetabolic states where accelerated aerobic glycolysis may contribute (trauma, burns, sepsis), conditions with increased muscle activity (seizures) and during exogenous lactate administration (lactate-buffered haemofiltration fluid). In many of these patients (e.g. patients with seizures) very high blood lactate concentrations have no prognostic implications because the acidosis is rapidly cleared.

CARDIAC DYSFUNCTION – ASSOCIATION, CAUSE OR RESULT OF LACTIC ACIDOSIS

Cardiac dysfunction is common in shocked patients with lactic acidosis and it has often been considered that therapies for lactic acidosis would improve cardiac function. However, cardiac dysfunction in these patients is probably instead due to other factors, with cytokines (TNF-α, interleukins) being the major cause in septic shock, with lactic acidosis a consequence or association rather than a cause of cardiac dysfunction. In lactic acidosis, some clinicians recommend normalisation of arterial pH based on two assumptions: (1) that acidosis causes cardiac dysfunction, and (2) that patients are better with 'normal' laboratory values.[59] Both of these assumptions are incorrect in most critically ill patients. While early research in isolated muscle, isolated heart preparations, animal models and clinical case reports supported the view that acidosis decreased cardiac function and decreased the haemodynamic response to catecholamines, later large animal studies in which preload, afterload and heart rate were carefully controlled found only marginal effects of lactic acidosis on contractility.[2,60] Also, laboratory reports of deceased cardiac function during acidosis studied an arterial pH much lower (pH 6.6–6.9) than that usually observed in critically ill patients.[61] Increasing experience with permissive hypercapnia on ARDS and asthma has supported the view that patients with respiratory acidosis have fewer complications and better outcomes when normal values are not targeted. Perhaps surprisingly, the major haemodynamic effect of acute hypercapnic acidosis in ARDS and asthma was increased cardiac output and vasodilation, not cardiac depression.[62] Therefore, targeting normal values in lactic acidosis is also unlikely in itself to be beneficial, and may be harmful.

MANAGEMENT

GENERAL

The principles of management of patients with lactic acidosis are to diagnose and correct the underlying condition (where possible), and restore adequate tissue oxygen delivery. In critically ill patients, lactic acidosis is often an indicator of major patient pathology. Therefore the main focus is to identify and treat the cause rapidly. A clinical examination and search for occult sepsis, inadequate resuscitation, localised ischaemia or cardiovascular failure are urgently required. In each case, after diagnosis and initial management, lactic acidosis may then be used as an ongoing monitor of disease progression or resolution.

TREAT THE PRIMARY DISORDER

Specific therapies and supports must be directed at each underlying cause. In hypovolaemic and cardiogenic shock, restoration of an adequate global oxygen delivery is required. Vasoconstrictors may worsen tissue perfusion and should only follow adequate intravascular volume and appropriate cardiac support. In septic shock, antibiotics appropriate to cover all likely sources of infections are a priority and in patients with possible ischaemic gut, surgery may be required for both diagnosis and therapy. Postsurgical gastrointestinal leaks may sometimes be difficult to diagnose, may not be detectable on computed tomography and require early laparotomy. In status epilepticus, lactic acidosis is a result of muscle activity and rapid use of effective anticonvulsants is indicated. In diabetic ketoacidosis, insulin, appropriate fluid and treatment of precipitants enable resolution of all metabolic abnormalities, including associated lactic acidosis. In thiamine deficiency, highlighted during a nationwide American shortage of multivitamins for patients receiving total parenteral nutrition,[63] high-dose intravenous thiamine corrected both the vasodilated shock and associated lactic acidosis. In acute severe asthma, lactic acidosis is commonly a result of high-dose intravenous beta-agonist therapy.[43] Salbutamol dose reduction usually resolves the problem. In vasodilated patients after cardiopulmonary bypass, lactic acidosis may also be related to beta-agonist therapy and resolves after substitution of intravenous epinephrine with norepinephrine. In these cases, lactic acidosis is not related to decreased tissue perfusion and adverse effects upon prognosis have not been noted. Patients with human immunodeficiency virus (HIV) receiving nucleoside analogue reverse transcriptase inhibitor (NRTI) therapy have a high incidence of hyperlactaemia (8.3%), which can progress to a rapidly fatal metabolic lactic acidosis syndrome. These patients with NRTI-induced mitochondrial dysfunction require withdrawal of the therapy (if lactate >5 mmol/L) and close monitoring.[64]

HYPERVENTILATION

Hyperventilation is a normal compensatory response to metabolic acidosis in conscious patients. Therefore in mechanically ventilated patients with lactic acidosis, clinicians will usually use some hyperventilation to correct acidaemia partially. Clearly in patients with pulmonary pathology, hyperventilation may be difficult or inappropriate, and in some patients, hyperventilation increases intrathoracic pressure, decreases venous return, decreases cardiac output and exacerbates the cause of lactic acidosis.

BICARBONATE

The use of bicarbonate therapy for the treatment of lactic acidosis continues to be controversial.[2,59,65,66] It was thought that correction of the acidosis through the administration of bicarbonate might reverse depressed cardiac performance; however, there is no evidence in critically ill patients that lactic acidosis depresses cardiac function, and laboratory studies report minimal depression in large animals.[60,67] Further, not all studies have actually demonstrated a rise in pH after the administration of bicarbonate.[68] One reason for these findings is that sodium bicarbonate also has adverse effects including acute hypercapnia and ionised hypocalcaemia,[61] which outweighs potential benefits in patients. Hypercapnia may increase intracellular acidosis (CO_2 crosses cell membranes rapidly) and hypocalcaemia decreases myocardial contractility.[69] Other side-effects of bicarbonate occur because bicarbonate is a hypertonic solution and include acute intravascular volume overload and cardiac depression. In addition, bicarbonate increases lactate production by increasing the activity of the rate-limiting enzyme phosphofructokinase, shifts the haemoglobin–oxygen dissociation curve, increases oxygen affinity of haemoglobin and thereby decreases oxygen delivery to tissues.

While some clinicians continue to use bicarbonate in patients with a pH<7.20, the most recent Surviving Sepsis guidelines published in 2008 strongly recommend against the use of bicarbonate when treating hypoperfusion-induced lactic acidaemia in patients with a pH≥7.15,[70] whereas others have recommended a lower target pH of 7.00 or less.[66] There are no large randomised controlled trials of the use of bicarbonate in lactic acidosis, and the only two randomised crossover studies in critically ill patients with lactic acidosis and shock found no improvement in cardiac function or any other beneficial effects of pH correction.[61,71] As such, bicarbonate has never been shown to be beneficial in any clinical trial of patients with lactic acidosis and its use in these patients is not recommended, regardless of the degree of acidaemia.[2]

However, there are two specific subgroups of patients with lactic acidosis in whom bicarbonate may be considered. Patients with pulmonary hypertension and right heart failure (e.g. lung transplant recipients) may have pulmonary vasoconstriction, which is exacerbated by acidosis. In these patients, although there are other useful therapies including inhaled nitric oxide and partial pH correction, it may improve right heart function. Secondly, patients with significant ischaemic heart disease and lactic acidosis may be at increased risk of major arrhythmias because severe acidosis lowers the myocardial threshold for arrhythmias. In both of these subgroups, slow bicarbonate infusions to keep the arterial pH above 7.15 may be justified.

ALTERNATIVE THERAPIES

CARBICARB®

Carbicarb® is an equimolar mixture of sodium carbonate and sodium bicarbonate that does not generate carbon dioxide and may therefore have fewer adverse effects than bicarbonate.[72] There is limited clinical research associated with Carbicarb®, and though it has been shown to increase intracellular pH and have fewer haemodynamic adverse effects than bicarbonate (in animal models), it does not address the underlying cause of lactic acidosis and is not in clinical usage.

DICHLOROACETATE

Dichloroacetate (DCA) stimulates the phosphate dehydrogenase complex, the rate-limiting enzyme that regulates entry of pyruvate into the tricarboxylic acid cycle, and thereby facilitates the oxidation of lactate. Although it has been shown to increase arterial pH and decrease lactate concentrations,[73] a large multicentre randomised clinical trial in patients with lactic acidosis found no benefits for either haemodynamics or patient outcome.[74] This study is the best evidence currently available to support the view that correction of lactic acidosis in critically ill patients without improving the underlying primary disorder has no overall impact on patient outcome. DCA is not available commercially.

TRIS/THAM

Tris-hydroxymethyl aminomethane (THAM) is a commercially available weak alkali rarely used as a clinical therapy because of concerns about side-effects that include hyperkalaemia, hypoglycaemia, extravasation-related necrosis and neonatal hepatic necrosis. In acute lung injury, THAM has been demonstrated to be an effective buffer in ventilated patients as it is not associated with an increased CO_2 load and is capable of ameliorating some of the haemodynamic effects of hypercapnia.[75,76] However, it is unclear whether buffering of hypercapnic acidosis in acute lung injury patients is of any benefit. A trial of a single dose of sodium bicarbonate compared with THAM in ICU patients with a mild metabolic acidosis found that both had similar alkalising effects, although the effect of sodium bicarbonate was longer lasting. As THAM did not increase Pa_{CO_2}, it was recommended in patients with mixed acidosis with high Pa_{CO_2} levels.[77] There is no evidence to show that administration of THAM in patients with lactic acidosis improves outcome.

DIALYSIS/HAEMOFILTRATION

Haemofiltration and continuous renal replacement therapies (CRRT) have been promoted as treatments for lactic acidosis, with several theoretical advantages. Bicarbonate-based haemodialysis can assist in treatment of acidosis through diffusion of bicarbonate from the dialysate into the serum without the risk of volume overload, hypernatraemia or hyperosmolality. Studies have shown improvements in acid–base balance with bicarbonate-based CRRT,[78,79] although controlled clinical trials showing an improvement in outcome are lacking. A study of 10 critically ill patients with acute renal failure and stable lactate concentrations found that, following an infusion of sodium lactate, bicarbonate-buffered haemofiltration was ineffective, contributing to less than 3% of lactate clearance.[80] They concluded that continuous veno-venous haemofiltration with dialysis cannot meet lactate overproduction.[80]

However, in lactate-intolerant patients (i.e. those with shock-induced lactic acidosis and/or liver disease), the use of lactate-based dialysis fluid may overload the patient's metabolic capacity for lactate, particularly if high-volume haemofiltration is employed.[81] In these patients, bicarbonate-based replacement fluid should be chosen. In addition, there are some case reports that high-volume renal replacement therapy may be beneficial in severe MALA,[82,83] as it efficiently removes metformin by diffusion through the dialysis membrane; however, no controlled studies have been published.

Access the complete references list online at http://www.expertconsult.com

7. Nguyen HB, Rivers EP, Knoblich BP, et al. Early lactate clearance is associated with improved outcome in severe sepsis and septic shock. Crit Care Med 2004;32(8):1637–42.
29. Laffey JG, Honan D, Hopkins N, et al. Hypercapnic acidosis attenuates endotoxin-induced acute lung injury. Am J Respir Crit Care Med 2004;169(1): 46–56.
60. Cooper DJ, Werner HA, Walley KR. Bicarbonate does not increase left ventricular contractility during L-lactic acidemia in pigs. Am J Respir Crit Care Med 1993;148(2):317–22.
61. Cooper DJ, Walley KR, Wiggs BR, et al. Bicarbonate does not improve hemodynamics in critically iii patients who have lactic acidosis: a prospective, controlled clinical study. Ann Intern Med 1990;112(7): 492–8.
70. Dellinger RP, Levy MM, Carlet JM, et al. Surviving Sepsis Campaign: international guidelines for management of severe sepsis and septic shock: 2008. Intensive Care Med 2008;34(1):17–60.
71. Mathieu D, Neviere R, Billard V, et al. Effects of bicarbonate therapy on hemodynamics and tissue oxygenation in patients with lactic acidosis: a prospective, controlled clinical study. Crit Care Med 1991;19(11):1352–6.
74. Stacpoole PW, Wright EC, Baumgartner TG, et al. A controlled clinical trial of dichloroacetate for treatment of lactic acidosis in adults. New Engl J Med 1992;327(22):1564–9.

Part Three

Acute Coronary Care

20

Acute cardiac syndromes, investigations and interventions

Bradley Power

Cardiovascular disease (CVD) accounts for 1 in 3 deaths in Western industrialised society, with coronary artery disease (CAD) being responsible for about half of these.[1] In persons over age 40, acute myocardial infarction (MI) is the cause of approximately 20% of all deaths. Up to 70–80% of these deaths occur outside hospital. Of those who die acutely, 50–65% have no previous history of cardiac disease. Of patients admitted to hospital, early mortality is 5–7%[2–4] (much higher in at-risk groups) and may rise to 9–11% by 12 months.[2] Lowering in-hospital and longer-term mortality from CAD requires us to identify rapidly patients who are at risk and to implement evidence-based treatment regimens.

MYOCARDIAL INFARCTION

MI is present when there is evidence of myocardial necrosis in a clinical setting consistent with myocardial ischaemia. Diagnosis is usually made on the basis of clinical suspicion, although tests such as electrocardiography (ECG) and biomarkers, echocardiography or autopsy findings are required to confirm the diagnosis.

Acute MI can occur in association with or result from a number of different pathological and epidemiological mechanisms (**Box 20.1**).[5] Each mechanism may have a different long-term prognosis despite similar biomarker and ECG changes. The pattern of MI may be different in an emergency department (ED) population to that in a general intensive care unit (ICU) population. Such classifications may be clinically important when applying the results of clinical trials to clinical practice in different patient groups. Although there can be significant overlap, small amounts of myocardial necrosis can occur with heart failure, arrhythmias, pulmonary embolism or post cardiac procedures; these are perhaps best labelled 'myocardial injury'.[5]

ACUTE CORONARY SYNDROMES (ACS) (**BOX 20.2**)

ACS represent the largest group of patients developing MI. They describe the spectrum of patients who present with chest discomfort or other symptoms caused by acute myocardial ischaemia. ACS can be further divided into acute MI and unstable angina (USA). Both are invariably caused by recent thrombus formation on pre-existing coronary artery plaque leading to impaired myocardial oxygen supply. In this sense they differ from stable angina, which is usually precipitated by increased myocardial oxygen demand with severe background coronary artery narrowing. Both represent medical emergencies and are one of the most frequent causes of hospital and coronary care unit (CCU) admission.

An immediate clinical imperative is to identify those patients with ST-segment elevation (STE) as rapid reperfusion therapy is strongly indicated in this group.

AETIOLOGY AND RISK FACTORS

Atheroma deposits in the walls of coronary arteries provide the substrate for the development of ACS. Modification of risk factors is one of the most important means of decreasing the prevalence and mortality from CVD and MI. About 85% of patients presenting with their first myocardial infarction have at least one risk factor.

Cessation of smoking, lowering plasma cholesterol (diet and medications) and adoption of a more active lifestyle can all help prevent the development of CAD. Treatment of high-risk hypertensive patients produces a large and early reduction in stroke incidence (30–40%) and mortality, and a significant fall in MI (20–25%) and also heart failure (>50%).[6,7]

PATHOPHYSIOLOGY

Formation of thrombus upon disrupted, fissured or eroded atheromatous plaque is the usual precipitant of an ACS.[5,8–10] Atherosclerotic plaque formation is probably initiated by injury to the vessel wall that may commence even as early as childhood. Highly activated macrophages are attracted to the site of injury and differentiate into tissue macrophages. Macrophages incorporate bloodstream lipids into the connective tissue fibres of the plaque, forming a thrombogenic soft lipid core. Plaque development is slow, but is rapidly accelerated in people with risk factors.

'Vulnerable plaque' is often rich in lipid and covered by a thin fibrin cap. The cause of plaque rupture or fissuring is unknown but exposes thrombogenic lipid and collagen, which are potent activators of platelets.

Box 20.1 Universal classification of myocardial infarction

Type 1: Spontaneous myocardial infarction
Spontaneous myocardial infarction related to ischaemia due to a primary coronary event such as plaque erosion *and/or* rupture, fissuring, or dissection. The patient may have severe CAD but on occasion non-obstructive or no CAD.

Type 2: Myocardial infarction secondary to an ischaemic imbalance
In instances of myocardial injury with necrosis where a condition other than CAD contributes to an imbalance between myocardial oxygen supply and/or demand, e.g. coronary endothelial dysfunction, coronary artery spasm, coronary embolism, tachy-/brady-arrhythmias, anaemia, respiratory failure, hypotension, and hypertension with or without LVH.

Type 3: Myocardial infarction resulting in death when biomarker values are unavailable
Cardiac death with symptoms suggestive of myocardial ischaemia, and presumed new ischaemlc changes or new LBBB, but death occurring before blood samples could be obtained, before cardiac biomarkers could rise or on rare cases biomarkers were not collected.

Type 4a: Myocardial infarction related to percutaneous coronary intervention (PCI)
Significant cardiac biomarker rise from normal or by more than 20% if previously elevated. In addition, either:

i. symptoms of myocardial ischaemia, *or*
ii. new ischaemic ECG changes or LBBB, *or*
iii. angiographic loss of patency or persistent flow abnormalities, or embolization, *or*
iv. imaging demonstration of loss of viable myocardium or regional wall motion abnormality.

Type 4b: Myocardial infarction related to stent thrombosis
Myocardial infarction associated with stent thrombosis detected by coronary angiography or autopsy in setting of myocardial ischaemia and with a significant rise and/or fall of biomarkers.

Type 5: Myocardial infarction related to coronary artery bypass grafting (CABG)
Myocardial infarction associated with CABG arbitrarily defined by elevation of cardiac biomarker values from normal baseline to above 10 times the URL. In addition, either:

i. new pathological Q waves or LBBB, *or*
ii. angiographic documented new graft or new native coronary artery occlusion, *or*
iii. imaging evidence of new loss of viable myocardium or new regional wall motion abnormality.

Adapted from Thygesen K, Alpert JS, Jaffe AS, et al. Third universal definition of myocardial infarction. Eur Heart J 2012;33(20):2551.[5] *doi:10.1093/eurheartj/ehs184.* Modified with permission of Oxford University Press (UK) © European Society of Cardiology.

Development of thrombus upon this eroded plaque results from: (1) platelet adherence and activation, and (2) coagulation pathway activation.

Although many pathways initiate platelet activation, the final common pathway of thrombus formation is via activation of the glycoprotein (GP) IIb/IIIa receptor,

Box 20.2 Classification of acute coronary syndromes

Acute coronary syndrome (ACS)
A spectrum of clinical conditions characterised by acute chest pain or myocardial ischaemia. Pain is of recent origin or is more frequent, severe or prolonged than known angina, is more difficult to control with medication or occurs at rest or with minimal exertion.

ACS includes myocardial infarction with ST-segment elevation (STEMI), myocardial infarction in the absence of ST-segment elevation (NSTEMI) and unstable angina. An initial clinical subdivision of ACS is made on the presence or absence of ECG ST-segment elevation.

STEMI
Patients presenting with ST-segment elevation ACS will invariably display initial or subsequent troponin elevation, although the extent of myocardial infarction and complications may be significantly moderated by intervention.

NSTEACS
Patients who present without ST-segment elevation, may later (after testing of biomarkers) be determined to have:

i. *NSTEMI:* cardiac biomarkers elevated indicating myocardial infarction
ii. *Unstable angina:* no evidence of cardiac biomarker elevation.

the platelet surface membrane receptor for fibrinogen. Activated GP IIb/IIIa receptors cross-link fibrinogen between activated platelets, promoting the formation of platelet thrombi. Platelets aggregate to form 'white thrombus'; however, this thrombus is seldom totally occluding. Activation of coagulation pathways by exposed lipid and fibrin, as well as by the now-activated platelets, leads ultimately to thrombin activation and the laying-down of fibrin clot. Red cells are enmeshed in this so-called 'red thrombus' complex, which surrounds the 'white thrombus'. Sudden artery occlusion by thrombus may thus complicate even only moderate-sized plaque; 70% of ACS patients may have a <50% stenotic lesion and in only 14% is the underlying stenosis >70% of the lumen diameter (**Fig. 20.1**).

These processes have immediate relevance to treatment:

- Antiplatelet agents prevent platelet adherence and heaping, which limits and even reverses the development of 'white thrombus'. These agents may target the adenosine diphosphate (ADP) receptor (e.g. clopidogrel, prasugrel) or may inhibit cyclo-oxygenase (e.g. aspirin). Although aspirin has been the major antiplatelet agent and blocks synthesis of thromboxane A_2, it fails to block platelet activation by thrombin, ADP and collagen.[11]
- Fibrinolytic agents lyse 'red thrombus' but are not active against 'white thrombus'.
- Antithrombin agents (e.g. heparins) may limit thrombin activation. Current thrombolytic agents lyse fibrin and red cell thrombus, but paradoxically may increase surface thrombin activation.

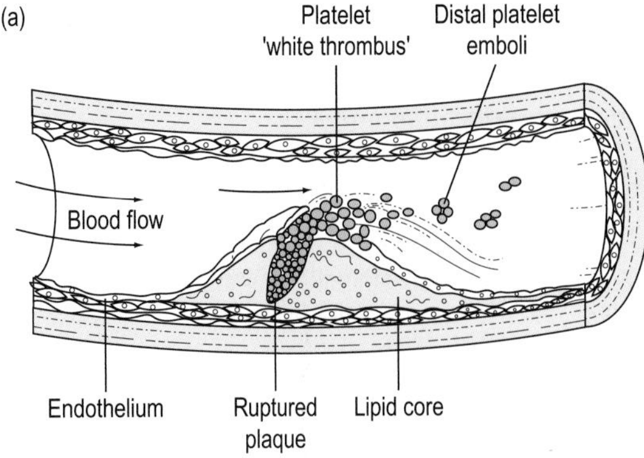

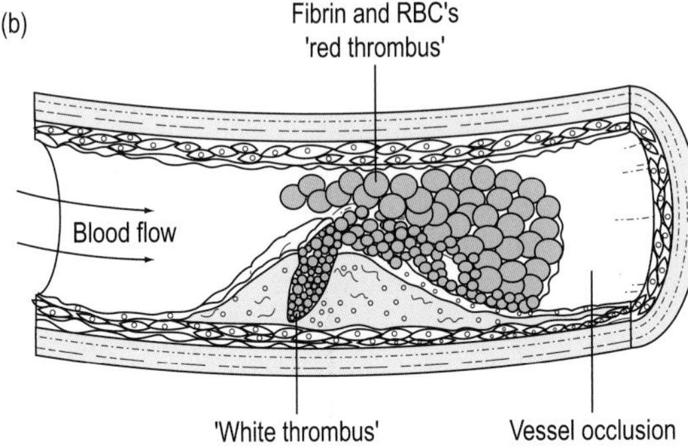

Figure 20.1 (a) Plaque rupture exposes thrombogenic lipid. 'White thrombus' is formed by adherent activated platelets. Coronary artery narrowing, distal platelet embolisation or arterial spasm can cause ischaemic myocardial pain and possible myocardial necrosis. This lesion is unstable and may lead to thrombin activation. 'White thrombus' is not removed by thrombolytic therapy. (b) Thrombin activation leads to a mesh of fibrin and red blood cells (RBCs) or 'red thrombus'. Arterial occlusion may result and, in arteries without adequate collateral circulation, myocardial necrosis follows. Complete arterial occlusion is suggested by ST-segment elevation on the electrocardiogram. Prompt reperfusion with thrombolytic therapy or with invasive coronary procedures may prevent extensive myocardial necrosis.

Totally occluding thrombus causes myocardial necrosis unless there is good collateral flow or the thrombus is rapidly cleared.[10] Occlusion is often accompanied by ST-segment elevation (STE) on the ECG. If thrombus is largely 'white thrombus', with minimal or non-occlusive red thrombus, STE is far less likely. Non-occlusive thrombus may be asymptomatic, may cause USA or MI, especially if spasm or distal embolisation of thrombus occurs. Although non-occlusive thrombus is less likely to be associated with early or sudden death, it is indicative of unstable plaque and is strongly associated with re-infarction and death in following months.

Ischaemic necrosis results in cellular disruption, loss of function, thinning and softening of the affected myocardium with an increase in ventricular compliance. As fibrosis takes place compliance is decreased. With time, there is often expansion of the infarcted segment and compensatory hypertrophy of unaffected myocardial cells (i.e. ventricular remodelling[10]). This can commence early after infarction, affecting overall ventricular function and prognosis.

Infarct size determines:

- left ventricular (LV) systolic function impairment
- stroke volume decrease
- ventricular filling pressure rise (leads to pulmonary congestion and hypotension that may impair coronary perfusion pressures and exacerbate the myocardial ischaemia)
- LV diastolic dysfunction.

CLINICAL PRESENTATION[4,5,12]

The diagnosis of myocardial ischaemia is usually made (suspected) on the basis of clinical history and ECG.[4,5]

HISTORY

Patients with myocardial ischaemia can present with chest pain or pressure, syncope, palpitations, dyspnoea or sudden death. Prodromal symptoms of unstable angina (USA) occur in the days preceding infarction in 20–60% of patients.

Typically, the pain of acute MI:

- is severe, constant and retrosternal, spreading across the chest
- lasts for more than 20 minutes and is without a clear precipitant
- may radiate to the throat and jaw, down the ulnar aspect of both arms and to the interscapular area.

Sweating, nausea, pallor, dyspnoea and anxiety are common.

The pain of USA may be similar but milder in nature. Features that may suggest it to be ischaemic are:[4]

- waxing and waning characteristics
- reproducibility upon minimal exertion or with emotion
- association with autonomic symptoms.

The pain may sometimes be atypical:

- epigastric (leading to possible misdiagnosis)
- confined to the jaw, arms, wrists or interscapular region
- burning or a 'pressure-like' sensation
- sharp or stabbing in nature
- reproduced by chest pressure.

These features do not necessarily exclude infarction.[5] Differential diagnosis includes:

- aortic dissection
- pericarditis.

Atypical or silent presentations are common: 25% of STEMI (ST-segment elevation myocardial infarction) patients and 45% of NSTEMI (non-ST-segment elevation myocardial infarction) patients may present without classic chest discomfort and are less likely to receive definitive treatment.[12] This presentation is more common in patients who are elderly, diabetic, have hypertension, who smoke or who take non-steroidal anti-inflammatory agents.

The assessment of clinical symptoms alone is insufficient for risk stratification and severity of pain does not usually correlate with the extent of infarction.

PHYSICAL EXAMINATION

Examination of patients with USA is often unremarkable. With more severe infarction and extensive myocardial injury, signs of autonomic activation (pallor, sweating, agitation, clamminess) as well as heart failure and even shock may be apparent. Pericardial friction rubs occur frequently after MI but are usually transient.

LV failure is associated with a higher mortality. Signs include gallop rhythm, tachycardia, tachypnoea and basal crackles. A fourth heart sound is often heard, but a third heart sound usually indicates a large infarction with extensive muscle damage. A systolic murmur may be present and may be transient or persistent. These murmurs can have prognostic significance and usually result from mitral regurgitation, due to either papillary muscle dysfunction or LV dilatation.

Cardiogenic shock, hypotension, oliguria and other features of low cardiac output are associated with particularly poor outcome. Shock may be present without hypotension and may develop many hours after onset of symptoms.[13] Right ventricle (RV) infarction results in hypotension and marked elevation of the jugular venous pressure (also seen with major LV dysfunction, usually in association with marked pulmonary venous congestion).

Conditions with similar presentations that do not benefit from thrombolysis are:

- pericarditis (auscultate for pericardial rub)
- aortic dissection (arterial pulses are compared; review chest X-ray if concerned).

INVESTIGATIONS

The presence of MI should also be qualified by:[5]

- anatomical location and size
- causation (e.g. MI Type 1–5) (see Box 20.1)
- time from occurrence (acute, early, late).

Technological advances allow accurate detection of very small infarcts (myocardial necrosis <1.0 g).

ELECTROCARDIOGRAPHY[14,15]

All patients presenting with symptoms suggestive of MI should have an ECG performed and interpreted within 10 minutes of arrival. The ECG is considered the initial single most important test for diagnosing and guiding the emergency treatment of MI. Patients experiencing myocardial ischaemia may have initial ECGs that reveal significant ST-segment elevation (STEACS) or that lack significant ST-segment elevation (NSTEACS). Serial ECGs may give information about the site, size and possible therapies.

Acute and complete occlusion of a coronary artery usually leads to serial ECG changes in leads subtending the area of ischaemia, where the:

- number of leads involved broadly reflects the extent of myocardium involved
- height of initial STE is modestly correlated with the degree of ischaemia
- acute resolution of STE correlates well with reperfusion.

Identification of classical acute and early changes where STEMI is present identifies patients in whom reperfusion therapy may interrupt, prevent or minimise myocardial necrosis (**Fig. 20.2**). These changes are not stereotyped and may vary significantly but include:

- *hyperacute* (0–20 minutes): tall, peaking T-waves and progressive upward coving and elevation of ST-segments
- *acute* (minutes to hours): persisting STE, gradual loss of R-wave in the infarcted area. ST-segments begin to fall and there is progressive inversion of T-waves
- *early* (hours to days): loss of R-wave and development of pathological Q-waves in area of ischaemia.

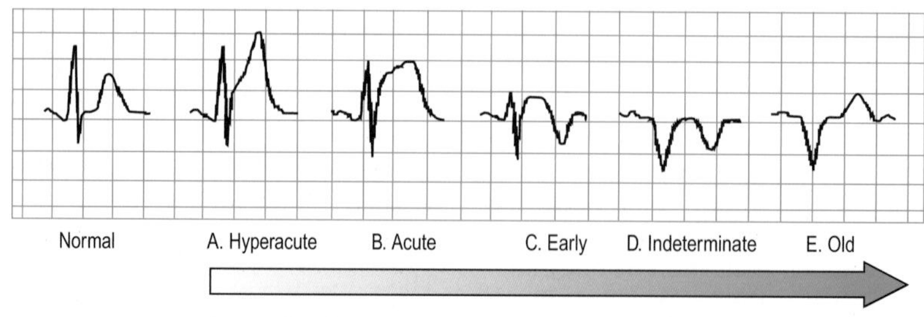

Figure 20.2 Total acute coronary occlusion leads to serial electrocardiogram changes. The evolution is variable and may be interrupted or altered by successful reperfusion. ST-segment elevation is an early and relatively specific indicator of the need for acute reperfusion in patients with acute coronary syndrome.

Return of ST-segments to baseline. Persistence of T-wave inversion
- *indeterminate* (days to weeks): pathological Q-waves with persisting T-wave inversion. ST-segments normalise (unless there is aneurysm)
- *old* (weeks to months): persisting deep Q-waves with normalised ST-segments and T-waves.

Clinical skill is needed to identify those ECG changes that are probably due to MI (true positive but also false negative). Other causes of STE and T-wave changes that should *not* receive thrombolytic therapy are shown in **Box 20.3**.[5,16]

Takotsubo syndrome is characterised by precordial ST-segment elevation, apical ballooning on echocardiography but normal vessels on angiography. It may follow the onset of recent severe stress and may cause up to 1–2% of STEMI. It has been recognised in critical illness.

Patients with ACS but without significant ST-segment elevation (generically, non-ST-segment elevation ACS (non-STEACS or NSTEACS), until further subdivided by biomarker studies) may still be at high risk of infarction and death. They probably have active, non-occluding thrombus or, if it is occluding, then some collateral flow is present. ECGs in these patients may be normal or display:[14,15]

- ST-segment depression
- STE (insufficient to meet thrombolysis criteria)
- T-wave inversion or 'normalisation' of previous inverted T-waves.

LOCALISATION OF INFARCTION[14,15]

The left anterior descending (LAD) coronary artery supplies the anterior two-thirds of the interventricular septum (septal perforators), the anterior and lateral wall of the LV (diagonal branches) and sometimes part of the RV. The left circumflex artery supplies the LV lateral (anterolateral marginal branches) and posterior walls, and occasionally its inferior aspect (posterior LV arteries: 15% of patients) and the posterior septum. The right coronary artery (RCA) supplies the RV wall, and usually the posterior septum and inferior (diaphragmatic) wall of the left ventricle (posterior LV arteries; 85% of people). The RCA is 'dominant' (as opposed to the circumflex) if it gives rise to the posterior descending coronary artery (PDA) (**Fig. 20.3**).

It is usual to use the ECG in initial clinical assessments to 'localise' the area of myocardial ischaemia. The pattern of lead involvement may assist with localisation of the MI (**Table 20.1**).[14,15] There is a reasonable correlation between the site of infarction as defined by the ECG, the occluded or 'culprit' coronary artery, and the infarcted region of myocardium. However, ECG localisation may differ from angiographic, echocardiographic and autopsy findings, especially where there is collateral circulation or previous coronary artery bypass grafting (CABG). Anterior wall infarctions usually result from occlusion of the LAD; inferior, true posterior (although the infarcted region may in truth be lateral)[15] and RV infarctions result from occlusion of the RCA or circumflex arteries.[14,15]

Common ECG patterns of infarction are shown in **Figure 20.4a, b**. Approximately 40–50% of patients present with anterior infarction and 50% with inferior infarction. Anterior wall infarctions may be extensive or localised (septal, anterior, lateral). Inferior infarctions may involve extension to the lateral, posterior or RV myocardium. Standard ECGs generally only record from anterior body leads and thus important ECG patterns that must not be missed are as follows.[14,17]

- True or 'strictly' posterior infarction involves 'mirror' changes in leads V_1 and V_2 and is important to diagnose because the amount of threatened myocardium is similar to that of inferior infarction. Usually there might be ST-elevation in inferior leads II, III, AVF that might not have met diagnostic criteria for reperfusion. These patients should receive reperfusion therapy, especially when non-standard posterior chest leads (V_7–V_9) show ST-elevation, even in the absence of ST-elevation in any of the standard 12-lead ECG leads. Such infarctions are usually actually lateral rather than posterior but the term 'posterior' is still retained.[14,17]
- RV infarction is usually concurrent with inferior wall infarction and very rare in isolation. A V_4R lead (V_4 lead in an equivalent position on the right anterior chest wall) is sensitive and specific for RV infarction and should be considered in patients with inferior MI.
- Resting ECG changes revealing significant ST-segment depression in eight or more body surface

Box 20.3 Electrocardiogram patterns mimicking ST-segment elevation myocardial infarction

Normal variant (non-ischaemic STE mainly V2–V3)
Early repolarisation (notched J-point mainly in anterolateral leads)
Metabolic disturbance (mainly hyperkalaemia, hypercalcaemia)
Drug toxicity
Brugada syndrome
Pre-excitation (Wolff–Parkinson–White syndrome)
Pericarditis
Myocarditis
Previous (old) myocardial infarction
LV aneurysm
Spontaneously reperfused myocardium
Apical ballooning syndrome (Takotsubo or 'broken heart') multiple causes, e.g. severe emotion, physical stress

Data from Thygesen K, Alpert JS, Jaffe AS, et al. Third universal definition of myocardial infarction. Eur Heart J 2012;33(20):2551,[5] and Pollak, P. and Brady W. Electrocardiographic patterns mimicking ST segment elevation myocardial infarction. Cardiol Clin 2012;30(4):601–15.[16]

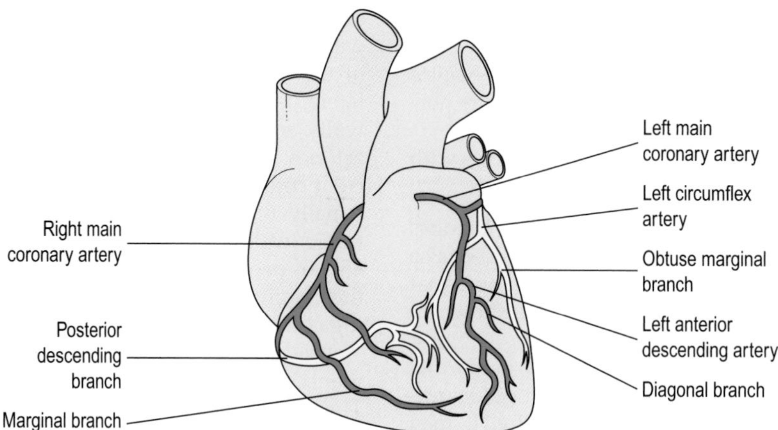

Figure 20.3 Coronary artery anatomy. The left anterior descending artery (LAD) supplies the anterior two-thirds of the interventricular septum (septal perforators), anterior and lateral wall of the left ventricle (LV: diagonal branches) and sometimes part of the right ventricle (RV). Circumflex (Cx) supplies the LV lateral (anterolateral marginal branches) and posterior walls, and occasionally its inferior aspect (posterior LV arteries: 15% of patients) and the posterior septum. The right coronary artery (RCA) supplies the RV wall, and usually the posterior septum and inferior (diaphragmatic) wall of the LV (posterior LV arteries; 85% of people). The RCA is 'dominant' (as opposed to the circumflex) if it gives rise to the posterior descending coronary artery (PDA) and the posterior left ventricular arteries.

Table 20.1 Electrocardiogram patterns of myocardial injury

ANTERIOR WALL	ST-SEGMENT ELEVATION	
'Extensive anterior' (antero-lateral)	V_1–V_6, I, aVL	Proximal LAD occlusion
Septal	V_1–V_3, disappearance of septum Q in leads V_5,V_6	LAD-septal branches
Anterior (localised or true)	V_2–V_5, I, aVL	Diagonal (supplies anterior LV wall) Occasionally marginal branch of CX
Lateral	V_5,V_6, I, aVL,	Distal LAD or circumflex
INFERIOR WALL		
Inferior (localised)	II, III, aVF	RCA (80%) or post-lateral branch of CX (20%)
Inferior (extended)	II, III, aVF ***plus***	
Infero-lateral	I, aVL, V_5, V_6	RCA or dominant CX
Infero-posterior	V_7, V_8, V_9 with ST depression V_1–V_2	RCA post descending branch or postero-lateral branch of CX
Right ventricular	V_1, V_3R, V_4R	Proximal RCA
*Posterior (localised)	V_7, V_8, V_9. (Elevation II, III, aVF may not be marked) Initial V_1,V_2 ST depression may evolve to tall R waves	RCA

The sensitivity, specificity and predictive value of these patterns in determining the culprit artery (as subsequently determined by angiography) are not perfect. This is especially true of occlusions of the RCA and CX.
*Posterior infarctions are usually identified as lateral on angiography but guidelines suggest that the name be retained. Lack of ST elevation on standard leads may lead to failure to appreciate that they are a STEMI and will benefit from reperfusion therapy. Clinicians should also be aware of novel patterns of ischaemia and 'STEMI equivalents' that may include 'Wellens phenomenon', STE elevation in aVR, ST changes in presence of LBBB and the de Winter ST/T complex.
RCA=right coronary artery; LAD,=left anterior descending coronary artery; CX=circumflex coronary artery.

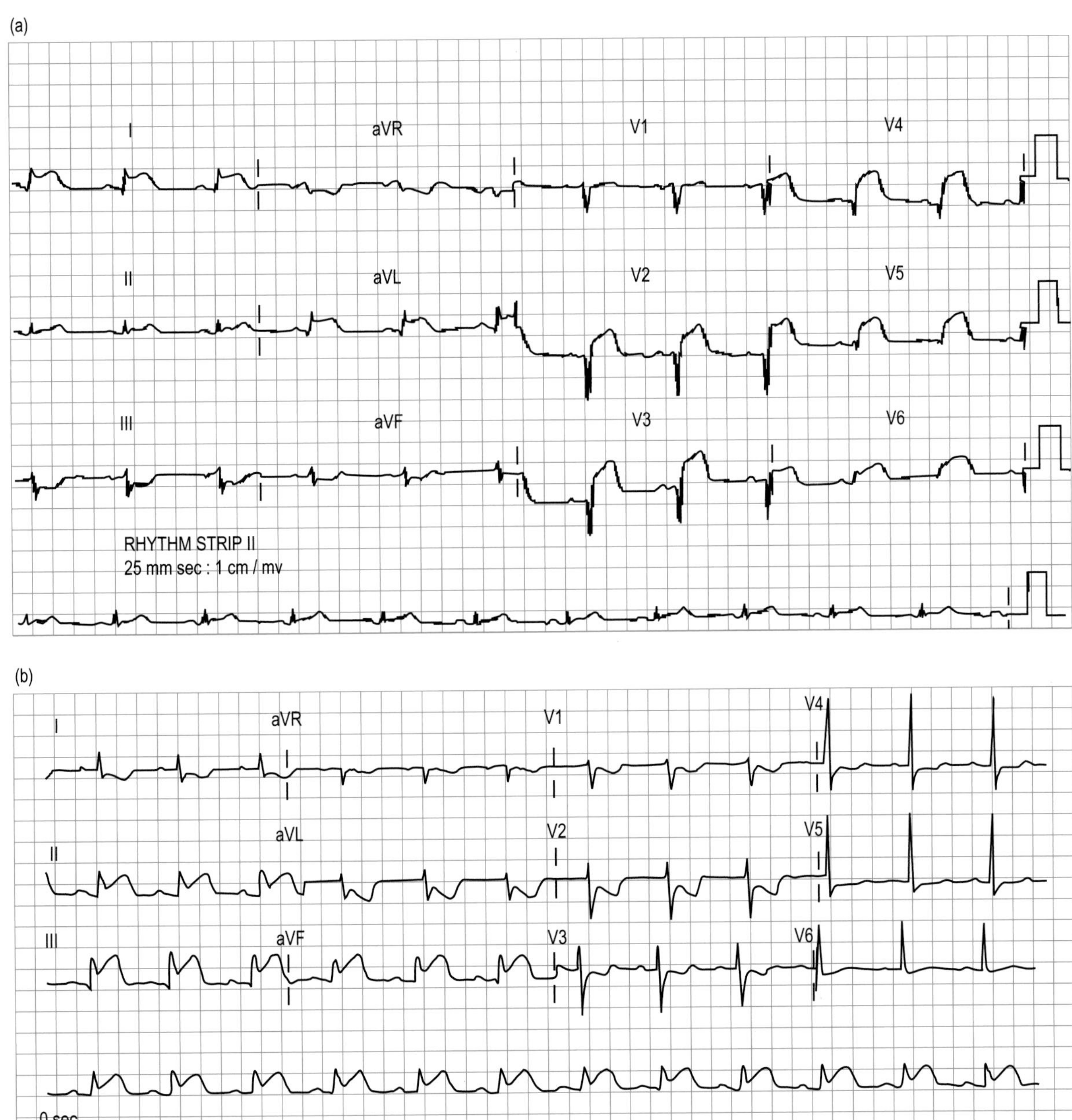

Figure 20.4 (a) Evolving antero-lateral MI. There is ST-segment elevation (STE) in anterior leads V_2–V_6 and lateral leads I, aVL. There is loss of anterior R wave height, and reciprocal ST-segment depression in leads III and aVF. If within time frames or if shocked, urgent reperfusion is indicated. (b) Acute inferior myocardial infarction (STE in the inferior leads II, III and aVF). There is ST depression in leads I, aVL, V_1 and V_2. The addition of right-sided (V_4R) and posterior leads would help identify the presence of RV and posterior infarction (STE). Reciprocal ST-segment depression in leads remote from the site of infarction is a highly sensitive indicator of myocardial infarction. It may be seen in 70% of inferior and 30% of anterior infarctions.

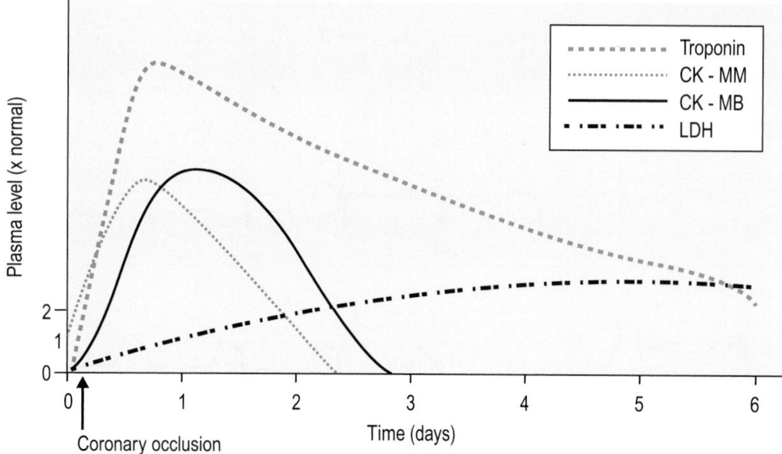

Figure 20.5 Serum biochemical marker changes after acute myocardial infarction. The sensitivity and specificity of cardiac troponins makes them useful for the early diagnosis of myocardial infarction. Their delayed fall may allow diagnosis where presentation is late. CK or CK-MB is useful if re-infarction with secondary biomarker rise is queried. LDH=lactate dehydrogenase.

leads coupled with STE in aVR and/or V_1 are highly suggestive of multivessel or left main coronary artery obstruction.[15]

- The specific pattern of deep T-wave inversion in V_2–V_4 with QT interval prolongation may suggest severe proximal LAD disease. It may occur after chest pain but be associated with imminent occlusion.[15]
- A normal ECG may be present in 15–20% of NSTEMI and does not exclude MI, although a normal ECG during pain is unusual.[14] Despite the absence of STE, a small percentage of patients progressively lose R-wave height and develop evidence of Q-waves and a small number progress to cardiogenic shock. The resting ECG does not have sufficient predictive value to stratify patients with NSTEACS reliably into those with infarction (NSTEMI) and those without (USA). Cardiac biomarkers are necessary to confirm myocardial cellular injury and meet diagnostic criteria for MI.

CARDIAC BIOCHEMICAL MARKERS (TROPONINS)[5] (FIG. 20.5)

The cardiac troponin (cTN) complex has three isoforms, two (cTnT and cTnI) of which are exclusively expressed (highly specific) in cardiac myocytes. Myocardial necrosis produces an initial release of troponin within the cell cytosol. Diffusion of this cytosolic troponin allows detection approximately 4–6 hours post infarct, with a peak usually at 12–24 hours. In acute injury there is a gradual return to normal within 7–14 days. This long tail on levels is thought to be due to secondary degradation of myofibrils with extended ongoing release. Renal failure prolongs excretion.

- High sensitivity and specificity of cardiac troponins has made them the gold standard for the confirmation of myocardial necrosis. Elevated levels should be taken as evidence of myocardial injury and, in the correct setting, as confirmation of MI.[5]
- Troponins should be checked in all patients with ACS. An acute rise and fall is usually desired to separate it from other causes of troponin elevation.
- cTn levels are more sensitive than creatinine kinase (CK). A third of people previously considered to have USA are now redefined as MI.[14,18]
- Troponins do not differentiate the cause of the myocardial injury (e.g. ischaemia, myocarditis, trauma), thus clinical context must always be considered.[5]

Troponin levels thus allow early and sensitive detection of myocardial necrosis. Troponins have significant clinical utility in guiding diagnosis and therapeutic planning.

- There is a strong correlation between troponin level, intracoronary thrombus and amount of threatened or ischaemic myocardium.
- Troponins identify groups who will derive benefit from therapies such as low-molecular-weight heparins (LMWHs), glycoprotein inhibitors (GPIs) and early percutaneous coronary intervention (PCI).

Troponins in critical illness[19,20]

The elevated levels of troponin in Type 1 MI (see Box 20.1) correlate well with risk stratification and predicted response to therapy. Cardiac-specific troponins are frequently elevated in critical illness (up to 40–50% of patients), including but not confined to sepsis, pulmonary embolus and renal insufficiency.[20] They fit the pattern of Type 2 MI, are of cardiac origin and are indicative of myocardial injury, but not necessarily of 'unstable plaque'. Their elevation does correspond with adverse outcomes.

A study of >15 000 adult major non-cardiac surgical patients revealed that 11.6% developed postoperative troponin elevations that had a strong association with 30-day mortality,[19] both in-hospital and post-discharge (45% a vascular and 55% a non-vascular cause of death). Whether the underlying aetiology is unstable plaque

(Type 1 MI) or supply demand ischaemia (Type 2 MI) is unknown. These patients are often excluded from ACS trials and the post-surgery risk–benefit of therapies such as aspirin, clopidogrel, LMWHs and PCI is not known. Clinical context is necessary to decide those likely to have significant underlying CAD that may require acute or subsequent intervention.

ECHOCARDIOGRAPHY[21] (SEE CH. 27)

Two-dimensional transthoracic echocardiography with colour Doppler has good clinical utility as a non-invasive investigation during admission for an ACS. Its primary role is in assessing the degree of regional and global LV dysfunction.

Echocardiography detects regional wall motion abnormalities (RWMAs), which can help confirm or exclude the diagnosis of MI in the small percentage of cases where diagnosis is uncertain (e.g. left bundle branch block (LBBB) or old infarction with atypical presentations). RWMA and loss of wall thickening with contraction are often present in these cases if due to ischaemia, whereas their absence suggests that ischaemia is not acute. It is useful for excluding differential diagnoses (e.g. aortic dissection or pericardial effusions), again in a small percentage of patients.[5]

Echocardiography is useful subsequently and in ICU populations to:

- assess infarct size, especially if thrombolysis has interfered with biomarker measurement
- diagnose RV infarction and infarct extension
- allow bedside assessment of LV and RV function
- diagnose specific complications (e.g. mitral regurgitation, pericardial effusion, mural thrombus and myocardial rupture, including ventricular septal defect).

Transoesophageal echocardiography has an increasing role in the therapy of cardiogenic shock and complicated myocardial infarction.

Dynamic or graded intravenous (i.v.) dobutamine stress echocardiography (2–10 days after MI) can assess myocardial viability and distinguish non-viable myocardium from stunned myocardium. Superiority to standard exercise testing has not been proven.

RADIONUCLIDE STUDIES[22]

Practical problems limit the use of radionucleotide angiography in the ED diagnosis of ACS. Nevertheless, rest technetium-99n-sestamibi myocardial perfusion single-photon emission computed tomography (SPECT) is validated, excluding ACS in patients presenting to EDs with chest pain. The negative predictive value for excluding MI may exceed 99% and for excluding future cardiac events may be greater than 97%. Dynamic or functional radionuclide studies (Thallium-201 or SPECT) are useful in post-infarction risk stratification and are able to detect 'threatened myocardium'.

STRESS TESTING

Stress testing may be useful in risk stratification and diagnosis of stable angina. Following infarction, the following may be of use:

- submaximal stress testing (to a heart rate of 120 beats/min), pre discharge, upon patients with an uncomplicated course
- maximal symptom-limited stress test 3–6 weeks post infarction.

CORONARY ANGIOGRAPHY AND LEFT VENTRICULOGRAPHY

Coronary angiography will also allow detection of other coronary artery disease and an assessment of LV function. It is the gold standard for the diagnosis (and often treatment) of CAD; however, the timing and need for this are determined by clinical risk. In the appropriate clinical setting, coronary angiography will usually identify a 'culprit artery' subtending an area of regional wall motion abnormality and additionally may allow definitive treatment of this abnormality. These indications are discussed later.

RISK STRATIFICATION OF ACUTE CORONARY SYNDROME (FIG. 20.6)[4]

An immediate goal is to identify patients with STEMI, who will then benefit from reperfusion therapy. This is almost always done on the basis of the presenting ECG.

STEMI

STEMI (including new, presumed new LBBB) with persistent pain is the most acutely lethal form of ACS and is usually due to complete occlusion of a coronary artery (>90% of patients).[18] It is an indication for reperfusion therapy. Such therapy may be successful and significantly reduce the size of the potential infarction, although some rise in troponin is usually inevitable. Patients who develop STE after admission should also then be stratified to this group.

Meta-analysis of trials involving nearly 60 000 patients revealed LBBB or STE on admission to be a strong indicator of benefits from reperfusion. Patients on trial entry with anterior STE had an absolute benefit of 37 lives saved per 1000 patients, patients with inferior STE 8 lives saved, and those in other locations 27 lives saved per 1000 patients treated.[23]

Guidelines advise early reperfusion therapy for ACS patients presenting with LBBB (new or presumed new) and that misdiagnosis is associated with high morbidity. Correct diagnosis is difficult as current data suggest that this group may be heterogeneous with multiple co-morbid conditions. Thus, perhaps only one-third of patients who present with LBBB may ultimately be shown to have ACS (occluded culprit artery), one-third non-ACS cardiac disease and perhaps one-third have non-cardiac disease. Non-pharmacological reperfusion

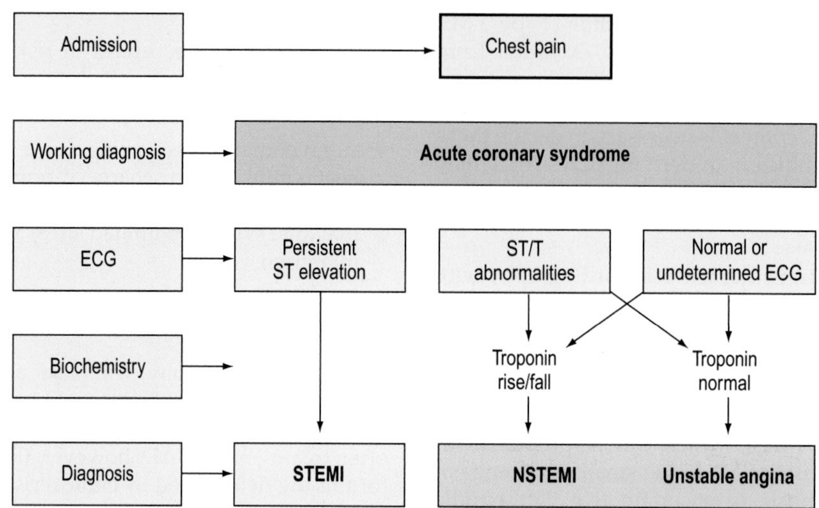

Figure 20.6 The spectrum of ACS. PCI=percutaneous coronary intervention; ECG=electrocardiogram; NSTEMI=non-ST-elevation myocardial infarction; STEMI=ST-elevation myocardial infarction. Physicians should obtain, interpret and stratify patients with ACS within10 minutes of arrival. STE in this clinical setting is usually due to complete coronary occlusion and most patients will ultimately have some biomarker elevation (STEMI). Rapid and sustained coronary artery reperfusion (PCI or fibrinolytic therapy) may significantly decrease myocardial damage. Well-organised systems of care should be in place to minimise delays. In patients without STE (non-STEACS), serial biomarker measurements may define those patients with elevated levels (NSTEMI) and those with ACS but normal biomarkers (unstable angina). Clinical review and further tests may lead to a non-ischaemic cause of chest pain in some patients. Subsequent echocardiography and imaging may help define the extent of injury, coronary anatomy pathology and its clinical importance. *(Adapted from Hamm et al, 2011[4] with permission. doi:10.1093/eurheartj/ehr236 'Adapted with permission of Oxford University Press (UK) © European Society of Cardiology' http://www.escardio.org/guidelines.)*

methods are thus perhaps favoured where the diagnosis is uncertain.[17,24]

Considerable variability in mortality risk exists among patients with STE. Readily available bedside clinical risk score tools may give insight into predicted 30-day mortality (**Fig. 20.7**).[25]

NSTEACS

Patients have ischaemic chest pain but have 'non-specific' ECG changes (normal, ST-segment depression or minimal elevation, T-wave inversion). After serial biomarker testing, these patients will later prove to have either USA if troponins remain normal or NSTEMI (elevated troponin). In contrast to fibrinolyis in STEMI, fibrinolysis in patients with ST-segment depression resulted in an excess of 14 deaths per 1000 patients treated and in patients with normal ECGs an excess of 7 deaths per 1000 patients.[23,26] Only 35–75% of patients have evidence of coronary thrombus formation and thrombolytic therapy is not beneficial in this group. Indeed, it is associated with worse outcomes.[18,23,27]

The therapy of NSTEMI aligns more clinically with that of USA than with that of STEMI. These two conditions, both forms of NSTEACS, represent a spectrum of disease and require common treatments directed at platelet inactivation and 'plaque stabilisation'. The term 'NSTEACS' recognises that they are clinically indistinguishable at presentation. Despite the heterogeneous nature of this group of patients and variable prognoses, early stratification using both ECG and troponins with simple clinical variables may define risk and guide evidence-based therapy (**Fig. 20.8**).[28] The more severe the ischaemia, the higher is the indication for more aggressive anticoagulation and invasive procedures.

Figure 20.9 displays the incidence of major coronary events over the following 6 months in patients presenting with and without STE. ST-segment depression has lesser early mortality but a similar or higher mortality at 6 months and at 10 years than those presenting with STE.[29]

Q-wave MI (QwMI) or non-Q-wave MI (NqwMI) are older terms used to describe MI. The 10-year mortality of NqwMI (70%) is 10% higher than that of QwMI.

IMMEDIATE MANAGEMENT OF ACUTE CORONARY SYNDROMES

PREHOSPITAL CARE

Fifty per cent of deaths from MI occur within the first hour of symptom onset. These deaths are usually due to ventricular fibrillation (VF). Treatment is defibrillation.

Review of trials comparing prehospital to in-hospital thrombolysis in highly selected patients suggests improvement in 30-day mortality (17% decrease, 95% CI 2–29%).

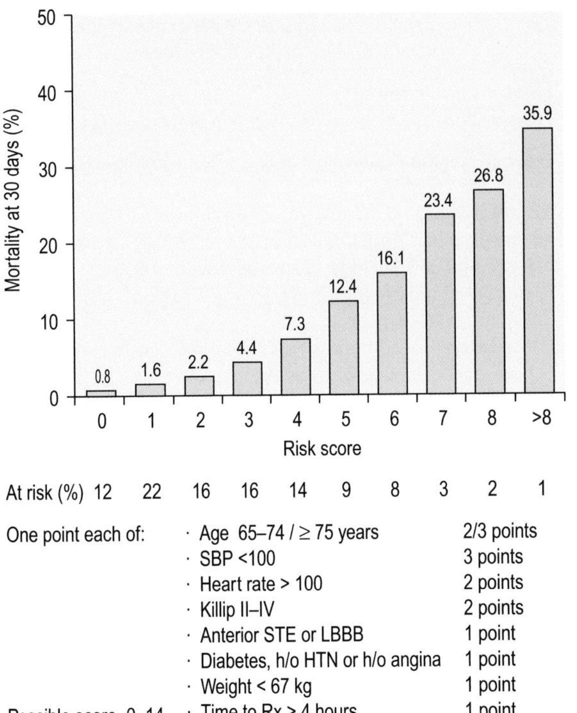

Figure 20.7 STEMI-TIMI: TIMI (thrombolysis in myocardial infarction) risk score for STEMI is a simple bedside evaluation for predicting 30-day mortality. STE=ST elevation; h/o=history of. *(From Morrow et al, 2000,*[25] *with permission.).*

IMMEDIATE HOSPITAL CARE

1. Cardiac monitoring.
2. Oxygen[18,30] (2–4 L/min via facemask or nasal prongs) is recommended for breathless or hypoxic patients although benefits of routine use in uncomplicated ACS are uncertain.[26,31]
3. ECG (12-lead) should be taken within 5 minutes of arrival.
4. Aspirin at 160–325 mg should be chewed and swallowed on arrival. Clopidogrel or prasugrel is given if there is aspirin sensitivity or high risk.[18,30] Dual antiplatelet therapy is usually recommended.
5. Sublingual nitroglycerine (GTN) may have beneficial effects. Side-effects include hypotensive reactions and a hypotensive bradycardic response (the Bezold–Jarisch reflex).
6. Venous access is usually established.
7. Pain relief should be provided. Pain produces catecholamines, which increase ischaemia. GTN, reassurance and small incremental boluses (1–2 mg) of morphine can be given. Admission NSAIDs should be ceased immediately as use in the week prior to admission is associated with increased risk of death and cardiac complications.[18,32] Pain relief is best served by rapid reperfusion.[33]

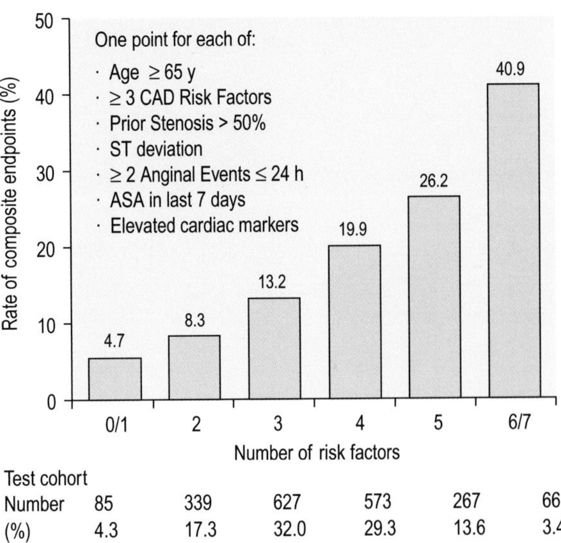

Test cohort						
Number	85	339	627	573	267	66
(%)	4.3	17.3	32.0	29.3	13.6	3.4

Figure 20.8 NSTEMI-TIMI: the thrombolysis in myocardial infarction (TIMI) score is used to estimate the risk of the composite end-point of death, MI, or need for urgent cardiac catheterisation (vertical axis) at 14 days in patients with USA or NSTEMI. Each risk factor is worth 1 point for a maximum score of 7. CAD=coronary artery disease. *(Adapted from Antman et al, 2000.*[28]*)*

8. Rapidly identify ACS patients with STE or new and presumed new LBBB (**Box 20.4**).[30,33] Emergent reperfusion therapy is of critical importance ('Time is muscle'). Hospital protocols with evidence-based goals should exist and outline the strategies to achieve them.
9. Emergent angioplasty (or rapid transfer to a centre capable of this) is generally superior to thrombolytic therapy (see following). Thrombolysis should generally be performed where the benefits of urgent PCI cannot be obtained.
10. Pulmonary oedema is treated with upright posture, i.v. furosemide, GTN or i.v. nitrates and, if severe, with continuous positive airway pressure ventilation.
11. Beta-adrenergic blockers (oral) should be commenced in haemodynamically stable patients as soon as possible (usually after thrombolytic therapy has been given or before PCI) but only where contraindications do not exist.
12. Prophylactic antiarrhythmics are *not* administered.

ACUTE MANAGEMENT OF STEMI (**FIG. 20.10**)[30]

REPERFUSION THERAPY

Prompt reperfusion therapy (mechanical or pharmacological) to establish coronary artery flow is the 'gold standard' for STEMI therapy and is far superior to non-reperfusion management.

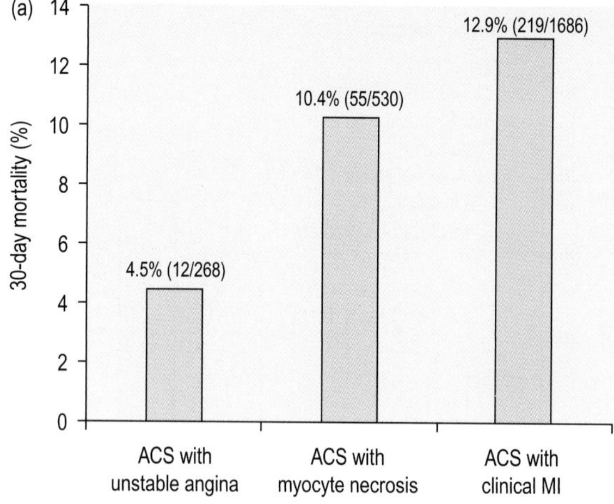

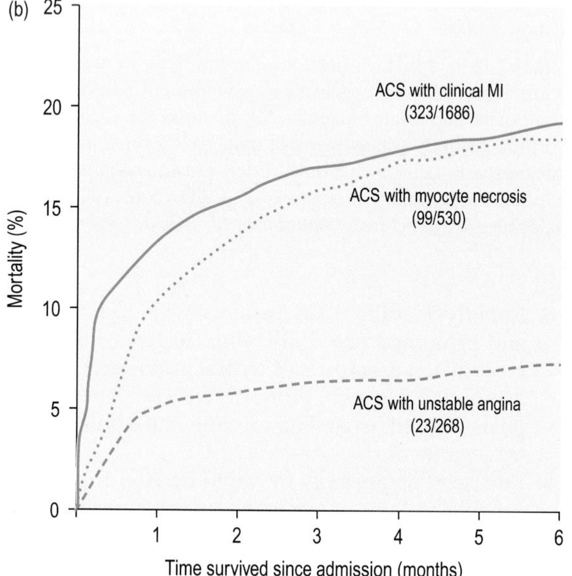

Figure 20.9 (a) Thirty-day mortality according to British Cardiac Society category. (b) Kaplan–Meier survival area curves for events from admission to 6 months. ACS=acute coronary syndrome. *(Reproduced from Das R, Kilcullen N, Morrell C et al. The British Cardiac Society Working Group definition of myocardial infarction: implications for practice. Heart 2006; 92:21–26,[29] with permission.)*

Reperfusion therapy should be considered for all patients presenting within 12 hours of onset of STEMI.[18,30]

Both primary PCI and fibrinolysis are proven treatments for STEMI, maximal benefit being achieved when they are given early. The timeliness of reperfusion treatment is a strong predictor of overall mortality.

Box 20.4 Typical indications for reperfusion therapy in acute myocardial infarction

Reperfusion therapy

Presentation ≤12 hours with ACS, unrelieved by GTN, *and*

New ST segment elevation in 2 or more contiguous leads with the cut-off points:
≥2 mV in men, >0.15 mV in women in leads V_2–V_3 and/or ≥1 mV in other leads, *or*
New-onset LBBB (include presumed new-onset), *or*
Posterior infarction (dominant R wave and ST depression ≥2 mV in V_1–V_2), *or*
Presentation 12–24 hours after onset of ACS with continuing pain and evidence of evolving infarction

Posterior myocardial infarction is an important presentation of STEMI where STE is not present in standard chest leads. STEMI (2–4% of cases) may present with new, presumednew LBBB although many patients who present with LBBB will not have an occluded culprit artery perhaps favouring PCI over thrombolysis.

Neeland IJ, Kontos MC, de Lemos JA. Evolving considerations in the management of patients with left bundle branch block and suspected myocardial infarction. J Am Coll Cardiol 2012;60(2):96–105.[24]

Age is strongly related to mortality in MI, often reflecting co-morbid illness.[28] Although elderly (>75 years) patients may receive a smaller relative mortality reduction than younger patients (<55 years), high baseline mortality in the elderly sees a threefold increase in lives saved (34 lives per 1000 treated versus 11 per 1000 in younger).[34]

Restoration of patency reduces infarct size, preserves LV function, reduces mortality and prolongs survival.

Strategies to achieve reperfusion can include:

- PCI (e.g. angioplasty with or without stent insertion)
- fibrinolytic (thrombolytic) therapy
- urgent CABG.

PRIMARY PERCUTANEOUS TRANSLUMINAL CORONARY INTERVENTION

- Primary PCI is far superior to thrombolytic therapy when delivered in centres of excellence and without delay with reduced short-term mortality (5.3% versus 7.4%), non-fatal re-infarction (2.5% versus 6.8%) and stroke (1.0 versus 2.0%).[35,36] TIMI-3 flow may be restored in 95% of patients compared with 54% after thrombolysis.
- The survival benefit of primary PCI compared with thrombolytic therapy is of the order of 20 extra lives saved per 1000 patients treated.[35] These benefits are not uniform and are significantly influenced by its better outcomes in high-risk patients (heart failure, cardiogenic shock, elderly, late presentations).

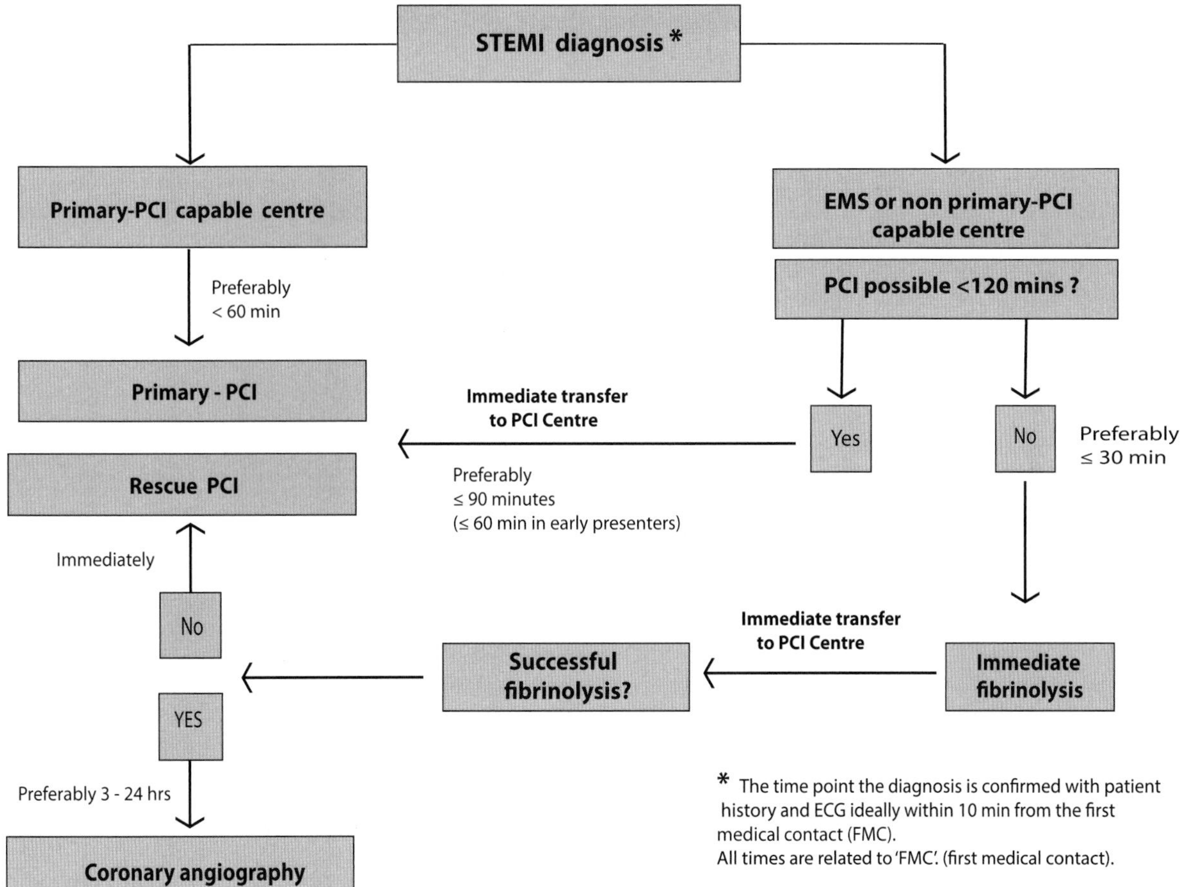

Figure 20.10 Prehospital and in-hospital management and reperfusion strategies within 24 h of FMC. Cath=catheterisation laboratory; EMS=emergency medical system; FMC=first medical contact; PCI=percutaneous coronary intervention; STEMI=ST-segment elevation myocardial infarction. *(Steg P.G., James SK, Atar D, et al. ESC Guidelines for the management of acute myocardial infarction in patients presenting with ST-segment elevation: The Task Force on the management of ST-segment elevation acute myocardial infarction of the European Society of Cardiology (ESC). Eur Heart J, 2012.* ***33****(20):2569–619. doi:10.1093/eurheartj/ehs215. Modified with permission of Oxford University Press (UK) © European Society of Cardiology.)*

Emergency PCI can be divided into:

- primary PCI
- pharmaco-invasive therapy (pharmacological perfusion followed by PCI)
- rescue PCI after failed pharmacological reperfusion.

Urgent PCI in STEMI is strongly indicated (level 1 evidence) in patients with:[18,30]

- presentation to cardiological centres of excellence
- contraindications to thrombolysis
- high risk but with predicted small or moderate benefit from thrombolytic therapy (e.g. elderly, diabetic and with presentation beyond 3 hours)
- cardiogenic shock even up to 12–36 hours after infarction[37] (see Ch. 24)
- failed thrombolysis
- previous CABG.

Very few patients have contraindications to PCI, the major risk factor being complications from adjunctive antiplatelet or antithrombin therapy. Caution is needed in those at risk of contrast-associated renal failure.[38,39] Primary PCI is limited by the risk of abrupt vessel closure (early) and late stenosis. Coronary stenting is superior to balloon angioplasty in preventing restenosis although survival and re-infarction benefits are less than in elective stent procedures.[13,40]

THROMBOLYTIC THERAPY

Thrombolytic therapy retains an important role in the acute treatment of STEMI because prompt access to PCI cannot always be provided.

- Thrombolytic therapy versus non-reperfusion treatment for STEMI results in significant mortality reduction (10.9% versus 13.4%; RRR 19%), a saving of approximately 20 lives per 1000 patients treated.[18,23]
- Outcomes are critically dependent upon time from symptom onset to administration. A goal after hospital arrival is 'door to needle time' of less than 30 minutes. Prehospital thrombolysis in highly selected patients is associated with reduced mortality compared with in-hospital thrombolysis (17% RRR).[30]
- Largest benefits are seen in anterior infarction (3.7% absolute mortality reduction), and less in inferior infarction (0.8% reduction).[23,41]

Thrombolysis within 6 hours of symptom onset prevents 30 deaths per 1000 patients treated; within 7–12 hours, 20 deaths per 1000 patients treated are prevented. There is no overall benefit for therapy beyond this time. Up to 40 deaths per 1000 could be prevented (RRR 50%) if treatment was given in the first hour.[23]

Thrombolytic agents (fibrinolytic agents)

Fibrinolytic agents (plasminogen activators) are divided into two major groups:

1. *Non-fibrin-specific:* these catalyse systemic fibrinolysis (e.g. streptokinase).[42]
2. *Fibrin-specific:* these produce limited plasminogen conversion in the absence of fibrinogen. Current agents include alteplase (tPA), reteplase (r-PA) and tenecteplase (TNK).

Disadvantages of fibrinolytic agents include that they take 30–45 minutes on average to reperfuse an occluded artery and complete reperfusion is achieved in only 60% of patients.

Development has sought to introduce agents that are more fibrin specific (more direct anti-thrombus action and induce less systemic fibrinolysis), have more resistance to plasminogen-activator inhibitor, or have a longer half-life (TNK) allowing bolus rather than infusion administration and with an acceptable rate of bleeding. Secondary fibrinolytic agents developed (t-PA) gave better patency rates than streptokinase and usually became the 'control arm' for subsequent trials.

Fibrin-specific agents (TNK, alteplase, reteplase) are recommended over non-fibrin-specific agents. Their shorter duration of action generally requires the concomitant early administration of UFH or LMWH.[30]

Major and minor contraindications are shown in **Table 20.2**.

Side-effects and choice of agent[30,38]

Bleeding complications are the most serious and important complication of thrombolysis. About 1% of patients may suffer an early cerebral haemorrhage. Risk factors are advanced age, significant admission systolic and diastolic hypertension, female gender, prior cerebrovascular disease and low weight. Major non-cerebral bleeds that require transfusion or significant intervention may occur in 4–13% of patients.

Failure to adjust the dose of fibrinolytic correctly to body weight may be associated with increased mortality and intracerebral haemorrhage.[38,39]

PRIMARY PCI VERSUS THROMBOLYTIC THERAPY

Despite the advantages of PCI over thrombolysis, many patients present to centres that do not offer primary PCI. Given the advantage of PCI over thrombolysis, the benefit of transfer to such a centre can be significant. Well-developed systems need to be in place to minimise transport delays.[30,40]

- Patients best suited for transfer for PCI are STEMI patients with high-risk features, those with high bleeding risk or other contraindications to

Table 20.2 Contraindications and cautions for fibrinolytic use in myocardial infarction (advisory following clinical consideration)

ABSOLUTE	RELATIVE (ADVISORY FOLLOWING CLINICAL CONSIDERATION)
• Previous haemorrhagic stroke • Other stroke or cerebrovascular accident ≤6 months • Intracranial neoplasm • Active internal bleeding ≤2 weeks (menses excluded) • Aortic dissection, known or suspected	• Severe uncontrolled hypertension on presentation (≥180/110 mmHg) • Oral anticoagulation therapy (INR > 2.5); known bleeding diathesis • Recent major trauma, surgery (≤4 weeks) including head trauma • Previous allergic reaction to drug to be used • Traumatic CPR • Active peptic ulcer disease • Pregnancy • Recent streptokinase; use different agent (risk of allergy, antibodies may reduce effectiveness) • History of prior CVA or intracerebral pathology not covered in contraindications • Chronic hypertension

PCI is generally the desired treatment in all of the above. INR=international normalised ratio; CPR=cardiopulmonary resuscitation; CVA=cerebrovascular accident.
Specialist advice should be sought urgently where doubt exists and PCI is not available. Patients with contraindication may still benefit from urgent PCI and indeed it is usually the preferred option.

fibrinolytic therapy or those presenting late (more than 3 hours after onset of symptoms).[38,43]

- Patients best suited for fibrinolytic therapy are those who present early and with low bleeding risk given that deleterious delays in reperfusion may worsen outcome. Current results from thrombolytic therapy in patients presenting early (<3 hours post onset) are very good as fresh clots seem more likely to be lysed.

The duration of symptoms and the time to achieve transfer are important modulating factors.[38,43] The advantages of more reliable revascularisation from PCI can be lost for many if transfer is not expedient and if delay is longer than 60–120 minutes.[38,43,44] The significance of transfer for an individual patient will vary significantly depending upon baseline risk.

Invasive strategy (PCI) is clearly superior to thrombolysis if:[18]

- ineligible for thrombolytic therapy
- cardiogenic shock or severe heart failure
- haemodynamically significant ventricular arrhythmias
- skilled PCI lab is available with surgical back-up:
  - medical contact-to-balloon or door-to-balloon is <90 minutes
- transfer can be achieved in <120 minutes and ideally <60 minutes
- diagnosis is uncertain not definite (e.g. ABS, myocarditis, pericarditis).

Other indicators that transfer to an expert centre for PCI should be considered are:

- high risk from STEMI
- age >75 years. PCI benefit over thrombolysis may be 1% at age 65, 6.9% at age >85[34]
- extensive anterior infarction with late presentation
- high risk of bleeding
- previous MI or CABG
- Killip class (see Table 20.4) is ≥3
- late presentation
- symptom onset was > 3 hours ago.

Fibrinolysis may be preferred if:[18,30,38]

- transfer to a centre for PCI may be harmful to patients where:
  - early presentation (3 hours from symptom onset and delay to invasive strategy)
  - invasive strategy is not an option (e.g. catheterisation lab occupied, not available)
  - delay to invasive strategy (e.g. prolonged transport time with delay likely greater than 60–120 minutes).

COMBINATIONS OF PCI AND THROMBOLYSIS[18,33,38,40,45]

Lack of universal access to acute PCI infarction requires many patients to receive fibrinolytic treatment. Given that urgent PCI is generally superior, various studies have been performed to provide PCI soon after fibrinolysis or to give fibrinolytic or other therapy to provide a bridge until PCI is available.

- There is little evidence that routine *immediate* PCI after fibrinolysis (<2–3 hours) confers benefit. Indeed this approach appears to be harmful.
- It is reasonable to transfer all patients following fibrinolytic therapy to a PCI-capable centre in anticipation of possible inadequate reperfusion as up to 20% who achieve reperfusion may re-infarct (see Fig. 20.10).[30] Repeat fibrinolytic therapy does not appear to provide benefit.
- Urgent PCI where there is evidence of failed reperfusion ('rescue PCI') has been shown to reduce re-infarction and heart failure with a tendency to improved survival.[46] Up to 40–50% of STEMI patients treated with fibrinolytics may have evidence of suspected inadequate reperfusion (ongoing STE or, less reliably, ongoing chest pain). Most benefit from rescue PCI is likely seen in patients with large myocardium at risk, those who remain haemodynamically unstable or in cardiogenic shock. Case-by-case assessment is required.
- Facilitated thrombolysis and pharmaco-invasive therapy[40,47] is a strategy of thrombolysis (full or adjusted dose) or significant antiplatelet or anticoagulant therapy followed as soon as possible by PCI (on site or after rapid transfer) regardless of whether there is evidence of failure to reperfuse. Results are variable.

ADJUNCTIVE THERAPY USED WITH REPERFUSION TREATMENTS (**FIG. 20.11**)

Early adjunctive therapy is necessary after thrombolysis as about 50% of patients fail to obtain or sustain coronary artery patency. The underlying artery remains unstable, evidenced by angiographic reocclusion in 30% and recurrence of ischaemia in 20%. Coronary arteries that have been dilated or have undergone stenting may similarly remain unstable.

Adjunctive therapies in the short term will thus largely be directed at platelet aggregation and the coagulation cascade in an attempt to decrease vessel or stent thrombosis. Therapies may also be directed at 'plaque stabilisation', myocardial ischaemia and arrhythmias. Improvement in adjunctive or supportive reperfusion therapies has been the major driver of improved outcomes from reperfusion strategies.

Compliance with guidelines for administration of these therapies significantly improves outcomes.

ASPIRIN AND CLOPIDOGREL

All patients undergoing reperfusion therapy for STEMI (PCI or fibrinolysis) should be given dual anti-platelet therapy (DAPT, aspirin and an ADP blocker, commonly aspirin and clopidogrel) unless contraindicated.[30,33]

Aspirin is one of the most significant and cost-effective treatments for STEMI. It prevents synthesis of

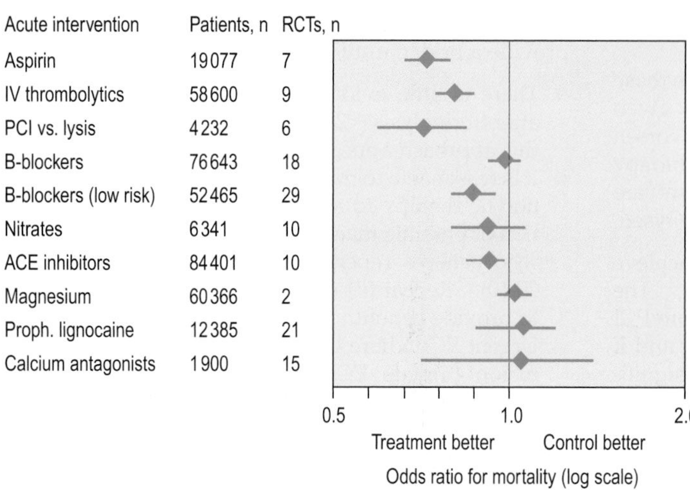

Figure 20.11 Effect of acute (early) adjunctive interventions upon mortality following MI. Results are from meta-analyses and various trials. Urgent percutaneous coronary intervention has not been compared to placebo but offers superior results to thrombolysis when performed at PCI centres within appropriate time frames. Beta blockers should only be used after exclusion of contra-indications. ACE=angiotensin-converting enzyme; RCT=randomised controlled trial; PCI=percutaneous coronary intervention.

thromboxane A_2, a potent stimulator of platelet aggregation and vasoconstriction. Given acutely in the ISIS-2 study it reduced absolute mortality by 2.4% (RRR 23%) and gave a nearly 50% RRR in re-infarction and stroke. It was comparable to the benefit from streptokinase and the combination had an additive benefit.[41,48] Treatment for a mean duration of 1 month resulted in approximately 25 fewer deaths and 10–15 fewer episodes of non-fatal re-infarction and non-fatal stroke for every 1000 patients treated.[48] It does not appear to increase bleeding and benefit is still present after 10 years. Similar benefit from aspirin is seen in patients who do not receive reperfusion.[39]

Clopidogrel confers significant additional benefit to patients who have received fibrinolytic therapy. Given in conjunction with thrombolytics and aspirin, it reduces the risk of early vessel reocclusion without a significant rise in bleeding. Clopidogrel added to aspirin and continued in patients not undergoing reperfusion therapy also lowered mortality rate (7.5% vs 8.1%) and the composite of death, re-infarction or stroke (9.2% vs 10.1%, 9 less events per 1000 patients). Benefit from this DAPT therapy is present across a wide range of MI severity and age groups and bleeding is not significantly increased.[39,43,49,50] Substitution of prasugrel or ticagrelor for clopidogrel following fibrinolysis is not currently advocated.[30]

DAPT is strongly indicated in STEMI patients undergoing primary PCI. Patients who undergo PCI and have a stent inserted benefit if they have received clopidogrel. Benefit is less evident in patients who undergo PCI but do not have a stent placed, and bleeding is problematic.

Newer ADP inhibitors such as prasugrel and ticagrelor have more rapid onset and predictable pharmacology than clopidogrel and are increasingly preferred. Caution is advised where there is increased risk of bleeding (advanced age, previous CVA, low body weight, liver disease) or need for CABG.

GLYCOPROTEIN IIB/IIIA INHIBITORS

Glycoprotein IIb/IIIa inhibitors (GPIs) include abciximab, eptifibatide and tirofiban and were particularly useful when stents were being placed. They have largely been replaced in the treatment of acute STEMI by P2Y12 antiplatelet agents. They may still retain some role in STEMI where a stent is to be placed, the lesion is complex, the patient is haemodynamically unstable and the absorption of oral agents is uncertain.[43,51,52] Historical trials of GPIs in combination with full-dose thrombolytics found increased bleeding. Trials in combination with half-dose thrombolytics were also disappointing, with increased bleeding (especially in the elderly) but no survival benefit. In STEMI patients who do not receive reperfusion therapy, GPIs do not appear to confer benefit.[39,43,50,52]

UNFRACTIONATED HEPARIN (UFH, STANDARD) AND LOW-MOLECULAR-WEIGHT HEPARIN

Antithrombin therapy is generally given in combination with PCI or with fibrin-specific fibrinolytic agents. Exposed or ruptured plaque leads to activation of thrombin.

The net benefit-to-risk ratio of using thrombin inhibitors in MI is not clear, however. Prior to the use of fibrinolytics and aspirin, a limited number of small trials suggested that UFH reduced mortality (from 13.1% to 9.2%, 20–25% RR reduction) but patient numbers were small. With the introduction of fibrinolytics and aspirin, UFH administration was continued, reflecting the basis on which the drugs were trialled and licensed. Heparin effect seemed to be more modest in this setting. Few trials (1239 patients) examined whether UFH added survival benefit to patients already treated with both thrombolytics and aspirin. At most, UFH benefits seems to be small (perhaps 5 lives saved per 1000 patients treated) and bleeding can be problematic.[39,41,53] UFH has been the comparator in studies of LMWHs. Four anticoagulants are currently used clinically (UFH, LMWH, bivalirudin and fondaparinux).

Current recommendations thus are:

- Patients undergoing thrombolysis with fibrin-specific agents require an anti-thrombin agent for 24–48 hours. Weight-adjusted intravenous UFH is still used but there has been a strong shift to the use of LMWH (e.g. enoxaparin).[38,53–56] Meta-analysis suggests an advantage of enoxaparin over UFH. Among STEMI patients treated with enoxaparin, approximately 21 deaths or MI events were prevented for every 1000 patients, at the cost of an increase of 4 non-fatal major bleeds.[55] Clinical assessment of bleeding risk may still affect treatment.[38] Streptokinase-treated patients usually receive heparin only when there is a high thromboembolic risk. Fondaparinux may be an alternative agent in non-PCI STEMI treated patients.
- LMWH (preferred) or UFH are recognised treatments for STEMI patients undergoing primary PCI.[30] There is evidence that intravenous enoxaparin (0.5 mg/kg) is superior to UFH with lower mortality and less bleeding.[30,57]
- Bivalirudin (a direct antithrombin inhibitor) is an alternative treatment for primary PCI in STEMI.[30,57]
- Fondaparinux (pentasaccharide factor Xa inhibitor) is associated with a peculiar problem of end-catheter thrombosis during PCI requiring concomitant use of intravenous enoxaparin and is not recommended for primary PCI in STEMI.[30,57]
- UFH or LMWH or fondaparinux administration is indicated in patients who present late or cannot undergo reperfusion therapy.

BETA BLOCKERS[30,33,58]

Pre-thrombolysis era trials demonstrated benefit from early beta-blocker therapy (intravenous and oral) leading to their aggressive use. Post-thrombolysis trials have demonstrated less benefit and even harm in some patient groups.[18,33,58] Early intravenous beta-blocker therapy in acute MI reduces the risk of re-infarction and VF, but increases the risk of early cardiogenic shock with increased mortality (COMMIT Study).[58] There is substantial net hazard in haemodynamically unstable patients and moderate net benefit in those more relatively stable patients.[58] They are best avoided but may have a role for the targeted treatment of specific problems such as hypertension or tachycardia, although it is wise to assess LV function, perhaps with echocardiography.

- Patients with MI who have contraindications such as pulmonary oedema, shock, hypotension, bradycardia, advanced atrio-ventricular block or asthma[18,30,33] should not receive early beta blockade.
- Haemodynamically stable patients should commence oral beta blockers within 24 hours of the onset of symptoms, introduction being gradual or delayed for 24 hours if there is concern.

OTHER THERAPIES

Although the initial doses of ACE inhibitor may cause hypotension, the early introduction of ACE inhibitors (within the first 48 hours of STEMI) is generally well tolerated and is associated with a small reduction in 30-day mortality, this being evident in the first week.[30] Nitrates may be beneficial for the treatment of recurrent angina, but may be harmful if hypotension occurs or prevents the use of more proven therapies such as ACEI or beta blockers. Glucose–insulin–potassium therapies have not been shown to provide 'cardio-protection' and complicating hyperglycaemia, hypokalaemia and fluid gain may be harmful.

COMPLICATIONS OF MI

ARRHYTHMIAS[30] *(SEE CH. 22)*

Rhythm disturbance occurs in nearly all patients following acute MI and is most likely within the first few hours of onset and during reperfusion. There has been a decline in the incidence of VF from approximately 4.5% of admissions to 1% of admissions with MI. Post-MI arrhythmias are best prevented by rapid revascularisation, maintenance of electrolytes and treatment of heart failure.

- Correct hypoxia, hypovolaemia or acid–base disturbances.
- Maintain serum potassium in the normal range (4.0–5.0 mmol/L).[18,59]
- Maintain the serum magnesium level.

Prophylactic beta blockers reduce the incidence of VF. Prophylactic lidocaine is associated with increased mortality and is reserved for the treatment of life-threatening ventricular arrhythmias. Prophylactic or routine i.v. magnesium is not of proven value.[18] Asymptomatic ventricular arrhythmias do not necessarily benefit from intervention.

POSTINFARCTION ANGINA AND REINFARCTION[8,26,30]

Postinfarction angina (STEMI or NSTEMI) usually results from decreased myocardial oxygen supply due to re-occlusion or spasm of a transiently patent coronary artery. It is usually an indication for consideration of revascularisation. Ischaemia may occur in the infarct related or other vessels and if severe may result in infarct extension. Simple factors such as tachycardia, hypertension, anaemia and fever should be corrected and aggressive treatment with antiplatelet agents, nitrates and beta blockers is indicated. Ongoing pain with ECG changes is indicative of high risk. Insertion of an intra-aortic balloon pump may help improve symptoms, minimise ischaemia and may bridge for

Table 20.3 Mechanical complications of myocardial infarction

	CVP	PAOP	CO	OTHER FINDINGS ON PAC	ECHOCARDIOGRAPHY
Mechanical complications					
Free wall rupture	↑	↑	↓↓	Usually tamponade physiology: RA mean, RV and PA end-diastolic, and PAOP pressures are elevated and within 5 mmHg (0.665 kPa) of one another	Pericardial effusion with tamponade and RV diastolic collapse; may visualise pseudoaneurysm
Acute ventricular septal defect	↑	↑	↓↓	Left-to-right shunt with oxygen step-up at RV level; V waves may be seen in PAOP tracing	Visualisation of left-to-right shunting with colour Doppler, can sometimes visualise defect as well
Acute mitral regurgitation	↑↑	↑↑	↓↓	V waves in PAOP tracing	Regurgitant jet apparent on colour Doppler; can diagnose papillary muscle rupture with flail leaflet
RV infarction	↑↑	↓ or normal	↓↓		RV dysfunction
Pump failure (cardiogenic shock)	↑↑	↑↑	↓↓		Decreased overall LV performance; regional wall motion abnormalities; dyskinetic or aneurysmal segments may be seen

Echocardiography has largely replaced the need for insertion of a pulmonary artery catheter although information for a PAC shown here is useful in understanding physiology. Coronary angiography and studies may be required to determine coronary anatomy and may provide additional data.
CVP=central venous pressure; PAOP=pulmonary artery occlusion pressure; CO=cardiac output; PAC=pulmonary artery catheterisation; RV=right ventricle; RA=right atrium; PA=pulmonary artery.

further PCI or CABG. Re-infarction in the 10 days following STEMI occurs in up to 5–10% of patients.

CARDIAC FAILURE (SEE CH. 24) AND CARDIOGENIC SHOCK (**TABLE 20.3**)[13,18,30,37,60,61]

There is a strong association between severity of LV dysfunction post MI and prognosis, well defined by the use of the Killip classification (**Table 20.4**).[62–64] LV dysfunction with the clinical signs of failure occurs in up to 30–40% of patients post STEMI and is associated with a mortality of 20–40%. It usually develops when the abnormally contracting segment exceeds 30% of the LV circumference: cardiogenic shock or death results when it exceeds 40%. It is more common in the setting of previous infarction, and is associated with a poor short- and long-term prognosis. With large MI there is progressive thinning of affected myocardium, with stretching and dilatation of the ventricle, and sometimes frank aneurysm formation. Goals of treatment are:

- correction of hypoxia
- clinical and echo-guided fluid therapy; avoidance of anaemia
- preload reduction with diuretics and nitrates; inotropes if needed
- avoidance of negative inotropes including beta blockers
- measured introduction of ACE inhibitors
- clinical determination as to whether they should follow a 'cardiogenic shock pathway'.

Table 20.4 Killip classification of severity of infarction based on clinical assessment and its correlation with hospital mortality in 1967[64] and 30-day mortality in 1993[63]

KILLIP CLASS		CASE FATALITY (%) KILLIP & KIMBALL[64]	GUSTO[63]
Class 1	No failure	6	5
Class 2	Mild to moderate heart failure (S3, rales <50% lung fields)	17	14
Class 3	Severe heart failure (S3, rales >50% lung fields)	38	32
Class 4	Cardiogenic shock	81	58

There is a strong correlation between the degree of left ventricular dysfunction and mortality in ACS.
Reproduced from Thompson P. Coronary Care Manual, 2nd edn, with permission.[62]

Angiotensin-converting enzyme (ACE) inhibitors appear to limit dilatation, preserve LV function and improve prognosis. Benefits are maximal in those with poor LV function. ACE inhibitors are thus recommended for all patients with significant LV dysfunction and are usually started early following MI.

Cardiogenic shock complicates up to 10% of STEMI and also 2–3% of NSTEMI. Although sometimes present on admission, it often does not arise for some hours. Mortality from cardiogenic shock remains very high (55–70%) and is the major cause of hospital mortality from STEMI. The presence of shock is usually evidenced by:

- SBP <90 mmHg (11.97 kPa) or a significant fall from baseline
- cardiac index <2.2 litres/min/m^2 after correction of hypoxia and hypovolaemia
- evidence of tissue perfusion (metabolic acidosis, oliguria, confusion).

In patients who manifest cardiogenic shock, 10% arrive at hospital in shock, but 90% develop it after hospitalisation. More than 60% have at least 75% stenosis of all three coronary arteries including the LAD.[60] Patients may have 'stunned' myocardium that is capable of improvement with revascularisation and initial intensive medical support. Revascularisation with PCI or CABG is preferred to thrombolysis and medical management; the benefits are still present beyond 5 years (survival 32.8% vs 19.6%).[37] Many patients require intubation and ventilation for management. Cardiac support therapy may include balloon counterpulsation and support with inotropes that may include dobutamine, milrinone and levosimendan.

The presence of right ventricle infarction[61] should be considered in any patient with inferior MI (review lead V_4R and echocardiogram). It is associated with significantly increased mortality. In its severest form, it is a cause of cardiogenic shock.[61] The triad of hypotension, clear lung fields and elevated JVP is seen in only 25% of patients. Treatment principles are different to those for LV dysfunction. Patients with RV infarction often require:

- volume loading and maintenance of filling pressures (clinical and echo assessment); diuretic therapy, afterload reduction and unrecognised hypovolaemia may aggravate hypotension and renal insufficiency in these patients
- maintenance of atrioventricular synchrony by aggressive treatment of atrial fibrillation and consideration of atrial and ventricular lead placement when pacing is required
- inotropic therapy.

Although 80% of cases of cardiogenic shock are due to extensive myocardial necrosis, mechanical complications including mitral regurgitation, ventricular rupture, tamponade and myocardial rupture may be causative. The different physiology of these causes is outlined in Table 20.3.

MITRAL REGURGITATION (MR)[18,65,66]

Transient functional mitral regurgitation is common after MI, LV wall dysfunction causing modification of the subvalvular apparatus and incomplete closure of the valve. This may be asymptomatic and silent detected in up to 30% of patients on echocardiography or may be associated with a soft murmur. Catastrophic papillary muscle rupture, usually 1–4 days post MI, may be associated with mortality of 75–95%, better haemodynamic tolerance being present in incomplete ruptures. Posterior leaflet rupture is most common as it receives its blood supply from the dominant coronary artery (usually the RCA), whereas the anterior leaflet has a dual blood supply. The infarction may be small and localised. A decrescendo systolic murmur may be present rather than the typical pansystolic murmur of chronic regurgitation; however, murmurs may be soft owing to equalisation of pressures between the LV and left atrium with severe regurgitation.[30]

MR can complicate even relatively small MI and the diagnosis should be considered in shocked patients, particularly women and those with NSTEMI, inferoposterior MI and pulmonary oedema.[66] Catastrophic MR requires surgery. Non-surgical and surgical mortality are high. Pharmacological and mechanical afterload reduction often provides a bridge. Where MR is severe and concomitant CABG is required, surgery is indicated. Where MR is significant but CABG is not required, the value of surgery is less certain.[65]

CARDIAC RUPTURE[10,18,30,67,68]

Rupture of the interventricular septum occurred historically in 1–2% of MI, but has fallen to an incidence of 0.2% in the post-thrombolysis era, usually in large infarctions (60% of cases). Anterior and inferior infarctions are equally represented and single-vessel disease is not uncommon. It is often heralded by a new long systolic murmur, which initially may be soft or absent and the patient may not be haemodynamically compromised; 22% may have had silent infarction. Diagnosis is best confirmed by echocardiography, helping to exclude the differential diagnosis of mitral valve rupture. Almost always there is progressive clinical deterioration (untreated mortality of 54% at 1 week and 92% at 1 year). Surgical repair is considered as soon as the diagnosis is made; intra-aortic balloon counterpulsation often provides a bridge to surgery. LV free wall rupture is usually catastrophic, resulting in pulseless electrical activity and death. Subacute rupture (leaking blood is contained by pericardium forming a false aneurysm) is less common and may mimic re-infarction. It requires urgent detection and surgery. Risk factors are advanced age, first infarction (lack of fibrosis) and acute hypertension, but chronic hypertension may be protective (hypertrophy).

SYSTEMIC EMBOLI[10,69]

Embolic (ischaemic) stroke occurs in approximately 1% of patients during their hospital admission and in 2% by 12 months. Most of these cases occur following extensive anterior MI.

- 30–40% of anterior Q-wave MIs may be complicated by mural thrombus (echocardiography). Embolisation is most frequent with large or protruding emboli and is uncommon following inferior infarction.
- 5–10% of these may undergo embolisation, usually within the first 10 days.

Anticoagulation therapy is usually recommended for ≥3 months (initial heparin, then warfarin) if mural thrombus is proven or if there is extensive anterior regional wall motion abnormality. Clinicians should have a high index of suspicion in the presence of large anterior infarction and routine echocardiography is recommended. Patients with poor LV function remain at long-term risk of embolic stroke. Current guidelines recommend continuation of warfarin for 3 months; however, the major impact on stroke prevention appears to result from optimisation of cardiovascular risk factors such as hypertension and lipids.[69]

POST-MI INJURY SYNDROME (DRESSLER'S SYNDROME) AND PERICARDITIS

A pericardial rub may develop 24–72 hours after large, usually anterior MI. Associated pain may mimic ischaemia and biomarkers and echocardiography may be useful in excluding post-infarction angina. Small pericardial effusions may be present. Dressler's syndrome is a now uncommon, later-presenting pericarditis thought to be an immunopathic response to myocardial necrosis. It is characterised by fever, pleuropericardial pain and rub, arthralgia and elevated inflammatory markers.

MANAGEMENT OF UNSTABLE ANGINA AND NSTEMI (NSTEACS)

NSTEACS often result from the development of non-occluding thrombus upon unstable plaque. Superimposed vasospasm and microembolisation may aggravate myocardial ischaemia. Therapies are directed at 'white thrombus' and plaque stabilisation, and at reduction of myocardial oxygen demand.

General principles of treatment are:

- immediate pharmacological relief of ischaemic symptoms
- immediate introduction of antiplatelet therapy, usually in conjunction with an antithrombin agent, to stabilise plaque white thrombus and prevent complete artery occlusion
- assessment of benefits of early invasive versus medical therapy (early PCI).

Thrombolytic agents are generally contraindicated in the treatment of NSTEACS; their routine administration is associated with poorer outcome.[23]

The causes of NSTEAC vessel instability and the cause of ischaemia are far more diverse than those of STEMI. Accordingly the results of interventions are far more diverse. Treatment decisions and their risk–benefit are often guided by scoring systems.

EARLY INVASIVE VERSUS MEDICAL THERAPY IN NSTEACS[8,26]

Although medical therapy is introduced to all patients, keen observation should be continued for signs of instability that suggest an invasive approach is appropriate. Prior to the introduction of potent antiplatelet inhibitors as 'upstream therapy' and coronary stents, early invasive strategies were associated with minimal benefit or with adverse outcome despite their theoretical attractiveness. The development of better adjunctive agents (principally GP inhibitors) has led to the recognition that early invasive strategies are associated with reduced rates of MI and death in many groups.

Scoring systems are available to guide therapy. They are ideally based on simple and readily available clinical information. The GRACE and TIMI risk scores predict both in-hospital and post-discharge 6-month mortality.[25,28]

The benefits of PCI are dependent upon the baseline risk to the patient. Emergent PCI is demonstrated to offer clinical benefit to patients with high-risk features such as elevated troponins, recurrent chest pain and recurrent ECG changes.

ANTI-ISCHAEMIC AGENTS

- Sublingual *nitrates* (300–600 μg usually given in two doses at least some minutes apart) may provide immediate relief of symptoms. Where pain or ECG changes are ongoing, nitrate infusions produce better pain control and decrease of ST-segment depression, suggesting lessening of ischaemia.[8] Clinical features determine dosing.
- *Beta blockers* require similar precautions to those outlined in the treatment of STEMI and intravenous beta blockade again should only be targeted to specific goals (e.g. control of tachycardia, hypertension). Long-term oral beta blockade is likely to be a mainstay of therapy.
- *Calcium channel blockers* (non-hydropyridine agents such as diltiazem or verapamil)[26] may provide symptom relief of recurrent ischaemia when beta blockers and nitrates have been fully used or where there are contraindications to beta blockers. Left ventricular failure is generally a contraindication.

ANTIPLATELET THERAPIES

Antiplatelet therapy is the cornerstone of treatment in both the acute and long-term treatment of NSTEACS. It should be started as soon as the diagnosis of NSTEACS is suspected.

The current standard of care for such patients includes dual antiplatelet therapy (DAPT) usually with aspirin and an adenosine diphosphate (ADP)-receptor antagonist, regardless of whether an invasive procedure is planned or not. It is indicated acutely and for 12 months after.

1. *Aspirin* has similar long-term benefits to those seen following STEMI and should be continued lifelong. Long-term low-dose (75–100 mg/day) is as effective as high-dose aspirin (300–325 mg/day) but is associated with lower rates of bleeding. Up to 10% of patients may have resistance to aspirin.[11]
2. *P2Y12-receptor antagonists* or *ADP receptor antagonists* include clopidogrel, prasugrel and ticagrelor. *Clopidogrel* (in combination with aspirin) was demonstrated in the 'CURE' study[70] to produce a 20% reduction in adverse events when commenced early and continued. Reduction was mainly in MI. Clopidogrel, however, has a slow onset of action that is then prolonged due to irreversible platelet binding. Some 4–30% of patients maintain significant platelet reactivity that is associated with risk of adverse cardiac events.[43,50,71] Newer *P2Y12* antagonists including *prasugrel* and *ticagrelor* do not require metabolic activation and also provide more extensive block. They show superiority to clopidogrel in PCI but at the expense of increased bleeding. They may be a preferred treatment where appropriate risk of stroke, advanced age and low weight is considered.[72] The role of these agents in non-PCI patients is under study but is likely to expand.
3. *GP IIb/IIIa inhibitors* include abciximab, tirofiban and eptifibatide. The more aggressive use of agents such as clopidogrel has seen their benefit decline. They probably retain some value in high-risk NSTEACS patients undergoing PCI. Given as 'medical treatment' they have not demonstrated significant benefit. Benefit is largely confined to patients undergoing PCI.[4,50] The direct antithrombin bivalirudin may provide similar benefits with lower risk of bleeding.

ANTITHROMBINS AND ANTICOAGULANTS[4,8,26]

- Anticoagulants are used in NSTEACS to inhibit thrombin production or activity and decrease thrombus complications.[4] Addition of UFH to aspirin therapy produces a significant reduction in recurrent angina, and subsequent MI.[73]
- Review of head-to-head studies of LMWHs compared with UFH show minimal difference between their outcomes (less difference than when used in STEMI).[73] Their simplicity, lack of need for monitoring and acceptable safety profile may favour their administration. They are generally preferred except perhaps where surgery is anticipated. Fondaparinux may also be used when a 'conservative' management approach is intended.
- Fondaparinux (requires bolus enoxaparin at time of PCI) and bivalirudin (requires concomitant heparin or antiplatelet therapy) are alternative anticoagulant treatments in NSTEMI patients undergoing an early invasive approach.

ONGOING AND DISCHARGE CARE OF ACS (SECONDARY PREVENTION) (FIG. 20.12)

A number of therapies have been studied in the long-term (secondary) treatment of ACS. These treatments are very similar for STEMI and NSTEACS:

1. *Aspirin:* is indicated at a dose of 100 mg per day unless there are contraindications and should be continued lifelong. In the first 2 years after MI, aspirin therapy results in an absolute decrease of approximately 36 vascular events (vascular death or non-fatal MI or stroke) for every 1000 patients treated.[48]
2. *Clopidogrel:* is generally continued throughout the hospital stay in both STEMI and NSTEMI.[33] Clopidogrel is generally continued for all STEMI patients without contraindications whether they

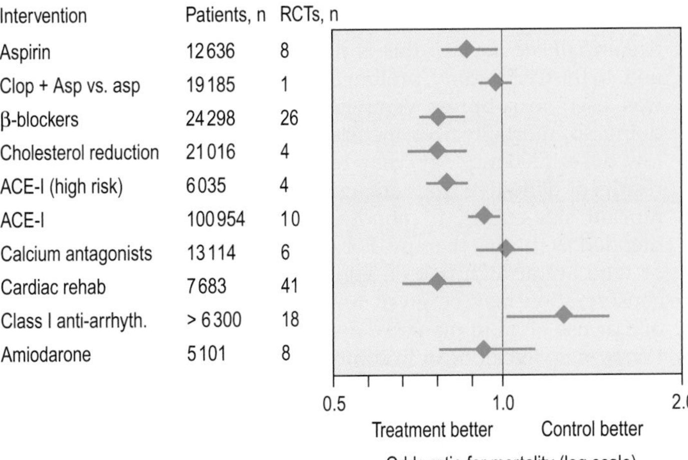

Intervention
Patients, n
RCTs, n
Aspirin 12636 8
Clop + Asp vs. asp 19185 1
β-blockers 24298 26
Cholesterol reduction 21016 4
ACE-I (high risk) 6035 4
ACE-I 100954 10
Calcium antagonists 13114 6
Cardiac rehab 7683 41
Class I anti-arrhyth. > 6300 18
Amiodarone 5101 8
0.5
1.0
2.0
Treatment better
Control better
Odds ratio for mortality (log scale)

Figure 20.12 Late intervention in acute myocardial infarction. Effect of various adjunctive treatments continued following hospital discharge. Results are from meta-analyses and various trials. Treatments may confer benefit for both STEMI and NSTEACS. DAPT benefit is dependent upon the presence and nature of stents as well as background bleeding risk. ACE=angiotensin-converting enzyme; RCT=randomised controlled trial; Clop=clopidogrel; Asp=aspirin.

have received PCI, thrombolysis or no reperfusion therapy. Given in conjunction with aspirin, clopidogrel is proven to be of benefit when administered long term to patients at high risk of future cardiovascular events (the CURE study), although it is associated with an increased risk of bleeding. Clopidogrel is also a useful treatment in patients with aspirin resistance. Presence and type of stent may determine whether clopidogrel or a P2Y12-receptor antagonists is continued longer.

3. *Beta blockers:* administered orally following discharge they are associated with significant re-infarction and survival benefit.
4. *Inhibitors of the renin–angiotensin–aldosterone system (RAAS):* patients with anterior MI and ejection fraction <40% maintained on long-term ACE inhibitor therapy may experience a 20% sustained RR in mortality (that is additive to aspirin and beta blockers) and a significant reduction in the incidence of LV failure.[30,74] In patients intolerant of ACE inhibitors, an ACE receptor blocker may be used. Aldosterone antagonists such as spironolactone and eplerenone may also be used in patients with severe LV dysfunction but caution is taken in the setting of RAAS inhibitor use and renal dysfunction as severe hyperkalaemia may occur[30] (see Ch. 24).
5. *Lipid-lowering agents:* all patients with ACS should commence statins in hospital. Benefit is maximal (and not confined to myocardial events) in patients with elevated cholesterol and other risk factors, but benefit is present at all cholesterol levels. Intensive statin therapy has an advantage (lower all-cause mortality) over less-intensive lipid reduction. Commencement of statins within the first day has benefits over later commencement.[75]
6. *Other anti-ischaemia agents*: routine use of calcium channel blockers does not appear to reduce recurrent myocardial infarction nor decrease mortality. They may be of symptomatic use in patients intolerant of beta blockers or where there is a clinical need such as hypertension or arrhythmia.[30] Carvedilol may be of benefit in patients with ACS.
7. *Antiarrhythmic therapy:* this is not routinely continued. In the CAST study, prolonged flecainide therapy was used to suppress ventricular ectopy. Despite doing so, mortality was increased. Amiodarone in low doses (200 mg/day) may reduce mortality, but results of definitive trials are awaited and it has significant side-effects. It cannot currently be recommended as routine therapy. For patients with actual, or who are at high risk of, ventricular arrhythmia, consideration may be given to long-term amiodarone or use of an implantable defibrillator.
8. *Warfarin:* given alone or in combination with aspirin is associated with lower rates of a composite of 'death, re-infarction and thromboembolic stroke'. Concerns about bleeding (especially in the elderly) see its clinical application restricted.[76] Warfarin is useful for patients with severe ventricular dysfunction, atrial fibrillation or a prothrombotic tendency.[18]
9. *Lifestyle advice:* this is most important and all patients should cease smoking and receive advice on exercise and diet. Blood pressure control and appropriate treatment of diabetes are of high importance.[7,77]

MYOCARDIAL INFARCTION IN THE INTENSIVE CARE UNIT

Myocardial ischaemia is a common problem in the ICU. It also commonly complicates perioperative care of major surgery, with mortality of up to 15–25%. Of concern, studies have shown that a rise in troponin level following non-cardiac surgery is associated with significant 30-day mortality. The problem is what to do about this. Diagnostic criteria are uncertain but a system has been proposed by Devereaux et al.[78] There are few randomised controlled trials to guide therapy of postoperative infarction, or infarction complicating the care of the critically ill. Many patients with such presentations were excluded from trials of ACS therapy.

The pathophysiology of postoperative infarction and infarction in ICU patients is probably different to that of ACS.[79] Studies suggest that, in the presence of severe ischaemia, left main disease and triple-vessel disease are common and that ischaemia is secondary to oxygen supply-and-demand problems (Type 2 MI) rather than thrombosis. However, data on this are conflicting.[79] The absence of thrombosis as an underlying pathological mechanism in many suggests that standard aggressive 'antithrombus' therapies will have different risk–benefit profiles, and that harm is exacerbated by the often high bleeding risk of these patients.

The patient with significant STE and haemodynamic instability in the ICU presents a difficult problem. Echocardiography may be useful in providing information about RWMA and the amount of myocardium at risk. Thrombolysis is usually precluded by bleeding risk and by uncertainty regarding the causative process. Angiography will allow diagnosis and intervention if necessary; however, the use of adjunctive therapy (short- and intermediate-term) may be associated with significant bleeding. Reversible factors such as hypoxia, severe anaemia, anxiety and tachycardia must all be controlled where possible. Hypotension may limit the ability to administer beta blockers and control tachycardia.

APICAL BALLOONING SYNDROME ('TAKOTSUBO SYNDROME')[80–83]

Apical ballooning syndrome (ABS) characteristically presents as acute LV dysfunction usually triggered by emotional or physical stress. It usually presents with chest pain that can mimic ACS. Although there is no flow-limiting lesion precipitating ischaemia, the biomarkers and ECG may suggest ischaemia. Echocardiography may display LVWMA affecting the apical and often the mid-ventricular region with sparing of the basal region. The hypercontractile basal myocardium can generate LV outflow tract obstruction.

Its presence is being increasingly recognised; 1–2% of patients presenting with an initial diagnosis of ACS are recognised to have ABS. Symptoms are like those of ACS and 1/3 have STE. Ninety per cent of patients are postmenopausal women, 70% have a clear emotional or physical trigger but only <3% are younger than 50 years. Diagnostic criteria have been devised, but management and the need for investigation are often clinically determined by the need to exclude vessel occlusion. Major complications in severe ABS include congestive cardiac failure, hypotension, cardiogenic shock, arrhythmia, LV thrombus and mitral regurgitation (systolic anterior motion due to outflow tract obstruction). Mortality may be 1–2%.

Treatment is usually supportive. Echocardiography will help determine if PCI is needed, this being preferable to thrombolysis. With regards to aetiology, elevated catecholamine levels related to severe stress are clearly implicated. A theoretically plausible, but unproven, theory is that there is a higher concentration of β-receptors in apical myocardium with decreasing levels from apex to base. There may be a resulting greater contractile response in apical myocardium than in basal myocardium whilst, paradoxically, high catecholamine levels may be negatively inotropic.[81]

BLEEDING COMPLICATIONS POST REPERFUSION THERAPY

The increased use of aggressive fibrinolytic regimens and of adjunctive reperfusion agents has led to troublesome bleeding in some patients. Many patients presenting for elective or emergent non-cardiac surgery have also been exposed to these agents. Some knowledge of reversal of these agents is necessary.[4,30,84]

1. *GPIIb/IIIa blockers*: abciximab, a chimeric monoclonal antibody, has a short half-life, but antiplatelet activity is still prolonged at 24–48 hours. Fortunately transfused platelets are not affected and will assist with bleeding reversal. The newer agents tirofiban and eptifibitide have very short half-lives when renal function is normal and antiplatelet action returns to normal 4–8 hours after discontinuation. During this period, however, antiplatelet action is profound. It is suggested that, at peak blood levels, administration of fresh frozen plasma (8 units) and platelets (2 units) is probably necessary to reverse antiplatelet action.[84]
2. *Clopidogrel*: it is recommended that clopidogrel and newer inhibitors be ceased at least 5 days before elective CABG, but this is not always possible in emergent surgery or in unstable cases. Major bleeding rates may approach 10% in these cases. Pharmacology suggests that platelet transfusions are necessary to moderate this but dose is unknown.[84]
3. *LMWHs:* reversal of LMWHs with protamine is variable and incomplete, even with doses of 100 mg. Protamine may reverse up to 60% of LMWH action. Although it may reverse 100% of the anti-IIa activity, it has far less effect on anti-Xa activity. It is suggested that doses of protamine should equal doses of enoxaparin administered on a milligram-per-milligram scale.[84]
4. *Fibrinolytic agents*: in the setting of life-threatening bleeding, large doses of cryoprecipitate (10–20 units) may be required to replete fibrinogen (target >1 g/L) and coagulation factors (especially factor VIII). Fresh frozen plasma may supplement factor V and VIII levels. Platelet transfusions at high dose may replace platelets and supplement factor V levels; ε-aminocaproic acid at a dose of 5 g (0.1 g/kg) over 30–60 minutes followed by continuous infusion (0.5–1.0 g/h) may assist with bleeding control. Fibrinolytic reversal carries the risk of culprit coronary artery reocclusion.[84]

OUTCOME OF MYOCARDIAL INFARCTION

The in-hospital mortality from acute MI has been steadily decreasing over the past three decades from 15% to 30% in the 1970s to approximately 10% in 1980 and now to around 8–9% in the new millennium.[2-4] Despite improved mortality, 60% of all deaths occur within the first hour (usually from VF), usually before reaching a medical facility.[4,36] Modern management of acute MI has undoubtedly contributed to decreased mortality. Further significant reductions in mortality must come from management strategies within the first hours of the onset of symptoms.

The major in-hospital changes are likely to come from:[3,30]

- better hospital organisation to increase access to PCI
- increased rates of PCI or thrombolysis in eligible patients
- increased use of adjuvant therapies and discharge medications.

The role of reperfusion therapy cannot be underestimated. In one study, the in-hospital mortality was 5.7% for those who received thrombolysis but 14.8% for those who were eligible for but did not receive such therapy (9.3% versus 18% in eligible women who did not receive therapy, 10.5% versus 19% in eligible elderly). Up to 24% of eligible patients do not receive reperfusion therapy.[3,36,44]

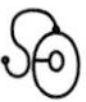

Access the complete references list online at http://www.expertconsult.com

4. Hamm CW, Bassand JP, Agewall S, et al. ESC Guidelines for the management of acute coronary syndromes in patients presenting without persistent ST-segment elevation: The Task Force for the management of acute coronary syndromes (ACS) in patients presenting without persistent ST-segment elevation of the European Society of Cardiology (ESC). Eur Heart J 2011;32(23):2999–3054.
5. Thygesen K, Alpert JS, Jaffe AS, et al. Third universal definition of myocardial infarction. Eur Heart J 2012;33(20):2551–67.
13. Gurm HS, Bates ER. Cardiogenic shock complicating myocardial infarction. Crit Care Clin 2007;23(4):759–77, vi.
14. Nikus K, Pahlm O, Wagner G, et al. Electrocardiographic classification of acute coronary syndromes: a review by a committee of the International Society for Holter and Non-Invasive Electrocardiology. J Electrocardiol 2010;43(2):91–103.
30. Steg PG, James SK, Atar D, et al. ESC Guidelines for the management of acute myocardial infarction in patients presenting with ST-segment elevation: The Task Force on the management of ST-segment elevation acute myocardial infarction of the European Society of Cardiology (ESC). Eur Heart J 2012; 33(20):2569–619.
38. Boden WE, Eagle K, Granger CB. Reperfusion strategies in acute ST-segment elevation myocardial infarction: a comprehensive review of contemporary management options. J Am Coll Cardiol 2007; 50(10):917–29.
45. Hanna EB, Hennebry TA, Abu-Fadel MS. Combined reperfusion strategies in ST-segment elevation MI: Rationale and current role. Cleve Clin J Med 2010;77(9):629–38.
60. Kumar A. Hemodynamically complicated ST-segment elevation myocardial infarction: presentation and treatment. Future Cardiol 2010;6(5):591–602.
61. Goldstein JA. Acute right ventricular infarction. Cardiol Clin 2012;30(2):219–32.
71. Menozzi A, Lina D, Conte G, et al. Antiplatelet therapy in acute coronary syndromes. Expert Opin Pharmacother 2012;13(1):27–42.

21

Adult cardiopulmonary resuscitation

Peter T Morley

The incidence and outcomes of cardiac arrests appear not to have changed dramatically over a number of decades. However, despite the appearance that outcomes from cardiac arrests are not improving, there are some bright spots where consistent improvement has been observed.[1,2] There are many potential reasons for these improvements, but the most likely are related to early detection, improved delivery of good CPR, and improved post-resuscitation care.

PREVALENCE AND OUTCOMES OF CARDIAC ARRESTS

Approximately 75% of deaths from cardiac arrests occur in the pre-hospital setting. Cardiac arrests in the community occur at approximately 50–150/100 000 person years.[3] The incidence of cardiac arrests is dramatically affected by the definition of the denominator (e.g. all cardiac arrests (89/100 000 person years) versus those with a presumed cardiac cause and where resuscitation was attempted (31/100 000 person years)[3]).

In-hospital cardiac arrests occur at approximately 1–5/1000 admissions,[4] with a similar denominator effect (as the majority of in-hospital cardiac deaths are expected and occur without attempts at resuscitation).

The majority of cardiac arrests in both pre- and in-hospital settings appear to be of cardiac origin, but the underlying causes, co-morbidities and presenting rhythms vary significantly between studies.

Outcomes of cardiac arrests are variable depending on the origin of the report, and are also critically dependent on the denominator.[3] The best outcomes from a cardiac arrest (near 100%) occur in the electrophysiology laboratory (where ventricular fibrillation (VF) is often deliberately induced). The outcomes from in-hospital cardiac arrest are surprisingly good (hospital discharge as high as 42%) despite significant co-morbidities, and are probably related to their early detection, the early arrival of the advanced life support team, and the detection and treatment of reversible causes.[5]

INTERNATIONAL REVIEW PROCESS

Since the formation of the International Liaison Committee On Resuscitation (ILCOR) in 1992, a cooperative international evaluation of the resuscitation science has resulted in the publication of international guidelines in 2000, and international consensus documents on resuscitation science in 2005 and 2010.[6] The process for the 2010 consensus on resuscitation science involved the review of 277 topics by 313 international contributors,[7] with the completion of 411 worksheets (available at www.ilcor.org). The published guidelines of the major resuscitation councils throughout the world (including the American Heart Association, and the European Resuscitation Council) are based on this consensus on science document. In 2010, Australasian guidelines were published,[8] cobadged by the Australian Resuscitation Council and the New Zealand Resuscitation Council, under the auspices of the Australian and New Zealand Council on Rescuscitation (ANZCOR).

The international science review process continues to be refined and a new consensus on resuscitation science document is planned for publication in 2015.

IMPORTANCE OF CHAIN OF SURVIVAL

The term chain of survival has been used to define the important links in the chain for the resuscitation process. The key links, which apply to both in- and out-of-hospital cardiac arrests, are: early recognition and the summoning of help, early basic life support, early access to defibrillation, and early advanced life support including post-resuscitation care.[6]

RECENT CHANGES TO GUIDELINES

As a result of the science review published in 2010,[6] a number of important changes have been made to the guidelines for both basic and advanced life support. In summary the basic life support changes include: commencing CPR where the victim is unresponsive and not breathing normally; commencing CPR with compressions rather than initial breaths; and an increased depth of compressions (>5 cm).[9] The advanced life support priorities include: focusing on the provision of good, uninterrupted CPR (including charging the defibrillator during compressions), and identifying reversible causes and specific circumstances where the standard ALS algorithm may need to be modified.[8,10]

These changes are discussed in more detail in the sections that follow.

BASIC LIFE SUPPORT (BLS)

The general flow of basic life support management is outlined in the 2010 Basic Life Support flow chart of ANZCOR (**Fig. 21.1**).[8]

COMMENCEMENT OF CARDIOPULMONARY RESUSCITATION

The current BLS guidelines recommend that CPR be commenced if the victim is unresponsive and not breathing normally.[8,9] An appropriately trained ALS provider can check for a central pulse (e.g. carotid) for up to 10 seconds during this period of assessment, but this should not delay CPR. It is now recommended that CPR should start with compressions.[8,9]

EXTERNAL CARDIAC COMPRESSION

SITE OF COMPRESSION

The desired compression point for CPR in adults remains over the lower half of the sternum. Compressions that are provided higher than this become less effective, and compressions lower than this are also less effective and have an increased risk of damage to intra-abdominal organs.

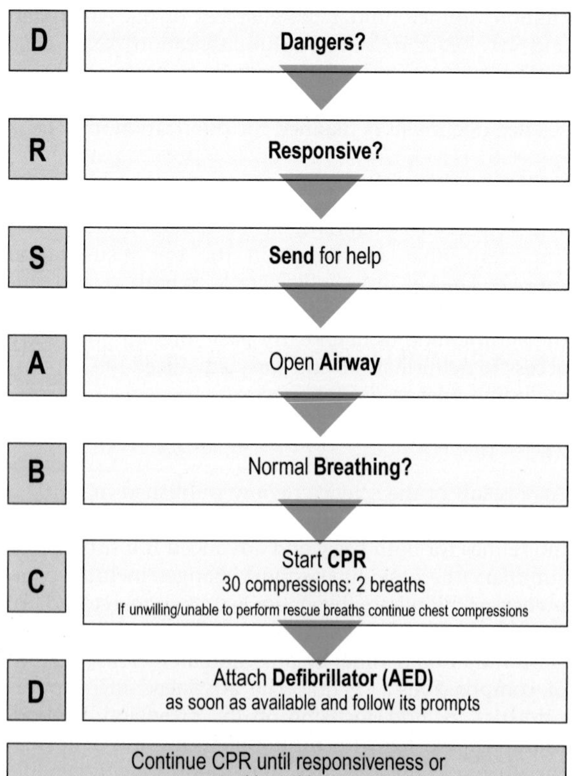

D
Dangers?
R
Responsive?
S
Send for help
A
Open Airway
B
Normal Breathing?
C
Start CPR
30 compressions: 2 breaths
If unwilling/unable to perform rescue breaths continue chest compressions
D
Attach Defibrillator (AED)
as soon as available and follow its prompts
Continue CPR until responsiveness or
normal breathing return

Figure 21.1 Basic life support flow chart. *Reproduced with permission from the Australian Resuscitation Council (www.resus.org.au).*[8]

RATE OF COMPRESSION

The optimal rate of cardiac compression during cardiac arrest in adults has not yet been determined.[2] In a recent human study,[11] lower rates (e.g. <80/min) were associated with worse outcomes and higher rates (>120/min) with more fatigue, and shallower compressions.[12] It is recommended that chest compressions should be performed at a rate of approximately 100 compressions/min.[8]

DEPTH OF COMPRESSION

The recommended compression depth for adults is now at least 5 cm.[8,9] It is still recommended that when performing chest compressions in adults (or infants or children) the chest should be compressed approximately one-third of its depth. In adults this facilitates delivery of at least 5 cm of compression.[8,13]

MINIMISE INTERRUPTIONS TO COMPRESSIONS

Interruptions in chest compressions ('hands-off time') are common, often prolonged, and are associated with a decrease in coronary perfusion pressure and a deceased likelihood of defibrillation success.[14] These adverse effects commence within 10 seconds of stopping CPR, but appear to be at least partially reversible with the recommencement of chest compressions. It is recommended that chest compressions be commenced as soon as the victim is confirmed to be unresponsive and not breathing normally.[8,9] The frequency and duration of interruptions in compressions for rhythm recognition or specific interventions (such as ventilations, charging the defibrillator, defibrillation, or intubation) should be kept to a minimum.

COMPRESSION : VENTILATION RATIO

The minute ventilation requirements during cardiac arrest are less than that in the non-arrested state as the cardiac output is reduced to approximately one-third of normal. A single compression:ventilation ratio of 30:2 remains recommended for adult BLS before the airway is secured (irrespective of the number of rescuers). This approach increases the number of compressions given per minute, minimises interruptions to chest compressions, and simplifies instruction for teaching and skills retention. The tidal breath should be delivered within 1 second, and the desired tidal volume to be delivered is one that results in a visible chest rise.[8]

MONITORING THE QUALITY OF CPR

A number of different techniques are available to monitor the quality of CPR, some of which are more

Box 21.1 Utility of end-tidal carbon dioxide monitoring during cardiac arrest[29]

Cardiovascular (absolute value of $ETCO_2$)
Falls immediately at the onset of cardiac arrest
Increases immediately with chest compressions
Provides a linear correlation with cardiac index
Allows early detection of ROSC (sudden increase)

Respiratory ($ETCO_2$ waveform)
Allows assessment of endotracheal tube placement
Allows assessment of expiratory flow limitation

Prognosis (absolute value of $ETCO_2$)
Predicts successful resuscitation

applicable to advanced life support.[10] Simple monitoring techniques include observing of the rate, depth and positioning of chest compressions, the rate and depth of ventilation, and palpating central pulses. Waveform capnography should be considered for all arrests (**Box 21.1**).[8] Additional monitoring techniques that can be used include: mechanical devices (e.g. for monitoring the depth of compressions) and new monitor/defibrillators (e.g. for monitoring the depth and rate of compressions and ventilation). Feedback from these devices has improved the quality of CPR but have not yet been translated into improvement in other outcomes.[15]

Feedback after cardiac arrests, as part of quality improvement, has been associated with improved cardiac arrest performance.[16]

'COMPRESSION-ONLY' CPR

Increasing anxiety about the performance of mouth-to-mouth ventilation has required the consideration of an alternative approach to traditional bystander CPR. A number of animal and human studies have suggested that ventilation may not be necessary during the initial phase of resuscitation from an arrest of a cardiac cause. Recent studies have shown benefits with conventional CPR in a number of settings (e.g. witnessed arrests,[17] and arrests with a non-cardiac aetiology[18]).

Despite the limited data to support 'compression-only' CPR, it is recommended that if rescuers are unable, not trained, or unwilling to perform mouth-to-mouth ventilation (rescue breathing) then they should perform 'compression only' CPR, as 'any attempt at resuscitation is better than no attempt'.[8]

DEFIBRILLATION

Defibrillation remains the definitive treatment for shockable rhythms such as pulseless ventricular tachycardia or ventricular fibrillation. Successful defibrillation requires an appropriate combination of defibrillator waveform and energy level.[8]

EARLY DEFIBRILLATION VS CPR BEFORE DEFIBRILLATION

The timing of defibrillation with regard to other interventions appears crucial. The traditional approach to the treatment of a shockable rhythm during cardiac arrest has been to perform defibrillation as soon as possible. In the scenario of recent-onset VF, this still holds, and the best outcomes are associated with defibrillation within 3 minutes (e.g. in electrophysiology labs or coronary care units). However, in situations where the VF has persisted for more than a few minutes, an initial period of CPR could be considered before defibrillation.[19]

WAVEFORM FOR DEFIBRILLATION

No specific defibrillator waveform (either monophasic or biphasic) is consistently associated with a greater incidence of return of spontaneous circulation (ROSC) or increased hospital discharge rates from cardiac arrest due to ventricular fibrillation. Defibrillation with biphasic waveforms (either truncated exponential or rectilinear), using equal or lower energy levels, appears at least as effective as monophasic waveforms for termination of VF.[20]

ENERGY LEVELS

Recommendations for energy levels to be used for defibrillation vary according to the type of defibrillator (and the specific waveform) that the rescuers are using. Current recommendations are based on maximising the likelihood of the success of each shock. The recommended energy level for defibrillation in adults where monophasic defibrillators are used is 360 J for all shocks. When using biphasic waveforms, the energy level should be set at 200 J for all shocks unless there exist relevant clinical data for the specific defibrillator suggesting that an alternative energy level provides adequate shock success (e.g. >90%). There is no consistent evidence (e.g. survival benefit) to suggest that an escalation of energy levels is required for subsequent shocks.[21]

MANUAL DEFIBRILLATION OR AUTOMATED EXTERNAL DEFIBRILLATOR

Automated external defibrillators provide an opportunity for untrained bystanders and BLS providers to defibrillate a shockable rhythm. In the hands of skilled healthcare providors, manual defibrillation should be used whenever possible as the delays inherent in the use of an AED may be detrimental.[22]

SINGLE-SHOCK TECHNIQUE

The use of a single-shock strategy for defibrillation is recommended (i.e. deliver a single shock and then immediately commence CPR). This strategy minimises the interruptions to chest compressions that occur during defibrillation attempts.

The Australian Resuscitation Council does, however, recommend the consideration of a stacked shock strategy (up to three shocks as necessary) in specific circumstances: patients with a perfusing rhythm who develop a shockable rhythm, in a witnessed and monitored setting, where a manual defibrillator is immediately available (e.g. first shock able to be delivered within 20 seconds) and the time required for rhythm recognition and charging of the defibrillator is short (e.g. <10 seconds). All subsequent shocks should be given using a single-shock strategy.[8]

PADS OR PADDLES

Self-adhesive defibrillation pads are safe and effective for defibrillation, can facilitate pacing and allow charging during compressions.[20] If there are concerns about contact or success of defibrillation, then paddles can be used, but they require the use of conductive gel pads and the application of sufficient firm pressure to maximise electrical contact.[8]

ADVANCED LIFE SUPPORT

Advanced life support has an established role in the management of cardiac arrests. Interestingly, in of itself, the provision of ALS (apart from defibrillation) has not been specifically demonstrated to be associated with improved outcomes. A number of ALS techniques are listed below; some of these are available only in the in-hospital setting.

ADVANCED LIFE SUPPORT FLOW CHART

The recommended sequence of treatment to be followed is outlined in the 2010 Advanced Life Support flow chart of ANZCOR[8] (**Fig. 21.2**). This flow chart is based on ILCOR's universal algorithm[6] and is designed for use as an aide memoire and a teaching tool.

PRECORDIAL THUMP

The provision of a precordial thump may be considered in a monitored arrest due to pulseless ventricular tachycardia if a defibrillator is not immediately available. The technique is not without risks, however, and should not delay defibrillation.

A precordial thump is no longer recommended for ventricular fibrillation.[8]

CHEST COMPRESSIONS

The provision of good basic life support is an essential part of the advanced life support management of both shockable and non-shockable rhythms. Interruptions to chest compressions for definitive procedures or interventions should be kept as brief as possible.[9,23] Chest compressions should be continued up until defibrillation, including during charging of the defibrillator.[10,24] CPR should also be commenced again immediately following defibrillation (without checking the rhythm), and continued for at least 2 minutes unless signs of life return (the victim becomes responsive or starts breathing). Even if defibrillation has successfully reverted the rhythm into one that could generate a pulse, in the vast majority of cases this is not initially associated with an output. Immediate compressions in these situations avoid the detrimental effects of prolonged interruptions in compressions and maintain the coronary perfusion.[20] After each 2 minutes of CPR (or if signs of life return), the underlying rhythm should be checked, and if a rhythm compatible with a return of spontaneous circulation is observed at that time then a central pulse should also be checked.

AIRWAY MANAGEMENT DURING CPR

There are no data to support the routine use of any specific approach to airway management during cardiac arrest.[10] Despite this, endotracheal intubation remains the gold standard for airway maintenance and airway protection during CPR.[8] If the victim is unconscious and has no gag reflex, and a trained operator is available, endotracheal intubation should be performed at the first appropriate opportunity.[25] The endotracheal tube provides optimal isolation and patency of the airway, allows suctioning of the airway and also provides access for the delivery of some drugs (e.g. epinephrine (adrenaline), lidocaine and atropine). However, attempts at endotracheal intubation should not interrupt cardiac compressions for more than 20 seconds. The routine use of an endotracheal tube during cardiac arrest management has not been shown to improve outcomes, and without adequate training and experience the incidence of complications, such as unrecognised oesophageal intubation, is unacceptably high. A large number of supraglottic airway devices have been trialled as alternatives to the endotracheal tube.[26] The training and experience of the resuscitation team members, and availability of such devices, will determine the appropriate choice of airway adjunct.

VENTILATION DURING CPR

A compression:ventilation ratio of 30:2 is recommended before the airway is secured, and after the airway is secured the recommended ventilation rate is 8–10/minute.[10] One way to provide this, and to minimise interruptions to compressions is to use a compression:ventilation ratio of 15:1 once the airway is secured.[8] Hyperventilation during cardiac arrest is associated with increased intrathoracic pressure, decreased coronary and cerebral perfusion, and, at least

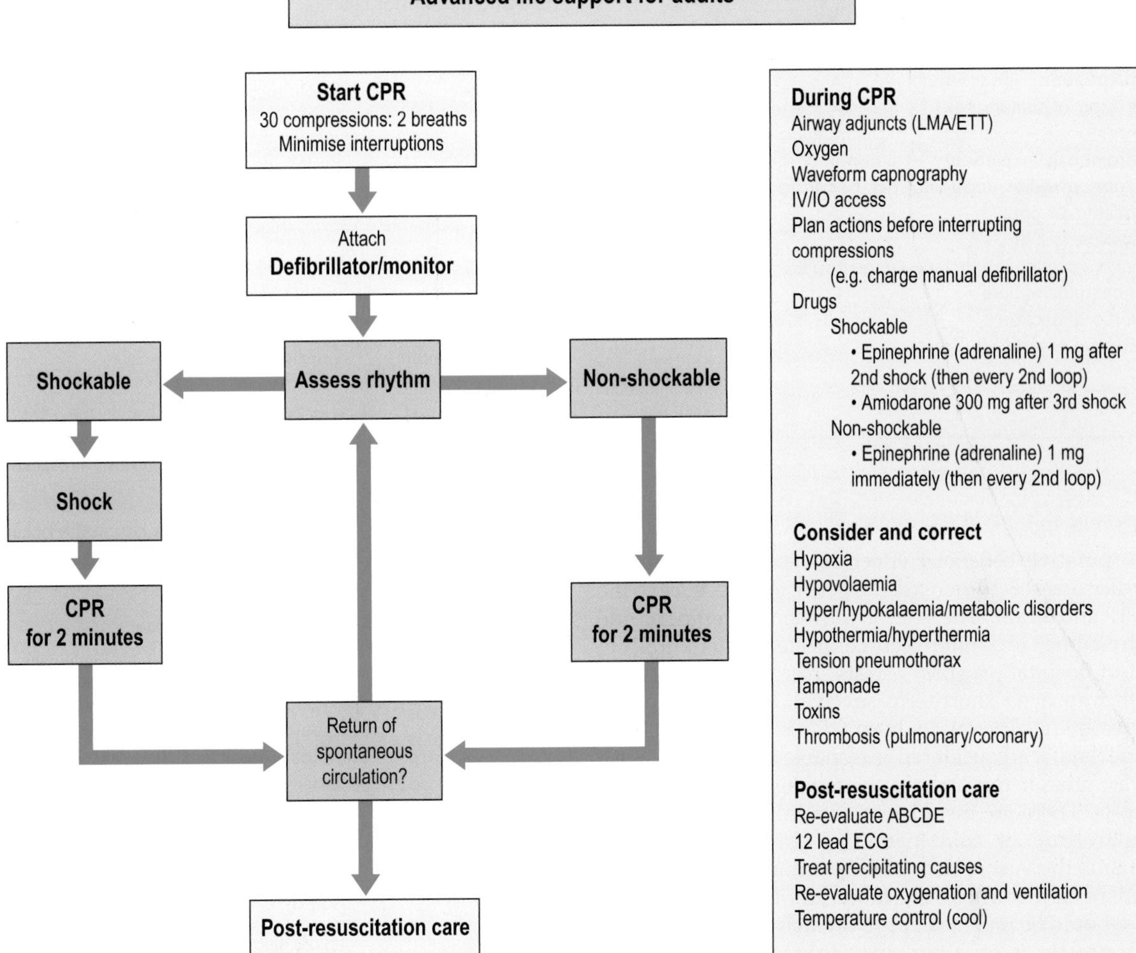

Figure 21.2 Advanced life support flow chart. *Reproduced with permission from the Australian Resuscitation Council (www.resus.org.au).*[8]

in animals, a decreased rate of return of spontaneous circulation.[27] If there is a concern about potential gas trapping, a period of disconnection from the ventilation circuit may be beneficial.[8] The tidal volume recommended is one that results in a visible chest rise.[8]

IDENTIFICATION OF REVERSIBLE CAUSES

Irrespective of the initial or subsequent rhythms, cardiac arrests can be precipitated or perpetuated by a number of conditions that if not detected and corrected may decrease the likelihood of successful resuscitation.[5] These 'reversible causes' are categorised in the ALS algorithm as the '4Hs and 4Ts' (www.resus.org.au; see 4Ts'[8] (Fig. 21.2, 'Consider and correct')). A number of techniques are available to assist in the diagnosis and exclusion of these conditions. These include a good history, a careful clinical examination, and some specific investigations and interventions. Echocardiography can potentially diagnose (or help exclude) a number of cardiac and non-cardiac reversible causes[28] (**Box 21.2**). Transoesophageal echocardiography requires a more skilled technician, but useful information can be obtained after minimal training with the transthoracic approach.[29]

MEDICATIONS DURING CPR

Although various drugs are recommended for use during the management of cardiac arrests, there are no placebo-controlled studies that show that the routine use of any drugs at any stage during human cardiac arrest increase survival to hospital discharge.[8] The intraosseous route should be considered for administration of medications if venous access is not immediately available.[30]

Box 21.2 Potentially useful diagnoses detectable by echocardiography[29]

Hypovolaemia*
Tamponade* (pericardial)
Tension pneumothorax*
Thrombosis – pulmonary* (thromboembolism)
Thrombosis – coronary* (regional or global wall motion abnormalities, including lack of cardiac motion)
Pacemaker capture
Unexpected VF
Acute valvular insufficiency (e.g. papillary muscle rupture)
Ventricular rupture
Aortic dissection
Massive pleural effusion

*Reversible causes listed in the '4Hs and 4Ts' (www.resus.org.au) (Fig. 21.2).

VASOPRESSORS

The putative beneficial effect of vasopressors during cardiac arrest is to increase the perfusion pressure to the heart and brain. The use of intravenous epinephrine (adrenaline) in randomised controlled trials enrolling out-of-hospital cardiac arrests has been associated with improved short-term survival, but no definitive increase in survival to hospital discharge.[31,32] Given these data, it is considered reasonable to continue to use a vasopressor routinely in the management of cardiac arrests. There are insufficient data to support any particular drug or combination of drugs. Epinephrine remains the vasopressor of choice during the management of cardiac arrest. The initial adult dose is 1 mg and this should be repeated approximately every 4 minutes. Vasopressin is an alternative drug, but studies have been unable to demonstrate that it has any consistent benefits.[33]

ANTI-ARRHYTHMICS

No anti-arrhythmic drug has been shown to improve long-term survival compared with placebo for the management of cardiac arrests.[8] However, administration of amiodarone (300 mg or 5 mg/kg) for shock refractory ventricular fibrillation has been associated with an increased survival to hospital when compared with either placebo or lidocaine. Either amiodarone or lidocaine (but not both) should be considered in those patients still in ventricular fibrillation after repeated attempts at defibrillation (including attempted defibrillation after the administration of epinephrine) have failed (i.e. immediately after the third shock).[8]

OTHER MEDICATIONS

Other medications that should be considered during cardiac arrest are those that address the underlying cause. These include electrolytes (such as magnesium or potassium), atropine, sodium bicarbonate and other specific 'antidotes' (see **Table 21.1**).[34,35]

Table 21.1 Cardiac arrest medications in specific circumstances

MEDICATION	POTENTIAL INDICATIONS
Atropine	Cholinergic/cardiac glycoside toxicity
Anti-venom	Snake, funnel-web spider, box jellyfish venom
Benzodiazepines	Sympathomimetic toxicity
Calcium	Hypocalcaemia, hypermagnesaemia, hyperkalaemia, beta-blocker/calcium channel blocker toxicity
Digoxin-specific antibodies	Cardiac glycoside toxicity
Flumazenil	Benzodiazepine toxicity
Epinephrine (adrenaline)	Beta-blocker/calcium channel blocker toxicity
Glucagon	Beta-blocker/calcium channel blocker toxicity
High-dose insulin/ dextrose	Beta-blocker/calcium channel blocker toxicity
Lipid emulsion	Local anaesthetic agents
Magnesium	Hypomagnesaemia, hypokalaemia, hypercalcaemia, tricyclic antidepressant/cardiac glycoside toxicity, torsade de pointes
Naloxone	Opioid toxicity
Potassium	Hypokalaemia
Pyridoxine	Isoniazid toxicity
Sodium bicarbonate	Hyperkalaemia, tricyclic antidepressant/sodium-channel-blocker toxicity

ADJUNCTS TO CPR

Many technologies and techniques have been evaluated as adjuncts to CPR in an attempt to improve survival in the management of cardiac arrests, but none has been consistently associated with improved outcomes.[36] Active-compression decompression (ACD) CPR is the most widely evaluated technique, but by itself has not been associated with improved long-term survival. The combination of ACD-CPR with an impedance threshold device was associated with improved neurological survival in one recently published trial in out-of-hospital cardiac arrests.[37] An automated version of ACD-CPR (LUCAS), and a modification of vest CPR (the load-distributing band) are both currently being evaluated in controlled trials. There has also been a resurgence of interest in extracorporeal techniques, especially as short-term rescue.[38] At this stage there is still insufficient supportive evidence to recommend the routine use of any of these adjunctive techniques.[8,10]

Mechanical devices (such as LUCAS or the load-distributing band) may, however, be useful alternatives to manual CPR in situations where tradional CPR is difficult or hazardous (e.g. during transport, or during interventions).[10,39]

POST-RESUSCITATION CARE

The missing link in research in resuscitation has for a long time been the period of care after the return of spontaneous circulation. Survival after cardiac arrest is largely dependent on the patient's co-morbidities and the initial hypoxic insults to the heart and brain. However, survival is also influenced by subsequent complications (including secondary insults and the ensuing systemic inflammatory response[40]), and possibly differences in post-resuscitation care[41] (**Box 21.3**).

RESUSCITATION CENTRES

An increasing body of evidence suggests that there may be benefits in transporting the victims of out-of-hospital cardiac arrests to a centre that is equipped to provide all of the desired components of post-arrest care (including percutaneous coronary interventions and therapeutic hypothermia).[42,43]

Box 21.3 Key factors to consider after resuscitation from cardiac arrest[8]

Immediate tasks
Re-evaluate ABCDE
12-lead ECG
Treat precipitating causes
Re-evaluate oxygenation and ventilation
Temperature control (cool)

Early goals
Continue respiratory support
Maintain cerebral perfusion
Treat and prevent cardiac arrhythmias
Determine and treat the cause of the arrest

Specific tasks
Maintain haemodynamics (SBP>100 mmHg (13 kPa))
Maintain adequate oxygenation (Sa_{O_2} 94–98%)
Maintain normal pH and normocarbia (e.g. Pa_{CO_2} 35–40 mmHg (4.5–5.2 kPa))
Treat hyperglycaemia (>10 mmol/L), but avoid hypoglycaemia
Consider therapeutic hypothermia (unless contraindicated)
Maintain appropriate sedation
Treat seizures
Continue search to identify underlying cause(s) and trauma related to resuscitation
Consider specific treatment for underlying cause (e.g. percutaneous coronary intervention, thrombolytics)
Consider prophylactic antiarrhythmics
Consider transfer to resuscitation centre

THERAPEUTIC HYPOTHERMIA

It is recommended that unconscious but haemodynamically stable survivors of out-of-hospital cardiac arrests due to ventricular fibrillation should be cooled to 32–34°C for 12–24 hours. A period of induced hypothermia should also be considered for cardiac arrests due to other rhythms, as well as in-hospital arrests.[8,10,44] (See Ch. 50 for further details.)

OTHER FACTORS IN POST-RESUSCITATION CARE

Factors other than therapeutic hypothermia are important in the post-arrest period. Attention should be given to good supportive care, including maintenance of cerebral perfusion, provision of adequate oxygenation, ventilation to normocarbia, avoidance of hyperglycaemia and treatment of seizures. Norwegian investigators were able to double their survival to hospital discharge (with a favourable neurological outcome) for out-of-hospital cardiac arrests by introducing a standardised post-resuscitation protocol. This protocol focused on vital organ function including the use of therapeutic hypothermia, percutaneous coronary interventions (PCI), and the control of haemodynamics (MAP>65 mmHg (8.5 kPa)), blood glucose (5–8 mmol/L), ventilation (normocapnia) and seizures.[45]

OXYGENATION

Traditional approaches to resuscitation have included the routine use of 100% oxygen. Data from animal and neonatal studies have suggested that this may be associated with adverse outcomes.[8] The adult cardiac arrest evidence regarding effects of oxygenation is accumulating, but is of low quality and remains controversial.[46,47] It seems reasonable, however, to titrate the Fi_{O_2} to target an acceptable Sa_{O_2} (e.g. 94–98%) as soon as the patient is stable.[8]

VENTILATION

Numerous studies in animals and humans have demonstrated the potential harm of cerebral ischaemia induced by hypocapnia after cardiac arrest. There are no data to support the targeting of a specific Pa_{CO_2} after resuscitation from cardiac arrest, but data extrapolated from patients with brain injury however, imply that ventilation to normocarbia (e.g. Pa_{CO_2} 35–40 mmHg (4.5-5.2 kPa)) is appropriate.[8] Arterial blood gas measurements should be used to titrate ventilation in the immediate post-resuscitation period, rather than the use of end-tidal CO_2 levels as there may be disparity.[8]

BLOOD PRESSURE CONTROL

There is limited human evidence to support specific haemodynamic goals after cardiac arrest. Reported successful blood pressure goals have varied from a period of relative hypertension (MAP 90–100 mmHg[48]

(11.7–13 kPa)), to more standard goals (MAP>65–70[45]). It is recommended to aim for a blood pressure equal to the patient's usual blood pressure or a systolic pressure greater than 100 mmHg.[8]

GLUCOSE CONTROL

Despite the early promise of improved outcomes with tight blood glucose control, subsequent studies have demonstrated this approach to be potentially harmful.[49] Blood glucose should be monitored frequently after cardiac arrest. Hyperglycemia (>10 mmol/L) should be treated with insulin, but hypoglycemia should be avoided.[8]

PERCUTANEOUS CORONARY INTERVENTION

Thrombolysis and percutaneous coronary interventions (PCI) are the mainstay of management after acute coronary syndromes. PCI has been used successfully when indicated in the early period after recovery of spontaneous circulation, and should be considered as part of routine post-arrest care in patients with ST elevation or a new left-bundle branch block.[50] Clinical findings of coma in patients prior to PCI are commonly present in out-of-hospital cardiac arrest (OHCA) patients, and these should not be a contraindication to consider immediate angiography and PCI. It is also reasonable to perform immediate angiography and PCI in selected patients, despite the absence of ST-segment elevation on the ECG or prior clinical findings such as chest pain.[51]

Therapeutic hypothermia is recommended in combination with primary PCI, and should be started as early as possible, preferably prior to initiation of PCI.

TREATMENT OF SEIZURES

Seizures are relatively common after cardiac arrest (3–44% incidence),[10] and in the post-arrest period they may be refractory to multiple medications. It is reasonable to intstitute prompt and aggressive treatment of seizures, but there is no definitive evidence to suggest that this approach (or preventative therapy) improves outcomes.[10]

OTHER FACTORS

The search should be continued to identify and treat underlying causes of the arrest. Trauma related to the resuscitation is relatively common, and should be identified and treated as appropriate.[8]

It may be reasonable to continue an infusion of an antiarrhythmic drug that successfully restored a stable rhythm during resuscitation (e.g. lidocaine 2–4 mg/min or amiodarone 0.6 mg/kg/h for 12–24 hours). If no antiarrhythmic drug was used during resuscitation from a shockable rhythm, an antiarrhythmic drug may be considered to prevent recurrent VF.

The placement and sterility of devices inserted during the arrest should also be reviewed.[8]

PROGNOSTICATION

It is impossible to predict accurately the degree of neurological recovery during or immediately after a cardiac arrest.

In adult patients who are comatose after cardiac arrest, who have not been treated with hypothermia and who do not have confounding factors (such as hypotension, sedatives or neuromuscular blockers), the absence of both pupillary light and corneal reflexes at 72 hours after arrest reliably predicts a poor outcome.[10] The absence of vestibulo-ocular reflexes at 24 hours and a GCS motor score of 2 or less at 72 hours are less reliable. Other clinical signs, including myoclonus, are not recommended to be used for predicting poor outcome.[52] After 24 hours, bilateral absence of the N20 cortical response to median nerve stimulation predicts poor outcome in comatose cardiac arrest survivors not treated with therapeutic hypothermia.

Accurate prediction of neurological outcome has become increasingly difficult since therapeutic hypothermia has been used in the post-arrest period.[10,53] A Glasgow Motor Score of 2 or less at 3 days after sustained return of spontaneous circulation and the presence of status epilepticus are potentially unreliable prognosticators of poor outcome in POST-cardiac arrest patients treated with therapeutic hypothermia. Given the limited available evidence, decisions to limit care should not be made based on the results of a single prognostication tool.[8,53]

The use of EEG, neuroimaging and biochemical markers may provide additional information, but at this stage are not sufficiently reliable to be used definitively for prognostication.[54]

MAINTENANCE OF ALS SKILLS

Many studies have confirmed that knowledge and skills related to ALS start to deteriorate relatively quickly (e.g. within 6 months).[55] New approaches to ALS teaching are required to ensure all staff maintain their skills. One successful approach has been to provide 6 minutes of practice every month.[56]

SUMMARY

Improved outcomes after cardiac arrest have been demonstrated in many centres over the past decade. This is almost certainly due to improvements made within each link of the chain of survival. These include: earlier recognition and activation of the emergency response (both pre-hospital and in-hospital), provision of good-quality basic life support (including minimising interruptions to chest compressions), optimised defibrillation, early and appropriate advanced life support with attention to identifying and treating underlying causes, and an increased focus on care in the critical post-resuscitation period.

Access the complete references list online at http://www.expertconsult.com

3. Finn JC, Jacobs IG, Holman CD, et al. Outcomes of out-of-hospital cardiac arrest patients in Perth, Western Australia, 1996–1999. Resuscitation 2001; 51(3):247–55.
5. Saarinen S, Nurmi J, Toivio T, et al. Does appropriate treatment of the primary underlying cause of PEA during resuscitation improve patients' survival? Resuscitation 2012;83(7):819–22.
6. Hazinski MF, Nolan JP, Billi JE, et al. Part 1: Executive summary: 2010 International Consensus on Cardiopulmonary Resuscitation and Emergency Cardiovascular Care Science With Treatment Recommendations. Circulation 2010;122(16 Suppl 2):S250–75.
8. Australian Resuscitation Council. [Homepage] 2012. Online. Available: www.resus.org.au.
35. Smith SW. Drugs and pharmaceuticals: management of intoxication and antidotes. EXS 2010;100:397–460.
40. Neumar RW, Nolan JP, Adrie C, et al. Post-cardiac arrest syndrome: epidemiology, pathophysiology, treatment, and prognostication. A consensus statement from the International Liaison Committee on Resuscitation (American Heart Association, Australian and New Zealand Council on Resuscitation, European Resuscitation Council, Heart and Stroke Foundation of Canada, InterAmerican Heart Foundation, Resuscitation Council of Asia, and the Resuscitation Council of Southern Africa); the American Heart Association Emergency Cardiovascular Care Committee; the Council on Cardiovascular Surgery and Anesthesia; the Council on Cardiopulmonary, Perioperative, and Critical Care; the Council on Clinical Cardiology; and the Stroke Council. Circulation 2008;118(23):2452–83.
44. Walters JH, Morley PT, Nolan JP. The role of hypothermia in post-cardiac arrest patients with return of spontaneous circulation: A systematic review. Resuscitation 2011;82(5):508–16.
45. Tomte O, Andersen GO, Jacobsen D, et al. Strong and weak aspects of an established post-resuscitation treatment protocol, a five-year observational study. Resuscitation 2011;82(9):1186–93.
51. Kern KB, Rahman O. Emergent percutaneous coronary intervention for resuscitated victims of out-of-hospital cardiac arrest. Catheter Cardiovasc Interv 2010;75(4):616–24.
54. Oddo M, Rossetti AO. Predicting neurological outcome after cardiac arrest. Curr Opin Crit Care 2011;17(3):254–9.

22

Management of cardiac arrhythmias

Andrew Holt

CARDIAC ELECTROPHYSIOLOGY

The electrophysiological properties of cardiac cells are important in understanding cardiac arrhythmias and their management. Cardiac cells undergo cyclical depolarisation and repolarisation to form an action potential. The shape and duration of each action potential are determined by the activity of ion channel protein complexes on the myocyte surface (**Table 22.1**).[1]

Ion channels are large glycoproteins that span the membrane bilayer with accessory subunits that contribute to pore structure or modulate function. Channel activation forms pores that permit rapid transit of ions creating ionic currents that determines the magnitude and rate of change of myocyte membrane potential.

Ion channels:

- are generally highly selective for certain ions
- activation control or 'gating' can be voltage or ligand binding
- most are voltage gated and modulated by ligand gating
- have 'rectifying' properties whereby they conduct ions more effectively in one direction.

Many of the ion channels are the molecular targets for antiarrhythmic drugs. The differential distribution of ion channel populations within the heart allows drugs to have preferential activity on different parts of the heart.

I_f 'pacemaker' channels are confined to the SA node and new drugs with specific I_f blocking activity such as ivabradine have been shown to be beneficial in angina and heart failure by slowing the heart rate without negative effects on ventricular contractility.

I_K channels responsible for potassium ion (K^+) repolarisation currents (I_K) vary throughout the heart with the rapidly activating forms, I_{Kur}, being confined to the atrium. Vernakalant, a new K channel blocker has predominant activity on the I_{Kur} channel and therefore predominant atrial activity.

Ion channel function can be affected by:

- genetic mutations of channel proteins
- changes in functional expression of channel protein genes
- acute ischaemia
- autonomic tone
- myocardial scarring
- electrolyte concentration.

The spectrum of cardiac action potentials varies from *fast-response* cells – conducting and contractile myocytes (**Fig. 22.1a**) – to *slow-response* cells of pacemaker myocytes – sinoatrial (SA) and atrioventricular (AV) nodes (Fig. 22.1b). Fast myocytes lose their characteristic action potential and behave more like slow myocytes when ischaemic. The action potential is divided into five phases and ion channel currents vary between fast- and slow-response cells (**Fig. 22.2**).

PHASE 0

In fast myocytes (see Fig. 22.1a) rapid depolarisation I_{Na} current occurs owing to activation of voltage-gated sodium ion (Na^+) channels. Activation is initiated in an all-or-none response once the threshold is reached. The Na^+ channels are inactivated as membrane potential rises to +30 mV and remain inactivated until repolarisation occurs. Rapidity of depolarisation determines speed of conduction. In slow-response myocytes depolarisation does not involve Na^+ channels and the slower rate of depolarisation is due to a slow inward calcium ion (Ca^{2+}) current via $I_{Ca\text{-}L}$ and $I_{Ca\text{-}T}$ voltage-dependent Ca^{2+} channels.

PHASE 1

Early rapid incomplete repolarisation to approximately 0 mV occurs owing to activation of transient outward current from I_{TO1} and I_{TO2} K^+ channels. Slow myocytes do not exhibit phase 1 or 2 characteristics (see Fig. 22.1b).

PHASE 2

The prolonged plateau repolarisation of fast myocytes is a consequence of low membrane conductance to all ions. The decreasing inward Ca^{2+} current of $I_{Ca\text{-}L}$ and $I_{Ca\text{-}T}$ Ca^{2+} channels is initially balanced and then overcome by the outward K^+ current of the delayed rectifiers or the I_k family of K^+ channels. During this phase the rise in calcium ion concentration ($[Ca^{2+}]_i$) is the trigger to release sarcoplasmic reticulum stores of Ca^{2+} and initiate the contractile process.

Table 22.1 Characteristics of cardiac ionic channels

ION	CHANNEL	
		INWARD CURRENT/DEPOLARISATION
Sodium Na_v	I_{Na}	• Present in atria, His–Purkinje and ventricle • Absent in sinoatrial and AV node • Generates phase 0 rapid depolarisation current • Drives action potential propagation
Calcium Ca_v	$I_{Ca\text{-}L}$	• Predominate Ca^{2+} channel • Contributes to phase 2 plateau • Produces depolarisation and propagation in SA and AV nodes • Triggers Ca^{2+} release from sarcoplasmic reticulum
	$I_{Ca\text{-}T}$	• Predominates in pacemaker cells • Contributes to later stages of phase 4 in pacemaker cells
Non-selective cation	I_f	• Predominately Na • Absent in ventricular cells • Activated by polarisation • Generates phase 4 depolarisation of pacemaker function • Strongly modulated by neurotransmitters
		OUTWARD CURRENT/REPOLARISATION
Potassium K_v	I_{to}	• Activated rapidly after depolarisation • Fast I_{to1} and slow I_{to2} variants • Responsible for phase 1 rapid early repolarisation • Predominate distribution subepicardial • Distribution creates heterogeneous repolarisation
	I_K	• Delayed rectifiers • Slow activation kinetics • Major repolarising current • Variants with slow I_{Ks}, rapid I_{Kr} and ultra-rapid I_{Kur} activation • I_K populations are not characterised in the SA node • I_{Kur} are not present in the ventricle • I_{Kur} along with I_{to} contributes to earlier repolarisation and shorter action potentials of atrial cells
	I_{K1}	• Inward rectifier • Current responsible for maintaining resting potential near K^+ equilibrium • Shuts off during depolarisation • Absence in SA node enables small currents to control pacemaker rates

PHASE 3

Relatively rapid repolarisation occurs as outward K^+ current of the delayed rectifiers increases. The I_{kr} K^+ channel, one of the I_k delayed rectifiers, is the common mechanism whereby antiarrhythmic drugs prolong the action potential and refractoriness.

PHASE 4

This is a stable electrical state in fast non-pacemaker myocytes owing to inward rectifier I_{K1} channels maintaining resting membrane potential near K^+ equilibrium and the absence of I_f pacemaker channels. In slow pacemaker myocytes the resting membrane potential (RMP) slowly depolarises owing to absence of I_{K1} channels and progressive activation of I_f pacemaker channels until the action potential threshold is reached (see Fig. 22.1b).

Fast-response and slow-response myocytes also have important differences in properties of refractoriness. In fast myocytes, Na^+ channels are progressively reactivated during phase 3 repolarisation as the membrane potential becomes more negative. When an extra stimulus occurs during phase 3, the magnitude of the resulting inward Na^+ current and likelihood of impulse propagation depend on the number of reactivated Na^+ channels. Refractoriness is therefore determined by the voltage-dependent recovery of Na^+ channels. The absolute refractory period (see Fig. 22.1) is that minimum time needed for recovery of sufficient Na^+ channels for a stimulus to result in impulse propagation. However, once propagation in fast myocytes occurs, conduction velocity is normal. In contrast, slow-response or Ca^{2+} channel-dependent myocytes exhibit time-dependent refractoriness. Even after full repolarisation, further time is needed before all Ca^{2+} channels are reactivated. Stimuli during this period produce reduced Ca^{2+} current and the propagation velocity of any resulting impulse is reduced. The conduction velocity independence of

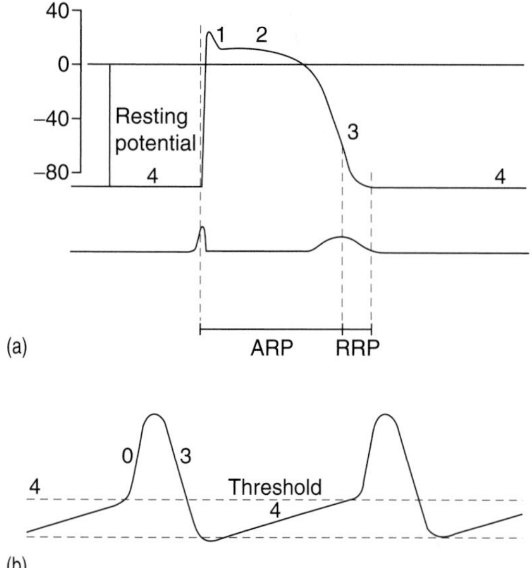

Figure 22.1 (a) Action potential in a fast-response, non-pacemaker myocyte: phases 0–4, resting membrane potential −80 mV, absolute refractory period (ARP) and relative refractory period (RRP). (b) Action potential in a slow-response, pacemaker myocyte. The spontaneous upward slope of phase 4, on reaching threshold potential, results in an action potential.

premature action potentials with fast-response myocytes is lost in the setting of Na^+ channel-blocking drugs or ischaemia because they behave increasingly like slow-response myocytes with resulting slowed impulse conduction.

RECEPTOR MODULATION OF CHANNEL FUNCTION

The autonomic nervous system is an important modulator of cardiac rhythm via effects on channel function. Beta-adrenergic receptor–effector-coupling system modulates channel function via cyclic adenosine monophosphate (AMP) phosphorylation of peptides associated with channels resulting in the following:

- $I_{Ca\text{-}L}$ increases Ca^{2+} current and contractility
- I_f activation threshold is changed to a more positive level
- I_K accelerates K^+ current repolarisation and increases AV node conduction.

Muscurinic M_2 receptor activation inhibits cyclic AMP effects and purinergic A_1 receptor activation slows K^+ current and AV conduction.

GENETIC BASIS TO ARRHYTHMIA[2]

In the absence of structural abnormalities of the heart, primary electrical disease is associated with mutations in ion channel genes. The long-QT syndrome (LQTS) (see below), short-QT syndrome, Brugada syndrome (idiopathic ventricular fibrillation, VF) and catecholaminergic polymorphic ventricular tachycardia (VT), and all causes of sudden cardiac death (SCD) in the young are examples of primary electrical disease where genetic mutations encoding for ion channel proteins have been characterised.

Inheritable forms of structural ventricular disease are associated with atrial arrhythmias and SCD. Examples include hypertrophic and dilated cardiomyopathies and arrhythmogenic right ventricular dysplasia, which are linked to mutations in sarcomeric, cytoskeletal and intercellular junction proteins, respectively.

The risk of cardiac arrhythmias and SCD in the setting of acquired structural heart disease such as ischaemic heart disease is in part genetically determined. Studies demonstrate an increased risk of SCD in patients who have a parental history of cardiac arrest.

MOLECULAR BASIS TO ARRHYTHMIA[2]

Structural and electrical remodeling in response to myocardial injury, altered haemodynamic loads and changes in neurohumoral signalling lead to alterations in:

- ion channel function
- intracellular calcium handling
- intercellular communication
- composition of intercellular matrix.

All of these factors lead to heterogeneous slowing of conduction velocity and prolonged refractoriness.

Tachycardia remodelling of the atrium is associated with:

- reduced functional expression of L-type Ca^{2+} channels, intracellular Ca^{2+} overload and shortening action potential duration.

Heart failure is associated with:

- down-regulation of each of the major repolarising K^+ currents, prolonging repolarisation and resulting in susceptibility to early-after-depolarisation (EAD)-mediated arrhythmia. As these changes are heterogeneous they also create the substrate for re-entrant arrhythmias
- reduced Na^+ channel density decreasing conduction velocity
- increased expression of Na^+–Ca^{2+} exchanger protein, leading to intracellular Ca^{2+} overload and predisposition to delayed-after-depolarisation (DAD)-mediated arrhythmia.

Intercellular ion channels or connexins at gap junctions are decreased and redistributed from the intercalated disc to lateral cell borders, slowing conduction velocity and uncoupling myocytes.

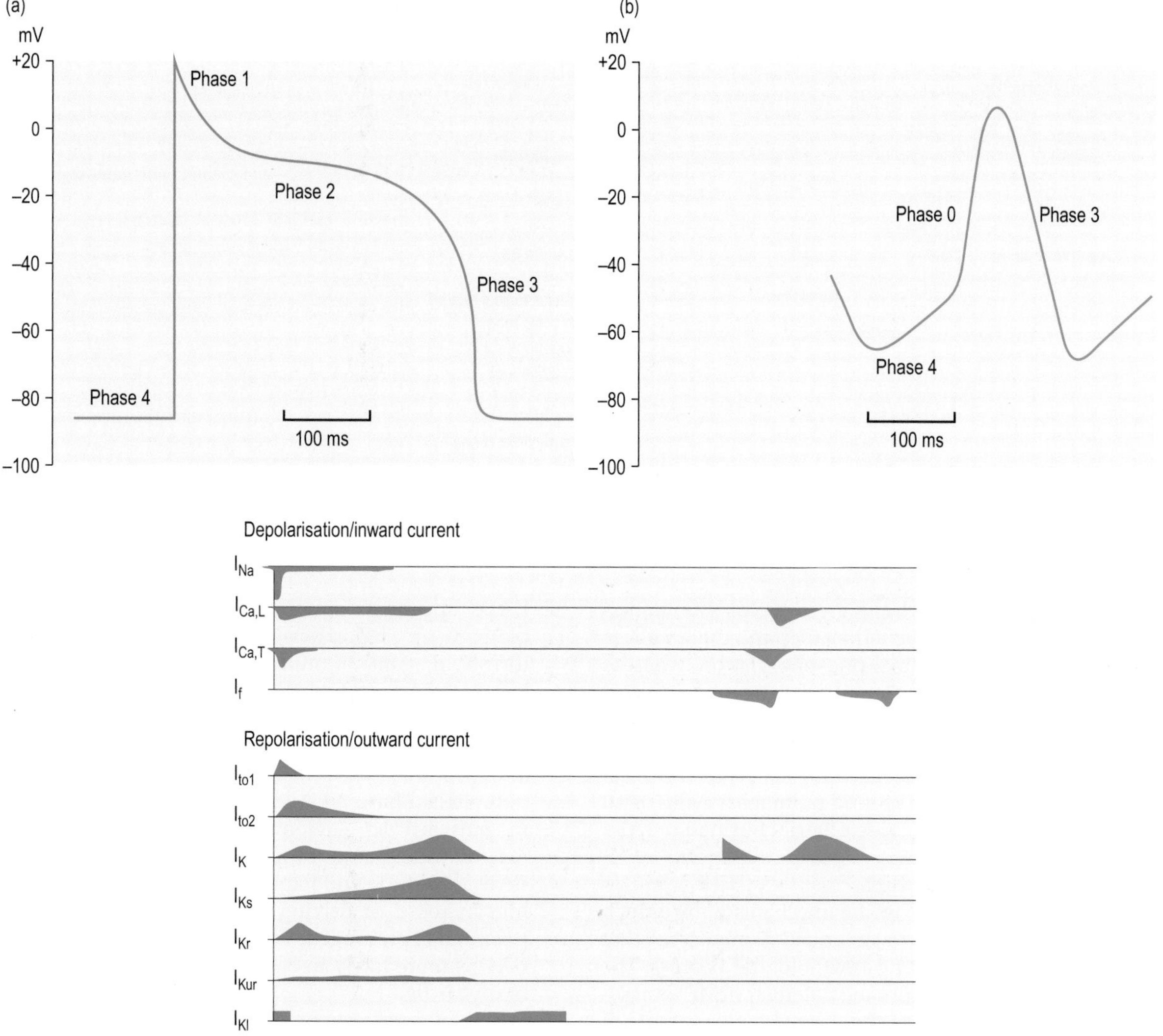

Figure 22.2 Temporal relationship between action potential and ionic channel activation for: (a) fast-response ventricular myocytes and (b) slow-response pacemaker myocytes.

Myocardial infarction scar produces:

- heterogeneous action potential duration with zones of healing myocytes with shortened action potential and surrounding hypertrophic myocytes with prolonged action potentials
- potential anatomical circuits due to fibrous tissue separating myocyte bundles.

ARRHYTHMOGENIC MECHANISMS[3–5]

Many factors in isolation or combination give rise to the substrate of arrhythmogenesis (**Fig. 22.3**). Arrhythmia may arise from abnormalities of impulse generation or conduction. **Table 22.2** demonstrates the relationship between mechanism and type of arrhythmia, and desired antiarrhythmic effect.

ABNORMAL IMPULSE GENERATION (TABLE 22.3)

ENHANCED NORMAL AUTOMATICITY

Automaticity is the property of spontaneous impulse generation by cardiac myocytes. This results from spontaneous depolarisation during phase 4. In the SA node and subsidiary pacemaker myocytes phase 4 spontaneous depolarisation results from an inward current, predominantly Na^+ via the non-selective cation channel I_f. SA node discharge rate is influenced by changes to

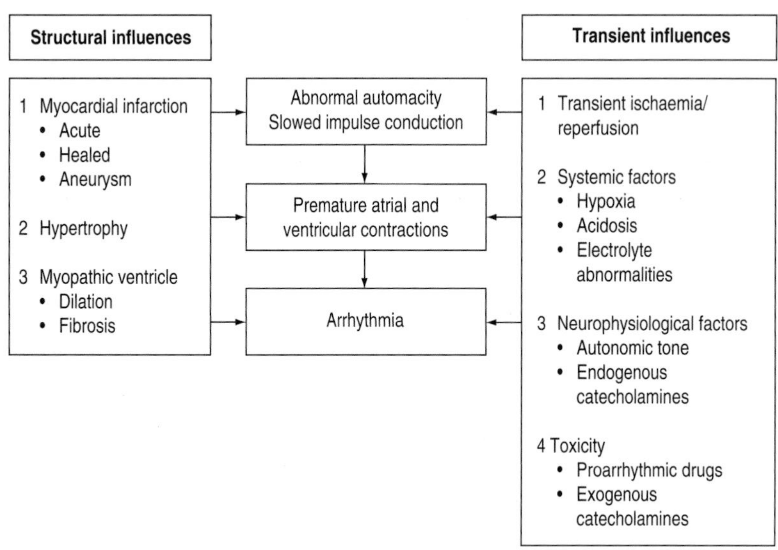

Figure 22.3 Factors that combine to form the substrate of arrhythmogenesis.

channel activity. Beta-adrenergic receptor stimulation increases both I_f and $I_{Ca\text{-}T}$ conductance and rate of phase 4 depolarisation by channel phosphorylation, whereas M_2 receptor increases I_k activity during phase 3 and early phase 4 to hyperpolarise myocytes, increasing time to reach depolarisation threshold.

Enhanced normal automaticity of subsidiary atrial pacemakers, for example around pulmonary veins, is an increasingly recognised cause of atrial fibrillation (AF).

ABNORMAL AUTOMATICITY

Abnormal automaticity is the mechanism by which spontaneous impulses are generated in myocytes that are partially depolarised by a pathological process. The less negative resting membrane potential (RMP) is associated with inactivation of the normal ionic currents of phase 4 depolarisation and the pacemaker current results from inward Na^+ and Ca^{2+} currents and is not readily susceptible to overdrive suppression from normal pacemaker activity. Due to this less negative membrane potential, these abnormal automatic myocytes inactivate the phase 0 fast inward Na^+ current, resulting in an impaired rate of impulse conduction (as well as contractility), which further contributes to arrhythmia. In this setting, Ca^{2+} carries the major inward current on depolarisation in these myocytes.

TRIGGERED ACTIVITY

Abnormal impulse generation from triggered activity originates from oscillations in the membrane potential that are initiated or triggered by a preceding action potential. There are two types of oscillations: EAD and DAD. EAD occurs during phase 2 or 3 of the action potential, whereas DAD occurs after the termination of depolarisation. The signal-averaged electrocardiograph (ECG) can detect after-depolarisations.

1. EADs appear as sub-threshold humps during the plateau or depolarisation phases. On reaching threshold, single or multiple action potentials can be induced. Plateau EADs are caused by an increased inward Ca^{2+} current (at this level of membrane potential, fast inward Na^+ channels are inactivated) and produce slow rising and propagating action potentials. Phase 3 EADs are caused by a reduction in outward K^+ currents and produce relatively rapidly rising and propagating action potentials. EAD amplitude and likelihood of triggered arrhythmia increase as driving rate decreases and action potential is prolonged. Tachyarrhythmia induced by EAD is more likely to occur on the background of a bradycardia.
2. DADs are produced by Na^+–Ca^{2+} exchanger current-induced oscillations in inward calcium current. These oscillations are caused by $[Ca^{2+}]_i$ overload saturating sarcoplasmic reticulum sequestration mechanisms, thereby leading to Ca^{2+}-induced Ca^{2+} release. Unlike EADs, DADs depend on previous rapid rhythm for their initiation.

ABNORMAL IMPULSE CONDUCTION[6]

Normal cardiac rhythm is dependent on orderly homogeneous conduction throughout atrial and ventricular tissue. This orderly homogeneity of impulse conduction can be lost by abnormal physical barriers to conduction such as infarction scars or functional disturbances in action potential leading to heterogeneity of impulse propagation. Magnitude and rate of depolarisation, presence of slow-response myocyte characteristics and rapidity of repolarisation influence speed of propagation. Functional disturbances in these properties are readily produced by channel receptor

Table 22.2 Classification of mechanisms of arrhythmia and desired antiarrhythmic drug action[3]

MECHANISM OF ARRHYTHMIA	ARRHYTHMIA	ANTIARRHYTHMIC EFFECT	REPRESENTATIVE DRUGS
AUTOMATICITY ENHANCED			
Normal	Inappropriate sinus tachycardia Unifocal atrial tachycardia	Decrease phase 4 depolarisation	Beta blocker Sodium channel blockers
Abnormal	Unifocal atrial tachycardia Accelerated idioventricular rhythms VT post myocardial infarction	Hyperpolarise or decrease phase 4 depolarisation	Calcium or sodium channel blockers M_2 agonists (muscarinic receptor)
TRIGGERED ACTIVITY			
Early after-depolarisation (EAD)	Torsade de pointes Digitalis-induced arrhythmias Some VT	Shorten action potential or suppress EAD	Increase heart rate with beta agonists or vagolytic agents, calcium channel blockers, beta blockers or magnesium
Delayed after-depolarisation (DAD)		Decrease calcium overload or suppress DAD	Calcium or sodium channel blockers, beta blockers, adenosine
RE-ENTRY: SODIUM CHANNEL DEPENDENT			
Long excitable gap	Afl type 1 Circus movement tachycardia in Wolff–Parkinson–White syndrome (WPW) Monomorphic VT	Depress conduction and excitability Prolong refractory period	Sodium channel blockers Potassium channel blockers
Short excitable gap	Afl type 2 Atrial fibrillation Circus movement tachycardia in WPW Polymorphic and monomorphic VT Bundle branch re-entry Ventricular fibrillation		
RE-ENTRY: CALCIUM CHANNEL DEPENDENT			
	Atrioventricular nodal re-entrant tachycardia Circus movement tachycardia in WPW VT	Depress conduction and excitability	Calcium channel blockers

Table 22.3 Causes of abnormal impulse generation

Enhanced normal automaticity	Adrenergic stimulation
Abnormal automaticity	Ischaemia
Early after-depolarisations	Hypoxia Hypercapnia Catecholamines Class IA antiarrhythmic drugs Class III antiarrhythmic drugs Other drugs that prolong repolarisation
Delayed after-depolarisations	Digoxin toxicity Increased intracellular Na^+ Decreased extracellular K^+ Increased intracellular Ca^{2+} Intracellular Ca^{2+} overload due to myocardial infarction or reperfusion after ischaemia

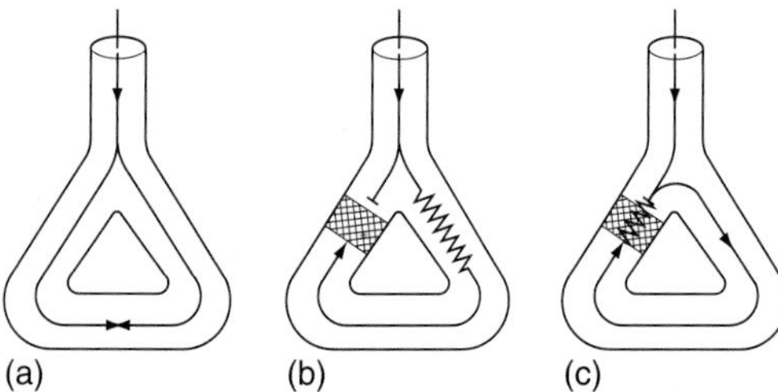

Figure 22.4 Re-entrant excitation. (a) Normal cardiac impulse conduction results in the impulse being extinguished. (b) Conduction down one limb is blocked by segment of refractory tissue (excitable gap). (c) The impulse is conducted back up the limb and arrives at the excitable gap, which has recovered from refractoriness and retrograde conduction is complete. If geometry and electrical properties are favourable, the excitable gap circulates around the re-entry loop and arrhythmia is initiated.

activation, ischaemia, hypertrophy and channel genetic mutation or expression.

Heterogeneity of impulse conduction may cause an arrhythmia by the phenomenon of re-entry. Re-entry describes the re-excitation of an area or entire heart by a circulating impulse. Although the classic 'bifurcating Purkinje fibre' model of Schmitt and Erlanger has given way to a much more complex picture, the essential electrophysiological requirements for re-entrant excitation remain. Requirements for re-entry are (**Fig. 22.4**):

- conduction block in one limb of the circuit
- slowed conduction in the other limb
- the impulse returns back along the limb initially blocked to re-enter and re-excite the pathway proximal to the block and complete the re-entry pathway.

When these properties are present, the chance of a circulating impulse producing re-entrant excitation depends on pathway geometry, the electrical properties and length of the depressed area and conduction velocity within each component. The segment of the re-entry pathway that is initially refractory and therefore blocks conduction down one limb and then recovers in time to conduct the return impulse is termed the 'excitable gap'. Therefore, the generation and subsequent maintenance of a circuit depend on this excitable gap of non-refractory tissue circulating between the advancing depolarising wave front and the repolarising tail. The resulting re-entrant impulse can be self-terminating; causing ectopic beats, or leads to atrial or ventricular tachyarrhythmia.

Risk of re-entry can be further modeled and quantified. Cardiac wavelength (λ) is the physical distance an electrical impulse travels in one refractory period; λ equals conduction velocity×refractory period (or action potential duration). Re-entry is critically dependent on the λ being shorter than the potential reentrant pathway. If λ exceeds the path length then the advancing impulse encroaches on the refractory tail and re-entry is terminated. Reducing λ (decreasing conduction velocity or refractory period) promotes re-entry circuits.

Re-entry may be terminated by:

- *increasing conduction velocity:* the excitable gap is abolished by the wave front arriving too early and meeting refractory tissue
- *increasing refractory period:* the excitable gap is lost
- *slowing conduction:* a unidirectional block can be converted into a complete block.

Ordered re-entry occurs along anatomical pathways which are 'macroscopic' loops (macro-re-entry), as in Wolff–Parkinson–White (WPW) syndrome. Functional circuits can be created following myocardial infarction, resulting in VT. 'Microscopic' loops (micro-re-entry) occur at the level of single fibres where antegrade and retrograde impulse propagation occurs in parallel fibres. Random re-entry refers to the generation of a circulating impulse, not from a fixed circuit but from constantly changing electrophysiologically distinct fibres or pathways created by the circulating impulse, resulting in AF or VF.

The cellular properties that lead to impaired conduction include:

- inactivation of the phase 0 fast Na^+ channels, which reduces both the magnitude and rate of propagation of any resultant action potential
- intercellular uncoupling, which increases resistance to action potential propagation and slows conduction. Intercellular coupling is reduced by ischaemia, $[Ca^{2+}]_i$ overload, acidosis and reduced expression of intercellular ion channel connexin proteins in diseases such as chronic heart failure.

ELECTROPHYSIOLOGICAL EFFECTS OF ISCHAEMIA

Both hypoxia and acidosis are implicated in the production of a less negative RMP in ischaemia. A rise in extracellular K^+ results from impairment of the adenosine triphosphate (ATP)-dependent K^+ inward channels. As $[K^+]_o/[K^+]_i$ is the major determinant of the RMP, intracellular K^+ loss results in a less negative RMP.

The consequences of this are:

- abnormal automaticity
- inactivation of the fast inward Na^+ channels, which slows the conduction velocity.

ELECTROLYTE ABNORMALITIES AND ARRHYTHMIA[7]

POTASSIUM

Hyper- and hypokalaemia both cause arrhythmia mediated by the resultant changes in RMP (**Table 22.4**).

Table 22.4 Arrhythmogenic effects of potassium disturbance

	ARRHYTHMOGENIC EFFECTS	ELECTROCARDIOGRAM CHANGES	ARRHYTHMIA
HYPERKALAEMIA	Less negative RMP Inactivation of fast Na^+ channels Slowed conduction velocity	Peaked T-waves Widening of P-wave and QRS complex	Sinus node suppression Atrioventricular block Ventricular fibrillation
HYPOKALAEMIA	Prolongation of rapid repolarisation Hyperpolarisation of RMP Increased pacemaker activity in Purkinje and ventricular fibres	U-waves ST-segment and T-wave changes	Atrial and ventricular ectopy Atrial and ventricular tachyarrhythmia Ventricular fibrillation

RMP=resting membrane potential.

In ischaemia, hyperkalaemia at the local tissue level caused by a pathological extracellular shift of K^+ is the major factor contributing to ventricular arrhythmia in this setting. In hypokalaemia, the dispersion of pacemaker activity and the effect on repolarisation are similar to the electrophysiological effects of cardiac glycosides and beta-adrenergic agonists, and it is not surprising that a combination of these factors is associated with an increased incidence of arrhythmia. The increased risk of death in hypertensive patients treated with thiazide diuretics has been attributed to hypokalaemia (and possibly hypomagnesaemia)-induced arrhythmia (Multiple Risk Factor Intervention Trial). Thiazide-induced hypokalaemia ventricular ectopy is worsened by exercise.[8] Hypokalaemia is associated with VF and VT following acute myocardial infarction (AMI). The increased incidence of VF/with a serum K^+ less than 3.5 mmol/L is clearly established and the probability of VT increases as the serum K^+ decreases. During AMI the incidence of VF/VT was 15% at 4.5 mmol/L, 38% at 3.5 mmol/L, 55% at 3.0 mmol/L and 67% at 2.5 mmol/L.[9]

MAGNESIUM

The antiarrhythmic properties of Mg^{2+} are clearly established, but a causal relationship between hypomagnesaemia and arrhythmia is largely circumstantial. Decreased extracellular Mg^{2+} by itself has little effect on the electrophysiological properties of myocytes or the ECG. Hypomagnesaemia has been implicated in the genesis of VT/VF in patients with hypertension and heart failure receiving thiazide or loop diuretics, acute alcohol intoxication or withdrawal and possibly with AMI. The product of K^+ and Mg^{2+} is the best predictor of arrhythmia in hypertensive patients taking thiazide diuretics.[10]

AUTONOMIC NERVOUS SYSTEM AND VENTRICULAR ARRHYTHMIA[11]

The autonomic nervous system, particularly vagal tone, has a significant effect on the occurrence of post myocardial infarction VF, as seen by the following:

- High vagal tone is associated with better outcome and less susceptibility to exercise-induced VF with new ischaemia in animal models.
- Post myocardial infarction exercise training results in an increased vagal tone, which inhibits induceable VF.
- Implantable electrical vagal stimulation and muscarinic agents, including edrophonium, are protective.
- The protection is not heart rate related as the protection remains even when atrial pacing is used to maintain the heart rate.
- The administration of atropine increases the likelihood of developing VF.

Vagal tone can be measured by variability in the heart rate (RR interval) or blood pressure rise induced by the pressor agent phenylephrine. Heart rate variability is considered a measure of tonic vagal activity whereas the phenylephrine method is considered a measure of magnitude of the vagal reflex in response to stimulus. A reduced vagal tone has been found post infarction in humans, which returns to normal over a 3–6-month period. There is no relationship between vagal tone and ejection fraction and the origin of reduced vagal tone post infarction appears to be due to afferent stimulation in response to necrotic tissue and impaired cardiac contractile geometry. This reduced vagal tone has also been shown to be predictive of mortality and inductility of arrhythmia at electrophysiological study (EPS).

HETEROGENEITY OF REPOLARISATION: T-WAVE ALTERNANS[12]

Regional differences in repolarisation are associated with preconditions for conduction block, re-entry and life-threatening arrhythmias. This heterogeneity is seen in settings of impaired sarcoplasmic reticulum uptake of Ca^{2+} during ischaemia, drug proarrhythmia and congenital prolonged QT syndromes. In addition to prolonged QTc, ECG changes show variability of T-waves. This variability can manifest as visible T-wave alternans (TWA), defined as a beat-to-beat alternation in the morphology and amplitude of the ST segment or T-wave (**Fig. 22.5**).

Computerised analytical methods for detecting non-visual TWA in the microvolt range have been developed for predicting risk of ventricular tachyarrhythmia, sudden death and need for implantable cardioverter-defibrillators. The utility of TWA appears to be better than left ventricular function. TWA can be quantified as the moving average of beat-to-beat variation in T-wave amplitude (**Fig. 22.6**).

TWA may find a role in guiding drug therapy as a marker of antiarrhythmic effect and proarrhythmia.

PROARRHYTHMIC EFFECTS OF ANTIARRHYTHMIC DRUGS[13,14]

Accompanying proarrhythmia with the use of antiarrhythmic drugs is increasingly recognised. The 'quinidine syncope' due to VF and polymorphic VT at therapeutic concentrations was also seen with disopyramide. The Cardiac Arrhythmia Suppression Trial (CAST) clearly defined the magnitude of this deleterious side-effect in drugs that were previously perceived to be of benefit.[15] This study, which involved flecainide, encainide and morizicine (a class IA drug), was terminated early because of adverse outcome in the flecainide and encainide groups (relative risk of arrhythmic death or non-fatal cardiac arrest of 3.6, 95% confidence interval (CI) 1.7–8.5). Proarrhythmia is reported between 5.9% and 15.8% depending on agent, clinical setting and definition of proarrhythmia, and now considered ubiquitous with all antiarrhythmic drugs.

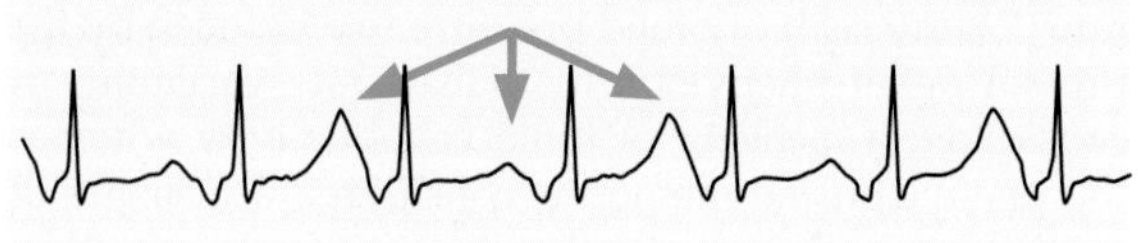

Figure 22.5 Visible T-wave alternans and prolonged QT associated with heterogeneity of repolarisation.

Proarrhythmia has been defined as an increase in frequency of ventricular ectopic beat (VEB) or aggravation of the target arrhythmia on Holter monitor or exercise test. Manifestations of proarrhythmia not only include VEB, monomorphic and polymorphic VT and VF, but also bradyarrhythmias and Afl with 1:1 AV conduction. Most proarrhythmic events occur soon after starting the drug, but late arrhythmias are also a significant problem.

Proarrhythmia appears to be correlated with the degree of drug-induced QT prolongation, T-wave variability and characteristics of sodium channel blockade by the agent involved. Sodium-channel-blocking agents with a long time constant for recovery of the sodium channel blockade cause more pronounced blockade, even at slow heart rates, slow conduction to a greater extent and are associated with greater proarrhythmia. Agents with a short time constant of sodium channel blockade, where sodium channel blockade is more pronounced at fast heart rates (e.g. class IB: lidocaine and mexiletine), are less proarrhythmic than drugs with long time constants (e.g. class IC: flecainide and propafenone). Class III drugs and quinidine proarrhythmia correlate with degree of QT prolongation.

The mechanism of drug proarrhythmia is probably via both slowing of conduction and abnormal automaticity. Paradoxically slowing conduction, which may block a re-entry circuit, may also create the very substrate needed for re-entry, unidirectional block and an excitable gap. The existence of a re-entrant circuit requires the circulating wave front of the impulse not to catch up with the refractory tissue behind the

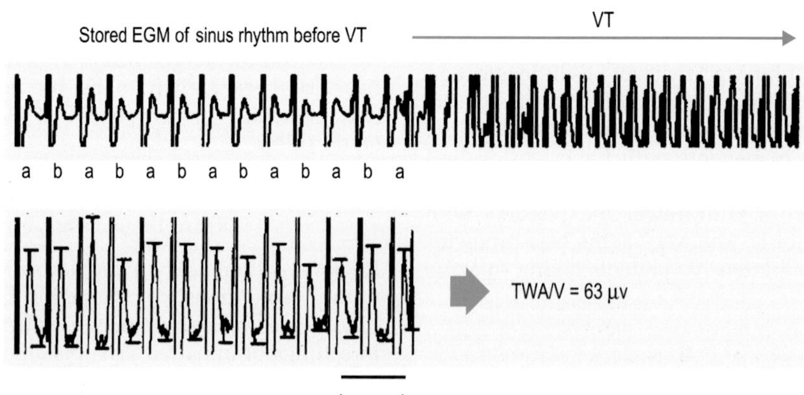

Figure 22.6 Example of heterogeneous repolarisation resulting in beat-to-beat microvolt fluctuation in T-wave amplitude measured by the Modified Moving Average method at 63 microvolts heralds the onset of ventricular tachycardia. *(From American Heart Association, with permission.)*

tail. Re-entry is more likely to occur with a shorter refractory period and reduced conduction velocity (**Fig. 22.7**).[11]

Increasing conduction velocity is an ideal antiarrhythmic property but there are no antiarrhythmic drugs that accelerate conduction. However antiarrhythmic drugs readily slow conduction and the degree of conduction slowing and therefore proarrhythmia tendency correlates with the potency of antiarrhythmic properties.

Prolonging the refractory period is also an ideal antiarrhythmic property, which increases the likelihood of abolishing any excitable gap by ensuring the wave front of a re-entrant circuit meets refractory tissue. The potency of class IA and III antiarrhythmic agents is dependent on the prolongation of the refractory period. This property is also protective against proarrhythmia due to re-entry mechanism. The effect of class IB agents on shortening the refractory period will contribute to proarrhythmia by this mechanism in this class.

Surface mapping of the heart has been used to quantify proarrhythmic effect. The scale of potency of proarrhythmia has been found to be:

flecainide > propafenone > quinidine > disopyramide > procainamide > mexiletine > lidocaine > sotalol.

Amiodarone was not included in this study but presumably its proarrhythmic potential is similar to other class III agents and less than the class I agents.

Antiarrhythmic drugs are effective at suppressing abnormal automaticity, with the exception of triggered automaticity due to EAD. Class IA, class III and many non-antiarrhythmic drugs can produce proarrhythmia via EAD. These drugs increase not only the frequency of EAD, but also the likelihood of them leading to triggered tachyarrhythmia. Slowing repolarisation, which leads to QT prolongation and slower heart rate, is central to this increased frequency and sensitivity to EAD. EAD manifests as prominent and bizarre T-U waves on the ECG and, if triggered activity results, VEB and ventricular tachyarrhythmia may occur. Torsade de pointes is the classical resulting arrhythmia, although less classical polymorphic VT and VF can result. Risk of proarrhythmia via this mechanism correlates with the degree of QT prolongation.

All antiarrhythmic drugs are capable of producing bradyarrhythmia via decreasing normal automaticity and slowing conduction. Digoxin can be proarrhythmic via the production of triggered activity due to DAD.

Antiarrhythmic drug proarrhythmia is facilitated by several factors, which are frequently found in patients on antiarrhythmic drugs or with heart disease (**Box 22.1**).

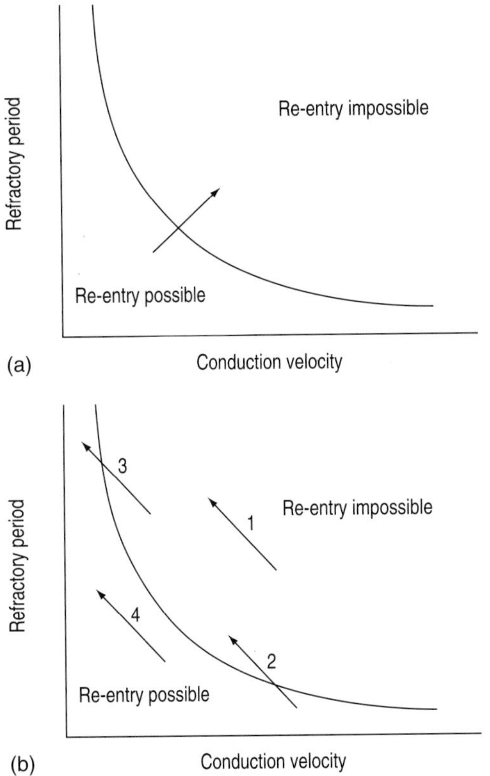

Figure 22.7 (a) Graph of refractory period of an excitable gap versus its conduction velocity around a theoretical re-entrant circuit. When conduction velocity is high enough so that refractory period of excitable gap exceeds circuit time, re-entry is impossible. Arrow demonstrates the action of an 'ideal' antiarrhythmic drug, which prolongs the refractory period and increases conduction velocity. (b) With antiarrhythmic drugs that increase the refractory period and slow conduction, the net effect of an antiarrhythmic drug may have no effect on proarrhythmia (arrows 1 and 4), decrease proarrhythmia (arrow 2) or increase proarrhythmia (arrow 3) depending on properties of a potential re-entrant circuit. *(Adapted from Schwartz PJ, La Rovere MT, Vanoli E. Autonomic nervous system and sudden cardiac death. Circulation 1992;85(Suppl 1):77–91, with permission.)*

Box 22.1 Factors facilitating antiarrhythmic drug proarrhythmia[13]

- Toxic blood levels due to excessive dose or reduced clearance from old age, heart failure, renal disease or hepatic disease
- Severe left ventricular dysfunction; ejection fraction less than 35%
- Pre-existing arrhythmia or arrhythmia substrate
- Digoxin therapy
- Hypokalaemia or hypomagnesaemia
- Bradycardia
- Combinations of antiarrhythmic drugs and concomitant drugs with similar toxicity

MANAGEMENT OF THE PATIENT WITH A CARDIAC ARRHYTHMIA

HISTORY AND PHYSICAL EXAMINATION

A careful history is important. Specific questions should confirm or exclude palpitations, syncope, chest pain, shortness of breath, ischaemic heart disease (especially previous myocardial infarction), congestive cardiac failure, valvular heart disease, thyrotoxicosis and diuretic therapy without adequate potassium supplements. A family history is helpful for arrhythmias associated with inherited disorders (e.g. LQTS and hypertrophic obstructive cardiomyopathy). The physical examination looks for underlying structural heart disease and signs to assist diagnosis, and assesses haemodynamic consequences of the arrhythmia.

VAGAL MANOEUVRES

Vagal manoeuvres may be undertaken during examination. These reflexly increase vagal tone, thereby prolonging AV node conduction and refractoriness. The effect may be:

- transient slowing of sinus tachycardia as SA nodal discharge rate is slowed
- termination of AV nodal re-entry tachycardia (AVNRT) and AV re-entry tachycardia (AVRT)
- unmasking (but not reversion) of atrial tachycardia, flutter (**Fig. 22.8**) and fibrillation.

VT is not affected. Carotid sinus massage has been most commonly used. Valsalva manoeuvre or iced water to the face may be useful. Eyeball pressure should be avoided as eye damage may result.

Increasingly the Valsalva manoeuvre is recommended. Maximum vagal effect is achieved with supine positioning and a Valsalva manoeuvre of 15 seconds duration and a pressure of 40 mmHg (5.32 kPa) with an open glottis. An adequate Valsalva manoeuvre method can be achieved by getting the patient to blow into a 10 mL syringe in an attempt to move the plunger.

INVESTIGATIONS

A 12-lead ECG should be recorded with a longer rhythm strip (usually lead II or V_1). If P-waves are not visible, atrial activity may be recorded using an oesophageal electrode or pacing lead, or via a central venous catheter or the right atrial injectate port of a pulmonary artery catheter, using 20% saline and a bedside monitor.[16]

Holter monitoring requires prolonged (usually 24–72 hours), non-invasive, ambulatory ECG monitoring, sometimes combined with exercise testing. EPS, which involves invasive electrophysiological testing with programmed electrical stimulation, attempts to reproduce the spontaneously occurring arrhythmia.[17,18] EPS is not clearly superior to Holter monitoring in evaluating drug treatment for ventricular arrhythmias. Other investigative techniques being studied include signal-averaged ECG, heart rate variability and electrical alternans measurement.[11,19]

MANAGEMENT OF SPECIFIC ARRHYTHMIAS

Treatment has two aspects: acute termination of the arrhythmia and long-term prophylaxis. The decision whether to treat depends on the rhythm diagnosis, haemodynamic consequences, aetiology of the arrhythmia and the prognosis (e.g. risks of sudden death or long-term complications).

ECTOPIC BEATS

These are premature impulses originating from the atria, AV junction or ventricles. The coupling interval (time between the ectopic and the preceding beat) is shorter than the cycle duration of the dominant rhythm.

PREMATURE VENTRICULAR ECTOPIC BEATS

These are also known as ventricular premature beats and ventricular premature complexes. The ventricle is not activated by the normal rapidly conducting bundle branches, and a wide QRS complex results from slow ventricular conduction.

ECG

There is no preceding P-wave.

- Premature complexes occur before the next expected QRS.
- QRS is wide (>120 ms).

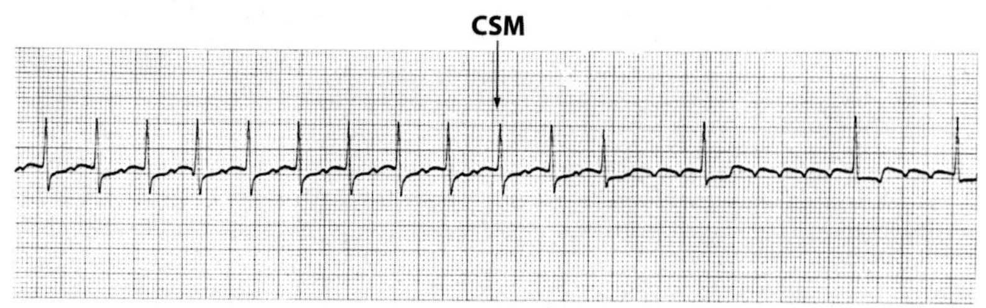

Figure 22.8 Atrial flutter with 2:1 atrioventricular (AV) block. Carotid sinus massage (CSM) increases AV block to 4:1 then 6:1.

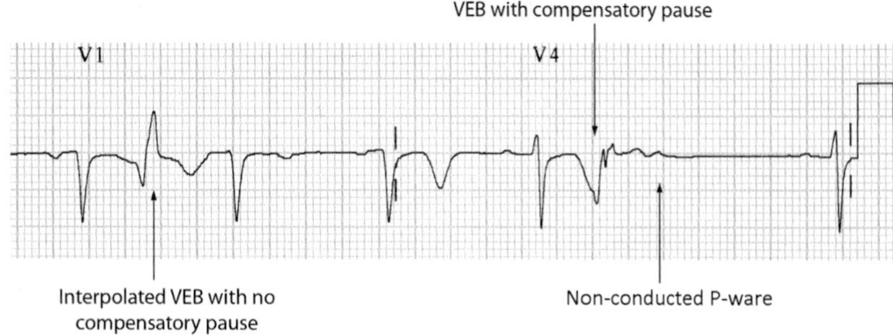

Figure 22.9 Sinus rhythm with an interpolated ventricular ectopic beat (VEB) without a compensatory pause and a VEB with a following non-conducted P-wave, resulting in a compensatory pause.

- T-wave of opposite polarity to the QRS (**Fig. 22.9**).
- VEB is not conducted retrogradely to the SA node.
- SA node is therefore not reset, and there is temporary AV dissociation with a full compensatory pause; the interval between the normal QRS complexes on either side of the VEB will usually be twice that of the dominant sinus rhythm.

Occasionally VEBs may not produce any pause, and are said to be interpolated (see Fig. 22.9). Interpolated VEBs occur when the background sinus rhythm is slow. The retrograde conduction into the AV node renders it partially refractory to the next impulse and its conduction through the AV node is slowed and the PR interval is prolonged. A VEB following each sinus beat is ventricular bigeminy. Ventricular trigeminy refers to recurring sequences of a VEB followed by two sinus beats. Two VEBs in succession are a couplet, and three, a triplet.

CLINICAL

Even when frequent, complex, or in short runs of non-sustained VT, VEBs are not associated with risk of sudden death in asymptomatic healthy adults.[20] However, there is increased risk of cardiovascular death with:

- *exercise-induced VEB:* risk of death 2.53 (95% CI 1.65–3.88)[21]
- *AMI and VEB:* frequent and complex VEBs often precede VF or sustained VT and are a marker of risk of subsequent SCD.

Apart from ischaemic heart disease, VEB may be associated with cardiomyopathy, valvular disease, myocarditis and non-cardiac precipitating factors (e.g. electrolyte and acid–base disturbances, hypoxia and drugs such as digoxin).

TREATMENT

Drug treatment of VEB is rarely indicated and may be dangerous.

- Correct potassium and magnesium.
- Severely symptomatic patients with frequent complex VEB may benefit from judicious beta blockade.
- The underlying cause of VEB is often more clinically relevant than the arrhythmia. Following myocardial infarction, beta-adrenergic blockers, which are indicated for long-term benefit, will also likely suppress VEB.
- Prophylactic lidocaine following AMI will increase total mortality and has been abandoned.[22,23]
- Attempts at long-term VEB suppression with class IC agents (flecainide and encainide), even if successful, increase mortality.[15]

Box 22.2 Classification of supraventricular tachycardia

Atrioventricular (AV) node dependent
AV nodal re-entry tachycardia: re-entry within the AV node
AV re-entry tachycardia: re-entry includes accessory pathway between atria and ventricles
Accelerated idionodal rhythm: increased automaticity of AV node
AV node independent
Atrial flutter: re-entry confined to atria
Atrial fibrillation: multiple re-entry circuits confined to atria
Unifocal atrial tachycardia: usually due to increased automaticity
Multifocal atrial tachycardia: increased automaticity or triggered activity
Others: sinus node re-entry tachycardia

SUPRAVENTRICULAR TACHYCARDIAS[24,25] (BOX 22.2)

Supraventricular tachycardia (SVT) is any tachycardia that requires atrial or AV nodal tissue for initiation and maintenance.

- SVTs are usually conducted rapidly through the bundle branches so that QRS complexes are narrow.
- All narrow-complex tachycardia are SVT and wide-complex tachycardia are usually ventricular.
- However, SVT may be wide complex in the setting of bundle branch block (BBB) and pre-excitation.

A clinically useful classification divides SVTs into AV node-dependent and AV node-independent. Distinguishing between AV node-dependent and independent SVTs can be difficult. Vagal manoeuvres or drugs that prolong AV nodal refractoriness (e.g. adenosine) may assist in diagnosis:

- Temporary AV block with unchanged atrial rate indicates AV node independence.
- Slowing or reversion of the tachycardia diagnoses AV dependence.

AV NODE-DEPENDENT SVT

In these SVTs, sometimes referred to as junctional tachycardia, the re-entry circuit or ectopic focus involves the AV node or junction. Blocking the AV node with drugs such as adenosine or vagal manoeuvres will terminate these SVTs.

AV NODE-INDEPENDENT SVT

Also referred to as atrial tachycardia, the atrial tissue only is required for the initiation and maintenance of the tachycardia. Blocking the AV node will not terminate these SVTs; it will merely slow the ventricular rate.

AV NODAL RE-ENTRY TACHYCARDIA (AVNRT) (**FIG. 22.10**)

Re-entry tachycardia is confined to the AV node. Antegrade conduction to the ventricles usually occurs over the slow pathway and retrograde conduction over the fast pathway.

ECG

There is regular narrow-complex tachycardia (140–220 beats/min) with abrupt onset and termination. P-waves are not usually observed as they are buried in the QRS complexes (**Fig. 22.11**).

CLINICAL

AVNRT is a common arrhythmia that is not usually associated with structural heart disease. The major symptom is palpitations.

TREATMENT

Vagal manoeuvres slow conduction through the AV node and may 'break' the tachycardia. If vagal manoeuvres fail, adenosine is the drug of choice and nearly all AVNRT will revert with adenosine.[23,26] Verapamil has been used in the past, but causes hypotension, which may be prolonged if cardiac function is depressed or patients are receiving beta-adrenergic blockers. Sotalol, amiodarone and flecainide may also be effective but are rarely used. Rapid atrial pacing will usually terminate AVNRT but is rarely needed.

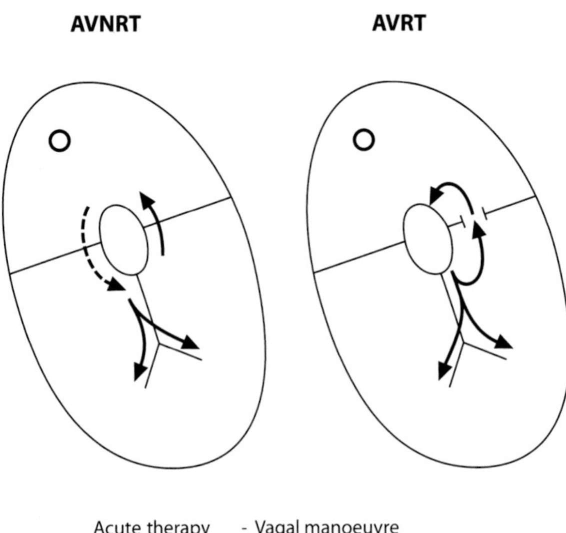

Acute therapy
- Vagal manoeuvre
- Adenosine

Chronic therapy
- Catheter ablation
- β blockers
- Class Ic
- Class III

Figure 22.10 Atrioventricular nodal re-entry tachycardia (AVNRT) has both pathways in the AV node. The conduction occurs over the slow pathway and retrogradely over the fast pathway. AV re-entry tachycardia (AVRT) involves antegrade conduction through the AV node and retrograde conduction through an accessory pathway.

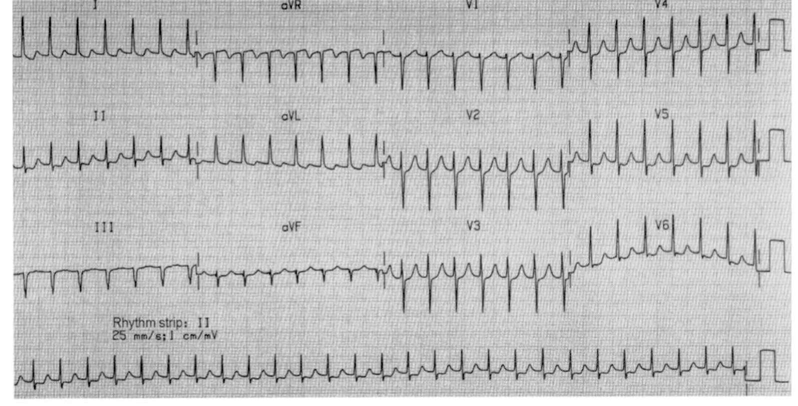

Figure 22.11 Atrioventricular nodal re-entry tachycardia (AVNRT). Narrow QRS tachycardia at 160 beats/min. P-waves are not apparent and are buried in the QRS complex.

Cardioversion is occasionally necessary when drugs are ineffective or when severe haemodynamic instability is present.

PREVENTION

Troublesome recurring episodes of AVNRT can be cured by radiofrequency ablation, using a transvenous catheter to interrupt the re-entrant circuit permanently.[27]

AV RE-ENTRY TACHYCARDIA (SEE FIG. 22.10)

The re-entry pathway consists of the AV node and an accessory pathway, which bypasses the AV node. The accessory pathway may be evident during sinus rhythm, with the ECG showing pre-excitation: short PR interval, delta wave and widening of the QRS (see WPW, below, under Pre-excitation syndrome). However, in 25% of cases, the accessory pathway conducts only retrogradely from ventricle to atria and the ECG pre-excitation will be concealed in sinus rhythm. Orthodromic AVRT, with antegrade nodal and retrograde accessory pathway circuit, is the most common regular SVT in patients with accessory pathway.

ECG

The ECG is similar to AVNRT. The length of the re-entry circuit is, however, greater and the accessory AV pathway is some distance from the AV node. It therefore takes longer for the impulse to be conducted backwards to the atria, and so the retrograde P-wave usually occurs after the QRS, sometimes at some distance, and is inverted in leads II, III and aVF (**Figs 22.12** and **22.13**).

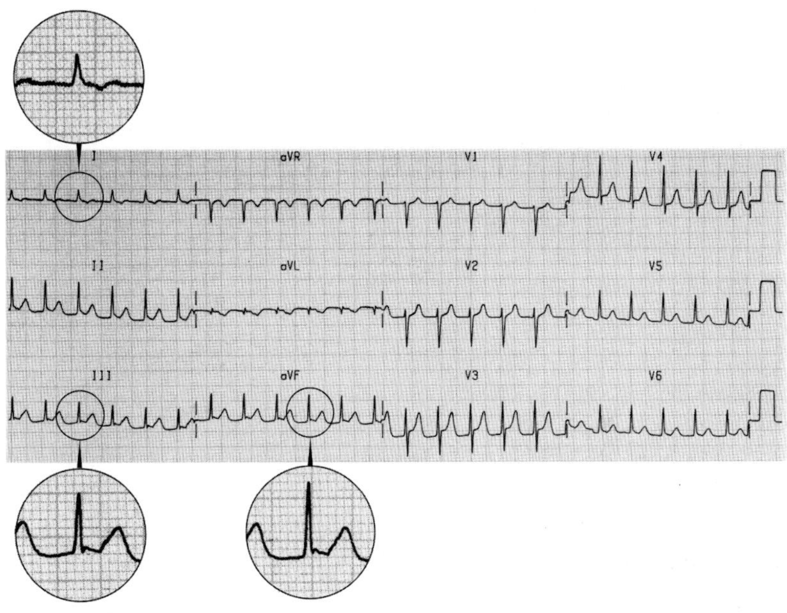

Figure 22.12 Atrioventricular re-entry tachycardia (AVRT). Narrow QRS tachycardia at 135 beats/min. Inverted P-wave in leads I, II, III and aVF just following the QRS complex.

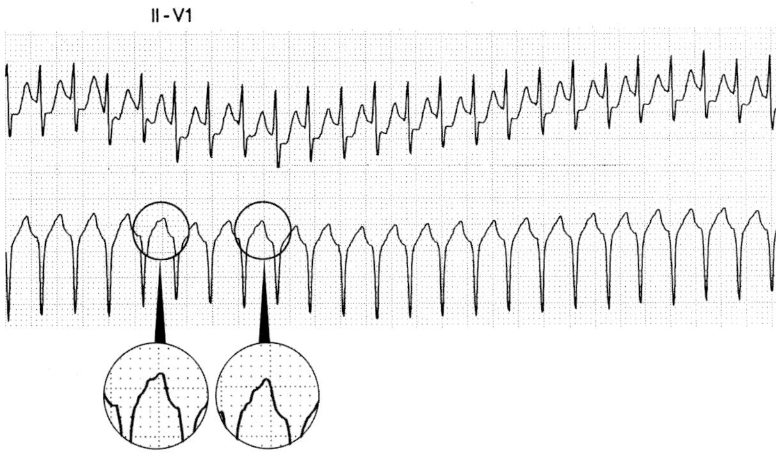

Figure 22.13 Atrioventricular re-entry tachycardia (AVRT). Rate is 214 beats/min. P-wave deflection is just seen on the upslope of the T-wave in lead V_1.

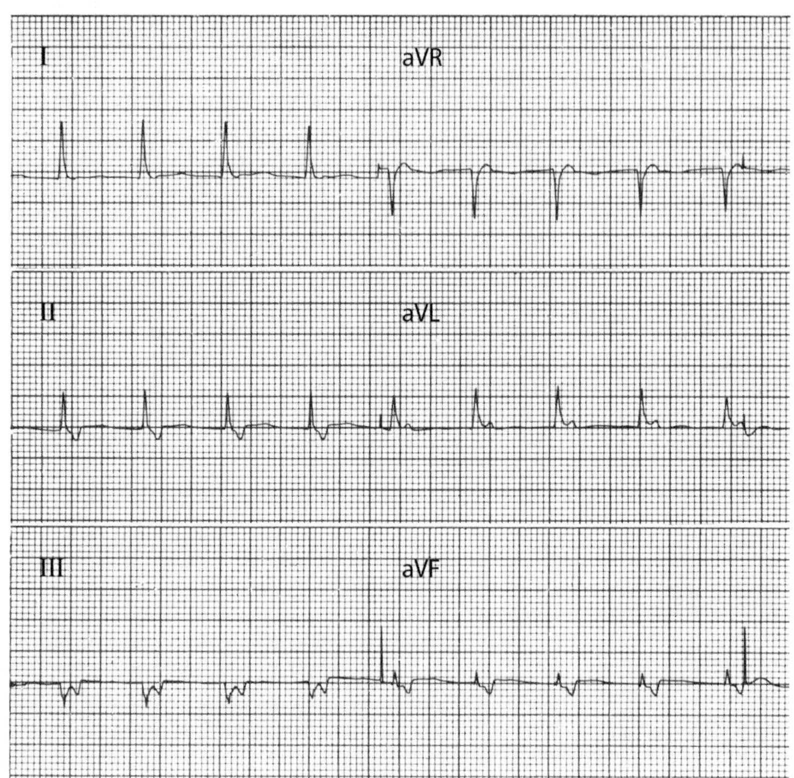

Figure 22.14 Accelerated idionodal rhythm: 105 beats/min. Inverted P-wave is immediately following the QRS complex in leads II, III and aVF.

CLINICAL

AVRT is similar to AVNRT, although antegrade conduction over the accessory pathway may be very rapid with WPW, if AF occurs.

TREATMENT[23,26]

Acute treatment is identical to AVNRT, but verapamil should be avoided in WPW syndrome, as it may block the AV node, facilitating very rapid conduction to the ventricles via the accessory pathway.[28]

PREVENTION

Drugs such as sotalol and flecainide may prevent recurrence of the tachycardia. Radiofrequency ablation of the accessory pathway is usually curative.[27]

ACCELERATED IDIONODAL RHYTHM

Increased automaticity of the AV junction (above the inherent discharge rate of 40–60 beats/min) is the usual cause of this arrhythmia. The often-used term 'non-paroxysmal AV junctional tachycardia' is cumbersome and misleading: junctional rate is commonly 60–100 beats/min, not strictly a tachycardia. AV dissociation is often present, but there may be synchronisation of the two pacemakers - so-called isorhythmic dissociation.

ECG

There are narrow complexes on the ECG at a regular rate (60–130 beats/min) (**Fig. 22.14**), often with independent atrial activity. With isorhythmic dissociation, the P-wave is either fixed relative to the QRS complex (usually just after) or oscillates to and fro across the QRS in a rhythmical manner.

CLINICAL

It may be observed in normal persons, but is often associated with structural heart disease, especially following inferior myocardial infarction. Digoxin intoxication is another important cause.

TREATMENT

In most cases, the rhythm is transient and well tolerated, and no treatment is required. Treatment is otherwise directed towards the underlying cause.

UNIFOCAL ATRIAL TACHYCARDIA

This is sometimes called ectopic atrial tachycardia to distinguish it from the atrial tachycardia (referring collectively to unifocal atrial tachycardia, Afl and AF). However, it is inappropriate to call atrial tachycardia paroxysmal atrial tachycardia. Paroxysmal, by definition, indicates an abrupt onset and termination, which

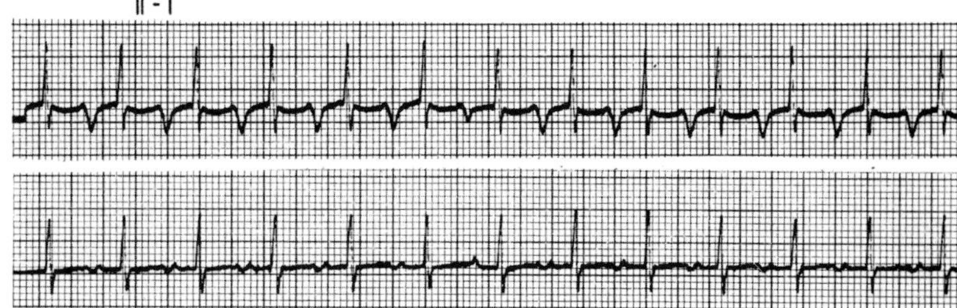

Figure 22.15 Unifocal atrial tachycardia with 1 : 1 atrioventricular conduction; rate is 140 beats/min. Large, inverted P-waves are seen in lead II.

applies less commonly to unifocal atrial tachycardia. Vagal manoeuvres will not terminate this arrhythmia, but AV block may be induced, or increased if already present.

ECG

P-wave morphology is abnormal but monomorphic. Atrial rate is often 130–160 beats/min, and may occasionally exceed 200 beats/min. Atrial rate distinguishes unifocal atrial tachycardia from atrial flutter (Afl), with Afl greater than 250 beats/min. The QRS complexes will usually be narrow (**Fig. 22.15**). AV block is common (**Fig. 22.16**).

CLINICAL

Digitalis intoxication is the most common cause, especially when AV block is present. Other causes include myocardial infarction, chronic lung disease and metabolic disturbances.

TREATMENT[23]

If applicable, digitalis is stopped and the toxicity treated. Otherwise digoxin may be used to control the ventricular rate. Beta-adrenergic blockers or amiodarone are alternatives. Rapid atrial pacing may be ineffective if the arrhythmia is due to increased automaticity, although it may increase AV block, thereby slowing ventricular rate. Synchronised DC shock may be necessary, but is avoided if digitalis intoxication is suspected.

MULTIFOCAL ATRIAL TACHYCARDIA[29]

Multifocal atrial tachycardia (MAT) is defined as an atrial rhythm, with a rate greater than 100 beats/min, with organised, discrete non-sinus P-waves having at least three different forms in the same ECG trace. The baseline between P-waves is isoelectric, and the PP, PR and RR intervals are irregular. This is an uncommon arrhythmia, also known as chaotic or mixed atrial tachycardia.

ECG

There are irregular atrial rates, usually 100–130 beats/min, with varying P-wave morphology (at least three different P-wave morphologies and varying PR interval) and some degree of AV block (**Fig. 22.17**). Most P-waves are conducted to the ventricles, usually with narrow QRS complexes.

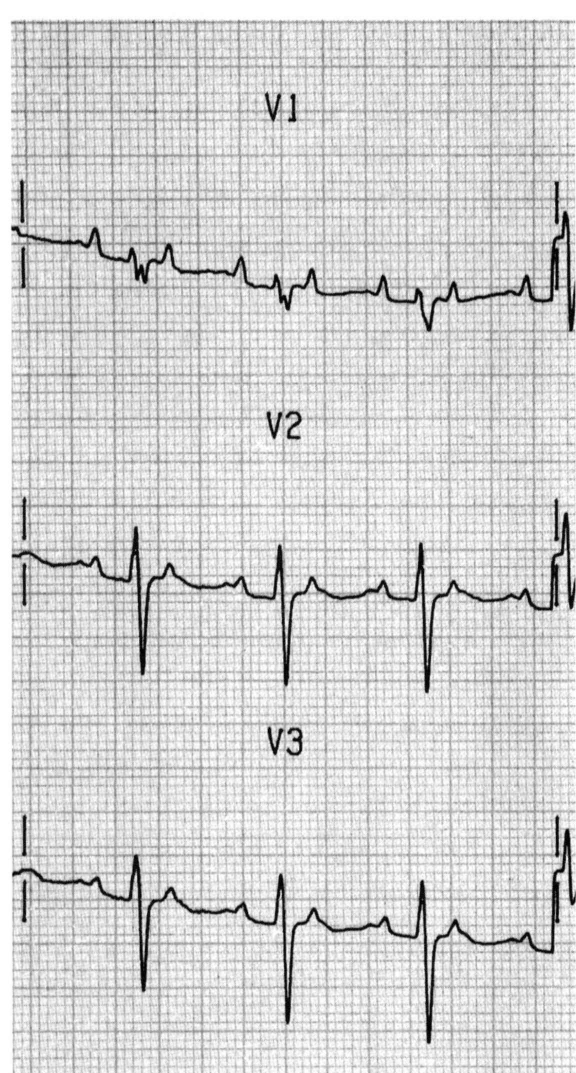

Figure 22.16 Unifocal atrial tachycardia with 2 : 1 atrioventricular conduction. Atrial rate is 170 beats/min.

CLINICAL

MAT is often misdiagnosed and inappropriately treated as AF. This rhythm occurs most commonly in critically ill elderly patients with chronic lung disease and cor pulmonale, and is associated with a very high mortality

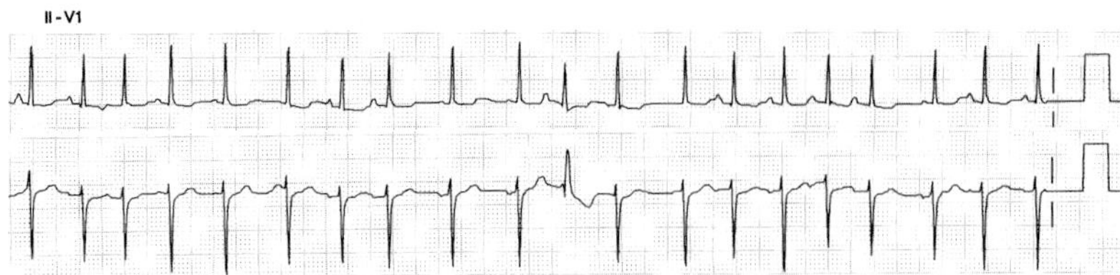

Figure 22.17 Multifocal atrial tachycardia with the rate about 130 beats/min. There is varying P-wave morphology and PR intervals. Note the wide complex preceded by a P-wave. The aberrant intraventricular conduction is related to the long–short cycle length sequence.

from underlying disease. Theophylline has been implicated as a precipitating cause, and rarely digoxin.

TREATMENT

Treatment should correct the underlying cause (e.g. treatment of cardiorespiratory failure, electrolyte and acid-base abnormalities and theophylline toxicity). Spontaneous reversion is common, and few patients require antiarrhythmic therapy. Magnesium is the drug of choice for acute control.[30] Beta blockers are probably more effective than diltiazem, but because of the common association of MAT with obstructive lung disease have limited utility.[31] Digoxin and cardioversion are ineffective, which highlights the need to differentiate MAT from AF. Longer-term control is best achieved with diltiazem in patients with good left ventricular (LV) function and amiodarone in those without.

ATRIAL FLUTTER[32,33]

Afl is an intra-atrial macro-re-entrant arrhythmia with an impulse and contraction wave circulating the atrium at rates of 250–350 beats/min, and in most cases, close to 300 beats/min. Afl occurs at about one-tenth the frequency of AF, often coexisting with AF, with 56% eventually developing AF. Afl is more common in males and incidence increases with age. Conditions associated with Afl are shown in **Box 22.3**.

AV conduction in Afl is usually 2:1, resulting in a regular rhythm, but conduction may be irregular. Rarely 1:1 AV conduction can occur and may be lethal.

Afl is classified according to the anatomical pathway of the circuit. Right atrial cavotricuspid-isthmus-dependent flutter involving a circuit bounded by tricuspid orifice, vena cavae orifices, Eustachian and crista terminalis, is overwhelmingly most common. From a left anterior oblique view, this counter-clock-wise circuit makes up 90% of Afl cases and is classically referred to as 'typical'. Circuits can also be clock-wise, involve the right atrium but with different circuits relating to scars or be located in the left atrium.

ECG

'Typical' Afl waves (characteristic sawtooth appearance with no isoelectric baseline) are best seen in V_1, and are negative in inferior leads with positive waves in V_1 that transition to negative in V_6 (**Fig. 22.18**). Rapid QRS waves may obscure typical flutter waves, and vagal manoeuvres may unmask them (see Fig. 22.8). AV conduction block (usually 2:1) is usually present, so that alternate flutter waves are conducted to the ventricles, with a ventricular rate close to 150 beats/min. Frequently flutter waves are not obvious and a ventricular rate of 150 beats/min leads to the presumption of Afl (**Fig. 22.19**). 'Non-typical' Afl, normally associated with scar or structural abnormalies often results in greater atrial and ventricular rates (**Fig. 22.20**). Treatment with drugs that affect AV node conduction may lead to higher degrees of AV block (**Fig. 22.21**) and/or variable AV block with irregular QRS duration. Afl with 1:1 conduction is associated with sympathetic overactivity, class I antiarrhythmic drugs (which slow atrial discharge rate to around 200 beats/min, thereby allowing each atrial impulse to be conducted) or Wolff–Parkinson–White syndrome and a short antegrade refractory period of the accessory pathway (**Fig. 22.22**). QRS complexes are usually narrow, as conduction through the bundle branches is normal.

Box 22.3 Conditions associated with atrial flutter

- Valvular heart disease
- Myocardial infarction
- Pericardial disease
- Cardiac tumours
- Hypertrophic cardiomyopathy
- Congenital heart disease
- Post surgical repair of congenital heart disease
- Post cardiothoracic surgery
- Post major non-cardiac surgery
- Severe pulmonary disease
- Pulmonary embolus
- Thyrotoxicosis
- Acute alcohol intoxication

TREATMENT[23,33]

Drug therapy has proven to be notoriously unsuccessful for Afl and large doses of AV blockers are often needed for rate control. Although no drug will reliably terminate Afl, ibutilide and dofetilide have been shown to be most likely to result in pharmacological reversion.

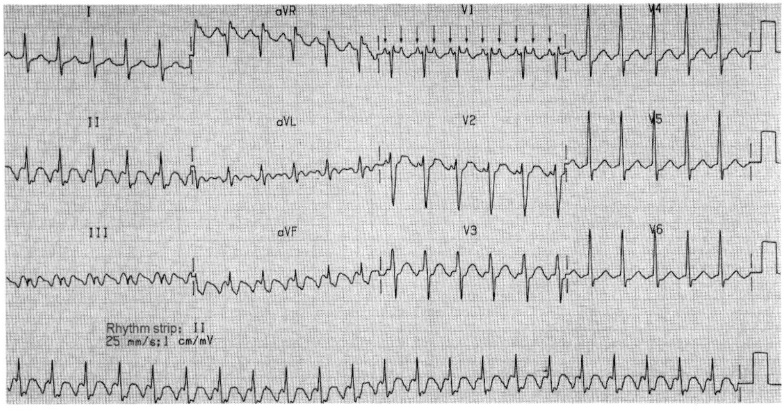

Figure 22.18 Atrial flutter with 2:1 atrioventricular conduction. Atrial rate is 270 beats/min (arrows V_1) and ventricular 135 beats/min. Characteristic 'sawtooth' inverted flutter waves are evident in leads II, III and aVF.

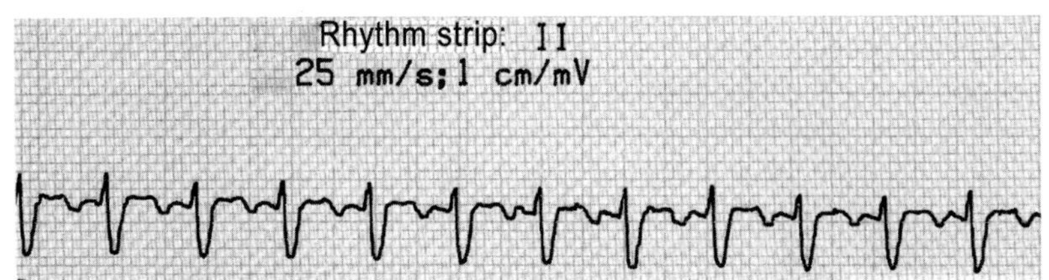

Figure 22.19 Atrial flutter with 2:1 atrioventricular (AV) conduction. Inverted flutter waves are difficult to differentiate from T-waves. Rate of 144 beats/min confirms atrial flutter with 2:1 AV conduction.

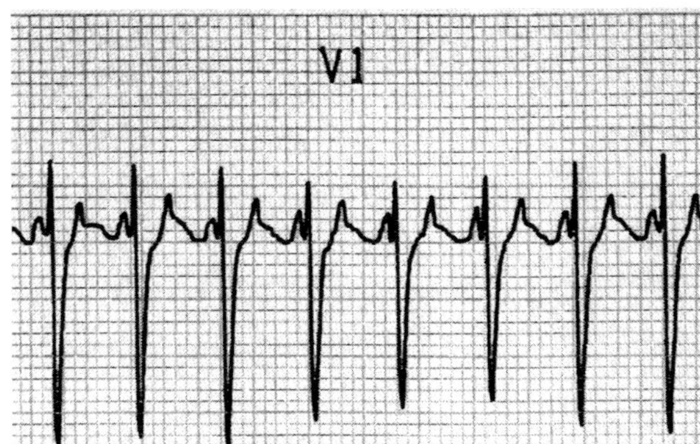

Figure 22.20 Atrial flutter with 2:1 atrioventricular conduction. Type II atrial flutter is confirmed by the rapid atrial rate of 380 beats/min.

Flecainide and procainamide may also occasionally be effective at terminating Afl. Initial attempts at slowing ventricular rate by drugs that will increase the degree of AV block are worthwhile in the first instance. Drugs such as digoxin, diltiazem, beta-adrenergic blockers, sotalol and amiodarone may be tried; the choice depends on LV function. It is important to remember class IA and IC drugs may lead to 1:1 AV conduction. Class I drugs should probably be avoided unless ventricular response has been slowed with calcium channel or beta-adrenergic blocking drugs.

Synchronised DC cardioversion, often with low energies (25–50 J), is a reliable treatment option and is often required. Rapid atrial pacing faster than the flutter rate will terminate 'typical' Afl in most patients.

Anticoagulation guidelines are the same as those for AF, although there are less supporting data.

PREVENTION

Prevention is difficult. Drugs used include sotalol and amiodarone at low doses. Class IC agents (e.g. flecainide) may be used in patients without significant structural heart disease. Increasingly, recurrent or refractory Afl may be cured by radiofrequency ablation, which creates a linear lesion between the inferior tricuspid annulus and the Eustachian ridge at the anterior margin of the inferior vena cava to interrupt the re-entry circuit.[27] 'Typical' Afl is most amendable to circuit ablation.

ATRIAL FIBRILLATION[34,35]

AF is the most common arrhythmia requiring treatment and/or hospital admission. The incidence increases with age: 5% of individuals over 70 years have this arrhythmia. There is also an age-independent increase in frequency owing to increasing obesity and obstructive sleep apnoea. LV dyfunction increases risk of AF (4.5-fold in men and 5.9 in women) with atrial stretch and fibrosis causing electrical and atrial ionic channel remodelling.

AF is common in:

- congestive cardiac failure (40%)
- coronary artery bypass grafting (25–50%)
- critically ill patients (15%).

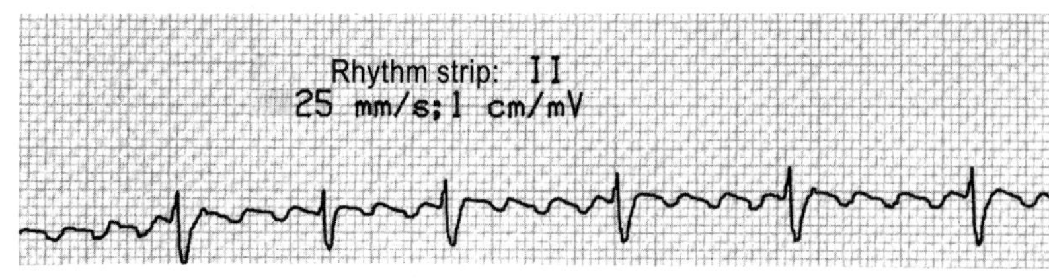

Figure 22.21 Atrial flutter varying between 3:1 and 4:1 atrioventricular (AV) conduction due to drug effect slowing AV node conduction.

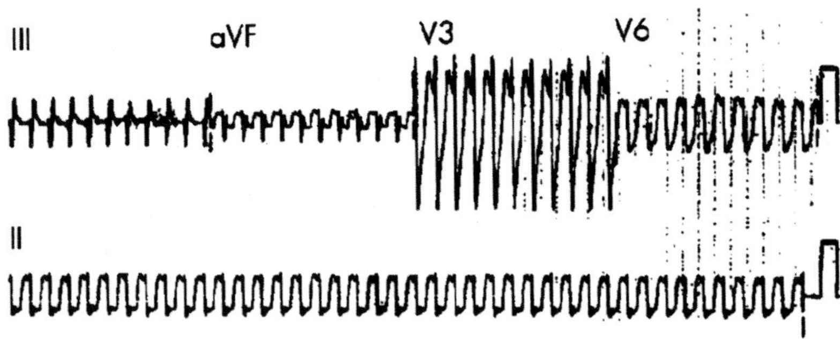

Figure 22.22 Atrial flutter with 1:1 conduction with a rate of 240 beats/min. Up-sloping of ST segment is easily mistaken as part of the QRS complex, giving the appearance of a broad QRS tachycardia in some leads. Lead III shows true narrow width of QRS complex.

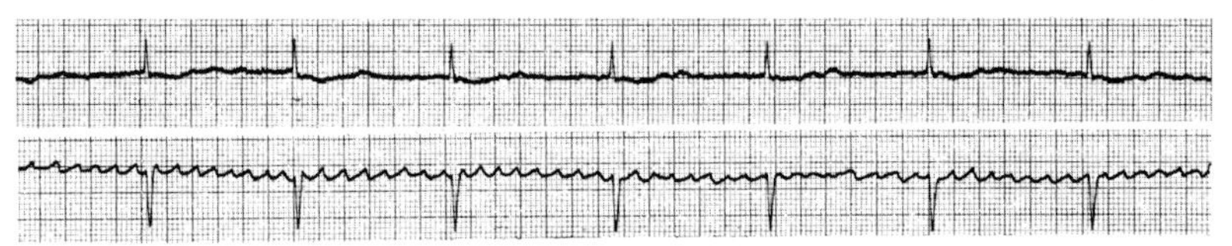

Figure 22.23 Atrial fibrillation. Irregular fibrillation waves with varying amplitude and morphology.

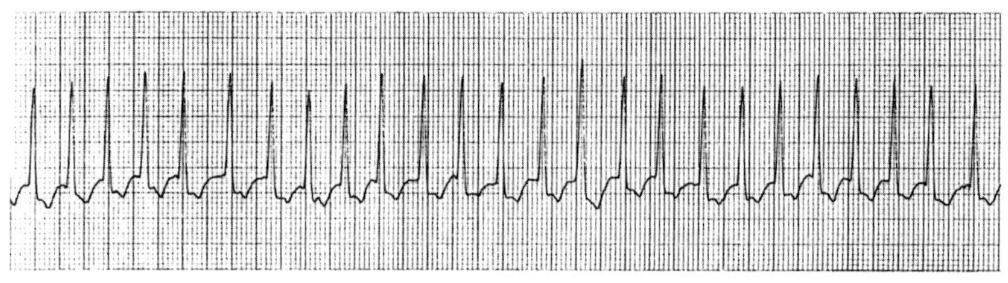

Figure 22.24 Atrial fibrillation with rapid ventricular rate. Ventricular irregularity and fibrillation waves are less evident when the rate is rapid.

Idiopathic or lone AF (i.e. with no structural heart disease or precipitating factor) in someone aged less than 60 years has an excellent prognosis; however, AF developing after cardiac surgery, for instance, is associated with increased stroke, life-threatening arrhythmias and longer hospital stays.

ECG

Atrial activity is chaotic with rapid (350–600 beats/min) and irregular depolarisation varying in amplitude and morphology (fibrillation waves). Ventricular response is irregularly irregular (**Fig. 22.23**). Most atrial impulses are not conducted to the ventricles; resulting in an untreated ventricular rate of 100–180 beats/min. QRS complexes will usually be narrow. When the ventricular rate is very rapid or very slow, ventricular irregularity may be missed (**Fig. 22.24**).

CLINICAL

AF is more common in patients with underlying heart disease (particularly those with a dilated left atrium) and abnormal atrial electrophysiology. Causes include ischaemic and valvular heart disease, pericarditis, hypertension, cardiac failure, thyrotoxicosis and alcohol abuse. AF may also occur after cardiac surgery and thoracotomy. AF can be chronic, or intermittent with paroxysmal attacks. Chronic AF has a poorer prognosis.

AF is associated with:

- *adverse haemodynamic effects:* rapid ventricular rate and loss of atrial systole may increase pulmonary capillary wedge pressure, while stroke volume and cardiac output decline
- systemic embolism and stroke
- *tachycardiomyopathy:* reversible global cardiomyopathy secondary to rapid heart rate. Assessing LV

function with echocardiogram before and after AV node ablation for AF refractory to medical therapy suggests that 10% of patients with AF have AF-induced tachycardiomyopathy.[36]

TREATMENT[23,37,38]

The goals of treatment include ventricular rate control, conversion to sinus rhythm, maintenance of sinus rhythm and anticoagulation where appropriate. There is increasing evidence available on the 'rate versus rhythm' control debate. Results from several recent major studies have challenged the previous belief that achievement of sinus rhythm is important in the long term (**Table 22.5**). When comparing control of ventricular rate versus reversion to sinus rhythm no clear survival benefit is apparent. However composite end-points of death, stroke and recurrent hospitalisation favour rate control only.[39–42]

The possible reasons why rhythm control has not been shown to be superior include:

- trials have included predominantly elderly high-risk patients
- sinus rhythm is difficult to achieve (39–63%)
- rate control strategies can result in sinus rhythm in up to 35% of patients
- underlying heart disease that initiates the AF persists
- there may be antiarrhythmic drug side-effects
- anticoagulation is still required even if rhythm control is successful.

However, rhythm control (if possible) appears superior in patients with LV dysfunction, with both amiodarone and dofetilide reducing mortality when sinus rhythm is achieved.[43,44] The paucity of data in younger patients (less than 60 years) favours initial attempts at rhythm control, particularly in those with structurally normal hearts, in the hope that progressive atrial electrical and anatomical remodelling is prevented.

RECENT ONSET OR PAROXYSMAL AF

*VENTRICULAR RATE CONTROL (**TABLE 22.6**)*

The urgency of ventricular rate control depends on the clinical situation and spontaneous reversion of AF is common. Treatment may not be necessary, and a reasonable strategy is based on clinical status:

- Haemodynamically unstable with rapid ventricular rate requires immediate synchronised DC shock (in addition to drug therapy) to control rate urgently.
- Haemodynamically stable, symptomatic with depressed LV function: semi-urgent synchronised DC shock or drug therapy, digoxin or amiodarone to control ventricular rate.
- Haemodynamically stable, symptomatic, normal LV function: control of ventricular response with beta-adrenergic blockers, diltiazem, digoxin (digoxin has poor control with exertion and other settings with increased sympathetic tone), magnesium (short-term), amiodarone or sotalol.
- Haemodynamically stable, with no structural heart disease and minimal or no symptoms: no immediate treatment is an option. Most cases will revert spontaneously within 24 hours. Single-dose flecainide for paroxymal AF has been recommended

Table 22.5 Atrial fibrillation rate versus rhythm control debate

STUDY	NUMBER	FOLLOW-UP (MONTHS)	AGE (YEARS)	AMIODARONE USE (%)	SINUS RHYTHM (%)	WARFARIN (%)	THROMBOEMBOLISM (%)	MORTALITY (%)
AFFIRM[39]		42						
Rate control	2027		70±9	10	35	85	6	21
Rhythm control	2033		70±9	70	63	70	7.5	24
RACE[40]		27						
Rate control	256		68±9	–	10	96	5.5	17
Rhythm control	266		68±9	–	39	86	7.9	13
STAF[41]		22						
Rate control	100		65±9	0	0	–	0.6	5
Rhythm control	100		66±9	0	–	–	3.1	2.5
PIAF[42]		12						
Rate control	125		61±9	0	10	100	–	1.6
Rhythm control	125		60±10	100	56	100	–	1.6

AFFIRM=Atrial Fibrillation Follow-up Investigation of Rhythm Management; RACE=Rate Control versus Electrical Cardioversion of persistent atrial fibrillation; STAF=Strategies of Treatment of Atrial Fibrillation; PIAF=Pharmacological Intervention in Atrial Fibrillation.

Table 22.6 Drugs for ventricular rate control in atrial fibrillation

	ACUTE	CHRONIC
STABLE	BETA BLOCKERS Metoprolol 2.5–5 mg i.v. bolus over 2 min – up to 3 doses Esmolol 50–200 μg/kg/min i.v. *NON*-DIHYDROPYRIDINE CALCIUM CHANNEL ANTAGONISTS Verapamil 0.0375–0.15 mg/kg i.v. over 2 min	Metoprolol ER 100–200 mg oral daily Atenolol 25–100 mg oral daily Bisoprolol 2.5–10 mg oral daily Verapamil 40 mg oral b.d. up to 360 mg ER oral daily Diltiazem 60 mg oral t.d.s. up to 360 mg ER oral daily
UNSTABLE: HYPOTENSION HEART FAILURE	Digoxin 0.5–1.0 mg i.v. Amiodarone 5 mg/kg i.v. over 1 h	Digoxin 0.125–0.50 mg oral daily Amiodarone 100–200 mg oral daily Dronedarone 400 mg oral b.d.

Table 22.7 Drugs for pharmacological conversion of recent-onset atrial fibrillation

DRUG	DOSE	FEATURES
Amiodarone	5 mg/kg i.v. over 1 h	Will slow ventricular rate Conversion delayed Amiodarone 80–90%, placebo 40–60% at 24 h Suitable structural heart disease and heart failure
Flecainide	2 mg/kg i.v. over 10 min 200–300 mg oral	Not suitable for structural heart disease or heart failure 67–92% conversion at 6 h Majority within 1 h of i.v. dose May prolong QT Risk of atrial flutter and 1 : 1 conduction
Ibutilide	1 mg i.v. over 10 min Further dose after 10 min	50% conversion within 90 min Risk of QT prolongation and torsades de points high
Propafenone	2 mg/kg i.v. over 10 min	Not suitable for structural heart disease or heart failure 41–91% conversion within 3 hours May prolong QT Risk of atrial flutter and 1 : 1 conduction
Vernakalant	3 mg/kg i.v. over 10 min Further 2 mg/kg if required	Suitable for structural heart disease and heart failure Rapid in approximately 10 min in responders 50% conversion rate 99% of responders remain in sinus rhythm at 24 h after single dose Well tolerated

(contraindicated in patients with structural heart disease).[45]

- If pre-excitation is suspected beta-adrenergic blockers, non-dihydropyridine calcium channel antagonists, digoxin and adenosine are contraindicated and amiodarone and class I drugs are indicated.

Ideal rate control can be defined as a resting heart rate of ≤80 beats/min, peak rate of ≤110 beats/min with 6-minute walk and an average of 100 beats/min.

CONVERSION TO SINUS RHYTHM

Antiarrhythmic drugs or DC shock cardioversion can be used. The likelihood of short- and long-term success depends on the clinical situation. Conversion to sinus rhythm is more important in young patients and those with heart failure. Maintenance of sinus rhythm is problematic: sinus rhythm at 1 year is 60% with amiodarone and 40% with sotalol, and associated with significant drug cardiac and extracardiac toxicities. The risk of stroke and need for antithrombotic therapy due to frequent AF recurrences, which may be asymptomatic, remain. Achieving sinus rhythm (especially greater than 60 years) is less important than previously thought.[39]

Pharmacological conversion of recent-onset AF is variously successful depending on the clinical setting and agent used (**Table 22.7**). Ibutilide, propafenone and vernakalant have rapid conversion rates, compared

Table 22.8 Drugs for long-term rhythm control in atrial fibrillation

DRUGS	DOSE	CONTRAINDICATIONS AND PRECAUTIONS	ECG CRITERIA FOR LOWERING DOSE OR DISCONTINUATION	AV NODE SLOWING OF PAROXYSMAL AF
Disopyramide	100–250 mg t.d.s.	Systolic heart failure QT-prolonging drugs	QT>500 ms	None
Flecainide Flecainide XL	100–200 mg b.d. 200 mg daily	Creatinine clearance <50 mL/min Coronary artery disease Reduced LV ejection fraction Conduction delay	QRS duration increase >25% over baseline	None
Propafenone Propafenone SR	150–300 mg t.d.s. 225–425 mg b.d.	Coronary artery disease Reduced LV ejection fraction Conduction delay Creatinine clearance <50 mL/min	QRS duration increase >25% over baseline	Slight
Sotalol	80–160 mg b.d.	LV hypertrophy Systolic heart failure Pre-existing QT prolongation Hypokalaemia Creatinine clearance <50 mL/min	QT>500 ms	Yes
Amiodarone	600 mg daily, 4 weeks, 400 mg daily, 4 weeks then 200 mg daily	QT prolonging drugs Warfarin dose adjustment	QT>500 ms	Yes
Dronedarone	400 mg b.d.	Heart failure NYHA Class III–IV QT prolonging drugs CYP3A4 inhibitors Creatinine clearance <30 mL/min	QT>500 ms	Yes

with flecainide and amiodarone the slowest. Amiodarone, ilbutilide and vernakalent are suitable in heart failure. All have risk of QT prolongation and proarrhythmia, with ibutilide being the worst and vernakalant the best, although there are anecdotal case reports of ventricular arrhythmias with the latter.[46–48]

Although long-term treatment goals increasingly favour chronic rate control (see Table 22.6), antiarrhythmic drugs are still used to promote long-term rhythm control (**Table 22.8**). All have many contraindications and precautions, with amiodarone the best from a cardiac perspective and worst from an extracardiac point of view. The dilemma of long-term antiarrhythmic treatment in AF is highlighted by the diametrically opposite effects that dronedarone has been shown to produce in this setting.[49] In ATHENA, dronedarone decreased all cause, cardiovascular and presumed arrhythmia mortality, stroke and heart failure, whereas in PALLAS all these outcomes were worse. In PALLAS all patients had 'permanent' AF and there was twice the baseline incidence of heart failure. Benefit would appear to be crucially dependent upon securing sinus rhythm, absence of structural substrate for proarrhythmia and cardiac reserve to tolerate the drug.

DC SHOCK CARDIOVERSION

DC shock cardioversion is indicated either before 24–48 hours or after appropriate anticoagulation protocol. Combining DC shock with antiarrhythmic drugs to promote maintenance of sinus rhythm is favoured; especially if risk factors for relapse exist. Cardioversion is less likely to be successful if:

- AF has been present for over 1 year
- left atrial size is greater than 45 mm
- untreated conditions are present (e.g. thyrotoxicosis, valvular heart disease and heart failure).

Critically ill patients who are septic, postoperative or on drugs such as catecholamines are likely to relapse.

ANTICOAGULATION AND CARDIOVERSION[50,51]

Loss of atrial contraction with AF is associated with stasis of blood flow and formation of blood clots in the left atrium, particularly the atrial appendage. Reversion to sinus rhythm and return of more effective atrial contraction may cause expulsion of any atrial clots and systemic emboli. Once AF has been present for more than 48 hours – some authors stipulate 24 hours – the risk of systemic emboli is significant and anticoagulation is required prior to DC shock cardioversion. The current recommended period of anticoagulation prior to DC shock cardioversion is 3 weeks. This 3-week period can be shortened to 1 day for heparin and 5 days for warfarin if the left atrium can be demonstrated free of clot using transoesophageal echocardiography. With this accelerated approach, heparin dose should be titrated to an activated partial thromboplastin time 2–3 times control or warfarin to produce an international normalised ratio (INR) of 2.0–3.0. In many clinical situations such as recent surgery or other bleeding risks, anticoagulation is contraindicated and elective cardioversion should be delayed until recommended anticoagulation cover is safe. Following successful cardioversion to sinus rhythm the risk of systemic embolism continues as the propensity to form atrial clot remains owing to atrial contractile stunning and anticoagulation should be continued for 4–6 weeks.

ATRIAL FIBRILLATION ABLATION THERAPY

Ablation techniques for AF have been continuously refined since the original Maze III surgical procedure, which involved numerous atrial incisions to form a maze-like pattern of scarring, blocking propagation of arrhythmia. The utility of this procedure was limited because it was surgical, with longer bypass times, postoperative bleeding and impaired atrial contractility. The magnitude of this original procedure was based on the belief that the entire atrium was involved in the initiation and maintenance of the fibrillatory conduction. This may be true for long-standing AF but paroxysmal AF appears to originate primarily at the junction of the left atrium and pulmonary veins. AF in 94% of patients is initiated by rapid discharges from one or more foci at or near the pulmonary vein orifices.[52] Atrial tissue in this area has heterogeneous electrophysiological properties and there is also clustering of vagal inputs, which creates substrate for rapid discharges that initiate micro-re-entrant circuits or 'rotors'. These high-frquency periodic rotors send spiral wave fronts of activation into surrounding atria. Localised ablation of a single dominant foci and rotor is inadequate as there are usually multiple foci.

There is renewed interest in surgical AF ablation therapy in conjunction with cardiac surgery. Complications have been reduced with energy (cryotherapy, radiofrequency) rather than incisions and the extent of lesions reduced. The minimum lesion set is now considered to be encirclement of pulmonary veins, linear lesion from the inferior pulmonary vein to mitral annulus and from the coronary sinus to the inferior vena cava.

Left atrial catheter (transatrial septum) AF ablation isolating all four pulmonary veins using radiofrquency is being heralded as the possible AF cure. Results are improving as all pulmonary veins are now isolated and the encircling lesion is clear of the pulmonary vein antrum (reducing pulmonary vein stenosis). Success rates of 81% (75–88%) free of AF and off drugs are reported. Success appears long term as any recurrence occurs early. A further 10–20% may become responsive to antiarrhythmic drugs which were previously ineffective. Repeating the procedure can increase success to >90% with failure only in patients found to have extensive atrial scarring (predicting and excluding patients with this extensive atrial scarring is a major future challenge). Although not yet the universal cure, the results are two- to threefold better than antiarrhythmic drugs alone.

Complication rates are also falling associated with:

- intracardiac echocardiography ensuring safer transeptal puncture and positioning of isolating lesions clear of the pulmonary vein antra
- higher levels of procedural anticoagulation
- strict limitations on radiofrequency energy output.

Transient ischaemic attacks, strokes, tamponade/perforation and symptomatic pulmonary vein stenosis are all well below 1% respectively. Proarrhythmia resulting from re-entrant tachycardia from incomplete ablative lesions is more common. Some are advocating ablation as first-line treatment whereas most are selecting younger patients (less than 70 years) with paroxysmal AF for whom antiarrhythmic therapy has failed, left atrial diameter is less than 5 cm and ejection fraction is greater than 40%.[27] Head-to-head studies comparing ablation and antiarrhythmic drugs are appearing with suggested survival benefit, improved quality of life, reduced adverse effects and cost-effectiveness after approximately 3 years with catheter AF ablation therapy.[53,54]

ANTICOAGULATION FOR CHRONIC ATRIAL FIBRILLATION[35]

VALVULAR ATRIAL FIBRILLATION

A 17-fold increased risk of embolic stroke with rheumatic mitral valve disease requires warfarin (INR 2–3). With prosthetic valves there is a similar target range of INR, though the exact level is dependent on the type of valve.

NON-VALVULAR ATRIAL FIBRILLATION

The risk of stroke has been determined by the $CHADS_2$ score (assign 1 point for congestive heart failure, hypertension, age=75 years and diabetes mellitus, and 2 points for stroke/TIA).[55] The $CHADS_2$ score has been further developed to the CHA_2DS_2VASc score to improve risk stratification of patients at moderate risk by doubling points to 2 for age ≥75 and including

Table 22.9 CHA_2DS_2VASc score and stroke risk stratification

	$CHA_2DS_2VAS_C$ SCORE	
RISK FACTOR		*SCORE*
Congestive heart failure LV dysfunction ejection fraction≤40%	C	1
Hypertension	H	1
Age≥75	A_2	2
Diabetes mellitus	D	1
Previous stroke, TIA or systemic embolism	S_2	2
Vascular disease – myocardial infarction, complex aortic plaque, prior peripheral revascularisation, amputation or angiographic evidence	V	1
Age 65–74	A	1
Female sex	S	1
Maximum score		**9**

	ADJUSTED STROKE RATE ACCORDING TO $CHA_2DS_2VAS_C$ SCORE
$CHA_2DS_2VAS_C$ SCORE	*ADJUSTED STROKE RATE %/YEAR**
0	0
1	1.3
2	2.2
3	3.2
4	4.1
5	6.7
6	9.8
7	9.6
8	6.7
9	15.2

*Based on Lip et al. Stroke 2010;41(12):2731–8.[56]

vascular disease (prior myocardial infarction, peripheral artery disease determined by prior revascularisation, amputation or angiographic evidence and aortic plaque, age 65–74 and female sex) (**Table 22.9**).

The treatment options are discussed below.

WARFARIN

Adjusted-dose warfarin reduces relative risk of stroke by 62%. The absolute risk reduction is 2.8% per year for primary and 8.4% per year for secondary prevention, although intracranial haemorrhage occurs (0.3% per year). Low-dose warfarin (INR 1.5–2.0) is less effective than an INR of 2.0–3.0 but has fewer haemorrhagic complications. Embolic stroke rate doubles as INR falls from 2.0 to 1.7, and is markedly higher at an INR of 1.3 compared with 2.0.[50,57]

ASPIRIN

Aspirin has reduced efficacy when compared with warfarin, with a 22% relative risk reduction and an absolute risk reduction of 1.5% and 2.5% per year for primary and secondary prevention. Warfarin compared with aspirin for AF will prevent 23 strokes and result in nine additional major bleeds per 1000 patients per year.

CLOPIDOGRIL PLUS ASPIRIN

Although warfarin is better under ideal circumstances, poor INR control will readily erode this benefit.

WARFARIN COMBINED WITH ANTIPLATELET THERAPY

There is no benefit over warfarin alone.

DABIGATRAN ETEXILATE

This direct thrombin inhibitor is a new anticoagulant that is likely to have an increasing role in AF anticoagulation with the benefit of fixed dosing not requiring monitoring. In non-valvular AF, dabigatran 150 mg b.d. had a 35% reduction in stroke and systemic embolism compared with warfarin. There was a similar rate of major bleeding, although intracranial haemorrhage was reduced by 59%. The lower dose of 110 mg b.d. had similar embolic efficacy to warfarin but with reduced bleeding. Dabigatran clearance is importantly influenced by creatinine clearance of less than 50 mL/min and rapid reversal is problematic.

RECOMMENDATIONS FOR ANTICOAGULATION IN PATIENTS WITH ATRIAL FIBRILLATION

Non-valvular AF

INR adjusted warfarin (2.0–3.0 target 2.5) or aspirin according to CHA_2DS_2VASc score and HAS-BLED score (**Tables 22.10** and **22.11**).

Dabigatran may be substituted for warfarin, depending on risk of bleeding. Risk of bleeding can be determined by the HAS-BLED score. With a HAS-BLED score of 0–2, dabigatran 150 mg bd gives superior embolic prevention with reduced intracranial haemorrhage. With a HAS-BLED score of ≥3, 110 mg b.d. gives similar efficacy to warfarin, but reduced haemorrhagic complications.

Valvular AF

Warfarin is indicated. Direct thrombin inhibitors are yet to be studied in this situation.

Risk of haemorrhage is reduced by keeping INR=3, systolic blood pressure <135 mmHg (17.95 kPa) and avoiding antiplatelet drugs.

Table 22.10 Approach to thromboprophylaxis in patients with atrial fibrillation.

CHA_2DS_2VASC SCORE	RECOMMENDED ANTITHROMBOTIC THERAPY
≥2	Oral anticoagulation – warfarin INR 2.0–3.0 Target 2.5 – dabigatran – HAS-BLED score 0–2: dabigatran 150 mg b.d. <2: dabigatran 110 mg b.d.
1	Either oral anticoagular – warfarin INR 2.0–3.0 Target 2.5 – dabigatran 110 mg b.d., *or* – aspirin 75–325 mg daily Prefer oral anticoagulation rather than aspirin
0	Either aspirin 75–325 mg daily, *or* No antithrombotic therapy Prefer no antithrombotic therapy rather than aspirin

Table 22.11 HAS-BLED bleeding risk score

H	Hypertension – systolic >160 mmHg (21.3 kPa)	1
A	Abnormal renal or liver function (1 point each) – chronic dialysis, renal transplant or creatinine ≥200 µmol/L – cirrhosis, bilirubin >2×upper limit of normal or liver enzymes >3×upper limit of normal	1 or 2
S	Stroke	1
B	Bleeding – previous history of bleeding, abnormal coagulation or anaemia	1
L	Labile INRs Unstable or high INRs, poor time in therapeutic range <60%	1
E	Elderly >65 years	1
D	Drugs or alcohol – antiplatelet agents, non-steroid anti-inflammatory drugs – alcohol abuse	1 or 2
	Maximum score	9

Temporary cessation of anticoagulation for AF with surgery is a common problem. Valvular AF requires heparin or enoxiparin until surgery and recommencement of heparin/enoxiparin, then warfarin as soon as safely possible. Non-valvular CHA_2DS_2VASc score <2

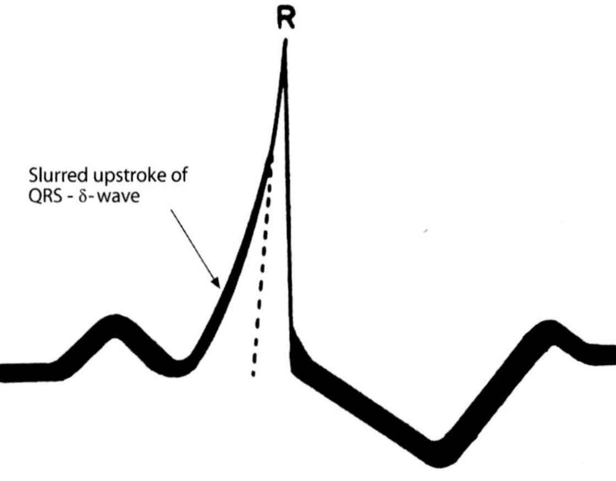

Figure 22.25 Ventricular pre-excitation via accessory pathway giving rise to a slurred upstroke and widened QRS complex.

can have anticoagulation withheld with minimal risk. Non-valvular CHA_2DS_2VASc score of ≥2 is increasingly managed as valvular AF.

Angioplasty and stenting of coronary arteries require aspirin and clopidogrel to maintain stent patency. Stenting in patients already on warfarin for AF is a common problem.

RECOMMENDATIONS FOR AF PATIENTS REQUIRING CORONARY ARTERY STENTING

- Non-valvular CHA_2DS_2VASc score <2: cease warfarin as aspirin and clopidorel are started.
- Valvular AF and non-valvular with CHA_2DS_2VASc score ≥2: add aspirin and clopidogrel to continued warfarin treatment.

PRE-EXCITATION SYNDROME

Pre-excitation syndromes have an additional or accessory AV pathway. The term 'WPW syndrome' is usually applied when tachyarrhythmia is present.

ECG

During sinus rhythm, an atrial impulse will reach the ventricles via both the AV node and the accessory AV pathway. The latter conducts the atrial impulse to the ventricles before the AV node, resulting in ventricular pre-excitation and a short PR interval. On reaching the ventricles, the pre-excitation impulse is not conducted via the specialised conducting system. Hence, early ventricular activation will be slowed, resulting in a slurred upstroke of the QRS complex, the so-called delta (δ) wave (**Fig. 22.25**). The abnormal ventricular activation also gives rise to secondary S-T segment and T-wave abnormalities. δ-wave polarity in a 12-lead ECG may help localise the anatomical position of the accessory pathway. Type A WPW is characterised by upright QRS deflections in the right precordial leads

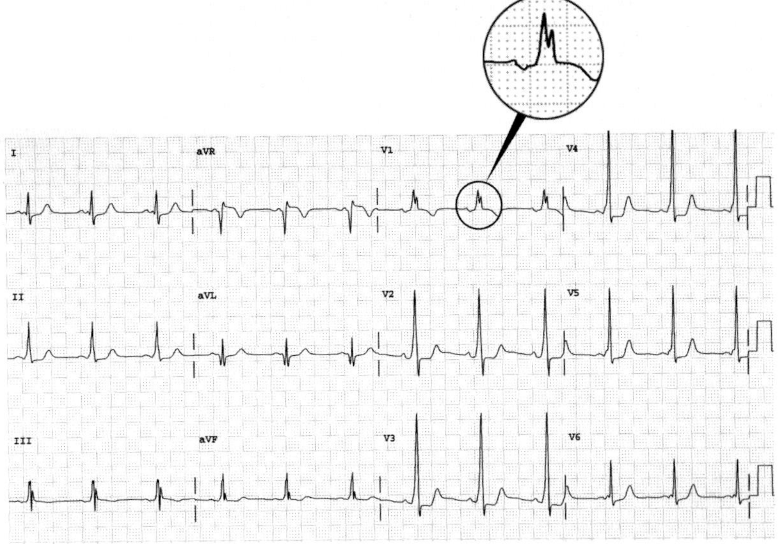

Figure 22.26 Type A Wolff–Parkinson–White syndrome with positive R-waves in the right precordial leads, short PR interval and δ-wave giving rise to a wide QRS complex.

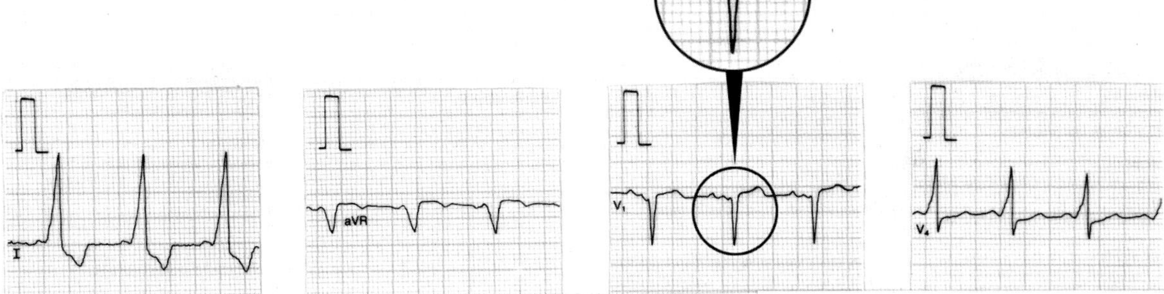

Figure 22.27 Type B Wolff–Parkinson–White syndrome with a negative QRS deflection in V_1.

(tall R-waves in V_1 and V_2) (**Fig. 22.26**). In type A WPW the accessory pathway is usually situated on the left with pre-excitation of the left ventricle. Type B WPW has a dominantly negative QRS complex in V_1 and the accessory pathway tends to be on the right with pre-excitation of the right ventricle (**Fig. 22.27**).

CLINICAL

AVRT or AF can occur with WPW. During AVRT, the re-entry impulse usually travels down the AV node and back up the accessory pathway. Ventricular activation is via the normal conducting pathways and the QRS will be narrow. Occasionally, the re-entry impulse may pass in the opposite direction (down the accessory pathway and up the AV node), resulting in a wide QRS-complex tachycardia due to abnormal slow ventricular activation. Treatment is the same as for AVRT (i.e. i.v. adenosine). AF is uncommon in WPW, but may be life-threatening. Most impulses are conducted via the accessory pathway, leading to wide QRS complexes. The ECG of WPW with AF usually shows rapid, irregular QRS complexes with variable QRS width (**Fig. 22.28**).

Ventricular response is very rapid, leading to hypotension or cardiogenic shock. This arrhythmia may degenerate to VF.

TREATMENT[23]

Treatment usually involves synchronised DC shock. Antiarrhythmic drugs may be used when patients are haemodynamically stable and the ventricular rate is not excessively rapid.

- Drugs that prolong the refractory period of the accessory pathway are useful (e.g. sotalol, amiodarone, flecainide and procainamide).
- Drugs that shorten the refractory period (e.g. digoxin) are contraindicated as they may accelerate ventricular rate.

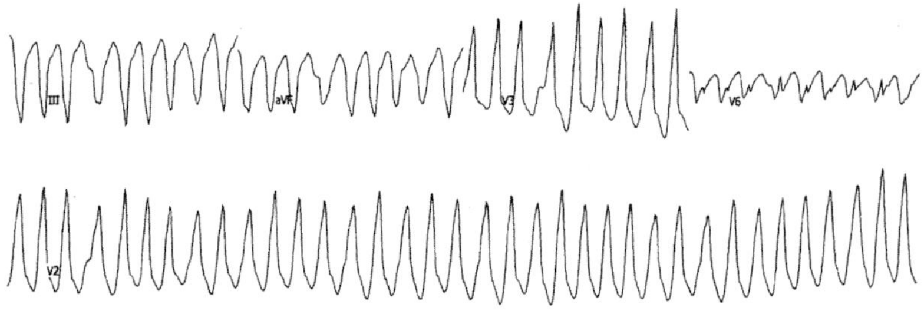

Figure 22.28 Wolff–Parkinson–White syndrome with atrial fibrillation. Rapid rate and irregularity of the broad QRS complexes help to distinguish from ventricular tachycardia.

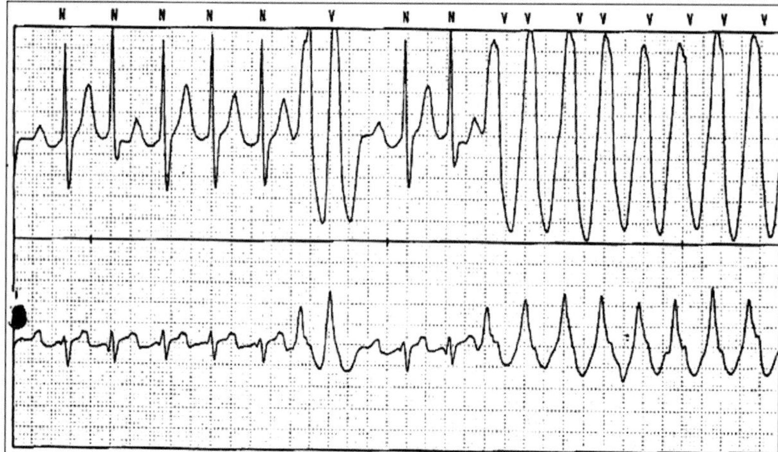

Figure 22.29 Monomorphic ventricular tachycardia preceded by a ventricular couplet.

- Verapamil and lidocaine may increase the ventricular rate during AF, and are also best avoided.[28]
- Beta-adrenergic blockers have no effect on the refractory period of the accessory pathway.

Long-term management by radiofrequency ablation of the accessory pathway is effective in selected patients.[23]

VENTRICULAR TACHYCARDIA

VT is defined as three or more VEBs at a rate greater than 130 beats/min, and may exceed 300 beats/min. VT lasting over 30 seconds is considered to be sustained. Non-sustained VT may not cause symptoms, but is associated with increased mortality in certain patients (e.g. after myocardial infarction). VT may be monomorphic (i.e. the same QRS morphology) (**Fig. 22.29**) or polymorphic (varying QRS morphology).

MONOMORPHIC VENTRICULAR TACHYCARDIA

This is the most common form of VT. It is commonly associated with previous myocardial infarction, and often causes symptoms (e.g. palpitations, shortness of breath, chest pain or syncope). It may result in cardiac arrest, due to the tachycardia itself or degeneration into VF. The most common mechanism is re-entry secondary to inhomogeneous activation of the myocardium and slow conduction through scar tissue from a previous myocardial infarction. AV dissociation (i.e. independent atrial and ventricular activity) (**Fig. 22.30**) is present in about 75% of instances, whereas retrograde ventricle to atrial conduction occurs in about 25%. AV dissociation is virtually diagnostic for VT during a wide-complex tachycardia, but ECG recognition of independent (and slower) atrial activity can be difficult (**Fig. 22.31**). VT is the most common cause of a wide-complex tachycardia (QRS>120 ms) and any such tachycardia should be considered VT until proven otherwise. Mistakes in diagnosis are common: SVT with aberrant conduction is often mistaken for VT. Inappropriate treatment based on incorrect diagnosis can have disastrous consequences.

ECG

Older criteria (e.g. QRS>140 ms and extreme electrical axis changes) are unhelpful in rhythm diagnosis.[58] ECG criteria initially proposed by Wellens and revised by Brugada et al permit accurate diagnosis in four sequential steps (**Fig. 22.32**).[59–61]

The sensitivity of these four consecutive steps was 0.987, with a specificity of 0.965.

- *Step 1:* is a RS complex present in any precordial lead? (QR, QRS, QS, monophasic R and rSR are not considered RS complexes.) If not (**Fig. 22.33**), the diagnosis is VT.
- *Step 2:* if a RS is present, then measure the duration of the R-to-S nadir (lowest part of the S-wave). If this

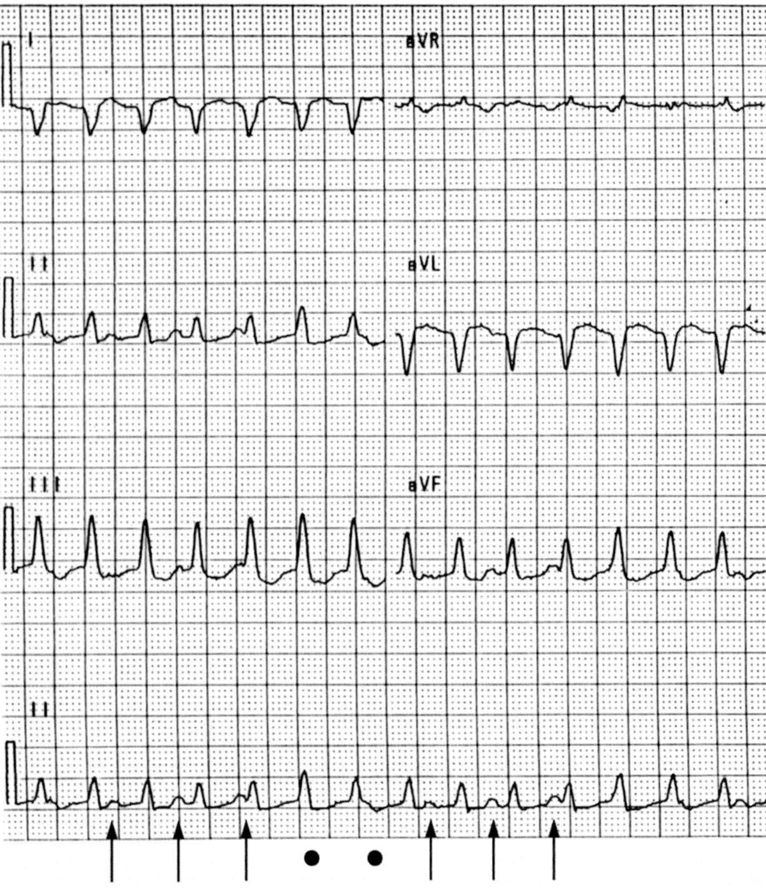

Figure 22.30 Ventricular tachycardia with obvious arteriovenous dissociation and independent P-waves are highlighted with arrows in lead II.

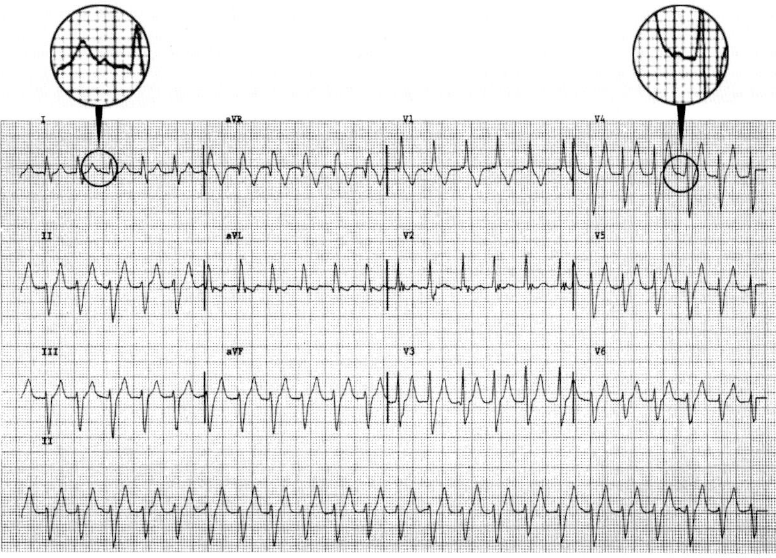

Figure 22.31 Ventricular tachycardia. Independent atrial activity can be difficult to see. Dissociated P-waves can just be seen in leads I and V_4.

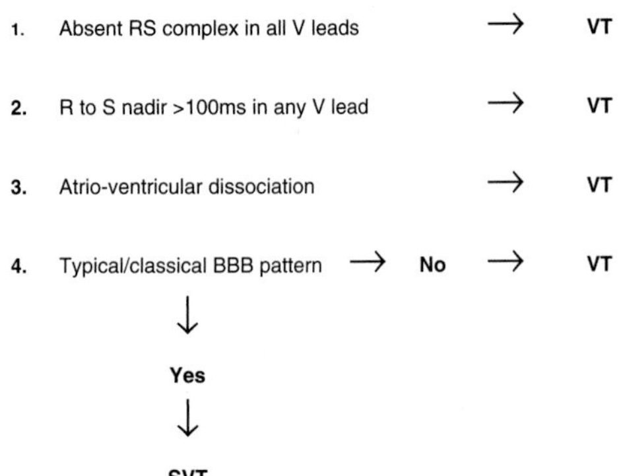
1. Absent RS complex in all V leads → VT
2. R to S nadir >100ms in any V lead → VT
3. Atrio-ventricular dissociation → VT
4. Typical/classical BBB pattern → No → VT
↓
Yes
↓
SVT

Figure 22.32 Algorithm proposed by Brugada et al[59] to diagnose ventricular tachycardia in the setting of a broad QRS-complex tachycardia.

duration is >100 ms in any V lead (**Fig. 22.34**), the rhythm is VT.

- *Step 3:* if RS<100 ms, then AV dissociation is searched for (more QRS complexes than P-waves; see Figs 22.30 and 22.31). Indirect evidence of AV dissociation such as capture or fusion beats may be present. Capture beats occur when atrial sinus impulses reach the AV node when it is no longer refractory from retrograde conduction of ventricular discharges: the AV node and ventricle are then 'captured' by the sinus impulse. The resultant QRS will occur earlier than the next expected VT complex and the QRS morphology will be that of the 'normal' underlying complexes for that patient. Similarly, a sinus impulse can penetrate the AV and 'fuse' with an already depolarising ventricle from the ectopic focus initiating the VT. The resulting QRS morphology of a fusion beat will be variable and depend on the relative contribution of the supraventricular and

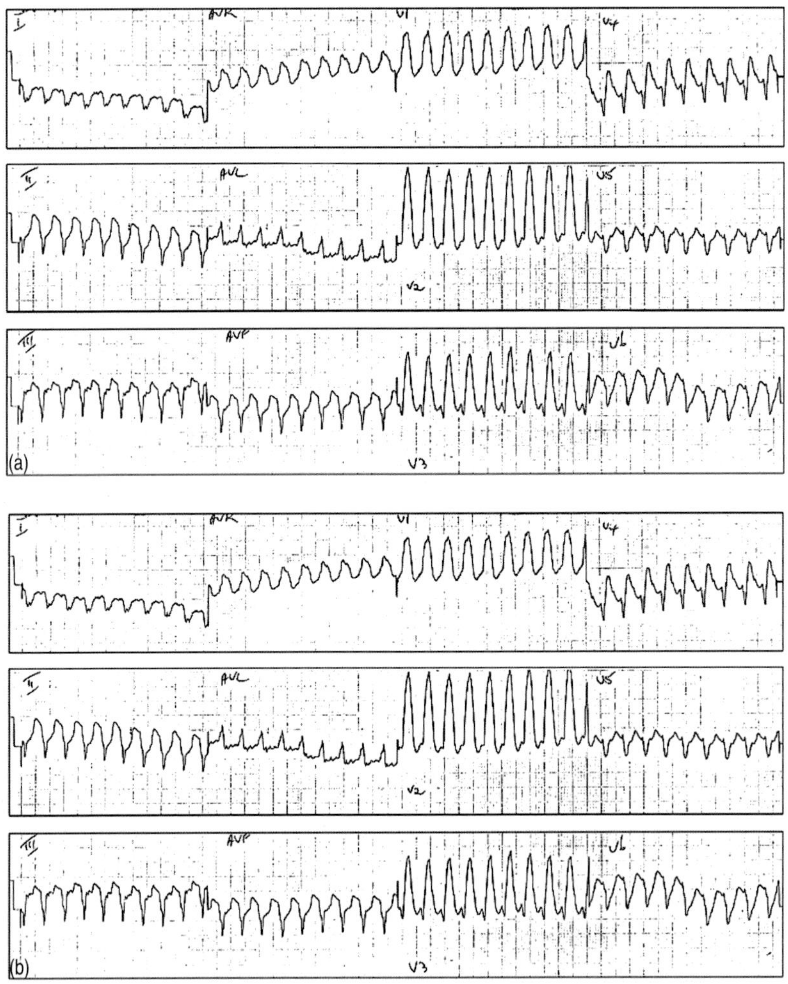

Figure 22.33 (a, b) Ventricular tachycardia. Broad QRS-complex tachycardia with absence of RS complex in all precordial leads.

Figure 22.34 Ventricular tachycardia. Time duration of R to the nadir of the negative S-wave is 120 ms. Note also independent P-waves in lead V_1.

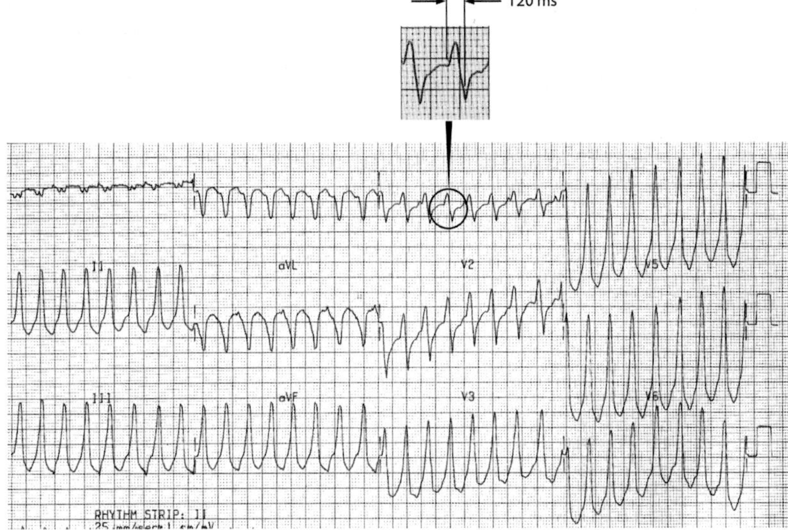

ventricular impulses to ventricular activation. Even a single capture or fusion beat confirms AV dissociation and VT (**Fig. 22.35**).

- *Step 4:* if AV dissociation is not present, then decide whether the wide QRS has a right or left BBB pattern. If the BBB is typical in both V_1 and V_6 leads, the rhythm is supraventricular in origin (see the section on BBB, below). If there are any atypical features, the rhythm is considered to be VT (see Figs 22.39 and 22.40, below).

Termination of a wide-complex tachycardia by i.v. adenosine strongly suggests the arrhythmia as SVT. However, adenosine in this setting has the risk of destabilising VT when blood pressure is barely compensated by vasodilatation or acceleration of accessory pathway conduction, and is not recommended by International Liaison Committee on Resuscitation (ILCOR) as a diagnostic strategy in wide-complex tachycardia.[23] Demonstration of AV dissociation by intracardiac ECG from a central venous catheter or a transvenous pacing lead signifies VT.

CLINICAL

The major cause of VT is significant coronary artery disease. Other causes include cardiomyopathy, myocarditis and valvular heart disease. Symptoms will depend on the ventricular rate, duration of tachycardia and underlying cardiac function. There are not necessarily any haemodynamic differences between VT and SVT with aberrant conduction but haemodynamic instability mandates management as for VT.

TREATMENT[23,62]

DC shock is indicated if a patient is haemodynamically unstable. Antiarrhythmic drug trial is indicated in haemodynamically stable VT.

- Amiodarone may terminate VT; there is less negative inotropic action but delayed effect.
- Sotalol and procainamide are more effective than lidocaine but are associated with significant myocardial depression.
- Although traditionally indicated, there are now doubts about the efficacy of lidocaine.

If drugs are ineffective, synchronised DC shock is indicated. Rapid right ventricular pacing may also be effective.

Long-term prevention of VT and sudden death is difficult. Sotalol guided by Holter ECG or electrophysiological testing, and empirical (i.e. non-guided) amiodarone are superior to other drugs in preventing arrhythmia recurrences. Empirical beta-adrenergic blockers also have a role. Implantable defibrillators can recognise and automatically terminate VT by rapid ventricular pacing or, if this fails, by internal DC cardioversion, which may be life-saving.

POLYMORPHIC VENTRICULAR TACHYCARDIA AND TORSADE DE POINTES

This arrhythmia has QRS complexes at 200 beats/min or greater, which change in amplitude and axis so that they appear to twist around the baseline (**Fig. 22.36**). Torsade de pointes usually has prolonged QT during sinus rhythm, and U-waves are often present (see section on long-QT syndrome, below). However, polymorphic VT may be associated with a normal QT interval in settings such as myocardial ischaemia, infarction or post cardiac surgery.

TREATMENT

Polymorphic VT associated with a normal QT interval during sinus rhythm (e.g. following AMI) should be

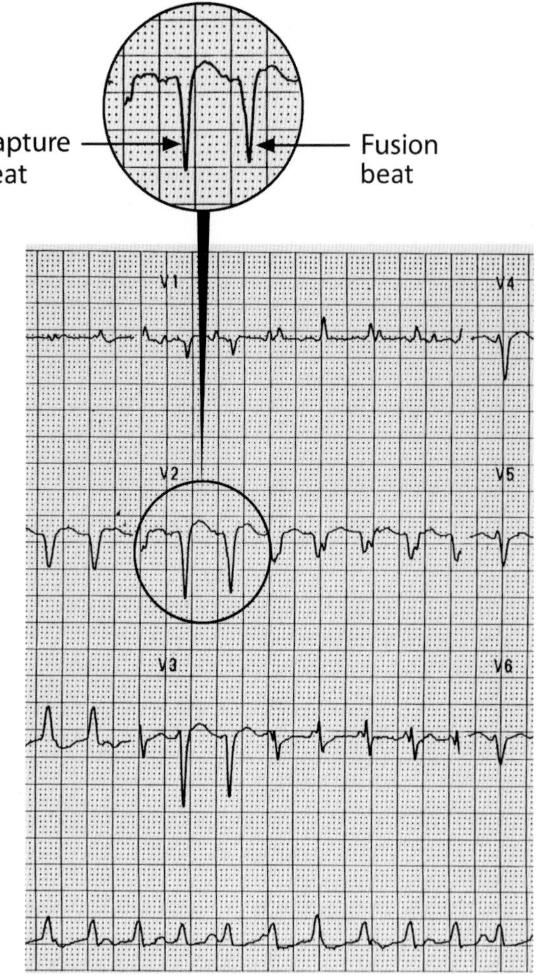

Figure 22.35 Ventricular tachycardia with a highlighted premature capture beat followed by a fusion beat showing transitional QRS morphology between the underlying normal QRS and VT complex. Note also independent P-waves.

treated in the same way as monomorphic VT. (See section on treatment of long-QT and polymorphic VT, below.)

ACCELERATED IDIOVENTRICULAR RHYTHM (AIVR)

This is often inappropriately called slow VT. Increased automaticity is probably the mechanism responsible for this relatively benign arrhythmia.

ECG

There is a wide QRS with a rate of 60–110 beats/min (**Fig. 22.37**). Sinus rate is often only slightly slower than the arrhythmia, so the dominant rhythm may be intermittent AIVR and sinus rhythm. Fusion beats are therefore common.

CLINICAL

The rhythm is commonly encountered in inferior myocardial infarction. AIVR may be misdiagnosed as VT. Occasionally, AIVR causes haemodynamic deterioration, usually due to loss of atrial systole. Increasing the atrial rate with either atropine or atrial pacing may then be necessary.

VENTRICULAR FIBRILLATION

VF always causes haemodynamic collapse, loss of consciousness and death if not immediately treated. Of patients resuscitated from VF, 20–30% have sustained an AMI, and 75% have coronary artery disease. VF (and VT) unassociated with AMI is likely to be recurrent; 50% die within 3 years.

ECG

The ECG shows irregular waves of varying morphology and amplitude (**Fig. 22.38**).

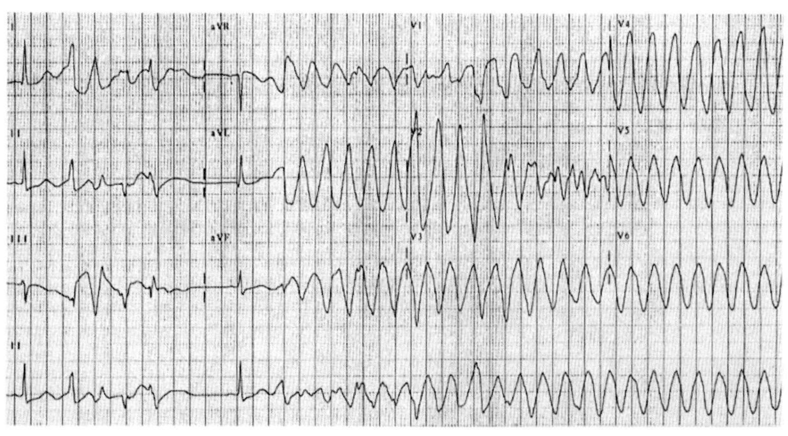

Figure 22.36 Torsade de pointes preceded by multifocal ventricular ectopic beats.

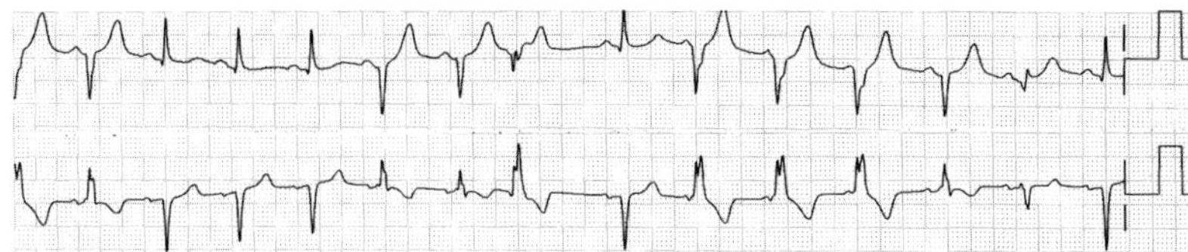

Figure 22.37 Sinus rhythm with short runs of accelerated idioventricular rhythm. Note frequent fusion beats as sinus rate is similar to the accelerated idioventricular rate.

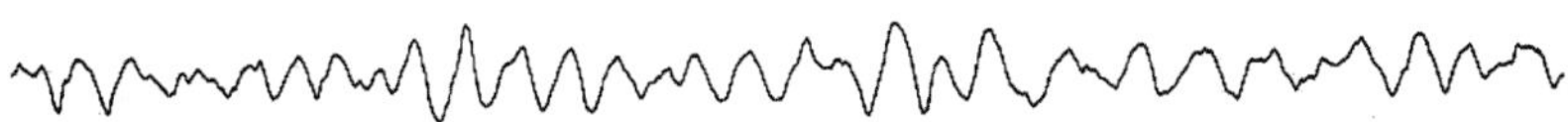

Figure 22.38 Ventricular fibrillation with waves of varying morphology and amplitude.

CLINICAL

VF is usually associated with ischaemic heart disease, although other causes include cardiomyopathy, antiarrhythmic drugs, severe hypoxia and non-synchronised DC cardioversion.

TREATMENT[62]

Give an immediate non-synchronised DC shock at 200 J and, if ineffective, repeated at 200–360 and 360 J (or biphasic equivalent). Time should not be wasted with basic life support if immediate defibrillation can be delivered.

If DC shock sequence fails, basic and advanced life support aiming to maximise coronary blood flow with chest compressions and vasopressors is crucial to cardiac success. Until recently, any role of antiarrhythmic drugs in DC shock-resistant VF has been traditional rather than proven. Recommendations have varied from lidocaine and bretyllium to amiodarone. The ILCOR currently recommends consideration of a range of antiarrhythmic drugs, including amiodarone, lidocaine, magnesium and procainamide. Recent studies indicate amiodarone as the drug of choice for DC shock-resistant VF. Amiodarone (300 mg) was superior to lidocaine and, in another study, 5 mg/kg followed by 2.5 mg/kg if required was superior to lidocaine. There is an incidence of bradycardia and hypotension but no difference in adverse effect profile between lidocaine and this sizeable amiodarone dose.[63,64] After return of circulation, appropriate antiarrhythmic therapy is less clear but the role of lidocaine continues to disappear. Precipitating factors should be sought and treated (for long-term management issues, see the section on sudden cardiac death, below).

RIGHT BUNDLE BRANCH BLOCK (**FIG. 22.39**)

In right BBB (RBBB) the normal rapid coordinated depolarisation of the right ventricle is lost due to conduction block in the right branch of the bundle of His. There is normal rapid depolarisation of the septum and the initial deflection of the QRS is not altered. The activation of the free wall of the left ventricle is also normal. However the final activation of the free wall of the right ventricle is slow and anomalous, leading to a broad QRS.

ECG

The ECG shows wide QRS (>120 ms) and the QRS morphology in the right ventricular leads V_1 and V_2 is often M shaped. This results in two R-waves, with the smaller of the R-waves being designated 'r' and the larger 'R'. The classical pattern is the M-shaped rSR in V_1 or V_2 and a broad S-wave in LV leads, especially I and V_6. In V_1 the R-wave is greater in amplitude than the R-wave. In V_6 the R-wave is greater than any S-wave present. Partial RBBB is identical, except the QRS duration is 110–120 ms.

CLINICAL

RBBB may be a normal variant, but may occur with massive pulmonary embolism, right ventricular hypertrophy, ischaemic heart disease and congenital heart disease (note that myocardial infarction can be diagnosed in the presence of RBBB).

LEFT BUNDLE BRANCH BLOCK (**FIG. 22.40**)

In left BBB (LBBB), there is delayed and anomalous activation of the interventricular septum from right to left (i.e. in the opposite direction to normal) and the free wall of the left ventricle.

ECG

There is a wide QRS (>120 ms) and in V_1 the characteristic morphology shows an rS or QS. In V_6 there are primary and secondary R-waves (RR′), often resulting in M-shaped or plateau morphology. Q-waves are never seen in LV leads (V_4–V_6) (note that myocardial infarction cannot usually be diagnosed in the presence of LBBB). Partial LBBB is similar, except that the QRS duration is 110–120 ms.

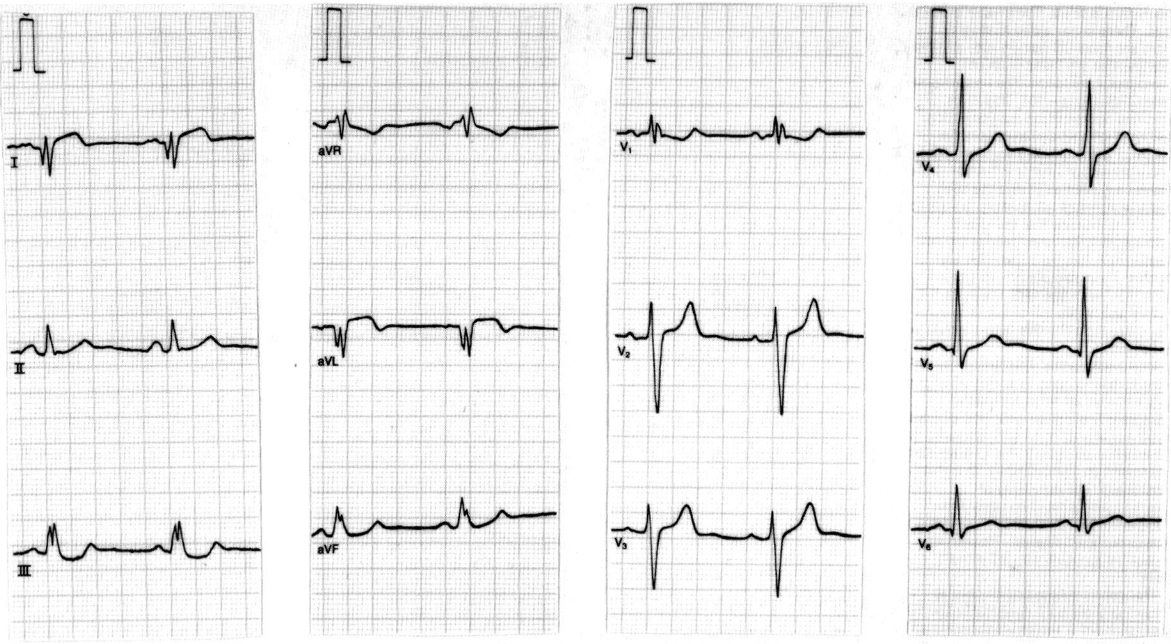

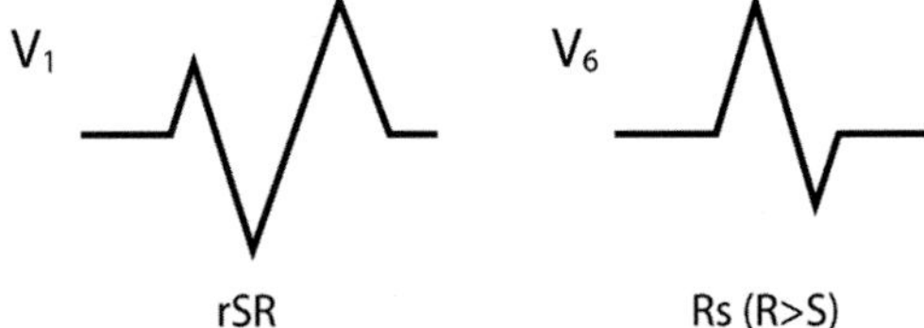

Figure 22.39 Right bundle branch block (RBBB) with characteristic M-shaped rSR complex in lead V_1 and Rs complex in V_6.

CLINICAL

LBBB is often associated with heart disease such as coronary artery disease, cardiomyopathy or LV hypertrophy. LBBB makes diagnosis of myocardial infarction difficult and the development of a new LBBB fulfils ECG criteria of acute infarction.

HEMIBLOCKS

The left branch of the bundle of His divides into the left anterosuperior division supplying the anterior superior lateral wall of the left ventricle and the posteroinferior division supplying the posterior inferior diaphragmatic surface of the left ventricle. Although block can occur in either division it is more common in the anterosuperior division, as it is more vulnerable to disease processes due to its longer course and thinner dimension. The anterosuperior division runs close to the aortic valve and tends to be involved in degenerative processes affecting this valve. The posteroinferior division is shorter and thicker and, unlike the anterosuperior division, has a double blood supply.

LEFT ANTERIOR HEMIBLOCK

There is left-axis deviation (usually lead I predominantly positive, leads II and III predominantly negative) with initial R-wave in inferior leads (II, III, aVF).

LEFT POSTERIOR HEMIBLOCK

There is usually right-axis deviation (lead I predominantly negative and lead III predominantly positive). Other causes of right-axis deviation (e.g. right ventricular hypertrophy) need to be excluded.

CLINICAL

RBBB with either left anterior hemiblock (**Fig. 22.41**) or left posterior hemiblock indicates an extensive conduction defect and a poor prognosis (high risk of complete heart block), especially in AMI.

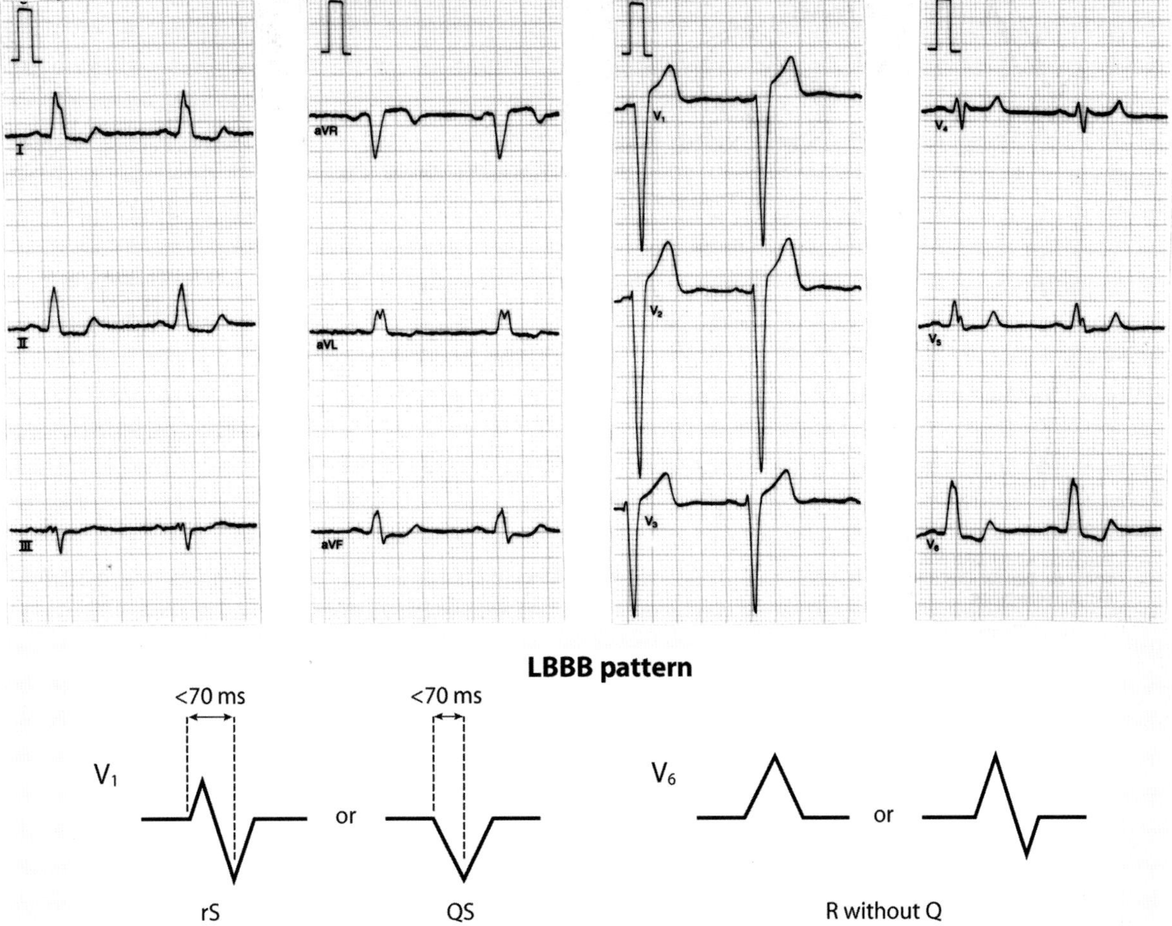

Figure 22.40 Left bundle branch block (LBBB).

HYPERKALAEMIA

A high serum K^+ can produce ECG changes (**Fig. 22.42**). Early changes consist of tall peaked T-waves with reduced P-wave amplitude. Progressive widening of the QRS may be confused with BBB. Cardiac arrest may eventually occur.

ATRIOVENTRICULAR BLOCK[62]

AV block is a delay or failure of impulse conduction from the atria to the ventricles. AV block is classified according to whether conduction of atrial impulses is delayed (first degree), blocked intermittently (second degree) or blocked completely (third degree).

FIRST-DEGREE AV BLOCK

ECG

PR interval (measured from the onset of the P-wave to the onset of the QRS) exceeds 200 ms (**Fig. 22.43**). Each P-wave is followed by a QRS. PR intervals may be prolonged to such a degree that the P-wave is buried in the previous T-wave or even QRS.

CLINICAL

First-degree AV block is commonly associated with increased vagal tone, and occasionally with drugs (especially digoxin), ischaemic heart disease (particularly inferior myocardial infarction) and rheumatic fever. It usually causes no symptoms and requires no treatment. If associated with digoxin, the drug should be ceased or the dose decreased.

SECOND-DEGREE AV BLOCK

Second-degree AV block is characterised by intermittent failure of AV conduction and is classified into Mobitz types I and II. Second-degree AV block can occur in SVTs; however, the conduction block is a physiological 'protective' mechanism in the setting of rapid atrial impulses.

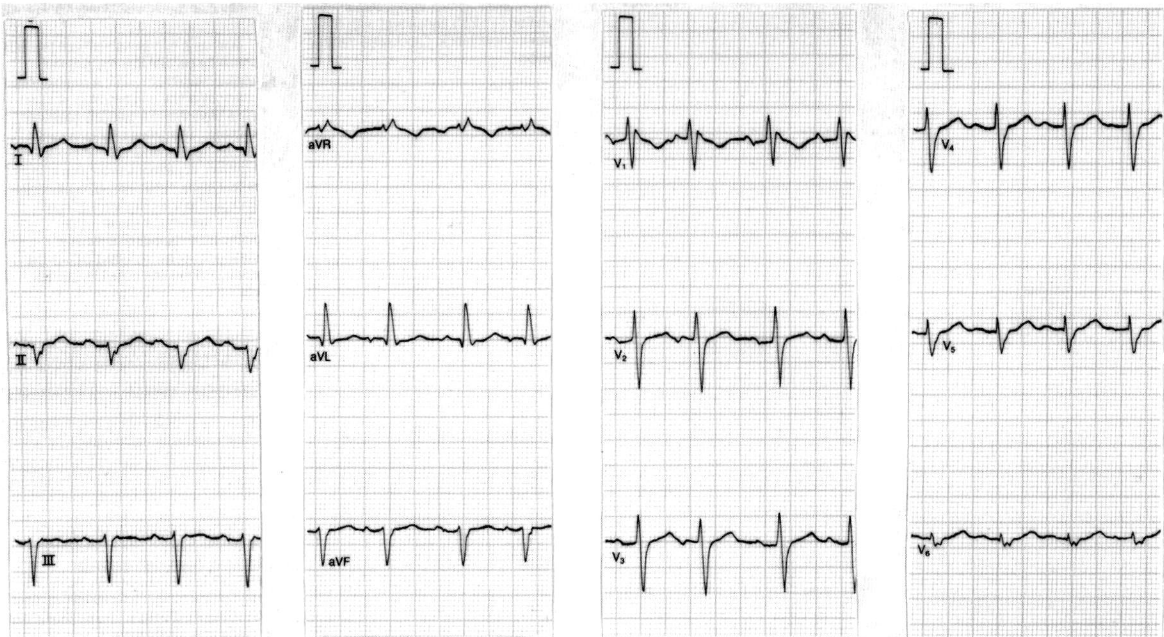

Figure 22.41 Right bundle branch block with left anterior hemiblock. There is left-axis deviation (mean frontal axis of –75°) and small R-waves in II, III and aVF.

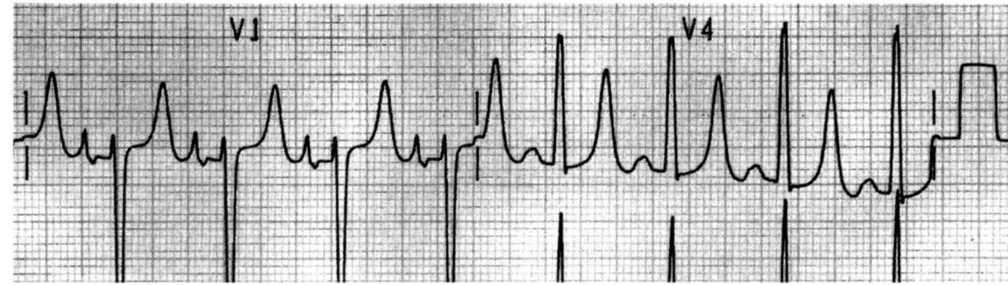

Figure 22.42 Sinus rhythm with peaked 'tent-shaped' T-waves in a patient with a serum potassium of 7.6 mmol/L.

MOBITZ TYPE I (WENCKEBACH)

Delay in AV conduction increases with each atrial impulse until an atrial impulse fails to conduct. This is usually a repetitive pattern, which may or may not begin with first-degree AV block. The level of AV block in type 1 is usually in the AV node itself and can be physiological (increased vagal tone) as well as pathological.

ECG

There is progressive lengthening of the PR interval over successive cardiac cycles, culminating in a non-conducted P-wave, resulting in a missed beat (**Fig. 22.44**). Type 1 is common in fit healthy people in the presence of high levels of resting vagal tone (**Fig. 22.45**).

CLINICAL

The condition is generally benign and does not carry the adverse likelihood of progression to complete AV block, although it may occur with inferior infarction. Treatment is rarely necessary.

MOBITZ TYPE II

There is intermittent failure of conduction of atrial impulses to the ventricles without preceding increases in the PR interval. The ratio of conducted to non-conducted atrial impulses varies; for example, every second or fourth atrial impulse may be conducted (i.e. 2:1 or 4:1 second-degree AV block). The lesion causing type II is usually situated in the bundle of His and is always pathological.

ECG

PR interval remains constant prior to the blocked P-wave. There is always a constant P-QRS-wave ratio: the P-waves are two (**Fig. 22.46**), three (rare) or four times more frequent than QRS-waves.

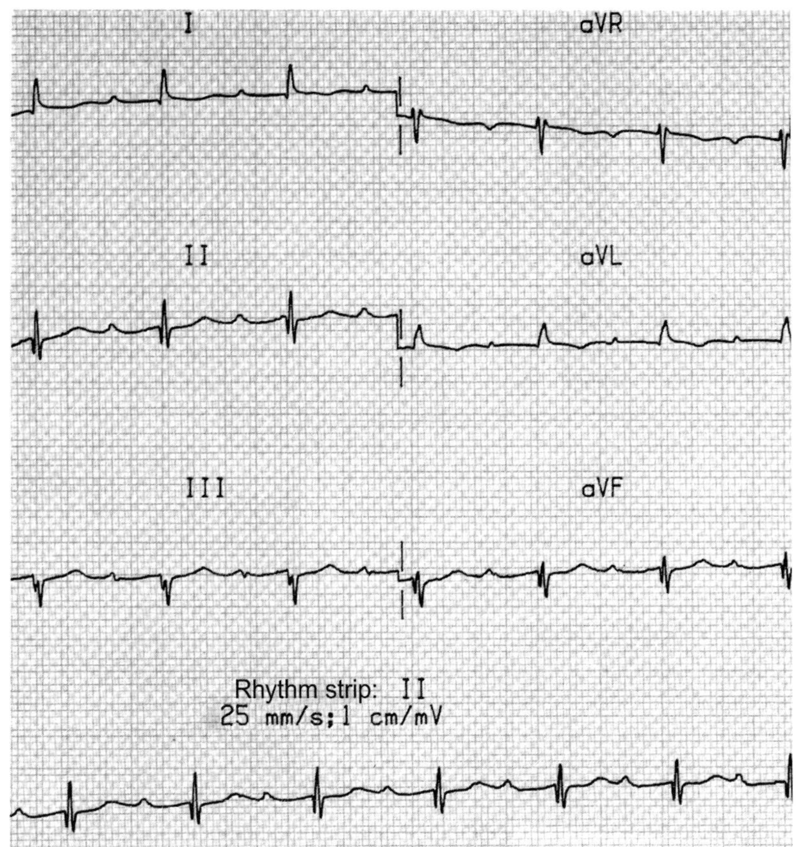

Figure 22.43 Sinus rhythm with first-degree AV block. The PR interval is 360 ms. Note inferior-wall myocardial infarction with Q-waves in II, III and aVF.

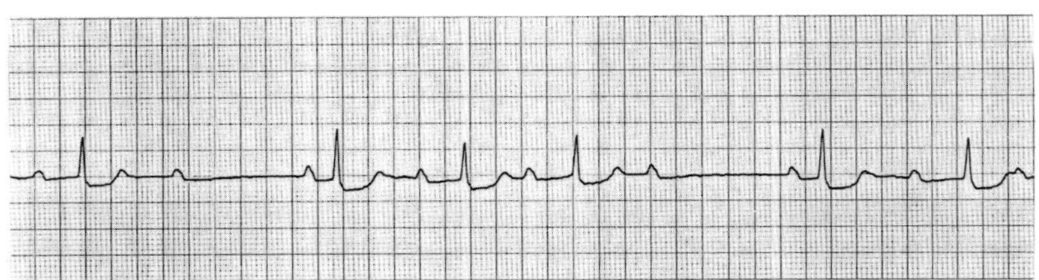

Figure 22.44 Mobitz type I (Wenckebach) second-degree arteriovenous block. Progressive lengthening of PR interval results in the failure of the second and sixth P-wave to be conducted.

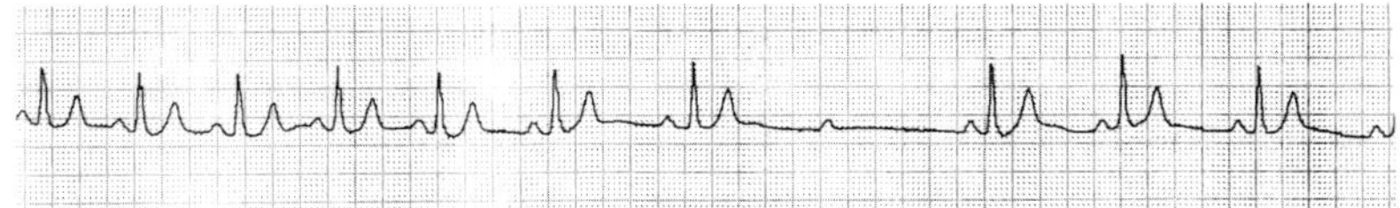

Figure 22.45 Intermittent type I second-degree arteriovenous block in a healthy male with obvious background sinus arrhythmia. Constant PR interval of 0.14 s suddenly increases to 0.22 s and next P-wave is not conducted.

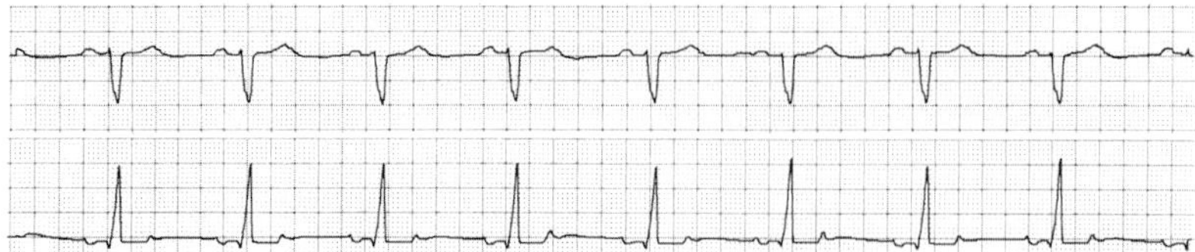

Figure 22.46 Mobitz type II second-degree arteriovenous (AV) block. Persistent 2 : 1 AV block with the atrial rate at 108 beats/min and the ventricular rate 54 beats/min.

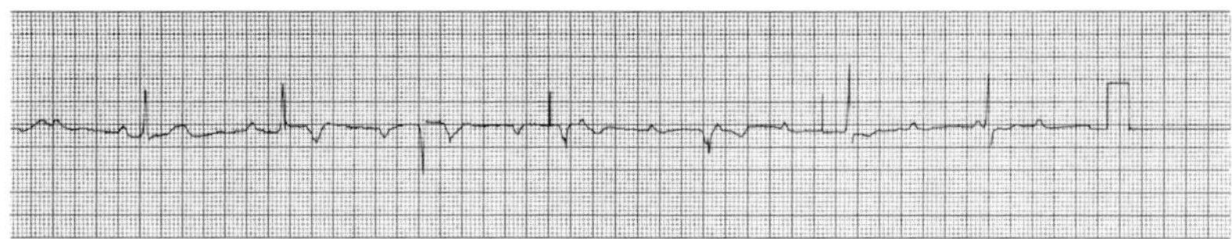

Figure 22.47 Leads I, aVR, V_1 and V_4 showing third-degree arteriovenous block. Complete dissociation of atrial activity at a rate of 107 beats/min and the ventricular rate at 46 beats/min. The escape rhythm is junctional (high up in the bundle of His) with a narrow QRS morphology.

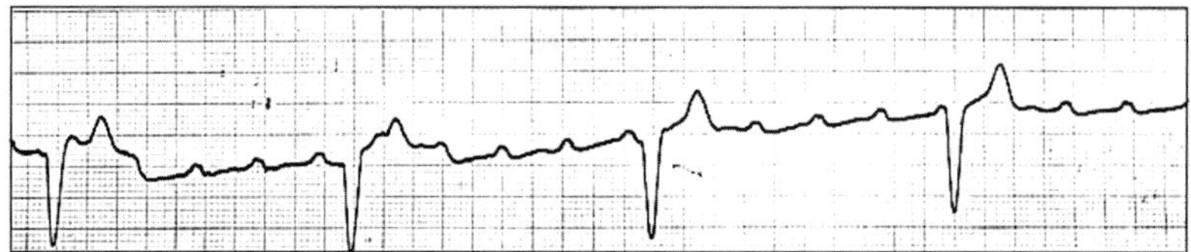

Figure 22.48 Third-degree arteriovenous block with an atrial rhythm at 135 beats/min and a broad distal ventricular escape rhythm which is unstable at a rate of 30 beats/min.

CLINICAL

It is likely to be associated with structural heart disease. Slower symptomatic ventricular rates may require pacing. The AV block may be intermittent or persistent. The adverse prognosis relates to the frequency of progression to complete AV block.

THIRD-DEGREE (COMPLETE) AV BLOCK

This rhythm occurs when no atrial impulses are conducted to the ventricles; atrial and ventricular contractions are dissociated. The SA node usually continues to depolarise the atria, whereas ventricular activation depends on a standby escape pacemaker located below the block. The escape pacemaker may be close to the His bundle (narrow QRS, stable pacemaker usually 40–60 beats/min) (**Fig. 22.47**), or more distal in ventricular tissue (wide QRS, relatively unstable pacemaker with a rate of 20–40 beats/min) (**Fig. 22.48**). If no ectopic escape pacemaker emerges, ventricular asystole will occur, resulting in a Stokes–Adams attack, or death if the episode is prolonged. Torsade de pointes may also occur associated with the bradycardia.

ECG

The ECG shows normal regular P-waves completely dissociated from QRS complexes. The QRS rate is always significantly slower than the P-wave rate and may be very slow at times.

CLINICAL

Idiopathic fibrosis of the conduction system is the most common cause. Other causes include myocardial infarction, valvular heart disease, cardiac surgery and a congenital form of complete heart block. Cardiac pacing is usually required to increase heart rate and cardiac output. Congenital forms often have a relatively fast escape ventricular rate, and patients may remain asymptomatic for many years.

SICK-SINUS SYNDROME

This consists of a number of sinus node abnormalities, including inappropriate sinus bradycardia, SA blocks or sinus arrest. When sinus bradycardia or SA block occurs, junctional escape rhythms are common. There may also be abnormalities of AV conduction. Paroxysms of AF or Afl may alternate with episodes of bradycardia (bradycardia–tachycardia syndrome) (**Fig. 22.49**).

CLINICAL

The bradycardias associated with sick-sinus syndrome (SSS) may result in syncope or near-syncope. SSS is

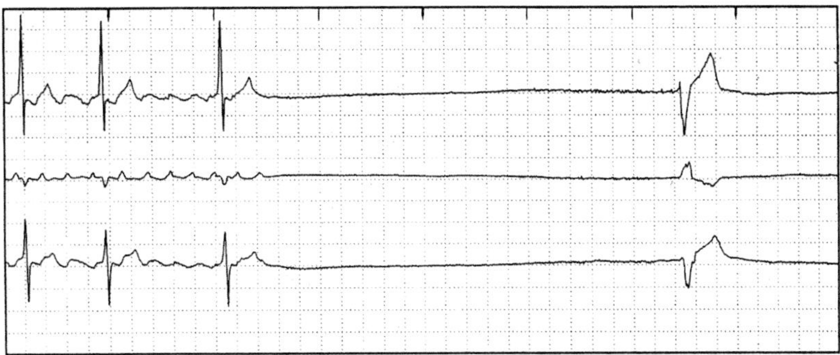

Figure 22.49 Characteristic findings in sick-sinus syndrome. Episodic atrial tachycardias (atrial flutter with variable block in this instance) with periods of sinus arrest and very slow ventricular escape rhythm upon spontaneous termination. CSM, carotid sinus massage.

often not associated with structural heart disease, but may occur with ischaemic and congenital heart disease.

TREATMENT

Cardiac pacing is usually required to control bradycardia symptoms. Atropine and low-dose isoproterenol may be useful prior to pacing, in the haemodynamically compromised patient. Bradycardia–tachycardia syndrome may require both pacing (for the bradycardia) and antiarrhythmic drugs (for the tachycardia). Anticoagulation needs to be considered if episodes of AF occur.

CRITICALLY ILL PATIENTS AND ARRHYTHMIA[65]

In the general population of critically ill patients, excluding acute coronary syndromes and cardiac surgical patients, arrhythmia is common. The documented incidence is as high as 78%; however, the incidence of arrhythmia that requires treatment is much lower, at 15–30%. SVT is by far the most common arrhythmia that requires treatment. AF, Afl and unifocal atrial tachycardias are the most frequent, in descending order. These SVTs are rarely the cause of admission but develop early in the admission, the majority by day 2. In critically ill patients, SVTs often result in:

- adverse myocardial oxygen supply–demand balance
- compromised blood pressure, cardiac output and systemic oxygen delivery
- impaired end-organ function such as oliguria and worsening gas exchange.

The development of SVT in a critically ill patient is associated with a significant increase in mortality, especially in patients with sepsis and respiratory failure. Incidence of SVT is increased with:

- elderly patients
- evidence or past history of heart disease
- haemodynamic features of diastolic failure with elevated pulmonary artery occlusion pressure
- catecholamine infusion
- severe sepsis.

The actual dose of the catecholamine infusion does not appear to be important and, although electrolyte disturbances are common in critically ill patients, low plasma potassium and magnesium levels do not appear to be important predictors of SVT development. The incidence of SVT, particularly AF, is so high in elderly patients with heart disease on a catecholamine infusion that consideration of prophylactic strategies is worthwhile.

Risk of in-hospital stroke is increased in critically ill patients with new-onset AF, odds ratio 2.70 and greater focus on the need for embolic prophylaxis is needed.[66]

TREATMENT OF SUPRAVENTRICULAR TACHYCARDIA IN CRITICALLY ILL PATIENTS

Continuing arrhythmogenic and chronotropic factors make rate control difficult.

- Digoxin often results in poor rate control due to persisting endogenous and exogenous sympathomimetic tone. The inotropic and vasopressor effects of acute digitalisation are beneficial. Digoxin (10 μg/kg) has been shown to provide superior circulatory support to dopamine at 8 μg/kg per min in septic patients.[67]
- Irrespective of plasma levels, magnesium has been shown to be effective at rate control; however, hypotension due to vasodilatation can be seen.
- Amiodarone is particularly effective and has allowed reliable acute rate control over a period of days in critically ill patients with circulatory shock requiring catecholamine infusions.[68] It can cause hypotension if patients are rapidly loaded. In another study, magnesium was at least as effective as amiodarone in rate control and time to reversion to sinus rhythm.[69]
- Other agents, such as diltiazem, sotalol and procainamide, are associated with prohibitive myocardial depression and hypotension.

Urgent cardioversion is indicated in unstable patients. The likelihood of remaining in sinus rhythm in the setting of high endogenous and exogenous sympathomimetic tone is low without concomitant use of an antiarrhythmic drug. Cardioversion is best reserved for hastening onset of sinus rhythm once a drug like amiodarone has controlled rate. Cardioversion should at least be attempted within 24–48 hours of onset in the hope that embolic and anticoagulation issues are avoided.

MYOCARDIAL INFARCTION AND ARRHYTHMIA[23]

Arrhythmia is common following AMI. While early arrhythmia contributes significantly to mortality, treatment is largely expectant and secondary to re-establishing coronary blood flow, minimising infarct size and treating ongoing ischaemia and heart failure. Late ventricular arrhythmia is particularly challenging, as selecting patients at risk is difficult and treatment options are limited.

MANAGEMENT OF ACUTE MYOCARDIAL INFARCTION AND ARRHYTHMIA CONTROL

Modern management of AMI, although targeted to prevent or reduce infarct size, has also been very effective in reducing arrhythmia incidence and sequelae. Numerous studies have documented transient ventricular arrhythmias at the time of reperfusion resulting from thrombolysis and acute angioplasty. However, the most common arrhythmias seen in this setting are VEB, AIVR and non-sustained VT, rather than VF or sustained VT.

Meta-analysis of thrombolytic trials has shown no increase in early VF following thrombolytic therapy in the first 24 hours. The likelihood of developing VF at any time during a hospital episode is reduced following thrombolytic therapy but the risk of developing VT is increased. The mechanism of reperfusion arrhythmia is believed to be related to intracellular calcium overload and the resulting triggered activity in the form of DAD. Dipyridamole, which inhibits the cellular uptake of adenosine, has been shown to be effective in preventing and treating reperfusion ventricular arrhythmia.

Prior to the introduction of thrombolytic therapy, beta-adrenergic receptor blockers significantly reduced the incidence of early VEB and VF. However, following routine use of thrombolytic therapy, the benefit of beta blockers relates to a reduction in post-infarction ischaemia and subsequent infarction.

The early work demonstrating survival benefit of magnesium was initially thought to be due to the prevention of arrhythmia.[70] However, the Leicester Intravenous Magnesium Intervention Trial (LIMIT-2) found the improved survival not to be related to a reduction in arrhythmia.[71] Subsequent studies in the thrombolytic era have failed to show any benefit at all with magnesium, although debate regarding optimal time of administration persists. Magnesium may have a role in patients in whom beta-adrenergic blockers or thrombolytic therapy are contraindicated.

ELECTROLYTE CONCENTRATIONS AND ARRHYTHMIA FOLLOWING ACUTE MYOCARDIAL INFARCTION

Serum potassium following AMI is negatively correlated with the incidence of VEB and VT, with the probability of VT falling until serum potassium exceeds 4.5 mmol/L.[9] There is no evidence that magnesium levels in this setting have any effect on ventricular arrhythmia. Nonetheless, ILCOR recommendations not only include the maintenance of serum potassium greater than 4.0 mmol/L, but also serum magnesium levels greater than 1.0 mmol/L.

BRADYARRHYTHMIAS POST ACUTE MYOCARDIAL INFARCTION

One-third of patients with AMI develop sinus bradycardia because of increased vagal tone. In inferior infarcts due to occlusion of the right coronary artery, bradyarrhythmia is due to ischaemia of the SA and AV nodes. Reperfusion of the right coronary artery can also lead to sinus bradycardia and heart block that is due to accumulation of adenosine in nodal tissue. Bradycardia in this setting is resistant to atropine.

Second- or third-degree AV block occurs in approximately 20% of AMI patients. High-degree AV block occurs early when present, with 42% presenting with AV block and most, 66%, developing in the first 24 h. Similar to all post-AMI arrhythmias, thrombolytic therapy has reduced the incidence down to 12%. When present, high-degree AV block is associated with an increased mortality. However, high-degree AV block is not an independent predictor, but rather a marker of extensive infarction and LV dysfunction.

Treatment is only indicated for sinus bradycardia associated with symptoms, hypotension or signs of poor cardiac output. Most often, first- and second-degree block also do not need treatment. Mobitz type I second-degree block may require treatment and atropine is indicated. However, in Mobitz type II, atropine usually has no effect on infranodal block and may precipitate third-degree block by increasing sinus rate and enhancing block. Atropine may improve heart rate with AV block occurring at the AV node, as demonstrated by a narrow QRS complex, by improving AV conduction or accelerating escape rhythm. Atropine is not indicated for infranodal third-degree block, which is diagnosed by the presence of a new wide QRS complex. When required, atropine is administered, 0.5–1.0 mg every 3 minutes until signs or symptoms are resolved, up to a maximum of 0.03–0.04 mg/kg. If atropine is not indicated or effective, cardiac pacing is required (**Box 22.4**). Transcutaneous pacing is indicated for initial management as a bridge until a transvenous temporary pacing wire can be inserted safely and with appropriate sterile technique. With the ready availability of transcutaneous pacing, i.v. catecholamines for

Box 22.4 Indications for pacing following myocardial infarction

Haemodynamically unstable bradycardia (<50 beats/min)
Mobitz type II second-degree atrioventricular block
Third-degree heart block
Bilateral bundle branch block
Left anterior fascicular block
New left bundle branch block
Bundle branch block and first-degree atrioventricular block

bradyarrhythmias are to be avoided in the setting of AMI.

ATRIAL FIBRILLATION POST ACUTE MYOCARDIAL INFARCTION

New-onset AF occurs in 10–15% of AMI. The incidence increases with age, large infarcts, LV hypertrophy and congestive cardiac failure. It is also related to atrial infarction with occlusion of the right coronary artery proximal to the sinus node branch or circumflex proximal to the left atrial circumflex branch. Later in the course of myocardial infarction, AF is related to postinfarct pericarditis.

Thrombolytic therapy has reduced the incidence of AF. In the setting of AMI, AF is usually self-limiting and requires no treatment. If rapid ventricular rates are associated with further ischaemic symptoms or haemodynamic compromise, cardioversion is indicated. Beta blockers, which are indicated in the treatment of AMI anyway, are the initial treatment of choice. Digoxin is not indicated in the setting of acute ischaemia as the likelihood of triggered activity associated with intracellular calcium overload is increased. AF following AMI is associated with an increase in mortality. Systemic emboli following AMI are three times more likely with AF and 50% occur in the first 24 hours of onset of AF. For this reason, sustained AF is an indication for anticoagulation prior to the normal 48-hour period following AMI.

VENTRICULAR ARRHYTHMIA POST ACUTE MYOCARDIAL INFARCTION[22,72,73]

VF/VT is the leading cause of mortality following AMI. Fifty per cent of patients dying from AMI do so prehospital due to VF/VT. Pre-hospital mortality is being reduced by improved community education, wider application of basic life support and availability of an automated external defibrillator (AED). Following admission to hospital, LV failure is the most common cause of death.

The major risk period for VF is the first 4 hours following onset of symptoms, with 4–18% of patients having VF in this period. Once admitted to hospital, 5% develop VF, mostly in this first 4-hour period. VF in this early 4-hour period is termed 'primary VF'. VF later in the course of an AMI, usually associated with LV failure or cardiogenic shock, is called 'secondary VF'.

Thrombolytic therapy has reduced VF incidence. The Gruppo Italiano per lo Studio della Streptochinasi nell'infarto miocardico (GISSI) study[72] found an incidence of primary VF of 3.6% and secondary VF of 0.6%. The overall incidence of ventricular arrhythmia in the Global Utilization of Streptokinase and Tissue plasminogen activator to treat Occluded arteries (GUSTO-1) report was VF, 4.1%, VT, 3.5% and both, 2.7%.

Primary VF increases in-hospital mortality and complications but not long-term mortality. Complex ventricular arrhythmias, defined as multiform VEB, couplets and non-sustained VT, occur in 35–40% of patients during hospital stay. They occur equally with Q-wave and non-Q-wave infarction. Complex ventricular arrhythmia is a risk factor for subsequent VF/VT and SCD, particularly in non-Q-wave infarction. Polymorphous VT is less common after AMI and does not appear to be related to QT prolongation or electrolyte disturbances in the reported cases.

Lidocaine reduces primary VF by 33% but mortality is increased by a similar amount such that there is no net benefit and the third International Study of Infarct Survival (ISIS-3) reported an overall trend to increased mortality.[74] Being more selective as to which patients receive lidocaine has not been possible, as only 50% of patients who develop VF have 'warning' ventricular arrhythmia. In the 'percutaneous coronary intervention or thrombolytic and beta-blocker' era of treatment of AMI, the use of prophylactic lidocaine, or any other antiarrhythmic drug, to prevent VF will have even less benefit. There are no conclusive data to support the use of lidocaine to prevent recurrent VF in those patients who have already suffered an episode of VF. Despite this, a short period of 6–24 hours of lidocaine has been advocated.

Patients who survive a late or secondary episode of VF/VT following myocardial infarction require full evaluation for preventive strategies, as do survivors of SCD. All survivors of a myocardial infarction are at an increased risk for SCD but accurate prediction is not feasible. Risk factors that have been shown to be associated with increased risk of a subsequent episode of VF/VT after myocardial infarction include:

- age
- Holter monitoring and demonstration of non-sustained VT, couplets and frequent VEB (i.e. >10 beats/min)
- impaired LV function (i.e. ejection fraction less than 30–40%)
- signal-average ECG and detection of delayed afterpotentials. In patients presenting with SCD after myocardial infarction, 68–87% have an abnormal signal-average ECG. However, the positive predictive value is poor, at 15–25%

- demonstrated inducibility of VT postinfarction is associated with increased risk of SCD. However, the positive predictive value is again poor, at 20–30%.

Combinations of these risk factors have been evaluated to predict risk after infarction. The combination of delayed potentials on signal-average ECG, LV ejection fraction of less than 40% and non-sustained VT on Holter monitor has been shown to be associated with up to 50% risk of SCD. Currently, there is no agreement on which patients require primary preventive strategies for VF/VT following myocardial infarction.

Using frequent VEB to identify patients at risk following myocardial infarction has been extensively used. There have been 54 randomised trials reported involving more than 20 000 patients using 11 different class I agents.

Class I agents showed no overall benefit on all-cause mortality and class IC agents have excess mortality despite arrhythmia suppression.[15]

Class II antiarrhythmics, beta blockers, have an established and broadening role, with recent evidence showing significant benefit.[75]

Class III agents lack a consistent class effect. Sotalol (Survival with oral D-sotalol: SWORD) was found to increase all-cause mortality and arrhythmia deaths.[76] Amiodarone (Canadian Amiodarone Myocardial Infarction Arrhythmia Trial: CAMIAT) reduces all-cause mortality in patients with frequent VEB post myocardial infarction,[77] but another study (European Myocardial Infarction Amiodarone Trial: EMIAT) evaluated amiodarone in patients with ejection fraction less than 40% and found no effect on all-cause mortality but a 35% reduction in arrhythmia deaths.[78] Subsequent analysis of combined CAMIAT and EMIAT data has emphasised the importance of beta blockers. The combination of amiodarone and beta blockers in these post-infarct patients was better than either drug alone.[79]

CARDIOTHORACIC SURGERY AND ARRHYTHMIA

SVT AFTER CARDIOTHORACIC SURGERY[80]

AF predominates, with Afl and unifocal atrial tachyarrhythmia also commonly occurring after coronary artery bypass grafting, with an incidence of 11–40% and in over 50% following valvular surgery. In addition to mechanisms found in non-surgical patients, pericardial inflammation or effusion, increased catecholamine production and postoperative autonomic changes are implicated. Major risk factors include:

- previous history of AF
- increasing age
- postoperative withdrawal of beta-blocker therapy.

Extent of coronary artery disease, postoperative ischaemia, duration of aortic cross-clamping or cardiopulmonary bypass and method of myocardial protection do not influence incidence. SVT post cardiothoracic surgery is not a benign event, with the major consequence being thromboembolic complications. Stroke occurs following coronary artery bypass grafting in 1–6% of patients and postoperative atrial tachyarrhythmia increase the incidence threefold. Other adverse effects include:

- haemodynamic instability
- prolonged inotropic support
- need for intra-aortic balloon pump
- reoperation for bleeding
- longer and more expensive critical care unit and hospital episodes.

PREVENTION OF SUPRAVENTRICULAR TACHYCARDIA[81,82]

Preoperative beta-blocker treatment should be continued postoperatively. Beta blockers consistently reduce SVT across many studies with differing agents.

Amiodarone prophylaxis after elective cardiac surgery reduced postoperative AF from 53% to 25%. Diltiazem has also been shown to be effective at SVT prevention and there was associated improvement in haemodynamic variables and rates of myocardial ischaemia. Verapamil is not effective. Esmolol was found to be more effective than diltiazem. Sotalol is also effective but problematic bradycardia and hypotension are greater.[83] Atorvastatin is also effective.[84]

There is no relation between SVT incidence and serum magnesium levels and there are conflicting data relating to the efficacy of prophylactic magnesium. Digoxin has no role in prevention.

TREATMENT OF SUPRAVENTRICULAR TACHYCARDIA

Treatment is aimed at control of ventricular rate, prevention of thromboembolism and cardioversion.

Digoxin, atenolol, diltiazem and magnesium are appropriate choices to control rate.

In persisting AF, the timing of electrical cardioversion is debatable. Early electrical cardioversion, inside 24–48 hours, avoids the need for anticoagulation but is associated with a significant recurrence rate as postoperative arrhythmogenic factors remain. In persistent or recurrent AF, sotalol and amiodarone, depending on myocardial function, are suitable antiarrhythmic drugs and should be continued for 6–12 weeks following cardioversion.

Timing of safe anticoagulation following cardiac surgery is also debatable. Many advocate delaying anticoagulation till 72 hours post surgery, which may be greater than 24–48 hours after onset of SVT. Most cardiac surgical patients receive aspirin and low-dose heparin in the early postoperative period, which is likely to reduce risk. However, it is worth noting that, in other AF settings, 325 mg of aspirin decreased thromboembolic events but 75 mg did not.

VENTRICULAR ARRHYTHMIA FOLLOWING CARDIAC SURGERY

Ventricular arrhythmia requiring treatment, DC shock or drug therapy is common following cardiac surgery and occurs in 23% of patients.[85] Arrhythmias requiring DC shock occur in the first 36 hours and are associated with:

- advanced age
- failure to use an internal mammary artery conduit (which is likely to reflect preoperative assessment of high risk)
- SVT.

The incidence was not related to previous myocardial infarction, ejection fraction of less than 50%, prolonged operative time, perioperative myocardial infarction or reduced number of vessels bypassed. In patients undergoing coronary artery bypass, grafting patients at high risk for sudden death, LV ejection fraction less than 36% and abnormalities on signal-averaged ECG had a 6.3% incidence of sustained VT and 4.3% VF.

VEBs are common early on return from surgery, with frequent or complex ectopy associated with adrenergic effects of emerging from anaesthesia and hypokalaemia. The threshold to treat these arrhythmias varies with clinicians. Potassium must be regularly checked and maintained above 4 mmol/L.

If there is accompanying emergent hypertension, in addition to the antiarrhythmic action, the vasodilating properties of magnesium provide an ideal profile at this stage. Patients with VT/VF reverting with DC shock who are haemodynamically stable should have prophylactic antiarrhythmic cover until adrenergic stimulation associated with awakening and weaning from mechanical ventilation is past. Lidocaine has been the agent of choice, but magnesium, amiodarone and sotalol are all more effective. Maintaining antiarrhythmic levels of magnesium may not be conducive to weaning from ventilation. Extrapolating from post myocardial infarct data would support the conversion to beta blockers if there were no contraindications.

A smaller proportion of patients develop malignant VF/VT, most often in association with poor LV function and a postoperative low-cardiac-output state requiring catecholamine infusions. In this setting, ventricular arrhythmia is common, often initiated by short-coupling polymorphous VT (normal QT_c), due to ongoing ischaemia or reperfusion of ischaemic heart.

- High-dose amiodarone may work best in combination with antiarrhythmic levels of magnesium (1.8–2.0 mmol/L) or lidocaine.
- Many of these patients need an intra-aortic balloon pump to defend coronary artery perfusion pressure not only because of the likely poor LV function and low-output state, but also to minimise the adverse affects of antiarrhythmic drugs and recurrent DC shocks.
- Pacing may be required to counteract bradyarrhythmia associated with escalating doses of antiarrhythmic drugs. Pacing at faster rates (90–110 beats/min, which may not be ideal from a cardiac-output point of view) may be protective against recurrent episodes by promoting homogeneity of depolarisation and suppression of abnormal automaticity. The presence of epicardial or transvenous pacing wires also enables bedside-programmed stimulation and overdrive pacing for termination of recurrent VT, which has fewer deleterious effects than recurrent DC shocks.

LONG-QT SYNDROME[86,87]

The traditional criteria of prolonged QT needs to be corrected for heart rate (QT_c, Bazett's formula, QT divided by the square root of the RR interval) and a QT_c greater than 0.44 ms. Borderline QT_c is common and stems from miscalculation in the setting of atypical T-waves and prominent U-waves. The recommended method to determine the end of the T-wave is by intersecting the tangent to the steepest slope of the last limb of the T-wave and the baseline (**Fig. 22.50**). The diagnosis of 'borderline LQTS' is common with QT_c in the range of 440–470 ms. QT_c should also be adjusted for age and gender with females an average 10 ms longer. There is significant overlap between the normal population and patients with congenital LQTS; 25–35% of congenital LQTS have a QT_c<440 ms (**Fig. 22.51**).

The causes of LQTS can be divided into acquired and congenital (**Box 22.5**). Most drugs that cause LQTS do so by binding to the HERG or alpha subunit of the I_{Kr} potassium channel and reducing repolarisation current. Unlike other I_K potassium channels, the HERG subunit of I_{Kr} is very sensitive to unintended drug binding owing to aromatic amino acids positioned in such a way as to block the channel. Common to all causes is a prolongation of repolarisation, which creates the substrate for random re-entry giving rise to polymorphous VT (classically of the torsade de pointes type), particularly under conditions of acute adrenergic arousal.

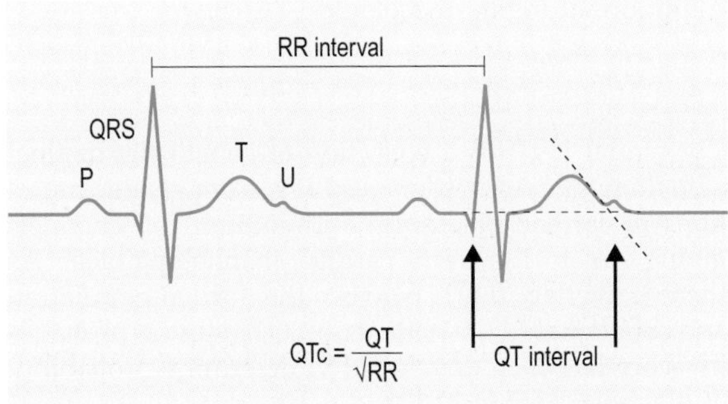

Figure 22.50 Determining QTc using the 'tangent method'.

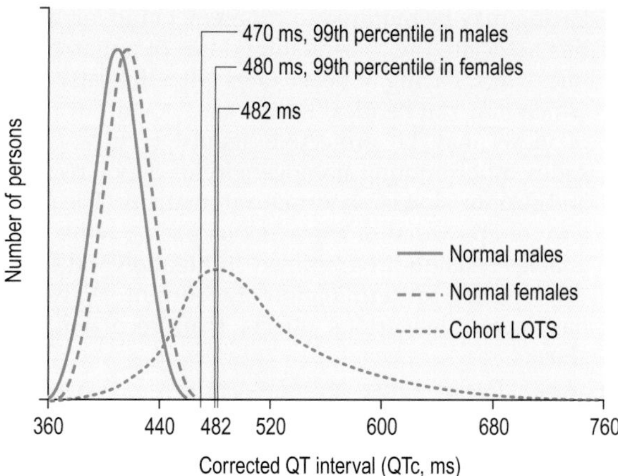

Figure 22.51 Distribution of QTc values (adapted from Johnson et al[87]). 99th percentile males 470 ms. 99th percentile females 480 ms. There is significant overlap of these 'normal' QTc persons and a cohort of mutation-positive patients, mean QTc 482 ms. *(From Taggart NW, Haglund CM, Tester DJ, et al. Circulation 2007;115:2613–20,[106] with permission.)*

Action potential prolongation results from either enhancing depolarisation (sodium (Na) channel, I_{Na}) or reducing repolarisation current (delayed rectifier potassium (K) currents, I_{Kr} and I_{Ks}).

There is less capacity to respond to additional stresses that impair repolarisation such as hypokalaemia, hypomagnesaemia and drugs with class III action.

Prolonged action potential in LQTS predisposes to arrhythmia in two ways:

1. Extended plateau phase of action potential results in susceptibility to EAD-initiated arrhythmia. EADs are due to re-opening of L-type calcium channels, the activity of which is increased by adrenergic stimulation, which explains the association between sudden cardiac death and exercise and excitement in LQTS.
2. Heterogeneity of prolonged action potential creates spatial dispersion of repolarisation, leading to regions of refractory block and substrate for re-entrant arrhythmia. This mechanism appears important in pharmacological LQTS.

CONGENITAL LQTS[88]

Congenital LQTS is a collection of genetically distinct arrhythmogenic disorders resulting from genetic mutations in cardiac potassium and sodium ion channels giving rise to the term 'cardiac channelopathies'. As there is overlap in QT_c between the normal population and congenital LQTS patients, a LQTS clinical probability score has been developed to determine probability of diagnosis (**Table 22.12**).

Congenital LQTS results from mutations in genes coding for cardiac proteins including ion channels, accessory subunits and modulatory proteins (**Table 22.13**).

Box 22.5 Causes of long-QT syndrome

Acquired
Drugs
- Class IA antiarrhythmic drugs
- Quinidine, procainamide
- Class III antiarrhythmic drugs
- Amiodarone, sotalol
- Tricyclic antidepressants
- Macrolide antibiotics
- Phenothiazines
- Antihistamines
- Cisapride

Myocardial ischaemia/infarction
Hypokalaemia
Cardiomyopathy
Acute myocarditis
Mitral valve prolapse
Acute cerebral injury
Hypothermia

Congenital
Familial
90%
Linked to a DNA marker on the short arm of chromosome 11
Autosomal-dominant in most cases
Some cases linked to congenital deafness and autosomal-recessive
Non-familial – related to new gene mutation
Sporadic: 10%

CLINICAL FEATURES[89]

Prevalence is estimated to be 1 in 2500–5000.

Thirty per cent of patients with congenital LQTS present with unexplained syncope or aborted sudden death (which is often not the first episode). The majority (60%) are identified when family members are screened after syncope or cardiac arrest in a family member. Ten per cent are detected on routine evaluation of ECG. The majority of episodes of syncope or sudden death (60%) are precipitated by emotions, physical activity or auditory stimuli causing acute adrenergic arousal. The degree of QT_c prolongation is not predictive of syncope or sudden death.

MANAGEMENT

The first line of management of polymorphous VT with shock is DC shock, with magnesium being the antiarrhythmic of choice.[90]

- Unresponsive rhythms or recurrence despite magnesium require pharmacological intervention (isoproterenol (isoprenaline) or epinephrine (adrenaline) depending on blood pressure) or electrical pacing.
- Factors associated with acquired LQTS need to be identified and eliminated.

Table 22.12 LQTS clinical probability score

FINDING	POINTS
HISTORY	
Syncope	
– without stress	1
– with stress	2
Congenital deafness	0.5
Family history of LQTS	1
Unexplained sudden death in a first-degree family member <age 30	0.5
ECG	
QTc by Bazett's formula	
450–459 ms in males	1
460–479 ms	2
≥480 ms	3
Torsades des pointes	2
T-wave alternans	1
≥3 leads with notched T-waves	1
Bradycardia <2nd centile for age	0.5
PROBABILITY SCORE	≤1 low probability >1 to <4 intermediate probability ≥4 high probability

Schwarlz PJ, Moss AJ, Vincent GM, et al. Diagnostic criteria for the long QT syndrome. An Update. Circulation 1993; 88:782–4.[107]

Table 22.13 Classification of congenital LQTS

TYPE	GENE MUTATION/ PROTEIN	FEATURES
LQT1	KCNQ1 α–subunit of I_{KS}	Reduced function of I_{KS} decreases repolarising current Most common at 30–35% but less severe When homozygous associated with congenital deafness
LQT2	KCNH2/h ERG α–subunit of I_{Kr}	Reduced function of I_{Kr} decreases repolarising current 25–30%
LQT3	SCN5A α–subunit of I_{Na}	Increased function of I_{Na} prolonging depolarising Na current Mutations in SCN5A also cause Brugada syndrome, cardiac conduction disease and dilated cardiomyopathy
LQT4	Anchor protein ankyrin B	Ankyrin B anchors ion channels in the cell
LQT5	KCNE1 β–subunit of I_{Ks}	Reduced function of I_{Ks} Homozygous leads to Jervell and Lange–Nielson syndrome Congenital deafness
LQT6	KCNE2 β–subunit of I_{Kr}	Reduced function of I_{Kr}
LQT7	K-channel I_{KI}	Anderson–Tauvel syndrome Associated skeletal deformities
LQT8	C_{AV} CACNAlc $I_{ca\text{-}L}$	Calcium channel is distributed widely Timothy's syndrome Multiple clinical manifestations

Strategies for prevention of recurrence in congenital LQTS depend on the presentation. Patients who present with or have a history of syncope or aborted sudden death have a high risk of recurrence (5% per year). Beta blockers are the first line of treatment with the goal of reducing the exercise heart rate to less than 130 beats/min. Symptomatic bradycardia following adequate beta blockade requires a permanent pacemaker. Patients with recurrence despite these measures and those with an early malignant course need stellate sympathetic ganglionectomy. In 5% of these high-risk patients triple therapy fails and an implantable defibrillator is required. Asymptomatic patients with incidental LQTS (<0.5% per year) and asymptomatic family members (0.5% per year) have a very low risk of syncope or sudden death. It is also very rare for the first episode to be fatal in these two groups so prophylactic measures are generally not required and close follow-up is sufficient.

Class IA, IC and III drugs may increase QT interval and should be avoided in polymorphous VT and torsade de pointes.

SUDDEN CARDIAC DEATH[91]

Arrhythmic causes of SCD can be divided into three categories:

1. *VT or VF:* this is most common.
2. *SVT with a very rapid ventricular rate:* this is usually associated with the development of AF or flutter in the presence of an accessory AV connection (but can occasionally be due to enhanced conduction over the normal AV conduction system).
3. *Bradycardia or asystole:* this is usually the result of an inadequate escape pacemaker mechanism associated with either a high-degree AV block or severe sinus node dysfunction. In addition, some patients with sinus node dysfunction have paroxysmal supraventricular arrhythmia (tachycardia–bradycardia syndrome) that on termination results in an exaggerated overdrive suppression of both the sinus node and escape pacemakers such that the prolonged pause evolves into asystole or VF.

The causes of these arrhythmias can be divided into three general categories:

1. *Ischaemic heart disease:* AMI or old myocardial infarction scar
2. *Non-ischaemic heart disease:* cardiomyopathy, valvular heart disease, congenital heart disease, ventricular hypertrophy and cardiac trauma
3. *No apparent structural heart disease:* primary electrical disease, electrolyte abnormalities, LQT syndromes and drugs.

Contributing factors are often multifactorial, particularly the combination of structural heart disease, proarrhythmic drugs and electrolyte abnormalities.

EVALUATION OF A SURVIVOR OF SCD

Primary prevention of SCD has been disappointing owing to difficulties in selecting patients at risk. Regardless of the aetiology of the SCD, the reported recurrence rate is high, at least 30–40% at 1 year. Therefore, in-hospital assessment is critical to establish the underlying cause and to guide therapy.

CORONARY ARTERY DISEASE AND SUDDEN CARDIAC DEATH

Extensive atherosclerotic coronary artery disease is the most common pathological finding in survivors and non-survivors of SCD. Fewer than 30% have evidence of a recent AMI. A larger proportion (up to 50%) has evidence of coronary artery thrombosis or plaque fissuring and rupture. In those patients not having an AMI, the majority (75%) has a coronary artery stenosis (> 50% of lumen), and 60% have three-vessel disease. Approximately 50% have evidence of an old myocardial infarction. The fact that the typical pathological background for SCD is severe epicardial coronary artery disease, with or without an old myocardial infarction and evidence of a new ischaemic syndrome, underlines the central role that coronary artery disease plays in SCD.

INVESTIGATIONS[17–19]

- *Chest X-ray:* cardiac size, presence of pulmonary oedema.
- *12-lead ECG:* acute ischaemia, previous infarction, ventricular aneurysm or LV hypertrophy. Abnormalities of rate, rhythm, conduction or sinus node dysfunction. PR interval, QRS complex duration or QT interval. Changes of electrolyte abnormalities.
- *Plasma electrolytes:* potassium, magnesium and calcium. Potassium levels may be difficult to interpret after a period of resuscitation.
- *Cardiac enzymes:* serial troponin T, creatinine phosphokinase with myocardial band fractionation and lactate dehydrogenase to establish the presence of a recent AMI.
- *Plasma blood levels of drugs that affect cardiac rhythm or conduction:* while proarrhythmic effects of drugs are more likely at high levels, it should be emphasised that proarrhythmia can occur at normal or low plasma drug levels.
- *Toxicology screen:* substance abuse or drug overdose (cocaine, psychotropic drugs), particularly in patients without overt structural heart disease.
- *24-hour Holter monitor ECG:* quantitative analysis of frequency of arrhythmia and to detect silent myocardial ischaemia.
- *Assessment of LV function:* LV ejection fraction. Gated pool scan gives a better estimate of global LV systolic function, but echocardiogram will give added diagnostic information such as valvular disease and myocardial hypertrophy. Both studies will detect segmental wall motion abnormalities.
- *Exercise tolerance test:* standard exercise ECG or thallium-201 scans. Echocardiogram immediately following exercise may be as informative.
- *Signal-average ECG:* averages between 100 and 400 heart beats, for identification of low-amplitude electrical signals, such as after-depolarisations. These are found in the terminal portion of the QRS complex and cannot be seen on the 12-lead ECG. Associated with an increased risk of spontaneous and inducible ventricular arrhythmia.
- *Cardiac catheterisation and coronary angiogram:* to quantify the degree of coronary artery disease.
- *EPS:* virtually always indicated to document and characterise ventricular tachyarrhythmia. The initial baseline EPS should be performed in the absence of any antiarrhythmic drugs. Inducibility of sustained ventricular arrhythmias at EPS is associated with worse outlook, with a 5-year risk of SCD of 32% versus 24% in those without inducible arrhythmia, and is an indication for an implantable defibrillator. The inducibility of VT/VF is less common in survivors of SCD (44%) than patients who present with recurrent sustained VT. In patients with sustained monomorphic haemodynamically stable VT, EPS mapping techniques are used to determine the possibility of surgical or catheter ablation. EPS is also important in other causes of SCD other than VT/VF. Patients with ventricular pre-excitation (WPW syndrome) require localisation of the accessory pathway. Propensity to develop complete heart block can be assessed by a His-bundle ECG.

PREVENTION OF RECURRENT VENTRICULAR ARRHYTHMIA IN SURVIVORS OF SUDDEN CARDIAC DEATH

MYOCARDIAL REVASCULARISATION AND SUDDEN CARDIAC DEATH

The Coronary Artery Surgery Study (CASS) registry looked at 13476 patients with significant operable coronary artery disease and showed an incidence of SCD of 5.2% in the medical arm compared with 1.8% in those assigned to surgery.[92] The precise mechanism of the benefit of surgery in primary prevention is unclear but is probably associated with prevention of ischaemia rather than arrhythmia control. In summary, the near-universal practice of surgical coronary revascularisation in SCD survivors with critical stenoses is based upon this primary prevention data (and the central role that ischaemia and infarction are known to play in arrhythmia substrate) rather than data demonstrating arrhythmia control.

ANTIARRHYTHMIC DRUGS AND SUDDEN CARDIAC DEATH[15,76–79]

The CAST study has clearly demonstrated the poor results of antiarrhythmic drug therapy alone in the prevention of arrhythmic SCD. Data from studies in survivors of SCD using amiodarone are conflicting, but generally poor, even with EPS confirmation of lack of inducibility. Certainly patients with an ejection fraction less than 30% do poorly on amiodarone alone. The primary role of antiarrhythmic drugs in the secondary prevention of SCD has all but disappeared, but amiodarone may be indicated if there is demonstrable suppression of inducible VT at EPS and the patient has an ejection fraction greater than 30–40%.

SURGICAL AND CATHETER ABLATION TECHNIQUES AND SUDDEN CARDIAC DEATH[27]

As most sustained ventricular arrhythmias arise from a scar within the myocardium, surgical attempts were made to excise these areas completely. Catheter ablation techniques for VT are suitable for the minority of patients with haemodynamically stable VT who can withstand prolonged mapping procedures. Currently, the success rates for ablative techniques are such that a significant number still need additional preventive therapies.

IMPLANTABLE CARDIOVERTER DEFIBRILLATORS AND SUDDEN CARDIAC DEATH

The reduction in SCD and overall cardiac mortality with implantable cardioverter defibrillators (ICDs) has been so spectacular and the results of previous therapies so poor that ICDs were initially introduced with little randomised controlled data. More recently controlled studies have shown:

- reduction in 3-year mortality by 31% compared to antiarrhythmic drug therapy in SCD survivors[93]
- reduced risk of death in patients with poor LV function following myocardial infarction[94]
- improved survival in patients with hypertrophic cardiomyopathy.[95]

However, no survival benefit was shown in high-risk patients following coronary artery bypass surgery.

Table 22.14 Mortality data for the various treatment regimens for sudden cardiac death

	SUDDEN DEATH (%)	TOTAL MORTALITY (%)
Implantable cardioverter defibrillator	3.5	13.6
Empirical amiodarone	12	34
Electrophysiological study-directed drug treatment	14	24
Surgery	3.7	37

Representative data from several studies are shown in **Table 22.14**. The benefit of ICD on survival persists for at least 8 years. Current indications are expanding, but the benefit is clear in the following groups of survivors of SCD and patients with documented VT/VF outside the early post-infarct phase:

- non-inducible VT/VF at EPS
- inducible VT/VF resistant to treatment
- VT/VF in patients with LV ejection fractions less than or equal to 30% regardless of results of EPS-directed drug therapy.

Further developments currently taking place include:

- transvenous catheter placement and subcutaneous patch avoiding the need for thoracotomy
- dual-chamber sensing to improve discrimination between SVT and VT that can be difficult on rate criteria alone, particularly in patients with intraventricular conduction delay
- technological advances reducing size, cost and increasing battery life.

Although one of the proposed advantages of ICD is the avoidance of antiarrhythmic drug side-effects, particularly the myocardial depressant effects, current practice usually combines ICD with low-dose amiodarone. This enables improved arrhythmia control by reducing atrial tachyarrhythmia and slowing VT rate, and prolonging battery life by reducing the frequency of arrhythmia. The role of ICD in the management algorithms of SCD is shown in **Figures 22.52** and **22.53**. Given the current lack of available ICD, some advocate restriction to patients less than 75 years. With wider availability of ICD, fewer patients will be managed on drug-only strategies in the future.

CLASSIFICATION OF ANTIARRHYTHMIC DRUGS

The time-honoured physiologically based classification of antiarrhythmic drugs is the Vaughan-Williams

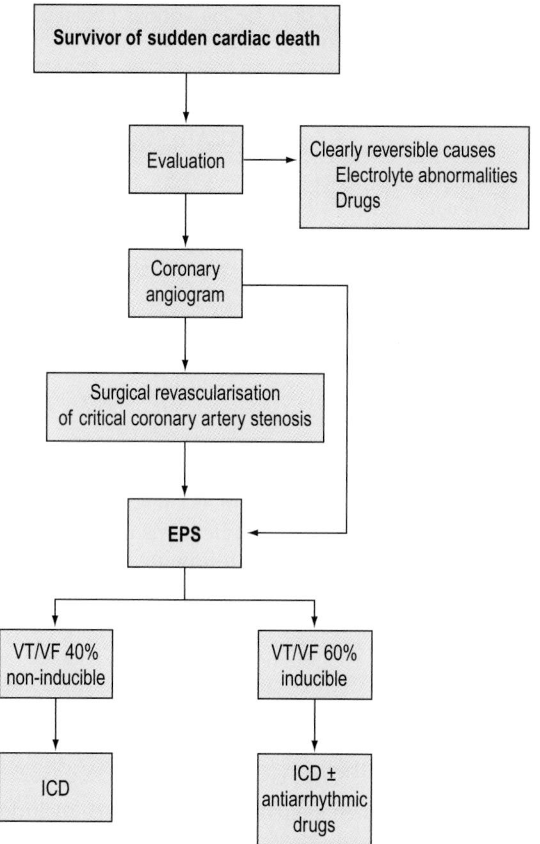

Figure 22.52 Management algorithm of a survivor of sudden cardiac death. This algorithm does not include the option of an antiarrhythmic drug alone in patients with intact left ventricular function who initially have inducible ventricular tachycardia/fibrillation (VT/VF) that is subsequently found to be suppressible on a drug with electrophysiological studies (EPS). ICD, implantable cardioverter defibrillator.

classification (**Table 22.15**), which has been modified over the years. This classification is a hybrid, with classes I and IV representing ion channel blockers, class II representing a receptor blocker and class III representing a change in an electrophysiological variable. The prolongation of repolarisation, the defining effect of class III agents, can be produced by a block of any one of several K^+ ionic channels (the delayed rectifier potassium current I_{Kr} responsible for phase 3 repolarisation is the ionic channel target of most class III agents) or from modification of Na^+ or Ca^+ channel function. This classification is also incomplete and does not include cholinergic agonists, digitalis, magnesium and adenosine. For this reason, an alternative classification has been advocated based upon molecular targets for drug action that include ion channels, receptors and pumps/carriers (**Table 22.16**).[3]

Table 22.15 Vaughan-Williams classification of antiarrhythmic drugs

CLASS	MECHANISM OF ACTION	EFFECT ON ACTION POTENTIAL	INDICATIVE DRUGS
Class I	Sodium channel blockers	Depresses rate of phase 0 depolarisation	
Class IA		Prolongs repolarisation	Procainamide Disopyramide Quinidine
Class IB		Shortens repolarisation	Lidocaine Mexiletine Phenytoin
Class IC		Minimal effect on repolarisation	Flecainide Encainide Propafenone
Class II	β-adrenergic receptor blockers		Propranolol Atenolol Metoprolol Esmolol
Class III	Potassium channel blockers	Prolongs repolarisation	Amiodarone Dronedarone Sotalol Ibutilide Vernakalant Bretylium
Class IV	Calcium channel blockers		Verapamil Diltiazem

ANTIARRHYTHMIC DRUGS[74]

DIGOXIN

Digoxin is a muscurinic subtype 2 receptor (M_2) agonist and a highly potent Na^+/K^+-ATPase pump-blocking agent. Digoxin exerts its antiarrhythmic activity predominantly at the AV node where at lower doses conduction is slowed by the M_2 vagotonic effect. This effect is easily reversed by enhanced sympathetic tone in the setting of exercise, critical illness and postoperative state. At higher concentrations, digoxin has a direct effect on AV node conduction by the Na^+/K^+-ATPase pump blockade and is more resistant to sympathomimetic effects. The decrease in $[K^+]_i$ and increase in $[Na^+]_i$ results in hyperpolarisation, shortening of atrial action potential and an increase in AV nodal refractoriness. There is also increased availability of intracellular Na^+ for the Na^+–Ca^{2+} exchanger, increasing $[Ca^{2+}]_i$ which results in the positive inotropic effects of digoxin, making it an ideal agent in the setting of LV dysfunction. However, the positive inotropic effects

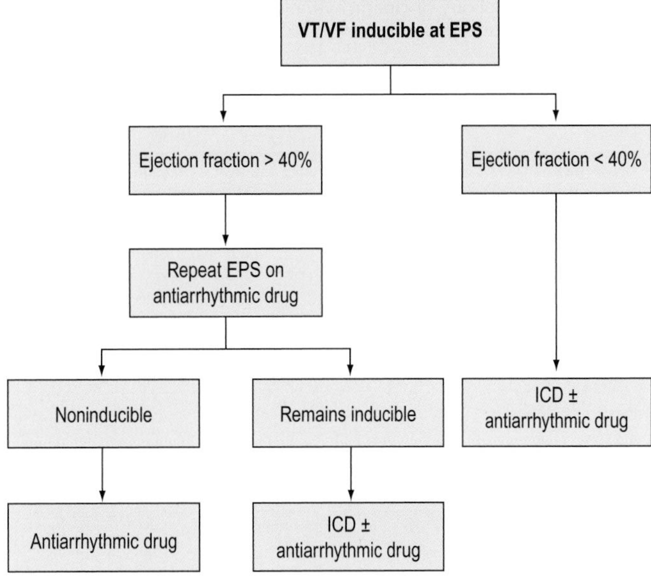

Figure 22.53 Patients found to have inducible ventricular tachycardia (VT) or fibrillation (VF) at electrophysiological studies (EPS), with an ejection fraction >40% and subsequent drug suppression of their VT/VF, can be managed on antiarrhythmic drugs alone.

of Na^+/K^+-ATPase blockade are deleterious in the setting of myocardial ischaemia and other causes of diastolic dysfunction. Digoxin also has weak vasopressor properties when administered as a slow bolus.[6] The major ECG effects of digoxin are PR prolongation and a non-specific alteration in ventricular repolarisation with characteristic reverse-tick S-T segments.

INDICATIONS AND DOSE

- *AF:* slowing of ventricular rate only
- *Loading dose:* 15 μg/kg i.v., typically administered over 30–60 min, but can be given faster
- *Maintenance dose*: depends on renal function.

PLASMA LEVELS

Oral bioavailabiliy can be reduced, especially if intestinal microflora-altering antibiotics are co-administered. Therapeutic levels are 0.5–2.0 ng/mL. Plasma levels must be measured during the post-distribution phase some 6–8 hours after dose. The elimination half-life is 36 hours with normal renal function. Difference between therapeutic and toxic levels can be reduced by hypokalaemia, hypomagnesaemia, hypercalcaemia, hypoxia, cardiac surgery and myocardial ischaemia. Many drugs increase digoxin plasma levels by competing with the renal P-glycoprotein-mediated transport, or by reducing renal blood flow or function.

CONTRAINDICATIONS

Relative contraindications include myocardial ischaemia/infarction, diastolic heart failure due to hypertrophy and ischaemia, renal failure and hyperkalaemia, planned DC shock cardioversion and tachycardia-bradycardia syndromes. Co-administration with other drugs that effect AV nodal conduction, typically beta-adrenergic and calcium channel blockers requires caution.

ADVERSE EFFECTS

The same increase in $[Ca]_i$ responsible for the positive inotropic effects of digoxin also forms the basis for toxicity arrhythmia. The increased inward calcium current is responsible for DAD-initiated arrhythmia. Digoxin toxicity can cause virtually any arrhythmia:

- DAD-related tachycardia with impairment of sinus node or AV nodal function
- unifocal atrial tachycardia with AV block is 'classic'
- ventricular bigeminy and various degrees of AV block occur.

With advanced toxicity severe hyperkalaemia due to poisoning of Na^+/K^+-ATPase results. Profound bradycardia, which may be unresponsive to pacing, develops.

Any serious toxicity arrhythmia should be treated with antidigoxin Fab fragments. Magnesium is the drug of choice for digoxin-toxic tachyarrhythmia. Digoxin, particularly at toxic levels, increases risk of VF precipitated by DC shock. Digoxin toxicity is associated with nausea, disturbances in cognitive function and blurred or yellow vision (xanthopsia).

BETA-ADRENERGIC BLOCKERS

Beta-adrenergic blocking or class II antiarrhythmic drugs have differing properties such as relative cardioselectivity (atenolol, metoprolol), non-cardioselectivity (propranolol), intrinsic sympathomimetic activity (pindolol), lipid solubility and

Table 22.16 Actions of antiarrhythmic drugs on membrane channels, receptors and ionic pumps in the heart

	CHANNELS										
	NA^+			K^+		CA^{2+}	RECEPTORS				PUMPS
DRUG	*FAST*	*MED*	*SLOW*	I_{KS}/I_{KR}	I_{KUR}		α	β	M_2	P	*NA^+/K^+ ATPASE*
Lidocaine	+										
Mexiletine	+										
Phenytoin	+										
Procainamide		+++		++							
Disopyramide		+++		++							
Quinidine		+++		++			+		+		
Propafenone		+++						++			
Flecainide			+++	+							
Encainide			+++								
Bretylium				+++			+/−	+/−			
Sotalol				+++				+++			
Amiodarone	+			+++		+	++	++			
Dronedarone	+			+++		+	++	++			
Ibutilide				+++							
Dofetilide				+++							
Vernakalant	+				+++						
Verapamil	+					+++	++				
Diltiazem						++	+				
Propranolol	+							+++			
Metoprolol								+++			
Esmolol								+++			
Atropine									+++		
Adenosine										A	
Digoxin									A		+++
Magnesium						+					A

Sodium channel blockers are subdivided into drugs with fast, medium and slow time constant for recovery from block. Receptors: α-, β-adrenoreceptors, M_2=muscarinic subtype 2; P=A_1 purinergic. Relative blocking potency: +=low; ++=moderate; +++=high; +/−=partial agonist/antagonist; A=agonist.

central activity (metoprolol, propranolol) and membrane-depressant effects (propranolol). The antiarrhythmic properties appear to be a class effect and no agent has been shown to be superior. There are data to suggest that the survival benefit of beta-adrenergic blockers post myocardial infarction may relate to some extent to the central modulation of autonomic tone of the more lipid-soluble agents. The direct membrane-stabilising or 'quinidine-like' effect of propranolol requires doses far greater than those used clinically and is of negligible clinical significance. Beta-adrenergic blockers competitively inhibit catecholamine binding at the beta-adrenergic receptor sites, which reduces the phase 4 slope of the action potential of pacemaker cells, prolongs their refractoriness and slows conduction in the AV node. Refractoriness and conduction in the His–Purkinje system are unchanged. Beta-adrenergic blockers are most effective in arrhythmia associated with increased cardiac adrenergic stimulation (postoperative states, sepsis, thyrotoxicosis, phaeochromocytoma, exercise or emotion).

INDICATIONS

Supraventricular tachycardia

Beta-adrenergic blockers may terminate SVT when the AV node is an intrinsic part of the re-entry circuit (AVNRT and AVRT); adenosine is more effective. AF and Afl do not revert with beta-adrenergic blockers, but the ventricular rate will be slowed. Beta-adrenergic blockers are effective at preventing SVT following cardiac surgery. Studies involving propranolol and atenolol have produced the best results. Beta-adrenergic blockers are effective in MAT, but, as this arrhythmia is most often seen in patients with severe chronic airflow limitation and cor pulmonale, their utility is limited.[31]

Ventricular arrhythmias

Beta-adrenergic blockers are ineffective for the emergency treatment of sustained VT. Empiric prophylactic administration of beta-adrenergic blockers appears to be as effective in ventricular arrhythmia prevention as electrophysiologically guided drug methods. However, ventricular arrhythmia most often occurs in the setting of poor LV dysfunction and beta-adrenergic blockers are either poorly tolerated or contraindicated.

Myocardial infarction

Survival in patients with AMI treated with thrombolytics is probably improved by early i.v. beta-adrenergic blockade. There may be other benefits such as decreased incidence of VF and relief of chest pain. Long-term beta-adrenergic blockade reduces mortality following myocardial infarction, the benefit being greatest in those at highest risk for sudden death. However, suppression of ventricular ectopy is not a requisite for benefit. Drugs with intrinsic sympathomimetic activity have not been shown to improve survival after AMI.

ATENOLOL

Atenolol does not have significant central action due to poor lipid solubility and is eliminated predominantly by the kidneys with an elimination half-life of 7–9 hours. Care is required in patients with poor or deteriorating renal function.

- *Loading dose i.v.:* 5 mg every 10 min, maximum 10 mg
- *Loading dose oral:* 50–100 mg
- *Maintenance dose oral:* 50–200 mg/day
- *ISIS-1 post-MI regimen:* 5 mg i.v. over 5 min, repeated 10 min later if heart rate exceeds 60 beats/min. If heart rate exceeds 40 beats/min 10 min later, oral 50 mg atenolol and continue at 100 mg daily
- *SVT prophylaxis following cardiac surgery:* 5 mg i.v. within 3 hours of surgery, repeated 24 hours later, followed by oral 50 mg daily for 6 days.

METOPROLOL

Metoprolol is lipid-soluble and has significant central action. It is eliminated by the liver with an elimination half-life of 3–4 hours.

- *Loading dose i.v.:* 1–2 mg/min, maximum dose of 15–20 mg
- *Loading dose oral:* 100–200 mg
- *Maintenance dose oral:* 50–100 mg/12-hourly.

PROPRANOLOL

Propranolol has been one of the most studied beta-adrenergic blockers for SVT prophylaxis following cardiac surgery.

- *Dose:* 10 mg orally 6-hourly starting the morning after surgery.

ESMOLOL

Esmolol is an ultrashort-acting cardioselective beta-adrenergic blocker, which is especially useful for rapid control of ventricular rate in AF or Afl. Esmolol has also been shown to prevent postoperative SVT. The distribution half-life is 2 minutes and the elimination half-life is 9 minutes. Esmolol is rapidly metabolised by hydrolysis of the ester linkage, chiefly by the esterases in the cytosol of red blood cells and not by plasma cholinesterases or red cell membrane acetyl-cholinesterase:

- *Loading dose i.v.:* 500 μg/kg over 1 min
- *Maintenance dose i.v.:* 50 μg/kg per min for 4 min. If satisfactory rate control is not achieved, the loading dose should be repeated and the maintenance dose increased to 100 μg/kg per min. If control is still not achieved after a further 4 min, then the procedure is repeated with 50 μg/kg per min increments in the maintenance infusion until 300 μg/kg per min is reached. Further increases in infusion rate are unlikely to be successful.

CONTRAINDICATIONS

Reversible airways disease and poor LV function are two common relative contraindications, which limit the utility of beta-adrenergic blockers in patients with cardiac disease. Beta-adrenergic blockers may also be poorly tolerated in diabetics and patients with severe peripheral vascular disease.

ADVERSE EFFECTS

Beta-adrenergic blockers, particularly those that are centrally acting, are often poorly tolerated in the long term. These effects include fatigue, hypotension, bradycardia, dry mouth, dizziness, headache and cold extremities.

CALCIUM CHANNEL BLOCKERS

Calcium channel blockers or class IV antiarrhythmic drugs block the slow calcium channels in cardiac tissue. Verapamil and diltiazem have similar electrophysiological properties. The dihydropyridine group of calcium channel blockers, which include nifedipine, does not have any significant electrophysiological properties. Calcium channel blockers depress the slope of diastolic depolarisation in the SA node cells, the rate of rise of the phase 0 and action potential amplitude in the SA and AV nodal cells. They also slow conduction and prolong the refractory period of the AV node, which results in their main antiarrhythmic actions. Refractoriness of atrial, ventricular and accessory pathway tissue is unchanged. The sinus rate does not usually change significantly because calcium channel blockers induce peripheral vasodilatation, which causes reflex sympathetic stimulation of SA node. Verapamil particularity has marked negative inotropic actions and hypotension is often seen; however, cardiac index is generally maintained because of afterload reduction. Diltiazem has a less negative inotropic effect than verapamil.

INDICATIONS

- *SVT:* calcium channel blockers are effective if the AV node is an integral part of the arrhythmia circuit. Verapamil has been superseded by adenosine for the first line of treatment for these with AVNRT and AVRT
- *AF and Afl:* slow ventricular response in AF and Afl, but termination of the arrhythmia is uncommon. Verapamil may prolong episodes of AF through a proarrhythmic effect
- *MAT*[31]: calcium channel blockers are effective
- *SVT following cardiac surgery:* diltiazem has been shown not only to reduce, but also to decrease incidence of ventricular arrhythmia and postoperative ischaemia
- *AF associated with the WPW syndrome:* calcium channel blockers may increase the ventricular response and should be avoided if this is suspected.[28]

In general, calcium channel blockers should not be given to patients with a wide-complex tachycardia not only because of the risk of accelerating accessory pathway conduction, but also because their myocardial depressant effects can result in cardiovascular collapse in the setting of VT and pre-existing myocardial dysfunction.

VERAPAMIL

Verapamil is cleared by the liver with an elimination half-life of 3–8 h. Therapeutic plasma concentration is 0.1–0.15 mg/L. With the availability of adenosine and the better tolerance of diltiazem, the use of verapamil has fallen substantially:

- *Loading dose i.v.:* 1 mg/min to a maximum of 10–15 mg or 0.15 mg/kg
- *Maintenance dose i.v.:* 5 mg/kg per min
- *Maintenance dose oral:* 80–120 mg 6–8-hourly.

DILTIAZEM

Diltiazem is cleared by the liver with an elimination half-life of 3.5 hours. There is reduced oral absorption and extensive first-pass hepatic metabolism: only 40% of oral dose is available compared with i.v.:

- *Loading dose i.v.:* 0.25 mg/kg, followed by 0.35 mg/kg if required
- *Maintenance dose i.v.:* 5–15 mg per hour
- *Maintenance dose oral:* 60–120 mg 6–8-hourly
- *SVT prophylaxis following cardiac surgery:* 0.1 mg/kg per hour, starting at onset of bypass and continuing for 24 hours. The dose can be titrated up for blood pressure control.

MAGNESIUM

Magnesium is an emerging antiarrhythmic agent with a range of indications; however, as an antiarrhythmic agent, magnesium has largely defied classification. Magnesium has many reported electrophysiological effects, including blocking voltage-dependent L-type Ca^{2+} channels. Magnesium is a necessary cofactor for the membrane enzyme Na^+/K^+-ATPase that provides energy for the membrane Na/K channels.[96] Consequences of magnesium deficiency are as follows:

- Intracellular potassium falls and intracellular sodium rises, leading to a reduction in RMP.
- Intracellular sodium is elevated, increasing the availability of sodium for the Na/Ca counter transport mechanism.
- The resulting elevation in intracellular calcium predisposes to DAD-triggered activity.

Magnesium administration reduces the availability of intracellular Na^+ and therefore this Ca^{2+} inward current. The dependency of normal membrane potassium gradients on magnesium is demonstrated by the inability to correct intracellular potassium deficiency with the administration of potassium in the setting of hypomagnesaemia. The antiarrhythmic properties of supra-normal levels of magnesium associated with pharmacological doses of magnesium appear to be largely due to augmentation of this physiological role of magnesium. Therefore, magnesium may be best classified as a Na/K pump agonist.

Magnesium in pharmacological doses decreases RMP, resulting in a reduction in automaticity. However, once depolarisation occurs, the maximum rate of depolarisation and action potential amplitude is increased, thereby improving conduction. Action potential duration is increased, thereby increasing the absolute refractory period and reducing relative refractory period. The net result is a reduction in the vulnerable period and more synchronous conduction. All of these electrophysiological effects are augmented in the setting of increased extracellular potassium. It is not surprising that the utility of magnesium appears greatest in the setting of ischaemia where loss of potassium from the cell is a major consequence. A secondary effect is the reduction in the availability of intracellular sodium to contribute to inward calcium flux, producing triggered activity. Magnesium has also been shown to elevate VF and ectopy threshold.[97]

INDICATIONS

- Acute rate control of AF, and has been shown to be as effective as amiodarone in the short term[69]
- Prevent postoperative SVT following cardiac surgery with varying efficacy
- Acute control of MAT
- Ventricular arrhythmia associated with triggered activity, such as torsade de pointes and digoxin toxicity[90]
- Drug-induced polymorphous VT, particularly that caused by class I agents, can also be terminated with magnesium
- Appears very effective at controlling transient ventricular arrhythmia in the setting of ischaemia such as post-infarct and cardiac surgery.

DOSE

- *AF rate and MAT control:* 0.15 mmol/kg as slow i.v. push. Subsequent dose recommendation has varied from 60 mmol to 0.1 mmol/kg per hour for 24 hours. Magnesium levels following 0.1 mmol/kg per hour were 1.92±0.49 mmol/L at 24 hours
- *SVT prophylaxis following cardiac surgery:* 20–25 mmol per day for 4 days
- *Transient ventricular arrhythmia:* 10 mmol as a slow i.v. push, repeated if required
- *LIMIT-2 post myocardial infarction dose:* 8 mmol bolus over 5 min, followed by 65 mmol over 24 hours. Mean plasma level 1.55 (SD 0.44) mmol/L.[71]

PLASMA LEVELS

Observational data would suggest that plasma levels of magnesium required for potent antiarrhythmic action are at least 1.8 mmol/L.

ADVERSE EFFECTS

- When administered too rapidly, magnesium can cause hypotension by excessive peripheral vasodilatation; this is associated with an unpleasant hot-flush sensation.
- Prolonged administration or excessive dosing can produce plasma levels associated with skeletal muscle weakness, which can be clinically significant in acute-on-chronic respiratory failure.
- Excessive action can be seen if magnesium is used in the setting of hyperkalaemia, resulting in bradyarrhythmia and heart block.

PROCAINAMIDE

Procainamide is a class IA antiarrhythmic drug with potent Na^+ channel-blocking activity and intermediate K^+ channel-blocking activity. The Na^+ channel-blocking action has an intermediate time constant of recovery. Procainamide has similar electrophysiological and ECG effects to quinidine but lacks vagolytic and alpha-adrenergic blocking activity:

- decreases automaticity
- increases refractory period
- slows conduction.

Procainamide is metabolised to *N*-acetyl procainamide. *N*-acetyl procainamide lacks Na^+ channel-blocking activity, but is equipotent in K^+ channel blockade and prolongation of action potential. The increasing effect of greater refractoriness and QT prolongation with chronic procainamide therapy relates to increased contribution of *N*-acetyl procainamide.

CLINICAL USE

Procainamide is used to treat both atrial and ventricular arrhythmias.

- Intravenous procainamide is more effective than lidocaine for terminating VT.
- Procainamide controls ventricular rate in AF and Afl.
- It is effective for conversion of AVNRT, AVRT and possibly AF and Afl.
- It controls rapid ventricular rate owing to accessory pathway conduction in pre-excitation syndromes and for wide-complex tachycardia that cannot be distinguished as being SVT or VT.

The need to infuse slowly to avoid hypotension is the major barrier to wider use in life-threatening arrhythmia. Maintenance therapy with procainamide is not widely used due to its side-effect profile:

- *Loading dose i.v.:* 6–17 mg/kg at 20 mg/min until there is arrhythmia control, hypotension ensues or QRS duration increases by more than 50%. Up to 50 mg/min has been used in urgent situations
- *Maintenance dose i.v:* 1–4 mg/min
- *Plasma levels:* *N*-acetyl procainamide has a longer duration of action
- *Adverse effects:* as with quinidine, the ventricular response may be accelerated if given for SVT; QT-interval prolongation and torsade de pointes may also occur.

A reversible lupus-like syndrome develops in 20–30% of patients receiving procainamide long term. Other side-effects include gastrointestinal disturbances (less common than with quinidine), central nervous system manifestations and cardiac depression.

LIDOCAINE

Lidocaine, long considered an important antiarrhythmic drug for ventricular tachyarrhythmia, is now relegated to lower-choice options or missing from most treatment algorithms. Na^+ channel-blocking effect is increased in myocardial ischaemia and is unproven outside acute ischaemia settings. It has no effect on SA node automaticity, but it depresses automaticity in other pacemaker tissues. Normally, lidocaine has little or no effect on conduction. The ECG shows no changes in sinus rate, PR interval, QRS width or QT interval with lidocaine.

CLINICAL USE

Lidocaine has reducing importance.

- It is ineffective against SVT.
- Amiodarone has taken over as the antiarrhythmic of choice for DC shock-resistant VF.[63,64]
- Lidocaine increases the current required for defibrillation, increases the likelihood of post DC shock asystole and therefore is detrimental during an episode of VF.
- Prophylaxis to prevent VF in AMI can no longer be recommended.

Extensive first-pass hepatic metabolism precludes oral use of lidocaine; i.v. dose should be reduced by 30–50% in severe liver disease or heart failure. The distribution half-life is about 8 min, and the elimination half-life is 1.5 h in normal patients (but may be increased >10 hours in severe heart failure or shock). An initial bolus of i.v. lidocaine 1.5–2.0 mg/kg over 1–2 min, followed by an infusion of 4 mg/min for 1 hours, then 2 mg/min for 2 hours, and thereafter 1–2 mg/min, is recommended. Increasing the maintenance infusion rate without an additional bolus requires about 6 hours (four elimination half-lives) to reach a steady state. If the initial bolus is ineffective, another bolus of 1 mg/kg may be given after 5 min. Another dosage regimen is 1.5–2.0 mg/kg initially, and 0.8 mg/kg at 8-minute intervals for three doses (i.e. three distribution half-lives), and thereafter 1–2 mg/min by infusion. The half-life of lidocaine increases after 24–48 hours as the drug in effect inhibits its own hepatic metabolism and dose reduction is required.

ADVERSE EFFECTS

Central nervous system toxicity with high plasma concentrations is the most common adverse effect (e.g. dizziness, paraesthesia, confusion, and coma and convulsions). Uncommonly, AV block or cardiac depression may occur. Cimetidine reduces lidocaine clearance, potentially causing toxic drug concentrations.

FLECAINIDE

Flecainide exhibits rate-dependent Na^+ channel blockade with slow time constant of recovery, with marked slowing of conduction in all cardiac tissue, and little prolongation of refractoriness.

CLINICAL USE

- May revert AVNRT and AVRT, although adenosine and verapamil are more widely used
- Useful in SVT, including AF and possibly Afl, particularly in the setting of accessory pathway syndromes
- Flecainide has been given in life-threatening VT.

Flecainide can be administered i.v. or orally. If flecainide is deemed necessary for prophylaxis of ventricular arrhythmias, therapy should start with ECG monitoring. In CAST, suppression of VEBs after myocardial infarction with flecainide was associated with increased mortality:[15]

- *Dose:* i.v. loading 2 mg/kg at 10 mg/min
- *Oral maintenance:* 100–200 mg 12-hourly.

ADVERSE EFFECTS

- Depression of cardiac contractility – flecainide is usually contraindicated in patients with abnormal LV function as it can worsen or precipitate heart failure.
- Conduction block – avoid in high-degree AV block unless a pacemaker is in situ.
- Flecainide increases pacing capture threshold.
- Proarrhythmic events are common, especially in patients with depressed LV function, and may be life-threatening.
- Torsade de pointes may occur, even in patients without structural heart disease.
- Incessant VT may be induced, unresponsive to any therapy, including cardioversion.
- Although flecainide depresses intracardiac conduction, a paradoxical increase in ventricular rate may occur with Afl or AF.
- Central nervous system effects include visual disturbances, dizziness and nausea.

PROPAFENONE

Propafenone is a class IC agent and has a structure similar to flecainide. The electrophysiological, haemodynamic and side-effect profile is also similar to flecainide and encainide. The I_{Na} blocking profile of propafenone has a fast time-constant resulting in greater activity at faster rates and less risk of bradycardia. In addition, propafenone has non-selective beta-blocking properties and can produce bronchoconstriction. Similar to flecainide, propafenone could be considered in both ventricular and SVT arrhythmia in the setting of normal LV function. Use of long-term propafenone should probably be limited because of its class IC profile, even though it was not included in the CAST study and contraindicated in structural heart disease because of proarrhythmia.

Propafenone is metabolised by the liver and the rate can vary significantly between patients. The short terminal half-life requires at least t.d.s. administration.

- *Dose:* i.v. 2 mg/kg at 10 mg/min; oral starting at 450–900 mg/day decreasing to 300 mg/day in three divided doses.

AMIODARONE

Amiodarone is a potent antiarrhythmic agent with a complex electrophysiological and pharmacological profile. The appealing broad spectrum and haemodynamic stability of amiodarone have resulted in it emerging as the most frequently used antiarrhythmic in critically ill patients. In this setting short-term use predominates and the formidable side-effect profile is much less significant. Amiodarone:

- prolongs action potential duration
- increases the refractoriness of all cardiac tissue
- has Na^+ channel blockade (class I), antiadrenergic (class II), calcium channel blockade (class IV) and antifibrillatory effects. The Na^+ channel blockade of amiodarone has a fast time constant for recovery
- QT prolongation reflects a global prolongation of repolarisation and is closely associated with its antiarrhythmic effects.

When given i.v., amiodarone has little immediate class III effect: the major action is on the AV node, causing a delay in intranodal conduction and a prolongation of refractoriness. This probably explains why i.v. amiodarone controls the ventricular rate in recent-onset AF, but is less effective for termination of this arrhythmia. Administration i.v. causes some cardiac depression, the magnitude depending on rate of administration and pre-existing LV function. Cardiac index is often unchanged because of its vasodilator properties.

CLINICAL USE

It is effective in suppressing both supraventricular and ventricular tachyarrhythmia.

SUPRAVENTRICULAR TACHYCARDIA

Amiodarone is effective in terminating and suppressing recurrences of AVNRT and AVRT tachycardia, although adenosine (for acute reversion) or verapamil (acute termination and long-term prophylaxis) is superior. Amiodarone i.v. is less effective in reverting Afl or AF, but the ventricular rate will slow. Administration over a longer time span (days to weeks) may be more effective in reverting recent-onset AF. In preventing recurrence of AF after reversion, amiodarone is comparable in efficacy to quinidine and flecainide but superior to sotalol and propafenone.[48]

DOSE

- Lower doses than that required for ventricular arrhythmia are usually sufficient
- *AVNRT and AVRT reversion or AF and Afl rate control:* 3–5 mg/kg i.v. over 10–60 min depending on blood pressure and myocardial function, followed by 0.35–0.5 mg/kg per hour. Poor rate control can be improved with additional 1–2 mg/kg boluses
- *Postoperative AF prophylaxis:* 200 mg orally 8-hourly for 5 days, followed by daily until hospital discharge
- *Long-term SVT control or AF rate control:* 100–200 mg/day orally will usually suffice.

VENTRICULAR TACHYARRHYTHMIAS

Amiodarone i.v. may be effective in treating life-threatening ventricular tachyarrhythmia refractory to other drugs, especially in myocardial infarction and poor LV function. Amiodarone's efficacy in DC shock-resistant VF further confirms a prominent role in this setting.[63,64] Long-term oral amiodarone is useful in controlling symptomatic VT and VF, especially when other conventional antiarrhythmics have failed. The absence of negative inotropic effect is useful in those with severely depressed LV function, but its many adverse effects limit widespread use. The Cardiac Arrest in Seattle, Conventional versus Amiodarone Drug Evaluation (CASCADE) study demonstrated that empirical amiodarone treatment was superior to guided (non-invasive Holter or EPS) class I drugs in survivors of VF not associated with AMI. Amiodarone prevented arrhythmia recurrence and decreased the incidence of sudden death. Amiodarone, presumably because it is better tolerated in patients with poor LV function and having less proarrhythmia, can be considered as first-line drug to prevent life-threatening ventricular tachyarrhythmias.[77–79] The rate of arrhythmia control is often slower with ventricular arrhythmia and may take several days to achieve. This delay appears to be independent of dose. The pharmacodynamic basis for this relates to the fact that much of the class III or K^+ channel-blocking activity is due to the amiodarone metabolite, desethylamiodarone, whereas the predominant actions of acute administration of amiodarone are due to its class I and class II activity. The full potency of the class III activity requires several days, at least, for the effects of desethylamiodarone to appear.

DOSE

- *Haemodynamic stable VT:* 5–7 mg/kg over 30–60 min, followed by 0.5–0.6 mg/kg per hour
- *DC shock-resistant VF:* 5 mg/kg, followed by 2.5 mg/kg if required[64]
- *Long-term prevention of ventricular arrhythmia:* oral loading with 1200 mg/day for 1–2 weeks, reducing to 400–600 mg/day and then 100–400 mg/day after 2–3 months. The dose should probably not be

reduced below 400 mg/day with life-threatening ventricular arrhythmia.

MYOCARDIAL INFARCTION

Data are limited at present, but amiodarone may improve long-term survival in patients after myocardial infarction.

PHARMACOKINETICS

Oral bioavailability of amiodarone is variable at 40–70%, with a delayed onset of action (days to weeks); however loading doses reduce this interval. Initial i.v. dose recommendations were 5–7 mg/kg over 30 min, followed by 50 mg/h. The kinetics of amiodarone has been modelled to four compartments when given acutely. Following a slow i.v. bolus over 15 min, amiodarone is rapidly distributed to the active compartment ($t_{1/2}\alpha$=4.2 min), with demonstrable prolongation of QTc and antiarrhythmic effect within 2–5 min. Subsequently, amiodarone is progressively redistributed to 'deeper' compartments ($t_{1/2}\beta$=36.6 min, $t_{1/2}\gamma$=4.5 h and $t_{1/2}\delta$=33.6 h).[98] This is in contrast to the very prolonged terminal half-life - greater than 50 days - after long-term treatment. This redistribution of amiodarone explains why repeated boluses are often required in the first 24–48 hours of treatment. Transient loading-dose hypotension due to myocardial depression or vasodilatation is dose-, rate- and patient-dependent. A loading dose of 5 mg/kg over 20 min resulted in significant further myocardial depression and a fall in cardiac index, whereas in patients without evidence of heart failure, 5 mg/kg over 1 minute resulted in hypotension due to systemic vasodilatation and an increase in cardiac index.[99,100]

MONITORING

Plasma amiodarone concentrations have poor correlation with arrhythmia control, and therapeutic levels, 1.0–2.5 mg/L, have the greatest utility for avoidance of adverse effects in long-term treatment.

ADVERSE EFFECTS

Adverse effects will occur in the majority of patients if they receive amiodarone for long enough. Most are reversible when the drug is discontinued. Adverse effects include:

- *Dermatological:* photosensitivity, bluish/grey skin discoloration (slate-blue skin)
- *Eye:* corneal microdeposits (almost 100%) with little or no clinical significance
- *Gastrointestinal disturbances*
- *Hypo- and hyperthyroidism*
- *Liver dysfunction:* asymptomatic increases in liver enzymes are common, and do not require amiodarone cessation unless enzymes are 2–3 times normal; hepatitis is rare
- *Neuropathy, myopathy and cerebellar abnormalities*
- *Pulmonary toxicity:* unexpected acute respiratory distress syndrome has been reported in patients on amiodarone undergoing procedures such as uncomplicated cardiopulmonary bypass surgery and pulmonary angiography. These observations suggest that amiodarone may predispose the lung to acute injury. Pulmonary toxicity is the most serious adverse effect, with a reported incidence of 10% at 3 years. Amiodarone pulmonary toxicity has been reported in one case after 13 days and 11.2 g cumulative dose and 11.2 g over 2 weeks in another. Patients on long-term amiodarone need regular respiratory function testing and decreased carbon monoxide diffusion of 15% below baseline requires dose modification or cessation. The severe syndrome of shortness of breath, cough and fever with pulmonary crepitations and widespread pulmonary infiltrates on chest X-ray has a mortality of 10%. Immediate discontinuation is necessary. Use of steroids is controversial.

Amiodarone interacts with other drugs, potentiating warfarin, digoxin and other antiarrhythmic agents. When administered concurrently, doses of these drugs should be reduced accordingly. On the positive side, long-term amiodarone is unlikely to precipitate or worsen heart failure and proarrhythmia is uncommon.

DRONEDARONE[49,101]

Dronedarone is an amiodarone analogue designed to reduce the lipophilicity of the molecule to reduce the pharmacokinetic complexity and toxicity. The iodine moieties have also been eliminated to prevent thyroid dysfunction.

Dronedarone is a multi-channel blocker, blocking I_{Na}, I_K and $I_{Ca\text{-}L}$ channels with a predominant electrophysiological effect of prolonging repolarisation or class III. It also has antiadrenergic properties.

Dronedarone decreases the recurrence of AF, controls rate with recurrences (heart reduction of 12.3 beats/min compared with placebo), especially with exercise. Secquential major studies evaluating dronedarone highlight the importance of variable outcome in differing patient populations. In comparing dronedarone with placebo the ATHENA study found dronedarone reduced all-cause mortality, cardiovascular admissions by 24%, death from cardiac arrhythmias, HR 0.55 (0.34–0.88) and stroke rate in addition to delaying recurrence of AF/Afl. Whereas in the PALLAS study (patients with permanent AF) all these outcomes were worse and the ANDROMEDA study (patients with poor LV function) was stopped due to increased mortality due to worsening heart failure. Meta-analysis of all placebo-controlled trials does show dronedarone has reduced mortality, but maintenance of sinus rhythm and absence of LV dysfunction is important to confer this mortality benefit. Dronedarone is currently contraindicated in patients with NYHA class III or IV heart failure.

In comparing dronedarone to amiodarone the picture is even less clear. In the DIONYSOS study (post electrical cardioversion) there was increased AF recurrence, dronedarone 63.5% and amiodarone 42% at 7 months, although drug discontinuation was higher with amiodarone. Meta-analysis of studies comparing the two drugs confirms greater efficacy for amiodarone maintaining sinus rhythm (HR 0.49; 0.37–0.63) but greater drug discontinuation rates and a trend to increased all-cause mortality with amiodarone. Dronedarone may have reduced torsade de pointes arrhythmia. The increased efficacy of amiodarone may relate to its lipophilicity giving higher tissue levels or the increased activity of its major metabolite, desethylamiodarone compared with *N*-debutyldronedarone.

Dronedarone has poor oral bioavailability, 15%, which can be variable, increasing by a factor of three if taken with food. It is extensively metabolised by cytochrome P450 CYP3A4 (inhibitors can result in marked elevation in plasma levels) to the metabolite *N*-debutyldronedarone, which is much less potent. The elimination half-life is 24 hours. Serum digoxin levels are increased due to inhibition of P-glycoprotein mediated intestinal and renal excretion.

- *Dose:* 400 mg oral b.d. with steady state in 7 days.

Although long-term data are lacking, there has been no evidence of thyroid dysfunction or pulmonary toxicity.

SOTALOL

Sotalol prolongs action potential duration, thereby prolonging the effective refractory period in the atria, ventricles, AV node and accessory AV pathways. It is also a potent non-cardio-selective beta-adrenergic blocker (class II). Sotalol also has antifibrillatory actions that are superior to those of conventional beta blockers. It can worsen heart failure in patients with depressed LV function. The negative inotropic beta-blocking effect is slightly offset by a weak positive inotropic effect owing to prolongation of the action potential (resulting in more time for calcium influx into contracting myocardial cells).

CLINICAL USE

Higher doses of sotalol are required to prolong cardiac repolarisation than to cause beta blockade. Sotalol may be administered i.v. or orally, and is excreted by the kidneys (elimination half-life 15 hours); i.v. dose is 0.5–1.5 mg/kg over 5–20 min. Oral therapy is initiated at 80 mg 12-hourly and increased to 160 mg 12-hourly, although doses of 320 mg 12-hourly have been administered.

SUPRAVENTRICULAR TACHYCARDIA

- Effective in AVNRT and AVRT, although adenosine and verapamil are superior. Long-term sotalol will prevent recurrences of these arrhythmias
- Probably ineffective for reversion of AF/Afl, but is effective in preventing recurrence of AF after cardioversion. If AF recurs, heart rate is likely to be well controlled with sotalol
- Prevents postoperative SVT.

VENTRICULAR ARRHYTHMIAS

Sotalol is superior to lidocaine to terminate sustained VT, and should be considered a first-line drug in patients without heart failure. Oral sotalol is more effective than class I drugs for the long-term prevention of VT or VF. Guided (Holter or EPS) sotalol and empirical amiodarone are first-line drugs to prevent recurrences of VT and VF over the long term; however, the worse outcome with sotalol in SWORD has significantly reduced the role of sotalol in this setting.[76]

ADVERSE EFFECTS

Side effects of sotalol are mainly due to beta blockade (e.g. bronchospasm, heart failure or AV conduction problems) and prolongation of QT proarrhythmia (e.g. torsade de pointes, similar 2% incidence as quinidine, which may occur early during drug titration or later during long-term treatment).

IBUTILIDE

Ibutilide is an I_{Kr} K^+ channel blocker, which prolongs action potential and increases the refractory period. This agent, with class III effect, is recommended for acute pharmacological conversion of AF and Afl, or as an adjunct to improve success of DC shock cardioversion. The success rate for ibutilide alone is higher for Afl (50–70%) than that with AF (30–50%) and, as expected, efficacy is greatest in short-term AF/Afl without structural heart disease. The major role of ibutilide appears to be cardioversion pretreatment to facilitate reversion to sinus rhythm from AF.[46] Ibutilide has minimal effect on blood pressure and heart rate and the major adverse effect is proarrhythmia, with torsade de pointes occurring in 3–6% of patients. For this reason, patients should be monitored for at least 6 h after administration. Ibutilide has a short duration of action and other antiarrhythmic drugs are required to maintain sinus rhythm.

DOSE

For patients weighing more than 60 kg, 1 mg over 10 min, which can be repeated 10 min later if unsuccessful. In patients weighing less than 60 kg, 0.01 mg/kg is given as initial dose.

DOFETILIDE

Dofetilide is one of the latest class III I_{Kr} K^+ channel blockers being investigated in the hope of finding an antiarrhythmic drug for long-term use with amiodarone's efficacy but without its side-effect profile.

Dofetilide's emerging role is again in pharmacological cardioversion of AF and Afl (superior to sotalol, similar to amiodarone but inferior to ibutilide) in about 30% of patients. Prevention of recurrence is similar to amiodarone and long-term oral therapy is not associated with increased mortality in post-MI and heart failure patients. It also appears safe in patients with LV dysfunction. Early (first 3 days) proarrhythmia (3.3% of patients developed torsade de pointes) also necessitates monitoring with commencement of therapy.[43,47,102,103]

DOSE

Recommended dose is 500 mg orally 12-hourly. Dose requires adjustment for renal function and QT-interval monitoring (QT_c interval >500 ms necessitates cessation) for a minimum of 3 days.

VERNAKALANT[104]

Vernakalant, a pyrrolidine compound, is a new multichannel blocker with I_K- and I_{Na}-blocking activity, with I_K blockade predominating (class III agent). The unique profile of vernakalant I_K blockade is the relative specificity for the atria and minimal effect on the ventricle. This specificity relates to differential activity on the various I_K channel isoforms, with I_{Kur} blockade being much greater compared with the modest activity at I_{Kr} channels. I_{Kur} channels are the 'ultra-rapid' I_K channels confined to the atria that are responsible for the fast early phase of repolarisation that results in the shorter action potential of atrial cells. Vernakalant therefore specifically prolongs atrial refractory period and slows atrial conduction with a rate-dependent profile.

Vernakalant in non-surgical, short-duration AF (ACT I and ACT III studies, duration less than 7 days) achieved sinus rhythm in 51.7% and 51.2% (placebo 4 and 3.6%) within 90 minutes, generally less than 10 minutes (median time to conversion 10 and 11 minutes). The i.v. dose of 3 mg/kg over 10 minutes, followed by a further 2 mg/kg over 10 minutes if conversion did not occur within 15 minutes of the first dose, produced not only rapid but durable conversion with 99% of responders remaining in sinus rhythm at 24 hours. Vernakalant was not effective in Afl, with a conversion rate of only 7%.

A similar cohort (AVRO study) comparing vernakalant (same dose as ACT I and III) with amiodarone (5 mg/kg over 1 hour followed by 50 mg over the next hour), again in recent-onset AF, found vernakalant again superior at 90 minutes with a conversion rate of 51.7 versus 5.2%. However at 4 hours amiodarone was catching up with 22.6 versus 54.4% conversion, with amiodarone recognised to have a longer onset of action.

In post-cardiac surgical patients who developed AF, having been in sinus rhythm preoperatively (ACT II study), vernakalant was superior to placebo with rapid conversion rates (47 versus 14%) and times (median time 12.4 minutes). However, unlike non-surgical patients, in this cohort responders were less durable with only 60% remaining in sinus rhythm at 24 hours. In all studies vernakalant had no effect on success rates with subsequent attempts at electrical cardioversion.

Vernakalant is extensively metabolised by the liver and subsequently excreted in the urine. The acute kinetics of vernakalant is not affected by congestive cardiac failure, renal or hepatic impairment.

Vernakalant is well tolerated with serious side-effects of hypotension and bradycardia during infusion infrequent (7.6%, placebo 5.1%), slightly higher than the rates of hypotension with amiodarone.

Although vernakalant may be seen as agent of choice for rapid pharmacological conversion of recent onset of AF, <7 days (the greater efficacy of ibutilide is eroded by risk of polymorphous ventricular arrhythmia), the superior conversion rate over amiodarone would appear to be lost at 24 hours and beyond, with amiodarone also likely to be a better agent to control ventricular rate in non-responders with greater AV-blocking activity.

ADENOSINE

Adenosine stimulates specific A_1 receptors present on the surface of cardiac cells, thereby influencing adenosine-sensitive K^+ channel cyclic adenosine monophosphate production. It slows the sinus rate and prolongs AV node conduction, usually causing transient high-degree AV block. The half-life of adenosine is usually less than 2 min as it is taken up by red blood cells and deaminated in the plasma. This ultrashort half-life is a major advantage over other antiarrhythmic drugs. The effects of adenosine, both antiarrhythmic and haemodynamic, can be antagonised by methylxanthines, especially theophylline and caffeine. Dipyridamole, an adenosine uptake blocker, potentiates the effect of adenosine. Adenosine effects are prolonged in patients on carbamazepine and in denervated transplanted hearts.

CLINICAL USE

- *AVNRT and AVRT tachycardia:* adenosine is the drug of choice. Expected reversion rates exceed 90%.[26] The AV nodal-blocking actions of adenosine may unmask atrial activity (e.g. flutter waves in Afl).
- Diagnosis of a wide-complex tachycardia may be assisted by the use of adenosine.
- SVT with intraventricular conduction block will terminate with adenosine, whereas few VTs will revert. Whether adenosine should be used routinely to discriminate between VT and SVT with aberrant conduction in haemodynamically stable wide-complex tachycardia is unclear. Potential for haemodynamic collapse in VT is real and ILCOR advises against.

Adenosine will not revert AF. Ventricular rate may transiently increase when AF is associated with the WPW syndrome.

Adenosine is given as a rapid bolus through a large peripheral or central vein followed by a saline flush, at intervals less than 60 seconds. The usual dose is 6 mg, followed by 12 mg if response is ineffective. Another 18 mg can be given if the last dose was well tolerated.

ADVERSE EFFECTS

Most patients experience transient side-effects such as flushing, shortness of breath and chest discomfort. Adenosine should not be given to asthmatic patients as bronchospasm may result.

DIRECT CURRENT CARDIOVERSION[105]

DC cardioversion/defibrillation is an important treatment option in tachyarrhythmia. In addition to its emergency role in cardiac arrest from VF or VT, urgent DC cardioversion is indicated in haemodynamically unstable VT and sustained SVT that precipitate angina, heart failure or hypotension. More elective DC cardioversion is indicated in haemodynamically stable VT following a trial of antiarrhythmic drug therapy. Cardioversion is most commonly used in AF/Afl once potential precipitants have been eliminated and, again, usually after antiarrhythmic drug treatment to prevent further episodes. Digoxin toxicity is a relative contraindication to DC cardioversion, which should also be used with care in patients on digoxin.

MECHANISM OF ACTION

DC shocks need to produce a current density that depolarises a critical mass of myocardium, thereby leaving insufficient myocardium to maintain the re-entrant tachycardia and prevent recurrence. For VF and AF, the critical mass involves the entire ventricles or atria, whereas for the more organised tachyarrhythmia, VT and Afl, which involve specific re-entrant circuits, regional depolarisation in the path of their circulating wave fronts is all that is required. DC shocks also prolong the refractoriness of myocardium and this effect will contribute to the arrhythmia termination and prevention of immediate recurrence.

ELECTRICAL ENERGY

Even though the goal is to achieve a certain current through the entire heart, atria or a region depending on the arrhythmia, DC shocks are prescribed as energy measured in joules (J) or watt-seconds. Obviously it would make more sense to be able to deliver a set current. This would prevent delivering inappropriately low currents in patients with high impedance and excessive current flow causing myocardial damage in patients with low impedance. Clinical studies to determine current doses are under way for defibrillation and cardioversion. The optimal current for VF using monophasic damped sinusoidal (MDS) waveform for cardioversion waveform appears to be 30–40 A. Current dosage for biphasic waveform is not available.

CURRENT WAVEFORM

Modern defibrillators deliver a current, the magnitude of which depends on the prescribed energy and thoracic impedance. This current can be delivered in a number of different waveforms.

MDS defibrillators deliver current that is in a single direction or polarity. They can be further characterised by the rate at which the current pulse returns to zero. MDS waveforms return to zero gradually, whereas truncated exponential waveforms return instantaneously. Recent evidence suggests that biphasic waveform for cardioversion (BTE) provides equal efficacy at lower electrical energies. A sequence of two current pulses is generated; the polarity of the second is in the direction opposite to the first. Biphasic waveforms with lower shock energies are associated with fewer ST-segment changes and less post-resuscitation myocardial dysfunction and have an ILCOR class IIa recommendation.

THORACIC IMPEDANCE

The magnitude of current flow is dependent on the resistance to current flow or thoracic impedance. The average adult thoracic impedance is 70–80 Ω. Factors that determine thoracic impedance include:

- energy selection
- electrode size
- electrode composition
- paddle-to-skin coupling
- distance between electrodes
- number of previous shocks
- time interval between previous and present shock
- pressure on electrodes
- phase of ventilation
- patient's body build
- recent sternotomy.

Conductive gel reduces impedance, while hair trapping air between skin and paddle and self-adhesive monitor/defibrillator electrode pads may increase it. There is no clear relationship between body size and energy requirements but compensation for patient-to-patient differences in impedance can be achieved by changes in duration and voltage of shocks, or by a process called burping, which involves releasing the residual membrane charge.

PADDLE POSITION AND SIZE

ILCOR recommends standard placement of the sternum paddle just to the right of the upper sternal border below the clavicle and the apex paddle to the left of the nipple, with the centre of the paddle in the mid-axillary line. Permanent pacemakers and ICD must be avoided as shock may cause malfunction or block current going to the heart. Inevitably, some current passes down the pacemaker lead and it is necessary to check pacing threshold post-shock. Other alternative paddle placements can enable avoidance of pacemakers and ICD or perhaps improve current direction. Using self-adhesive electrodes, the sternum electrode can be placed posterior to the heart on the right infrascapular region and the apex on the left precordium. The use of right parasternal and left posterior infrascapula has been advocated for AF because this configuration provides an optimal vector of current delivery to the atria. Large electrodes or paddles have less impedance; however, excessively large electrodes may result in less transmyocardial current flow. The minimum recommended electrode size is 50 cm^2, with the sum of both electrodes exceeding 150 cm^2.

SYNCHRONISED CARDIOVERSION

With cardioversion of atrial tachyarrhythmia and VT, when time permits, synchronisation of DC shock with the R-wave of the QRS complex is required to reduce the possibility of inducing VF by delivering the shock during the relatively refractory portion of the T-wave of the cardiac cycle. Synchronisation in VT may be difficult and misleading because of the wide complex or polymorphous nature. Synchronisation should not delay DC shock in pulseless VT or VT associated with unconsciousness, hypotension or severe pulmonary oedema.

DIRECT CURRENT SHOCK DOSAGE

Recommendations for energy doses are changing, as biphasic waveform generators become more widely available. Where studied, BTE shocks have been consistently as effective as higher-energy MDS shocks. Recommended doses are always a balance between the energy likely to generate a critical current flow and that not likely to cause functional and morphological damage. Electrical energies greater than 400 J have been reported to cause myocardial necrosis.

- *VF and pulseless VT:* escalating MDS shocks, starting at 200 J, then 200–300 J and, finally, 360 J. Evidence for sequential escalation of the energy dose is not strong and repeated shocks at the same energy result in increasing current delivery as impedance falls. Repeated non-escalating lower-energy BTE shocks, in the range of 150–175 J, are as effective as escalating MDS recommendations.
- *VT:* energy dose for cardioversion of VT depends on morphology and rate. For monomorphic VT, synchronised 100 J MDS is the starting energy. For polymorphic VT, synchronised if possible, 200 J MDS is the starting energy and for both stepwise increases if the first shock fails.
- *AF:* initial energy is synchronised 100–200 J MDS and stepwise increases if first shock fails. Despite obvious concerns for myocardial injury, mega dose energy at 720 J has been used with success in large patients with AF refractory to 360 J, without evidence of myocardial injury. Constant-current, rectilinear biphasic waveforms appear to be more effective in cardioverting AF. This biphasic waveform at the low energy of 120 J was superior to 200 J MDS.
- *Afl, AVNRT and AVRT:* these atrial tachyarrhythmias require least energy and the initial recommended energy is synchronised 50–100 J MDS.

SEDATION

A separate doctor expert in managing the airway must perform sedation for cardioversion. The dose of the sedating agent is titrated on the basis of patient factors and type of arrhythmia. Patients with poor myocardial function not only need reduced dose, but also onset time is slower because of low cardiac output. Sensitive tachyarrhythmias such as Afl require only low doses, whereas AF is likely to need higher and repeated doses as higher energy and repeated shocks may be necessary. Cardioversions should be performed with standard resuscitation equipment available and pre-oxygenation is crucial.

DIGOXIN AND CARDIOVERSION

Digoxin toxicity results in a significant reduction in the threshold for inducing ventricular arrhythmia with DC shock. If digoxin toxicity is a possibility, then reconsideration of the need for cardioversion or at least careful titration of energy is required. Clinical experience would suggest the latter procedure of starting with 10 J MDS, and a stepwise increase thereafter increases safety of DC shock in this setting.

ANTICOAGULATION FOR CARDIOVERSION[105]

Cardioversion of AF and, to a lesser extent, Afl is associated with catastrophic thromboembolism, especially stroke. Early studies suggested an incidence of up to 6.3% without anticoagulation. It is accepted that the likelihood of clots forming in the left atrium after 48 hours in AF and for these to be dislodged when sinus rhythm is restored is so high that anticoagulation is indicated prior to cardioversion in AF.

Anticoagulation for 3–4 weeks before cardioversion reduced the risk of embolism by 80%. The risk of thromboembolism following cardioversion continues for a period.

- Echocardiographic findings suggestive of atrial thrombi formation occur in up to 35% of patients post cardioversion.
- Left atrial appendage emptying velocities often decrease despite the development of coordinated electrical activity after cardioversion, presumably because of stunning of mechanical function.

Prolonged AF greater than 48 hours requires anticoagulation for 3 weeks prior to cardioversion and warfarin therapy for at least another 4 weeks depending on risk of recurrence of AF.

Transoesophageal echocardiography, which allows detection of thrombi in the left atrial appendage with much greater accuracy, has been found to be a safe means of expediting cardioversion. Anticoagulation with heparin for 1 day or warfarin for 5 days prior to demonstrating the left atrium to be free of thrombi by transoesophageal echocardiography, then 4 weeks of warfarin following cardioversion, was as effective in preventing emboli as the conventional longer anticoagulation regimen. However, there was a significant reduction in major haemorrhagic events in the transoesophageal echocardiography-guided, shorter lead-in anticoagulation strategy.

Access the complete references list online at http://www.expertconsult.com

1. Nerbonne JM, Kass RS. Molecular physiology of cardiac repolarization. Physiol Rev 2005;85:1205–53.
3. Task Force of the Working Group on Arrhythmias of the European Society of Cardiology. The Sicilian gambit: a new approach to the classification of antiarrhythmic drugs based on their actions on arrhythmogenic mechanisms. Circulation 1991;84:1831–51.
23. Field JM, Hazinski MF, Sayre MR, et al. Part 1: Executive Summary: 2010 American Heart Association Guidelines for Cardiopulmonary Resuscitation and Emergency Cardiovascular Care. Circulation 2010;122:S640–56.
33. Lee KW, Yang Y, Scheinman MM. Atrial flutter: A review of its history, mechanisms, clinical features and current therapy. Curr Prob Cardiol 2005;30:121–68.
66. Walkey AJ, Wiener RS, Ghobrial JM, et al. Incident stroke and mortality associated with new-onset atrial fibrillation in patients hospitalized with severe sepsis. JAMA 2011;306:2248–55.
87. Johnson JN, Ackerman M. QTc: how long is too long? Br J Sports Med 2009;43:657–62.
101. Dobrev D, Nattel S. New antiarrhythmic drugs for treatment of atrial fibrillation. Lancet 2010;375:1212–23.

23

Cardiac pacing and implantable cardioverter defibrillators

Aaisha Opel and Oliver R Segal

Cardiac pacing has rapidly evolved since its introduction by Zoll in 1952.[1] The first pacemaker was an external device designed by John Hopps in 1950. This was followed by the insertion of an internal device in 1958 by Elmqvist and Senning. The technological knowledge gained in pacing has assisted in the even more rapidly advancing field of implantable cardioverter defibrillators (ICDs). Although implantation and follow-up of permanent pacemakers and ICDs are in the domain of appropriately trained cardiologists, intensive care physicians should be familiar with such devices as a significant number of critically ill patients will have cardiac rhythm devices. It is also essential, when urgent pacing is required, that the intensivist is skilled in aspects of temporary pacing, including lead insertion and testing.

Cardiac pacing repetitively delivers very low electrical energies to the heart, initiating and maintaining cardiac rhythm. Pacing may be temporary, with an external pulse generator, or permanent, with an implanted pulse generator. More recently, a hybrid approach has been developed using a standard permanent pacemaker generator and lead but externalising the generator outside the body. This is useful for patients needing long-term temporary pacing (e.g. those with systemic or device-related infection or those with long-term causes of temporary bradycardia such as Guillain–Barré syndrome or its variant Miller–Fisher syndrome). Pacing is usually used to treat bradycardia, but rapid atrial or ventricular pacing can also be used to terminate both supraventricular (SVT) and ventricular tachycardias (VT).

More recently, the indications for pacing have expanded beyond symptomatic bradycardia and include conditions such as the long QT syndrome, hypertrophic obstructive cardiomyopathy (HOCM) and congestive cardiac failure.

PACING SITES

TRANSVENOUS ENDOCARDIAL PLACEMENT

Pacing leads are passed via a vein to the endocardial surface of the right atrium (RA), the right ventricle (RV), or both chambers. In patients with heart failure, an additional lead is passed to the left ventricular coronary veins via the coronary sinus (which drains into the right atrium). Balloon-flotation pacing catheters for temporary pacing are less stable and are generally reserved for emergency pacing purposes.

EPICARDIAL PLACEMENT

This is mainly used in conjunction with cardiac surgery, where electrodes are attached directly to the epicardial surface of the atrium and/or ventricle and pass out through the skin in the epigastrium. These are useful after cardiac surgery, particularly after valve surgery, but rapidly deteriorate postoperatively and are typically no longer functional after 5–10 days.

TRANSCUTANEOUS EXTERNAL PACING

Transcutaneous pacing can be instigated rapidly in an emergency by personnel unskilled in transvenous pacing. However, this is a temporary measure. Patches are applied anterolaterally or anteroposteriorly, over the heart. Conscious patients can experience significant pain due to pectoral muscle contraction and may require analgesia or sedation.

Other pacing modalities such as the transoesophageal route are used rarely, except in paediatrics.

PERMANENT PACING

INDICATIONS FOR PERMANENT PACING

Guidelines for permanent pacing are published by a joint American taskforce and updated fairly regularly.[2] They recommend the following pacing indications, stratified according to the likely benefit. (Please note that the vast majority of pacing indications have only levels of evidence C (expert consensus) or B (limited non-randomised trials of small numbers of patients) as pacing predated modern randomised controlled trials.)

1. *Class I:* benefit clearly outweighs risks – treatment should be performed:
    a. in second- or third-degree atrioventricular (AV) block with:
        - *symptoms* and bradycardia
        - pauses greater than 3 seconds or rate less than 40 beats per minute whilst awake, even without symptoms

- postoperative or post-AV node ablation
- neuromuscular disease, with or without symptoms

b. in sinus node dysfunction with documented bradycardia *and symptoms*
c. in recurrent syncope due to spontaneous carotid sinus stimulation or carotid sinus pressure and pauses greater than 3 seconds
d. in chronotropic incompetence *with symptoms*
e. in pause-dependent ventricular tachycardia.

2. *Class IIa–IIb:* benefit outweighs risks – reasonable to perform procedure or procedure can be considered:
   a. in asymptomatic complete AV block with average ventricular rate 40 beats/min in an awake patient
   b. in asymptomatic Mobitz type II second-degree AV block with narrow QRS
   c. in asymptomatic sinus bradycardia with heart rate <40 beats/min
   d. in first-degree heart block (>300 ms) in patients with depressed left ventricular function and symptoms of left ventricular failure.
3. *Class III:* risks clearly outweigh the benefits – pacing should not be performed:
   a. in asymptomatic first-degree heart block
   b. in reversible AV block secondary to drug toxicity.
4. Other indications: non-bradycardia indications for pacing include pacing to improve haemodynamics. Evolving indications include the following:[2,3]
   a. *Heart failure*: patients with heart failure, severe left ventricular impairment and left bundle branch block (LBBB) may benefit from restoring synchronous ventricular contraction through pacing the RV and left ventricle (LV) at the same time – known as biventricular pacing. Such cardiac resynchronisation therapy (CRT) improves symptoms of heart failure and survival in about two-thirds of these patients. Patients who benefit most are those in sinus rhythm, have QRS widths greater than 150 ms and NYHA class II–IV heart failure symptoms.[4,5] Some patients with dys-synchronous LV contraction on echocardiography but narrow QRS width can also benefit. The use of CRT via a permanently implantable biventricular pacemaker (the LV lead is usually passed via a tributary of the coronary sinus to the epicardial surface of the LV) has gained widespread acceptance for treatment of heart failure, together with appropriate medications. Temporary biventricular pacing with a temporary transvenous pacemaker lead passed to a coronary vein via the coronary sinus has been used successfully in cardiogenic shock and high-degree AV block.[6] Permanent devices combining CRT and ICDs, known as CRT-D, are used in those who fulfil CRT criteria and have an indication for an ICD.
   b. *Hypertrophic cardiomyopathy (HCM)*: pacing can be used in symptomatic patients with a high gradient in the left ventricle. Right ventricular apical pacing causes dys-synchronous ventricular activation and can decrease LV gradient and systolic anterior motion (SAM) of the mitral valve. However, the evidence to support this is weak (currently a class IIb indication) and is probably helpful in only a small proportion of suitable patients.

PACEMAKER MODES

The Heart Rhythm Society (HRS), previously known as the North American Society of Pacing and Electrophysiology (NASPE), and Heart Rhythm UK, previously the British Pacing and Electrophysiology Group (BPEG), developed the NBG code[7] for pacing. This is a generic code used to identify modes of pacing (**Table 23.1**). The code was updated in 2002 to include multisite pacing therapy (position V)[8]:

- *Position I:* refers to the chamber(s) paced: A=atrium, V=ventricle, and D=dual chamber, i.e. both A and V.
- *Position II:* refers to chamber(s) in which sensing occurs: A=atrium, V=ventricle, and D=dual chamber, i.e. both A and V, O=no sensing.
- *Position III:* refers to the pacemaker's response to a sensed event. This may be:
  - I (inhibition) – a pacemaker's discharge is inhibited (switched off) by a sensed signal, for example, VVI, where ventricular pacing is inhibited by spontaneous ventricular activity.

Table 23.1 The North American and British Group (NBG) pacemaker code

POSITION I	POSITION II	POSITION III	POSITION IV	POSITION V
Chamber(s) paced	Chamber(s) sensed	Response to sensing	Rate modulation	Multisite pacing
O=none	O=none	O=none	O=none	O=none
A=atrium	A=atrium	T=triggered	R=rate modulation	A=atrium
V=ventricle	V=ventricle	I=inhibited		V=ventricle
D=dual	D=dual	D=dual		D=dual

Note: Positions I–III are used exclusively for antibradycardia function.
(Reproduced from Bernstein AD, Daubert JC, Fletcher RD, et al. Pacing. Clin Electrophysiol 2002;25:260.)

- T (triggered) – a pacemaker's discharge is triggered by a sensed signal.
- D (dual) – both T and I responses can occur. This designation is reserved for dual-chamber systems. A depolarisation sensed in the atrium inhibits the atrial output but triggers ventricular pacing. There is, however, a delay (the AV interval) between the sensed atrial depolarisation and the triggered ventricular pacing, which mimics the normal P–R interval. If a spontaneous ventricular depolarisation is sensed, ventricular pacing is inhibited.
- O – no action.

- *Position IV:* refers to *R* or rate response and is only relevant to permanent pacing systems. An *R* indicates that the pacemaker incorporates a sensor(s) to vary the pacing rate independent of intrinsic cardiac activity. The sensor(s)[9] increases or decreases the heart rate according to the body's metabolic needs. They are useful for patients with impaired sinus node function, chronotropic incompetence (when heart rate does not increase appropriately with exercise) and patients with atrial fibrillation and complete heart block or slow ventricular rates. Two different sensors are widely used:
  1. Activity sensors with vibration detectors (accelerometer or piezoelectric crystal) increase heart rate when movement is detected. They have the disadvantage that they may respond to non-physiological stimuli (e.g. pacing rate increase may occur when the patient is using an electrical drill).
  2. Minute ventilation sensors (respiratory rate times tidal volume, which is estimated by measuring impedance differences between the pacing electrode and the pacemaker unit) rely on minute volume changes to alter the pacing rate. This sensor may occasionally inappropriately accelerate the pacing rate (e.g. in a mechanically ventilated patient requiring a large minute volume). Changing the 'upper rate' limit of the pacemaker or switching the rate-adaptive function 'off' will usually solve the problem. Other sensors, such as ventricular paced Q–T interval systems, are also used in clinical practice. Recently rate-adaptive systems with dual sensors, where one sensor cross-checks the other and only responds if both sensors are receiving consistent data, have become available. All modern permanent pacemakers are programmable and the degree of rate response can be modified to optimise heart rate with exercise.
- *Position V:* is used to indicate whether multisite pacing is present
  O = none of the cardiac chambers
  A = atrium
  V = one or both ventricles
  D = any combination of atria and ventricles.

For example, the code for a patient with dual-chamber, rate-responsive pacing (DDDR) and biventricular pacing is DDDRV.

SPECIFIC PACING MODES

The three-position code (**Fig. 23.1**) is adequate to describe emergency temporary pacing and most forms of permanent pacing in the intensive care unit (ICU) (**Table 23.2**).

SINGLE-CHAMBER PACING

1. *AOO and VOO (asynchronous atrial and ventricular) pacing:* in this mode there is no ability to sense cardiac activity (**Fig. 23.2**) and it is useful during and after cardiac surgery or when a patient is exposed to external sources of noise (e.g. surgical diathermy or MRI scanning).
2. *AAI (atrial demand) pacing:* this is indicated in patients with sinus bradycardia and intact AV conduction. It is reserved for patients in whom the risk of developing AV block is thought to be low.
3. *VVI (ventricular demand) pacing (**Fig.** 23.3):* this is the most commonly used mode and the mode of choice in life-threatening bradyarrhythmias. Spontaneous cardiac rhythm is sensed and a minimum ventricular rate is programmed to prevent symptoms or in the ICU setting to also optimise cardiac output. There is a low risk of pacemaker-induced ventricular tachyarrhythmia (**Fig. 23.4**), but AV synchrony is lost, which may depress cardiac output and blood pressure.

DUAL-CHAMBER PACING

Two sets of electrodes are required (atrial and ventricular).

1. *DDD pacing:* there is pacing and sensing in both chambers (**Fig. 23.5**). An atrial impulse will trigger a ventricular output if none is seen after the programmed AV delay and will simultaneously inhibit an atrial output. If the impulse is conducted normally to the ventricle, ventricular pacing is inhibited. An upper rate limit is programmed to prevent the pacemaker tracking fast atrial rates (e.g. in atrial flutter or tachycardia). The response to DDD pacing depends on the underlying cardiac rhythm:
   a. atrial bradycardia with intact AV conduction – atrial pacing
   b. normal sinus rhythm with high-degree AV block – tracking of P-waves and ventricular pacing
   c. sinus bradycardia with AV block – sequential atrial and ventricular pacing
   d. normal sinus rhythm and AV conduction – inhibition of both atrial and ventricular pacing.

   Pacemaker-mediated tachycardia (PMT), or 'endless-loop' tachycardia,[10] can occur in

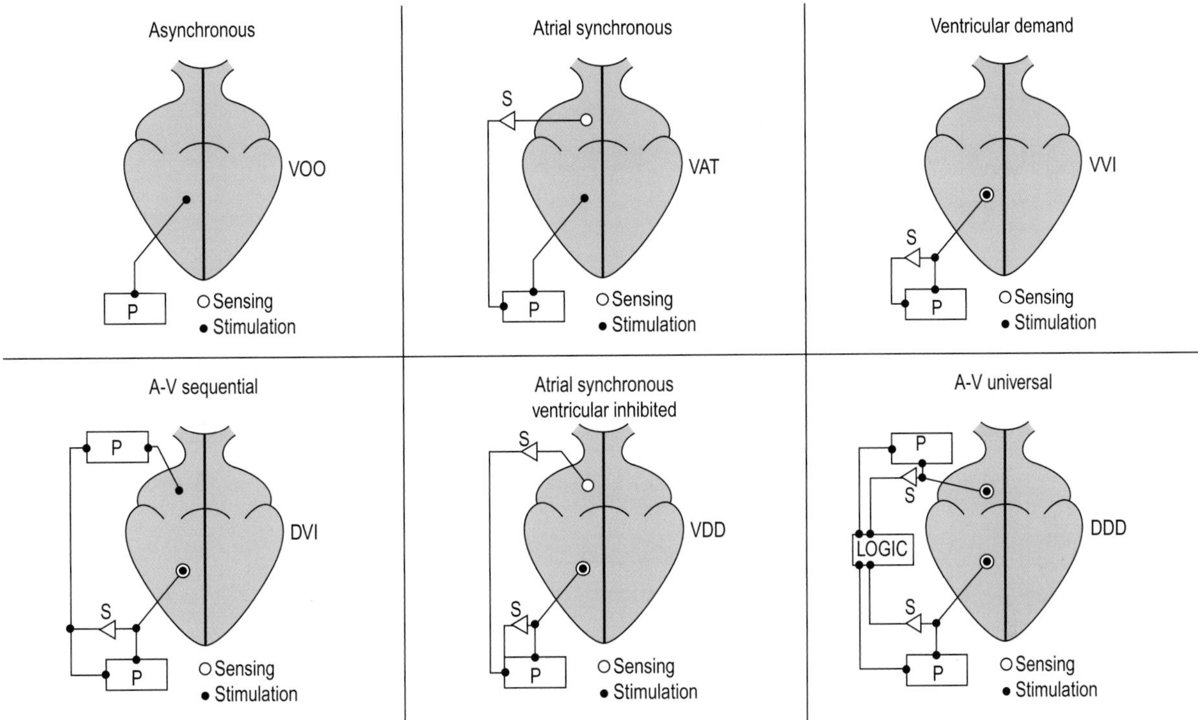

Figure 23.1 Examples of pacemaker modes and their three-position (letter) codes. P=pacemaker; S=sensing.

Table 23.2 Examples of pacemaker modes

MODE	
VOO	Paces the ventricle, no sensing, fixed-rate, asynchronous Usually only used for pacemaker testing, during use of diathermy and 'emergency' pacing
VVI	Paces the ventricle, senses ventricular activity, ventricular activity inhibits the pacemaker Ventricular demand
AAI	Paces the atrium, senses atrial activity, atrial activity inhibits the pacemaker Atrial demand Indicated in sinus bradycardia with intact AV conduction
DDD	Paces and senses both atrium and ventricle: atrial activity triggers ventricular pacing
DDI	Paces and senses both atrium and ventricle Atrial activity not tracked; thus atrial tachyarrhythmias do not trigger rapid atrial pacing AV sequential, non-P synchronous Useful for sinus bradycardia with AV block and intermittent atrial tachyarrhythmias

dual-chamber pacing systems where a ventricular premature beat (**Fig. 23.6**) conducted retrogradely to the atria is sensed and ventricular pacing is triggered resulting in an endless loop: the circuit's anterograde limb is the pacemaker, and the retrograde limb is via the AV node. This can be prevented by programming a blanking period after a ventricular-paced beat so that retrograde atrial activity is not sensed. The blanking period is known as the post-ventricular atrial refractory period, or PVARP, and is found on all modern pacemakers. An alternative is to switch to an asynchronous (non-sensing) mode or programming to DDI mode.

2. *DDI pacing (AV sequential, non-P-wave synchronous):* in this mode sensing occurs in both atrium and ventricle, but sensed atrial events do not trigger ventricular pacing. Imagine it as a patient with separate VVI and AAI pacemakers that cannot talk to each other. PMT or endless-loop tachycardia cannot occur in

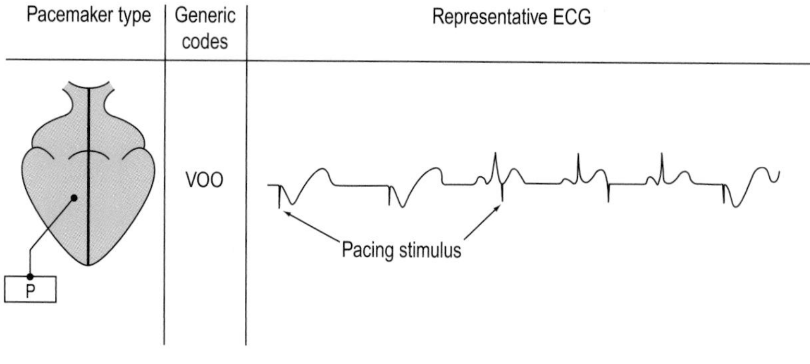

Figure 23.2 Fixed-rate ventricular pacing VOO. P=pacemaker.

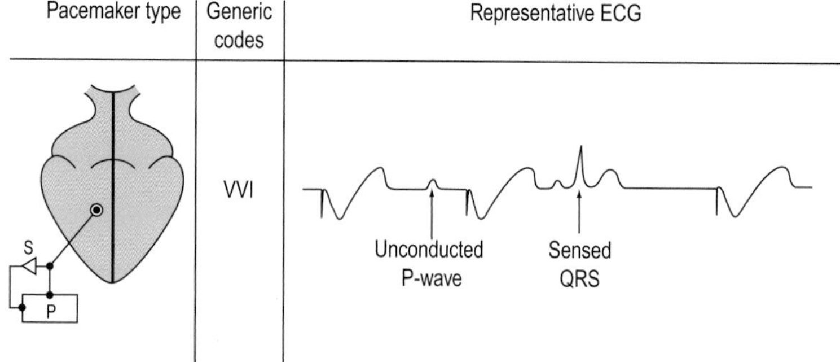

Figure 23.3 Ventricular demand pacing VVI. P=pacemaker; S=sensing.

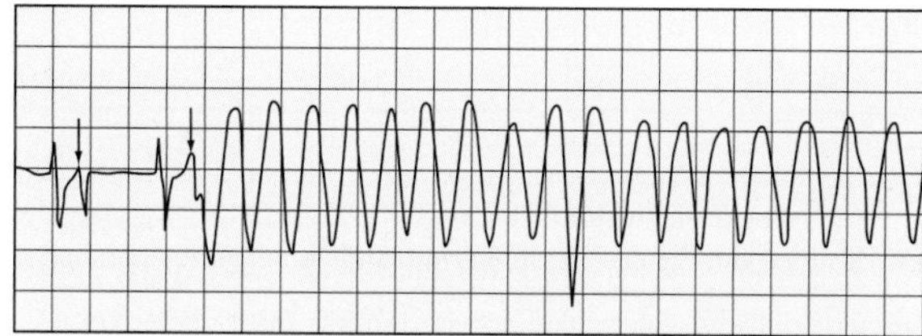

Figure 23.4 Non-sensing of QRS (see first two beats). Pacing spikes (arrows) fall on the T-wave with subsequent pacemaker-induced ventricular tachycardia.

DDI and neither will tracking of rapid atrial rates. For this reason, modern pacemakers programmed DDD will switch to DDI when an atrial tachyarrhythmia is detected (e.g. atrial fibrillation). When this happens the pacemaker will simply pace the ventricle at its back-up rate and not track the tachycardia.

HAEMODYNAMICS OF CARDIAC PACING AND THE AV INTERVAL

In the normal heart, cardiac output increases three- to fourfold during exercise, mainly due to increased heart rate and stroke volume and the ability of pacemakers to increase heart rate is therefore paramount. Nevertheless, loss of AV synchrony (i.e. the normal activation sequence of atria contracting first and then the ventricles) will decrease cardiac output by up to 25%,[11] most commonly in atrial fibrillation. Many permanent pacemakers are rate-adaptive. When temporary pacing is used, especially in the ICU setting, higher than normal lower rates may be needed if oxygen delivery is inadequate. For life-threatening bradyarrhythmias, increasing heart rate with VVI mode pacing is the treatment of choice and heart rate modulation with exercise is required only for permanent pacemaker patients.

During VVI and VVIR pacing, the atria and ventricles beat independently and AV synchrony is lost. This can have deleterious effects, known collectively as 'pacemaker syndrome'.[12] It can occur with any pacing mode where AV dissociation occurs and blood pressure, stroke volume and cardiac output may fall with the onset of pacing. Another feature is due to the atria contracting against closed tricuspid and mitral valves causing regurgitation of blood into the neck via the jugular veins. This is felt as uncomfortable neck pulsations. The pacemaker syndrome can be eliminated by restoring AV synchrony.

However, and somewhat counterintuitively, dual-chamber pacing has not been shown to improve mortality even though haemodynamics are usually superior to VVI pacing.[13] It does though appear to lower the incidence of AF.[3]

Changing the programmed AV interval of a dual-chamber pacemaker can affect the amount of ventricular pacing that is seen and also the haemodynamics, for the reasons outlined above. If this interval is programmed short (e.g. 80 ms), it will promote ventricular

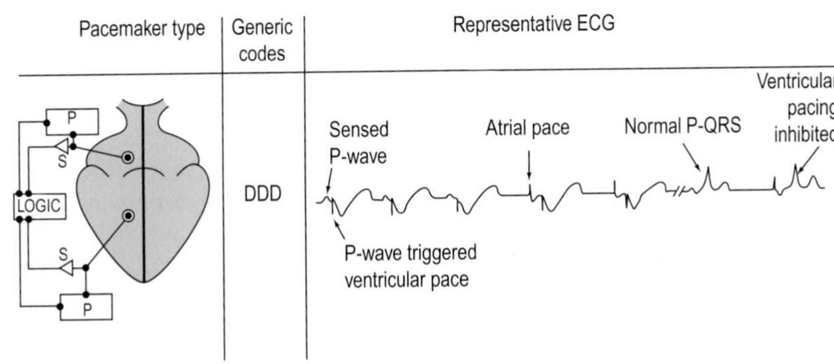

Figure 23.5 DDD pacing. P=pacing; S=sensing.

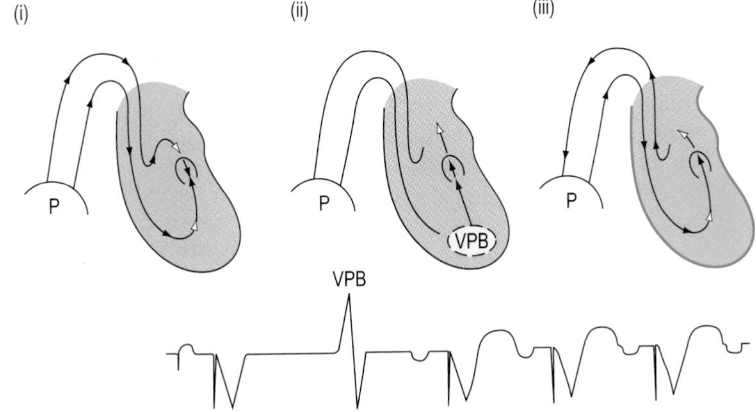

Figure 23.6 Pacemaker-mediated 'endless-loop' tachycardia: (i) under normal conditions (first beat) there is no conduction from the ventricles to the atria because of ventriculo-atrial (VA) block or because the atrial and ventricular impulses collide and extinguish each other in the atrioventricular node; (ii) if a ventricular premature beat (VPB) is conducted retrogradely to the atria (second beat), inducing an inverted 'p'-wave, this may be sensed by the pacemaker (P) which then triggers a ventricular paced beat (third beat); (iii) if the paced ventricular beat is then retrogradely conducted from the ventricle to the atria and sensed, an 'endless loop' may occur (beats 4, 5); that is, pace ventricle VA conduction 'p' wave (sensed) ventricular pace, and so forth.

pacing. If it is programmed long (e.g. 250 ms), it will promote intrinsic ventricular activity (if present). The correct AV interval will depend on patients' clinical state and their intrinsic AV conduction and inter-atrial conduction (the time to conduct between the RA and LA). Promoting ventricular pacing may be a good thing if it improves haemodynamics, but promoting intrinsic conduction is often better especially if the intrinsic AV delay is not very long. Adjusting the AV interval in the patient with poor cardiac output or low oxygen delivery can be optimised using echocardiography or thermodilution assessment of cardiac output.

TEMPORARY PACING

INDICATIONS FOR TEMPORARY PACING

Temporary cardiac pacing is indicated for:

- any sustained symptomatic bradycardia not promptly responding to medical treatment
- malignant ventricular arrhythmias secondary to bradycardia
- second- or third-degree AV block with haemodynamic compromise
- asystole.

The decision to pace is based on bradycardia causing haemodynamic deterioration, and not on the specific rhythm disturbance. For example, pacing is indicated in a patient with atrial fibrillation and a ventricular rate of 40 beats per minute associated with a blood pressure of 70/40 mmHg (9.3/5.3 kPa), cardiac failure and oliguria, but not in an asymptomatic, normotensive patient with the same rhythm or even a patient with an inferior myocardial infarction, complete heart block and a ventricular rate of 45 beats per minute with a narrow QRS complex.

Temporary pacing is indicated for the treatment of heart block or sinus bradycardia after cardiac surgery. In high-risk patients (e.g. aortic or mitral valve replacement), prophylactic epicardial electrodes are attached during surgery. DDD epicardial pacing has been shown to increase cardiac output at any given heart rate compared with VVI pacing.[14] Temporary perioperative cardiac-pacing strategies to increase stroke volume and cardiac output include optimisation of AV delay and rarely multisite pacing.[15] Temporary pacing may be required in patients with inferior myocardial infarction or during coronary angioplasty, particularly of the right coronary, which supplies the SA and AV nodes. Asymptomatic patients with bifascicular block do not require prophylactic pacing prior to general anaesthesia, although transcutaneous pacing should be available, but should be considered for all patients with trifascicular block (bifascicular block and prolonged PR interval). Patients with Mobitz type II or third-degree AV block should be paced prior to general anaesthesia and surgery.

Caution should be exercised in patients with acute myocardial infarction as many will have received antiplatelet agents. Transcutaneous pacing prevents the need for transvenous pacing, but should only be used as an emergency in high-risk patients.

TEMPORARY LEADS AVAILABLE

VENTRICULAR PACING LEADS

There are different types of temporary pacing lead available with different degrees of rigidity and French size. The commonest calibres will be 4–6 F. These leads are relatively stiff and can be shaped before advancing through a sheath, but are still flexible enough to be manipulated under fluoroscopic control to the correct position in the RV. Balloon-flotation leads can, in theory, float into a stable position in the RV and are useful if fluoroscopy is not available in emergent situations, or as back-up when transferring patients to centres for permanent pacing. There are also active fixation temporary pacing leads, which have a fixed screw at the distal tip. This screw can be inserted into myocardium by rotating the lead body. Care should be taken with these leads as the risk of perforation is higher than for passive leads.

ATRIAL PACING LEADS

Leads designed specifically for placement in the right atrium have a preformed J-shaped tip designed to hook into the RA appendage. This site is often best for lead stability, low pacing thresholds and good sensing.

TECHNIQUE OF TEMPORARY TRANSVENOUS PACING

VENTRICULAR PACING

A sterile technique is mandatory in an environment with good fluoroscopic imaging, non-invasive cardiac monitoring and resuscitation facilities. In emergencies, transcutaneous pacing (VVI) can be implemented first while transvenous VVI pacing is being prepared. A bipolar lead introduced under fluoroscopic control is most commonly used.

Vascular access

The Seldinger technique is employed to access a central vein with a 5 or 6 French sheath. The sheath has a haemostatic valve, which prevents blood loss at the time of lead insertion. Percutaneous insertion via the right internal jugular vein probably offers least complications with ease of manipulation and stability of the lead. However, the subclavian vein approach is often used as it allows more freedom for arm and neck movement, but there is a slightly greater risk of pneumothorax. Patients likely to need permanent pacing later in their treatment should have the left subclavian vein saved for this purpose. Antecubital veins are associated with lead instability and thrombophlebitis. The femoral vein can be used. It is usually quick and easy to insert a ventricular pacing wire from this route, but the patient must remain lying flat. Lead stability is probably less good than superior routes and there is higher risk of infection and deep-vein thrombosis. Femoral temporary pacing is useful over a short period of time, for instance to cover a surgical procedure in a patient with trifascicular block or those who have received thrombolytic agents but should not be used for longer-term pacing if possible.

Positioning the pacing lead

The pacing lead is manipulated under fluoroscopic control in the posteroanterior (PA) position close to the apex of the RV (**Fig. 23.7**). This position offers the greatest stability, but the true apex should be avoided as it is thin and the risk of perforation is higher. As the lead crosses the tricuspid valve to the RV, it is usual to see ventricular ectopy (VE). However, if continuous, the lead should be pulled back to the right atrium. In the

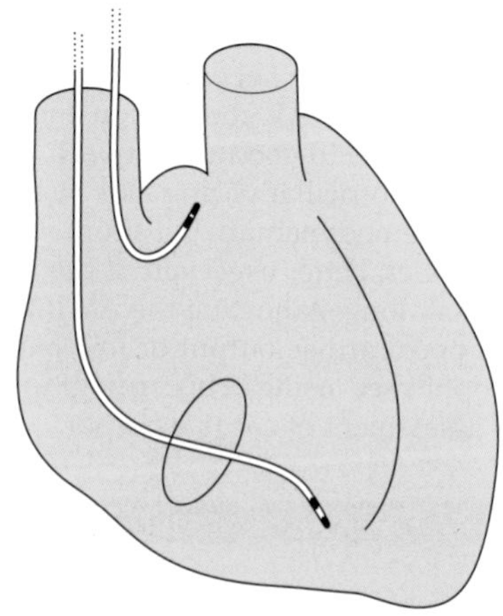

Figure 23.7 Characteristic appearance of temporary transvenous pacing leads ideally positioned in the right atrium (right atrial appendage) and apex of right ventricle.

absence of VE, the lead position should be confirmed in the left anterior oblique (LAO) position to ensure it is not in the coronary sinus or a posterior vein. Manipulation of the lead is achieved by clockwise and counterclockwise torque in combination with simultaneous advancement and retraction of the lead. Temporary pacing leads are relatively stiff and perforation can occur, especially if leads are seen to buckle whilst advancing, but it is also important to ensure sufficient slack in the lead to avoid the loss of position with subsequent patient movement.

Once in a satisfactory position, the lead should be tested electrically for sensing, pacing and diaphragmatic capture (see below). It should be sutured to the skin at two different sites: one where it exits the skin, and a second to a loop formed with the lead. A chest X-ray should be obtained to exclude pneumothorax and to confirm satisfactory positioning.

ATRIAL PACING

J-shaped atrial leads are designed to be advanced and hooked into the right atrial appendage. The appendage is an anterior structure, which is superior to the right atrium. Once the tip is advanced into the appendage orifice, retraction of the lead will hook the tip into the appendage body and a side-to-side motion of the lead tip may be seen if the patient is in sinus rhythm. The correct position is best confirmed by a lateral chest X-ray.

DUAL-CHAMBER PACING

Modern external pacing boxes are available (**Fig. 23.8**) that will pace in all modes. These units are small, easy to use and can fit into a small pouch suitable for mobile patients.

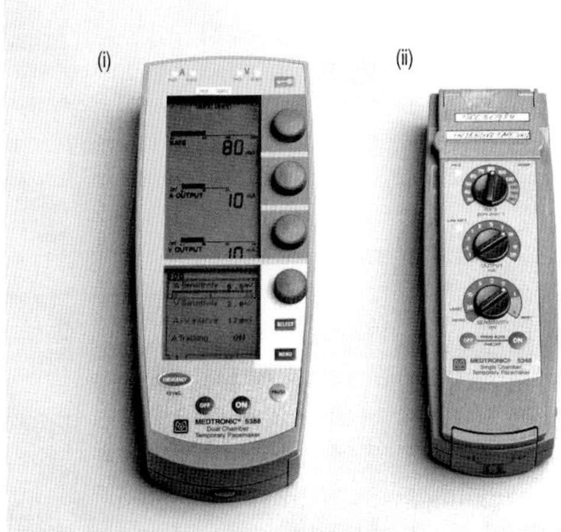

Figure 23.8 External pacemakers. Medtronic, Inc. (i) Model 5388 (dual-chamber); (ii) model 5348 (single-chamber). Both are capable of rapid pacing for certain tachycardias.

Troubleshooting

Lead does not cross the tricuspid valve Looping the lead in the right atrium and then applying counterclockwise torque will help prolapse it into the RV.

Lead cannot be advanced to the RV apex Withdrawing the lead after advancing it to the RV outflow tract (RVOT) may help the tip fall towards the apex. A small amount of torque may aid the process. Alternatively, the lead may need to be shaped with a different degree of curve.

If this manoeuvre does not help, a more basal position on the inferior wall can be used. The RVOT should be used only if the patient is asystolic as lead stability is poor here with passive leads.

Lead advances only towards the RVOT Ensure that this is not in the coronary sinus by checking that it does not curve posteriorly in the LAO position. If it is not, apply a slightly posteriorly facing curve to the distal tip of the lead and try again.

Testing the pacing leads

Modern temporary pacing boxes are sophisticated devices, which can perform checks of sensing as well as pacing threshold. Checking the sensitivity of a pacing lead electrogram is a very important step. Sensitivity, or sensing, is simply calculation of the amplitude of the sensed electrograms. Large electrograms are easy to sense and small ones are not and undersensing may occur. Undersensing will cause inappropriate delivery of a pacing stimulus. If this occurs on or near a T-wave, this can lead to ventricular fibrillation (VF). On most boxes sensing is indicated by a flashing light or other digital marker. The sensitivity dial is slowly rotated from a low value to a higher one until sensing stops. This represents the sensitivity of the sensed electrograms. A higher value is better than a lower one. The sensitivity is programmed to allow continuous sensing of all intrinsic signals.

Pacing threshold The rate should be set at least 10 beats per minute faster than the intrinsic heart rate, or at 60 beats per minute if the patient has a profound bradycardia. The pacing output should be set at 5 V and sensitivity at 1 mA. The box is switched on and ventricular capture confirmed by the presence of a pacing spike immediately followed by a broad QRS of LBBB morphology at the same rate as that set on the box.

The output is slowly decreased until consistent capture is lost. It is then increased until capture returns. This is the pacing threshold and ideally should be less than 1 V. However, if another stable position cannot be found then a higher threshold may be acceptable. In those with no underlying rhythm or profound bradycardia, loss of capture will lead to asystole – in which case the output should be rapidly increased until capture returns. The stability of the wire is checked in its position just above the pacing threshold by asking the patient to take deep breaths, cough and sniff whilst looking for loss of capture and viewing the wire fluoroscopically. Diaphragmatic capture is checked in leads on the inferior RV wall by pacing at the maximum output, usually 10 V, and feeling the abdomen or fluoroscopically screening the diaphragm. If diaphragmatic capture occurs, the lead must be repositioned.

If a threshold of less than 1 V is achieved, the pacing rate is set to the desired rate to achieve adequate cardiac output or 40 beats per minute if intermittent back-up pacing is required. The voltage is usually set to three times the pacing threshold to allow sufficient safety margin, or at least 3 V. Temporary pacing is programmed in VVI mode to allow sensing of spontaneous ventricular activity and to inhibit pacing.

Complications of temporary pacing[16]

Temporary pacing should have a low complication rate. However, it is rare nowadays for operators to gain regular experience at insertion and similarly training may also be inadequate. Several studies from the UK report complications in a third to a half of cases.[17,18] Thus, temporary transvenous pacing is best avoided where possible; rather, insertion of a permanent system at the earliest opportunity is best, and in many centres this now happens out of 'normal' working hours. Complications include:

- pneumothorax, haemothorax, arterial puncture, AV fistula and perforation of the RV or RA leading to cardiac tamponade
- undersensing, leading to inappropriate pacing and pacemaker-induced arrhythmias; oversensing (of extrinsic or intrinsic noise), with pacemaker inhibition and loss of cardiac output; failure to capture due to poor or unstable lead position, increasing pacing threshold with chronicity of lead
- diaphragmatic capture (may be associated with RV perforation)
- thrombus of the central vein and importantly infection, especially with leads older than 7 days.

How to manage abrupt failure to pace

A life-threatening situation may arise if a temporary pacemaker fails suddenly. The following is an ordered approach to such an emergency:

1. Make sure the pacemaker box is switched on and connected to the pacing lead(s).
2. The pacemaker output should be increased to its maximum setting (usually 10 V or 20 mA).
3. Asynchronous DOO/VOO mode(s) should be selected to prevent oversensing.
4. If pacing still fails, connect the pacemaker directly to the pacing lead bypassing the connecting wire (if present), as occasionally connecting wires may be faulty.
5. Consider replacing the pacemaker box or its batteries.
6. External transcutaneous pacing should be immediately available and commenced while a new pacing system is inserted.
7. Cardiopulmonary resuscitation and positive chronotropic drugs such as atropine, isoproterenol (isoprenaline) or epinephrine (adrenaline) should be available.

PACEMAKER PROGRAMMING

Multiple parameters can be programmed on both modern temporary and permanent pacing systems. All pacing practitioners, and this includes physicians who implant temporary systems, should be familiar with programming the mode, rate, pacing output and sensitivity of a pacing system and should also be able to diagnose and troubleshoot basic pacing problems like undersensing and oversensing. If dual-chamber pacing systems are used, programming the AV delay should be performed to optimise cardiac output and cardiac function (perhaps using echocardiographic guidance). Programming permanent pacing systems is more complicated than for temporary systems and should be performed only by individuals qualified to do so. Internationally recognised pacing qualifications include the IBHRE and EHRA examinations awarded by the Heart Rhythm Society and the European Heart Rhythm Association, respectively.

NOISE AND ELECTROMAGNETIC INTERFERENCE

Any signal sensed by a pacemaker will lead to pacing being inhibited or triggered (e.g. in dual-chamber systems). These signals will include noise, or electrical artefact sensed by a pacing system. Noise is characterised as intrinsic (from within the patient) or extrinsic, from outside the patient. Sources of intrinsic noise include lead fracture, fluid in the generator header and diaphragmatic and skeletal myopotentials. Extrinsic noise includes electromagnetic interference (EMI) (e.g. from a nearby electrical device or its trailing wires and surgical diathermy). Other sources include MRI scanners (patients with some modern permanent pacemakers can be safely scanned in MRI scanners) or electronic devices placed over the pacemaker generator (e.g. mobile telephones or MP3 players). Noise can be misinterpreted by ICDs as VT or VF and can result in inappropriate therapy and shocks.

MRI scanning is sometimes necessary in patients with non-MRI-safe pacing systems or ICDs. Recent studies have demonstrated that MRI scanning can be performed safely in selected patients with these types of system,[19] but this must be performed in collaboration with a pacing expert and the risks presented by MRI must be outweighed by the diagnostic benefit of the scan on a case-by-case basis.

CARDIOVERSION/DEFIBRILLATION IN PATIENTS WITH A PERMANENT PACEMAKER (OR ICD)

To avoid damage to the pacemaker device, shocking pads should be placed in the anterior–posterior position and at least 10 cm from the unit. The pacemaker (or ICD) should be checked before and afterwards. In patients with a temporary transvenous pacemaker, the external unit and leads should be kept well away from the pads.

DIATHERMY

Bipolar diathermy should be used whenever possible and the pacemaker programmed to an asynchronous mode in pacing-dependent patients. In an emergency (e.g. asystole in a patient whose pacemaker is inhibited by diathermy), placing a magnet over the pacemaker generator will result in asynchronous pacing at 'magnet' rate (magnet rate varies according to pacemaker manufacturer). ICDs do not have a magnet rate; placing a magnet over an ICD will switch off its therapies (i.e. antitachycardia pacing and shocks) but ICD therapies should be switched off before using diathermy. After surgery the pacemaker or ICD should be tested and reprogrammed appropriately.

CARDIAC PACING IN TACHYARRHYTHMIAS

Although pacemakers are not usually inserted for the treatment of atrial arrhythmias, AVNRT or AVRT, these rhythms may be treated safely and effectively by rapid pacing and/or premature electrical stimulation where a device is already present. They can also be used for treatment of VT, but rapid VT should be managed with DC cardioversion. Rapid cardiac pacing has advantages over DC cardioversion (**Box 23.1**) and drug therapy (**Box 23.2**), but is of no value in sinus tachycardia, AF and VF (**Box 23.3**). Pacing at rates of 80–100 beats per minute can be used to try to suppress ventricular and supraventricular rhythms as well as torsade de pointes in patients with the congenital long QT syndrome.

VENTRICULAR TACHYCARDIA

Ventricular burst pacing is a simple and often effective technique to pace VT. The ventricle is paced at a rate starting at about 120% of the VT rate for 8–10 beats (**Fig. 23.9**). If this fails (**Fig. 23.10**), increasing the pacing rate and/or the number of paced beats in the train should be tried cautiously. Slow VTs particularly are very stable and often require very long pacing trains. Potential complications include accelerating the VT rate, which can precipitate VF. Trained personnel, a defibrillator and resuscitation facilities must be available to perform this safely.

Box 23.1 Pacing versus cardioversion for the treatment of tachyarrhythmias

- Pacing may assist in rhythm diagnosis
- Pacing may be used (cautiously) in digitalis intoxication
- Pacing does not require a general anaesthetic
- Pacing avoids complications of DC shock, especially myocardial depression
- Repeated reversions are easier with pacing
- Standby pacing is immediately available if bradycardia or asystole occurs after electrical reversion

Box 23.2 Pacing versus drug therapy for the treatment of tachyarrhythmias

- Pacing may aid in arrhythmia diagnosis
- Pacing avoids drug-induced cardiac depression and other drug side-effects
- Pacing can be used when drug therapy has failed
- Termination of the tachycardia with pacing is often immediate
- Standby pacing is immediately available

Box 23.3 Indications for rapid cardiac pacing in suitable arrhythmias

- Failure of drug therapy
- Recurrent arrhythmias
- Contraindication for cardioversion (e.g. digitalis intoxication)
- Aid to arrhythmia diagnosis (e.g. wide-complex tachycardia to differentiate ventricular tachycardia from supraventricular tachycardia)

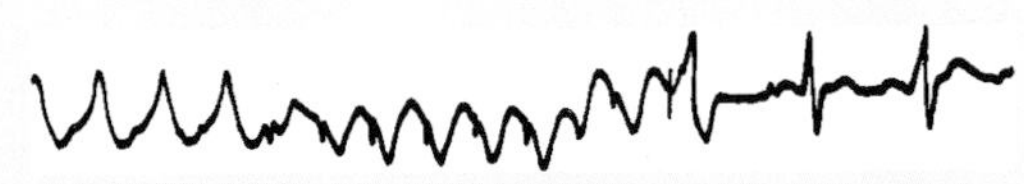

Figure 23.9 Wide-complex tachycardia. Ventricular burst pacing with ventricular capture results in normal sinus rhythm on cessation of pacing.

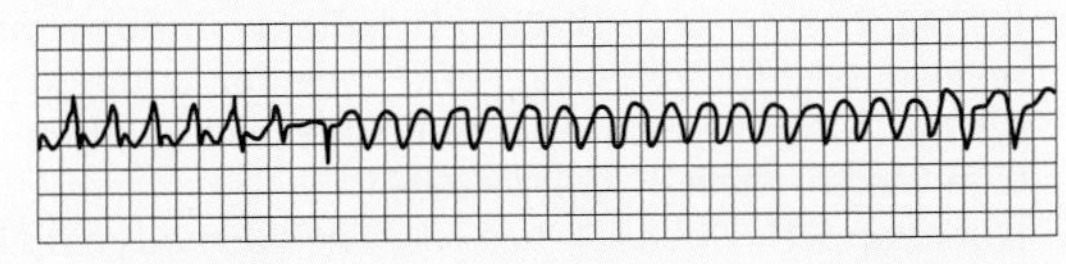

Figure 23.10 Wide-complex tachycardia is followed by ventricular burst pacing. When pacing is discontinued, a wide-complex tachycardia of opposite polarity is precipitated.

IMPLANTABLE CARDIOVERTER DEFIBRILLATORS (ICD)[2]

This is an implantable device that recognises and tries to terminate VT and VF through antitachycardia pacing and shocks, respectively. Guidelines are published for ICD implantation.[14] ICDs are of proven survival benefit and a class I indication in patients who have survived VF or haemodynamically unstable VT not due to a transient or reversible cause (e.g. an electrolyte imbalance). ICD implantation is also indicated for patients with structural heart disease and spontaneous sustained VT, whether haemodynamically stable or unstable. ICDs are also now used prophylactically in high-risk patients (i.e. those with severely impaired LV function) and are especially efficacious in patients with previous myocardial infarction.[20]

Most ICD systems are implanted transvenously and can perform antitachycardia pacing as well as normal permanent pacing, if necessary. Single- or dual-chamber ICDs may be implanted. The addition of an atrial lead gives another piece of information for the ICD to use to diagnose a tachycardia as VT rather than an SVT, but has not conclusively been shown to do this better than single-chamber devices. ICDs continuously monitor the patient's heart rate and deliver therapy when the heart rate exceeds the programmed detection rate. Devices are programmed with different tachycardia zones, stratified according to rate:

1. *VF zone:* for rates usually faster than 200 beats per minute. High-energy shocks are delivered if detection criteria are met, but antitachycardia pacing can be delivered while the device is charging in case it is a very fast VT. Shocks are biphasic as these are more efficient and require lower energies than monophasic waveforms and can be programmed below the maximum output if the programmer wishes to save device battery life.
2. *Fast VT zone:* for rates between 170 and 200 beats per minute – several attempts of antitachycardia pacing are usually programmed initially, of increasing aggressiveness. This is followed by shocks if unsuccessful.
3. *Slow VT zone:* for rates between 150 and 170 beats per minute. This is similar to the fast VT zone, but even more weighted to antitachycardia pacing.

COMPLICATIONS

Occasionally, ICDs can deliver multiple discharges in short sequence and this is a clinical emergency. Shocks may be appropriate or inappropriate. Frequent malignant ventricular arrhythmias may result in multiple appropriate discharges. If the multiple shocks are successful in defibrillating the patient during an arrhythmia 'storm', the ICD device may be deactivated and antiarrhythmic drugs or even general anaesthesia initiated. This will save device battery longevity and be much more comfortable for the patient. If shocks are inappropriate, for example for atrial fibrillation or lead fracture, the ICD needs to be reprogrammed or should be switched off.

Access the complete references list online at http://www.expertconsult.com

2. Epstein AE, DiMarco JP, Ellenbogen KA, et al. ACC/AHA/HRS 2008 guidelines for device-based therapy of cardiac rhythm abnormalities. J Am Coll Cardiol 2008;51(21):e1–e62.
4. Cleland JGF, Daubert JC, Erdmann E, et al. The effect of cardiac resynchronisation therapy on morbidity and mortality in heart failure (CARE-HF). N Eng J of Med 2005;352:1539–49.
7. Bernstein AD, Camm AJ, Fletcher RD, et al. The NASPE/BPEG generic pacemaker code for antibradyarrhythmic and adaptive rate pacing and antitachyarrhythmic devices. Pace 1987;107:794–9.
8. Bernstein AD, Daubert JC, Fletcher RD, et al. North American Society of Pacing and Electrophysiology/British Pacing and Electrophysiology Group: the revised NASPE/BPEG generic code for antibradycardia, adaptive-rate, and multisite pacing. Pacing Clin Electrophysiol 2002;25:260–4.
11. Donovan KD, Dobb GJ, Lee KY. The haemodynamic importance of maintaining atrioventricular synchrony during cardiac pacing in critically ill patients. Crit Care Med 1991;19:320–6.
13. Toff WD, Skehan JD, De Bono DP, et al. The United Kingdom Pacing and Cardiovascular Events (UKPACE) trial: United Kingdom Pacing and Cardiovascular Events. Heart 1997;78:221–3.
15. Spotnitz HM. Optimizing temporary perioperative cardiac pacing. J Thorac Cardiovasc Surg 2005;129: 5–8.
20. Moss AJ, Zareba W, Hall WJ, et al. Prophylactic implantation of a defibrillator in patients with myocardial infarction and reduced ejection fraction. N Engl J Med 2002;346:877–83.

FURTHER READING

Chow AWC, Buxton AE. Implantable Cardiac Pacemakers and Defibrillators: All You Wanted to Know. Malden, MA: Blackwell; 2006.

Ellenbogen KA, Wood MA. Cardiac Pacing and ICDs. 5th ed. Chichester, UK: Wiley-Blackwell; 2008.

Hayes DL, Lloyd MA. Cardiac Pacing and Defibrillation: A Clinical Approach. Elmsford, NY: Blackwell; 2000.

Roland X, Stroobandt S, Barold S, et al. Sinnaeve Implantable Cardioverter-defibrillators Step by Step: An Illustrated Guide. Chichester, UK: Wiley-Blackwell; 2009.

Timperley J, Leeson P, Mitchell ARJ, et al. Pacemakers and ICDs (Oxford Specialist Handbooks in Cardiology). Oxford, UK: OUP; 2008.

24

Acute heart failure

Nicholas Ioannou, Pratik Sinha and David Treacher

The pattern of heart failure seen in the community, outpatients clinics and specialist cardiac wards is dominated by the acute coronary syndromes and chronic heart failure, predominantly caused by ischaemic heart disease and hypertension.[1,2] Heart failure is the commonest cause of hospital admission in people over 65 years of age and it has been estimated that in North America and Europe over 15 million patients have heart failure and 1.5 million new cases are diagnosed each year.[3] Patients present with chest pain, palpitations, shortness of breath, fatigue and oedema and will usually have single-organ failure. Management focuses on reducing cardiac work to relieve symptoms and prevent further myocardial damage.

Patients either admitted with or who develop acute heart failure on the intensive care unit (ICU) frequently have overt or occult underlying coronary artery disease, but will usually have significant other organ dysfunction. Management in this setting focuses on both improving global and regional oxygen delivery and maintaining perfusion pressure, often with the use of drugs that stimulate rather than rest the myocardium.[4,5] The resolution of this apparent paradox requires that for each patient management should attempt to achieve the frequently difficult balance between the best interests of the myocardium and the circulatory requirements of the other vital organs. The critical care physician should target the minimum necessary oxygen delivery and arterial pressure to maintain other organ function at maximum cardiac efficiency (e.g. ensuring adequate fluid resuscitation before starting beta agonists) so that cardiac work and the risk of myocardial ischaemia and necrosis from exuberant beta agonist use are minimised and the cardiologist should consider the wider circulation and other organ requirements when instituting strategies to protect the myocardium.

DIAGNOSIS OF ACUTE HEART FAILURE

The diagnosis of acute heart failure in critically ill patients can be more difficult than is commonly recognised. Although the underlying pathology in most patients with acute heart failure on intensive care will be coronary artery disease, other diagnoses must be considered (**Box 24.1**).

It is also important to reassess critically the patient referred with a diagnosis of acute heart failure to decide whether this is indeed the primary problem. The history, examination and initial investigations with routine blood tests, electrocardiogram (ECG) and chest X-ray may be compatible with this diagnosis but many such patients are elderly with multiple co-morbidities, and deciding whether the patient is suffering from a primary myocardial pathology as opposed to a pulmonary problem or indeed systemic sepsis[6] can be difficult. Equally, patients believed to have a primary respiratory problem may fail to wean from ventilatory support because of a failure to realise that they have left ventricular failure with a high left atrial pressure and incipient pulmonary oedema, causing a reduction in pulmonary compliance, an increased work of breathing and respiratory distress when ventilatory support is withdrawn.

Further investigations that can help to confirm or refute an initial diagnosis of acute heart failure are echocardiography and the measurement of biomarkers such as natriuretic peptides and cardiac troponins.

ECHOCARDIOGRAPHY (SEE CH. 27)

Echocardiography is an extremely valuable investigation in the management of the critically ill patient with acute heart failure[7] and the modern critical care physician should at least be able to perform a basic examination. Transthoracic echocardiography (TTE) is non-invasive and can be performed rapidly at the bedside. The images obtained with TTE may be suboptimal in ventilated patients but experienced operators can achieve considerable improvement using microbubble contrast techniques.[8] If transthoracic views are difficult to obtain or if better resolution is required (e.g. for the detection of small vegetations) then transoesophageal echocardiography (TOE) should be considered. TOE gives excellent views of the aorta (dissection flaps), the left atrial appendage and left heart valves; however, right heart structures and the apex of the left ventricle are less well imaged.

Echocardiography will frequently establish the underlying cardiac pathology and can be used to monitor the response to treatment. It will:

1. Identify pericardial effusions and determine whether ventricular filling is impaired (tamponade) and whether drainage is indicated. However, ultimately tamponade is a clinical diagnosis based on the full haemodynamic picture in the context of pericardial fluid demonstrated on the echocardiogram. Many of the diagnostic features related to alterations with respiration are affected by positive-pressure ventilation and drainage may be appropriate even if such classic echocardiographic criteria are not present. Even small effusions may cause tamponade since it is the rate of accumulation of fluid rather than the amount of fluid that determines the degree of cardiac compromise.
2. Identify obstruction to cardiac filling from other intrathoracic space-occupying lesions that increase intrathoracic pressure, particularly in ventilated patients (pleural effusion, alveolar gas trapping in asthma).
3. Assess adequacy of *volume* preload of left ventricle, particularly in the context of raised preload *pressures* and monitor response to fluid challenge.
4. Identify primary valvular heart disease (critical aortic stenosis, acute mitral regurgitation from papillary muscle rupture, acute endocarditis) when urgent surgery is indicated and distinguish this from functional valvular regurgitation due to primary ventricular disease for which surgery could be lethal.
5. Identify septal defects, regional wall motion abnormalities and aneurysmal dilatation from recent or previous myocardial infarction.
6. Identify the presence of intracardiac thrombus or clot.
7. Identify increased end-systolic and diastolic dimensions, indicating ventricular contractile failure; termed systolic dysfunction or heart failure with reduced ejection fraction (HF-REF).[9] However, the use of ejection fraction as an index of ventricular dysfunction can be misleading, especially in patients on inotropic drugs.
8. Identify diastolic dysfunction as a consequence of impaired ventricular relaxation, also termed heart failure with preserved ejection fraction (HF-PEF).[9] Preserved ejection fraction in this context does not necessarily equate to an adequate cardiac output[10] and high-pressure preload measurements may fail to reflect the true volume preload and the potential need for extra fluid volume.
9. Identify pulmonary hypertension associated with tricuspid regurgitation when an estimate of pulmonary artery (PA) systolic pressure can be made.
10. Identify right ventricular size and function and discriminate between pressure and volume overload of the right ventricle. The presence of right ventricular dysfunction can also be used to diagnose and risk stratify patients presenting with suspected acute pulmonary embolism (PE).

Box 24.1 Causes of acute heart failure on the intensive care unit

Coronary artery disease
Cardiac arrhythmias – atrial fibrillation
Infection – systemic sepsis, viral myocarditis
Mechanical – endocarditis, pulmonary emboli, valve problems, septal defects, tamponade, high intrathoracic pressure with inadequate preload
Drugs – beta blockers, calcium antagonists, cytotoxic therapy (e.g. doxorubicin), alcohol, cocaine
Hypoxaemia
Metabolic – acidaemia, thiamine deficiency, thyrotoxicosis, hypocalcaemia, hypophosphataemia
Myocardial contusion – blunt thoracic trauma
Myocardial infiltration – tumour, sarcoidosis, amyloidosis
Vasculitis – rare
Neuromuscular conditions – Duchenne muscular dystrophy, Friedrich's ataxia, myotonic dystrophy

MEASUREMENT OF NATRIURETIC PEPTIDES AND CARDIAC TROPONINS

Myocardial injury and the development of acute heart failure are common but frequently unrecognised complications of critical illness occurring not only in patients with an overt acute coronary syndrome but also in other conditions such as sepsis and major pulmonary embolism.[11] Relying on blood tests alone to establish a diagnosis or to plan management is inadvisable but, when interpreted in conjunction with the wider clinical picture, natriuretic peptides and cardiac troponins appear to be sensitive markers of myocardial stress and necrosis and to have significant prognostic significance.

NATRIURETIC PEPTIDES

B-type natriuretic peptide (BNP) and *N*-terminal pro B-type natriuretic peptide (NT-proBNP) are the most commonly measured natriuretic peptides in clinical practice. BNP was first isolated from porcine brain[12] and was originally termed brain natriuretic peptide; however, the major source was subsequently shown to be from the ventricular myocardium. The main stimulus for natriuretic peptide synthesis and release is myocardial wall stress; cardiac myocytes release the prohormone proBNP, which is subsequently cleaved into biologically active BNP and the inactive *N*-terminal fragment (NT-proBNP). Although natriuretic peptide release appears to be related to end-diastolic volume and pressure, it does not reliably differentiate between HF-REF and HF-PEF or accurately predict ejection fraction or filling pressures.[13] Measurement of BNP and NT-proBNP in the emergency department may discriminate patients with heart failure from those with pulmonary or other non-cardiac causes for acute dyspnoea and has been shown to reduce rates of ICU admission, length of hospital stay and cost.[14] Studies have demonstrated that, at a cut-off of 100 pg/mL, BNP has a sensitivity of 90% and a specificity greater than 70% as a test for excluding heart failure.[15] Similar data have also been reported for NT-proBNP.[16] Measurement of natriuretic peptides is now recommended by international guidelines for the management of heart failure.[9,17,18] Furthermore, BNP has also been shown to be a marker of myocardial dysfunction and prognosis in severe sepsis.[19]

CARDIAC TROPONINS

Troponins are regulatory proteins that form part of the thin filament of the myocyte contractile apparatus (in addition to actin and tropomyosin); three subunits have been identified: (i) TnI, which binds actin to inhibit actin–myosin interaction, (ii) TnT, which binds tropomyosin, and (iii) TnC, which binds calcium ions resulting in a conformational change in the troponin–tropomyosin complex thus exposing myosin-binding sites. The cardiac isoforms, cTnI and cTnT, are specific to the heart and can be measured in the blood after myocyte necrosis with 50% release by 4 hours, peaking at 12–24 hours and remaining elevated for up to 10 days. They are far more sensitive than traditional cardiac enzyme tests such as creatine kinase and have substantially changed the definition, diagnosis and management of acute myocardial infarction. Cardiac troponins may be released in conditions other than acute coronary ischaemia[20] such as sepsis and after chemotherapy and in the absence of evidence of myocardial necrosis, as in acute heart failure or major PE, where it is believed that the acute ventricular dilatation causes increased membrane permeability. Raised troponin levels are also associated with increased morbidity and mortality in surgical ICU patients[21] and in patients presenting with acute decompensated heart failure.[22]

Elevated levels of cardiac troponins, BNP and NT-proBNP, may also be detected in the presence of right ventricular dysfunction following an acute PE. They can be used to risk stratify patients owing to their high negative predictive value for in-hospital death and adverse events. In haemodynamically stable patients, normal values indicate a lower risk of adverse outcome; therefore less aggressive therapy may be warranted.[23-25]

Raised levels of these markers, indicating early myocardial stress, may have an important role in alerting the clinician to impending myocardial failure and the need to review the use of drugs that stimulate the myocardium and to consider the introduction of a beta blocker, particularly in the context of tachycardia.

It should be remembered that, for critically ill patients with acute heart failure not resulting from primary myocardial infarction, if the precipitating cause is successfully treated without significant myocardial necrosis occurring the acute heart failure will resolve, cardiac function will return to its premorbid state and the prognosis will be improved.

The remainder of this chapter addresses the assessment and principles of management of ventricular function in patients admitted to the ICU with acute heart failure. This inevitably involves reference to circulatory failure and the state of the peripheral circulation, but the more detailed aspects of oxygen delivery and control of the regional and microcirculation are considered elsewhere[26] (see Chs 15 and 16), as are the acute coronary syndromes[2] (see Ch. 20) and chronic heart failure.[1]

CIRCULATORY FAILURE OR 'SHOCK'

The principal function of the heart is the generation of the energy necessary to perfuse the lungs with venous blood and to propel the oxygenated arterial blood through the systemic circulation at a rate and pressure that ensure that the fluctuating metabolic requirements of the various organs are met at rest and during exercise. This should be performed at maximum efficiency so that the work performed is not at the cost of unnecessarily high myocardial energy expenditure and the risk of myocardial ischaemia is minimised.

Failure to maintain an adequate oxygen supply to the tissues with the consequent development of anaerobic cellular metabolism defines circulatory failure or 'shock', a term that benefits from brevity but little else since it implies neither cause nor prognosis, but its use is now widespread and inescapable. **Box 24.2** classifies circulatory 'shock'.

In considering these causes of circulatory failure, several points require emphasis:

1. Acute heart failure resulting in cardiogenic shock is not a pathological diagnosis but a collective term

Box 24.2 Major categories of circulatory failure or 'shock'

Cardiogenic – myocardial infarction, myocarditis, vasculitis, valve dysfunction (e.g. critical aortic stenosis, mitral regurgitation, acute endocarditis), post cardiac bypass surgery, drug overdose (beta blockers, calcium antagonists)
Hypovolaemic – haemorrhage, burns, gastrointestinal fluid loss
Obstructive – pulmonary embolus, cardiac tamponade, tension pneumothorax
Anaphylactic – drugs, blood transfusion, insect sting
Septic – bacterial infection, non-infective inflammatory conditions (e.g. pancreatitis, burns, trauma)
Neurogenic – intracranial haemorrhage, brainstem compression, spinal cord injury

that embraces all causes of myocardial failure. Treatment must focus on the underlying diagnosis.

2. Patients admitted to ICU may have acute heart failure either as the primary reason for admission (e.g. severe myocardial infarction), or develop it as part of multiple-organ failure triggered by an extracardiac cause, frequently the delayed or ineffective treatment of severe sepsis.
3. Pre-existing cardiac disease, usually ischaemic heart disease, is an important factor in determining the physiological response to critical illness. Several studies investigating the effect of manipulating oxygen delivery have demonstrated the poor prognosis associated with the inability of the heart to achieve a hyperdynamic response to critical illness either spontaneously or with volume loading and inotropic support.[4,5] Preoperative assessment with cardiopulmonary exercise testing is probably appropriate for all patients undergoing major surgery as a means of identifying those with poor physiological reserve so that the true risk of surgery can be identified and perioperative management planned accordingly.
4. Although hypotension is often considered to be the cardinal sign of circulatory failure, other global features (persistent tachycardia, confusion, tachypnoea, impaired peripheral perfusion, progressive metabolic acidaemia) occur earlier since the body has powerful homeostatic mechanisms that maintain pressure at the expense of flow.
5. The heart must provide its own blood supply and, if coronary blood flow does not match myocardial oxygen requirements, coronary ischaemia develops and cardiac and global circulatory failure may ensue.[27]
6. The primary problem in hypovolaemic, cardiogenic and obstructive shock is a progressive decline in cardiac output (CO) and global oxygen delivery, which, if not corrected, leads to secondary failure of the peripheral circulation and progressive organ dysfunction. In septic, anaphylactic and neurogenic shock, however, the primary problem is the loss of control of the peripheral circulation resulting in systemic hypotension and disordered distribution of blood flow, although CO and global oxygen delivery are usually increased.[28]
7. Although a primary cause for the circulatory failure may be identified, other causes may contribute to the evolution of the final pathology. For example, in septic shock the initial and major derangement is peripheral; it is characterised by microcirculatory chaos triggered by cytokine release, white-cell activation, disruption of the coagulation cascade resulting in microthrombi that occlude the microvasculature and endothelial disruption resulting in interstitial oedema. This same process occurs in the coronary microvasculature impairing myocyte function. There is also widespread loss of fluid from the intravascular to the extravascular space, resulting in hypovolaemia. The primary peripheral circulatory failure may therefore be compounded by both cardiogenic and hypovolaemic shock.
8. 'Early' and 'late' shock are terms that reflect the association between the duration and severity of the circulatory derangement and prognosis. Early intervention in circulatory shock has a major impact on survival.[29] If treatment is delayed until organ failure is established, the underlying pathological processes are frequently irreversible.
9. Although not a true 'mixed' venous sample, the oxygen saturation of blood taken from an internal jugular ($S_{cv}O_2$) or subclavian cannula has been shown to be valuable in assessing whether global oxygen delivery (DO_2) is adequate for global tissue oxygen consumption. A value < 70% should prompt consideration of whether a fluid challenge or other strategy to increase DO_2 is indicated. A value > 70% is not necessarily reassuring in patients with established hyperdynamic shock as this may reflect an inability of the tissues to extract and utilise oxygen.

ASSESSMENT OF VENTRICULAR FUNCTION

Making the considerable assumption that the circulation can be analysed as a constant-flow, fixed-compliance system, six key measurements traditionally define ventricular performance:

- right and left atrial pressures (RAP, LAP) or ventricular preload
- mean systemic and pulmonary arterial pressures (MAP, PAP) or ventricular afterload
- heart rate (HR)
- CO (Q_t).

Table 24.1 illustrates typical values in normal subjects and in the common causes of circulatory failure with calculation of the associated vascular resistances and oxygen delivery. The values quoted are merely examples that indicate the pattern of circulatory derangement produced by these pathologies: pre-existing cardiopulmonary disease and the severity of the condition will affect the precise figures obtained in individual cases and the response to vasoactive therapy.

Stroke volume (SV) is calculated from CO and heart rate:

$$SV = Q_t / HR \tag{24.1}$$

Three factors determine stroke volume: (1) preload, (2) afterload, and (3) myocardial contractility.

VENTRICULAR PRELOAD

Ventricular preload, traditionally assessed from atrial filling pressures, determines the end-diastolic ventricular volume, which, according to Starling's law of the heart and depending on ventricular contractility,

Table 24.1 Measurements in a normal 75 kg adult and in various conditions causing circulatory 'shock'

	RAP (mmHg)	LAP (mmHg)	mPAP (mmHg)	MAP (mmHg)	HR (per min)	CARDIAC OUTPUT (L/min)	SVR*	PVR*	STROKE WORK (g.m)		VENOUS COMPLIANCE (mL/mmHg)	CaO_2 (mL/100mL)	DO_2 (mL/min)
									LV	*RV*			
Normal	5	10	15	90	70	5.0	17	1.0	78	9.7	300	20	1000
Major haemorrhage	0	3	10	80	100	3.2	25	2.2	34	4.4	40	16	512
Left ventricular failure	7	19	23	90	100	3.6	23	1.1	35	7.8	80	18	648
Cardiac tamponade	14	16	19	65	110	2.3	22	1.3	14	1.4	50	20	460
Major PE	10	6	35	70	110	2.6	23	11.2	21	8.0	40	16	416
Exacerbation of COAD	10	9	35	80	100	6.5	11	4.0	63	22.1	150	13	845
Septic shock:													
(i) pre-volume	2	7	17	49	130	4.2	11	2.4	18	6.6	350	15	630
(ii) post-volume	10	14	25	68	120	8.0	7	1.4	49	13.6	200	14	1120

Typical circulatory measurements in a normal adult and in various cardiorespiratory conditions that may cause shock. The severity of the condition and pre-existing cardiorespiratory disease will affect the precise figures obtained in individual cases.

Pressures referenced to zero at 5th intercostal space, mid-axillary line in supine patient. LV=left ventricle; RV=right ventricle; CaO_2=arterial oxygen content; DO_2=global oxygen delivery; mPAP/MAP=mean pulmonary artery/arterial pressure.

SVR*/PVR*=systemic/pulmonary vascular resistance×80 to give SI units: dyn·s·cm^{-5}.

dictates the stroke work generated by each ventricle at the next cardiac contraction. The resulting stroke volume depends on the resistance or afterload that confronts the ventricle.[30]

On the general ward the jugular venous pressure (JVP) is measured from the sternal angle; however, in the ICU vascular pressures are measured from the mid-axillary line in the fifth intercostal space. From this reference point, in the supine position, the normal RAP is between 4 and 8 mmHg and the LAP is between 8 and 12 mmHg. Relative changes in either the contractility of the two ventricles or the respective vascular resistances will change the relationship between the atrial pressures, which must then be independently assessed.

The predominant factor determining preload is venous return, which depends on the intravascular volume and venous tone, which is controlled by the autonomic nervous system, circulating catecholamine levels and local factors, particularly PO_2, PCO_2 and pH.

The systemic venous bed is the major intravascular capacitance or reservoir of the circulation with a compliance that can vary from 30 to over 300 mL/mmHg and which provides a buffer against the effects of intravascular volume loss. It also explains the response observed in major haemorrhage and subsequent transfusion. As volume is lost, venous tone increases, preventing the large falls in atrial filling pressures and CO that would otherwise occur. If the equivalent volume is returned over the subsequent few hours the RAP gradually returns to normal as the intravascular volume is restored and the reflex increase in sympathetic tone abates. However, rapid re-infusion of the same volume does not allow sufficient time for the venous and arteriolar tone to fall and may result in the LAP rising to a level that precipitates pulmonary oedema, although the intravascular volume has only been returned to the pre-haemorrhage level and left ventricular function is normal (**Fig. 24.1**).

If the preload is low and either blood pressure or CO is inadequate, the priority is volume loading to restore intravascular volume and venous return.

Raised preload pressures reflect: (1) high intravascular volume, (2) impaired myocardial contractility, or (3) increased afterload.

Preload may be reduced by:

- removing volume from the circulation (diuretics, venesection, haemofiltration) or increasing the capacity of the vascular bed with venodilator therapy (e.g. glyceryl trinitrate, morphine[31])
- improving contractility
- reducing afterload.[32]

In assessing preload, end-diastolic *volume* rather than pressure is relevant and when interpreting atrial *pressures* as measures of preload, two points must be considered:

1. Intravascular pressure (*P*v) measurements are misleading if the intrathoracic pressure (*P*t) is raised since the true distending pressure that determines ventricular end-diastolic volume is the transmural pressure (*P*v–*P*t). This is particularly relevant if there is significant alveolar gas trapping generating intrinsic positive end-expiratory pressure (PEEP), as seen in asthma; in positive-pressure ventilation with high PEEP levels; and when an inverse inspiratory-to-expiratory time ratio is used.[33,34]
2. When the ventricle is poorly compliant, as in diastolic dysfunction, the end-diastolic pressure–volume relationship ceases to exhibit the approximately linear relationship over the normal physiological range of ventricular filling volumes (**Fig. 24.2**). Under these conditions, *pressure* will not necessarily reflect the adequacy of *volume* preload.

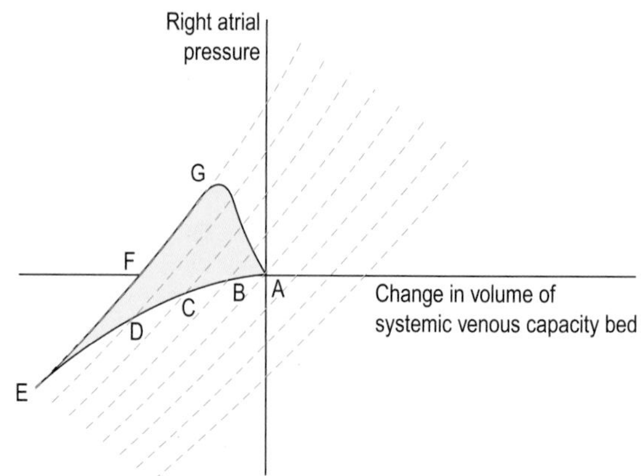

Figure 24.1 Venous compliance curves: each dotted line represents a line of constant venous compliance ranging from low compliance (increased tone) on the left to increased compliance (reduced tone) on the right. Line ABCDE shows the effect of progressive haemorrhage with the reduction in venous compliance limiting the fall in atrial pressure. Line EFGA shows the effect of rapid reinfusion of the same volume that was removed, but at a rate that does not allow the sympathetically mediated increase in venous tone to abate. Each dotted line represents a line of constant venous compliance ranging from minimum on the left to diminished venous tone on the right.

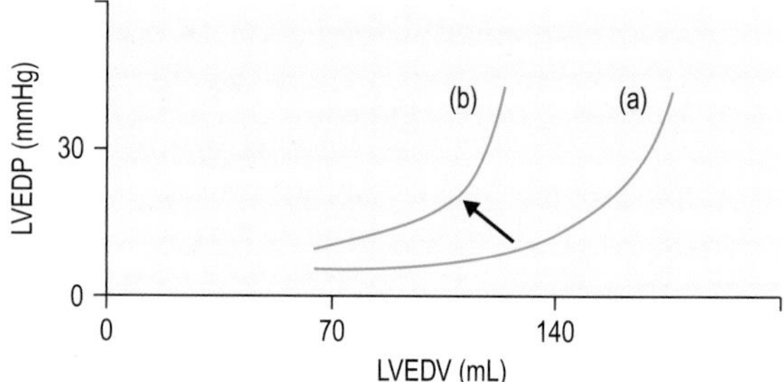

Figure 24.2 End-diastolic pressure–volume relationship (EDPVR) curves: (a) normal heart; (b) diastolic dysfunction. In the context of reduced ventricular compliance the EDPVR curve shifts upward and to the left. *(Modified from Brandis K. The Physiology Viva.[35])*

Box 24.3 Calculation of ventricular afterload and stroke work

$$\text{Systemic vascular resistance (SVR)} = [(\text{MAP} - \text{RAP})/\text{Qt}] \times 80 \text{ dyn.s.cm}^{-5}$$
$$= [(90-5)/5] \times 80 = 1360 \text{ dyn.s.cm}^{-5}$$
$$\text{SVRI} = \text{SVR} \times \text{BSA} = 1360 \times 1.65 = 2244 \text{ dyn.s.cm}^{-5}.\text{m}^{-2}$$
$$\text{Pulmonary vascular resistance (PVR)} = [(\text{mPAP} - \text{LAP})/\text{Q}_t] \times 80 \text{ dyn.s.cm}^{-5}$$
$$= [(15-10)/5] \times 80 = 80 \text{ dyn.s.cm}^{-5}$$
$$\text{PVRI} = \text{PVR} \times \text{BSA} = 80 \times 1.65 = 132 \text{ dyn.s.cm}^{-5}.\text{m}^{-2}$$
$$\text{Stroke volume (SV)} = \text{Qt/HR} = 72 \text{ mL}$$
$$\text{Stroke volume index (SVI)} = 72/1.65 = 44 \text{ mL/m}^2$$
$$\text{Ventricular stroke work (VSW)} = \text{SV} \times (\text{afterload} - \text{preload})$$
$$\text{LVSW} = \text{SV} \times (\text{MAP} - \text{LAP}) \times 0.0136 \text{ g.m}$$
$$= 72 \times (90-10) \times 0.0136 = 78 \text{ g.m}$$
$$\text{LVSWI} = 78/1.65 = 47 \text{ g.m/m}^2$$
$$\text{RVSW} = \text{SV} \times (\text{mPAP} - \text{RAP}) \times 0.0136 \text{ g.m}$$
$$= 72 \times (15-5) \times 0.0136 = 10 \text{ g.m}$$
$$\text{RVSWI} = 10/1.65 = 6 \text{ g.m/m}^2$$

MAP = mean arterial pressure; mPAP, = mean pulmonary artery pressure. Pressures are measured in mmHg, cardiac output (Q_t) in L/min. Values for resistance and stroke work are frequently indexed using the patient's body surface area (BSA) derived from height and weight. In calculating ventricular stroke work, 0.0136 converts to SI units of g.m. Example calculations assume a normal 75 kg individual with BSA 1.65 m^2.

Alternative methods of assessing ventricular preload are discussed later in this chapter under 'Assessment of intravascular volume status' and in Chapter 16.

VENTRICULAR AFTERLOAD

The vascular resistance against which each ventricle works is calculated, by analogy with Ohm's law, as the pressure gradient across the vascular bed divided by the CO (**Box 24.3**).

Circulatory management requires a clear understanding of this relationship between pressure, flow and resistance. If ventricular work is constant, increased vascular resistances produce higher pressures but with a lower CO. A systemic dilator such as sodium nitroprusside will reduce systemic resistance and blood pressure and increase CO. Although such manipulation is attractive in increasing CO for the same cardiac work, it is important to maintain a blood pressure that ensures appropriate distribution of blood flow and a diastolic pressure sufficient to maintain coronary artery perfusion, particularly in patients with known ischaemic heart disease or pre-existing hypertension.

The effects of some of the commonly used vasoactive agents are shown in **Table 24.2** and considered in more detail later (see Chs 90 and 91).

VENTRICULAR CONTRACTILITY AND EFFICIENCY

The work that the ventricle performs under given loading conditions defines contractility. For each ventricle it may be expressed mathematically as the gradient and intercept of the relationship between atrial filling pressure and stroke work (**Fig. 24.3**). The resulting stroke volume varies with the resistance of the vascular bed into which the ventricle is ejecting. Although the right ventricle generates a much smaller stroke work, the afterload (pulmonary vascular resistance) against which it ejects is correspondingly lower as the right and left ventricular stroke volumes must necessarily be the same over time.

The work generated by each ventricle with each heart beat is the ventricular stroke work and is calculated as shown in **Box 24.3**.

Consideration of ventricular work is important since optimum circulatory management requires that the necessary pressures and flows to maintain satisfactory organ perfusion and oxygen delivery are achieved at maximum cardiac efficiency (i.e. for the minimum ventricular work to avoid myocardial ischaemia). Furthermore, left ventricular efficiency is the ratio of work output to energy input and may be less than 20% in patients with acute heart failure, with over 80% of energy lost as heat.

If circulatory failure is due to impaired myocardial contractility, as defined by a 'flattened' stroke work/filling pressure equation (see **Fig. 24.3**), the atrial pressures will often already be raised. Provided such pressures reflect volume preload, further increases are not helpful since the ventricle becomes increasingly distended with high wall tension, as predicted by Laplace's law:

$$\text{wall tension} = (\text{intraventricular pressure} \times \text{radius}) \div (\text{wall thickness} \times 2) \qquad (24.2)$$

This increase in wall tension compromises myocardial blood supply, particularly epicardial to endocardial blood flow, resulting in endocardial ischaemia, further impairment of ventricular contractility and the risk of pulmonary oedema developing.

The remaining therapeutic options are:

- *Reduce afterload* using an arteriolar dilator (nitrates, alpha blocker, phosphodiesterase inhibitor,

Table 24.2 Circulatory effects of commonly used vasoactive drug infusions

DRUG	RECEPTORS/ MECHANISM OF ACTION	CARDIAC CONTRACTILITY	HEART RATE	BLOOD PRESSURE	CARDIAC OUTPUT	SPLANCHNIC BLOOD FLOW	SVR	PVR
Dopamine								
(<5 μg/kg/min)	DA, β1	+	0/+	0/+	+	0/+	0/+	0/+
(>5 μg/kg/min)	β1, α1, DA	++	+	+	++	0	+	+
Epinephrine	β1, β2, α1	++	++	++	+++	–	+	+
Norepinephrine	α1, β1	0/+	0	++	0/–	0/–	++	++
Isoproterenol (isoprenaline)	β1, β2	+	++	+/0	0/+	0/+	–	–
Dobutamine	β1, β2, α1	++	+	–/0/+	++	0	–	–
Levosimendan	Sensitises cTnC, ATP-sensitive K^+ channels	++	0/+	0/–	++	0	–	–
Dopexamine	β2, DA, β1	+	+	0/–	+	+	–	–
Glyceryl trinitrate	Via NO	0	0/+	–	+	+	–	–
Nitroprusside	Via NO	0	0/+	–	+	+	–	–
Milrinone	PDE-3 enzyme inhibitor	+	+	–	++	0/+	–	–
Nitric oxide (inhaled)	Via NO	0	0	0	0/+	0	0	–
Prostacyclin	Prostacyclin receptor (IP)	0	0/+	–	+	+	–	–

+=increase; 0=no change; –=decrease. These effects are guidelines only. The response will depend on the circulatory state of the patient when the drug is started.

angiotensin-converting enzyme (ACE) inhibitor), although this strategy is frequently limited by the resulting fall in systemic pressure.[36]

- *Increase myocardial contractility*, either by removing negatively inotropic influences (acidaemia, hyperkalaemia, drugs, e.g. beta blockers) or by using a positive inotrope, which may be defined as an agent that increases the gradient of the stroke work to filling pressure relationship, resulting in a larger stroke volume for the same pre- and afterload pressures. When considering the use of an inotropic agent (see **Table 24.2**), the adverse effects of vasoactive agents on ventricular efficiency, metabolic rate and regional distribution of flow should be considered.

HEART RATE AND RHYTHM

In cardiac failure the stroke volume is usually constant for rates up to 100/min and thereafter falls as restriction of diastolic filling time limits end-diastolic volume. Increasing the heart rate from 70 to 90/min will increase CO by almost 30%. Achieving this with a chronotrope such as the β_1-agonist isoprotenerol (isoprenaline) increases myocardial work and oxygen consumption and also ventricular irritability. In patients with ischaemic heart disease and particularly after a recent myocardial infarction, atrial or atrioventricular sequential pacing (which maintains coordinated atrial contraction in heart block) improves haemodynamics without stimulating myocardial metabolism and increasing myocardial irritability.[37]

Heart rates above 110/min, particularly with an irregular rhythm, should be controlled by either drugs or DC cardioversion after ensuring that plasma potassium and magnesium levels have been corrected. If the rhythm is supraventricular and unstable with intermittent periods of sinus rhythm, pharmacological control is indicated using either digoxin or amiodarone. Digoxin is appropriate for atrial fibrillation and has a temporary positive inotropic effect.[38] However, amiodarone is suitable for all supraventricular rhythms and is more likely to restore sinus rhythm. A meta-analysis showed that, used prophylactically, it reduced the rate of arrhythmic episodes and sudden death in patients with recent myocardial infarction or congestive cardiac failure.[39] It is, however, a negative inotrope and this can be significant in the patient with severe heart failure.

A fixed rate of 150/min suggests atrial flutter and should prompt careful inspection of the ECG and a trial of adenosine. A persistent sinus tachycardia unexplained by fever may be due to hypovolaemia, pain or anxiety.

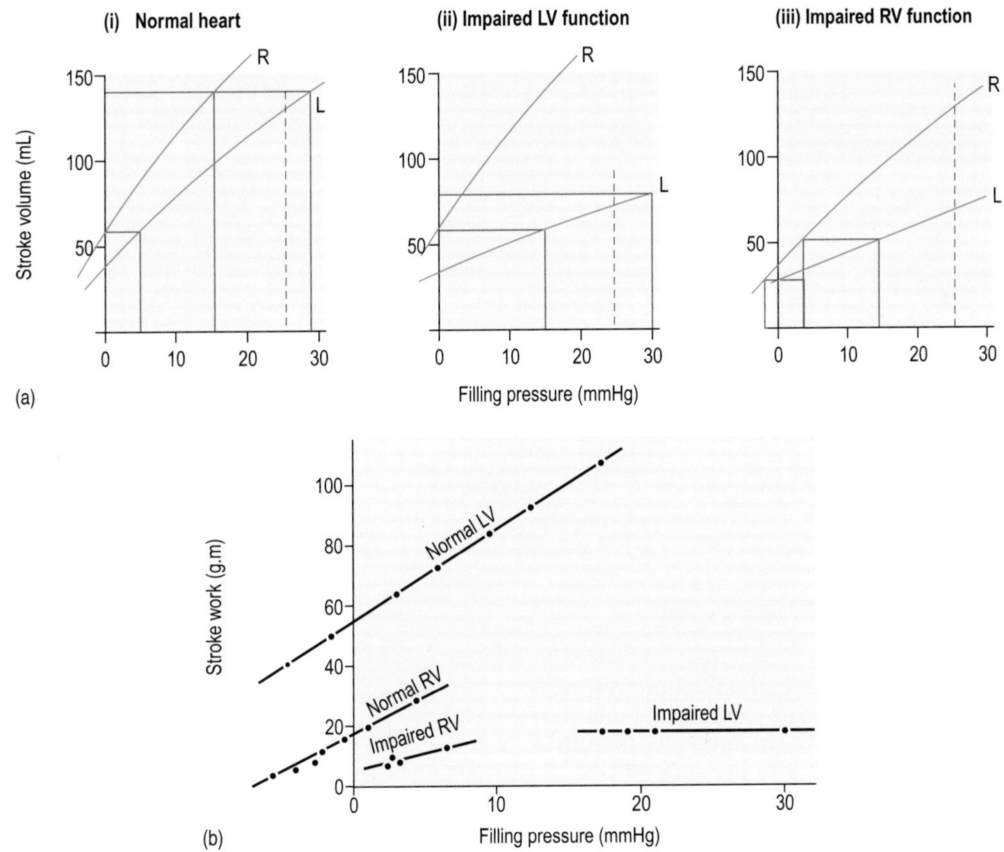

Figure 24.3 Ventricular function curves: (a) relationship between stroke volume (ml) and atrial filling pressure for left (L) and right (R) ventricles in patients with normal and impaired ventricular function; (b) relationship between stroke work (g.m) and atrial filling pressure (in mmHg) for the left (L) and right (R) ventricles for a normal subject and a patient with severe left and right ventricular failure.

ASSESSMENT OF MYOCARDIAL FUNCTION

Of the six key circulatory variables that define ventricular function, three (RAP, MAP and HR) can be assessed clinically and are routinely monitored in ICU patients. However, additional monitoring, traditionally using the PA catheter, is required to *measure* the other three variables (LAP, PAP and Q_t) in order to answer the following questions:

1. Is further intravascular volume indicated?
2. Is CO too low and compromising global oxygen delivery?
3. Is dilator, constrictor or inotropic therapy appropriate?

It is certainly not always necessary to use invasive monitoring. Initial management can be based on clinical assessment of intravascular volume and CO. The discipline of committing to an estimate of these key variables ensures that both the analysis of the circulation and the approach to treatment are logical. Further monitoring should be instituted if the initial management does not produce clinical improvement. Alternative, less invasive methods are available for assessing CO such as oesophageal Doppler,[40] lithium dilution,[41] continuous CO by pulse contour analysis (PiCCO) and echocardiography[7] – techniques that can also provide data on the volume rather than pressure preload of the left ventricle. **Table 24.3** lists some features of the techniques available for measuring cardiac output and whether they provide information on left ventricular preload. Further details of circulatory monitoring and these other techniques are described in the section on haemodynamic monitoring (see Ch. 16). A recent International Consensus Conference produced guidelines for the haemodynamic monitoring and management of patients with shock.[42]

KEY POINTS WHEN ASSESSING CARDIAC FUNCTION

- Pressure is no guarantee of flow.
- Trends and changes are more important than a single observation.

Table 24.3 Comparison of methods for assessing cardiac output

METHOD	INVASION/RISK	VENTRICULAR PRELOAD ASSESSED	COMPLEXITY	MEASUREMENT ERROR	COST
Indicator dilution					
Thermodilution (using PA catheter)	+++	From 'wedge' pressure	++	+	++
Fick	+++	No	+++	+	++
Indocyanine green	+++	No	++	+	++
Lithium	++	Yes	+	+	+
Respired gas					
Modified Fick	+	No	++	++	+
Inert gas rebreathing	+	Yes	+++	++	+
Doppler (oesophageal)	+	Yes	++	++	+++
Echocardiography	0	Yes	++	+++	+
Impedance cardiography	0	No	++	++	+
Pulse contour analysis	+	Yes (ITBV)	+	++	+
Clinical assessment	0	Yes	+	++	0

- Dynamic tests (e.g. assessing stroke volume response or a change in pulse pressure or stroke volume variation to a fluid challenge) are more revealing than static tests (e.g. central venous pressure, MAP).
- Monitoring devices may be complex with many potential sources of error, e.g. 'blocked' catheters, failure to re-level the transducer after a change in the patient's position. Readings should always be interpreted with care and in conjunction with clinical assessment.
- Invasive monitoring has its own hazards (infection, trauma, immobility) and should be removed if no longer required.

PULMONARY ARTERY CATHETERISATION

This remains a widely used method for measurement of left atrial and PA pressures and assessment of CO using the thermodilution technique. Although generally viewed as the 'gold standard' for determining CO, the error is at least 10%, even with fastidious attention to technical detail.

Inflation of the balloon at the end of the catheter provides a PA occlusion pressure (or pulmonary capillary wedge pressure), which reflects left atrial pressure provided there are no significant pulmonary vascular bed abnormalities, as occur in chronic obstructive airways disease and long-standing mitral valve disease. Despite obtaining a good-quality wedge tracing, the measurement must be interpreted with caution since increased intrathoracic pressure and diastolic dysfunction make this pressure measurement an unreliable index of true left ventricular volume preload.

The focus on 'goal-directed therapy' led to the widespread use of PA catheters, but their indiscriminate use was challenged by a multicentre case-controlled study suggesting that patients managed with a PA catheter had a poorer outcome than those managed without such intervention.[43] This study probably reflected the enthusiasm for inappropriate goal-directed therapy prevalent at that time, poor training in the use of the catheter and an inability of clinicians to respond appropriately to the data obtained.[44] More recent evidence suggests neither harm nor benefit with the use of a PA catheter and a risk–benefit assessment should be made on an individual patient basis prior to its use.

Box 24.4 lists the indications for PA catheterisation in heart failure. Other aspects of haemodynamic monitoring are discussed in Chapter 16.

Box 24.4 Indications for pulmonary arterial catheterisation in patients with heart failure

Failure to improve with initial circulatory management and uncertainty about adequacy of cardiac output and relationship between atrial filling pressures

Assessment of left ventricular preload when the relationship between right and left atrial pressures is uncertain owing to recent myocardial infarction, valvular abnormalities or high pulmonary vascular resistance. A low wedge pressure indicates that further volume is indicated, but a high value does not necessarily exclude the need for further volume

Measurement of cardiac output by thermodilution to direct appropriate choice of vasoactive drug and to manipulate therapy, particularly when high doses are being used

Need to monitor pulmonary arterial pressures and assess right ventricular function

ASSESSMENT OF INTRAVASCULAR VOLUME STATUS

CLINICAL

This is conventionally based on measurement of the right atrial filling pressure and the assumption that a normal relationship exists between the atrial filling pressures, which is not necessarily valid in the critically ill patient particularly in cardiogenic shock. Although values < 12 mmHg suggest hypovolaemia, higher levels are more difficult to interpret particularly in the ventilated patient. The RAP should therefore be interpreted carefully and in light of other clinical evidence. However, such static tests for assessing the intravascular volume are less valuable than dynamic tests, such as the fluid challenge and the effect of positive-pressure ventilation, which assess the circulatory response to an intervention.

Intravascular volume depletion is suggested if hypotension is precipitated by sedation, analgesia and postural change. In the patient receiving positive-pressure ventilation, respiratory fluctuation in the arterial pressure tracing also suggests relative hypovolaemia. This is confirmed if brief disconnection from the ventilator causes the blood pressure to rise and venous pressure to fall; the measurement off the ventilator more accurately reflects the ventricular end-diastolic *transmural* pressure. This manoeuvre is relatively contraindicated in patients with acute respiratory distress syndrome as loss of positive end-expiratory pressure may cause widespread alveolar collapse.

FLUID CHALLENGE

If hypovolaemia is suspected, a fluid challenge should be administered and the impact on blood pressure, flow and preload observed. In the volume-depleted patient blood pressure and flow will increase with only a small, transient increase in filling pressure. While pulmonary gas exchange remains satisfactory there is less anxiety about giving further fluid. Sufficient volume will have been given when either the target pressures are achieved and the evidence of poor peripheral perfusion and organ dysfunction has resolved, or when there is a sustained rise in filling pressures to a level above which there is a risk of pulmonary oedema developing. An objective assessment of the effect of such a fluid challenge can also be made by looking for a ≥ 10% rise in stroke volume.

Deciding the appropriate fluid volume to give in sepsis can be difficult and frequently represents a balance between giving sufficient volume to prevent the use of excessive doses of constricting inotropes and giving excessive amounts with consequent tissue oedema and deterioration in pulmonary gas exchange.

If there is concern about administering a fluid challenge, an assessment of fluid responsiveness in critically ill patients can be made by passive leg raising; the legs are elevated to 45° from the horizontal resulting in a reversible fluid challenge as venous blood is diverted to the central circulation (Trendelenberg positioning of the bed may also be used to simulate this manoeuvre).

VALSALVA MANOEUVRE

The effect of changes in intrathoracic pressure can be used to assess intrathoracic blood volume and provide an estimate of true left ventricular preload. **Figure 24.4** shows the classic Valsalva response in a normal subject and in a patient with a high intrathoracic blood volume. If a normal-type trace is observed on the monitor, further volume is indicated, whereas a square-wave response indicates an adequate left ventricular volume preload.[45] This response can be quantified by calculating the ratio of the pulse pressure during phase 2 of the manoeuvre to the baseline value. This correlates with measurements of pulmonary capillary wedge pressure[46] and can be applied at the bedside in sedated, ventilated patients.[47] However, if the patient is breathing spontaneously, this test is difficult both to perform and to interpret.

ECHOCARDIOGRAPHY

Echocardiography is useful in identifying inadequate volume preload and the need for further fluid resuscitation, particularly when the preload pressures are high, as may occur with diastolic dysfunction. Performing serial studies to assess the response to therapy (fluid challenge, starting vasoactive therapy, changing ventilator settings) can be particularly valuable.

MANAGEMENT OF CARDIAC FUNCTION IN THE CRITICALLY ILL

Circulatory management should be regularly reviewed in the critically ill patient. Following initial assessment and with knowledge of the primary diagnosis, the need for extra monitoring should be decided, provisional targets should be set for fluid balance, ventricular preload, mean and diastolic arterial pressures and a management plan agreed on how to achieve these goals. Generally a MAP>65 mmHg with diastolic pressure>50 mmHg is acceptable but adequate cerebral, coronary, splanchnic and renal perfusion may require higher pressures, particularly in the elderly patient with pre-existing hypertension or widespread atheroma.

CORRECTION OF METABOLIC FACTORS

The following metabolic factors should be promptly corrected:

- *hypoxaemia:* PO_2<8 kPa
- *acidaemia:* pH<7.20
- *hyperkalaemia:* K^+>5.5 mmol/L

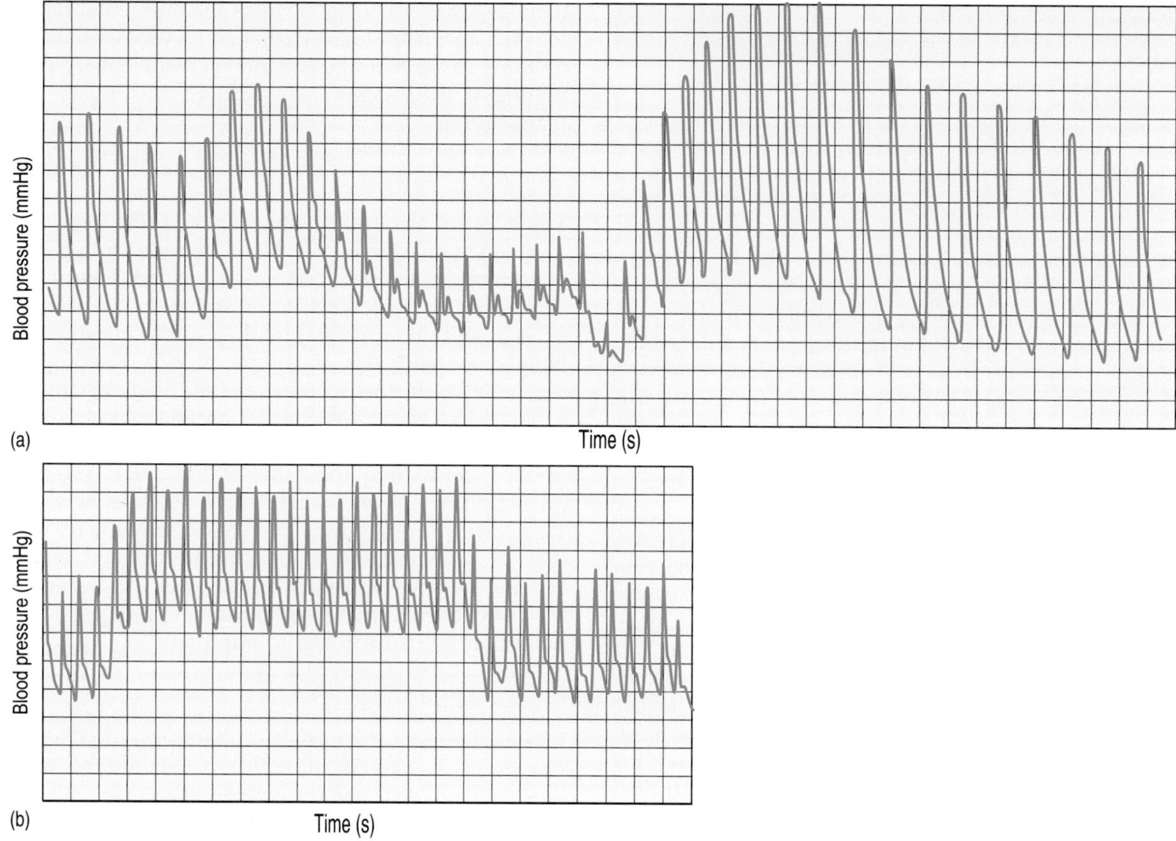

Figure 24.4 Valsalva traces (arterial waveforms): the Valsalva manoeuvre is performed by applying a pressure of at least 30 mmHg (judged from an RA trace) for 12–15 seconds. (a) Normal pulse pressure response. (b) Square-wave pulse pressure response.

- *hypomagnesaemia:* Mg^{2+}<0.9 mmol/L
- *hypocalcaemia:* ionised Ca^{2+}<1.0 mmol/L
- *hypophosphataemia:* PO_4^-<0.8 mmol/L
- *anaemia:* Hb<90 g/L
- *thiamine deficiency:* malnutrition, excess alcohol, diuretic or digoxin treatment.

Metabolic acidaemia with pH<7.20 or base deficit >10 mmol/L should be corrected since myocardial contractility increases linearly with rising pH to values >7.40. The suggestion that sodium bicarbonate should not be used as it produces a damaging paradoxical intracellular acidosis is misleading since the experiments demonstrating this effect were performed in vitro using non-physiological solutions, within a closed system that allowed no correction for any rise in carbon dioxide concentration and in which the sodium bicarbonate was given by bolus rather than by slow infusion.[48] The case for using bicarbonate to correct a metabolic acidaemia in the clinical setting has been recognised[49] and is supported by studies looking at the use of bicarbonate rather than lactate as the buffer solution in haemofiltration.[50] **Figure 24.5** shows the effect of correcting a severe metabolic acidaemia on CO by changing from lactate to bicarbonate haemofiltration.

Although a prospective randomised study demonstrated an improved survival for critically patients if haemoglobin concentration was maintained at 70–90 g/L rather than at 100–120 g/L, this did not apply to the elderly and those with coronary artery disease, in whom the haemoglobin level should be maintained >90 g/L.[51]

Patients with poor dietary thiamine (vitamin B1) intake, chronic alcohol abuse and those on chronic furosemide or digoxin therapy are at risk of thiamine deficiency, resulting in impaired myocardial function. Oral thiamine improves left ventricular function in these patients.[52,53]

SELECTION OF APPROPRIATE VASOACTIVE AGENTS (SEE CH. 90)

The choice of vasoactive agent when treating acute heart failure represents a balance between the global

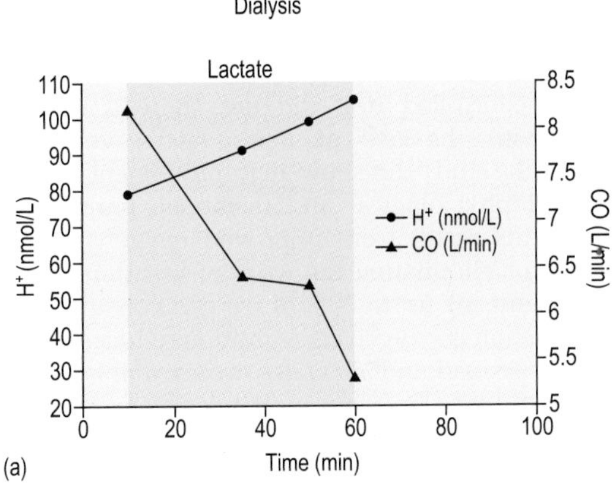

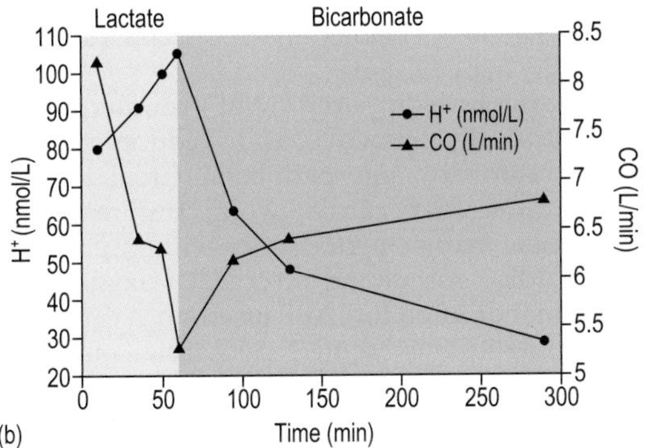

Figure 24.5 Effect of dialysis: (a) rising hydrogen ions and falling CO with lactate buffer dialysis; (b) change to bicarbonate buffer – there is falling hydrogen ion concentration and a rising cardiac output.

circulatory requirements and those of a stressed myocardium. The properties of commonly used agents are shown in **Table 24.2**.

The impact of these drugs in individual patients will be influenced by the *baseline state of the circulation*, i.e. if either intensely constricted or dilated, the same drug will potentially produce different effects on pressure, flow and its distribution. The initial choice of vasoactive agent will depend on the MAP, CO and derived systemic vascular resistance (SVR). For example:

- *CO and MAP are both low with a high SVR:* an inotropic and dilating (inodilator) effect is required and dobutamine or milrinone would be appropriate. Levosimendan would also be a suitable choice in this setting. If CO rises but MAP falls, as may happen with dobutamine, milrinone and levosimendan, and a more powerful inotropic effect is required, epinephrine (adrenaline) may be appropriate. However, increasing doses of epinephrine risk myocardial ischaemia, ventricular irritability, splanchnic ischaemia and the development of hyperlactataemia.[54] Consequently, it may be more appropriate to use norepinephrine (noradrenaline) to maintain MAP when inodilating drugs are being administered.
- *MAP and SVR are low with high CO:* this is frequently seen in sepsis: arteriolar constriction with norepinephrine (noradrenaline) is indicated after adequate volume resuscitation.
- *MAP is at or above target but CO is low with raised SVR:* a dilating agent (nitrate, e.g. glyceryl trinitrate) or an inodilator is appropriate.

When pulmonary vascular resistance and RAP are acutely raised, a pulmonary vasodilator to offload the right ventricle and maintain CO is required but hypotension may result from concomitant systemic arteriolar dilatation and hypoxaemia can develop owing to increased ventilation–perfusion mismatch.

Dopamine has been widely used in the erroneous belief that it selectively improves renal blood flow. However, if the patient has been fully volume resuscitated and a modest inotropic effect with only a small increase in SVR and a natriuretic effect are required, then a low-dose dopamine infusion (<5 μg/kg/min) may be considered.[55] A recent randomised controlled trial demonstrated a greater number of adverse events with the use of dopamine compared with norepinephrine (noradrenaline) in patients with shock. Moreover, in a predefined sub-group of patients with cardiogenic shock mortality was higher in patients treated with dopamine.[56]

Dopexamine is used to improve splanchnic blood flow but, despite reported benefits when used with volume loading in perioperative patients,[57,58] there is little evidence of outcome benefit in established shock.

Patients with chronic heart failure and those receiving long-term beta-agonist infusion often develop tolerance with reduced catecholamine receptor responsiveness, resulting in less effect in raising intracellular cyclic adenosine monophosphate (cAMP) levels and increasing myocardial contractility. Phosphodiesterase inhibitors (milrinone, enoximone) offer an alternative strategy. Milrinone competitively inhibits the phosphodiesterase III isoenzyme, responsible for the breakdown of cAMP, thereby increasing intracellular cAMP levels and improving myocardial contractility independent of β-receptor stimulation. There is also improvement in ventricular diastolic relaxation and a reduction in pulmonary vascular resistance. However, these agents are powerful vasodilators and hypotension frequently limits their use or requires a norepinephrine infusion.

Levosimendan is an intracellular calcium sensitiser and thus bypasses the receptors through which other inotropic agents act. It binds to and sensitises cTnC to calcium without raising intracellular calcium, thus improving cardiac performance and contractility during systole without impairing ventricular relaxation during diastole. Administered as a continuous infusion

(0.1 μg/kg/min) over 24 hours, it has a long-lasting, pharmacologically active metabolite, which results in any improvement in myocardial contractility being sustained for several days.[59,60] Levosimendan also causes vasodilation of vascular smooth muscle due to its action on adenosine triphosphate (ATP)-sensitive potassium channels found in the myocardium, peripheral blood vessels and coronary arteries. Consequently, dose-dependent hypotension may occur although the reduction in preload and afterload and improved coronary blood flow will be beneficial to the failing heart. In the patient with severe heart failure already on inotropic drugs, treatment should start with a low-dose infusion (0.05 μg/kg/min) and no loading dose should be given. Levosimendan may be used concomitantly with beta blockers owing to its site of action, which does not involve beta-adrenergic receptors. Its role in severe acutely decompensated heart failure and cardiogenic shock following acute myocardial infarction appears promising; however, levosimendan remains unlicensed in several countries worldwide and the available evidence to date does not consistently confirm a significant mortality benefit.[61–63]

BETA BLOCKADE

Several studies have demonstrated a reduction in mortality and number of hospitalisations in patients with chronic heart failure treated with beta blockers.[64–66] Furthermore, large studies have demonstrated their benefit early after acute myocardial infarction.[67] Conversely, there is conflicting evidence regarding the perioperative role of beta blockers, and their use should be limited to high-risk patients in order to minimise adverse events.[68]

Although beta blockers are usually commenced in stable patients with heart failure, there is good evidence that they may be safely initiated in patients recovering from recent decompensation or in fact continued at a reduced dose during an episode of decompensation.[69,70]

If tachycardia develops or persists during an episode of acute decompensated heart failure, it may be appropriate to consider a trial of a beta blocker but it is advisable to start with a small dose of a short-acting drug such as metoprolol or a low-dose esmolol infusion. If this beta-blocker 'challenge' is successful then the beneficial effects will include an increased time for ventricular filling, improved coronary perfusion and reduced myocardial oxygen demand.

MECHANICAL SUPPORT FOR THE HEART

Continuous positive airway pressure (CPAP), non-invasive positive pressure ventilation (NIPPV) and invasive mechanical ventilation are commonly used to provide support for patients with acute cardiogenic pulmonary oedema. A recent systematic review concluded that non-invasive ventilation, in particular CPAP, reduced hospital mortality, endotracheal intubation and ICU length of stay.[71] However, a large randomised controlled trial did not show a mortality benefit with the use of non-invasive ventilation, although the study did show an improvement in symptoms and physiological and metabolic parameters.[72] The benefits result from improved oxygenation and reducing or eliminating the work of breathing, which may account for up to 30% of oxygen consumption.[73] This reduction in oxygen consumption reduces left ventricular workload and alleviates myocardial ischaemia. When instituting invasive mechanical ventilation the clinician must be prepared to give volume and even inotropic or vasopressor support as the sedation and other anaesthetic agents given for intubation will reduce endogenous levels of catecholamines, producing arteriolar and venular dilatation and potentially catastrophic hypotension.

Intra-aortic balloon pump (IABP) counterpulsation is physiologically attractive as it reduces afterload, improves coronary and peripheral circulatory perfusion and decreases cardiac work. This results in a more efficient cardiac performance with improvement in both cardiac output and myocardial oxygenation.[74] A common indication for IABP insertion is cardiogenic shock complicating acute myocardial infarction, however a recent randomised controlled trial has questioned the benefit of the IABP in this setting; the study demonstrated that there was no significant difference in 30-day mortality in the IABP and the no IABP groups.[75] Other indications for IABP support include weaning from cardiopulmonary bypass, high-risk percutaneous coronary intervention (although current evidence does not support the routine insertion of IABP in this setting)[76] and as a 'bridging therapy' to cardiac transplantation. The main absolute contraindications to IABP insertion are moderate-to-severe aortic regurgitation and aortic dissection and complications include limb ischaemia, bleeding and infection.

Extracorporeal membrane oxygenation (ECMO) is a technology that has developed from the cardiopulmonary bypass circuit and in a venoarterial (VA) configuration can provide short-term circulatory support in addition to respiratory support. VA ECMO has been used perioperatively in cardiac surgery, in refractory cardiogenic shock and during cardiopulmonary arrest.[77]

Ventricular assist devices (VADs) are mechanical systems that provide circulatory support for patients with both acute and chronic severe heart failure. Support can be provided for the left ventricle, the right ventricle or both. VADs can temporarily take over myocardial function and are usually indicated only if all other treatment options have been explored and improvement in myocardial function can be anticipated.[78] VADs are currently used as a 'bridge' to myocardial recovery in acute heart failure following cardiac surgery or recent myocardial infarction, or when there is a realistic prospect of cardiac transplantation. However, with recent advances in VAD technology a role appears to be emerging for these devices as a 'destination therapy', in patients with end-stage chronic heart failure who are not eligible for cardiac transplantation.[79] Complications associated with VADS can be significant and include device failure, bleeding, infection, thromboembolism and stroke.

CARDIOGENIC SHOCK AFTER ACUTE MYOCARDIAL INFARCTION

Cardiogenic shock occurs in 5–10% of patients following acute myocardial infarction and the mortality rate remains significantly high at 50–80% with medical treatment alone.[80] In patients admitted to intensive care with cardiogenic shock, the following additional points should be noted:

- The effects of management on myocardial oxygenation must be considered as well as global circulatory targets.
- Although the patient may be ventilated on ICU, therapies demonstrated to improve myocardial salvage must not be overlooked or delayed. Emphasis should be placed on early revascularisation therapy and patients should undergo urgent coronary angiography to allow angioplasty and stenting if appropriate. The benefits of aspirin are significant if given in the early hours after infarction; if necessary the aspirin can be given rectally. A beta blocker[67] and an ACE inhibitor[81] should be started as soon as clinically possible but bradycardia, heart block, hypotension and impairment of renal function may cause delay. Once stable, patients with left ventricular dysfunction and heart failure should also be started on an aldosterone receptor antagonist such as spironolactone[82] or eplerenone.[83,84]
- In patients admitted following an out-of-hospital cardiorespiratory arrest, therapeutic hypothermia (cooling to 32–34°C) has been shown to be beneficial,[85,86] but if planned this should not prevent other interventions such as primary angioplasty being performed if appropriate. It must also be realised that monitoring the patient is more complex in the hypothermic patient since paralysis is often necessary to prevent shivering, most of the techniques for CO measurement are invalidated and both bedside assessment of the circulation and interpretation of acid–base and lactate data are difficult.
- It is important to recognise:
  - right ventricular infarction (ST elevation in lead V_4R) since further monitoring may be necessary to ensure appropriate volume loading and to direct therapy to offload the right ventricle[87]
  - the development of either a ventricular septal defect or mitral regurgitation from papillary rupture as urgent surgery may be indicated.[88]

PULMONARY HYPERTENSION

Pulmonary hypertension (PH) is a frequently encountered pathophysiological disorder in ICU and is associated with high mortality.[89] **Box 24.5** summarises the most recent clinical classification of PH.[90] The classification splits PH into groups according to underlying cause and therefore likely to have similar treatment

Box 24.5 Clinical classification of pulmonary hypertension[90]

1. Pulmonary arterial hypertension (PAH)
   1.1 Idiopathic
   1.2 Familial
      1.2.1 BMPR2
      1.2.2 ALK1, endoglin (with or without hereditary haemorrhagic telangiectasia)
      1.2.3 Unknown
   1.3 Drug and toxin induced
   1.4 Associated with:
      1.4.1 Connective tissue diseases
      1.4.2 HIV infection
      1.4.3 Portal hypertension
      1.4.4 Congenital heart diseases
      1.4.5 Schistosomiasis
      1.4.6 Chronic haemolytic anemia
   1.5 Persistent pulmonary hypertension of the newborn
1. Pulmonary veno-occlusive disease and/or pulmonary capillary haemangiomatosis
2. Pulmonary hypertension due to left heart disease
   2.1 Systolic dysfunction
   2.2 Diastolic dysfunction
   2.3 Valvular disease
3. Pulmonary hypertension due to lung diseases and/or hypoxia
   3.1 Chronic obstructive pulmonary disease
   3.2 Interstitial lung disease
   3.3 Other pulmonary diseases with mixed restrictive and obstructive pattern
   3.4 Sleep-disordered breathing
   3.5 Alveolar hypoventilation disorders
   3.6 Chronic exposure to high altitude
   3.7 Developmental abnormalities
4. Chronic thromboembolic pulmonary hypertension
5. PH with unclear and/or multifactorial mechanisms
   5.1 Haematological disorders: myeloproliferative disorders, splenectomy
   5.2 Systemic disorders: sarcoidosis, pulmonary Langerhans cell histiocytosis, lymphangioleiomyomatosis, neurofibromatosis, vasculitis
   5.3 Metabolic disorders: glycogen storage disease, Gaucher disease, thyroid disorders
   5.4 Others: tumoural obstruction, fibrosing mediastinitis, chronic renal failure on dialysis

ALK-1 = activin receptor-like kinase 1 gene; PAH = pulmonary arterial hypertension; BMPR2 = bone morphogenetic protein receptor type 2; HIV = human immunodeficiency virus.

strategies. An important distinction to note is that group 1 PH or pulmonary arterial hypertension (PAH), previously known as primary pulmonary hypertension, includes a set of disorders where PH is the primary problem. In contrast, all other classification groups are due to conditions that lead to PH as result of cardiac dysfunction, abnormalities in the lung parenchyma, chest wall abnormalities, or mechanical obstruction of the pulmonary vasculature.

PH is defined as a mean pulmonary arterial pressure (mPAP) greater than 25 mmHg on right heart catheterisation whilst the patient is at rest.[91] In the critical care setting, common pathological conditions leading to PH include severe respiratory failure,[92] ARDS,[93] left-sided heart failure leading to increased left atrial pressures,[94] massive pulmonary embolism,[95] mechanical ventilation,[96] and following cardiac and thoracic surgery.[97] The presence of PH in many of these conditions is associated with increased mortality.[93–95,97] In addition several factors including sepsis, cardiac arrhythmias, and treatment failure can precipitate acute exacerbations of chronic PAH leading to ICU admissions. Sepsis in these patients is associated with poor outcome.[98]

Several disorders lead to PH in ICU yet there are no consensus or international guidelines that exist to assist with the management of these patients. Detailed reviews addressing PH[99–101] and PAH[101,102] in the critical care setting fail to make authoritative recommendations mainly as a result of paucity of data. Therefore management of PH relies on extrapolated data from animal studies, surgical patients, local expertise and biological plausibility of interventions.

PATHOPHYSIOLOGY

An understanding of the pathophysiological changes seen in patients with PH is essential to understand the available treatment strategies and the likelihood of their success. Invariably the most crucial manifestation of PH is right ventricular (RV) dysfunction. Under normal conditions RV outflow is to a high-compliance, low-pressure and low-resistance system. The thin-walled RV is highly sensitive to small increases in the pulmonary vascular resistance (PVR) leading to ventricular dilation, an increase in end-systolic volume, and reduced ejection fraction and pulmonary blood flow. This in turn results in a reduction in cardiac output (CO). In the initial stages the RV responds by enhancing contractility in order to maintain CO.[103] Further increases in RV afterload overwhelm these compensatory mechanisms resulting in reduced cardiac output and systemic circulatory failure. The intimate anatomical relationship of the two ventricles sharing a septum and both being bound by tight pericardial fibres leads to interdependence. In the setting of increased afterload the dilated RV loses its normal shape and pushes the septum towards the left ventricle thereby compromising LV filling and output.[104,105] RV dilatation can also lead to tricuspid regurgitation further lowering cardiac output. In addition to these anatomical considerations, fall in systemic blood pressure can compromise RV perfusion thereby leading to ischaemia and further RV dysfunction. Unlike the LV, under normal conditions coronary perfusion to the RV is maintained throughout the cardiac cycle. As RV pressure increases there is a decrease in the perfusion pressure gradient between the aorta and the RV during systole, thereby limiting coronary perfusion mainly to diastole.[106]

CLINICAL ASPECTS

Key to the management of patients with PH is diagnosis of underlying cause and, if feasible, treatment should focus on prompt reversal of the cause. Like most other disorders requiring critical care the maxim of good ICU care is applicable to these patients also. The discussion that follows looks at treatment strategies specific to PH and the associated RV dysfunction.

MONITORING

The gold standard for diagnosing and monitoring PH in the ICU remains the PA catheter. Invasiveness of the procedure and a lack of evidence supporting a benefit in the general ICU population have meant that the use of the PA catheter has declined in the critical care setting.[107,108] Furthermore, the use of PA catheters specifically in PH has not been studied. Echocardiography is increasingly being used in ICU and can provide clinicians with much of the information needed to manage such patients. It has the added benefit of being non-invasive and provides information on RV and LV structure and function, pericardial effusions and tricuspid incompetence.[100] A recent systematic review, however, found only modest correlation between pulmonary pressures determined by echocardiography and those measured by right heart catheterisation.[109] The virtues of echocardiography in PH in ICU populations have not been studied and ultimately local expertise is likely to dictate local practice.

MANAGEMENT

The need for adequate oxygenation applies to most critically ill patients but assumes greater importance in PH. RV myocardial oxygen demands are increased in severe PH and hypoxia may increase PVR by precipitating hypoxic pulmonary vasoconstriction. In many cases mechanical ventilation may be unavoidable; however, it comes at a cost. Positive-pressure ventilation has adverse effects on RV afterload and along with administration of sedatives can further compromise CO. Ventilatory strategies should focus on maintaining adequate oxygenation whilst avoiding high plateau pressures.

Fluid resuscitation of patients with PH is extremely challenging. The RV predominantly relies on adequate filling to maintain cardiac output. Conversely, RV dilation as a consequence of volume overload can lead to inefficiency of RV function and can also encroach into LV filling space. In patients with evidence of RV overload and septal bowing, aggressive fluid removal should be considered as it may improve cardiac output as a consequence of improved LV filling.

Maintenance of sinus rhythm in these patients will improve RV end-diastolic volume and cardiac output. Where possible cardioversion should be performed in patients with tachyarrhythmias. In those patients where this cannot be achieved the focus should be on rate control to optimise ventricular filling time.

Vasopressors and inotropes

The goal of using vasoactive drugs in patients with RV dysfunction secondary to PH is to maintain an adequate CO whilst avoiding increases in PVR and cardiac arrhythmias. In the face of systemic hypotension norepinephrine, a powerful systemic vasoconstrictor, should be considered in these patients. Improving systemic blood pressure has the additional benefit of improving coronary perfusion. However, norepinephrine also causes pulmonary vasoconstriction. In an animal model of acute PH, administration of norepinephrine restored systemic blood pressure and increased PAP.[110] Overall the effect was to improve both RV contractility and cardiac output. In the same study, animals treated with dobutamine showed a greater improvement in RV contractility in comparison with norepinephrine. The dobutamine treated animals also showed a greater reduction in mPAP. In clinical studies dobutamine has been shown to improve RV performance in ischaemic failure.[111] Evidence from these studies suggest that low-dose dobutamine may be useful in acute PH complicated by RV failure. Increases in myocardial oxygen demand and tachyarrhythmias may preclude dobutamine use in all patients with PH.

In another animal study the use of levosimendan and dobutamine in PH was compared. Improvement in RV contractility was similar after administration of both drugs; of the two agents levosimendan was superior at reducing PVR.[112] Small observational studies in humans have shown a similar trend of improved RV contractility and reduced PVR following administration of levosimendan in patients with cardiogenic shock.[113] In theory, levosimendan appears to be a promising alternative to dobutamine with the additional benefit of PVR reduction without increasing oxygen consumption.

Phosphodiesterase-3 (PDE-3) inhibitors such as milrinone and amrinone have inotropic and vasodilating properties. They can improve cardiac output by reducing PVR and increasing RV contractility. PDE-3 inhibitors have been shown to successfully reduce PVR and improve RV contractility in animal models of pulmonary hypertension[114,115] and in patients undergoing cardiac surgery.[116] Treatment with milrinone may require additional vasopressor support, given its propensity for systemic vasodilatation. Inhaled milrinone has shown promise as a therapy to selectively reduce PVR in heart transplant patients[117] and in an animal model of PH,[118] but its use is currently experimental.

Pulmonary vasodilators

Several pulmonary vasodilators are available and the choice of therapy and route of administration usually depend on the side-effects of the drug and the condition of the patient. Intravenous agents can lead to systemic haemodynamic instability and inhaled vasodilators may be more favourable in the ICU setting.[100]

Inhaled nitric oxide (INO) increases production of cyclic guanosine monophosphate (cGMP) and is a potent pulmonary vasodilator. It results in reversal of hypoxic pulmonary vasoconstriction, reduction in PVR and improved oxygenation. INO has been shown to reduce PVR and improve RV stroke work in postoperative cardiothoracic patients with PH.[119,120] Methaemoglobinaemia, NO_2 production and rebound pulmonary hypertension after abrupt cessation are adverse effects associated with INO use.

Inhaled and intravenous prostaglandins are also used as vasodilators in pulmonary hypertension. Inhaled prostacyclin use is associated with significant reduction in mPAP and improvement in ICU patients with PH.[121] There are, however, considerable associated side-effects in this population. Inhaled iloprost, a synthetic prostacyclin analogue, has been shown to reduce mPAP and improve RV function in PH post cardiopulmonary bypass. There was also a significant reduction in PVR to SVR ratio.[122] In a small single-centre study in post-heart-and-lung-transplant patients, inhaled prostacyclin showed similar efficacy to INO in managing PH.[123]

Phosphodiesterase-5 (PDE-5) inhibitors stop the degradation of cGMP leading to vasodilation. In patients with chronic PAH oral sildenafil, a selective PDE-5 inhibitor, has been shown to reduce mPAP[124] and improve cardiac output by reducing PVR.[125] Sildenafil has also been used as bridge to avoid rebound hypotension following INO withdrawal in post-cardiac-surgery patients.[126] Following haemodynamic stabilisation there may be a role for sildenafil in reducing PVR in the critical care setting.

Mechanical devices

In patients where all other treatment options have been exhausted, lung transplantation may be the only viable option. Case studies have reported the use of RV assist devices in patients with PH. Extracorporeal life support, in the form of veno-arterial extracorporeal membrane oxygenation or pumpless lung assist devices inserted into the pulmonary circulation, has also been described as a bridge to transplantation.[99]

SUMMARY

PH and consequent RV dysfunction are frequently encountered in the ICU with a high associated mortality rate. Prompt identification of the underlying cause and its treatment should be the main focus of management. There is very little evidence for the use of specific treatments in the ICU setting and a 'one-size fits all' approach is unlikely to work given the varied aetiology. A few general principles such as optimising fluid status, optimising heart rate and rhythm, avoiding high-pressure ventilation, maintaining coronary perfusion by optimising systemic pressure, inotropic support for RV dysfunction, and inhaled pulmonary vasodilation may be applied where appropriate. Choice of individual therapies should be guided by an understanding of their mechanism of action and the expected physiological response in an individual patient. The response should be monitored closely to avoid adverse events and to optimise therapy.

Access the complete references list online at http://www.expertconsult.com

3. Redfield MM. Heart failure – an epidemic of uncertain proportions. N Engl J Med 2002;347:1442–4.
9. ESC guidelines for the diagnosis and treatment of acute and chronic heart failure 2012: The Task Force for the Diagnosis and Treatment of Acute and Chronic Heart Failure 2012 of the European Society of Cardiology. Developed in collaboration with the Heart Failure Association (HFA) of the ESC. Eur J Heart Fail 2012;14(8):803–69.
13. Omland T. Advances in congestive heart failure management in the intensive care unit: B-type natriuretic peptides in evaluation of acute heart failure. Crit Care Med 2008;36(1 Suppl):S17–27.
22. Peacock WF 4th, De Marco T, Fonarow GC, et al. Cardiac troponin and outcome in acute heart failure. N Engl J Med 2008;358(20):2117–26.
33. Cournand A, Motley HL, Werko L, et al. Physiological studies of the effects of intermittent positive pressure breathing on cardiac output in man. Am J Physiol 1948;152–62.
42. Antonelli M, Levy M, Andrews PJD, et al. Haemodynamic monitoring in shock and implications for management. International Consensus Conference, Paris, France, April 2006. Intens Care Med 2007; 33:575–90.
45. Sharpey-Schafer EP. Effects of Valsalva's manoeuvre on the normal and failing circulation. Br Med J 1955;1:693–5.
56. De Backer D, Biston P, Devriendt J, et al. Comparison of dopamine and norepinephrine in the treatment of shock. N Engl J Med 2010;362(9):779–89.
61. Follath F, Cleland JG, Just H, et al. Efficacy and safety of intravenous levosimendan compared with dobutamine in severe low-output heart failure (the LIDO study): a randomised double-blind trial. Lancet 2002;360(9328):196–202.
72. Gray A, Goodacre S, Newby DE et al. Noninvasive ventilation in acute cardiogenic pulmonary edema. N Engl J Med 2008;359(2):142–51.
75. Thiele H, Zeymer U, Neumann FJ, et al. Intraaortic balloon support for myocardial infarction with cardiogenic shock. N Engl J Med 2012;367(14):1287–96.
80. Babaev A, Frederick PD, Pasta DJ, et al. Trends in management and outcomes of patients with acute myocardial infarction complicated by cardiogenic shock. JAMA 2005;294(4):448–54.
92. Zapol WM, Snider MT. Pulmonary hypertension in severe acute respiratory failure. N Engl J Med 1977; 296(9):476–80.
94. Guazzi M, Arena R. Pulmonary hypertension with left-sided heart disease. Nature Rev Cardiol 2010; 7(11): 648–59.
99. Hoeper MM, Granton J. Intensive care unit management of patients with severe pulmonary hypertension and right heart failure. Am J Respir Crit Care Med 2011;184(10):1114–24.
102. Delcroix M, Naeije R. Optimising the management of pulmonary arterial hypertension patients: emergency treatments. Eur Respir Rev 2010;19(117):204–11.
113. Russ MA, Prondzinsky R, Carter JM, et al. Right ventricular function in myocardial infarction complicated by cardiogenic shock: improvement with levosimendan. Crit Care Med 2009;37(12):3017–23.
124. Galie N, Ghofrani HA, Torbicki A, et al; Sildenafil Use in Pulmonary Arterial Hypertension (SUPER) Study Group. Sildenafil citrate therapy for pulmonary arterial hypertension. N Engl J Med 2005; 353(20):2148–57.

25 Valvular and congenital heart disease and bacterial endocarditis

Mary White and Susanna Price

Valvular heart disease (VHD) is less common than coronary artery disease, hypertension and heart failure; none the less it remains a significant health care issue worldwide.[1,2] In developing countries rheumatic heart disease (RhHD) predominates; however, over the preceding half century in industrialised nations the predominance of VHD has shifted from a rheumatic to degenerative aetiology.[3] These changes in the burden of VHD have been accompanied by significant developments in interventions, including transcatheter procedures for valve implantation and repair.[4] Additionally, advances in surgical and interventional cardiology techniques have resulted in increasing numbers of patients with congenital heart disease surviving to adulthood.[5] Thus valvular and congenital heart disease are increasingly likely to be present in the critical care patient population, and knowledge of the underlying pathophysiology, clinical presentation and management are important for the intensive care clinician.

GENERAL PRINCIPLES: VALVULAR HEART DISEASE

The prevalence of VHD is 2.5%, increasing significantly with age (<65 years <2%, 66–75 years 8.5%, >75 years 13.2%).[6] The commonest aetiologies are degenerative and rheumatic (RhHD), with others (endocarditis, inflammatory, congenital) accounting for fewer than 10% of cases. Whereas degenerative valve disease predominates in industrialised nations, the prevalence of RhHD remains significant, particularly in the elderly. In developing countries improved socioeconomic conditions together with antibiotic prophylaxis have contributed to the reduction in incidence of rheumatic fever; however, RhHD remains an important cause of mortality and morbidity in young adults, accounting for 350–500 000 deaths per annum in Asia alone.[6] VHD (left-sided) may be a primary cause of intensive care admission, or an incidental finding that may significantly alter management of the critically ill patient. Characteristics of left-sided valve disease are shown in **Table 25.1**.

Right-sided VHD is rarely a cause for critical care admission, and then generally due to associated pathology (i.e. sepsis in endocarditis) rather than the haemodynamic effects of the valve lesion.

Approximately 28% of patients with VHD have had previous valve replacement. Adequate and appropriate anticoagulation is paramount to the management of patients with previous mechanical valve replacement as subtherapeutic anticoagulation, even for 24 hours, may lead to thrombosis presenting as acute cardiovascular collapse. The differential diagnosis is pannus formation, although thrombosis is classically associated with a more acute, severe presentation, and the two may coexist. Current recommendations are for surgical intervention, with thrombolysis being reserved for patients in extremis in whom surgery is contraindicated. Additional considerations include avoidance of bacteraemia, and indwelling cannulae should be removed as soon as possible. When severe heart failure (HF) is diagnosed in any patient with a prosthetic valve, prosthesis malfunction must be presumed until proven otherwise.[7]

Evaluation of VHD includes obtaining a history to determine symptomatology and co-morbidities, and clinical examination to determine the presence/severity of the lesion(s) and associated features. Chest radiography (CXR) and electrocardiography may indicate pulmonary venous/arterial hypertension/congestion, cardiomegaly or conducting system disease/ventricular hypertrophy/associated arrhythmia. Echocardiography remains the key investigation to confirm the diagnosis and severity of VHD, together with the patient's prognosis. Although the features associated with significant VHD are well described in the outpatient population there are challenges when assessing critically ill patients (see Ch. 27). Other investigations are important in risk stratification and planning of patient intervention; however, they are not generally relevant to the ICU patient population.

Postoperative management of VHD is primarily determined by the degree of ventricular dysfunction (both right and left) and pulmonary hypertension (PHT). In long and complex surgery, RV myocardial protection is particularly challenging, and postoperative interventions are directed to managing the RV and pulmonary circulation (see Ch. 26). No assumptions should be made regarding postoperative ventricular function, and where haemodynamics are not optimal postoperatively then repeated expert echocardiography is mandated. Similarly, where there is potential for

Table 25.1 Characteristics of left-sided valve disease in the Euro Heart Survey[1]

VARIABLES	AORTIC STENOSIS (N=1197)	AORTIC REGURGITATION (N=369)	MITRAL STENOSIS (N=336)	MITRAL REGURGITATION (N=877)
DEMOGRAPHIC CHARACTERISTICS				
Mean age (years)	69±12	58±16	58±13	65±14
Age >70 years (%)	56	25	18	44
Male (%)	57	74	19	52
Aetiology				
Degenerative (%)	81.9	50.3	12.5	61.3
Rheumatic (%)	11.2	15.2	85.4	14.2
Endocarditis (%)	0.8	7.5	0.6	3.5
Inflammatory (%)	0.1	4.1	0	0.8
Congenital (%)	5.4	15.2	0.6	4.8
Ischaemic (%)	0	0	0	7.3
Other (%)	0.6	7.7	0.9	8.1

From Lung B, Baron G, Butchart EG, et al. A prospective survey of patients with valvular heart disease in Europe: the Euro Heart Survey on Valvular Heart Disease. Eur Heart J 2003;24:1231–1243.

coronary artery compromise (i.e. mitral valve/aortic root surgery) where haemodynamic instability occurs there should be a low threshold for imaging the coronary tree. Postoperative haemodynamic assessment should not rely solely upon CO monitoring, but must include repeated physiological echocardiographic studies to determine the effects (beneficial or detrimental) of any intervention. Where standard interventions fail, appropriate and timely referral for mechanical support is paramount (see Ch. 16).

AORTIC VALVE DISEASE: AORTIC STENOSIS (AS)

In AS, obstruction to LV ejection results in development of LV hypertrophy, and eventually dilatation and failure. Coronary artery disease coexists in 30–50% of elderly patients with AS, and may result in disproportionate LV dysfunction.[8] Calcific AS is a chronic, progressive disease with a long latent period during which patients remain asymptomatic. When asymptomatic the 2-year event-free survival rate is 20–50%.[9–12] Once symptoms supervene, 5-year survival falls to 15–50%. Typical symptoms include syncope, dyspnoea and exertional angina. Clinical examination may reveal a slow-rising small volume pulse, LV heave and soft A2. An ejection systolic murmur radiating to the carotids is characteristic, but may be absent in critical AS. Features of secondary PHT may also be present. ECG features are non-specific, but include LVH. CXR may show a normal cardiothoracic ratio, valvular calcification and/or post-stenotic dilatation of the ascending aorta. The diagnosis is confirmed with echocardiography (see Ch. 27).

Patients with severe AS may be admitted to the ICU with haemodynamic instability, or AS may be an incidental finding in a critically ill patient. AS requiring ICU admission is usually severe and may be previously undiagnosed due to the gradual onset of symptoms. Patients may present in a low CO state, this may be related to the onset of arrhythmia, myocardial infarction or a late/misdiagnosis.

MANAGEMENT

AS severe enough to be the primary cause for ICU admission is a mechanical problem, and unless there is a contraindication, the patient requires aortic valve replacement (AVR). If the patient is not a candidate for AVR the prognosis is extremely poor. Here, balloon aortic valvuloplasty (BAV) may be considered in order to improve haemodynamics and as a bridge to definitive intervention.[13] Recently transcatheter aortic valve implantation (TAVI) has been developed for patients in whom conventional surgery is judged too high risk; however, haemodynamic instability is currently considered a relative contraindication.[4]

Supporting the patient with critical AS on the ICU is challenging. Stroke volume/CO are limited, and the potential to develop myocardial ischaemia (due to mismatch of myocardial oxygen supply and demand from the hypertrophied LV) with consequent catastrophic haemodynamic deterioration is high. Positive inotropic agents will potentially exacerbate this mismatch and may provoke arrhythmias, and pressors may be required to maintain coronary perfusion pressure. Intra-aortic balloon counterpulsation (IABP) may improve coronary artery perfusion and reduce myocardial oxygen consumption, particularly in patients with coexistent coronary artery disease. Vasoactive agents should be used with caution and under close haemodynamic monitoring. Although vasodilators are generally relatively contraindicated in this patient population, they are potentially beneficial where the SVR is high. Atrial fibrillation (AF) is poorly tolerated; electrolyte imbalance should be aggressively corrected, and a low threshold maintained for institution of antiarrhythmic therapy.[14]

AORTIC REGURGITATION

Aortic regurgitation (AR) is generally well tolerated unless of acute onset in the presence of a hypertrophied LV, or very severe. The haemodynamic consequences are of LV volume overload, resulting in high filling pressures and pulmonary oedema, and a low CO state. As with AS, AR as a primary cause of ICU admission is likely to be severe.[15]

Symptoms of long-standing significant AR include fatigue and dyspnoea; however, acute severe AR may occur in patients with minimal prodrome. Clinical findings include tachycardia with a normal/low volume pulse in a patient with a low CO state, together with features of pulmonary oedema. An audible S3 should be expected. As with AS, the classical findings may be absent in catastrophically severe AR, as the pulse may not be collapsing and the early diastolic murmur may be absent owing to its short duration. Features relating to the underlying pathology (dissection/endocarditis) may also be apparent. CXR may show cardiomegaly and pulmonary oedema, and the electrocardiogram features of associated pathology (i.e. LVH in a patient with hypertension and aortic dissection). Unlike AS, severe AR may be well tolerated, and it is key to identify features that suggest that it is the haemodynamic burden of regurgitation that has precipitated the ICU admission. Here echocardiography is diagnostic (see Ch. 27).

Where surgical intervention is considered, the requirement for preoperative coronary angiography should be carefully evaluated, as the risk of vegetation embolisation during catheter manipulation may outweigh the potential benefits. Here coronary CT may be of use. Aortic root abscess should be presumed to be present in patients with aortic endocarditis until proven otherwise. Daily 12-lead ECG and continuous monitoring is required. PR interval, prolongation, increasing QRS duration and/or a change in axis suggest the diagnosis. These patients are at risk of rapid progression to high-grade AV block and temporary pacing may be required pending surgery.[7]

MANAGEMENT

Haemodynamic consequences of severe acute AR relate to low CO state, high LV filling pressures and low coronary perfusion pressure (perfusion of the left coronary system is diastolic), with more severe AR being associated with a worse outcome. Where premature MV closure is identified on echocardiography, performance of emergency surgery reduces mortality from 80% to 20%.[16] Attempts to increase coronary perfusion pressure using pressor agents may simply increase LV afterload, resulting in worsening of regurgitation, and IABP is contraindicated. Vasodilation in an attempt to reduce afterload is generally precluded by the low diastolic pressures. Bradycardia will increase the regurgitant volume (by increasing diastolic duration). Conversely patients may respond to manoeuvres that increase heart rate; however, positively chronotropic agents are often vasodilators and this may limit their utility.[7]

The definitive treatment for AR severe enough to precipitate ICU admission is AVR. In patients with known/suspected endocarditis, sudden deterioration requiring ICU admission should prompt investigations to exclude fistula formation, complete heart block or myocardial infarction secondary to coronary embolism. With aortic root abscess, urgent surgical referral is essential.[17]

Moderate AR is generally well tolerated. Clinical features are usually characteristic and the main concern in ICU is to avoid development of endocarditis. Haemodynamic management should include avoidance of bradycardia and a reduction in afterload whilst maintaining diastolic blood pressure to ensure adequate coronary perfusion pressure.

AORTIC VALVE REPLACEMENT (AVR)

The haemodynamic postoperative management in patients immediately post-AVR generally relates to the underlying ventricular disease rather than the valve itself. Patients at risk of haemodynamic instability in the immediate postoperative ICU course include those with significant LV systolic dysfunction and/or hypertrophy, RV dysfunction and/or PHT. Where haemodynamic instability occurs, it is vital to diagnose the underlying cause and monitor the effects of any interventions, as some may paradoxically worsen the clinical status of the patient (**Table 25.2**).

Anticoagulation and/or antiplatelet agents should be prescribed on an individual patient basis. In all patients post-AVR, the potential for bradyarrhythmias should prompt daily interrogation of their temporary pacing system, together with determination of their underlying rhythm. Appropriate referral for consideration for additional pacing (no underlying rhythm) and/or permanent pacing should be according to local/national guidelines.[18]

Table 25.2 Aortic valve replacement – interventions

	POTENTIAL INTERVENTIONS	NOTES
LV systolic dysfunction	• Positive inotrope(s) • Consider early mechanical circulatory support if indicated	• May be underdiagnosed if over-reliance on EF/FS; long-axis function should be assessed • May be revealed postoperatively due to challenges in myocardial preservation (esp. with coexisting CAD) • Standard referral practice varies internationally but indications exist (INTERMACS)
LV hypertrophy	• Avoidance of positive inotrope(s) • Maintenance of AV synchrony • Low threshold for antiarrhythmic agents	• May increase myocardial *VQ* mismatch • May cause LVOTO and paradoxical fall in CO • Tolerate AF poorly
RV dysfunction	• Standard for RV failure, including positive inotropic agents, RV-protective ventilation, aggressive treatment of causes of increased RV afterload	• May limit CO by causing LVOTO in presence of significant LVH • May be significant, especially in the presence of PHT
Pulmonary hypertension	• Standard for PHT on the ICU: pulmonary vasodilators, avoidance of pulmonary vasoconstrictors	• Systemic application of pulmonary vasodilators may cause significant haemodynamic instability • Pulmonary vasoconstrictors may be unavoidable in presence of significant LVH
Valve malfunction	• Surgical discussion	• Suspect if hyperdynamic ventricle in presence of low-CO state • Care in interpreting echo gradients immediately postoperatively (see Ch.27)
Tamponade	• Surgical discussion with a view to re-exploration	• TTE potentially misleading, TEE indicated (see Ch.27) • Low threshold for surgical re-exploration

EF/FS=ejection fraction/fractional shortening; LVOTO=left ventricular outflow tract obstruction; INTERMACS=Interagency Registry for Mechanically Assisted Circulatory Support.

MITRAL VALVE DISEASE: MITRAL REGURGITATION (MR)

MR results in volume overload of the LV, leading eventually to dilatation and failure, together with PHT and subsequently RV failure. MR is classified as either primary (intrinsic lesion affecting components of the valve apparatus) or secondary/functional (leaflets are structurally normal; MR results from distortion of the subvalvular apparatus, secondary to LV enlargement and remodelling).[7] When MR is the primary indication for ICU admission it is likely to be severe.[19] As sedation and ventilation reduce the severity of MR, it should also be considered as a possible differential in patients who fail to wean from mechanical ventilation.

Acute MR secondary to papillary rupture, infective endocarditis or trauma should be considered in patients presenting with acute pulmonary oedema and/or cardiogenic shock, together with the relevant clinical history. In acute, severe MR the presentation is of a low CO state, with classical clinical features often absent as the murmur may be soft/inaudible. Chronic MR is more common – examination revealing tachycardia, a displaced LV apex, the presence of S3 and a pan-systolic murmur. Echocardiographic features confirm the diagnosis, underlying cause and severity of regurgitation (see Ch. 27).

MANAGEMENT

In the absence of intervention to address the underlying valve lesion, acute MR is poorly tolerated and associated with a dismal prognosis. The estimated all-cause 5-year mortality in severe chronic MR is 22±3%. Predictors of poor outcome include age, AF, MR severity, PHT, LA dilatation, increased LV end-systolic dimensions and a low LV ejection fraction. Management options for severe MR are surgical (repair/replacement) or, where surgery is contraindicated, medical management (or possibly percutaneous mitral repair).[19,20]

There is no randomised controlled trial comparing MV repair and replacement; however, repair has a lower perioperative mortality, improved survival, better preservation of postoperative LV function and lower long-term mortality. Predictors of postoperative outcome are age, AF, preoperative LV function, PHT and reparability of the valve.[21] The timing of surgery in acute severe primary MR remains controversial.

Although papillary muscle rupture requires urgent surgical intervention, typically valve replacement, patients with chordal rupture may be stabilised for 24–48 hours allowing the LV to adapt to the increased volume load.[19] Supportive therapy includes IPPV, IABP, inotropes and vasodilators and renal replacement therapy as indicated.[22] Surgery is indicated in patients with symptomatic severe primary MR (LVEF>30% and LVESD<55 mm, left ventricular end-systolic diameter), and should be considered in those with severe LV dysfunction refractory to medical therapy, with high likelihood of durable repair and low co-morbidity.[7]

Operative mortality in secondary MR is higher than primary, and is associated with a worse long-term prognosis. Severe ischaemic MR is not usually improved by revascularisation alone, and residual regurgitation postoperatively is associated with increased mortality.[23,24] Indications for surgical intervention in severe secondary MR include those with an LVEF>30% undergoing CABG. Surgery should be considered in those who remain symptomatic despite optimal medical therapy (including CRT), and in those where the LVEF<30% with an option for revascularisation and evidence of myocardial viability.[7] In patients with no surgical option and severe secondary MR despite optimal medical therapy, percutaneous intervention may be considered (currently endovascular edge-to-edge repair) in appropriate centres.[7]

In all patients, optimisation of medical therapy is essential, and where HF is present should be in accordance with published guidelines. These include ACE inhibitors, beta blockers, aldosterone antagonists and, where indicated, resynchronisation therapy.[22]

MITRAL STENOSIS

In mitral stenosis (MS) obstruction to LV inflow results in gradual elevation of left atrial pressure, progressive pulmonary venous and arterial hypertension, and subsequent RV failure. The commonest cause worldwide is RhHD; however, rarer causes include systemic lupus erythematosus, left atrial myxoma and severe annular calcification. Rheumatic MS is a chronic progressive disease with a long latent period, and is well tolerated until it becomes severe. ICU admission is usually precipitated by the onset of AF, or any condition that results in an increase in circulating volume (i.e. pregnancy).[25]

Symptoms of MS include exertional dyspnoea, recurrent bronchitis, fatigue and haemoptysis. Clinical features include mitral facies, a small volume pulse (often AF), a parasternal heave, tapping apex, loud S1 with a rumbling mid-diastolic murmur, and palpable (and loud) P2. In a patient in extremis, the mid-diastolic murmur may be absent owing to the low CO state. In the critical care population MS may mimic ARDS (bilateral pulmonary infiltrates and poor gas exchange). The ECG may demonstrate P mitrale, and CXR an enlarged left atrium; however, echocardiography is pivotal to make the diagnosis, grade the severity of stenosis and that of associated PHT and RV dysfunction, together with assessment of other valves that are commonly also involved in the disease process (see Ch. 27).

MANAGEMENT

As with all valvular lesions, where the primary indication for admission to ICU, MS is likely to be severe, and intervention (surgical or transcatheter) should be performed only in those with clinically significant MS (valve area <1.5 cm^2).[26] Percutaneous mitral commissurotomy (PMC) is the procedure of choice when surgery is contraindicated, or as a bridge to surgery in high-risk, critically ill patients. Outcome predictors include age, functional class, PHT and coronary artery disease (CAD). PMC achieves good results in >80% of patients, with a periprocedural mortality of 0.5–4%, haemopericardium 0.5–10%, embolism 0.5–5% and severe MV regurgitation in 2–10%.[27] Surgical options are MV replacement/repair, with an operative mortality of 3–10%. In pregnant patients with MV area <1.5 cm^2, symptomatic MS should be treated with beta blockers and diuretics; however, in cases of persistent dyspnoea or pulmonary artery hypertension despite medical therapy, PMC can be considered after the 20th week in an experienced centre, with anticoagulant therapy in high-risk patients.[28]

All patients with severe MS are at high risk of thrombus formation and those in AF should be anticoagulated with a target INR of 2.5–3. In patients with sinus rhythm, anticoagulation is indicated where there has been prior embolism or a thrombus is present in the LA.[7,29] In patients with less severe MS, symptomatic relief of dyspnoea can be achieved with diuretics and/or long-acting nitrates. Beta blockers or heart-rate-regulating calcium channel blockers can improve exercise tolerance.

MITRAL VALVE REPLACEMENT

Postoperative management of MV surgery is usually uncomplicated; however, there are a number of scenarios that, when present, can be challenging to manage in the postoperative phase (**Box 25.1**).[30]

Box 25.1 Postoperative complications in mitral valve replacement

Valve-related complications	General complications
MV repair	Generalised LV dysfunction
LVOT obstruction (SAM, systolic anterior motion)	Circumflex coronary artery disruption
Acute failure	PHT
MV replacement	RV dysfunction
Para-prosthetic regurgitation	Tamponade
Prosthetic block	

The main challenge post-MV surgery relates to the degree of PHT (which may be fixed) and associated RV dysfunction (exacerbated by cardiopulmonary bypass). Management of the right-sided circulation is discussed in Chapter 26.

ADULT CONGENITAL HEART DISEASE

Adult congenital heart disease (ACHD) is common (8 per 1000 live births).[31] Currently, approximately 90% of children born with heart defects survive to adulthood, and adult patients in the US now outnumber their pediatric counterparts.[32] ACHD is generally classified according to its complexity. In the critically ill population, increasing complexity is associated with higher ICU morbidity and mortality.[33] When considering a patient in the more acute scenarios, ACHD is classified according to the underlying pathophysiology. In all patients, expert input should be sought regarding investigation and management as soon as possible after hospital/ICU admission.

CONGENITAL SHUNT LESIONS

The physiological changes associated with shunts are determined primarily by the size of the defect and alterations in systemic and pulmonary vascular resistance (SVR/ PVR, **Box 25.2**).

ATRIAL SEPTAL DEFECTS

Formation of the atrial septum occurs from the growth and partial reabsorption of two tissue membranes; the septum primum and secundum. The foramen ovale is the opening between the upper and lower limbs of the septum secundum, allowing shunting of blood from the right to left atrium in utero. Immediately postpartum there is functional closure of the foramen ovale, facilitated by a decrease in RA and increase in LA pressure. Subsequently these anatomically fuse to complete the formation of the interatrial septum. In 20–25% of people, there is incomplete fusion resulting in a patent foramen ovale.[31] Although the magnitude of shunt is not usually significant, this may result in paradoxical embolisation and, in the critically ill ventilated patient, right–left shunting may be the cause of disproportionate hypoxaemia.

Other abnormalities of atrial septation result in a range of defects, the commonest being secundum ASD, which is more frequently seen in females and occurs in 20% patients with trisomy 21. Other variants include involvement of the superior vena cava (superior sinus venosus defect), inferior vena cava (inferior sinus venosus defect) and/or abnormal pulmonary venous drainage. Primum ASDs may be associated with abnormalities of the atrio-ventricular valves and ventricular septal defects (AVSD). Flow across the defect occurs in both systole and diastole, with a predominant left–right shunt in adults. Patients with a significant ASD exhibit signs and symptoms of biatrial volume and RV overload; however, the direction and magnitude of the shunt are variable and age-dependent. In all patients, there may be PHT of a severity independent of the volume of shunt.

Box 25.2 Shunts

Left–right shunt	Right–left shunt
Atrial septal defect	*Tetralogy of Fallot
Ventricular septal defect	*Transposition of great vessels
Truncus arteriosus	*Double-outlet RV
*Total anomalous pulmonary venous connection	*Single ventricle
ALCAPA	

*Requires interatrial and/or interventricular connections for the patient to survive ex utero.

ALCAPA=anomalous left coronary artery from pulmonary artery.

VENTRICULAR SEPTAL DEFECTS

Ventricular septal defect (VSD) is the most common form of congenital heart defect in children (20% of CHD), resulting from abnormal ventricular septation. The type of VSD is defined by the anatomical position (perimembranous, muscular, inlet or outlet), the size of shunt and whether there is resistance to flow between the two chambers (restrictive).[34]

In patients with a VSD, blood flow has two possible pathways: through the usual outflow tract of that ventricle or across the defect to the outflow tract of the other ventricle. Thus, the direction and volume of flow across a VSD is dependent on:

- *relative resistance of each pathway*
- *size of VSD:* the smaller the defect, the higher is the resistance, limiting the interventricular shunt. Conversely in a large, non-restrictive VSD with normal PVR, the sum of resistors from LV to pulmonary artery is very low compared with resistance to flow across the defect, resulting in significant left–right systolic flow across the VSD
- *elevation of PVR in the presence of a large VSD:* the sum of the resistors may approximate the aortic resistance and net shunting will be minimal
- *pulmonary resistance higher than systemic resistance:* the shunt will be right–left regardless of the size of the VSD.

A left–right shunt at ventricular level reduces the LV (and hence cardiac) output by the amount of the shunt. Compensatory mechanisms act to increase intravascular volume until LV end-diastolic volume is sufficient to achieve both a normal CO and the proportionate left–right shunt resulting in a significant LV volume overload. High LV volume elevates LA filling pressures and may cause pulmonary congestion at rest and/or during exertion. Although the volume of diastolic flow across a VSD is generally minimal, it is an indicator of significant LV disease.

A secondary effect of a larger VSD is the transmission of LV pressure to the pulmonary vascular bed, with the ventricles becoming functionally a common chamber. In the absence of RV obstruction, the pressure in the pulmonary artery equals that in the aorta. The combination of volume and pressure overload contributes to the development of pulmonary vascular disease with reverse shunting (Eisenmenger syndrome).[35]

PATENT DUCTUS ARTERIOSUS

The ductus arteriosus (DA) is an arterial structure connecting the aorta and main pulmonary artery. In utero it allows blood flow from the PA to bypass the non-functioning lungs to return to the placenta via the descending aorta. Usually it closes within 72 hours of birth. If the DA is not completely obliterated, an arterial connection remains between the systemic and pulmonary circulations - patent ductus arteriosus (PDA).

Shunt direction and volume depend on the relative resistance to flow in each direction. In most patients, as systemic resistance is higher than pulmonary, the result is left-to-right flow. The size of the PDA is the principal determinant of the volume of flow. With large PDAs the LV end-diastolic volume must increase to allow the stroke volume to supply both the normal CO and the left-to-right shunt. LA pressures rise and pulmonary venous congestion may limit exertion. There is flow in both diastole and systole and this diastolic flow may result in impaired coronary and splanchnic perfusion.[36]

CONGENITAL OBSTRUCTIVE LESIONS

Under normal conditions the ventricular outflow tracts, semilunar valves and great vessels present no/minimal obstruction to flow. Narrowing of any of these pathways reduces distal flow, and the increase in afterload may result in ventricular hypertrophy, reduced compliance, and higher filling pressures. Symptoms are related to the severity of the obstruction and the side of the heart involved.[37]

INCREASED RV AFTERLOAD

The RV response to increased afterload is to develop hypertrophy and increase systolic pressure. In CHD stenotic lesions are generally well tolerated until they become severe.

Subvalvular pulmonary obstruction in adults is most frequently a residuum of earlier surgical intervention (i.e. for tetralogy of Fallot), but can be found in adult patients with CHD. Severe subvalvular obstruction may rarely present de novo in adults with a double-chambered RV. However, the diagnosis presents most frequently in childhood as a complex that includes the subvalvular muscular obstruction and a perimembranous VSD.

Valvular pulmonary stenosis (PS) is present in 8–10% of patients with CHD. In mild PS (<30 mmHg (4 kPa)), the natural history in patients who have not undergone surgery is indistinguishable from controls. Moderate gradients, whilst well tolerated in children, become more important in adults, possibly owing to progressively decreasing ventricular compliance. More severe obstructive gradients increase RV afterload, resulting in chamber hypertrophy. Clinical presentation of symptomatic patients includes exercise intolerance and arrhythmia.

Supravalvular PS can occur as an isolated abnormality, associated with complex cardiac malformations (i.e. tetralogy of Fallot), fetal teratogenic exposure (i.e. rubella/toxoplasmosis), genetic syndromes (i.e. Noonan's/William's syndromes), or as a result of scarring from previous surgery, including PA banding or arterial switch for transposition of the great arteries. The haemodynamic burden is identical to that of valvular PS.[38]

INCREASED LV AFTERLOAD

Minor degrees of left-sided obstruction are well tolerated; however, when severe, symptoms supervene. There is a tendency for young patients with CHD to under-report symptoms, and a careful history together with objective assessment is important.

Subvalvular AS comprises a spectrum of pathologies affecting the LV outflow tract ranging from a discrete subaortic membrane to hypertrophic cardiomyopathy. Regardless of the presenting anatomical features, each of these lesions tends to be progressive during childhood. The principal effect is increased ventricular afterload, with potential hypertrophy, arrhythmia, reduced chamber compliance and pulmonary venous congestion.

Coarctation is a congenital narrowing of the aorta, accounting for 5–8% of CHD. The obstruction classically occurs just distal to the origin of the left subclavian artery (site of the previous DA). This fixed obstruction, together with maintenance of flow, results in significant proximal hypertension. Over time, alternate pathways develop between the ascending and descending aorta (collaterals), resulting in the classical CXR finding of rib notching. Significant collaterals may mask the severity of obstruction. Coarctation is associated with a bicuspid valve in 50–85% of patients.[39]

ICU MANAGEMENT OF PATIENTS WITH ACHD

Although the principles of resuscitation in this patient population generally differ little from those with acquired heart disease, management of the acutely unwell ACHD patient is challenging, presenting potential pitfalls in examination, assessment and intervention. Expert advice should be sought at the earliest opportunity. The most common acute presentations are arrhythmia, HF and endocarditis. The main principles guiding ICU management of these patients are to understand:

- the cardiopulmonary anatomy – including any previous interventions: knowledge of the primary lesion, subsequent surgery/interventions and presence of residual haemodynamic lesions (dynamic/fixed)
- the normal physiology - including haemoglobin/haematocrit, oxygen saturation, systemic and pulmonary blood pressure and 12-lead ECG
- how supportive and therapeutic interventions might affect the circulation (beneficial and/or detrimental)
- the specific reason for deterioration/admission.

Common pathologies associated with ACHD that may impact on ICU care are outlined in **Table 25.3**.

In addition, many tenets of critical care management may be particularly harmful in this patient population and should be applied carefully, including volume loading, sedation, positive-pressure ventilation, normal parameters for transfusion and oxygen supplementation. Although the ICU management of such patients is highly specialised, certain presentations merit particular consideration, as they occur relatively frequently in

Table 25.3 Pathologies associated with ACHD

CARDIOVASCULAR	PULMONARY	GASTROINTESTINAL/RENAL/ENDOCRINE
ABSENT OR ABNORMAL CONNECTIONS	INTUBATION	ASSOCIATED ANATOMICAL DEFECTS
• Expected (Fontan/TCPC total cavopulmonary connection) • Unexpected (LSVC left superior caval vein)	• Craniofacial abnormalities in associated syndromes may complicate	• Associated asplenia • GI or renal malformation
MULTIPLE PREVIOUS CANNULATION	ASSOCIATED CONGENITAL PULMONARY DISEASE	CYANOTIC CONGENITAL HEART DISEASE
• Challenging vascular access	• Hypoplastic lung • Severe congenital V/Q mismatch	• Associated renal impairment common
POTENTIAL/ACTUAL RIGHT–LEFT SHUNTING	LUNG REPERFUSION INJURY POSTOPERATIVELY	ENTERAL FEEDING
• Air filters required on lines	• ARDS/ALI-like picture • Unilateral/bilateral	• Severe RHF may necessitate low feeding rates
CO MEASUREMENT	PULMONARY HYPERTENSION	TOLERANCE TO FLUID LOADING/ RESTRICTION
• Intracardiac shunt may complicate • No PA/R-sided connection • Small aorta may invalidate OD	• May not need treating per se • In presence of an inadequate CO, iNO, PC and sildenafil	• Univentricular circulations require relatively full circulation • Acute RH dilatation may occur (i.e. Ebstein's anomaly)
TRANSVENOUS PACING	TRACHEOSTOMY	LIVER FUNCTION
• No access to RV (i.e. Fontan/TCPC) • ECG interpretation • Atrial re-entry may mimic sinus tachycardia	• Presence of collateral blood vessels, abnormal neck anatomy • Previous cardiac surgery • Phrenic nerve palsy	• Abnormal LFTs common postoperatively and associated with increased mortality • Thyroid function • Commonly abnormal in ACHD
DIFFERENTIAL EFFECTS OF VASOACTIVE DRUGS ON SYSTEMIC/ PULMONARY VASCULATURE	DIFFICULTY WITH VENTILATORY WEANING	HAEMOGLOBIN
• Unpredictable • May affect CO and saturations	• Associated congenital musculoskeletal deformities not uncommon	• Cyanotic ACHD associated with erythrocytosis may necessitate more liberal transfusion policy

Adapted from Griffiths M, Cordingley J, Price S, editors. 2010. Cardiovascular Critical Care. Wiley Blackwell BMJ Books. ISBN-13: 978-1405148573, with permission.

the emergency setting. ICU mortality in ACHD medical admissions is high (36% in non-arrhythmia cases). As with the non-ACHD population, where no potentially reversible cause for deterioration exists and there is no prospect of intervention, the appropriateness of ICU admission should be considered.[40]

ARRHYTHMIA

The diagnosis of arrhythmia can be challenging, in particular in patients with massive atrial enlargement. Here, atrial tachycardia may mimic sinus tachycardia, and interrogation of an implanted pacemaker or careful comparison with previous ECGs may be required to make the diagnosis. Cardioversion to a malignant rhythm is not uncommon and, as in some patients there may be no transvenous access to the heart, transcutaneous pacing should be immediately available. Amiodarone is frequently prescribed in ACHD, and thyroid function tests should be performed on the diagnosis of a tachycardia or bradycardia, or hospital admission with decompensation of a previously stable patient.[38]

HEART FAILURE

Causes of HF in the ACHD population include impaired LV and RV function (which may be subpulmonary or systemic), volume overload, arrhythmia, excessive shunt and stenotic lesions. Although the principles of management appear similar to those with acquired heart disease, management of the systemic RV and that of the univentricular heart are particularly challenging, and do differ significantly, thus expert advice should be sought.[38]

HAEMOPTYSIS

Haemoptysis in patients with PHT should always be considered a serious event and early transfer to high-level care should be considered, particularly as the most frequent cause of death is related to inability to protect the airway, rather than blood loss per se. Haemopytsis may be attributed to bronchitis, bleeding diathesis, pulmonary artery rupture, pulmonary embolism, tracheaoesophageal fistula or rupture of aorto-pulmonary collaterals. In Eisenmenger physiology, haemoptysis accounts for up to 15% of deaths. Investigations include: CXR, bronchoscopy, CT angiography and embolisation, which may be life saving.[38]

CYANOTIC ACHD

As these patients have a relatively good prognosis the diagnosis is not a contraindication per se to ICU admission. The physiology reflects the body's response to prolonged cyanosis, and includes a rightward shift in the oxyhaemoglobin dissociation curve, increase in CO and increased haemocrit (erythrocytosis). Routine venesection is not recommended as iron deficiency is common, although it may be considered where there are symptoms/signs of hyperviscosity. Appropriate volume replacement is important to avoid haemodynamic collapse. Clotting abnormalities have been documented, including abnormal PT/PTT and deficiency in factors V, VII, VIIII and IX. When measuring the INR, citrate bottles adjusted for the haemocrit must be used. Thrombocytopenia occurs, but only rarely requires treatment. Renal dysfunction is common and may manifest as proteinuria, hyperuricaemia or renal impairment. Thus, contrast should be used only in patients who are well-hydrated, and the contrast load minimised. Any abnormal neurology, and/or persistent headache in cyanotic ACHD patients, should prompt a high index of suspicion for cerebral abscess/haemorrhage.[38]

INFECTIVE ENDOCARDITIS

If untreated, infective endocarditis (IE) is potentially lethal,[41] accounting for up to 1% of all severe hospital sepsis and carrying a hospital mortality of 33%. Despite advances in diagnostics and medical therapy, the incidence has remained relatively static, possibly owing to increased degenerative valvular disease, intravenous drug abuse, numbers of patients with intravascular devices, exposure to nosocomial disease and an increasing number of patients receiving haemodialysis therapy. Previous invasive procedures are considered more common as a cause than dental procedures and consequently the recommendations for antibiotic prophylaxis have changed. Currently *Staphylococcus aureus* is the commonest causative organism.[41]

CLINICAL PRESENTATION

General malaise, weight loss, night sweats and low-grade fever are reported as common symptoms; however, the clinical presentation is often very non-specific. Clinical signs include splinter haemorrhages in nail beds and conjunctiva, clubbing, splenomegaly, anaemia and signs of embolisation, together with features of valvular dysfunction. Regurgitant murmurs are often present and when in combination with symptoms and signs associated HF are a poor prognostic sign. Additional predictors of poor outcome include: age, prosthetic endocarditis, diabetes mellitus, significant co-morbidity, renal failure, stroke, septic shock, periannular complications, and *S. aureus*/fungal/Gram-negative bacilli as the causative organism. Blood cultures remain the cornerstone of diagnosis, confirmed by expert echocardiography,[42] including transoesophageal echocardiogram (TOE) where indicated (see Ch. 27). Although the Duke criteria are useful for classification, they do not replace clinical judgement.[43] In patients who abuse intravenous drugs, endocarditis with pulmonary embolisation is frequently misdiagnosed as pneumonia. Similarly, in those with prosthetic endocarditis (PVE) associated with significant left-sided paraprosthetic regurgitation, the resultant infected pulmonary oedema may also be misdiagnosed as pneumonia. Culture-negative endocarditis (clinical, echocardiographic and ECG findings suggestive, but no organisms cultured) should raise the suspicion of previous antimicrobial therapy or fastidious organisms/Q fever as the cause.[43]

MANAGEMENT

Controversy remains regarding timing of antimicrobial therapy, with some suggesting that the results of positive cultures should be awaited prior to initiation of treatment. The commonest community-acquired organism in native valve endocarditis (NVE) is *S. aureus*. Antimicrobial treatment should be according to the ESC/EACTS guidelines, modified according to local knowledge where appropriate.[43]

Surgery is undertaken in approximately half of patients with IE and is indicated in patients with high-risk features that make the possibility of cure with antibiotic treatment unlikely, and who do not have co-morbid conditions or complications that make the prospect of recovery remote. Age per se is not a contraindication. The three main indications for early surgery in endocarditis are HF (commonest and most severe complication), uncontrolled infection (most commonly associated with perivalvular extension/difficult-to-treat organisms), and prevention of embolisation (highest in the first 2 weeks). Unless surgery is contraindicated the presence of any one or more of these features demands early surgical intervention in patients with NVE. Complicated PVE, staphylococcal PVE and PVE occurring early postoperatively are associated with worse prognosis if managed without surgery, and must be managed aggressively.

Access the complete references list online at http://www.expertconsult.com

4. Moat NE, Ludman P, de Belder MA, et al. Long-term outcome after transcatheter aortic valve implantation in high-risk patients with severe aortic stenosis: the U.K. TAVI (United Kingdom Transcatheter Aortic Valve Implantation) Registry. J Am Coll Cardiol 2011;58(20):2130–8.
6. Lung B, Vahanian A. Epidemiology of valvular heart disease in the adult. Nat Rev Cardiology 2011;8: 162–72.
7. The Joint Task Force on the Management of Valvular Heart Disease of the European Society of Cardiology (ESC) and the European Association for Cardiothoracic Surgery (EACTS). Guidelines on the management of valvular heart disease (version 2012). Eur J Cardiothoracic Surg 2012;42(4):S1–S44.
15. Vahanian A, Lung B, Pierard L, et al. Valvular heart disease. The ESC Textbook of Cardiovascular Medicine. 2nd ed. Malden/Oxford/Victoria: Blackwell Publishing; 2009. p. 625–70.
17. Levy F, Laurent M, Monin JL, et al. Aortic valve replacement for low-flow/low-gradient aortic stenosis operative risk stratification and long-term outcome: a European multicentre study. J Am Coll Cardiol 2008;51:1466–72.
18. The Task Force for Cardiac Pacing and Cardiac Resynchronization Therapy of the European Society of Cardiology. Developed in Collaboration with the European Heart Rhythm Association. Guidelines for cardiac pacing and cardiac resynchronization therapy. Eur Heart Journal 2007;28:2256–95.
22. The Task Force for the Diagnosis and Treatment of Acute and Chronic Heart Failure 2012 of the European Society of Cardiology. Developed in collaboration with the Heart Failure Association (HFA) of the ESC. Guidelines for the diagnosis and treatment of acute and chronic heart failure 2012. Eur Heart J 2012;33:1787–847.
24. The Society of Thoracic Surgeons. Adult cardiac surgery database, executive summary, 10 years STS report. Online. Available: http://www.sts.org/sites/default/files/documents/pdf/ndb2010/1stHarvestExecutiveSummary%5B1%5D.pdf
27. Cruz-Gonzalez I, Sanchez-Ledesma M, Sanchez PL, et al. Predicting success and long-term outcomes of percutaneous mitral valvuloplasty: a multifactorial score. Am J Med 2009;122:581.e11–e19.
33. The Task Force on the Management of Grown-up Congenital Heart Disease of the European Society of Cardiology (ESC) Endorsed by the Association for European Paediatric Cardiology (AEPC). ESC Guidelines for the management of grown-up congenital heart disease (new version 2010). European Heart Journal 2010;31:2915–57.
43. The Task Force on the Prevention, Diagnosis, and Treatment of Infective Endocarditis of the European Society of Cardiology (ESC). Guidelines on the prevention, diagnosis, and treatment of infective endocarditis. Eur Heart Journal 2009;30:2369–413.

26

Intensive care after cardiac surgery

Raymond F Raper

Coronary artery bypass surgery is one of the most frequently undertaken surgical procedures. Because of the prevalence of cardiac disease, cardiac surgery has significant health and economic implications. Intensive care may account for up to 40% of the total hospital costs for these patients and much of the short-term morbidity and mortality is based on perioperative events.

The overall mortality following cardiac surgery is low (approximately 3%). However, this ranges from less than 1% for elective coronary artery bypass grafting to more than 30% for more complicated surgery in patients with significant myocardial dysfunction and associated disorders. Intensive care management following cardiac surgery usually involves a short period of recovery before discharge to the ward. For a small percentage of patients, however, at least potentially remediable complications may require the complete intensive care armamentarium, with a highly significant impact on the intensive care unit (ICU) and hospital budgets and resources.

ORGANISATION

The convergence of large numbers of patients with very similar problems in the cardiac ICU provides an ideal environment for the standardisation of care based on protocols and clinical pathways. One of the traps of postoperative cardiac care is that the sameness of the patients tends to obscure their particularity. Individual patient assessment must carefully address the multisystemic manifestations of cardiovascular and degenerative diseases.

Cardiac surgery involves a continuum of care from presentation to post-discharge management and rehabilitation. The intensive care specialist must be involved in this continuum, rather than functioning in isolation from surgeons, anaesthetists, cardiologists and even family practitioners.

The postoperative stage is largely set by the preoperative and operative phases of management. A component of postoperative management is active participation both in principle and in particular in patient selection and preparation, as well as in the conduct of anaesthesia and surgery. Relevant aspects include suitability and preparation for surgery, advanced care planning and more technical issues such as temperature management, invasive monitoring, haemodynamic management and transport. Movement from the operating theatre to the ICU and later to the ward will appear seamless only if the management systems have been well coordinated in advance.

Changing patterns of practice are resulting in the management of older patients with more co-morbid pathologies. Newer procedures are now being offered to patients previously considered inoperable. Patient and family expectations of surgery are expanding. This, together with greater expectation for regular and detailed communication, will increasingly impact on intensive care practice.

CARDIOVASCULAR MANAGEMENT

The first step in the intensive care management of the newly arrived patient who has undergone cardiac surgery involves a simple transfer of ventilation, monitoring and drug administration from transport to ICU systems. This should be structured to minimise disruption.

- Confirm integrity and position of endotracheal and gastric tubes and intravascular catheters.
- Re-establish mechanical ventilation of both lungs.
- Undertake chest radiography to assess lung expansion, pleural integrity and catheter placement.
- Perform early 12-lead electrocardiography to exclude or identify acute ischaemia.

Management is conveniently dictated by standardised protocols, which should cover investigations, fluid and electrolyte management, vasoactive and other drug administration and mechanical ventilation. Standardisation is probably more important than the particulars of the protocol, which might vary considerably among institutions. Optimal cardiovascular management requires a sound knowledge of normal and abnormal cardiovascular physiology. It also requires an understanding of the haemodynamic changes usually seen in the postoperative patient (**Fig. 26.1**).[1]

MONITORING

Electrocardiography and continuous invasive blood pressure and central venous pressure monitoring are

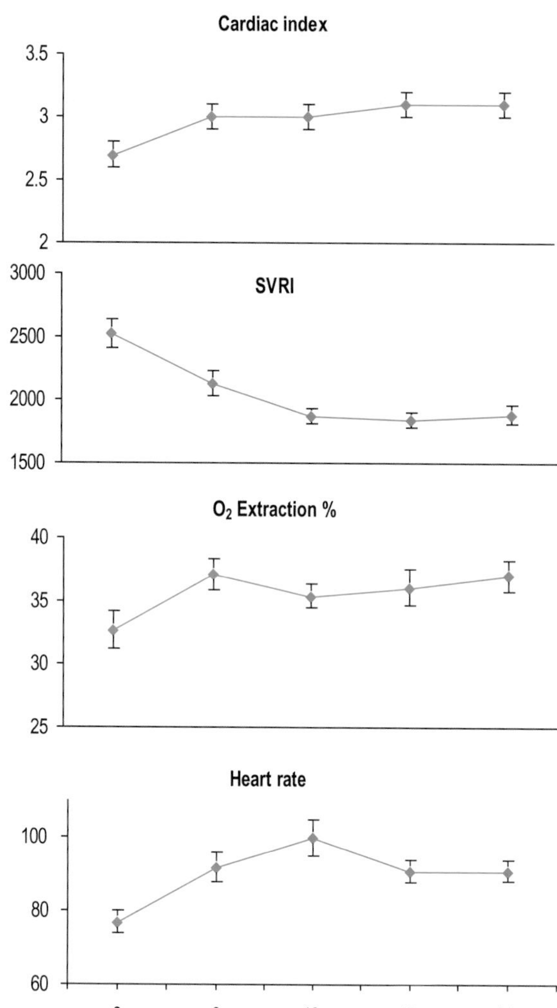

Figure 26.1 Haemodynamic changes following cardiac surgery. SVRI = systemic vascular resistance index.

standard. Flotation pulmonary artery (PA) catheterisation has become somewhat controversial. It is now reasonably well established that PA catheterisation is safe but may not alter outcomes.[2]

- Surgery can be safely undertaken at least in low-risk patients without PA catheterisation.[3]
- Collateral evidence supports PA catheter use in more complicated cases.
- It is essential that the known limitations and complications of PA catheters are considered in usage and interpretation.[4]

Cardiac output measurement by pulse contour analysis and a variety of ultrasound techniques are becoming more commonplace. A precise role for these techniques is not established, especially in the postsurgical patient, where Doppler-enabling windows may be difficult to obtain. Pulse contour analysis is invalid in the presence of intra-aortic counterpulsation. Nevertheless, these techniques and continuous mixed venous saturation monitoring are attractive and very useful in individual patients.

Transoesophageal echocardiography is now almost routine in the operating theatre, at least for more complicated patients. The technique is less suitable for monitoring in the ICU, but is helpful in the diagnosis and management of cardiovascular instability in postoperative patients.

FLUID AND ELECTROLYTE MANAGEMENT

Despite generous intraoperative fluid administration, effective hypovolaemia is common in the early postoperative period, especially as warming with associated vasodilatation occurs.

RESUSCITATION FLUID

- Use of isotonic fluid is essential.
- No benefit for any particular resuscitation fluid has been established. The suggestion that albumin may not be safe has been essentially dispelled.[5]
- Larger volumes of crystalloid than colloid solutions are required.
- An excessively positive fluid balance may increase perioperative complications.

Polyuria is frequently observed in the early postoperative period, possibly related to hypothermia, haemodilution and the after-effects of non-pulsatile cardiopulmonary bypass on stretch and baroreceptors. This usually settles within the first 6 hours, but often necessitates considerable volume replacement in the meantime.

POTASSIUM AND MAGNESIUM HOMEOSTASIS

Hypomagnesaemia and hypokalaemia are frequent in the early postoperative stage. These are exacerbated by polyuria. Late hyperkalaemia is also quite common, especially in patients with renal impairment or prior angiotensin-converting enzyme (ACE) inhibitor administration. Treatment for hyperkalaemia is rarely required in the absence of significant renal impairment. Especially in patients with atrial or ventricular ectopy or tachydysrhythmias, potassium and magnesium levels must be maintained in the high normal range.

Calcium homeostasis is generally not threatened by cardiopulmonary bypass. Massive transfusion, however, frequently causes hypocalcaemia. Ionised calcium levels are now easily monitored by point-of-care blood gas analysers.

HYPOTENSION

Hypotension is both a consequence and a cause of myocardial dysfunction. The major causes include:

- hypovolaemia
- vasodilation

Box 26.1 Low cardiac output

Preload
- Hypovolaemia, including haemorrhage
- Tamponade, pericardial constriction
- Left ventricular diastolic dysfunction
  - Hypertrophy
  - Ischaemia
  - Oedema
  - Hypertrophic or restrictive cardiomyopathy
  - Pulmonary hypertension
  - Right ventricular failure

Afterload
- Excessive vasoconstriction
- Aortic stenosis
- Functional left ventricular obstruction
  - Obstructive cardiomyopathy
  - Systolic anterior motion of the mitral valve

Myocardial function
- Mechanical (ventricular septal defect, valve pathology)
- Cardiomyopathy
- Ischaemia, postischaemic stunning
- Metabolic, electrolyte abnormalities, pharmacological depression

- pericardial tamponade
- heart failure.

Other causes of low cardiac output state (**Box 26.1**) should be considered and excluded. Whatever the cause, hypotension frequently causes myocardial ischaemia and consequent heart failure, especially if it occurs in the first 12–24 hours postoperatively. Angiography during this time almost always shows a significant reduction in the calibre of native coronary arteries, indicating increased coronary resistance and, presumably, altered coronary vasodilator reserve. Treatment of hypotension is urgent if a spiral of ischaemia and heart failure is to be averted.

MANAGEMENT

Successful management of hypotension depends on:

- rapid diagnostic assessment
- diagnosis-specific intervention.

Context is very helpful. Early hypotension in patients with well-preserved ventricular function and no obvious ischaemia usually responds well to fluid administration. Patients with poor ventricular function and increasing inotrope requirement are likely to have a more sinister pathophysiology.

Vasoconstrictors may be useful in breaking the cycle of hypotension–ischaemia–hypotension, but must be used cautiously in patients with impaired ventricular function, and especially in patients with major vascular or aortic pathology, for whom a hypertensive overshoot may be catastrophic.

HYPERTENSION

Complications associated with hypertension include:

- bleeding
- heart failure
- vascular (especially aortic) injury
- myocardial ischaemia.

Significant postoperative hypertension is more common in patients having a history of hypertension and with cessation of beta blockade, but is reasonably common in the early postoperative period. Both absolute pressure and dp/dt are important factors in vascular injury. Vascular resistance declines over the first few hours (see Fig. 26.1) so that therapy during this period is best undertaken with agents with a short duration of action. Nitroglycerine is theoretically more appropriate than nitroprusside because of the possibility of coronary steal with the latter agent.[6] In practice, this is almost never apparent and nitroprusside appears to be more effective. Simple measures such as the provision of adequate analgesia and sedation should also be considered.

The target blood pressure varies with the indication. Excessive reduction of blood pressure risks reducing myocardial oxygen supply more than demand. Under most circumstances, a mean arterial pressure between 90 and 100 mmHg (12.0 and 13.5 kPa) seems optimal.[7] Much lower target pressures may be applicable for the management of heart failure or in the presence of a vulnerable aorta, such as occurs with aortic trauma, dissection or aneurysm. Reduction of dp/dt with beta blockade is more important than absolute blood pressure control in the management of aortic dissection.

LOW CARDIAC OUTPUT

The aetiology of a low cardiac output following heart surgery is diverse (see Box 26.1). The most common causes include:

- intravascular volume depletion
- systolic heart failure
- pericardial tamponade.

Transient, reversible myocardial depression may follow an episode of acute ischaemia (preoperative or intraoperative) and is especially problematic where intraoperative myocardial protection has been difficult or suboptimal. Recognition of a low-output state in the absence of invasive monitoring may be difficult. Many of the usual signs of low output are also consequences of anaesthesia and surgery. Tachycardia may be obscured by drugs, hypothermia and heart disease, and even lactic acidosis may be an unreliable marker in this patient group.[1]

In the early postoperative period, a relatively low cardiac output may not warrant intervention, providing tissue oxygen delivery is adequate. Since beta blockade is beneficial in the postoperative cardiac patient, beta agonists should not be used unquestioningly. Nevertheless, optimisation of cardiac function may confer some benefit[8] and intervention is clearly required when tissue oxygen delivery is inadequate.

MANAGEMENT OPTIONS

1. Establish the diagnosis, including aetiology. Distinguishing tamponade from heart failure may require cardiac imaging with transthoracic or transoesophageal echocardiography. This should be the first recourse when uncertainty remains following conventional haemodynamic assessment. Tamponade may not be detectable using transthoracic echocardiography in the early phase after surgery.[9] The principal role of echocardiography is thus the investigation of possible alternative diagnoses.
2. Correct all easily reversible factors, including hypovolaemia, tamponade, acute myocardial ischaemia, electrolyte abnormalities and dysrhythmias.
3. Vasodilators are helpful in the presence of hypertension and ventricular dilatation. Postsurgical vasodilation after the first 4–8 hours often obviates any ongoing role for these agents.
4. Inotropic agents: because of the associated vasodilatation, ino-constricting agents are frequently required, alone or in combination. Issues to consider include:
   a. Dobutamine is an essentially pure β_1-agonist. In the management of acute heart failure, it has been associated with an increase in mortality.[10]
   b. Norepinephrine (noradrenaline) is a potent vasoconstrictor. It is commonly used to manage vasodilation but should probably not be used alone in the presence of a low cardiac output.
   c. Vasopressin has no clearly established role in postoperative cardiac surgery, but does reduce the level of norepinephrine (noradrenaline) required and may thus spare the myocardium from excessive beta stimulation.
   d. Epinephrine (adrenaline) is a potent ino-constrictor but its metabolic effects (especially lactic acidosis) and relative tachycardia make usage in cardiac surgical patients problematic.[11]
   e. Milrinone is a phosphodiesterase inhibitor with a long duration of action and potent vasodilating properties. These make milrinone relatively difficult to introduce and to wean. It has similar haemodynamic effects to dobutamine and is associated with increased atrial fibrillation. Overall benefit is not established.[12] It may be a useful inotropic agent in patients with β-receptor down-regulation.
   f. Levosimendan is a calcium-sensitising agent. It offers little overall benefit in the treatment of heart failure[13] but may be beneficial in the perioperative period.[14]
5. Intra-aortic balloon counterpulsation (IABC; see below).
6. Ventricular assist devices (VAD) are expensive and technically far more demanding than IABC. The refinement of extracorporeal membrane oxygenation (ECMO) circuits has increased their use for short-term cardiac support. When instituted for failure to wean from bypass, the outlook is generally poor.[15,16] Most published VAD data relate to non-surgical patients in whom the role of heart assist devices is increasingly established both as a 'bridge to transplant' and as 'destination therapy'.
7. Delayed sternal closure has an established role in improving outcome after cardiac surgery.[17] Cardiac output is increased and inotropic requirement reduced. Subsequent sternal closure has an acceptably low complication rate. The sternum may be left open following an initial attempt at closure or re-opened with later deterioration. Sternal retraction may be required.
8. Mechanical ventilation is generally continued throughout the period of low output. This reduces cardiac workload by removing the work of breathing. Positive intrathoracic pressure reduces left ventricular afterload, which is beneficial to the dilated left ventricle. Positive pressure may be detrimental, however, in the presence of diastolic ventricular dysfunction or hypovolaemia, where the reduction in venous return may further reduce ventricular preload.

INTRA-AORTIC BALLOON COUNTERPULSATION

IABC has an established role in support of cardiac surgery. Its two actions are: (1) augmentation of diastolic coronary perfusion pressure; and (2) left ventricular afterload reduction. This is achieved by balloon inflation (30–50 mL capacity) within the aorta during diastole and rapid deflation of the balloon immediately before aortic valve opening. The catheter is usually inserted using a Seldinger technique, but can be placed by femoral artery cutdown or directly into the descending thoracic aorta. Timing of inflation and deflation is critical to optimal function. This is best achieved using the pressure waveform and a 1:2 ratio (**Fig. 26.2**).

Inflation is timed to coincide with the dicrotic notch. Deflation is timed to occur as late as possible in diastole, ensuring that the IABC end-diastolic pressure is lower than the patient's end-diastolic pressure. IABC increases cardiac index and coronary perfusion and reduces left ventricular filling pressure, myocardial lactate production and oxygen extraction percentage.

Indications for IABC are summarised in **Box 26.2**.

IABC has an established role in the management of reversible myocardial dysfunction especially in the context of myocardial revascularisation (surgical or endovascular). There is a probable benefit in high-risk surgical patients undergoing elective

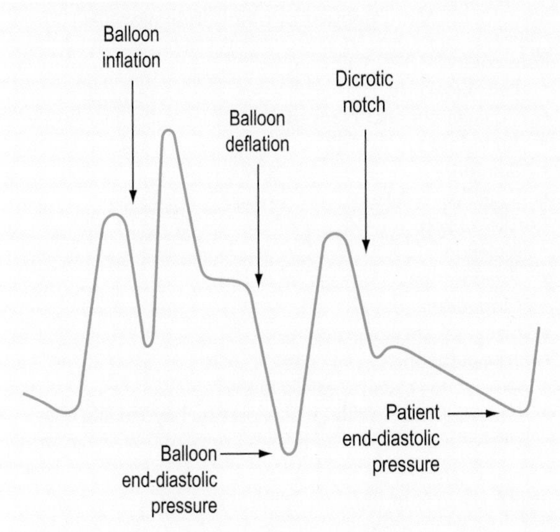

Figure 26.2 Intra-aortic balloon counterpulsation pressure waveform. Inflation is timed to coincide with the dicrotic notch. Deflation is timed to occur as late as possible in diastole, ensuring that the IABC end-diastolic pressure is lower than the patient's end-diastolic pressure.

Box 26.2 Indications for intra-aortic balloon counterpulsation

Prophylactic
- Cardiac surgery
  - Two of: left main >70%, left ventricular ejection fraction <0.4, unstable angina, reoperation
  - Failure to wean from cardiopulmonary bypass
- Non-cardiac procedures in the presence of severe left ventricular impairment, unstable angina

Cardiogenic shock
- *Reversible* myocardial depression
- Support for reperfusion, revascularisation
- Bridge to transplant

revascularisation.[18] IABC is not helpful, however, in the management of cardiogenic shock from irremediable causes except as a bridge to transplant. Complications include:

- limb ischaemia (6–16%)
- vascular trauma, dissection
- infection (cutdown>percutaneous)
- balloon rupture
- bleeding
- thrombocytopenia
- malposition, vascular obstruction
- malfunction, failure to unwrap.

Limb ischaemia is the most frequent complication and optimal management requires early recognition based on routine, systematic observation.

ISCHAEMIA

Postoperative myocardial ischaemia predicts a more complicated course.[19] Recognition is enhanced by automated multilead ST analysis with confirmatory electrocardiography, although diagnosis may be difficult in the presence of preoperative electrocardiographic abnormalities.

Ischaemia may be due to graft failure. Remedial options include coronary angiography and/or reoperation. Angiography offers the potential for tailored reoperation or non-operative intervention. Management decisions may be influenced by surgical factors such as the availability of further conduit and the state of the native arteries. Thus close liaison among ICU personnel, cardiologists and surgeons is essential.

DIASTOLIC DYSFUNCTION

Ventricular hypertrophy is the commonest cause of diastolic dysfunction, and is exacerbated by poor myocardial protection during surgical procedures. Myocardial ischaemia, right ventricular (RV) dilatation and pericardial abnormalities (including tamponade) can also reduce left ventricular volume in spite of elevated filling pressures.[20] Recognition and management can be very difficult.

Diagnosis generally requires:

- demonstration of small ventricular volumes (using echocardiography or other techniques)
- the presence of increased filling pressures.

MANAGEMENT

- Treatable causes should be addressed.
- Blood volume must be maintained, with blood transfusion where necessary.
- Maintenance of sinus rhythm is helpful, if not essential.
- Atrial pacing at an enhanced heart rate is often beneficial since the stroke volume is fixed and the diastolic filling time is already foreshortened.
- β-agonists and milrinone improve diastolic relaxation and hence ventricular compliance.

DYSRHYTHMIAS

Ventricular and supraventricular dysrhythmias are common. Prevention and treatment of electrolyte abnormalities may be prophylactic. New occurrence of complex ventricular dysrhythmias should stimulate a search for causal ischaemia and graft malfunction.

- Ventricular fibrillation and pulseless ventricular tachycardia require rapid defibrillation, preferably before external cardiac massage, which may cause mechanical injury post sternotomy. If haemodynamic stability cannot be rapidly restored, open cardiac massage should be instituted.

- Facilities for atrioventricular pacing are essential as transient heart block is common.

ATRIAL FIBRILLATION (AF)

AF is the most common complication of cardiac surgery.[21,22] Its incidence varies from 10 to 40% in patients undergoing coronary artery surgery and up to 50% with some valvular procedures. Predisposing factors include a history of AF, valvular heart disease (especially mitral valve pathology), increasing age and prolonged P-wave duration. AF can be effectively treated and its recurrence prevented with intraoperative radiofrequency ablation and left atrial reduction during cardiac surgery.[23] There may also be some long-term survival benefit.[24] AF is probably less frequently observed following 'off-pump' surgery, and is most frequently encountered around the second and third post-operative days, but may occur weeks after surgery and hospital discharge.

AF is a potentially serious complication. Apart from discomfort, it may provoke or complicate haemodynamic instability. The major complication of AF, however, is stroke, with an increased risk of approximately three-fold. Based on echocardiography, there is the potential for embolic stroke within 3 days of onset of AF.

AF is also associated with:

- increase in inotrope usage
- increased use of IABC
- increased reoperation for bleeding
- prolonged ICU and hospital stay
- increased costs.

Several strategies are beneficial in preventing AF:[25]

- beta blockade
- amiodarone
- sotalol[26]
- diltiazem
- biatrial pacing
- dexamethasone
- colchicine [27]
- statins.[28]

Treatment should be tempered with an understanding that spontaneous reversion to sinus rhythm is frequent. A treatment strategy is summarised in **Box 26.3**.

- Beta blockade is best established.
- Digitalis is not more effective than placebo at reverting AF and may not be helpful in ventricular rate control in the presence of catecholamine stimulation.
- Anti-coagulation should be considered where AF persists for longer than 48 hours and in all cases where elective cardioversion is undertaken.
- Early cardioversion tends to be ineffective and potentially harmful. Although officially recommended in the presence of instability, this is not based on any empirical evidence.

Box 26.3 Management of atrial fibrillation (AF)

Rate control
- Beta blockade
- Calcium channel blockers
- Amiodarone
- Sotalol
- Digitalis

Cardioversion
- Ibuletide
- Amiodarone
- Magnesium
- Electrical cardioversion

Anticoagulation
- Always for elective cardioversion
- Consider if atrial fibrillation persists beyond 48 hours

RIGHT VENTRICULAR DYSFUNCTION

RV failure following cardiac surgery is reasonably common. Aetiological factors include:

- direct RV ischaemia or infarction
- poor myocardial protection
- anteriorly placed RV
- bypass-related pulmonary hypertension.

Management involves:

- volume resuscitation
- maintenance of RV perfusion pressure with vasoconstrictors
- IABC as required
- inotrope administration
- RV afterload reduction.

Useful afterload-reducing agents include nitric oxide, prostaglandins and sildenafil. Conventional vasodilators tend to produce excessive systemic vasodilatation. Occasionally, RV balloon counterpulsation or an RV assist device may be required. Delayed sternal closure has an established role.

EMERGENCY REOPERATION

Emergency resternotomy is indicated as part of resuscitation when haemodynamic stability cannot be rapidly re-established with conventional means.[29,30] Advantages compared with closed-chest resuscitation include:

- establishment of the cause of instability
- correction of the cause (e.g. tamponade, kinked graft)
- more effective cardiac massage
- direct establishment of atrial and ventricular pacing.

Resternotomy also enables the re-establishment of cardiopulmonary bypass and regrafting or correction of mechanical abnormalities as required. Infectious complications of emergency resternotomy are probably increased, but the incidence is not prohibitive.

RESPIRATORY MANAGEMENT

Postoperative mechanical ventilation remains routine in cardiac surgical patients. Immediate extubation appears to offer little patient benefit,[31] but may be expedient. Neither is routine prolongation of ventilation beneficial. Extubation can be safely undertaken with simple protocols. Reintubation is rarely required, but is more likely in older patients with pre-existing lung and vascular disease and impaired ventricular function. Reoperative surgery and bleeding requiring massive transfusion also increase the likelihood of early extubation failure.

Hypoxia is very common in the early postoperative period. It is mostly attributable to atelectasis and responds well to simple measures such as positive end-expiratory pressure (PEEP), prolonged inspiration and simple recruitment manoeuvres. Atelectasis is a consequence of cardiopulmonary bypass and intraoperative ventilation with high inspired oxygen and without PEEP. Long-term sequelae are rare. Incentive spirometry and chest physiotherapy are commonly utilised in the postoperative period, without good supportive evidence. Early mobilisation appears most beneficial. Adequate analgesia facilitates physiotherapy and mobilisation. Non-steroidal agents may increase the risk of complications.[32]

More sinister causes of hypoxia include severe heart failure and hypoxaemic respiratory failure (acute respiratory distress syndrome, ARDS). The aetiology of ARDS is diverse, but includes shock, massive blood product administration and cardiopulmonary bypass itself. Management is not particular to this group of patients. Occasionally, profound hypoxia accompanies minor atelectasis with moderate pulmonary hypertension. Patent foramen ovale (which is seen in 10–15% of the normal population) with right-to-left intracardiac shunt is the likely mechanism.

Clinically detected pulmonary embolism is an uncommon complication of cardiac surgery, probably due to bypass-induced platelet dysfunction, routine postoperative antiplatelet therapy and thromboprophylaxis.[33] Asymptomatic thromboembolism may be significantly more common, however.[34,35] Contrary to earlier beliefs, 'off-pump' surgery may not be associated with an increase in prothrombotic tendency or a need for a more aggressive thromboprophylaxis regimen.[36]

POSTOPERATIVE COMPLICATIONS

BLEEDING AND TRANSFUSION

Excessive postoperative bleeding is a major cause of increased morbidity and mortality. Mechanisms are complex and include preoperative anticoagulation, thrombolysis and antiplatelet therapy as well as activation of haemostatic mechanisms, including fibrinolysis. 'Off-pump' surgery may be associated with excessive bleeding because of administration of anticoagulant and antiplatelet therapy out of fear of early graft closure. There is increasing evidence that transfusion is associated with excessive complications, including death, and that transfusion rates vary amongst institutions.[37]

Most studies of pharmacological strategies to minimise postoperative blood loss have involved preoperative or intraoperative intervention. Extrapolation to the postoperative phase is intuitive rather than established. Aprotinin and the lysine analogues aminocaproic acid and tranexamic acid reduce bleeding and exposure to blood and blood products. Aprotinin has been associated with an increased risk of serious end-organ damage.[38] Desmopressin is probably less effective and has been associated with an increased risk of myocardial infarction.[39]

Effective postoperative measures include reversal of residual heparin (including 'heparin rebound') and correction of coagulopathy with blood products. A systematic approach to operative and postoperative blood conservation, including point-of-care testing to guide therapy, can significantly reduce bleeding and transfusion and resultant complications.[40] Application of PEEP has been shown to be effective in some studies, but not others. Retransfusion of shed blood reduces autologous transfusion requirements without apparent side-effects. Controlled tamponade with discontinuation of drain suction and even clamping of drains has also been reported.[41] Activated factor VII may be effective in controlling bleeding, but may result in increased risk of stroke.[42] Finally, a restrictive transfusion strategy can reduce exposure to transfusion without increased risk.[43]

RENAL FAILURE

Depending on definition and patient groups, acute renal failure is observed in 1–5% of patients undergoing cardiac surgery. Risk factors include increasing age, heart failure, prolonged bypass, diabetes, pre-existing renal impairment and postoperative shock. Surgery without cardiopulmonary bypass may be relatively protective and other potentially modifiable factors include anaemia, blood transfusion and reexploration.[44] Morbidity, mortality and costs are significantly increased. Effective preventive strategies beyond careful haemodynamic management and minimisation of associated nephrotoxic insults have not been established. Nevertheless, attention to urine output in the presence of known risk factors appears warranted.

SHIVERING

Shivering is frequent following cardiac surgery. Mechanisms are complex and not entirely related to core temperature. Shivering causes a significant increase in metabolic rate and hence cardiac workload. This is especially important in the patient with impaired cardiac function and limited reserve. Effective preventive agents include dexamethasone, clonidine, high-dose morphine and external warming. Pethidine and tramadol effectively reduce the duration of shivering. Short-term neuromuscular blockade is occasionally required.

STERNAL INFECTION

Deep sternal wound infection is uncommon (0.5–2.5%). Associated morbidity and mortality are significant. Risk factors have been variously reported but consistently include diabetes, obesity and use of internal mammary arteries, especially if bilateral. Other contributing factors include prolonged surgery, chronic lung disease, male sex, low postoperative cardiac output, blood transfusion, sternal reopening and dialysis. Close control of blood sugar levels in diabetics[45] and preoperative nasal and oropharyngeal decontamination[46] may help prevent infection.

NEUROLOGICAL COMPLICATIONS

Neurological complications of cardiac surgery include neuropsychiatric deterioration as a consequence of cardiopulmonary bypass, delirium and a range of peripheral neuropathies, the most frequent of which is unilateral phrenic nerve palsy. Paraplegia is a recognised complication of thoracic aortic surgery.

The most devastating neurological complication is cerebral infarction. The incidence varies with patient selection, but ranges from 1 to 5%. The pathophysiology is mostly embolic. Risk factors include carotid artery stenosis, hypertension, AF, aortic atheroma, impaired ventricular function and peripheral vascular disease. 'Off-pump' and especially 'anaortic' surgery (no aortic manipulation) are protective[47] and other operative techniques may also reduce the incidence.

GASTROINTESTINAL COMPLICATIONS

Peptic ulcer disease, pancreatitis, cholecystitis, gut ischaemia, ileus and hepatic dysfunction are uncommon (<1%) after cardiac surgery. Morbidity, however, is quite high. Risk factors include increased age, more complicated surgery and postoperative shock. The incidence of gastrointestinal complications may be reduced with 'off-pump' surgery.

LONG-TERM CONSIDERATIONS

Patients surviving cardiac surgery have a continuing risk of disease progression. It is important that effective secondary prevention strategies be considered or recommenced in the postoperative period. Initiatives with proven long-term benefit in patients with ischaemic heart disease include antiplatelet therapy, beta blockade, ACE inhibitors, lipid-lowering statins and exercise. Treatment for hypertension, diabetes and other intercurrent disorders should also be reinstituted.

A small percentage of patients require long-term ICU management for a variety of complications. Excellent long-term survival and quality of life are possible in this group of patients, especially if the prolonged ICU stay results from pulmonary complications rather than severe heart failure or neurological dysfunction.

Box 26.4 Risk factors for cardiac patients undergoing non-cardiac surgery*

- High-risk surgery (abdominal, thoracic, major vascular)
- History of ischaemic heart disease
- History of congestive heart failure
- History of cerebrovascular disease
- Treatment with insulin
- Renal impairment

*High risk: three or more factors.

NON-CARDIAC SURGERY

Non-cardiac surgery poses a significant risk to the patient with cardiac disease. Postoperative cardiac complications result in significantly increased immediate and late mortality. Simple preoperative assessment enables risk stratification, which might lead to deferment or cancellation of non-essential surgery. Indications for specific investigations and treatments are probably not different in the preoperative patient. However, this might be the first time that a cardiac assessment has been undertaken and hence significant cardiac pathology identified. Risk factors are summarised in **Box 26.4**. Cumulative factors are more than additive. Patients undergoing vascular procedures have a high risk of associated coronary artery disease and should be carefully assessed preoperatively. Perioperative risk can be modified by anaesthetic technique and by optimal medical (or surgical) management of heart disease, which might include myocardial revascularisation.

The principles of postoperative management are the same as those outlined for the cardiac surgical patient. The period of risk for cardiac complications extends for some days after surgery and close monitoring to identify and manage events during this time is desirable in high-risk patients. The immediate perioperative period poses risks associated with anaesthesia, bleeding, fluid and electrolyte imbalance, haemodynamic instability and temperature abnormalities. These can be effectively managed. Early reinstitution of protective treatment (aspirin, beta blockers, ACE inhibition, statins, antihypertensive therapy) may protect against later complications.

Access the complete references list online at http://www.expertconsult.com

12. Jebelli M, Ghazinoor M, Mandegar MH, et al. Effect of milrinone on short-term outcome of patients with myocardial dysfunction undergoing coronary artery bypass graft: A randomized controlled trial. Cardiol J 2010;17:73–8.
14. Landoni G, Mizzi A, Biondi-Zoccai G, et al. Reducing mortality in cardiac surgery with levosimendan: a meta-analysis of randomized controlled trials. J Cardiothorac Vasc Anesth 2010;24:51–7.
18. Theologou T, Bashir M, Rengarajan A, et al. Preoperative intra aortic balloon pumps in patients undergoing coronary artery bypass grafting. Cochrane Database Systematic Rev 2011;1:CD004472. Online. Available: http://onlinelibrary.wiley.com/doi/10.1002/14651858.CD004472.pub3/abstract.
24. Attaran S, Saleh HZ, Ward A, et al. Does the outcome improve after radiofrequency ablation for atrial fibrilation in patients undergoing cardiac surgery? A propensity-matched comparison. Eur J Cardiothorac Surg 2012;41:806–10.
28. Chopra V, Wesorick D, Sussman J, et al. Effect of perioperative statins on death, myocardial infarction, atrial fibrillation, and length of stay. A systematic review and meta-analysis. Arch Surg 2012;147:181–9.
40. Moskowitz DM, McCullogh JN, Shander A, et al. The impact of blood conservation on outcomes in cardiac surgery: is it safe and effective? Ann Thorac Surg 2010;90:451–8.
44. Karkouti K, Duminda N, Wijeysundera MD, et al. Acute kidney injury after cardiac surgery. Focus on modifiable risk factors. Circulation 2009;119:495–502.
47. Misfield M, Potger K, Ross DE, et al. 'Anaortic' off-pump coronary artery bypass grafting significantly reduces neurological complications compared to off-pump and conventional on-pump surgery with aortic manipulation. Thorac Cardiovasc Surg 2010;58:408–14.

27

Echocardiography in the intensive care unit

Guido Tavazzi and Susanna Price

Historically exclusively the domain of the cardiologist, there has been gradual adoption of echocardiography by other specialties. Transoesophageal echocardiography is now considered mandatory for much of cardiac surgery and is predominantly performed by cardiothoracic anaesthetists. Echocardiography is recommended in international guidelines for investigation of non-traumatic cardiac arrest, and transversal ultrasound is widely used in emergency and trauma medicine.[1] In intensive care, concerns regarding safety of the pulmonary artery catheter, together with development of alternative cardiac output monitoring, and demonstration that echocardiography yields information additional to the pulmonary artery catheter has led to an increase in its use.[2] It is thus inevitable that echocardiography for the assessment and diagnosis of critically ill patients will increase, and therefore intensivists should have knowledge of the principles and limitations of the technique, together with its relevant application(s) in the ICU setting.

PRINCIPLES OF ECHOCARDIOGRAPHY[3]

Ultrasound is generated by application of an alternating current across piezoelectric crystals, the resulting vibration generating a longitudinal wave. The same crystals act as receivers of returning, reflected ultrasound waves, and vibrations induced by these returning waves are used to generate images. Ultrasound can be refracted, reflected and/or attenuated, allowing discrimination between adjacent tissues by virtue of their different acoustic properties. Diagnostic ultrasound frequencies are 1–12 MHz.

Ultrasound is therefore a sound wave comprising longitudinal waves of compression and decompression of the transmitting medium (air/water/soft tissue/blood) travelling at a fixed velocity. As a longitudinal wave, ultrasound is defined by its amplitude, wavelength and cycle duration. One important difference between ultrasound and audible sound is that at higher frequencies ultrasound tends to move in straight lines, and can be reflected and focused. Although some properties differ between ultrasound and audible sound, important principles apply to both. First, the relationship between the wavelength, its velocity and frequency is determined by the equation $\lambda = V/f$, where λ is wavelength, V the velocity of ultrasound through tissues, and f the frequency of the transducer. As V is relatively fixed in soft tissues, the resolution of images is determined by manipulation of the other two factors: a higher frequency probe resulting in a shorter wavelength and better resolution, but at the expense of greater attenuation and reduced penetration. Spatial and temporal resolution determine the image quality, where axial resolution is limited by wavelength, and temporal resolution is determined by frame rate and in turn by the number of pulses/scan line, the number of scan lines/sector and the sector depth and width. Ultrasound is additionally reflected by small objects, and does not propagate easily in gaseous media. This is particularly relevant in echocardiography, as the heart shares the thoracic cavity with the lungs, and thus there are only certain windows where the heart may be visualised.

A number of echocardiographic modalities and techniques are available, and their principles, pitfalls and potential critical care uses are outlined in **Table 27.1**.

PRINCIPLES OF ICU ECHOCARDIOGRAPHY

As with any investigation, ICU echocardiography should be undertaken within existing clinical governance structures, with clear guidelines for infection control/consent/acquisition/storage, reporting and review of images.[4] The imaging technique of choice in the ICU is transthoracic echocardiogram (TTE) unless this is impractical, technically impossible or there is a primary indication for transoesophageal echocardiogram (TOE). Challenges in obtaining adequate TTE views in immobile, ventilated patients are well documented. Here, left-sided contrast can improve the diagnostic yield, even in the hands of inexperienced operators.[5]

TOE should not be performed under sedation in hypoxic patients or those unable to protect their airway. ICU TOE will therefore generally be undertaken in intubated, ventilated patients. Prior to TOE, coagulation and platelet results should be known and correction considered. If oesophageal intubation is difficult and/or coagulation is suboptimal, it should be performed under direct laryngoscopic vision. As patients are often haemodynamically unstable a designated

Table 27.1 Principles and major pitfalls of echocardiographic techniques

DEVELOPMENT	PRINCIPLE	PITFALLS/LIMITATIONS	BENEFITS	ICU USAGE
A-mode	Received energy at a certain time displayed as amplitude	Obsolete	Obsolete	Obsolete
B-mode	Display of A-mode as brightness	Obsolete	Obsolete	Obsolete
M-mode	Display of B-mode over time	Difficult to interpret Angulation of cardiac chambers leads to inaccuracy	High temporal resolution	Wall thickness, TAPSE, MAPSE, premature closure of MV, SAM MV, early closure AV, FS/EF, RV diastolic collapse, volaemia
2D	Electronic/mechanical sweep of M-mode, reconstructed to provide real-time 2D images of anatomical structures	Temporal resolution less than M-mode Inaccurate positioning may lead to misinterpretation of chamber size	Images easily interpretable	Structural disease: chambers, valves, extracardiac structures
CW Doppler	Simultaneous transmission and receiving of US	Increasing incident angle leads to underestimation of velocities No spatial resolution along length of interrogation	Determines maximum velocity along length of interrogation	TR, PASP, pressure difference between any two chambers
PW Doppler	Emission of US and depth set by time to receive As change in velocity small, phase shift used	Incident angle dependent Limited velocity resolution	Determines velocity at specific point	LAP, CO, MPI, t-IVT
Colour Doppler	Based on PW Doppler principles Multiple sample volumes with blood flow velocity and direction colour coded Generally BART (blue away, red towards)	Need high-quality 2D images	Identification of normal/ abnormal blood flow Facilitates alignment of CW Doppler	Valvular regurgitation, intracardiac shunts
TOE	Miniaturised US mounted on modified endoscope	Invasive	High resolution, easy imaging	Prosthetic valve endocarditis, intracardiac masses, inadequate TTE views Intraoperative imaging
R-sided contrast	US reflection of saline/ blood interface Bubbles absorbed by pulmonary circulation	Adequate 2D imaging required	Safe, easy to perform and interpret	Intracardiac shunt (?differentiation from intrapulmonary)
TDI	As PW Doppler, but with filters set to detect low velocity	Incident angle dependent If poor image quality/low velocities difficult to interpret	Easier to measure than M-mode	Estimation LAP

Continued

Table 27.1 Principles and major pitfalls of echocardiographic techniques—cont'd

DEVELOPMENT	PRINCIPLE	PITFALLS/LIMITATIONS	BENEFITS	ICU USAGE
3D	Multiple PE crystals simultaneously transmitting and receiving	Need high-quality 2D images	Images that resemble real structures	Limited: mostly cardiology/cardiac surgery 3D EF if images adequate
Strain/strain rate	Deformation of adjacent parts of myocardial tissue based on TDI measurements for gradient of velocities	Incident angle dependent Translocation of tissue confound Load dependent	Identification of ventricular dysfunction not apparent by other means	Research tool, dyssynchrony Ventricular contractility
Speckle tracking	Tracking signature blocks of myocardial tissue	Need high-quality 2D images	Avoids incident angle Identification of all 4 vectors of LV movement	Research tool, dyssynchrony Ventricular contractility
HCU	Miniaturised device to facilitate usage	Quality of images, restriction of functionality	Small and portable	Cardiac arrest Basic echocardiography
Contrast	US reflective agents that pass through pulmonary circulation	Side effects, caution in low EF, high PAP	Improved endocardial border delineation Demonstration of coronary perfusion	EF Infarction i/c masses
ICE	Miniaturised US catheter	Cost	High resolution	Interventional cardiology
Disposable TOE	Miniaturised US probe	Cost, single plane, resolution, limited functionality	Size, duration of usage	Proposed as monitor

A-mode=amplitude mode, B-mode=brightness mode; M-mode=motion mode; TAPSE=tricuspid annular plane systolic excursion; MAPSE=mitral annular plane systolic excursion; MV=mitral valve; SAM=systolic anterior motion; AV=aortic valve; FS=fractional shortening; EF=ejection fraction; RV=right ventricle; US=ultrasound; CW=continuous wave; TR=tricuspid regurgitation; PASP=pulmonary artery systolic pressure; PW=pulse wave; LAP=left atrial pressure; CO=cardiac output; MP=myocardial performance index; t-IVT=total isovolumic time; TTE=transthoracic echocardiography; PE=piezoelectric; TDI=tissue Doppler imaging; HCU=hand-carried ultrasound; ICE=intracardiac echocardiography; i/c=intracardiac; TOE=transoesophageal echocardiography.

intensivist/anaesthetist should manage the airway, ensure haemodynamic stability, and where required modify the haemodynamics according to those required by the operator.

Challenges in ICU echocardiography relate not only to difficulties in image acquisition; but also the confounding effects of sedation, positive-pressure ventilation, pharmacological/mechanical circulatory support, loading conditions, and changes in the metabolic milieu.[4] The critical care echocardiographer must consider all these factors before accurate interpretation is possible, and remember that normal values for indices commonly measured in the non-critical care setting may not be applicable to the ICU population.

INDICATIONS FOR ICU ECHOCARDIOGRAPHY

Although the commonest reason to request an ICU echocardiogram is to assess LV function, indications for ICU echocardiography should rather be to answer a specific clinical question; monitoring effects of therapeutic interventions, formulating a diagnosis and/or suggesting interventions whereby cardiac output (CO) can be improved. The potential scope for ICU echocardiography outlined in the literature is summarised in **Table 27.2**. The most important role is first to rule out/diagnose potentially treatable cardiac disease, either leading to ICU admission, or contributing to the patient's clinical status. When significant cardiac pathology has been excluded, echocardiography should then be used to evaluate the patient's haemodynamics and monitor the effects of interventions.

DIAGNOSTIC ECHOCARDIOGRAPHY

Cardiac pathology may either be the primary reason for ICU admission, in which case it is likely to be severe, or otherwise an incidental finding, contributing to morbidity. Echocardiography should diagnose/exclude significant ventricular disease (including myocardial ischaemia/infarction or complications thereof),

Table 27.2 Indications for echocardiography in the critically ill

EMERGENCY AND ACUTE MEDICINE/ICM	INTENSIVE CARE MEDICINE
• Penetrating trauma, blunt trauma • Postcardiotomy due to cardiac surgery • Hypotension, shock of unknown origin • Unconsciousness, unresponsiveness • Acute severe dyspnoea • Syncope in young adults • Vein thrombosis • AMI and its mechanical complications • Atypical chest pain: suspected aortic dissection, suspected aortic abdominal/thoracic aneurysm, non-traumatic cardiac rupture • Iatrogenic complications from invasive procedures (e.g. pacemaker insertion, PCI, EP) • Great vessel disease	• Systolic function and RWMA abnormalities • Diastolic function • Hypovolaemia and volume responsiveness • Tamponade and pericardial disease • The sepsis syndromes • Preload, afterload and filling status • Acute cor pulmonale • Hypoxaemia • Complications of AMI • Chest trauma • Assessment of shock • Failure to wean from mechanical ventilation • Haemodynamic measurements • Position of cannulae for extracorporeal support
CARDIAC ARREST	
• Underlying rhythm: pulseless electrical activity/EMD/VF • Underlying cause: hypovolaemia/tension pneumothorax/tamponade/coronary thrombosis/pulmonary embolism • Guidance of intervention: volaemia/drainage of tamponade • Early detection of ROSC • Bradycardia–asystole, pacemaker–ECG • Performance of CPR • Effectiveness of chest compressions • Post-arrest hypotension/low CO state: adaptation of vasopressors/inotropes/volaemia	

RWMA=regional wall motion abnormalities; AMI=acute myocardial infarction; EP=electrophysiological; PCI=percutaneous cardiac intervention; EMD=electromechanical dissociation; VF=ventricular fibrillation; ROSC=return of spontaneous circulation; ECG=electrocardiogram; CPR=cardiopulmonary resuscitation; CO=cardiac output.

valvular disease, non-valvular obstruction to flow (LV outflow tract obstruction, pulmonary embolism) and/or pericardial pathology[4] (**Table 27.3**).

VENTRICULAR FUNCTION

Although commonly performed, standard measurements of ventricular function are rarely helpful beyond the initial diagnostic study as values may change significantly with volume loading, ventilation, inodilator therapy and other ICU interventions. Further, the RV is often neglected, and normal values for ventricular function (right and left) in the ICU are poorly defined.

LEFT VENTRICLE

LV contractility is complex, with systolic function comprising minor and long-axis contraction, rotational and differential basal and apical rotational vectors, and diastolic function an equally complex, active process.[3] A number of techniques exist to assess LV function, including measurement of dimensions and volumes in two/three dimensions, wall thickness and motion, assessment of filling patterns and measurement of myocardial deformation. None assesses all components of contractility, and all are variably load and inotropy dependent; therefore measured values should be interpreted with caution in the critically ill.

LV systolic function

Traditionally, assessment of LV contractility has depended upon linear measurement of changes in LV internal dimensions (fractional shortening, FS) or differences between systolic and diastolic areas/volumes in the minor axis (ejection fraction, EF), rather than thickening of the myocardium per se. Nevertheless, in cardiology, values have been correlated with prognosis in numerous pathological processes. Experienced echocardiographers can visually estimate EF by eyeballing alone; however, of note, normal values of FS/EF are unknown for the critically ill patient population, and remain highly variable depending upon ICU interventions as well as the inherent contractility of the myocardium. Although three-dimensional (3D) assessment of EF may be superior to 2D measurements, they are equally load dependent.[6]

In addition to global function there may be regional functional abnormalities, which may manifest as myocardial thinning (normal 6–12 mm), and/or abnormal motion (hypokinesis/akinesis/dyskinesis). In order to assess the myocardium comprehensively it is divided into 17 segments, each of which is individually evaluated, and any wall motion abnormalities correlated with the relevant coronary artery territories.[3] Positive inotropic agents may induce ischaemia (hence their use for stress echocardiography) with consequent

Table 27.3 Clinical and echocardiographic findings on the ICU

CLINICAL FINDING	CARDIAC CAUSE	ECHOCARDIOGRAPHIC FINDING	NOTES
Low CO unresponsive to inotropes	Valvular disease	Any severe stenotic or regurgitant lesion	Difficult to assess in ICU Sequential stenotic lesions may mask severity of individual lesions
	Intrinsic cardiac disease	HOCM/LVH with LVOTO Large VSD/ASD Severe LV/RV dysfunction	See text
	Extrinsic cardiac disease	Tamponade, pericardial effusion, pericardial disease	NB Postoperative cardiac surgical patients (see text)
Oliguria	Underfilling	Low transmitral/tricuspid velocities Small ventricular volumes Apposition of LV papillary muscles in systole	If severe LVH papillary apposition may be unreliable sign
	Intrinsic cardiac disease	Poor LV function, severe AS	High LAP demonstrated
	Pericardial disease	Pericardial effusion, pericardial tamponade, pericardial constriction	NB Postoperative cardiac surgical patients (see text)
Increased filling pressures (left-sided)	Impaired LV	Increased E > A ratio (corrected for age), short IVRT	See text for detailed explanation
	MV disease	Significant MS or MR	MR: dynamic ventricle, increased forward velocities (>1 m/s), short-duration and low-velocity (<3 m/s) regurgitant jet
Increased filling pressures (right-sided)	Secondary to left-sided disease	Significant AS, AR, MS, MR/LV disease	
	Impaired RV	Reduced TAPSE	Any reduction in association with PHT is significant Mild impairment after CABG is normal
	TR	Annular dilatation or endocarditis	If severe, RV dynamic with increased forward velocities (>1 m/s), short-duration and low-velocity regurgitant jet
Sepsis/SIRS	LV/RV dysfunction	Ventricular dilatation, systolic/diastolic dysfunction	Changes controversial and may be masked by inotropes
	Source of sepsis	Endocarditis	
Endocarditis	Native/prosthetic valve, pacemaker wires, extracardiac 'endocarditis'	Vegetations, paraprosthetic leaks, aortic root abscess	Vegetations rare in prosthetic valve endocarditis
Pulmonary hypertension	Acute PE	Dilated RV, severe TR	May rarely demonstrate intracardiac thrombus
	Post-pneumonectomy	Displaced heart, increased pulmonary acceleration time	Views often difficult even with TOE
	Mitral valve disease	Significant MS or MR (2D, PW, CW and colour Doppler)	Severe MR in ICU may be difficult to diagnose (see text)
Failure to wean from ventilator	Intrinsic cardiac disease	Ischaemia, severe MR, HOCM, LV/RV dysfunction	Stress echo may be necessary to make diagnosis
CVA/embolic event	Intracardiac thrombus	LA appendage, RA, apical LV thrombus Endocarditis	Exclude intracardiac shunt with contrast study
Cyanosis	Intracardiac shunting	Positive contrast study	Use agitated blood/saline. Perform Valsalva manoeuvre

CO=cardiac output; ICU=intensive care unit; HOCM=hypertrophic obstructive cardiomyopathy; LVH=left ventricular hypertrophy; LVOTO=left ventricular outflow tract obstruction; VSD=ventricular septal defect; ASD=atrial septal defect; LV=left ventricle; RV=right ventricle; AS=aortic stenosis; LAP=left atrial pressure; IVRT=isovolumic relaxation time; MV=mitral valve; MS=mitral stenosis; MR=mitral regurgitation; AR=aortic regurgitation; TAPSE=tricuspid annular plane systolic excursion; PHT=pulmonary hypertension; CABG=coronary artery bypass graft; TR=tricuspid regurgitation; PE=pulmonary embolism; TOE=transoesophageal echocardiography; PW=pulse wave; CW=continuous wave; LA=left atrium; CVA=cerebrovascular accident.

Adapted from Price S, Prout J, Jaggar SI, et al. 'Tamponade' following cardiac surgery: terminology and echocardiography may both mislead. Eur J Cardiothorac Surg 2004; 26:1156-1160.

induction of abnormalities in myocardial motion. Thus any ICU echocardiogram should be interpreted in the context of the level of inotropic support, and where abnormalities in contractility conform to known coronary artery territories, ischaemia/infarction should be suspected.

Although the majority of LV myocardial fibres are arranged circumferentially, longitudinal fibres situated in the subepicardium and subendocardium play a major role in maintaining normal function, accounting for long-axis (LAX) movement of the base with respect to the apex of the heart. LAX function has three components: amplitude, velocity and timing, and is measured using M-mode (mitral annular plane systolic excursion, MAPSE) and velocities of this motion assessed using tissue Doppler imaging (TDI).[7,8] As these fibres are subendocardial, they are exquisitely sensitive to ischaemia. Regional abnormalities in MAPSE correlate with infarction demonstrated on myocardial perfusion imaging, and may occur in the presence of dobutamine before the appearance of standard regional wall motion abnormalities and/or ECG changes.[9]

LV diastolic function[3,10]

In the normal heart, LV filling is biphasic, with early passive flow (E-wave) and late flow from atrial contraction (A-wave). Derived measures of diastolic function include isovolumic relaxation time (IVRT, time from aortic valve closure to mitral valve opening, normal 70–110 ms), ratio of peak velocities (E/A, normal 0.75–1.40), and E-wave deceleration time (normal 160–240 ms; **Fig. 27.1a**). Where diastolic dysfunction occurs (in either ageing and/or ventricular disease) there may be progressive prolongation of the IVRT (>110 ms) resulting in a lower early-diastolic pressure difference between LA and LV, an E-wave consequently

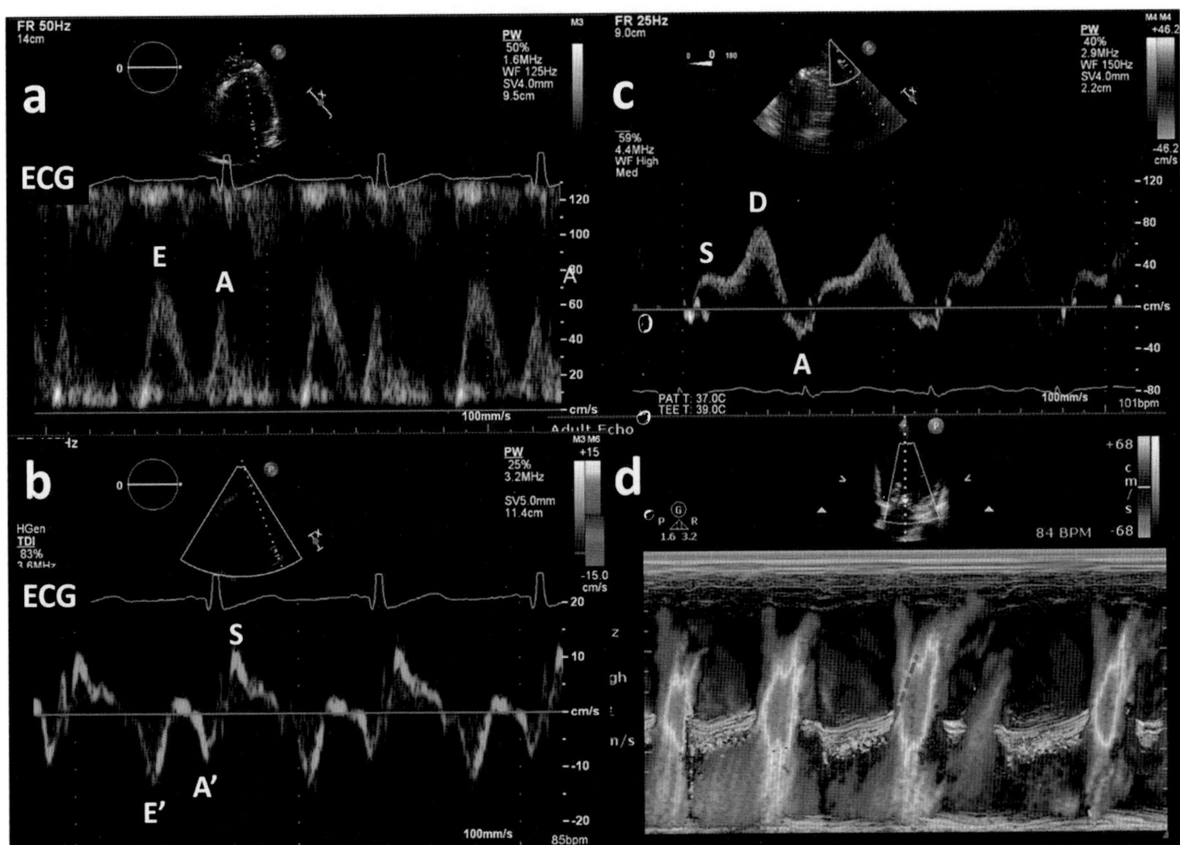

Figure 27.1 Methods for estimation of left atrial pressure using different types of Doppler. (a) PW Doppler across mitral valve showing dominant E wave, normal E deceleration time in a young patient with normal ejection fraction. (b) Tissue Doppler imaging of the lateral wall of the left ventricle, with systolic (S), E′ and A′ waves from the same patient as shown in (a). E/E′ is <10, indicating the left atrial pressure is not elevated. (c) PW Doppler of the pulmonary veins (TOE) with systolic (S), diastolic (D) and atrial (A) components in a patient with elevated left atrial pressure (suppression of the early S wave, with dominant D wave). (d) colour Doppler showing an M-mode of the inflow of the mitral valve, with the fastest aliasing velocity (red line). For explanation, see text. PW = pulse wave; TOE = trans-oesophageal echocardiography; ECG = electrocardiogram.

of lower velocity, a longer deceleration time (>240 ms) and an A-wave of progressively higher velocity. Thus, as normal values are age, inotropy, and filling dependent, as well as varying with pathology, interpretation in critically ill patients is challenging. Colour flow propagation velocity (CFPV; Fig. 27.1d), as determined by colour M-mode Doppler, has been proposed as a measurement to diagnose LV diastolic dysfunction (<50 cm/s indicating diastolic disease). Closely related to the time constant of isovolumic relaxation (Tau), CFPV is independent of heart rate, and relatively preload insensitive; however, TTE image quality on the ICU may limit its use. Finally, tissue Doppler imaging (TDI) of the myocardium at the base of the heart may assist in the diagnosis. Here early myocardial tissue velocities (E′) correlate with invasively measured Tau, thus providing a measure of myocardial relaxation (E′ of ≥10 cm/s is normal relaxation, <10 cm/s is impaired, and <5 cm/s is severely impaired; Fig. 27.1b,c).

RIGHT VENTRICLE

The RV is exquisitely sensitive to increases in afterload and reduction in coronary perfusion, and fails due to one or both of these factors, readily demonstrated using echocardiography.[11] In the ICU, RV dysfunction is commonly secondary to pulmonary disease/ventilation and/or LV dysfunction, where again echocardiography is pivotal for diagnosis. A range of techniques is used to assess RV function, including M-mode, PW Doppler and TDI.

RV systolic function

Due to its complex geometry, assessment of RV volumes using 2D echocardiography is challenging, with poor reproducibility. Normal RV wall thickness is 3.3 + 0.6 mm, and is smaller than the LV (RVEDA/LVED< 0.6).[3] Measurement of the longitudinal annular movement of the RV free wall using M-mode (tricuspid annular plane systolic excursion, TAPSE) correlates well with radionuclide and cardiac magnetic resonance assessment of RV function.[12] Normal TAPSE is 2 cm (**Fig. 27.2d**), falling after cardiac surgery to 1.5 cm,[12] and any reduction in TAPSE in the setting of pulmonary hypertension indicates significant RV dysfunction; an amplitude of <1 cm implies severe impairment. 3D echocardiography for assessment of RV function has a potential role, as although reportedly systematically underestimating RV volumes it is demonstrably superior to 2D for assessing contractility.[13]

RV diastolic function

The principles of assessment of LV diastolic function theoretically apply equally to the RV, although the isovolumic phases of the cardiac cycle are shorter, and more ill defined, transtricuspid velocities are lower, and subject to significant respiratory variation. RV restriction is common (43–50% ICU patients) and diagnosed by demonstrating forward flow across the pulmonary valve in late diastole (**Fig. 27.3a**).[14] Positive-pressure ventilation may abolish this pulmonary arterial diastolic wave, making the diagnosis more challenging. Further confounding factors include the presence of LV restriction, elevation of pulmonary arterial diastolic pressures, tachycardia and requirement for high ventilatory pressures.

GLOBAL MEASURES

A number of measures of systolic and diastolic (global) ventricular function have been proposed, the myocardial performance (Tei) index and total isovolumic time (t-IVT). The Tei index combines systolic and diastolic Doppler assessment, is simple to calculate, reproducible, independent of heart rate, blood pressure and characterised by low interobserver and intraobserver variability, and can be calculated for both the right and left heart (Tei=IVCT+IVRT/ET, normal LV=0.37± 0.05, normal RV=0.28±0.04).[3,15] Although predictive of mortality and morbidity in numerous cardiac pathologies, it is load and activation dependent, and is not well validated in the ICU. t-IVT is a marker of global ventricular electromechanical dyssynchrony, and effectively wasted time during the cardiac cycle (t-IVT=60-total filling time-total ejection time, normal <14 s/min).[3,16] Although also not well validated in the ICU setting, an abnormally prolonged t-IVT should prompt a search for the underlying cause (ischaemia/ ventricular dyssynchrony) and provide guidance for interventions to optimise CO. In selected patients, SV and CO can be increased by echocardiographically guided optimisation of pacing (36–43% increase), identified by demonstration of a prolonged t-IVT (up to 23% cardiothoracic patients).[17]

VALVULAR FUNCTION[3,18–19]

Valvular heart disease as a primary cause of ICU admission is likely to be severe, and affecting the left-sided valves. Pulmonary and tricuspid valvular disease rarely causes acute illness mandating ICU admission, unless associated with endocarditis.. The epidemiology and clinical manifestations of valvular heart disease relevant to intensive care are described in Chapter 25.

AORTIC STENOSIS

The echocardiographic diagnosis of aortic stenosis (AS) depends upon a number of features, including the presence of immobile valve leaflets, and demonstration of a significant increase in blood velocity as it crosses the narrowed valve orifice (high gradient). Echocardiographic features of severe AS are shown in **Table 27.4**.[18] Where LV function is poor and CO low, the increase in velocities across the aortic valve may be correspondingly low, and significant AS missed. Although there are no agreed values for what constitutes significant AS in the critically ill patient, a ×4 step-up in velocity across the valve probably indicates severe AS. TOE is

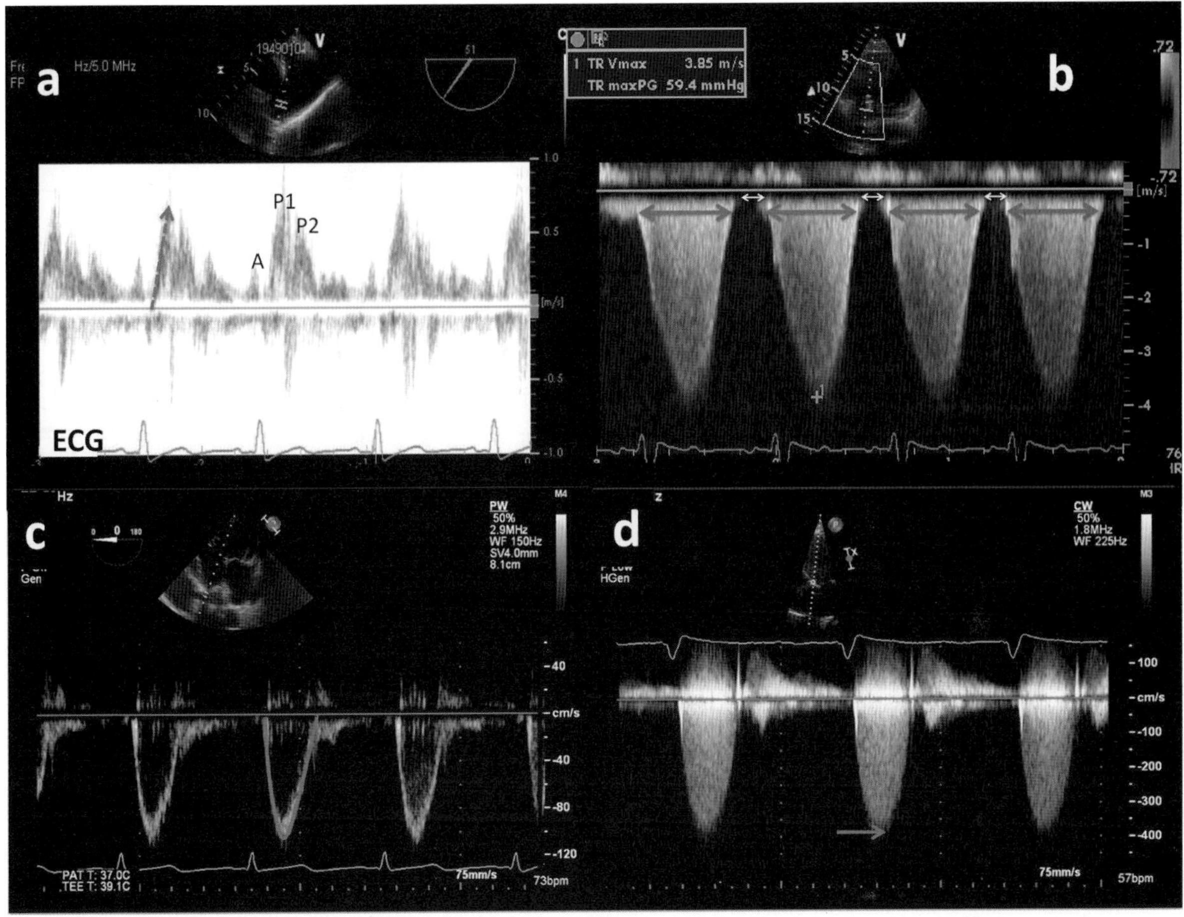

Figure 27.2 Echocardiographic features of pericardial collections (a) TTE parasternal long axis view in a patient with pleural and pericardial collections. The anatomical limits of the pericardial collection (P) are demonstrated with it appearing anterior to the descending aorta (*). The pleural collection (PL) can extend posterior to the descending aorta. The parietal pericardium (arrowed) is clearly seen between the two. Intra-cardiac shunting on echocardiography. (b) TTE subcostal view evidence of diastolic collapse on M-mode subcostal view. (c) 2D TOE showing a secundum ASD in a hypoxic patient with peumonia referred for extracorporeal membrane oxygenation. The left atrium is at the to of the image and shunting across the defect is clearly seen on colour Doppler (arrowed). Contrast TTE (apical 4-chamber view) in a patient with a large PFO. Here, the right heart is fully opacified with bubbles, and the LV partially opacified. (d) Evaluation of the RV systolic function: movement of the annulus with respect to the apex is measured using M-mode taken from the apical 4 chamber view (TTE), and demonstrated over time for (a) right ventricle, TAPSE. LV=left ventricle; P=pericardial collection; PL=pleural collection; RA=right atrium; RV=right ventricle; LA=left atrium; LV=left ventricle.

generally not indicated to confirm the diagnosis (Fig. 27.3d); however, an expert opinion should be sought regarding the TTE findings, as stress echocardiography may be indicated. Relevant additional echocardiographic findings include the degree of LV hypertrophy and dysfunction, pulmonary hypertension and the presence of concomitant valve disease (in particular in the presence of rheumatic AS or endocarditis).

AORTIC REGURGITATION

Aortic regurgitation (AR) is diagnosed using echocardiography by demonstration of a volume-loaded, dilated LV, and regurgitant jet using colour Doppler, confirmed using CW Doppler, together with inspection of the valve leaflets/aortic root. The diagnosis should be suspected in a patient with a low CO state associated with a hyperdynamic LV. Severe AR results in high forward velocities across the aortic valve, diastolic regurgitant velocities falling to <2 m/s at end-diastole, and holodiastolic flow reversal in the descending aorta. Echocardiographic features of severe AR are shown in Table 27.4.[18] Where AR is catastrophic, aortic velocities may reach zero before end-diastole, followed by diastolic MR. Here, M-mode of the mitral valve demonstrates premature closure.

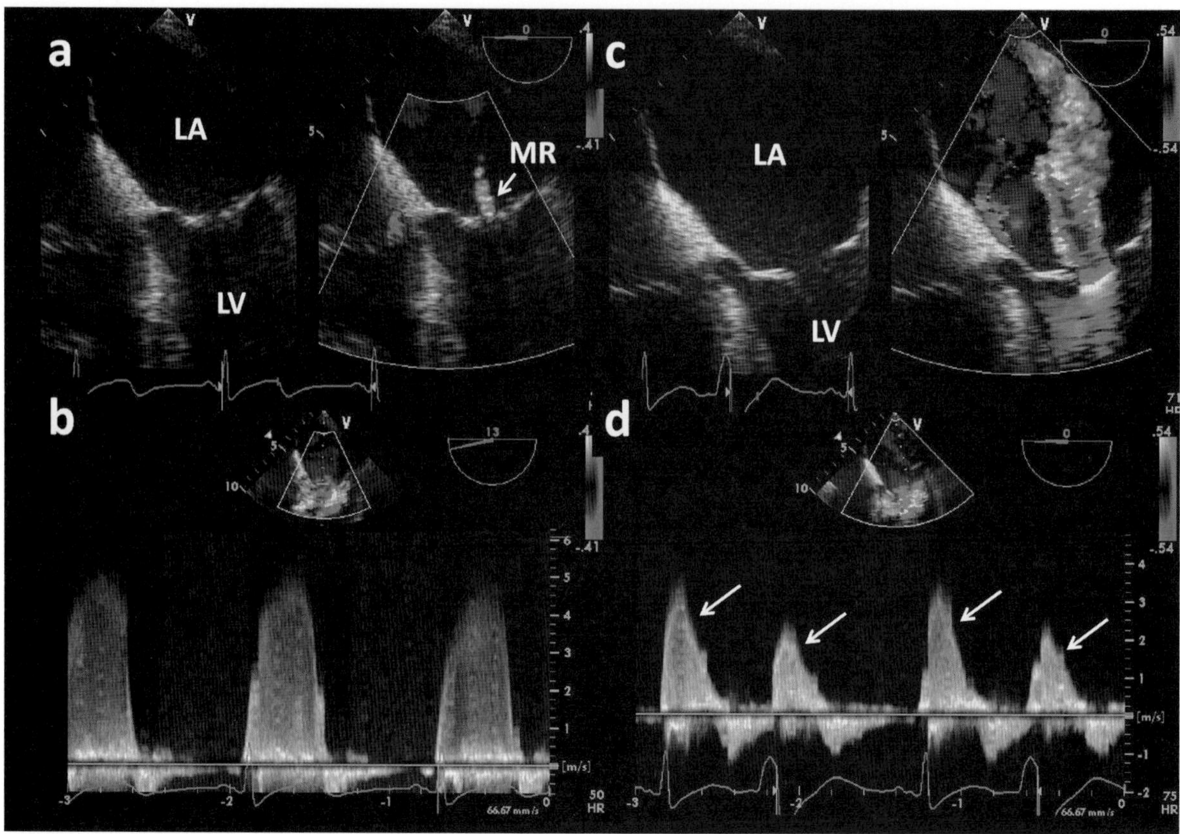

Figure 27.3 Doppler echocardiographic features of pulmonary hypertension and high pulmonary vascular resistance. (a) TOE showing PW Doppler across the pulmonary artery in a patient with severe pulmonary hypertension. The pulmonary acceleration time (time from onset to peak of forward flow, dotted arrow) is short, indicative of a high pulmonary vascular resistance. The presence of a double component of the pulmonary systolic wave (P1 and P2) is expression of high pressure. The pre-systolic pulmonary arterial wave (A) is indicative of RV restrictive physiology, corresponding to forward flow in late diastole as a result of atrial contraction (p wave on the ECG). (b) CW Doppler across the tricuspid valve in pulmonary hypertension showing TR. The peak systolic velocity between RV and RA is 3.9 m/s, corresponding to a peak gradient of 59.4 mmHg. Right atrial pressure was 20 mmHg, therefore calculated PASP is 59.4+20=19.4 mmHg. In addition, the TR is long (540 ms, solid red arrows), due to prolonged RV activation, and therefore limiting the time available in diastole for RV filling (white arrows). See text for full explanation. For orientation a miniaturised 2D figure is shown at the top of each image. ECG=electrocardiogram; TOE=transoesophageal echo; PW=pulse wave; RV=right ventricle; CW=continuous wave; TR=tricuspid regurgitation. Doppler evaluation of flow from the left heart. (c) PW Doppler with sample volume positioned in the left ventricle outflow tract, just below the aortic valve (shown by the parallel lines in the miniature 2D image at the top of the figure). The flow is laminar and moving from the LV to the descending aorta, away from the probe (flow is negative to respect to the baseline on Doppler trace). Tracing the envelope (shown in red) gives the velocity-time integral which when multiplied by the LVOT area gives the stroke volume. (d) CW Doppler across the LVOT and aortic valve in a patient with aortic stenosis (sample line dotted in miniature 2D image at the top of the figure). Peak velocity (arrowed in red) is 4 m/s, corresponding to a peak velocity of 64 mmHg (for explanation see text). ECG=electrocardiogram; PW=pulse wave; 2D=two dimension; LV=left ventricle; LVOT=left ventricular outflow tract; CW=continuous wave.

Care should be taken in the presence of significant LV disease, as equalisation of aortic and LV pressures at end-diastole measured by Doppler may occur owing to either very low aortic pressures (severe AR) or very high LV end-diastolic pressures (severe LV disease). Furthermore, the two entities may coexist. Where severe AR is diagnosed, echocardiography should be used to demonstrate the underlying cause and its complications, including endocarditis (vegetations/root abscess/abnormal communications/involvement of other valves) and dissection (anatomy of the dissection/coronary artery involvement/pericardial collection). In patients with suspected dissection, undertaking TOE should be integrated with surgical decision making/

Table 27.4 Echocardiographic parameters in severe valvular disease

	SEVERE STENOSIS	
	AORTIC STENOSIS	MITRAL STENOSIS
Valve area (cm^2)	<1.0	<1.0
Indexed valve area (cm^2/m^2 BSA)	<0.6	–
Mean gradient (mmHg) (kPa)	>40 (>5.32)	>10 (>1.33)
Maximum jet velocity (m/s)	>4.0	–
Velocity ratio	<0.25	–
	SEVERE REGURGITATION	
	AORTIC REGURGITATION	*MITRAL REGURGITATION*
Valve morphology	Abnormal/flail/large coaptation defect	Flail leaflet/ruptured papillary muscle/large coaptation defect
Colour flow regurgitant jet	Large in central jets, variable in eccentric jets	Very large central jet or eccentric jet adhering, swirling and reaching the posterior wall of the left atrium
CW signal of regurgitant jet	Dense	Dense, triangular
Other	Holodiastolic flow reversal in descending aorta (EDV >20 cm/s)	Large flow convergence zone

BSA=body surface area; CW=continuous wave; EDV=end-diastolic velocity.
Adapted from ESC/ESCTS guidelines on valvular heart disease (EHJ 2012).[18]

timing, as the risk of catastrophic haemodynamic destabilisation/progression of the dissection is significant. Depending upon local protocols, another imaging modality may be used to confirm the diagnosis, and TOE limited to intraoperative use.

MITRAL REGURGITATION

Quantification of mitral regurgitation (MR) is challenging, and confounded by the effects of positive-pressure ventilation and the use of vasoactive agents, as these may significantly alter the degree of regurgitation. Severe MR is diagnosed by demonstration of a dynamic, volume-overloaded LV in the presence of a low CO state plus a characteristic regurgitant jet on CW Doppler that is short, with a low velocity (<3 m/s) and high forward transmitral velocities (>160 cm/s). Echocardiographic features of severe MR are shown in Table 27.4.[18] In catastrophic MR, regurgitant flow may not be well visualised with colour Doppler, and PW Doppler across the valve may show low-velocity, sinusoidal, laminar flow. In assessing MV disease, the whole valve apparatus should be evaluated (leaflets, annulus and LV) and leaflets systematically analysed according to the Carpentier classification.[3,18,19] Care should be taken when assessing the MV following a penetrating chest wound, as a longitudinal injury to the anterior leaflet may result in its appearing structurally normal, despite having a significant defect. Secondary (functional) MR may be dynamic, and if suspected stress echocardiography should be considered. Where severe MR of any aetiology is suspected in a critically ill patient, expert TOE should be performed (**Fig. 27.4**).

In a small group of patients with left bundle branch block (LBBB), ventricular filling is temporally limited by the duration of MR, which may be only mild in terms of regurgitant volume. Here any increase in heart rate may result in further shortening of ventricular filling time, thereby limiting SV and CO.[20] In the outpatient setting, optimally timed AV delay pacing (using echocardiography) may increase SV significantly, although this has not yet been systematically demonstrated in the ICU setting.

MITRAL STENOSIS

The echocardiographic diagnosis of mitral stenosis (MS) depends upon demonstration of a structural abnormality of the leaflets (and/or subvalvular apparatus), together with an increase in blood velocity across the valve measured using Doppler. Thus, the diagnosis of MS may be challenging when the CO is low and echocardiographic transvalvular velocities are correspondingly low. Echocardiographic features of severe MS are shown in Table 27.4.[18] Additional findings that support the diagnosis include significant LA dilatation, pulmonary hypertension, RV dysfunction, and rheumatic involvement of other valves. Where diagnosed, expert TOE examination should be performed to determine the structural abnormalities of the valve and potential suitability for balloon mitral valvuloplasty, including presence/absence of left atrial thrombus.

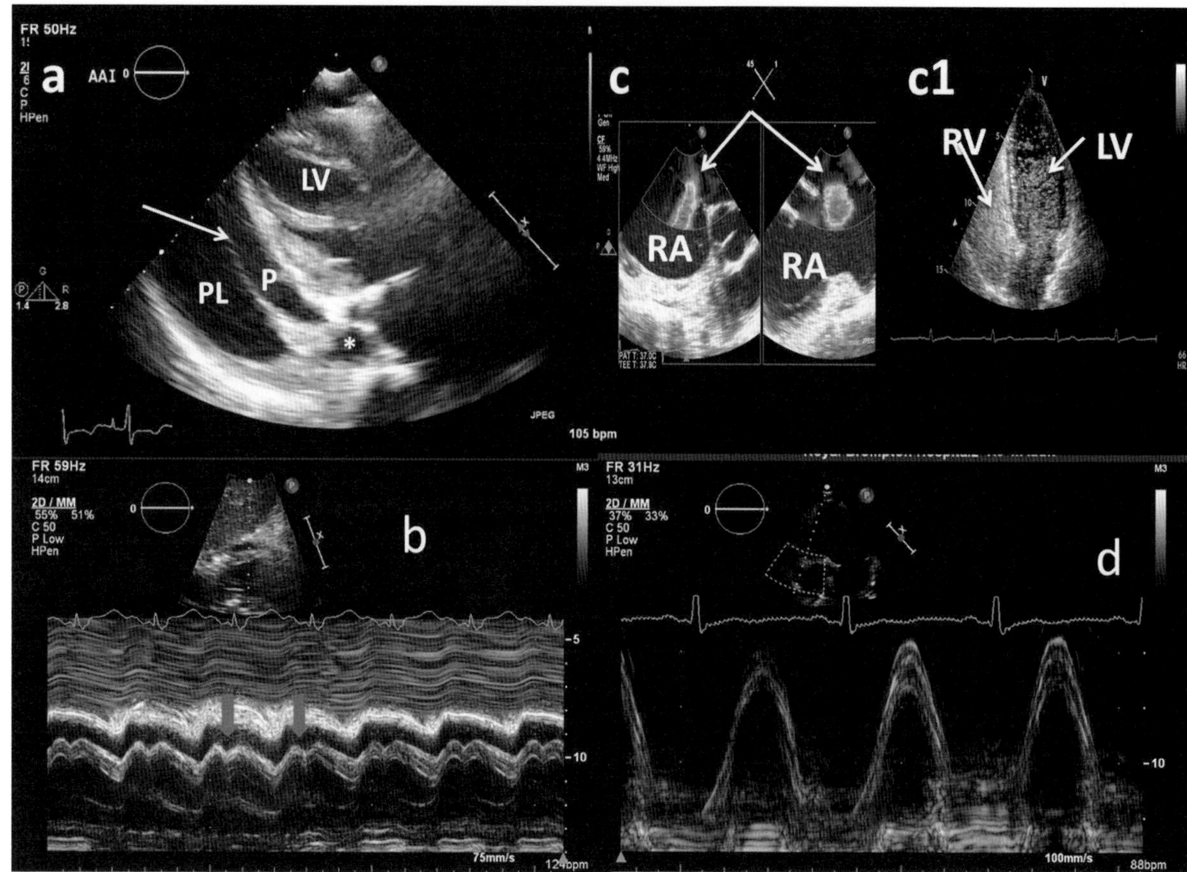

Figure 27.4 Echocardiographic features of dynamic MR under rest conditions (a & b) and after pressor and volume loading (c & d). (a) TOE mid-oesophageal 4-chamber view, focusing on the MV in systole. A small jet of MR is seen between the two central leaflets of the MV. (b) The corresponding CW regurgitant Doppler trace with a high velocity (5 m/s) and dome-like appearance. (c) after volume and pressor loading the MV leaflets no longer coapt (seen on the 2D image, left) and there is a corresponding broad jet of MR which is laminar and reaches the back of the LA. (d) CW Doppler of MR from (c) is shown, with a fall in MR velocities (despite increase in systemic pressures) and change in shape to triangular demonstrating the V-wave cutoff sign (arrowed). LA=left atrium; LV=left ventricle; MR=mitral regurgitation; TOE=transoesophageal echocardiography; MV=mitral valve; 2D=two dimensional.

PROSTHETIC VALVE MALFUNCTION

Significant prosthetic valve malfunction may result from either obstruction (pannus/thrombus) or regurgitation (paravalvular/valvular), which may be due to leaflet degeneration (biological prostheses) or endocarditis. Echocardiographic features include demonstration of a volume-overloaded LV, and/or evidence of normalisation of septal motion on TTE, together with direct evidence of valve malfunction (stenosis/regurgitation). Suspected infection of a prosthesis is an indication for expert TOE. In contrast to native valve endocarditis, it is unusual to see vegetations on a mechanical valve as infection tends to destroy the suture line rather than lead to the development of large masses.[3,18] The ability of echocardiography to differentiate between endocarditis and valve leaflet degeneration in bioprosthetic valvular regurgitation is limited, particularly where there is significant leaflet calcification; however, the presence of paraprosthetic regurgitation/abscesses supports the diagnosis of infection. Similarly, echocardiography is not the imaging modality of choice when differentiating between pannus and thrombus; here CT has been shown to be superior.

PERICARDIAL DISEASE

The pericardium comprises two layers, containing approximately 50 mL pericardial fluid (normal intrapericardial pressure –2 to 2 mmHg (–0.266 to 0.266 kPa)). Intrapericardial pressure falls with intrapleural pressure during inspiration (spontaneous ventilation) with a fall in right-sided cardiac pressures, and corresponding increase in right heart velocities. These effects are frequently exaggerated in patients with clinically significant pericardial disease, the most common of which is tamponade. Although primarily a clinical diagnosis, echocardiography can be used to confirm the diagnosis and to guide pericardiocentesis.

TAMPONADE

Tamponade is variably defined, but is an impairment of cardiac filling due to a rise in intrapericardial pressure, irrespective of the volume of pericardial collection. Hence, a small, rapidly accumulating collection may have profound haemodynamic effects, and by contrast a slowly accumulating, large collection may be associated with a modest rise in intrapericardial pressure and no haemodynamic effects. The first stage in echocardiographic diagnosis of tamponade is to demonstrate a collection within the pericardial space (Fig. 27.2a). This should be described according to its size, site and consistency. The second stage is to demonstrate the haemodynamic effects of the collection (Fig. 27.2b).[3] These all depend upon the pressure effects upon the relevant cardiac chamber, and may be modified in the presence of cardiac disease.

When the pericardial pressure exceeds that of a cardiac chamber, echocardiography may show chamber collapse; those with the lowest pressure are most vulnerable. Additionally, as pressures differ during the cardiac cycle, the vulnerability of each depends upon the phase of the cardiac cycle. Hence sequential demonstration of RV early-diastolic collapse, RA late-diastolic collapse, LA late-diastolic collapse and LV early-diastolic collapse may be seen as tamponade progresses. The sensitivity and specificity of these signs are variable, with RV diastolic collapse specific (85–100%) but less sensitive (60–90%) than sustained (>30% cycle) diastolic collapse of the RA. Additional features that support the diagnosis include a swinging heart, pseudosystolic anterior motion of the MV, and demonstration of fixed, dilated caval veins.

With the heart encased within a non-expansile collection, the normal respiratory variation in transvalvular flows will be exaggerated, demonstrated readily using echocardiography. Thus, in spontaneous ventilation, during inspiration as intrathoracic pressure falls, this results in an increase in venous return to the right heart, and this results in a shift of the interventricular septum, and a fall in left-sided flows. This exaggerated variation (>25% tricuspid or >15% mitral) is regarded as abnormal, and corresponds to the clinical sign of pulsus paradoxus. Positive-pressure ventilation reverses the effect.

HAEMODYNAMICS[3,21]

In addition to its role in diagnosis of underlying cardiac disease, echocardiography can be used as an adjunct for assessment of haemodynamics. It is important to note that echocardiography cannot measure pressures per se, but rather the velocity of blood moving from one chamber to another as a result of a pressure difference between the two chambers. Any pressure measurements are therefore derived, and should be interpreted with care.

CARDIAC OUTPUT AND STROKE VOLUME

Stroke volume (SV) is measured using echocardiography by multiplying the velocity–time integral (VTI, also known as stroke distance, normal 20 cm) by the cross-sectional area of the relevant outflow tract at that point (LV or RV). VTI is measured using PW Doppler (Fig. 27.3c) immediately (5–10 mm) proximal to either the aortic or pulmonary valve, and the relevant outflow tract dimension measured at the same point. The greatest source of error is calculation of the cross-sectional area as images may be suboptimal, the outflow tract non-circular, and any error in radial measurement will be magnified (area $=\pi r^2$). As outflow tract dimensions measured do not vary over the short term, trends in VTI may be used to monitor changes in SV.

LEFT ATRIAL PRESSURES

A number of echocardiographic techniques either alone or in combination can be used to estimate left atrial pressure (LAP). These range from the use of traditional techniques (M-mode and phonocardiography) to more complex and modern applications (TDI).

As LAP rises, the pattern of transmitral flow changes. Thus, where there is severe reduction in ventricular (or pericardial) compliance the increase in filling pressure causes abnormalities in LV filling. Here, as LAP increases, equalisation of atrial and ventricular pressures occurs early, the mitral valve opens earlier than normal (short IVRT is <60 ms), the increased LAP increases the transmitral gradient in early-diastole (increasing E-wave peak) with rapid equalisation of ventricular and atrial pressures (short E deceleration time <160 ms).[3,10] Further, because of the high LVEDP, little/no filling occurs with atrial contraction and the A-wave is markedly reduced or absent – restrictive physiology. However, because of the conflicting effects of ageing and pathology, none of these parameters can be used alone to estimate LAP.

Combining transmitral Doppler (blood velocities) with TDI (tissue velocities) has been shown to improve the correlation with LAP. Here, the ratio E/E′ is calculated, with a ratio <10 corresponding to LAP<15 mmHg (2 kPa), and ratio >15 corresponding to LAP>18 mmHg (2.4 kPa); however, a number of controversies exist, and as correlation between 11–14 is poor, additional parameters should be used, generally in combination.[3,21,22] Thus, using PW Doppler indices, mitral E/A<1.4, pulmonary vein S/D > 0.65 and EF > 44% have been shown to predict PAOP<18 mmHg (2.4 kPa), and/or using TDI and colour Doppler, a lateral E/E′<8.0 or E/*V*p<1.7 predicted a PAOP<18 mmHg (2.4 kPa) (sensitivity of 83% and 80%, and specificity of 88% and 100%) (Fig. 27.1).[23]

PULMONARY ARTERY PRESSURES

Pulmonary artery systolic pressure (PASP) can be estimated by measuring maximal tricuspid regurgitation (TR) velocity using CW Doppler, and applying the simplified Bernoulli equation to convert this number into a pressure (RV pressure=4×(peak TR velocity)^2). Estimated right atrial pressure (RAP) is then added to calculate PASP. Care is needed in severe RV dysfunction, as PASP may be significantly underestimated by this technique; further, PASP may fall owing to progressive RV failure. In the absence of TR, the pulmonary regurgitation (PR) trace can be interrogated to estimate PA diastolic pressure (4×(PR end-diastolic velocity)^2 + RAP) and mean PA pressure (4×(PR peak velocity)^2). Finally, increased PVR is suggested by a short pulmonary acceleration time (<80 ms) and is calculated using the ratio of peak TR velocity to the RVOT VTI ($PVR=TR/VTI_{RVOT}\times10 + 0.16$).[3,21]

RIGHT ATRIAL PRESSURES

Where invasive measurement of RAP is not available, echocardiography may be used to estimate its value, by measurement of IVC size (<20 mm vs >20 mm), degree of IVC inspiratory collapse (<50% vs >50%) and hepatic vein dimension (normal vs dilated).[3] However, their validity in the ICU population is questionable.

VOLUME RESPONSIVENESS

Echocardiography allows assessment of the patient's volume status, complementary to invasive haemodynamic measurements.[3,4,21] Echocardiographic volume status assessment is based on static values (single-measure dimensions and flows) and dynamic indices (variation in flows and dimensions after dynamic manoeuvres).

STATIC PARAMETERS

Estimation of preload- and volume-responsiveness using static measurements is generally unreliable. However, the following parameters have been suggested to indicate severe hypovolaemia in the critically ill: first, a small, hyperkinetic LV (in the presence of a normal RV) with end-systolic cavity obliteration, secondly LV end-diastolic area <5.5 cm^2/m^2 BSA and thirdly a small IVC (<10 mm) with inspiratory collapse (spontaneously breathing patients), or a small IVC at end-expiration with variable respiratory change (mechanically ventilated patients). In this scenario, though, the correlation between IVC dimensions and RAP is poor. LAP does not correlate with volume responsiveness, but demonstration of abnormally high pressures with a restrictive filling pattern should signal caution in volume resuscitation.

DYNAMIC PARAMETERS

These include a number of measures (including effects of mechanical ventilation and passive leg raising on cardiac function/filling status) to predict a potential increase in SV in response to filling. Passive leg raising has been proposed to predict fluid responsiveness in spontaneously breathing patients; however, sensitivity and specificity are relatively low, and the number and nature of confounding factors (intra-abdominal pressure, hypovolaemia, arrhythmia) probably limit its usefulness in the ICU population.

Cyclical changes in intrathoracic pressure induced by mechanical ventilation result in corresponding cyclical changes in right and left heart filling, and hence in SV (if the patient is on the ascending part of the Frank–Starling curve). Thus, respiratory variations in VTI may be used as an index of fluid responsiveness (cut-off 18% variation VTI, 12% variation peak LVOT velocity; **Fig. 27.5**) and are comparable with the techniques of systolic pressure, SV and pulse pressure variation measured using other monitors.[3,4,21,24] In addition, respiratory variation in SVC and IVC dimensions have been proposed to predict fluid responsiveness. An IVC distensibility index (maximum–minimum/minimum) >18% (12% normalised to mean value) has been suggested to predict a significant increase in SV in response to fluid challenge. In contrast, a high SVC collapsibility index (maximum–minimum/maximum) >36% predicts a positive response to volume expansion (≥15% increase in SV) with sensitivity 90% and specificity 100%. A number of caveats exist when interpreting dynamic volume responsiveness: patients must be in sinus rhythm, fully mechanically ventilated, with no spontaneous breathing effort. Further, the effects of lung protective ventilatory strategies may lead to false-negative values, and false-positive results may be seen in patients with RV disease.

ECHOCARDIOGRAPHY IN SPECIFIC SCENARIOS

A number of clinical scenarios/questions may be raised in the critically ill that potentially require focused echocardiography, rather than a fully comprehensive study. The ICU echocardiographer must know the potential pitfalls and coexisting pathologies in order to make a relevant assessment.

MYOCARDIAL ISCHAEMIA/INFARCTION

Echocardiography is included in the universal definition of myocardial infarction (MI), and suspicion of a mechanical complication of MI is a class IA indication for echocardiography.[19] Generally the extent of infarction/ischaemia should be demonstrated and

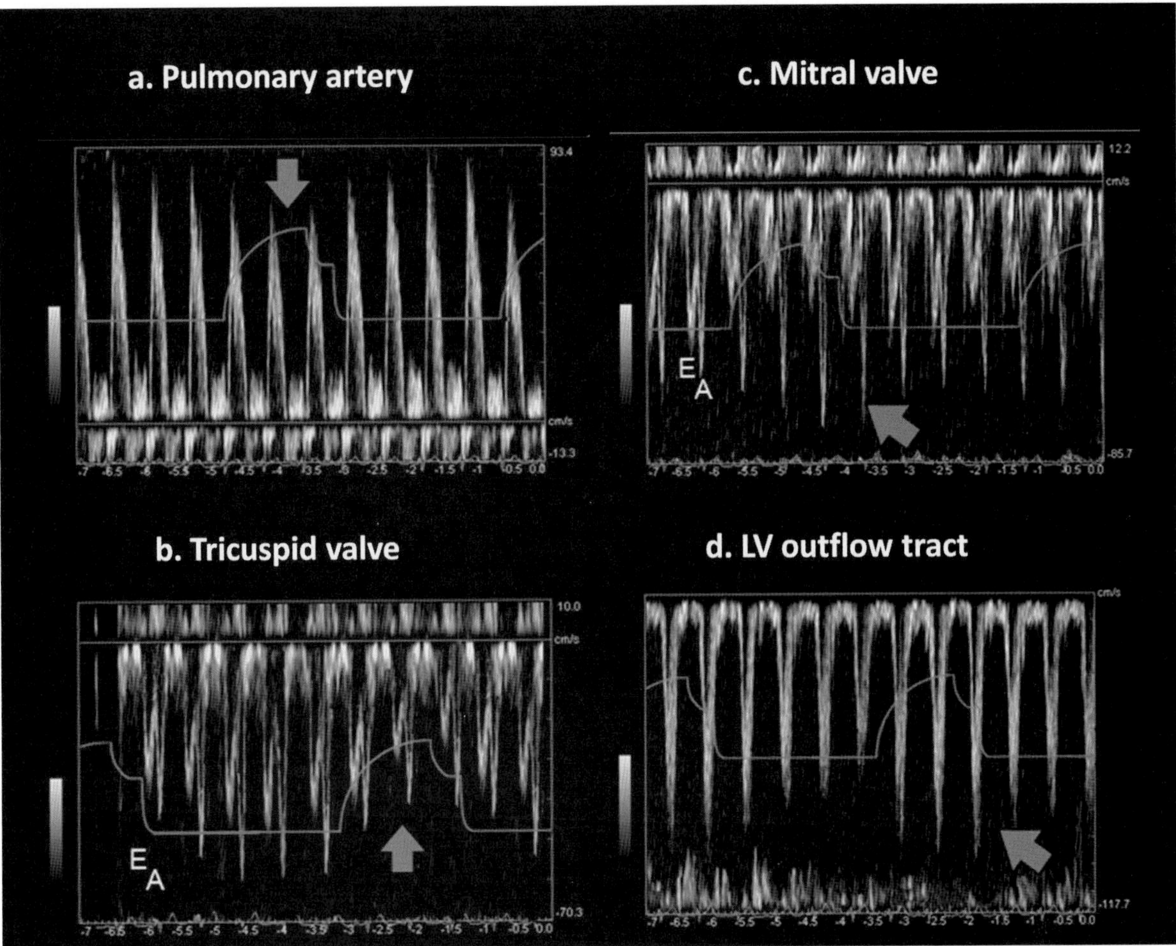

Figure 27.5 Variation in transvalvular flows in response to positive pressure ventilation measured using PW Doppler echocardiography, and superimposed ventilatory pressure waves shown in green. On the left of the figure, changes in right heart velocities are shown, and on the right, changes in left heart velocities. During inspiration there is a fall in peak velocity across the (a) pulmonary and (b) tricuspid valves. After inspiration there is a corresponding progressive fall in (c) transmitral and (d) LV outflow tract velocities (arrowed). For full explanation, see text. LV=left ventricle. Image courtesy of G. Via, Italy.

complications (MR, ventricular septal rupture (VSR)/cardiac rupture/RV infarction) actively excluded.

MR may result from complete/partial papillary muscle rupture, which is usually very severe. More common is posterior leaflet restriction due to inferior/posterior infarction/ischaemia, with associated functional MR, which may be dynamic, presenting as failure to wean from mechanical ventilatory support. Here a targeted echocardiogram performed when the patient is clinically compromised is indicated, and/or stress echocardiography (dobutamine+volume loading/pressor agents).

VSR is now a relatively uncommon complication, but should be suspected in patients post MI presenting with cardiogenic shock. Imaging may be challenging as rupture may occur at any point in the septum, the defects may be multiple, but are generally easily appreciated using colour Doppler. Care should be taken in interpreting LV function, as it may appear deceptively good (due to offloading to the RV), and additional assessment must include RV function, MR and PASP. A small amount of fluid in the pericardial space is common following transmural MI, rarely causing haemodynamic compromise. By contrast LV free wall rupture may occur, resulting in a very rapidly accumulating collection and catastrophic tamponade. RV infarction should be suspected in patients with occlusion of the proximal right coronary artery, and function assessed using standard parameters, together with measurement of PASP, LV function and exclusion of right–left shunting through a PFO. Differentiation between RV infarction and pulmonary embolism (PE) can be challenging, but suggested by the absence of pulmonary hypertension and coexistence of LV postero-inferior hypokinesia.

ACUTE COR PULMONALE (ACP)

This is characterised by a sudden severe increase in RV afterload resulting in acute RV dilatation and failure. Major causes of ACP include acute pulmonary embolism and ARDS.

PULMONARY EMBOLISM (PE)

The definitive diagnosis is made by demonstration of thrombi/masses in the pulmonary arteries, although in the majority of cases echocardiography provides only indirect signs of PE. These include pulmonary hypertension, signs of RV systolic overload (septal dyskinesia), diastolic overload, RV free wall hypokinesia and moderate–severe TR.[3,25] Pre-existing pulmonary hypertension is suggested by RV hypertrophy and PASP > 60 mmHg (7.98 kPa).

ACUTE RESPIRATORY DISTRESS SYNDROME

ACP occurs relatively commonly in this patient population, and has been shown to correlate with increased mortality. Where the diagnosis of ARDS/ALI is made, mechanical ventilation may have unfavourable effects on RV function, owing to altered pulmonary dynamics and secondary increase in alveolar pressure and PVR. Due to introduction of more lung-protective ventilatory strategies this is less frequently seen; however, a mild degree of RV dysfunction is common and, where present, ventilation can be altered to minimise plateau and positive end-expiratory pressures.[26] Diagnosis of RV dysfunction is important in patients with lung injury considered for mechanical circulatory support, as it may preclude the use of shunt-inducing devices (interventional lung assist/veno-venous extracorporeal membrane oxygenation).

HYPOXAEMIA

Echocardiography may be used in the diagnosis and management of hypoxaemic patients on the ICU, including establishing the differential diagnosis (cardiogenic vs non-cardiac), assessment of secondary effects of pulmonary pathology on cardiac performance, diagnosis of a low CO state and/or diagnosis of anatomical shunt (intracardiac or intrapulmonary).

Many ICU factors increase right-sided pressures, leading to right–left intracardiac shunting across an atrial septal defect/patent foramen ovale (Fig. 27.2c). Intrapulmonary shunts are independent of right-sided pressure, and have been described in ARDS, pneumonia, thoracic trauma and hepatic cirrhosis. The choice of technique to demonstrate shunting depends upon clinical context, quality of imaging and need for detection of intrapulmonary shunt; however, TOE is generally superior. Diagnosis depends on a positive agitated saline contrast study (intracardiac; microbubbles pass into the LA immediately vs intrapulmonary; delayed appearance microbubbles via pulmonary veins; (Fig. 27.2c)), visualisation of the relevant structural abnormality and colour Doppler confirmation. Provocative manoeuvres (i.e. Valsalva) may be required, and in the presence of high LAP a shunt may be missed.

WEANING FROM MECHANICAL VENTILATION

Discontinuation of positive-pressure ventilation increases LV afterload and preload, and significantly increases the rate–pressure product. In patients with cardiac disease this may result in the left and/or right heart being unable to match the increased work, leading to rising LAP, pulmonary oedema, and/or RV dysfunction. Echocardiography can diagnose a cardiovascular contribution to weaning failure, and suggest interventions to facilitate successful withdrawal of mechanical ventilatory support. A baseline echocardiogram should be performed at the start of the weaning trial, and evidence of inotropy, lusitropy, chronotropy (negative/positive), preload and afterload mismatch should be actively sought. Additionally evidence of increasing LAP, myocardial ischaemia, decrease in LV/RV global function and/or worsening atrioventricular valvular regurgitation suggests a cardiac contribution to failure to wean.

SEPSIS SYNDROMES

Echocardiography plays a key role in the management of the septic ICU patient by guiding haemodynamic management and excluding cardiac causes for sepsis. Sepsis-related LV dysfunction is well recognised, with global and regional wall motion abnormalities described in up to 60% of patients.[27,28] RV dysfunction develops in up to 30% of patients, either in isolation or associated with LV dysfunction.[29] Ventricular dysfunction can be masked by vasodilatation and/or inadequate preload and should be reassessed after haemodynamic optimisation.[4,30] Emerging evidence in the paediatric literature suggests strain/strain rate imaging may detect significant abnormalities in ventricular function in septic shock that are not detectable by conventional echocardiography.[31]

Echocardiography may reveal a cardiac source of sepsis related to either native/prosthetic valve infection or indwelling catheters/implanted devices. The diagnosis of endocarditis is made on the basis of a well-established set of diagnostic criteria, of which echocardiography is one of the major factors. Three echocardiographic findings are important: mobile echodense mass(es) attached to valvular/mural endocardium/implanted material, fistulae/abscess formation, and/or new disruption/dehiscence of a prosthetic valve. TOE has a higher sensitivity and specificity, and is mandated where prosthetic valve endocarditis is suspected, to identify major complications and guide surgical planning.[3,18,19]

CATECHOLAMINE-INDUCED LV DYSFUNCTION

Excessive catecholamine use may result in myocardial ischaemia or Takotsubo cardiomyopathy.[32] These can be readily diagnosed using echocardiography. In addition, catecholamines may result in dynamic LV outflow tract obstruction diagnosed by demonstration of cavity/outflow tract obliteration using 2D echocardiography together with high outflow velocities on CW Doppler.[3,4]

CHEST TRAUMA[3]

There are several considerations in the ICU echocardiography in this patient population. When tamponade is suspected TTE provides a rapid diagnosis, otherwise it has a relatively low diagnostic yield compared with TOE. A wide range of abnormalities have been described following chest trauma, and where time permits a comprehensive study should be performed to diagnose/exclude: pericardial/pleural collections, aortic and mitral valve disruption, aortic disruption (high sensitivity and specificity with TOE), VSR, coronary artery disruption (ischaemia and/or fistulae) and myocardial contusion.

TAMPONADE POST-CARDIAC SURGERY[33]

Collections may accumulate rapidly, but be small, localised and difficult to demonstrate using TTE owing to persistent presence of air in the mediastinum immediately postoperatively. Diagnosis relying on TTE misses ≤50% cases, and TOE should be considered. As tamponade is a clinical diagnosis, in the presence of suggestive features re-exploration is the investigation of choice.

CONCLUSIONS

The potential scope for ICU echocardiography is huge, and expanding. In the near future, all practitioners involved in acute care will have the skills necessary for basic, focused echocardiography, in particular as US extends into the medical student curriculum.[34] Comprehensive echocardiography in the critically ill is challenging, and although cardiology-based echocardiographers may possess the full range of echocardiographic techniques, they will not necessarily have the ICU knowledge necessary to put them into clinical context. Similarly, although increasing numbers of intensivists are undergoing training in echocardiography, they may not have access to the full range of echocardiographic techniques required, although it is important to remember that the older techniques have much to offer and can be applied in a sophisticated manner within the pathophysiological context of the intensive care unit. With cardiologists returning to cardiac ICU, and intensivists embracing the technique of echocardiography, the potential for future collaborative research in this field is clear.

Access the complete references list online at http://www.expertconsult.com

4. Price S, Via G, Sloth E, et al. World Interactive Network Focused On Critical UltraSound ECHO-ICU Group. Echocardiography practice, training and accreditation in the intensive care: document for the World Interactive Network Focused on Critical Ultrasound (WINFOCUS). Cardiovasc Ultrasound 2008;6:49.
10. Gibson DG, Francis DP. Clinical assessment of left ventricular diastolic function. Heart 2003;89:231–8.
11. Haddad F, Hunt SA, Rosenthal DN, et al. Right ventricular function in cardiovascular disease, part I: Anatomy, physiology, aging, and functional assessment of the right ventricle. Circulation 2008;117:1436–48.
18. Joint Task Force on the Management of Valvular Heart Disease of the European Society of Cardiology (ESC); European Association for Cardio-Thoracic Surgery (EACTS); Vahanian A, Alfieri O, Andreotti F, et al. Guidelines on the management of valvular heart disease (version 2012). Eur Heart J 2012; 33:(19):2451–96.
19. Galiuto L, Badano L, Fox K, et al. The EAE Textbook of Echocardiography. New York: Oxford University Press; 2011.
21. De Backer D, Cholley B, Slama M, et al. Haemodynamic monitoring using echocardiography in the critically ill. Berlin: Springer; 2011.
23. Vignon P, AitHssain A, François B, et al. Echocardiographic assessment of pulmonary artery occlusion pressure in ventilated patients: a transoesophageal study. Crit Care 2008;12(1):R18. Epub 2008 Feb 19.

Part Four

Respiratory Failure

28

Oxygen therapy

Adrian J Wagstaff

In humans, uptake of environmental oxygen via the lungs provides necessary substrate for energy production. This is a key ingredient to survival. Aerobic respiration is the most efficient mechanism for adenosine triphosphate (ATP) production by oxidative phosphorylation and serves as the fuel to maintain cellular homeostasis and metabolism. Absence or lack of ATP leads to loss of cellular integrity initially followed by cellular and later organism death. A substantial part of critical care is targeted at treating and/or preventing hypoxia, yet in recent years the risks of hyperoxia leading to organ damage have become better understood. Thus an understanding of the common pathways and significance of cellular hypoxia is vital to providing appropriate and safe support and treatment to the acutely unwell patient.

PHYSIOLOGY OF OXYGEN DELIVERY

The transfer of a gas across a membrane relies on physical principles and is summarised by Fick's first law of diffusion[1]:

$$O_2 \text{ diffusion} = K \times A/T \times \Delta P \qquad (28.1)$$

where K is the diffusion constant for a particular gas, A is the surface of a membrane; T is the membrane's thickness and ΔP the difference in partial pressure across the membrane. As oxygen is poorly soluble in water, diffusion alone became insufficient to deliver oxygen to the cells, and novel methods of delivery have evolved, most notably the cardiovascular system.[2] This provided the means to deliver oxygen around the body.

OXYGEN DELIVERY

Transport of oxygen to the cells can thus be divided into six simple steps reliant only on the laws of physics: (1) convection of oxygen from the environment into the body (ventilation); (2) diffusion of oxygen into the blood (oxygen uptake): (3) reversible chemical bonding with haemoglobin; (4) convective transport of oxygen to the tissues (cardiac output): (5) diffusion into the cells and organelles; (6) the redox state of the cell. This chain of events is oxygen delivery or more correctly oxygen flux ($\dot{D}_{O_2}$).

Step 1: convection – ventilation The first step occurs in the lung in the form of pulmonary ventilation. At sea level the partial pressure of oxygen in environmental air is approximately 160 mmHg (21.3 kPa). On inspiration the air is humidified and mixed with exhaled carbon dioxide (CO_2) such that at the alveolus the P_{AO_2} is 100 mmHg (13.3 kPa). This will vary in different environments and different conditions (**Table 28.1**). Much of oxygen therapy is based on increasing oxygen delivery into the lungs whether by masks or other devices.

Step 2: diffusion – alveolus to blood Oxygen within the alveolus diffuses across the alveolar–capillary membrane. The average thickness of the alveolar capillary membrane is 0.3 μm and the surface area of the respiratory membrane between 50 and 100 m^2. This leads to a Pa_{O_2} in the pulmonary capillaries of approximately 90 mmHg (12 kPa). Herein lies many of the problems seen in the critically ill where two mechanisms predominate: (1) the thickness and barrier effect of the space between alveolus and capillary - usually a minor issue, and (2) the relationship between perfusion and ventilation at alveolar level (*V/Q* ratio) - in ARDS intrapulmonary shunt is the predominant cause of hypoxaemia.

Step 3: haemoglobin binding Oxygen is poorly soluble in water, having a solubility of 0.003082 g/100 g H_2O. Having diffused across the alveolar capillary membrane, the oxygen binds rapidly to the respiratory pigment haemoglobin. The saturation of haemoglobin with oxygen (Sa_{O_2}):P_{O_2} relationship is not linear and forms a sigmoidal shape (**Fig. 28.1**). The P50 is the Pa_{O_2} at which 50% of the haemoglobin is saturated. Various factors are known to alter the affinity of haemoglobin for oxygen (**Table 28.2**). These have teleological advantages as for example, a low pH or high CO_2 at tissue level could imply tissue hypoxia, and the reduction in oxygen-binding affinity increases oxygen availability. Similarly hyperthermia (fever), hypercarbia and an increase in the concentration of 2,3-diphosphoglycerate (2,3 DPG) all move the curve to the right and increase oxygen availability. 2,3-DPG is a by-product of glycolysis and therefore binds haemoglobin in predominantly hypoxic tissues, facilitating a release of oxygen. Conversely hypocarbia, alkalosis and low concentrations of 2,3-DPG result in a leftward shift of the curve and a

Table 28.1 Clinical significance of some Pa_{O_2} and Sa_{O_2} values

Pa_{O_2}		Sa_{O_2}	
MMHG	KPA	(%)	CLINICAL SIGNIFICANCE
160	20.0	99	Inspired air at sea level
97	12.9	97	Young normal man
80	10.6	95	Young normal man asleep Old normal man awake Inspired air at 19000 ft (5800 m)
70	9.3	93	Lower limit of normal
60	8.0	90	Respiratory failure (mild); shoulder of O_2 dissociation curve
50	6.7	85	Respiratory failure (significant); admit to hospital
40	5.3	75	Venous blood – normal Arterial blood – respiratory failure (severe). Acclimatised man at rest at 9000 ft (2750 m)
30	4.0	60	Unconscious if not acclimatised
26	3.5	50	P50 of haemoglobin
20	2.7	36	Acclimatised mountaineer exercising at 19000 ft (5800 m); hypoxic death

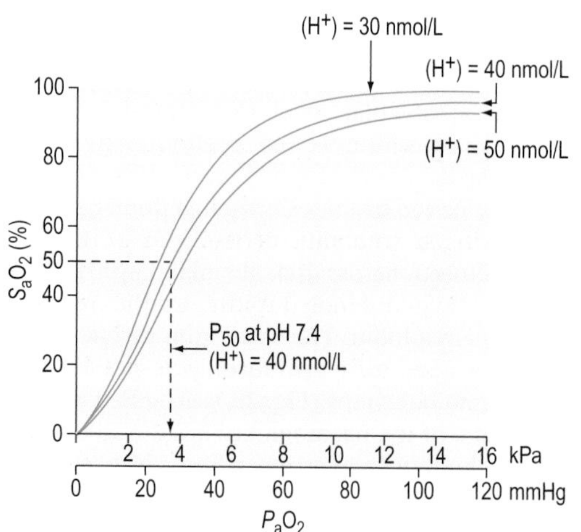

Figure 28.1 Haemoglobin oxygen dissociation curve. Normal curve at 40 nmol/L and shifts to left and right.

higher affinity for binding for any given P_{O_2}. Systemic interventions such as alteration in P_{CO_2} or pH will influence the curve and therefore oxygen dissociation and availability.

Step 4: convection – cardiovascular In humans the cardiovascular system is the solitary delivery system of

Table 28.2 Factors influencing the position of the oxygen dissociation curve

FACTORS INCREASING P50 (CURVE SHIFTS TO THE RIGHT)	FACTORS DECREASING P50 (CURVE SHIFTS TO THE LEFT)
Hyperthermia	Hypothermia
Decreased pH (acidaemia)	Increased pH (alkalaemia)
Increased P_{CO_2} (Bohr effect)	Decreased P_{CO_2}
Increased 2,3 DPG	Decreased 2,3 DPG Fetal haemoglobin Carbon monoxide Methaemoglobin

oxygen to the cells. This is achieved by the convection (bulk flow) of oxygen, predominantly bound to haemoglobin (21 mL/100 mL) from the lungs via the heart and out into the systemic circulation by way of the arteries. These branch down to form the capillaries where the oxygen is offloaded to the tissues. Convection of oxygen by the cardiovascular system is influenced centrally by the cardiac output (CO) and peripherally by local control of the regional perfusion of the tissues.

Oxygen delivery also relies on its concentration in the blood (Ca_{O_2}). This is calculated by the formula[3]:

$$Ca_{O_2} = (Hb(g/dL) \times 1.39 \times Sa_{O_2}(\%)) + (0.003 \times Pa_{O_2}) \quad (28.2)$$

Each gram of haemoglobin binds 1.39 mL of oxygen. Thus changes in Sa_{O_2} and haemoglobin concentration are important in determining the oxygen concentration. Delivery of oxygen is therefore summarised by the formula:

$$\text{delivery of oxygen } (\dot{D}_{O_2})\text{ mL/min} = 10 \times \text{CO (L/min)} \times Ca_{O_2} \quad (28.3)$$

Normal resting $\dot{D}_{O_2}$ is approximately 1000 mL/min. Oxygen consumption ($\dot{V}_{O_2}$) at rest is about 250 mL/min:

$$\text{oxygen consumption } (\dot{V}_{O_2})\text{ mL/min} = 10 \times \text{CO (L/min)} \times (Ca_{O_2} - C\bar{v}_{O_2}) \quad (28.4)$$

where $C\bar{v}_{O_2}$ is calculated as $(1.39 \times [Hb] \times S\bar{v}_{O_2}) + (0.003 \times P\bar{v}_{O_2})$. It can be seen that the amount of oxygen extracted is about 25% of that delivered at rest and that there is a large reserve. This obviously varies between organs. This ratio is referred to as the oxygen extraction ratio: $OER = \dot{V}_{O_2} / \dot{D}_{O_2}$.

During exercise this can increase by up to 70–80% at maximum. Oxygen that is not removed by the tissues returns to the heart and lungs. Globally the difference between that delivered and that returning is the consumption. This model can also be used to look at regional consumption. Hence the saturation of mixed venous blood ($S\bar{v}_{O_2}$) which is all the returning blood, or

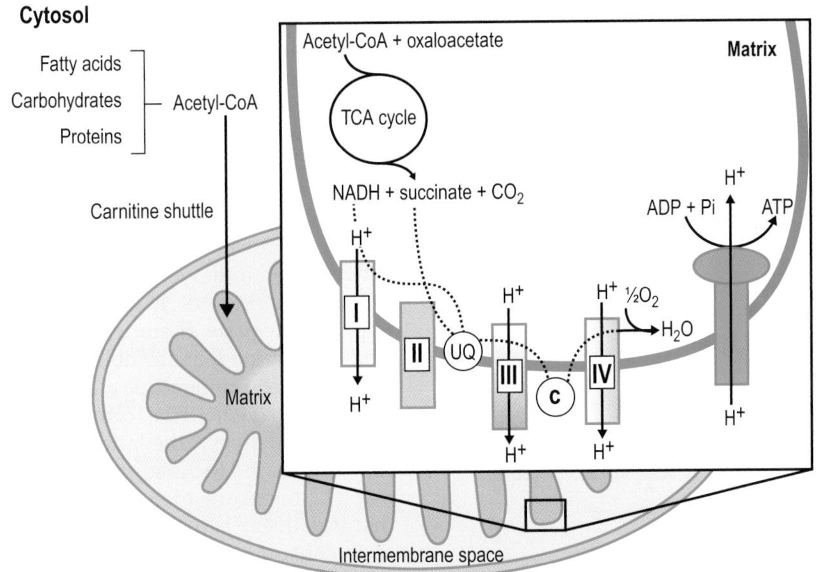

Figure 28.2 Schematic representation of the mitochondrion. Detail of the electron transport chain within the inner mitochondrial membrane is shown. *(After van Boxel[4].)*

central venous blood (most of the returning blood), can be used as an indicator of global $\dot{V}_{O_2}$ and indirectly the adequacy of $\dot{D}_{O_2}$. If oxygen delivery by the microcirculation and cellular oxygen uptake are adequate, then a $S\bar{v}_{O_2}$ value of 65% usually indicates that global $\dot{D}_{O_2}$ is appropriate. Lower values may indicate increased uptake, but more often reduced or inadequate delivery. Mixed venous blood is useful for measurement of global $\dot{D}_{O_2}$, but it usually requires the presence of a pulmonary artery catheter. The use of central venous saturations has become an alternative surrogate that is usually adequate and considerably more practical. The body cannot store large amounts of oxygen (although the lungs and myoglobin can act as short-term reservoirs) so is dependent on a continuous supply. The excess ability to increase $\dot{D}_{O_2}$ to match changes in $\dot{V}_{O_2}$ is an adaptation that permits sudden changes in demand, such as exercise where $\dot{V}_{O_2}$ can sometimes exceed 1500 mL/min.

Step 5: diffusion – blood to mitochondrion Ninety per cent of cellular aerobic metabolism takes place in the mitochondria. The rate of diffusion of oxygen from bound oxyhaemoglobin to the mitochondria follows similar principles to the diffusion of oxygen into the blood from the alveoli: (1) Fick's law of diffusion, where ΔP depends on $\dot{D}_{O_2}$ and the rate of cellular uptake and utilisation, and (2) the position of the oxygen haemoglobin dissociation curve. Once delivered to the cell, oxygen generates ATP by the electron transport chain, utilising the reducing power of NADH and $FADH_2$ generated from the citric acid cycle.[4] The movement of electrons through the chain requires a terminal electron acceptor. This is molecular oxygen, which combines with the electrons and protons to form water. Without oxygen, the proton motive force generated by the electron chain would not exist and phosphorylation of ADP to ATP would cease (**Fig. 28.2**).[5]

Originally at approximately 160 mmHg (21.3 kPa), the partial pressure of oxygen (P_{O_2}) at the mouth can fall to as low as 1 mmHg (0.133 kPa) in some mitochondria. Below this value, cellular demands for oxygen outweigh its delivery, and ATP production may be reduced.

Step 6 – the redox state of the cell Oxygen delivery from atmosphere to cell is conventionally considered a cascade, implying that a high concentration at one end cascades down and increases oxygen in the cell. Though this will increase oxygen potentially available to the cell, the driving force for it to enter the cell and mitochondrion is the gradient between the partial pressures of oxygen within and outside the cell. Increased oxygen utilisation reduces that tension and increases that gradient; conversely, adequate oxygen in the cell will reduce the gradient until oxygen will not diffuse. Hence the cell itself determines how much oxygen it uses by creating the gradient that 'sucks in' oxygen – and not a cascade. Similarly it is the ATP/ADP ratio and probably hydrogen ion concentration that drives ATP production and modifies oxygen requirement (i.e. the cell is largely autonomous and uses what it needs).[6] Whereas adequate oxygen delivery is important, excess oxygen is at least theoretically of no benefit.

PATHOLOGY OF OXYGEN DELIVERY ($\dot{D}_{O_2}$)

Failure of oxygen delivery to the cells leads rapidly to cellular dysfunction, and can lead to cellular death and organ dysfunction culminating in the organism's death. $\dot{V}_{O_2}$ drives the $\dot{D}_{O_2}$ requirement, and failure of $\dot{D}_{O_2}$ to match $\dot{V}_{O_2}$ results in reduction in aerobic metabolism and energy production, necessitating ATP production by the less-efficient glycolytic pathway. The level of $\dot{D}_{O_2}$ at which $\dot{V}_{O_2}$ begins to decline has been termed the 'critical $\dot{D}_{O_2}$' and is approximately 300 mL/min in an adult (**Fig. 28.3**).[7] 'Shock' is the usual term used in this situation, defined loosely as failure of delivery of oxygen to match the demand of tissue. Commonly this refers to failure of the circulation, but low $\dot{D}_{O_2}$ can result from several pathological mechanisms that can occur singly or in combination (**Table 28.3**).

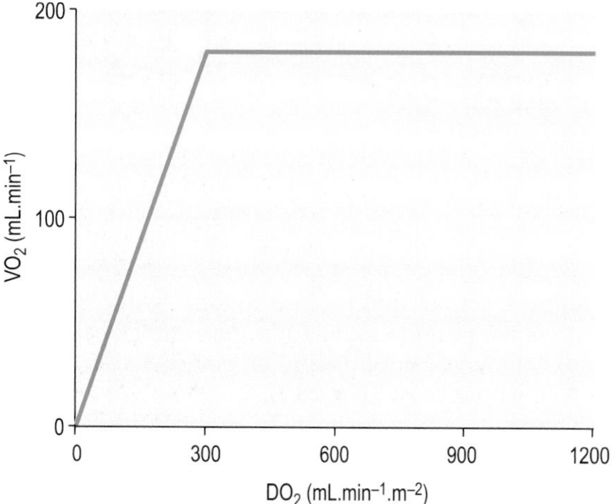

Figure 28.3 The normal relationship between $\dot{V}_{O_2}$ and $\dot{D}_{O_2}$. Above the value of 'critical $\dot{D}_{O_2}$' $\dot{V}_{O_2}$ is independent of oxygen delivery. Below this value and $\dot{V}_{O_2}$ becomes supply dependent and may be amenable to therapeutic interventions.

The impact of a low $\dot{D}_{O_2}$ can be worsened by increased oxygen demand. The metabolic rate increases with exercise, inflammation, sepsis, pyrexia, thyrotoxicosis, shivering, seizures, agitation, anxiety and pain.[8] Therapeutic interventions such as adrenergic drugs (e.g. epinephrine[9]) and certain feeding strategies can also lead to and increased $\dot{V}_{O_2}$. In critical illness, where oxygen delivery is considered to be in jeopardy, there has been considerable interest in the relationship between $\dot{D}_{O_2}$ and $\dot{V}_{O_2}$ (see Fig. 28.3). The presence of signs or markers of tissue hypoxia such as acidosis imply inadequate tissue oxygenation. This could be from either inadequate delivery failing to meet consumption requirements or reduced ability of the tissues to extract oxygen. The former could be corrected by increasing delivery; the latter is more difficult. Historically this has led to the strategy for delivering 'supranormal' $\dot{D}_{O_2}$ to ensure adequate supply.[10,11] It is irrefutable that if delivery is inadequate it should be corrected to meet consumption, but unless different measurement techniques are used mathematical linkage occurs so as one increases so does the other.[12,13] Further, the inotropes used to increase delivery also increase consumption. As discussed later, hyperoxia also has directly detrimental effects.

Clinical studies clearly show that adequate resuscitation to meet oxygen requirements is sensible. In the critically ill going beyond this is not helpful[14,15] although there may still be a place for supra-optimal values in the high-risk surgical patient.[10,11] In the acute situation the combined use of markers of tissue hypoxia, such as acidosis and lactate in conjunction with surrogates of oxygen delivery such as Scv_{O_2} and standard haemodynamic measurements of an adequate circulation, have proved beneficial.[16,17] So-called early goal-directed therapy is now included in published and recently updated guidelines for the treatment of severe sepsis

Table 28.3 Types of hypoxia

TYPE OF HYPOXIA	PATHOPHYSIOLOGY	EXAMPLES
Hypoxic hypoxia	Reduced supply of oxygen to the body leading to a low arterial oxygen tension	1. Low environmental oxygen (e.g. altitude) 2. Ventilatory failure (respiratory arrest, drug overdose, neuromuscular disease) 3. Pulmonary shunt: (a) anatomical – VSD with R–L flow (b) physiological – pneumonia, pneumothorax, pulmonary oedema, asthma
Anaemic hypoxia	The arterial oxygen tension is normal, but the circulating haemoglobin is reduced or functionally impaired	Massive haemorrhage, severe anaemia, carbon monoxide poisoning, methaemaglobinaemia
Stagnant hypoxia	Failure of transport of sufficient oxygen due to inadequate circulation	Left ventricular failure, pulmonary embolism, hypovolaemia, hypothermia
Histotoxic hypoxia	Impairment of cellular metabolism of oxygen despite adequate delivery	Cyanide poisoning, arsenic poisoning, alcohol intoxication

Table 28.4 Early goal-directed therapy: a summary of D_{O_2} parameters set to achieve in first 6 hours of the diagnosis of severe sepsis with associated hypotension and a plasma lactate concentration of ≥4 mmol/L

VARIABLE	PARAMETERS
Arterial oxygen saturation (Sa_{O_2})	≥93%
Central venous pressure (CVP)	8–12 mmHg (1.06–1.6 kPa)
Mean arterial pressure (MAP)	65–90 mmHg (8.65–11.97 kPa)
Urine output (UO)	≥0.5 mL/kg/h
Mixed venous oxygen saturations (Sv_{O_2}) or central venous oxygen saturations (Scv_{O_2})	≥70%
Haematocrit	≥30%

After Rivers et al.[16]

(**Table 28.4**).[18] The benefits of this new approach may well have as much to do with the prompt and aggressive improvements in haemodynamics and resuscitation as the values obtained. Timing is probably the significant difference compared with other applications of the 'supranormal' technique. Targeted oxygen delivery is a major debate that is still evolving (**Box 28.1**). Oxygen delivery can be improved in a variety of ways from the ambient inspired oxygen through the lungs and cardiovascular system to the cell itself, but once at the cell the ability to manipulate delivery ceases.

CELLULAR HYPOXIA

In environments where the $\dot{D}_{O_2}$ is reduced, human cells can tolerate hypoxia to a certain extent by adapting 'hibernation' strategies to reduce metabolic rate, increased oxygen extraction from surrounding tissues and enzyme adaptations that allow continuing metabolism at low P_{O_2}.[19] Anaerobic metabolism is actively utilised by some tissues. In low oxygen concentrations, both myocardial and vascular endothelium up-regulate glycolytic enzymes and glucose transport proteins.[20] Research performed in humans at altitude in order to mimic hypoxic stress suggests that, though $\dot{D}_{O_2}$ is preserved, $\dot{V}_{O_2}$ is reduced.[21] This may be due to reduced oxygen uptake at a microcirculatory level, reduced cellular oxygen consumption or an improvement in the efficiency of ATP production. These theories may be evidenced by the recovery of critical illness multi-organ failure, in which function may be compromised in the short term without long-term structural damage,[22] and in vitro studies of mitochondria, which demonstrate more efficient ATP production when exposed to hypoxic environments.[23] The ability of humans to tolerate and then acclimatise to altitude mainly by a reduction in $\dot{V}_{O_2}$ may explain why many critical care strategies

Box 28.1 Summary of targeted oxygen delivery

Goal-directed therapy

- Supraoptimal values in the critically ill – not recommended
- Perioperative optimisation with supranormal values – possibly useful but controversial
- Resuscitation against markers of peripheral oxygen use such as Scv_{O_2} and lactate (early goal-directed therapy) – currently advocated

to increase Pa_{O_2} (e.g. inhaled nitric oxide) fail to convey any survival benefit. Indeed, accepting a Pa_{O_2}/Sa_{O_2} below 'normal' levels does not appear to significantly reduce survival and may reduce the risk of oxygen toxicity.[23]

REGIONAL HYPOXIA

Much of what has been discussed describes effects of oxygen delivery and uptake for the body as a whole. The reality is far more complex, as not only can the $\dot{D}_{O_2}$ of each organ system be manipulated to meet demand, but also, within each organ, regional demands may vary and can be varied. Few of the clinical methods commonly used for assessing $\dot{D}_{O_2}$ can identify changes in either organ or regional $\dot{D}_{O_2}$. Thus it is possible in critical illness for tissue hypoxia to exist with associated organ dysfunction despite normal global $\dot{D}_{O_2}$ and $S\bar{v}_{O_2}$ values.[24]

The effects of disordered or diverted regional blood flow can be important. For example, in shock splanchnic blood flow is often reduced, with the potential for ischaemia. Clearly detection of gut ischaemia could be used to influence management of oxygen delivery and hopefully reduce the likelihood of multi-organ failure.[25] The control of regional blood flow is itself complex. Methods of increasing global $\dot{D}_{O_2}$ in the hope that this will optimise all tissues often necessitates the use of vasoactive drugs (vasopressors, inotropes and vasodilators). Paradoxically, although such therapy can influence regional flow it may not necessarily be in the direction sought in individual regions.

DIAGNOSIS AND MONITORING OF $\dot{D}_{O_2}$

Early recognition and treatment of oxygen delivery failure is important for preserving organ function.[16] Clinical assessment of $\dot{D}_{O_2}$ and $\dot{V}_{O_2}$ (e.g. heart rate, blood pressure or urine output) can be misleading. Particularly in the young patient, the ability of the OER increase to as high as 70–80% can mean that such variables can change only late in the evolution of diminished $\dot{D}_{O_2}$. However, the assessment of an effective cardiac output (ECO) - normal heart rate, blood pressure and peripheral perfusion with signs of organ function and normal oxygen saturation - must not be excluded in favour of more technical quantitative methods. Rather, the technical values must be considered in the clinical context. All assessments of $\dot{D}_{O_2}$, clinical or technical, require continuous re-evaluation to ensure that treatments being planned or administered are appropriate for the patient's current condition.

Sa_{O_2} AND Pa_{O_2}

Both these measures are included in the Ca_{O_2} equation (28.2), and their importance is clear. However, what is a 'safe' Sa_{O_2} and/or Pa_{O_2} can be difficult to define. Measured systemically, they do not alone reflect tissue oxygenation, and oxygen extraction mechanisms vary between organs. In general, however, supplementary oxygen is required when Pa_{O_2} falls below 60 mmHg (8 kPa) or the Sa_{O_2} is below 88%. Table 28.1 lists the clinical significance of common Pa_{O_2} and Sa_{O_2} values.

ACID–BASE BALANCE

Many intensive care units use acid–base balance as a simple bedside indicator of global $\dot{D}_{O_2}$. The presence of acidosis and a base deficit of less than −2 may be used to detect evidence of inadequate $\dot{D}_{O_2}$ presuming this reflects lactate accumulation. However, plasma lactate concentration is an unreliable indicator of tissue hypoxia; it represents the balance between production and consumption so if used in isolation or as a single value to assess $\dot{D}_{O_2}$ can easily mislead.[26] The use of lactate as a marker of $\dot{D}_{O_2} / \dot{V}_{O_2}$ balance is best used as a trend using serial measurements.

$S\bar{v}_{O_2}$ / Scv_{O_2}

In critical illness a falling $\dot{D}_{O_2}$ can be compensated for by an increase in oxygen extraction. This leads to a lower oxygen saturation of haemoglobin returning to the right side of the heart. Analysis of this saturation either in vivo (fibreoptic oximetry) or in vitro (oximetry) allows assessment of the OER. Classically, a low $S\bar{v}_{O_2}$ (< 70%) in the face of a normal Sa_{O_2}, implies tissue hypoperfusion secondary to a low CO, either hypovolaemia or pump failure. It could, however, indicate very high $\dot{V}_{O_2}$ as may occur with hyperthermia. Conversely a raised $S\bar{v}_{O_2}$ (> 75%) will imply low demand (e.g. hypothermia, or a cellular utilisation problem), easily explained in cyanide poisoning when the oxidative phosphorylation mechanism is inhibited, but much more difficult to rationalise when seen (commonly) in sepsis. In a very low output state it could indicate total failure of peripheral perfusion and therefore no oxygen usage. Scv_{O_2} is a reasonable surrogate for $S\bar{v}_{O_2}$ and reduces the need for the more complex pulmonary artery catheter.[17,27] Whichever method of venous oxygen saturation is used, it must be in conjunction with other markers of adequacy of oxygen delivery and clinical context, as outlined in Table 28.4.

MEASUREMENT OF REGIONAL $\dot{D}_{O_2}$

Most assessments of $\dot{D}_{O_2}$ are global and do not reflect regional differences between organs or even different tissues within an organ. Current methods of non-invasively assessing individual organ or tissue oxygenation are limited; measurements are difficult, require specialised techniques and are not widely available. Currently only gastric tonometry and near-infrared spectroscopy (NIRS) have clinical applications in the detection of organ hypoxia.[25] Novel techniques such as palladium porphyrin phosphorescence-based techniques are being evaluated in animals, but require improvement as palladium is itself cytotoxic.[28] Cellular oxygenation measurement methods are also in development.[29]

OXYGEN THERAPY APPARATUS AND DEVICES

In the hypoxic self-ventilating patient, delivery of oxygen to the alveoli is usually achieved by increasing the environmental oxygen fraction (Fi_{O_2}). Most commonly this involves the application of one of the many varieties of oxygen mask to the face, such that it covers the nose and mouth. There are other methods (e.g. nasal cannulae), but each needs to fulfil the same basic requirements.

Most of the simpler devices (e.g. plastic masks, nasal cannulae) deliver oxygen at relatively low oxygen flow rates relative to peak inspiratory flows (25–100+ L/min). The final Fi_{O_2} delivered is heavily influenced by the entrainment of environmental air, which dilutes the set Fi_{O_2}. From a physical principle perspective, the actual concentration of oxygen delivered is determined by the interaction between the delivery system and the patient's breathing pattern. The Fi_{O_2} that reaches the alveolus is therefore unpredictable. Factors that influence this can broadly be divided up into patient factors and device factors (**Box 28.2**).[30]

In the hypoxic patient it is common to find significant increases of inspiratory flow rates as well as an absence of the respiratory pause. This can result in the actual Fi_{O_2} at the alveolus being significantly less than that thought to be delivered. This is due to a greater proportion of the inhaled gas being entrained air when the patient's inspiratory flow rate increases. The normal peak inspiratory flow rate (PIFR) is 25–35 L/min; in

Box 28.2 Factors that influence the Fi_{O_2} delivered to a patient by oxygen delivery devices[30]

Patient factors	Device factors
Inspiratory flow rate	Oxygen flow rate
Presence of a respiratory pause	Volume of mask
Tidal volume	Air vent size
	Tightness of fit

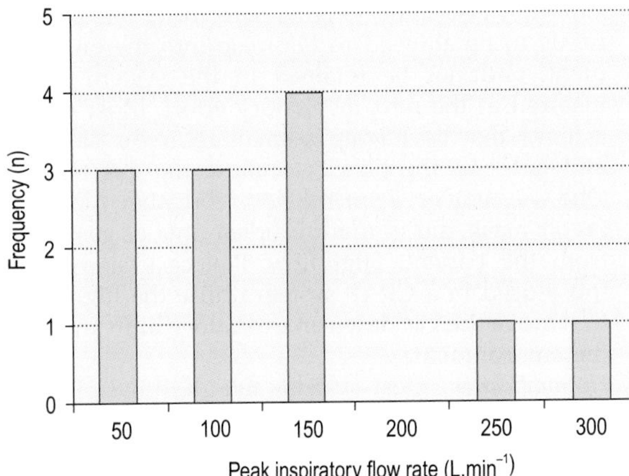

Figure 28.4. Spirometric peak inspiratory flow rates (PIFR) taken from a group of 12 critical care patients with respiratory distress and hypoxia. Most of the patients have a PIFR below 150 L/min. However, two patients exceed 200 L/min. This will have a negative effect on the concentration of oxygen delivered from a variable performance system (e.g. Hudson).[30]

critical illness this can increase eightfold (**Fig. 28.4**).[31] The greater the inspiratory flow rate, the lower is the alveolar Fi_{O_2}. This is particularly true for the variable performance-type masks, but is seen even in the more 'reliable' Venturi-type masks particularly when higher Fi_{O_2} inserts are used. The presence of a valve-controlled reservoir bag on a 'non-rebreather' semi-rigid plastic mask should compensate for high inspiratory flows – hence the belief that such masks can deliver 100% oxygen. This is not the case though, and in models of human ventilation such masks do not seem to confer significant extra oxygen delivery ability above that of semi-rigid plastic masks without a reservoir bag (**Figs 28.5** and **28.6**).[32] The failure of oxygen masks to deliver the desired Fi_{O_2} can be improved either by having a high enough oxygen flow rate and reservoir to compensate for the high inspiratory flow rate e.g. high-flow nasal cannulae such as the Vapotherm®, or by sealing the upper airway (nose and mouth) from the environment (e.g. the CPAP mask). Indeed, there is evidence supporting the hypothesis that some of the improvement in oxygenation seen with CPAP ventilation may be due to the eradication of entrainment of environmental air rather than the positive airway pressure exerted by the CPAP valve.[32]

In summary, the use of non-sealing oxygen masks and cannulae should be guided by the patient's requirements and response to therapy, rather than a belief that the concentration being delivered is that reaching the alveolus. This can be particularly important in the treatment of patients whose ventilatory drive is sensitive to P_{O_2} levels.

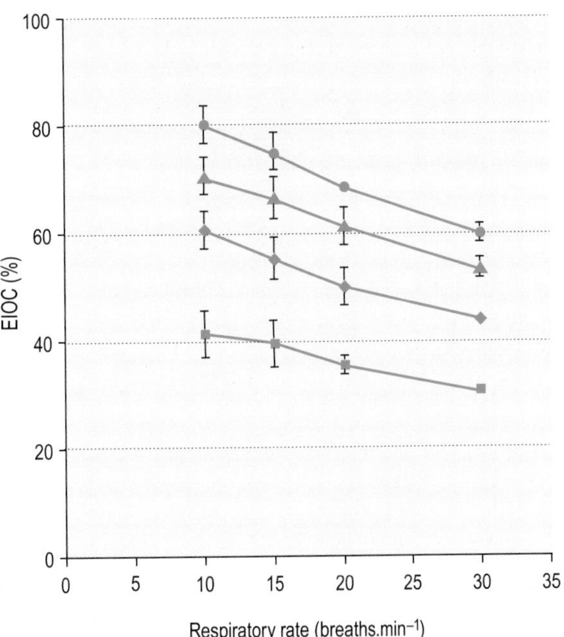

Figure 28.5 The performance of a Hudson mask on a model of human ventilation at a tidal volume of 500mLs and four oxygen flow rates (2 L/min (□), 6 L/min (◇), 10 L/min (△) and 15 L/min (○)). As the respiratory rate increases, the effective inspired oxygen concentration (EIOC) deteriorates.[31]

OXYGEN DELIVERY DEVICES

Methods of delivering oxygen to conscious patients with no instrumentation to their airway can broadly be divided into four categories: (1) variable performance systems, (2) fixed performance systems, (3) high-flow systems, and (4) others. With the exception of the intravascular devices, all comprises similar component parts:

1. *Oxygen supply:* oxygen can be delivered from pressurised cylinders, hospital supply from cylinder banks or a vacuum-insulated evaporator (VIE), or an oxygen concentrator.
2. *Oxygen flow control:* oxygen supplied to the device is controlled by some sort of valve, often with an associated flow meter (e.g. OHE ball valve flow meter).
3. *Connecting tubing:* both from the supply to the flow control and from the flow control to the device, the type and size of the tubing are important. Small-bore tubing can limit oxygen flow when high flow is intended. In some systems the connecting tubing can also act as a reservoir – e.g. Ayre's T-piece. Some devices require specialised tubing with appropriate end attachments – such as the Schräeder valves required for connecting to the wall oxygen supply.

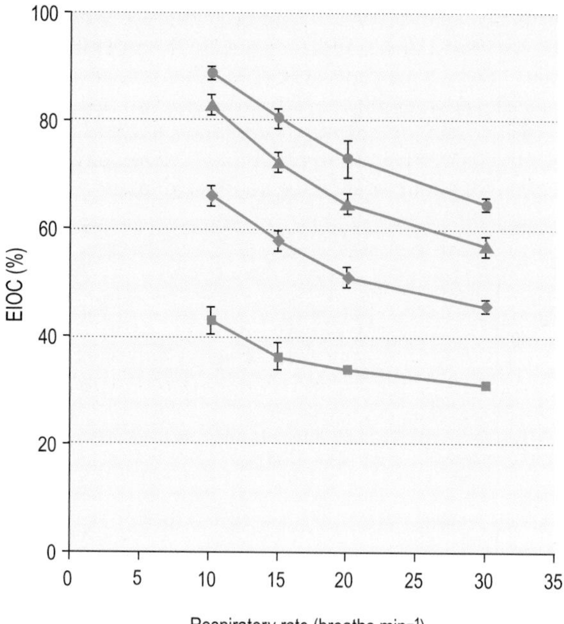

Figure 28.6 The performance of a Hudson non-rebreather mask on a model of human ventilation at a tidal volume of 500 mL and four oxygen flow rates (2 L/min (□), 6 L/min (◇), 10 L/min (△) and 15 L/min (○)). As the respiratory rate increases, the effective inspired oxygen concentration (EIOC) deteriorates. Note also how the curves of the graph are similar to the Hudson mask without the reservoir bag, implying no superiority with its addition.[31]

4. *Reservoir:* all oxygen delivery devices have some sort of reservoir. In a simple oxygen mask it is the mask itself. Some low-flow CPAP circuits have a balloon reservoir. The nasal cannulae utilise the nasopharynx as a reservoir. An oxygen tent uses the volume of the tent as a large reservoir. The effectiveness of the reservoir in 'storing' oxygen ready for the next inspiratory effort is one of the important factors in governing its ability to deliver the desired oxygen concentration. The oxygen tent is a good example of the effectiveness of a large reservoir, as it eliminates air entrainment whatever the patient's PIFR. Thus the oxygen flow rate does not have to be high, but just enough to ensure that CO_2 re-breathing is abolished. Indeed it is the retention of CO_2 that can be the major problem if gas is expired into the reservoir.
5. *Patient attachment:* the patient is connected to the oxygen supply and reservoir such that the device delivers oxygen to the airway – either by directly covering the upper airway (e.g. plastic mask/head box), intranasally, or by increasing the oxygen concentration in the wider environment as in an oxygen tent.
6. *Expired gas facility:* expired gas from the patient needs to be allowed to dissipate into the environment, and not be retained in the system to be inspired at the next inspiratory effort. Most masks achieve this by having a small reservoir capacity and holes in the plastic to allow the gas to exit. One-way valves, as in the non-rebreather type reservoir mask, aid in unidirectional flow of gas away from the patient. High-flow T-piece systems like those used in a CPAP system utilise the high flow to remove the gas down an expiratory limb and into the environment.
7. *Humidification:* most systems use the physiological humidification properties of the nasopharynx and trachea. However, high-flow systems may overcome this leading to drying of the airway and secretions, which can be uncomfortable and undesirable. Artificial humidification (and warming) should be employed using devices such as a water bath or heat and moisture exchanger (HME).
8. *Oxygen monitor:* some systems have an oxygen monitor incorporated in the apparatus (e.g. a fuel cell). This allows the much more accurate monitoring of Fi_{O_2}, but this is dependent on where in the system it is placed, and also adds bulk and expense to the oxygen delivery method.

VARIABLE PERFORMANCE SYSTEMS

Typically these are non-sealed mask or nasal cannulae systems, which deliver oxygen at low gas flows (2–15 L/min). The reservoir is usually small, consisting of the volume of the mask in the case of the semi-rigid type, or the nasopharynx as in the nasal cannulae. The entrainment of environmental air is important in their delivery capability and has to be considered when being used.

Nasal cannulae The proximity of the reservoir – the nasopharynx – means that these systems are particularly sensitive to changes in inspiratory flow rate and particularly the loss of the respiratory pause. However for mild hypoxia, they are tolerated well by patients who can eat and drink with them in situ. They can cause drying of the nasal mucosa when used at higher flow rates, and newer systems are available that can humidify and warm the inspired oxygen. They are cheap and easy to use with no risk of CO_2 retention.

Simple semi-rigid plastic masks (e.g. Hudson, MC) The most commonly used type of oxygen mask, these are cheap and easy to administer. The reservoir comprises the mask, and rebreathing of CO_2 can therefore occur if used at oxygen flow rates below 4 L/min. A maximum Fi_{O_2} of only 0.6–0.7 can be achieved, which will be lower in the presence of respiratory distress.

Tracheostomy masks These semi-rigid plastic masks act in the same way as their facial counterparts. However, the delivery they achieve is very dependent on the presence of an endotracheal tube and the inflation status of its cuff. If absent or if the cuff is deflated then air from the nasopharynx will mix with that being delivered to the tracheostomy, and further dilute the Fi_{O_2}.

T-piece system These simple systems, consisting of an inspiratory limb and expiratory limb forming the bar of the 'T', can be used with endotracheal tubes (oral, nasal or tracheostomy) or with a sealed CPAP-type mask. The oxygen flow rate needs to be high enough to match the patient's PIFR so as to prevent rebreathing of expired gas and thus potential entrainment of air from the expiratory limb. The seal of the mask or tube cuff is important also to prevent entrainment of air.

FIXED PERFORMANCE SYSTEMS

These systems are so called because their delivery of oxygen is independent of the patient factors outlined above.

Venturi-type masks Oxygen concentration is determined by the Venturi principle: oxygen passing through a small orifice entrains air to a predictable dilution. The Fi_{O_2} is adjusted by changing the Venturi 'valve' and setting the appropriate oxygen flow rate. Although the Venturi effect can deliver 40–60 L/min, this is possible only at the lower Fi_{O_2} valves (e.g. at Fi_{O_2} of 0.24 the flow rate is approximately 53 L/min at an inflow of 2 L/min), and oxygen flow rate falls as the Fi_{O_2} increases. Thus, in respiratory distress associated with hypoxia, the reduction in oxygen flow rate can lead to failure despite a higher Fi_{O_2} setting. The larger orifice leads to the system behaving more like a simple mask.

Anaesthetic breathing circuits Non-rebreathing systems have one-way valves (e.g. Ambu-bag) and usually closed mask systems so they deliver what is set. Non-rebreathing systems (e.g. Mapleson A, B, C, D and E) depend on the gas flows to ensure no rebreathing. No air entrainment is possible but rebreathing occurs readily at low flows (most require flows > 150 mL/kg).

HIGH-FLOW SYSTEMS

As alluded to above, the T-piece system can act as a fixed-performance system if the oxygen flow rate is sufficiently high. Other high-flow systems exist (e.g. Vapotherm®) that use flow rates up to 30 L/min nasally. They require humidification and heating of the inspired gas to allow patient tolerance.

Positive-pressure devices Non-invasive positive pressure (NIPPV) delivers oxygen with some element of positive pressure exerted during the respiratory cycle. It does not require instrumentation of the airway, and is delivered either by tight fitting mask to the face, nose or as a helmet. The simplest CPAP system is a T-piece with a positive-pressure valve attached to the expiratory limb, as with a Mapleson E system. Other methods are also available; some utilise a balloon reservoir rather than a high-flow oxygen generator (Mapleson A). CPAP helps improve functional residual capacity and compliance.[34] There is no air entrainment, which contributes to the initial rapid improvement. Theoretically the positive pressure aids alveolar recruitment. A potential problem with the T-piece CPAP systems is that the oxygen flow rate has to be adjusted to the patient's PIFR so as to prevent closure of the valve, increasing the inspiratory work of breathing. Other methods of non-invasive positive-pressure ventilation such as bilevel positive airway pressure (BIPAP) deliver oxygen at flows that should match the patient's demand.

OTHER METHODS OF OXYGEN DELIVERY

Intravascular oxygenation has been used, but not extensively - particularly in the self-ventilating patient population. Extracorporeal membrane oxygenation (ECMO) supporting the lung has recently grown in use secondary to a landmark study and recent influenza pandemics.[35,36]

MANAGEMENT OF OXYGEN THERAPY

In the correct situations, oxygen is a life-saving drug/therapy. It remains part of the initial resuscitation and ongoing management of the critically unwell. In the UK at any one time 15–17% of all hospital inpatients will be receiving oxygen.[37] However, oxygen can have detrimental effects in certain patient groups and/or situations and this may result in significant morbidity or mortality. In the UK, the British Thoracic Society published guidelines for the emergency use of supplemental oxygen in 2008 and, to date, these remain the most comprehensive.[38]

RESPIRATORY FAILURE

Identifying patients that require oxygen therapy is vital. Supplemental oxygen is required to treat most causes of hypoxia, yet different patient groups may have different resting oxygen concentrations. For example, patients with cyanotic heart disease or chronic neuromuscular disorders may have a Sa_{O_2} of 80%, yet have adapted to tolerate these oxygen tensions. The normal values of Pa_{O_2} and Sa_{O_2} in healthy volunteers are summarised in **Table 28.5**.[39] In many cases of critical illness, low oxygen tensions are due to hypoxic hypoxia. This may be as a result of reduced environmental oxygen such as that seen at altitude, pulmonary oedema or pneumonia resulting in ventilation–perfusion mismatch and intrapulmonary shunt. This is so called Type I respiratory failure where ventilation is intact, but gas transfer or haemoglobin saturation is impaired. It is defined as a Pa_{O_2}<8kPa (60 mmHg) with a normal or low Pa_{CO_2}.[39] Broadly speaking, hypoxia in any of these situations will be improved by increasing inhaled oxygen concentrations. However, caution must be taken when dealing with ventilatory or Type II respiratory failure. The differentiation of the two types of respiratory failure is made using the Pa_{CO_2}. The normal value is 4.6–6.1kPa (34–46 mmHg) and hypoxic patients with Pa_{CO_2} concentrations above this range should be considered as being in Type II respiratory failure. Many

Table 28.5 Mean (SD) Pa_{O_2} and Sa_{O_2} values (with range) in kPa and mmHg. Values shown for seated healthy men and women, non-smoking volunteers at sea level[39]

AGE (YEARS)	MEAN Pa_{O_2} (kPa and mmHg)	RANGE ±2SD Pa_{O_2} (kPa and mmHg)	MEAN Sa_{O_2} (%)	Sa_{O_2} ±2 SD
18–24	13.4 (0.71) 99.9 (5.3)	11.98–14.82 89.3–110.5	96.9 (0.4)	96.1–97.7
25–34	13.4 (0.66) 99.8 (4.9)	12.08–14.72 90–109.6	96.7 (0.7)	95.3–98.1
35–44	13.18 (1.02) 98.3 (7.6)	11.14–15.22 83.1–113.5	96.7 (0.6)	95.5–97.9
45–54	13.0 (1.07) 97 (8)	10.86–15.14 81–113	96.5 (1)	94.4–98.5
55–64	12.09 (0.6) 90.2 (4.5)	10.89–13.29 81.2–99.2	95.1 (0.7)	94.5–97.3
>64	11.89 (1.43) 88.7 (10.7)	9.02–14.76 67.3–110.1	95.5 (1.4)	92.7–98.3

causes of ventilatory failure are not affected by the oxygen tension in the blood (e.g. Guillain–Barré, opioid overdose). However, with commoner causes such as acute exacerbations of chronic obstructive pulmonary disease (COPD) and acute severe asthma, the patient's ventilation can be sensitive to oxygen therapy.

TARGETED OXYGEN THERAPY

The need for oxygen to prevent tissue hypoxia and cellular dysfunction is clear. However, it is not possible to define a single level of hypoxaemia that is dangerous to all patients. Some patients with chronic lung disease may be accustomed to living with an Sa_{O_2} of 80%, whereas others with acute organ failure may be harmed by short-term exposure to an Sa_{O_2} of < 90%.[38] So the level of hypoxaemia has to be given context not just in severity, but also in time and evidence of negative physiological effect. There is no evidence that saturations above normal result in benefit. Rather, hyperoxia can have adverse effects. As a rule of thumb, maintaining Sa_{O_2} above 90% in critically ill patients is considered best practice, and permits a margin of error.[38,40,41] Those patients at risk of hypercapnic Type II respiratory failure should be managed with a little more caution and their Sa_{O_2} target should be set between 88% and 92%. Their further management will be discussed in Chapter 30.

MONITORING

All patients demonstrating hypoxia and the need for oxygen therapy should have a full medical history and physical examination. Focus should be placed on pre-existing respiratory or cardiac disease to ensure correct interpretation of the technical data as well as appropriate oxygen targets being set. Pulse oximetry is extremely valuable as a non-invasive measure of arterial oxygenation. Calibrated on normal subjects, their readings must be treated with caution when below 80%, but are accurate above 88%. They may have decreased accuracy in the critically ill, but the mean difference is within 1.3%.[42] Whereas pulse oximetry is an excellent tool for assessing Sa_{O_2} it gives no data regarding pH and/or Pa_{CO_2} as a marker of ventilatory function or the haemoglobin concentration. Thus it cannot be used as a monitor of ventilation, or an absolute assessment of Ca_{O_2}. Thus in scenarios where hypoxaemia is suspected, an arterial blood gas should be performed and interpreted (Chs 18 and 91). Arterial blood gas analysis is the gold standard for assessing respiratory failure. Usually assessed from aspirating blood from a systemic artery, ear-lobe specimens also have utility in assessing Pa_{CO_2} and pH, at less discomfort to the patient. They are, however, less accurate and less precise at lower oxygen tensions.[43,44] An algorithm for the introduction and monitoring of oxygen therapy in acute hypoxia is summarised in **Figure 28.7**.

HAZARDS OF OXYGEN THERAPY

SUPPLY

Medical oxygen supply is a compressed gas. Pipeline supply to the 'wall' is usually at 4 bars of pressure (3040 mmHg). The cylinder supply when full is 137 bar (104 120 mmHg). As such, there are important risks when using oxygen as explosion is a risk. Direct administration of oxygen at delivery pressures carries a real risk of barotrauma to the airway and alveoli, if not governed by an appropriate pressure-limiting valve (e.g. OHE flow meter).

Oxygen also supports combustion. The possibility of sparks in an oxygen-rich environment must be avoided. Patients must not smoke cigarettes when receiving oxygen therapy, even via nasal cannula. Another example is to ensure that oxygen supplies are removed

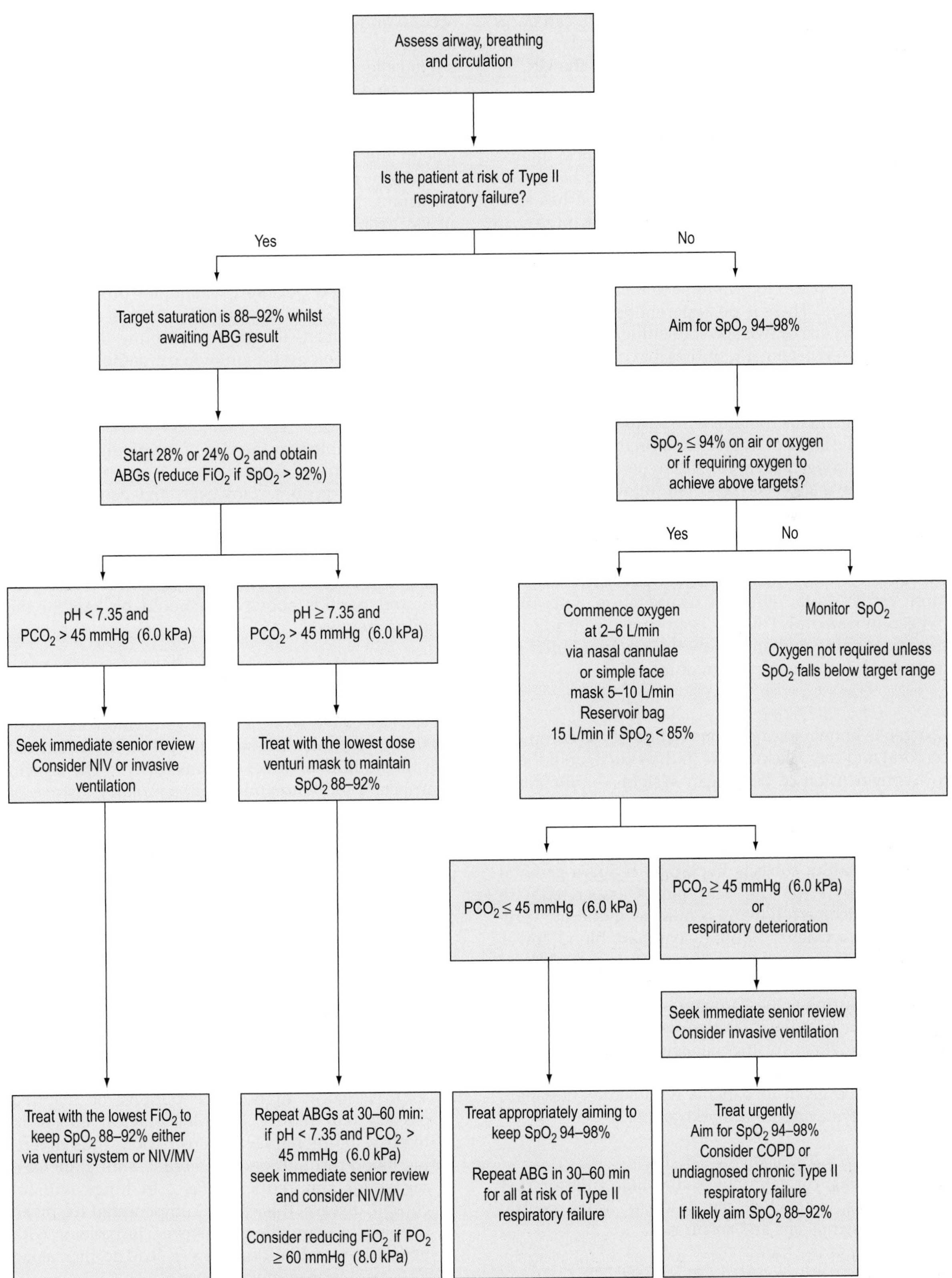

Figure 28.7 Oxygen prescription for acutely hypoxaemic patients in hospital. Any increase in F_{IO_2} must be followed by repeat ABGs in 1 hour or sooner. ABG=arterial blood gas; NIV=non-invasive ventilation; MV=mechanical ventilation. *(Modified from the BTS guidelines 2008.[38])*

or turned off when defibrillating, as a spark can occur in such situations. A recent ICU fire secondary to an oxygen cylinder explosion was reported in the UK.[45]

OXYGEN TOXICITY

Despite being a naturally occurring substance, the use of oxygen in a medical environment should be considered pharmacotherapy. As with all drugs, it has side-effects in overdose. There has been a great interest in the potential toxic effects of oxygen in recent years. As is evident from the above management of oxygen therapy, there needs to be a limit to the concentrations of oxygen used. There is no apparent benefit in hyperoxia except in one or two specific settings. Indeed in the critical care environment studies have shown that a high Pa_{O_2} level within the first 24 hours is an independent risk factor for hospital mortality.[46] This finding remains contentious though, with further studies demonstrating the effect of hypoxia as a predictor of mortality, but no strong effect seen with hyperoxia.[47] Adverse outcomes have also been reported following treatment of post-cardiac-arrest patients with hyperoxia.[48] These findings also have not been reproduced by further studies, but there is still evidence of a U-shaped mortality curve for Pa_{O_2} in this group of patients.[49] What is more certain is the effect of resuscitation with 100% oxygen in neonates. This has been shown to lead to an excess mortality and air is now the recommended gas to be used in the resuscitation of infants.[50]

VASOCONSTRICTION

Oxygen is known to cause constriction of the coronary, cerebral and renal vasculature and, as such, could lead to hypoperfusion of key organ systems - potentially reducing $\dot{D}_{O_2}$ when an increase is desired. This hazard would only be played off against a very moderate increase in Ca_{O_2} assuming all the haemoglobin is saturated. In healthy subjects hyperoxia reduces cerebral blood flow by 11–33%.[51,52] This may be associated with a worse outcome following a mild to moderate cerebrovascular accident.[52] Similarly coronary blood flow is reduced in the presence of hyperoxaemia (8–29% in healthy subjects).[53] This may promote myocardial ischaemia during acute coronary syndromes, possibly increasing myocardial infarction size.[54] This has led UK national guidelines for the management of acute coronary syndromes to stipulate that supplementary oxygen should *not* be given to patients with acute chest pain unless there is evidence of hypoxaemia.[55]

CNS TOXICITY (PAUL BERT EFFECT)

Seen in diving, oxygen delivered at high pressure (>3 atmospheres, ≈300 kPa) can lead to acute central nervous system signs and seizures.

LUNG TOXICITY (LORRIANE SMITH EFFECT)

Exposure to a high Fi_{O_2} results in pulmonary injury. It is known that a progressive reduction in compliance occurs and is associated with interstitial oedema, leading to fibrosis. The mechanism remains unclear, but is believed to involve direct cellular damage to the lung tissue by highly reactive oxygen free radicals. High concentrations of oxygen produce a higher concentration of reactive oxygen species (ROS) that overwhelm the normal scavenging mechanism lining the respiratory tract. This possibly associated with loss of surfactant, and increase in sympathetic activity and airway collapse due to the lack of other non-respiratory gases leads to lung damage. Evidence for this mechanism is supported by the worsening of lung damage seen in paraquat poisoning. Paraquat produces large amounts of ROS, and the administration of supplemental oxygen worsens its effects. Detecting this problem as the sole aetiology for pulmonary pathology can be difficult, especially as the usual indications for oxygen therapy usually imply some form of pulmonary pathology.

It is reasonable that the risk of oxygen-induced pulmonary toxicity is dependent on concentration and duration of exposure. However, the concentration/duration that constitutes 'likely to cause toxicity' is not clear. In some subjects long exposure times and high concentrations do not lead to problems. In general, patients should remain below an Fi_{O_2} of 0.5 where possible, and periods above this should be kept to the minimum required.

BRONCHO-PULMONARY DYSPLASIA (BPD)

First described in 1967, this is a form of chronic lung disease associated with neonatal ventilation; its pathophysiology includes the same factors as the adult, but with the additional effect of immaturity.[56] The advent of surfactant in the treatment of respiratory distress of the newborn and the addition of maternal steroid therapy to promote pulmonary development have lowered the incidence and reduced the severity of the disease.

OTHER PULMONARY EFFECTS

Supplemental oxygen also has other more predictable physiological effects within the lungs that may not been seen as truly toxicological, but cause problems in themselves. The greatest is the effect of oxygen on ventilation, especially in those at risk of Type II respiratory failure.

I. *V/Q mismatch:* high concentrations of inspired oxygen will reduce the physiological effects of hypoxic pulmonary vasoconstriction, thus diverting blood through poorly ventilated lung, increasing shunt and reducing Pa_{O_2}. In lungs without chronic disease, this can be compensated for by an increase in ventilation. However, in patients with borderline ventilation, this can lead to increasing Pa_{CO_2} and worsening acidaemia.

II. *Ventilatory drive:* hypoxia below 8 kPa (60 mmHg) leads to an increase in ventilation. Values above this level have little impact on ventilation. It remains contentious whether this mechanism is important when rises in Pa_{CO_2} are seen in patients with COPD.[57,58]

III. *Haldane effect:* increasing Fi_{O_2} decreases the CO_2 buffering capacity of haemoglobin, thus potentially leading to an increase in Pa_{CO_2} and acidaemia.

IV. *Absorption atelectasis:* in the presence of small-airway obstruction, high alveolar oxygen concentrations result in rapid absorption of gas, causing collapse of the alveoli and reduction in the diffusion surface area. This has been demonstrated even at an Fi_{O_2} of 0.5.[59]

V. *Higher density of oxygen compared with air:* oxygen is more dense than air and thus breathing high concentrations at increased viscosity increases the work of breathing. This effect is probably negligible in patients with normal underlying lungs and neuromuscular function, but can be significant in those with chronic disease.

RETINOPATHY OF PREMATURITY

Previously referred to as retrolental fibroplasia, retinopathy of prematurity (ROP) was first described in 1942. It is a vasoproliferative disorder of the eye affecting premature neonates. Similar to the lungs, the completion of development of the retinal vasculature is late in gestation (32–34 weeks).[60] In the 1950s an epidemic of ROP was described and a causal link to uncontrolled oxygen therapy was made.[61] Improved monitoring of oxygen therapy reduced the incidence of ROP, but was associated with an increase in perinatal mortality secondary to respiratory failure.[62] Subsequently, and despite good oxygen control, ROP continues to occur. This is now most likely due to the increased survival of increasingly premature low-birth-weight infants[63] rather than high Pa_{O_2} alone. This suggests both oxygen- and non-oxygen-related factors. ROP is a biphasic disease where the relatively hyperoxic environment following delivery initially leads to a slowing or even cessation of retinal vascular development of the premature infant. Additional oxygen may further contribute to this problem by affecting the expression of vascular growth factors. The second phase of the disease is a hypoxic-induced neovascularisation, similar to that seen in diabetic retinopathy. This leads to fibrous scarring with risk of retinal detachment. How much oxygen is too much remains contentious and further research is required.[64]

HYPEROXIC AND HYPERBARIC OXYGEN THERAPY

As stated above there are very few indications for increasing the Pa_{O_2} above 'normal', approximately 13 kPa (100 mmHg). Indeed it is likely to be harmful. However, there exist some data to support its use in certain conditions, the majority of which do not involve the critical care physician. These include the treatment of cluster headache, reduction in oxidative stress in colonic surgery and prevention of desaturation during endoscopy.[65–68] The use of hyperoxia to treat postoperative nausea and vomiting and prevent postoperative wound infections lacks high-quality evidence.[66]

ACUTE CARBON MONOXIDE POISONING

Carbon monoxide poisoning as a condition necessitating hyperoxic therapy attracts particular attention. A common consequence of house fires, it binds to haemoglobin with an affinity 210 times that of oxygen. Its half-life in air is 320 minutes, but this can be reduced to 90 minutes by giving the patient 100% oxygen, or 23 minutes with the addition of 3 atmospheres (≈300 kPa) of hyperbaric therapy. Competitive dissociation of carbon monoxide from the haem-binding site and provision of dissolved oxygen to the tissues is believed to combine to reduce the sequelae of carbon monoxide poisoning, but the mechanisms are likely to be more complex.[69] Some studies have suggested both acute and longer-term benefit,[70,71] but others have been unable to conclude significant improvement.[72,73] Recent investigations have attempted to distinguish those patients more likely to benefit from hyperbaric oxygen therapy. Factors such as increasing age (>35 years), an exposure time of >24 hours, an associated loss of consciousness and carboxyhaemoglobin levels greater than 25% appear to result in an increased incidence of neurological sequelae, and probably benefit from hyperbaric oxygen.[74] Geographical distance to an appropriate centre often has a significant influence on hyperbaric usage in the acute setting, but mobile units and some evidence that late therapy may be of benefit should not necessarily preclude its usage.[75,76]

HYPERBARIC OXYGEN

As alluded to in the treatment of carbon monoxide poisoning, oxygen can be delivered to patients at higher than atmospheric pressure (2–3 atmospheres). This serves to increase the amount of oxygen carried in the plasma, rather than bound to haemoglobin. This follows Henry's law that states: 'At a constant temperature, the amount of a given gas dissolved in a given type and volume of liquid is proportional to the partial pressure of that gas in equilibrium with that liquid.' As the partial pressure of oxygen in the environment rises, so to does the amount of oxygen dissolved in the plasma. Consequently, the contribution of the Pa_{O_2} in the Ca_{O_2} formula (28.2) increases. At rest the metabolic demands of an average person can be met by dissolved oxygen alone when breathing 100% at 3 atmospheres.

Hyperbaric oxygen therapy can be delivered either in a monoplace chamber designed for one individual, or in multiplace chambers for 2–10 people. The chambers encompass the whole body, and gas is piped from source, heated and humidified. The common indications and complications of hyperbaric oxygen therapy are listed in **Boxes 28.3 and 28.4**, respectively.[77,78]

Box 28.3 Recognised indications for hyperbaric oxygen therapy[77,78]

Primary therapy	Adjunctive therapy
Carbon monoxide poisoning	Radiation tissue damage
Air or gas embolism	Crush injuries
Decompression sickness (the 'bends')	Compromised skin flaps or grafts
Osteoradionecrosis	Refractory osteomyelitis
Clostridial myositis and myonecrosis	Intracranial abscess
	Chronic wound healing

Box 28.4 Complications of hyperbaric oxygen therapy

- *barotrauma:* middle ear and sinuses, rupture of the oval or round window, gastrointestinal distension, tooth displacement and pain, gas embolism on decompression
- *oxygen toxicity (as above):* especially a problem in the critically ill who may be on high concentrations for longer periods[78]
- *generalised seizures:* Paul Bert effect
- *visual problems:* acute myopia, cataract formation.

Access the complete references list online at http://www.expertconsult.com

4. van Boxel G, Doherty WL, Parmar M. Cellular oxygen utilization in health and sepsis. CEACCP 2012; 12(4):207–12.
17. Dellinger RP, Levy MM, Rhodes A, et al; Surviving Sepsis Campaign Guidelines Committee including the Pediatric Subgroup. Surviving Sepsis Campaign: International Guidelines for Management of Severe Sepsis and Septic Shock: 2012. Crit Care Med 2013; 41(2):580–637.
20. Grocott MP, Martin DS, Levett DZ, et al; Caudwell Xtreme Everest Research Group. Arterial blood gases and oxygen content in climbers on Mount Everest. N Engl J Med 2009;360(2):140–9.
31. Wagstaff TAJ, Soni N. Performance of six types of oxygen delivery devices at varying respiratory rates. Anaesthesia 2007;62(5):492–503.
37. O'Driscoll BR, Howard LS, Davison AG. BTS guideline for emergency oxygen use in adult patients. Thorax 2008;63(Suppl. 6):vi1–68.
46. de Jonge E, Peelen L, Keijzers PJ, et al. Association between administered oxygen, arterial partial oxygen pressure and mortality in mechanically ventilated intensive care unit patients. Crit Care 2008;12(6): R156.
69. Weaver LK. Clinical practice. Carbon monoxide poisoning. N Engl J Med 2009;360(12):1217–25.

29

Airway management and acute airway obstruction

Gavin M Joynt and Gordon YS Choi

The primary objective of airway management is to clear or bypass the obstructed airway and protect the lungs from soiling. Acute upper airway obstruction is a life-threatening emergency, resulting from a wide range of pathophysiological processes. Rapid assessment and establishment of a patent airway are vital, often in the absence of a specific diagnosis. As no single airway management modality is universally applicable, the intensive care unit (ICU) physician must be capable of performing a variety of airway management techniques (**Fig. 29.1**).

AIRWAY MANAGEMENT TECHNIQUES

Airway management techniques can be considered non-invasive or invasive, depending on whether instrumentation occurs above or below the glottis, and is surgical or non-surgical (**Table 29.1**). Definitive techniques secure the trachea and provide some protection from macroscopic aspiration and soiling. Although most airway management in ICU is still achieved by bag-and-mask ventilation and direct laryngoscopic tracheal intubation, the use of fibreoptic bronchoscopy and video laryngoscopy is increasingly common, especially in special circumstances. Management of failed intubation and ventilation by various alternative techniques (e.g. laryngeal mask airway (LMA) and cricothyroidotomy) is now well described.[1,2]

The technique of choice will depend on each situation and is a consequence of the interaction of patient factors and the clinician's experience (**Table 29.2**). Other factors include availability of help, levels of training and supervision and accessibility of equipment. A portable storage unit with a wide choice of equipment appropriate for difficult airway management is necessary in the ICU (**Box 29.1**).

NON-INVASIVE TECHNIQUES

BAG-MASK VENTILATION

As with most airway management techniques, mask ventilation is a basic skill that requires time and experience to master. It should be learned using mannikins, simulators and practice in the controlled environment of the operating theatre so that when used in the emergency setting in ICU the skill is well established. The bag may be a self-inflating resuscitator, or one attached to an anaesthetic circuit. Most resuscitators require a reservoir bag in series with the self-inflating bag that ensures a high oxygen concentration can be delivered. The addition of positive end-expiratory pressure (PEEP) may improve arterial oxygenation and overcome airway obstruction due to laryngospasm.

Some considerations when performing mask ventilation include the following:

- *Inadequate ventilation:* the seal of the mask against the face may be inadequate and good hand positioning is essential. Ventilation of edentulous patients may be aided by improving hand position or special masks. Two operators are recommended if a mask face leak is excessive: one to hold the mask and the other to manipulate the bag-mask resuscitator.
- *Hyperventilation:* unnecessary hyperventilation may occasionally cause dynamic pulmonary hyperinflation and cardiovascular compromise.
- *Gastric insufflation:* this increases the risk of vomiting and aspiration. Carefully applied cricoid pressure may prevent gastric gas insufflation.
- *Pulmonary aspiration:* in the emergency situation with a full stomach, mask ventilation with cricoid pressure may be necessary until the airway can be secured. Passage of a nasogastric tube to aspirate gastric contents may be successful, but emptying cannot be guaranteed and vomiting may be induced.

ORO- AND NASOPHARYNGEAL AIRWAYS

In the unconscious patient, functional obstruction may occur because of loss of muscular tone and inspiratory airway narrowing at the soft palate, epiglottis and tongue base. An oropharyngeal airway device may establish an adequate airway for spontaneous or bag-mask ventilation when proper head positioning is insufficient. It is inserted with the concavity facing the palate and then rotated 180° into the proper position as it is advanced. Complications include mucosal trauma, worsening the obstruction by pressing the epiglottis against the laryngeal outlet if the tongue displaces posteriorly, and occasionally laryngospasm. The following sizes (length from flange to tip) are recommended: large adult: 100 mm (Guedel size 5), medium adult: 90 mm (Guedel size 4), and small adult: 80 mm (Guedel size 3).

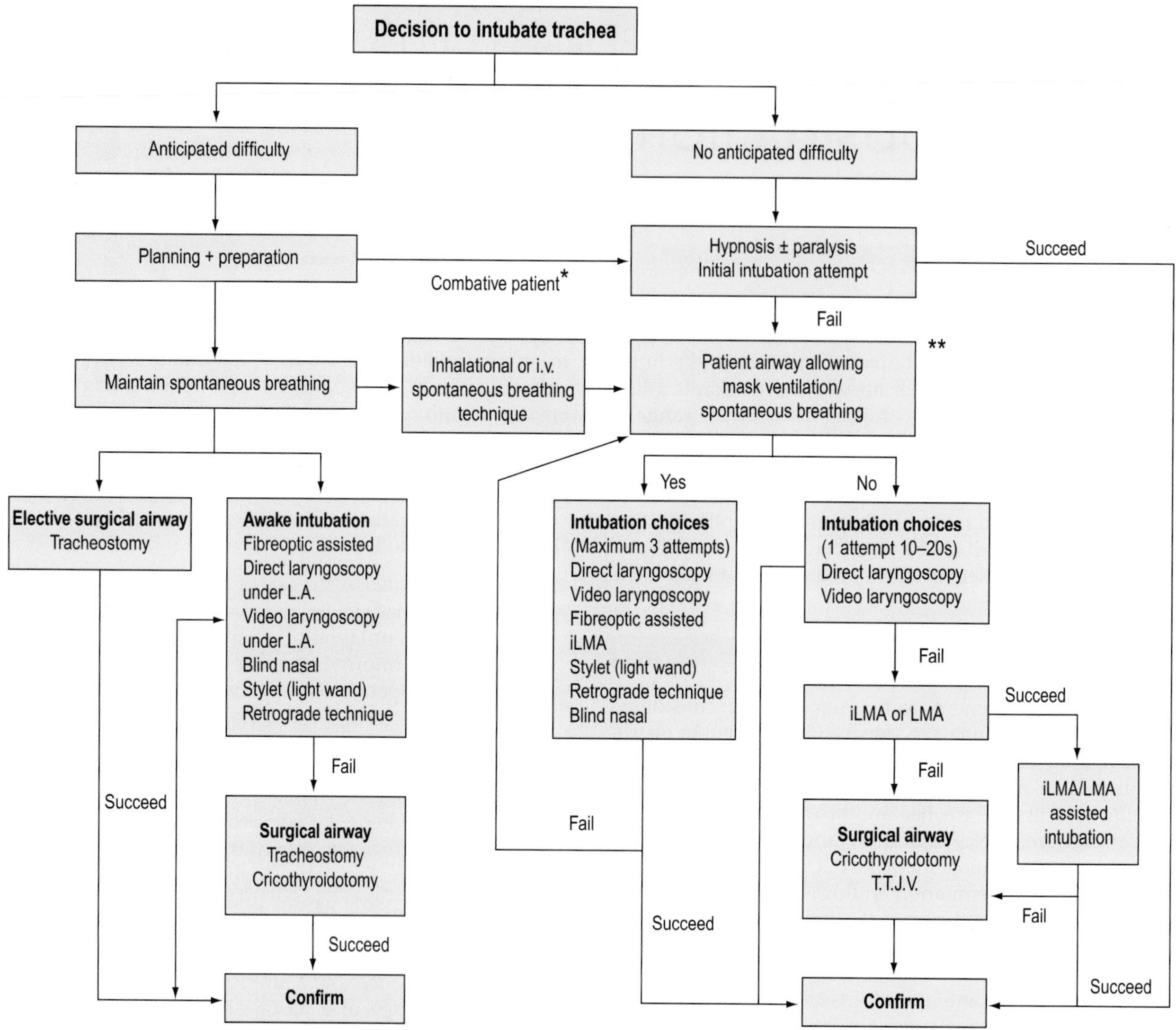

Figure 29.1 Difficult airway algorithm (see text). LA=local anaesthetic; iLMA=intubating laryngeal mask airway; LMA=laryngeal mask airway; TTJV=transtracheal jet ventilation.

A nasopharyngeal airway is a soft rubber or plastic tube inserted into the nostril and advanced along the floor of the nose (in the direction of the occiput). It is better tolerated by semiconscious patients than the oropharyngeal airway. Complications include epistaxis, aspiration and, rarely, laryngospasm and oesophageal placement.

LARYNGEAL MASK AIRWAY (LMA) AND INTUBATING LMA (ILMA)

The LMA is a reusable device that consists of a silicone rubber tube connected to a distal elliptical spoon-shaped mask with an inflatable rim, which is positioned blindly into the pharynx to form a low-pressure seal against the laryngeal inlet.[3] There are a variety of sizes for use in children and adults. LMAs are useful to achieve non-definitive airway patency in many emergency situations (see Fig. 29.1), and can be used to provide limited positive-pressure ventilation.

Once positioned the LMA can be used to guide the passage of stylets, bougies, the bronchoscope or even an endotracheal tube into the trachea.[4] The intubating LMA (FasTrach) is a modification of the LMA with several features to facilitate intubation once the LMA is placed.[5] There is a guiding ramp and epiglottic elevating bar at the aperture to direct the endotracheal tube to the glottis. It also has an anatomically curved, rigid shaft and handle to allow easy and firm manipulation during placement and when the endotracheal tube is passed.[6]

Table 29.1 Characteristics of airway management techniques

TECHNIQUE	EXPERIENCE REQUIRED	TIME REQUIRED	DEFINITIVE
NON-INVASIVE			
Bag-and-mask	+	Seconds	–
LMA and ILMA	+	1 min	–
Combitube	–	1 min	+
INVASIVE (NON-SURGICAL)			
Endotracheal intubation			
Direct laryngoscopy	+	Variable	+
Bronchoscopic	+	Several minutes	+
Video laryngoscopy	+	Variable	+
Retrograde	–	Minutes	+
INVASIVE (SURGICAL)			
Jet ventilation	–	Minutes	–
Cricothyroidotomy			
Percutaneous	–	Minutes	±
Surgical	+	1 min	+
Tracheostomy			
Percutaneous	+	Minutes	+
Surgical	+	Minutes	+

LMA=laryngeal mask airway; ILMA =intubating laryngeal mask airway.

The LMA is prepared for insertion by deflating and smoothing out the cuffed rim to be wrinkle-free, and the posterior surface is lubricated with water-soluble jelly. The patient is positioned as for endotracheal intubation, with slight flexion of the neck and extension of the atlanto-occipital joint (sniffing-the-morning-air position). The LMA is inserted with the tip of the cuff continuously applied to the hard palate, and with the right index finger guiding the tube to the back of the tongue until a firm resistance is encountered. The cuff is then inflated with 20–40 mL of air (adult sizes) before attachment of the breathing circuit. The successful use of LMA requires some familiarity with the equipment and technique, and at least simulated exposure is strongly recommended. Contraindications for using the LMA include inability to open the mouth, pharyngeal pathology, airway obstruction at or below the larynx, low pulmonary compliance or high airway resistance. Complications include aspiration, gastric insufflation, partial airway obstruction, coughing, laryngospasm, postextubation stridor and kinking of the shaft of the LMA.

COMBITUBE (OESOPHAGEAL–TRACHEAL DOUBLE-LUMEN AIRWAY)

The oesophageal–tracheal Combitube is a double-lumen tube that is blindly inserted into the oropharynx up to the indicated markings.[7] The oesophageal lumen has a stopper at the distal end and side perforations at the pharyngeal level whereas the tracheal lumen has a hole at the distal end. It has two cuffs, a distal one and a proximal pharyngeal balloon. The patient is ventilated through the oesophageal lumen initially as the Combitube usually enters the oesophagus,[7] with the distal cuff sealing the oesophagus and the proximal balloon sealing the pharynx. Gas exits the perforations and enters the pharynx and larynx. In the event of failure of ventilation, the tracheal lumen is ventilated and the distal cuff seals the trachea.

Table 29.2 Application of airway management techniques

	DIFFICULT DIRECT LARYNGOSCOPIC INTUBATION	DIFFICULT SPONTANEOUS/MASK VENTILATION
Awake	Fibreoptic bronchoscopic intubation Blind nasal intubation Retrograde intubation	Percutaneous cricothyroidotomy* Surgical tracheostomy*
Anaesthetised or comatose (empty stomach)	Bag-and-mask ventilation Direct laryngoscopic intubation Different blade choices Video laryngoscopy Fibreoptic bronchoscopic intubation Intubating LMA/LMA Lighted stylet Blind nasal intubation	Laryngeal mask airway Transtracheal jet ventilation Rigid ventilating bronchoscope Percutaneous cricothyroidotomy Surgical tracheostomy
(full stomach)	Consider cricoid pressure Consider ProSeal LMA Combitube	Percutaneous cricothyroidotomy Surgical tracheostomy Combitube

Examples of common alternatives are given. The technique chosen will depend on clinician preference.
* Under local anaesthesia. LMA=laryngeal mask airway.

Box 29.1 Suggested contents of a portable storage facility for difficult airway management

Masks
Face and nasal masks of differing make and size variety
Airways
Oropharyngeal airways
Nasopharyngeal airways
Airway intubator guide for oral endoscopic intubation
Laryngeal mask airway (LMA) and intubating LMA with appropriate endotracheal tubes
Rigid laryngoscope with a variety of designs and sizes
Short handle or variable angle (Patil–Syracuse) laryngoscope
Curved blades: Macintosh, Bizarri–Guiffrida
Straight blades: Miller
Bent blade: Belscope
Articulating tip blade: McCoy
Video laryngoscope
Disposable
Non-disposable
Endotracheal tubes of assorted size
Murphy tubes
Microlaryngoscopy tubes
Endotracheal tube stylets
Gum elastic bougie (Eschmann stylet)
Malleable stylet
Tube changer, hollow tube changer (jet stylet)
Lighted stylet (light wand)
Fibreoptic intubation equipment
Patil endoscopic mask for oral endoscopic intubation
Fibreoptic endoscopes with light source, adult and paediatric-sized
Device for emergency non-surgical airway ventilation
Combitube
Emergency surgical airway access
Percutaneous cricothyroidotomy set
Transtracheal jet ventilation – cannula and high-pressure O_2 source connectors
Regulated central wall O_2 pressure (Sanders-type injector)
Unregulated central wall O_2 pressure
Exhaled carbon dioxide monitor
Capnometer/capnograph
Chemical indicators

Although demonstrated to be useful in the prehospital setting, its role in resuscitation and management of the difficult airway in the ICU environment is yet to be established. Barotrauma, especially oesophageal rupture, has been reported.

INVASIVE TECHNIQUES

ENDOTRACHEAL INTUBATION

Endotracheal intubation remains the 'gold standard' airway management technique, allowing for spontaneous and positive-pressure ventilation, with good macroscopic protection from aspiration. Indications include acute airway obstruction, facilitation of tracheal suctioning, protection of the airway in those without protective reflexes and respiratory failure requiring ventilatory support with high inspired concentrations of oxygen and PEEP.

Prior to proceeding with an intubation attempt, regardless of the technique chosen, pre-oxygenation, as well as preparation and checking of all relevant equipment, is essential. Difficult airway management equipment (see Box 29.1) should also be accessible within a few minutes. Food, vomitus, blood or sputum may obstruct the airway and suction should always be available. Suction apparatus should generate at least 300 mmHg (40 kPa) and 30 L/min. Excessively vigorous suctioning should be avoided as it can cause laryngospasm, vagal stimulation, mucosal injury and bleeding.

Direct laryngoscopy

Although essential for all intensivists, direct laryngoscopy is a difficult skill to master.[8] If multiple intubation attempts are required, the maximum interruption to ventilation should be about 30 seconds. Adequate ventilation and oxygenation must be provided between attempts. Minimum monitoring should consist of continuous-pulse oximetry, electrocardiogram (ECG) and blood pressure. The BURP (Backward, Upward, Rightward Pressure) technique may be helpful to bring the vocal cords into the field of vision. Endotracheal tube size describes the internal diameter and, where possible, 8.0–9.0 mm in adult males and 7.5–8.0 mm in adult females are generally used to facilitate sputum clearance, minimise airway resistance and allow access for fibreoptic bronchoscopy. Special purpose tubes include double-lumen tubes to facilitate lung isolation, spiral imbedded tubes, and laser-resistant tubes.

The route of intubation may be orotracheal or nasotracheal. The orotracheal route is generally recommended because it may be associated with fewer complications.[9] However, nasotracheal intubation allows easier tube fixation and avoids the risk of tube occlusion from biting. It is contraindicated in the presence of fracture of the base of the skull. Other complications include epistaxis, turbinate cartilage and nasal septal damage during insertion.

Stylet guide (introducer)

The 'anterior larynx' can often be more easily intubated if a gum elastic bougie is advanced in the midline and directed anteriorly into the trachea. The endotracheal tube is then advanced over the guide. Clinical signs of correct tracheal placement of the guide include coughing, resistance felt before the guide is fully advanced (usually at 45 cm or less from the lips because of resistance at the carina or bronchus) and a sensation of clicks from the tracheal rings. A number of alternative intubating guides are available, including the hollow endotracheal tube changer, which can be attached to a side-stream capnometer, or to an oxygen source. The lighted stylet is less commonly used and has a light at the distal end that results in a characteristic midline transillumination appearance when the light enters the larynx.

Rigid indirect fibreoptic instruments

Video-laryngoscopes are newer devices that generate a view of the glottis from near the laryngoscope tip. When used for difficult airway management, they produce similar or better intubation success rates compared with direct laryngoscopy, and reduce cervical spine movement during laryngoscopy.[10] Limitations do exist for each particular device, and both training and operator experience contribute to successful use. Although increasingly available, there is insufficient evidence supporting the routine use of video-laryngoscopy as a replacement for traditional direct laryngoscopy.[10]

Fibreoptic bronchoscopic technique

This technique offers advantages of direct visualisation, immediate diagnosis of upper airway lesions and immobility of the neck during the procedure.[11] It also allows reasonably comfortable intubation of a cooperative, awake patient under local anaesthesia, and use of the sitting position. Experience and skill are necessary, especially for dealing with emergent situations, but success rates >96% are expected.[12] Fibreoptic intubation may also be performed in anaesthetised patients, using a modified facemask with diaphragm for oral intubation. Nasal intubation is usually performed through an endotracheal tube placed in the nasopharynx, with the tip just above the glottis. The fibreoptic bronchoscope tip is guided into the trachea and the tube is advanced over the bronchoscope. Correct placement is visually checked before the scope is removed. In ICU the fibreoptic bronchoscope can be used to improve the safety of airway procedures such as endotracheal tube changes and percutaneous tracheostomy.[13,14] A number of specially designed oral airways are available to assist oral fibreoptic intubation (e.g. the Ovassapian, Williams, or Berman airway). The most common cause of failure is obstructed vision from blood or secretions.

Blind nasal intubation

Blind nasal intubation is sometimes considered in spontaneously breathing patients. Possible indications include inability to open the mouth (e.g. mandibular fracture or temporomandibular joint pathology), and cervical spine and faciomaxillary injury. Contraindications include bleeding disorders, nasal airway obstruction, skull base fracture and pre-existing sinusitis. Operator proficiency is required.

Retrograde intubation technique

A J-tip guidewire (length required in adults approximately 70 cm) is introduced percutaneously through the cricothyroid membrane, and advanced into the retropharynx. The tip is retrieved from the oral cavity, and the wire is used to guide an oral endotracheal tube past the obstruction and into the trachea.[15] The procedure is a relatively simple and safe alternative if other techniques fail or are not possible. Commercial kits are available.

Confirmation of tracheal tube placement

Confirmation of correct intratracheal tube placement is essential. Direct visualisation and measurement of expired CO_2 by capnography are the most reliable methods.[16] Capnography may produce false-positive results with the first few breaths after oesophageal intubation (i.e. detectable PE_{CO_2}), if gastric insufflation from mask ventilation has occurred. A false-negative (decreased PE_{CO_2}, despite correct position) may occur with cardiac arrest and low-cardiac-output states. Position can also be reliably confirmed by the use of self-inflating oesophageal detectors. Other clinical signs, such as auscultation of breath sounds over both sides of the chest and epigastrium, visualisation of condensed water vapour in the tube and chest wall movement are less reliable. The use of capnography is further discussed in Chapter 38.

Complications of endotracheal intubation

These may be classified into those occurring during intubation (e.g. incorrect tube placement, laryngeal trauma, deleterious cardiovascular response to laryngoscopy and intubation, increase in intracranial pressure, hypoxaemia and aspiration), while the tube is in place (e.g. blockage, dislodgment, tube deformation, damage to larynx and complications of mechanical ventilation), and following extubation (e.g. aspiration and postextubation airway obstruction, laryngeal and tracheal stenosis). As few ICU patients can be adequately starved prior to intubation, the use of cricoid pressure, provided it does not obscure the glottic view, is usually required to reduce the risk of aspiration. Hypotension in ICU patients is common immediately following intubation because of drug-induced myocardial depression, decrease in peripheral vascular resistance and sympathetic stimulation, and reduced venous return after positive-pressure ventilation. Fluid administration and the use of vasopressor drugs may be required. Special techniques should be used to minimise side-effects such as cardiovascular responses and increases in intracranial pressure when appropriate.

TRANSTRACHEAL JET VENTILATION (TTJV)

Percutaneous TTJV, using a large-bore intravenous (i.v.) catheter inserted through the cricothyroid membrane, can be used to provide temporary ventilation when other techniques have failed.[17] Ventilation through the cannula with a standard manual resuscitator bag is inadequate, and a jet injector system is necessary. A high-pressure (up to 50 psi or 344 kPa) oxygen source is required for adequate ventilation through a 14 FG i.v. cannula. Expiratory gases must be able to escape via the glottis. Appropriate chest movements during expiration must be noted. The consequence of expiratory obstruction is severe and potentially fatal barotrauma.

Complications may be caused by insertion of the i.v. cannula (e.g. bleeding and oesophageal perforation), use of high-pressure gases (e.g. hyperinflation, barotrauma), catheter kinking or displacement (the latter causing potentially catastrophic subcutaneous emphysema) and failure to protect the airway (i.e. aspiration).

CRICOTHYROIDOTOMY

Cricothyroidotomy, by surgery or percutaneously, is a reliable, relatively easy way of providing an emergency airway.[18] It is the method of choice if severe or complete upper airway obstruction exists. The simplest, fastest and most proven method uses a horizontal incision through the cricothyroid membrane (with the space held wide open by the scalpel handle or forceps), followed by insertion of a small tracheostomy or endotracheal tube (**Fig. 29.2**). Commercial cricothyroidotomy sets, using the Seldinger technique, are available. A tube with internal diameter of 3.0 mm will allow adequate gas flow for self-inflating bag ventilation provided supplemental oxygen is used. Since the diameter of the cricothyroid space is 9 by 30 mm, tubes of 8.5 mm outer diameter or less should avoid laryngeal and vocal cord damage. Complications such as subglottic stenosis (1.6%), thyroid fracture, haemorrhage and pneumothorax are acceptably low. Cricothyroidotomy is generally contraindicated in complete laryngotracheal disruption and age <12 years.

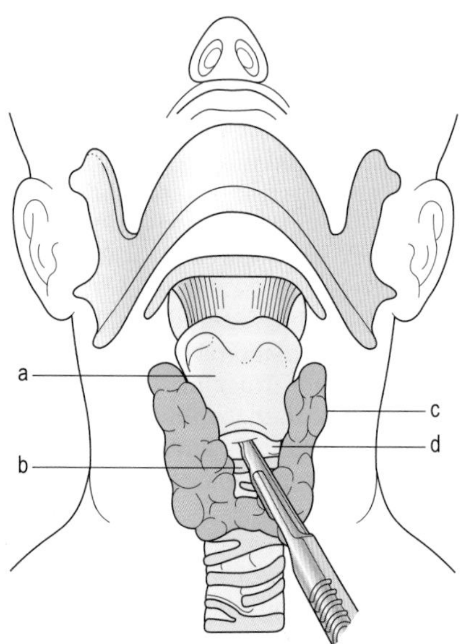

Figure 29.2 Cricothyroidotomy performed with a scalpel: (a) thyroid cartilage; (b) cricoid cartilage; (c) thyroid gland; (d) cricoid membrane, usually easily palpable subcutaneously.

TRACHEOSTOMY

There is little agreement on the indications, best technique or optimal timing of tracheostomy in ICU patients. Suggested indications for tracheostomy include:[19]

- bypass of glottic and supraglottic obstruction
- access for tracheal toilet
- provision of a more comfortable airway for prolonged ventilatory support
- protection of the airways from aspiration.

In uncomplicated patients, percutaneous tracheostomy performed by an intensivist at the bedside is at least as safe as surgical tracheostomy performed in the operating room, and is probably associated with a lower incidence of infectious complications.[20,21] Convenience and cost savings have made percutaneous tracheostomy the procedure of choice in many institutions. Ciaglia's percutaneous technique was described in 1985.[22] After making an adequate skin incision and using blunt dissection with forceps, the endotracheal tube is first withdrawn so that its cuff lies just above the vocal cords. The operator confirms tube position to be above the stoma site by palpation of the trachea. A J-wire is placed in the trachea through a needle inserted through the membrane above or below the second tracheal ring.

Curved dilators can be used to enlarge the stoma. A tracheostomy tube is then inserted into the trachea and the endotracheal tube removed. A modified tapered dilator to avoid the use of multiple dilators is quicker to use, but may cause more tracheal wall injuries and ring fractures. The Griggs technique utilises a Kelly forceps, modified to allow it to be guided by the J-wire, to dilate the tract before insertion of the tracheostomy tube.[23] The speed and safety of the two techniques are similar, although the Griggs technique may cause marginally more bleeding and cannula insertion may be more difficult.[24] Fibreoptic bronchoscopy during percutaneous tracheostomy may help to prevent incorrect guidewire placement and tracheal ring rupture or herniation, but definitive evidence supporting its routine use is lacking.[25]

Minitracheostomy describes the percutaneous insertion of a small 4 mm non-cuffed tracheostomy tube through the cricothyroid membrane or trachea, mainly to facilitate suctioning in patients with poor cough ability. Complications of tracheostomy are listed in **Box 29.2**.

LOCAL ANAESTHESIA

Instrumentation of the upper airway in awake patients requires good local anaesthesia to increase comfort, improve cooperation, attenuate cardiovascular responses and reduce the risk of laryngospasm. Rapid transcricoid injection, 'spray as you go' with a fibreoptic bronchoscope,

Table 29.3 Local anaesthesia of the upper airway in adults

TECHNIQUE	DRUG DOSAGE
NERVE BLOCK	
Internal branch of superior laryngeal nerve	Lidocaine 1–2% (2 mL/side)
Glossopharyngeal nerve	Lidocaine 1–2% (3 mL/side)
TOPICAL ANAESTHESIA OF THE TONGUE AND OROPHARYNX	
Gargle	Lidocaine viscous 4% (5 mL)
Commercial lidocaine spray	Lidocaine 10% (5–10 sprays=50–100 mg)
Nebulised	Lidocaine 4%
Spray as you go	Lidocaine 1–2%
TOPICAL ANAESTHESIA OF THE NASAL MUCOSA	
Cocaine spray or paste	Cocaine 4–5% (0.5–2 mL)
Gel	Lidocaine 2% gel (5 mL)
Commercial lidocaine spray	Lidocaine 10% (10 sprays=100 mg)
Lidocaine laryngeal mask airway+phenylephrine spray	Lidocaine 3%+phenylephrine 0.25% (0.5 mL)
TOPICAL ANAESTHESIA OF GLOTTIS AND TRACHEA	
Spray-as-you-go through bronchoscope	Lidocaine 1–4% (3 mg/kg)
Cricothyroid membrane puncture	Lidocaine 2% (5 mL)
Nebulised	Lidocaine 4% (4 mL)±phenylephrine 1% (1 mL)

Box 29.2 Complications of tracheostomy

Immediate

- Procedural complications
  - Haemorrhage
  - Surgical emphysema, pneumothorax, air embolism
  - Cricoid cartilage damage
- Misplacement in pretracheal tissues or right main bronchus
- Compression of tube lumen by cuff herniation
- Occlusion of the tip against the carina or tracheal wall

Delayed

- Blockage with secretions
- Infection of the tracheostomy site, tracheobronchial tree, and larynx
- Pressure on tracheal wall from the tracheostomy tube or cuff
  - Mucosal ulceration and perforation
  - Deep erosion into the innominate artery
  - Tracheo-oesophageal fistula

Late

- Granulomata of the trachea
- Tracheal and laryngeal stenosis
- Persistent sinus at tracheostomy site
- Tracheomalacia and tracheal dilatation

or nebulised lidocaine to the nares, posterior pharynx and tongue is effective (**Table 29.3**).[26] Nerve block techniques may improve analgesia but are not essential. Systemic absorption of topically applied lidocaine (maximum dose 4 mg/kg) is variable, and the clinician should be alert for signs and symptoms of toxicity.

THE DIFFICULT AIRWAY

The difficult airway has been described as one in which a conventionally trained anaesthesiologist experiences difficulty with mask ventilation, tracheal intubation or both. Difficult intubations may be expected in 1–3% of patients presenting for general anaesthesia, and the incidence is likely to be considerably higher in ICU patients.

More than 85% of difficult intubations can be managed successfully by experienced clinicians without resorting to a surgical solution. The experience of the operator is probably the most important factor determining success or failure. Experience implies greater manual skills, better anticipation of problems, use of preprepared strategies, and familiarity with multiple techniques. Thus, training of intensivists must specifically include a variety of airway management strategies and skills.

ASSISTANCE AND ENVIRONMENT

The patient's condition may rapidly deteriorate as a consequence of a poorly managed airway emergency. The most senior help available should be immediately summoned. If the situation allows, the patient should be moved to the best location for emergency airway interventions, usually the operating theatre or ICU, and difficult airway equipment requested (see Box 29.1). A senior assistant can help in gaining i.v. access, administering drugs, setting up equipment and managing the airway. A skilled intensivist or ear, nose and throat surgeon (gowned and standing by) can help to provide a surgical airway or perform rigid bronchoscopy to remove foreign bodies.

ANTICIPATING AND GRADING A DIFFICULT AIRWAY

Intubation difficulty can be anticipated or predicted by the following (although the sensitivity and specificity of individual features and classifications tend to be low):

1. Anatomical or pathological features of difficult intubation in subjects who otherwise appear normal:
   a. short neck, especially if obese or muscular (a thyromental distance <6 cm)
   b. limited neck and jaw movements (e.g. as a result of trismus, osteoarthritis, ankylosing spondylitis, rheumatoid arthritis or perioral scarring)
   c. protruding teeth, small mouth, long high curved palate or receding lower jaw
   d. space-occupying lesions of the oropharynx and larynx
   e. congenital conditions with any of the above features (e.g. Marfan's syndrome).
2. Mallampatti classification[27] of visualising the oropharyngeal structures (a cooperative sitting patient is required for this assessment, and class >2 predicts possible difficulty):
   a. class 1: visible soft palate, uvula, fauces and pillars
   b. class 2: visible soft palate, uvula and fauces
   c. class 3: visible soft palate and base of uvula
   d. class 4: soft palate is not visible.
3. The degree of difficulty experienced visualising the larynx by direct laryngoscopy should be recorded and is commonly graded by the classification of Cormack and Lehane:[28]
   a. grade I: complete glottis is visible
   b. grade II: anterior glottis is not visible
   c. grade III: epiglottis but not glottis is visible
   d. grade IV: epiglottis is not visible.

FAILED INTUBATION AND VENTILATION ALGORITHMS

A preformulated plan in the event of failed intubation and/or ventilation is essential and a number have been described. The algorithm shown in Figure 29.1 is an example. Effective implementation depends on the appropriate use of the algorithm and airway techniques described above.

If the initial attempt at intubation fails, call for help immediately. Repeated attempts at direct laryngoscopy should be avoided unless a more experienced operator intervenes, or a potentially helpful manoeuvre has been carried out (e.g. significant repositioning, externally applied laryngeal pressure or change of laryngoscope blade). Hypoxia will quickly result if the patient is inadequately ventilated between attempts. In addition, oedema and bleeding caused by repeated attempts may impair both mask ventilation and the use of alternative techniques such as fibreoptic intubation. When indicated to prevent hypoxia a surgical airway should not be delayed (see Figs 29.1 and 29.2).

UPPER AIRWAY OBSTRUCTION

ANATOMY AND PATHOPHYSIOLOGY

The upper airway begins at the nose and mouth, and ends at the carina. Obstruction is likely to occur at sites of anatomical narrowing, such as the hypopharynx at the base of the tongue, and the false and true vocal cords at the laryngeal opening. Sites of airway obstruction are classified as supraglottic (above the true cords), glottic (involving the true vocal cords) or infraglottic (below the true cords and above the carina).

The upper airway can also be divided into intrathoracic and extrathoracic portions, which behave differently during inspiration and expiration. The intrathoracic airway dilates during inspiration because it is 'pulled outwards' by negative intrapleural pressure. Positive intrapleural pressure during expiration causes compression and narrowing. Conversely the compliant extrathoracic airway, unexposed to intrapleural pressure, collapses during inspiration and expands during expiration. Recalling this phenomenon helps the understanding of typical clinical signs, imaging and flow–volume loops.

AETIOLOGY

Acute upper airway obstruction may result from functional or mechanical causes (**Box 29.3**). Functional causes include central nervous system and neuromuscular dysfunction. Mechanical causes may occur within the lumen, in the wall or extrinsic to the airway.

CLINICAL PRESENTATION

The signs of sudden complete upper airway obstruction are characteristic and progress rapidly. The victim cannot breathe, speak or cough, and may hold the throat between the thumb and index finger – the universal choking sign.[29] Agitation, panic and vigorous breathing efforts are rapidly followed by cyanosis. Respiratory efforts diminish as consciousness is lost, and death results within 2–5 minutes if obstruction is not relieved. Lethargy, diminishing respiratory efforts and loss of consciousness are late signs of hypoxaemia and hypercarbia. Bradycardia and hypotension herald impending cardiac arrest.

Signs of partial airway obstruction include voice changes and coughing, progressing to drooling, gagging, choking, noisy respiration and inspiratory stridor. Paradoxical chest wall movements and intercostal and supraclavicular retractions may be marked in severe obstruction. Powerful respiratory efforts may produce dermal ecchymoses and subcutaneous emphysema. Respiratory decompensation may be of rapid onset, and progress to complete obstruction.

SPECIAL EVALUATION OR INVESTIGATIONS

If the patient remains stable, specific diagnostic evaluation may be undertaken, provided advanced airway

Box 29.3 Clinical conditions associated with acute upper airway obstruction

Functional causes

Central nervous system depression
- Head injury, cerebrovascular accident, cardiorespiratory arrest, shock, hypoxia, drug overdose, metabolic encephalopathies

Peripheral nervous system and neuromuscular abnormalities
- Recurrent laryngeal nerve palsy (postoperative, inflammatory or tumour infiltration), obstructive sleep apnoea, laryngospasm, myasthenia gravis, Guillain–Barré polyneuritis, hypocalcaemic vocal cord spasm

Mechanical causes

Foreign body aspiration

Infections
- Epiglottitis, retropharyngeal cellulitis or abscess, Ludwig's angina, diphtheria and tetanus, bacterial tracheitis, laryngotracheobronchitis

Laryngeal oedema
- Allergic laryngeal oedema, angiotensin-converting enzyme inhibitor associated, hereditary angioedema, acquired C1 esterase deficiency

Haemorrhage and haematoma
- Postoperative, anticoagulation therapy, inherited or acquired coagulation factor deficiency

Trauma

Burns
- Inhalational thermal injury, ingestion of toxic chemical and caustic agents

Neoplasm
- Pharyngeal, laryngeal and tracheobronchial carcinoma, vocal cord polyposis

Congenital
- Vascular rings, laryngeal webs, laryngocele

Miscellaneous
- Cricoarytenoid arthritis, achalasia of the oesophagus, hysterical stridor, myxoedema

management facilities and skilled personnel are immediately available.

LARYNGOSCOPY AND BRONCHOSCOPY

Indirect laryngoscopy in a stable, cooperative patient is useful to diagnose foreign bodies, retropharyngeal or laryngeal masses and other glottic pathology.

Assessment with a flexible fibreoptic bronchoscope or laryngoscope is the evaluation method of choice in ICU patients and enables direct visualisation of upper airway anatomy and function. The procedure can be performed without transporting the patient and risking complete obstruction. It can be applied to an awake, spontaneously breathing patient and, with care, should not worsen the obstruction. Definitive airway control by intubation can usually be achieved. Disadvantages are the need for a skilled operator and a cooperative patient, and a reduced visual field limits effectiveness if blood and secretions are copious.

Direct laryngoscopy enables forceps removal of foreign bodies and high-volume suctioning of blood, vomitus and secretions. Endotracheal intubation can rapidly be achieved under direct vision. A disadvantage is the need for general anaesthesia or good local analgesia (often difficult in the emergency setting). Direct laryngoscopy can be traumatic, and may worsen soft-tissue bleeding and oedema.

RADIOGRAPHIC IMAGING

Patients with potentially unstable airways should not be transported from a 'safe' environment like the emergency room, operating theatre or ICU for radiological investigation until the airway is secure. Anteroposterior and lateral plain neck X-rays may be useful to detect radiopaque foreign bodies. Computed tomography (CT), preferably with three-dimensional post-processing, may provide detailed diagnostic information and prognostic at initial evaluation in stable patients, or in those in whom the airway has been secured.[30,31] Although magnetic resonance imaging (MRI) has been used to image the upper airway, its use in acute airway obstruction is unproven.

GAS FLOW MEASUREMENT

Flow–volume loop measurement reveals characteristic patterns corresponding to different types and position of pathological lesions (**Fig. 29.3**).[32]

MANAGEMENT

Simplified algorithms to assist the management of partial and complete upper airway obstruction are shown in **Figures 29.4** and **29.5** respectively. Improvisation may be required for certain difficult problems. The chosen technique should be an appropriate one in which the clinician has reasonable skill and experience. Special techniques in patients with suspected cervical spine instability are discussed in Chapter 78.

1. Supplemental oxygen (100%) is immediately administered and adequate help summoned.
2. A choice of equipment for definitive airway control must be available and ready for use (see Box 29.1).
3. In adults i.v. access should be secured.
4. Initiate continuous monitoring of vital signs and pulse oximetry.
5. The risk and benefit of patient transport before securing the airway must be carefully considered.

AIRWAY MANAGEMENT TECHNIQUES IN AIRWAY OBSTRUCTION

THE UNCONSCIOUS PATIENT

If the upper airway is obstructed by the tongue and retropharyngeal tissues in an unconscious patient, airway patency is initially achieved by using standard airway manoeuvres[33] and oropharyngeal and

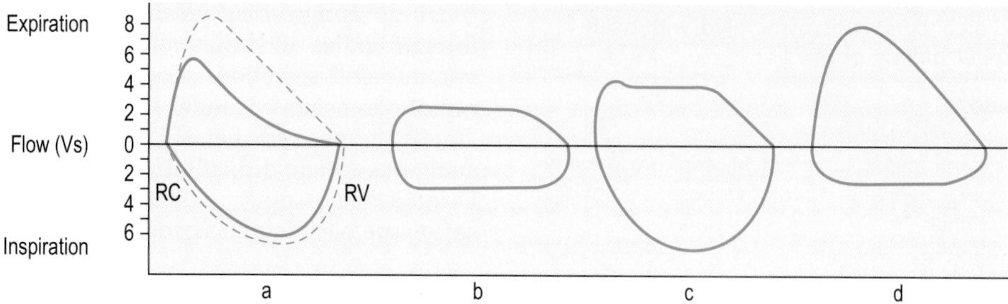

Figure 29.3 Flow–volume loops. Patterns resulting from different pathological lesions: (a) lower airway obstruction (e.g. chronic obstructive pulmonary disease or asthma); (b) fixed, non-variable upper airway obstruction (e.g. fibrous ring in trachea); (c) variable upper airway obstruction, intrathoracic (e.g. tumour in the lower trachea); (d) variable upper airway obstruction, extrathoracic (e.g. vocal cord tumour or paralysis).

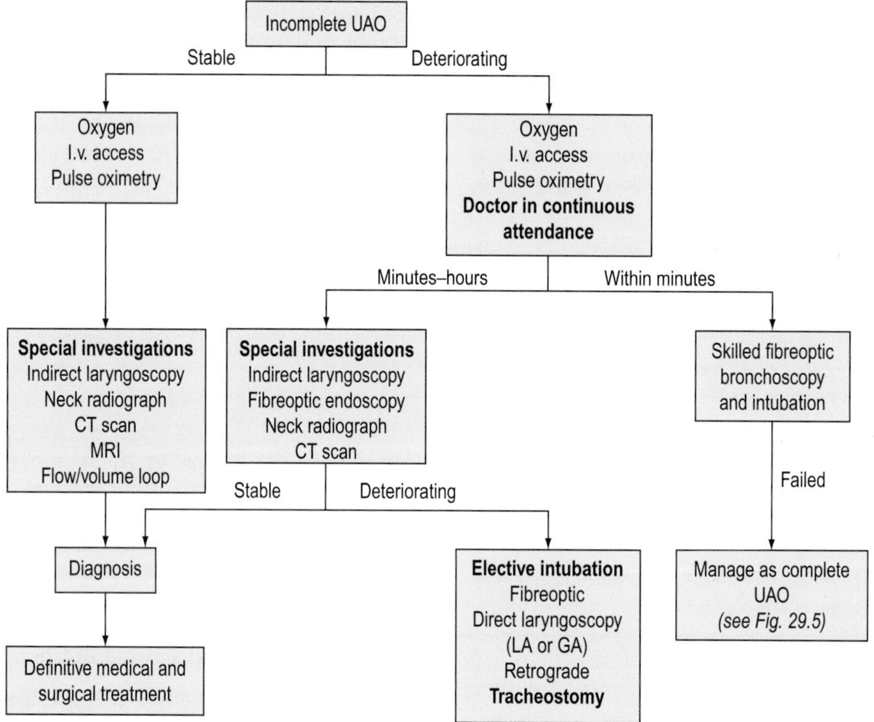

Figure 29.4 Management of partial upper airway obstruction (UAO). i.v.=intravenous; CT=computerised tomography; MRI=magnetic resonance imaging; LA=local anaesthesia; GA=general anaesthesia.

nasopharyngeal airways. Definitive airway control should follow if consciousness does not immediately return.

ENDOTRACHEAL INTUBATION

1. *Direct laryngoscopic intubation* is the method of choice for the unconscious, apnoeic patient as it allows rapid evaluation of any supraglottic problem and immediate airway security. *Video laryngoscopy* is an alternative in experienced hands. Both can also be attempted in an awake patient after careful application of local anaesthesia. Although there is some risk of loss of the airway after local anaesthesia, complete loss of the airway under general anaesthesia is common and may be catastrophic.
2. *Awake fibreoptic intubation* in a spontaneously breathing patient is usually safe, but requires a skilled operator. The procedure will take 2–10 minutes or longer,[34] and urgency of the case must be assessed beforehand with this timeframe in mind. Alternatives should be initiated if the obstruction progresses or if intubation fails after a reasonable time. The following points may assist visualisation in acute upper airway obstruction:

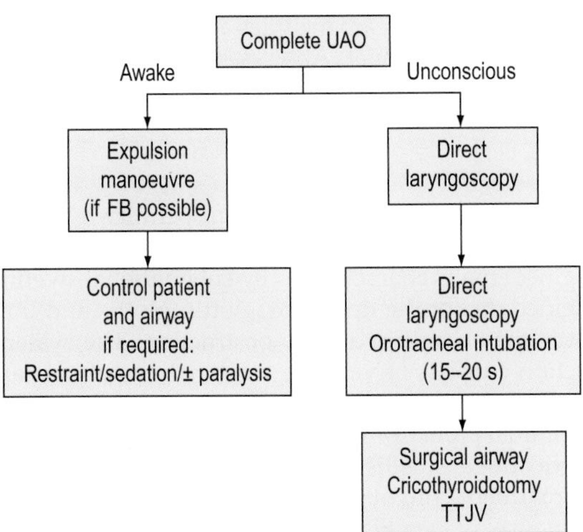

Figure 29.5 Management of complete upper airway obstruction (UAO). Attempts at orotracheal intubation should not take longer than 10–20 seconds. FB=foreign body; TTJV=transtracheal jet ventilation.

a. The procedure should be clearly explained to the patient.
b. Good local anaesthesia and mucosal vasoconstrictors are important (see Table 29.3).
c. If desired, the suction port of the fibrescope can be used to insufflate 100% oxygen or apply local anaesthetic. This also clears the fibrescope tip of secretions. Additional large-bore suction catheters may help. Failure is most commonly due to excessive secretions and bleeding.

3. *Blind nasotracheal intubation* may be considered by experienced operators. Once endotracheal intubation is safely accomplished and confirmed, secure fixation of the endotracheal tube is mandatory. The patient's upper limbs may need to be restrained to avoid self-extubation.

SURGICAL AIRWAYS

A surgical airway is indicated when endotracheal intubation is not possible, or when an unstable cervical spine is threatened by available airway techniques. It is the last line of defence against hypoxia. In airway obstruction, options include the following:

1. *Cricothyroidotomy:* this is the method of choice if severe or complete upper airway obstruction exists.
2. *Percutaneous transtracheal jet ventilation*: the technique must not be used in complete upper airway obstruction because expiratory obstruction can cause severe and potentially fatal barotrauma.
3. *Tracheostomy*: in the emergency setting this is rarely required, although surgical tracheostomy under local anaesthesia may be reasonable under some controlled conditions (see Fig. 29.4).

COMMON CLINICAL CONDITIONS AND THEIR MANAGEMENT

FOREIGN-BODY OBSTRUCTION

Foreign-body obstruction is the most common cause of acute airway obstruction. The elderly, especially those in institutions, are at risk. The use of dentures, alcohol and depressant drugs increases risk. Fatal food asphyxiation or 'café coronary' should be considered in any acute respiratory arrest where the victim cannot be ventilated.[35]

Those still able to cough or speak clearly should be given the opportunity to expel the foreign body spontaneously. Expulsion of the foreign body can be attempted with the Heimlich manoeuvre.[29] From behind, the rescuer encircles his or her arms around the victim, placing the thumb of one fist between the umbilicus and xiphisternum. The fist is gripped by the other hand, and an inward, upward thrust is applied. Chest thrusts (rescuer's arms should encircle the chest, and a fist placed over midsternum) may be of use in pregnancy and obesity. Unwanted effects, such as vomiting, aspiration, fractured ribs, barotrauma and ruptured organs, have been reported. Extract visible solid material with a finger sweep only in unconscious patients.[33] If these manoeuvres fail, management immediately proceeds as shown in Figures 29.4 and 29.5.

EXTRINSIC AIRWAY COMPRESSION

Extrinsic space-occupying lesions can cause upper airway obstruction. Compression from haematomas may be associated with trauma, neck surgery, central venous catheterisation, anticoagulants and congenital or acquired coagulopathies. Haematomas following surgery should immediately be evacuated by removing skin and tissue sutures. If this fails, an artificial airway must be secured immediately. In patients with coagulation abnormalities, intubation is preferred over a surgical airway. Most haematomas secondary to coagulopathy do not require surgical intervention, and resolve with conservative therapy (i.e. vitamin K and blood component therapy).

Partial airway obstruction caused by retropharyngeal abscess is best managed by drainage under local anaesthesia. Gentle fibreoptic examination and intubation or direct laryngoscopy and intubation may be considered. Risks are related to inadvertent rupture of the abscess, with subsequent flooding of the airway. Ludwig's angina is a mixed infection of the floor of the mouth resulting in an inflammatory mass in the space between the tongue and the muscles and anterior neck fascia. The supraglottic airway is compressed and becomes narrowed.[36] Direct laryngoscopy is difficult, as the tongue cannot be anteriorly displaced. Awake fibreoptic-guided intubation and a surgical airway, along with antibiotic therapy, are management options.

INTRINSIC AIRWAY COMPRESSION

Burn inhalation and ingestion injury

Patients with large burn area (more than 40%), or with severe facial burns or inhalation injury (soot in the nostrils, burns of the tongue and pharynx, stridor or hoarseness) are at risk of developing progressive supraglottic oedema, usually within 24–48 hours. Such patients may require early prophylactic tracheal intubation. Assessment of injury and need for tracheal intubation can best be decided by frequently repeated awake fibreoptic laryngoscopy, together with close clinical observation.[37] Ingestion of hot fluids or corrosive agents can also cause delayed oedema and airway swelling and should be managed similarly.[38]

Adult epiglottitis

Epiglottitis is an uncommon but increasingly recognised infectious disease in adults.[39] It involves the epiglottis and supraglottic larynx, causing swelling with consequent airway obstruction. *Haemophilus influenzae* and *H. parainfluenzae*, *Streptococcus pneumoniae*, haemolytic streptococci and *Staphylococcus aureus* are common causative organisms. Clinical features are sudden onset of sore throat (pain often greater than suggested by clinical findings), muffled voice, dysphagia, stridor, dyspnoea and respiratory distress. Systemic toxaemia is common. Gentle indirect laryngoscopy, fibreoptic laryngoscopy or lateral neck X-ray confirms the diagnosis. Reported mortality in adults ranges from 0% to 7%. [40]

Airway management is controversial.[40,41] Some experts recommend securing a definitive airway on presentation whereas others suggest close observation in ICU. There are, however, reports of sudden obstruction and death with the latter approach.[40] Onset of dyspnoea, dysphonia, stridor, a rapid clinical course and diabetes may predict the need for intubation.[42] Tracheal intubation and tracheostomy are acceptable, but tracheal intubation may result in better long-term outcome.

Prior to securing the airway, patient positioning is important, and changing from a sitting to supine position may induce complete obstruction. In more stable patients, awake fibreoptic intubation is preferable if a skilled operator is available. Endotracheal intubation under general anaesthesia following gaseous induction is often recommended. Obstruction can occur, even when this procedure is undertaken by a skilled anaesthetist in the operating room.[41] A skilled assistant, scrubbed and ready to secure a surgical airway, may prevent disaster. Rapid-sequence induction using muscle relaxants is dangerous and should be avoided. Tracheostomy under local anaesthesia is a safe alternative.

Airway management is followed by antibiotics and supportive care. Cefotaxime 2 g i.v. 6-hourly or ampicillin 1–2 g i.v. 6-hourly *plus* chloramphenicol 50 mg/kg per day are empirical regimens. Patient factors, local bacterial sensitivities and cultures of blood and epiglottal swabs may influence the antibiotic choice. Supportive care includes adequate sedation and tracheobronchial toilet. Abscesses should be surgically drained. There is no good evidence supporting the use of steroids.

Angioedema

Allergic responses involving the upper airway may be localised or part of a systemic anaphylactic reaction. Angioedema is characterised by subepithelial swelling. Angioedema of the lips, supraglottis, glottis and infraglottis may result in airway obstruction. The systemic reaction consists of variable combinations of urticaria, bronchospasm, shock, cardiovascular collapse and abdominal pain. Common causative agents are Hymenoptera stings, shellfish ingestion and drugs.

Treatment consists of immediately ensuring an adequate airway (see Figs 29.4 and 29.5), and administration of oxygen, epinephrine (adrenaline), histamine antagonists and steroids. Close observation in case of relapse for at least 24 hours after severe reactions is necessary. As it is likely to recur, the patient should be followed-up and fully investigated.

Hereditary angioedema is a rare, inherited disorder of the complement system, caused by functionless or low levels of C1 esterase inhibitor.[43] Non-pruritic, usually non-painful angioedema involving skin and subcutaneous tissue occurs in various locations, including the upper airway.[44] Precipitating causes include stress, physical exertion and localised trauma (including dental or maxillofacial surgery and laryngoscopy). Acute attacks do not respond to epinephrine, antihistamines or corticosteroids. Management consists of establishing a secure airway and infusion of C1 esterase inhibitor concentrate (25 U/kg) which has an onset of action of 30–120 minutes.[44,45] If not available, fresh frozen plasma (2–4 units) may be considered.

Stanozolol 2 mg daily or danazol 200 mg/day has been shown to be effective in decreasing frequency and severity of attacks with reduced side-effects.[46] Antifibrinolytic agents (e.g. tranexamic acid) are less effective. Guidelines recommend use of C1-inhibitor concentrate for preoperative prophylaxis or, if this is unavailable, the dose of attenuated androgen should be doubled for 5 days before and 2 days after the procedure. Icatibant acetate, a subcutaneous synthetic peptide blocker of the bradykinin-2 receptor, and ecallantide, a subcutaneous recombinant protein kallikrein antagonist, have both recently become available for the symptomatic treatment of hereditary angioedema.[46] Angiotensin-converting enzyme inhibitor-related angioedema is increasingly seen and is possibly the result of reduced bradykinin metabolism.[47] Treatment focuses on airway support.

Postextubation laryngeal oedema

Laryngeal oedema following extubation occurs in about 20% of adults, but is severe enough to precipitate re-intubation in only 1–5%. The risk of postextubation oedema may be increased by excessive airway manipulation, traumatic intubation, high cuff pressures and duration of tracheal intubation greater than 36 hours (however, after 1 week the risk appears to decline again). Prophylactic use of corticosteroids (e.g. methylprednisolone initiated 12 hours before planned extubation at 20 mg i.v. 4-hourly with the last dose immediately prior to tube removal) has been shown to reduce the incidence of postextubation laryngeal oedema and subsequent re-intubation.[48] Treatment in adults is conservative, with close observation and humidified oxygen therapy. Nebulised plain epinephrine (1–2 mL 1:1000 solution diluted with 2 mL saline or undiluted 1:1000 solution 4–5 mL) or racemic epinephrine (0.25–0.5 mL 2.25% solution in 2–4 mL saline) have been used. Nebulisation may need to be repeated every 30–60 minutes.

Postobstruction pulmonary oedema

Postobstruction pulmonary oedema, also known as negative-pressure pulmonary oedema, may occur after general anaesthesia (incidence 0.05–0.1%) or after relief of acute upper airway obstruction (incidence 11%).[49] This appears to be related to the markedly decreased intrathoracic pressure caused by forced inspiration against a closed upper airway, resulting in transudation of fluid from pulmonary capillaries to the interstitium. In addition, increased venous return may increase pulmonary blood flow and pressure, further worsening oedema. Hypoxia, the hyperadrenergic stress state, and increased ventricular afterload may also affect capillary hydrostatic pressure, although pulmonary capillary occlusion pressure is often normal. The oedema usually occurs within minutes after the relief of the obstruction, but may be delayed several hours.[50] Management includes the application of continuous positive-airways pressure or positive pressure ventilation with PEEP, maintenance of airway patency, oxygen therapy, diuretics, morphine and fluid restriction.

Access the complete references list online at http://www.expertconsult.com

3. Brain AIJ. The laryngeal mask: a new concept in airway management. Br J Anaesth 1983;55:801–5.
6. Ferson DZ, Rosenblatt WH, Johansen MJ, et al. Use of the intubating LMA-Fastrach in 254 patients with difficult-to-manage airways. Anesthesiology 2001;95:1175–81.
10. Niforopoulou P, Pantazopoulos I, Demestiha T, et al. Video-laryngoscopes in the adult airway management: a topical review of the literature. Acta Anaesthesiol Scand 2010;54:1050–61.
20. Delaney A, Bagshaw SM, Nalos M. Percutaneous dilatational tracheostomy versus surgical tracheostomy in critically ill patients: a systematic review and meta-analysis. Crit Care 2006;10:R55.
22. Ciaglia P, Firsching R, Syniec C. Elective percutaneous dilatational tracheostomy. Chest 1985;87:715–19.
32. Miller RD, Hyatt RE. Evaluation of obstructing lesions of the trachea and larynx by flow volume loops. Am Rev Respir Dis 1973;108:475–81.
42. Katori H, Tsukuda M. Acute epiglottitis: analysis of factors associated with airway intervention. J Laryngol Otol 2005;119:967–72.
46. Longhurst H, Cicardi M. Hereditary angio-oedema. Lancet 2012;379(9814):474–81.
48. François B, Bellissant E, Gissot V, et al. 12-h pretreatment with methylprednisolone versus placebo for prevention of postextubation laryngeal oedema: a randomised double-blind trial. Lancet 2007;369(9567):1083–9.
50. Udeshi A, Cantie SM, Pierre E. Postobstructive pulmonary edema. J Crit Care 2010;25:508.e1–5.

30

Acute respiratory failure in chronic obstructive pulmonary disease

Matthew T Naughton and David V Tuxen

The term chronic obstructive pulmonary disease (COPD) is applied to patients with chronic bronchitis and/or emphysema. COPD affects up to 10% of the adult population aged >40 years and is the fourth most common cause of death worldwide.[1,2] It is increasing in prevalence particularly in women,[1,2] and is commonly associated with cardiovascular disease, depression, gastro-oesophageal reflux, osteoporosis and cancer.[3,4] Severity of COPD can be easily assessed objectively by spirometry[5] (**Table 30.1**) and functionally based upon dyspnoea and exercise capacity[6] (**Table 30.2**).

An acute exacerbation of COPD (AECOPD) is defined as 'an event in the natural course of the disease characterised by change in dyspnoea, cough or sputum'.[4] AECOPD is the commonest admission diagnosis in UK general hospitals (~16% of admissions).[4] Patients with an AECOPD have an in-hospital mortality of 3–8%, and a 30-day mortality of 14–26% (compared with 8% for myocardial infarction).[2–4,7–9] Cautious oxygen delivery and non-invasive ventilatory (NIV) support have been the major advances in therapy in the past decade, which have resulted in a reduced need for invasive mechanical ventilation (IMV) and improved survival. The need for either IMV or NIV ventilatory support in AECOPD varies considerably across continents: for example in the UK, IMV and NIV are used in 1% and 11% of admissions respectively,[8] whereas in the USA they are used in 3% and 5% of admissions respectively.[9]

AETIOLOGY

The causes of COPD can be divided into environmental and host factors. Environmental factors include tobacco smoke, air pollution, indoor fumes (e.g. indoor cooking with solid biomass fuel) and poor socioeconomic status. The biggest single factor in over 95% of patients with COPD is tobacco smoking (**Fig. 30.1**). However, only approximately 15% of smokers develop COPD. Marijuana smoking may cause premature and quite advanced bullous emphysema compared with tobacco smokers, owing to extremely hot and toxic inhaled smoke held at peak inspiration for prolonged periods of time.[3] Host factors are the balance between circulating proteases and antiproteases (e.g. α-1 antitrypsin deficiency) and the intake of antioxidant vitamins (A, C, E).[10]

PATHOPHYSIOLOGY

Reduced expiratory air flow in COPD is due to both increased airway resistance and reduced lung elastic recoil. Airway resistance is increased by mucosal oedema and hypertrophy, secretions, bronchospasm, airway tortuosity and air-flow turbulence and loss of lung parenchymal elastic tissues that normally support the small airways. Loss of lung elastic recoil pressure is due both to loss of lung elastin and to loss of alveolar surface tension from alveolar wall destruction.

Reduced lung elastic recoil decreases expiratory air flow by reducing the alveolar pressure driving expiratory air flow and by reducing the intraluminal airway pressure, which normally distends small airways during expiration. Forced expiration increases alveolar driving pressure, but also causes dynamic airway compression resulting in no improvement or sometimes reduction in expiratory air flow. These factors are present in varying proportions, depending on the degree of chronic bronchitis and emphysema and the individual patient.

Air-flow limitation results in prolonged expiration, pulmonary hyperinflation, inspiratory muscle disadvantage, increased work of breathing and the sensation of dyspnoea. All these factors are worsened during an exacerbation of COPD.

Pulmonary hyperinflation has both static and dynamic components. The static component remains at the end of an expiratory period long enough for all expiratory air flow to cease (30–120 s), enabling the lungs and chest wall to reach their static functional residual capacity (FRC). This component of hyperinflation is due to loss of parenchymal elastic recoil, chest wall adaptation[11] and airway closure, which occurs throughout expiration. Dynamic pulmonary hyperinflation is the further increase in hyperinflation due to slow expiratory air flow not allowing completion of expiration before the arrival of the next breath. The extent of dynamic hyperinflation depends on the severity of air-flow obstruction, the amount inspired (tidal volume) and the expiratory time.[12] Chest wall hyperinflation leads to suboptimal muscle length–tension

Table 30.1 Global Initiative for Obstructive Lung Disease (GOLD) criteria for COPD severity based upon spirometry[5]

	FEV_1/FVC (%)	FEV_1 (% PREDICTED)
1	<70	>80
2	<70	50–80
3	<70	30–50
4	<70	<30

Table 30.2 The body mass index, airflow obstruction, dyspnoea and exercise capacity (BODE) index (maximum is 10)[6]*

SCORE	0	1	2	3
FEV_1 (% predicted)	>65	50–64	36–49	<35
Six-minute walk distance	>350	250–350	150–250	<150
Modified MRC dyspnoea score	0–1	2	3	4
Body mass index	>21	<21		

*The 4-year survival rates are 80% for a score of 2, 70% for 3–4, 60% for 5–6 and 20% for scores 7–10.
Modified Medical Research Council (MRC) score is from zero (no dyspnoea) to 4 (extreme dyspnoea upon getting dressed or leaving the house). FEV_1=forced expiratory volume in 1 second.

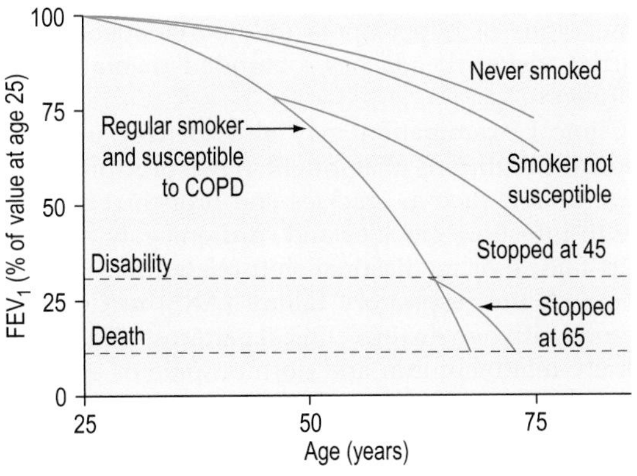

Figure 30.1 Decline in lung function with age in different smoking categories. FEV_1=forced expiratory volume in 1 second; COPD=chronic obstructive pulmonary disease.

relationships and mechanical disadvantage, thereby predisposing patients to respiratory muscle fatigue as the work of breathing increases, particularly if associated with myopathic situations (steroids, electrolyte disturbances).[13,14] Minor reductions in lung function due to infection, mild cardiac failure or atelectasis increase the work of breathing, due to increases in both respiratory impedance and dead space. With acute changes in workload, rapid decompensation with ventilatory failure and acute hypercapnia may occur.

Although chronic hypercapnia, as a consequence of reducing minute ventilation, is a fatigue-sparing mechanism that occurs in some patients, this is usually accompanied by renal compensation with retention of bicarbonate ions to correct the low pH. This has the additional effect of reducing the respiratory distress caused by hypercapnic acidosis. Central respiratory drive may also be impaired, or poorly responsive to physiological triggers – hypoxaemia or hypercapnia – and lead to chronic hypercapnia. This may occur in the setting of sleep (i.e. obstructive sleep apnoea),[11] obesity or drugs (e.g. sedatives, antiepileptics, alcohol).

Hypoxia and vascular wall changes lead to pulmonary vasoconstriction, pulmonary hypertension, cor pulmonale, *V/Q* mismatching and the development of shunts.

CHRONIC BRONCHITIS OR EMPHYSEMA?

The value of labelling patients as chronic bronchitis or emphysema is uncertain as the two disease processes usually coexist and the principles of management are similar. Five pathophysiological processes may be present to varying degrees in each patient with COPD: (1) inflammatory airway narrowing (bronchiolitis), (2) loss of connective tissues tethering airways, (3) loss of alveoli and capillaries, (4) hyperinflation, and (5) increased pulmonary vascular resistance. Early/mild COPD tends to be dominated by bronchiolitis with a minimal component of emphysema, whereas when COPD becomes severe the reverse is true. However, recognition that COPD is dominated by one of these patterns is helpful with regard to clinical pattern and prognosis.

PRECIPITANTS OF ACUTE RESPIRATORY FAILURE

In approximately 50% of patients there is an infective cause, in 25% heart failure and in the remaining 25% retained secretions, air pollution, coexistent medical problems (e.g. pulmonary embolus, medication compliance or side-effects) or no cause can be identified (**Box 30.1**).[14,15]

INFECTION

The most common bacterial isolates are *Streptococcus pneumoniae* and *Haemophilus influenzae* in 80% of exacerbations. *S. viridans*, *Moraxella* (previously *Branhamella*) *catarrhalis*, *Mycoplasma pneumoniae* and *Pseudomonas aeruginosa* may also be found. Viruses can be isolated in 20–30% of exacerbations and include rhinovirus, influenza and parainfluenza viruses, coronaviruses and occasionally adenovirus, and respiratory syncytial virus. Whether these organisms are pathogens or colonisers is often unclear. Background microbiological agents are identified in 48% of stable COPD, compared

Box 30.1 Precipitants of acute respiratory failure in chronic obstructive pulmonary disease

Infective (including aspiration)
Left ventricular failure (systolic and diastolic failure)
Sputum retention (postoperative, traumatic)
Pulmonary embolism
Pneumothoraces and bullae
Uncontrolled oxygen
Sedation
Medication – non-compliance or side-effects
Nutritional (K, PO4, Mg deficiency, CHO excess)
Sleep apnoea

with 70% during an AECOPD.[16,17] Pneumonia has been estimated to account for 20% of presentations requiring mechanical ventilation.[4]

HEART FAILURE

Left ventricular (LV) systolic failure may result from coexisting ischaemic heart disease, fluid overload, tachyarrhythmias or biventricular failure secondary to cor pulmonale. LV diastolic failure occurs commonly and is precipitated by hypoxaemia, tachycardia, pericardial constraint due to intrinsic positive end-expiratory pressure ($PEEP_i$) or right ventricular (RV) dilation.[11,18,19] Increased work of breathing related to COPD will also increase by up to 10-fold the amount of blood flow to the respiratory pump muscles,[20] thereby causing an increased demand upon the overall cardiac output. In patients with borderline cardiac status, this may precipitate heart failure. The components of RV and LV failure can be accurately distinguished by Doppler echocardiography. Pulmonary congestion can be difficult to diagnose because of the abnormal breath sounds and chest X-ray appearance that are commonly present in COPD. In a recent publication, 51% of patients with acute exacerbation of COPD had echocardiographic evidence of left heart failure (systolic 11%, diastolic 32%, systolic and diastolic 7%).[11] A further study of CT and MR scanning and echocardiography in a large community population (15% of whom had COPD) identified that severity of emphysema on CT scanning indirectly correlated with left ventricular end-diastolic volume, stroke volume and cardiac output.[18] These authors concluded that increasing severity of COPD was associated with worsening cardiac function.

UNCONTROLLED OXYGEN

This may precipitate acute hypercapnia in patients with more severe COPD, due to: (1) shunting blood to low-*V/Q* lung units and increasing dead space, (2) loss of hypoxic drive, (3) dissociation of CO_2 from Hb molecule (Haldane effect), and (4) anxiolysis and reduction in tachypnoea.[21] Major randomised controlled trials have indicated significant reductions in need for IMV, hospital length of stay and mortality with controlled (or targeted at a specific Sp_{O_2} range – e.g. 88–92%) oxygen therapy compared with uncontrolled oxygen therapy in ambulances,[22] emergency rooms[23] and hospital wards.[8]

DIAGNOSIS AND ASSESSMENT

The clinical examination findings of COPD should be confirmed and severity quantified by spirometry (see Tables 30.1 and 30.2). In mild stable disease (e.g. forced expiratory volume in 1 second (FEV_1) >50% predicted normal), an expiratory wheeze on forced expiration and mild exertional dyspnoea may be the only symptoms.

In moderate-severity COPD (e.g. FEV_1 30–50% predicted normal), modest to severe exertional dyspnoea is associated with clinical signs of hyperinflation (ptosed upper border of liver beyond the 4th intercostal space anteriorly and loss of cardiac percussion) and signs of increased work of breathing (use of accessory muscles and tracheal tug).

In severe stable COPD (e.g. FEV_1<30% predicted normal), marked accessory muscle use is associated with tachypnoea at rest, pursed-lip breathing, hypoxaemia and signs of pulmonary hypertension (RV heave, loud and palpable pulmonary second sound and elevated a-wave in jugular venous pressure (JVP)) and cor pulmonale (elevated JVP, hepatomegaly, ankle swelling).

In severe unstable COPD, there is marked tachypnoea at rest, hypoxaemia and tachycardia, and, in some, signs of hypercapnia (dilated cutaneous veins, blurred vision, headaches, obtunded mentation, and confusion).

Clinical examination may also identify associated medical conditions that might have precipitated the exacerbation such as crackles and bronchial breathing due to infection, crackles and cardiomegaly related to heart failure or mediastinal shift related to a pneumothorax. Acute respiratory failure (ARF) in COPD can present with two distinct clinical patterns[15] (**Table 30.3**), namely relatively thin and normocapnic or obese and hypercapnic.

Basic investigations such as spirometry are very useful for confirming a clinical diagnosis and determining severity of disease. An FEV_1/VC ratio <70% with an FEV_1 of 50–80% predicted normal without a bronchodilator response usually indicates mild COPD. A significant bronchodilator response, which implies asthma, is regarded as a 12% or greater increase and 200 mL increase in either FEV_1 or VC. An FEV_1 30–50% predicted normal indicates moderately severe COPD and FEV_1<30% predicted normal indicates severe COPD.[5]

Flow–volume curves usually demonstrate reduced expiratory flow rates at various lung volumes and the characteristic concave expiratory flow pattern. Lung volumes measured by either helium dilution or plethysmography show elevated total lung capacity, FRC and residual volume. Characteristically, the residual

Table 30.3 Clinical differences between normocapnic and hypercapnic chronic obstructive pulmonary disease

NORMOCAPNIC (Pa_{CO_2} 35–45 MMHG)	HYPERCAPNIC (Pa_{CO_2} >45 MMHG)
Emphysema > chronic bronchitis	Chronic bronchitis > emphysema
Thin	Obese
Pursed-lip breathing	Central nervous system depression: consider the role of oxygen therapy
Accessory muscle use	Alcohol, sedatives, analgesics
Hyperinflated	Sleep-related hypoventilation
Right heart failure late	Right heart failure early

volume/total lung capacity ratio is >40% in COPD and represents intrathoracic gas trapping. The total lung carbon monoxide (TLCO) uptake is a measurement of alveolar surface area and its reduction approximates the amount of emphysema present (usually <80% predicted normal).

A chest X-ray will commonly show hyperinflated lung fields, as suggested by 10 ribs visible posteriorly, six ribs visible anteriorly or large air space anterior to heart (>⅓ of the length of the sternum), flattened diaphragms (best seen on lateral chest X-ray) and a paucity of lung markings. Pulmonary hypertension is manifested by enlarged proximal and attenuated distal vascular markings and by RV and atrial enlargement. Lung bullae may be evident.

A high-resolution computed tomographic (CT) scan of the chest (1–2 mm slices) can demonstrate characteristic appearance and regional distribution of emphysema. It can also assess any coexistent bronchiectasis, LV failure[24] and pulmonary fibrosis. Such scans are less sensitive than standard chest CT scans (1 cm slice) for detecting pulmonary lesions (e.g. neoplasms). Nuclear ventilation perfusion scans can also provide a characteristic appearance of COPD.

An electrocardiogram (ECG) is commonly normal but may show features of right atrial or RV hypertrophy and RV strain, including P pulmonale, right-axis deviation, dominant R-waves in V1–2, right bundle-branch block, ST depression and T-wave flattening or inversion in V1–3. These changes may be chronic or may develop acutely if there is significant increase in pulmonary vascular resistance during the illness. The ECG may also show coexistent ischaemic heart disease, tachycardia and atrial fibrillation. Occasionally, continuous ECG monitoring is required to identify transient arrhythmias, which may also precipitate acute deterioration. Plasma brain natriuretic peptide (BNP) levels may also assist in the diagnosis of heart failure (elevated BNP) from pulmonary causes (low BNP) in patients under 70 years free of renal impairment.[25]

DIFFERENTIAL DIAGNOSIS

The history of *chronic asthma* is one of long-term dyspnoea, wheeze and cough, usually at night or upon exercise, beginning in childhood with clear-cut precipitating agents (e.g. weather, dust, pets, drugs) and a favourable response to either steroids or inhaled β_2-agonists. Late-onset asthma (>40 years of age) is not uncommon and is often associated with recurrent gastro-oesophageal reflux. In both forms of asthma, TLCO is normal. There is usually a bronchodilator response in the FEV_1 if the patient has unstable asthma. In patients in whom asthma is considered but lung function tests are normal, the FEV_1 response to an inhalational challenge (e.g. methacholine or hypertonic saline) may assist in discriminating asthma from other causes of dyspnoea.

Bronchiolitis obliterans is a condition that presents as a fixed air-flow obstruction following a viral illness, inhalation of toxic fumes, following bone marrow or heart/lung transplantation, or related to drugs (e.g. penicillamine). It generally begins as a cough some weeks after insult and insidious onset of dyspnoea. There is a broad spectrum of radiological appearances from normal to reticulonodular to diffuse nodular. Lung tissue via bronchoscopy or by thoracoscopy is required for diagnosis. Histologically, there is a characteristic chronic bronchiolar inflammation appearance, and if granulation tissue extends into the alveoli it is referred to as bronchiolitis obliterans or organising pneumonia. Removal of the offending agent and instigation of steroids are generally associated with a favourable prognosis.

Bronchiectasis is often associated with fixed mild to moderate air-flow obstruction. A chronic productive cough (daily for 2 consecutive years) is characteristic. Clinical features such as clubbing, localised pulmonary crackles and a characteristic appearance on high-resolution CT, with dilated or plugged small airways at least twice the size of accompanying blood vessel, assist in the diagnosis.

Congestive heart failure (CHF) may be a differential diagnosis of COPD, or simply coexist, as both disorders are common in smokers.[11] Orthopnoea and paroxysmal nocturnal dyspnoea are features that correlate with heart failure severity. A past history of myocardial ischaemia or atrial fibrillation should alert one to the possibility of heart failure. An echocardiogram and high-resolution CT (looking for shift in interstitial oedema with changes in posture from supine to prone)[24] are sensitive markers of CHF.

ASSESSMENT OF RESPIRATORY FAILURE

An acute exacerbation of COPD (AECOPD) is defined as 'an event in the natural course of the disease characterised by change in dyspnoea, cough or sputum'.[4]

Arterial blood gases are mandatory to assess hypoxia, hypercapnia and acid–base status. Chronic hypercapnia may be recognised by a bicarbonate level

>30 mmol/L and a base excess >4 mmol/L indicating renal compensation. However, other causes of high serum bicarbonate need to be excluded (e.g. diuretic therapy, high-dose steroids or high-volume gastric fluid loss), or chronic hypercapnia may be incorrectly assumed and the severity of COPD overestimated. Renal compensation for chronic hypercapnia will increase the serum bicarbonate by approximately 4 mmol/L for each 10 mmHg (1.33 kPa) of chronic Pa_{CO_2} rise above 40 mmHg (5.3 kPa), in order to return pH to the low-normal range. Irrespective of the COPD patient's usual Pa_{CO_2} level, an acute increase in Pa_{CO_2} leads to a decreased arterial pH. This indicates that compensatory mechanisms are exhausted and there is an increased risk of respiratory collapse. The agreement between arterial and peripheral venous blood gases in terms of pH or Pa_{CO_2} is extremely poor (±0.1 and ±25 mmHg (0.013 and 3.25 kPa) respectively).[26] Thus the use of peripheral venous blood gases to assess respiratory failure should be used with great caution.

MANAGEMENT OF RESPIRATORY FAILURE

NON-VENTILATORY MANAGEMENT

OXYGEN THERAPY

Oxygen given by low-flow intranasal cannulae or 24–35% Venturi mask should be titrated to achieve a saturation (Sp_{O_2}) of 88–92% as these levels will avoid significant increases in Pa_{CO_2} in the majority of COPD patients with ARF. Increases in Pa_{CO_2} are most common in patients with initial Pa_{CO_2}>50 mmHg (6.5 kPa) and pH<7.35.[27] Excessive oxygen therapy is the cause of increased hypercapnia in a third of acidotic AECOPD patients.[8] For this reason, ABGs should be repeated 1 hour following initiation of oxygen therapy, as with NIV, to ensure an optimal direction of improvement in the underlying AECOPD. If the rise in Pa_{CO_2} is excessive (>10 mmHg or 1.33 kPa), then Fi_{O_2} should be reduced, titrating Sp_{O_2} to 2–3% below the previous value, and arterial blood gases should be repeated. If no Pa_{CO_2} rise occurs with oxygen therapy, then a higher Sp_{O_2} may be targeted with repeat ABG.

Inadequate reversal of hypoxia (e.g. Sp_{O_2}<85%) is suggestive of an additional problem such as pneumonia, pulmonary oedema or embolus, or a pneumothorax. Investigation of this should commence and a higher O_2 delivery system should be used (see Ch. 28). Although high levels of O_2 should be avoided, reversal of hypoxia is important and O_2 should not be withheld in the presence of hypercapnia, or withdrawn if it worsens.

BRONCHODILATORS

Bronchodilators are routinely given in all acute exacerbations of COPD because a small reversible component of air-flow obstruction is common, and bronchodilators improve mucociliary clearance of secretions. A large meta-analysis of 22 large randomised controlled long-term trials of ambulatory COPD patients involving anticholinergics and/or β_2-agonists (short- and long-acting) over 3–60 months indicated that anticholinergics are more favourable than placebo in terms of acute exacerbations and hospitalisations.[3,28] There were no favourable advantages with β_2-agonists compared with placebo for acute exacerbations or hospitalisations, and placebo was better than β_2-agonists in terms of respiratory death.[28] There is a cardiovascular risk if given in excessive doses.[29]

Anticholinergic agents, such as ipratropium bromide, have been shown to have a similar or greater bronchodilator action than β-agonists in COPD,[4,5] and also to have fewer side-effects and no tachyphylaxis. Anticholinergic agents should be used routinely in AECOPD. An ipratropium bromide nebule of 0.5 mg in 2 mL should be nebulised initially 2-hourly, then every 4–6 hours. Long-term use of ipratropium bromide has been shown to reduce the incidence of exacerbations[23] and is therefore recommended for chronic use in ambulatory COPD. Long-acting anticholinergics (e.g. tiotropium) offer potential of once-daily dosing.

Nebulised β-agonists are also effective bronchodilators in COPD,[4,5] although they may cause tachycardia, tremor, mild reductions in potassium and Pa_{CO_2} (due to pulmonary vasodilatation) and tachyphylaxis. As in asthma, lactic acidosis may also occur with excessive β-agonists, either nebulised or intravenous. Nebulised β-agonists (e.g. salbutamol, terbutaline or fenoterol) given 2–4-hourly should be used routinely in combination with ipratropium. This combination has been shown to be more effective than either agent alone. Parenteral sympathomimetic agents are not recommended for routine use. In stable patients, long-term use of β-agonists may improve symptoms of dyspnoea, particularly in the subgroup of COPD with an objective bronchodilator response.

STEROIDS

In acute exacerbations of COPD, short-term steroids have been shown to improve air-flow obstruction[30] including those patients requiring mechanical ventilation for COPD.[31] Doses similar to those for acute asthma should be used. Methylprednisolone 0.5 mg/kg, given 6-hourly for 72 hours, was used in the study by Albert et al,[30] demonstrating benefit in patients with an exacerbation of COPD. Current American Thoracic Society guidelines recommend the equivalent to oral prednisolone at 0.5 mg/kg body weight for up to 10 days, then ceasing; however, this will depend upon the response to treatment, and their premorbid use.[5] Steroids should be avoided if the deterioration is clearly due to bacterial pneumonia without bronchospasm.

Longer-term oral steroids in COPD are associated with a substantial increased risk of side-effects (osteoporosis, diabetes, peptic ulcer, myopathy, systemic hypertension, fluid retention, weight gain), and are therefore not recommended.[5] A small group of patients (15%) may demonstrate a significant bronchodilator response; coexistent asthma is likely in these patients and longer-term high-dose (usually inhaled) steroids may be necessary. In the majority of patients, long-term inhaled steroids do not improve lung function or survival; however, they may improve quality of life and reduce admissions.[5]

ANTIBIOTICS

Antibiotics have an accepted role in the treatment of infection-induced exacerbations of COPD.[4] Amoxicillin is a suitable first-line agent against *Haemophilus influenzae* and *Streptococcus pneumoniae* for outpatient exacerbations. Serious exacerbations requiring hospital admission require newer agents such as ciprofloxacin or a third-generation cephalosporin. Antibiotics for pneumonia are discussed elsewhere in this volume.

AMINOPHYLLINE

Aminophylline is a weak bronchodilator in COPD. It improves diaphragm contractility, stimulates respiratory drive, improves mucociliary transport and right heart function, is anti-inflammatory and is a weak diuretic.[32,33] Some studies have shown no benefit and significant side-effects,[34] whereas others have shown small benefit[35] in stable COPD. For an exacerbation, aminophylline (loading dose 5–6 mg/kg i.v. over 30 minutes, followed by an infusion of 0.5 mg/kg per hour). Serum theophylline levels must be monitored regularly to reduce risk of toxicity.

ANTICOAGULANTS

Subcutaneous heparin (e.g. 5000 units b.d.) is recommended as a prophylactic measure against venous thromboembolism. There is no evidence for warfarinisation in COPD patients with pulmonary hypertension.

ELECTROLYTE CORRECTION

Electrolyte correction is important. Hypophosphataemia,[13] hypomagnesaemia,[36] hypocalcaemia[14] and hypokalaemia may impair respiratory muscle function. Hyponatraemia may occur with inappropriate antidiuretic hormone release or with excess use of diuretics and inappropriate intravenous fluids.

NUTRITION

Nutrition is important, as patients with severe COPD are often undernourished – a subnormal BMI is a risk factor for mortality in COPD. Excessive carbohydrate calories should be avoided as this increases CO_2 production (by >15%) and may worsen respiratory failure. Low-carbohydrate/high-fat combinations are preferred in ARF during spontaneous ventilation.

CHEST PHYSIOTHERAPY

Chest physiotherapy should be initiated and regularly repeated as both a curative and preventive measure. Encouragement of coughing and deep breathing are the two most important factors. 'Bubble positive expiratory pressure (PEP)' is an inexpensive method of assisting sputum clearance in patients with retained secretions or those having difficulty expectorating.

NEBULISED MUCOLYTIC AGENTS

Nebulised mucolytic agents, such as *N*-acetylcysteine, continue to be proposed, although their benefit has never been established in acute exacerbations of COPD. Oral mucolytics have been shown to reduce cough frequency and severity in stable COPD.[37]

NON-INVASIVE VENTILATION (NIV)

NIV, a technique in which ventilatory support is provided via a nasal or facial mask without endotracheal intubation, is now a routine standard of care for AECOPD. When applied well, NIV has the same physiological effect as IMV.[38] Two landmark randomised controlled trials in intensive care wards in 1995[39] and in general medical wards in 2001[40] clearly indicated a role for NIV in hypercapnic AECOPD. Since then, there have been several randomised controlled trials and meta-analyses of NIV in hypercapnic AECOPD which have demonstrated improved respiratory physiology, reduced mortality (up to 12 months), reduced iatrogenic complications, reduced need for intubation and mechanical ventilation and reduced length of stay in hospital.[8,9,41,42] All studies have shown good tolerance of the technique (>80% of patients), with few side-effects, improvements in both oxygenation and Pa_{CO_2} compared with medically treated control patients.

Two important reviews of acute NIV use in AECOPD from the USA and the UK have been recently been published. In the USA between 1998 and 2008, the use of NIV increased (from 1.0 to 4.5% of all admissions) and IMV decreased (from 6.0 to 3.5%) with NIV eclipsing IMV in 2008.[9] Associated with this significant change in pattern of ventilatory support was an overall reduction in mortality in those started on NIV or IMV early.[9] In the UK, during a 3-month snapshot of 232 hospitals during 2008, 11% of all admissions with AECOPD received NIV.[8] Oxygen toxicity was found to occur in a third of hypercapnic AECOPD.[8] In both USA and UK studies, NIV failure with transfer to IMV was associated with greatest mortality (estimated to be ~30 (USA)–40 (UK)%) compared with successfully used NIV (6 (USA)–11 (UK)%) and non-hypercapnic COPD (~3% USA, 5% UK).

The goal of NIV is: (1) to unload respiratory muscles and augment ventilation and oxygenation, reduce CO_2 and correct acidosis until the underlying problem can be reversed; (2) when applied intermittently, to offset the adverse effects of sleep- or position-induced adverse changes to ventilation, increased upper airway resistance and lung volume.

Indications for NIV are a deterioration of COPD with: (1) acute dyspnoea; (2) respiratory rate >28 breaths/min; (3) Pa_{CO_2}>45 mmHg (5.85 kPa) with a pH<7.35, despite optimal medical treatment and not related to excessive supplemental oxygen. Although these indications are for mild exacerbations, most randomised studies have used these as entry guidelines.[8,41,42] Initial guidelines recommended NIV use to be limited to patients with pH in the range 7.25–7.35; however, recent evidence suggests that NIV is useful even in those patients with lower pH values (to as low as 7.0) and associated more severe hypercapnia (as high as 140 mmHg (18.2 kPa)).[43]

Included in the indications are recently extubated patients in whom NIV has been shown to reduce re-intubation rates significantly.[44,45] Recently NIV has been advocated for use in patients with hypoxic respiratory failure,[46] but success is significantly less in the setting of hypoxaemia and either normocapnia or hypocapnia. NIV may also have a role in some patients where mechanical ventilation is considered inappropriate.

Side-effects of NIV include discomfort, intolerance, skin necrosis, gastric distension and aspiration. Pressure support has been reported as better tolerated than assist/control.[47] End-of-life plans should be considered in all patients with AECOPD, particularly those undergoing NIV, as ~20% of patients will fail to respond or deteriorate. This period of time on NIV can be used to assess resuscitation status.

INVASIVE MECHANICAL VENTILATION

When respiratory failure progresses despite aggressive conservative management, including NIV, invasive mechanical ventilatory (IMV) support may be necessary. The decision to ventilate requires careful consideration in some patients who may have near-end-stage lung disease and whose quality of life may not justify aggressive treatment. This decision requires consideration of the outcome of ARF.

An episode of ARF further decreases survival (**Fig. 30.2**). ARF precipitated only by bronchitis has a better outcome, whereas ARF due to more serious causes such as pneumonia, LV failure and pulmonary embolus has a worse outcome, and studies including all such outcomes have lower survival rates.

If ARF requires IMV, survival decreases further still (see Fig. 30.2). Although only 1[8] to 3.5%[9] of patients with AECOPD require IMV, and 4.5[9] to 11%[8] need NIV, the short-term survival in this more severe subset is still good, with a hospital survival rate in some series as

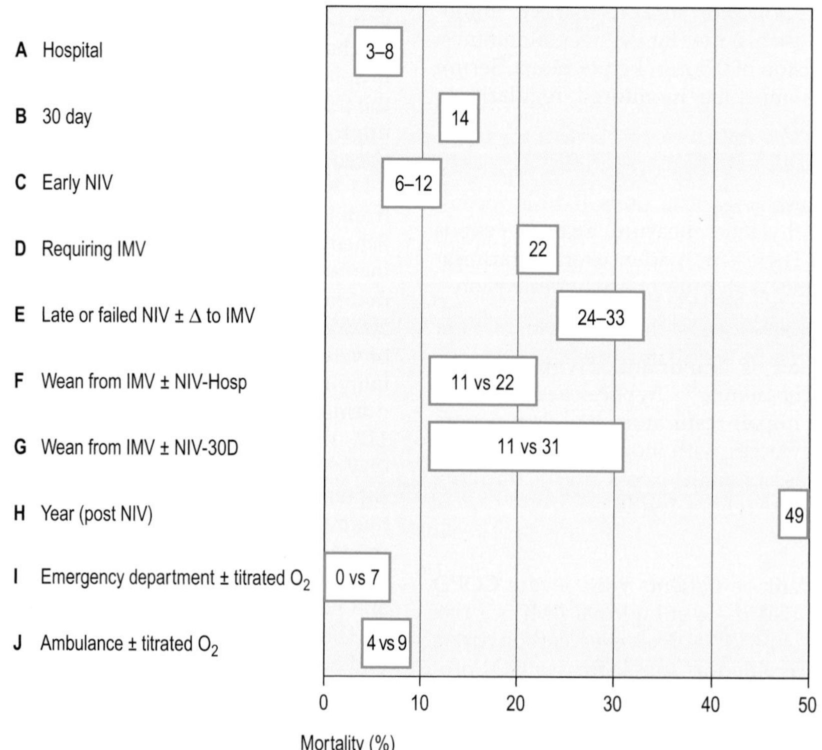

Figure 30.2 Estimated mortality for groups of patients with acute exacerbations of COPD. A and B groups: refer to in-hospital and 30-day mortality;[8,9] C group: refers to early institution of NIV;[8,9] D group: refers to patients requiring IMV;[9] E group: refers to hypercapnic AECOPD patients either failing NIV and needing IMV, or those identified late as requiring NIV;[8,9] F and G groups: weaned from IMV and randomised to either immediate NIV or not (i.e. randomised controlled trial) with in-hospital and 30-day mortality;[44] H group: 1-year mortality post NIV;[7] I and J groups: effect of titrated versus untitrated oxygen at emergency department[23] and ambulance.[22]

high as 90%, but 2- and 3-year survival is significantly lower. The severity of ARF and the severity of underlying COPD based on FEV_1, lifestyle score and dyspnoea score are also predictors of outcome. Lifestyle and dyspnoea categories may be the most useful factors in the decision to withhold IMV. Lifestyle categories 3 (housebound and at least partly dependent) and 4 (bed- or chair-bound) indicate both a poor outcome[48] and quality of life that may not justify aggressive treatment.

Thus IMV may be withheld in end-stage lung disease, when low survival, poor quality of life or permanent ventilator dependence is likely. If end-stage lung disease is suspected but there is insufficient information, then a brief trial of aggressive therapy, including IMV, should be undertaken and subsequently withdrawn if unsuccessful. Despite this, most patients with COPD who present with ARF do not have end-stage disease and, although their immediate problems may be life threatening, their short-term outcome is sufficiently good to justify full active treatment.

INVASIVE MECHANICAL VENTILATION TECHNIQUE

The goals of IMV in COPD are to support ventilation while reversible components improve, to allow respiratory muscle to rest and recover whilst preventing wasting from total inactivity and to minimise dynamic hyperinflation. This is usually best accomplished with low-level ventilatory support. Patients requiring low-level support may be commenced on 8–15 cmH_2O pressure support, with 3–8 cmH_2O PEEP. Patients who are completely exhausted, post arrest, comatose or not tolerating pressure support alone should be commenced or transferred to synchronised intermittent mandatory ventilation mode.

Excessive dynamic hyperinflation must be avoided by using a low-minute ventilation – 115/mL per kg is a guideline[6] – and allowing adequate time for expiration. This should be achieved by the use of a small tidal volume (8 mL/kg) and a ventilator rate <14 breaths/min.[12] Dynamic hyperinflation can be assessed clinically by visualising the expiratory flow–time curve, and by measuring plateau airway pressure (P_{plat}) or $PEEP_i$. P_{plat} should be measured by applying an end-inspiratory pause of 0.5 seconds. This should be applied only following a single breath as it shortens expiratory time and if it is applied to a series of breaths it increases dynamic hyperinflation, resulting in an increased P_{plat} level and increased risk to the patient. If P_{plat} is >25 cmH_2O, there is likely to be excessive dynamic hyperinflation, and the ventilator rate should be reduced. However, P_{plat} may be high without dynamic hyperinflation if chest wall compliance is low. Intrinsic PEEP measured as a prolonged end-expiratory pause more directly assesses dynamic hyperinflation. Provided $PEEP_i$ is accurately measured, it is a useful tool to follow dynamic hyperinflation. In severe air-flow limitation it may be necessary to accept low levels of $PEEP_i$, but as $PEEP_i$ rises above 8–10 cmH_2O further prolongation of expiratory time must be considered. Although still controversial, the use of a high inspiratory flow rate is recommended[12,49] as it results in a shorter inspiratory time and hence a longer expiratory time for a given ventilatory rate. It has been shown to reduce dynamic hyperinflation and alveolar pressure[12] further and to improve gas exchange.[49]

If dynamic hyperinflation is excessive and causing circulatory compromise or risk of barotrauma, then minute ventilation should be decreased, hypercapnic acidosis accepted and spontaneous ventilation, which will only increase dynamic hyperinflation, should be discouraged by sedation. Muscle relaxants should be avoided unless essential. When dynamic hyperinflation is critical during controlled mechanical ventilation, $PEEP_i$ increases pulmonary hyperinflation and should not be applied.[50]

If dynamic hyperinflation is not excessive then spontaneous ventilation should be encouraged to promote ongoing respiratory muscle activity and to minimise wasting. Flow-by, pressure support and low-level CPAP may all reduce the work of spontaneous breathing and promote a better ventilatory pattern. CPAP approximately equal to the level of $PEEP_i$ is most commonly recommended.[51] Care must be taken with all of these supports as each can increase dynamic hyperinflation by a different mechanism, leading to circulatory compromise or risk of barotrauma. Flow-by increases resistance through the expiratory valve, pressure support increases tidal volume and may increase inspiratory time, and CPAP reduces threshold load and makes ventilator triggering easier in patients with PEEPi.

WEANING FROM INVASIVE MECHANICAL VENTILATION

Approximately 6–20% of patients on IMV support fail weaning and place themselves in a high mortality and morbidity group[44,45] (see Ch. 31). Numerous criteria have been proposed to assess the capacity of the patient to wean;[52] however, the predictive value of any of these individual criteria is limited. The simple criterion of patient respiration rate/tidal volume <100 breaths/min per litre had the best predictive value for weaning success, but the advantage of this overly simple clinical assessment during weaning is uncertain. Other indications to extubate COPD patients safely include Fi_{O_2}<40%; Pa_{O_2}/Fi_{O_2}>200, PEEP 5 cmH_2O, cardiovascular stability, afebrile, pH>7.35, Pa_{CO_2}<50 mmHg (6.5 kPa), GCS>10 and, if available to be measured, static compliance >25 mL/cmH_2O.[44] Some patients unable to achieve these criteria may require weaning with Pa_{CO_2} 50–65 mmHg (6.5–8.45 kPa) with a bicarbonate level of >30 mmol/L allowed or encouraged to reduce the work of breathing and achieve a less abnormal pH. Following extubation, weaning can be continued with immediate placement upon NIV, which is associated with reduced re-intubation rates, lower ICU and hospital length of stay and mortality and morbidity.[44,45] Synchronisation of NIV, especially during sleep, is crucial and may require polysomnography.[53]

TRACHEOSTOMY

Tracheostomy may be beneficial in a small group of patients who have failed extubation despite NIV, or who have successfully weaned but are unable to adequately clear secretions, or who have required long-term ventilatory support. After 10 days of endotracheal intubation, the risk of laryngeal trauma and sepsis increases.

A tracheostomy allows long-term ventilatory support, sputum clearance, protection of the upper airway from oral secretions and, off mechanical ventilation, reduced dead space and upper-airway resistance. Compared with naso/orotracheal intubation, tracheostomy is much less intrusive and therefore less sedation is required. Also, it allows direct access to the large airways for the purpose of suctioning and bronchoscopy. However, patients are unable to generate sufficient upper-airway seal to cough, and as such may have ongoing atelectasis until tracheostomy removal and the development of an effective cough. Usually a nasoenteric feeding tube is required. Consider percutaneous endoscopic gastrostomy (PEG) tube feeding if long-term tracheostomy is being considered to avoid nasal trauma and infection and to reduce oesophagitis. Minimal occlusion tracheostomy cuff pressures (usually <20 cmH_2O) should be checked 8-hourly. Adequate humidification and the use of tracheostomies with an inner cannula is recommended to allow for inner tube cleaning or replacement to avoid occlusion by dried secretions.

Consider removing the tracheostomy when:

- the oxygenation requirement is low (e.g. Fi_{O_2}<40%)
- the patient does not require ventilatory support or requires only intermittent low-level ventilatory support and non-invasive ventilatory support is available
- the patient is cooperative and has a good capacity to cough and can, for example, clear secretions via the tracheostomy tube
- the patient has a low suction frequency requirement (<2–4-hourly).

Before tracheostomy removal, always ensure the patient is able to protect the upper airway from aspiration and can swallow safely and there is an absence of upper-airway obstruction (e.g. no granulation tissue or tracheal stenosis).

POST-INTENSIVE-UNIT CARE

REASSESSMENT OF POTENTIAL PRECIPATING CAUSES

COPD is commonly associated with cardiovascular disease, depression (and social isolation), and occult malignancy – all of which may need further management following an admission. Lung function assessment is crucial post admission and regular follow-up.[3,4]

Assessment for long-term oxygen therapy should be undertaken (Pa_{O_2}<55 mmHg (7.15 kPa), or <60 mmHg (7.8 kPa) with cor pulmonale) as there are two trials indicating a survival benefit.[54,55] Current smoking is a contraindication to domiciliary oxygen therapy due to the risk of fire. This can be checked by assessing carboxyhaemoglobin values on ABG (>2% suggests smoking) or urinary cotinine levels.

Assessment of underlying obstructive sleep apnoea (COPD and OSA=overlap syndrome) should be considered. Treatment of this combination with CPAP is associated with an improved survival and exacerbation-free survival over a 9.5-year period according to a large, although uncontrolled, Spanish trial.[56] Habitual snoring, witnessed apnoeas, obesity (BMI>30), large neck size (>45 cm) and crowded oropharynx (Mallampati grade 3–4) provide clues of the possibility of underlying OSA.

DOMICILIARY NOCTURNAL NON-INVASIVE VENTILATORY SUPPORT

In COPD patients with chronic hypercapnia, avoidance of excessive domiciliary oxygen therapy is advised. Whether long-term domiciliary nocturnal NIV is required in this group is less clear. In the two largest studies,[57,58] improved physiology (sleep quality and ABG) were noted overnight without changes in FEV1 and a borderline improvement in survival. Long-term NIV has also been associated with improved ventilation perfusion matching.[29] Patients may benefit from domiciliary NIV if they have the following: (a) confirmed COPD diagnosis with optimal medical treatment and reversal of coexistent medical problems, (b) chronic hypercapnia, (c) at least two admissions with acute acidotic hypercapnia that responded to NIV, (d) demonstration of sleep-related hypoventilation (e.g. total sleep time hypoxic (Sp_{O_2}<90%) >30% plus a rise in Pa_{CO_2} of >5 mmHg (0.65 kPa)), (e) 1-month trial of domiciliary NIV with objective adherence and improved quality of life and (f) an improvement in physiological markers (e.g. awake Pa_{CO_2} or 6-minute walk distance).

REHABILITATION

Rehabilitation should be considered for all patients with COPD, particularly those following ARF. There are numerous randomised controlled trials showing improvements in exercise physiology, lung function, quality of life and reduced hospitalisation rates.[59] The change in 6-minute walk distance with rehabilitation is a powerful predictor of improved survival and significant patient motivator.[60]

VACCINATION AND ANTIBIOTICS

Two large trials have recently advocated the use of macrolide antibiotics (erythromycin[16] or azithromycin[17]) for stable COPD. Both studies, conducted over a

12-month period, indicated a significant reduction in exacerbations, probably via anti-inflammatory and antibacterial effects. However, this benefit needed to be offset against potential for greater long-term microbiological resistance and side effects such as hearing loss. Vaccination should be considered in all patients with COPD when stable. Annual influenza and 5-yearly pneumococcal vaccination are recommended.[4]

DOMICILIARY OXYGEN

Based upon two studies conducted in the 1970s–80s indicating a mortality benefit,[54,55] supplemental oxygen should be provided to patients with advanced COPD who: (a) are optimally controlled medically, (b) do not smoke, and (c) have Pa_{O_2}<55 mmHg (7.15 kPa) or Pa_{O_2}<60 mmHg (7.8 kPa) with cor pulmonale. Great caution should be undertaken to avoid excessive oxygen at home when stable (aim for overnight oximetry of 88–92%) and during acute exacerbations.[8,22,23]

LUNG TRANSPLANTATION

Lung transplantation is another palliative surgical procedure for patients with advanced disabling COPD who are aged <65 years, are not ventilator dependent, are on less than 10 mg prednisolone/day and are free of significant coexistent disease.[61] The current 1-, 2- and 5-year international survival figures are 75, 66 and 50% respectively. Common complications are systemic hypertension, bronchiolitis obliterans, acute rejection, viral infection with cytomegalovirus and neoplasms.

PROGNOSIS

Patients with sufficiently severe COPD to warrant hospital admission incur an inpatient mortality of 8%, and 90-day mortality of 15% in the UK.[8,9] Predictors of mortality were performance status, age and admission urea, albumin, pH, Pa_{CO_2} and Sp_{O_2} plus the presence of respiratory physicians involved in the care.[62]Although in-hospital mortality for hypercapnic COPD patients may reach 62%,[63] in an Australian report in-hospital mortality for hypercapnic COPD patients treated with NIV was 11% and all deaths were with palliative intent, which followed time to allow for patient and family discussions.[43] In Hong Kong, acute hypercapnic COPD patients have a 12-month re-admission rate of 80% and a 49% 1-year mortality.[7] The body-mass index, air-flow obstruction, dyspnoea and exercise capacity (BODE) index is a 10-point scale made up from the following four variables: (1) body mass index, (2) air-flow obstruction, (3) severity of dyspnoea, and (4) exercise capacity, and has been found to be very useful in predicting survival in ambulatory patients with COPD[6] (see Table 30.2).

Access the complete references list online at http://www.expertconsult.com

4. Wedzicha JA, Seemungal TA. COPD exacerbations: defining their cause and prevention. Lancet 2007; 370(9589):786–96.
5. Pauwels RA, Buist AS, Calverley PM, et al. Global strategy for the diagnosis, management, and prevention of chronic obstructive pulmonary disease. NHLBI/WHO Global Initiative for Chronic Obstructive Lung Disease (GOLD) Workshop summary. Am J Respir Crit Care Med 2001;163(5):1256–76.
8. Roberts CM, Stone RA, Buckingham RJ, et al. Acidosis, non-invasive ventilation and mortality in hospitalised COPD exacerbations. Thorax 2010; 66(1):43–8.
9. Chandra D, Stamm JA, Taylor B, et al. Outcomes of noninvasive ventilation for acute exacerbations of chronic obstructive pulmonary disease in the United States, 1998-2008. Am J Respir Crit Care Med 2012; 185(2):152–9.
20. Malhotra A, Schwartz DR, Ayas N, et al. Treatment of oxygen-induced hypercapnia. Lancet 2001; 357(9259):884–5.
38. Elliott MW, Nava S. Noninvasive ventilation for acute exacerbations of chronic obstructive pulmonary disease: 'Don't think twice, it's alright!' Am J Respir Crit Care Med 2012;185(2):121–3.

31

Mechanical ventilation

Andrew D Bersten

Mechanical ventilation for acute respiratory failure (ARF) is now routine in the ICU. The 1952 Copenhagen polio epidemic introduced the notion of organised areas (ICU) for the provision of positive-pressure ventilation,[1] which was usually applied through a tracheostomy that had been inserted to allow suction of secretions. However, methods of ventilatory assistance without intubation had proliferated prior to the polio epidemic (both negative-pressure chest wall devices and positive-pressure face-mask devices), and current trends are to an increased use of non-invasive ventilation (NIV) in patients with respiratory failure.[2]

Almost all of the ventilatory modes that are conventionally applied during *intubated* ventilation (IV) can be applied *non-invasively*; however, IV remains the primary mode of respiratory assistance in critically ill patients. There is also an increasing number of patients receiving chronic ventilatory assistance, but, since the majority of these use chronic NIV, this chapter is primarily directed at intubated mechanical ventilation for both ARF and acute-on-chronic respiratory failure.

A PHYSIOLOGICAL APPROACH

During normal spontaneous breathing, contraction of the respiratory muscles overcomes both the elastic recoil and resistance of the respiratory system (lung and chest wall). A fall in regional pleural pressure results in alveolar inflation due to the resultant pressure gradient. Expiration is usually passive, but the expiratory muscles may assist the elastic recoil of the respiratory system.

The work (W) performed by the respiratory muscles (W_{mus}) can be measured from the relationship between pressure (P) and volume (V), and partitioned into elastic (W_{el}) and resistive (W_{res}) work:

$$W_{mus} = W_{el} + W_{res} \qquad (31.1)$$

Inertial work is negligible, and usually ignored; furthermore equation 31.1 does not explicitly describe the elastic work required to initiate inspiration when intrinsic PEEP ($PEEP_i$) is present.

Because volume is constant in equation 31.1, it can be simplified to:

$$P_{mus} = P_{el} + P_{res} \qquad (31.2)$$

It follows that during positive-pressure ventilatory assistance, where P_{ao} is the ventilatory pressure applied at the airway:

$$P_{ao} + P_{mus} = P_{el} + P_{res} \qquad (31.3)$$

and that when the work is solely applied by the ventilator with no respiratory muscle contraction (controlled mechanical ventilation):

$$P_{ao} = P_{el} + P_{res} \qquad (31.4)$$

This nomenclature allows physiological discussion of the different ventilatory modes from controlled ventilation to spontaneous, unassisted ventilation, and introduces the equation of motion that is used in the estimation of respiratory mechanics (Ch. 38):

$$P_{ao} = E_{rs} \bullet V + R_{rs} \bullet \dot{V} + P_o \qquad (31.5)$$

where E_{rs} is the respiratory system (lung and chest wall) elastance (the inverse of compliance), R_{rs} is the respiratory system resistance, $\dot{V}$ is the gas flow rate, and P_o is the total PEEP (the sum of extrinsic PEEP ($PEEP_e$) and $PEEP_i$). $PEEP_i$ imposes a threshold load - additional elastic work, as inspiratory muscle contraction must occur without $\dot{V}$ until P_{ao} falls below atmospheric pressure (see below, patient–ventilator interaction).

MODES OF VENTILATION

CONTROLLED MECHANICAL VENTILATION (CMV)

The simplest form of positive-pressure breath occurs in a relaxed subject, and the ventilator provides a constant gas flow during inspiration. The volume delivered will depend upon the inspiratory time (T_i), and P_{ao} during inspiration will reflect E_{rs} and R_{rs} (**Fig. 31.1**). Expiration is a passive, and usually exponential, decline in volume to the relaxation volume of the respiratory system, also termed the functional residual capacity (FRC).

CMV is the most basic form of mechanical ventilation; however, it is extremely useful, and still commonly used. Preset minute ventilation is made up from a fixed respiratory rate (f) and tidal volume (V_T). Provided that there are not large variations in alveolar dead space, this maintains a preset alveolar ventilation (V_A) and CO_2 clearance. Consequently, CMV is useful in conditions

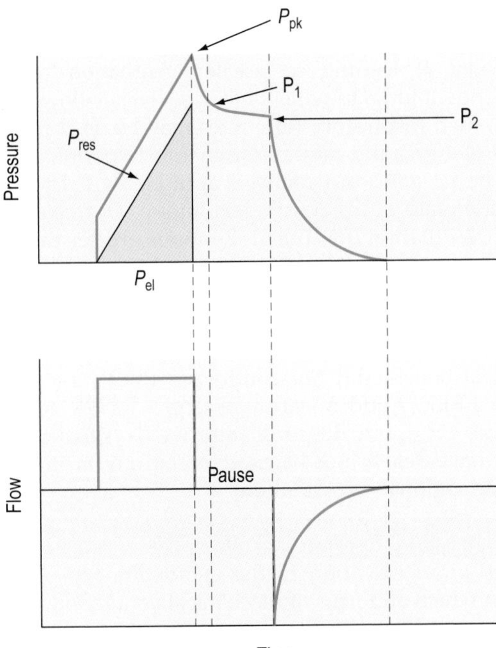

Figure 31.1 Schematic diagram of a volume-controlled breath with constant inspiratory flow. A period of no inspiratory gas flow has been interposed before expiration (pause) to illustrate dissipation of lung resistance as airways resistance (fall from P_{pk} to P_1) and tissue resistance (fall from P_1 to P_2). The inspiratory pressure due to the elastic properties of the respiratory system is illustrated as the filled area (P_{el}), and the lung resistive pressure is labelled as P_{res}. (See text for more detail.)

where there is alveolar hypoventilation (e.g. respiratory muscle weakness), when Pa_{CO_2} needs to be maintained in a fixed range (e.g. raised intracranial pressure) or when the work of breathing must be minimised (e.g. severe cardiorespiratory failure). Because CMV may not match respiratory drive, and spontaneous, supported or assisted breaths are not possible during CMV, sedation and sometimes muscle paralysis may be needed. CMV is usually combined with PEEP$_e$, which can recruit collapsed lung and reduce intrapulmonary shunt. The components are discussed below.

TIDAL VOLUME (V_T)

Larger V_T, typically 12–15 mL/kg, or intermittent recruitment manoeuvres (sighs) prevent progressive atelectasis and intrapulmonary shunt during general anaesthesia.[3] However, this may result in excessive lung stretch, particularly in patients with acute respiratory distress syndrome (ARDS), leading to ventilator-induced lung injury (VILI). For example in ARDS V_T of 6 mL/kg versus 12 mL/kg predicted body weight (i.e. often 4–5 mL/kg versus 9–10 mL/kg true weight) reduced mortality from 40% to 31%.[4] Consequently, lower V_T should be strongly considered during CMV, and other forms of ventilatory assistance, in patients with ARDS; however, greater levels of PEEP are usually required. Whereas the reduction in V_T is particularly applicable to ARDS, excessive lung stretch will be less likely in other patient cohorts that are able to ventilate a greater proportion of the lung (see Ch. 33, Acute Respiratory Distress Syndrome). Intermediate V_T offers more efficient V_A when ventilator support is required for obstructive lung disease as the anatomical dead space fraction is lower.

RESPIRATORY RATE (F)

The desired minute ventilation can be selected from the product of V_T and f. Common CMV rates are 10–20 breaths per minute in adults. Sufficient expiratory time (T_e) must be allowed to minimise dynamic hyperinflation and PEEP$_i$. Although high f (up to 35 breaths per minute) was allowed in the ARDS Network protocol, and the low V_T, low mortality group had a mean f of ~30 breaths per minute,[5] laboratory data suggest a possible additive role of high f in VILI.[5]

INSPIRATORY FLOW PATTERN

The simplest form of CMV uses a constant inspiratory $\dot{V}$ ($\dot{V}_I$) and, in combination with T_i, a preset volume is delivered. This is also called volume-controlled ventilation (VCV); some ventilators use V_T and T_i to set $\dot{V}_I$. Alternative $\dot{V}_I$ patterns that are commonly available with VCV include a ramped descending flow pattern and a sine pattern. When a time preset inspiratory pressure is delivered this is termed pressure-controlled ventilation (PCV).

Although there are no convincing outcome data differentiating these different modes of CMV, PCV is increasingly used when the peak airway pressure (P_{pk}) is high with VCV. However, the alveolar distending pressure, which is usually inferred from the plateau pressure (P_{plat}), is no different provided that T_i and V_T are the same.[6] During PCV, P_{res} is dissipated during inspiration so P_{pk} and P_{plat} are equal, and during VCV P_{res} accounts for the difference between P_{pk} and P_{plat} (**Fig. 31.2**). Similarly, different CMV $\dot{V}_I$ patterns will alter P_{pk} without changing P_{plat} or mean airway pressure (P_{mean}) when T_i and V_T are constant. In ARDS patients, comparing VCV and PCV there was no difference in haemodynamics, oxygenation, recruited lung volume or distribution of regional ventilation.[7] Although PCV may dissipate viscoelastic strain earlier,[7] high $\dot{V}_I$ may cause or exacerbate VILI,[8] which may explain why some animal models have found PCV, which inherently has a high early $\dot{V}_I$, to be injurious compared with VCV.

Pressure-regulated volume control (PRVC) is a form of CMV where the V_T is preset, and achieved at a minimum pressure using a decelerating flow pattern.

INSPIRATORY PAUSE

An end-inspiratory pause allows examination of the decay in P_{pk}, and measurement of P_{plat} (see Ch. 38), and

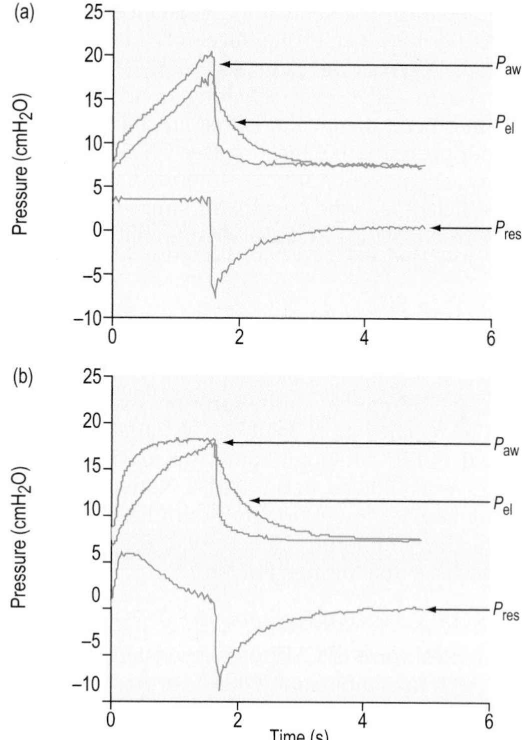

Figure 31.2 Actual pressure–time data from a patient with ARDS ventilated with volume-controlled ventilation (panel a), and then with pressure-controlled ventilation (panel b); tidal volume, I:E ratio and respiratory rate are constant. The airway pressure (P_{aw}, bold line) has been broken down to its components, P_{el} and P_{res} (see Fig. 31.1). Although there is no inspiratory pause, there is marked similarity between panel a and Figure 31.1, with the inspiratory difference between P_{aw} and P_{el} due to a constant P_{res}. In panel b, the decelerating inspiratory flow pattern seen with pressure-controlled ventilation results in dissipation of P_{res} by end inspiration. Consequently, during pressure-controlled ventilation $P_{aw} \approx P_{plat}$ obtained during volume-controlled ventilation. In other words, for the same ventilator settings there is no difference in the elastic distending pressure.

may alter the distribution of ventilation. If T_i and V_T are maintained constant there is no improvement in oxygenation, and a more rapid $\dot{V}_I$ will be needed. Theoretically, during an end-inspiratory pause 32% of the total energy loss within the respiratory system will be dissipated,[9] which may significantly reduce the forces driving expiration, potentially exacerbating gas trapping in patients with severe air-flow limitation.

INSPIRATORY TIME, EXPIRATORY TIME, I:E RATIO

The combination of V_T and inspiratory $\dot{V}$ will determine T_i, which in combination with f sets T_e. A typical T_i is 0.8–1.2 s; with a V_T of 500 mL and inspiratory $\dot{V}$ of 0.5 L/s the T_i is 1.0 seconds. During spontaneous ventilation, the distribution of ventilation at low $\dot{V}$ is determined by regional E, and at high inspiratory $\dot{V}$ by regional R leading to greater ventilation of non-dependent lung. In patients with severe air-flow limitation, high inspiratory flow rates may be used in order to prolong T_e and minimise dynamic hyperinflation.[10]

The I:E ratio is usually set at or below 1:2 to allow an adequate T_e for passive expiration. During inverse ratio ventilation (IRV) the I:E ratio is greater than 1:1. The putative benefits of a prolonged T_i include higher expiratory $\dot{V}$ and improved mucus clearance,[11] and recruitment of long time-constant alveoli, and a short T_e results in gas trapping and PEEP$_i$. Early reports of clinical benefit did not control for PEEP$_i$, and, when total PEEP, f and V_T are constant,[7,8] PCIRV tends to reduce Pa_{CO_2} but does not improve oxygenation, and may have deleterious haemodynamic effects and exaggerate regional overinflation.[7]

POSITIVE END-EXPIRATORY PRESSURE (PEEP)

PEEP is an elevation in the end-expiratory pressure upon which all forms of mechanical ventilation may be imposed. When PEEP is maintained throughout the respiratory cycle in a spontaneously breathing subject, the term constant positive airway pressure (CPAP) is used. The primary role of PEEP is to maintain recruitment of collapsed lung, increase FRC and minimise intrapulmonary shunt. PEEP may also improve oxygenation by redistributing lung water from the alveolus to the interstitium and, although there is no direct effect of PEEP to reduce extravascular lung water, this may occur in patients with left ventricular failure due to a reduction in venous return and left ventricular afterload. Furthermore, inadequate PEEP may contribute to VILI by promoting tidal opening and closing of alveoli. PEEP levels of 5–15 cmH_2O are commonly used, and levels up to 25 cmH_2O may be required in patients with severe ARDS. Although meta-analysis of three large multicentre trials[12] found no benefit of higher PEEP levels in ARDS, mortality was lower in more hypoxaemic patients and there were fewer rescue therapies required, suggesting individual titration may need to be considered.

PEEP titration in ARDS is complex (see Ch. 33, Acute Respiratory Distress Syndrome), and should aim to improve oxygenation and minimise VILI. Since PEEP reduces venous return, cardiac output and O_2 delivery may fall despite an improvement in P_{ao}; indeed this concept has been used to optimise PEEP in ARF.[13] However, in addition to recruitment, increasing PEEP may lead to overinflation of non-dependent alveoli that are already aerated at end expiration.[14,15] Patients with focal ARDS are a particular risk group as recruitment is limited; VILI can be minimised when PEEP is reduced below standard levels.[16] In general, overinflation and VILI are less likely if alveolar distending pressure is kept $<$30–35 cmH_2O, or the change in driving pressure is $<$2 cmH_2O when V_T is constant.[17]

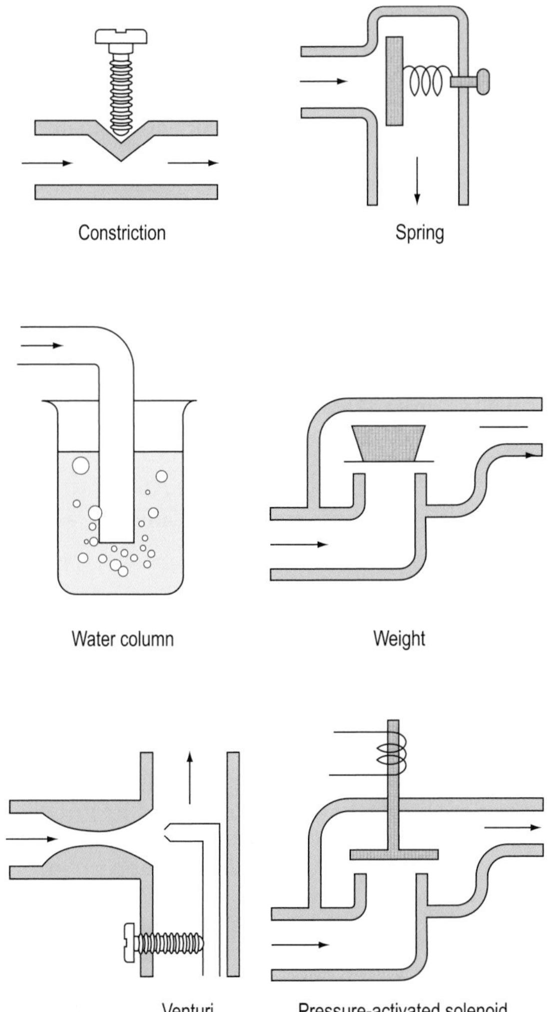

Figure 31.3 Positive end-expiratory pressure values.

$PEEP_e$ is applied by placing a resistance in the expiratory circuit (**Fig. 31.3**), with most ventilators using a solenoid valve. Independent of the technique, a threshold resistor is preferred since it offers minimal resistance to flow once its opening P is reached. This will minimise expiratory work, and avoid barotrauma during coughing or straining.

$PEEP_i$ is an elevation in the static recoil pressure of the respiratory system above $PEEP_e$ at end expiration. $PEEP_i$ arises due to an inadequate T_e, usually in the setting of severe air-flow obstruction. However, it may be a desired end-point during IRV. The sum of $PEEP_e$ and $PEEP_i$ is the total PEEP ($PEEP_{tot}$). The distribution of $PEEP_i$ is likely to be less uniform than an equivalent $PEEP_e$; this may not have the same physiological effects. When patients with severe air-flow obstruction are triggering ventilation, $PEEP_e$ less than $PEEP_i$ may be applied to reduce elastic work (see below, patient–ventilator interaction).

FRACTIONAL INSPIRED OXYGEN CONCENTRATION (Fi_{O_2})

Adequate arterial oxygen saturation is achieved through a combination of minute ventilation, PEEP and Fi_{O_2} adjustment. Even patients with normal respiratory systems usually need an $Fi_{O_2} > 0.21$, due to ventilation–perfusion mismatch secondary to positive-pressure ventilation. In patients with ARF it is common to start with an Fi_{O_2} of 1 and titrate down as PEEP and minute ventilation are adjusted. Because high Fi_{O_2}s are damaging to the lung, and nitrogen washout may exacerbate atelectasis, it is reasonable to aim at an $Fi_{O_2} \leq 0.6$.

SIGH

Many ventilators have the ability to intermittently deliver a breath at least twice V_T. Sighs may reduce atelectasis, in part, through release of pulmonary surfactant,[18] resulting in recruitment and improved oxygenation in ARDS.[19] However, if sighs or recruitment manoeuvres are used, care must be taken to avoid recurrent excessive lung stretch.

ASSIST-CONTROL VENTILATION (ACV)

During ACV, in addition to the set f, patient effort can trigger a standard CMV breath (**Fig. 31.4**). This allows greater patient comfort, and V_T is controlled at a safe level; however, there may be little reduction in respiratory work compared to an unassisted breath at low $\dot{V}_I$, because the respiratory muscles continue to contract through much of the breath.[20] The equivalent PCV breath is termed pressure assist-control ventilation (PACV). Differences between triggering modes will be discussed below (patient–ventilator interaction).

INTERMITTENT MANDATORY VENTILATION (IMV), SYNCHRONISED IMV (SIMV)

IMV was introduced over 20 years ago to aid weaning from CMV by allowing the patient to take 'unimpeded' breaths while still receiving a background of controlled breaths. Proposed advantages include a reduction in sedation, lower mean intrathoracic pressure with less barotrauma and adverse haemodynamic consequences, improved intrapulmonary gas distribution, continued use of respiratory muscles and faster weaning. During SIMV T_i is partitioned into patient-initiated and true spontaneous breaths to avoid breath stacking. However, during spontaneous breaths the work of breathing imposed by the endotracheal tube, circuit and ventilator must be overcome.[21] In weaning studies comparing SIMV with T-piece trials and pressure support ventilation (PSV), SIMV is the slowest.[22] Many clinicians add PSV during gradual reduction in respiratory rate with SIMV to overcome the added

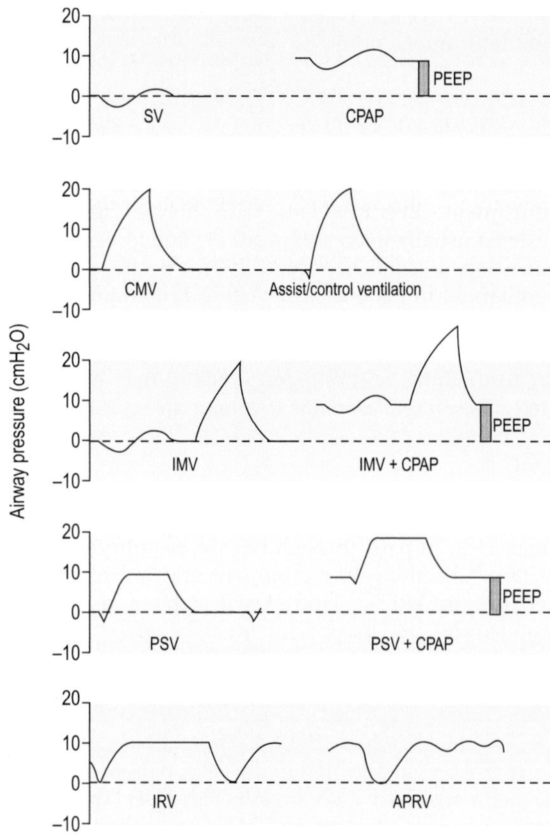

Figure 31.4 Schematic representation of airway pressure versus time for a variety of forms of ventilatory assistance. SV=spontaneous ventilation; CPAP=continuous positive airway pressure; PEEP=positive end-expiratory pressure; CMV=controlled mechanical ventilation; IMV=intermittent mandatory ventilation; PSV=pressure support ventilation; IRV=inverse-ratio ventilation; APRV=airway pressure release ventilation.

respiratory work imposed by the circuit and endotracheal tube; however, this approach has not been formally compared with other weaning techniques, and upper airway oedema following extubation increases extubated W_{res} similar to that imposed by the endotracheal tube prior to extubation.[23]

PRESSURE SUPPORT VENTILATION (PSV)

During PSV, each patient-triggered breath is supported by gas flow to achieve a preset pressure, usually designated to be above the $PEEP_e$. This can be explained by referring to the equation of motion where:

$$P_{mus} + P_{ao} = E_{rs} \bullet V + R_{rs} \bullet \dot{V} + P_o \quad (31.6)$$

During PSV, P_{ao} is the targeted variable by the ventilator, which leads to a significant and important reduction in P_{mus} and work of breathing.[24] The detection of neural expiration varies between ventilators, but commonly relies upon a fall in the inspiratory $\dot{V}$ to either 25% of the initial flow rate or to less than 5 L/min; some ventilators allow titration of the percentage reduction in initial flow to allow improved patient–ventilator synchrony. PSV may also be titrated to offset the work imposed by the circuit and endotracheal tube. The absolute level required to offset this will vary with endotracheal tube size and inspiratory $\dot{V}$,[25] but is commonly 5–10 cmH_2O.[26] PSV can be used during weaning, or as a form of variable ventilatory support with pressures of 15–20 cmH_2O commonly used. Disadvantages include variable V_T, and hence minute ventilation, the potential to deliver an excessive V_T (common in patients recovering from ARDS) and patient–ventilator asynchrony, which is common with high levels of PSV (see below).

Volume-assured pressure support (VAPS) is a mode of adaptive PSV where breath-to-breath logic achieves a preset V_T.

PROPORTIONAL ASSIST VENTILATION (PAV)

PAV is a form of partial ventilatory support where inspiratory P is applied in proportion to patient effort. Because this allows the breathing pattern and minute ventilation to be matched to patient effort, it is only suitable if respiratory drive is normal or elevated. In concept this should optimise the patient–ventilator interaction; however, the prescription of PAV requires a greater level of physiological understanding than similar forms of partial ventilatory support such as PSV, since there is no target P, V, or $\dot{V}$. PAV is usually prescribed using volume assist (VA) and flow assist (FA), with V and $\dot{V}$ measured continuously. VA generates greater P as V increases leading to elastic unloading, and FA generates greater P as $\dot{V}$ increases leading to resistive unloading. Not surprisingly the units of VA are cmH_2O/L (i.e. an elastance term) and those for FA are $cmH_2O/L/s$ (i.e. a resistance term). This can be illustrated by referring to equation 31.6:

$$P_{mus} + P_{ao} = E_{rs} \bullet V + R_{rs} \bullet \dot{V} + P_o$$

where P_{ao} is determined by PAV, where PAV=VA+FA, so:

$$P_{mus} + \mathrm{VA} \bullet V + \mathrm{FA} \bullet \dot{V} = Ers \bullet V + R_{rs} \bullet \dot{V} + P_o \quad (31.7)$$

$$\text{consequently} \quad P_{mus} = (E_{rs} - \mathrm{VA}) \bullet V + (R_{rs} - \mathrm{FA}) \bullet \dot{V} + P_o \quad (31.8)$$

If E_{rs} and R_{rs} are known, PAV can, at least in principle, be targeted to reduce a specified proportion of either, or both, elastic and resistive respiratory work. For example, when VA and FA are adjusted to counterbalance E_{rs} and R_{rs} so as to achieve normal values, minute ventilation increases, and respiratory drive and work decrease; if $PEEP_i$ is present, work can be further reduce by applying $PEEP_e$.[27] Respiratory mechanics are relatively hard to estimate in spontaneously breathing patients, although they are now offered on some ventilators their accuracy has been questioned,[28] which may reduce the validity of adjusting PAV according to estimated load (PAV+). Consequently, PAV is often titrated to patient comfort. Despite a growing body of data demonstrating reduced work of breathing, and improved patient–ventilator synchrony with PAV, it is a more difficult technique to use, and definitive studies showing a clinically important outcome difference are awaited.

NEURALLY ADJUSTED VENTILATORY ASSISTANCE (NAVA)

During NAVA a modified nasogastric tube is used to record diaphragmatic electrical activity, which is used to control the assisting level of inspiratory pressure. This short-circuits trigger and feedback functions with improved patient–ventilator interaction, less asynchrony and less overassistance compared with PSV.[29] NAVA may also improve oxygenation, perhaps by allowing more variable V_T consistent with the concept of biological variability. Although NAVA is available on some commercial ventilators its use is limited, and there are no data showing a clinically important benefit.

BILEVEL VENTILATION

Also described as biphasic positive airway pressure (BIPAP), this is a ventilatory mode where two levels of airway pressure are provided. Cycling between these two levels of airway pressure may be time cycled or triggered by ventilatory effort, in which case inspiratory positive airway pressure (IPAP) and expiratory positive airway pressure (EPAP) are set; however, this is no different to equivalent support with PSV and PEEP. Patient-triggered bilevel ventilation is most commonly used during NIV.

AIRWAY PRESSURE RELEASE VENTILATION (APRV)

During APRV spontaneous breathing is possible in addition to time-triggered and time-cycled biphasic pressure levels (high and low CPAP). Usually the time cycling provides a prolonged T_i aimed at recruiting slow time constant air spaces. Minute ventilation and CO_2 excretion are augmented by brief (1–1.5 s) periodic cycling to the lower level of CPAP. As the augmented V_T is dependent upon elastance of the respiratory system, it will be smaller in patients with 'stiff' respiratory systems. APRV without spontaneous breathing has a similar pressure profile to PCIRV.

APRV offers a number of benefits and is usually applied during IV. The prolonged T_i is usually associated with improved oxygenation at a similar or lower P_{aw} to conventional ventilation. Spontaneous respiratory efforts may: (1) improve matching of ventilation and perfusion due to increased dependent aeration, (2) increase venous return and hence cardiac output or pulmonary blood flow in infants following cardiac surgery[30] and (3) promote reduced sedation. However, randomised clinical trials have not shown improved outcomes,[31] unsupported spontaneous breaths may increase left ventricular afterload and promote ventilator–patient asynchrony and, as slow time constant air spaces are also slow to empty, APRV is contraindicated in COPD and asthma.

HIGH-FREQUENCY VENTILATION (HFV)

HFV encompasses techniques where small V_T (1–3 ml/kg) are delivered at high f (100–600/min). This offers reduced tidal lung stretch and reduced VILI. Hazards include inadequate humidification and gas trapping in patients with severe air-flow limitation. High-frequency jet ventilation (HFJV) utilises dry gas from a high-pressure source delivered into an intratracheal catheter or specifically manufactured endotracheal tube. Although HFJV has been used with improvement in gas exchange in adults with ARDS,[32] high-frequency oscillation (HFO) has received more interest including neonatal, paediatric and adult use.

HFO uses oscillatory flow within the airway to provide active inspiration and expiration at rates of 3–10 Hz. There are a number of putative mechanisms of gas exchange in addition to the more usual bulk flow seen during CMV and SV.[33] Ventilation and V_T are determined by the driving pressure, which controls the reciprocating flow, and by $1/f$. Oxygenation is determined by the mean P_{aw} sometimes in combination with recruitment manoeuvres which influence the volume of recruited lung. Typically the mean P_{aw} is set 5 cmH_2O above the CMV value.[34] Although the mean P_{aw} during HFO is theoretically dissipated with lower alveolar pressures, and this appears to be the case in homogeneous lung injury, damaged regions of the lung with low compliance, and hence short time constants, may be exposed to alveolar pressures approaching mean P_{aw},[35] resulting in regional VILI.

Although oxygenation is improved in both infants and patients with ARDS, definitive outcome data are currently awaited. HFO appears to be equivalent to CMV in preterm infants with similar mortality and chronic lung disease.[36] In ARDS randomised trials have been relatively small and have arguably targeted improved oxygenation rather than lung protection. A meta-analysis of these has suggested reduced mortality with HFO;[28] however, the largest trial included in this analysis administered a V_T of around 10.6 mL/kg predicted body weight in the control CMV group[37] making interpretation difficult. Two large trials with appropriate strategies are currently well under way and should clarify this issue.

LIQUID VENTILATION

Perfluorocarbons have a high solubility for both O_2 and CO_2, and reduce surface tension, somewhat analagous to pulmonary surfactant. Partial liquid ventilation is now the most common method of administration, with perfluorocarbon equal to the functional residual capacity administered via the endotracheal tube. The non-dependent lung is still ventilated, and may have increased blood flow due to compression of the pulmonary circulation in the dependent lung by the perfluorocarbon. Together with the perfluorocarbon-mediated reduction in surface tension, alveoli are recruited and oxygenation improved. However, when PEEP is applied the perfluorocarbon may be pushed distally and overdistend dependent alveoli.

Small clinical studies have reported improved gas exchange and respiratory mechanics after administration of perfluorocarbons;[38] however, a moderately large clinical study (n=311) found that patients receiving conventional ventilation compared with both low- and high-dose perflourocarbons had more ventilator-free days and tended to reduced mortality.[39] Consequently, liquid ventilation cannot be recommended.

INDICATIONS AND OBJECTIVES OF MECHANICAL VENTILATION[40]

Institution of mechanical ventilation is a clinical decision; it can only be supported by parameters such as blood gases or measures of respiratory muscle function. Even then, the decision to choose IV over NIV will be influenced by numerous factors including the indication and its likely course. Often there will be an indication for intubation (**Box 31.1**) and mechanical ventilation; however, if intubation is required to overcome upper airway obstruction no ventilatory assistance may be needed despite the increase in respiratory work imposed by the endotracheal or tracheostomy tube.[18] Once the decision has been made to proceed to ventilatory support the choice of mode should be based on a physiological approach, local expertise, and simplicity.

Patients who are likely to need ventilatory assistance (e.g. acute severe asthma) should be considered for early ICU admission since this will allow faster responses and avoid cardiorespiratory arrest. Specific issues and methods of ventilatory assistance are dealt with in the chapters on ARDS, asthma, COPD and non-invasive ventilation. In patients with traumatic brain injury IV is commonly required to protect the airway and to assist control of ICP, similarly patients with severe pancreatitis or serious abdominal infection may need prolonged IV to maintain an adequate FRC, reduce work of breathing, protect their airway and allow suctioning of secretions.

Box 31.1 Indications and objectives of intubated mechanical ventilation

Endotracheal intubation or tracheostomy
- For airway protection (e.g. coma)
- For suction of secretions
- To assist sedation and neuromuscular paralysis (e.g. to ↓$\dot{V}_{O_2}$ ↓ *respiratory distress*)
- To overcome upper-airway obstruction

Mechanical ventilation
- To manipulate alveolar ventilation (V_A) and Pa_{CO_2} (e.g. reverse respiratory acidosis, ↓ cerebral blood flow and intracranial pressure)
- To ↑ Sa_{O_2} and Pa_{O_2} (by ↑ functional residual capacity, ↑end-inspiratory lung volume, ↑V_A, ↑ Fi_{O_2})
- To ↓ work of breathing (e.g. to overcome respiratory muscle fatigue)
- To ↑ functional residual capacity (e.g. ↑ Pa_{O_2}, ↓ ventilator-induced injury)
- To stabilise the chest wall in severe chest injury

INITIATION OF INTUBATED MECHANICAL VENTILATION

A manual resuscitation circuit, mechanical ventilator and equipment for safe endotracheal intubation (Ch. 29) should be available. Initial ventilator settings are commonly set to achieve adequate oxygenation and V_A; however, this will depend upon the patient's condition. Common settings are: V_T 6–8 mL/kg, f 10–20 breaths/min, PEEP 5 cmH_2O, and Fi_{O_2} 1.0, and these will need to be adjusted according to the specific pathophysiology and response.

MANUAL RESUSCITATION CIRCUITS

Manual resuscitation circuits are primarily used to provide emergency ventilation when spontaneous effort is absent or inadequate. They may be used with a face or laryngeal mask, or an endotracheal tube. Occasionally they are used to provide a high inspired O_2 concentration during spontaneous breathing; however, this may impose significant additional respiratory work.[41] In the ICU they are commonly used for preoxygenation and manual lung inflation.

Their basic design includes a fresh gas flow of O_2, a reservoir bag and valves to allow spontaneous or positive-pressure breathing. Most manual resuscitation circuits use a self-inflating reservoir bag since this allows the circuit to be used by unskilled personnel and does not require a fresh gas flow. However, circuits using reservoir bags that are not self-inflating are still used in some institutions since they allow a better manual assessment of the respiratory mechanics, the 'educated hand', and it is clear when there is an inadequate seal with a mask. Oxygen-powered manually triggered devices have been used for many years; however, this has declined markedly since high $\dot{V}$ and P may lead to barotrauma or gastric inflation.

Self-inflating reservoir bags use a series of one-way valves to allow fresh gas flow oxygen and entrained air to fill the bag. Inspired oxygen fractions as high as 0.8 may be achieved with neonatal or paediatric bags when an additional reservoir bag is used to allow fresh gas flow filling during expiration, after the bag has refilled.[42] However, lower Fi_{O_2}s (~0.6) will be obtained with both conventional O_2 flow rates of 8–15 L/min, and usual V_T and *f*, with an adult bag. Generally the valves are simple flap or duckbill in nature, and both positive pressure and spontaneous ventilation are possible. The reservoir bag volume in adults is typically 1600 mL, and V_T can be judged from chest wall movement. It is essential these devices use standard 15/22 mm connectors to allow rapid connection to standard endotracheal tubes and ventilator circuits.

COMPLICATIONS OF MECHANICAL VENTILATION (Box 31.2)[26]

Although mechanical ventilation may be vital, it also introduces numerous potential complications. Monitoring includes a high nurse: patient ratio (usually 1:1), ventilator alarms, and pulse oximetry. Capnography is required to confirm endotracheal tube placement, both at the time of intubation and during ventilatory support, and may be used to monitor the adequacy of V_A; however, expired CO_2 is strongly influenced by factors that alter alveolar dead space such as cardiac output. Intermittent blood gases, $PEEP_i$, airway pressures in volume-preset modes and V_T in pressure-preset modes should be recorded. Individual patients may benefit from more extensive monitoring of their respiratory mechanics or tissue oxygenation.

The patient's airway (i.e. patency, presence of leaks and nature and amount of secretions), breathing (i.e. rate, volume, oxygenation), and circulation (i.e. pulse, blood pressure and urine output) must be monitored. Ventilatory and circuit alarms should be adjusted to monitor an appropriate range of *V*, *P* and temperature. This should alert adjacent staff to changes in *P* and/or *V* that may be caused by an occluded endotracheal tube, tension pneumothorax or circuit disconnection. These alarms may be temporarily disabled while the cause is detected, but never permanently disabled. Sudden difficulties with high *P* during volume-preset ventilation or oxygenation must initiate an immediate search for the cause. This should start with the patency of the airway, followed by a structured approach both to the circuit and ventilator, and to factors altering the *E* and *R* of the lung and chest wall such as bronchospasm, secretions, pneumothorax and asynchronous breathing. In addition to careful clinical examination an urgent chest radiograph and bronchoscopy may be required.

Mechanical ventilation is also associated with a marked increase in the incidence of nosocomial pneumonia due to a reduction in the natural defenses of the respiratory tract, and this represents an important advantage offered by NIV. In patients successfully managed with NIV, Girou and colleagues reported a reduction in the incidence of nosocomial pneumonia, associated with improved survival, compared to IV.[43] Erect versus semirecumbent posture[44] also reduces the incidence of ventilator-associated pneumonia.

Whereas lung overdistension may result in alveolar rupture leading to pulmonary interstitial air, pneumomediastinum or pneumothorax, it may also lead to diffuse alveolar damage similar to that found in ARDS. Both are termed VILI, and V_T reduction leads to a marked decrease in ARDS mortality, due to a reduction in multiple organ dysfunction[5] (Ch. 33). Laboratory data suggest that inadequate PEEP with tidal recruitment and derecruitment of alveoli also leads to VILI; however, this has not been proven in a clinical trial. Finally, patient–ventilator asynchrony may result in wasted respiratory work, impaired gas exchange and respiratory distress (see below).

Positive-pressure ventilation elevates intrathoracic pressure, which reduces venous return, right ventricular preload and cardiac output. The impact is reduced by hypervolaemia, and partial ventilatory support

Box 31.2 Complications of intubation and mechanical ventilation

Equipment
- Malfunction or disconnection
- Incorrectly set or prescribed
- Contamination

Pulmonary
- Airway intubation (e.g. damage to teeth, vocal cords, trachea; see Ch. 29)
- Ventilator-associated pneumonia (reduced lung defence; see Ch. 36)
- Ventilator-associated lung injury (e.g. diffuse lung injury due to regional overdistension or tidal recruitment of alveoli)
- Overt barotrauma (e.g. pneumothorax)
- O_2 toxicity
- Patient–ventilator asynchrony

Circulation
- ↓ Right ventricular preload →↓ cardiac output
- ↑ Right ventricular afterload (if the lung is overdistended)
- ↓ Splanchnic blood flow with high levels of positive end-expiratory pressure (PEEP) or mean P_{aw}
- ↑ Intracranial pressure with high levels of PEEP or mean P_{aw}
- Fluid retention due to ↓ cardiac output →↓ renal blood flow

Other
- Gut distension (air swallowing, hypomotility)
- Mucosal ulceration and bleeding
- Peripheral and respiratory muscle weakness (see Ch. 57)
- Sleep disturbance, agitation and fear (which may be prolonged after recovery)
- Neuropsychiatric complications

where patient effort and a reduction in pleural pressure augments venous return. Secondary effects include a reduction in regional organ blood flow leading to fluid retention by the kidney, and possibly impaired hepatic function. This latter effect is seen only at high levels of PEEP where an increase in resistance to venous return and a reduction in cardiac output may combine to reduce hepatic blood flow.

Sleep disturbance, delirium and discomfort are common in mechanically ventilated patients. These effects may be reduced with analgesia and sedation until weaning is planned; however, it is also important not to prolong mechanical ventilation due to excessive use of sedatives, which may also depress blood pressure and spontaneous respiratory effort. A recent large clinical trial found no advantage of daily sedation over continuous infusion of sedation targeted to the lowest effective dose.[45] Both methods offer early mobilisation in ventilated subjects, shorter duration of ventilation, reduced delirium, ICU and hospital length of stay, and improved mortality and functional outcomes.[46,47] However, this direction must be balanced with strategies such as use of neuromuscular blockers in the first 48 hours of mechanical ventilation in ARDS, which reduced mortality,[48] which prevent or reduce asynchronous ventilatory effort.

Although pulmonary function has generally recovered by 12 months, complex neuropsychological and physical sequelae persist to at least 5 years in surviving ARDS patients.[49] Cognitive impairment has been associated with hypotension, hypoxaemia and hyperglcaemia. In addition anxiety, depression and post-traumatic stress disorder are common and appear to be associated with the severity of illness, duration of mechanical ventilation and premorbid factors including depression. All of these issues are increasingly important as improvements in care and greater numbers of patients treated result in more survivors from critical illness. Of particular note it appears that early interventions can be effective, but that late interventions fail to improve outcomes.

WITHDRAWAL (WEANING) FROM MECHANICAL VENTILATION

Once the underlying process necessitating mechanical ventilation has started to resolve, withdrawal of ventilatory support should be considered; increased duration of ventilation leads to a progressive rise in complications such as ventilator-associated pneumonia. However, other important parameters that must be considered include the neuromuscular state of the patient (ability to initiate a spontaneous breath), adequacy of oxygenation (typically low requirements for PEEP (5–8 cmH$_2$O) and Fi_{O_2} (<0.4–0.5]), and cardiovascular stability.[50] Once a patient is considered suitable to wean, a secondary question is whether an artificial airway is still required for airway protection or suction of secretions. Many patients can rapidly make the transition from mechanical ventilation to extubation, but ~20% of patients fail weaning despite meeting clinical criteria.[21] Advanced age, prolonged mechanical ventilation and chronic obstructive pulmonary disease all increase the likelihood that weaning will be difficult.[21]

Weaning failure is usually associated with an increase in respiratory drive, and respiratory rate and a fall in V_T, which contributes to hypercapnea;[51] about 10% of patients fail due to central respiratory depression. Various indices such as maximal inspiratory pressure (MIP), minute ventilation (V_E), f, V_T, f/V_T ratio and the CROP index have been investigated as predictors of weaning failure (**Table 31.1**). They are rarely used alone and careful clinical assessment is often adequate, yielding a re-intubation rate as low as 3%,[52] and none of these indices assess airway function following extubation. Although the typical threshold value for the rapid shallow breathing index (f/V_T ratio) is >105, a large recent multicentre study reported progressive increase in risk as this increased with a threshold of 57; in addition a positive fluid balance immediately prior to extubation was a significant risk factor for re-intubation.[53] Consequently, weaning indices should not necessarily delay extubation or a weaning trial. However, they

Table 31.1 Sample of measurements that have been used to predict successful outcome from weaning in critically ill patients*

PARAMETER	TYPICAL THRESHOLD VALUE†	COMMENT
V_E	≤15 L/min	Moderate to high sensitivity, low specificity
MIP	≤–15 cmH$_2$O	High sensitivity, low specificity
CROP index#	≥13	Moderate to high sensitivity, modest specificity
DURING A SPONTANEOUS BREATHING TRIAL		
f	≤38 breaths/min	High sensitivity, low specificity
V_T	≥325 mL (4 mL/kg)	High sensitivity, low specificity
f/V_T	≤105	High sensitivity, moderate specificity

#CROP index=$(C_{dyn} \times MIP \times [Pa_{O_2}/PA_{O_2}]/f)$.[22]
Abbreviations: MIP=maximal inspiratory pressure; CROP=compliance, respiratory rate, oxygenation, maximal inspiratory pressure.
*See reference 50 for further detail.
†Although threshold values are often used, the data are not dichotomous. For example, as the f/V_T ratio increases, so does the rate of re-intubation.[53]

may quantitate important issues in the general clinical assessment, and may be directly relevant for a given patient. For example, frequent small V_T, an inadequate vital capacity (less than 8–12 mL/kg), large minute ventilation (≥15 L/min), depressed respiratory drive, and reduced respiratory muscle strength (MIP≤ –15 cmH_2O), or drive should be strongly factored into deciding whether a patient is ready to safely undergo a trial of weaning.

Direct comparisons between T-piece trials, PSV and SIMV as weaning techniques have been performed in patients previously failing a 2-hour trial of spontaneous breathing. In the study by Brochard and colleagues,[54] PSV led to fewer failures and a shorter weaning period. In contrast Esteban and coworkers[55] found that a once-daily trial of spontaneous breathing resulted in the shortest duration of mechanical ventilation; however, a relatively high proportion of patients required re-intubation (22.6%). Viewed together these studies suggest that weaning was slower with SIMV,[19] although SIMV with PSV was not studied, and that either PSV or a T-piece trial are the preferred methods for weaning. Since low levels of PSV can help compensate for the additional work of breathing attributable to the endotracheal tube and circuit, some clinicians use low levels of PSV (5–7 cmH_2O) during weaning or during a spontaneous breathing trial. However, the work of breathing following extubation is usually higher than expected, probably due to upper airway oedema and dysfunction, so that work is similar to that during a T-piece trial.[22,23]

Re-intubation is relatively common, with reported rates of 15%, and is associated with a 7–11 fold increased risk of hospital death.[19] Although this may reflect extubation of sicker patients, there does appear to be a specific effect of extubation failure on outcome perhaps due to the risks of re-intubation itself along with its haemodynamic consequences, and an increased risk of infection. Thille and co-workers[56] reported that 27% of patients developed pneumonia, and that 50% of patients died following re-intubation. They identified age >65 years and underlying cardiorespiratory disease as risk factors for extubation failure. Unplanned extubations were associated with higher endotracheal tube position on chest radiograph. Hence, an important goal during mechanical ventilation will be to proceed to early and expeditious extubation with a low reintubation rate.

PATIENT–VENTILATOR INTERACTION

During partial ventilatory support or spontaneous breathing, the ventilator should match neural drive; however, suboptimal patient–ventilator interaction, also termed asynchrony, is common, frequently not diagnosed and is associated with prolonged mechanical ventilation, increased length of stay both in hospital and in the ICU, and with increased mortality when more than 30% of breaths are asynchronous.[57] Clinical signs of asynchrony include agitation, diaphoresis, tachycardia, hypertension and failure of weaning or NIV. Once this pattern is identified it is crucial that airway complications (partial obstruction, displacement) or a major change in the clinical state (e.g. pneumothorax, acute pulmonary oedema) are excluded before considering problems with patient–ventilator interaction.

Although both PAV and NAVA reduce asynchrony, they are complex and less commonly used. Recognition and management of asynchrony are assisted by a physiological approach to the respiratory cycle: (a) triggering of inspiration, (b) inspiration and (c) cessation of inspiration. Difficulties at each of these phases will lead to changes in respiratory drive and effort that may be expressed throughout the respiratory cycle. Careful bedside observation of the patient–ventilator interaction is essential as isolated observation of P, V and $\dot{V}$ waveforms displayed by the ventilator leads to under recognition of asynchrony. In one series[58] ineffective triggering accounted for most of the asynchronous episodes with autocycling the next most common cause. Prevalence of asynchrony increased with PSV≥12 cmH_2O, large V_T and low respiratory rates in part reflecting dynamic hyperinflation and $PEEP_i$.

TRIGGERING OF INSPIRATION

1. $PEEP_i$ is an important hindrance to the triggering of inspiration in patients with severe air-flow limitation, since their inspiratory muscles must first reduce P_{ao} below ambient pressure.[59] Consequently P_{mus} must exceed $PEEP_i$ prior to triggering an assisted breath usually by either reducing airway pressure (pressure trigger) or reducing circuit flow (flow trigger). This inspiratory threshold load may be up to 40% of the total inspiratory work in acute respiratory failure when dynamic hyperinflation is present, and commonly results in ineffective triggering. Triggering can be markedly improved and respiratory work reduced by low levels of $PEEP_e$;[37,60] commonly 80–90% of dynamic $PEEP_i$[61] if this is measured.
2. Patient effort may be sensed, and the ventilator cycled (triggered) to inspiratory assistance, by changes in any of P_{ao}, flow, volume, shape-signal and detection of neural drive (NAVA). During pressure triggering a fall in P_{ao} is usually sensed at the expiratory block of the ventilator. Sensing at the Y-piece is not superior since there is a similar delay in sensing as the transducer is usually sited in the ventilator with a similar or greater length of gas tubing. Flow triggering senses a fall in continuous circuit flow, and was introduced as a method of reducing inspiratory work. However, there has been a marked improvement of both pressure and flow triggering in modern ventilators with the trigger time delay falling from ~400 ms to <60 ms in most modern ventilators,[62] and a similar improvement in the maximum fall in

airway pressure;[63] consequently ventilator triggering contributes about 5% of respiratory effort. Attempts to improve the trigger function by oversetting the pressure sensitivity (<–0.5 cmH_2O) may lead to autocycling, which may also occur with overset flow triggering. This is due to the *P* and $\dot{V}$ effects of cardiac oscillations, hiccups, circuit rainout or mask leak with NIV, and has been reported as a cause of apparent respiratory effort in brain-dead patients.[64] Flow triggering reduces the risk of autocycling at a given trigger sensitivity, and reduces respiratory effort a small amount compared with pressure triggering; however, it does not alter the frequency of ineffective efforts, or patient effort following triggering.[55] A combination of shape-signal and volume triggering is used on the Vision (Philips Respironics) ventilator; the increased sensitivity of shape-signal triggering reduces effort but increases autocycling.[55]

INSPIRATION

Once inspiration is triggered or sensed by the ventilator, $\dot{V}$ is determined by *P*, *Ti* or $\dot{V}$. For example during PSV ventilation a target *P* is held until expiration is sensed, and during ACV $\dot{V}$ is held for a set T_i. During ACV there may be continued inspiratory effort, and since inspiratory $\dot{V}$ is fixed, this will be reflected by a scalloping of the P_{ao}–*T* graph if $\dot{V}$ is inadequate. Again this may be illustrated using the equation of motion:

$$P_{mus} + P_{ao} = E_{rs} \bullet V + R_{rs} \bullet \dot{V} + P_o \qquad (31.9)$$

P_{mus} will reflect the difference between P_{ao} due to *E*, *R* and P_o and the observed P_{ao}. In contrast, during *P*-cycled ventilation (PACV) greater patient effort is rewarded and inspiratory work is lower than during equivalent ACV.[65]

Modern ventilators allow adjustment of inspiratory $\dot{V}$ and $\dot{V}$ pattern, and the rate of rise of P_{ao}. Low inspiratory $\dot{V}$ rates during ACV results in significant inspiratory work, but this may be markedly reduced by increasing inspiratory $\dot{V}$ to 65 L/min.[66] However, these issues are quite complex, and *f* increases (probably due to a lower respiratory tract reflex) as $\dot{V}_I$ increases,[67] reducing *Te*, which may contribute to dynamic hyperinflation in patients with severe air-flow obstruction. During PSV and PACV, many ventilators allow adjustment of the rate of rise of *P* to its target. Although an excessively steep *P* ramp leads to earlier attainment of the *P* target and greater early $\dot{V}$ rates, this is associated with increased dyspnoea and effort, as is too flat a *P* ramp.[55]

CESSATION OF INSPIRATION

During PSV, an increase in airway resistance will result in a longer expiratory time constant and a delayed fall in $\dot{V}_I$. Since this is the usual trigger for cycling to expiration, the ventilator may continue to provide $\dot{V}_I$ while the patient desires to exhale. This commonly leads to recruitment of expiratory muscles, detected both clinically and as a transient rise in the end-inspiratory P_{ao}.[68] Some modern ventilators allow control of the fall in $\dot{V}_I$ that is sensed as end inspiration; the default is usually a reduction of $\dot{V}_I$ to 25% of the peak $\dot{V}_I$ rate. When airway resistance is high a higher cycling threshold (e.g. 45%) can reduce T_i, V_T and $PEEP_i$ with reduced trigger effort. However, this may result in premature termination of inspiration in ARDS where the time constant is short. High levels of PSV (≥20 cmH_2O), weak respiratory muscles and mask leak with NIV are other common causes of asynchrony at the termination of inspiration. In this last group, PACV, which is time cycled, allows improved patient–ventilator synchrony at end-inspiration compared with PSV.[69]

High V_T, commonly associated with high levels of PSV often precedes wasted efforts due to shortened T_e and $PEEP_i$. As asynchrony is reduced with less PSV, the optimum level of PSV will occur when there is minimal increase in *f* and P_{mus}. This typically occurs at a PSV of 13 cmH_2O with V_T 6 ml/kg and T_i 0.8 seconds.[70]

Access the complete references list online at http://www.expertconsult.com

4. [No authors listed] Ventilation with lower tidal volumes as compared with traditional volumes for acute lung injury and the acute respiratory distress syndrome. The Acute Respiratory Distress Syndrome Network. N Engl J Med 2000;342:1301–8.
12. Briel M, Meade M, Mercat A, et al. Higher vs lower positive end-expiratory pressure in patients with acute lung injury and acute respiratory distress syndrome: systematic review and meta-analysis. JAMA 2010;303:865–73.
16. Grasso S, Stripoli T, De Michele M, et al. ARDSnet ventilatory protocol and alveolar hyperinflation:role of positive end-expiratory pressure. Am J Respir Crit Care Med 2007;176:761–17.
56. Thille AW, Harrois A, Schortgen F, et al. Outcomes of extubation failure in medical intensive care unit patients. Crit Care Med 2011;39:2612–18.
60. Petrof BJ, Legare M, Goldberg P, et al. Continuous positive airway pressure reduces work of breathing and dyspnea during weaning form mechanical ventilation in severe chronic obstructive pulmonary disease. Am Rev Respir Dis 1990;141:281–9.

32

Humidification and inhalation therapy

Steven T Galluccio and Andrew D Bersten

The upper airway normally warms, moistens and filters inspired gas. When these functions are impaired by disease, or when the nasopharynx is bypassed by endotracheal intubation, artificial humidification of inspired gases must be provided.

PHYSICAL PRINCIPLES

Humidity, the amount of water vapour in a gas, may be expressed as:

- *absolute humidity (AH):* the total mass of water vapour in a given volume of gas at a given temperature (g/m^3)
- *relative humidity (RH):* the actual mass of water vapour (per volume of gas) as a percentage of the mass of saturated water vapour, at a given temperature. Saturated water vapour exerts a saturated vapour pressure (SVP). As the SVP has an exponential relation with temperature (**Table 32.1**), addition of further water vapour to the gas can only occur with a rise in temperature
- *partial pressure.*

PHYSIOLOGY

Clearance of surface liquids and particles from the lung depends on beating cilia, airway mucus and transepithelial water flux. Airway mucus is derived from secretions from goblet cells, submucosal glands and Clara cells, and from capillary transudate. Conducting airways are lined with pseudostratified, ciliated columnar epithelium and numerous fluid-secreting glands. As the airway descends, the epithelium becomes stratified, and then cuboidal and partially ciliated, with very few secretory glands at the terminal airways. The cilia beat in a watery (sol) layer over which is a viscous mucous layer (gel), and move a superficial layer of mucus from deep within the lung toward the glottis (at a rate of 10 mm/min at 37°C and 100% RH). Both cilia function and mucus composition are influenced by temperature and adequate humidification.

The nasal mucosa has a large surface area with an extensive vascular network that humidifies and warms inhaled gas more effectively than during mouth breathing. Heating and humidification of dry gas are progressive down the airway, with an isothermic saturation boundary (i.e. 100% RH at 37°C or AH of 43 g/m^3) just below the carina.[1] Under resting conditions, approximately 250 mL of water and 1.5 kJ (350 kcal) of energy are lost from the respiratory tract in a day. A proportion (10–25%) is returned to the mucosa during expiration due to condensation.

The minimal moisture level to maintain ciliary function and mucus clearance is uncertain. Although reproducing an isothermic saturation boundary at the carina may be ideal, it does not seem essential in all situations. Mucus flow is markedly reduced when RH at 37°C falls below 75% (AH of 32 g/m^3), and ceases when RH is 50% (AH of 22 g/m^3).[2] This suggests that an AH exceeding 33 g/m^3 is needed to maintain normal function. Mucociliary function is also impaired by upper respiratory tract infection, chronic bronchitis, cystic fibrosis, bronchiectasis, immotile cilia syndrome, dehydration, hyperventilation, general anaesthetics, opioids, atropine and exposure to noxious gases. High fractional inspired oxygen concentrations (Fi_{O_2}) may lead to acute tracheobronchitis, with depressed tracheal mucus velocity within 3 hours.[3] Inhaled β_2-adrenergic agonists increase mucociliary clearance by augmenting ciliary beat frequency, and mucus and water secretion.[4]

CLINICAL APPLICATIONS OF HUMIDIFICATION

TRACHEAL INTUBATION

The need for humidification during endotracheal intubation and tracheostomy is unquestioned. As the upper airway is bypassed, RH of inspired gas falls below 50% with adverse effects, including:[5]

- increased mucus viscosity
- depressed ciliary function
- cytological damage to the tracheobronchial epithelium, including mucosal ulceration, tracheal inflammation and necrotising tracheobronchitis[6]
- microatelectasis from obstruction of small airways, and reduced surfactant leading to reduced lung compliance
- airway obstruction due to tenacious or inspissated sputum with increased airway resistance.

Metaplasia of the tracheal epithelium occurs over weeks to months in patients with a permanent tracheostomy.

Table 32.1 Relationship of temperature and saturated vapour pressure

TEMPERATURE (°C)	SATURATED VAPOUR PRESSURE (mmHg)	(kPa)	ABSOLUTE HUMIDITY (g/m³)
0	4.6	0.6	4.8
10	9.2	1.2	9.3
20	17.5	2.3	17.1
30	31.3	4.2	30.4
34	39.9	5.3	37.5
37	47.1	6.3	43.4
40	55.3	7.4	51.7
46	78.0	10.4	68.7

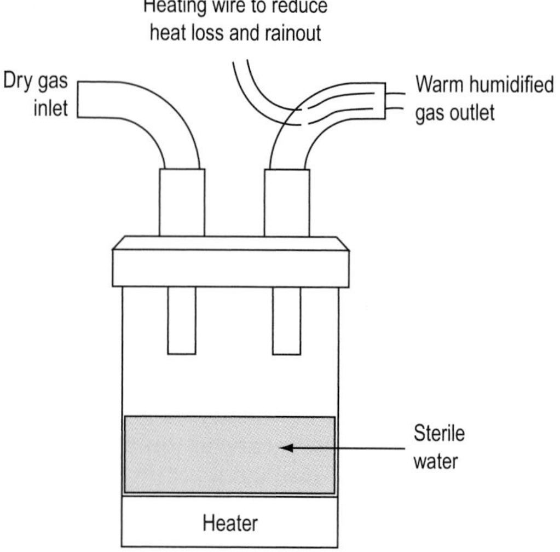

Figure 32.1 Hot-water 'blow-by' humidifier.

These patients do not usually require humidified gas, suggesting that humidification occurs lower down the respiratory tree. Nevertheless, humidification of inspired gas may be needed during an acute respiratory tract infection.

HEAT EXCHANGE

The respiratory tract is an important avenue to adjust body temperature by heat exchange. Humidification of gases reduces the fall in body temperature associated with anaesthesia and surgery.[5] Excessive heat from humidification may produce mucosal damage, hyperthermia and overhumidification.[7] However, if water content is not excessive, mucociliary clearance is unaffected up to temperatures of 42°C. Overhumidification may increase secretions and impair mucociliary clearance and surfactant activity, resulting in atelectasis.[6]

IDEAL HUMIDIFICATION

The basic requirements of a humidifier should include the following features:[8]

- the inspired gas is delivered into the trachea at 32–36°C with a water content of 30–43 g/m³
- the set temperature remains constant and does not fluctuate
- humidification and temperature remain unaffected by a large range of fresh gas flows, especially high flows
- the device is simple to use and to service
- humidification can be provided for air, oxygen or any mixture of inspired gas, including anaesthetic agents
- the humidifier can be used with spontaneous or controlled ventilation
- there are safety mechanisms, with alarms, against overheating, overhydration and electrocution
- the resistance, compliance and dead-space characteristics do not adversely affect spontaneous breathing modes
- the sterility of the inspired gas is not compromised.

METHODS AND DEVICES

WATER-BATH HUMIDIFIERS

Inspired gas is passed over or through a water reservoir to achieve humidification. Their efficiency is dependent on ambient temperature and the surface area available for gas vaporisation.

Cold-water humidifiers

These units are simple and inexpensive, but are inefficient, with a water content of around 9 g/m³ (i.e. about 50% RH at ambient temperatures). They are also a potential source of microbiological contamination. Routine use of cold-water humidifiers to deliver oxygen with simple facemasks is both unnecessary and at risk of suggesting the gas is adequately humidified.

Hot-water humidifiers (Figs 32.1 and 32.2)

Inspired gas is passed over (blow-by humidifier) or through (bubble or cascade humidifier) a heated-water reservoir. Gas leaving the reservoir theoretically contains high water content. The water bath temperature is thermostatically controlled (e.g. at 45–60°C) to compensate for cooling along the inspiratory tubing targeting an inspired RH of 100% at 37°C. A heated wire may be sited in the inspiratory tubing to maintain preset gas temperature and humidity. It is commonly believed that hot-water humidifiers do not produce aerosols, but microdroplets (mostly less than 5 μm diameter) have

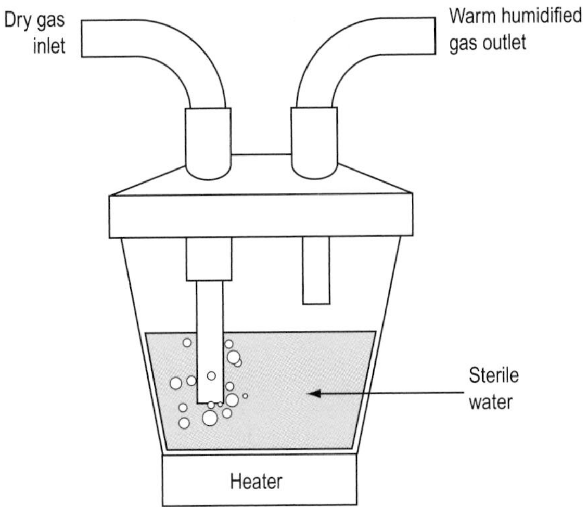

Figure 32.2 Hot-water 'cascade' or 'bubble' humidifier.

been reported with bubble humidifiers,[9] and this may be a potential source of infection.

Fisher–Paykel humidifier This is a commonly used blow-by humidifier. The delivery hose is heated by an insulated heating wire to achieve a manual preset inspired temperature. Audible alarms indicate disconnection and variations over 2°C from the set delivery temperature. The heater base is protected from overheating by a thermostat set at 47°C. If this fails, another safety thermostat operates at 70°C. A disposable humidification chamber is filled manually with water or by a gravity-feed set. To minimise rainout, the chamber outlet can be set at a temperature below the delivery hose outlet temperature; 2–3°C is usually adequate and does not compromise RH. Temperature alarms are fixed at 41°C and 29.5°C, with a back-up safety set at 66°C for the delivery chamber.

Although these humidifiers are often regarded as providing optimal humidification in ventilated patients, their performance is lower than expected both in practice and under optimal conditions in bench studies.[10] Under conditions of high ambient and/or high ventilator output temperature, the inlet temperature to the humidification chamber can be high enough that the heater base operates at a low enough temperature that humidification is impaired, with reduction in inspired water content.[10] The automatic compensation now available on this humidifier helps compensate for poor performance, which can also be prevented by setting the chamber outlet and hose to 40°C. High minute ventilation is well tolerated, but a small decrease in water content output has also been found with higher respiratory rates.[11]

HEAT AND MOISTURE EXCHANGERS

HMEs are popular intensive care unit (ICU) humidifiers due to their simplicity and increased efficiency. Modern HMEs are light with a small dead space (30–95 mL), but show great heterogeneity in humidity output, often not matching manufacturer-claimed performance.[12]

Hygroscopic HMEs adsorb moisture on to a foam or paper-like material that is chemically coated (often calcium chloride or lithium chloride), and this tends to increase their efficiency (i.e. AH around 30 g/m^3) compared with hydrophobic HMEs (i.e. AH 20–25 g/m^3).[13–18] Such hydrophobic HMEs possess antimicrobial properties and may act as a microbial filter (HMEF). These filters can have efficiencies greater than 99.9 977%,[19] i.e. less than 23 out of 1 million bacteria will pass through (filters that can exclude all virus particles are not currently available). Modern HMEs include both hydroscopic and hydrophobic properties. However, since nosocomial pneumonia is primarily due to aspiration of oropharyngeal secretions followed by secondary ventilator tubing colonisation, HMEs have not been shown to reduce the frequency of nosocomial pneumonia more than hot-water humidifiers when compared during prolonged ventilation.[19–21]

The efficiency of older HMEs decreases with time;[11] however, modern HMEs may retain their ability to humidify for prolonged periods with minimal change in resistance (a measure of tube patency and thus adequacy of humidification).[22,23] In patients undergoing invasive ventilation for a mean duration greater than 1 week there was no difference in endotracheal tube resistance between HME and active humidification.[23] However, allocation of humidification device was not randomised but based on perceived clinical need. Consequently, HMEs that achieve relatively high AH may be suitable for long-term mechanical ventilation in selected patients, particularly as the majority of reported HME complications (e.g. thick secretions and endotracheal tube occlusion) occur with units of lower humidification levels.[24–26] Nevertheless, HMEs increase dead space and imposed work of breathing, and cannot match the humidification offered by hot-water humidifiers, which remain the 'gold standard', particularly if secretions are thick or bloody, minute ventilation is high,[16,19,27] or in children and neonates.

COMPLICATIONS OF HUMIDIFICATION

INADEQUATE HUMIDIFICATION

An AH exceeding 30 g/m^3 is recommended in respiratory care.[27] Inadequate humidification is usually a problem only with HMEs. With hot-water humidifiers, however, efficiency is reduced by increasing gas flow rates and rainout. A decrease of about 1°C occurs for each 10 cm of tubing beyond the end of the delivery hose (i.e. the Y-connector and right-angled connector), and should be catered for. Inadequate humidification in high-frequency ventilation can be overcome by using superheated humidification of the entrained gas with a temperature thermistor built into the endotracheal tube.[24,28]

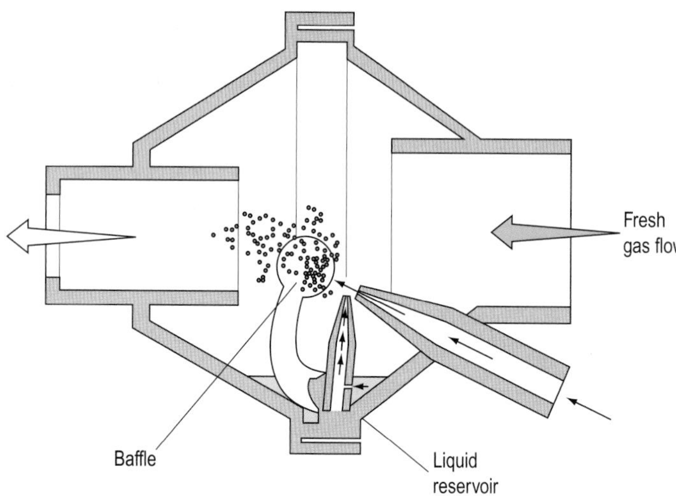

Figure 32.3 Sidestream nebuliser.

OVERHUMIDIFICATION

Overheating malfunction of hot-water humidifiers may cause a rise in core temperature, water intoxication, impaired mucociliary clearance and airway burns.[7]

IMPOSED WORK OF BREATHING

The work of breathing imposed by a humidifier is primarily resistive work and increases with inspiratory flow rate; the progressive increase in water content of HMEs is also associated with increased resistance.[29] The Fisher–Paykel humidifier imposes relatively low work compared with a bubble humidifier,[30] and HMEs typically have a resistance of 2.5 cmH_2O/L per second.[16]

INFECTION

Humidifiers do not appear to be an important factor in nosocomial respiratory tract infection. Although water reservoirs represent a good culture medium for bacteria such as *Pseudomonas* species, it is rare to culture bacteria from humidifiers, and is usually preceded by colonisation of the circuit by the patient's own flora within the first 24 hours of use.[31,32] Indeed, the incidence of nosocomial pneumonia is reported to be higher (due to outside contamination) if the circuit is changed too frequently (every 24 or 48 h).[32,33]

HUMIDIFICATION DURING NON-INVASIVE VENTILATION (NIV)

The hygrometric effects of NIV depend upon several factors, including type of ventilator (conventional versus turbine), V_T, peak inspiratory flow rates, Fi_{O_2} and degree of mask leak.[34,35] NIV applied without artificial humidification has been associated with accumulation of dried secretions in the oropharynx with subsequent aspiration, difficult intubation or frank airway obstruction.[36] In healthy volunteers, a delivered AH of at least 15 mgH_2O/L was necessary to ensure comfort during NIV.[37] This level is achievable with either passive or active humidification, but a higher humidity output may be required for patients with respiratory failure. Although there is a lack of robust data, current guidelines advocate the use of heated humidification over HMEs.[27]

HUMIDIFICATION FOR OXYGEN THERAPY DURING SPONTANEOUS BREATHING

Despite the ubiquity of oxygen therapy, there is no evidence to guide the addition of humidification for spontaneously breathing patients. There is no particular oxygen flow rate or duration of exposure that mandates artificial humidification. However, patient discomfort during high-flow oxygen therapy is improved with the use of heated humidification compared with bubble humidifiers or no artificial humidification at all.[38,39] It is unknown to what extent patient discomfort signals inadequate humidification and the potential for complications such as deranged mucociliary transport or increased airway resistance.

INHALATION THERAPY

Therapeutic aerosols are particles suspended in gas that are inhaled and deposited within the respiratory tract. Numerous factors, including particle size, inertia and physical nature, gravity, volume and pattern of ventilation, temperature and humidity, airway geometry, lung disease and the delivery system, alter aerosol deposition. In general, particles of diameter 40 μm deposit in the upper airway, those of 8–15 μm deposit in bronchi and bronchioles, those of 3–5 μm deposit in peripheral conducting airways and those of 0.8–3.0 μm settle in lung parenchyma. Optimal particle size will depend on the clinical indication and agent used. Obviously, if an HME with filtration characteristics is being used, the aerosol needs to be delivered proximal to the filter.

AEROSOL DELIVERY

Therapeutic aerosols may be delivered by nebuliser (jet, ultrasonic or vibrating mesh), metered-dose inhaler (MDI) or dry-particle inhaler (DPI). Although each of these methods tends to be less efficient in ventilated patients, provided that care is taken to optimise their performance, each can provide equivalent clinical effect.

NEBULISERS[40]

The most common jet nebulisers are sidestream nebulisers. These use an extrinsic gas flow through a narrow orifice, to create a pressure gradient that draws the drug mixture from a liquid reservoir (i.e. Bernoulli's principle; **Fig. 32.3**). The gas is then directed at a baffle to reduce the mean particle size. This extrinsic gas flow (usually 3–10 L/min) adds to the inspiratory flow, and may increase patient tidal volume unless the ventilator automatically compensates, or the preset tidal volume is adjusted. Further, this additional gas flow may impair ventilator triggering since it may prevent the development of a negative pressure or necessary reduction in continuous flow needed. Mainstream nebulisers employ inspiratory gas flow to actuate nebulisation. These are commonly large-volume water nebulisers that entrain air to achieve fresh gas flow rates of 20–30 L/min.

Ultrasonic nebulisers use high-frequency sound waves (typically 1 MHz) to create an aerosol above a liquid reservoir, to produce small uniform droplets (<5 μm) and a high mist density (i.e. 100–200 g/m^3). Tidal volume is not altered; however, ultrasonic nebulisers may cause overhydration and increased airway resistance. Further drawbacks in the critical care setting include: size, poor battery life, and the potential for drug inactivation by ultrasonic waves and heating.[40,41]

More recent nebuliser designs have utilised a vibrating mesh or plate. Medication in solution or suspension is forced through multiple apertures in the mesh or plate to produce an aerosol. A variety of vibrating mesh nebulisers are commercially available; common features include aerosol generation with high fine-particle fraction and overall higher drug output with minimal residual volume compared with jet nebulisers; additional benefits over ultrasonic types are the lack of heating effect or potential for drug degradation.[40]

Nebuliser aerosol deposition is highly variable, with significant rainout in the ventilatory circuit, endotracheal tube and large conducting airways. In a bench study delivery ranged from 6% of nebuliser charge to 37% depending upon humidification and breath activation; parallel in vivo data were similar but found a 20-fold difference in drug delivery.[42] Numerous factors have been shown to improve aerosol deposition, but only some of these are commonly practised. For example, although heating and humidification reduce aerosol deposition ≈50% due to increase in both droplet size and rainout, regular circuit disconnection and exclusion of humidification prior to nebulisation are not practical. However, placement of the nebuliser in the inspiratory limb of the circuit less than 30 cm from the endotracheal tube allows this tubing to act as a spacer or aerosol-holding chamber. This reduces aerosol velocity and losses due to impaction. Inspiratory activation of the nebuliser increases deposition by two- and threefold under dry and humidified conditions respectively;[41] use of a large chamber fill, tidal volume of 500 mL or more and minimisation of turbulent inspiratory flow (low flow rate, prolonged inspiratory time) also augment aerosol delivery.[39]

METERED-DOSE INHALERS

MDIs contain drug in ethanolic solution with a hydrofluoroalkane (HFA) propellant, allowing a relatively fixed volume (i.e. dose) to be delivered with each actuation (e.g. 100 μg for salbutamol and 20 μg for ipratropium).[40,43] Aerosol delivery is approximately 4–6% in ventilated adults, but increases to 11% when a spacer chamber is used, which is similar to optimal no-spacer values reported in the ambulant population.[44] Similar to nebulisers, absence of humidification, inspiratory limb position, inspiratory activation and minimisation of turbulence by lowering inspiratory flow rate and prolonging inspiratory time will increase aerosol delivery. It is important to avoid use of an elbow adapter, because this has been associated with dramatic reductions in aerosol delivery and efficacy.

DRY-POWDERED INHALERS

DPIs are commonly used in ambulant practice. Their use is not recommended in patients undergoing mechanical ventilation since they are breath actuated (requiring inspiratory flow rates close to 60 L/min) and, moreover, circuit humidification can cause powder clumping with impeded aerosol formation.[45]

CLINICAL APPLICATIONS OF INHALATION THERAPY

HUMIDIFICATION

Humidifiers produce gas with a water content dictated by temperature and water vapour pressure, whereas nebulisers produce gas with a water content determined by the aerosol content. The latter can provide water to the respiratory tract, particularly if the water reservoir is heated to increase mist density. However, the risk of infection is increased, as droplets can carry bacteria to the alveoli. Consequently, only sterile water should be used to fill the reservoir, and all units should be regularly changed and sterilised.

MUCOLYTICS

The role of mucolytics to reduce viscosity of secretions in critically ill patients is unknown. Oral mucolytics such as acetylcysteine reduce exacerbations of chronic bronchitis and chronic obstructive pulmonary disease (COPD), although this appears to be isolated to subjects not receiving inhaled steroids.[46] It is uncertain if this interaction applies to newer thiol derivatives (such as erdosteine[47] and carbocisteine[48]), which are also associated with reduced COPD exacerbations. Case reports of recombinant human DNase appear promising when standard regimens fail to clear thick secretions[44] but the main evidence base for DNase utility is in bronchiectasis specifically due to cystic fibrosis.[49]

BRONCHODILATOR THERAPY

Optimal aerosol delivery and bronchodilator response are extremely important in critically ill patients with severe air-flow limitation, and this can be achieved using either a nebuliser or MDI technique provided that care is taken to optimise performance. Efficacy of MDI administration is optimised by use of a spacer with actuation synchronised with the onset of inspiration.[40] The response can be judged clinically, and in ventilated patients monitored by changes in peak-to-plateau airway pressure gradient, calculated airways resistance and intrinsic PEEP. Numerous studies show effective bronchodilatation with β_2-agonists and anticholinergic agents such as ipratropium in ventilated patients, and their combination is more effective than a single agent alone.[44]

Bronchodilator dosing

Standard doses of salbutamol for acute asthma are 2.5–5 mg administered by a nebuliser or 4–6 puffs of an MDI (400–600 μg), but the bronchodilator response can be shorter lasting than in ambulatory subjects. Consequently, dosing should be 3–4-hourly. Ipatropium is usually administered as 0.5 mg by a nebuliser or four puffs (80 μg) of an MDI. Higher or more frequent drug dosing is often effective when there is severe, reversible air-flow obstruction, and continuous nebulisation of a β_2-agonist may be used in acute severe asthma until there has been a clinical response. If the patient is moribund with minimal ventilation or is unable to tolerate nebulisation, parenteral administration should be considered; however, under most circumstances there is no particular benefit with this route.[50]

NON-INVASIVE VENTILATION (NIV)

Optimal bronchodilator therapy for patients requiring NIV, particularly for acute exacerbations of COPD, is unknown. It is preferable not to interrupt NIV for this purpose and both nebulisers and MDIs appear effective during NIV.[44] Despite the potential for increased loss of nebulised drug in a high-gas-flow continuous positive-airways pressure circuit, good bronchodilator response with salbutamol has been reported in this setting.[51]

INHALED CORTICOSTEROIDS

Inhaled corticosteroids are recommended in persistent asthma[52] and severe chronic obstructive pulmonary disease with frequent exacerbations.[53] However, in acute episodes of these conditions, inhalational delivery does not preclude the need for systemic corticosteroid therapy.[54] Small-particle inhaled corticosteroids offer the theoretical benefit of improved total and peripheral lung distribution.[55] For example, ciclesonide has a mass median aerodynamic diameter (MMAD or particle size) of 1.1 μm versus a MMAD of 3.5 μm with CFC-propelled beclometasone.[55] Improvement in clinical end-points with these new formulations, particularly in mechanically ventilated patients, remains to be demonstrated.

DELIVERY OF ANTIBIOTICS AND ANTIVIRAL AGENTS

Aerosolised antibiotics have been contentious for many years; however, the potential to achieve high concentrations of antibiotics at the site of infection while minimising adverse effects remains appealing. In animal models of bronchopneumonia inhaled amikacin[56] and ceftazidime[57] achieved 3–30 times increases in lung tissue concentrations and better sterilisation of lung compared with intravenous administration. In humans, gentamicin by conventional intravenous dosing has been shown to reach only subinhibitory concentrations in the alveolar lining fluid.[58]

Numerous studies in patients with cystic fibrosis have shown a reduction in sputum volume and density of bacteria, and improved lung function with reduced risk of hospitalisation when inhaled aminoglycosides are used.[59,60] Similar results, including a reduction of markers of airway inflammation, have been reported with bronchiectasis,[61,62] and in mechanically ventilated patients with chronic respiratory failure.[63]

Three recent randomised controlled trials of adjunctive aerosolised antibiotics in ventilator-associated tracheobronchitis (VAT) and/or VAP have shown positive outcomes with reduction in the Clinical Pulmonary Infection Score, facilitation of weaning, or reduction in systemic antibiotic use.[64–66] Treatment protocols included amikacin 400 mg daily,[64] gentamicin 80 mg 8-hourly,[65] and vancomycin 120 mg 8-hourly.[66] The presumption of emerging bacterial resistance with increased aerosolised antibiotic use, akin to the known risk with systemic delivery, is not confirmed by the available data.[67] Paradoxically, emergence of resistance may be reduced via higher pathogen eradication rates, earlier intervention in treating VAT and reduced exposure to systemic therapy.[68]

Other antimicrobials that have been safely nebulised include colistin (polymyxin), aztreonam, amphotericin B and pentamidine. However, inhaled amphotericin may result in bronchospasm. Aerosolised ribavirin has limited evidence of benefit for respiratory syncytial virus infection.[69,70] Ribavirin deposition in the circuit may cause valve malfunction, and concerns of teratogenicity in health care personnel have dictated its use with care.[70]

SPUTUM INDUCTION

Nebulised 3% saline is effective in sputum induction for diagnosing *P. jirovecii* pneumonia in patients with the acquired immunodeficiency syndrome (AIDS). The need for bronchoscopy can be obviated[71] with specificity of sputum induction approaching 100% and sensitivity of at least 55%.[72]

Sputum induction has been used to diagnose a number of other infections, and appears to be safe in patients with severe air-flow limitation.[73]

SURFACTANT THERAPY

Surfactant preparations have been delivered by instillation and as an aerosol in neonates with respiratory distress syndrome, and in adults with ARDS. Aerosolised surfactant could theoretically achieve more uniform distribution and avoid problems of instilling liquid into injured lungs. However, large amounts are needed for lung deposition, and preferential distribution occurs to less-damaged lung areas that receive better ventilation.[74] Clinical studies of exogenous surfactant in adult ARDS have not shown any mortality benefit, although novel preparations are currently being tested.[75]

INHALED NITRIC OXIDE

The therapeutic potential of inhaled nitric oxide (iNO) lies as a selective pulmonary vasodilator with minimal systemic side effects. iNO improves outcomes in newborns with persistent pulmonary hypertension.[76] In adult patients with ARDS, iNO results in an improvement in oxygenation in about 60–80% of patients with a 10% reduction in pulmonary arterial pressure.[77] However, these physiological benefits have not translated into effects on mortality or duration of mechanical ventilation.[78]

PROSTANOIDS[44]

Inhaled prostanoids target selective pulmonary vasodilatation to well-aerated areas, leading to similar improvements in oxygenation as iNO in patients with the acute respiratory distress syndrome. When delivered systemically these agents lead to impaired oxygenation and to hypotension due to non-selective pulmonary and systemic vasodilatation respectively. Iloprost (a synthetic epoprostenol/prostacyclin analogue) has a longer half-life (about 20–30 minutes compared with 3 minutes for prostacyclin), and is sometimes used for chronic pulmonary hypertension (2.5–5 mg 6–9 times per day), and similar doses can be used in mechanically ventilated patients. Treprostinil has a longer half-life still, allowing four times daily dosing.[79]

INHALED HELIUM MIXTURES

Helium is 7.2 and 8 times less dense than air and oxygen respectively. This property is useful in the setting of increased airways resistance as less turbulent and more efficient laminar flow is encouraged. Therefore, albeit an inert gas without any direct anatomical effect, helium can improve dynamic respiratory mechanics and reduce work of breathing. Effect size relates to the relative helium concentration, in practice at least 60–70% helium is required, limiting applicability to patients able to tolerate Fi_{O_2} of 30–40%. Helium–oxygen mixtures (heliox) potentially have a role in managing obstructive disease of both the upper and lower airways.[77] However, clinical use of heliox remains controversial and without evidence-based guidelines. In patients with COPD exacerbations, an open-label, randomised trial of 65% helium in oxygen versus Fi_{O_2} of 0.35 during NIV failed to demonstrate any significant improvement in duration of NIV or need to progress to intubation.[80] A larger multicentre study is currently under way.[81]

It should be noted that heliox as the driving gas in a ventilator circuit will influence the delivery of other inhaled agents. For example, aerosolised drug output from a MDI is increased, whereas output from a nebuliser is decreased.[77] As a further consideration, heliox may improve particle distribution to the peripheral small airways, perhaps as a function of reduced turbulence.[82]

Access the complete references list online at http://www.expertconsult.com

12. Lellouche F, Taillé S, Lefrançois F, et al. Humidification performance of 48 passive airway humidifiers: comparison with manufacturer data. Chest 2009;135:276–86.
20. Gillies KM, Todd DA, Lockwood C. Heated humidification versus heat and moisture exchangers for ventilated adults and children. Cochrane Database Syst Rev 2010;14:CD004711.
27. Restrepo RD, Walsh BK. Humidification during invasive and noninvasive mechanical ventilation: 2012. Resp Care 2012;57:782–8.
40. Dhand R, Guntur VP. How best to deliver aerosol medications to mechanically ventilated patients. Clin Chest Med 2008;29:277–96.
68. Palmer LB. Aerosolized antibiotics in the intensive care unit. Clin Chest Med 2011;32:559–74.
77. Gentile MA. Inhaled medical gases: more to breathe than oxygen. Resp Care 2011;56:1341–57.

33

Acute respiratory distress syndrome

Andrew D Bersten

The acute respiratory distress syndrome (ARDS) was first described in 1967 by Ashbaugh and colleagues as the 'acute onset of tachypnea, hypoxemia and loss of compliance after a variety of stimuli'.[1] Continued research examining the underlying mechanisms and management strategies is now translating into improved outcome.

DEFINITIONS

The ARDS Definition Task Force (the Berlin definition[2]) has recently revised the long-standing 1994 American–European Consensus Conference (AECC) definition[3] (**Table 33.1**). ARDS still refers to acute hypoxaemic respiratory failure due to bilateral and diffuse alveolar damage, and is now classified as mild, moderate and severe based on the Pa_{O_2}/Fi_{O_2} ratio (Table 33.1). The broad term 'acute lung injury' (ALI), which referred to cases with a Pa_{O_2}/Fi_{O_2} ratio <300, has been replaced and many concerns addressed. A minimum positive end-expiratory pressure (PEEP) of 5 cmH_2O is specified, and chest radiograph criteria and exclusion of hydrostatic oedema clarified, including examples. The lung injury score (LIS),[4] which uses a four-point score attributed to ranges of Pa_{O_2}/Fi_{O_2} ratio, PEEP, respiratory system compliance and the number of quadrants involved on chest radiograph has also been used to quantify severity of ARDS; however, as neither lung compliance nor dead space improved the predictive ability of the Berlin definition, the LIS may become less pertinent.

CHEST RADIOGRAPH AND CHEST CT IN ARDS

The intent of chest imaging is to exclude opacities due to pleural effusion, nodules, masses, collapse and pleural thickening, and that the infiltrate must be bilateral and consistent with pulmonary oedema.[2] Autopsy and chest radiographs of ARDS show a uniform process affecting both lungs. However, chest CT[5] has demonstrated marked heterogeneity of lung inflation in ARDS with a dorsal, dependent increase in lung density, and relatively normal inflation of ventral lung. In addition, CT frequently reveals previously undiagnosed pneumothorax, pneumomediastinum and pleural effusion. After the second week of mechanical ventilation CT scans may demonstrate altered lung architecture and emphysematous cysts or pneumatoceles.

CT numbers or Hounsfield units can be assigned to each voxel (~2000 alveoli in a standard 10-mm slice).[5] These data can then be used to assess what proportion of a region of interest is non-aerated, poorly aerated, normally aerated, or hyperinflated. Whole-lung CT allows (a) reconstruction of the upper and lower lobes (the middle lobe is difficult to separate), (b) the same section of lung to be studied at different levels of inflation or PEEP (the lung also moves in a cepahalo-caudad direction with respiration), and (c) a broader picture of the lung to be obtained (lung damage is heterogeneous in ARDS). However, whole-lung CT demands considerable exposure to ionising radiation, and different information, perhaps more pertinent to mechanical ventilation is obtained from dynamic CT.

Clinical assessment of chest CT is discussed in Chapter 39, and CT findings in ARDS are discussed below under Clinical management.

EPIDEMIOLOGY

Estimates of the incidence and outcome from ARDS vary widely due to differences in the definitions used, case-mix and local factors. Using the AECC definition the Australian incidence was 34 per 100 000 for ALI and 28 per 100 000 for ARDS;[6] recent US estimates were 79 and 59 per 100 000 respectively[7] – both much greater than many previous estimates. The Australian data equate to 1 in 10 non-cardiothoracic ICU patients developing ARDS, which reflects the tendency for clinicians to underestimate its incidence. However, the incidence of ARDS appears to be decreasing likely due to improvements in health care such as use of protective ventilation strategies, reduced transfusion-associated ALI (TRALI) and better management of sepsis.[8]

For many years the mortality for ARDS was reported to be ~60%; the Australian multicentre data reported mortality rates of 32% for ALI, and 34% for ARDS,[6] with US mortality rates a little higher at 38.5% and 41%.[7] Particular diagnostic groups such as multiple trauma have a lower mortality rate than other causes of ARDS, and patients with ARDS who have chronic liver disease, non-pulmonary organ dysfunction, sepsis or age greater than 70 years (hazard ratio 2.5)[9] have a higher risk of

Table 33.1 Criteria and classification of ARDS

	AECC DEFINITION#	BERLIN DEFINITION*
Onset	Acute (not defined) onset No risk factor formally defined	Within 7 days of a known risk factor (See Box 33.1)
Chest imaging	Bilateral opacities on chest radiograph	Bilateral opacities consistent with pulmonary oedema on either chest radiograph or CT
Pulmonary oedema	PAOP≤18 mmHg when measured or no clinical evidence of raised left atrial pressure	Non-hydrostatic oedema; not fully explained by heart failure or fluid overload Echocardiography or another objective measure may be required
Classification	ALI $Pa_{O_2}/Fi_{O_2} \leq 300$ ARDS $Pa_{O_2}/Fi_{O_2} \leq 200$	Mild $200 < Pa_{O_2}/Fi_{O_2} \leq 300$ Moderate $100 < Pa_{O_2}/Fi_{O_2} \leq 200$ Severe $Pa_{O_2}/Fi_{O_2} \leq 100$

#No minimum ventilatory setting defined for Pa_{O_2}/Fi_{O_2} data
*Based on oxygenation measured on a minimum of 5 cmH_2O PEEP. For the mild classification only, oxygenation can also be assessed during non-invasive ventilation. For the moderate and severe classification the patient must be receiving intubated ventilatory assistance.

death. Clinical trial outcomes report low mortality rates in the control arm in part due to the exclusion of patients with limited life expectancy; consequently many factors need to be considered when assessing outcome prediction.

PULMONARY FUNCTION IN SURVIVORS

Respiratory function continues to improve after discontinuation of mechanical ventilation, and usually returns towards normal by 6–12 months.[10,11] Although a variety of abnormal pulmonary function tests may be found, impaired diffusing capacity is the most common. This is rarely symptomatic, but occasional patients have severe restrictive disease, and this is correlated with their cumulative LIS.[11]

QUALITY OF LIFE IN SURVIVORS

Compared with disease-matched ICU patients who do not develop ARDS, patients with ARDS have a more severe reduction in both pulmonary and general health-related quality of life.[12] Many patients have reduction in exercise tolerance that may be attributable to associated critical illness neuropathy and myopathy; nerve entrapment syndromes, contractures, postural hypotension, and heterotopic calcification may play a role in a minority.[10] When followed for 5 years in a young and severe cohort (median age 45 years) with relatively few prior comorbidities, there was persistent functional impairment with little improvement after 12 months.[13] Depression, anxiety and post-traumatic stress disorder are also common (20–50% of survivors). Finally, most survivors have cognitive impairments such as slowed mental processing, or impaired memory or concentration, and these correlate with the duration of ventilation, hyperglycaemia and variability in blood glucose, and the period and severity of desaturation <90%.[14,15]

Box 33.1 Clinical risk factors for ARDS

Direct	Indirect
Pneumonia	Non-pulmonary sepsis
Aspiration of gastric contents	Multiple trauma
Lung contusion	Massive transfusion
Fat embolism	Pancreatitis
Near drowning	Cardiopulmonary bypass
Inhalational injury	
Reperfusion injury	

In an analysis of survivors of the ARDS Network Fluid and Catheter Trial (FACTT),[16] Mikkelsen and co-workers[17] found that over half the subjects suffered from cognitive dysfunction and from psychological disability, and that these parameters were associated with lower Pa_{O_2}, enrolment in the restrictive fluid arm, and hypoglycaemia. Taken together these data caution against permissive hypoxaemia as a strategy to reduce ventilator-induced lung injury (VILI), and suggest that quality of survival is an important additional outcome for clinical trials.

PATIENTS AT RISK FOR ARDS

About one-third of critically ill patients exposed to either a direct or indirect risk factor (**Box 33.1**) develop ARDS, most within 6–48 hours. Multiple risk factors such as low pH, chronic alcohol abuse or chronic lung disease substantially increase the incidence of ARDS in at-risk patients. Diabetes reduces the risk of developing ARDS.[18]

PATHOGENESIS

Although it is well accepted that diffuse alveolar damage with: (a) pulmonary oedema due to damage of the alveolocapillary barrier, (b) a complex inflammatory infiltrate and (c) surfactant dysfunction,[19] are essential components of ARDS, the sequence of events is uncertain and probably depends upon the precipitating insult and host response. For example in endotoxin-induced lung injury, hypoxaemia and reduced lung compliance occur well before recruitment of neutrophils or an increase in lung weight due to an increase in permeability.[20] In addition, typical of early ARDS, surfactant turnover is dramatically increased prior to these changes. Furthermore, epithelial lining fluid sampled immediately following intubation in patients with ARDS has markedly increased concentrations of type III procollagen peptide,[21] suggestive of fibrosing alveolitis extremely early in the course of lung damage.

THE ALVEOLOCAPILLARY BARRIER

The normal lung consists of 300 million alveoli with alveolar gas separated from the pulmonary microcirculation by the extremely thin alveolocapillary barrier (0.1–0.2 μm thick). Since the endothelial pore size is 6.5–7.5 nm, and the epithelial pore size is almost one-tenth that at 0.5–0.9 nm, the epithelium is the major barrier to protein flux.[22] The surface area of the alveoli is estimated to be 50–100 m^2, which is made up predominantly of alveolar type I cells, with the metabolically active type II cells accounting for ~10% of the surface area. In turn, these cells are covered by the epithelial lining fluid with an estimated volume of 20 mL, ~10% of which is surfactant, the rest being filtered plasma water and low-molecular-weight proteins and a small number of cells, mainly alveolar macrophages and lymphocytes.

In ARDS the alveolocapillary barrier is damaged with bidirectional leakage of fluid and protein into the alveolus and leakage of surfactant proteins and alveolar cytokines into the plasma. Total protein content in bronchoalveolar lavage (BAL) fluid is 20–100 times that found in both healthy subjects and ventilated subjects without cardiorespiratory disease.[23,24] There is also disruption of the epithelial barrier, surfactant dysfunction and proliferation of alveolar type II cells as the progenitor of type I cells. Indirect causes of ARDS cause pulmonary endothelial injury, followed by recruitment of inflammatory cells and then epithelial damage, whereas direct causes of ARDS cause epithelial injury and secondary recruitment of inflammatory cells. The outcome of these processes must reflect a balance between repair and fibrosing alveolitis.

CELL TYPES INVOLVED

The large surface area of pulmonary epithelium and endothelium including the associated microcirculation, myofibroblasts, and both alveolar macrophages and recruited neutrophils are all important components of acute lung injury. BAL fluid has a marked increase in cell count; alveolar macrophage numbers are increased about twofold, but as a fraction of the cell count falls from around 90% to 20–40% of the cell count due to a greater increase in neutrophils from around 1% to 50–80% of the cell count. In addition microparticles, tiny vesicles potentially derived from most of these cell types, are found in both BAL fluid and blood and may play an important role in both lung damage and repair.[25] A temporal trend towards more normal neutrophil and alveolar macrophage ratios in BAL fluid is associated with survival.

NEUTROPHILS

Neutrophils are the most abundant cell type found in both the epithelial lining fluid (e.g. BAL fluid), and alveoli in histological specimens from early in the course of ARDS. Although neutrophil migration across the endothelium and then the epithelium does not cause injury, when activated neutrophils are pro-inflammatory and pro-apoptotic, and release reactive oxygen species, cytokines, eicosanoids and a variety of proteases that may make an important contribution to basement membrane damage, increased permeability and direct cell damage. Following bone marrow demargination, activated neutrophils adhere to the endothelium on their passage to the alveolus, and this may be accompanied by an early, transient leucopenia. Although neutrophils have an important role in host defence due to their bactericidal activity, there is a marked (50–1000-fold) increase in the release of cytotoxic compounds when they are activated by adherence to the endothelium, epithelium or contact with interstitial extracellular matrix proteins.[26] The factors involved in adhesion of neutrophils are complex and involve the integrin family of proteins, selectins and a number of adhesion molecules.

In models of ARDS, antibodies to adhesion molecules (e.g. CD11b/CD18 antibodies) ameliorate lung injury, suggesting a crucial and central role of this cell type. However, ARDS occurs in neutropenic patients, and was not more common when granulocyte colony-stimulating factor was administered to patients with pneumonia.[27] Clearly, other cell types play an important role, and neutrophil chemoattractants such as IL-8 must be present in the lung prior to neutrophil accumulation.

ALVEOLAR MACROPHAGES

Alveolar macrophages are the most common cell type normally found in BAL fluid, and together with interstitial macrophages play an important role in host defence and modulation of fibrosis. They are capable of releasing IL-6 and a host of mediators similar to the activated neutrophil, including TNF-α and IL-8 in response to stretch,[28] and may amplify lung injury. Macrophages also release factors such as TGF-α and PDGF that stimulate fibroblast proliferation, deposition of collagen and glycosaminoglycans, angiogenesis and lung fibrosis.

A study using different cell markers found that there appear to be different pools of alveolar macrophages termed the M1 and M2 phenotype.[29] The M1 phenotype is characterised as a resident alveolar macrophage that is pro-inflammatory, and the M2 phenotype appears to represent recruited monocytes and be central to lung repair and fibrosis depending upon timing, local milieu and cross talk with other cell types. This may account for the observation that ARDS survivors progressively increase alveolar macrophage number; however, any conclusion awaits further work examining alveolar macrophage phenotypes and clinical outcomes.

EPITHELIUM

Alveolar epithelial type II cells are extremely metabolically active; they manufacture and release surfactant, along with type I cells control alveolar water clearance through epithelial Na channels and Na^{+}/K^{+} ATP-ase, express cytokines, which in turn interact with surfactant production, and are the progenitor of type I cells following injury. In response to both stretch and endotoxin, type II cells express IL-8 and TNF-α, with the latter cytokine augmenting Na^{+}, and hence water, egress from the alveolus.[30] Damage to the epithelium leads to dysfunctional surfactant release and impaired resolution of alveolar oedema which both reduces vectorial transport of Na^{+} in part through down-regulation of ion transport genes, and up-regulates gene expression of Il-8, TNF-α and IL-β.[31]

Epithelial biomarkers include surfactant protein B (SP-B), which is predictive of ARDS,[32] and SP-D, and the receptor for advanced glycation end-products (RAGE) both of which have been associated with severity and outcome of ARDS.

ENDOTHELIUM

Pulmonary endothelial cells express a variety of adhesion molecules and COX-2, secrete endothelin and cytokines including IL-8,[33] stimulate procoagulant activity and 'cross talk' with the alveolar macrophages and type II cells. In addition to generalised endothelial activation, the endothelium is subject to mechanical stress both secondary to vascular pressure, and its association with the alveolus. Plasma levels of von Willebrand factor antigen are both predictive of and associated with outcomes from ARDS[34]; however, as it is synthesised by all vascular endothelial cells it is a non-specific biomarker.

Microvascular thrombosis is common in ARDS, associated with inflammation, and contributes to pulmonary hypertension and wasted ventilation. Platelet aggregation contributes through release of thromboxane A_2, serotonin, lysosomal enzymes, and platelet-activating factor. Impaired fibrinolysis also contributes to these changes, and abnormal plasma levels of protein C and plasminogen activator inhibitor-1 are associated with outcome and organ failure in ARDS. Lung injury also leads to expression of the coagulation factor X on pulmonary epithelium, which appears to be a direct link between coagulation and pulmonary fibrosis.[35]

CHEMOKINES IN ARDS

The expression and secretion of chemokines (chemoattractant cytokines) at sites of inflammation is a key proximal step in initiating the inflammatory cascade. IL-8-induced chemotaxis and activation of neutrophils are elevated in ARDS BAL fluid both within hours of the initiating insult and before recruitment of neutrophils, and in a manner that reflects subsequent morbidity and mortality. IL-8 antibodies prevent recruitment of neutrophils and protect the lung. Indeed, the recruitment and retention of neutrophils requires the generation and maintenance of a localised chemotactic/haptotactic gradient.[36]

MEDIATORS IN ARDS[37]

Inflammation is usually a redundant process so that numerous mediators, including cytokines, chemokines, complement, reactive oxygen species, eicosanoids, platelet-activating factor, nitric oxide, proteases, growth factors and lysosomal enzymes, derived from a number of different cell types, play important roles in the pathophysiology of ARDS. As the alveolocapillary barrier becomes injured these are no longer compartmentalised in the alveolus, and many of these proteins have been measured in blood as well as in the epithelial lining fluid. Care must be taken when interpreting these data as immunological levels may not reflect biological activity, inhibitors or binding proteins may complex with the active protein or epitope and interfere with immunological detection, and the ultimate biological effect will depend upon a balance of pro-inflammatory and anti-inflammatory effects.

Of the pro-inflammatory mediators, TNF-α, IL-1β, IL–6 and IL-8 are the most important. However, even greater increases are found in their cognate receptors or antagonists such as the counter-regulatory cytokine IL-10, so that their biological impact is markedly reduced.[38] Blood or epithelial lining fluid levels are associated with mortality, but are rarely used clinically.

RESOLUTION OF ARDS AND THE DEVELOPMENT OF FIBROSING ALVEOLITIS

Although histological evidence of fibrosing alveolitis (mesenchymal cells and new vessels in alveoli) is not usually found until at least 5 days following the onset of ARDS, elevated levels of type III procollagen peptide are found in the epithelial lining fluid soon after diagnosis;[21] both oedema fluid and plasma levels are associated with mortality.

Clinical resolution of ARDS usually occurs provided that both the underlying cause is promptly and effectively treated, and that appropriate supportive care is provided. Alveolar oedema resolves with active transport of Na^+ by the type II cells followed by passive clearance of water through transcellular aquaporin channels; repair of the alveolocapillary barrier is associated with improved outcome. Type II cells proliferate and cover the denuded epithelium before differentiating into type I cells.

Both host response and the clinical course of ARDS influence lung remodelling in ARDS. Cross-talk between type II cells and alveolar macrophages, probably the M2 phenotype, along with epithelial mesenchymal transition – a process where reactive oxygen species, hypoxia, TGF-β and mechanical stress lead to altered epithelial transcription – are central to interstitial responses. Epithelial cells assume characteristics of mesenchymal cells with loss of polarity, increased resistance to apoptosis, and increased migration (into the interstitium) where they lay down a fibrotic matrix.[39]

CLINICAL MANAGEMENT OF ARDS

The factors leading to ARDS must be promptly and appropriately treated. This includes diagnosis and treatment of infection with drainage of collections and appropriate antimicrobial agents, recognition and rapid resuscitation from shock, splinting of fractures, and careful supportive care. Prevention of deep venous thrombosis, stress ulceration, nosocomial infection, and malnutrition, often with enteral nutrition, must all be considered.

Early mobilisation of mechanically ventilated patients accompanied by appropriate levels of analgesia and sedation is feasible and safe, and offers shorter duration of ventilation, reduced delirium, ICU and hospital length of stay, and improved mortality and functional outcomes.[40,41] However, this must be balanced with strategies such as use of neuromuscular blockers in the first 48 hours of mechanical ventilation in ARDS, which reduced mortality,[42] possibly through prevention or reduction of asynchronous ventilatory effort.

MECHANICAL VENTILATION

Acute hypoxaemic respiratory failure,[43] and an increase in the work of breathing, usually mandates mechanical ventilation (**Table 33.2**). The role of non-invasive ventilation in ARDS is contentious; there are no large definitive studies, and although some groups report encouraging results these are usually in patients with mild ARDS.[44] Failure of NIV is common, associated with greater complication rates and mortality, perhaps due to delayed intubation.[45-47] If non-invasive ventilation is considered in ARDS it requires particular care (see Ch. 37).

The method and delivery of ventilatory support must take into account both the pathophysiology of ARDS and ventilator-induced lung injury (VILI). The ARDS Network randomised 861 ALI patients from 75 ICUs to receive either a tidal volume (V_T) of 12 or 6 mL/kg predicted body weight.[48] Mortality was reduced by 22%, from 40% to 31%, in the lower V_T group. There was a strict PEEP and F_{IO_2} protocol, and patients were ventilated with assist-control ventilation

Table 33.2 Pathophysiology of acute lung injury (ALI) and adult respiratory distress syndrome (ARDS)

FEATURE	CAUSE(S)
Hypoxaemia	True shunt (perfusion of non-ventilated airspaces) Impaired hypoxic pulmonary vasoconstriction V/Q mismatch is a minor component
↑Dependent densities (CT)	Surfactant dysfunction alveolar instability
(Collapse/consolidation)	Exaggeration of normal compression of dependent lung due to ↑weight (↑lung water, inflammation)
↑Elastance (↓compliance)	Surfactant dysfunction (↑specific elastance) ↓Lung volume ('baby lung') ↑Chest wall elastance Fibrosing alveolitis (late)
↑Minute volume requirement	↑Alveolar dead space (VD_{phys} V_t often 0.4–0.7) ↑V_{CO_2}
↑Work of breathing	↑Elastance ↑Minute volume requirement
Pulmonary hypertension	Pulmonary vasoconstriction (thromboxane A_2, endothelin) Pulmonary microvascular thrombosis Fibrosing alveolitis Positive end-expiratory pressure

to avoid excessive spontaneous V_T. Similar data with improved long-term survival are found in routine clinical practice[49]; however, it is the concept of lung protection rather than an exact V_T formula that is important.[50] As Hager and colleagues[51] found that lower V_T ventilation was protective across all quartiles of plateau pressure (P_{plat}) in the ARDS Network trial, with no safe upper limit of P_{plat}, it appears that the key variable is lower V_T rather than control of static airway pressure.

AVOIDANCE OF OVERSTRETCH AND INADEQUATE RECRUITMENT

The increase in dependent lung density found on chest CT, due to non-aerated and poorly aerated lung, reduces the volume of aerated lung available for tidal inflation (baby lung). Both PEEP and tidal recruitment will increase aeration of some of these air spaces, but a V_T that is not reduced in proportion to the reduction in aerated lung may lead to overstretch of aerated lung parenchyma and further diffuse alveolar damage. This is termed volutrauma as increased airway pressure (P_{aw}) despite low V_T, due to decreased chest wall compliance, causes minimal damage compared with high V_T, high P_{aw} ventilation.[52] Atelectrauma refers to injury due to repeated opening and closing of air spaces during tidal inflation. Both volutrauma and atelectrauma result in alveolar inflammation and elevated alveolar cytokines (biotrauma), which may 'spill' into the systemic circulation.[53] However, as CT scans performed during ARDS Network protective ventilation show that tidal inflation occurs primarily in either normally aerated or overinflated compartments, with little tidal recruitment,[54] and PET-CT scans suggest that overinflation but not tidal recruitment is inflammatory,[55] overstretch appears to be the dominant mechanism causing VILI.

OVERSTRETCH

The normal lung is fully inflated at a transpulmonary pressure of ~25–30 cmH_2O. Consequently, a maximum P_{plat}, an estimate of the elastic distending pressure, of 30 cmH_2O has been recommended.[48] However, overinflation may occur at much lower elastic distending pressures (18–26 cmH_2O).[52,56]

The transpulmonary pressure may be lower than expected for a given P_{plat} in patients with a high chest wall elastance (e.g. obesity, abdominal compartment syndrome, after abdominal or thoracic surgery). While placement of an oesophageal balloon (see Ch. 38) allows measurement of the transpulmonary pressure and may allow better titration of PEEP,[57] it must be correctly placed, have an adequate occlusion pressure ratio, and measurements are preferably performed in a semi-sitting position in order to lift the mediastinum off the oesophagus.

Finally, inspiratory muscle contraction through reduction of intrapleural pressure lowers P_{plat}, potentially avoiding simple detection of an excessive transpulmonary pressure. This is particularly common when pressure support ventilation is used as a primary mode of ventilatory support; V_T that would produce an unacceptably high P_{plat} during mechanical ventilation will produce the same volutrauma during a spontaneous or supported mode of ventilation, and should be avoided. Provided the same V_T is generated, spontaneous ventilation does not reduce VILI compared to controlled ventilation.[58]

Static or dynamic volume-pressure curves or quantitative chest CT can be used to infer overinflation, though chest CT cannot determine overstretch.[5] Consequently, unless particular expertise is available, V_T limitation is currently the most practical approach.

ADEQUATE PEEP

PEEP improves Pa_{O_2} by recruiting alveoli and increasing functional residual capacity. Because PEEP may reduce cardiac output by impairing venous return, Suter and coworkers suggested that at best PEEP the oxygen delivery (oxygen content × flow) was highest, and that this coincided with greatest compliance.[59] PEEP is commonly titrated to a particular Pa_{O_2}/Fi_{O_2} ratio such as the ARDS Network protocol.[48] However, the amount of lung available for recruitment is extremely variable,[60] and does not differ comparing pulmonary with extrapulmonary ARDS.[61] Factors such as the duration, late ARDS being less recruitable, and phenotype influence whether PEEP leads to alveolar recruitment, overinflation or a balance of both. Based on chest imaging, ARDS can be subdivided into focal, intermediate and diffuse phenotypes, with progressive increase in the amount of recruitable lung.[62,63] Applying ARDS Network ventilation to focal ARDS (about ⅓ of most cohorts) leads to high lung stress, with increased cytokine release, which can be ameliorated by using lower levels of PEEP.[64]

The lower inflection point of a volume–pressure curve has been used to set PEEP; early studies suggested that this reflected recruitment of collapsed alveoli. However, in patients with ARDS, recruitment occurs well above the lower inflection point, often along the entire volume–pressure curve and above the upper inflection point.[65,66] Concurrently, there is frequently evidence of overstretching and hyperinflation on CT scans[36,67] or dynamic volume–pressure analysis.[56] Meta-analysis of major clinical trials using protective V_T and comparing higher and lower PEEP scales[68] did not find an overall improvement in outcome with higher PEEP, although rescue therapies were required less often. However, patients with mild ARDS tended to have worse outcomes with higher PEEP, and those with moderate to severe ARDS had better outcomes.

These data suggest individual patients may benefit from a tailored approach. Although routine CT analysis has been advocated by some, it is cumbersome and has not been shown to influence outcome; non-invasive bedside alternatives are under investigation. Consequently, PEEP titration is often a compromise aiming to minimise both atelectrauma and volutrauma.[69] Reasonable approaches to PEEP titration include: (a) the use of a scale similar to the ARDS Network protocol, (b) titration of PEEP to Pa_{O_2} aiming for a PEEP of ~15 cmH_2O, or (c) measuring elastic mechanics at the bedside. Consistent with Suter's early observation,[59] both nadir elastance after a recruitment manoeuvre,[70] or minimal change in driving pressure[56] (see also Ch. 38), offer bedside methods to individualise PEEP.

In patients at risk for ARDS prophylactic PEEP (8 cmH_2O) was not protective.[71]

Recruitment manoeuvres and open lung ventilation

Open lung ventilation refers to an approach where the lung is maximally recruited, usually through application of higher PEEP, recruitment manoeuvres, and efforts to minimise derecruitment. In theory increased lung volume will result in less tidal overinflation, and improved outcome. However, despite alveolar recruitment with open lung ventilation, overinflation may occur in previously normally aerated lung.[72] The recruitment manoeuvre may be followed by a marked improvement in oxygenation; however, this is not a consistent finding, and hypotension may occur due to reduced venous return if there is inadequate fluid loading.

During a typical recruitment manoeuvre a high level of CPAP (30–40 cmH_2O) is applied for 30–40 seconds in an apnoeic patient, followed by return to a lower level of PEEP and controlled ventilation. This may be suboptimal; an alternative for example is a staircase recruitment manoeuvre where airway pressure is sequentially increased every 2 minutes, and then decreased until oxygenation deteriorates.[73] A number of small trials have shown improvement in oxygenation following recruitment manoeuvres; however, the largest clinical trial[74] failed to show an effect. Grasso and colleagues[75] found that recruitment manoeuvres were effective only early in ARDS and with lower levels of baseline PEEP, which probably explains the variable responses reported.

In addition to physical recruitment of alveoli, lung stretch above resting V_T is the most powerful physiological stimulus for release of pulmonary surfactant from type II cells. This is associated with a decrease in lung elastance and improved Pa_{O_2} in the isolated perfused lung,[76] and is a possible explanation for the improvement in oxygenation, recruited lung volume and elastance reported with addition of three sigh breaths in patients with ARDS.[77] Similarly, in models of lung injury biologically variable or fractal V_T is associated with less lung damage with lower alveolar levels of IL-8,[78] improved oxygenation and lung elastance, and greater surfactant release.[79] These data caution against monotonous low V_T ventilation, and suggest that intermittent or variable lung stretch may reduce lung injury.

MODE OF VENTILATION

Non-invasive ventilation should not be routinely used in ARDS (see Ch. 37) and most patients require intubated mechanical ventilation. Following intubation, controlled ventilation allows immediate reduction in the work of breathing, and application of PEEP and a controlled Fi_{O_2}. Later in the clinical course assisted or supported modes of ventilation may allow better patient–ventilator interaction (see Ch. 31), and possibly improved oxygenation through better $\dot{V}/\dot{Q}$ mismatch as a result of diaphragmatic contraction.[80] Withdrawal or weaning from mechanical ventilation is discussed in Chapter 31.

An advantage of assist-control ventilation (as used in the ARDS Network study) is that spontaneous effort generates a controlled V_T. Care should be taken with synchronised intermittent mandatory ventilation (SIMV), particularly if pressure support is added to SIMV, as excessive V_T may occur during supported breaths. There is an increasing tendency to use pressure-controlled ventilation (PC) or pressure-regulated volume control (PRVC) as P_{pk} is lower than volume-controlled (VC) ventilation with a constant inspiratory flow pattern. However, the decelerating flow pattern of PC or PRVC means that most of the resistive pressure (P_{res}) during inspiration is dissipated by end inspiration, which is in contrast to VC with a constant inspiratory flow pattern where P_{res} is dissipated at end inspiration (see Fig. 31.2). Consequently, with PC and PRVC $P_{pk} \approx P_{plat}$ which is the same as P_{plat} during VC.[81] Both oxygenation, haemodynamic stability and mean airway pressure are no different between PC and VC, and a moderate-sized randomised study found no difference in outcome.[82] However, there may be differences in lung stress due to greater viscoelastic build-up with VC.[83]

Inverse ratio ventilation, often together with PC, has been used in ARDS. However, when $PEEP_i$ and total PEEP are taken into account, apart from a small decrease in Pa_{O_2}, there are no advantages with inverse ratio ventilation. Mean airway pressure is higher with a greater risk of both haemodynamic consequences, and regional hyperinflation.[81] Consequently, an inspiratory to expiratory ratio greater than 1:1 is recommended.

A number of other modes of ventilation (see Ch. 31) including airway pressure release ventilation (APRV) and high-frequency oscillation (HFO) have been proposed for use in ARDS. Randomised clinical trials have not shown improved outcomes with APRV,[84] despite potential physiological benefits. The small V_T used with HFO are appealing, and some centres use HFO as rescue therapy when conventional ventilatory strategies are failing, while others would consider venovenous extracorporeal membrane oxygenation (ECMO; see Ch. 41). Definitive clinical trials of both trials are underway and awaited.

TARGET BLOOD GASES

As discussed above there are many variables that need to be considered when choosing target blood gases in ARDS. For example if a patient also has a traumatic brain injury, it may be inappropriate to accept hypercapnia.

Oxygenation targets and F_{IO_2}

There must be a compromise between the major determinants of oxygenation including the extent of poorly or non-aerated lung, hypoxic pulmonary vasoconstriction and mixed venous oxygen saturation, and the target Pa_{O_2}. The association between cognitive impairment and arterial saturation (Sa_{O_2}) <90%[14] suggests that a $Sa_{O_2} \geq 90\%$, usually a $Pa_{O_2} > 60$ mmHg, is a reasonable target. Because positive-pressure ventilation may reduce cardiac output it is also important to consider tissue oxygenation.

In addition to PEEP, increased F_{IO_2} is used to improve Sa_{O_2}. However, high F_{IO_2} may also cause tissue injury including diffuse alveolar damage. The balance between increased airway pressure and F_{IO_2} is unknown, but high F_{IO_2} is generally regarded as being less damaging.[85] In part this is because diffuse alveolar damage itself protects the lung against hyperoxia, perhaps through prior induction of scavengers for reactive oxygen species.[86] A reasonable compromise is to start ventilation at a F_{IO_2} of 1 and to titrate down, aiming for a $F_{IO_2} \leq 0.6$. In patients with extreme hypoxaemia, additional measures such as inhaled nitric oxide (iNO) and prone positioning may be tried, along with a lower Sa_{O_2} target.

Carbon dioxide target

Low V_T strategies will result in elevations in Pa_{CO_2} unless minute ventilation is augmented by an increase in respiratory rate. The ARDS Network protocol aimed at normocapnia, with a maximum respiratory rate of 35, to minimise respiratory acidosis.[48] This exposes the lung to more repeated tidal stretch, and may result in dynamic hyperinflation due to a shortened expiratory time.[87] In addition, allowing the Pa_{CO_2} to rise above normal may not be harmful in many patients.

If hypercapnic acidosis occurs slowly, intracellular acidosis is well compensated, and the associated increase in sympathetic tone may augment cardiac output and blood pressure. Although the respiratory acidosis may worsen pulmonary hypertension and induce myocardial arrhythmias these effects are often small, particularly if there has been time for metabolic compensation. In addition, in an ischaemia–reperfusion model of ARDS, therapeutic hypercapnia reduced lung injury and apoptosis.[88] However, clinical studies of permissive hypercapnia must be undertaken before therapeutic hypercapnia is considered. Hypercapnia should be avoided in patients with or at risk from raised intracranial pressure.

ADDITIONAL MEASURES TO IMPROVE OXYGENATION

PRONE POSTURE

In ~70% of patients with ARDS, prone positioning will result in a significant increase in Pa_{O_2}, with a modest increase in Pa_{O_2} sustained in the supine position.[89] The mechanisms involved include recruitment of dorsal lung, with concurrent ventral collapse; however, perfusion is more evenly distributed leading to better $\dot{V}/\dot{Q}$ matching. Recent meta-analysis[90] did not show an improvement in overall mortality; however, when studies only enrolling patients with moderate and severe ARDS were examined, prone position was associated with reduced ICU mortality without increased airway complications. Meta-regression revealed a trend to better results with longer periods of prone position. These data support the use of prone positioning as rescue therapy in life-threatening hypoxaemia.

MANIPULATION OF THE PULMONARY CIRCULATION

Inhaled nitric oxide (iNO) and aerosolised prostacyclin (PGI_2) may be used to reduce pulmonary shunt and right ventricular afterload by reducing pulmonary artery impedance. When hypoxic pulmonary vasoconstriction is active, there is redistribution of pulmonary blood flow away from the poorly ventilated dependent areas to more normally ventilated lung leading to an increase in Pa_{O_2}. Both iNO and PGI_2 are delivered to well-ventilated lung; both vasodilate the local pulmonary circulation and augment the effects of hypoxic pulmonary vasoconstriction. Intravenous almitrine is a selective pulmonary vasoconstrictor that reinforces hypoxic pulmonary vasoconstriction and, although this may improve oxygenation alone, there is a synergistic effect with iNO.

Inhaled NO or PGI_2 may also be used to reduce right ventricular afterload; however, a consequent increase in cardiac output is rare in ARDS. Intravenous PGI_2 will improve cardiac output in ARDS, though there is non-specific pulmonary vasodilation with increased blood flow through poorly ventilated lung zones, resulting in deterioration in oxygenation.

Inhaled nitric oxide

Nitric oxide is an endothelium-derived smooth muscle relaxant. It also has other important physiological roles including neurotransmission, host defence, platelet aggregation leucocyte adhesion, and bronchodilation. Doses as low as 60 parts per billion iNO may improve oxygenation, however, commonly used doses in ARDS are 1–60 parts per million, with the higher doses required for reduction in pulmonary artery pressure. A rise in Pa_{O_2} exceeding 20% is generally regarded as a positive response; iNO should be continued at the minimum effective dose.

Inhaled NO may be delivered continuously or using intermittent inspiratory injection. Delivery is usually in the form of medical grade NO/N_2, and this should be adequately mixed to avoid delivery of variable NO concentrations. It is recommended that inspiratory NO and NO_2 concentrations are measured, either by an electrochemical method or by chemiluminescence. The electrochemical method is accurate to 1 p.p.m., which is adequate for clinical use, and is less expensive. Local environmental levels of NO and NO_2 are low and predominantly influenced by atmospheric concentrations; however, it is still common practice to scavenge expired gas. Binding to haemoglobin in the pulmonary circulation rapidly inactivates NO, and systemic effects are reported only following high concentrations of iNO. Systemic methaemoglobin levels may be monitored, and are generally less than 5% during clinical use of iNO, but they should be compared with a baseline level. Nitric oxide may cause lung toxicity through combination with oxygen free radicals, and through metabolism of NO to NO_2; however, these do not appear to be major clinical problems.

Only 40–70% of patients with ARDS have improved oxygenation with iNO (responders), and this is likely due to active hypoxic pulmonary vasoconstriction in the remainder. Addition of i.v. almitrine can have an additive effect on oxygenation, and may improve the number of responders. Clinical trials[91] have shown no improvement in mortality or reversal of ARDS, and an increased risk of renal impairment. However, iNO transiently improves oxygenation (as compared with placebo or no iNO), which has been sustained beyond 12–24 hours in some trials. As constant dosing of iNO leads to both increased sensitivity and apparent tachyphylaxis,[92] subsequent investigation needs to consider different dose regimens. Currently iNO cannot be recommended for routine use in ARDS; however, in some patients with severe hypoxaemia, perhaps in combination with almitrine, iNO will provide temporary rescue.

Inhaled prostacyclin

PGI_2 (up to 50 ng/kg/min) improves oxygenation as effectively as iNO in ARDS patients,[93] and may reduce pulmonary hypertension. It is continuously jet nebulised due to its short half-life (2–3 minutes). Potential advantages include increased surfactant release from stretched type II cells, avoidance of the potential complications of iNO, and minimal toxicity. However, PGI_2 is dissolved in an alkaline glycine buffer, which alone can result in airway inflammation, and the sticky nature of the aerosol can result in expiratory valve obstruction. Iloprost is a derivative of PGI_2 with similar activity, a longer duration of action, without an alkaline buffer. Neither agent has been shown to improve outcome in ARDS patients.

PHARMACOLOGICAL THERAPY

There is no proven pharmacological therapy for ARDS despite numerous studies. However, the lack of a protective ventilation strategy in many of these studies may have masked a drug effect.

SURFACTANT REPLACEMENT THERAPY

Surfactant dysfunction is an important and early abnormality contributing to lung damage in ARDS.[19,94] Pulmonary surfactant reduces surface tension promoting alveolar stability, reducing work of breathing and lung water. In addition surfactant has important roles in lung host defence. Reactive oxygen species, phospholipases and increased protein permeability lead to inhibition of surfactant function. In addition, composition is abnormal, and turnover markedly increased. Ventilator-induced lung injury is difficult to demonstrate without surfactant dysfunction.[94] Consequently, there has been considerable interest in exogenous surfactant replacement therapy.

Exogenous surfactant therapy has an established role in neonatal respiratory distress syndrome. In paediatric ARDS, particularly that due to direct lung injury, clinical trials have been promising. However, in adults results have been disappointing; subgroup analysis of recombinant surfactant protein-C-based surfactant administered intratracheally improved oxygenation in direct ARDS without an improvement in mortality.[95] However, subsequent research in this cohort failed to confirm these data, perhaps owing to inactivation of the surfactant during administration.[96]

GLUCOCORTICOIDS

Glucocorticoids may have a role in ARDS through their reduction of the intense inflammatory response and their potential to reduce fibroproliferation and collagen deposition, by faster degradation of fibroblast procollagen mRNA. Preventative steroids increase the incidence of ARDS and, although there may be a greater number of ventilator-free days and the possibility of a reduction in mortality,[97,98] neuromuscular complications, and increased mortality when steroids are administered more than 13 days after the onset of ARDS,[99] argue against their routine use.

KETOCONAZOLE

Ketoconazole is an antifungal drug that also inhibits thromboxane synthase and 5-lipo-oxygenase. However, promising results from small studies in at-risk patients have not been confirmed in a larger treatment trial.[100]

OTHER PHARMACOLOGICAL THERAPIES

Numerous other therapies including cytokine antagonism, non-steroidal anti-inflammatory drugs, scavengers of reactive oxygen species, and lisofylline[101] have been trialled without success. The complex balance of inflammation and repair in ARDS, and the critical additional damage secondary to VILI, may explain these results. However, studies in less heterogeneous groups with minimisation of VILI using standardised ventilation protocols, together with a growing understanding of ARDS, offer potential pharmacological therapies.

Access the complete references list online at http://www.expertconsult.com

2. The ARDS Definition Task Force. Acute respiratory distress syndrome: the Berlin definition. JAMA 2012;307:2526–33.
13. Herridge MS, Tansey CM, Matte A, et al. Functional disability 5 years after acute respiratory distress syndrome. N Engl J Med 2011;364:1293–304.
23. Steinberg KP, Milberg JA, Martin TR, et al. Evolution of bronchoalveolar cell populations in the adult respiratory distress syndrome. Am J Respir Crit Care Med 1994;150:113–22.
52. Dreyfuss D, Saumon G. Ventilator-induced lung injury: Lessons from experimental studies. Am J Respir Crit Care Med 1998;157:294–323.
69. Rouby JJ, Lu Q, Goldstein I. Selecting the right level of psitive end-expiratory pressure in patients with acute respiratory distress syndrome. Am J Respir Crit Care Med 2002;165:1182–6.

34

Pulmonary embolism

Andrew R Davies and David V Pilcher

Pulmonary embolism (PE) is a commonly considered but relatively uncommonly diagnosed condition in hospitalised patients. It is important to have an adequate understanding of the pathophysiology as well as a rapid and reliable strategy of investigation and management. This is particularly important in intensive care unit (ICU) patients where diagnosis can be difficult and PE may be life threatening, with mortality rates in haemodynamically unstable patients being about 30%.[1]

Early deaths in PE are usually the result of acute right ventricular (RV) failure and cardiogenic shock. After the first few days, mortality is less common and mostly determined by recurrent thromboembolic events and the underlying disease state.

AETIOLOGY

Deep venous thrombosis (DVT) and PE are components of a single disease termed venous thromboembolism (VTE). Embolisation of DVT to the pulmonary arteries leads to PE. The incidence of VTE in the population is about 1 in 1000 per year and is more common both with advancing age and in males.

Most PE results from DVT of the lower limbs, pelvic veins or inferior vena cava (IVC), although DVT of the upper limbs, right atrium or ventricle does occur. Up to 40% of patients with DVT develop PE, although if the DVT is isolated to below the knee then clinically obvious PE is rare.

Predisposing risk factors for VTE involve one or more components of Virchow's triad: (1) venous stasis, (2) vein wall injury, and (3) hypercoagulability of blood. The main factors are immobility (from any cause), surgery, trauma, malignancy, pregnancy and thrombophilia (see **Box 34.1**).

VTE can be recurrent, which should prompt investigation for thrombophilia. This is a group of inherited conditions associated with a high incidence of VTE. The most important of these is activated protein C resistance, which is mediated by the factor V Leiden mutation. Up to 50% of patients with recurrent VTE episodes (as well as 20% of patients with a single episode) have this condition; however, its association appears to be greater with DVT than with PE.[2] Up to 5% of patients with VTE develop chronic pulmonary hypertension.[3]

PATHOPHYSIOLOGY

The effects of PE range from being incidental and clinically irrelevant to causing severe obstruction to the pulmonary circulation and sudden death. Pulmonary arterial obstruction and the subsequent release of vasoactive substances such as serotonin and thromboxane A_2 from platelets lead to elevated pulmonary vascular resistance and acute pulmonary hypertension.

Acute pulmonary hypertension increases RV afterload and RV wall tension, which leads to RV dilatation and dysfunction, with coronary ischaemia being a major contributing mechanism.[4] In massive PE, the combination of coronary ischaemia, RV systolic failure, paradoxical interventricular septal shift and pericardial constraint leads to left ventricular (LV) dysfunction and obstructive shock. In patients with underlying cardiorespiratory disease, a small PE can have profound consequences.

Pulmonary arterial obstruction causes a mismatch between lung ventilation and perfusion, which leads to hypoxaemia. The ventilation of lung units that have reduced or no perfusion causes increased dead-space ventilation and an increase in the end-tidal to arterial CO_2 gradient. Alveolar hyperventilation also occurs, leading to hypocapnia. Increased right atrial pressure can open a patent foramen ovale, which may result in right-to-left shunting, manifested as either refractory hypoxaemia or paradoxical (arterial) embolisation, commonly to the brain, leading to cerebral infarction.

CLINICAL PRESENTATION

PE is relatively uncommon in critically ill patients despite the frequent presence of risk factors for VTE. However, when PE does occur the diagnosis is frequently overlooked or is difficult to confirm because several more prevalent cardiopulmonary diseases, including heart failure, pneumonia and chronic lung diseases, have similar clinical features. Up to one in six patients have the diagnosis made more than 10 days after symptom onset.[5]

Clinical assessment should raise the suspicion of PE but is neither sensitive nor specific enough to reliably confirm or exclude the diagnosis on its own. A number of clinical decision rule (CDR) systems have been

Box 34.1 Risk factors for venous thromboembolism

Primary hypercoagulable states (thrombophilia)
Antithrombin III deficiency
Protein C deficiency
Protein S deficiency
Resistance to activated protein C (inherited factor V Leiden mutation)
Hyperhomocysteinaemia
Lupus anticoagulant (antiphospholipid antibody)
Secondary hypercoagulable states
Immobility
Surgery
Trauma
Malignancy
Pregnancy and the puerperium
Obesity
Smoking
Oestrogen-containing oral contraception or hormone replacement therapy
Indwelling catheters in great veins and the right heart
Burns
Patients with limb paralysis (e.g. spinal injuries)
Heart failure
Increasing age

developed, the most widely reported of which are the Wells' score and the Geneva score.[6] These CDRs use a combination of symptoms, signs and risk factors to stratify patients into different disease probability categories. CDRs provide accurate and reproducible determinations of probability and outcome for use in a diagnostic or therapeutic strategy. Patients can therefore have their probability determined as unlikely (in whom PE can be safely ruled out with a negative D-dimer result)[7] or likely (in whom an imaging test is required and in whom prompt anticoagulant therapy should be considered). The differential diagnoses are listed in **Box 34.2**.

SYMPTOMS

Dyspnoea, pleuritic chest pain, and haemoptysis are the classic symptoms of PE. Most patients will have at least one of these symptoms, with dyspnoea being the most common. The combination of pleuritic chest pain and haemoptysis reflects a late presentation where pulmonary infarction has occurred. If syncope occurs, and there is no other obvious cause, it is likely that this is a massive PE. A family history of venous thrombosis makes an inherited thrombophilia likely.

PHYSICAL SIGNS

Physical signs can be absent, but the most frequent sign is tachypnoea. Others include tachycardia, fever and signs of RV dysfunction (raised jugular venous pressure, parasternal heave and loud pulmonary component of the second heart sound). In massive PE, signs may include hypotension, pale mottled skin and peripheral or even central cyanosis. It is important to examine for signs of DVT, particularly in the legs.

Box 34.2 Differential diagnosis of pulmonary embolism

Acute myocardial infarction
Acute coronary syndrome
Acute pulmonary oedema
Pneumonia
Asthma or exacerbation of chronic obstructive pulmonary disease
Pericardial tamponade
Pleural effusion
Fat or amniotic fluid embolism
Pneumothorax
Aortic dissection
Rib fracture
Musculoskeletal pain
Anxiety

INVESTIGATIONS

The diagnosis of PE requires a high level of clinical suspicion and the appropriate use of investigations. The aim of these investigations is to confirm or exclude the presence of PE, but also to stratify treatment accordingly. The optimal investigation strategy depends upon the individual patient and institution; however, multidetector computed tomographic pulmonary angiography (CTPA) scanning is now the imaging test of first choice. A suggested investigation algorithm is shown in **Figure 34.1**.

D-DIMER

The serum D-dimer level, which becomes elevated when acute thrombus formation occurs, is useful for exclusion of VTE, particularly when it is normal and combined with a low-risk clinical assessment.[8] Because of its sensitivity, negative D-dimer tests, particularly using enzyme-linked immunosorbent assays (ELISA), enzyme-linked immunofluorescence assays (ELFA) and latex quantitative assays, are highly predictive of the absence of both DVT and PE.

A high D-dimer concentration is also an independent predictive factor associated with mortality.[9] Unfortunately, D-dimer levels are often elevated in ICU patients for reasons including infection, inflammation, cancer, surgery and trauma, acute coronary syndrome, stroke, peripheral artery disease or ruptured aneurysm. D-dimer tests should be used with caution in patients who are elderly (as the upper limit of normal increases with age), who have prolonged symptoms and who are already receiving therapeutic anticoagulant therapy.

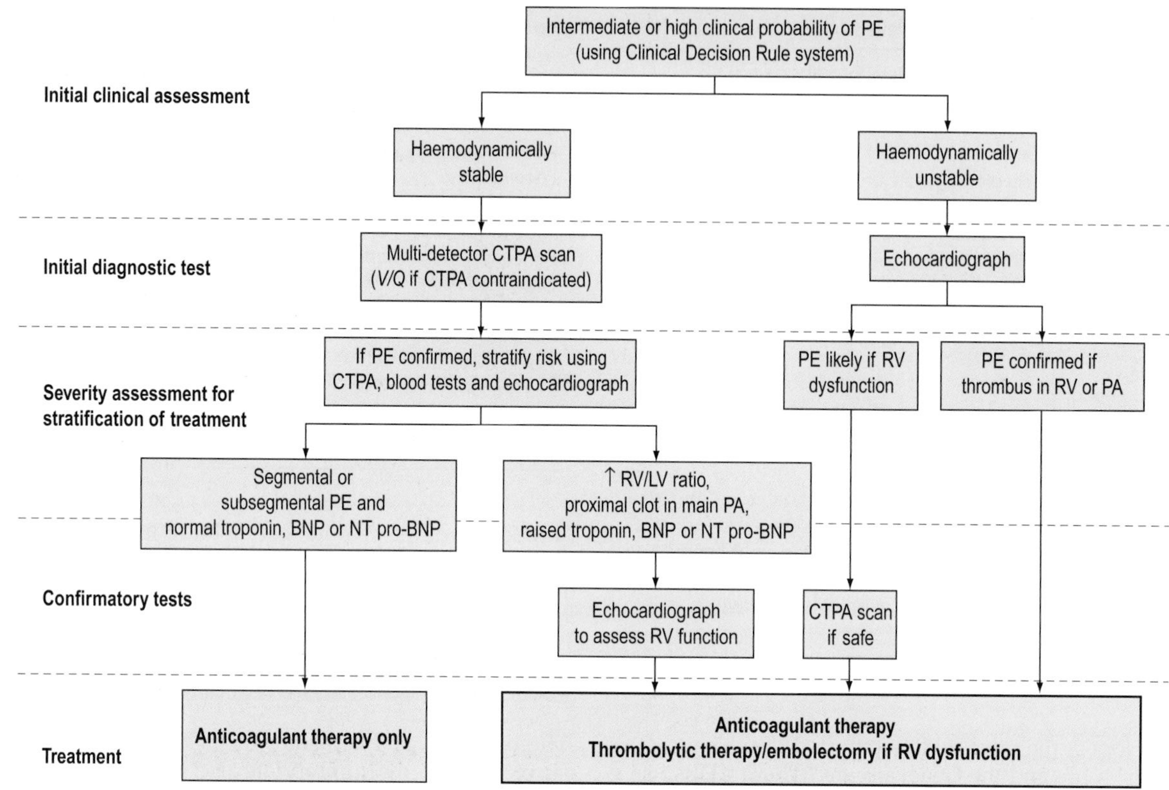

Figure 34.1 Suggested investigation and treatment algorithm for pulmonary embolism (PE). CTPA=computed tomographic pulmonary angiography; *V/Q*=ventilation/perfusion scan; RV=right ventricular; PA=pulmonary artery; BNP=brain natriuretic peptide; RV/LV=right ventricle/left ventricle; IVC=inferior vena cava.

TROPONIN, BRAIN NATRIURETIC PEPTIDE (BNP) AND NT-TERMINAL PRO-BNP

Although of little use for confirming or excluding the diagnosis, measurement of troponin, BNP or NT-pro-BNP can assist in risk stratification of patients with diagnosed PE. A raised troponin is associated with haemodynamic instability in patients with non-massive PE independently of clinical, echocardiographic and laboratory findings.[10] Raised troponin also predicts a higher mortality.[11] Low levels of BNP and NT-pro-BNP have been shown to correlate with an uneventful course in patients with known PE.[12] NT-pro-BNP appears to be a better predictor of outcome than troponin.[13]

ARTERIAL BLOOD GASES

A normal arterial blood gas profile does not exclude the diagnosis of PE; however, hypoxaemia (with a widened alveolar–arterial oxygen gradient), hypocapnia and an increased end-tidal CO_2 gradient should raise the suspicion of PE, even if these are common findings in critically ill patients for other reasons. Metabolic acidosis may be present if shock from a large PE occurs.

ELECTROCARDIOGRAPH

A normal electrocardiograph (ECG) is found in about one-third of patients. Apart from sinus tachycardia (which is non-specific), the most frequent ECG abnormalities are non-specific S–T depression and T-wave inversion in the anterior leads, reflecting right heart strain. The pattern of a deep S-wave in lead I and a Q-wave and inverted T-wave in lead III (S1Q3T3) is classical, but infrequently present. Other possible ECG abnormalities include left- or right-axis deviation, P pulmonale, right bundle-branch block and atrial arrhythmias. The ECG is also useful in excluding acute myocardial infarction and pericarditis.

CHEST X-RAY

The chest X-ray is often normal or only slightly abnormal, with non-specific signs such as cardiac enlargement, pleural effusion, elevated hemidiaphragm, atelectasis and localised infiltrates. More specific findings, including focal oligaemia, a peripheral wedge-shaped density above the diaphragm and an enlarged right descending pulmonary artery, are uncommon and difficult for non-radiologists to identify. The chest

X-ray is also useful in identifying an alternative diagnosis such as pneumothorax, pneumonia, acute pulmonary oedema, rib fracture and pleural effusion.

IMAGING TESTS INCLUDING CTPA SCAN

Imaging is required in any patient with a high or likely clinical probability. As the technology has improved, CTPA scanning, especially the multidetector scanner (MD-CTPA),[14] has now largely replaced lung ventilation–perfusion (*V*/*Q*) scanning as the cost-effective and clinically reliable imaging procedure of choice in patients with suspected PE.[15] This is because the CTPA scan has the advantages of greater diagnostic accuracy, ready availability at most hospitals, more rapid image acquisition time, and the possibility of making an alternative diagnosis. High-resolution images to the level of segmental and in some cases subsegmental pulmonary arteries can be obtained in a short time period (often a single breath-hold). When compared with conventional angiography it appears reliable, with excellent sensitivity, specificity and accuracy.[16] It is therefore recommended that the CTPA scan should be the principal imaging test for patients with high and moderate probability of PE.

Although inconclusive CTPA scans occur in around 10%, a negative CTPA result means that withholding anticoagulant therapy is safe.[17] An emerging problem of CTPA scanning, however, is the increased detection (around 10%) of small peripheral emboli in subsegmental pulmonary arteries due to better visualisation of these arteries. The clinical significance of these findings in critically ill patients is unknown; however, these are usually unlikely to lead to a bad outcome if left untreated.

The CTPA scan can also be used to assess the severity of PE. An increased RV/LV ratio[18] and clot in the proximal branches of the pulmonary artery[19] correlate with the clinical severity of PE. Severity stratification is further increased by combining CTPA scanning with other tests such as troponin[10] and BNP or NT-Pro-BNP.[12] CTPA scanning may also identify the causative DVT in the veins of the legs, pelvis and abdomen or detect alternative or additional diagnoses such as a pulmonary mass, pneumonia, emphysema, pneumothorax, pleural effusion or mediastinal adenopathy (**Fig. 34.2**).

Despite the increased use of the CTPA scan, the *V*/*Q* scan retains a role when CTPA is either unavailable or contraindicated (e.g. significant renal

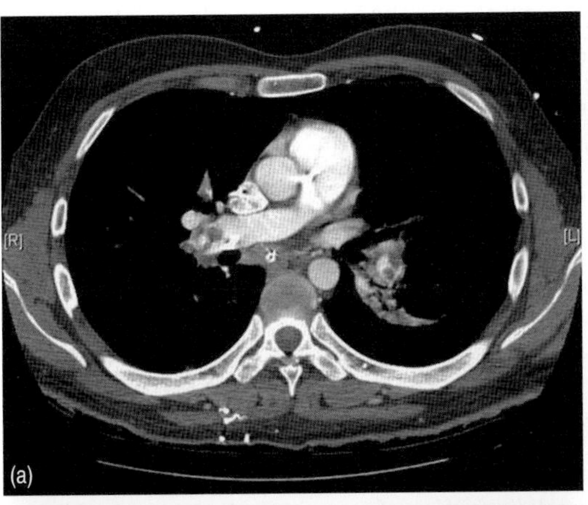

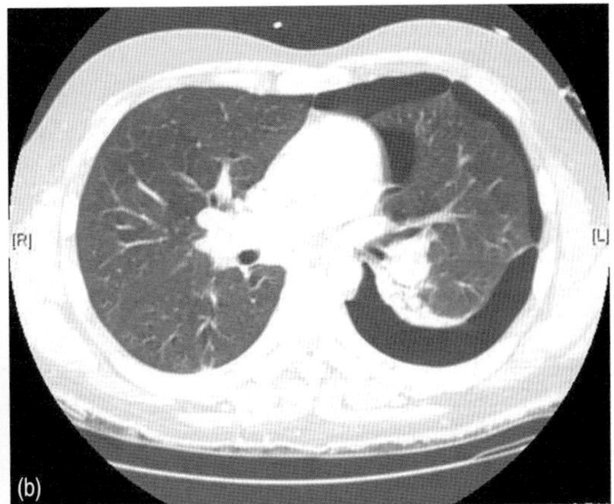

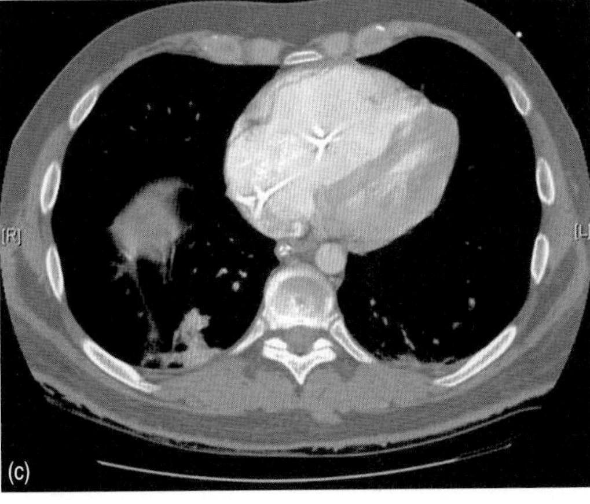

Figure 34.2 Computed tomography (CT) scanning and pulmonary embolism (PE). Three CT images from the same patient demonstrating the ability of CT to detect pulmonary emboli, assess severity and confirm additional diagnoses. (a) (mediastinal window): filling defects in the right pulmonary artery and inferior branch of the left pulmonary artery. A pulmonary artery catheter is also in situ. (b) (lung window): a left pneumothorax with pleural adhesions, and a small area of left-sided posterior consolidation. (c) (mediastinal window): dilatation of the right ventricle relative to the left ventricle.

impairment, anaphylaxis to intravenous contrast or pregnancy).[20] *V/Q* scanning also allows quantification of regional blood flow within the lungs, which may be required in the assessment of chronic pulmonary venous embolism.

PE may also be diagnosed by gadolinium-enhanced magnetic resonance pulmonary angiography (MRA). In some series as many as 25% of examinations have been regarded as non-interpretable.[21]

ECHOCARDIOGRAPHY

Because of its portability, echocardiography has the greatest usefulness in critically ill patients with probable PE. Many patients with PE have an echocardiographic abnormality, the most common being RV dilatation, RV hypokinesis, paradoxical interventricular septal motion toward the LV, tricuspid regurgitation and pulmonary hypertension. The pattern of RV hypokinesis with apical sparing is considered pathognomonic for PE.[22] The presence of RV dysfunction correlates with mortality.[23] However, it must be noted that a negative echocardiography does not exclude PE.

Transthoracic echocardiography will also allow estimation of pulmonary arterial pressure, identification of intracardiac thrombi (which usually requires surgical embolectomy) and aids in differential diagnosis by excluding aortic dissection and pericardial tamponade. Transoesophageal echocardiography has the additional benefit of directly identifying embolus in the proximal pulmonary arteries, which is common in patients with haemodynamically significant PE.

Echocardiography has its best application in haemodynamically unstable patients, where it can be rapidly brought to the patient. If the patient has RV dilatation and hypokinesis in the right clinical setting, PE is extremely likely.

DIAGNOSIS OF DVT USING ULTRASOUND

Doppler ultrasound has been recommended to search for DVT in the leg veins, from where over 90% of emboli originate. If a leg DVT is confirmed, anticoagulation is required unless the DVT is entirely below the knee, where the associated morbidity is low. Ultrasound is highly accurate in symptomatic or proximal DVT, although in asymptomatic patients ultrasound is much less likely to find DVT, meaning the absence of a DVT does not exclude PE. The best use of ultrasound is when a CTPA scan is contraindicated.[24]

INVESTIGATION STRATEGY IN HAEMODYNAMICALLY STABLE PATIENTS

- A CTPA scan is the preferred initial test and, if positive, the patient should be stratified into high or moderate risk. The presence of clot within pulmonary arteries confirms the diagnosis of PE.
- An echocardiograph should then be considered to assess RV dysfunction for high-risk patients who have:
  - clot within proximal pulmonary arteries
  - raised RV/LV ratio (i.e. >0.9–1.0)
  - raised troponin, BNP or NT-pro-BNP.
- If a CTPA scan is not possible (contraindicated or unavailable), an alternative investigation, such as a *V/Q* scan, MRA or ultrasound should be considered.
- None of these tests excludes PE, but a negative result in a haemodynamically stable patient means that the outcome without anticoagulation is unlikely to be poor.

INVESTIGATION STRATEGY IN HAEMODYNAMICALLY UNSTABLE PATIENTS

- An echocardiograph (preferably transoesophageal) should be the first test performed.
- If the patient has acute RV dilatation and visible embolus, PE is confirmed.
- If there is RV dilatation but no visible embolus, then a CTPA scan is required depending on how unstable the patient is.
- If there is no RV dilatation, the haemodynamic instability is unlikely to be due to PE (although this cannot be excluded completely). Efforts towards finding an alternative diagnosis are the priority.
- If echocardiography is not readily available, a CTPA scan should be performed.

MANAGEMENT

MANAGEMENT PRINCIPLES

Once PE has been confirmed patients at all levels of severity should receive anticoagulation with either unfractionated or low-molecular-weight heparin (LMWH) to prevent further embolisation. In more severe cases of PE, however, the key principle is embolus destruction to maximise a more rapid effect on relief of RV dysfunction. To assist in planning management, it is important to grade the severity of PE. Prediction models based on clinical findings at diagnosis may be useful for the prognostic assessment of patients with acute PE. The Pulmonary Embolism Severity Index is the most extensively validated prognostic clinical score[25] and a simplified version of this has been recently developed.[26] The place of these in critical illness is yet to be determined and it may be that a combination of a predictive scoring system with a diagnostic test is the most useful.[27]

MASSIVE PE (HAEMODYNAMICALLY UNSTABLE)

Patients with PE and hypotension have an approximately 30% mortality rate despite treatment.[1] If cardiopulmonary resuscitation is required, this increases to

65%. These patients have the most to benefit from a strategy that includes attempts at urgent embolus destruction (with thrombolytic therapy or embolectomy), concurrent haemodynamic support and prevention of further embolisation.

SUBMASSIVE PE (HAEMODYNAMICALLY UNSTABLE WITH EVIDENCE OF RV DYSFUNCTION)

Patients with PE and evidence of RV dysfunction have higher mortality (around 15%) and recurrence rates than those with normal RV function.[23] They also develop shock and RV thrombi more frequently. These patients require prevention of further embolisation but also warrant strong consideration of embolus destruction using thrombolytic therapy. Thrombolytic drugs appear to improve outcomes,[28] although this appears to be at the expense of a higher bleeding risk.[29] The presence of RV dysfunction (to meet the submassive classification) can be confirmed using echocardiogram but can also be inferred from evidence of RV dilatation on CTPA scanning or by raised troponin, BNP and NT-pro-BNP, all of which have been shown to predict higher mortality.[30]

MILD PE (HAEMODYNAMICALLY STABLE WITH NO RV DYSFUNCTION)

Patients with PE who have normal blood pressure and normal RV function (determined by echocardiography or CTPA scan) have a low risk of death or recurrence. The predominant management goal is prevention of further embolisation using anticoagulant therapy, as treatment focused on embolus destruction is unlikely to confer additional benefits.

In summary, the major principles of management are therefore:

- prevention of further embolisation (for all of massive, submassive and mild PE)
- embolus destruction (for massive and submassive PE)
- concurrent haemodynamic support (only required in massive PE).

A suggested management strategy is outlined in Figure 34.1.

PREVENTION OF FURTHER EMBOLISATION

ANTICOAGULANT THERAPY

Heparin has been known to prevent recurrence and reduce the mortality from PE for over 40 years. LMWHs are as effective and safe as unfractionated heparin[31] and may even be better.[32] LMWHs offer several advantages over unfractionated heparin, including a longer half-life, increased bioavailability, a more predictable dose-response and fewer requirements for monitoring and dose adjustments. They should be readily used in the stable patient with PE.

Table 34.1 Weight-based dosing of intravenous heparin

INITIAL DOSING			
Loading 80 units/kg			
Maintenance infusion 18 units/kg per hour			
Perform APTT in 6 hours			
SUBSEQUENT DOSE ADJUSTMENTS			
APTT	DOSE CHANGE (UNITS/KG PER HOUR)	ADDITIONAL ACTION	NEXT APTT
<35 seconds	+4	Rebolus of 80 units/kg	6 hours
35–45 seconds	+2	Rebolus of 40 units/kg	6 hours
46–70 seconds	Nil	Nothing	6 hours
71–90 seconds	−2	Nothing	6 hours
>90 seconds	−3	Stop infusion for 1 hour	6 hours

Adapted from Raschke et al.[33]
APTT = activated partial thromboplastin time.

Unfractionated heparin should be used in patients with renal impairment, and following thrombolytic therapy or embolectomy, as it can be easily and rapidly reversed. Intravenous unfractionated heparin should be administered after a bolus and initial monitoring should be with 6-hourly activated partial thromboplastin time (APTT) testing. Since subtherapeutic levels of anticoagulant therapy increase the risk of recurrence, it is important to achieve therapeutic heparinisation rapidly. Weight-based dosing of heparin should be used as target anticoagulation levels are reached sooner[33] (**Table 34.1**).

The predominant complications of both unfractionated heparin and LMWHs are bleeding related. These include bleeding peptic ulcer, stroke, retroperitoneal haematoma and postsurgical wound haemorrhage. Heparin-induced thrombotic thrombocytopenia syndrome (HITTS) can also occur. Bleeding complications and HITTS appear to be less common when LMWHs are being used. A number of conditions are considered to be relative contraindications to anticoagulant therapy. These include active peptic ulceration, recent surgery, recent trauma and recent cerebral haemorrhage. In each individual patient the risk-to-benefit ratio (taking into account the severity of the PE) should be considered before anticoagulation is withheld from the patient.

Oral anticoagulants should be started as soon as possible so that LMWH or unfractionated heparin can eventually be ceased. For warfarin, this is generally when the international normalised ratio is >2.0. Although warfarin has been commonly used as the long-standing anticoagulant of choice, adverse events leading to hospitalisation remain common.[34] New oral anticoagulants, including rivaroxaban (which competitively binds activated factor X) and dabigatran (a direct inhibitor of thrombin) have been developed.[35,36] These drugs have more rapid onset of action and more predictable anticoagulant effects meaning fixed dosages and no routine laboratory coagulation monitoring. Large studies have found that rivaroxaban is non-inferior to a LMWH/warfarin combination[37] and dabigatran is non-inferior to warfarin.[38] The place of these drugs in critically ill patients with PE remains unknown.

INFERIOR VENA CAVA FILTER

Inferior vena caval (IVC) filters are another method used to prevent further embolisation. They may also be useful as primary prevention, although safety and efficacy have not been firmly established. IVC filters are indicated for patients in whom anticoagulation is contraindicated and those who experience recurrent PE despite adequate anticoagulation.[39] They may have a role in patients with massive or submassive PE who have undergone open surgical embolectomy or thrombolysis. Insertion is usually performed percutaneously in a radiology department, but it can be done at the bedside. They lower early recurrence rates but increase long-term DVT recurrence rates.[40] Newer retrievable designs may be more efficacious and more safe if removed at the appropriate time.

Absolute indications include:

- new or recurrent PE despite anticoagulation
- contraindications to anticoagulation
- complications resulting from anticoagulation.

Other recommended indications include:

- patients with extensive DVT
- patients following a surgical embolectomy
- patients following thrombolytic therapy.

EMBOLUS DESTRUCTION

THROMBOLYTIC THERAPY

Intravenous thrombolytic drugs result in dramatic and immediate haemodynamic improvement in some patients by dissolving the embolus and rapidly reducing pulmonary arterial obstruction. Experimental studies, clinical observations and randomised trials have consistently demonstrated the favourable effects of thrombolytic therapy on angiographic, haemodynamic and scintigraphic parameters of patients with acute PE, although comparisons with patients who received heparin have essentially revealed similar degrees of embolus resolution after a few days to a week.

A large multicentre patient registry found that patients receiving thrombolytic therapy (clearly on an ad hoc basis) for PE had lower rates of mortality and recurrence than patients receiving heparin.[41] Despite this, no randomised study has demonstrated that thrombolytic therapy improves survival over standard anticoagulation, most likely because studies have been underpowered. A meta-analysis found that thrombolytic therapy for PE was associated with a non-significant reduction in recurrent PE or death when compared with heparin.[29] A significant survival benefit in favour of thrombolytic therapy was demonstrable when analysis was restricted to those studies that included massive PE.

It is therefore recommended that once the diagnosis has been confirmed thrombolytic therapy should be given without delay to patients with massive PE unless there is a clear contraindication.[42] Around 90% of patients should respond to thrombolytic therapy.[43] The clinical benefits and relative underuse of this therapy have been recently highlighted using non-randomised data.[44]

There is also justification for the use of thrombolytic therapy in patients with submassive PE as a randomised study found a significant reduction in the requirement for emergency escalation of treatment, although without an effect on survival.[28] It would also seem appropriate to give thrombolytic therapy to patients with demonstrable intracardiac thrombus.

There is a large array of thrombolytic drugs with few comparative studies. Although there may be slight differences between thrombolytic drugs, the choice of drug is less important than the choice to give thrombolytic therapy at all. Suggested doses are recommended in **Table 34.2**, and this can be administered through either a peripheral or a central venous catheter. In contrast to acute myocardial infarction, thrombolytic therapy may be useful in PE when given up to 14 days after symptoms begin.[45] Once the thrombolytic therapy has been administered, heparin should be commenced.

Haemorrhagic complications are not uncommon and can significantly affect patient morbidity; however it is difficult to predict those patients who are at the highest risk for bleeding. Major clinically significant bleeding can occur in up to 10% of patients, although cerebral haemorrhage is fortunately uncommon

Table 34.2 Recommended doses of thrombolytic drugs for pulmonary embolism

Urokinase	4400 units/kg bolus (over 10 minutes) followed by 4400 units/kg per hour for 12 hours
Streptokinase	250 000 unit bolus (over 15 minutes) followed by 100 000 units/hour for 24 hours
Alteplase	10 mg bolus followed by 90 mg over 2 hours
Reteplase	10 unit boluses 30 minutes apart

(0.9%).[46] Recent surgery is not an absolute contraindication and patients should have their individualised risks and the benefits weighed up; in shocked patients with massive PE the balance appears to be in favour of thrombolytic therapy for almost all patients.

If bleeding occurs, the thrombolytic therapy should be ceased, fresh frozen plasma should be given to replace coagulation factors and an antifibrinolytic drug (such as aprotinin) should be commenced.

SURGICAL EMBOLECTOMY

The merit of surgical pulmonary embolectomy, which has traditionally been seen as a life-saving option for moribund patients with massive PE, has been questioned since the advent of reliable thrombolytic therapy. Embolectomy surgery results vary widely and there has traditionally been an associated perioperative mortality of 25–50%. There is little reliable evidence comparing embolectomy and thrombolytic therapy. Mortality rates have been found to be lower when using a surgical approach combining rapid diagnosis, prompt surgical intervention and a high frequency of concurrent IVC filter placement.[47]

Surgical embolectomy should therefore be strongly considered in patients with PE and hypotension who have absolute contraindications to thrombolytic therapy, or if thrombolytic therapy has failed.[42] It may also be useful when patients have free-floating intracardiac thrombus.

PERCUTANEOUS EMBOLECTOMY

Percutaneous pulmonary embolectomy methods include either embolus extraction techniques (pure percutaneous embolectomy) or embolus disruption techniques (including catheter-directed thrombolytic therapy and percutaneous thrombus fragmentation techniques).[48] Success rates have been over 80% with reasonable complication rates, mostly from single-centre case series.[49] Randomised studies comparing percutaneous embolectomy with systemic thrombolytic therapy or systemic anticoagulation have not been done, so for now percutaneous embolectomy should be considered in patients with contraindications to systemic thrombolytic therapy who are in specialised centres.

CONCURRENT HAEMODYNAMIC SUPPORT

Shocked patients with PE (massive PE) need urgent haemodynamic support in addition to attempts at embolus destruction and prevention of further embolisation.

INTRAVENOUS FLUIDS

Volume loading can improve haemodynamic status in patients with massive PE, although if excessive then fluid therapy may worsen RV function, which can in turn affect LV function and become detrimental.[50] Cautious administration of small amounts of intravenous fluid should occur.

VASOPRESSORS

Ischaemia in the coronary circulation is an important factor in the haemodynamic instability of massive PE.[4] Embolus destruction (with thrombolytic therapy or embolectomy) should have the greatest effect on ischaemia reduction. However, elevation of the blood pressure and reduction in pulmonary and RV pressures may also be helpful, based on the rationale that the RV coronary perfusion pressure (RVCPP) can be severely impaired in massive PE.

RVCPP is estimated by the formula:

$$\mathrm{RVCPP} = \mathrm{MAP} - \mathrm{RVPm} \qquad (34.1)$$

where MAP is the mean arterial pressure and RVPm is the mean RV pressure, all in mmHg.

RVPm can then be estimated by the formula:

$$\mathrm{RVPm} = \mathrm{CVP} + 1/3\,(\mathrm{PAPs} - \mathrm{CVP}) \qquad (34.2)$$

where CVP is the central venous pressure and PAPs is the systolic pulmonary arterial pressure, all in mmHg.

When RVCPP falls as low as 30 mmHg (4 kPa) (normal being around 70–80 mmHg (9.31–10.64 kPa)), RV myocardial blood flow falls substantially and this contributes significantly to severe RV failure and shock. Efforts to elevate the MAP or reduce the PAPs should increase the RVCPP and therefore improve coronary blood flow to relieve ischaemia. Haemodynamic support for the shock state due to massive PE should therefore predominantly involve vasopressor drugs as these will predominantly increase MAP, and therefore RVCPP.

Norepinephrine (noradrenaline) is preferred to a pure alpha agonist such as phenylephrine, as cardiac output and RV myocardial blood flow effects are greater owing to the added beta-adrenoceptor agonist action. Dopamine, epinephrine (adrenaline) and vasopressin are reasonable alternatives to norepinephrine.

Although systemic vasodilators might improve the cardiac output in massive PE, they may be harmful overall as the MAP will either fall or remain constant at best and therefore the RVCPP will not increase. Isoprenaline, dobutamine, nitroglycerin, nitroprusside or milrinone should be considered only if the MAP is adequate and treatment is focused on cardiac output or pulmonary artery pressure.

Extracorporeal membrane oxygenation (ECMO) is an extreme but alternative form of mechanical assistance that may be available in more specialised institutions.[51] It should be considered for patients with PE who have had cardiopulmonary arrest or have very severe shock.

SELECTIVE PULMONARY VASODILATORS

Inhaled nitric oxide may be useful in patients with massive PE[51] by selectively decreasing pulmonary arterial pressure with minimal effect on systemic haemodynamics. It may also assist in the severely hypoxaemic patient. Inhaled prostacyclin is an alternative.[52]

OTHER MANAGEMENT ISSUES

Oxygen should be supplemented to target adequate oxygen saturation. High flows may be required because of hyperventilation and the increased dead space. Intubation and mechanical ventilation are often necessary in patients with massive PE.

If chest pain is prominent, morphine should be administered. To guide resuscitation, it is useful to have at least a central venous catheter, particularly before thrombolytic therapy is given. Although there is increased risk of bleeding owing to the concurrent administration of thrombolytic therapy and/or anticoagulant therapy in these patients, this is probably outweighed by the importance of secure venous access and monitoring of the circulation in patients with haemodynamic compromise due to PE.

PREVENTION

Prophylaxis is probably the most important management aspect of VTE. All ICU patients should have an adequate assessment as to whether prophylaxis is warranted, although most should receive it using pharmacological thromboprophylaxis.[39] Careful attention to the intervention and dose is required, as omission of prophylaxis[53] and failure of prophylaxis[54] are common.

LMWHs have challenged traditional prophylaxis with fixed low-dose subcutaneous unfractionated heparin such that both are suggested alternatives for the prevention of VTE in critically ill patients.[39] Both therapies seem comparable for prophylaxis of DVT; however, rates of PE and HITTS were lower in a recent large study.[55]

Mechanical approaches (including graduated-compression stockings and intermittent pneumatic compression devices)[56] seem best utilised in patients who are bleeding or at major risk of bleeding. When bleeding risk decreases, pharmacological thromboprophylaxis should be commenced.

Access the complete references list online at http://www.expertconsult.com

23. Konstantinides S, Goldhaber SZ. Pulmonary embolism: risk assessment and management. Eur Heart J 2012;33(24):3014–22. doi: 10.1093/eurheartj/ehs258. Epub 2012 Sep 7.
28. Konstantinides S, Geibel A, Heusel G, et al. Heparin plus alteplase compared with heparin alone in patients with submassive pulmonary embolism. N Engl J Med 2002;347(15):1143–50.
29. Wan S, Quinlan DJ, Agnelli G, et al. Thrombolysis compared with heparin for the initial treatment of pulmonary embolism: a meta-analysis of the randomized controlled trials. Circulation 2004;110(6):744–9.
39. Kahn SR, Lim W, Dunn AS, et al. Prevention of VTE in nonsurgical patients: Antithrombotic Therapy and Prevention of Thrombosis, 9th ed: American College of Chest Physicians Evidence-Based Clinical Practice Guidelines. Chest 2012;141(2 Suppl):e195S–226S.
42. Kearon C, Akl EA, Comerota AJ, et al. Antithrombotic therapy for VTE disease: Antithrombotic Therapy and Prevention of Thrombosis, 9th ed: American College of Chest Physicians Evidence-Based Clinical Practice Guidelines. Chest 2012;141(2 Suppl):e419S–94S.
44. Stein PD, Matta F. Thrombolytic therapy in unstable patients with acute pulmonary embolism: saves lives but underused. Am J Med 2012;125(5):465–70.
55. Cook D, Meade M, Guyatt G, et al. Dalteparin versus unfractionated heparin in critically ill patients. N Engl J Med 2011;364(14):1305–14.

35

Acute severe asthma

David V Tuxen and Matthew T Naughton

Acute severe asthma is a medical emergency associated with a significant morbidity and mortality. Many of the adverse outcomes are attributed to underestimation of severity with delayed and/or inadequate treatment[1-3] and are potentially preventable.

The worldwide prevalence of asthma varies widely (2–37 % in children),[4] but is increasing worldwide[5-7] with life-threatening episodes affecting an estimated 0.5% of asthmatics per year.[8] Australia, New Zealand and UK have amongst the highest incidences.[6,7] In Australia, 9% have asthma as a long-term condition[9] and up to 40% of children have asthma symptoms at some time.[5] Although the prevalence of asthma is increasing, many countries have achieved reductions hospital presentations and admissions,[10,11] reduced intensive care admissions and reduced overall asthma mortality.[10,11] Improved community management of asthma,[1,2] more widespread use of inhaled corticosteroids[3] and other preventative measures such as action plans have been given the credit for these improvements. Improved intensive care asthma management has resulted in less requirement for mechanical ventilation and decreasing mechanical ventilation mortality (**Fig. 35.1**).[10,11] These changes have resulted in the group of asthma patients who require mechanical ventilation having more severe asthma, that is more refractory to treatment and more difficult to manage.[12,13] Despite reducing admissions, significant and potentially preventable mortality continues to occur in those patients who do require intensive care or mechanical ventilation[12,14,15]

CLINICAL DEFINITION

Asthma has been defined as a lung disease with the following characteristics[16]: (i) airway obstruction that is reversible (completely or partially) either spontaneously or with treatment, (ii) airway inflammation, and (iii) increased airway responsiveness to a variety of stimuli. Exacerbations of asthma are characterised by increasing dyspnoea, cough, wheeze, chest tightness and decreased expiratory air flow. Status asthmaticus has had varying definitions. However, for practical purposes, any patient not responding to initial doses of nebulised bronchodilators should be considered to have status asthmaticus.[17]

'Difficult' (as opposed to 'severe') asthma is another term in which patients can present with mild, moderate or severe asthmatic symptoms. Characterisations can include: (a) discordance between symptoms and objective markers of asthma such as lung function or arterial blood gases, (b) severe asthma despite treatment that should be effective, (c) a disconnection between patient expectations and effective outcomes.[18] Commonly, there is poor compliance, psychosocial adversity and secondary gain with continued symptoms. Significant anxiety, social and adverse family circumstances frequently coexist. Differential diagnoses include hyperventilation syndromes, vocal cord dysfunction, COPD or lack of adherence to treatments (estimated to occur in two-thirds of patients presenting). An alternative description includes poor perceivers or over-reactors. These patients are difficult because sometimes they present with severe life-threatening asthma, yet experience would suggest this to be preventable if the usual medication were taken.

AETIOLOGY

The pathogenesis of asthma is complex with both genetic and environmental influences. The increase in asthma prevalence has been attributed to the 'hygiene hypothesis',[19] which suggests that reduced exposure to childhood infections as a result of antibiotics and hygienic lifestyle promotes an imbalance in T-cell phenotype leading to inflammatory cytokine overproduction. IgE-dependent mechanisms appear to be particularly important in generating the characteristic state of airway inflammation and bronchial hyperreactivity with the allergens in the local environment dictating the specificity of the antibody response.[20] Triggers of acute asthma can be non-specific (cold air, exercise, atmospheric pollutants), specific allergens (housemite, pollen, animal danders), modifiers of airway control (aspirin, beta blockers), or stress or emotion. No precipitant can be identified in over 30% of patients.

A wide range of risk factors for life-threatening asthmatic episodes and/or the need for mechanical ventilation are now recognised. First is *underestimation of severity*, with delayed and/or inadequate treatment by managing doctors and/or the patient.[1-3] Secondly, *patient behaviour factors* that are associated with the

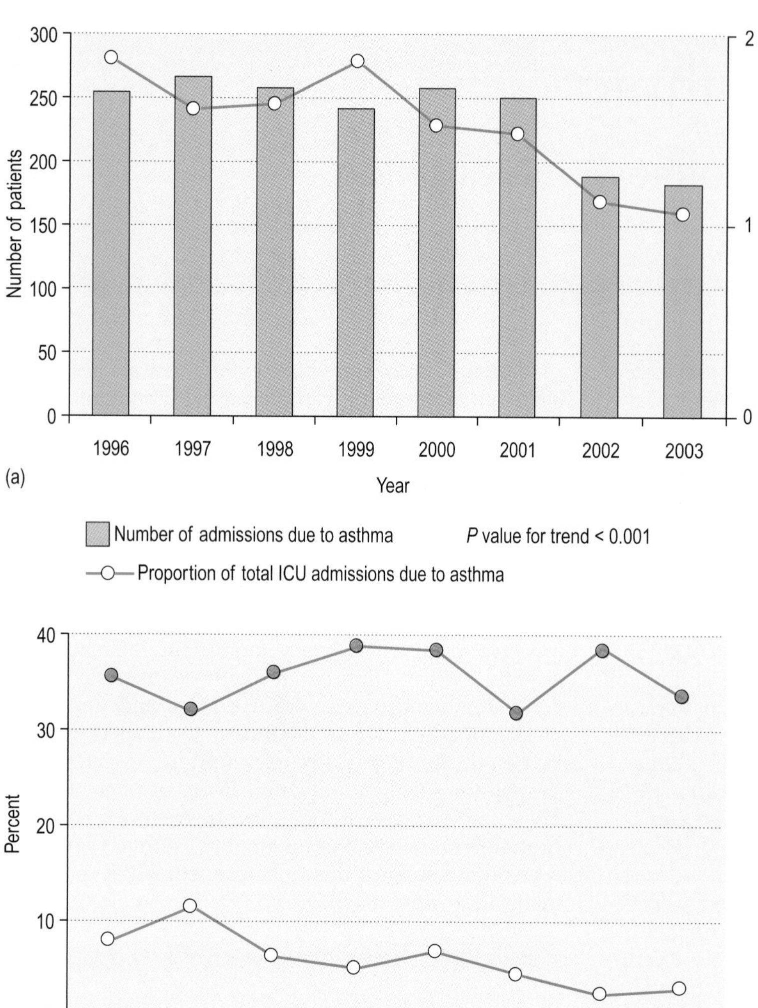

Figure 35.1 ICU admissions, mechanical ventilation and mortality due to asthma in Australia from 1996 to 2003. *(Modified from Stow P, Pilcher D, Wilson J, et al.[10])*

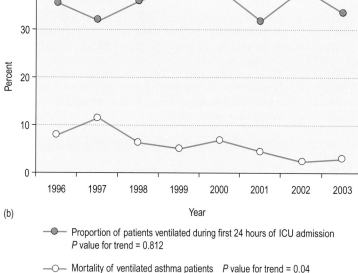

requirement for mechanical ventilation are smoking (and illicit drugs), poor treatment compliance, prior treatment with beta agonists without inhaled steroids.[12,21] Low socioeconomic status has also been recognised as a risk factor. Thirdly, *genetic polymorphism* (the IL4RA*576R allele) is now recognised as a significant factor related to fatal or near-fatal asthma attacks.[13,22] Other functional factors linked to severe asthma attacks include airway remodelling, down-regulation of β-receptors, and lack of steroid responsiveness.[13] Diminished perception of dyspnoea in some patients with acute severe asthma leads to delayed interventions.[13,23]

PATHOPHYSIOLOGY

The post-mortem airway pathology of patients who die from acute asthma includes bronchial wall thickening from oedema and inflammatory cell infiltrate, hypertrophy and hyperplasia of bronchial smooth muscle and submucosal glands, deposition of collagen beneath the epithelial basement membrane and prominent intraluminal secretions. These secretions may narrow or occlude the small airways, and post-mortem studies frequently report extensive plugging and atelectasis.[24,25] When interpreting the latter findings it is important to remember that during life in very severe asthma the lungs are hyperinflated to close to total lung capacity (TLC) by maximal inspiratory effort and to beyond TLC during mechanical ventilation. At this time radiological atelectasis is rare, suggesting that most airways are communicating at these high lung volumes, even if airways are very narrowed. Only at death does the prolonged apnoea allow lung deflation, widespread airway closure and alveolar gas absorption to give the post-mortem appearance of extensive complete occlusion that was not present to the same degree during life.

In some deaths bronchial mucus is absent; in these cases airway obstruction may be mainly due to intense smooth bronchoconstriction. This observation may account for two patterns of progression of asthma:

1. Acute severe asthma is the more common group (80–90%), with progression of symptoms over many hours or days, often with a background of poor control and recurrent presentations. Most patients in this group are female, with upper respiratory infections are frequent triggers; it responds more slowly to treatment, which may reflect greater contribution from mucous inspissation and chronic bronchial wall inflammation with eosinophilia.[23,26]
2. 'Hyperacute', 'fulminating', 'asphyxic' or 'sudden onset' severe asthma is where the interval between onset of symptoms and intubation is less than 3 hours.[23,26–28] This presentation is less common (approximately 10–20% of life threatening presentations), tends to occur in younger patients with relatively normal lung function but high bronchial reactivity, and the majority of patients are male. Massive respiratory allergen exposure, cold air or exercise and psychosocial stress are the most frequent triggers.[23] This group characteristically has neutrophilic inflammation, typically responds quickly to bronchodilators and is thought to be mainly due to bronchial smooth muscle contraction.

The characteristic pathology of asthma leads to increased airway resistance and dynamic pulmonary hyperinflation. This has a number of consequences:

- *Increased work of breathing* results from increased airway resistance and reduced pulmonary compliance as a result of high lung volumes. When asthma is severe, dynamic hyperinflation may bring the lung volume close to total lung capacity.[29] This causes a severe mechanical disadvantage of inspiratory muscles with diaphragm flattening and results in a large inspiratory muscle effort affecting a small change in inspiratory pressure. The final outcome can be respiratory muscle failure with insufficient alveolar ventilation and consequent hypercapnia.[30]
- *Ventilation–perfusion mismatch* is the result of airway narrowing and closure. This leads to impaired gas exchange and increases the minute ventilation requirement, further adding to the work of breathing.[30]
- *Adverse cardiopulmonary interactions* are seen when the marked changes in lung volume and pleural pressure impact on the function of both left and right ventricles.[31,32] Spontaneous breathing during acute asthma can generate inspiratory pressures as low as -35 cmH_2O.[31,32] This increases venous return to the right ventricle (RV) and increases RV volume during inspiration. However, increased RV afterload as a result of hypoxic pulmonary vasoconstriction, acidosis and increased lung volume[31,32] and increased pulmonary capacitance decrease return to the left ventricle (LV). These negative intrapleural pressures also cause increased LV afterload[31,32] and increased RV afterload with septal shift reduces LV volume[31,32] further reducing LV output during inspiration. Pulsus paradoxus is the most direct result of these cardiopulmonary interactions in severe asthma. This is a decrease in systolic blood pressure during inspiration of >10 mmHg (1.33 kPa), typically 15–25 mmHg (2–3.33kPa), normal ≤5 mmHg (0.66kPa). The degree of pulsus paradoxus may not correlate with the severity of asthma as it may be reduced by inspiratory muscle weakness or fatigue.

CLINICAL FEATURES AND ASSESSMENT OF SEVERITY

The symptoms of asthma are well known and include wheeze, cough, dyspnoea, and chest discomfort or tightness. Triage and assessment of severity of the acute asthma attack are crucial. Underestimation or non-measurement of asthma severity is associated with increased mortality.[33,34] Assessment has two key features: assessment of initial severity and ongoing assessment of response to treatment:

History Any history of prior intubation and mechanical ventilation for asthma is a predictor for life-threatening asthma.[33,34] A history of poor asthma control, multiple recent medical presentations for asthma and poor response to prior treatments are recognised risk factors. Other risk factors are listed above (see Aetiology).

Physical examination The general appearance and level of distress can be an important indicator of severity (**Table 35.1**). Use of accessory muscles, suprasternal retraction, markedly diminished breath sounds or a silent chest, central cyanosis, inability to speak, a disturbance in the level of consciousness, upright posture and diaphoresis all suggest a severe attack.[35] A respiratory rate >30/min, pulse rate >120/min and pulsus paradoxus of >15 mmHg (2 kPa) are associated with severe asthma though their absence does not preclude life-threatening asthma. Patients with diminished perception of dyspnoea may mask severe asthma and lead to underestimation of severity.[13,23]

Ventilatory function tests The patient may not be able to perform these due to breathlessness. However, FEV_1 and peak expiratory flow rate (PEFR) are useful

Table 35.1 Assessment of asthma severity

	MILD	MODERATE	SEVERE
Conscious state	Alert, relaxed	Anxious, difficulty sleeping	Agitated, delirious
Speech	Sentences	Phrases	Words
Accessory muscles	Nil	Mild	Significant sitting upright
Wheeze	Moderate	Loud	Loud or silent
Pulse rate (BPM)	<100	100–120	>120
Peak expiratory flow (% predicted)	>80%	60–80%	<60%
Pa_{CO_2} (mmHg) (kPa)	<45 (5.98)	<45 (5.98)	>45 (5.98)

Pulsus paradoxus when present indicates severe asthma; however, it is an unreliable test.

indicators of severity and response to treatment when done serially. An FEV_1<1.0 litre or PEFR<100 L/min indicates very severe asthma at significant risk of requiring mechanical ventilation. In some patients forced expiration may worsen symptoms; these measurements should cease if this occurs.[36]

Pulse oximetry Pulse oximetry is usually readily available and provides a rapid assessment of oxygenation. It is also very valuable in regulation oxygen therapy, both for avoiding hypoxia (Sp_{O_2}>90%)[37] and for avoiding potential side-effects of hyperoxia (Sp_{O_2}<95%).[38] Of course, pulse oximetry cannot assess arterial P_{CO_2} or acid–base state and so does not replace the need for blood gases.

Arterial blood gases Arterial hypoxaemia is almost invariably present in a patient with severe asthma breathing room air though it usually responds well to low-level oxygen supplementation (28–35%).[37] Blood gases should not delay initiation of treatment, and are not required in mild asthma or moderate asthma that is responding well to treatment. They are very important in severe asthma, or moderate asthma with inadequate treatment response. The Pa_{CO_2} is an important measure of severity and, if hypercapnia is present, an important guide to treatment response.

Ventilation is initially increased in an acute attack leading to hypocapnia and a respiratory alkalosis.[37] As the asthmatic attack worsens, the work of breathing, V/Q mismatch and adverse cardiopulmonary interactions all increase, and the minute ventilation required to maintain the same alveolar ventilation and Pa_{CO_2} increases. Eventually the patient is incapable of meeting this demand and the Pa_{CO_2} rises. The presence of hypercarbic acidosis is associated with a FEV_1 of <20% predicted and reliably indicates that asthma is severe. A metabolic acidosis may also be present, and this is most commonly due to lactic acidosis[39] associated with intravenous or continuous nebulised beta agonists.[40,41]

Chest X-ray Although not generally helpful in assessing severity,[42] a chest X-ray should be performed when asthma is severe or refractory to treatment, when barotrauma or lower respiratory tract infection is suspected or when the diagnosis is in doubt. It is not required in milder attacks that respond well to treatment.

Assessment of treatment response Repeated evaluation of the patient's response to treatment is a valuable tool in assessing severity of acute asthma. The response to the first 2 hours of treatment is an important predictor of outcome.[43] Adverse events are associated with underestimation of severity, inadequate observation after initial assessment and under treatment. Ongoing evaluation of response to therapy is critical. This evaluation should include repeated assessments of: (i) appearance and physical indicators of severity (see Table 35.1); (ii) objective measurements – FEV1 or PEFR, heart rate, respiratory rate, pulsus paradoxus; (iii) Sp_{O_2} and oxygen requirements; (iv) progress of Pa_{CO_2} or metabolic acidosis if present on blood gases.

Admission to intensive care is preferred if the above criteria suggest severe asthma. Indications for immediate admission to intensive care include respiratory arrest, altered mental status, dysrhythmias or associated myocardial ischaemia.

DIFFERENTIAL DIAGNOSIS

The diagnosis of asthma is usually obvious. However, wheeze and dyspnoea may be caused by other illnesses including left ventricular failure, aspiration, upper airway obstruction, inhaled foreign body, pulmonary embolism or hyperventilation syndromes. Wheeze and dyspnoea arising in hospitalised patients who were not admitted with asthma are less likely to be due to asthma. Clues to another or additional diagnosis include: (i) no past history of asthma; (ii) sudden onset following vomiting or food intake; (iii) focal or asymmetrical chest auscultation findings; (iv) risk factors for thromboembolism; (v) onset during hospitalisation when admitted with another condition.

MANAGEMENT

ESTABLISHED TREATMENTS

Initial therapy of acute severe asthma should include the following.

OXYGEN

Hypoxaemia contributes to life-threatening events that complicate acute severe asthma.[44] Humidified supplemental oxygen should be titrated to achieve a Sp_{O_2}>90%. The risk of oxygen-induced increasing hypercapnia with coexisting chronic air-flow limitation or pre-existing chronic hypercapnia is a well-known reason to maintain a lower Sp_{O_2} (eg. 90–92%). This phenomenon was not believed to be relevant to the majority of patients with acute asthma; however, there is now emerging evidence that hyperoxia may be harmful to a more widespread group[45] by releasing pulmonary hypoxic vasoconstriction, worsening V/Q matching and increasing hypercapnia. A recent randomised controlled trial[38] showed a decrease in Pa_{CO_2} in a group receiving 28% O_2 and an increase in Pa_{CO_2} in a group receiving 100% Fi_{O_2}.

BETA AGONISTS

Short-acting beta agonists remain the first-line bronchodilator therapy of choice.[4,46–48] Agents include salbutamol (albuterol), terbutaline, isoproterenol (isoprenaline) and epinephrine (adrenaline). Salbutamol is generally the agent of first choice as it has relative β_2-selectivity, with decreased β_1-mediated cardiac toxicity. Long-acting beta agonists such as salmeterol have no role in status asthmaticus owing to slow onset of action and association with fatalities in this setting.[17] Beta agonists cause bronchodilatation by stimulation of β_2-receptors on airway smooth muscle and may reduce bronchial mucosal oedema.[49]

The standard approach is to start with nebulised salbutamol in high and repeated doses.[50] The typical adult dose is 5–10 mg (in 2.5 to 5.0 mL diluent volume) every 2–4 hours, but more frequent doses with a higher total dose are often required in severe asthma. It should be noted that less than 10% of the nebulised drug reaches the lung even under ideal conditions.[51] Continuous nebulisation appears to be superior to intermittent doses and is commonly used at the beginning of treatment in severe asthma.[17,52] The nebuliser should be driven by oxygen with the flow at 10–12 L/min and a reservoir volume of 2–4 mL so as to produce particles in the desired 1–3 μm range.[53] The total dose should be modulated by response to treatment and the level of toxic side-effects.

Beta agonists can also be delivered by metered dose inhaler (MDI). There are data to suggest that, in non-intubated patients, MDIs combined with a spacing device are as effective as or more effective than nebulisers and are cheaper to use.[54,55] In intubated patients both nebulisers and MDIs have been used effectively.[56] Two-thirds of acutely presenting patients will respond well to inhaled beta agonists[57] irrespective of the method of administration. The remaining one-third are refractory even to high doses and usually require longer periods of intense treatment including multiple other agents.

Intravenous beta agonists remain controversial. There is no clear evidence of benefit[58] and significant side-effects. Despite this, intravenous beta agonists have a theoretical benefit of additional access to lung units with severe air-flow obstruction and poor nebulised drug delivery and some studies have demonstrated improved response when intravenous beta agonist is used.[59] Intravenous beta agonists continue to be considered if the patient is not responding to continuous nebulisation.[60] The typical dose is 5–20 μg/min, but doses >10 μg/min should be used with caution because of side-effects, which should be monitored closely. Salbutamol 100–300 μg may also be given intravenously to non-intubated patients in extremis or delivered down an endotracheal tube should there be no time to gain i.v. access.

Side-effects of beta agonists include tachycardia, dysrhythmias, hypertension, hypotension, tremor, hypokalaemia, worsening of ventilation–perfusion mismatch and hyperglycaemia,[61] but the most common side-effect of parenteral beta agonists occasionally seen with continuous nebulised beta agonists is lactic acidosis. This occurs in over 70% of patients, has an onset within 2–4 hours of commencing an infusion or following a intravenous statim doses, levels may reach 4–12 mmol/L and may significantly add to a respiratory acidosis and respiratory distress.[41,62,63] Parenteral infusions should be initially limited to 10 μg/min and statim doses should not exceed 250 μg. Serum bicarbonate and lactate should be regularly monitored. If lactic acidosis becomes significant, the salbutamol infusion should be reduced or ceased. Lactic acidosis will generally resolve within 4–6 hours of infusion cessation and is seldom a problem with infusions in place for more than 24 hours.

Long-term high-dose beta-agonist use has been associated with increased mortality,[64] but whether high-dose beta agonists are a marker of disease severity, an indicator of suboptimal inhaled steroids or a direct cause of death is unclear. These concerns do not apply in the treatment of the acute asthma attack.

ANTICHOLINERGICS

Anticholinergics cause bronchodilatation by decreasing parasympathetic-mediated cholinergic bronchomotor tone.[65] Ipratropium bromide is the most commonly used anticholinergic for asthma and is a quaternary derivative of atropine. Although some conclude there is insufficient evidence,[66] a number of studies and meta-analyses suggest clear additional benefit and few side-effects when ipratropium bromide is added to the beta-agonist regimen.[67,68] Ipratropium is now widely used as first-line therapy for acute severe asthma in conjunction with beta-agonist therapy. Preservative-induced bronchoconstriction has been reported in a few patients and can be prevented by using preservative-free solutions.[69] The bronchodilatation effect of ipratropium bromide appeared to be maximal with a dose of 250 μg when studied in children between 9 and 17 years of age. The optimal dose is not known in adults; a reasonable regimen would be to add 500 μg of ipratropium bromide to the salbutamol nebuliser every 2- 6 hours; however, initial dose intervals as low as 10–20 minutes have been recommended.[70]

CORTICOSTEROIDS

The role of corticosteroids in the acute asthma attack has been well established. Systemic steroids should be considered in all but mild exacerbations of asthma.[48] Their benefits include increased β-responsiveness of airway smooth muscle, decreased inflammatory cell response and decreased mucus secretion. Early treatment with corticosteroids has been shown to decrease the likelihood of hospitalisation and decrease the mortality rate from acute asthma. Systematic reviews[48,71] suggest that effects commence within 6–12 hours, that oral is as effective as intravenous, and that there is little evidence of benefit for initial daily doses exceeding 800 mg/day of hydrocortisone (160 mg/day methylprednisolone) given in four divided doses.

Inhaled steroids have established long-term benefit and are believed to be a major factor in asthma mortality reduction.[1-3] Although some believe there is insufficient evidence,[66] there are data that inhaled steroids may also have a role during an acute attack[72,73] and it appears reasonable to use them routinely from day one as they may also enable more rapid dose reduction of parenteral steroids, potentially reducing side-effects.

Parenteral corticosteroid dose reductions should commence after 1–3 days according to the severity of the attack, the degree of chronic inflammation and the response to treatment and should be converted to a reducing dose of oral steroids within 4–7 days (e.g. oral prednisolone starting at 40–60 mg per day).

Side-effects of corticosteroids include hyperglycaemia, hypokalaemia, hypertension, acute psychosis and myopathy,[74,75] though they are usually well tolerated acutely. The immunosuppressive effects can increase the risk of infections including *Legionella*, *Pneumocystis carinii* and varicella[76,77] especially when the patient is on long-term corticosteroids. Allergic reactions including anaphylaxis have been reported with the use of most corticosteroid preparations.[78]

AMINOPHYLLINE

There have been conflicting reports regarding the efficacy of aminophylline in acute asthma ranging from no benefit[78] to improved lung function and improved outcome.[79] However, it is accepted that aminophylline is an inferior bronchodilator, with a narrow therapeutic range and frequent side-effects[80] including headache, nausea, vomiting and restlessness, with cardiac arrhythmias and convulsions that can occur at serum levels above 200 μmol/L (40 mg/L).

As a result, aminophylline is not a first-line treatment.[47,48,60,66] Aminophylline may be given to patients with acute asthma who are not showing a favourable response to full treatment with first-line agents. Careful administration and monitoring are required with an initial loading dose of 3 mg/kg (maximum 6 mg/kg, omitted if the patient is already taking oral theophylline) and an infusion of 0.5 mg/kg/h. This should be reduced in patients with cirrhosis, cardiac failure or chronic obstructive airways disease and in patients taking cimetidine, erythromycin or antiviral vaccines. Drug levels should be taken after a loading dose (if given), and then 24 hours later aiming for a level of 30–80 μmol/L (5–12 mg/L). Levels should be repeated daily thereafter until stability has been achieved. The duration should be based on the response to treatment.

NON-ESTABLISHED TREATMENTS

A number of other therapies have reported benefit in acute severe asthma, but their role in addition to full standard therapy has not been clearly established and they are not advocated for routine use. However, these modes of therapy can be considered in the patient who is in extremis or remaining severe despite conventional treatment.

EPINEPHRINE

Epinephrine has some theoretical advantages over pure β_2-agonists in that its additional α-agonist actions of vasoconstriction and mucosal shrinkage may improve airway calibre. However, in practice, nebulised or subcutaneous epinephrine has not been shown to confer any advantage over nebulised β_2-agonists and is not recommended because of its cardiac side-effects.[70] It may be tried in the patient who is failing to respond to conventional treatment. The nebulised dose is 2–4 mg in 2–4 mL (1% solution, 0.05 mL/kg) 1–4-hourly. The subcutaneous dose is 0.2–0.5 mg (0.2–0.5 mL of 1:1000 epinephrine) repeated if necessary 2–3 times at 30-minute intervals. Epinephrine by infusion may avert mechanical ventilation in very severe cases, but should be used with caution with ECG monitoring and preferably with central venous access. An initial i.v. dose of 0.2–1.0 mg (2–10 mL of 1:10 000 epinephrine) is given slowly over 3–5 minutes. This may be followed by a continuous infusion of 1–20 μg/min, which is weaned when the acute attack subsides.[81]

MAGNESIUM SULPHATE

Magnesium sulphate is postulated to block calcium channels, and possibly acetylcholine release at the neuromuscular junction, leading to smooth muscle relaxation and bronchodilatation. It appeared to be well tolerated in early studies, and a number of some prospective randomised, double-blind, prospective trials of adding intravenous or nebulised magnesium sulphate to conventional therapy in adults with acute asthma were performed. Some showed benefit whereas others showed no benefit.

Three meta-analyses[82-84] did not support routine use of magnesium and it is not recommended for acute asthma. If given, recommended doses are 5–10 mmol (1.25–2.5 g, 2.5–5.0 mL of 50% solution) given slowly over 20 minutes, but doses up to 40–80 mmol (10–20 g) have been given.[85] Side-effects include hypotension, flushing, sedation, weakness, areflexia, respiratory depression and cardiac arrhythmias seen at higher serum levels (>5 mmol/dL or 12 mg/dL). Serum concentrations should be measured if repeated or high doses are used.

HELIOX

Inhalation of a helium:oxygen mixture reduces gas density and turbulence with reduced air-flow resistance. The most effective gas mixture is 70% helium (30% oxygen) and the minimum concentration likely to provide benefit is 60% helium. Work of breathing is decreased and pulmonary access of inhaled bronchodilators may be improved.[86,87] Small case-series and reports have suggested benefit from heliox, randomised prospective trials have both positive and negative results.[88,89] Meta-analyses[90,91] have shown trends towards improved aspects of lung function but insufficient evidence to recommend use of heliox in severe asthma. However, it otherwise appears safe and may be tried in critical asthma to avert intubation or during difficult mechanical ventilation provided the patient can tolerate 30–40% O_2.

ANAESTHETIC AGENTS

Ketamine, a dissociative anaesthetic agent, has been used in severe asthma.[92] It may cause bronchodilatation by both sympathomimetic potentiation and a direct effect on airway smooth muscle.[93] Small case-series have suggested some benefit, although a small randomised controlled trial found no benefit with ketamine in the treatment of acute severe asthma[94] – ketamine may be a useful induction agent for endotracheal intubation (dose 1–2 mg/kg) as it may ameliorate the bronchoconstrictor response to intubation. It has been used as a continuous infusion in the dose range of 0.5–2 mg/kg/h[94,95] to treat refractory asthma. Side-effects include increased bronchial secretions, a hyperdynamic cardiovascular response and hallucinations; the hallucinations can be reduced with concomitant benzodiazepines.

The volatile inhalational agents including halothane, isoflurane and enflurane have been used in mechanically ventilated patients with severe asthma.[96] Clinical data are limited to small case-series, and side-effects include direct myocardial depression, arrhythmias and hypotension.[97] The volatile anaesthetic agents should be used with great care and usually only as a prelude to or during invasive ventilation. An anaesthetic machine or custom-fitted ventilator is required for safe administration.

LEUKOTRIENE ANTAGONISTS

Leukotriene antagonists have shown benefit in chronic asthma[98] and there is some evidence of benefit in acute asthma.[99,100] There is insufficient evidence and the benefits were of insufficient magnitude to recommend these agents for acute severe asthma.[66] However, some authors do not exclude them from use in patients refractory to all standard treatments.[101]

BRONCHOALVEOLAR LAVAGE

Bronchoalveolar lavage has been used in severe refractory asthma to clear mucous plugging during mechanical ventilation.[102] It can transiently worsen bronchospasm and hypoxaemia and should be used when air-flow obstruction has stabilised. It may have a role in ventilated patients with resistant mucus impaction, but it is rarely used.

THERAPIES NOT RECOMMENDED

Antibiotics are not routinely indicated[103] unless there is clear evidence of infection. Antihistamines are not effective. Inhaled mucolytics have been shown to have no benefit and may worsen air-flow obstruction. Sedation is unsafe in acute asthma. There is a clear association between their use and avoidable deaths.[104] Patients with severe asthma should not be sedated unless being intubated and ventilated, or in carefully monitored circumstances.

VENTILATION IN ASTHMA

DYNAMIC HYPERINFLATION

In all degrees of air-flow obstruction, slow expiratory air flow results in incomplete exhalation of gas during normal expiratory times. Gas is trapped in the lungs by the arrival of the next breath and the lungs are unable to return their normal passive relaxation volume (functional residual capacity, FRC). Incomplete exhalation of each successive breath causes progressive accumulation of trapped gas called dynamic hyperinflation (DHI, **Fig. 35.2**),[105] which continues until an equilibrium point is reached where the exhaled volume increases to match the inspired volume.[105] This equilibrium occurs because increasing lung volume increases small airway calibre and lung elastic recoil pressure, both of which improve expiratory air flow and allow the inspired tidal volume to be exhaled in the expiratory time available. There are three primary determinants of this equilibrium point: the volume inspired (V_t), the time for expiration (t_e which depends on both the ventilator rate or cycle time and the inspiratory flow or inspiratory time, t_i) and, of course, the severity of air-flow obstruction (the time constant of the lung). The first two determinants are controlled by the ventilator settings and compound to the minute ventilation (V_e) making this the most important determinant of DHI.

Gas trapped at the end of expiration exerts a positive pressure on the alveoli; this pressure is intrinsic positive end-expiratory pressure ($PEEP_i$) or auto-PEEP.[105,106] During expiration, sequential closure of the most severely obstructed airways occurs with only the less obstructed airways remaining in communication with

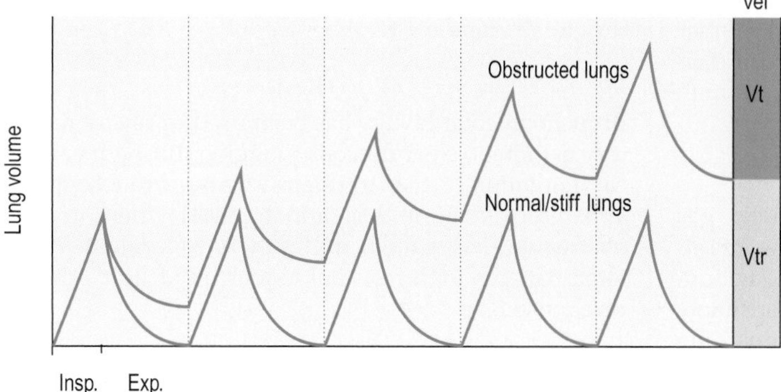

Figure 35.2 Dynamic hyperinflation. The volume history of normal or acutely injured lungs compared with that of obstructed lungs when commenced on controlled mechanical ventilation. This shows initial lung volume to be at the passive relaxation volume of the respiratory system or functional residual capacity (FRC).

the central airway at the end of tidal expiration.[107] As a consequence, measured $PEEP_i$ underestimates the true magnitude of $PEEP_i$ and is recognised as being insensitive to changes in severity.[107]

In mild air-flow obstruction, this process is adaptive as it allows the desired minute ventilation, which could not be achieved at FRC, to be achieved at a higher lung volume (**Fig. 35.3**, mild AO'). As asthma becomes more severe (Fig. 35.3, 'mod AO') the static FRC that would be reached with a long expiratory time is elevated above the normal FRC by airway closure (static hyperinflation) and DHI further increases lung volume to a level where work of breathing is increased by lower lung compliance and respiratory muscles become less efficient from shortening and mechanical disadvantage. At this level some degree of dyspnoea is expected. When asthma is severe enough to risk requiring mechanical ventilation, static hyperinflation may increase FRC by 50%[108] and very little DHI is required to reach total lung capacity (Fig. 35.3, 'severe AO'). In this circumstance, the minute ventilation required to maintain normocapnia would cause hyperinflation beyond normal total lung capacity. During spontaneous ventilation, the patient with severe asthma is unable to exceed total lung capacity (Fig. 35.3), has a much lower maximum minute ventilation capacity and as a result must become hypercapnic even at maximum respiratory effort with no fatigue.[17] When mechanical ventilation is commenced, increased tidal volume and rate delivery is easily able to increase minute ventilation and DHI well beyond normal total lung capacity (Fig. 35.3).[105] The consequences of this are commonly hypotension (due to increased intrathoracic pressure and decreased venous return) and barotrauma.[29,105,108,109]

NON-INVASIVE VENTILATION (NIV)

Non-invasive ventilation (NIV) has been widely used for a variety of respiratory problems.[110] In severe asthma there are a number of potential benefits. Externally applied PEEP may help overcome $PEEP_i$ due to gas trapping and thus reduce the inspiratory threshold work of breathing. Augmentation of inspiration with NIV may further decrease the work of inspiration and increase tidal volume and minute ventilation. If tidal volume is increased with a shorter inspiratory time, then increased minute ventilation can occur without a proportional increase in dynamic hyperinflation. Both inspiratory augmentation and PEEP may facilitate airspace opening, thus reducing V/Q mismatch.[111,112]

The role of NIV is well established in chronic obstructive pulmonary disease where a number of randomised trials have shown benefit.[113,114] Although there have been no large randomised trials in acute asthma, there is increasing evidence of benefit from NIV for this indication with all studies reporting positive outcome.[115,116] Non-randomised studies have reported improvements in respiratory acidosis and respiratory rate following the introduction of NIV, and low requirements for invasive ventilation. In small prospectively randomised studies of acute asthma, Sokorovski et al[116] showed better lung function and decreased hospitalisation rate and Gupta et al[117] found accelerated the improvement in lung function, decreased inhaled bronchodilator requirement, and shortened ICU and hospital stay. In a retrospective cohort study, Murase et al[118] found that NIV reduced the rate of endotracheal intubation from 18% (9/50) to 3.5% (2/57, p=0.01).

There have been multiple reviews of NIV for acute severe asthma.[119–122] All concluded there is limited evidence for some benefits, insufficient data to be conclusive and that larger trials are needed. Where opinions were given, all recommended use if NIV in selected patients with asthma.[120–122] A trial of NIV in patients with acute severe asthma and risk of respiratory decompensation is now warranted in patients who are cooperative and can tolerate the facemask. Indications for use are: (i) moderate to severe dyspnoea or respiratory distress, (ii) hypercapnic acidosis, and (iii) respiratory rate >25, accessory muscle use or paradoxical breathing.[112] Contraindications to NIV include cardiac or respiratory arrest, a decreased conscious state, severe upper gastrointestinal bleeding, haemodynamic instability, facial trauma or surgery, inability to protect the airway and clear secretions and high risk of aspiration.[111]

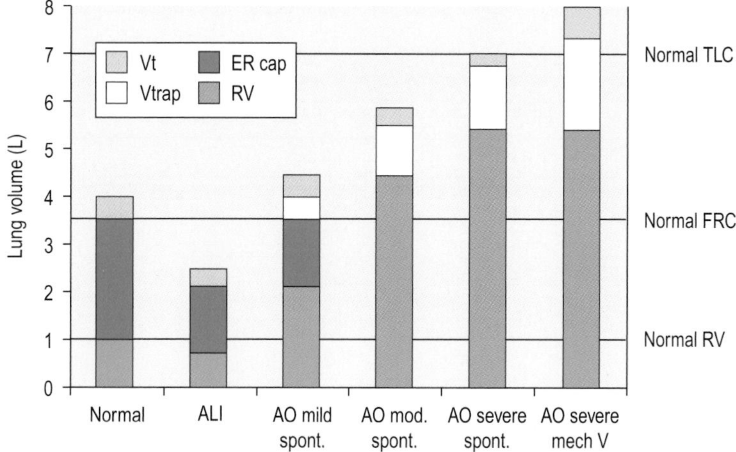

Figure 35.3 Comparison of lung volumes in patients with normal lungs, acute lung injury (ALI), and mild, moderate and severe air-flow obstruction (AO). Severe AO is shown during both spontaneous ventilation (Spont) and mechanical ventilation (Mech V). TLC=total lung capacity. Functional residual capacity (FRC) is the static lung volume at the end of expiratory flow (60-90 seconds in severe AO). Expiratory reserve capacity (ER Cap) is the additional gas expired with expiratory effort after FRC has been reached. Residual volume (RV) is the minimum lung volume possible after prolonged expiration and maximum expiratory effort. V_{trap} is the gas trapped by dynamic hyperinflation during tidal ventilation.

Nasal masks are usually not suitable in acute respiratory failure and facemasks of full-face masks fitted to achieve comfort and a reliable seal are usually best.

NIV should be commenced with 5 cmH_2O CPAP (expiratory positive airway pressure, EPAP 5 cmH_2O) and 8–10 cmH_2O pressure support (inspiratory positive airway pressure IPAP 13–15 cmH_2O). The aim is a respiratory rate <25 breaths/minute and an exhaled tidal volume of 7 mL/kg. CPAP may be increased to 7 or 10 cmH_2O if there is difficulty initiating inspiration, or pressure support may be increased if tidal volume is low or respiratory rate remains high. It is not possible to reliably achieve total pressures (IPAP) >20 cmH_2O. NIV should be undertaken in an area familiar with its use and where close observation is available.

Complications of NIV include nasal bridge ulceration, mask discomfort, nasal congestion, gastric insufflation, aspiration, hypotension and pneumothorax.[112] However, hypotension and pneumothorax are uncommon compared with their risk during mechanical ventilation.

INVASIVE VENTILATION

Invasive mechanical ventilation in acute severe asthma may be life saving, but can be associated with significant morbidity and mortality[108] (**Table 35.2**). Institution of invasive ventilation with endotracheal intubation carries the risk of inadvertent pulmonary hyperinflation[105,106,108] and potential aggravation of bronchospasm and a significant part of the morbidity and mortality has been attributed to pulmonary hyperinflation.[105,106,108] Despite these risks, the incidence of mechanical ventilation for asthma is decreasing and mortality of patients ventilated for asthma is also decreasing in some series[10,11] (see Fig. 35.1, Table 35.2).

The decision to intubate depends on both the clinical status of the patient and the natural history of the type of asthma present. Hyperacute asthma may present with marked hypercapnia (Pa_{CO_2} > 60 mmHg (7.98 kPa)) due to mechanical limitations of ventilation as a result of dynamic hyperinflation. Such patients may not initially be fatigued and may respond rapidly to treatment, thereby avoiding mechanical ventilation. Acute severe asthma that has been progressing for days may have less hypercapnia but will often respond poorly to treatment. The Pa_{CO_2} may rise despite maximal treatment owing to fatigue and the patient may require intubation at a lower Pa_{CO_2}. The general principles are to use NIV early but to avoid mechanical ventilation if safe to do so.

The decision to intubate is based primarily on the degree of respiratory distress as assessed by an experienced clinician and the patient themselves. A patient with a high Pa_{CO_2} (e.g. >70 mmHg (9.31 kPa)) who is dyspnoeic but not distressed and who may respond to full treatment over a few hours needs close observation but not immediate intubation. Patients are often able to tolerate hypercapnia without requiring invasive ventilation.[123] A patient with a lower Pa_{CO_2} (e.g. 50–60 mmHg (6.66–7.98 kPa)) who has been unwell for days, who has a deteriorating status despite treatment and significant respiratory distress is likely to need intubation. A patient who complains of respiratory exhaustion is likely to need intubation. Absolute indications for intubation include cardiac or respiratory arrest, severe hypoxia or rapid deterioration of conscious state.[17,61]

Table 35.2 Comparison of reported mortality associated with the mechanical ventilation of patients with severe asthma over the last five decades

				MORTALITY (%)		
DECADE	NO. PAPERS	NO. EPISODES	NO. DEAD	*MEAN*	*MINIMUM*	*MAXIMUM*
1960s	8	125	18	14.4	0	27
1970s	7	183	31	16.9	6	38
1980s	10	382	46	12.0	0	36
1990s	12	571	61	10.7	0	26
2000s	5	950	65	6.8	4	21

Once the decision to intubate has been made, a safe option is to perform rapid sequence intubation using the orotracheal approach. A large as possible endotracheal tube should be used to reduce the work of breathing and to reduce the risk of tube occlusion by the tenacious secretions that often occur with asthma. Once the endotracheal tube is in place, slow hand ventilation (8–10 breaths/minute) should maintain oxygenation until the ventilator can be connected.

INITIAL VENTILATOR SETTINGS

The principles of initial mechanical ventilation are avoid excessive DHI[29,105,108,109,124] and to avoid excessive hypoventilation (**Fig. 35.4**) by commencing with a minute ventilation <115 ml/kg/min (<8 L/min in a 70 kg patient) best achieved with a tidal volume of 5–7 mL/kg, a respiratory rate of 10–12 breaths/min and a short inspiratory time to ensure an expiratory time ≥4 seconds.[29,105,108,109,124] This degree of hypoventilation will usually result in hypercapnic acidosis and continued respiratory distress necessitating heavy sedation, and sometimes requires 1–2 bolus doses of a neuromuscular-blocking agent.

The use of volume-controlled ventilation is most established for this ventilatory pattern. In volume control, a high inspiratory flow rate (70–100 L/min) is required to achieve a short inspiratory time. This will result in a high peak airway pressure (PIP) but this will lower DHI and P_{plat} and reduce barotrauma compared with lower inspiratory flow rates[105,108] Pressure-controlled or assisted modes have been used[125] without adverse consequences. The theoretical advantage of a safe pressure limit in pressure modes is offset by the fact that equilibrium with the set safe pressure cannot be reached during the short inspiratory times required and thus either a higher pressure must be set or more than necessary hypoventilation may occur. It is not clear whether one mode is superior to the other.

If significant hypotension occurs this should be treated by reducing the respiratory rate, (thereby reducing dynamic hyperinflation) and volume loading.

PEEP

The role of extrinsic PEEP during mechanical ventilation of the patient with severe asthma requires careful consideration. During spontaneous breathing, CPAP has been shown to reduce facilitate the initiation of the next breath and reduce the work of breathing in many patients with severe air-flow obstruction. However, during initial controlled hypoventilation when there is an excessive level of PEEPi and dynamic hyperinflation and work of breathing is not an issue, early work has shown that extrinsic PEEP will further increase lung volumes. As this conferred no benefit and risk of detriment it was recommended that extrinsic PEEP should not be used.[109] More recently some research has suggested that low-level PEEP may improve the distribution of ventilation (as does hyperinflation) and reduce Pa_{CO_2}[126] and one study[127] has found that extrinsic PEEP may paradoxically reduce hyperinflation in some patients ventilated with air-flow obstruction. The uncertain benefit and unpredictable responses to PEEP in these latter studies continue to suggest that extrinsic PEEP should not be routinely used during controlled ventilation for severe air-flow obstruction.[126]

ASSESSMENT OF DYNAMIC HYPERINFLATION

Once mechanical ventilation has started, the degree of DHI should be assessed by measurement of *plateau airway pressure* (P_{plat}). This is the airway pressure after transient expiratory occlusion at the end of inspiration. This may be achieved by an end-inspiratory hold function on most current ventilators, which delays the commencement of the next breath (Fig. 35.4a), or by applying a 0.5 s 'plateau', which does not delay the onset of the next breath. The latter should be applied for a single breath only as application for several breaths in a row will decrease expiratory time and progressively increase DHI. This is the most easily measured estimate of average alveolar pressure at the end of inspiration and is directly proportional to the degree of hyperinflation and should be maintained at <25 cmH_2O.[105,108]

In patients with severe asthma, P_{plat} of 25 cmH2O correlated with an average end-inspiratory lung volume of <20 mL/kg (1.4 L in a 70 kg patient, Figs 35.2 and 35.3) above FRC. This has been shown to be a good predictor of complications during mechanical ventilation[108] and to correlate with a total lung volume at total lung capacity.[29]

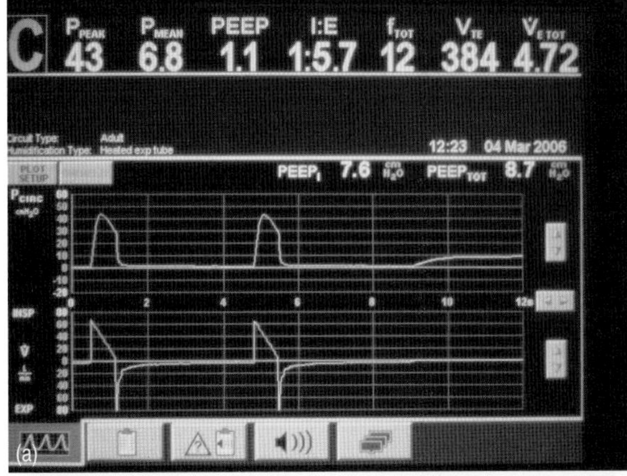

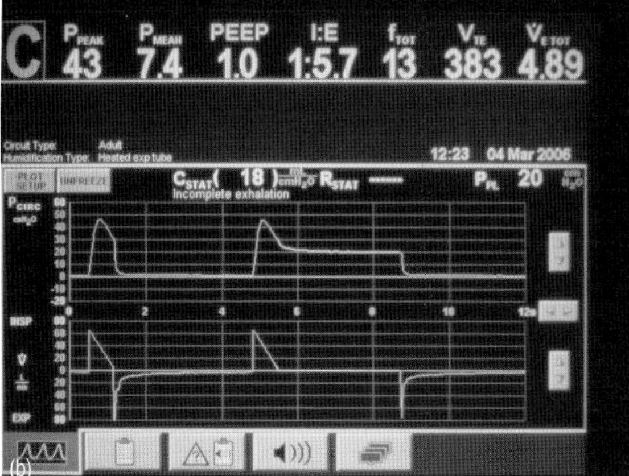

Figure 35.4 (a) The ventilator circuit pressure and flow traces versus time during controlled ventilation of a patient with severe air-flow obstruction. Note the use of a low rate, low V_t, a high inspiratory flow rate (V_i 80 L/min) and hence a short inspiratory time (t_e < 1 second). This causes a high peak airway pressure but allows a long expiratory time (>4 seconds). Expiratory flow is low throughout expiration and appears close to baseline at the onset of the next breath (2nd on screen). Suggesting minimal gas trapping but when a $PEEP_i$ manoeuvre is done (end-expiratory pause) these is a surprising degree of $PEEP_i$ present (7.6 cmH2O). (b) The ventilator circuit pressure and flow traces versus time during controlled ventilation of the same patient in part a. When a P_{plat} manoeuvre is done (end-inspiratory pause) the P_{plat} is safe (20 cmH2O) with this ventilator pattern despite the degree of PEEPi present. Note the low P_{plat} despite the high peak airway pressure.

Intrinsic PEEP ($PEEP_i$) is the airway pressure during occlusion of expiratory flow at the end of expiration (Fig. 35.4b). This is also an automated end-inspiratory hold function on most current ventilators. However, this measurement is known to underestimate true $PEEP_i$, as a consequence of small-airway closure during expiration resulting in many higher-pressure alveoli not communicating with the central airway at the end of expiration.[107] Because of this, $PEEP_i$ can be used to show the presence of DHI but is not recommended to regulate the mechanical ventilation. Ideally $PEEP_i$ should be <12 cmH_2O although the exact safe level is unknown..

Assessment of the change in blood pressure and central venous pressure should be made during a period of transient ventilator disconnection (1–2 min) or transient ventilator rate reduction (4–6 breaths/min for 2–4 min). If DHI has been suppressing circulation then a significant increase in blood pressure and reduction in central venous pressure will occur.

ADJUSTMENT OF VENTILATION

Ventilatory patterns with excessive minute ventilation risk hypotension and barotrauma and are associated with a high mortality. Use of profound hypoventilation will guarantee avoidance of these complications but usually necessitates heavy sedation and neuromuscular blockade (**Fig. 35.5**). This, in association with parenteral steroids, has a high probability of myopathy,[74,128,129] which may cause severe prolonged disability. To minimise the risk of both these complications, DHI should be carefully assessed and the minimum amount of hypoventilation used to achieve a safe level of DHI (see Fig. 35.5) in association with less sedation and minimal or no use of neuromuscular-blocking agents.

Ventilation should be adjusted based on assessment of DHI, not on Pa_{CO_2} *or pH.* If P_{plat} is >25 cmH_2O or circulatory suppression is present, the ventilator rate should be reduced.[105,130] If P_{plat} is low, ventilation can be liberalised by increasing the ventilator rate or reducing sedation and allowing spontaneous ventilation. Hypercapnia is usually present but is well tolerated[131] and does not appear to depress cardiac function. There is no evidence of benefit from sodium bicarbonate but it may reduce acidaemia-induced respiratory distress and may be given if the pH is less than 7.1.

When air-flow obstruction improves (decreasing P_{plat} and $PEEP_i$), sedation may be decreased, ventilator rate reduced and spontaneous ventilation assisted with pressure support ventilation. Pressure support of 10–16 cmH_2O may be used. Once spontaneous ventilation has commenced and when DHI is no longer critical, 3–7 cmH_2O CPAP may be introduced to assist ventilator triggering and reduce the work of breathing.

COMPLICATIONS OF INVASIVE VENTILATION IN ASTHMA

Hypotension may be caused by sedation, DHI, pneumothoraces or arrhythmias.[105,108] Hypovolaemia may be a contributory factor but is rarely a cause. Hypotension may be mild or life threatening.[132] Hypotension due to DHI may be diagnosed by recovery of blood pressure during apnoea of 60 seconds (the 'apnoea test')[132] or by a longer period of low ventilator rate (4–6 breaths/min for 2–4 min). If this occurs, ventilation should be continued at a lower rate.

Circulatory arrest with apparent electromechanical dissociation (EMD) is a recognised complication that may

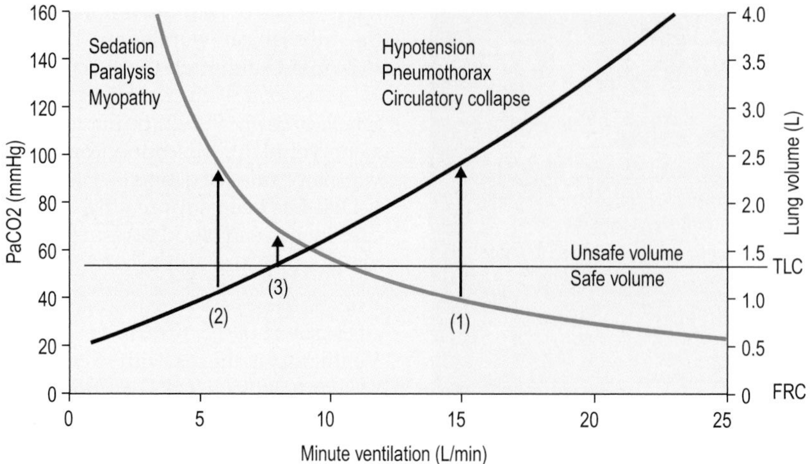

Figure 35.5 The effects of minute ventilation on Pa_{CO_2} and end-inspiratory lung volume above FRC in a typical patient with severe asthma. (1) The minute ventilation required for normocapnia, (2) profound hypoventilation, (3) optimal hypoventilation.

occur within 10 minutes of intubation and can lead to death or severe cerebral ischaemic injury if not managed correctly.[132–134] Standard mechanical ventilation recommendations (minute ventilation 115 mL/kg/min) have been estimated to be safe for 80% of patients requiring mechanical ventilation for acute severe asthma, with the remaining 20% requiring a small to moderate reduction in minute ventilation to return DHI to a safe level.[108] A small percentage of patients with unusually severe asthma can rapidly develop excessive DHI during initial uncontrolled mechanical ventilation leading to EMD, sometimes despite 'safe' levels of minute ventilation. If the cause of this is not immediately recognised, it can lead to prolonged and unnecessary CPR, unsafe procedures such as intercostal vascular access needles or pericardial taps and risk cerebral injury and death.[132–134] When this occurs, immediate disconnection from ventilation for 60–90 seconds (the 'apnoea test', above) or profound hypoventilation (2–3 breaths/min)[61] will diagnose and improve this situation. An even smaller percentage of patients may remain hypotensive despite profound hypoventilation with marked hypercapnia, fluid loading and inotropes. These patients may require heliox delivered by the mechanical ventilator[135] or extracorporeal membrane oxygenation.[134,136–138]

Pneumothoraces were common before the advent of protective ventilatory strategies. DHI during mechanical ventilation was probably the major causative factor involved.[105,108] Pneumothoraces may also occur in association with subclavian central venous catheter insertion and as a consequence of intercostal needle insertion for suspected tension pneumothorax during circulatory arrest (above). Asthma continues to remain one of the three most common conditions (with ARDS and interstitial lung disease) associated with barotrauma during mechanical ventilation with a risk rate of 6.3% compared with an overall risk rate of 2.9% for all mechanically ventilated patients.[139] The presence of severe air-flow obstruction prevents lung collapse and favours gas loss through the ruptured alveoli, with the result that tension is almost always present in the pneumothorax. Once a unilateral tension pneumothorax is present, this will necessarily reduce ventilation to that lung and redistribute ventilation to the contralateral lung thereby further increasing DHI in the second lung and bilateral tension pneumothoraces may result with severe adverse consequences.

As soon as a tension pneumothorax is suspected, the ventilator rate should be immediately reduced to decrease the risk to the second lung. Clinical diagnosis of a tension pneumothorax can be difficult as the lungs in severe asthma are already overexpanded and hyper-resonant with poor air entry. An urgent chest X-ray is always advisable for confirmation prior to intercostal catheter insertion unless severe hypotension is present. Intercostal catheters should always be inserted by blunt dissection. If intercostal needles are inserted for suspected pneumothorax, an intercostal catheter should always be inserted soon thereafter because if a tension pneumothorax was not present it is highly likely after the intercostal needles.

Acute necrotising myopathy is a serious complication that may occur in patients who are invasively ventilated for asthma and receive neuromuscular-blocking agents or very deep sedation.[74,128,129,140,141] It is characterised by weakness with electromyographic evidence of myopathy and increased serum creatine kinase levels. Muscle biopsy reveals two patterns: myonecrosis with muscle cell vacuolisation or predominant type II fibre atrophy.[74,140] Recovery can be slow with prolonged weaning from mechanical ventilation, the need for rehabilitation. Incomplete recovery after 12 months has been reported in a few patients.[141,142] The aetiology of the myopathy appears to be a combination of the effects of corticosteroids and neuromuscular-blocking agents (NMBA) with the duration of paralysis a strong predictor of myopathy.[141,142] The type of NMBA used seems to

Box 35.1 **Key points**

1. Asthma prevalence in the community is increasing but admissions to hospital and intensive care are decreasing
2. Acute severe asthma is a life-threatening medical emergency both on presentation and during mechanical ventilation
3. Underestimation of severity and under-treatment are the biggest contributors to asthma mortality
4. Patients who do require mechanical ventilation have more severe asthma refractory to treatment and are more difficult to ventilate
5. Intravenous and continuous nebulised salbutamol can cause significant lactic acidosis
6. Mechanical ventilation can easily cause excessive dynamic hyperinflation leading to hypotension and pneumothorax
7. Mechanical ventilation needs careful regulation with initial V_e<115 mL/kg/min (8 L/min) and P_{plat}<25 mmHg (3.32 kPa)
8. Very severe dynamic hyperinflation can lead to cardiorespiratory collapse diagnosed by an apnoea test
9. Neuromuscular-blocking agents and heavy sedation can lead to severe necrotising myopathy
10. Following intensive care, asthma requires full treatment including inhaled steroids, a management plan and careful follow-up.

make no difference to the incidence of myopathy.[140] Effective paralysis by deep sedation without the use of NMBAs also confers the risk of severe weakness in this patient group.[143] Gehlbach et al[15] found that the risk factors for prolonged mechanical ventilation were female gender, use of NMBAs, requirement for inhaled corticosteroids prior to admission and a high illness severity score (APACHE II). The relative contributions of corticosteroids versus NMBAs in the causation of myopathy are unclear. It seems wise to minimise the dose of parenteral corticosteroids with early introduction of nebulised agents, to minimise or avoid NMBAs if possible and minimise deep sedation.

MORTALITY, LONG-TERM OUTCOME AND FOLLOW-UP

In a summary of 37 papers reporting the outcomes of 1260 patients requiring mechanical ventilation for asthma in the four decades prior to the year 2000,[62] there was an overall mortality of 12.4% with a progressive reduction in reported mortality during that period (see Table 35.2). A selection of reports[10,12,14,15,21] published since 2000 have shown continued reduction in overall mortality (see Table 35.2) but with mortalities as high as 21% still occurring in one series.[14] The largest and most comprehensive recent series[10] reported 1899 patients admitted to 22 Australian intensive care units over an 8-year period (1996–2003). This series reported a requirement for mechanical ventilation for 36% of patients admitted with severe asthma and a progressive reduction in annual mortality of the ventilated patients from 10% to 3% over the 8-year period.

The need for invasive ventilation increases the risk of death[10,14,144] and survivors of these near-fatal episodes of asthma have an increased risk of intensive care re-admission and an increased risk of death after hospital discharge.[33,34] For these reasons, patients who have an episode of asthma severe enough to require hospitalisation, particularly intensive care admission, need careful follow-up. This should include active identification and avoidance of precipitants, aggressive bronchodilator therapy including inhaled steroids, regular medical review, regular measurement of lung function, management plans for a deteriorating status, and ready access to emergency services. Patients with difficult asthma may benefit from detailed psychological and sometimes speech therapy assessment.[18]

Access the complete references list online at http://www.expertconsult.com

10. Stow P, Pilcher D, Wilson J, et al. Improved outcomes from acute severe asthma in Australian intensive care units (1996–2003). Thorax 2007;62(10):842–7.
15. Gehlbach B, Kress JP, Kahn J, et al. Correlates of prolonged hospitalization in inner-city ICU patients receiving noninvasive and invasive positive pressure ventilation for status asthmaticus. Chest 2002;122(5):1709–14.
18. Harrison BD. Difficult asthma in adults: recognition and approaches to management. Intern Med J 2005; 35(9):543–7.
23. Restrepo RD, Peters J. Near-fatal asthma: recognition and management. Curr Opin Pulm Med 2008;14(1):13–23.
33. McFadden ER Jr. Acute severe asthma. Am J Respir Crit Care Med 2003;168(7):740–59.
74. Douglass J, Tuxen D, Horne M, et al. Myopathy in severe asthma. Am Rev Respir Dis 1992;146(2): 517–19.
105. Tuxen D, Lane S. The effects of ventilatory pattern on hyperinflation, airway pressures, and circulation in mechanical ventilation of patients with severe airflow obstruction. Am Rev Respir Dis 1987;136:872–9.
108. Williams T, Tuxen D, Scheinkestel C, et al. Risk factors for morbidity in mechanically ventilated patients with acute severe asthma. Am Rev Respir Dis 1992;146(3):607–15.
117. Gupta D, Nath A, Agarwal R, et al. A prospective randomized controlled trial on the efficacy of non-invasive ventilation in severe acute asthma. Respir Care 2010;55(5):536–43.

36

Pneumonia

Kai Man Chan and Charles D Gomersall

The management of pneumonia is based on four findings and premises:

- Pneumonia is associated with a wide range of largely non-specific clinical features.[1]
- Pneumonia can be caused by over 100 organisms.
- The relationship between specific clinical features and aetiological organism is insufficiently strong to allow a clinical diagnosis of the causative organism.[2]
- Early administration of appropriate antibiotics is important.[2]

The net result is that the differential diagnosis is wide and treatment should be started before the aetiological agent is known. The differential diagnosis and the likely causative organisms can be narrowed by using epidemiological clues, the most important of which are whether the pneumonia is community-acquired or healthcare-associated and whether the patient is immunocompromised. Note that the flora and antibiotic resistance patterns vary from country to country, hospital to hospital and even ICU to ICU within a hospital and this must be taken into account.

COMMUNITY-ACQUIRED PNEUMONIA

Evidence-based guidelines have been issued by the British Thoracic Society,[3] the Infectious Diseases Society of America (IDSA) and American Thoracic Society (ATS)[2] and the European Respiratory Society.[4] Links to these and other pneumonia-related guidelines can be found at the following 'link page': http://www.aic.cuhk.edu.hk/web8/Pneumonia%20guidelines.htm.

DEFINITION

An acute infection of the pulmonary parenchyma that is associated with at least some symptoms of acute infection, accompanied by an acute infiltrate on a chest radiograph (CXR), or auscultatory findings consistent with pneumonia (e.g. altered breath sounds, localised crackles) in a patient not hospitalised or residing in a long-term care facility for ≥14 days prior to the onset of symptoms.

The overall incidence is 3–40 per 1000 inhabitants per year, with 40–60% requiring hospital admission. Overall, 10% of patients are admitted to ICU. The overall mortality of hospitalised patient is approximately 10%.[5]

AETIOLOGY

Table 36.1 gives possible aetiological agents based on epidemiological clues. *Streptococcus pneumoniae* is the most commonly isolated organism. The next most common bacterial pathogens in patients admitted to ICU are: *Legionella* species, *Haemophilus influenzae,* Enterobacteriaceae species, *Staphylococcus aureus* and *Pseudomonas* species.[2]

CLINICAL PRESENTATION

Pneumonia produces both systemic and respiratory manifestations. Common clinical findings include fever, sweats, rigors, cough, sputum production, pleuritic chest pain, dyspnoea, tachypnoea, pleural rub and inspiratory crackles. Classic signs of consolidation occur in less than 25% of cases. Multi-organ dysfunction or failure may occur depending on the type and severity of pneumonia.

The diagnosis of pneumonia may be more difficult in the elderly. Although the vast majority of elderly patients with pneumonia have respiratory symptoms and signs, over 50% may also have non-respiratory symptoms and over a third may have no systemic signs of infection.

INVESTIGATIONS[2,4]

Investigations should not delay administration of antibiotics as delays are associated with an increase in mortality.[2] Important investigations include:

1. Chest X-ray (CXR)
2. Arterial blood gases or oximetry
3. Full blood count
4. Serum creatinine, urea and electrolytes
5. Liver function tests
6. Blood cultures (×2) prior to the administration of antimicrobials
7. Sputum (if immediately available) for urgent Gram stain and culture. The usefulness of sputum tests remains debatable because of contamination by upper respiratory tract commensals. However, a

Table 36.1 Possible aetiological agents based on epidemiological clues[2,3,9,7]

EXPOSURE	ORGANISM
EXPOSURE TO ANIMALS	
Handling turkeys, chickens, ducks or psittacine birds or their excreta	*Chlamydia psittaci*
Exposure to birds in countries in which avian flu has been identified in birds	Influenza A H5N1
Handling infected parturient cats, cattle, goats or sheep or their hides	*Coxiella burneti*
Handling infected wool	*Bacillus anthracis*
Handling infected cattle, pigs, goats or sheep or their milk	*Brucella* spp.
Insect bite. Transmission from rodents and wild animals (e.g. rabbits) to laboratory workers, farmers and hunters	*Francisella tularensis*
Insect bites or scratches; transmission from infected rodents or cats to laboratory workers and hunters	*Yersinia pestis*
Contact with infected horses (very rare)	*Pseudomonas mallei*
Exposure to mice or mice droppings	Hantavirus
GEOGRAPHICAL FACTORS	
Immigration from or residence in countries with high prevalence of TB	*Mycobacterium tuberculosis*
North America; contact with infected bats or birds or their excreta; excavation in endemic areas	*Histoplasma capsulatum*
South-west USA	*Coccidiodes* species, Hantavirus
USA; inhalation of spores from soil	*Blastomyces dermatitidis*
Asia, Pacific, Caribbean, north Australia. Contact with local animals or contaminated skin abrasions	*Burkholderia pseudomallei*
HOST FACTORS	
Diabetic ketoacidosis	*Streptococcus pneumoniae, Staphylococcus aureus*
Alcoholism	*Strep. pneumoniae, S. aureus, Klebsiella pneumoniae,* oral anaerobes, *M. tuberculosis, Acinetobacter* spp.
Chronic obstructive pulmonary disease or smoking	*Strep. pneumoniae, Haemophilus influenzae, Moraxella catarrhalis, Chlamydia pneumoniae, Legionella* spp., *Pseudomonas aeruginosa*
Sickle cell disease	*Strep. pneumoniae*
Pneumonia complicating whooping cough	*Bordatella pertussis*
Pneumonia complicating influenza	*Strep. pneumoniae, S. aureus,* CA-MRSA
Pneumonia severe enough to necessitate artificial ventilation	*Strep. pneumoniae, Legionella* spp., *S. aureus, Haemophilus influenzae, Mycoplasma pneumoniae,* enteric Gram-negative bacilli, *Chlamydia pneumoniae, M. tuberculosis,* viral infection, endemic fungi
Nursing home residency	Treat as healthcare-associated pneumonia
Poor dental hygiene	Anaerobes
Suspected large-volume aspiration	Oral anaerobes, Gram-negative enteric bacteria
Structural disease of lung (e.g. bronchiectasis, cystic fibrosis)	*P. aeruginosa, Burkholderia cepacia, S. aureus*

Table 36.1 Possible aetiological agents based on epidemiological clues—cont'd

EXPOSURE	ORGANISM
Lung abscess	Community-acquired meticillin-resistant *S. aureus*, oral anaerobes, endemic fungi, *M. tuberculosis*, atypical mycobacteria
Endobronchial obstruction	Anaerobes, *Strep. pneumoniae, H. influenzae, S. aureus*
Intravenous drug addict	*S. aureus*, CA-MRSA, anaerobes, *M. tuberculosis, Strep. pneumoniae*
End-stage renal failure	CA-MRSA
OTHERS	
Epidemic	*M. pneumoniae*, influenza virus
Air-conditioning cooling towers, hot tubs or hotel or cruise ship stay in previous 2 weeks	*Legionella pneumophilia*
Presentation of a cluster of cases over a very short period of time	Bioterrorist agents: *B. anthracis, F. tularensis, Y. pestis*

single or predominant organism on a Gram stain of a fresh sample or a heavy growth on culture of purulent sputum is likely to be the organism responsible. The finding of many polymorphonuclear cells (PMN) with no bacteria in a patient who has not already received antibiotics can reliably exclude infection by most ordinary bacterial pathogens. Specimens should be obtained by deep cough and be grossly purulent. Ideally the specimen should be obtained before treatment with antimicrobials, if this does not delay administration of antibiotics, and be transported to the laboratory immediately for prompt processing to minimise the chance of missing fastidious organisms (e.g. *Strep. pneumoniae*). Acceptable specimens (in patients with normal or raised white blood cell counts) should contain >25 PMN per low-power field (LPF) and <10–25 squamous epithelial cells (SEC)/LPF or >10 PMN per SEC. These criteria should not be used for *Mycobacteria* and *Legionella* infection. Certain organisms are virtually always pathogens when recovered from respiratory secretions (**Box 36.1**). Patients with risk factors for tuberculosis (TB) (**Box 36.2**), and particularly those with cough for more than a month, other common symptoms of TB and suggestive radiographic changes, should have sputum examined for acid-fast bacilli. Sputum cannot be processed for culture for anaerobes owing to contamination by the endogenous anaerobic flora of the upper respiratory tract. In addition to the factors listed in Table 36.1, foul-smelling sputum, lung abscess and empyema should raise suspicion of anaerobic infection.

8. Aspiration of pleural fluid for Gram stain, culture, pH and leucocyte count – all patients with a pleural effusion >1 cm thick on a lateral decubitus chest X-ray.

Box 36.1 Organisms that are virtually always pathogens when recovered from respiratory secretions

Legionella
Chlamydia
TB
Influenza, para-influenza virus, RSV, adenovirus, hantavirus, SARS coronavirus
Stronglyloides stercoralis
Toxoplasma gondi
Histoplasma capsulatum
Coccidiodes immitis
Blastomycoses dermatitidis
Cryptococcus neoformans

Box 36.2 Risk factors for pulmonary tuberculosis

Living in or originating from a developing country
Age (<5 years, middle-aged and elderly men)
Alcoholism and/or drug addiction
HIV infection
Diabetes mellitus
Lodging-house dwellers
Immunosuppression
Close contact with smear-positive patients
Silicosis
Poverty and/or malnutrition
Previous gastrectomy
Smoking

9. Urinary *Legionella* antigen. This test is specific (>95%). In patients with severe Legionnaires disease sensitivity is 88–100% for *L. pneumophilia* serogroup 1 (the most commonly reported cause of *Legionella* infection). Thus a positive result is virtually

diagnostic of *Legionella* infection but a negative result does not exclude it. In areas (e.g. South Australia) where other *Legionella* species are more common, this test is less helpful.

10. Urinary pneumococcal antigen has moderate sensitivity (50–80%) and high specificity (>90%).
11. Microimmunofluorescence serology for *Chlamydia pneumoniae* IgM. A titre ≥1:16 is significant.
12. HIV serological status.

Other investigations should be considered in patients with risk factors for infection with unusual organisms. Bronchoalveolar lavage may be useful in immunocompromised patients, those who fail to respond to antibiotics, or those in whom sputum samples cannot be obtained.[6]

Molecular diagnosis (e.g. PCR-based methods) has the advantages of quick results (within 3 hours), enhanced sensitivity, independence from organism viability and hence previous antibiotics, and theoretical possibility for determination of antimicrobial susceptibility.[7] Of note, it is important to test for genes specific for the organism in question[10] and the sampling site remains important. PCR is most useful when performed on specimens from a normally sterile site. For example, PCR for *Pneumococcus* is positive in 62% of blood samples from adult patients with confirmed or probable pneumococcal pneumonia,[8] whereas blood cultures are positive in only 37%. For respiratory specimens under most circumstances, interpretation remains problematic due to low specificity related to floral contamination and colonisation. PCR assays are more sensitive than culture for *Mycoplasma* and *Chlamydia* species and at least as sensitive for *Legionella*.[7] PCR assays also detect *Legionella* strains other than serogroup 1. The BTS guidelines[3] recommend PCR of lower respiratory tract sample or, if unavailable, throat swab for the diagnosis of *Mycoplasma* pneumonia. PCR for *Chlamydophilia* should be performed when invasive respiratory samples were collected from patients with severe community-acquired pneumonia. The role of PCR in diagnosing PCP is mainly limited to non-HIV patients, in whom conventional microscopy and staining of induced sputum and BAL have a lower sensitivity than in HIV patients.[9]

MANAGEMENT

GENERAL SUPPORTIVE MEASURES

Intravenous fluids may be required to correct dehydration and provide maintenance fluid. A general approach should be made to organ support with an emphasis on correcting hypoxia.

ANTIMICROBIAL REGIMENS

Increased mortality among those who do not receive empirical antibiotics that cover the infecting pathogen(s) is well documented.[11] Each unit should have its own regimens tailored to the local flora and antibiotic resistance patterns. In the absence of such regimens the regimen outlined in **Figure 36.1** may be helpful. This

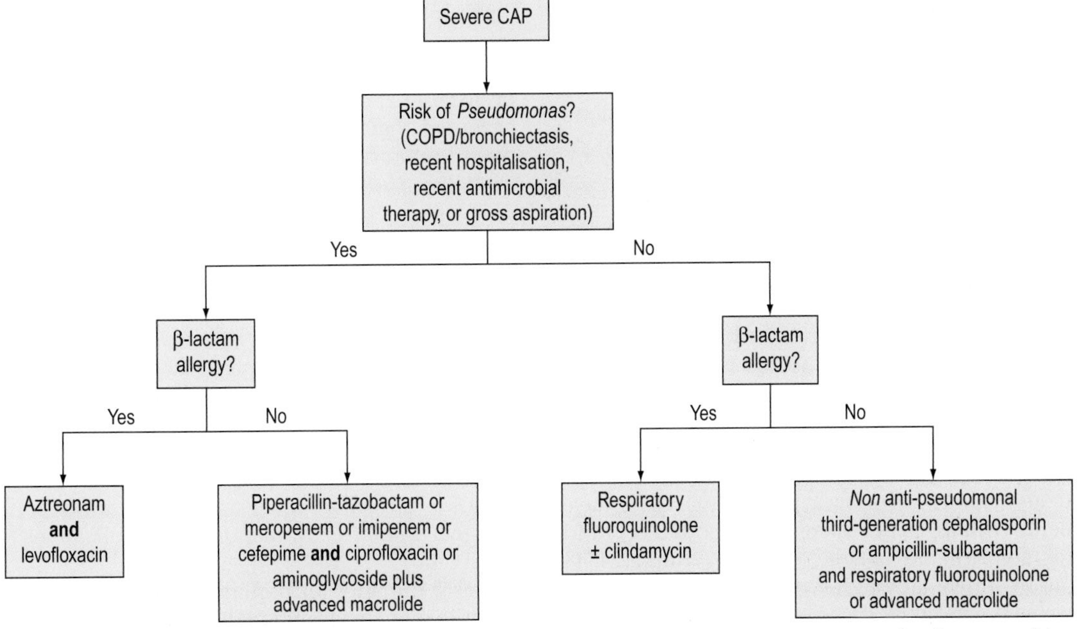

Figure 36.1 Antibiotic regimens for treatment of severe community-acquired pneumonia in critically ill patients.[2,4] Respiratory fluoroquinolones include moxifloxacin and levofloxacin. Advanced macrolides include azithromycin and clarithromycin. Non-antipseudomonal third-generation cephalosporins include cefotaxime and ceftriaxone.

should be modified in the light of risk factors (see Table 36.1). Quinolones may be less appropriate in areas with a high prevalence of TB as their use may mask concurrent TB infection. Appropriate antimicrobial therapy should be administered within 1 hour of diagnosis.[4,12] There is controversy regarding the appropriate change to empirical therapy based on microbiological findings.[2,4] Changing to narrower-spectrum antimicrobial cover may result in inadequate treatment of the 5–38% of patients with polymicrobial infection. Increasing evidence demonstrates improved outcome with combination antimicrobial as compared with monotherapy, particularly in severely ill patients with bacteraemic pneumococcal pneumonia.[5] Odds ratio of death was 1.5 to 6 for monotherapy as compared with combination therapy. Benefits were seen only in combination therapy with macrolide as part of the regimen, but not in combination with fluroquinolone regimen.[13] For the treatment of drug-resistant *Strep. pneumoniae* (DRSP) the regimens in Figure 36.1 are probably suitable for isolates with a penicillin MIC<4 mg/L.[2] If the MIC is ≥4 mg/L an antipneumococcal fluoroquinolone, vancomycin, teicoplanin or linezolid should be given.[4]

DURATION OF THERAPY

No clinical trial has specifically addressed this issue. Courses as short as 5 days may be sufficient.[14] IDSA/ATS guidelines recommend stopping after a minimum of 5 days if the patient is afebrile for 48–72 hours and organ dysfunction has largely resolved.[2] Short courses may be suboptimal for patients with bacteraemic *S. aureus* pneumonia, meningitis or endocarditis complicating pneumonia or infection with less common organisms (e.g. *Burkholderia pseudomallei* or fungi) or *Pseudomonas aeruginosa*. Procalcitonin may be useful to guide antibiotic therapy, but not all studies have demonstrated a benefit.[15]

RESPONSE TO THERAPY[2]

This can be assessed subjectively (a response is usually seen within 1–3 days of starting therapy) or objectively on the basis of respiratory symptoms, fever, oxygenation, WBC count, bacteriology, CXR changes, C-reactive protein reduction and procalcitonin reduction of 80–90% from peak value. The average time to defervescence varies with organism, severity and patient age (7 days in elderly patients, 2.5 days in young patients with pneumococcal pneumonia, 6–7 days in bacteraemic patients with pneumococcal pneumonia, 1–2 days in patients with *M. pneumoniae* pneumonia and 5 days in patients with *Legionella* pneumonia). Both blood and sputum cultures are usually negative within 24–48 hours of treatment although *P. aeruginosa* and *M. pneumoniae* may persist in the sputum despite effective therapy. CXR changes lag behind clinical changes with the speed of change depending on the organism, the age of the patient and the presence or absence of comorbid illnesses. The CXR of most young or middle-aged patients with bacteraemic pneumococcal pneumonia is clear by 4 weeks, but resolution is slower in elderly patients and patients with underlying illness, extensive pneumonia on presentation or *Legionella pneumophilia* pneumonia.

If the patient fails to respond consider the following questions:

- Has the patient got pneumonia?
- Are there host factors that explain the failure (e.g. obstruction of bronchus by a foreign body or tumour, inadequate host response)?
- Has a complication developed (e.g. empyema, superinfection, bronchiolitis obliterans organising pneumonia, metastatic abscess)?
- Is the right drug being given in an adequate dose by the right route?
- Is the organism resistant to the drug being given?
- Are there other organisms?
- Is the fever a drug fever?

Useful investigations include computerised tomography (CT) of the chest, thoracocentesis, bronchoalveolar lavage (**Table 36.2**) and transbronchial or open-lung biopsy.

PREDICTION OF ADVERSE OUTCOME AND ADMISSION TO ICU

Scoring systems have been developed to predict adverse outcome and ICU admission including pneumonia severity index (PSI), CURB-65, CRB-65, modified ATS major and minor criteria, SCAP prediction rule, SMART-COP, REA-ICU index and CAP-PIRO.[16] Although they may help identify the sicker patients they should not be used as a sole determinant of ICU admission as local admission criteria will be affected by local facilities, both in and outside ICU. It should be noted that none of the criteria has been prospectively demonstrated to avoid late transfers or lower mortality.

INFLUENZA PNEUMONIA

Influenza pneumonia may present with severe respiratory failure and multi-organ failure. However the pattern of organ failure appears to vary between strains with H5N1 being associated with a much higher mortality and a higher incidence of multi-organ failure than pandemic H1N1,[17] which itself presented differently to seasonal influenza. In particular, trophism for lower respiratory tract, a higher rate of ICU admission[18] and a higher rate of extrapulmonary complications[19] were observed.

Early initiation of oseltamivir is recommended for critically ill patients although there is no direct evidence of outcome benefit. Glucocorticoids do not appear to be useful and may prolong viral replication.[20] Bacterial superinfection should be considered, with Gram-positive cocci being most frequently isolated.[21]

Table 36.2 Procedure for obtaining microbiological samples using bronchoscopy and protected specimen brushing and/or bronchoalveolar lavage[35,49]

Infection control	In patients suspected of having a disease that is transmitted by the airborne route (e.g. tuberculosis): • the risk of transmission should be carefully weighed against the benefits of bronchoscopy, which may generate large numbers of airborne particles • perform bronchoscopy in a negative-pressure isolation room • consider the use of a muscle relaxant in ventilated patients, to prevent coughing • staff should wear personal protective equipment, which should include a fit-tested negative-pressure respirator (N95, FFP2 or above) as a minimum; use of a powered air-purifying respirator should be considered
General recommendations	Suction through the endotracheal tube should be performed before bronchoscopy Avoid suction or injection through the working channel of the bronchoscope Perform protected specimen brushing before bronchoalveolar lavage
Ventilated patients	Set F_{IO_2} at 1.0 Set peak pressure alarm at a level that allows adequate ventilation Titrate ventilator settings against exhaled tidal volume Consider neuromuscular blockade in addition to sedation in patients at high risk of complications who are undergoing prolonged bronchoscopy
Protected specimen brushing (PSB)	Sample the consolidated segment of lung at subsegmental level If purulent secretions are not seen advance the brush until it can no longer be seen, but avoid wedging it in a peripheral position Move brush back and forth and rotate it several times
Bronchoalveolar lavage (BAL)	Wedge tip of bronchoscope into a subsegment of the consolidated segment of lung Inject, aspirate and collect 20 mL of sterile isotonic saline. Do not use this sample for quantitative microbiology or identification of intracellular organisms. It can be used for other microbiological analysis Inject, aspirate and collect additional aliquots of 20–60 mL The total volume of saline injected should be 60–200 mL
Complications	Hypoxaemia (possibly less with smaller BAL volumes) Arrhythmia Transient worsening in pulmonary infiltrates Bleeding (particularly following PSB) Fever (more common after BAL)
Positive results	>5% of cells in cytocentrifuge preparations of BAL fluid contain intracellular bacteria OR $\geq 10^3$ colony-forming units/mL in PSB specimen OR $\geq 10^4$ colony-forming units/mL in BAL fluid

Although there are data demonstrating that surgical masks are as effective as N95 (FFP 2) masks in preventing transmission of seasonal influenza in non-ICU settings it is important to note that the capacity for airborne transmission (and hence the need for N95 masks) is dependent on the exact characteristics of the organism and the frequency of aerosol-generating procedures so these data should not be extrapolated to other influenza viruses and ICU settings.

HEALTHCARE-ASSOCIATED PNEUMONIA

Nosocomial pneumonia occurs in 0.5–5% of hospital patients, with a higher incidence in certain groups (e.g. postoperative patients and patients in ICU). Diagnosis may be difficult: the clinical features of pneumonia are non-specific and many non-infectious conditions (e.g. atelectasis, pulmonary embolus, aspiration, heart failure and cancer) can cause infiltrates on a chest X-ray. Identification of the organism responsible is even more difficult than in patients with community-acquired pneumonia owing to the high incidence of oropharyngeal colonisation by Gram-negative bacteria. Blood cultures are positive in only about 6% of cases of nosocomial pneumonia. Ventilator-associated pneumonia (VAP) is nosocomial pneumonia arising >48–72 hours after intubation. Reported incidence of VAP is between 10 and 20% for those receiving mechanical ventilation for more than 48 hours.[22] It is associated with a higher incidence of multi-drug-resistant organisms.[1]

PATHOGENESIS

Nosocomial pneumonia is thought to result from microaspiration of bacteria colonising the upper respiratory tract. Other routes of infection include macroaspiration of gastric contents, inhaled aerosols, haematogenous spread, spread from pleural space and direct inoculation from ICU personnel.

CLINICAL DIAGNOSIS

Diagnosis is based on time of onset (>48 hours after admission to a healthcare facility[1]), CXR changes (new or progressive infiltrates) and either clinical features and simple laboratory investigations or the results of quantitative microbiology. Using a clinical approach, pneumonia is diagnosed by the finding of a new infiltrate or a change in an infiltrate on chest radiograph and growth of pathogenic organisms from sputum plus one of the following: white-blood-cell (WBC) count greater than 12×10^5/L, core temperature ≥38.3°C, sputum Gram stain with scores of more than two on a scale of four of polymorphonuclear leucocytes and bacteria.

INVESTIGATIONS

These are broadly similar to those required in community-acquired pneumonia:

- *Chest X-ray:* although studies using a histological diagnosis as the gold standard have demonstrated that pneumonia may be present despite a normal CXR, most definitions of nosocomial pneumonia require the presence of new persistent infiltrates on a CXR.
- *Respiratory secretions:* considerable controversy surrounds the issue of whether invasive bronchoscopic sampling (Table 36.2) of respiratory secretions is necessary. Whether invasive sampling is employed or tracheal aspirates are used, empirical broad-spectrum antibiotics should be started while results are awaited. The results of microbiological analysis of respiratory secretions are used to either stop antibiotics or narrow the spectrum.[1] Although the use of an invasive strategy is associated with a higher likelihood of modification of initial antimicrobials,[23] the effect on important clinical outcome such as mortality, antibiotic-free days, and organ dysfunction is variable.[1] Although tracheal aspirates may predominantly reflect the organisms colonising the upper airway, they may be useful in indicating which organisms are not responsible for the pneumonia, thus allowing the antimicrobial cover to be narrowed.[1] This interpretation is based on the premise that the predominant route of infection is via the upper respiratory tract. From this it can be assumed that if the organism is not present in the upper respiratory tract the probability of it being present in the lung parenchyma is low. Certain organisms are virtually always pathogens when recovered from respiratory secretions (see Box 36.1).
- *Blood cultures:* identify the aetiological agent in 8–20% of patients. Bacteraemia is associated with a worse prognosis. In 50% of patients with severe hospital-acquired pneumonia and positive blood cultures there is another source of sepsis.

MANAGEMENT

Management is based on the finding that early treatment with antimicrobials that cover all likely pathogens results in a reduction in morbidity and mortality.[2] The initial selection of antimicrobials is made on the basis of epidemiological clues (**Fig. 36.2**, **Table 36.3**). Antimicrobials should be administered within 1 hour of diagnosis.[12] The results of microbiological investigations are used to narrow antimicrobial cover later. Treatment should be reassessed after 2–3 days or sooner if the patient deteriorates (**Fig. 36.3**). An outline of management based on an invasive approach is given in **Figure 36.4**.

DURATION OF THERAPY

Current ATS guidelines recommend 7 days' treatment provided the aetiological agent is not *P. aeruginosa* or other non-lactose fermenter and the patient has a good clinical response with resolution of clinical features of infection.[1] The outcome of patients who receive appropriate initial empirical therapy for ventilator-associated pneumonia for 8 days is similar to those who receive treatment for 15 days.[1]

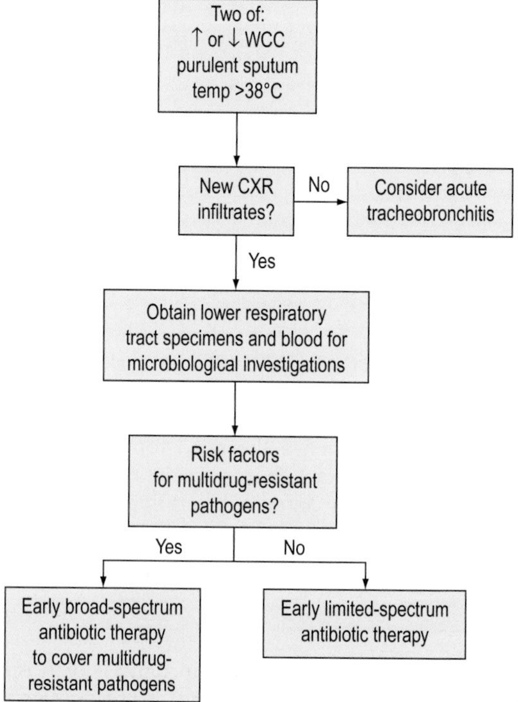

Figure 36.2 An outline of initial management of nosocomial pneumonia based on a non-invasive clinical approach.[1]

Table 36.3 Recommended initial empirical treatment for nosocomial pneumonia[1]

SITUATION	ANTIBIOTICS
No risk factors for multidrug-resistant pathogens	Ceftriaxone *or* Levofloxacin, moxifloxacin or ciprofloxacin *or* Ampicillin/sulbactam *or* Ertapenem
Antimicrobial therapy in previous 90 days *or* Current hospitalization for ≥5 days *or* High frequency of antibiotic resistance in the specific hospital unit *or* Hospitalisation for 2 days or more in previous 90 days *or* Residence in nursing home or extended care facility *or* Home infusion therapy (including antibiotics) *or* Chronic dialysis within 30 days *or* Home wound care *or* Family member with multidrug-resistant pathogen *or* Immunosuppression *or* Bronchiectasis	One of: Antipseudomonal cephalosporin (cefepime or ceftazidime) *or* Antipseudomonal carbapenem (meropenem or imipenem–cilastin) *or* ß-lactam/ß-lactamase inhibitor (e.g. piperacillin–tazobactam or cefaperazone–sulbactam) *plus* one of: Aminoglycoside *or* Antipseudomonal quinolone (levofloxacin or ciprofloxacin) *plus* one of the following for patients at high risk of meticillin-resistant *Staphylococcus aureus* (MRSA) infection: Linezolid *or* Vancomycin *or* Teicoplanin

The use of dual therapy is not well supported by evidence but it does reduce the probability that the pathogen is resistant to the drugs being given. If an extended spectrum β-lactamase-producing strain or an *Acinetobacter* sp. is suspected a carbapenem should be given. If *Legionella pneumophilia* is suspected use a quinolone. Risk factors for MRSA infection in areas with a high incidence of MRSA include diabetes mellitus, head trauma, coma and renal failure.

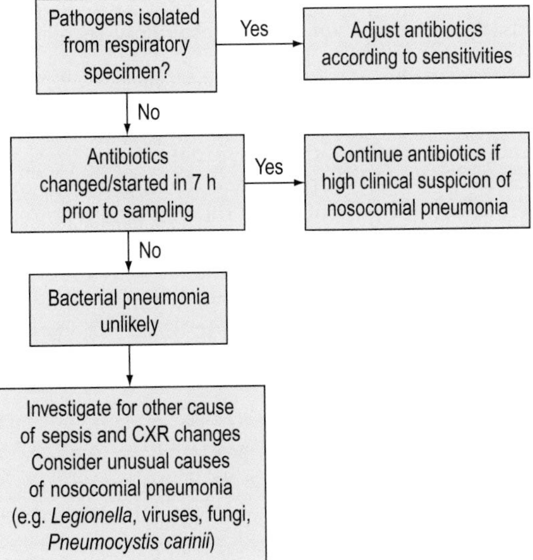

Figure 36.3 Subsequent management of nosocomial pneumonia based on a non-invasive clinical approach.[1]

RESPONSE TO THERAPY

Clinical improvement is usually not apparent for 48–72 hours and therapy should not be changed during this time. The CXR is of limited value for assessing response; initial deterioration is common and improvement often lags behind clinical response. However, a rapidly deteriorating CXR pattern with a >50% increase in size of infiltrate in 48 hours, new cavitation or a significant new pleural effusion should raise concern. If the patient fails to respond consider the diagnosis, host factors (e.g. immunosuppressed, debilitated), bacterial factors (e.g. virulent organism) and therapeutic factors (e.g. wrong drug, inadequate dose). Review the antibiotics and repeat cultures. It may be useful to broaden the antimicrobial cover while waiting for the results of investigations. Consider invasive sampling of respiratory secretions, computerised tomography or ultrasound of the chest (to look for an empyema or abscess), another source of infection, open-lung biopsy to establish diagnosis and aetiology, or administration of steroids.

MORTALITY AND MORBIDITY ATTRIBUTABLE TO VAP

Substantial morbidity and mortality associated with VAP have previously been reported.[22] However, a causal relationship is difficult to establish. It should be noted that patients who developed VAP tend to be more severely ill and at higher risk of death not only on ICU admission, but throughout the course of their illness. Most of the relevant studies were observational and failed to adequately control confounders like disease severity, evolution of disease progression, and ICU length of stay with mortality. In addition, significant heterogeneity exists among these studies. Although the presence of VAP is associated with a significantly longer ICU length of stay (mean of 6.1 days; 95% CI: 5.32–6.87) and increased healthcare cost,[22] more recent studies reported that mortality attributable to VAP tends to be small, if any.[24,25] The attributable mortality has been reported to be 1% on the 30th day of ICU and

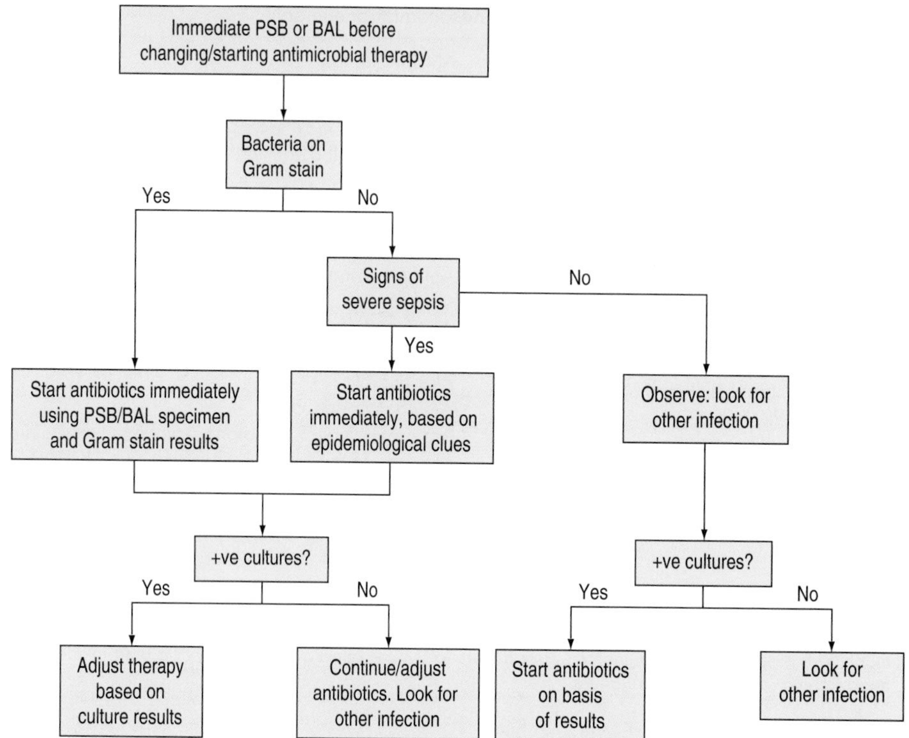

Figure 36.4 Management of suspected nosocomial pneumonia based on invasive sampling of respiratory secretions.

1.5% on the 60th day of ICU in a recent study using a multicentre high-quality database and incorporating novel statistical methodology to control evolution of severity of illness.[25]

PREVENTION

Several guidelines for prevention of ventilator-associated pneumonia and hospital-acquired pneumonia have been published.[26–30] Interventions can be divided into general infection control measures and specific measures. General measures include alcohol-based hand disinfection, hospital education programme on infection control, the use of microbiological surveillance and a programme to reduce antibiotic prescription. The major specific recommendations are summarised in **Table 36.4**. There is no evidence that 'bundles' of recommendations are more effective than the sum of the individual components.

TUBERCULOSIS

The main risk factors are listed in Box 36.2. Typical clinical features include fever, sweating, weight loss, lassitude, anorexia, cough productive of mucoid or purulent sputum, haemoptysis, chest wall pain, dyspnoea, localised wheeze and apical crackles. Patients may also present with unresolved pneumonia, pleural effusions, spontaneous pneumothorax and hoarseness or with enlarged cervical nodes or other manifestations of extrapulmonary disease. Clinical disease is seldom found in asymptomatic individuals, even those with strongly positive tuberculin test (Heaf grade III or IV). The outlook for patients with tuberculosis who require ICU admission is poor. In one retrospective study the in-hospital mortality for all patients with tuberculosis requiring ICU admission was 67% but in those with acute respiratory failure it rose to 81%.[31] The presentation and management of TB in HIV-positive patients are different (see below).

INVESTIGATION OF PULMONARY TUBERCULOSIS

IDENTIFICATION OF MYCOBACTERIA

Multiple[32,33] sputum samples should be collected, preferably on different days, for microscopy for acid-fast bacilli and culture. If sputum is not available bronchial washings taken at bronchoscopy and gastric lavage or aspirate samples should be obtained. Gastric aspirates need to be neutralised immediately on collection. Bronchoscopy and transbronchial biopsy may be useful in patients with suspected TB but negative sputum smear. Pleural biopsy is often helpful and mediastinoscopy is occasionally needed in patients with mediastinal lymphadenopathy. Part of any biopsy specimen should always be sent for culture. Nucleic acid amplification tests on sputum have sensitivity similar to culture in

Table 36.4 Strategies for prevention of ventilator-associated pneumonia

LEVELS OF RECOMMENDATIONS	SPECIFIC INTERVENTIONS	REMARKS
Universally recommended by all guidelines[27–30]	1. Semirecumbent position to 45°	At least 30–45°
	2. Avoidance of endotracheal intubation	
	3. Preference of oral tracheal route	
	4. New circuit for a new patient and no schedule change unless soiled or damaged	
	5. Avoidance of flushing of condensate into lower airway or in-line medication	
	6. HME changes no more frequently than 5–7 days	
	7. Continuous aspiration of subglottic suctioning	For patients expected to require mechanical ventilation for >72 hours
Generally recommended by most guidelines	1. Preferential use of non-invasive ventilation[27,28,30]	
	2. Avoidance of unplanned re-intubation[27,28,30]	
	3. Maintenance of endotracheal cuff pressure of about 20 mmHg (2.66 kPa)[27,28,30]	
	4. Closed suctioning[28,29]	No effect on VAP, mainly for staff safety
	5. Chlorhexidine oral decontamination[27,29,30]	
	6. Sedation vacation and weaning protocol[27,28]	
	7. Judicious use of stress ulcer prophylaxis[27,28,30]	
	8. Restrictive blood transfusion[28]	
Benefits less clear	1. Preference of HME over heated humidifier[28,30]	HME associated with reduction in VAP in patients ventilated for >7 days, lower cost
	2. Silver-sulfadiazine-coated endotracheal tube[27,28,30]	
	3. Early tracheostomy (within 7 days of mechanical ventilation)[29]	
	4. Selective decontamination of digestive tract (SDD)[27,28,30]	Mortality reduction demonstrated when topical antimicrobials combined with short-course systemic antibiotics, BSAC recommended SDD in patients expected to require mechanical ventilation for >48 hours, ETF discourage routine use due to concern of emergence of resistant organisms
Not yet reviewed by guidelines[50]	1. High-volume low-pressure ultrathin membrane endotracheal tube cuff with SSD	
	2. Ultrathin membrane cuff with tapered shape and SSD	
	3. Low-volume low-pressure endotracheal tube cuff with SSD	
	4. Balloon device for biofilm removal	
	5. Saline instillation before tracheal suctioning	

HME=heat moist exchanger; SSD=subglottic secretion drainage.

smear-negative patients with pulmonary tuberculosis but have the advantage of a much more rapid result. There is, however, a significant false-negative rate.[32]

CHEST X-RAY (CXR)

A normal CXR almost excludes TB (except in HIV-infected patients) but endobronchial lesions may not be apparent and early apical lesions can be missed. Common appearances include patchy/nodular shadowing in the upper zones (often bilateral), cavitation, calcification, hilar or mediastinal lymphadenopathy (may cause segmental or lobar collapse), pleural effusion, tuberculomas (dense round or oval shadows) and diffuse fine nodular shadowing throughout the lung fields in miliary TB. Inactivity of disease cannot be inferred from the CXR alone. This requires three negative sputum samples *and* failure of any lesion seen on CXR to progress. CXR appearances in HIV-positive patients with TB differ from those in non-HIV-infected patients.

TREATMENT OF PULMONARY TB[32–34]

The decision to initiate anti-TB treatment should be based on level of clinical suspicion, results of AFB smear and sometimes mycobacterial culture. If the initial clinical suspicion is strong and the patient is seriously ill attributable to possible TB, treatment should be initiated promptly, sometimes before the result of AFB smear. Subsequent positivity of AFB smear or nucleic acid amplification test provides support to the continuation of treatment. Combination chemotherapy consisting of four drugs is necessary for maximal efficacy. Treatment is divided into initial phase and continuation phase. The most commonly used initial regimen consists of 8 weeks of rifampicin 600 mg daily (450 mg for patients <50 kg), isoniazid 300 mg daily, pyrazinamide 2 g daily (1.5 g for patients <50 kg) and ethambutol 15 mg/kg daily as initial phase treatment. Ethambutol should be used only in patients who have reasonable visual acuity and who are able to appreciate and report visual disturbances. This mandates careful consideration in patients who require heavy sedation. Visual acuity and colour perception must be assessed (if ethambutol is to be used) and liver and renal function checked before treatment is started. Steroids are recommended for children with endobronchial disease and, possibly, for patients with tuberculous pleural effusions. Pyridoxine 10 mg daily should be given to prevent isoniazid-induced neuropathy to those at increased risk (e.g. patients with diabetes mellitus, chronic renal failure or malnutrition or alcoholic or HIV-positive patients). Negative AFB smear should not delay initial treatment if clinical suspicion remains high. Supporting features included chronic cough, weight loss, characteristic chest X-ray findings, emigration from a high-incidence country, no other immediate diagnosis, and positive tuberculin test.

INFECTION CONTROL

Patients admitted to an ICU with infectious TB or suspected of having active pulmonary TB should be managed in an isolation room with special ventilation characteristics, including negative pressure. Patients should be considered infectious if they are coughing or undergoing cough-inducing procedures or if they have positive AFB smears and they are not on or have just started chemotherapy, or have a poor clinical or bacteriological response to chemotherapy.[32,35] Patients with non-drug-resistant TB should be non-infectious after 2 weeks of treatment which includes rifampicin and isoniazid.[32] As TB spreads through aerosols it is probably appropriate to isolate patients who are intubated even if only their bronchial washings are smear-positive. Staff caring for patients who are smear-positive should wear personal protective equipment including a fit-tested negative-pressure respirator (N95, FFP2 or higher). Use of a powered air-purifying respirator should be considered when bronchoscopy is being performed.[35] Detailed infection control advice can be obtained via the 'link page' (http://www.aic.cuhk.edu.hk/web8/Pneumonia%20guidelines.htm.).

PNEUMONIA IN THE IMMUNOCOMPROMISED

The lungs are amongst the most frequent target organs for infectious complications in the immunocompromised. The incidence of pneumonia is highest amongst patients with haematological malignancies, bone marrow transplant (BMT) recipients and patients with AIDS.

The speed of progression of pneumonia, the CXR changes (**Table 36.5**) and the type of immune defect provide clues to the aetiology. Bacterial pneumonias progress rapidly (1–2 days) whereas fungal and protozoal pneumonias are less fulminant (several days to a week or more). Viral pneumonias are usually not fulminant, but on occasions may develop quite rapidly. Bronchoscopy is a major component of the investigation of these patients. Empirical management based on CXR appearances is outlined in Table 36.5. Early non-invasive ventilation may improve outcome amongst immunocompromised patients with fever and bilateral infiltrates.[36]

PNEUMOCYSTIS JIROVECI PNEUMONIA (PCP)[37]

The incidence of this common opportunistic infection has fallen substantially in patients with AIDS who are receiving prophylaxis and effective antiretroviral therapy, with most cases occurring in patients who are not receiving HIV care or among patients with advanced immunosuppression. The onset is usually insidious with dry cough, dyspnoea and fever on a background of fatigue and weight loss. Crackles in the chest are rare. Approximately 15% of patients have a concurrent cause for respiratory failure (e.g. Kaposi sarcoma, TB, bacterial pneumonia). Useful investigations are:

1. *CXR:* classical appearance is diffuse bilateral perihilar interstitial shadowing, but in the early stages this is very subtle and easily missed. The initial CXR is normal in 10%. In a further 10% the changes are atypical with focal consolidation or coarse patchy shadowing. None of the changes are specific for PCP and may be seen in other lung diseases associated with AIDS. Pleural effusions, hilar or mediastinal lymphadenopathy are unusual in PCP but common in mycobacterial infection or Kaposi's sarcoma or lymphoma.
2. *Induced sputum:* in this technique the patient inhales nebulised hypertonic saline from an ultrasonic nebuliser. This provokes bronchorrhoea and the patient

Table 36.5 Causes of CXR changes and empirical treatment of pneumonia in the immunocompromised

CHEST X-RAY APPEARANCE	CAUSES	EMPIRICAL TREATMENT FOR SUSPECTED PNEUMONIA
Diffuse infiltrate	CMV and other herpes viruses *Pneumocystis carinii* Bacteria *Aspergillus* (advanced) *Cryptococcus* (uncommon) Non-infectious causes, e.g. drug reaction, non-specific interstitial pneumonitis, radiation pneumonitis (uncommon), malignancy, leucoagglutinin reaction	Broad-spectrum antibiotics for at least 48 h (e.g. 3rd-generation cephalosporin and aminoglycoside) Co-trimoxazole Lung biopsy or lavage within 48 h or full 2-week course of co-trimoxazole (depends on patient tolerance of invasive procedure)
Focal infiltrate	Gram-negative rods *S. aureus* *Aspergillus* *Cryptococcus* *Nocardia* *Mucor.* *P. carinii* (uncommon) Tuberculosis Legionella Non-infectious causes (e.g. malignancy, non-specific interstitial pneumonitis, radiation pneumonitis)	Broad-spectrum antibiotics If response seen continue treatment for 2 weeks If disease progresses lung biopsy/aspirate within 48–72 hours or empirical trial of antifungal±macrolide

coughs up material containing cysts and trophozoites. The technique is time-consuming and requires meticulous technique and is less sensitive than bronchoscopy but less invasive. The possibility of concurrent tuberculosis should be considered and steps taken to minimise the risk of spread of infection.

3. Bronchoscopy with bronchoalveolar lavage leads to the diagnosis in over 90% of cases. Specimens should be sent for cytology. Transbronchial biopsy is not necessary in most cases. PCR using bronchial lavage specimens may be useful in non-HIV patients with suspected PCP.

Antipneumocystis treatment should be started as soon as the diagnosis is suspected. Treatment of choice is trimethoprim plus sulfamethoxazole (co-trimoxazole) 20 mg/kg/day+100 mg/kg/day for 3 weeks plus prednisolone 40 mg orally twice daily for 5 days followed by 20 mg twice daily for 5 days and then 20 mg per day until the end of PCP treatment. Side-effects of co-trimoxazole are common in HIV patients (nausea, vomiting, skin rash, myelotoxicity). The dose should be reduced by 25% if the WBC count falls. Patients who are intolerant of co-trimoxazole should be treated with:

- pentamidine 4 mg/kg/day i.v. or
- primaquine with clindamycin or
- trimetrexate with leucovorin (±oral dapsone).

Response to treatment is usually excellent, with a response time of 4–7 days. If the patient deteriorates or fails to improve: consider (re-)bronchoscopy (is the diagnosis correct?), treat co-pathogens and consider a short course of high-dose i.v. methylprednisolone and/or diuretics (patients often fluid-overloaded). Approximately 40% of patients with HIV-related PCP who require mechanical ventilation survive to hospital discharge.[38]

Initiation of antiretroviral therapy in patients presenting with HIV-related PCP is controversial. The Centers for Disease Control and Prevention (CDC) recommend against doing so in the acute phase, but recent data suggest that the outcome may be improved by initiation within the first 4 days of ICU admission.[39]

BACTERIAL PNEUMONIA[37]

This is the most common cause of acute respiratory failure in HIV-positive patients. Bacterial pneumonia is more common in HIV-infected patients than in the general population and tends to be more severe. *Strep. pneumoniae, H. influenza, Pseudomonas aeruginosa* and *S. aureus* are the commonest organisms. *Nocardia* and Gram negatives should also be considered. Atypical pathogens (e.g. *Legionella*) are rare. Response to appropriate antibiotics is usually good but may require protracted courses of antibiotics because of high tendency to relapse. Patients with severe immunodeficiency ($CD4^+$ T lymphocyte count <100/μL) and a history of *Pseudomonas* infection or bronchiectasis or neutropenia should receive antibiotics that cover *P. aeruginosa* as well as other Gram negatives. The possibility of concurrent PCP or tuberculosis should be excluded.

TUBERCULOSIS

TB may be the initial presentation of AIDS, particularly in sub-Saharan Africa. The pattern of TB in HIV patients depends on the degree of immunosuppression. In patients with $CD4^+$ T lymphocytes >350 cells/μL the clinical presentation is similar to TB in non-HIV-infected patients, although extrapulmonary disease is more common. In patients with $CD4^+$ T lymphocytes <350 cells/μL extrapulmonary disease (pleuritis, pericarditis, meningitis) is common. Severely immunocompromised patients ($CD4^+$ T lymphocytes <100 cells/μL) may present with severe systemic disease with high fever, rapid progression and systemic sepsis. In these patients lower and middle lobe disease is more common, miliary disease is common and cavitation is less common. Sputum smears and culture may be positive even with a normal CXR.

Response to treatment is usually rapid. Management of TB in HIV is complex owing to numerous drug interactions; consultation with an expert in treatment of HIV-related TB should be strongly considered. Complex interactions occur between rifamycins (e.g. rifampicin and rifabutin) and protease inhibitors and non-nucleoside reverse transcriptase inhibitors used to treat patients infected with HIV. The choice of rifampicin or rifabutin depends on a number of factors including the unique and synergistic adverse effects for each individual combination of rifampicin and anti-HIV drugs, and consultation with a physician with experience in treating both TB and HIV is advised.[40] IDSA-recommended dosage adjustment for patients receiving antiretrovirals and rifabutin[37] can be obtained via the 'link page' (http://www.aic.cuhk.edu.hk/web8/Pneumonia%20guidelines.htm.). The optimal time for initiating antiretroviral therapy in patients with TB is controversial. Early therapy may decrease HIV disease progression but may be associated with a high incidence of adverse effects and an immune reconstitution reaction.[37]

CMV PNEUMONITIS[41,42]

Risk of infection is highest following allogeneic stem cell transplantation, followed by lung transplantation, pancreas transplantation and then liver, heart and renal transplantation and advanced AIDS. If both the recipient and the donor are seronegative then the risk of both infection and disease are negligible. If the recipient is seropositive the risk of infection is approximately 70% but the risk of disease is only 20%, regardless of the serostatus of the donor. However if the recipient is seronegative and the donor is seropositive the risk of disease is 70%. If steroid pulses and antilymphocyte globulin are given for treatment of acute rejection the risk of developing disease is markedly increased. Infection may be the result of primary infection or reactivation of latent infection. It is clinically important, but often difficult to distinguish between CMV infection and CMV disease and a definitive diagnosis can be made only histologically. Detection of CMV-pp65 antigen in peripheral WBC and detection of CMV DNA or RNA in the blood by quantitative polymerase chain reaction are the most useful tests for demonstrating CMV disease. Using thresholds of 10/300 000–50/200 000 positive circulating peripheral WBC, the positive predictive value for CMV-pp65 ranges from 64% to 82% and the negative predictive value from 70% to 95%[43,44] Treatment consists of intravenous ganciclovir for at least 14 days. Foscarnet can be used if ganciclovir fails.

FUNGAL PNEUMONIA

Fungi are rare but important causes of pneumonia. They can be divided into two main groups based on the immune response required to combat infection with these organisms. Histoplasma, blastomycosis, coccidioidomycosis, paracoccidioidomycosis and *Cryptococcus* require specific cell-mediated immunity for their control and thus, in contrast to infections that are controlled by phagocytic activity, the diseases caused by these organisms can occur in otherwise healthy individuals although they cause much more severe illness in patients with impaired cell-mediated immunity (e.g. patients infected with HIV and organ transplant recipients). With the exception of *Cryptococcus* these organisms are rarely seen outside North America. *Aspergillus* and *Mucor* spores are killed by non-immune phagocytes and as a result these fungi rarely result in clinical illness in patients with normal neutrophil numbers and function.

CANDIDIASIS

This is effectively a combination of the two types of fungal infection in which impaired cell-mediated immunity predisposes to mucosal overgrowth with *Candida* but impaired phagocytic function or numbers is usually required before deep invasion of tissues occurs. Primary *Candida* pneumonia (i.e. isolated lung infection) is uncommon[41,45] and more commonly pulmonary lesions are only one manifestation of disseminated candidiasis. Even more common is benign colonisation of the airway with *Candida*. In most reported cases of primary *Candida* pneumonia amphotericin B has been used. In disseminated candidiasis treatment should be directed to treatment of disseminated disease rather than *Candida* pneumonia per se.[45]

INVASIVE ASPERGILLOSIS[46]

This is a highly lethal condition in the immunocompromised despite treatment and therefore investigation and treatment should be prompt and aggressive. It is associated with exposure to construction work. Definitive diagnosis requires both histological evidence of acute-angle branching, septated non-pigmented hyphae measuring 2–4 μm in width, and cultures yielding *Aspergillus* species from biopsy specimens of involved organs. Recovery of *Aspergillus* species from respiratory secretions in immunocompromised, but not immunocompetent, patients may indicate invasive disease with a positive predictive value as high as

80–90% in patients with leukaemia or bone marrow transplant recipients. Bronchoalveolar lavage with smear, culture and antigen detection has excellent specificity and reasonably good positive predictive value for invasive aspergillosis in immunocompromised patients. Although radiological features may give a clue to the diagnosis they are not sufficiently specific to be diagnostic.

In acutely ill immunocompromised patients intravenous therapy should be initiated if there is suggestive evidence of invasive aspergillosis while further investigations to confirm or refute the diagnosis are carried out. First-line therapy is voriconazole.[47] Echinocandins and amphotericin are alternatives.

PARAPNEUMONIC EFFUSION

This may be an uncomplicated effusion that resolves with appropriate treatment of the underlying pneumonia or a complicated effusion that develops into an empyema unless drained. Complicated effusions tend to develop 7–14 days after initial fluid formation. They are characterised by increasing pleural fluid volume, continued fever and pleural fluid of low pH (<7.3) that contains a large number of neutrophils and may reveal organisms on Gram staining or culture. An outline of management is given in **Figure 36.5**.

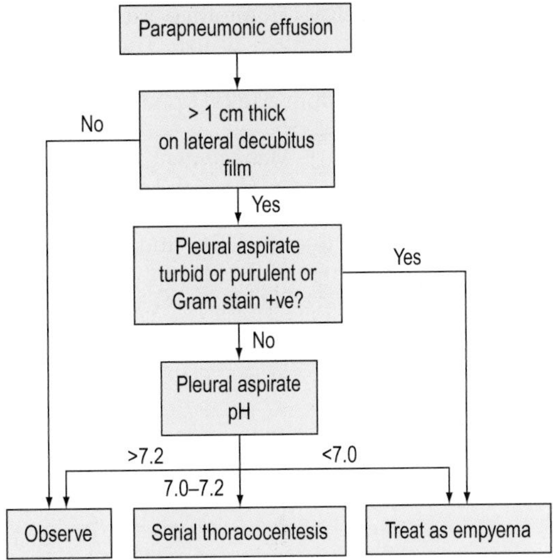

Figure 36.5 An approach to the management of parapneumonic effusions.

EMPYEMA[48]

DEFINITION

Collection of pus in the pleural space.

AETIOLOGY

Follows infection of the structures surrounding the pleural space, including subdiaphragmatic structures, and chest trauma, or may be associated with malignancy. Anaerobic bacteria, usually streptococci or Gram-negative rods, are responsible for 76% of cases.

DIAGNOSIS

The diagnosis is usually simple. The patient is usually septic and may have a productive cough and chest pain. The chest X-ray may show features suggestive of a pleural effusion and underlying consolidation but may also show an abscess cavity with a fluid level, in which case CT scanning will be required to distinguish between an abscess and an empyema. Ultrasound can be useful to confirm the presence of fluid in the pleural space and to determine whether it can be drained by needle aspiration or, if there is debris within the fluid, drainage using an intercostal drain. The diagnosis is confirmed by aspiration of pus.

TREATMENT

The mainstay of treatment is drainage either by intercostal drain or by surgical intervention. Patients who present before the pus is loculated and a fibrinous peel has formed on the lung can usually be treated by simple drainage. The combination with intrapleural fibrinolysis may be beneficial. Optimal surgical management, which consists of decortication (open or thoracoscopic), is indicated if the empyema is more advanced or if simple drainage fails. This is a major procedure and many patients with cardiac or chronic respiratory disease will not tolerate it. Alternatives for these patients are instillation of thrombolytics into the pleural space or thoracostomy. Antibiotics have only an adjunctive role. Broad-spectrum antibiotic regimens with anaerobic cover should be used until the results of microbiological analysis of the aspirated pus are available.

Acknowledgements

All tables and figures are reproduced from ICU web (www.aic.cuhk.edu.hk/web8) with permission of the authors.

Access the complete references list online at http://www.expertconsult.com

1. American Thoracic Society and Infectious Diseases Society of America. Guidelines for the management of adults with hospital-acquired, ventilator-associated, and healthcare associated pneumonia. Am J Respir Crit Care Med 2005;171:388–416.
2. Mandell LA, Wunderink RG, Anzueto A, et al. Infectious Diseases Society of America/American Thoracic Society consensus guidelines on the management of community-acquired pneumonia in adults. Clin Infect Dis 2007;44:S27–72.

3. Pneumonia Guidelines Committee of the BTS Standards of Care Committee. British Thoracic Society guidelines for the management of community acquired pneumonia in adults: update 2009. Thorax 2009;64(Suppl III):iii1–55.
16. Waterer GW, Rello J. Management of community-acquired pneumonia in adults. Am J Respir Crit Care Med 2011;183:157–64.
34. American Thoracic Society, CDC, and Infectious Diseases Society of America. Treatment of tuberculosis. Am J Respir Crit Care Med 2003;167:603–62.
49. Meduri GU, Chastre J. The standardization of bronchoscopic techniques for ventilator-associated pneumonia. Chest 1992;102:557S–64S.
50. Lorente L, Blot S. New issues and controversies in the prevention of ventilator-associated pneumonia. Am J Respir Crit Care Med 2010;182:870–6.

37

Non-invasive ventilation

Graeme J Duke and Andrew D Bersten

Non-invasive ventilation (NIV) is a valuable therapeutic option in the management of acute and chronic respiratory failure – for certain diagnoses it is the preferred option. The application of NIV predates the introduction of laryngoscopy (early 1900s) and the widespread use of positive-pressure mechanical ventilation via an endotracheal tube (MV) in the 1950s.[1] Successful use of NIV in acute respiratory failure was first published in 1936.[2]

NIV is defined as ventilatory support without an (invasive) endotracheal airway. It has an increasingly important role in the early management of reversible acute respiratory failure (ARF),[3,4] and in domiciliary management of chronic respiratory failure due to obstructive sleep apnoea (OSA) and neuromuscular disease.

NIV may be achieved either through the delivery of positive pressure to the airway (P_{ao}) or the application of a negative-pressure generator to the chest ('chest box' or cuirass) or body ('iron lung'). A conceptual framework is shown in **Figure 37.1**.

Negative-pressure generators may be used for the management of acute or chronic respiratory disease.[5] Major limitations to the use of negative-pressure generators include the induction of OSA, lack of fractional inspired oxygen (Fi_{O_2}) control, equipment bulk and size.[6] However, external negative-pressure generators suit some patients with chronic respiratory failure, particularly as there is no oral or nasal prosthesis. This chapter deals primarily with the use of positive-pressure NIV to treat ARF.

The clinical efficacy of NIV depends upon: (a) the mode used and (b) the nature and severity of the underlying respiratory pathophysiology. Correctly applied, NIV can reduce morbidity and mortality, whereas inappropriate application may delay definitive therapy and adversely affect outcome. An understanding of the physiological rationale for NIV will assist the clinician understand the indications and benefits, and predict the side-effects of the various NIV modes.[7,8] Several important aspects regarding ventilatory support are discussed in Chapter 31 (Mechanical ventilation), and this chapter will focus on those aspects specific to NIV.

PHYSIOLOGY OF NIV

The physiological benefits of NIV are similar to those of invasive ventilatory support. NIV can reverse many of the adverse physiological and mechanical derangements associated with ARF, through a combination of:

- augmentation of alveolar ventilation (V_A) to reverse respiratory acidosis and hypercarbia
- alveolar recruitment and increased Fi_{O_2} to reverse hypoxia
- reduction in work of breathing (W_{mus}) to reduce or prevent respiratory muscle insufficiency
- stabilisation of the chest wall in the presence of chest trauma or surgery
- reduction in left ventricular (LV) afterload that may lead to improved cardiac function
- reduction of right ventricular afterload and improved right ventricular function.[9]

In brief, the respiratory effort (pressure–volume work) required to achieve a desired minute volume (V_E) may be viewed as the summation of the individual forces that must be overcome to generate inspiratory flow, namely: elastic work (or 'stretch'; W_{el}), flow-resistive work (air-flow obstruction; W_{res}) and threshold work. Threshold work, the work required to overcome the effects of dynamic hyperinflation and intrinsic PEEP ($PEEP_i$) prior to triggering inspiratory assistance, is another form of elastic work and included as part of W_{el}. Since the volume component is constant the equation of motion can be written as:

$$P_{mus} = P_{el} + P_{res} \quad (37.1)$$

(See Ch. 31, Mechanical ventilation, for more detailed explanation.)

With the addition of a device for ventilatory support, the respiratory muscle effort (P_{mus}) required by the patient is equivalent to the difference between the applied P_{ao} and the total work required to maintain V_E:

$$P_{mus} = (P_{el} + P_{res}) - P_{ao} \quad (37.2)$$

This relationship may be rearranged into its individual components, as follows:

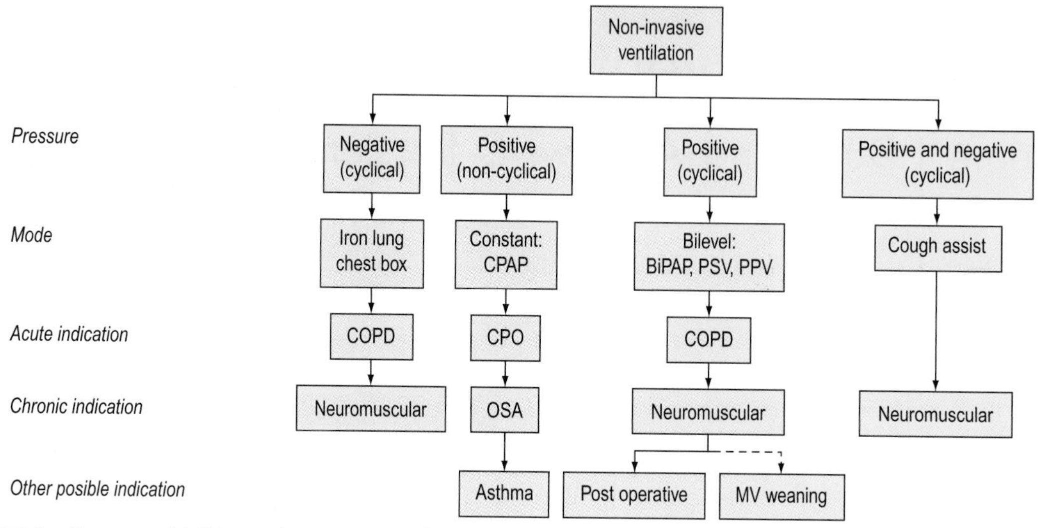

Figure 37.1 Conceptual NIV paradigm. (See text for definitions.)

$$P_{mus} + P_{ao} = E \bullet V + R \bullet \dot{V} + PEEP_i \qquad (37.3)$$

where E is the respiratory elastance (inverse of compliance), V is the volume of gas, R is the respiratory and circuit flow resistance, $\dot{V}$ is the inspiratory flow rate and $PEEP_i$ is the intrinsic PEEP

It is important to remember that breathing via a circuit will create additional air-flow resistance (R) adding to breathing work (P_{mus}), and thus attention to circuit design is important (see below).

$PEEP_i$ and dynamic hyperinflation are absent in the healthy lung, but common in the presence of tachypnoea and/or expiratory air-flow obstruction. During flow limitation, $PEEP_i$ impedes the onset (triggering) of inspiratory support modes (IPAP and PSV). This threshold load ($PEEP_i$) must be counterbalanced by either an equivalent amount of inspiratory effort or end-expiratory pressure before inspiratory flow can commence.

Respiratory failure occurs when the forces opposing inspiration – namely elastic (P_{el}), resistive (P_{res}) and threshold ($PEEP_i$) work – exceed the respiratory muscle effort (P_{mus}) required to maintain V_E. Hypermetabolic states (e.g. trauma, sepsis) increase basal V_E, whereas pulmonary and chest wall diseases increase respiratory workload and neuromuscular disease impairs respiratory muscle effort. NIV may prevent respiratory failure by counterbalancing the increased respiratory workload and/or reducing respiratory muscle effort, and thus maintain V_A.

Any invasive MV mode may be delivered non-invasively and four are commonly described in clinical research: continuous positive airway pressure (CPAP), PSV, bilevel or biphasic positive airway pressure (BIPAP), and pressure- or volume-limited intermittent positive-pressure ventilation. Other modes under investigation include high-frequency and proportional assist ventilation.

All NIV modalities utilise (semi-closed or) closed circuits and are thus capable of controlling and delivering high Fi_{O_2}. This is an important mechanism by which NIV improves oxygenation, independently of other mechanisms discussed below.

CONTINUOUS POSITIVE AIRWAY PRESSURE

CPAP is a form of NIV because it provides respiratory support even though the P_{ao} applied is constant throughout the respiratory cycle. This mode addresses a number of the objectives of ventilatory support, namely:

- reduction in the work of breathing by:
  - alveolar recruitment and reduction in elastic work
  - reducing threshold load created in the presence of $PEEP_i$
- reversing hypoxia through delivery of high Fi_{O_2}, alveolar recruitment, and reduction of intrapulmonary shunt
- reduction of left ventricular (LV) transmural pressure (afterload).[10,11]

INSPIRATORY POSITIVE AIRWAY PRESSURE (IPAP) AND PSV

Positive inspiratory airway pressure without expiratory pressure (e.g. PSV or IPAP), provides respiratory support by reducing both the elastic and resistive components of respiratory work resulting in:

- augmentation of tidal volume (V_E) and reduction in Pa_{CO_2}

- reduction in P_{mus} and diminish or prevent respiratory muscle insufficiency
- induction of pulmonary surfactant release through alveolar inflation above resting tidal volume.[12]

Bilevel positive airway pressure allows separate settings for inspiratory (IPAP) and expiratory (EPAP) airway pressure levels; it is conceptually similar to PSV plus CPAP.[13] Respiratory frequency is usually patient-dependent but may be mechanically time cycled and independent of patient effort.

CONTROLLED VENTILATION

NIV may also be administered as volume- or pressure-limited mechanical ventilation applied via a mask (instead of an endotracheal airway).

PATIENT–VENTILATOR INTERACTION

This is discussed in Chapter 31 (Mechanical ventilation), and subdivided into: (a) triggering of inspiration, (b) inspiration and (c) cessation of inspiration. The only aspect that is specific to NIV arises from mask leaks, which may interfere with the ability to sense the end of expiration because there is continued 'expiratory' gas flow.

NIV EQUIPMENT

Equipment design varies according to NIV mode and purpose (e.g. critical care or domiciliary setting), and significant variations in performance characteristics have been documented.[1,14] The important characteristics of an efficient NIV circuit include:

- high gas flow to match peak inspiratory air flow – high flows may be generated by a pressurised gas supply, a gas turbine, or a jet venturi mechanism: a device providing continuous flow imposes less circuit work than a demand flow device
- an expiratory resistor capable of maintaining the desired PEEP, yet offering a low resistance to expiratory flow to reduce fluctuations in the delivered P_{ao} – this may be a threshold resistor or flow resistor; the optimal position for the expiratory valve is as close to the patient's airway as possible
- short wide-bore tubing to reduce turbulence and flow resistance
- a flow or pressure sensor for identifying inspiratory effort and triggering the predetermined inspiratory pressure support (e.g. PSV or IPAP)
- ability to control and deliver a wide range of F_{IO_2}
- other desirable features include the facility to humidify inspired gases and to nebulise drugs. the provision for pressure-relief safety valves, battery back-up, apnoea back-up support, acoustic suppression and monitoring of volume and P_{ao} are important for hospital NIV equipment and less important for domiciliary (long-term) devices.

Several varieties of mask design are also available and the optimal configuration depends upon the purpose and mode of NIV, patient anatomy, and preference. These include intranasal, nasal, and oronasal, full-face and helmet (full-head) masks. Desirable features of a mask include lightweight and transparent materials affording a comfortable airtight seal, minimal dead space, and separate inspiratory and expiratory ports to minimise air-flow turbulence and rebreathing.[14,15] In lung model studies, expiratory ports over the nasal bridge reduce dead space,[16] which may prove to be clinically advantageous, and traditional orofacial masks have lower dead space than full-face masks or helmet designs.[17]

Mask discomfort, arising from the mask seal, air leaks, humidification, or claustrophobia, is a common cause of noncompliance. Masks that cover nose and mouth tend to produce more reliable and constant P_{ao} because they are unaffected by mouth breathing – a common problem in the critically ill patient. Nasal masks are less restrictive on the patient's ability to talk, eat/drink, and expectorate and therefore gain higher compliance in long-term and domiciliary applications. To effectively compensate for air leaks, nasal masks should be used with circuits capable of rapidly augmenting and delivering high flows (>100 L/min).

Fibreoptic bronchoscopy can be safely performed during NIV, using a full-face mask with at least two ports. One of these can be modified to provide a simple valve for insertion of the bronchoscope, and the other used for NIV. Provided there is adequate flow reserve during suction, this can be performed during any mode of NIV. This technique may allow both diagnostic and therapeutic bronchoscopic intervention without intubation even in critically ill patients.

COMPLICATIONS AND ASSESSMENT OF EFFICACY

Contraindications and complications specific to NIV are listed in **Box 37.1**. Acutely unwell patients requiring NIV should be managed in a critical care ward, or similar area with appropriately trained on-site medical and nursing staff. Although the development of sophisticated, portable non-invasive ventilators makes it easy to provide NIV in any environment, its benefits may diminish outside the critical care environment.[18,19]

Following the initial application of NIV reversal of hypoxia and reduction in respiratory effort is commonly observed irrespective of the underlying disease. Although these intermediate goals are important, they are a poor guide to the efficacy of NIV. More reliable clinical measures of NIV efficacy include reversal of hypercarbia, a sustained improvement in respiratory function and patient outcomes, such as a reduction in non-compliance, intubation, nosocomial pneumonia and mortality.

Box 37.1 Contraindications and complications of NIV

Contraindications

- Respiratory arrest
- Unprotected airway (coma, sedation)
- Upper airway obstruction
- Inability to clear secretions
- Untreated pneumothorax
- Marked haemodynamic instability

Complications

- Mask discomfort, patient intolerance
- Facial or ocular abrasions
- Nasal congestion, sinus pain
- Oronasal dryness
- ↑ Intraocular pressure (particularly in patients with glaucoma)
- ↑ Intracranial pressure (particularly in patients with neurotrauma)
- ↓ Blood pressure (if hypovolaemic)
- Aspiration pneumonia (rare)
- Aerophagy and gastric distension (uncommon; routine gastric decompression is unnecessary)

NIV AND ACUTE RESPIRATORY FAILURE (ARF)[1,18,20]

CARDIOGENIC PULMONARY OEDEMA (CPO)[1,8,21]

CPO is a common cause of severe reversible ARF. Since the 1930s, a number of investigators have documented the therapeutic benefits of all modes of NIV, particularly CPAP. CPO leads to an increase in elastic workload (P_{el}) and, to a less extent, resistive workload (P_{res}), an increase in lung water and impaired surfactant function. CPAP reverses hypoxia, recruits alveoli and reduces intrapulmonary shunt and LV afterload. Redistribution of extravascular lung water from alveoli to the interstitial space is aided by recruitment of alveoli and surfactant production.

Over 30 prospective randomised controlled trials of NIV in CPO have consistently demonstrated physiological improvements in hypoxic and hypercapnic respiratory failure, and a significant reduction in the need for intubation (95% CI RR=0.32–0.60), hospital length of stay, and improved survival (95% CI RR=0.44–0.92).[19] Even though the majority of these patients were managed in a critical care setting the average length of stay and duration of respiratory support was much shorter for NIV (9±11 hours) than those who required MV.[22]

The optimal mode of NIV in CPO appears to be CPAP. The optimal P_{ao} level remains to be resolved, although 10 cmH_2O appeared to be safe and effective in the majority of subjects. Although the addition of a differential inspiratory pressure (e.g. bilevel[23] and PSV[24,25]) may be as effective as CPAP in avoiding (95% CI RR=0.33–0.86) intubation it may not provide a survival benefit and may increase the rate of myocardial infarction[26,27] (95% CI RR=0.92–2.42).[21]

Benefits appear to be greater in those with acute coronary syndrome as the primary aetiology.[21] CPAP reduces preload and afterload[10,11] and myocardial catecholamine release[28] whereas the cyclical P_{ao} (of bilevel NIV) may cause fluctuation in preload and afterload during respiration.[1,29] Current evidence supports the routine use of mask-CPAP in moderate or severe CPO as standard therapy and as the first-line option for respiratory support.[18,30]

ARF IN CHRONIC OBSTRUCTIVE PULMONARY DISEASE (COPD)

COPD patients have an elevated resistive work (P_{res}), often coupled with an elevated basal V_E and elastic work (P_{el}) as a result of the pre-existing parenchymal damage. Threshold load ($PEEP_i$) is frequently present as a result of air-flow obstruction, and is exacerbated during ARF by further increased P_{res} and respiratory rate. Reversible ARF is a common complication of COPD.

The importance of NIV in hypercapnic ARF is now supported by at least 14 well-performed prospective randomised controlled studies[20,31–33] in over 600 patients. Most investigators have demonstrated a low incidence of side effects and a significant decrease in intubation rates and in-hospital mortality.[33] The meta-analysis of NIV trials reveals significant reductions in mortality (95% CI RR=0.35–0.76) and the need for intubation (95% CI RR=0.33–0.53) – the number of patients needed to avoid one intubation or death being as few as 4 and 10 respectively.[34] Risk reduction appears to be proportional to the severity of respiratory acidosis.[35] The incidence of nosocomial pneumonia is lower with NIV[36–38] and this may explain some of the survival benefit associated with NIV.[38]

Current evidence supports the use of NIV in hypercapnic ARF as a component of standard therapy in COPD subjects. This is supported by many respiratory medicine societies throughout the world[18,30,39] that 'patients hospitalised for exacerbations of COPD with rapid clinical deterioration should be considered for noninvasive positive pressure [ventilatory support] to prevent further deterioration in gas exchange, respiratory workload and the need for endotracheal intubation'.[18]

All modes of NIV have been shown to be effective but there are no comparative trials that address the question of optimal mode or pressure level.[18] Patients with ARF arising predominantly from reversible airflow obstruction (P_{res}) and/or threshold load are likely to respond to CPAP alone. Hypercapnic patients often have reduced alveolar ventilation or respiratory muscle insufficiency and are therefore likely to benefit from the addition of inspiratory support, such as PSV, IPAP, or NIPPV.

A trial of NIV is justified by the presence of respiratory acidosis (pH<7.37) or persistent breathlessness.[34,40] It is poorly tolerated in those without acidosis.

Inspiratory support (usually 5–20 cmH_2O) should be titrated to improve V_E as indicated by improvement in tidal volume and pH, and reduction in respiratory rate and/or Pa_{CO_2}. Low levels of CPAP or EPAP (4–8 cmH_2O) are usually required to counterbalance threshold load. Clinical observation and judgement are required to titrate this to a level that minimises the effort required to trigger inspiratory support (PSV or IPAP). Fi_{O_2} is titrated to reverse hypoxia.

Early predictors of NIV success in COPD patients include improvements in pH and Pa_{CO_2} (but not Pa_{O_2}) within the first 1–2 hours of therapy.[34,40] Predictors of NIV failure include persistent mask intolerance, severe acidosis (pH<7.25), tachypnoea (>35/min), impaired conscious state, and poor clinical response to initial therapy.[41] The bedside care plan should include a clear strategy for those patients who fail a trial of NIV. Mask intolerance, nursing workload, and failure rates are greater during NIV for COPD than those reported in CPO. These patients benefit from a critical care setting where expertise and equipment are available and reported outcomes appear better.[19,34]

Whilst reported success rates are high (70–90%), NIV failure (i.e. intubation) appears to increase with the severity of respiratory acidosis.[34,40] For the poorly compliant patient, reassurance and explanation together with a trial of different size and/or type of mask, or initiation with lower-pressure settings, and brief periods of NIV will sometimes assist. Low-dose anxiolytic drugs may be beneficial where anxiety is a recurrent precipitant of dyspnoea, but should be used with extreme caution because of their respiratory depressant side-effects.

Late failure (>48 h) occurs in 10–20% of patients[20,32,41] despite an initial improvement with NIV. This group of patients has a high mortality risk.[42] Whether this reflects the severity of the underlying disease or delayed initiation of MV remains unclear.

ASTHMA

Asthma is an acute inflammatory lung disease that increases resistive (P_{res}) and threshold ($PEEP_i$) respiratory work. Physiological and clinical improvement has been demonstrated in acute asthmatics with the application of CPAP[43–45] and bilevel NIV.[45–47] One randomised controlled trial of bilevel NIV titrated over 30 minutes resulted in significant improvement in $FEV_{1.0}$ and a lower hospital admission rate.[48]

The clinical role of NIV in the management of acute asthma and the benefit of differential inspiratory and expiratory pressures remains to be clarified. Nebulised drugs can be effectively delivered even in the presence of a high-flow NIV circuit.[49] Controlled clinical studies with robust end-points are awaited. We have found 5 cmH_2O CPAP to be effective in moderate to severe asthma not responding to steroids and continuous inhaled bronchodilators, and that mask intolerance is the most common cause for failure. If NIV is used in asthma this must be performed in a high-acuity environment where there appropriately skilled staff members are immediately available should the patient require urgent intubation.

ACUTE LUNG INJURY (ALI) AND ACUTE RESPIRATORY DISTRESS SYNDROME (ARDS)

Like CPO, ALI leads to an increase in elastic workload (P_{el}) and, to a lesser extent, resistive workload (P_{res}) arising from an increase in alveolar-capillary permeability, the release of inflammatory mediators, and impaired surfactant function. Even though the addition of PEEP is beneficial (during MV) for ALI or ARDS and NIV has a lower prevalence of nosocomial pneumonia,[36–38] current data do not support the routine use of NIV in non-cardiogenic pulmonary oedema and undifferentiated hypoxaemic acute respiratory failure.[50,51]

Despite numerous publications reporting the successful use of NIV in the setting of community-acquired pneumonia (without COPD) and other forms of ALI, the failure rate remains high.[33,50–55] This may reflect the differences in duration, severity, and the pathophysiology of pneumonia, ALI and ARDS compared with CPO. Apparent benefit may be due to the inclusion of subjects with cardiogenic pulmonary oedema[56] or COPD[57,58] – specific subgroups known to benefit from NIV.

PNEUMONIA IN THE IMMUNOCOMPROMISED PATIENT

MV is associated with high morbidity and mortality risks in immunocompromised patients with hypoxic respiratory failure.[58–61] These patients may benefit from an early trial NIV since this appears to be associated with improved hospital survival.[61] Whether NIV simply avoids a high-morbidity therapy (MV)[36] or identifies responders with a more readily reversible form of ARF is unclear. Nevertheless it seems reasonable, based on the current data, to offer NIV to these patients.[18,61] Once again, clear bedside guidelines should be established for the management of patients who fail a trial of NIV and those in whom MV is deemed inappropriate or futile because of its high associated mortality risk.[61]

POSTOPERATIVE AND POST-TRAUMATIC ARF

ARF in postoperative and trauma patients may arise from a number of reversible pathological processes associated with increases in elastic workload (P_{el}) and impaired respiratory muscle function (P_{mus}), including dependent atelectasis, impaired chest-wall mechanics, poor cough, nosocomial infection, aspiration pneumonitis and non-respiratory trauma or sepsis.

Mask CPAP consistently improves intermediate physiological parameters (e.g. oxygenation and respiratory rate) and reduces the risk of intubation in general surgical[62] and cardiothoracic patients[63] with mild post-operative hypoxic respiratory failure, but evidence for a survival benefit is lacking. NIV may improve survival in certain subgroups such as postoperative lung resection[64] but many of these patients have underlying COPD, and extrapolation of these results to non-COPD patients awaits further study.

Mask CPAP has been shown to be superior to MV in patients with isolated severe chest trauma,[65,66] but the benefit of NIV remains unclear. NIV is contraindicated in the presence of other significant injuries such as neurotrauma and intracranial hypertension, facial trauma or the presence of an untreated pneumothorax.

NIV-ASSISTED WEANING

Since NIV is effective in reducing the need for intubation and MV, it has been postulated that NIV may prevent re-intubation. NIV has therefore been recommended to expedite early weaning from MV[67] or as rescue therapy following failed[68] or accidental extubation. The putative advantages relate to reduction in the duration and the risks of MV (e.g. nosocomial pneumonia).

For COPD patients there appears to be a survival benefit[67–69] but it cannot be recommended in the non-COPD group, for whom NIV offers no benefit[18,70,71] or even increased mortality.[68] Although NIV is an option for post-extubation rescue therapy in the COPD subgroup, it is not a substitute for strategies to improve early access to NIV (in COPD and CPO) and improve weaning success and the risk of premature extubation.

NIV AND CHRONIC RESPIRATORY DISEASE

NIV is an important modality for short-term assistance and long-term treatment of severe chronic respiratory failure associated with obstructive and central sleep apnoea syndromes,[18,72] and chronic hypoventilation syndromes associated with extrapulmonary disease such as neuromuscular disease,[72] and thoracic deformities.[73,74] There appears to be less benefit in chronic parenchymal lung disease such as (stable) COPD[69,74–6] and cystic fibrosis (CF).[77]

These patients may require short-term respiratory support during an acute illness or as an aid to perioperative care in a critical care environment. NIV (plus mini-tracheostomy for secretion removal) may improve outcome compared with intubation and MV[73] but failure rates appear to be higher than in hypercapnic COPD.[76] Diagnosis of these underlying disorders during admission for treatment of severe ARF should prompt referral and assessment for long-term NIV.

NIV AND SLEEP APNOEA SYNDROMES[78,79]

Moderate or severe OSA results in nocturnal hypoventilation and episodic hypoxia that can lead to pulmonary and systemic hypertension, cardiac failure, and daytime hypercapnia and somnolence.[80,81] Many of these complications can be arrested or reversed through the appropriate use of nocturnal CPAP.[18,74,77] Patients with suspected sleep apnoea require accurate assessment by a respiratory physician, including sleep studies, prior to the routine use of domiciliary CPAP. Bilevel or controlled ventilation is required when there is inadequate central respiratory drive or increased elastic work. In many patients respiratory drive will improve, and they can then be managed with CPAP after a period of bilevel or controlled ventilation.

Intercurrent illness, surgery, or the use of sedatives and opioid analgesics, will increase the frequency and duration of hypopnoea, apnoea and hypoxia. CPAP should be available even for those patients who do not require admission to a critical care ward.

NIV AND CHRONIC HYPOVENTILATION SYNDROMES

Domiciliary NIV (predominantly using inspiratory support modes or NIPPV) should be considered in all patients presenting with severe chronic respiratory failure due to neuromuscular disease.[72,74,82] Early referral and consideration of domiciliary NIV are recommended because of improved outcomes[72,83,84] and quality of life. In CF patients it may have a role simply as a bridge to organ transplantation.[59,77] In direct contrast to the role of NIV in acute exacerbations of COPD, there is little or no benefit of domiciliary NIV in the presence of stable COPD[18,39,75,76] unless one of the former conditions coexists.

Assessment of these patients for domiciliary NIV includes respiratory function tests, blood gas analysis and sleep studies, together with trials of NIV modes and pressure settings. In general, indications for long-term NIV include the demonstration of symptomatic respiratory failure, daytime hypercapnia and a significantly reduced (<20% predicted) vital capacity. The use of nocturnal or intermittent NIV has been shown to improve daytime respiratory and cardiac function, to improve exercise endurance, to slow the progression of respiratory dysfunction, and to reduce the frequency of hospitalisation.[72,85]

Access the complete references list online at http://www.expertconsult.com

1. Mehta S, Hill NS. Noninvasive ventilation. State of the art. Am J Respir Crit Care Med 2001;163:540–77.
21. Weng C-L, Zhao Y-T, Liu Q-H, et al. Meta-analysis: noninvasive ventilation in acute cardiogenic pulmonary edema. Ann Intern Med 2010;152(9):590–600.
53. Ferrer M, Esquinas A, Leon M, et al. Noninvasive ventilation in severe hypoxemic respiratory failure: a randomized clinical trial. Am J Respir Crit Care Med 2003;168:1438–44.
61. Gristina GR, Antonelli M, Conti G, et al. Noninvasive versus invasive ventilation for acute respiratory failure in patients with hematologic malignancies: A 5-year multicenter observational survey. Critical Care Med 2011;39(10):2232–9.
62. Squadrone V, Coha M, Cerutti E, et al. Continuous positive airway pressure for treatment of postoperative hypoxemia: a randomized controlled trial. JAMA 2005;293:589–95.
70. Esteban A, Frutos-Vivar F, Ferguson ND, et al. Noninvasive positive-pressure ventilation for respiratory failure after extubation. New Engl J Med 2004;350(24):2452–60.

38

Respiratory monitoring

Andrew D Bersten

History and respiratory examination are particularly important in the critically ill patient. Particular attention should be directed at the respiratory rate (f), the most poorly documented vital sign, the quantity and nature of sputum, and evidence of excessive inspiratory and/or expiratory pleural pressure changes and effort, which include accessory muscle use, tracheal tug, supraclavicular and intercostal indrawing, paradoxical abdominal movement (which is suggestive of diaphragmatic fatigue[1]), and pulsus paradoxus. During spontaneous ventilation an excessive fall in blood pressure during inspiration (>10 mmHg) is found both in low-output states such as cardiac tamponade, cardiogenic shock, pulmonary embolism, hypovolaemic shock, and in acute respiratory failure. The fall in pleural pressure during spontaneous inspiration has a curvilinear relationship with the fall in blood pressure. However, as there is marked variation between individuals,[2] pulsus paradoxus is most useful in following trends. A reduction in the degree of paradox may reflect improvement with a fall in the negative pleural pressure needed for ventilation, or may reflect respiratory muscle insufficiency, and an inability to generate the same negative pleural pressure.

Additional information can be gained from blood gases and pulse oximetry (Ch. 18), and capnography, ventilatory pressures, and waveform analysis in patients receiving respiratory assistance. This chapter will focus on tests of respiratory function that are directly relevant to critically ill patients.

MONITORING GAS EXCHANGE

OXYGENATION

This is reviewed in Chapter 18, and is only briefly discussed here. Hypoxaemia may be due to a low partial pressure of inspired O_2 (rare), hypoventilation, diffusion impairment (rare), ventilation–perfusion ($\dot{V}/\dot{Q}$) mismatch, and shunt. Inert gas analysis has been used to quantitate $\dot{V}/\dot{Q}$ mismatch, and has demonstrated that hypoxaemia in ARDS is predominantly due to alveoli that are perfused but not ventilated (shunt),[3] consistent with CT scan evidence of increased dependent lung density. The alveolar gas equation is a common but less accurate method to assess hypoxaemia:

$$PA_{O_2} = \text{inspired } P_{O_2} - Pa_{CO_2} / \text{respiratory quotient} \quad (38.1)$$

where PA_{O_2} is the alveolar PO_2, and this is usually simplified to:

$$PA_{O_2} = (760 - 47) \times Fi_{O_2} - Pa_{CO_2} / 0.8 \quad (38.2)$$

where 760 is atmospheric pressure in mmHg, and 47 is the saturated vapour pressure of water at 37°C, since gas at the alveolus is fully humidified. The normal PA_{O_2} to Pa_{O_2} gradient is less than 15 mmHg, but increases to 25 mmHg in the elderly. This normal A–a gradient is due to some venous admixture through the lungs, and a small right-to-left shunt through both the bronchial veins, and the thebesian veins of the coronary circulation. This equation removes hypercarbia as a direct cause of hypoxaemia, and an increase in the A–a gradient will usually be due to $\dot{V}/\dot{Q}$ mismatch or right-to-left shunt. A commonly used alternative measure of hypoxaemia is the Pa_{O_2}/Fi_{O_2} ratio. However, this does not account for the effect of a raised Pa_{CO_2}, and both measures are influenced by a number of factors (e.g. cardiac output, Hb, Fi_{O_2}) in addition to the extent of venous admixture, which may be estimated from the intrapulmonary shunt equation:

$$\dot{Q}_s / \dot{Q}_t = Cc'_{O_2} - Ca_{O_2} / Cc'_{O_2} - Cv_{O_2} \quad (38.3)$$

where $\dot{Q}_s$ is the intrapulmonary shunt blood flow, $\dot{Q}_t$ is the total pulmonary blood flow, Cc'_{O_2} is the end-capillary O_2 content calculated from the PA_{O_2}, and Ca_{O_2} and Cv_{O_2} are the O_2 contents of arterial and mixed venous blood respectively.

CARBON DIOXIDE

Pa_{CO_2} is determined by alveolar ventilation ($\dot{V}_A$), and CO_2 production ($\dot{V}_{CO_2}$):

$$Pa_{CO_2}(\text{mmHg}) = \dot{V}_{CO_2}(\text{mL/min STPD}) \times 0.863 / \dot{V}_A(\text{L/min BTPS}) \quad (38.4)$$

where $\dot{V}_A$ is the minute ventilation ($\dot{V}_E$) minus the wasted or dead space ventilation ($\dot{V}_D$). The modified Bohr equation (assuming $PA_{CO_2} = Pa_{CO_2}$) calculates the proportion of the V_T that is wasted ventilation (i.e. physiological dead space; V_{Dphys}):

$$V_{Dphys} / V_T = Pa_{CO_2} - P\bar{E}CO_2 / Pa_{CO_2} \quad (38.5)$$

where $P\bar{E}_{CO_2}$ is the mixed expired P_{CO_2}, and V_{Dphys} is composed of anatomical dead space (V_{Danat}) and alveolar dead space (V_{Dalv}) – notionally due to alveoli that are ventilated but not perfused. Normally V_{Dalv} is minimal and V_{Danat} comprises 30% of V_T. Since the volume of an endotracheal tube is less than the mouth or nose, and pharynx, intubation may reduce V_{Danat}; however, when the connection from the endotracheal tube is taken into account there is little change in dead space. Positive pressure ventilation increases dead space by distension of the airways increasing V_{Danat}, and through a tendency to increase alveoli that are ventilated but not perfused. In patients with ARDS, marked increases in V_{Dalv} lead to marked increases in the V_{Dphys}/V_T ratio (exceeding 0.6), which is an independent prognostic factor.[4]

CAPNOGRAPHY

Capnography measures and displays exhaled CO_2 throughout the respiratory cycle, with sampling usually by a mainstream sensor as sidestream systems tend to become blocked by secretions. However, when capnography is used in non-intubated patients, sidestream sampling is commonly used (*e.g.* modified nasal cannulae). Infrared spectroscopy measures the fraction of energy absorbed and converts this to a percentage of CO_2 exhaled. During expiration the capnogram initially reads no CO_2, but as anatomical dead space is exhaled there is a rise in the exhaled CO_2 to a plateau, which falls to 0% CO_2 with the onset of inspiration. In patients with significant respiratory disease a plateau may never be achieved. The end-tidal CO_2 (PE'_{CO_2}) is the value at the end of the plateau, and is normally only slightly less than the Pa_{CO_2}. However, this gradient will increase when alveolar dead space (V_{Dalv}) increases, such as low cardiac output, pulmonary embolism and elevated alveolar pressure. Consequently the PE'_{CO_2} may not reflect Pa_{CO_2} in critically ill patients. Nevertheless, in a stable patient the gradient will be fairly constant, and can be used to guide $\dot{V}_E$ during transport,[5] and when other factors including the adequacy of minute ventilation are unchanged then sudden changes in the PE'_{CO_2} may provide an early signal. Indeed, PE'_{CO_2} directly correlates with cardiac output, and PE'_{CO_2} monitoring has been used to assess adequacy of cardiopulmonary resuscitation, and its prognosis.[6]

The presence of exhaled CO_2 confirms endotracheal tube placement, and is recommended even when the tube is seen to pass through the vocal cords,[7] since clinical assessment is not always reliable. Simple colorimetric devices may be used for this purpose. However, detection of expired CO_2 is not infallible[7] as false positives can rarely occur following ingestion of carbonated liquids, and false negatives may be due to extremely low pulmonary blood flow, or very large alveolar dead space such as pulmonary embolus or severe asthma. Monitoring with capnography is also recommended for transport[8] and respiratory monitoring[9] in critically ill patients, and should be available for every anaesthetised patient.[10]

GAS TRANSFER (DIFFUSING CAPACITY)

This is a test of the transfer of a gas, typically carbon monoxide (CO), across the alveolocapillary barrier. The transfer factor is calculated as:

$$\text{volume of CO taken up} / (PA_{CO} - Pc_{CO}) \quad (38.6)$$

and, as CO is so completely taken up by Hb, Pc_{CO} is taken as zero. This test is usually performed as an outpatient, is not usually measured in ICU, and diffusion abnormality is rarely a cause of hypoxaemia. The transfer factor is often corrected for lung volume since diseases such as emphysema and pulmonary fibrosis may affect both lung volume and diffusion. In chronic heart failure diffusing capacity is reduced and correlates with exercise performance and CHF severity and prognosis, due to a reduction in the volume of alveolar tissue and amount of blood participating in gas exchange.[11]

LUNG VOLUME AND CAPACITIES (Fig. 38.1)

The tidal volume (V_T) is the volume of gas inspired and expired with each breath, and the volume at end expiration is the functional residual capacity (FRC). The residual volume (RV) is the FRC minus the expiratory

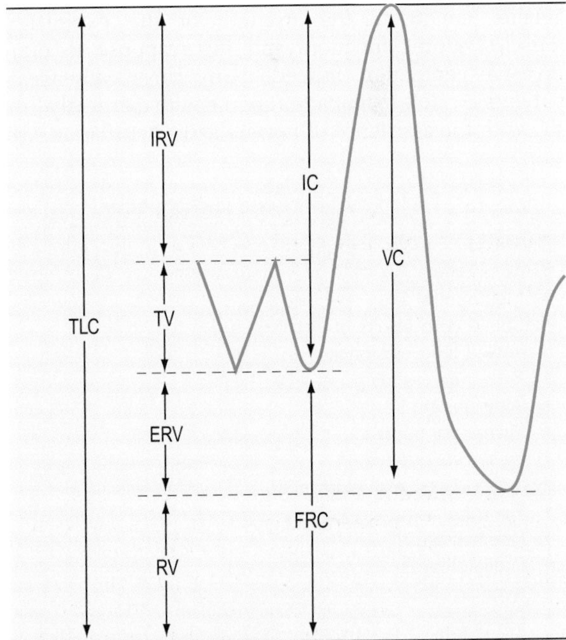

Figure 38.1 Lung volumes and capacities. TLC=total lung capacity; IRV=inspiratory reserve volume; TV=tidal volume; ERV=expiratory reserve volume; RV=residual volume; IC=inspiratory capacity; FRC=functional residual capacity; VC=vital capacity.

reserve volume (ERV). If a maximum inspiratory effort is made from FRC this is termed a vital capacity (VC) manoeuvre when the total lung capacity (TLC) is reached. Clinically, the most important of these are the FRC, V_T, and VC, and the latter two are easily measured using a spirometer or integrated from flow.

TIDAL VOLUME

Minute volume is composed of f and V_T; normally ~17 breaths/min and ~400 mL respectively in adults.[12] Rapid shallow breathing is common in patients with respiratory distress, and in those failing weaning. Although the f/V_T ratio>100 was initially shown to be highly predictive of weaning failure,[13] subsequent studies have reported varying results.

VITAL CAPACITY

At TLC inspiratory muscle forces are counterbalanced by elastic recoil of the lung and chest wall. Both these parameters and the size of the lung, which varies with body size and gender (**Box 38.1**), determine TLC. Vital capacity, the difference between TLC and FRC, is also reduced by factors that reduce FRC, *e.g.* increased abdominal chest wall elastance and premature airway closure in COPD. The normal VC is ~70 mL/kg; although reduction to 12–15 mL/kg has been suggested as an indication for mechanical ventilation, many other factors need to be considered including the patient's general condition, the strength of the expiratory muscles, glottic function, and the response to non-invasive ventilation. Indeed, many chronically weak patients are able to manage at home with extremely low VC with the assistance of non-invasive ventilation.

Box 38.1 Factors that decrease vital capacity

Decreased muscle strength
- Myopathy
- Neuropathy
- Spinal cord injury

Increased lung elastance
- Pulmonary oedema
- Atelectasis
- Pulmonary fibrosis
- Loss of lung tissue

Increased chest wall elastance
- Pleural effusion
- Haemothorax
- Pneumothorax
- Kyphoscoliosis
- Obesity
- Ascites

Reduced functional residual capacity
- Atelectasis
- Premature airway closure (e.g. chronic obstructive pulmonary disease)

FUNCTIONAL RESIDUAL CAPACITY

Direct measurement of FRC is rare in ICU. Anatomical rather than functional estimates can be derived from CT scan: however, techniques such as nitrogen or oxygen washout[14] are becoming available on modern ventilators. When FRC is less than the closing volume, the lung volume at which airway closure is present during expiration, there is a marked increase in $\dot{V}/\dot{Q}$ mismatch. Consequently, PEEP is commonly used to elevate FRC. Increases in lung volume above resting lung volume can be directly measured from a prolonged expiration to atmospheric pressure using either a spirometer or integration of flow,[15] or by repeated FRC measurements. FRC is decreased in ARDS and pulmonary oedema, in patients with abdominal distension, and following abdominal and thoracic surgery. Increased FRC places the diaphragm at a mechanical disadvantage, and is seen with severe air-flow limitation and dynamic overinflation, and when there is loss of elastic recoil (e.g. emphysema).

ELECTRICAL IMPEDANCE TOMOGRAPHY (EIT)

EIT uses impedance variation (as gas is a poor conductor) derived from multiple chest wall electrodes to monitor regional tidal ventilation. This is usually performed following a recruitment manoeuvre or change in PEEP setting.[16] Care must be taken to differentiate the diaphragm from collapsed lung, as the diaphragm moves cephalad both during expiration and at lower lung volumes. EIT can be calibrated to volume, and used to examine changes in end-expiratory lung volume but not FRC itself. PEEP may be adjusted to these changes and to indices of heterogeneity of ventilation; however, this does not define the balance between recruitment and overdistension. Currently EIT is a promising research tool, which may have application for tailoring ventilation.

MEASUREMENT OF LUNG MECHANICS

The forces the respiratory muscles must overcome during breathing are the elastic recoil of the lung and chest wall, and airway and tissue resistance. During controlled mechanical ventilation the ventilatory pressures reflect the work done to overcome these forces; however, during partial ventilatory support the pressure at the airway opening reflects both these forces and those generated by the respiratory muscles. Estimates of respiratory mechanics are often readily available, and can assist titration of ventilatory support.

ELASTIC PROPERTIES OF LUNG AND CHEST WALL

The respiratory system (RS) is composed of the lung (L), and chest wall (CW), which is comprised of the rib cage and abdomen. Although it is often convenient to consider respiratory system mechanics as implying information about the lung, abnormal chest wall compliance can markedly influence these measurements.[17–20]

The pressure gradient across the lung (P_L) that generates gas flow is equal to the difference between the pressure at the airway opening (P_{ao}) and the mean pleural pressure (P_{pl}), which is estimated as the oesophageal pressure (P_{es}):

$$P_L = P_{ao} - P_{es} \qquad (38.7)$$

Although the P_{es} is not always an accurate measure of the absolute P_{pl}, the change in P_{es} reflects the change in P_{pl}. However, this requires an appropriately positioned and functioning oesophageal balloon. In spontaneously breathing subjects a thin latex balloon sealed over a catheter is introduced into the lower third of the oesophagus and P_{es} and P_{ao} measured simultaneously during an end-expiratory airway occlusion. A well-positioned oesophageal balloon will have a ratio of $\Delta P_{es}/\Delta P_{ao}$ of ~1.[21] This technique is reliable in supine, intubated spontaneously breathing patients[22] and in paralysed subjects it appears that a similar pressure change, induced by manual rib cage pressure,[23] can be used to verify oesophageal balloon function.

Chest wall mechanics are derived from P_{es} referenced to atmospheric pressure and, in ventilated relaxed subjects, respiratory system mechanics are derived from P_{ao} referenced to atmospheric pressure. It is not surprising then that $P_{RS}=P_L+P_{CW}$. Finally, abdominal mechanics can be estimated as either intravesical or intragastric pressure. However, despite these provisos, useful information can be obtained from respiratory system mechanics.

Measuring the slope of the V–P relationship of the lung or respiratory system allows a simple estimate of the elastic properties of the lung. Since the E_{RS} is directly related to its components ($E_{RS}=E_L+E_{CW}$), it is preferred to compliance, which is inversely related: $1/C_{RS}=1/C_L+1/C_{CW}$. The normal E_{RS} is 10–15 cmH_2O/L and the normal C_{RS} is 60–100 mL/cmH_2O in ventilated patients.

MEASUREMENT OF ELASTANCE

Elastance and resistance are frequency dependent, and respiratory mechanics depend upon the volume and volume history of the lung.[24] With increasing frequency of breathing, total respiratory system resistance falls and elastance increases, and this is particularly obvious in patients with air-flow obstruction.[25,26] Consequently these factors must be taken into account when interpreting respiratory mechanics. In a passively ventilated subject P_{ao} is the sum of: (i) the pressure required to overcome airway, endotracheal tube and circuit resistance (P_{res}), (ii) the elastic pressure required to expand the lung and chest wall (P_{el}), (iii) the elastic recoil pressure at end expiration or total PEEP (P_o), and (iv) the inertial pressure required to generate gas flow (P_{inert}):

$$P_{ao} = P_{el} + P_{res} + P_o + P_{inert} \qquad (38.8)$$

Since the elastance (E), is equal to $\Delta P/\Delta V$, with the resistance (R) equal to $\Delta P/\Delta \dot{V}$, and ignoring the inertance,[27] this can be rewritten as the single-compartment equation of motion:

$$P_{ao} = E_{RS}V + R_{RS}\Delta\dot{V} + P_o \qquad (38.9)$$

Elastance can then be measured using either static techniques, where cessation of gas flow allows dissipation of P_{res}, or dynamic techniques, where flow is not interrupted.

END-INSPIRATORY OCCLUSION METHOD

The simplest estimate of E_{RS} can be made using a rapid end-inspiratory airway occlusion during a constant flow breath, provided that the respiratory muscles are relaxed (**Fig 38.2**). If a plateau is introduced at end inspiration there is a sudden initial pressure drop due to dissipation of flow resistance ($P_{pk}-P_1$) followed by a slower, secondary pressure drop to a plateau

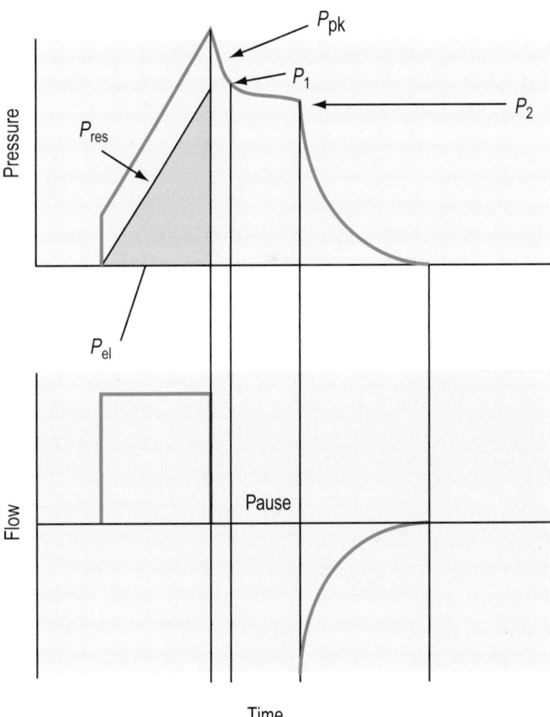

Figure 38.2 Schematic diagram of a volume-controlled breath with constant inspiratory flow. A period of no inspiratory gas flow has been interposed before expiration (pause) to illustrate dissipation of lung resistance as airways resistance (fall from P_{pk} to P_1) and tissue resistance (fall from P_1 to P_2). The inspiratory pressure due to the elastic properties of the respiratory system is illustrated as the filled area (P_{el}), and the lung resistive pressure is labeled as P_{res}. (See text for more detail.)

($P_{dif}=P_1-P_2$) due to stress relaxation. At least 1–2 seconds are taken for this plateau to be achieved, and P_2 is often called the plateau pressure; however, if P_{plat} is measured too soon it will lie somewhere between P_1 and P_2.

Stress adaptation

Stress relaxation of the respiratory system is due to both tissue viscoelasticity and time constant inequalities of the respiratory system (pendelluft). In the normal lung pendelluft has a minimal contribution to stress relaxation.[28] However, heterogeneity of regional resistance and elastance can markedly influence stress relaxation.[29] Pulmonary surfactant and its contribution to changes in surface tension, parenchymal factors including elastic fibres in the lung, contractile elements such as the alveolar duct muscle and changes in pulmonary blood volume have all been implicated in the viscoelastic properties of the lung. In the abnormal lung it is difficult to separate either of these factors or the role of pendelluft in stress adaptation.

Calculation of respiratory mechanics

Returning to Figure 38.2, it is now simple to estimate respiratory system resistance and elastance from P_{ao}. The static elastance ($E_{rs,st}$) and the dynamic elastance ($E_{rs,dyn}$) are calculated as:

$$E_{rs,st} = (P_2 - P_o) / V_T \tag{38.10}$$

$$E_{rs,dyn} = (P_1 - P_o) / V_T \tag{38.11}$$

where P_o is the total PEEP (extrinsic plus intrinsic PEEP). The difference between $P_{el,dyn}$ and $P_{el,st}$ is the effective recoil pressure of the respiratory system during mechanical ventilation. Consequently, additional work is performed during inspiration to overcome stress adaptation, and this is stored and dissipated during expiration. This contributes to the hysteresis seen in dynamic volume–pressure curves during mechanical ventilation, and to the generation of expiratory flow. This latter component may be important in patients with air-flow obstruction since the imposition of a pause at end inspiration results in a 32% dissipation of the total energy loss within the respiratory system.[30]

THE STATIC VOLUME–PRESSURE CURVE

The quasistatic volume–pressure (V–P) curve is infrequently performed, and the relevance of a measurement performed on a single occasion is questionable when lung mechanics are not constant. Various techniques have been described, but the overall concept is that incremental volume and pressure points are made after a sufficient period of no flow has allowed P_{res} to be dissipated. This allows definition of a sigmoidal-shaped curve with upper and lower inflection points, and a mid-section with relatively linear V–P relations, allowing inflation elastance to be measured as this slope at a given lung volume. If similar measures are made during deflation a deflation curve and its hysteresis can also be described.

The V–P curve provides an advantage over an end-inspiratory elastance as, with the latter, it is not possible to know which part of the V–P curve is being measured. Consequently this 'chord' elastance may span either inflection point, yielding a falsely high figure. The upper inflection point represents a sudden decrease in elastance with increasing volume, and this has been interpreted as lung overinflation. The lower inflection point represents a sudden decrease in elastance with increased volume, and this has been interpreted as recruitment of atelectatic air spaces. Ventilation between these two inflection points should minimise both shearing forces secondary to repetitive collapse and reopening of alveoli, and overstretch of alveoli. However, this interpretation of the V–P curve has been questioned. In patients with ARDS, recruitment occurs well above the lower inflection point, along the entire V–P curve and above the upper inflection point.[31, 32] An alternative interpretation is that the lower inflection point represents a zone of rapid recruitment, and that the upper inflection point is due to a reduced rate of recruitment.[33]

Conventionally the static V–P curve has been measured in paralysed ventilated patients with the 'super-syringe' method.[34] In a paralysed patient the respiratory system is progressively inflated from FRC in 100 mL steps up to ~1700 mL or a predefined pressure limit. After each step sufficient time is allowed for a well-defined plateau to become apparent (using a pause of 3–6 seconds). The effects of temperature, humidity, gas compression and ongoing gas exchange during the manoeuvre need to be taken into account,[35,36] and the volume history standardised before it is performed. Many patients become hypoxaemic following disconnection from the ventilator during the 60 seconds or so without PEEP. An alternative is to randomly insert a range of single-volume inflations, followed by a prolonged pause,[37] during normal mechanical ventilation at 0 cmH_2O PEEP. Advantages include simplicity, the patient is not disconnected from the ventilator, the volume history is the same for each measurement and gas exchange during the measurement is negligible. However, again, many patients will become hypoxaemic due to prolonged periods without PEEP (this procedure may take ~15 minutes), particularly following a small-volume breath. Finally, an automated low-flow V–P curve method allowing subtraction of P_{res} is available on some ventilators, takes around 20 seconds to perform, and correlates well with the static occlusion technique.[38,39]

THE DYNAMIC V–P CURVE

Dynamic P_{ao}, $\dot{V}$ and V are displayed by many ventilators, but the volume signal is not referenced to FRC and the signals are not readily available for quantitative analysis. However, $\dot{V}$ is readily measured with a heated pneumotachograph, and volume can then be derived by simple integration. If P_{ao} is also collected it is relatively simple to measure dynamic mechanics.

The dynamic V–P curve appears to show hysteresis, due to the effects of airway and tissue resistance; however, during tidal breathing even the static V–P does not show hysteresis.[40] In contrast to static V–P relations, dynamic mechanics are collected during normal ventilation so they do not interfere with patient care, and they provide a 'functional' description of respiratory mechanics. Indeed the 'effective' alveolar distending pressure is more accurately $P_{el,dyn}$, not $P_{el,st}$. Since dynamic mechanics are potentially continuous they could also be used to servo-control ventilatory strategies.

There are a number of ways to analyse dynamic V–P data. A line can be drawn between no-flow points at end inspiration and end expiration to determine elastance; however, this is relatively inaccurate as it is based on two points that can be hard to exactly identify. Multiple linear regression analysis is now the technique most commonly employed. The patient does not need to be paralysed[41] provided the respiratory muscles are not active during ventilation. The signal can also be split to allow analysis of inspiratory and expiratory mechanics.

Provided the model fit is acceptable, elastance and resistance are accurately and reproducibly calculated using the single compartment equation of motion:

$$P_{ao} = E_{RS}V + R_{RS}\Delta\dot{V} + P_o \qquad (38.12)$$

Static $PEEP_i$ is accurately calculated, as $P_o - PEEP_e$, when compared with either an end-expiratory airway occlusion method[42] or by direct measurement of end-expiratory alveolar pressure.[43] However, the single compartment model only approximates the respiratory system, and frequency and volume dependence of the derived mechanics are observed.

Changes in elastance during tidal breathing can be modeled with the stress index derived from power analysis of the P_{ao}–t curve ($P_{ao}=a^t+c$),[44] and addition of a volume-dependent term to the equation of motion:[14,45]

$$P_{ao} = (E_1 + E_2V)V + R_{RS}\Delta\dot{V} + P_o \qquad (38.13)$$

$$E_{rs} = E_1 + E_2V \qquad (38.14)$$

Since power analysis requires a constant inspiratory $\dot{V}$ pattern to discount resistive effects, it is not as versatile as the volume-dependent technique, which models resistance and can be applied to any inspiratory $\dot{V}$ pattern. Both measures correlate highly with each other suggesting they measure the same parameter.

High stress, and possibly overinflation, is inferred when the stress index is greater than 1.1 and when the volume-dependent elastance increases, which may be quantified:

$$\%E_2 = 100E_2V / E_{rs} \qquad (38.15)$$

A stress index below 0.9 and a negative volume dependence (negative $\%E_2$) suggest significant atelectasis during tidal breathing. Provided both V_T and $\dot{V}$ are constant, the change in driving pressure, either $P_{pk} - PEEP_{tot}$ or $P_1 - PEEP_{tot}$ 20–30 minutes following a change in PEEP is highly correlated with $\%E_2$.[14] Using the 95% predictive interval for these data, an increase in $\Delta P > 2$ cmH_2O, consistent with a significant increase in elastance, suggests high stress and overinflation. Similarly, the lowest E_{rs} during PEEP titration targets the best balance between recruitment and overinflation, and may be superior to the stress index or $\%E_2$ in laboratory models.[46]

Both the stress index and volume-dependent elastance also vary with stress relaxation, and high stress may not mean overinflation; in COPD bullous lung disease is due to a loss of lung tissue and elastic recoil. This may be measured on CT as hyperaerated; however, the associated wall stress may be high or low depending upon the degree of inflation.

INTERPRETATION OF ELASTANCE

Elastance may be increased due to a reduction in lung volume or to an increase in specific elastance, the product of E and FRC. Small body size, female gender, lung resection and reduced aerated lung volume (e.g. ARDS) are important factors in reducing effective lung volume. Specific elastance is increased in ARDS, pulmonary oedema and pulmonary fibrosis.

MEASUREMENT OF THE RESISTANCE OF THE LUNG AND CHEST WALL

Lung resistance (R_L) is the sum of airway (R_{aw}) and tissue resistance (R_{ti}). Resistance is flow-, volume- and frequency-dependent, and R_L decreases as f increases. It is also important to compare measurements at similar lung volumes since there is a hyperbolic relation between lung volume and R. This is particularly obvious in ARDS where the incremental administration of PEEP can result in a decrease in R_{aw} due to concurrent recruitment and an increase in lung volume. Indeed, although the absolute values are increased, when corrected for end-expiratory lung volume R_L, R_{aw} and R_{ti} are unchanged in ARDS,[15] although specific R_{ti} did increase with PEEP.[17] Finally, since gas flow may be a mixture of laminar and turbulent flow, resistance is often flow-dependent.

END-INSPIRATORY OCCLUSION TECHNIQUE

The total inspiratory R_{aw}, including the endotracheal tube and associated ventilatory apparatus, can be calculated in a relaxed patient following an inspiratory pause (see Fig. 38.2) as:

$$R_{aw} = (P_{pk} - P_1) / \dot{V} \qquad (38.16)$$

and R_L calculated by using P_2 instead of P_1. Since the endotracheal tube and apparatus will make a significant contribution to R_{aw} it is best to measure P_{ao} distal to the endotracheal tube with an intratracheal catheter. An alternative approach is to calculate and subtract endotracheal tube resistance using the Rohrer equation ($R=K_1+K_2\dot{V}$),[47] and this is now automatically included in some ventilators. However, as in vivo endotracheal tube resistance is often greater than in vitro resistance,[48] due to the effect of secretions and interaction with the tracheal wall, these corrections may be inaccurate. Despite these provisos, this simple measure of resistance, or the P_{pk} to P_{plat} difference at a constant $\dot{V}$, can be clinically useful in both the diagnosis and monitoring of air-flow obstruction.[49]

DYNAMIC TECHNIQUES

Total, inspiratory and expiratory R can also be estimated, using either multiple linear regression analysis or from linear interpolation of the V–P curve at a constant volume. However, this latter technique assumes a constant elastance during tidal inflation, and may be inaccurate because it relies on only two measurements. Finally, an average expiratory R can be calculated from the time constant (τ) derived from passive expiration if the E is known, since:

$$\tau = R / E \qquad (38.17)$$

However, the lung does not empty as a single compartment in patients with air-flow obstruction, and E is assumed to be constant over the tidal expiration.

OTHER MEASUREMENT TECHNIQUES

The interrupter technique consists of a series of short (100–200 ms) interruptions to relaxed expiration by a pneumatic valve.[50] This results in an expiratory plateau in P_{ao} following equilibration with alveolar pressure. From the V, P and $\dot{V}$ data the expiratory elastance and the expiratory P-$\dot{V}$ relationship are measured. This technique does not make assumptions about the behaviour of the respiratory system and can identify dynamic air-flow limitation.

Assuming that the respiratory system behaves linearly, it can be analysed following a forced-flow oscillation at the airway opening.[51] The resultant pressure waveform depends upon the impedance of the respiratory system, which can be analysed following Fourier analysis of the P and $\dot{V}$ waveforms into resistance and reactance. This will then allow measurement of R_{aw}, R_{ti}, E_{rs} and inertance, and information can be gained regarding small airways disease by examining R_{aw} at different oscillatory frequencies.

FORCED EXPIRATORY FLOW

Maximum expiratory flow rates from TLC, the forced vital capacity (FVC), the forced expiratory volume in the first second of expiration (FEV_1) and the peak expiratory flow rate (PEFR) are commonly measured in cooperative subjects with a spirometer or flow meter. The PEFR is cheap but is relatively effort-dependent, and is less specific and reliable than the FEV_1. It is most useful for office or home use. The normal PEFR is 450–700 L/min in males and 300–500 L/min in females. It is reduced with obstructive diseases, and gross muscle weakness.

The FEV_1 is usually expressed as a ratio of the FVC since both may be reduced in restrictive disease, with a normal ratio. The FEV_1 is normally 50–60 mL/kg and 70–83% of FVC. In asthma and COPD the FEV_1 is reduced out of proportion to the FVC to a ratio less than 70%.

MEASUREMENT OF INTRINSIC PEEP

$PEEP_i$ may (a) have unrecognised haemodynamic consequences,[52] (b) adds an elastic load to inspiratory work during assisted and supported ventilatory modes, which may be reduced by application of small amounts of $PEEP_e$,[53] and (c) reflects dynamic hyperinflation with the consequent risks of barotrauma[54] and right heart failure. If $PEEP_i$ is not taken into account during calculation of chord compliance an incorrect denominator is used, which may result in gross error.[55] As automated measures of mechanics do not account for $PEEP_i$, estimates of elastance must be corrected.

The two most commonly described techniques for measuring $PEEP_i$ are end-expiratory airway occlusion in a relaxed subject and the fall in oesophageal pressure during inspiration prior to initiation of inspiratory $\dot{V}$. However, these are not really comparable measures since static and dynamic $PEEP_i$ respectively, are measured. Static $PEEP_i$ is measured as the plateau P_{ao} that is reached following an end-expiratory occlusion; typically a plateau is reached in ~5 seconds, but this will be shorter in ARDS and longer in severe COPD. With the cessation of gas flow, alveolar pressure equilibrates with P_{ao}. Since the lung is composed of nonhomogeneous units this will represent the average static $PEEP_i$. All respiratory effort must be absent since muscle pressure will increase end-expiratory P_{ao}. End expiration must be accurately identified. This is most easily done by the ventilator itself either using an end-expiratory hold manoeuvre or by using the next inspiration, the onset of which is concurrent with expiratory valve closure, to close a valve that directs inspiratory flow to atmosphere and seals the circuit. Static $PEEP_i$ is a surrogate measure of dynamic hyperinflation, and this volume may be directly measured using a spirometer[52] or a pneumotachograph[14] during a prolonged expiration.

Dynamic $PEEP_i$ is measured as the pressure change required to initiate inflation. In ventilated subjects this will be the change in P_{ao} prior to initiation of inspiratory $\dot{V}$,[53] and in spontaneously breathing subjects the change in oesophageal[51] or transdiaphragmatic[56] pressure from their end-expiratory relaxation values prior to inspiratory $\dot{V}$. Measurement of dynamic $PEEP_i$ in spontaneously breathing subjects is not particularly straightforward. The changes in pressure are small and influenced by cardiogenic oscillations, which are preferably filtered out.[57] Furthermore, dynamic $PEEP_i$ is not constant, with breath-to-breath variation probably due to variation in the extent of dynamic hyperinflation. Many patients with air-flow obstruction have an active expiration that 'falsely' increases $PEEP_i$, at least with respect to its elastic load since cessation of active expiration does not require work.[58] Consequently, it is preferable to concurrently measure intragastric pressure as a measure of active expiration.

Finally, $PEEP_i$ can be measured as P_o from dynamic P, V and $\dot{V}$ data in ventilated subjects. This is thought to be a measure of dynamic $PEEP_i$ since static $PEEP_i$ systematically yields a slightly greater result,[42] with similar discrepancies reported between other dynamic measures of $PEEP_i$ and static $PEEP_{i.}$.[59,60] This systematic difference correlates with, and is thought to be due to, the viscoelastic properties and regional time constant inequalities of the respiratory system.[59] This has clinical significance as, although matching dynamic $PEEP_i$ with $PEEP_e$ reduces respiratory work through a decrease in elastic load,[53] it does not counterbalance these forces.

PATIENT–VENTILATOR ASYNCHRONY

Asynchrony between the patient and ventilator is more common than usually recognised during both intubated and non-invasive ventilatory support, and is often due to patient effort failing to trigger the ventilator. Clinical findings include agitation and anxiety, tachycardia, tachypnoea, and increased work of breathing. Careful observation of the patient–ventilator interaction, including waveforms, can be used to further identify and help match ventilatory assistance to neural drive.[61] (See also Ch. 31, Mechanical ventilation.)

INSPIRATION

TRIGGERING OF INSPIRATION

Ineffective respiratory efforts are best detected from the P_{es} waveform; however, this is rarely monitored. Ineffective triggering due to $PEEP_i$ may be detected from the expiratory $\dot{V}$ waveforms as an abrupt decrease in $\dot{V}$ at either the onset of inspiratory muscle activity or relaxation of the expiratory muscles. Monitoring of P_{ao} is less sensitive unless the circuit expiratory resistance is increased (e.g. HME or poorly functioning expiratory valve) so that small changes in expiratory $\dot{V}$ are reflected in P_{ao}. Sensing P_{ao} at the Y-piece does not offer any advantage as the pressure signal needs to travel the same distance via separate gas tubing to the ventilator expiratory block. Inadequate sensitivity may also lead to ineffective triggering with similar but more obvious waveform effects.

Autotriggering, a triggered assisted or supported breath without patient effort, may occur owing to excessively low trigger threshold or to P_{ao} or $\dot{V}$ distortion, as commonly seen with large cardiogenic oscillations, hiccups, condensate in tubing or a circuit leak. Again waveform analysis may help detect and manage the problem; for example, it may be necessary to reduce trigger sensitivity to prevent cardiogenic oscillations from being detected as inspiratory effort.

INSPIRATION

During an assisted volume control breath, P_{ao} may fall, often seen as a scalloped shape, if there is excessive inspiratory muscle effort as seen in $\dot{V}$ starvation. Expiratory muscle effort, as may be seen with an excessive V_T or prolonged inspiratory time (T_i), leads to a rise in P_{ao}. During an assisted pressure control breath or during pressure support, changes in patient effort are detected from the $\dot{V}$ waveform. Finally, excessively rapid development of the set delivered pressure, a rapid rise time, may be detected by an overshoot in P_{ao}; an excessively long rise time will be seen as a rounded inspiratory $\dot{V}$ profile, similar to that seen with continued inspiratory muscle effort.

CESSATION OF INSPIRATION

Mismatch of the mechanical and neural T_i can be detected from waveform changes at the cessation of inspiration.

Mechanical T_i shorter than neural T_i

There will be prolonged inspiratory muscle effort during early expiration; if this leads to a sufficient fall in P_{ao} or $\dot{V}$ an early triggered breath follows. During pressure-cycled ventilation this will lead to a second small I_T breath due to the high baseline lung volume, but in assist volume control P_{ao} will be excessive. Typically this is seen with a stiff respiratory system, $PEEP_i$ or inadequate pressure support.

Mechanical T_i longer than neural T_i

This leads to features of passive inflation such as a linear increase in P_{ao} during assist volume control ventilation; during pressure-cycled ventilation there may be an increase in P_{ao} due to loss of inspiratory effort, or an unexplained fall in $\dot{V}$.

EXPIRATION

Changes in P_{ao} during expiration are usually small unless expiratory circuit resistance is abnormally high. However, in patients with expiratory flow limitation the expiratory $\dot{V}$ waveform shows a typical 'tick' pattern; there is a rapid spike in expiratory flow due to dynamic compression of large conducting airways at the beginning of expiration, and this is followed by low, slowly declining expiratory $\dot{V}$ due to high $\dot{V}$ expiratory resistance. When $PEEP_i$ is present the expiratory $\dot{V}$ fails to cease prior to the inspiratory trigger; however, this may be difficult to detect due to the poor fidelity present on most commercial ventilators.

MONITORING NEUROMUSCULAR FUNCTION

INSPIRATORY OCCLUSION PRESSURE

The pressure 100 ms (P_{100} or $P_{0.1}$) after a random occlusion timed at the beginning of inspiration is a measure of respiratory drive. There is a large range of normal values (1.5–5 cmH_2O), but it is reproducible in an individual patient. In ventilated patients the $P_{0.1}$ correlates with the work of breathing during pressure support ventilation, and changes in the same direction as $PEEP_e$ is increased if work is reduced.[62] Consequently, $P_{0.1}$ may prove to be a useful method of titrating $PEEP_e$ in patients with dynamic hyperinflation; however, this is not valid when flow triggering is used.

MAXIMUM MOUTH PRESSURES

Maximum inspiratory (MIP) and expiratory (MEP) mouth pressures can be used to estimate the power of the respiratory muscles. MIP is usually measured in ventilated patients using a unidirectional expiratory valve for ~20 seconds.[63] This ensures the procedure is performed from a low lung volume and does not require patient cooperation. However, despite this the results are quite variable.[64] Normal values vary with age and gender; young females may exceed ~–90 cmH_2O, and young males ~–130 cmH_2O. A MIP<–20 cmH_2O is predictive of weaning failure; however, this is associated with too many false positives and negatives to be useful.[12] MEP may be useful in myopathic patients with expiratory muscle weakness. Transdiaphragmatic pressure is assessed using an oesophageal and gastric balloon to measure the pressure in these two cavities.

WORK OF BREATHING

The work of breathing (W_B) is the sum of elastic work (W_{el}), flow-resistive work (W_{res}) and inertial work (negligible), and can be estimated from V–P data during spontaneous or assisted ventilation. An oesophageal balloon is used to examine changes in pleural pressure, $\dot{V}$ is measured with a pneumotachograph, and volume is derived as its integral. Although conceptually W_B is the inspiratory area of a V–P loop, this needs to be referenced to the chest wall V–P curve, and the appropriate area measured from a Campbell diagram.[65]

The normal W_B is ~0.5 J/L of $\dot{V}_E$, and this may be significantly increased in patients with acute respiratory failure, and by additional work imposed by ventilatory apparatus including the endotracheal tube and connector, humidifier and ventilator circuit.[66] The consequences of a large increase in W_B may include an increase in the $\dot{V}O_2$ attributable to breathing ($\dot{V}O_{2\,resp}$), respiratory muscle insufficiency, CO_2 retention and acute respiratory failure. However, W_B is rarely measured outside of research projects since the Campbell diagram is a relatively tedious approach. Simplifications have been used, but these are not as accurate, and W_B only estimates energy expenditure during muscle shortening with relatively poor correlation with $\dot{V}O_{2\,resp}$.[67] Consequently, the pressure–time product (PTP), which does correlate with $\dot{V}O_{2\,resp}$,[68] is more commonly measured.[10]

PRESSURE–TIME PRODUCT

PTP is usually calculated from the oesophageal pressure–time integral during inspiration. In mechanically ventilated patients the oesophageal pressure during assisted breathing is compared with that during a controlled breath, or that pressure calculated from the chest wall elastance and lung volume.[10] However, the early correlation of $\dot{V}O_{2\,resp}$ with PTP used the transdiaphragmatic pressure in spontaneously breathing subjects.[65] Using either technique, importantly, the effort expended before $\dot{V}$ occurs due to $PEEP_i$ is measured, probably accounting for the better correlation of $\dot{V}O_{2\,resp}$ with PTP than W_B.[65] Although incremental pressure support ventilation may reduce PTP in COPD patients, the effect can be variable with some patients also showing evidence of expiratory muscle activity due to delayed sensing of neural expiration.[10]

Access the complete references list online at http://www.expertconsult.com

13. Yang K, Tobin MJ. A prospective study of indices predicting outcome of trials of weaning from mechanical ventilation. N Engl J Med 1991;324:1445–50.
29. Otis AB, McKerrow CB, Bartlett RA, et al. Mechanical factors in distribution of pulmonary ventilation. J Appl Physiol 1956;8:427–43.
46. Carvalho AR, Spieth PM, Pelosi P, et al. Ability of dynamic airway pressure curve profile and elastance for positive end-expiratory pressure titration. Intensive Care Med 2008;34:2291–9.
53. Petrof BJ, Legare M, Goldberg P, et al. Continuous positive airway pressure reduces work of breathing and dyspnea during weaning from mechanical ventilation in severe chronic obstructive pulmonary disease. Am Rev Respir Dis 1990;141:281–9.
61. Georgopoulos D, Prinianakis G, Kondili E. Bedside waveforms interpretation as a tool to identify patient-ventilator asynchronies. Intensive Care Med 2006;32:34–47.

39

Imaging the chest

Simon PG Padley

RADIOLOGICAL TECHNIQUES

Of the imaging techniques available for investigating patients in the intensive care unit (ICU), the chest radiograph remains the most important, with ultrasound being utilised in a selected group of patients. High-resolution and spiral computed tomography (CT) allow further investigation of these patients in certain situations.

CONVENTIONAL CHEST RADIOGRAPHY

Because of the advent of modern PACS (picture archiving and communication systems), digital chest radiographs are now readily available in the ICU shortly after acquisition, and may be compared with previous radiographs using multi-monitor display workstations. The views of the chest most frequently performed in the ambulant patient are the erect postero-anterior (PA) and lateral projections, taken with the patient breath-holding at total lung capacity. While portable or mobile chest radiography, as undertaken on an ICU, has the obvious advantage that the examination can be done without moving the patient from the ward, there are many disadvantages. These include:

- shorter focus–film distance causing magnification
- limited X-ray output necessitating long exposure times with resultant movement blurring
- difficulties with satisfactory patient positioning.

DIGITAL CHEST RADIOLOGY

In the ICU, digital chest radiographs may be obtained utilising conventional X-ray generators, but the image is acquired on a reusable capture. The digital information is then manipulated, displayed and stored in whatever format is desired. Digital radiographic systems are able to capture and display a standard-density image from a much wider range of exposures (**Fig. 39.1**).

COMPUTED TOMOGRAPHY

CT relies on differing absorption of X-rays by tissues with constituents of differing atomic number, so slight differences in X-ray absorption can be interpreted to produce a cross-sectional image. The components of a CT scanner are an X-ray tube, which rotates around the patient, and an array of X-ray detectors opposite the tube. The speed with which a CT scanner acquires an image depends upon the time it takes to rotate the anode around the patient. Modern CT machines have tube rotation times of as little as 0.25 seconds.

Spiral (also known as volume or helical) scanning entails sustained patient exposure by the rotating X-ray tube during continuous movement of the examination couch through the CT gantry aperture. In this way a continuous data set or 'spiral' of information may be acquired in a single breath-hold. The information is reconstructed into axial sections, perpendicular to the long axis of the patient, identical to conventional CT sections. Three-dimensional reconstructions of complex anatomical areas can also be produced.

When short rotation times are coupled with the ability to acquire multiple spirals simultaneously (currently up to 320 detector rows), the speed of these systems becomes so great that breath-holding or suspended ventilation is no longer necessary for high-quality imaging. Furthermore, the detector thickness that determines the minimum slice width of the reconstructed images is now commonly less than 1 mm.

INTRAVENOUS CONTRAST ENHANCEMENT

The inherent high contrast on CT between vessels and surrounding air in the lung, and vessels and surrounding fat within the mediastinum reduces the need for intravenous contrast enhancement in most instances. However, in some circumstances, for example to aid the distinction between hilar vessels and a soft-tissue mass or to detect a pulmonary artery embolus, contrast is required. The timing of the injection of contrast media depends on the technical attributes of the CT scanner. Rapid scanning protocols with automated injectors tend to improve contrast enhancement of vascular structures at the expense of enhancement of solid lesions because of the rapidity of scanning. With spiral CT, it is possible to achieve good opacification of all the thoracic vascular structures with small volumes of contrast media. Optimal contrast enhancement of the pulmonary arteries occurs 10–15 seconds after the start of contrast injection, usually at 5 mL/s by a power injector. Timing of image acquisition is vital for accurate

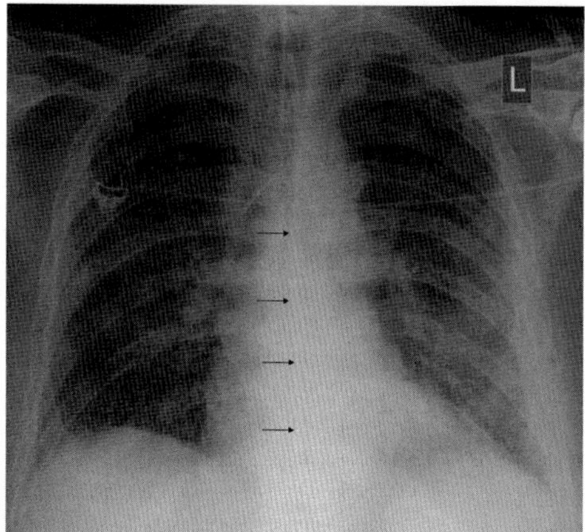

Figure 39.1 Digital radiograph. There is an endotracheal tube, a left internal jugular vein line and a nasogastric tube (arrows).

diagnosis of pulmonary embolism. However, when examining inflammatory lesions such as the reaction around an empyema, it may be necessary to delay scanning by 60 seconds to allow contrast to diffuse into the extravascular space.

HIGH-RESOLUTION COMPUTED TOMOGRAPHY (HRCT)

Narrow collimation images of the lung correlate closely with the macroscopic appearances of pathological specimens. In diffuse lung disease, HRCT allows a substantial improvement in diagnostic accuracy compared with chest radiography. Narrow-section images can be acquired either as part of a volumetric acquisition or as interspaced images, usually 1.5 mm thickness, obtained every 1 cm. The radiation burden to the patient of this interspace or sequential technique is considerably less than with volumetric scanning – typically by a factor of 10 times.

CLINICAL APPLICATIONS OF HRCT IN THE ICU PATIENT

HRCT is increasingly being used to confirm the impression of an abnormality seen on a chest radiograph. HRCT may also be used to achieve a histospecific diagnosis in some patients with obvious but non-specific radiographic abnormalities. Furthermore, HRCT has provided a number of useful insights into chest disease in the severely ill patient in an ICU setting.

HRCT in uncomplicated acute respiratory distress syndrome (ARDS)[1]

- HRCT reveals that the apparently homogeneous opacification apparent on the chest radiograph has an anterior-to-posterior graded increase in density – an appearance referred to as a gravitational gradient (**Fig. 39.2**).

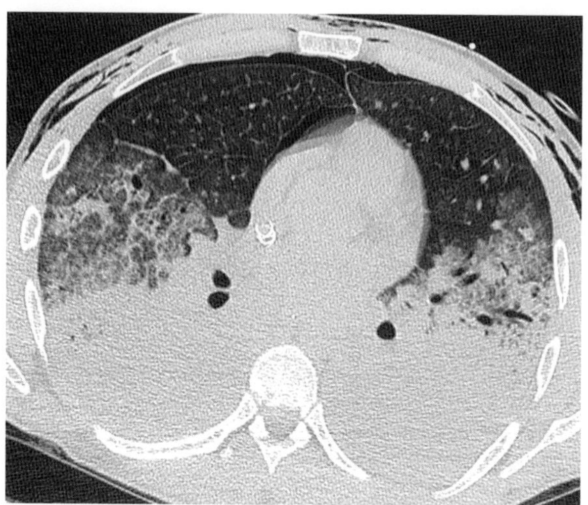

Figure 39.2 Computed tomography of a patient with acute respiratory distress syndrome. Note the marked anterior to posterior density gradient. The anterior lung is of almost normal density, becoming of ground-glass attenuation in the mid part of the lung before fading into consolidation posteriorly. There are small pneumothoraces bilaterally and surgical emphysema.

- HRCT demonstrates early dilatation of the smaller airways within areas of ground-glass density, an appearance that suggests development of fibrosis, and may prompt anti-inflammatory treatment.
- HRCT demonstrates that a shift from the supine to the prone position results in redistribution of the previously dependent dense parenchymal opacification to the now dependent anterior lung, a phenomenon that may be accompanied by improvements in patient oxygenation.

HRCT of complications of ARDS[2,3]

- Infection is common in ARDS. Diagnosis may be difficult. Radiographically there may be a lack of specific findings, often due to superimposition of changes attributable to ARDS. This is a particular problem in the critically ill patient when the usual indicators of pneumonia are also unreliable. Although the diagnosis may still be in question following HRCT, associated pneumonic changes such as abscess formation, empyema and mediastinal disease, as well as development of non-dependent areas of consolidation, are all useful pointers to superadded infection (see Fig. 39.2).
- Barotrauma – mediastinal and interstitial emphysema, as well as pneumothorax, are all increasingly common at higher levels of peak end-expiratory pressure (PEEP). The incidence of barotrauma has been reported to be as high as 50%.
- HRCT allows the exact location of loculated air collections to be defined.

NORMAL RADIOGRAPHIC ANATOMY

THE MEDIASTINUM, CENTRAL AIRWAYS AND HILAR STRUCTURES

Appreciation of abnormality requires a sound grasp of normal radiological anatomy. The mediastinum is delimited by the lungs on each side, the thoracic inlet above, the diaphragm below and the vertebral column posteriorly. Because the various structures that make up the mediastinum are superimposed on each other on the chest radiograph, they cannot be separately identified. Nevertheless, because a chest radiograph is usually the first imaging investigation, it is necessary to have an appreciation of the normal appearances of the mediastinum, together with variations due to the patient's body habitus and age. Key points include:

- Only the outline of the mediastinum and the air-containing trachea and bronchi (and sometimes oesophagus) are clearly seen on a normal chest radiograph.
- The right superior mediastinal border is formed by the right brachiocephalic vein and superior vena cava, and becomes less distinct as it reaches the thoracic inlet. The right side of the superior mediastinum can appear to be considerably widened in patients with an abundance of mediastinal fat.
- The left mediastinal border above the aortic arch is the result of summation of the left carotid and left subclavian arteries together with the left brachiocephalic and jugular veins.
- The left cardiac border comprises the left atrial appendage, which merges inferiorly with the left ventricle. The silhouette of the heart should always be sharply outlined. Any blurring of the border is due to loss of immediately adjacent aerated lung, usually by collapse or consolidation.
- The density of the heart shadow to the left and right of the vertebral column should be identical and any difference indicates pathology (e.g. an area of consolidation or a mass in a lower lobe).
- The trachea and main bronchi should be visible through the upper and middle mediastinum.
- In older individuals, the trachea may be displaced by a dilated aortic arch. In approximately 60% of normal subjects, the right wall of the trachea (the right paratracheal stripe) can be identified as a line of uniform thickness (less than 4 mm in width); when it is visible it excludes the presence of an adjacent space-occupying lesion, most usually lymphadenopathy.
- The carinal angle is usually less than 80°. Splaying of the carina is an insensitive sign of subcarinal disease, either in the form of massive subcarinal lymphadenopathy, or a markedly enlarged left atrium.
- The origins of the lobar bronchi, where they are projected over the mediastinal shadow, can usually be identified but the segmental bronchi within the lungs are not generally seen on plain radiography.
- Normal hilar shadows on a chest radiograph represent the summation of the pulmonary arteries and veins.
- The hila are approximately the same size and the left hilum normally lies between 0.5 cm and 1.5 cm above the level of the right hilum. The size and shape of the hila show remarkable variation in normal individuals, making subtle abnormalities difficult to identify.

THE PULMONARY FISSURES, VESSELS AND BRONCHI

The two lungs are separated by the four layers of pleura behind and in front of the mediastinum. The resulting posterior and anterior junction lines are often visible on chest radiographs as nearly vertical stripes, the posterior junction line lying higher than the anterior. The junction lines are not invariably seen and their presence or absence is not usually of significance (**Fig. 39.3**).

The upper and lower lobes of the left lung are separated by the major (or oblique) fissure. The upper, middle and lower lobes of the right lung are separated by the major fissure and the minor (horizontal or transverse) fissure. The minor fissure is visible in over half of normal PA chest radiographs. The major fissures are not visible on a frontal radiograph and are inconstantly identifiable on lateral radiographs. In a few individuals, fissures are incompletely developed - a point familiar to thoracic surgeons performing a lobectomy, because of incomplete cleavage between lobes. Accessory fissures are occasionally seen.

All of the branching structures seen within normal lungs on a chest radiograph represent pulmonary arteries or veins. It is often impossible to distinguish arteries from veins in the lung periphery. On a chest radiograph taken in the erect position, there is a gradual increase in the diameter of the vessels, at equidistant points from the hilum, travelling from lung apex to base; this gravity-dependent effect disappears if the patient is supine or in cardiac failure.

THE DIAPHRAGM AND THORACIC CAGE

The interface between aerated lung and the diaphragm is sharp and the highest point of each dome is normally medial to the midclavicular line. The right dome of the diaphragm is higher than the left by up to 2 cm in the erect position unless the left dome is elevated by air in the stomach (**Fig. 39.4**).

Filling-in or blunting of these costophrenic angles usually represents pleural disease, either pleural thickening or an effusion.

POSITIONING OF TUBES AND LINES[4]

CENTRAL VENOUS CATHETERS (CVC)

The end of a CVC needs to be intrathoracic, and is ideally in the superior vena cava. CVCs may be introduced via

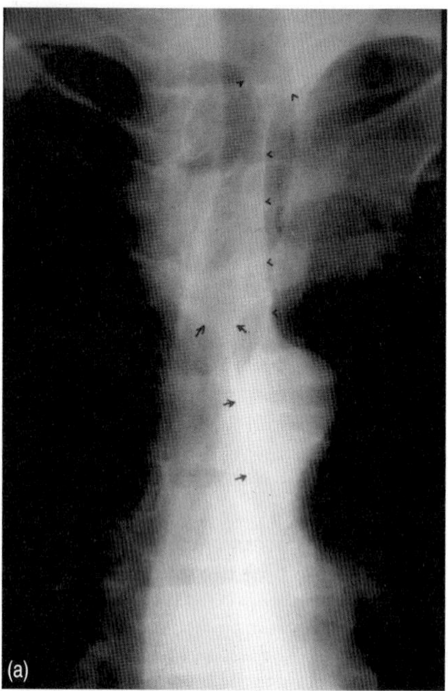

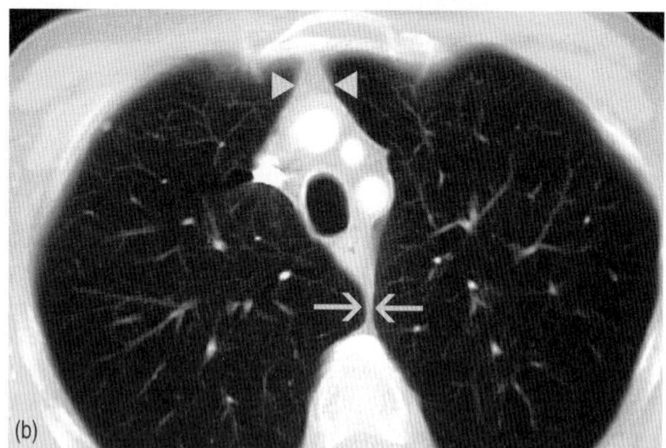

Figure 39.3 (a) Close-up of the mediastinum of a patient in whom both the anterior and posterior junction lines are evident. The anterior junction line is more inferior and slants from right to left (short arrows), whereas the posterior junction line is more vertical, superior and is delineated by the arrowheads. (b) Computed tomography scan through the upper mediastinum demonstrating the anterior (arrowheads) and posterior (arrows) junction lines in a different patient.

an antecubital, subclavian or jugular vein. Subclavian venous puncture carries a risk of pneumothorax and mediastinal haematoma. Rarely, perforation of the subclavian vein leads to fluid collecting in the mediastinum or pleura. All catheters have a potential risk of coiling, misplacement, knotting and fracture (**Fig. 39.5**). The tip should not abut the vessel wall at an obtuse angle.

PULMONARY ARTERY FLOTATION CATHETERS

Ideally the end of the catheter should be maintained less than 5–8 cm (2–3 inches) beyond the bifurcation of the main pulmonary artery in either the right or left pulmonary artery (see Fig. 39.5). When the pulmonary artery occlusion pressure is measured, the balloon is inflated, and the flow of blood carries the catheter tip peripherally, to an occluded position. After the measurement has been made the balloon is deflated and the catheter returns to a central position; otherwise there is a risk of pulmonary infarction. The inflation balloon is radiolucent. The balloon should normally be kept deflated.

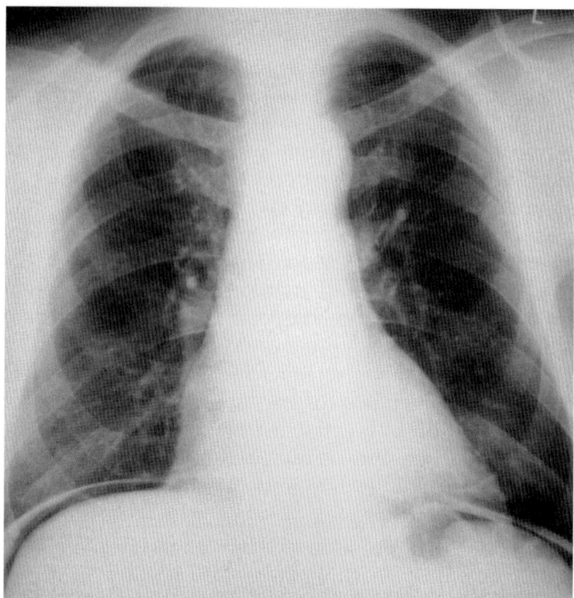

Figure 39.4 Erect chest radiograph of a patient with a pneumoperitoneum demonstrating the normal thickness in position of the hemidiaphragms. The right lies slightly higher than the left.

NASOGASTRIC TUBES

These should reach the stomach but may coil in the oesophagus or occasionally are inserted into the tracheobronchial tree (**Fig. 39.6**).

ENDOTRACHEAL TUBES

Extension and flexion of the neck may make the tip of an endotracheal tube move by as much as 5 cm. With the neck in neutral position the tip of the tube should ideally be about 4–5 cm above the carina. A tube that is inserted too far usually passes into the right bronchus, with the risk of non-ventilation or collapse of the left lung (**Fig. 39.7**).

TRACHEOSTOMY TUBES

The tube tip should be situated centrally in the airway at the level of T_3. Acute complications of tracheostomy include pneumothorax, pneumomediastinum and

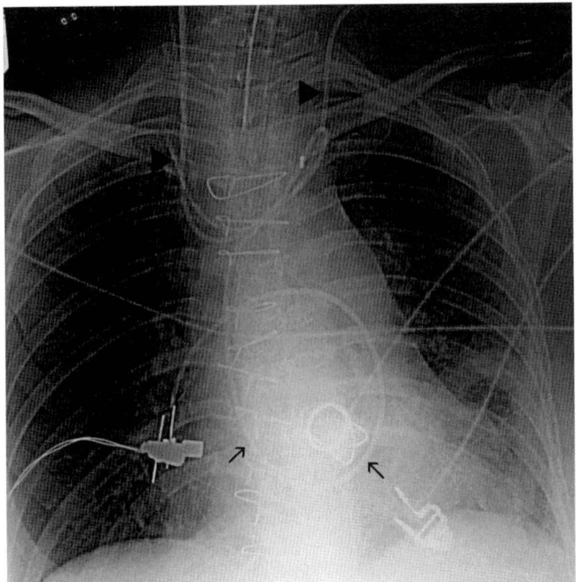

Figure 39.5 Intensive care unit patient with multiple tubes and lines in place. The endotracheal tube tip position is satisfactory, and there are sternotomy wires, an intra-aortic balloon pump (radiopaque tip) and a prosthetic heart valve. The central line inserted into the left internal jugular vein passes into the right internal jugular vein. The Swan–Ganz catheter, which has been inserted via the right internal jugular vein, loops into the left brachiocephalic vein, before taking a satisfactory course through the cardiac chambers (black arrows).

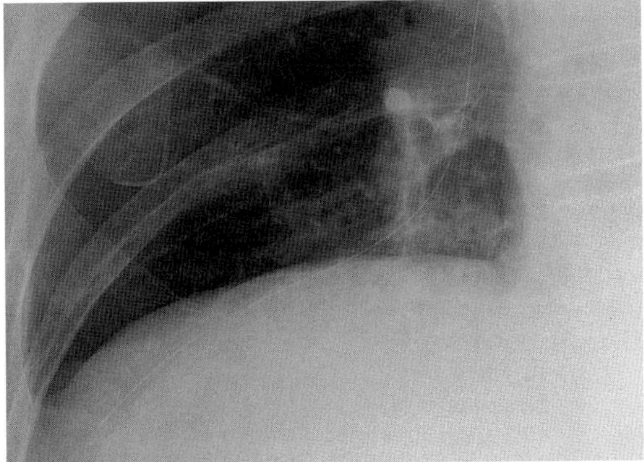

Figure 39.6 Misplaced nasogastric tube.

subcutaneous emphysema. Long-term complications include tracheal ulceration, stenosis and perforation.

PLEURAL TUBES

These are used to treat pleural effusions and pneumothoraces. A radiopaque line usually runs along pleural tubes, and is interrupted where there are side holes. It

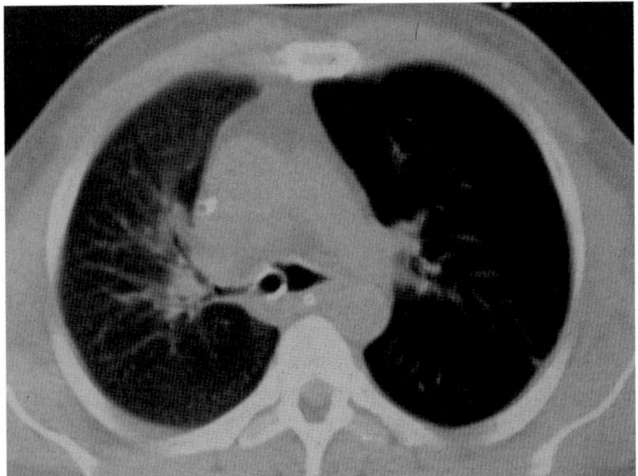

Figure 39.7 Endotracheal tube inserted into the right main bronchus as demonstrated on computed tomography. This image, obtained in expiration, demonstrates air trapping in the left lung.

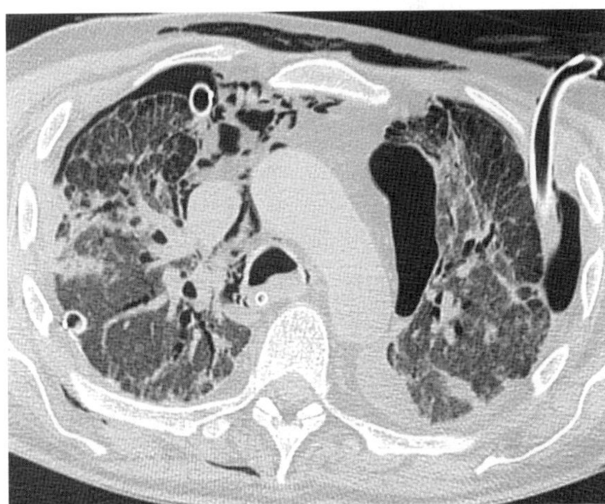

Figure 39.8 Computed tomography scan demonstrating bilateral pneumothoraces in a patient with acute respiratory distress syndrome. Note is made of bilateral chest drains.

is important to check that all the side holes are within the thorax. Tracks may remain on the chest X-ray following removal of chest tubes, causing tubular or ring shadows. When doubt remains about tube position, then CT scanning should be considered (**Fig. 39.8**).

MEDIASTINAL DRAINS

These are usually present following sternotomy. Apart from their position, they look like pleural tubes.

INTRA-AORTIC BALLOON PUMP

These are used in patients with cardiogenic shock, often following cardiac surgery. The ideal position of the catheter tip is just distal to the origin of the left subclavian artery (**Fig. 39.9**). If the catheter tip is advanced too far it may occlude the left subclavian artery, and if it is too distal the balloon may occlude branches of the abdominal aorta. The intra-aortic balloon pump may be visible only by its radiopaque tip (see Fig. 39.9).

PACEMAKERS

These may be permanent or temporary (**Fig. 39.10**). Temporary epicardial wires are sometimes inserted during cardiac surgery, and may be seen as thin, almost hair-like metallic opacities overlying the heart. Temporary pacing electrodes are usually inserted transvenously via a subclavian or jugular vein. If a patient is not being paced properly, a chest radiograph may reveal that the position of the electrode tip is unstable, or that a fracture in the wire has occurred.

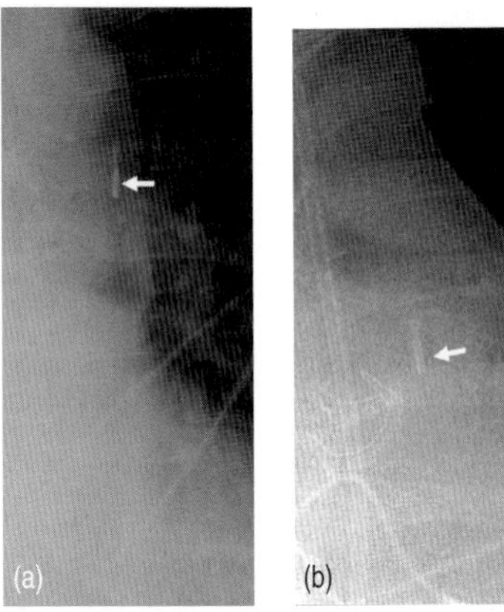

Figure 39.9 Intra-aortic balloon pump. Two chest radiographs demonstrating the tip of the balloon pump: (a) just distal to the origin of the left subclavian artery (arrow), and (b) further down the descending thoracic aorta (arrow).

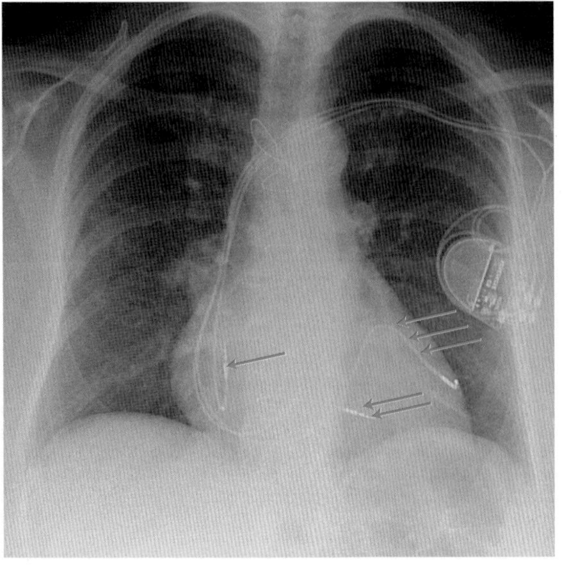

Figure 39.10 Biventricular pacemaker. Note the right atrial lead (arrow), right ventricular lead (double arrows) and coronary sinus lead (triple arrows).

RADIOGRAPHIC SIGNS OF PATHOLOGY

CONSOLIDATION

Consolidation, or synonymously air space shadowing, is due to opacification of the air-containing spaces of the lung, usually without a change in volume of the affected area. It is not possible to tell what the air space filling is due to in the absence of a clinical history, except perhaps for shadowing due to cardiogenic alveolar oedema, when there will be associated signs of cardiac failure. Typical features of all forms of consolidation (**Fig. 39.11**) include:

- ill-defined margins, except where it directly abuts a pleural surface
- sharply demarcated by fissures
- loss of vascular markings
- air bronchograms – the bronchi, usually invisible, may become apparent in negative contrast to the air space opacification
- acinar opacities, due to individual acini or secondary pulmonary lobules being opacified but still surrounded by normally aerated lung, usually seen at

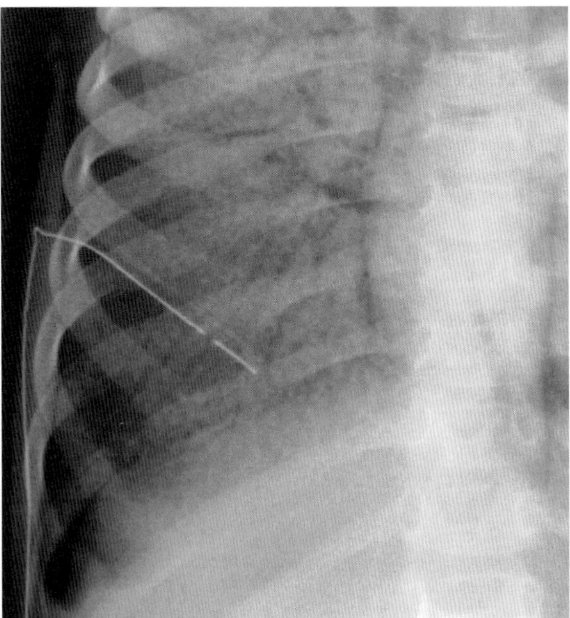

Figure 39.11 Close-up view of an area of consolidation adjacent to the right heart border, which is obscured. Air bronchograms can be identified passing through this area. A chest tube is in situ.

the periphery of a more confluent area of consolidation, and 0.5–1 cm in diameter
- ground-glass opacification, when consolidation has caused only partial filling of the air spaces
- silhouette sign – consolidation abutting a soft-tissue structure causes the silhouette of that structure to be lost.

When an area of consolidation undergoes necrosis, due to either infection or infarction, then liquefaction may result, and if there is either a gas-forming organism or communication with the bronchial tree then an air–fluid level may develop in addition to cavity formation.

COLLAPSE

When there is partial or complete volume loss in a lung or lobe this is referred to as collapse or atelectasis, implying a diminished volume of air in the lung with associated reduction of lung volume. There are several different mechanisms for lung or lobar collapse, for example relaxation or passive collapse, when fluid or air accumulates in the pleural space, cicatrisation collapse, when volume loss is associated with pulmonary fibrosis, adhesive collapse, as in ARDS, and resorption collapse, as in bronchial obstruction.

The radiographic appearance in pulmonary collapse depends upon a number of factors. These include the mechanism of collapse, the extent of collapse, the presence or absence of consolidation in the affected lung and the pre-existing state of the pleura. This latter factor includes the presence of underlying pleural tethering or thickening and the presence of pleural fluid.

The direct signs of collapse include:

- displacement of interlobar fissures
- loss of aeration resulting in increased density or the presence of the silhouette sign
- crowding of vessels and bronchi.

The indirect signs of collapse include:

- elevation of the hemidiaphragm, especially with lower lobe collapse
- mediastinal displacement, especially in upper lobe collapse
- hilar displacement, where the hilum is elevated in upper lobe collapse and depressed in lower lobe collapse
- compensatory hyperinflation of remaining normal lung, resulting in increased transradiancy or herniation across the midline from the normal side
- crowding of the ribs reflecting diminished overall volume of the affected hemithorax.

COMPLETE LUNG COLLAPSE

Complete collapse (**Fig. 39.12**) will cause complete opacification of the hemithorax, with displacement of the mediastinum to the affected side and elevation of the hemidiaphragm. Compensatory hyperinflation of the contralateral lung with herniation across the midline may be apparent. Herniation may occur in the retrosternal space, anterior to the ascending aorta, or may be posterior to the heart.

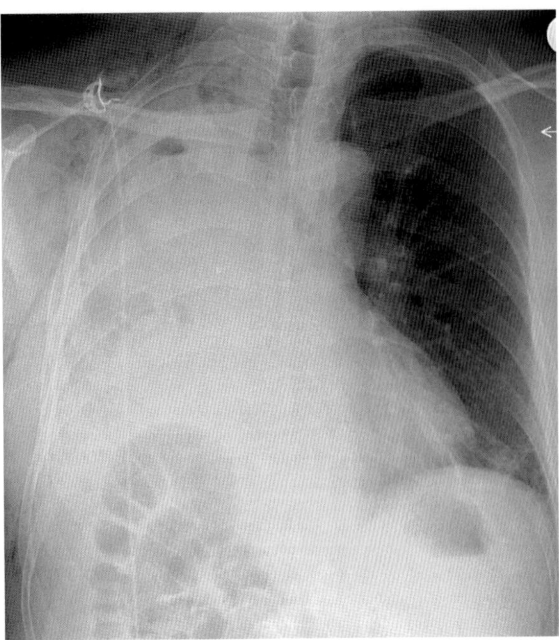

Figure 39.12 Complete lung collapse. There was an obstructing tumour in the right main bronchus. The right hemithorax is opaque, the mediastinum has shifted and the trachea is deviated to the right.

INDIVIDUAL OR COMBINED LOBAR COLLAPSE

In any situation, some or all of the signs may be present.

*Right upper lobe collapse (**Fig. 39.13**)*

- Horizontal fissure moves upwards and medially towards the superior mediastinum.
- Trachea deviates to the right.
- Compensatory hyperinflation of the right middle and lower lobes.

*Middle lobe collapse (**Fig. 39.14**)*

- Horizontal fissure and lower half of the oblique fissure move towards each other – best seen on the lateral projection.
- Frontal radiograph changes may be subtle, with obscuration of the right heart border.
- Indirect signs of volume loss are rarely obvious.

Right lower lobe collapse

- There is partial depression of the horizontal fissure.
- There is triangular opacity of the collapsed lower lobe on the frontal projection, usually obscuring the diaphragm but preserving the right heart border.

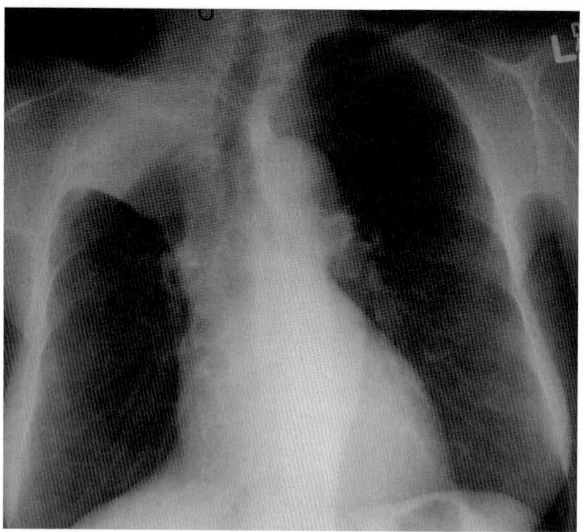

Figure 39.13 Right upper lobe collapse. The horizontal fissure has become elevated and the right upper lobe has become a wedge-shaped density extending from the hilum to the right lung apex. There is evidence of volume loss with shift of the trachea to the right side.

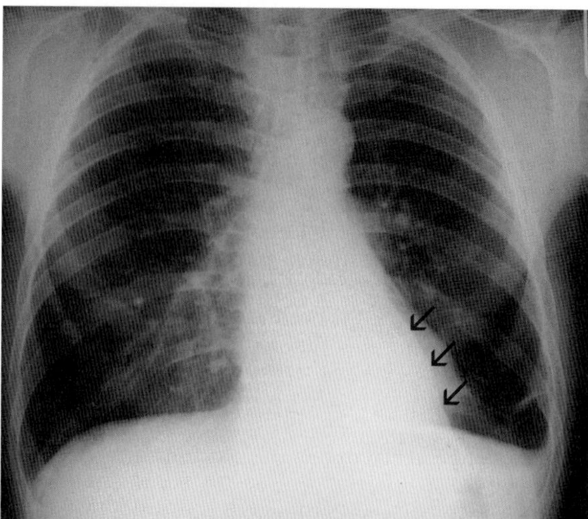

Figure 39.15 Left lower lobe collapse. The left lower lobe has become a wedge-shaped density behind the heart forming a double left heart border (arrows). The left hilar vessel to the lower lobe has disappeared as a result of collapse.

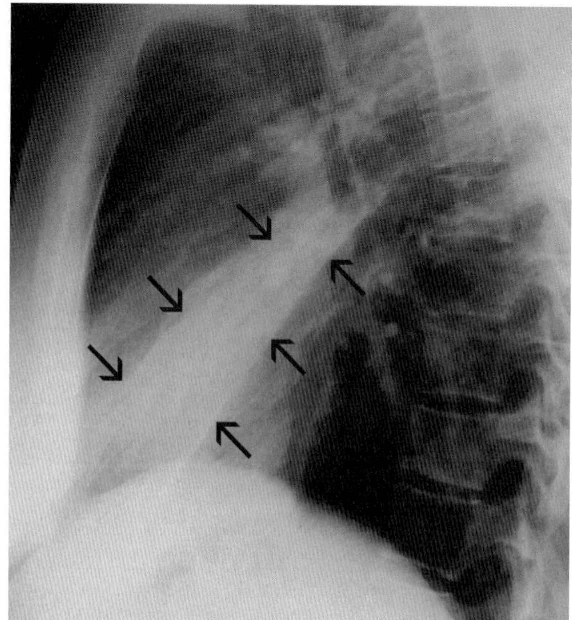

Figure 39.14 Middle lobe collapse. The horizontal fissure is depressed and demarcates the collapsed middle lobe as a wedge-shaped density best demonstrated on the lateral (arrows).

- Eventually a completely collapsed lower lobe may be so small that it flattens and merges with the mediastinum, producing a thin, wedge-shaped shadow.

*Left lower lobe collapse (**Fig. 39.15**)*

- Collapsed lobe may be obscured by the heart and a penetrated view may be required.
- Mediastinal structures and the diaphragm adjacent to the non-aerated lobe are obscured.
- Extreme volume loss may cause the lobe to be so small as to be invisible as a separate opacity.
- There is loss of lower lobe artery silhouette at the hilum.

Lingula collapse

- Is often involved in collapse of the left upper lobe.
- May collapse individually.
- Radiographic features are similar to those of middle lobe collapse.

*Left upper lobe collapse (**Fig. 39.16**)*

- Lateral view demonstrates anterior displacement of the entire oblique fissure, oriented almost parallel to the anterior chest wall, demarcating the posterior surface of the upper lobe as an elongated opacity extending from the apex almost reaching the diaphragm and lying anterior to the hilum.
- Eventually the upper lobe retracts posteriorly and loses contact with the anterior chest wall.

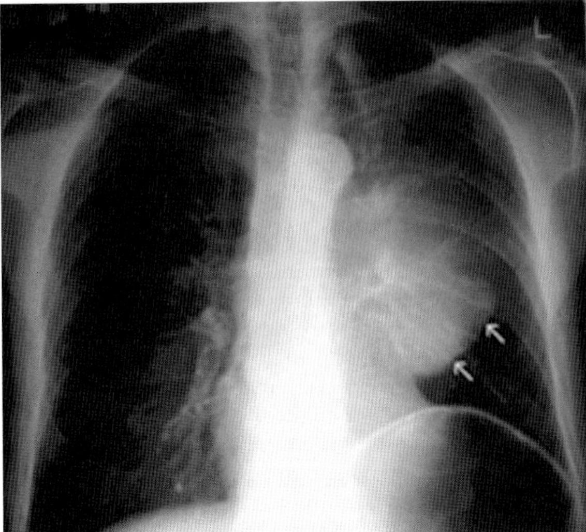

Figure 39.16 Left upper lobe collapse. A hazy opacity extends from the hilum towards the left lung apex. It is sharply demarcated inferiorly and laterally (white arrows) owing to the presence of a large tumour at the left hilum, which is obstructing the left upper lobe bronchus. Note the signs of volume loss, particularly the elevation of the left hemidiaphragm.

- Frontal radiograph demonstrates an ill-defined hazy opacity in the upper, mid and sometimes lower zones, with loss of hilar clarity.
- Hilum is often elevated, and the trachea deviated to the left.

COMBINED COLLAPSE

Right lower and middle lobe collapse is the most common pairing since a lesion may occur in the bronchus intermedius. The appearances are similar to right lower lobe collapse except that the horizontal fissure is not apparent, and the opacification reaches the lateral chest wall on the frontal radiograph, and similarly extends to the anterior chest wall on the lateral view.

Right upper and middle lobe collapse is much less common because of the distance between the origins of their bronchi, and can generally be taken to imply the presence of more than one lesion. This combination will produce appearances almost identical to those of left upper lobe collapse (see Fig. 39.16). On occasion isolated right upper lobe collapse will also produce appearances that are identical to left upper lobe collapse.

UNILATERAL INCREASED TRANSRADIANCY

The commonest causes are technical and include:

- patient rotation
- poor beam centring
- offset grid.

Pathological causes include:

- chest wall changes
- mastectomy
- congenital unilateral absence of pectoral muscles, known as Poland's syndrome
- reduced vascularity when interruption or significant reduction in the blood supply to one lung may cause that lung to be of increased transradiancy
- lung hyperexpansion due to air trapping or asymmetric emphysema.

When there is relative increased transradiancy of one hemithorax for which there is no obvious cause then the possibility of generalised increase in radiopacity of the opposite side should be considered – for example, the posterior layering of a pleural effusion in a supine patient. Usually hypertransradiancy due to technical factors can be identified by comparison of the soft tissues around the shoulder girdle, and particularly over the axillae.

ABNORMALITIES OF THE MEDIASTINUM

Pneumomediastinum or mediastinal emphysema is the presence of air between the tissue planes of the mediastinum (see section on Injuries to the mediastinum, below). Chest radiography may show vertical translucent streaks in the mediastinum, representing air separating the soft-tissue planes. The air may extend up into the neck and over the chest wall, causing subcutaneous emphysema, and also over the diaphragm. The mediastinal pleura may be displaced laterally and then be visible as a thin stripe alongside the mediastinum.

Acute mediastinitis is usually due to perforation of the oesophagus, pharynx or trachea and chest radiograph usually shows widening of the mediastinum and pneumomediastinum.

Mediastinal haemorrhage may occur from venous or arterial bleeding. The mediastinum appears widened, and blood may be seen tracking over the lung apices. It is imperative to identify a life-threatening cause such as aortic rupture.

Aortic dissection or aneurysmal dilatation may also cause widening of the mediastinal silhouette on chest radiography (**Fig. 39.17**).

PLEURAL FLUID

The most dependent recess of the pleural space is the posterior costophrenic angle and this is where a small effusion will tend to collect. As little as a few millilitres of fluid may be detected using decubitus views with a horizontal beam, ultrasound or CT. Larger volumes of fluid eventually fill in the costophrenic angle on the frontal view, and with increasing fluid a homogeneous opacity spreads upwards, obscuring the lung base (**Fig. 39.18**). The fluid usually demonstrates a concave upper edge, higher laterally than medially, and obscures the

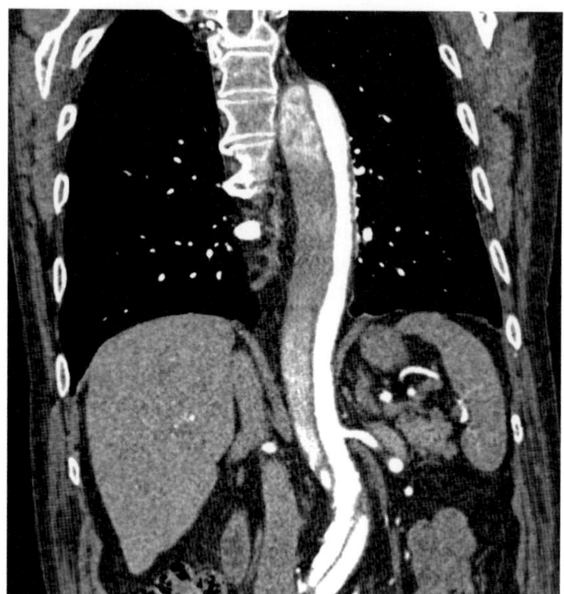

Figure 39.17 Aortic dissection. Coronal computed tomographic image showing intimal flap in the descending aorta.

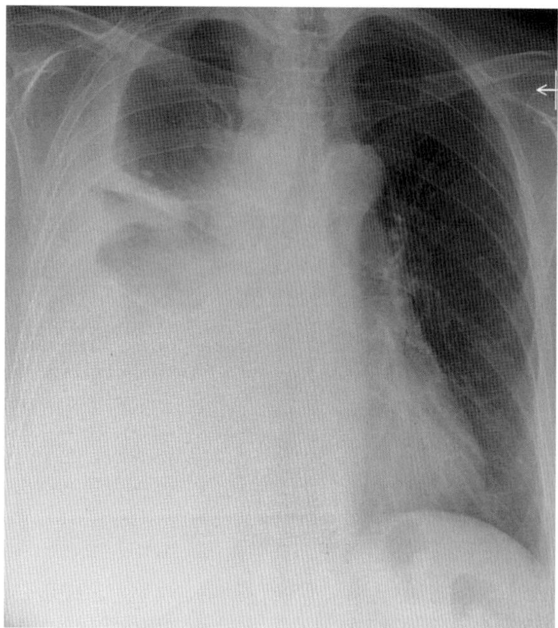

Figure 39.18 Large right pleural effusion. There is a typical configuration of the right upper border, a meniscus extending up the lateral chest wall.

diaphragm. Fluid may track into the fissures. A massive effusion may cause complete opacification of a hemithorax with passive atelectasis. The space-occupying effect of the effusion may push the mediastinum towards the opposite side, especially when the lung does not collapse significantly. Effusions in a supine patient redistribute into the paravertebral sulcus and produce an even increased density throughout that hemithorax.

Lamellar effusions are shallow collections between the lung surface and the visceral pleura, sometimes sparing the costophrenic angle, and occur early in heart failure.

Subpulmonary effusions accumulate between the diaphragm and undersurface of a lung, mimicking elevation of the hemidiaphragm, altering the diaphragmatic contour so the apex moves more laterally than usual. When left-sided, there is increased distance between the gastric air bubble and lung base.

Fluid may become loculated in the interlobar fissures and is most frequently seen in heart failure. Loculated interlobar effusions may disappear rapidly and are sometimes known as pulmonary pseudotumours.

Differentiation between a simple effusion and a complicated parapneumonic effusion or an empyema usually requires thoracentesis. Loculation is best demonstrated with ultrasound.

PNEUMOTHORAX

In an erect patient, air will usually collect at the apex (**Fig. 39.19**). The lung retracts towards the hilum and on a frontal chest film the sharp white line of the visceral pleura will be visible, separated from the chest wall by the radiolucent pleural space, which is devoid of lung markings. This should not be confused with a skin fold, which mostly occurs in supine or recumbent patients. The lung usually remains aerated, although perfusion is reduced in proportion to ventilation and therefore the radiodensity of the partially collapsed lung remains relatively normal. A large pneumothorax may lead to complete retraction of the lung, with some mediastinal shift towards the normal side. Since it is a medical emergency, tension pneumothorax is often treated before a chest radiograph is obtained. However, if a radiograph is taken in this situation it will show marked displacement of the mediastinum. Radiographically the lung may be squashed against the mediastinum, or herniate across the midline, and the ipsilateral hemidiaphragm may be depressed. A supine pneumothorax may produce increased transradiancy towards the diaphragm, and a deep sulcus sign.

COMPLICATIONS OF PNEUMOTHORAX

Pleural adhesions may limit the distribution of a pneumothorax and result in a loculated or encysted pneumothorax (see Fig. 39.8). The usual appearance is an ovoid air collection adjacent to the chest wall, and it may be radiographically indistinguishable from a thin-walled subpleural pulmonary cyst or bulla. Pleural adhesions are occasionally seen as line shadows stretching between the two pleural layers, preventing relaxation of the underlying lung. Rupture of an adhesion

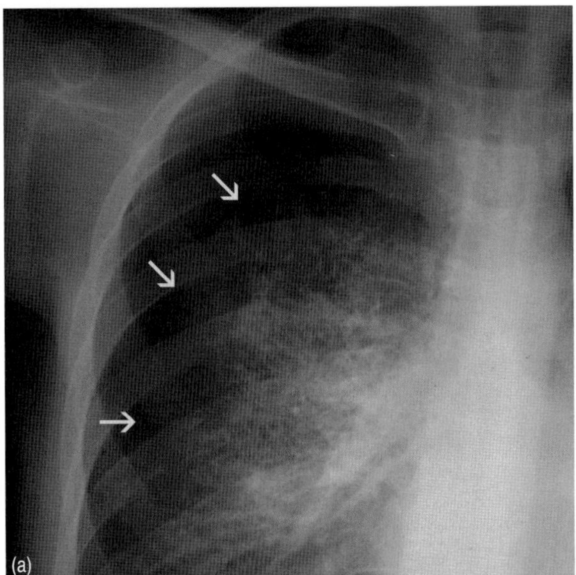

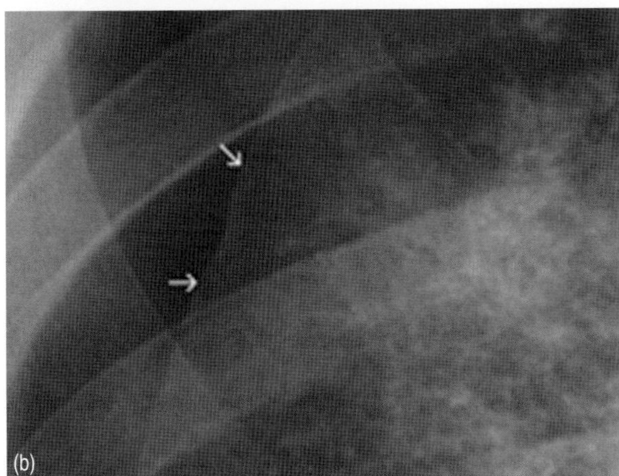

Figure 39.19 Pneumothorax. (a) This patient, with underlying lung abnormality, has developed a pneumothorax. The fine white line that represents the visceral pleura delineates the edge of the lung. (b) Close-up of the pleural line. Note how there are no vascular markings beyond this point.

may produce a haemopneumothorax. Collapse or consolidation of a lobe or lung in association with a pneumothorax is important because it may delay re-expansion of the lung.

Since the normal pleural space contains a small volume of fluid, blunting of the costophrenic angle by a short fluid level is commonly seen in a pneumothorax. In a small pneumothorax this fluid level may be the most obvious radiological sign. A larger fluid level usually signifies a complication and represents exudate, pus or blood, depending on the aetiology of the pneumothorax. A hydropneumothorax is a pneumothorax containing a significant amount of fluid (**Fig. 39.20**). On

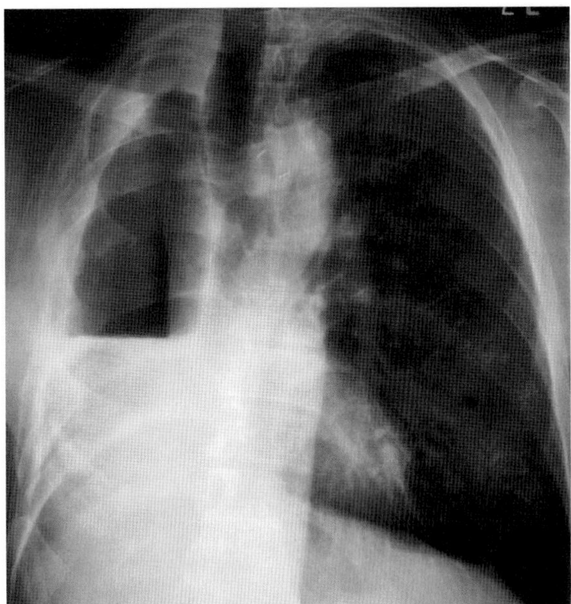

Figure 39.20 Hydropneumothorax developing in a patient who has had a previous pneumonectomy on the right for carcinoma. Spontaneous development of a bronchopleural fistula has occurred.

a radiograph obtained with a horizontal beam, a fluid level is evident. A hydro- or pyopneumothorax may arise as a result of a bronchopleural fistula, and may be a complication of surgery, tumour or infection.

PULMONARY EMBOLISM

CT diagnosis of pulmonary embolism is becoming routinely available, and depends upon the ability to acquire, within a single breath-hold, a volume of data large enough to include the entire thorax. This rapid acquisition allows excellent contrast opacification of the pulmonary arterial tree for the duration of the scan, revealing any thrombus within the central pulmonary vessels (**Fig. 39.21**). There are numerous studies evaluating helical and electron beam CT in the diagnosis of acute pulmonary embolus, with excellent reported sensitivity and specificity for the detection of clot down to the segmental level.[5–8] Most of these studies also allow other diagnoses to be made that explain the symptoms of chest pain or dyspnoea, even when no pulmonary embolism is present.

TRAUMA AND THE ICU PATIENT

SKELETAL INJURY[9]

Following trauma, rib fractures are common and may be single, multiple, unilateral or bilateral. In cases of chest trauma, the chest X-ray is more important in detecting a complication of rib fracture than the fracture

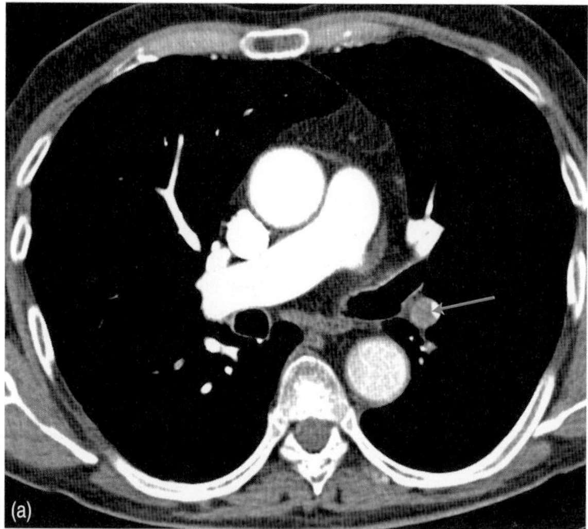

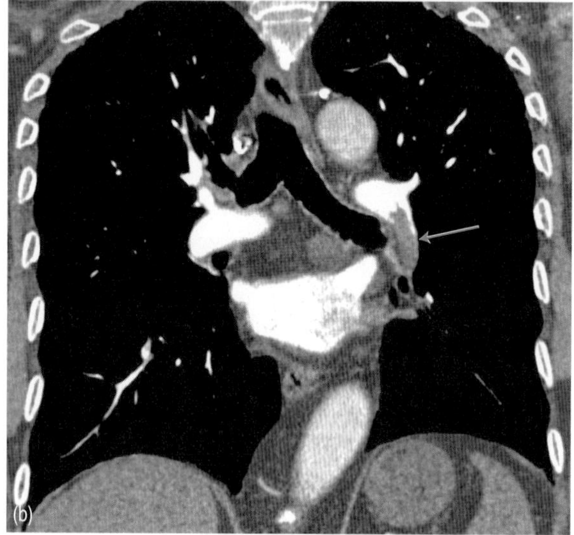

Figure 39.21 Pulmonary embolism: (a) axial and (b) coronal computed tomographic image of an embolus in the left lower lobe pulmonary artery (arrows).

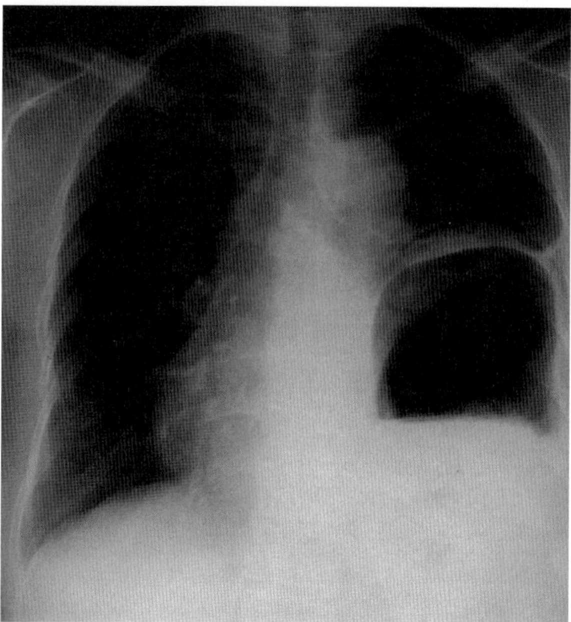

Figure 39.22 Ruptured left hemidiaphragm. Previous trauma resulted in rupture of the hemidiaphragm. A chest radiograph obtained some months later demonstrates herniation of the stomach into the left hemithorax.

itself. Fracture of one of the first three ribs is often associated with major intrathoracic injury, and fracture of the lower three ribs may be associated with important hepatic, splenic or renal injury. Complications of rib fracture include a flail segment, pneumothorax, haemothorax and subcutaneous emphysema. A flail segment is usually apparent clinically and radiologically. The fractured ends of ribs may penetrate underlying pleura and lung and cause a pneumothorax, haemothorax, haemopneumothorax or intrapulmonary haemorrhage. Air may also escape into the chest wall and cause subcutaneous emphysema. Fractures of the sternum usually require a lateral film or CT for visualisation. Fractures of the thoracic spine may be associated with a paraspinal shadow, which represents haematoma. Fractures of the clavicle may be associated with injury to the subclavian vessels or brachial plexus, and posterior dislocation of the clavicle at the sternoclavicular joint may cause injury to the trachea, oesophagus, great vessels or nerves of the superior mediastinum.

DIAPHRAGMATIC INJURY[10]

Laceration of the diaphragm may result from penetrating or non-penetrating trauma to the chest or abdomen. Rupture of the left hemidiaphragm is encountered more frequently in clinical practice than rupture on the right (**Fig. 39.22**). The typical plain film appearance is of obscuration of the affected hemidiaphragm and increased shadowing in the ipsilateral hemithorax due to herniation of stomach, omentum, bowel or solid viscera, although such herniation may be delayed. Ultrasound may demonstrate diaphragmatic laceration and free fluid in both the pleura and peritoneum. Barium studies may be useful to confirm herniation of stomach or bowel into the chest.

PLEURAL INJURY[9,11]

Pneumothorax may be a complication of rib fracture, and is then usually associated with a haemothorax. If no ribs are fractured, pneumothorax is secondary to a pneumomediastinum, pulmonary laceration or penetrating chest injury. Pneumothorax due to a penetrating injury is liable to develop increased pressure, resulting in a tension pneumothorax, which may require emergency decompression. Haemothorax may also occur with or without rib fractures, and is due to laceration of intercostal or pleural vessels. If a pneumothorax is also present a fluid level will be seen on a horizontal-beam film. Pleural effusion may also result from trauma. Open injuries to the pleura are prone to infection and development of an empyema.

INJURIES TO THE LUNG[9,11,12]

Pulmonary contusion is due to haemorrhagic exudation into the alveoli and interstitial spaces and appears as patchy, non-segmental consolidation within the first few hours of penetrating or non-penetrating trauma. There is usually improvement within 2 days and clearance within 3–4 days. Pulmonary lacerations may be obscured by pulmonary contusion, but, as this resolves, the laceration will become evident. If filled with blood it appears as a homogeneous round opacity, and if partly filled with blood it may show a fluid level (**Fig. 39.23**). Such pulmonary haematomas or blood cysts gradually decrease in size, but may take a few months to resolve completely. Fat embolism is a rare complication of multiple fractures, with poorly defined nodular opacities throughout both lungs, which resolve within a few days.

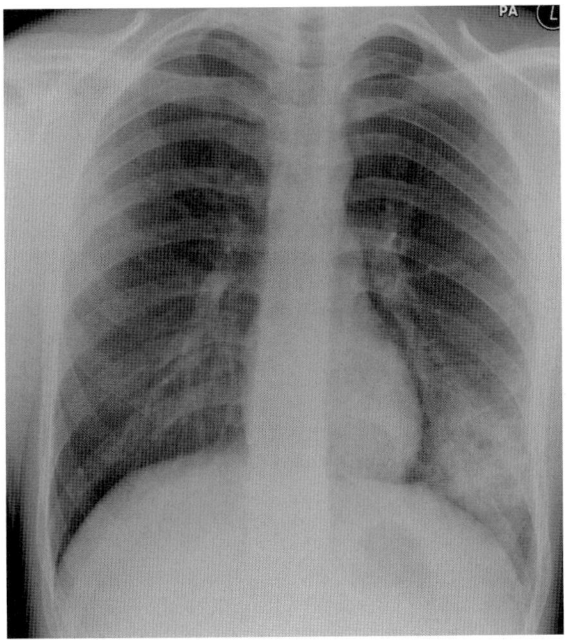

Figure 39.23 Pulmonary contusion. Left lower lobe air space opacity with a small amount of air within.

INJURIES TO THE TRACHEA AND BRONCHI[12,13]

Laceration or rupture of a major airway is an uncommon result of severe chest trauma. Fracture of the first three ribs and mediastinal emphysema and pneumothorax may also be evident. The injury is usually in the trachea just above the carina, or in a main bronchus just distal to the carina. If the bronchial sheath is preserved there may be no immediate signs or symptoms, but tracheostenosis or bronchiectasis may occur later. CT may be helpful in diagnosis, but bronchoscopy is the best diagnostic method in the acute stage.

INJURIES TO THE MEDIASTINUM[14]

Pneumomediastinum and mediastinal emphysema, discussed above, are the presence of air between the tissue planes of the mediastinum. Air may reach here as a result of pulmonary interstitial emphysema, perforation of the oesophagus, trachea or bronchus, or from a penetrating chest injury. Pulmonary interstitial emphysema is a result of alveolar wall rupture due to high intra-alveolar pressure, and may occur during violent coughing, severe asthma or crush injuries, or be due to positive-pressure ventilation. Air dissects centrally along the perivascular sheath to reach the mediastinum. Rarely, air may dissect into the mediastinum from a pneumoperitoneum. A pneumomediastinum may extend beyond the thoracic inlet into the neck, and over the chest wall. Pneumothorax is a common complication of pneumomediastinum, but the converse rarely occurs. Pneumomediastinum usually produces vertical translucent streaks in the mediastinum. This represents gas separating and outlining the soft-tissue planes and structures of the mediastinum. Gas shadows may extend up into the neck, or dissect extrapleurally over the diaphragm, or extend into the soft-tissue planes of the chest wall, causing subcutaneous emphysema. The mediastinal pleura may be displaced laterally, and become visible as a linear soft-tissue shadow parallel to the mediastinum. If mediastinal air collects beneath the pericardium the central part of the diaphragm may be visible, producing the 'continuous diaphragm' sign. Mediastinal haemorrhage may result from penetrating or non-penetrating trauma, and be due to venous or arterial bleeding. Many cases are probably unrecognised, as clinical and radiographic signs are absent. Important causes include automobile accidents, aortic rupture and dissection, and introduction of CVCs. There is usually bilateral mediastinal widening, but a localised haematoma may occur.

ACUTE AORTIC INJURY

Aortic rupture (**Fig. 39.24**)[15] is usually the result of an automobile accident. Most non-fatal aortic tears occur at the aortic isthmus, the site of the ligamentum arteriosum. Only 10–20% of patients survive the acute episode,

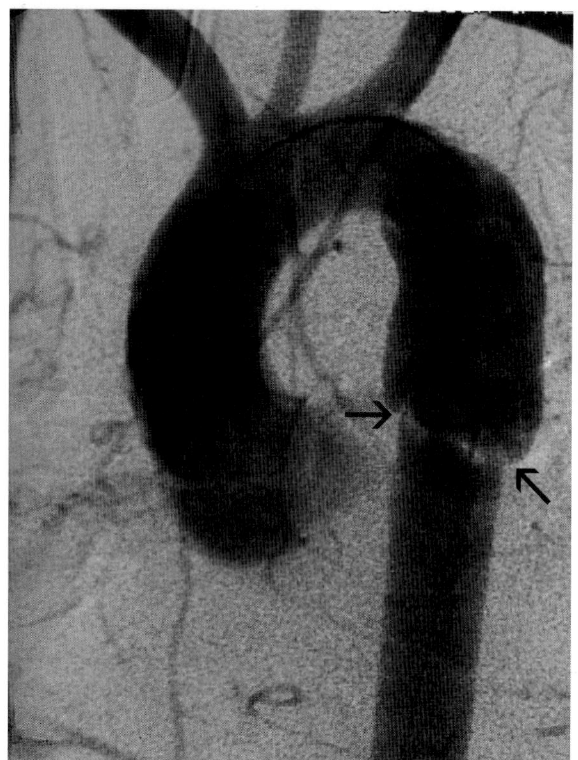

Figure 39.24 Arch aortogram demonstrating widening of the descending thoracic aorta due to aortic wall rupture. The point of return to normal calibre is demarcated by the arrows.

but a small number may develop a chronic aneurysm at the site of the tear. The commonest acute radiographic signs are widening of the superior mediastinum, and obscuration of the aortic knuckle. Other radiographic signs include deviation of the left main bronchus anteriorly, inferiorly and to the right, and rightward displacement of the trachea, a nasogastric tube or the right parasternal line. A left apical extrapleural cap or a left haemothorax may be visible. Although aortography is the definitive investigation, CT, transoesophageal echocardiography or magnetic resonance imaging may be diagnostic. In everyday practice, many departments will have emergency access to a CT scanner, but will not be centres of cardiothoracic surgery. A properly conducted CT scan demonstrating a normal mediastinum has a very high negative predictive value for aortic rupture. However, if CT is equivocal or shows a mediastinal haematoma then generally angiography will be required prior to surgery.

CARDIAC INJURY[16]

This is rare but may result from penetrating or blunt trauma. Penetrating injuries are usually rapidly fatal but may cause tamponade, ventricular aneurysm or septal defects. Blunt trauma may cause myocardial contusion and infarction and may be associated with transient or more permanent rhythm disturbance.

OESOPHAGEAL RUPTURE[17]

This is usually the result of instrumentation or surgery, but occasionally occurs in penetrating trauma, and is rarely spontaneous and due to sudden increase of intraoesophageal pressure (Boerhaave syndrome). Clinically there is acute mediastinitis; radiographically there are signs of pneumomediastinum, with or without a pneumothorax or hydropneumothorax, which is usually left-sided. The diagnosis should be confirmed by a swallow. This should initially be with water-soluble contrast medium in order to avoid the small risk of granuloma formation in the mediastinum that has been described following barium leakage. Chylothorax due to damage to the thoracic duct may become apparent hours or days after trauma. Thoracic surgery is the commonest cause.

THE POSTOPERATIVE CHEST

THORACIC COMPLICATIONS OF GENERAL SURGERY

ATELECTASIS

Atelectasis is the commonest pulmonary complication of thoracic or abdominal surgery. The chest X-ray usually shows elevation of the diaphragm, due to a poor inspiration. Linear opacities are present in the lower zones, and represent a combination of subsegmental volume loss and consolidation. The shadows usually appear about 24 hours postoperatively and resolve within 2–3 days.

PLEURAL EFFUSIONS

Pleural effusions are common immediately following abdominal surgery and usually resolve within 2 weeks. They may be associated with pulmonary infarction. Effusions due to subphrenic infection usually occur later.

PNEUMOTHORAX

Pneumothorax, when it complicates extrathoracic surgery, is usually a complication of positive-pressure ventilation or central venous line insertion. It may complicate nephrectomy.

ASPIRATION PNEUMONITIS

Aspiration pneumonitis is common during anaesthesia, but fortunately is usually insignificant. When significant, patchy consolidation appears within a few hours, usually basally or around the hila. Clearing occurs within a few days, unless there is superinfection.

PULMONARY OEDEMA

In the postoperative period, oedema may be cardiogenic or non-cardiogenic.

PNEUMONIA

Postoperative atelectasis and aspiration pneumonitis may be complicated by pneumonia. Postoperative pneumonias, therefore, tend to be associated with bilateral basal shadowing.

SUBPHRENIC ABSCESS

Subphrenic abscess usually produces elevation of the hemidiaphragm, pleural effusion and basal atelectasis. Loculated gas may be seen below the diaphragm, and fluoroscopy may show splinting of the diaphragm. Subphrenic abscess can be demonstrated by CT or ultrasound.

PULMONARY EMBOLISM

Pulmonary embolism may produce pulmonary shadowing, pleural effusion or elevation of the diaphragm, but is not excluded by a normal radiograph. In the ICU setting the radiological investigation of choice is spiral CT scanning.

THORACIC COMPLICATIONS OF CARDIAC SURGERY

Most cardiac operations are performed through a sternotomy incision, and wire sternal sutures are often seen on the postoperative films. Mitral valvotomy is now rarely performed via a thoracotomy incision, but this route is still used for surgery of coarctation of the aorta, patent ductus arteriosus, Blalock–Taussig shunts and pulmonary artery banding.

Widening of the cardiovascular silhouette is usual, and represents bleeding and oedema. Marked or progressive widening of the mediastinum suggests significant haemorrhage (**Fig. 39.25**). Some air commonly remains in the pericardium following cardiac surgery, so that the signs of pneumopericardium may be present.

Left basal shadowing is almost invariable, representing atelectasis. This shadowing usually resolves over a week or two. Small pleural effusions are also common in the immediate postoperative period.

Pneumoperitoneum is sometimes seen, due to involvement of the peritoneum by the sternotomy incision. It is of no pathological significance (see Fig. 39.4).

Violation of left or right pleural space may lead to a pneumothorax. Damage to a major lymphatic vessel may lead to a chylothorax or a more localised chyloma. Phrenic nerve damage may cause paresis or paralysis of a hemidiaphragm.

Surgical clips or other metallic markers have sometimes been used to mark the ends of coronary artery bypass grafts. Prosthetic heart valves are usually visible radiographically, but they may be difficult to see on an underpenetrated film.

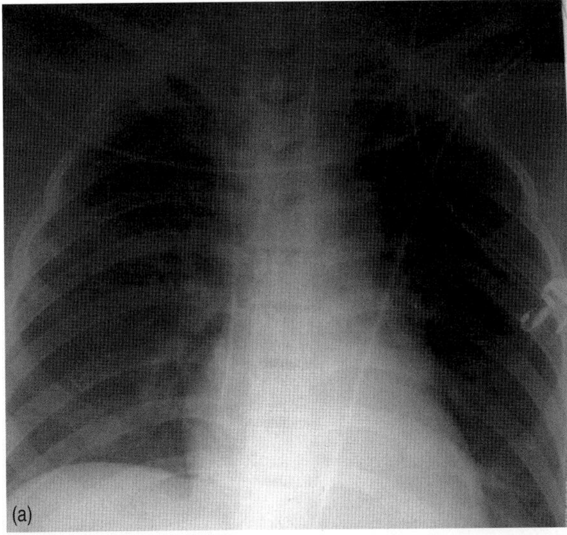

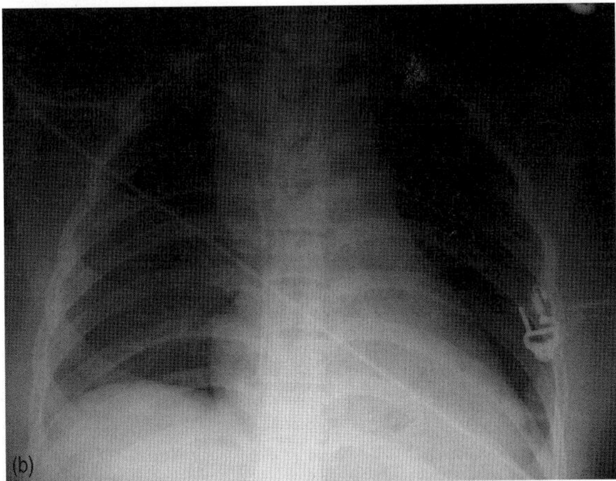

Figure 39.25 Following cardiac surgery (a) the postoperative chest radiograph appears satisfactory. A few hours later (b) the mediastinum has widened considerably, due to mediastinal haemorrhage.

Sternal dehiscence may be apparent radiographically by a linear lucency appearing in the sternum and alteration in position of the sternal sutures on consecutive films. The diagnosis is usually made clinically and may be associated with osteomyelitis. A first or second rib may be fractured when the sternum is spread apart. The importance of this observation is that it may explain chest pain in the postoperative period.

Acute mediastinitis may complicate mediastinal surgery, although it is more commonly associated with oesophageal perforation or surgery. Radiographically there may be mediastinal widening or pneumomediastinum, and these features are best assessed by CT scan.

Access the complete references list online at http://www.expertconsult.com

1. Sheard S, Rao P, Devaraj A. Imaging of acute respiratory distress syndrome. Respir Care 2012;57:607–12.
4. Knutstad K, Hager B, Hauser M. Radiologic diagnosis and management of complications related to central venous access. Acta Radiol 2003;44:508–16.
6. Henzler T, Barraza Jr JM, Nance Jr JW, et al. CT imaging of acute pulmonary embolism. J Cardiovasc Comput Tomogr 2011;5:3–11.
9. Peters S, Nicolas V, Heyer CM. Multidetector computed tomography-spectrum of blunt chest wall and lung injuries in polytraumatized patients. Clin Radiol 2010;65:333–8.
11. Miller LA. Chest wall, lung, and pleural space trauma. Radiol Clin North Am 2006;44:213–24.
12. Sangster GP, González-Beicos A, Carbo AI, et al. Blunt traumatic injuries of the lung parenchyma, pleura, thoracic wall, and intrathoracic airways: multidetector computer tomography imaging findings. Emerg Radiol 2007;14:297–310.
14. Euathrongchit J, Thoongsuwan N, Stern EJ. Nonvascular mediastinal trauma. Radiol Clin North Am 2006;44:251–817.

40

Ultrasound in the ICU

Ubbo F Wiersema

Over the past decade point-of-care ultrasound has become an integral part of intensive care practice. An increasing number of clinical applications have been developed that facilitate time-critical therapeutic decision making and invasive diagnostic procedures. This chapter will describe ultrasound techniques that have an established role in intensive care, and are readily acquired with a short period of training. Acquisition of ultrasound proficiency is best achieved with a combination of theoretical learning (basic physics of ultrasound, relevant anatomy, image interpretation), direct supervision of image acquisition, and practice.[1,2]

EQUIPMENT

The ideal ultrasound machine for intensive care applications is compact, easily transportable and robust. The console should be waterproof and able to withstand repeated disinfection procedures. To avoid transmission of nosocomial skin flora between patients the transducer, console and electrocardiograph leads (if used) should be disinfected (e.g. with alcohol-based wipes) after each examination.[3,4] Single-use coupling gel should be used instead of multi-use bottles.

Different transducers (probes) are designed for different applications:

- A low-frequency (3–5 MHz) phased array transducer (transthoracic echocardiography transducer) is suitable for chest and abdominal ultrasound.
- A mid-frequency (5–8 MHz) microconvex curved array transducer is also suitable for chest ultrasound and is sometimes useful for subclavian vein ultrasound.
- A high-frequency (6–13 MHz) linear array transducer is necessary for vascular access and ocular ultrasound.
- A low-frequency (2–5 MHz), large-footprint, curved array transducer provides optimal abdominal ultrasound imaging, but is not essential.

CHEST ULTRASOUND

Ultrasound waves are unable to penetrate aerated lung tissue. Historically, this has limited ultrasound of the chest largely to the evaluation of pleural effusions. In recent years, the recognition that analysis of ultrasound artefacts arising from the pleura can provide valuable information about underlying lung pathology has led to wider application of lung ultrasound.[3] Compared with chest radiography and computed tomography (CT), ultrasound is rapid, inexpensive and safe from ionising radiation. Almost all lung parenchymal pathology abuts the pleura and can thus be detected by ultrasound. Diagnostic accuracy of ultrasound compares favourably with CT, and significantly exceeds clinical examination and plain radiography.

EQUIPMENT

Several transducers can be used for chest ultrasound. The standard transthoracic echocardiography, phased array, low-frequency (3–5 MHz) transducer provides good depth penetration and sufficient resolution for most chest ultrasound applications. This transducer is ideally suited for evaluating pulmonary oedema and pleural effusions[5,6] and can therefore be used to complement echocardiographic assessment of cardiac function. A microconvex 5–8 MHz curved array transducer provides better artefact visualisation than lower-frequency transducers, but depth penetration may be insufficient for large patients. The microconvex design facilitates placement of the transducer between the ribs of thin patients.[3] A high-frequency linear array transducer (6–13 MHz) allows detailed pleural line analysis, and is optimal for pneumothorax detection (e.g. after venous cannulation) but has limited other applicability.

Imaging in 2D is adequate for most examinations. M-mode is useful for lung sliding analysis (see below). Doppler imaging is not required.[3]

EXAMINATION TECHNIQUE

Mechanically ventilated patients can usually be satisfactorily examined in the supine or semirecumbent position. Imaging of the posterior lungs is achieved by scanning along the posterior axillary line with the arm lifted out of the way over the anterior chest. A thorough examination of the lungs involves scanning bilaterally over four quadrants of the anterior chest wall (upper and lower zones laterally and medially), the upper and lower lateral chest wall (bounded by the anterior and posterior axillary lines), and upper, middle and lower zones of the posterior chest wall.[3,7] For a complete study each intercostal space, along multiple vertical lines, should be imaged.[5,6,8] The findings for each space can then be documented in tabulated form. Only the dorsal lung segments behind the scapulae cannot be examined by ultrasound.

Fluid-filled chest pathology (e.g. pleural effusions, atelectasis) is gravity-dependent and thus lies inferiorly. In contrast, aerated pathology (i.e. pneumothorax) is non-dependent, and lies superiorly. Detection of specific pathology should thus be directed accordingly, noting that in the supine patient the least dependent region is the basal anterior chest, which is where a small pneumothorax will collect.[7]

The examination sequence should commence with scanning of the lower lateral chest. Here identification of the diaphragm provides a useful landmark for further imaging. Subdiaphragmatic structures (liver, spleen and kidneys) may be identified to confirm the location of the diaphragm. Right-sided subdiaphragmatic structures are usually easier to visualise than left-sided structures. Diaphragmatic movement with tidal ventilation should be identified. The scanning depth should initially be set to 15–20 cm to evaluate basal lung pathology. The scanning depth can then be reduced to 10 cm (and use of a higher-frequency transducer considered) to facilitate artefact analysis and complete the examination over the whole chest wall.

For each region of interest the transducer should be placed between the rib spaces and aligned with the longitudinal axis of the patient. The orientation marker on the transducer should face cephalad. By convention the orientation marker is displayed on the upper left of the screen with abdominal ultrasound and displayed on the upper right of the screen with echocardiography. Choice of transducer and type of examination selected from the display menu will determine the default marker location on the screen.

IMAGE INTERPRETATION

For every region examined, image interpretation involves each of the following steps:

- identification of the pleural line between the ribs
- artefact analysis
- lung sliding analysis
- evaluation for pathology that can be directly visualised (e.g. pleural effusion, consolidation).

EXTRAPLEURAL LANDMARKS

In 2D mode, with the transducer aligned with the longitudinal axis of the patient, the ribs above and below the pleural space cast a dark shadow that extends down to the full depth of the image on the screen. Between the ribs, the pleural line can be identified as a bright (hyperechoic) horizontal line located 0.5 cm deep to the outer surface of the ribs (**Fig. 40.1**). The pleural line is the reference line for artefact analysis and lung sliding analysis.

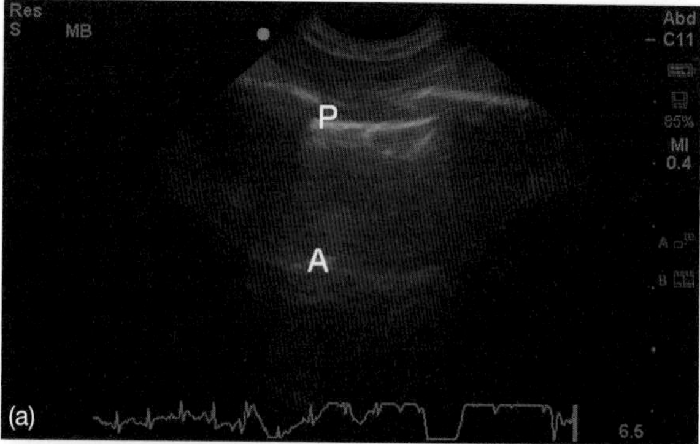

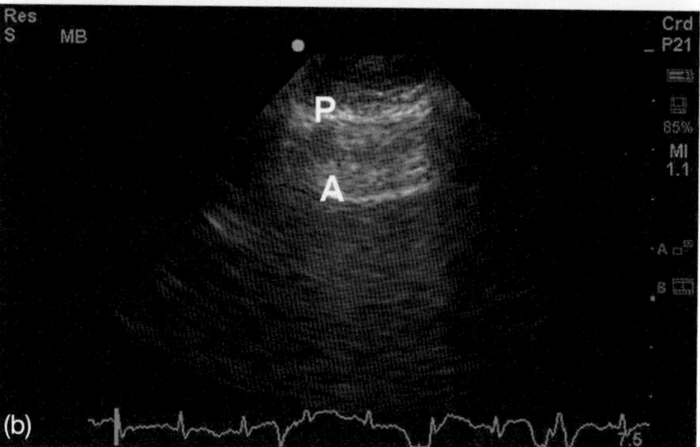

Figure 40.1 A lines demonstrated with a 5–8 MHz microconvex curved array transducer (a) and 1–5 MHz phased array transducer (b). Note the horizontal bright (hyperechoic) pleural line (P) and A line (A) flanked on each side by dark rib shadows.

ARTEFACT ANALYSIS

Ultrasound waves cannot be transmitted through aerated tissue. Normal lung parenchyma is thus not visible beyond the visceral pleura. The pleural line is formed by the reflection of ultrasound waves at the interface between the pleura and lung parenchyma (Fig. 40.1). All artefacts used for analysis of lung pathology (except E lines) arise from the pleural line.

- *A-line artefacts* (Fig. 40.1): these are bright horizontal repetitions of the pleural line due to reverberation artefacts, and are a normal finding.[3,9] The vertical distance between two adjacent A lines is the same as the distance between the skin and the pleural line. Usually only one or two A lines are visible depending on image gain and depth settings. A lines are so-called because they are reminiscent of the cross bar of the capital letter A framed by the diagonal shadows cast by the ribs.

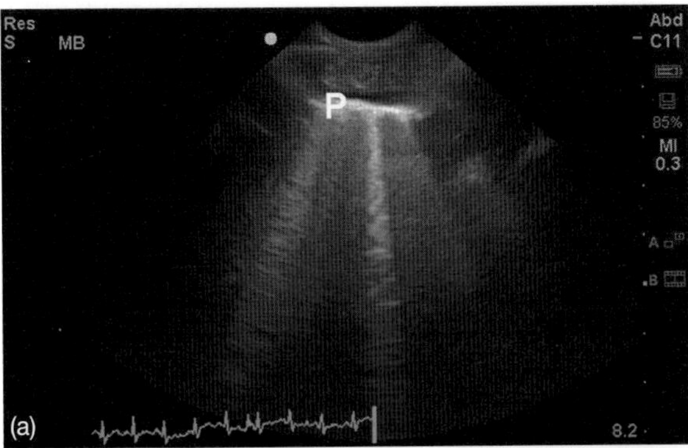

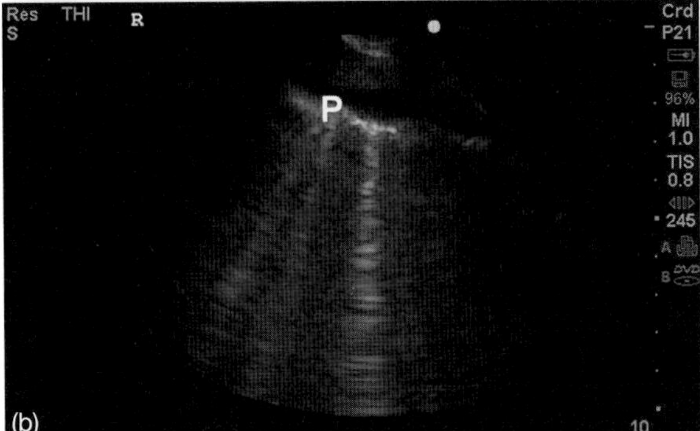

Figure 40.2 B lines demonstrated with 5–8 MHz microconvex curved array transducer (a) and 1–5 MHz phased array transducer (b). Note vertical bright (hyperechoic) lines originating at the pleural line (P) and extending to the bottom of the screen.

- *B-line artefacts* (**Fig. 40.2**): these were previously known as *comet-tail artefacts*[9] or *ultrasound lung comets*,[5] and are defined as discrete vertical bright lines originating at the pleural line and fanning out to the bottom of the screen without fading.[10] B lines arise from reverberation artefacts generated at the interface of fluid-filled or fibrosed interlobular septa abutting the visceral pleura.[9,11] The presence of multiple B lines, termed *'B pattern'*, erases the A-line artefact. With greater loss of aeration the B lines become more closely spaced, or confluent (*white-out*) (**Fig. 40.3**). B lines are equivalent to Kerley B lines seen on the chest radiograph although they may be present before radiographic changes are visible. Isolated B lines or short, ill-defined vertical artefacts are of uncertain significance.
- *E-line artefacts* (**Fig. 40.4**): these have a very similar appearance to B lines, but arise superficial to the pleural line.[3,7] They occur with subcutaneous emphysema where pockets of air create an air–tissue interface that generates reverberation artefacts. It is important to distinguish B lines from E lines by clearly identifying the origin of vertical artefacts in relation to the pleural line; although subcutaneous emphysema is usually easy to detect clinically.

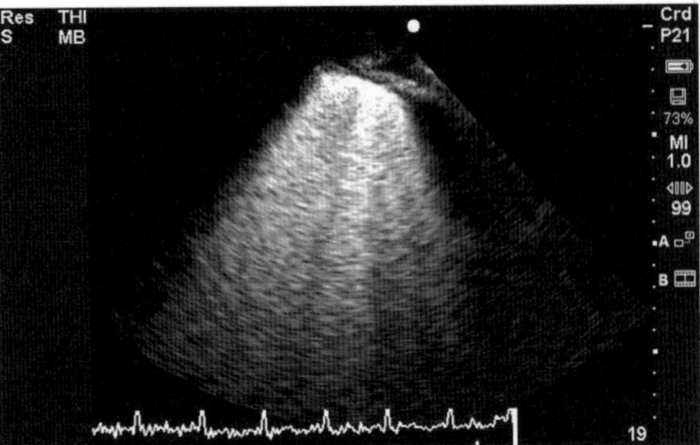

Figure 40.3 Confluent B lines creating a 'white out' appearance, demonstrated with a 1–5 MHz phased array transducer.

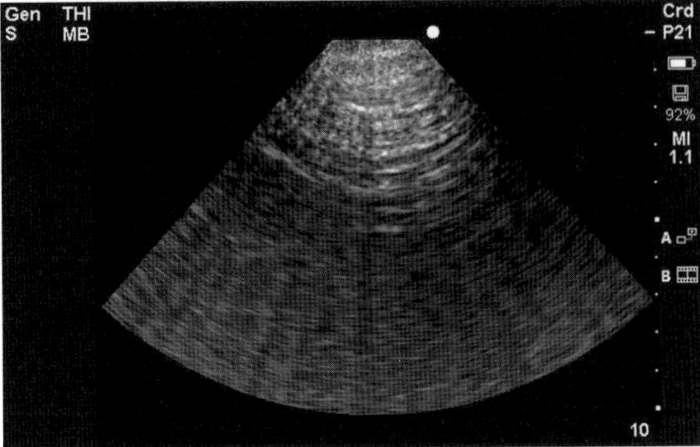

Figure 40.4 E lines demonstrated with a 1–5 MHz phased array transducer. Note the vertical bright (hyperechoic) lines originate above the pleural line, which is poorly defined.

LUNG SLIDING ANALYSIS

With tidal inflation of the normal lung, the visceral pleura slides against the parietal pleura. On ultrasound this is seen as movement below the pleural line. The movement is best appreciated using M-mode imaging, which shows an image reminiscent of the seashore: above the pleural line there are a series of horizontal lines created by extrapleural tissue static in time (the sea), and below the pleural line there is a grainy appearance due to reflection from moving visceral pleura (the beach) (**Fig. 40.5**).[3,7] The transducer must be held completely still on the chest wall. Diagnostic accuracy is improved if a higher-frequency transducer is used. Lung sliding is absent if the visceral pleura cannot be visualised because of air in the pleural space (pneumothorax) (**Fig. 40.6**), or if lung movement is abolished (e.g. pleural fibrosis, dense consolidation, atelectasis or apnoea). Lung sliding may appear absent in patients with chronic obstructive pulmonary disease, or at the apices with small volume tidal ventilation. The *lung pulse sign* (see section on atelectasis below) can be present only when lung sliding is absent (**Fig. 40.7**).[12]

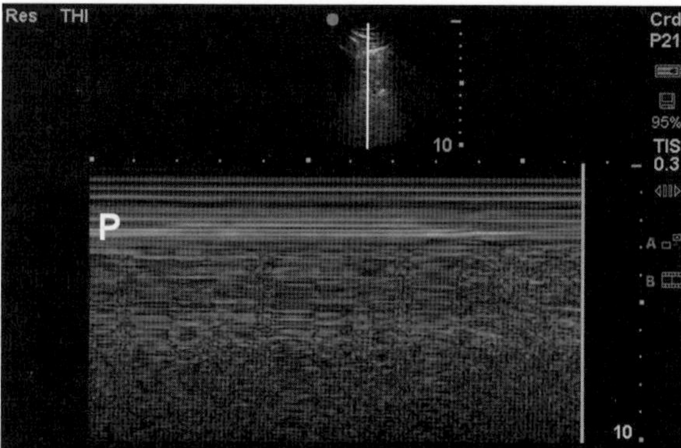

Figure 40.5 Lung sliding (sea shore sign) demonstrated with a 1–5 MHz phased array transducer in M-mode. Note the smooth horizontal lines above the pleural line (P) (extrapleural tissues static over time), and the 'sandy' appearance below the pleural line (due to artefact from visceral pleural sliding with tidal ventilation).

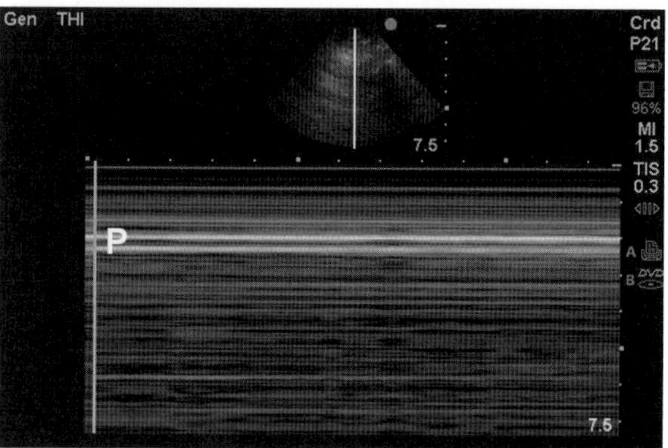

Figure 40.6 Absent lung sliding demonstrated with a 1–5 MHz phased array transducer in M-mode. Note the smooth horizontal lines above and below the bright (hyperechoic) pleural line (P).

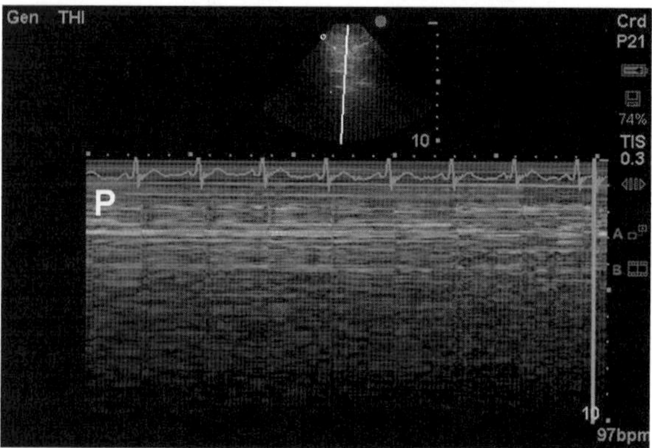

Figure 40.7 Lung pulse sign demonstrated with a 1–5 MHz phased array transducer in M-mode. Note the vertical lines below the pleural line (P) due to transmitted cardiac pulsations.

DIRECTLY VISUALISED PATHOLOGY

Ultrasound waves are able to penetrate non-aerated tissues. Thus pleural fluid, and non-aerated lung pathology (such as consolidation or complete atelectasis), can be readily visualised.

SPECIFIC PATHOLOGIES

The diagnostic accuracy of ultrasound is comparable to CT and superior to plain radiography for all the pathologies discussed below. Ultrasound is also sensitive to rapid changes in severity of disease and can thus be used to monitor disease progression and make timely clinical decisions.[13–15]

The ultrasound appearance of normal lung is characterised by the presence of A lines and lung sliding. About a quarter of normal individuals have one or two B lines at the lung bases[4,5,9] but other artefacts should be absent.

Pleural effusion

Ultrasound enables the detection of small pleural effusions (<50 mL) not visible on chest radiography. Ultrasound can also provides information about the nature of an effusion; septated pleural collections are better characterised with ultrasound than with CT.

Examination for pleural effusion commences with identification of the diaphragm on scanning over the lower lateral chest. The diaphragm appears as a smooth bright (hyperechoic) line overlying the abdominal contents (usually liver or spleen, with the kidneys deep and caudal to these). Pleural fluid manifests as a relatively homogeneous dark (hypoechoic) area between the diaphragm and parietal pleura (**Fig. 40.8**). As pleural fluid acts as an acoustic window, the lung surface (visceral

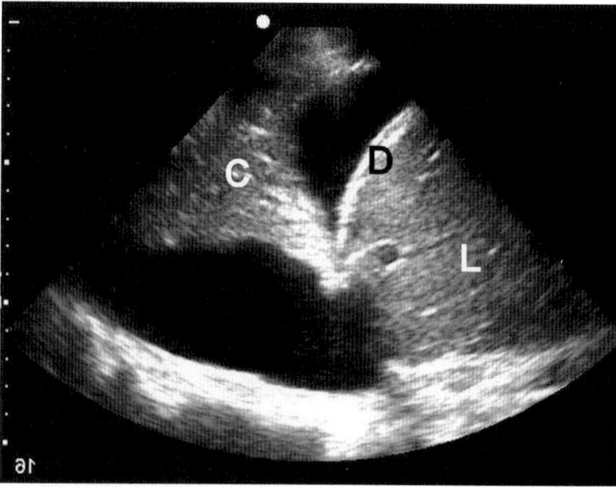

Figure 40.8 Liver (L), diaphragm (D), pleural effusion and collapsed/consolidated lung (C) demonstrated with a 1–5 MHz phased array transducer aligned with the longitudinal axis of the patient in the basal right mid-axillary line.

pleura) can be seen as a regular deep border to the effusion. Aerated lung will show a bright pleural line; often with B lines adjacent to the effusion. Normal lung will tend to float above an effusion, whereas collapsed or consolidated lung will float within a moderate or large effusion (Fig. 40.8). A small pleural effusion confined to the costophrenic angle may be difficult to detect. However, its presence can be inferred if the dome of the diaphragm, which is normally obscured by aerated lung, can be seen. Large effusions allow direct visualisation of mediastinal structures (e.g. aorta and great vessels) if sufficient depth is imaged.

Pleural effusion quantification Various techniques have been described to estimate the volume of pleural fluid.

Measurements are made scanning in the basal intercostal spaces of the posterior axillary line with the transducer aligned in a transverse plane. In supine mechanically ventilated patients, a posterior pleural separation >5 cm strongly predicts a drainage volume of >500 mL.[16] In semirecumbent (15°) mechanically ventilated patients the maximum pleural separation (in mm) multiplied by 20 gives an estimate of drainage volume (in mL).[17] Measurements can be made at either end-expiration or end-inspiration, but are not very reliable at estimating volumes of small or very large effusions. A multiplane method, is obtained by multiplying the longitudinal extent of the effusion by the cross-sectional area at mid length, increases measurement accuracy.[18] However, a precise volume measurement is rarely necessary for clinical decision making.

Nature of pleural effusion Ultrasound characteristics may indirectly suggest the nature of an effusion and can be used to guide the decision whether to perform thoracocentesis. On ultrasound the appearance of an effusion can be categorised as simple, with a uniformly anechoic (black) appearance; or complex, with echogenic material (bright dots), or septa visible within the effusion. Complex effusions can be classified as: complex non-septated with echogenic foci, complex septated, or homogeneously echogenic.[19]

Transudates typically appear anechoic (Fig. 40.8). In addition the low viscosity of a transudate allows substantial movement of lung tissue with tidal ventilation. This is best appreciated as a sinusoidal pattern of the lung surface line with M-mode during tidal ventilation.[3] The pleural line is usually smooth.

Exudates are usually but not always complex. On M-mode imaging there is minimal sinusoidal movement with tidal ventilation if the exudate is very viscous. The pleural line may appear thickened and irregular from pleural inflammation. A homogeneously echogenic pattern may be almost tissue-like in appearance and should not be mistaken for an area of consolidation (see below). In patients who clinically appear infected, a complex, relatively hyperechoic, septated, or homogeneously echogenic pattern suggests empyema. An anechoic or minimally hyperechoic pattern is unlikely to represent empyema.[19] Haemothoraces appear complex with septa and areas of differing echogenicity, depending on the age of the blood.

Thoracocentesis Ultrasound guidance of thoracocentesis decreases complications and improves fluid collection rates.[4] It allows identification of the optimal site for drainage, and measurement of the depth of the pleural space. Potential hazards such as the diaphragm or pleural adherences can be avoided, and the risk of intrafissural or intraparenchymal tube placement reduced. The decision to perform thoracocentesis is based on size, suspected nature of the effusion and clinical circumstances.

Alveolar consolidation

Consolidated lung (except bronchi) is not aerated and can therefore be directly visualised where it abuts the pleura, or where there is a pleural effusion between the chest wall and consolidated lung (**Fig. 40.9**).[12,20] Artefacts that arise from the pleural line are absent, although B lines may be seen at the edges of consolidated areas. Consolidation is rarely confined just to deeper lung tissue, almost always extending to involve peripheral lung tissue adjacent to pleura. The full extent of consolidation can thus usually be defined. In mechanically ventilated patients consolidation preferentially affects the basal posterior lung segments. By contrast, with community-acquired pneumonia consolidation may affect any lung region.

The echo-texture of consolidation resembles that of liver (hepatisation), although usually coarser in appearance (Fig. 40.9). When examining the right basal chest, care should be taken to distinguish between

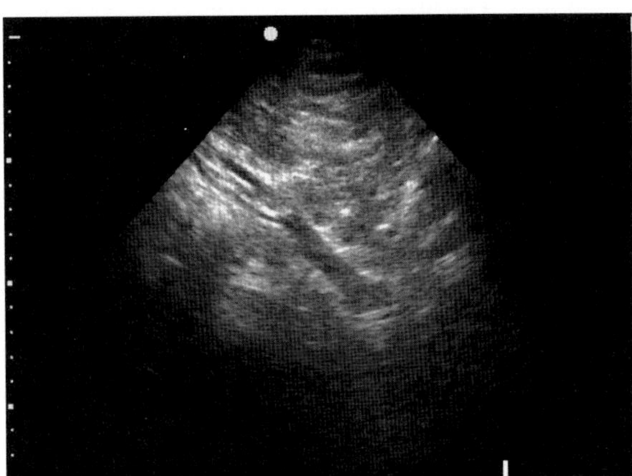

Figure 40.9 Consolidated lung demonstrated with a 1–5 MHz phased array transducer aligned with the longitudinal axis of the patient in the mid left mid-axillary line. Note the dark (hypoechoic) diagonal region representing the oblique fissure, and the bright (hyperechoic) punctiform air bronchograms.

Table 40.1 Lung ultrasound reaeration score[13,14]*

LUNG PATHOLOGY	DEGREE OF AERATION	ULTRASOUND FINDINGS
Normal lung	More aeration	A lines
Interstitial infiltrate	⇕	B lines
Alveolar–interstitial infiltrate		White out (confluent B lines)
Alveolar consolidation	Less aeration	Consolidation

*Loss of aeration may be due to oedema, inflammation or fibrosis.

consolidated lung and liver parenchyma by clearly identifying the diaphragm (Fig. 40.8). The borders of the consolidated area may be irregular at the junction with normal lung tissue, but will be regular if the full thickness of lung is affected.

Within consolidated lung, air bronchograms appear as bright (hyperechoic) punctiform or linear artefacts (Fig. 40.9). The air bronchogram artefact moves with respiration (dynamic air bronchogram), outwards (towards the transducer) with inspiration and inwards (away from the transducer) with expiration.[21] The dynamic air bronchogram distinguishes consolidation from resorptive atelectasis.[21]

Atelectasis

Resorptive atelectasis commonly affects the dependent lung regions of mechanically ventilated patients. On ultrasound the affected lung appears consolidated, but air bronchograms are static with respiration.[21]

Complete lobar collapse may occur with bronchial intubation or mucus plugging. This can be detected immediately on ultrasound by absence of lung sliding and the lung pulse sign.[12] These signs are best appreciated using M-mode imaging with a high-frequency transducer. The lung pulse sign consists of vibrations in the M-mode trace (below the pleural line) due to transmitted cardiac pulsations (see Fig. 40.7). Over time, progressive absorption of gas leads to the development of consolidated lung (resorptive atelectasis).

Alveolar–interstitial syndrome

Alveolar–interstitial syndrome encompasses disease processes with which there is predominant interstitial involvement, and partial loss of lung aeration. In the acute setting this is most often due to hydrostatic or capillary leak pulmonary oedema. Less common causes include interstitial fibrosis (interstitial pneumonia) and opportunistic infection (in immunocompromised patients). Ultrasound has a high diagnostic accuracy for alveolar–interstitial syndrome.[9]

On ultrasound the hallmark of alveolar–interstitial syndrome is the presence of multiple (at least three) B lines largely independent of patient positioning.[5,9] The ultrasound pattern of B lines corresponds to the degree of lung aeration.[14] In mild disease, where thickening is confined to interlobular septa, the B lines are characteristically 7 mm apart (measured at the pleural line) (see Fig. 40.2). With progressive pulmonary oedema and increasing alveolar flooding, or with fine fibrosis, B lines are more closely spaced (approximately 3 mm apart). In severe cases B lines become confluent creating a 'white-out' pattern (see Fig. 40.3); this pattern is equivalent to ground-glass opacification on CT.[4,9,22] Complete alveolar flooding is indistinguishable from primary alveolar consolidation.[14,22] With respiration the B lines move to-and-fro across the screen with lung sliding.

In acute alveolar–interstitial syndrome a number of ultrasound findings can be used to distinguish acute respiratory distress syndrome (ARDS) from cardiogenic pulmonary oedema.[22] ARDS is characterised by a non-uniform distribution of B lines, with areas of normal lung and areas of confluent B lines or white-out. Areas of consolidation are often present, particularly in the posterobasal regions. Lung sliding is reduced, or absent, in densely affected regions and the pleural line appears irregular, thickened and coarse when examined with a high-frequency transducer. In contrast, cardiogenic pulmonary oedema shows a homogeneous distribution of B lines. Consolidation is infrequent and pleural line abnormalities are absent. Pleural effusions are common.

With cardiogenic pulmonary oedema a *lung comet score* can be used to provide a semiquantitative measure of extravascular lung water. The score is obtained by adding together the number of B lines seen from each intercostal space examined over the anterior and lateral chest.[5,6,8] The number of B lines has been shown to correlate with functional class, and severity of systolic and diastolic left ventricular dysfunction on cardiac echocardiography.[6] Reduction in lung comet score occurs with resolution of interstitial oedema.[15] An absence of B lines is consistent with a low pulmonary artery occlusion pressure.[23,24] During fluid resuscitation, the new appearance of B lines heralds the development of interstitial oedema before radiographic changes are visible.

In ALI/ARDS a lung ultrasound *reaeration score* based on the severity of interstitial changes (**Table 40.1**) provides a semiquantitative measure of positive end-expiratory pressure induced lung recruitment.[14] The lung ultrasound reaeration score has also been used to evaluate resolution of ventilator-associated pneumonia with antibiotics.[13]

Pneumothorax

The diagnosis of pneumothorax by ultrasound requires more expertise than other aspects of chest ultrasound,[4] due to the reliance on artefact analysis and low incidence of pneumothorax. However, in experienced hands the diagnostic accuracy of ultrasound for occult pneumothorax, defined as pneumothorax visible on CT but not plain radiograph, matches that of CT.[7]

As free pneumothorax is non-dependent, signs of pneumothorax should be sought anteroapically in the semirecumbent patient or anterobasally in the supine patient. Where there is a pneumothorax the parietal and visceral pleura are separated by air through which ultrasound waves cannot penetrate. Thus any lung pathology, or artefacts abutting or arising at the visceral pleura, cannot be visualised; lung sliding, B lines and the lung pulse sign must be absent. However, the A-line sign is present, generated at the tissue/air interface of the parietal pleura. The combination of A lines, absent B lines, absent lung sliding and absent lung pulse sign is 100% sensitive, but not specific for pneumothorax. Detection of the edge of the pneumothorax, termed the *lung point sign*, confirms the diagnosis of pneumothorax and allows a rough assessment of its size.[7] With the transducer held perfectly still, using 2D mode, the lung is seen to slide in and out of view with tidal ventilation. This can also be appreciated using M-mode imaging, which shows alternating lung sliding and absent lung sliding. The lung point sign will be visualised anteriorly with an occult or small pneumothorax and more laterally with a moderate-sized pneumothorax.[7] The lung point sign will be absent with a large pneumothorax, where lung sliding is absent over the entire chest.[7] In mechanically ventilated patients, care should be taken to avoid mistaking a temporary cessation of lung sliding, due to a pause in ventilation, for true lung sliding; the lung pulse sign should be present with pauses in ventilation.

A false-positive diagnosis of pneumothorax is more likely in patients with chronic obstructive pulmonary disease. If clinical uncertainty remains then chest CT may be indicated. During cardiopulmonary resuscitation the exclusion of pneumothorax may be particularly difficult, because lung sliding will be absent unless there is effective ventilation, and the lung pulse sign will be absent during apnoeic periods because of the lack of cardiac contractility.

Subcutaneous emphysema is characterised by an air–liquid interface superficial to the pleural line. This creates E-line artefacts, which are similar in appearance to B lines but arise superficially to the pleural line (see Fig. 40.4). The presence of subcutaneous emphysema is suggestive of pneumothorax. Unfortunately, the presence of E lines precludes further ultrasound analysis for signs of pneumothorax or other lung pathology. In these circumstances other imaging techniques may be required depending on the clinical circumstances.

DIAPHRAGMATIC DYSFUNCTION

Ultrasound promises to be a simple and safe alternative to fluoroscopy or phrenic nerve conduction studies for the diagnosis of diaphragmatic dysfunction. Ultrasound techniques are based on the measurement of either the extent of diaphragmatic excursion with respiration viewed from the anterior or lateral upper abdomen, or changes in diaphragm thickness at the zone of apposition between the diaphragm and the basal, lateral chest wall.[25–27] Measurements can be made using 2D or M-mode.[25–27]

DIAGNOSTIC ALGORITHMS

A number of algorithms exist that incorporate chest ultrasound in the diagnostic assessment of patients with undifferentiated respiratory failure, shock, trauma (E-FAST) or cardiac arrest.

The Bedside Lung Ultrasound in Emergency (BLUE) protocol combines lung ultrasound with deep-vein ultrasound to facilitate a diagnosis in patients with acute respiratory failure.[28] A diagnosis of pulmonary embolus may be inferred from the combination of clear lungs and deep vein thrombosis on ultrasound, as direct diagnosis of pulmonary embolism with lung ultrasound is problematic.[29] Echocardiography can be added for a complete assessment of respiratory failure. For undifferentiated hypotension or shock, abdominal ultrasound is also added to detect free peritoneal fluid and abdominal aortic aneurysm.[30]

ABDOMINAL ULTRASOUND

A complete ultrasound examination of the abdomen requires radiological expertise. However, detection of haemoperitoneum (and haemopericardium) with Focused Assessment with Sonography in Trauma (FAST) is well established in emergency medicine,[31–33] and the same examination sequence can be readily applied to the intensive care patient to detect intraperitoneal fluid of any cause. Examples include detection of haemoperitoneum after abdominal surgery, or ascites in patients with chronic liver disease and portal hypertension. Once detected, if the ascites requires paracentesis the optimal location for needle puncture can be determined by scanning more widely over the abdomen.

Low-frequency curved or phased array transducers are suitable for the FAST examination. The examination sequence consists of four standard views:[31,32]

- *Right upper quadrant:* with the transducer in the mid axillary line, aligned with the longitudinal axis of the patient (orientation marker cephalad). Three potential spaces where fluid may collect are examined in turn by moving the transducer cephalad and caudad:

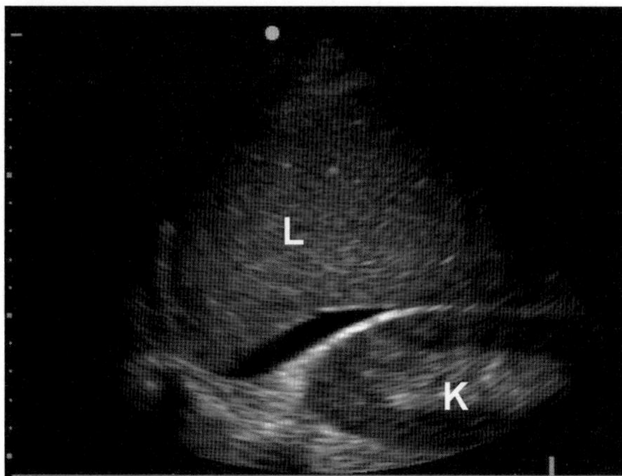

Figure 40.10 Right upper quadrant FAST scan (1–5 MHz phased array transducer) demonstrating free intraperitoneal fluid in the hepatorenal recess (Morison's pouch). Liver (L), kidney (K).

the subdiaphragmatic space, hepatorenal recess (Morison's pouch) and around the inferior pole of the kidney (**Fig. 40.10**). In the supine patient, the hepatorenal recess is the most dependent and sensitive site for detection of peritoneal fluid accumulation.

- *Left upper quadrant:* with the transducer aligned longitudinally along the posterior axillary line. The subdiaphragmatic, splenorenal and inferior renal pole regions are examined. Fluid is more likely to be detected subdiaphragmatically than in the splenorenal recess, because the phrenocolic ligament closely apposes the spleen and kidney.[30]
- *Pelvis:* with the transducer just cephalad to the symphysis pubis and directed caudally. Images should be obtained in both longitudinal and transverse planes. The pelvis view is difficult to obtain if the bladder is decompressed (urinary catheter in situ), because the filled bladder is used as an 'acoustic window' to the pelvic peritoneal spaces.
- *Subcostal cardiac view:* to detect pericardial effusion.

The Extended-FAST (E-FAST) examination adds focused lung ultrasound for the detection of traumatic haemothorax and pneumothorax.[32] The basal anterior chest is examined bilaterally (supine patient) for signs of pneumothorax, and the basal posterolateral chest is examined for pleural fluid (haemothorax).

ULTRASOUND-GUIDED VASCULAR CANNULATION

Central venous cannulation is an essential component of intensive care practice. With the traditional 'landmark technique' location of the vein for cannulation is based on identification of skin surface anatomical landmarks and palpation, and is reliant on normal anatomy and venous patency. Complications include failure to cannulate the vein, pneumothorax, arterial puncture, haematoma, haemothorax and nerve injury. Risk of complication depends on operator experience, urgency and patient comorbidities; with reported rates of 5–20%.[34] Inclusion of ultrasound with the procedure improves first-pass success, leads to lower complication rates and is advocated by patient safety practice recommendations.[34–38] Ultrasound can also be used to aid arterial cannulation.[39]

ULTRASOUND TECHNIQUE

For the ultrasound novice, learning the necessary skills to image the central veins requires only a short period of supervised training, although developing good hand–eye coordination for real-time imaging during cannulation may take longer.

A high-frequency (7–11 MHz) linear transducer provides optimal image resolution suitable for vascular structures close to the skin surface. The vertical imaging depth should be set to ensure complete visualisation of the vein to be cannulated and significant structures (e.g. artery) deep to the vein. To avoid left–right confusion, the orientation marker on the screen should match the orientation of the transducer on the patient.

Ultrasound can be used in an indirect or direct way to assist cannulation. With the indirect (static) approach, imaging is used only prior to skin preparation to confirm location and patency of the vein. This avoids the need for a sterile transducer cover, but doesn't account for distortion of anatomy during needle puncture and may increase the risk of needle damage to the posterior vessel wall.[38] This technique is best suited to cannulation of large superficially located veins. The direct (dynamic) approach involves real-time ultrasound guidance of needle insertion. The vein can be imaged in a transverse or longitudinal plane. Transverse imaging gives a better view of the anatomical relationships of the vein to surrounding structures (**Fig. 40.11**). However, the full depth of the needle may be difficult to visualise (**Fig. 40.12**).[36–41] Longitudinal imaging provides optimal visualisation of the entire length of the needle and its depth of insertion[41,42] but is technically more difficult than cannulation with transverse imaging.[36,38] The direct approach requires sterile gel and transducer cover.

VESSEL IDENTIFICATION

The anatomical position of the artery and vein may vary from the usual pattern, particularly in the neck. Certain characteristics are used to distinguish vein from artery and determine venous patency.[38] Veins are thin-walled, elliptical in cross-section and compressible with light external pressure (see Fig. 40.11). Arteries are thick-walled, circular in cross-section, and more pulsatile (during normal haemodynamic conditions). Veins are usually larger than the adjacent artery; however, the

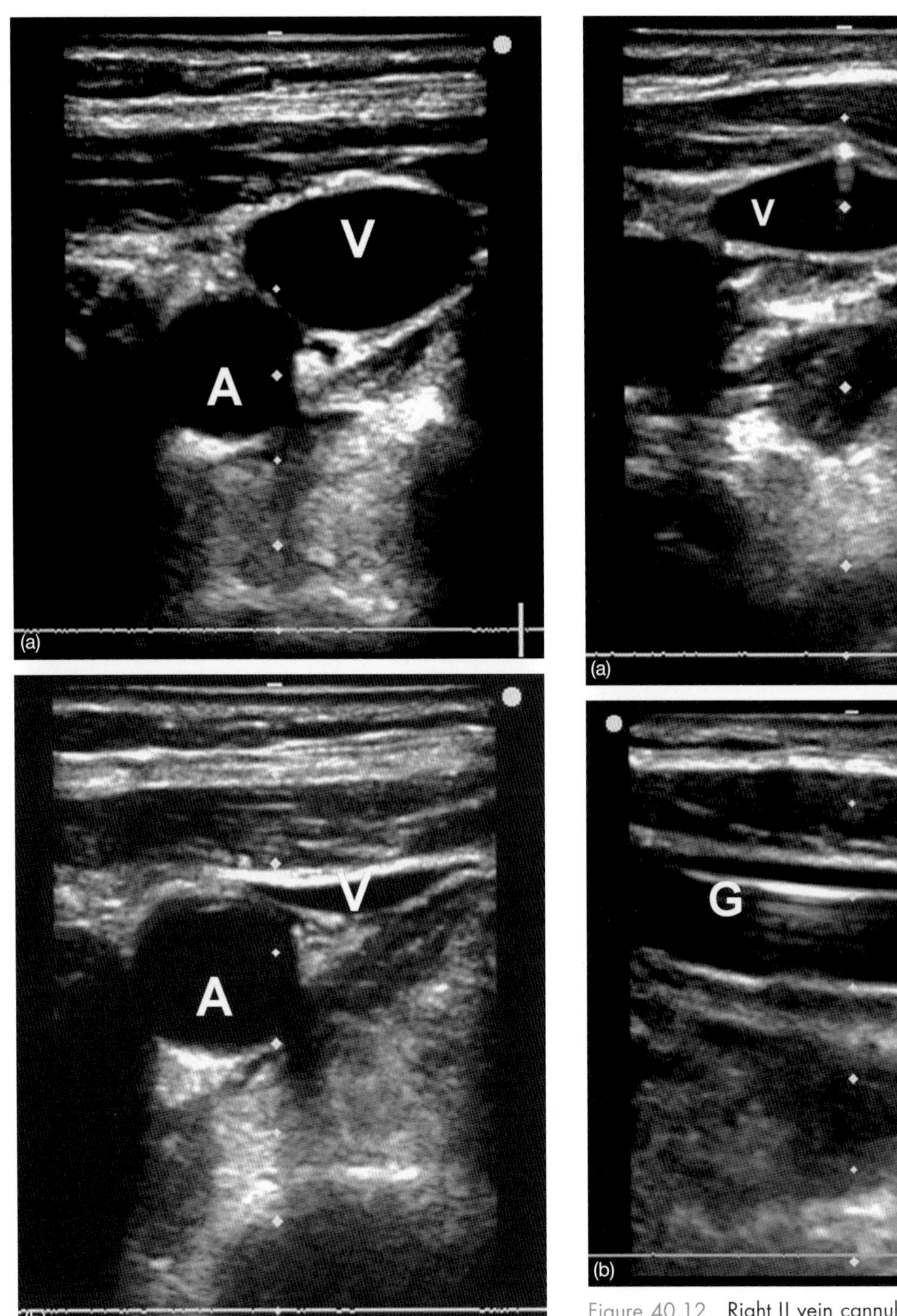

Figure 40.11 Right IJ vein (V) and carotid artery (A) imaged in a transverse (short axis) plane with a 6–13 MHz linear array transducer. The vein has an oval contour without external compression (a), but appears slit-like when light external compression is applied (b). The depth markers down the centre of the image are at half-centimetre intervals.

Figure 40.12 Right IJ vein cannulation demonstrated with a 6–13 MHz linear array transducer. In the transverse (short-axis) image (a) the needle is visualised in cross-section as a bright (hyperechoic) dot seen at the top of the vein (V). Note that in this still image it is not possible to determine which part of the needle shaft is being visualised and thus at what depth the needle tip is. The longitudinal (long-axis) image (b) shows the guidewire (G) within the vein (V).

internal jugular vein may appear smaller due to anatomical variation or hypovolaemia, and will appear slit-like in the hypovolaemic patient who is not in the Trendelenberg position. Colour flow Doppler demonstrates pulsatile arterial blood flow during systole. Venous blood flow is visible on colour flow Doppler during both systole and diastole if a low-velocity (Nyquist) scale is used.

Thrombus appears as an irregular filling defect that is often quite mobile. Thrombus downstream from the site where the vein is being scanned may not be visible, but its presence can be suspected if the vein is incompressible with light pressure. Absence of colour flow Doppler across part of the venous lumen may help to identify thrombus.

INTERNAL JUGULAR VEIN CANNULATION

Cannulation of the internal jugular (IJ) vein is ideally suited to ultrasound guidance because of the ease with which good images can be obtained, and the significant incidence of anatomical variants. The IJ vein is classically described as being located lateral to the carotid artery as it courses behind the sternocleidomastoid muscle between the anterior and posterior triangles of the neck. However, in a small proportion of patients the IJ vein runs medial to the carotid artery and in the majority of patients the vein overlies the artery to some extent.[36,38] The degree of overlap is increased by excessive head rotation away from the neutral position, and is more likely to occur with older age and obesity. In two-thirds of patients the right IJ is larger than the left IJ.[43] A quarter of patients have one IJ vein less than 0.4 cm^2 in cross-sectional area.[43] As anatomical variation is not predictable a priori from skin surface features, ultrasound should be used for IJ vein cannulation (**Box 40.1**).[34,36,38]

Box 40.1 A suggested approach to direct ultrasound guidance of IJ vein cannulation using the Seldinger method

1. Obtain informed consent for procedure
2. Place patient in Trendelenberg position with head slightly rotated away from the side to be cannulated
3. Image IJ vein to determine suitability for cannulation; presence of unsuitable anatomy or thrombus should prompt cannulation of an alternative site
4. Ensure appropriate ultrasound depth, marker position and gain settings
5. Prepare and drape sterile field
6. With the help of an assistant, apply sterile sheath over transducer with coupling gel inside sheath and separate sterile coupling gel outside sheath
7. Scan along the vein to determine the optimal site for venous puncture, i.e. easy to access with needle, large cross-sectional area and minimum overlap with the carotid artery. The degree of head rotation may need to be adjusted to minimise vessel overlap
8. For right-handed cannulation hold the transducer with the left hand
9. If imaging in a transverse (short-axis) plane, advance the needle incrementally and then adjust the transducer position each time to ensure visualisation of the needle tip (Fig. 40.12). With longitudinal (long-axis) imaging puncture the skin with the needle directly underneath one end of the transducer; adjust the needle direction (not the transducer position) to ensure that it remains visible on the screen as the needle advances. With either method, needle damage to the posterior wall of the vein may be less with a bevel-downward rather than bevel-upward approach[44]
10. Once venous blood is aspirated, place the transducer on the drapes and hold the needle with the left hand whilst removing the syringe from the needle with the right hand
11. Insert the guidewire into the needle with the right hand
12. Remove the needle over the guidewire and then scan over the vein to confirm satisfactory guidewire placement (Fig. 40.12)
13. Dilate and cannulate the vein over the guidewire to complete the procedure

SUBCLAVIAN VEIN CANNULATION

More consistent surface landmarks and less anatomical variation make the landmark technique for subclavian (SC) vein cannulation very reliable. However, if unsuccessful after two attempts, the risk of complications (pneumothorax, subclavian artery puncture) increases significantly with further attempts.[38] Ultrasound may be used to guide SC vein cannulation, but the clavicle often obscures a clear image of the vein. A microconvex transducer (which is easier to place under the clavicle than a linear transducer) sometimes improves visualisation of the vein. Alternatively cannulation can be attempted from a more lateral, axillary vein, approach, where the clavicle does not obscure imaging of the vein. This latter technique requires a steeper angle of needle entry with potential risk of pneumothorax, and should be attempted only under direct ultrasound guidance.[38] The axillary vein approach has been reported to be superior to the standard landmark technique in both novice and experienced operators.[45,46] Routine use of ultrasound for SC cannulation is not supported by current literature, but is recommended in high-risk patients to identify SC vein location and patency, or to guide an axillary vein approach.[38] Following the procedure, ultrasound can also be used to examine the lung for evidence of pneumothorax.

FEMORAL VEIN CANNULATION

The femoral vein can be reliably identified from surface landmarks and palpation of the femoral artery. The femoral vein is usually medial to the femoral artery, but significant vessel overlap may occur, particularly in children.[47] Ultrasound is recommended to identify vessel overlap and patency.[38]

OPTIC NERVE ULTRASOUND

Simple 2D ultrasound measurement of the diameter of the nerve sheath surrounding the optic nerve provides a rapid, non-invasive method of detecting elevated intracranial pressure (ICP). In patients presenting to hospital with suspected traumatic brain injury, ultrasound-measured optic nerve sheath diameter (ONSD) identifies patients with elevated ICP who warrant further neuroimaging.[48,49] Furthermore, with traumatic brain injury changes in ONSD correlate with changes in invasively measured ICP.[50, 51] However, invasive monitoring remains the gold standard for ICP measurement where this is not contraindicated by a risk of infection or haemorrhage. Validation of ultrasound ONSD is limited in other clinical settings, for example metabolic disorders (e.g. acute hepatic failure, diabetic ketoacidosis), or cerebrovascular disease (stroke syndromes).

The optic nerve sheath is a continuation of the meningeal layer surrounding the brain. Increases in ICP are transmitted by the cerebrospinal fluid through the perineural subarachnoid space to cause oedema and swelling of the optic nerve sheath that can be detected with ultrasound. The sheath is most porous and thus becomes most swollen 3 mm deep to the optic disk.

A high-frequency (10–15 MHz) linear transducer is used with the image depth set to 3–4 cm. A thick layer of acoustic gel is applied over the closed upper eyelids, with the patient lying supine or 20° head up. The transducer is then lightly placed over the upper, lateral eyelid, with the examiner's hand resting on the patient's forehead and the transducer held like a pencil. Care must be taken to ensure that no pressure is applied to the globe with the transducer. To reduce the risk of harmful effects (cavitation) of ultrasound acoustic output the mechanical index (MI) should be set to less than 0.23. The possibility of thermal damage is limited by scanning for less than 5 minutes.

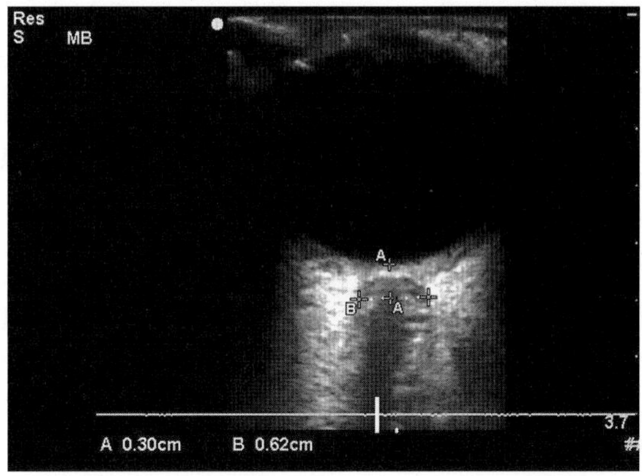

Figure 40.13 Globe and optic nerve demonstrated with a 6–13 MHz linear array transducer. Measurement of the optic nerve sheath diameter (vertical calliper) is demonstrated 3 mm deep (horizontal calliper) to the optic nerve head.

The optic nerve is seen as a hypoechogenic column beyond the globe and optic disk, surrounded bilaterally by the hyperechogenic optic nerve sheath (**Fig. 40.13**). With the optic nerve aligned directly opposite the transducer, the optic nerve sheath diameter is measured perpendicular to the vertical axis of the imaging plane, at a depth of 3 mm from the optic disk (see Fig. 40.11). At this depth detection of significant swelling is maximised, and distortion of ONSD measurement by artefactual shadowing is minimised. Several measurements should be taken in both longitudinal and transverse imaging planes, and the results averaged for each eye. Measured in this fashion normal values for ONSD are <5 mm. Values greater than 5.7–6.0 mm predict an elevated ICP (>20 cmH_2O) with good sensitivity and specificity.[49] Inaccuracies can arise if the transducer is orientated in a strictly axial imaging plane, with the optic nerve scanned along the visual axis. This results in a fusiform appearance of the optic nerve, and potentially unreliable ONSD measurements.[52] Imaging directly through the cornea and lens may also generate artefacts and reduce measurement reliability.

Access the complete references list online at http://www.expertconsult.com

3. Lichtenstein DA: Ultrasound in the management of thoracic disease. Crit Care Med 2007;35: S250–61.
10. Volpicelli G, Elbarbary M, Blavias M, et al. International evidence-based recommendations for point-of-care lung ultrasound. Intensive Care Med 2012;38: 577–91.
32. Kirkpatrick AW: Clinician-performed focused sonography for the resuscitation of trauma. Crit Care Med 2007;35:S162–72.
38. Troianos CA, Hartman GS, Glas KE, et al. Guidelines for performing ultrasound guided vascular cannulation: recommendations of the American society of echocardiography and the society of cardiovascular anesthesiologists. J Am Soc Echocardiogr 2011;24:1291–318.
49. Dubourg J, Javouhey E, Geeraerts T, et al. Ultrasonography of optic nerve sheath diameter for detection of raised intracranial pressure: a systematic review and meta-analysis. Intensive Care Med 2011; 37:1059–68.

41

Extracorporeal membrane oxygenation (ECMO)

Vincent Pellegrino

41.1 ECMO for respiratory failure

The management of severe lung injury remains a significant problem in critically ill patients. Despite the use of protective mechanical lung ventilation, the mortality of patients with severe acute respiratory distress syndrome (ARDS) remains high and increases with the severity of lung injury.[1,2] Protective lung ventilation in patients with severe ARDS may be limited by progressive hypoxaemia and hypercapnia despite recourse to adjunctive therapies that improve oxygenation, such as inhaled nitric oxide (NO) or prone positioning.

Veno-venous extracorporeal membrane oxygenation (VV ECMO) is an alternative form of lung support that provides non-pulmonary oxygen delivery and carbon dioxide removal, facilitates lung protective ventilation and provides time for lung recovery. Although previously predominately used as a neonatal and paediatric support, it is now increasingly being used in adults.[3]

Current ECMO systems are mobile, can facilitate inter-hospital patient transport even over long distances, can be instituted quickly and provide support over days to months.

DEFINITIONS

ECMO

EXTRACORPOREAL MEMBRANE OXYGENATION (ECMO)

This is a form of extracorporeal support comprising specialised *access cannula* to drain venous blood, an external circuit (*tubing*), a gas exchange device (*oxygenator*) where blood becomes enriched with oxygen (O_2) and has carbon dioxide (CO_2) removed, and a *return cannula* through which circuit blood returns to the patient. A pump drives the circuit blood flow and heat exchange is possible. A *fresh gas flow* is delivered to the oxygenator. ECMO can provide adequate oxygenation and CO_2 clearance in patients with minimal or absent native lung function. ECMO may achieve circuit blood flows up to approximately 7 litres of blood per minute.

MODE

The vessels from which ECMO circuit blood is obtained and returned define the *mode of ECMO*. Veno-venous ECMO (VV ECMO) is the ECMO mode used for respiratory support. Blood is removed from the great veins and returned to the right atrium and the patient's native circulation is powered entirely by the heart. Veno-arterial ECMO (VA ECMO) should not be used to support isolated respiratory failure.

CONFIGURATION

The *configuration of VV ECMO* refers to the manner in which the cannulae interact with the native circulation and is defined by the cannulae insertion sites, the type of cannula used and the tip positions (**Table 41.1.1**). *Access cannulae* drain blood from the venous system under negative pressure and may be either single-stage or multi-stage. Single-stage cannulae drain blood from a short region near the tip only. Multi-stage cannulae drain blood through side holes over a long length of the cannula, in addition to the tip, and allow a greater negative pressure in the circuit. For this reason they can provide higher circuit blood flow. *Return cannulae* deliver blood back to the patient under positive pressure from the ECMO circuit and expel blood only near the cannula tip (single stage). A double-lumen cannulae is available for adult VV ECMO support (Avalon Elite™) that contains both access and return lumens in a single cannula.[4]

$ECCO_2R$

Extracorporeal CO_2 removal ($ECCO_2R$) systems differ from ECMO. They use smaller cannulae, low-blood-flow extracorporeal circuits and oxygenators, and predominately remove CO_2.[5] Circuit blood flow is limited to less than 3 litres per minute and such systems cannot support patients with minimal lung function or severe hypoxaemia but can eliminate virtually all the CO_2 produced. By controlling CO_2, they facilitate protective lung ventilation.[6] Recently, a number of new $ECCO_2R$ systems have become available. Current $ECCO_2R$ systems may be pump-driven veno-venous systems with a membrane oxygenator (PALP™, Maquet or Hemolung RAS)[7,8] or be 'pumpless' and use an arterio-venous mode (iLA Membrane Ventilator® Novalung)[9] or utilise a dialysis membrane in addition to the gas exchange membrane (DECAPsmart®, Hemodec).[10]

Table 41.1.1 Configurations of VV ECMO

CONFIGURATION	INSERTION SITE	CANNULA TIP POSITION	CANNULA TYPE AND SIZE	ADVANTAGES / DISADVANTAGES
Femoro-femoral (fem-fem)	*Access:* Right or left femoral veins *Return:* Right or left femoral veins	*Access:* Hepatic IVC *Return:* Right atrium	*Access:* Multi- or single-stage (21–25F) *Return:* Single-stage (21–23F)	*Advantages:* Rapid to establish, safe, easy to secure and transport *Disadvantages:* Frequent problems with access insufficiency
Femoro/jugular–femoral[42] (high-flow)	*Access:* Femoral vein and right jugular vein *Return:* Femoral vein	*Access:* Hepatic IVC and SVC *Return:* Right atrium	*Access:* Multi- or single-stage (21–25F) and short single-stage cannula (17–19F) *Return:* Single-stage (19–23F)	*Advantages:* Can fully support severe respiratory failure even in large patients *Disadvantages:* Multiple cannulation required
Femoro-jugular (Fem-Jug)	*Access:* Femoral vein *Return:* Right jugular vein	*Access:* Hepatic IVC *Return:* SVC/right atrium	*Access:* Multi-stage (21–25F) *Return:* Short single-stage (19–21F)	*Advantages:* Full support and infrequent access insufficiency *Disadvantages* Longer to insert, difficult to secure and maintain dressing, decannulation risk
Dual-lumen/two-stage (Avalon)	Right jugular vein	*Access:* Hepatic IVC and SVC *Return:* Right atrium	31F	*Advantages:* Single cannulation, allows ambulation *Disadvantages* Difficult to secure and maintain dressings, high circuit pressures

In all cases, ECMO blood flow travels from the vena cavae to the atria (cavo-atrial flow) to minimise recirculation.

GAS EXCHANGE PRINCIPLES IN VV ECMO

OXYGEN DELIVERY

Delivery of oxygen to the circuit blood by the oxygenator is governed by the oxygen-carrying capacity of the blood. Current adult membrane oxygenators can oxygenate up to 7 litres of deoxygenated blood flow per minute. The quantity of oxygen that can be delivered to the patient on VV ECMO depends on the quantity of blood arriving at the oxygenator (circuit blood flow), the preoxygenator O_2 saturation and the haemoglobin. Additional fresh gas flow to the oxygenator cannot increase the oxygen delivery to the circuit blood. *In the presence of a large pulmonary shunt, the patient's arterial oxygen saturation will depend predominately on the proportion of deoxygenated venous return that can be captured by the VV ECMO circuit.* Capturing additional deoxygenated venous blood with VV ECMO will improve the arterial oxygen saturation. The oxygen consumption and haemoglobin will also affect the patient's arterial oxygen saturation in the presence of a large lung shunt.

CARBON DIOXIDE REMOVAL

Removal of CO_2 *by the membrane oxygenator is largely determined by the ratio of fresh gas flow to circuit blood flow in the oxygenator.* For a given circuit blood flow, increasing the fresh gas flow to the oxygenator will increase CO_2 removal. The fresh gas flow rate to the membrane oxygenator is titrated to achieve a desired partial pressure of CO_2 in the arterial blood. Normally, the ratio of fresh gas flow (L/min) to the circuit blood flow (L/min) at commencement of ECMO is approximately 1:1. With lung recovery, fresh gas flow can be gradually reduced while maintaining circuit blood flow. When the lung is capable of safely removing all CO_2 production, fresh gas flow is ceased to the oxygenator and extracorporeal respiration ceases.

RECIRCULATION

Optimal configuration of VV ECMO must ensure adequate separation between the access and return cannulae within the venous system in order to minimise *recirculation* of ECMO circuit blood flow.[11] Blood entering the oxygenator with high oxygen content, can accept little additional oxygen owing to the nature of the oxygen content curve. This will greatly reduce the quantity of oxygen delivery the patient can receive from the ECMO circuit and may be a cause of arterial hypoxaemia. Some degree of recirculation is inevitable, particularly at higher pump blood flow rates. Clinically significant recirculation results in a reduced colour difference between pre- and postoxygenator blood (both appear bright red) or an O_2 saturation of over 80% in the preoxygenator blood. In contrast, recirculation does not reduce CO_2 clearance.

HIGH OXYGEN CONSUMPTION

High cardiac output in conjunction with high oxygen consumption due to illness, patient size and fever may result in hypoxaemia, despite optimal VV ECMO configuration, and maximal circuit blood flow ≥7 L/min. This is associated with low preoxygenator oxygen saturation (<60%).

EQUIPMENT

Current generation blood pumps, membrane oxygenators and circuit coatings have improved the safety and reliability of ECMO.[12] This has allowed less-specialised bedside staffing and allowed ECMO care to be integrated into the scope of practice of ICU medical and nursing staff.[12] Major features are given below.

ROTARY PUMPS

Rotary pumps have largely superseded roller pumps and offer many advantages when used in circuits with low resistance to flow. These magnetically coupled pumps generate a rotational force, which drives blood radially within the pump head. A negative pressure is generated in the centre of the pump (inlet) and a positive pressure at the periphery (outlet). The pressure gradient within the pump head drives circuit blood flow, which is proportional to the rotational speed controlled by the operator. The pressure load across the circuit and the circuit resistance determine the actual circuit flow rate. The pressure load across a VV ECMO circuit is negligible as both access and return cannula are sited in the venous system. Pump head thrombosis, which can cause rapid and very severe haemolysis, is extremely rare with current rotary pump heads.

MEMBRANE OXYGENATORS

Membrane oxygenators made from polymethylpentene have markedly improved the safety and reliability of ECMO.[13] Plasma leak across the membrane seen in previous microporous membrane oxygenators has been eliminated. They allow high gas transfer with low resistance to blood flow and can be coated to minimise activation of coagulation. Acute oxygenator failure is now extremely rare.

SURFACE COATINGS

Surface coatings to reduce blood–surface interaction and activation of coagulation and inflammatory systems are present on all current ECMO components. The patient-centred benefits of one coating compared with another have not been established in ECMO.[14,15]

INDICATIONS AND PATIENT SELECTION

VV ECMO is indicated for life-threatening forms of acute respiratory failure where the risks of less-invasive support are considered greater than the risks of ECMO (**Fig. 41.1.1**). It is predominately used to provide support and allow time for recovery of the underlying condition where there is a reasonable expectation of long-term survival without severe disability. Cardiac function must be adequate, as VV ECMO provides no direct cardiac support. Adult ECMO outcomes for respiratory

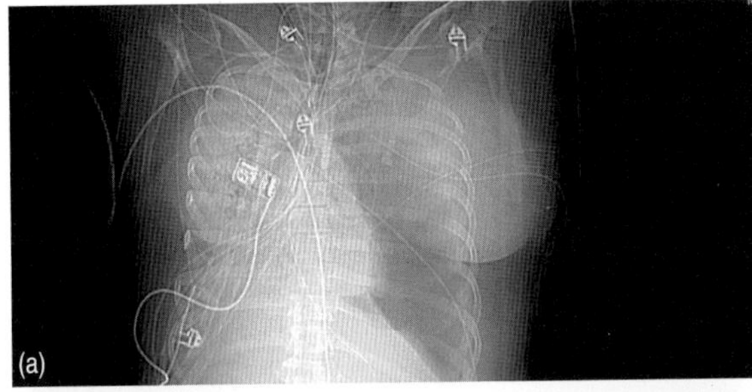

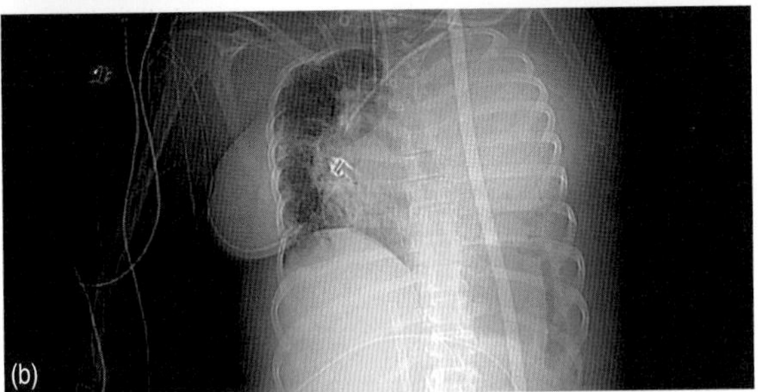

Figure 41.1.1 VV ECMO for severe respiratory failure secondary to influenza. The patient was commenced on VV ECMO urgently following the development of a tension pneumothorax during mechanical ventilation, which resulted in a cardiac arrest. (a) An extensive left-sided pneumothorax despite two intercostal catheters on day 1 of VV ECMO support with extensive right-sided consolidation. By day 8 (b) the pneumonitis had resolved and the patient could be weaned from extracorporeal gas exchange despite the development of extensive left-sided haemothorax during ECMO support, which resulted in lung necrosis (noted at thoracotomy) and ultimately death.

support from case series from specialised centres suggest that outcomes are improving.[16,17] Increasing clinical experience with ECMO support has helped define conditions that are more likely to be associated with successful outcome.[18]

Conditions where the use of VV ECMO is commonly associated with recovery and favourable outcomes (age <70) despite severe respiratory failure are:

- ARDS with primary lung injury from infection,[19] aspiration or direct trauma
- primary graft dysfunction following lung transplantation[20]
- pulmonary vasculitis (Goodpasture's, ANCA-associated, autoimmune).

Conditions where recovery is unlikely with the use of VV ECMO as a rescue therapy in the event of severe respiratory failure are:

- respiratory failure associated with long-term immunosuppression (heart, renal, bone marrow transplant recipients, HIV, graft-versus-host disease)
- respiratory failure associated with malignancy[21]
- chronic lung transplant rejection[22]
- severe septic shock where multiple advanced organ failure and purpura are present prior to the initiation of ECMO.

ECMO is also used as a bridge to lung transplantation in selected patients with advanced forms of irreversible respiratory failure.[23] ECMO should be used for known cases of irreversible end-stage respiratory failure (cystic fibrosis, interstitial lung disease, chronic obstructive airways disease) only after careful case selection by lung transplant centres.

The decision to institute ECMO for severe respiratory failure is often complex and clinical triggers and logistic factors must be considered when determining the need for and the timing of ECMO. These include:

- severity of lung injury
- adequate trial of less invasive interventions
- rate of lung injury progression
- need for inter-hospital transport
- risk of bleeding.

Clinical triggers for VV ECMO initiation in suitable patients[24] include:

- ratio of Pa_{O_2} mmHg to Fi_{O_2}<75 (Sa_{O_2}<90%)
- hypercapnia with pH<7.15 with safe mechanical ventilation settings (plateau pressure ≤35 mmHg (4.65 kPa) and tidal volume ≤6 mL/kg predicted body weight)
- extensive (3–4 quadrant) lung infiltrate consistent with acute lung injury

despite:

- optimising circulatory support (cardiac assessment with echocardiography) using inotropes or volume state therapy (where appropriate)
- trial of high PEEP (18–22) and recruitment manoeuvre (if not contraindicated)
- 2–12-hour trial of iNO or alternative pulmonary vasodilator (if available).

Rapidly progressive (6–12 hours) lung infiltrates and increasing ventilator requirements particularly in the early stages of hospital admission are often associated with a fulminate illness that reduces the time window when ECMO may be of benefit and generally favours the earlier use of ECMO.

ECMO is a mobile support that can be used across all patient transport modalities (road, fixed wing and helicopter) with very low rates of complications reported.[17,25–27] Unstable patients with severe respiratory failure requiring inter-hospital transport should be considered for ECMO.

CANNULATION FOR VV ECMO

ECMO cannulae can be safely inserted using a percutaneous dilation technique or by a surgical cut-down approach. Percutaneous dilation, which avoids skin cutting, can achieve a tight seal between skin, vessels and cannulae. This avoids bleeding associated with surgical dissection. It can also be performed quickly in a variety of settings without the need for surgical equipment or staffing.

Risks associated with 'blind' percutaneous cannulation for VV ECMO can be greatly reduced with the use of real-time vascular ultrasound and echocardiography guidance prior to and during percutaneous dilation and cannulae advancement. Ultrasound guidance and echocardiography are increasingly being adopted in numerous hospital departments and equipment is widely available. Image intensifiers can also help prevent complications associated with VV ECMO cannulation; however, they introduce additional patient transfers, require additional staffing, and may not be available in smaller centres (**Table 41.1.2**).

Utility of real-time vascular and cardiac ultrasound in VV ECMO[28] includes:

- cardiac assessment
  - cardiac function
  - detection of proximal pulmonary artery emboli
  - detection of pericardial collections and extrinsic cardiac compression
- identification of proximal vein thrombosis prior to cannulation (unilateral occlusive jugular vein thrombosis is a contraindication to contralateral jugular vein cannulation owing to the risk of cerebral oedema)
- anatomical assessment of the target vessel and branches
  - reduces carotid or femoral artery puncture
  - prevents inadvertent sapheno-femoral junction cannulation
  - identifies abnormal anatomy

Table 41.1.2 Potential major complications of cannulation for VV ECMO

COMPLICATION	CAUSE	PREVENTION
Haemorrhage	Perforation of venous system	• Real-time guidewire localisation • Ensuring guidewire continually has free movement through dilators during dilator insertion • Use 'soft' tapered dilators • Enter femoral vessel below inguinal ligament
	Cannula site bleeding	• Maintain tight skin/tissue seal with cannula • Avoid arterial puncture • Avoid transfixing the inguinal ligament • Avoid surgical dissection
Cardiac injury	Femoral dilator/cannula advanced into interatrial septum	• Image intensifier or echocardiography guidance
	Jugular dual-lumen dilator/cannula advanced into right ventricle	• Image intensifier or echocardiography guidance
Cannula malposition	Femoral access cannula in lower IVC	• Image intensifier or echocardiography guidance
	Jugular dual-lumen cannula tip in hepatic vein or right ventricle	• Image intensifier or echocardiography guidance • Adequate cannula securing

- maintenance of guidewire J-loop position in the right atrium
  - detects inadvertent guidewire entrapment ('kinking') during serial dilation
  - prevents excessive guidewire introduction and cardiac effects during cannula insertion
- guides optimal cannula tip placement
  - ensures femoral access cannulae are sited within the hepatic inferior vena cava
  - ensures return cannula sited in the right atrium without encroachment on the interatrial septum
  - ensures optimal positioning of dual-lumen VV cannula (Avalon Elite®) return port[29]
  - prevents dual-lumen VV cannula (Avalon Elite®) tip being sited in the hepatic vein.[29]

ECMO-SPECIFIC PATIENT CARE

MANAGEMENT OF CIRCUIT BLOOD FLOW SETTINGS

Rotary (constrained vortex) blood pumps generate circuit blood flow proportional to their pump speed and are afterload sensitive. In VV ECMO, afterload across the pump is low and stable provided there are no circuit obstructions. Generally, the pump operates in a pump-speed-controlled mode where pump speed is the set variable and resulting pump flow is measured. Pump speed settings are chosen to deliver sufficient circuit blood flow to achieve required oxygen delivery. Depending on patient size, oxygen consumption and lung shunt, circuit blood flow between 4 and 7 L/min will be required to achieve safe arterial oxygen saturations of over 85%, while maintaining safe lung ventilation.

MONITORING OF CIRCUIT PRESSURE

The pressure in the extracorporeal circuit becomes progressively more negative from drainage cannula tip to the inflow to the pump head. The maximal positive circuit pressure occurs at the outlet of the pump head and falls progressively to the return cannula. The oxygenator is located distal to the pump head and receives blood under positive pressure. The pressure change across the oxygenator can be measured safely and easily without introducing circuit connectors and gives an indication of clot burden within the oxygenator. One current-generation ECMO pump (Cardiohelp-HLS, Maquet) has integrated pressure monitoring of pre- and postoxygenator pressure in addition to negative-pressure monitoring at the pump head inlet.

ACCESS INSUFFICIENCY

As pump speed is increased, the negative pressure at the access cannulae inlet also becomes more negative. If venous return to the access (draining) ECMO cannula is inadequate for the degree of pump suction, venous 'suck-down' will occur and circuit blood flow will fall and become variable, usually with audible and visible effects on the inflow of the circuit (access insufficiency). This situation must be identified and rectified quickly (reducing pump speed) to prevent haemolysis and potential vascular injury.[30] Access insufficiency may prevent adequate circuit blood flow and oxygen delivery. Multi-stage access cannulae distribute the negative circuit pressure over a longer length of a vessel and deliver higher maximal blood flow than similar single-stage access cannulae.

Factors that increase the occurrence of access insufficiency include:

- femoral access cannula tip sited too low
- dual-lumen cannula not optimally sited
  - distal tip sited in the hepatic vein (instead of IVC)
  - catheter withdrawn and SVC access sited too high within the right brachiocephalic vein
- reduced venous return
  - blood or volume loss
  - vasodilation
  - raised intrathoracic or intra-abdominal pressure
- reduced venous capacitance
  - extrinsic right heart compression.

TITRATION OF FRESH GAS FLOW TO THE OXYGENATOR

Fresh gas flow (FGF) to the oxygenator maintains the diffusion gradients for O_2 delivery to, and CO_2 removal from, the circuit blood. Fresh gas flow can be composed of dry air–oxygen mix or pure O_2. The partial pressure of O_2 in the FGF determines the postoxygenator blood partial pressure O_2. The FGF rate determines the partial pressure of CO_2 in the postoxygenator and its rate is chosen to achieve a desired Pa_{CO_2} in the patient's arterial blood.

LUNG VENTILATION

Non-injurious lung ventilation is a primary goal of ECMO support in respiratory failure. Non-pulmonary gas exchange facilitates low pressure and volume strategies and a number of lung ventilation modes have been advocated during the different phases of ECMO support. PEEP levels are chosen to maintain lung aeration. Peak lung pressures can easily be maintained below 30 cmH_2O with ECMO support. Tidal volumes may be negligible despite normal distending pressures and remain much less than the anatomical dead space of the lung during ECMO support. Improving lung compliance and the return of physiological tidal volume herald lung recovery from acute lung injury.

WEANING

As lung recovery occurs it is standard to wean ECMO gas flow until it is off, at which point the patient is no longer receiving extracorporeal support. Cannulae are generally removed after a period of time off gas flow (usually 2–24 hours). There is no need to wean circuit blood flow below 3 L/min during weaning, which reduces the need for additional anticoagulation. Percutaneously inserted venous cannulae can be removed at the bedside (off anticoagulation) and skin sites compressed for 20 minutes.

In general, ECMO weaning and decannulation are performed in advance of airway extubation. Where ECMO is used in chronic respiratory failure conditions, it can be advantageous to extubate patients during ECMO support in order to maintain wakefulness and avoid the complications of sedation. Ambulant ECMO is highly desirable for cystic fibrosis patients being bridged to transplantation to maintain secretion clearance.[31] Whether ambulant ECMO provides additional benefit for patients with acute respiratory failure is currently uncertain.

ANTICOAGULATION

Anticoagulation for ECMO is given to reduce the rate of clot formation within the circuit, and reduce clot formation associated with cannulae.[32] Clotting is often seen in low-flow regions of the oxygenator but is not an indication for circuit change. It is generally accepted that systemic anticoagulation with heparin should be provided for all patients on ECMO *provided there is no bleeding and there is no anticipated or recent surgery*. Anticoagulation practices are based on patient bleeding risk profiles and VV ECMO can be successfully run for days without anticoagulation in order to arrest bleeding. Essential surgery can also be performed during ECMO support.[33]

ECMO-SPECIFIC PATIENT COMPLICATIONS

Prevention of complications is fundamental to successful ECMO care. Patients are at increased risk of bleeding, particularly from the injured lung, and have an increased risk of haemolysis. VV ECMO can provide great stability to the patient with severe respiratory failure, but may also induce dangerous complications if the circuit is breached (accidental decannulation, circuit rupture) or the blood pump fails. Staff training and beside resources to standardise decision-making are important components of successful ECMO programmes. Avoiding excessive sedation, provision of timely pressure care and physical therapy during VV ECMO support are becoming routine.

BLEEDING

Bleeding remains the main complication of ECMO; however, many sources of bleeding can be prevented. Cannulation site bleeding should be uncommon in VV ECMO if optimal percutaneous cannulation techniques are used and surgical dissection is avoided. Pulmonary bleeding is a frequent cause of death during VV ECMO support for respiratory failure.[34] Insertion of intercostal catheters during ECMO is an extremely high-risk intervention and should not be performed unless no other alternative remains. In particular, intercostal catheters should not be inserted for pneumothoraces or pleural fluid drainage unless they are massive or cause haemodynamic collapse.[35] During VV ECMO, pneumothoraces may be managed by increasing ECMO support and reducing pulmonary ventilation, without the need for tube insertion. Fibrinolysis and secondary consumptive coagulopathy can occur during ECMO particularly with older circuits and induce generalised bleeding. Monitoring of fibrinogen and D-dimer levels and elective ECMO circuit changes are required to control this process.

Therapies for managing severe bleeding during ECMO support are given in Subchapter 41.1.2 ECMO for cardiac failure.

HAEMOLYSIS

Haemolysis (repeated plasma free Hb >0.1g/dL) is extremely uncommon with current-generation circuits; however regular monitoring of plasma free Hb is still routine in many centres. Severe haemolysis (plasma free Hb >1.0 g/L or with hyperkalaemia or red urine) suggests pump head thrombosis and must be treated with an urgent circuit change.

AIR EMBOLISM

Air will rapidly enter the circuit during pump operation if there is any breach in the negative pressure region of the circuit. Taps and other potential breaches on the negative (pre-pump) side of the circuit should be avoided. Air that enters the circuit will de-prime the pump head (reducing circuit flow), accumulate in the oxygenator and may reach the return line and cause patient air embolism. Staff education and circuit design are essential preventative measures. De-airing the circuit following air embolism is technically challenging.

CLINICAL TRIALS

ECMO has been used since 1966 as a rescue therapy for severe acute respiratory failure that is refractory to mechanical ventilation.[36] The process of establishing the clinical efficacy for this practice has a long and fascinating history owing to the unique ethical[37] and logistical challenges inherent in this form of support and the patient populations with this disease. In the 1970s and 1980s, uncontrolled observational reports suggested clinical benefits with the use of extracorporeal support, but these were not realised in subsequent randomised controlled trials (RCTs).[38,39]

In 2001, the CESAR trial,[40] a prospective randomised adult ECMO trial conducted in the United Kingdom, commenced enrolment. The results were published in 2009, and the intention-to-treat analysis showed that significantly more patients allocated to consideration for treatment including ECMO survived to 6 months without disability compared with those allocated to conventional management. This result represented a relatively large treatment effect, albeit with borderline precision and with a sample size that was less than initially planned. Reasonable concerns with regard to the basis of the efficacy, the quality of respiratory care in the control arm and the generalisability of the findings outside the UK have been raised.[41]

Currently, a subsequent French multinational adult ECMO trial for severe respiratory failure is under way. Mechanical ventilation strategies for both arms demand protective lung ventilation (ClinicalTrials.gov Identifier: NCT01470703).

Access the complete references list online at http://www.expertconsult.com

1. Phua J, Badia JR, Adhikari NK, et al. Has mortality from acute respiratory distress syndrome decreased over time?: A systematic review. Am J Respir Crit Care Med 2009;179:220–7.
10. Terragni PP, Del Sorbo L, Mascia L, et al. Tidal volume lower than 6 ml/kg enhances lung protection: role of extracorporeal carbon dioxide removal. Anesthesiology 2009;111:826–35.
17. Forrest P, Ratchford J, Burns B, et al. Retrieval of critically ill adults using extracorporeal membrane oxygenation: an Australian experience. Intensive Care Med 2011;37:824–30.
18. Brogan TV, Thiagarajan RR, Rycus PT, et al. Extracorporeal membrane oxygenation in adults with severe respiratory failure: a multi-center database. Intensive Care Med 2009;35(12):2105–14.
19. Davies A, Jones D, Bailey M, et al. Extracorporeal membrane oxygenation for 2009 influenza A(H1N1) Acute respiratory distress syndrome. JAMA 2009; 302:1888–95.
24. Brodie D, Bacchetta M. Extracorporeal membrane oxygenation for ARDS in adults. N Engl J Med 2011;365:1905–14.
38. Zapol WM, Snider MT, Hill JD, et al. Extracorporeal membrane oxygenation in severe acute respiratory failure. A randomized prospective study. JAMA 1979;242:2193–6.
39. Morris AH, Wallace CJ, Menlove RL, et al. Randomized clinical trial of pressure-controlled inverse ratio ventilation and extracorporeal CO_2 removal for adult respiratory distress syndrome. Am J Respir Crit Care Med 1994;149:295–305.
40. Peek GJ, Mugford M, Tiruvoipati R, et al. Efficacy and economic assessment of conventional ventilatory support versus extracorporeal membrane oxygenation for severe adult respiratory failure (CESAR): a multicentre randomised controlled trial. Lancet 2009;374:1351–63.

41.2 ECMO for cardiac failure

Mortality from cardiogenic shock and refractory ventricular fibrillation is very high and frequently cannot be adequately managed with medical therapy. Veno-arterial extracorporeal membrane oxygenation (VA ECMO) is a rapidly deployable, short-term system for complete or partial support of the circulatory system. It can allow time for reversible forms of cardiac failure to recover and can prevent end-organ damage from under perfusion. It can provide organ support before, during or after therapeutic cardiovascular procedures. In patients with advanced chronic heart failure and secondary acute end-organ injury, it can provide a bridging support to longer-term devices and allow time for thorough case selection.

Traditionally, veno-arterial (VA) ECMO has been employed by surgical staff in the operative setting, but progressively it is being applied in non-operative settings by a number of trained specialists. Although previously predominately used as a neonatal and paediatric support, it is increasingly being used in adults.

Additional explanations of ECMO are given in the section on ECMO for respiratory support.

DEFINITIONS

MODE

Veno-arterial ECMO (VA ECMO) is the ECMO *mode* used for cardiac support. Blood is removed from the right atrium and adjacent veins and then returned to the aorta, bypassing the native heart and lungs. VA ECMO comprises a specialised *access cannula* to drain venous blood, an external circuit (*tubing*), a gas exchange device (*oxygenator*) where blood becomes enriched with oxygen and has carbon dioxide removed, and a *return cannula* through which circuit blood returns to the arterial system. A pump drives the circuit blood flow and heat exchange is possible. A *fresh gas flow* is delivered to the oxygenator. ECMO circuit flows are adequate to provide complete systemic perfusion (5–7 litres of blood per minute); however, it may not provide specific left ventricular 'unloading'.[1] Percutaneous cardiopulmonary bypass is another term for VA ECMO.

In veno-pulmonary artery (VPA) ECMO, venous blood is accessed from a large central vein and returned to the pulmonary arterial system via a specialised surgical conduit after it has passed through the oxygenator. It provides short-term right ventricular (and respiratory) support in the intraoperative setting following left ventricular assist device insertion.[2]

CONFIGURATION

The *configuration of VA ECMO* determines the manner in which the ECMO circuit interacts with the native circulation. Cannulae insertion sites and the tip positions define configuration. Broadly, there are three adult VA ECMO configurations (**Table 41.2.1**):

- femoro-femoral
- jugulo-subclavian[3]
- central (including V-PA ECMO).

DISTINCT FROM ECMO

Short-term *ventricular assist devices (VAD)* may employ similar cannulae, circuit tubing and pumps to ECMO, but do not include an oxygenator and are configured to provide single ventricular mechanical support only. Left VAD (LVAD) is configured using a left heart access cannula with an aortic return cannula. Right VAD (RVAD) is configured using right heart access with a pulmonary artery return. Biventricular VAD support configurations (BiVAD) are distinct from VA ECMO.

BLOOD FLOW PRINCIPLES

VA ECMO blood flow bypasses the native heart and lungs. Two arterial circulations may be identifiable during VA ECMO support. In contrast to VV ECMO, recirculation is not seen during VA ECMO support.

NATIVE CARDIAC OUTPUT

Native cardiac output produces pulsatile pulmonary and aortic blood flow during VA ECMO support. Cardiac function can vary from absent to near-complete during different phases of VA ECMO support. Oxygen and carbon dioxide (CO_2) gas tensions of the native cardiac output will reflect the pulmonary gas exchange and predominately be delivered to the coronary and cephalic circulations. Because CO_2 is only delivered to the lung by the native cardiac output, through the pulmonary circulation, airway CO_2 excretion is also indicative of native cardiac output.

CIRCUIT BLOOD FLOW

The distribution of the returning VA ECMO circuit blood within the arterial tree is dependent on the particular VA ECMO configuration, ECMO circuit blood flow and the native cardiac output. The gas tensions in the ECMO circuit blood flow reflect gas exchange across the oxygenator. During complete VA support, ECMO circuit blood flow provides all systemic perfusion and arterial gas tensions will be similar to post-oxygenator readings. In this state, the arterial waveform is non-pulsatile. As cardiac function returns, pulsatility will be seen and arterial gas tensions will reflect the proportion of native and circuit blood flow reaching the sampling site.

Table 41.2.1 Configurations of VA ECMO

CONFIGURATION	INSERTION SITE	CANNULA TIP POSITION	CANNULA TYPE AND SIZE	ADVANTAGES/ DISADVANTAGES
Femoro-femoral ECMO (Fem-fem)	*Access:* Femoral vein *Return:* Common femoral artery (with distal perfusion cannula)	*Access:* Right atrium *Return:* Iliac artery or distal aorta	*Access:* Multi-stage (19–25F) *Return:* Single stage (15–21F)	*Advantages:* Quick to deploy Surgery not required *Disadvantages:* High rate of limb ischaemia if distal perfusion cannula not used Unable to ambulate Allows cephalic differential hypoxaemia
Jugulo-subclavian ECMO[3]	*Access:* Right jugular vein *Return:* Right subclavian artery (tunnelled)	*Access:* Right atrium *Return:* Right subclavian artery (T-graft)	*Access:* Short single stage (19–23F) *Return:* Specialised graftable	*Advantages:* Allows ambulation and unrestricted sitting Reduces cephalic differential hypoxia *Disadvantages:* Right arm swelling or axillary plexus injury
Central ECMO (atrio-aortic)	*Access:* Sternotomy or tunnelled subcostally *Return:* Sternotomy or tunnelled subcostally	*Access:* Right atrium via atrial appendage *Return:* Proximal ascending aorta	Standard by-pass cannulae (access and return) inserted via sternotomy (36–46F) *or* Specialised long-term surgical (graftable) arterial cannula and malleable atrial cannula (tunnelled with closed sternum) (36–46F)	*Advantages:* Accessible during cardiac surgery Large cannula and lower circuit resistance *Disadvantages:* Surgical site bleeding Restricted patient movement and pressure area care Respiratory effects of sternotomy
Femoro-pulmonary artery ECMO (VPA ECMO)[2]	*Access:* Femoral vein *Return:* Tunnelled via chest wall	*Access:* Right atrium *Return:* Main pulmonary trunk	*Access:* Multi-stage (19–25F) *Return:* Specialised surgical graft and short single stage 19F cannula	*Advantages:* Maintains full LVAD flows Provides respiratory and right heart support Removal without surgery *Disadvantages:* Pulmonary artery vascular graft remains in situ

DIFFERENTIAL OXYGENATION DURING VA ECMO

A significant lung shunt in association with an improving native cardiac output can result in large degrees of differential oxygenation in patients supported with peripheral VA ECMO. With femoral arterial VA ECMO return, highly oxygenated blood is preferentially distributed to the caudal regions as native cardiac output improves while deoxygenated blood leaving the left ventricle predominately perfuses the coronary and cephalic circulations. For this reason, patients on peripheral VA ECMO should have arterial oxygenation monitored via the right arm.

CIRCUIT PRESSURE

The pressure gradient across a VA ECMO circuit is greater than in VV ECMO owing to the physiological systemic arteriovenous pressure. Consequently, in VA ECMO, it is normal to require higher pump speeds to achieve full support, and pressure monitoring in the circuit (see VV ECMO) will record higher pressures at the membrane and in the return line. Such high ECMO circuit pressure may limit the ability for the provision of continuous renal replacement via the ECMO circuit.

INDICATIONS AND PATIENT SELECTION

VA ECMO is indicated for life-threatening forms of cardiac failure where the risks of less invasive support are considered greater than the risks of ECMO and there is a reasonable expectation of long-term survival without severe disability. Currently ECMO is generally considered in patients up to the age of 70 without other chronic organ failures or terminal illnesses.

Common indications for VA ECMO support with a reasonable chance (>50%) of subsequent recovery and favourable outcomes include:

- acute fulminate myocarditis[4–6]
- cardiomyopathy (bridge to VAD)[7]
- AMI-cardiogenic shock prior to multiple organ failure[8]
- drug overdose with profound cardiac depression or arrhythmia[9–11]
- pulmonary embolism with cardiogenic shock[12]
- primary graft failure: post heart[13,14]/heart–lung transplant.

The use of ECMO for refractory 'in-hospital' cardiac arrest (with ECMO commenced within 60 minutes)[15–17] is associated with recovery rates of approximately 30% (alive to discharge), which both may be superior to standard treatment and may be improving over time.

Conditions where recovery is rare (<25%) despite the use of VA ECMO as a rescue therapy include:

- adult cardiogenic shock with established multi-organ failure
- adult septic shock with severe myocardial depression and multi-organ failure
- heart transplant with chronic rejection
- 'out of hospital' and prolonged cardiac arrest.[18]

Cardiac and vascular lesions that prevent the successful application of VA ECMO are:

- aortic dissection
- severe aortic regurgitation[19]
- severe mitral regurgitation.

ECMO is also used as a bridge to VAD and heart transplantation in selected patients with advanced forms of irreversible cardiac failure and pulmonary hypertension. Decisions regarding the choice of mechanical support modalities in this population should involve specialised transplant services.

CLINICAL TRIGGERS FOR VA ECMO INITIATION IN SUITABLE PATIENTS WITH CARDIOGENIC SHOCK

Due to the rapid onset of end-organ damage with cardiogenic shock and refractory arrest, the timing of VA ECMO initiation is critical in patient outcome. A guide to the clinical triggers and logistic factors to be considered when determining the timing of ECMO for a deteriorating patient with cardiogenic shock is given below:

- pharmacological support of cardiac index and blood pressure is likely to exacerbate the underlying primary cardiac illness (e.g. AMI-cardiogenic shock or recurrent VF)
- cardiac index and blood pressure inadequate despite pharmacological support:
  - moderate- or high-dose inotropes (epinephrine (adrenaline) >0.3 μg/kg/min equivalent) in combination with an IABP, vasopressors and positive-pressure ventilation for predominately left ventricular failure
  - moderate- or high-dose inotropes (epinephrine (adrenaline) >0.3 μg/kg/min equivalent) in combination with pulmonary artery vasodilator and/or systemic vasopressors for predominately right ventricular failure
- onset of secondary hepatic, renal or skin ischaemia despite pharmacological support
- lactate >5 mmol/L and rising despite pharmacological support.

VA ECMO is a mobile support that can be used across all patient transport modalities (road, fixed wing and helicopter) with very low rates of complications reported.[20] Time delays incurred with ECMO retrieval must be considered during assessment.

CANNULATION FOR VA ECMO

ECMO cannulae can be safely inserted using a percutaneous dilation technique or by a surgical cut-down approach. Percutaneous dilation, which avoids skin cutting, can achieve a tight seal between skin and cannulae. This avoids bleeding associated with surgical dissection. It can also be performed quickly in a variety of settings without the need for surgical equipment or staffing.[21]

Risks associated with 'blind' percutaneous cannulation for VA ECMO can be greatly reduced with the use of real-time vascular ultrasound and echocardiography guidance prior to and during percutaneous dilation and cannulae advancement. Ultrasound guidance and echocardiography are increasingly being adopted in numerous hospital departments and equipment is widely available. Image intensifiers can also help prevent complications associated with VV ECMO cannulation; however, this introduces additional patient transfers, requires additional staffing and may not be available in smaller centres.

UTILITY OF REAL-TIME VASCULAR AND CARDIAC ULTRASOUND IN VA ECMO[22]

- Cardiac assessment
  - Cardiac and valvular function

  - Detection of proximal pulmonary artery emboli
  - Detection of pericardial collections and extrinsic cardiac compression
  - Presence of aortic disease
  - Detection of intracardiac thrombosis
- Anatomical assessment of the target vessel and branches
  - Prevents inadvertent sapheno-femoral junction venous cannulation
  - Prevents inadvertent profunda femoris artery injury (arterial cannulation)
  - Identifies abnormal anatomy
- Immediate confirmation of needle entry in vein and confirmation of arterial cannulation prior to dilation (required during pulseless resuscitation)
- Maintenance of guide-wire J-loop position during dilation
  - Detects inadvertent guide-wire entrapment ('kinking') during serial dilation
  - Prevents excessive guide-wire introduction and cardiac effects during cannula insertion
- Guides optimal cannula tip placement
- Weaning study from VA ECMO[23]
  - LVOT blood flow assessment.

ECMO-SPECIFIC PATIENT CARE

ASSESSMENT OF NATIVE CARDIAC OUTPUT

This is approximately assessed at the bedside using the pulsatility of the arterial blood pressure and end-tidal CO_2 trace (**Fig. 41.2.1**). It can be measured from velocity–time integration of blood flow through the left ventricular outflow tract with echocardiography, but not by thermodilution due to partial loss of indicator into the ECMO circuit. Native cardiac output must be assessed regularly during VA ECMO support to titrate lung ventilation in order to avoid gross abnormalities in lung V/Q ratios. It is also important in assessing the adequacy of overall systemic perfusion.

MANAGEMENT OF CIRCUIT BLOOD FLOW SETTINGS

VA ECMO circuit blood flow settings are primarily chosen to achieve adequate overall systemic perfusion. ECMO circuit flow, which is continually measured, in combination with the native cardiac output equate to the total body blood flow. Adequate mechanical systemic perfusion allows inotropic support to be weaned or ceased and lowers myocardial work. Adequate mechanical circulatory support can allow safe performance of high-risk percutaneous cardiac procedures.

ACCESS INSUFFICIENCY

Access insufficiency can occur in all modes of ECMO and is described in the section on ECMO for respiratory failure.

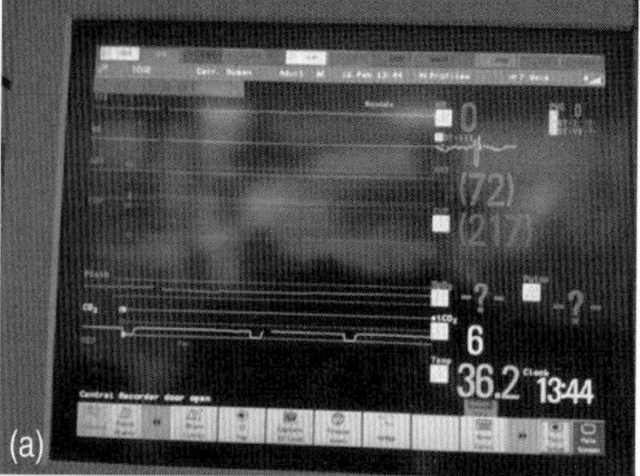

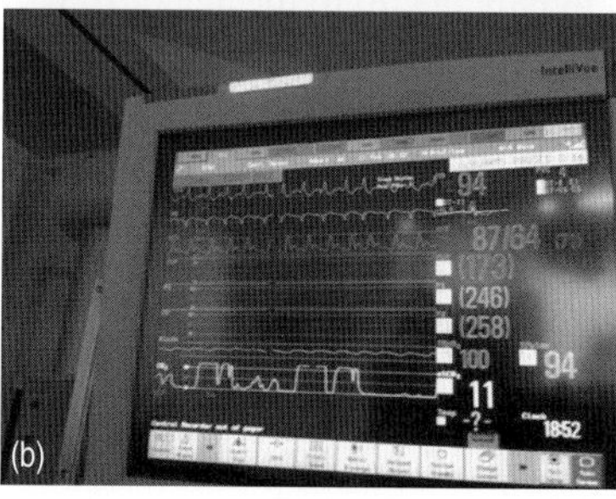

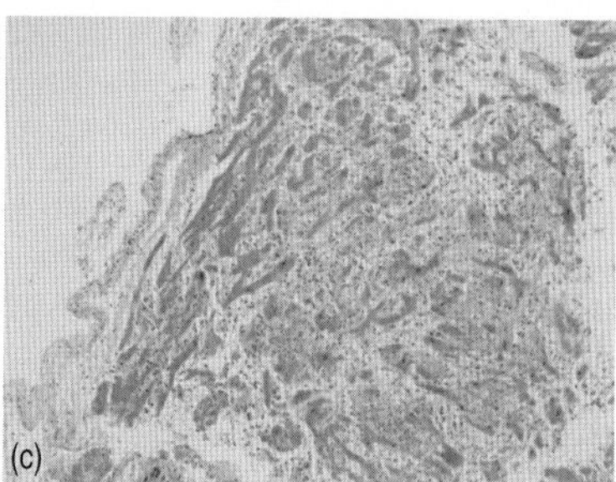

Figure 41.2.1 The stages of cardiac support with VA ECMO for a case of severe lymphocytic myocarditis. Arterial pulsatility was lost on day 1 following ECMO initiation for cardiogenic shock. On day 2 (a) after ECMO support the asystole and ventricular standstill were frequently seen for hours. By day 3 (b), pulsatility and end-tidal CO_2 signals returned with cardiac recovery following immunosuppressive therapy. The patient was decannulated by day 7 and extubated by day 9 and made a full recovery. (c) Cardiac biopsy on day 1 showing heavy lymphocytic infiltration.

TITRATION OF FRESH GAS FLOW TO THE OXYGENATOR

Fresh gas flow (FGF) to the oxygenator maintains the diffusion gradients for O_2 delivery to, and CO_2 removal from, the circuit blood (see ECMO for respiratory failure). Where VA ECMO provides partial circulatory support, significant CO_2 clearance will occur via the lungs and low rates of FGF to the oxygenator will be required to prevent respiratory alkalosis. Inadequate FGF during VA ECMO will prevent oxygenation of venous blood within the ECMO circuit and impose an extrapulmonary right-to-left shunt.

LUNG VENTILATION

Many patients on peripheral VA ECMO support do not require mechanical ventilation or sedation, in contrast to patients configured with central VA ECMO support. Positive-pressure ventilation is beneficial in the management of pulmonary oedema, which may develop during VA ECMO support where left ventricular failure is more severe than right ventricular failure. Mechanical lung ventilation may also form part of the management of a lung shunt, which becomes evident during VA ECMO as native cardiac function returns (see below).

PREVENTION OF DISTAL LIMB ISCHAEMIA

All patients with a peripheral ECMO arterial return catheter should have a *distal perfusion cannula* inserted to prevent limb ischaemia occurring as a result of the occlusive and compressive effects of the return cannula.[24] The presence of normal lower limb perfusion should not prevent the insertion as limb ischaemia may progress quickly. Distal perfusion cannulae are not required for specialised surgical cannulation using a 'T' graft.

DIFFERENTIAL HYPOXIA

Differential hypoxia occurs when hypoxaemic blood from the pulmonary circulation is ejected from the left heart while fully oxygenated blood enters the arterial circulation from the ECMO circuit. It develops during peripheral VA ECMO support as cardiac function returns when a large intrapulmonary shunt is present, and its development indicates cardiac recovery. It is not seen in central VA ECMO as the ECMO circuit blood enters the arterial tree at the proximal aorta. Its development can be anticipated in known cases of combined severe respiratory and cardiac failure, or it may only become apparent following successful resuscitation. Right subclavian artery return configuration will reduce the cerebral effects in peripheral ECMO, compared with femoral return.

Management includes weaning off any inotropic agents, treating the lung shunt with positive-pressure ventilation, PEEP, bronchoscopy, and inhaled nitric oxide if appropriate. Increasing the ECMO circuit blood flow should reduce the proportion of venous return able to reach the lungs. If severe hypoxaemia persists (Sa_{O_2}<85%) despite other measures, consideration of changing the mode of ECMO support from VA to VV should be considered.

LOSS OF PULSATILITY

The ability of the heart to open the aortic and pulmonary valves and contribute to cardiac output may be temporarily lost in severe forms of cardiac failure. The progressive loss of pulsatility during VA ECMO support may indicate extrinsic cardiac compression or progressive cardiac failure and urgent echocardiography is required to establish the cause. Extrinsic cardiac compression from bleeding is more common in the postoperative cardiac setting and must be managed surgically.

Severe myocardial failure with loss of pulsatility is associated with increased risk of intracardiac thrombosis with arterial embolisation. Management is aimed at preservation of some intracardiac blood flow and higher anticoagulation targets. Increased inotropic support, reduction in arterial pressure and reduced ECMO circuit blood flow may improve cardiac blood flow.

MANAGEMENT OF LEFT VENTRICULAR FAILURE

Pathology that results in a predominance of left ventricular heart failure, compared with right ventricular failure (e.g. massive left ventricular AMI), the presence of aortic or mitral valve regurgitation or high mean arterial pressure, can result in progressive distension of the left ventricle, and congestion of the pulmonary circulation and lungs during VA ECMO support. Non-surgical options for control of LVF during VA ECMO support include positive-pressure ventilation and high PEEP, reduction in mean arterial pressure and reducing or ceasing inotropic support. Surgical options include the addition of a left heart drainage cannula to the circuit, conversion from ECMO to a LVAD, or the use of minimally invasive transaortic valve axial pumps.[25–28]

PREVENTION AND MANAGEMENT OF BLEEDING

Prevention of bleeding remains the greatest challenge for ECMO patient care and preventative strategies are given in Chapter 41.1.1 on VV ECMO for respiratory failure. Surgical site bleeding is the most common cause of severe bleeding in VA ECMO. The management of severe bleeding during ECMO commonly involves the following responses and involvement of surgeons and specialist haematology support:

INITIAL RESPONSE TO BLEEDING

- Heparin should be ceased and not be recommenced until all bleeding has stopped for 12–24 hours.
- Aggressively replace all clotting element deficiencies:
  - cryoprecipitate until fibrinogen >1.5 g/dL
  - platelets until count is >80000 and normal maximal amplitude (MA) on a thromboelastogram (TEG)
  - FFP or human prothrombin complex (Prothrombinex™) until INR is <1.3 and there is normal reaction (R) time on TEG.

ADDITIONAL TREATMENTS IF THERE IS SEVERE OR REFRACTORY BLEEDING

- Fibrinolytic treatment[29]
- Factor VIIa treatment[30,31]
- Surgery.

Protamine is not given to bleeding patients with heparin-bonded circuits owing to the risk of acute circuit thrombosis.

ANTICOAGULATION

Anticoagulation for ECMO in the setting of severe cardiac failure reduces the risk of clot formation within the heart, extracorporeal circuit and cannulae. Heparin is the first-line therapy despite both its limitations and the spectrum of heparin-induced thrombocytopenia and thrombosis (HITTs). Most centres target anticoagulation values below those for management of thromboembolic disease. Definitive recommendations for the titration of heparin therapy are lacking. Activated clotting time (ACT), activated partial thromboplastin time (APTT) and thromboelastograms (TEG) are all used in different centres, but there remains poor correlation between tests and no relevant outcome data on which to base recommendations.[32]

HITTs is a rare, but potentially devastating, complication of heparin therapy during ECMO support. Case reports of successful management with the use of intravenous direct thrombin inhibitors (heparin ceased) exist.[33-35]

WEANING AND DECANNULATION

VA ECMO for cardiac failure generally runs for 3–12 days, which allows time for assessment of cardiac recovery or planning for alternative support if indicated. Cardiac recovery is suggested by improving pulsatility with low or no inotropic support. A formal echocardiographic weaning study is required to assess suitability for decannulation.[23] During a weaning study, haemodynamics, ventricular function and native cardiac output are monitored and measured at progressively lower ECMO circuit blood flow rates (to 1 L/min in adults). Adequate recruitment in the native cardiac output during weaning and haemodynamic stability support the decision to schedule decannulation. Central and peripheral configurations of VA ECMO require surgical repair of the artery after decannulation.

EXPECTED PATIENT OUTCOMES

The clinical effectiveness of VA ECMO for cardiogenic shock and refractory VF has not been evaluated in prospective clinical trials. A number of larger case series and cohort studies allow some assessment of the expected outcomes in the more common patient groups that received VA ECMO support. Successful patient outcomes from a complex intervention are likely to occur in centres with clinical leadership, training and competency programmes, adequate protocols and resources and governance programmes. The application of ECMO before end-organ damage and use in selected patients with either reversible conditions or suitable for longer-term treatment options will also probably be associated with improved outcomes.[36]

In addition the Extracorporeal Life Support Organization, which was established in 1989, maintains a registry of ECMO use in registered ECMO centres around the world. The ELSO registry provides annual outcome data for members (see www.elsonet.org) in addition to educational programmes and resources.

Access the complete references list online at http://www.expertconsult.com

8. Tsao NW, Shih CM, Yeh JS, et al. Extracorporeal membrane oxygenation-assisted primary percutaneous coronary intervention may improve survival of patients with acute myocardial infarction complicated by profound cardiogenic shock. J Crit Care 2012;27(5):530.e1–11.
12. Malekan R, Saunders PC, Yu CJ, et al. Peripheral extracorporeal membrane oxygenation: comprehensive therapy for high-risk massive pulmonary embolism. Ann Thorac Surg 2012;94:104–8.
17. Thiagarajan RR, Brogan TV, Scheurer MA, et al. Extracorporeal membrane oxygenation to support cardiopulmonary resuscitation in adults. Ann Thorac Surg 2009;87:778–85.
22. Platts DG, Sedgwick JF, Burstow DJ, et al. The role of echocardiography in the management of patients supported by extracorporeal membrane oxygenation. J Am Soc Echocardiogr 2012;25:131–41.
23. Aissaoui N, Luyt CE, Leprince P, et al. Predictors of successful extracorporeal membrane oxygenation (ECMO) weaning after assistance for refractory cardiogenic shock. Intensive Care Med 2011;37:1738–45.
32. Oliver WC. Anticoagulation and coagulation management for ECMO. Semin Cardiothorac Vasc Anesth 2009;13:154–75.

Part Five

Gastroenterological Emergencies and Surgery

42

Acute gastrointestinal bleeding

Joseph JY Sung

Acute gastrointestinal (GI) bleeding is a common admission to the intensive care unit (ICU) and a major cause of morbidity and mortality. Peptic ulcer disease accounts for 75% of upper GI bleeding.[1,2] Bleeding from varices, oesophagitis, duodenitis and Mallory–Weiss syndrome each account for between 5% and 15% of cases. About 20% of GI bleeding arises from the lower GI tract. Common aetiological causes for GI bleeding are listed in **Box 42.1**. Mortality from upper GI bleeding has remained at approximately 10% for decades, but recent reports suggest that mortality from ulcers bleeding has fallen substantially, to about 5%.[3] Furthermore, the majority of cases died of causes unrelated to bleeding, but rather to cardiopulmonary or multi-organ failure.[4] This observation emphasises the benefit of good supportive care in the intensive care unit for patients presenting with gastrointestinal bleeding. Variceal bleeding has a much higher mortality of about 30%. Risk factors for mortality include old age, associated medical problems, coagulopathy and the magnitude of bleeding.

UPPER GASTROINTESTINAL BLEEDING

CLINICAL PRESENTATION

The patient may or may not present with a history of upper GI problems. There may be pain but bleeding ulcers can be painless, especially in elderly patients and users of non-steroidal anti-inflammatory drugs. Frequently, the common symptoms of hypovolaemia such as tachycardia, pallor, sweating, cyanosis, mental confusion and oliguria are present, especially in massive GI bleeding. A history of vomiting and retching preceding haematemesis suggests Mallory–Weiss syndrome.

Haematemesis and melaena are the most common presentations of acute upper GI bleeding. Haematochezia is the passage of bright red or maroon blood from the rectum, in the form of pure blood or admixed with stool. It usually represents a lower intestinal source of bleeding, but can also be a feature of massive upper GI bleeding.

INVESTIGATION

ENDOSCOPY OR BARIUM STUDY

As history and physical examination are seldom useful in identifying the specific site of bleeding, investigations are necessary in most cases of GI bleeding. Endoscopy has replaced barium studies as the investigation of choice and recent studies show that endoscopy should be offered within 24 hours of presentation to hospital to provide optimal clinical outcome.[5]

Endoscopy is preferred to barium X-rays for the following reasons:

- Endoscopy allows more precise identification of the site and nature of bleeding.
- Endoscopic appearance often predicts the risk of recurrent bleeding from ulcer and varices (see below).
- Lesions such as gastritis, portal hypertensive gastropathy and duodenitis are difficult to diagnose by barium X-ray.
- Treatments such as injecting ulcers may be instigated during endoscopy (see below).
- Barium X-ray is notoriously unreliable in patients with previous gastric surgery.

However, endoscopy is not without potential problems and in particular can induce serious hypoxia in patients with cardiorespiratory diseases. Careful supervision with continuous monitoring of blood pressure, pulse and oxygen saturation with a pulse oximeter is mandatory. Oxygen should be administered by nasal cannula when necessary.

ANGIOGRAPHY

Angiography is seldom used for the diagnosis of upper GI bleeding. Theoretically, when the bleeding is very brisk (greater than 0.5 mL/minute), and obscures the endoscopic view, angiography may help to identify the sources of bleeding and may sometimes be used to embolise the bleeding point. In practice, however, most patients with this degree of haemorrhage should be considered for emergency laparotomy.

MANAGEMENT OF NON-VARICEAL UPPER GI BLEEDING

The goals of managing a patient with acute GI bleeding are, first, to resuscitate, second, to control active bleeding and, third, to prevent recurrence of haemorrhage.

RESUSCITATION

Blood and plasma expanders should be given through large-bore intravenous cannulae. Vital signs should be

Box 42.1 Common causes of acute gastrointestinal bleeding

Upper gastrointestinal bleeding
Peptic ulcers (DU : GU 3 : 1)
Varices (oesophageal varices : gastric varices 9 : 1)
Portal hypertensive gastropathy
Mallory–Weiss syndrome
Gastritis, duodenitis and oesophagitis
Lower gastrointestinal bleeding
Diverticular bleeding
Angiodysplasia and arteriovenous malformation
Colonic polyps or tumours
Meckel's diverticulum
Inflammatory bowel diseases

DU=duodenal ulcer; GU=gastrointestinal ulcer.

closely monitored. In patients with hypovolaemic shock, central venous pressure and hourly urine output should also be observed (see Ch. 15). Following adequate resuscitation, management is directed at identifying the lesion and distinguishing the high-risk patient, who is likely to require early endoscopic or surgical treatment.

THE HIGH-RISK PATIENT

Significant GI bleeding is indicated by syncope, haematemesis, systolic blood pressure below 100 mmHg (13.3 kPa), postural hypotension and a blood transfusion requirement of more than 4 units of blood in 12 hours, to maintain blood pressure. Patients over 60 years old and with multiple co-morbidities are at even higher risk.[3] Those admitted for other medical problems (e.g. heart or respiratory failure, or cerebrovascular bleed) and who have GI bleeding during hospitalisation also have a higher mortality.

THE HIGH-RISK ULCER

Peptic ulcers that are actively bleeding or have bled recently may show stigmata of haemorrhage on endoscopy. These include localised active bleeding (i.e. pulsatile, arterial spurting or simple oozing), an adherent blood clot, a protuberant vessel or a flat, pigmented spot on the ulcer base. Stigmata of haemorrhage are important predictors of recurrent bleeding (**Table 42.1**). The proximal postero-inferior wall of the duodenal bulb and the high lesser curve of the stomach are common sites for severe recurrent bleeding, probably owing to their respective large arteries (gastroduodenal and left gastric arteries).

Table 42.1 Stigmata of haemorrhage and risk of recurrent bleeding in peptic ulcers

STIGMATA OF HAEMORRHAGE	% RECURRENT BLEEDING
Spurter or oozer	85–90
Protuberant vessel	35–55
Adherent clot	30–40
Flat spot	5–10
None	5

TREATMENT

Pharmacological control

Acid-suppressing drugs such as H_2-receptor antagonists and proton pump inhibitors are very effective drugs to promote ulcer healing. An acidic environment impairs platelet function and haemostasis. Therefore, reducing the secretion of gastric acid should reduce bleeding and encourage ulcer healing. A recent study has shown that potent acid suppression using intravenous proton pump inhibitors reduces recurrent bleeding after endoscopic therapy.[6] Proton pump inhibitors should be recommended in high-risk peptic ulcer bleeding patients as an adjuvant to endoscopic therapy. In contrast, antifibrinolytic agents such as tranexamic acid have not been effective in reducing the operative rate and mortality of acute GI haemorrhage. Recent studies show that, in patients at high risk of recurrent bleeding, pharmacological control without endoscopic haemostasis is inadequate.[7] Thus a combination of endoscopic and pharmacological therapy offers the best therapy for ulcer-bleeding patients.[8,9]

Endoscopic therapy

Most patients with acute upper GI haemorrhage stop bleeding spontaneously and have an uneventful recovery. No specific intervention is required in these patients. Endoscopic haemostasis should be used in patients with a high risk of persistent or recurrent bleeding. In the last two decades, endoscopic haemostasis, with its high efficacy and low morbidity, has resulted in a dramatic decrease in emergency surgery, and has reduced the mortality of ulcer bleeding. The three most popular methods of haemostasis are as follows.

Epinephrine (adrenaline) injection

Endoscopic injection of epinephrine (1:10 000 dilution) at 0.5–1.0 mL aliquots (up to 10–15 mL) into and around the ulcer bleeding point has achieved successful haemostasis in over 90% of cases.[8] Debate exists as to whether the haemostatic effect is a result of local tamponade by the volume injected or vasoconstriction by epinephrine. Absorption of epinephrine into the systemic circulation has been documented, but without any significant effect on the haemodynamic status of the patient.[10] Epinephrine injection is an effective, cheap, portable and easy-to-learn method of haemostasis, and has acquired worldwide popularity.

Coaptive coagulation

This method uses direct pressure and heat energy (heater probe) or electrocoagulation (bipolar coagulation probe (BICAP)) to control ulcer bleeding. The depth of tissue injury induced by these devices is minimal, as the bleeding vessel is tamponaded prior to coagulation. The overall efficacy of the epinephrine injection, heater probe and BICAP probe methods are comparable.[11] Occasionally, it is not possible to obtain a view en face of the bleeding ulcers, particularly those on the lesser curve or on the posterior wall of the duodenal bulb. In these situations, direct pressure cannot be applied, and the failure rate of coaptive coagulation tends to be higher.

Haemoclips

Endoscopic clipping of a bleeding vessel is an appealing alternative treatment that has gained popularity in recent years. The advantage of haemoclips over thermocoagulation is that there is no tissue injury induced and hence the risk of perforation is reduced. Studies comparing haemoclips with injection and thermocoagulation have shown favourable results.[12,13] However, the application of haemoclips in certain sites, for example lesser curve, gastric fundus and posterior wall of the duodenum, is technically difficult. Loading of clips on to the application device is cumbersome and time-consuming and transfer of torque from the handle to the tip of the device is limited.

SURGERY

Surgery remains the definitive method of stopping haemorrhage, but there is little agreement on the exact indications and best timing for surgical intervention. These issues are even less clear now that endoscopic treatment is so effective. Accordingly, good cooperation among intensivists, gastroenterologists and surgeons is essential. Indications for surgery can be:

- arterial bleeding that cannot be controlled by endoscopic haemostasis
- massive transfusion (i.e. total of 6–8 units of blood) required to maintain blood pressure
- recurrent clinical bleeding after initial success in endoscopic haemostasis
- evidence suggestive of GI perforation.

Surgical procedures include underrunning of the ulcer, underrunning plus vagotomy and drainage, and various types of gastrectomy. The overall mortality of emergency surgery for GI bleeding is about 15–20%. In a study investigating the best salvage treatment for patients with recurrent bleeding after endoscopic therapy, surgery was found to be comparable to repeating endoscopic treatment in securing haemostasis.[14] However, morbidity is significantly higher in surgical patients than in endoscopic patients. Early surgery should be considered in patients with hypovolaemic shock and/or large peptic ulcer with protuberant vessels. A protocol to manage bleeding peptic ulcer is shown in **Figure 42.1**.[15]

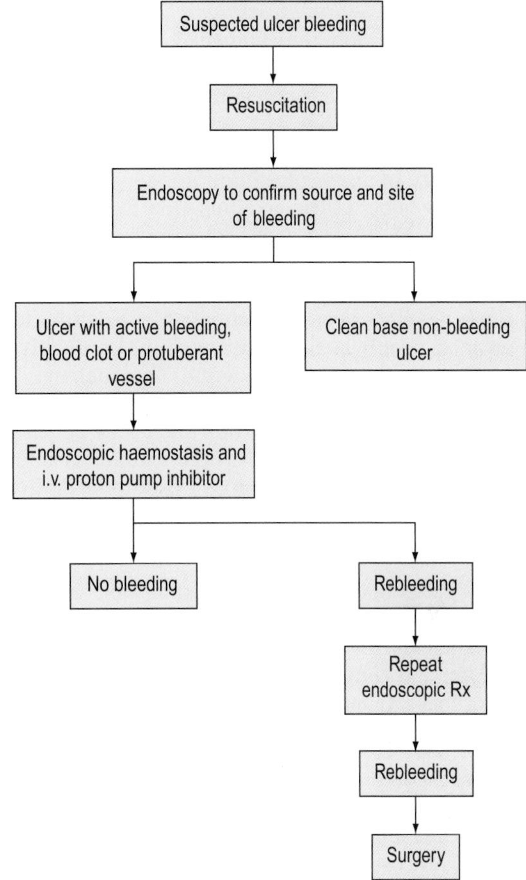

Figure 42.1 Management of peptic ulcer bleeding.

ACUTE STRESS ULCERATION

Acute stress ulceration is associated with shock, sepsis, burns, multiple trauma, head injuries, spinal injuries and respiratory, renal and hepatic failure. Bleeding may be occult or overt, from 'coffee-grounds' aspirates to frank haemorrhage. Lesions are most commonly seen in the gastric fundus, and range from mild erosions to acute ulcerations. The exact mechanism leading to acute mucosal erosion/ulceration in critically ill patients is still unclear. Hypoxia and hypoperfusion of the gastroduodenal mucosa are probably the most important factors, but haemodynamic instability, respiratory failure and coagulopathy are also strong independent factors in critically ill patients. The reported incidence of stress-related mucosal bleeding in ICU patients ranges from 8 to 45%.[16] It has been declining in the last decade as a result of highly effective management of hypotension and hypoxaemia.

PROPHYLAXIS AND TREATMENT

Significant ulcerations are managed as above. Minor bleeding and prophylactic treatment are considered together. Prophylactic treatment aims for gastric alkalinisation (gastric pH > 3.5), with the rationale that gastric acidity is the main cause of stress ulceration.[16] The incidence of stress ulceration appears to be lower with prophylactic gastric alkalinisation than with placebos, although an improvement in survival has not been shown.[17,18] Concerns have included gastric bacterial overgrowth and associated nosocomial pneumonia, but these have not been substantiated by existing data. On balance, prophylactic treatment should probably be reserved only for at-risk patients. The mainstay of prophylaxis and treatment for minor bleeding remains supportive - optimise oxygenation and tissue perfusion and control of infection. There is little consensus among critical care experts in the choice of prophylactic treatment used.[19,20] Drugs given include the following:

Antacids

Antacids given hourly via a nasogastric tube can maintain gastric alkalinisation. Gastric pH monitoring is necessary. Antacids contain magnesium, aluminium, calcium or sodium, and complications may arise from excessive intake of these minerals. Bowel stasis and diarrhoea can also be problems. They are used less commonly now.

Sucralfate

This is a basic aluminium salt of sucrose octasulphate. It is effective in healing ulcers by increasing mucus secretion, mucosal blood flow and local prostaglandin production. These effects promote mucosal resistance against acid and pepsin (i.e. they are cytoprotective). As it does not alter gastric pH, Gram-negative bacterial colonisation of gastric juice is less likely. The incidence of nosocomial pneumonia may be less with sucralfate than with antacids or H_2-receptor antagonists, but this is debatable and is offset by the potential risk of aspiration.[17] Sucralfate is given via a nasogastric tube as 1.0 g every 4–6 hours. Constipation is a side-effect, and aluminium toxicity may arise from renal dysfunction.

H_2-receptor antagonists

These drugs suppress acid secretion by competing for the histamine receptor on the parietal cell. Cimetidine is less potent and has interactions with anticonvulsants, theophyllines and warfarin. Famotidine and nizatidine are newer agents but have no particular advantage over ranitidine. The problem of H_2-receptor antagonists is the development of tachyphylaxis after the first day of administration, leading to reduction of effectiveness in acid suppression. At least one meta-analysis suggested that ranitidine did not confer any protection against stress ulcer in intensive care patients.[21]

Proton pump inhibitors

These are potent acid-suppressing agents as they block the final common pathway of acid secretion by the parietal cell, namely the proton pump. All proton pump inhibitors (omeprazole, lansoprazole, pantoprazole and rabeprazole) can be given as oral medications. Omeprazole and pantoprazole are also available in intravenous form for those who cannot be fed orally. In two non-randomised studies, intravenous omeprazole was shown to protect critically ill patients requiring ventilation from the development of stress-related mucosal bleeding from the upper GI tract.[20] As yet, there are no prospective data indicating which are the high-risk patients who might benefit from this treatment.

VARICEAL BLEEDING

Acute variceal bleeding is a serious complication of portal hypertension, with a high mortality. About 50% of patients with bleeding varices have had an earlier bleed during hospitalisation. The degree of liver failure, using Child–Pugh's classification (see Ch. 44), is the most important prognostic factor for early rebleeding and survival.

RESUSCITATION

Immediate resuscitation with whole blood and fluid is mandatory. Overtransfusion may cause a rebound increase in portal pressure (with a consequent increased risk of rebleeding) and must be avoided. Fresh frozen plasma and platelet concentrates transfusion may be indicated. A nasogastric cannula is often inserted for the removal of blood (and also drug administration). Forceful aspiration through the nasogastric tube should be discouraged as bleeding may be induced. Lactulose (15–30 mL every 4–6 hours) should be given to prevent or correct hepatic encephalopathy. A colonic wash-out can be used, but a magnesium-containing enema should be avoided in the presence of renal failure. Close attention must be given to haemodynamic monitoring.

When the patient is haemodynamically stable, upper GI endoscopy should be performed to identify the source of bleeding. Patients with portal hypertension could bleed from oesophageal or gastric varices, peptic ulcers or portal hypertensive gastropathy or combinations of these.

PHARMACOLOGICAL CONTROL

Vasopressin (0.2–0.4 U/min) used to be the most widely used agent to reduce portal blood pressure and control variceal bleeding. Adverse effects of vasopressin such as cardiac ischaemia (in about 10% of patients) and worsening coagulopathy (by release of plasminogen activator) have discouraged the use of this drug in recent years. Terlipressin, a triglycyl synthetic analogue of vasopressin, has a longer half-life and fewer cardiac side-effects and appears more effective and safe when used in combination with glyceryl trinitrate.[22] Infusion of somatostatin and its analogue (octreotide, vapreotide) reduces portal blood pressure and azygous blood flow. They are safe and effective vasoactive agents to be used in acute variceal bleeding.[23] The benefit is more pronounced if these vasoactive agents are given early, even before endoscopy.[22,24] Octreotide has also been shown to be effective when used as an adjuvant therapy in combination with endoscopic therapy.[25] Recurrent bleeding episodes and hence requirement of transfusion are significantly reduced. Activated factor VII has recently been tested for control of variceal bleeding. Despite its initial promise in correcting coagulopathy, this drug has not been found effective in controlling variceal bleeding.[26]

ENDOSCOPIC SCLEROTHERAPY

Endoscopic injection sclerotherapy is the mainstay of treatment. At endoscopy, sclerosants can be injected directly into the variceal columns (intravariceal injection) or into the mucosa adjacent to the varices (paravariceal injection) to cause venous thrombosis and inflammation, and tissue fibrosis. Commonly used sclerosants are ethanolamine oleate, sodium tetradecyl sulphate (1–3%), polidocanol and ethyl alcohol. None has appreciable advantage over the others and the choice is very much a personal preference of the endoscopist, and depends also on availability. Endoscopic sclerotherapy controls 80–90% of acute variceal bleeding. Complications such as ulcer formation, fever, chest pain and mediastinitis are common. Bleeding from gastric varices is more difficult to control by injection sclerotherapy because of difficult access.

Butylcyanoacrylate (Histoacryl®) has recently been used for gastric variceal injections, with a claimed superior haemostatic effect. It is mixed with lipiodol to delay the rate of polymerisation and allow radiological monitoring of the injection.

ENDOSCOPIC VARICEAL LIGATION

Endoscopic variceal ligation was introduced in the late 1980s as a mechanical method to control bleeding from varices. Rubber bands mounted on the banding device at the tip of the endoscope are released to strangulate the bleeding varices. Numerous studies comparing endoscopic variceal ligation with endoscopic sclerotherapy showed that the technique is as effective as injection sclerotherapy in acute bleeding. Procedure-related complications are significantly fewer, as there is no tissue chemical irritation. An overtube to facilitate banding avoids aspiration during the procedure, but may result in serious oesophageal injury if used improperly. The tunnel vision produced by the banding device as originally designed restricts visibility, and thus makes the procedure technically difficult when bleeding is heavy. With the introduction of multiple banding devices that are loaded with 5–10 rubber bands, and the use of transparent caps, the problems of overtube injury and tunnel vision have been overcome. In many centres, endoscopic variceal ligation has replaced injection sclerotherapy as the first choice for variceal haemorrhage. Many have combined the two endoscopic treatments together in an attempt to improve the outcome. Existing data so far do not suggest this combined therapy is any better, however, hence combined endoscopic therapy cannot be recommended.

BALLOON TAMPONADE

Variceal bleeding can be controlled by exerting pressure directly on the bleeding point using a balloon. The Sengstaken–Blackmore tube has been replaced by the four-lumen Minnesota tube, which allows aspiration of gastric and oesophageal contents. Inflation of the gastric balloon (by 250–350 mL of water) is often sufficient to stop the bleeding by occluding the feeding veins to the oesophageal varices. If bleeding continues, the oesophageal balloon can be inflated by air and kept at a pressure of 50–60 mmHg (6.7–8.0 kPa). Duration of using balloon tamponade should be limited to 24 hours to avoid tissue pressure necrosis. Because of available effective pharmacological and endoscopic therapies, balloon tamponade should be used only in the exceptional cases when these therapies fail to effect control of bleeding.

TRANSJUGULAR INTRAHEPATIC PORTOSYSTEMIC SHUNT (TIPS)

Using a transjugular approach, a catheter is inserted into the hepatic vein, and advanced under fluoroscopic guidance into a branch of the portal vein.[27] By means of a guidewire and dilators, a self-expandable metal stent is introduced to create an intrahepatic portosystemic shunt. In good hands, success can be achieved in over 90% of cases. This procedure significantly reduces portal blood pressure and thus bleeding from varices. Major complications include intra-abdominal haemorrhage and stent occlusion. Hepatic encephalopathy has been reported in 25–60% of patients. Nevertheless, this is an effective salvage treatment for uncontrolled variceal bleeding. Meta-analysis comparing TIPS with endoscopic therapy showed that the former has secure haemostasis but at the cost of increasing risk of hepatic encephalopathy.[28]

A number of markers of outcome after TIPS have been under investigation, including the Acute Physiology, Age and Chronic Health Evaluation (APACHE) score, presence of hyponatraemia and Child C liver disease, hepatic encephalopathy before TIPS, presence of ascites and serum albumin. Until a reliable marker of outcome can be identified, TIPS should be reserved for the subset of patients who continue to bleed or develop recurrent bleeding after endoscopic therapy. Unlike shunt surgery, TIPS will not reduce the chance of future liver transplantation.

SURGERY

Surgical treatments for variceal bleeding include direct devascularisation of the lower oesophagus plus the proximal stomach and a variety of surgical shunts. The role of surgery has diminished since the advent of endoscopic treatment and TIPS.[29] Surgery is now used

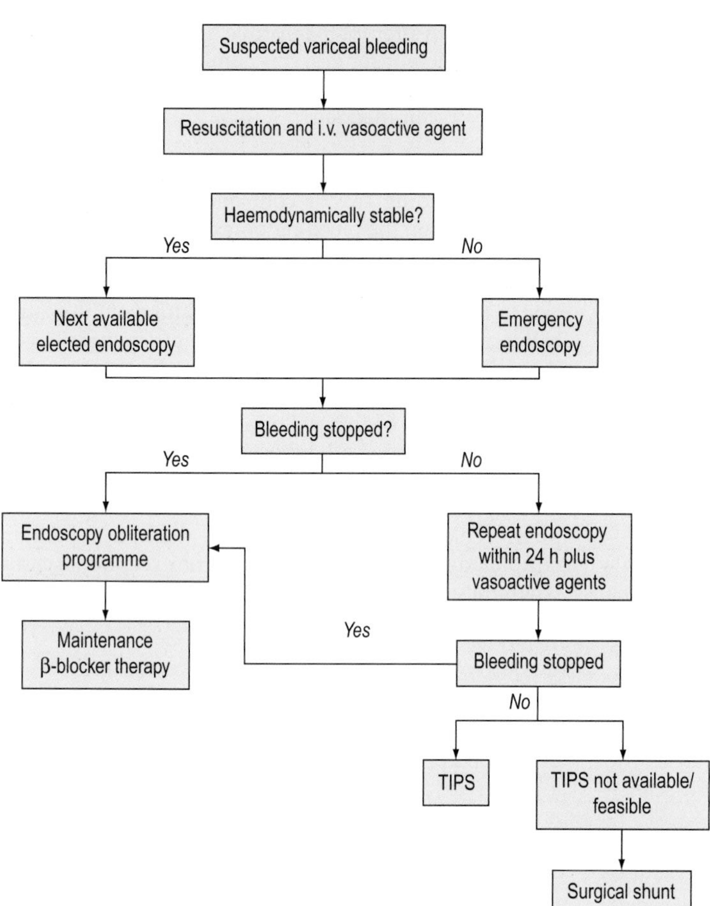

Figure 42.2 Management of variceal haemorrhage. TIPS=transjugular intrahepatic portosystemic shunt.

as a second-line treatment, when bleeding continues or recurs after two sessions of injection sclerotherapy or banding ligation. Both staple transection of the oesophagus and portocaval shunt surgery are highly effective emergency measures. Despite successful control of bleeding, long-term survival is not significantly improved. Hepatic encephalopathy is one of the major complications of shunting operations. Expectations that the Warren distal splenorenal shunt will preserve antegrade portal flow and avoid accelerated deterioration of liver function have not been realised. The Warren shunt is technically more difficult, especially if performed as an emergency. Choice of surgery should be carefully made in those who are potential transplant candidates, as it may complicate subsequent surgery. A protocol to manage variceal bleeding is shown in **Figure 42.2.**

LOWER GASTROINTESTINAL BLEEDING

Lower GI bleeding arises from a source distal to the ligament of Treitz. It accounts for 10–20% of acute GI bleeding. Common causes of colonic bleeding include diverticular haemorrhage and angiodysplasia (both occur on the right-sided colon), colonic polyps and carcinoma, and inflammatory bowel diseases.

CLINICAL PRESENTATION

Haematochezia (bright-red blood) is the most common presentation of lower GI bleeding. However, bleeding from small intestine and right colon may also present as melaena. Abdominal pain preceding a massive bleeding episode suggests either ischaemia or inflammatory bowel disease. Painless massive bleeding is common in diverticulosis, angiodysplasia or from a Meckel's diverticulum. In a patient with portal hypertension, haemorrhoids may present with massive haematochezia.

INVESTIGATIONS

Haemorrhoids and rectal tumour can easily be identified by proctosigmoidoscopy, which should always be performed. Since upper GI bleeding is about five times as common as lower GI bleeding, the former should be excluded. When both proctosigmoidoscopy and gastroscopy are negative, the lower GI tract should be examined by colonoscopy, angiography or radionucleotide scan. Barium enema plays no role in the management of acute rectal bleeding.

COLONOSCOPY

Patients with mild-to-moderate haematochezia can be examined safely by colonoscopy. Colonoscopy is difficult in an actively bleeding patient, and may carry an increased risk of perforation. Visualisation is often unsatisfactory due to the dark discoloration of blood. Colonoscopy yields much better results with adequate bowel preparation once bleeding has stopped. Therefore as a technique urgent/emergency colonoscopy does not seem to be necessary as it will not improve the outcome of patients with lower gastrointestinal bleeding.[30]

ANGIOGRAPHY OR RADIONUCLIDE SCAN

The diagnostic efficacy of radionuclide scan and angiography varies in different studies. ^{99m}Tc sulphur colloid is quickly removed from the bloodstream after injection. Its diagnostic yield is low because of its short circulatory half-life. ^{99m}Tc labelling of red cells prolongs the duration of radioactivity in the body. Red cell scan has been reported to detect the source of active bleeding in over 80% of cases.

Diagnostic angiography is helpful in two situations: (1) when the view of endoscopy is completely obscured by active haemorrhage; (2) in defining abnormal vasculatures, where angiography is more sensitive even if extravasation of contrast material is not seen. These lesions include angiodysplasia, arteriovenous malformation and various inherited vascular anomalies (e.g. Rendu–Osler–Weber syndrome, pseudoxanthoma elasticum and Ehlers–Danlos syndrome). Angiography may localise the site of bleeding in 80–85% of patients when the bleeding rate is more than 0.5 mL/min. Both superior and inferior mesenteric angiograms are often needed.

MANAGEMENT

ENDOSCOPY

Bleeding from vascular anomalies can be treated by electrocoagulation, heater probe and laser photocoagulation, unless the anomalies are too large or too diffuse. Bleeding colonic polyps can be removed by polypectomy or coagulated by hot biopsy forceps. Bleeding

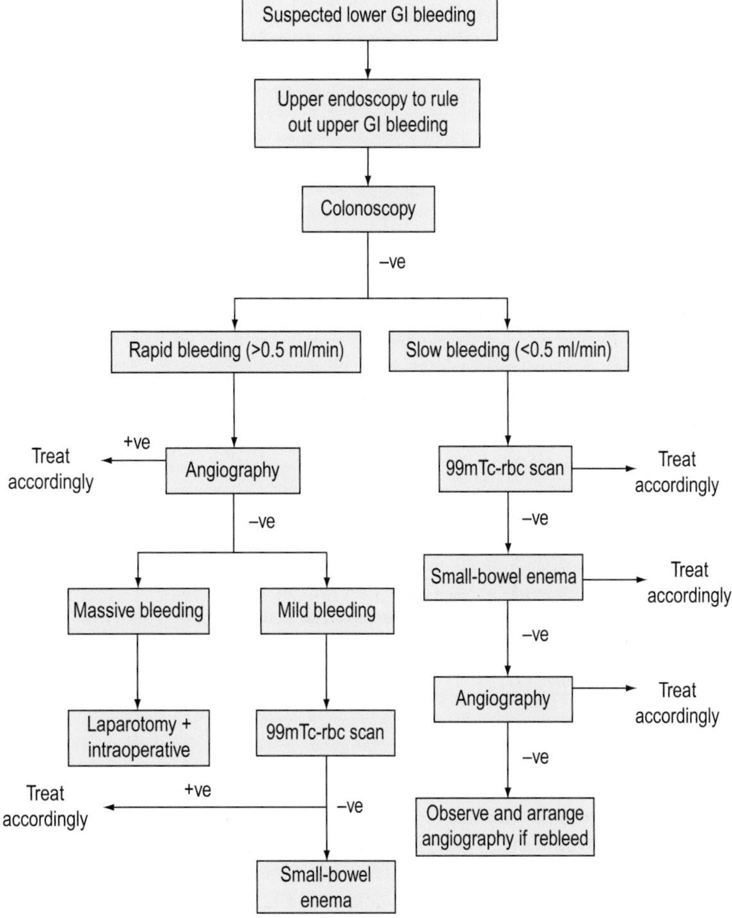

Figure 42.3 Management of lower gastrointestinal (GI) bleeding.

from colonic diverticula can also be controlled with thermocoagulation through colonoscopy.[31]

ANGIOGRAPHY

Angiographic intra-arterial infusion of vasopressin or occlusion of the bleeding artery with embolic agents such as an absorbable gelatin sponge (Gelfoam®) may be used in lower GI bleeding pathologies. Both diverticular bleeding and bleeding from angiodysplasia can be stopped by vasopressin infusion during angiography, but recurrence of bleeding frequently occurs with diverticular disease.

SURGERY

Diverticular bleeding usually arises from a relatively large vessel, and may be difficult to control with endoscopic or angiographic therapy. Partial resection of the colon is warranted after localisation of the bleeding site. Surgery is also indicated in vascular anomalies when endoscopic treatment fails. When an obvious and refractory massive lower GI bleeding is not identified by endoscopic or angiographic examinations, immediate laparotomy with possible subtotal colectomy should be offered. A protocol to manage lower GI bleeding is shown in **Figure 42.3.**

Access the complete references list online at http://www.expertconsult.com

4. Sung JJY, Tsoi KKF, Ma T, et al. Causes of mortality in patients with peptic ulcer bleeding: a prospective cohort study of 10,428 cases. Am J Gastroenterol 2010;105:84–9.
5. Tsoi KKF, Ma T, Sung JJY. Endoscopy for upper gastrointestinal bleeding: how urgent is it? Nat Rev Gastroenterol Hepatol 2009;6:463–9.
7. Lau JYW, Sung JJY, Lee KK, et al. Effect of intravenous omeprazole on recurrent bleeding after endoscopic treatment of bleeding peptic ulcers [see comment]. N Engl J Med 2000;343:310–16.
16. Cook DJ, Fuller HD, Guyatt GH, et al. Risk factors for gastrointestinal bleeding in critically ill patients. Canadian Critical Care Trials Group. N Engl J Med 1994;330:377–81.
22. Levacher S, Letoumelin P, Pateron D, et al. Early administration of terlipressin plus glyceryl trinitrate to control active upper gastrointestinal bleeding in cirrhotic patients. Lancet 1995;346:865–8.
26. Bosch J, Thabut D, Albillos A, et al. Recombinant factor VIIa for variceal bleeding in patients with advanced cirrhosis: a randomized controlled trial. Hepatology 2008;47:1604–14.
28. Papatheodoridis GV, Goulis J, Leandro G, et al. Transjugular intrahepatic portosystemic shunt compared with endoscopic treatment for prevention of variceal rebleeding: a meta-analysis. Hepatology 1999;30:612–22.
30. Laine L, Shah A. Randomized trial of urgent vs elective colonoscopy in patients hospitalized with lower GI bleeding. Am J Gastroenterol 2010;105:2636–41.

43

Severe acute pancreatitis

Duncan LA Wyncoll

Acute inflammation of the pancreas produces a spectrum of symptoms, which may be mild and self-limiting, or reflect severe disease that rapidly leads to multiple-organ failure and death. In a majority of patients a treatable underlying cause is identified. Although mild, interstitial, oedematous pancreatitis is more common, it is the more severe form – acute necrotising pancreatitis (ANP) – that accounts for the associated mortality. Two decades ago the mortality was frequently quoted to be 25–35%, even in the best centres.[1] However, more recently published series have suggested a lower mortality (15%).[2] Management of patients with severe ANP is time consuming, and labour and resource intensive. Long-term follow-up suggests that, although some survivors suffer permanent exocrine and endocrine insufficiency, most maintain a good quality of life.[3]

In the last 20 years there has been a gradual move towards aggressive supportive therapy for ANP. Numerous putative therapeutic interventions have been tried, but few have provided any objective evidence of clinical benefit.

AETIOLOGY

Biliary disease and alcohol remain the two commonest causes of acute pancreatitis worldwide, accounting for about 70% of cases. Although no discernible cause is found in many of the remaining cases, there are well-established associations with a number of infections, certain drugs, hyperlipidaemias and trauma. See **Box 43.1** for a more exhaustive list.

RANSON'S CRITERIA

Although the overall mortality rate for acute pancreatitis is approximately 5–10%, the vast majority of deaths occur in those with the severe form of the disease. Since 1974 the standard means of documenting the severity of disease and risk of mortality has been by Ranson's criteria (**Box 43.2**).[4] These factors were determined following the analysis of just 100 patients with predominantly alcohol-induced pancreatitis using clinical and laboratory data obtained at admission and after 48 hours, and the number of positive criteria should predict outcome. A decade later these criteria were re-evaluated and the first eight were found to be most predictive – this is now known as the Glasgow criteria, or Imrie score.[5]

SCORING

The Acute Physiology and Chronic Health Evaluation (APACHE) II scoring system has also been used in predicting the severity of pancreatitis, and can be used daily throughout the patient's hospital admission rather than solely within the first 48 hours, thus potentially documenting progress or deterioration. However, such scoring systems are complex to perform and have been evaluated only prospectively 24–48 hours after the onset of pancreatitis, which means that the criteria may not be valid for patients subsequently admitted to the intensive care unit (ICU). Those factors with most predictive value for mortality include advanced age, presence of renal or respiratory insufficiency and presence of shock.

The scoring of patients with acute pancreatitis is important for a number of reasons. Firstly, the clinician can be alerted early to the presence of potentially severe disease. Secondly, comparisons of severity can be made both within and between patient series; and thirdly, rational selection of patients can be made for inclusion in trials of potential new treatments or interventions. Unfortunately the scoring systems used at present are often inadequate in patients with severe ANP, which is sometimes characterised by rapidly progressive multiple-system organ dysfunction. In this setting the Ranson criteria and APACHE score do not take account of the effects of treatment upon measured parameters. The solution may be to use a combination of the Ranson score, the radiological scoring systems (see below) and a descriptive organ failure score such as the Sepsis-related Organ Failure Assessment.[6]

THE MANAGEMENT OF SEVERE PANCREATITIS

IMAGING

Dynamic contrast-enhanced computed tomography (CT) provides the best means of accurately visualising the pancreas and diagnosing pancreatitis and its local complications. It may also be used for guiding percutaneous catheter drainage.

Box 43.1 Aetiology of acute pancreatitis

Excess alcohol ingestion
Biliary tract disease
Idiopathic
Metabolic
Hyperlipidaemia
Hyperparathyroidism
Diabetic ketoacidosis
End-stage renal failure
Pregnancy
Post renal transplant
Mechanical disorders
Posttraumatic, postoperative, post endoscopic retrograde cholangiopancreatography
Penetrating duodenal ulcer
Duodenal obstruction
Infections
Human immunodeficiency virus, mumps, Epstein–Barr virus, *Mycoplasma, Legionella, Campylobacter*, ascariasis
Vascular
Necrotising vasculitis – systemic lupus erythematosus, thrombotic thrombocytopenia
Atheroma
Shock
Drugs
Azathioprine, thiazides, furosemide, tetracyclines, oestrogens, valproic acid, metronidazole, pentamidine, nitrofurantoin, erythromycin, methyldopa, ranitidine
Toxins
Scorpion venom, organophosphates, methyl alcohol

Box 43.2 Adverse prognostic factors in acute pancreatitis
Ranson's score[4]

On admission
Age >55 years
White cell count >16 000/mm^3
Glucose 11 mmol/L
Lactate dehydrogenase 400 IU/L
Aspartate transaminase >250 IU/L
Within 48 hours of hospitalisation
Decrease in haematocrit >10%
Increase in blood urea >1.8 mmol/L
Calcium <2 mmol/L
Pa_{O_2} <8 kPa
Base deficit >4 mmol/L
Fluid deficit >6 L

Risk factors	Mortality rate
0–2	<1%
3–4	≅15%
5–6	≅40%
>6	≅100%

Blamey et al.[5] found that only eight variables (not lactate dehydrogenase, base deficit and fluid deficit) were predictive and are often referred to as the Glasgow criteria or Imrie score.

In severe acute pancreatitis, there is lack of normal enhancement to contrast of all or part of the gland. This is consistent with pancreatic necrosis, defined as diffuse or focal areas of non-viable parenchyma. Microscopically, there is evidence of damage to the parenchymal network, acinar cells and pancreatic ductal system and necrosis of perilobular fat. Areas of necrosis are often multifocal, rarely involving the whole gland, and may be confined to the periphery with preservation of the core. Necrosis develops early in the course of the disease and is usually established 96 hours after the onset of symptoms. The extent of pancreatic necrosis and the degree of peripancreatic inflammation have been used to determine outcome. A grading system combining the two CT prognostic indicators (the extent of necrosis and the grade of peripancreatic inflammation) gives the 'CT severity index'.[7]

Most complications of acute pancreatitis occur in patients in whom the initial diagnosis is based upon peripancreatic fluid collections, and a strong correlation has been established between the CT depiction of necrosis and the development of complications and death.[8] In patients with necrosis in the pancreatic head, the outcome is as severe as when the entire pancreas is affected. By contrast, for patients with necrosis in only the distal portion of the gland, the outcome is usually good, with few complications. The mechanism may be that necrosis in the pancreatic head causes obstruction of the pancreatic duct, and produces a rise in pressure in the acinar cells leading to damage and leakage of activated destructive proteases.

Following the initial CT scan, repeated scanning is indicated if the patient's clinical condition deteriorates, usually through the development of pancreatic necrosis, abscess or pancreatic pseudocyst, haemorrhage, or colonic ischaemia or perforation.

Ultrasonography in acute pancreatitis is less useful since visualisation of the gland may be obscured by 'gas-filled' bowel. Moreover, the degree of necrosis, which determines prognosis, cannot be assessed. However, there may be a role for this mode of imaging in demonstrating gallstones, or in the subsequent management when ultrasound-guided fine-needle aspiration (FNA) of the pancreas or surrounding tissue may help to establish the presence of infection.

SURGERY IN SEVERE PANCREATITIS

In previous decades the role of surgery was a controversial area in the management of severe ANP. During the 1980s, most patients with acute pancreatitis of even moderate severity underwent operative intervention; this was particularly true for those patients thought to have infected pancreatic necrosis. The results were poor, with mortality rates in excess of 50%, although this was sometimes without ICU support. In the 1990s the concept of a conservative, non-surgical approach to severe ANP was developed. Targeted surgical intervention according to infection status, based on Gram stain and culture of ultrasound or CT-guided FNA, has refined this conservative approach with significantly better results.[9] The aim now is often to postpone surgery for as long as possible. Many centres report that a conservative approach and avoiding open necrosectomy result in lower mortality. Open surgery is reserved for concomitant intra-abdominal complications.

If severe acute pancreatitis is an unsuspected 'chance' finding at laparotomy, a T-tube should be inserted into the common bile duct, particularly if it has been explored and the opportunity taken for placement of a feeding jejunostomy tube. Some surgeons oppose this approach, as opening a hollow viscus risks peritonitis.

PANCREATIC ABSCESSES

Pancreatic abscesses are circumscribed collections of pus containing little or no pancreatic necrosis, which arise as a later consequence of severe acute pancreatitis or pancreatic trauma. They commonly occur about 3–4 weeks after the onset of severe pancreatitis, and a CT scan most accurately makes the diagnosis. If the appropriate expertise is available, percutaneous catheter drainage may be very successful. Some series report effective drainage of intra-abdominal collections with a single treatment in 70% of patients, increasing to 82% with a second attempt, although proceeding to open surgical drainage is more frequently required in pancreatic abscess, especially if complicated by yeast infection.[10]

ENDOSCOPIC RETROGRADE CHOLANGIOPANCREATOGRAPHY (ERCP)

ERCP represents an alternative approach, particularly for patients with severe biliary pancreatitis. A number of prospective randomised studies have been carried out to compare early ERCP with conservative treatment in acute biliary pancreatitis. Although the studies are not entirely consistent, ERCP and papillotomy seem to be beneficial in confirmed or suspected severe biliary pancreatitis if undertaken by a skilled operator, whereas in mild pancreatitis the risks of intervention probably outweigh the benefits. This observation is confirmed by both a systematic review of the five ERCP trials[11] and by the recommendations of the 2004 International Consensus Conference on the management of severe acute pancreatitis in the critically ill.[12]

TREATMENT WITH PHARMACOLOGICAL AGENTS

Theories regarding the pathogenesis of acute pancreatitis have promoted the concept that autodigestion of the gland and peripancreatic tissue by activated pancreatic enzymes is a central component. This has led to the suggestion that the reduction of pancreatic exocrine secretion, thereby 'resting the pancreas', might improve outcome. The problem is that the secretory status of the pancreas in severe ANP is not known. Consequently, it is not clear whether inhibition of secretion actually occurs or whether this is beneficial. Therapies designed to inhibit pancreatic secretion, such as H_2-blockers, atropine, calcitonin, glucagon and fluorouracil, do not alter the course of the disease. However, other pharmacological therapies, such as aprotonin and gabexate mesilate, both protease inhibitors, and somatostatin and octreotide, are still in widespread use in the hope of improving the outcome.

SOMATOSTATIN AND OCTREOTIDE

Somatostatin and its long-acting analogue octreotide are potent inhibitors of pancreatic secretion. They also stimulate activity of the reticuloendothelial system and play a regulatory role, mostly inhibitory, in the modulation of the immune response via autocrine and neuroendocrine pathways. Both are cytoprotective with respect to the pancreas.[13] Other effects include:

- Somatostatin also blocks the release of tumour necrosis factor and interferon-γ by peripheral mononuclear cells.
- Octreotide increases the phagocytotic activity of monocytes.

These actions may be important in the modulation of the pathogenesis of acute respiratory distress syndrome (ARDS) and septic shock, both of which can complicate severe ANP. Both agents are effective in experimental pancreatitis, and in the prevention of complications in patients undergoing surgery for chronic pancreatitis, but potential difficulties include:

- Pre-emptive administration is not possible in the acute situation.
- Both agents are powerful splanchnic vasoconstrictors.
- The development of pancreatic necrosis has been linked to hypoperfusion of the gland and vasoconstrictors worsen the histological severity of experimental pancreatitis.[14]

Consequently, these agents have both beneficial and detrimental effects. Systematic evaluation suggests that there is insufficient evidence to support the use of octreotide or somatostatin in the treatment of patients with moderate to severe acute pancreatitis.[15] Additionally, the therapeutic effect of octreotide, if present at all, is probably very small and therefore unlikely to have any significant impact on the management of ANP.

PROTEASE INHIBITORS

A further pathogenic mechanism involved in acute pancreatitis is autodigestion of the pancreas by the activation of proteases. More accurately, there is an imbalance between proteases and antiproteases. Aprotinin and gabexate mesilate are proteolytic enzyme inhibitors that act on serine proteases such as trypsin, phospholipase A_2, kallikrein, plasmin, thrombin and C1r and C1s esterases.

Numerous studies of the protease inhibitor gabexate mesilate in patients with variable severity of pancreatitis have now been undertaken. Taken together these show no significant reduction in mortality, length of stay or the need for surgery.[16]

The reason why these agents, in clinical practice, do not have the expected beneficial effect on outcome may be the lag time between the onset of pancreatitis and administration. Additionally, derangement to the microvascular control of the pancreas combined with increased vascular permeability may contribute. Continuous regional arterial infusion or intraperitoneal administration may be more advantageous, but so far trials using these modes of administration have only involved small numbers of patients. At present, there is insufficient evidence to recommend protease inhibitors in ANP.

ANTI-INFLAMMATORY THERAPY

Patients with ANP exhibit a generalised uncontrolled inflammatory response. Potentially there is a therapeutic window between the onset of symptoms and the development of organ failure during which anti-inflammatory therapy might be successful. Potential targets include tumour necrosis factor-α, interleukin (IL)-1β, IL-6, IL-8, IL-10, platelet-activating factor and intracellular adhesion molecules.[17] Although many have been studied in animals, there are limited human data.

It is also fascinating to observe that there is a constellation of changes in hypopituitary–adrenal axis hormone levels that strongly suggests that the existence of relative adrenocortical insufficiency in patients with ANP is very comparable to that of severe sepsis and multiple-organ failure.[18] There are currently no published trials of corticosteroid therapy in patients with ANP.

PROPHYLACTIC ANTIBIOTICS

Bacterial infection of necrotic pancreatic tissue occurs in approximately 50% of patients with ANP, and infection is the major cause of morbidity and mortality. Early studies investigating the role of prophylactic antibiotics in acute pancreatitis showed no benefit, but most included patients with mild disease and employed agents (e.g. ampicillin) with inefficient penetration of pancreatic tissue. Subsequent studies have still not clarified their role, and prophylactic use remains widespread but controversial.

Carbapenems have exceptional penetration into pancreatic tissues and broad activity against most of the common pathogens encountered in this disease. In the 1990s there was hope that this new class of antibiotic would prove more useful; and some of the early trials did suggest a modest benefit with imipenem.[19] The incidence of septic complications was significantly reduced in the treated group (12.2 versus 30.3%), although there was only a trend towards decreased mortality (7 versus 12%). However, the most recent systematic review, which included 14 trials (but still only 841 patients), suggested antibiotic prophylaxis was not associated with a statistically significant reduction in mortality (RR 0.74 [95% CI 0.50–1.07]), in the incidence of infected pancreatic necrosis (RR 0.78 [95% CI 0.60–1.02]) or in the incidence of non-pancreatic infections (RR 0.70 [95% CI 0.46–1.06]).[20] Of note though, in the majority of these trials, patients with severe ANP and overt shock *were excluded*, leaving open the possibility that prophylactic antibiotics may still have a role in the very sickest patients.

Patients with mild pancreatitis definitely do not benefit from antibiotics.

PROPHYLACTIC ANTIFUNGAL THERAPY

The incidence of fungal infection correlates with the extent of pancreatic necrosis, as well as the severity of disease on admission. Antibiotic administration has been claimed to promote fungal infection; however, up to 25% of patients with ANP who do not receive antibiotics also develop fungal infection with an associated mortality rate of up to 84%.[21] One small, randomised study suggested fluconazole reduced the rate of fungal infection, but had no effect on mortality. Advocates of prophylactic antifungal therapy argue that it may delay the need for surgery, which is associated with a better outcome.[22]

SELECTIVE DECONTAMINATION OF THE GUT

The original selective digestive decontamination (SDD) strategy contained three components: oropharyngeal and gastric decontamination with polymyxin E, tobramycin, and amphotericin B and intravenous cefotaxime for 4 days.[23] There is ongoing debate as to the effectiveness of this strategy and results are conflicting regarding any reduction in mortality, particularly when applied to a general critically ill population. However, more promising results have been seen in specific patient populations.

Severe acute pancreatitis may be one clinical situation that supports the hypothesis that gut hypoperfusion promotes bacterial translocation, leading to infection of the inflamed pancreas and peripancreatic tissue.[24] The only controlled trial of SDD in pancreatitis was performed in 102 patients[25] who were randomised to receive SDD: oral colistin, amphotericin and norfloxacin with addition of a daily dose of the three drugs given as a rectal enema and systemic cefotaxime until Gram-negative bacteria were successfully eliminated from the oral cavity and rectum. Surveillance samples were taken regularly to assess whether any subsequent infection was of exogenous or endogenous origin. There were 18 deaths (35%) in the control group, compared with 11 (22%) in the SDD group ($P < 0.05$). This difference was caused by a fall in late mortality due to significant reduction in the incidence of Gram-negative pancreatic infection. There was also a reduction in the mean number of laparotomies in the SDD patients. Since the SDD regimen used in this study incorporated intravenous cefotaxime it could be argued that the improvement in outcome was not due to the colistin, amphotericin or norfloxacin components, but merely due to a systemic antibiotic effect.

Meta-analyses and even large randomised controlled trials of this intervention continue to suggest clear trends towards a reduction in mortality in critically ill patients.[26] However, the perhaps unfounded fear of the emergence of resistant Gram-positive cocci prevents widespread adoption of this strategy.

NUTRITIONAL SUPPORT IN ACUTE NECROTISING PANCREATITIS

The provision of nutritional support for the patient with ANP is an essential component of supportive therapy, especially since many patients with pancreatitis are nutritionally depleted prior to their illness and face increased metabolic demands throughout the course of their disorder. Failure to reverse or prevent malnutrition, and a prolonged negative nitrogen balance, increases mortality rates. The route by which nutrition is administered is, none the less, still debated. In the last two decades there has been a trend away from the use of total parenteral nutrition (TPN) in favour of enteral nutrition (EN) in supporting the critically ill. Studies suggest that TPN started within 24 hours of admission to ICU, compared with a watch-and-wait policy and/or EN where tolerated is associated with increased infective complications and hospital length of stay.[27]

TOTAL PARENTERAL NUTRITION

Severe pancreatitis is still sometimes stated as an absolute contraindication to EN, and TPN is considered by some as 'standard' therapy by some physicians. This is largely because it is regarded as a way of 'resting the pancreas', based on the assumption that the necrotic pancreas is still a secretor of activated enzymes. In fact, the secretory state of the pancreas has never been prospectively studied in severe necrosis. Several retrospective and prospective evaluations of TPN in acute pancreatitis have failed to demonstrate conclusively an effect on survival, or on the incidence and severity of organ failure.

ENTERAL NUTRITION

An increasing number of reports on the use of EN in severe ANP confirm that it is safe and feasible for not all but the majority of patients. When EN is given it has been suggested that it should be delivered distal to the ligament of Treitz, below the area of the cholecystokinin (CCK) cells distal to the third part of the duodenum, as CCK stimulation may worsen the course of the disease. Intragastric delivery of nutrients may result in an increased volume of pancreatic protein and bicarbonate secretion. By contrast, jejunal nutrient delivery does not appear to increase pancreatic exocrine secretion.

Consequently, jejunal tube feeding as far distally as possible in the upper gastrointestinal tract conforms to the concept of 'pancreatic rest'. A number of comparisons of EN with TPN have been made in mild and severe acute pancreatitis, all suggesting that EN is well tolerated without adverse effects on the course of the disease.[28] Patients who received EN experienced fewer total complications and were at lower risk of developing septic complications than those receiving TPN.[29] EN seems to modulate the inflammatory and sepsis response beneficially, and if tolerated may be superior to TPN. In spite of the enthusiasm for EN of some clinicians, in ANP, where there is often an ileus and slow bowel transit time, some patients will not tolerate it. It is not uncommon to be faced with the option of no nutrition or TPN; in this situation TPN with normoglycaemic control should be used.

An international task force has recently made some recommendations,[30] which can be summarised as follows:

1. Most patients with mild or moderate uncomplicated pancreatitis do not benefit from nutritional support.
2. In moderate to severe pancreatitis, let hyperacute inflammation settle, then start a trial of EN via a jejunal tube.
3. In patients who require surgery for diagnosis or treatment, a jejunal tube should be placed, either pulled down from the stomach, or a separate jejunostomy.
4. TPN is indicated only if a 5–7-day trial of EN is not tolerated.
5. In all patients, whether fed enterally or parenterally, a protocol ensuring good glycaemic control is recommended.

CONCLUSION

The main determinant of outcome in severe acute pancreatitis is the extent of pancreatic necrosis and the subsequent risk for the development of infected necrosis. A thorough assessment using appropriate scoring systems and the early use of dynamic contrast-enhanced CT will highlight those patients likely to benefit from early critical care. Despite numerous suggested specific therapies there is still no incontrovertible evidence that any one confers a significant mortality benefit. However, general supportive measures should include vigorous replacement of fluid losses to correct circulating volume, correction of electrolyte and glucose abnormalities, and respiratory, cardiovascular and renal support as necessary. Patients with sterile necrosis should receive a broad-spectrum prophylactic antibiotic that adequately penetrates pancreatic tissue if they develop shock. Due attention should also be paid to nutritional support, for which a jejunal feeding tube with EN is recommended prior to initiation of TPN.

Access the complete references list online at http://www.expertconsult.com

2. Malangoni MA, Martin EL. Outcome of severe pancreatitis. Am J Surg 2005;189:273–7.
7. Bharwani N, Patel S, Prabhudesai S, et al. Acute pancreatitis: the role of imaging in diagnosis and management. Clin Radiol 2001;66:164–75.
11. Tse F, Yuan Y. Early routine endoscopic retrograde cholangiopancreatography strategy versus early conservative management strategy in acute gallstone pancreatitis. Cochrane Database Syst Rev 2012;(5): CD009779.
12. Nathens AB, Curtis JR, Beale RJ, et al. Management of the critically ill patient with severe acute pancreatitis. Crit Care Med 2004;32:2524–36.
18. De Waele JJ, Hoste EA, Baert D, et al. Relative adrenal insufficiency in patients with severe acute pancreatitis. Intensive Care Med. 2007;33:1754–60.
20. Wittau M, Mayer B, Scheele J, et al. Systematic review and meta-analysis of antibiotic prophylaxis in severe acute pancreatitis. Scand J Gastroenterol 2011;46: 261–70.
21. Trikudanathan G, Navaneethan U, Vege SS. Intra-abdominal fungal infections complicating acute pancreatitis: a review. Am J Gastroenterol 2011;106: 1188–92.
30. Mirtallo JM, Forbes A, McClave SA, et al. International consensus guidelines for nutrition therapy in pancreatitis. J Parenter Enteral Nutr 2012;36:284–91.

44

Liver failure

Christopher Willars and Julia Wendon

44.1 Acute hepatic failure

DEFINITIONS

The manner in which acute deteriorations in hepatic function are described is not uniform. In this chapter, we use the term *acute hepatic failure* to describe both *acute liver failure* (ALF) and *acute on chronic liver failure* (ACLF) – which are distinct clinical entities and which require very different management strategies.

ACUTE LIVER FAILURE

Acute liver failure (ALF) is a rare condition, with about 400 cases per year in the UK. ALF arises in the context of massive parenchymal injury and results in a multi-system disorder that is phenotypically similar to severe septic shock. Liver damage is manifest by coagulopathy and encephalopathy, which occurs within days or weeks of the liver injury. There is diversity in terms of aetiology and in terms of clinical progression.

Patients with ALF may initially appear relatively well, but progression to multi-organ failure is rapid. The key to a successful outcome lies in prompt recognition, resuscitation and referral to a specialist centre.

CLASSIFICATION

The clinical classification described by O'Grady et al[1] (**Table 44.1.1**) uses the time from jaundice to encephalopathy to differentiate between hyperacute, acute and subacute liver failure. It is particularly useful because it informs us of likely aetiology and clinical course.

Hyperacute liver failure progresses rapidly (the onset of encephalopathy is within 7 days of the development of jaundice) and is generally associated with profound coagulopathy, high-grade encephalopathy, severe organ dysfunction and a higher incidence of intracranial hypertension, but confers higher rates of spontaneous survival. The onset of encephalopathy often precedes clinical jaundice.

Acute liver failure has an intermediate course. Common aetiologies include the viral hepatitides and idiosyncratic drug reactions.

Subacute liver failure is associated with a later onset of encephalopathy, but with the worst outcomes in the absence of transplantation. Aetiology is frequently seronegative (idiopathic – the history suggests a viral or immune-mediated aetiology but all serological tests are negative) or drug related. Jaundice is inevitable but the transaminitis is often less pronounced than in acute and hyperacute presentations. Patients frequently present with established ascites and so may be clinically difficult to distinguish from those with chronic liver disease (CLD).

AETIOLOGY

Determination of the aetiology of ALF (**Box 44.1.1**) is important for prognostication and because specific therapy may be available. There is a wide geographical variation in the aetiology of ALF. Acetaminophen (paracetamol) toxicity is responsible for the majority of cases of ALF seen in the UK and the USA, whereas viral hepatitis is the most common cause of ALF worldwide (**Table 44.1.2**).

A good history and review of the results of blood tests over the preceding weeks are essential to making a diagnosis. Any new drug ingestion (prescribed, recreational or over the counter) should be considered a potential culprit and discontinued if possible. In addition any treatments that may be detrimental to liver recovery should be avoided.

DIAGNOSIS

A standardised investigative pathway ensures clinical consistency. *Laboratory tests* that may be useful in establishing a diagnosis are listed in **Table 44.1.3**. It is paramount that diagnosis proceeds in tandem with resuscitative measures.

Doppler ultrasound is very useful in determining patency of the hepatic artery, vein and portal vein. Budd–Chiari syndrome, ischaemic hepatitis, portal vein thrombosis and even tricuspid regurgitation may be apparent. *Ultrasound examination* of the liver parenchyma may reveal heterogeneity, fatty infiltration (reflectivity) and tumour. Splenomegaly and ascites are evident, if present.

Axial CT imaging provides additional information about other abdominal anatomy, lymphadenopathy and liver perfusion. Serial imaging in ALF may

Table 44.1.1 Classification of acute liver failure

DEFINITION	TIME (DAYS)	COMMONEST AETIOLOGIES
Hyperacute	<7 days	Acetaminophen overdose, hepatitis A and B
Acute	8–28 days	Hepatitis ABE, idiosyncratic drug reactions
Subacute	29 days–8 weeks	Idiosyncratic drug reaction, seronegative hepatitis

Box 44.1.1 Aetiology of ALF

Viral hepatitis
Hepatitis A, B, D, E, seronegative hepatitis
Herpes simplex, cytomegalovirus, chickenpox – usually limited to immunocompromised hosts
Drug-related
Acetaminophen
Antituberculous drugs
Recreational drugs (ecstasy, cocaine)
Idiosyncratic reactions (anticonvulsants, antibiotics, non-steroidal anti-inflammatory drugs (NSAIDs))
Aspirin in children may lead to Reye syndrome
Kava kava
Toxins
Carbon tetrachloride, phosphorous, *Amanita phalloides*, alcohol
Vascular events
Ischaemia, veno-occlusive disease, Budd–Chiari syndrome (hepatic vein thrombosis)
Hyperthermic liver injury
Pregnancy
Acute fatty liver of pregnancy, HELLP syndrome, liver rupture
Other
Wilson's disease, autoimmune, lymphoma, carcinoma, haemophagocytic syndrome. trauma

demonstrate a collapsing liver (**Fig. 44.1.1**). Nodularity of the liver should not be assumed to represent cirrhosis and chronic liver disease. The imaging pattern of subacute liver failure, with focal areas of collapse and regeneration, may be difficult to distinguish from cirrhosis.

Liver biopsy is rarely undertaken in the acute setting because of the high risk of bleeding. The contribution of histology to the assessment of ALF is controversial. Features suggestive of specific diagnoses such as Wilson's disease (cirrhosis) and autoimmune features may be evident and histology may be particularly useful if infiltration with tumour is suspected and a tissue diagnosis is required prior to consideration of systemic chemotherapy. However, in ALF, non-specific confluent necrosis is the commonest histological finding. Its

Table 44.1.2 Geographical distribution of aetiology in ALF

	UK	US	FRANCE	INDIA	JAPAN
Paracetamol	54	40	2	–	–
Drug induced	7	12	15	5	–
Seronegative	17	17	18	24	45
Hepatitis A/B	14	12	49	33	55
Hepatitis E	–	–	–	38	–
Other	8	19	16	–	–

severity has been used to assess prognosis: >50% necrosis is associated with poor prognosis. However, nodules of regeneration may occur randomly, particularly in subacute liver failure, and sampling error may thus make this a less than ideal tool for predicting outcome. The transjugular route is considered safest, although there is a risk of sampling error.

Echocardiography should be performed to exclude low cardiac output states as a cause of hypoxic hepatitis, and where transplantation is considered.

PARACETAMOL (ACETAMINOPHEN) TOXICITY

Paracetamol, taken intentionally or inadvertently, remains one of the commonest forms of acute hepatotoxicity. This incidence of paracetamol overdose has risen since the 1970s and in 1998 the Medicines Control Agency (UK) introduced legislation to limit its availability, and paracetamol is now sold as 16×500 mg tablets; a maximum of 8 g per packet.

Cytochrome P450 enzymes convert ~5% of acetaminophen to *N*-acetyl *p*-benzoquinone imine (NAPQI), a metabolite which is normally detoxified by conjugation with hepatic glutathione. Hepatocellular glutathione becomes rapidly depleted in overdose, and NAPQI persists, causing damage to cell membranes leading to hepatocyte death unless NAC (N-acetylcysteine or methionine is administrated in a timely fashion.

Following massive paracetamol ingestion, relatively small doses are absorbed and when NAC is administered early less than 1% of cases result in significant hepatotoxicity.

The recommended dosage schedule is 150 mg/kg in 5% dextrose over 15–60 minutes, followed by 50 mg/kg in 5% dextrose over 4 hours, and followed by 100 mg/kg in 5% dextrose over 16 hours. Ongoing administration at doses of 150 mg/kg over a 24-hour period may be indicated.

Even late administration of *N*-acetylcysteine (up to 36 hours after ingestion) may improve outcome. The risk factors listed in **Table 44.1.4**[2] confer a predisposition to paracetamol-induced hepatotoxicity:

The Prescott nomogram (**Fig. 44.1.2**) is used in the UK and Europe to determine the risk of acetaminophen

Table 44.1.3 Aetiology of acute liver failure and initial investigations

Hepatitis A (HAV)	Immunoglobulin M (IgM) anti-HAV
Hepatitis B+D (HBV, HDV)	HBsAg, IgM anti-core, HBeAg, HBeAb, HBV DNA, delta antibody
Hepatitis E (HEV)	IgM antibody
Seronegative hepatitis	All tests negative: diagnosis of exclusion
Paracetamol	Drug levels in blood and clinical pattern of disease – may be negative on third or subsequent days after overdose; markedly elevated aspartate and alanine serum transaminase (often >10 000)
Idiosyncratic drug reactions	Eosinophil count may be elevated, although most diagnoses are based on temporal relationship
Ecstasy	Blood, urine, hair analysis and history
Autoimmune	Autoantibodies, immunoglobulin profile
PREGNANCY-RELATED SYNDROMES	
Fatty liver	Uric acid elevated, neutrophilia, often first pregnancy, history, CT scan for rupture and assessment of vessels
HELLP syndrome	Platelet count, disseminated intravascular coagulation a prominent feature; CT scan as above
Liver rupture	May be seen in association with pre-eclampsia, fatty liver and HELLP
Wilson's disease	Urinary copper, ceruloplasmin (although low in many causes of acute liver failure), present up to second decade of life, Kayser–Fleischer rings, low alkaline phosphate levels
Amanita phalloides	History of ingestion of mushrooms, diarrhoea
Budd–Chiari syndrome	Ultrasound of vessels (HV signal lost, reverse flow in portal vein), CT angiography, ascites, prominent caudate lobe on imaging, haematological assessment
Malignancy	Imaging and histology; increased alkaline phosphate and LDH; often imaging may be interpreted as normal
Ischaemic hepatitis	Clinical context, marked elevation of transaminases (often >5000); may demonstrate dilated hepatic veins on ultrasound, echocardiogram
Heatstroke	Myoglobinuria and rhabdomyolysis are often prominent features

CT=computed tomography; HELLP=**h**aemolysis (microangiopathic haemolytic anaemia), **e**levated **l**iver enzymes and **l**ow **p**latelets; HIV=human immunodeficiency virus; LDH=lactate dehydrogenase.

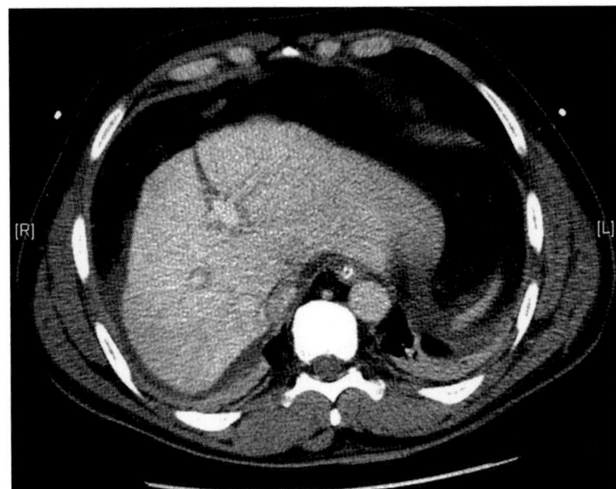

Figure 44.1.1 A collapsed liver in the case of a 42-year-old man with ALF.

Table 44.1.4 Risk factors for paracetamol hepatotoxicity

DECREASED HEPATIC GLUTATHIONE STORES	INDUCTION OF CYTOCHROME P450
Anorexia nervosa	Phenytoin
Bulimia	Carbamazepine
HIV	Rifampicin
Cystic fibrosis	Phenobarbital
Malnourishment	Long-term ethanol ingestion

Greene et al. Postgrad Med J 2005;81:204–16 (published by BMJ group).[2]

toxicity. It can be applied only to a single acute overdose presenting within 16–24 hours.

If in doubt, commence treatment. NAC administration can be life saving, and adverse reactions and unpleasant side-effects are rare.

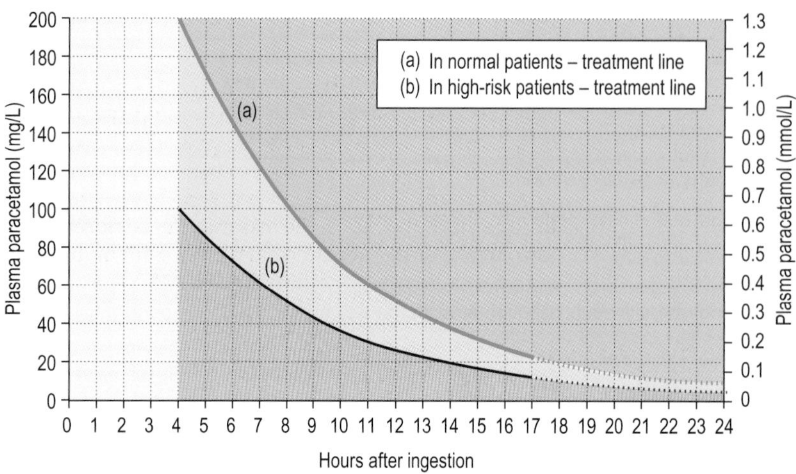

Figure 44.1.2 The Prescott nomogram.

It should be noted that negative paracetamol levels 16–24 hours after ingestion do not exclude the potential for hepatotoxicity. A staggered overdose is said to have occurred where there have been multiple ingestions over a period of time. Overdoses may be intentional or unintentional. Combined analgesics confer a risk of inadvertent overdose when they are abused for their narcotic content. A clear and detailed history is extremely important.

Patients with features of moderate or severe overdose should be managed in a critical care environment; the importance of early appropriate fluid resuscitation should not be underestimated. Contact should be made with a tertiary centre, and cases discussed with decision to transfer made in a timely fashion.

Early signs of nausea and vomiting after overdose are followed by signs of liver failure (see below) 48–72 hours after ingestion.

ACUTE VIRAL HEPATITIS

Acute viral hepatitis accounts for 40–70% of patients with ALF worldwide.

Acute hepatitis A (HAV) infection rarely leads to ALF (0.35% of infections), but continues to account for up to 10% of cases; morbidity increases with the age of infection. It is hoped that the prevalence will decrease with improving hygiene standards generally and the uptake of vaccination.

Acute hepatitis B (HBV) causes 25–75% of viral hepatitis-induced ALF. The liver injury is immunologically mediated with active destruction of infected hepatocytes. Diagnosis is by the presence of the IgM antibody (HBcAb) to hepatitis B core antigen. Hepatitis B surface antigen (HbsAg) is frequently negative by the time of presentation. Hepatitis B DNA should also be assayed. ALF may also be seen with hepatitis D, as either a co-infection or supra-infection.

Re-activation of hepatitis B is an increasing cause of ALF and should always be considered in a patient who has received steroids or chemotherapy. High-risk patients should be screened for sAg and HBV DNA and treated with antiviral agents if they are positive. This is a recognised problem in oncology and haematology but it is also a potential risk to patients in intensive care where steroids may be administered.

Hepatitis C (HCV) infection is commonly associated with chronic liver disease but *not* with ALF. It is detected by the presence of antibodies to HCV in serum. HCV-related cirrhosis will be discussed in detail in the subsequent chapter.

Hepatitis E (HEV), like hepatitis A, is transmitted via the faecal–oral route. It is particularly prevalent in the Indian subcontinent and Asia generally and is responsible for sporadic instances of ALF in the western world. It can be diagnosed by the detection of antibodies to HEV in serum.

Other viruses, such as herpes simplex 1 and 2, varicella zoster virus, cytomegalovirus, Epstein–Barr virus and measles virus, may all rarely cause ALF, but may be seen especially in the immunocompromised patient. Diagnosis is by serological and polymerase chain reaction (PCR) testing. Rift Valley fever, dengue, yellow fever, lassa fever and the haemorrhagic fevers should be considered in those who are at risk.

SERONEGATIVE HEPATITIS

Seronegative hepatitis (so called) is seen in patients in whom there are no identifiable viral causes or obvious candidate drugs. Such patients may present with a prodromal illness and with acute or subacute manifestations of the disease. Prognosis is less good than those with an identifiable virus and once they have poor prognostic criteria the chances of survival without liver transplant are exceptionally small. A subgroup may represent an acute autoimmune form of ALF, although many will not have any positive immune markers such as elevated IgG or positive smooth-muscle or liver kidney antibodies. The pattern of markers shows an increased incidence of autoantibody positivity in seronegative cases and viral cases with elevated IgM in viral causes.[3,4]

DRUG-INDUCED LIVER INJURY (DILI)

Drug-induced hepatitis is responsible for approximately 15–25% of cases of ALF. In some patients there appears to be a true hypersensitivity reaction, and symptoms develop after a sensitisation period of 1–5 weeks, recur promptly with re-administration of the drug and may be accompanied by fever, rash and eosinophilia. In others the clinical pattern is less acute. Some herbal remedies are implicated as putative hepatotoxins, but their role is made more difficult to assess by the variable nature of the constituent parts. Halothane hepatitis is now almost unheard of.

RECREATIONAL DRUGS AND LIVER FAILURE

Ecstasy (methylenedioxymethamphetamine) may cause ALF although, given the prevalence of exposure to the drug, the incidence is presumably low. Proposed mechanisms of injury include immune-mediated mechanisms and/or heatstroke. Cocaine use may result in ischaemic hepatitis. Yellow phosphorus, carbon tetrachloride, chloroform, trichloroethylene and xylene (glue sniffing) are very rare causes of ALF.

AMANITA PHALLOIDES

Mushroom poisoning can be seen even when only very small amounts have been ingested (e.g. *Amanita phalloides*). The initial presentation is often with diarrhoea. Patients subsequently develop signs of hepatic necrosis at 2–3 days after ingestion. The liver injury is caused by amatoxins. Forced diuresis may be helpful as large amounts of toxin are excreted in urine, but inadvertent dehydration may result in renal failure. Thioctic acid, silibinin (silybin) and penicillin have been advocated as therapy, but have not been subjected to controlled trials.

FULMINANT WILSON'S DISEASE

The characteristic features are those of cirrhosis, seen on imaging, with concomitant problems such as thrombocytopenia that may be long-standing, Kayser-Fleischer rings on examination and frequently non-immune-mediated haemolysis.

ACUTE BUDD–CHIARI SYNDROME (HEPATIC VENOUS OBSTRUCTION)

Hepatic venous obstruction (Budd-Chiari syndrome) may cause ALF. There are symptoms and signs of liver of necrosis, often with capsular pain from congestion and ascites. In Asia this may be associated with anatomical anomalies of the inferior vena cava, whereas in Europe and the USA the experience is normally of thrombosis of the hepatic veins, often with an underlying procoagulant condition (**Fig. 44.1.3**).

ISCHAEMIC HEPATITIS

Heat shock injury is now relatively rarely seen but ischaemic hepatitis remains relatively common. They are normally associated with a congested liver that is subjected to a secondary insult - hypoxia or decreased-flow arterial inflow. This is seen with hypoxaemic respiratory failure, cardiac arrhythmias and hypotension.

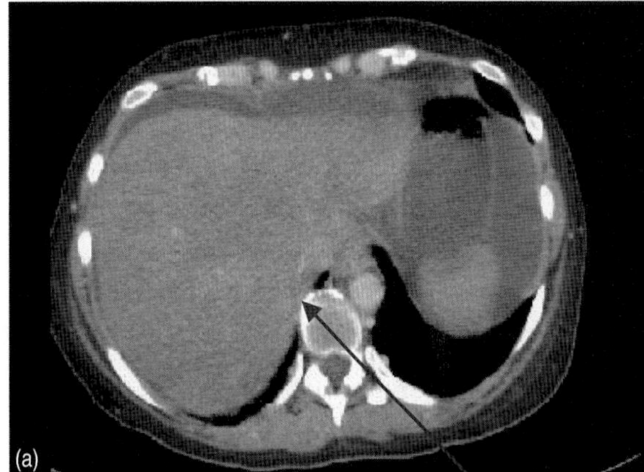

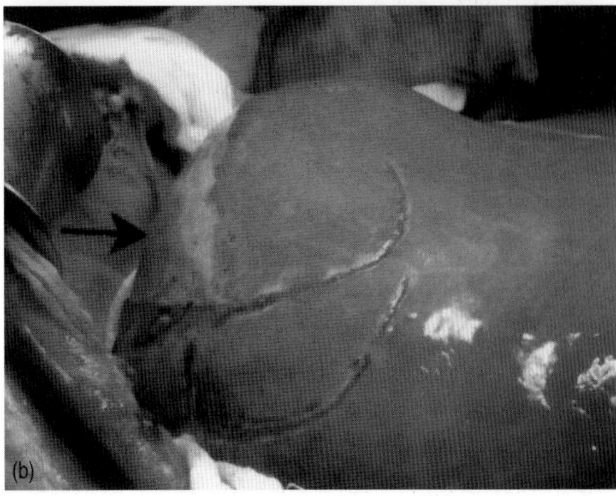

Figure 44.1.3 (a) Acute Budd–Chiari syndrome: The intrahepatic IVC is grossly attenuated. (b) Budd-Chiari liver: The arrow shows liver necrosis; ischaemic/infarcted liver.

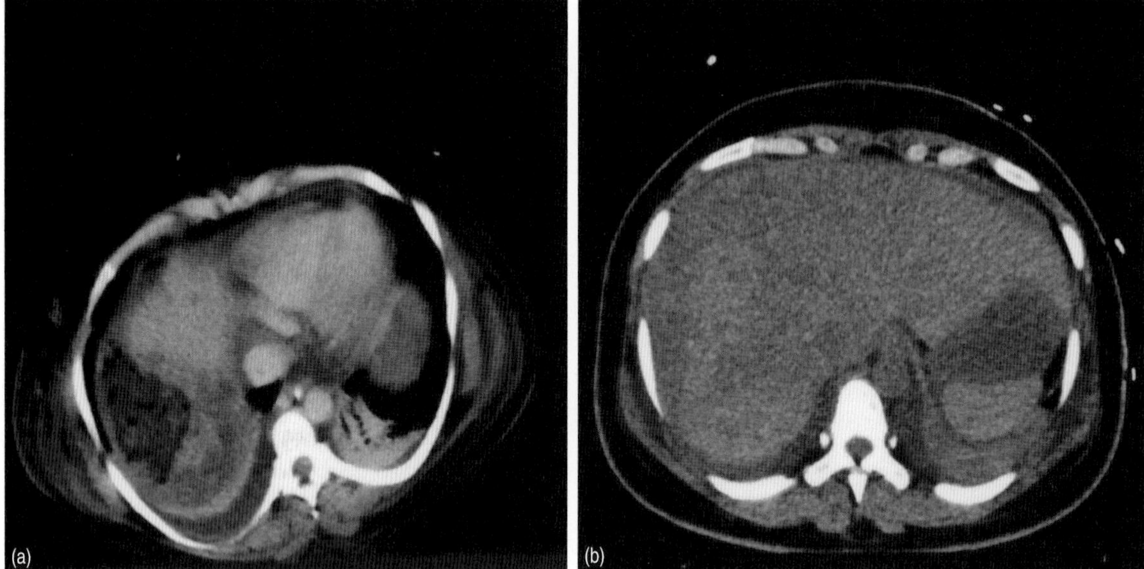

Figure 44.1.4 Liver CT in pregnancy-related liver disease demonstrating abnormal perfusion (a and b) with rupture, packing (a) and associated areas of infarction. Major bleeding into the liver.

PREGNANCY-RELATED ACUTE LIVER FAILURE

Pregnancy-related liver failure includes HELLP (**h**aemolysis (microangiopathic haemolytic anaemia), **e**levated **l**iver enzymes and **l**ow **p**latelets), acute fatty liver of pregnancy and liver rupture, often in association with pre-eclampsia. The prognosis of pregnancy-related ALF is usually good, although some develop severe liver injury with small-vessel disease, liver ruptures may require packing and occasionally transplantation is required (**Fig. 44.1.4**)

MALIGNANCY

Malignancy may also present with ALF, albeit rarely. The clinical pattern normally is that of elevated biliary enzymes in addition to the transaminases. This pattern of disease may be seen in those with hepatic lymphoma, often with an elevated lactate dehydrogenase or indeed with diffuse infiltration with other malignancies.

CLINICAL FEATURES

JAUNDICE

The classification above uses the time from jaundice to encephalopathy to describe ALF as either hyperacute, acute or subacute. In hyperacute liver failure (paracetamol toxicity, *Amanita* poisoning, acute viral hepatitis), encephalopathy may precede the onset of clinical jaundice.

Acute liver failure is frequently accompanied by a rapidly progressive syndrome of multi-organ failure requiring high levels of organ support.

HEPATIC ENCEPHALOPATHY

Hepatic encephalopathy is described by the modified Parsons–Smith scale (**Table 44.1.5**), which is based on functional impairment, changes in consciousness, cognitive function and behavior. The presence of encephalopathy is essential for a diagnosis of acute liver failure.

INTRACRANIAL HYPERTENSION

Hepatic encephalopathy is frequently complicated by cerebral oedema and intracranial hypertension with diminished cerebral perfusion and a risk of transtentorial herniation. The onset is rapid and allows little time for adaptive mechanisms (in contrast to patients with chronic liver disease where there is time for adaptation and control of cellular osmolarity). This has a significant implication in terms of the transfer of patients with ALF between hospitals. Intubation and ventilation with adequate sedation and implementation of neuroprotective strategies (see below) should be considered prior to transfer in any patient with progressive encephalopathy.

Patients with high-grade encephalopathy (coma) are at greatest risk of developing cerebral oedema. Elevated arterial ammonia levels, a higher MELD (model for end-stage liver disease) score, younger age, and requirement for vasopressor and renal replacement therapy are independent risk factors for hepatic encephalopathy and arterial ammonia levels >200 μmol/L are associated with cerebral herniation.[5,6]

Ammonia is produced by bacteria in the bowel and is taken up by cerebral astrocytes for deamination to

Table 44.1.5 Modified Parsons–Smith scale of hepatic encephalopathy

GRADE	CLINICAL FEATURES	NEUROLOGICAL SIGNS	GLASGOW COMA SCORE
0/subclinical	Normal	Seen only on neuropsychometric testing	15
1	Trivial lack of awareness, shortened attention span	Tremor, apraxia, incoordination	15
2	Lethargy, disorientation, personality change	Asterixis, ataxia, dysarthria	11–15
3	Confusion, somnolence to semi-stupor, responsive to stimuli	Asterixis, ataxia	8–11
4	Coma	±Decerebration	<8

glutamine. Water then moves into the intracellular compartment down its osmotic gradient. There are also induced changes in neurotransmitter synthesis and release, mitochondrial function and neuronal oxidative stress. The net result is astrocyte swelling and cerebral oedema.[7,8]

The association between the development of encephalopathy and markers of inflammation is well demonstrated, both in regard to systemic inflammatory response syndrome (SIRS) markers and inflammatory mediators such as tumour necrosis factor.[9,10] Curiously, a similar relationship between inflammation and encephalopathy is seen in patients with CLD.[11] What is not yet clear is whether treatments that modulate the inflammatory response will be of benefit. This and other avenues proposed from basic animal research may well result in several novel approaches to the treatment of cerebral oedema and possibly encephalopathy over the forthcoming years.

Blood–brain barrier injury, increased cerebral blood flow and hyperemia accompanying astrocyte swelling can potentiate cerebral oedema independently of astrocyte glutamine concentration. Thus, cerebral oedema may be vasogenic with inflammatory disruption of the blood–brain barrier or cytotoxic with osmotic dysregulation.

Blood flow is intimately coupled to cerebral metabolic rate, arterial oxygen and carbon dioxide tensions and acid–base status. The 'toxic liver hypothesis' describes the situation whereby there is a massive release of pro-inflammatory cytokines in association with the profound systemic inflammatory response and accumulation of toxic metabolites that accompanies acute liver failure. Altered cerebral blood flow and loss of autoregulation occurs in the face of this inflammatory milieu.

The Munro–Kellie hypothesis states that the intracranial cavity is essentially an incompressible box and that any increase in the volume of one of the intracranial components (blood, brain, CSF) must be accompanied by a decrease in the volume of another. CT studies have demonstrated effacement and ventricular attenuation are frequent radiological findings.

Diencephalic transtentorial herniation causes posterior cerebral artery insufficiency with temporal, thalamic, and occipital infarction; obstructive hydrocephalus; and brainstem ischaemia, compression and death.

The normal range for intracranial pressure is between 7–15 mmHg (0.93–2 kPa) in the supine adult. Many definitions of intracranial hypertension have been volunteered, but a pressure of >20 mmHg (2.66 kPa) for a period of 20 minutes should be considered worthy of treatment. The USALFG (US acute liver failure study group) recommend osmotic therapy for patients with an ICP >25 mmHg (3.33 kPa).[12]

The clinical management of the cerebral complications of ALF has been developed pragmatically and by the extrapolation of data from the neurosurgical literature. The use of intracranial pressure monitoring is controversial. Advocates would point out that clonus, brisk reflexes and hypertonicity can be detected clinically, but pupillary changes, systemic hypertension and reflex bradycardia are not apparent until intracranial hypertension is established, and that radiographic changes are non-specific. Sceptics would point out that there is no RCT evidence supporting an outcome benefit associated with intracranial pressure monitoring in ALF and that insertion confers a risk of intracranial haemorrhage. The USALFG found bleeding complications in up to 10% of patients, although many institutions use parenchymal monitors, which may be more accurate but confer a higher bleeding risk. At the authors' institution, standard practice is to use an epidural bolt – which may be slightly less accurate but confers a bleed rate of <1%. Bleeding associated with monitor insertion may be minimised by appropriate coagulation support at the time of placement. Some centres support coagulation at the time of insertion with plasma products and platelets whereas others use recombinant factor VII.

Standard practice in the authors' institution is that patients whose conscious level deteriorates to grade 3/4 coma are electively intubated, sedated and ventilated. A combination of opiate (e.g. fentanyl) and propofol is commonly used. The decision to move to ICP

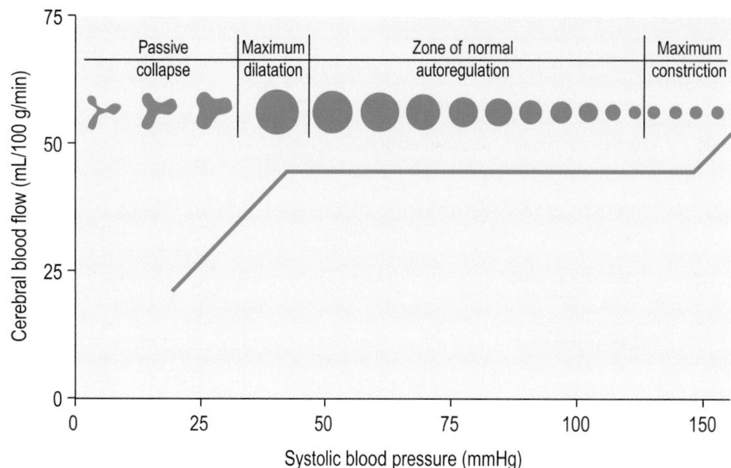

Figure 44.1.5 The relationship between SBP and CBF. Autoregulation may be lost, however, with flow pathologically dependent on pressure.

monitoring is highly individual and is supported by a hyperacute presentation, younger age and higher arterial ammonia levels (>150 mmol/L). Decision making is frequently supported by reverse jugular venous oximetry and Doppler estimation of middle cerebral arterial flow.

A cerebral perfusion pressure of >50 mmHg (6.66 kPa) has been suggested as optimal. It is of note that patients with ALF often do not autoregulate to pressure and consequently increases in blood pressure may be associated with increased cerebral blood flow and potentially increased ICP, particularly if they are at a critical point on their pressure–volume curve. Sustained cerebral perfusion pressures <40 mmHg (5.33 kPa) have been associated with very poor outcomes in some studies,[13] whereas others report good outcome despite periods of cerebral hypoperfusion (**Fig. 44.1.5**).

Invasive cardiovascular monitoring is mandatory (the authors advocate flow monitoring to guide fluid resuscitation). Norepinephrine (noradrenaline) and vasopressin are commonly used pressor agents. The use of terlipressin was associated with a rise in intracranial pressure in one study.[11]

In most patients, maintenance of P_{CO_2} 4.5–5.0 kPa is considered ideal. Cerebral blood flow is intimately coupled to arterial carbon dioxide tension and minute ventilation must therefore be carefully controlled. Lung injury/ARDS is relatively common and so protective ventilation strategies should be utilised.

Hyponatraemia and hyperammonaemia have been shown to be detrimental, whereas a randomised controlled trial showed benefit to the patients whose serum Na was maintained between 140 and 150 mmol/L. The use of hypertonic saline has been associated with a significant reduction in ICP, although the same study was not powered to detect a difference in outcome.

First-line treatment of a sustained rise in ICP remains mannitol 0.5 g/kg given as a bolus with an appropriate subsequent diuresis. It is essential that serum osmolarity is maintained at less than 320 mOsm to avoid damage to the blood–brain barrier and worsening of vasogenic oedema. Hypertonic saline is increasingly used in this setting.

Hypothermia has been shown to reduce cerebral blood flow, ICP and cerebral ammonia uptake.[14,15] The role of hypothermia as an early preventive intervention in grade III/IV coma is contentious and the results of controlled studies are awaited. Fever should be avoided.

Other treatment options that have been shown to be potentially beneficial are thiopental and intravenous indomethacin (0.5 mg/kg).[16] Potential monitoring and treatment algorithms, as used by this unit, are detailed in **Figure 44.1.6**.

SEPSIS

Sepsis is common in ALF and both culture-positive and negative SIRS are seen. Patients are functionally immunosuppressed in terms of impaired cell-mediated immunity, complement levels and phagocytosis.[17] Functional immmunoparesis can only be observed and depression of human leucocyte antigen (HLA) DR expression correlates with prognosis and severity of liver injury.[18,19] As such, scrupulous attention with regard to hand washing and line care needs to be applied to decrease the risk of nosocomial infection. Regular culture screens are required and antimicrobials are indicated in patients with any clinical suggestion of sepsis. Prophylactic intravenous antifungals should be considered, especially in those listed for transplantation. The choice of antimicrobial agent should be driven by local resistance patterns. Antimicrobial therapy should be reviewed in the light of culture results on a daily basis.

COAGULOPATHY

Coagulopathy is the hallmark of ALF, with prolongation predominantly of the prothrombin time and to lesser degrees the activated partial thromboplastin ratio

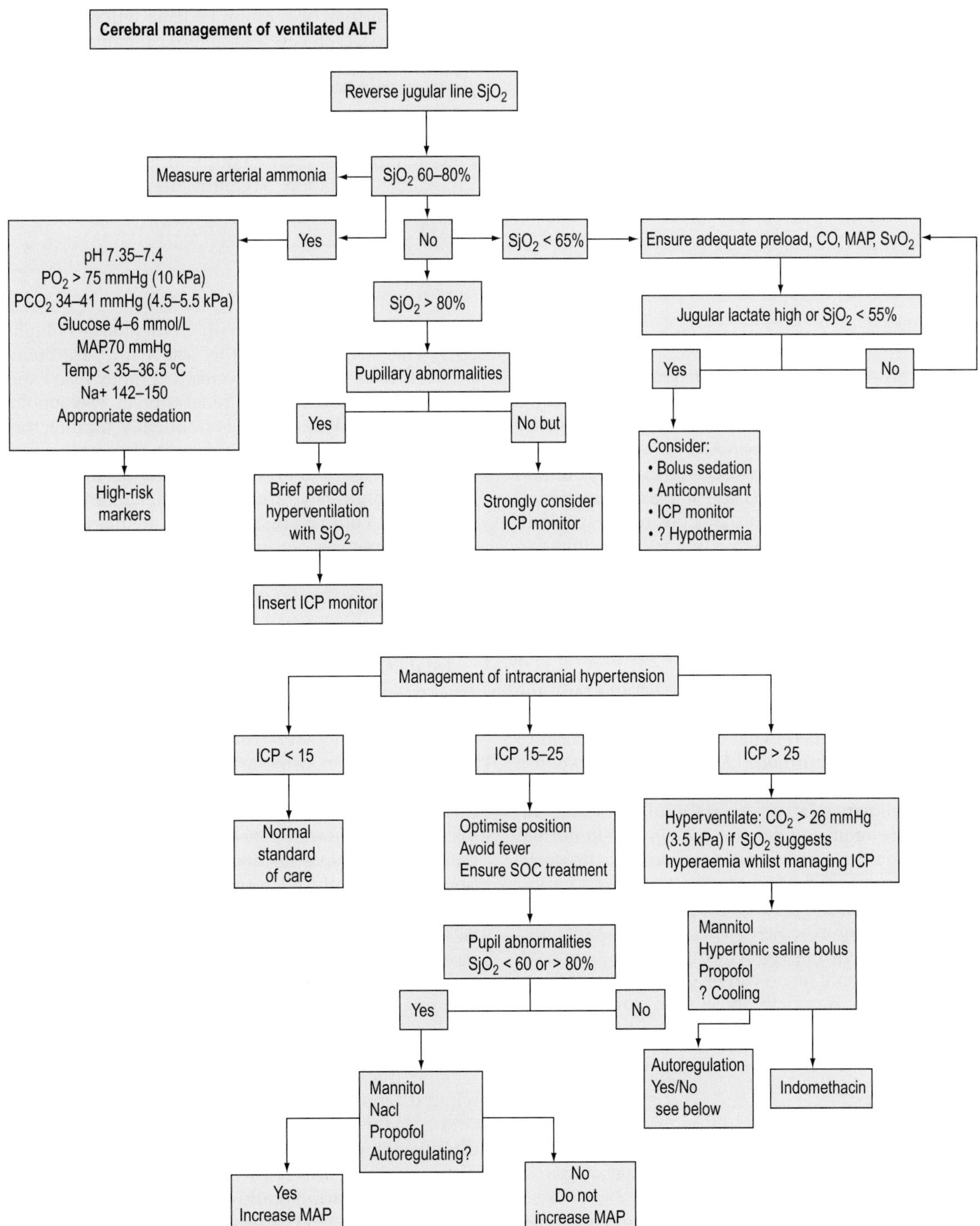

Figure 44.1.6 Treatment of raised intracranial pressure.

(APTR). In a small percentage of patients the coagulopathy will respond, at least partially, to vitamin K. Intravenous vitamin K 10 mg is normally administered. Thrombocytopenia is common and frequently consumptive in nature. Bleeding is rare, although may be seen in those with severe prolongation of APTR, low fibrinogen and severe thrombocytopenia. Coagulation or repletion of coagulation factors is necessary for clinical bleeding and prophylactically before major invasive procedures. Coagulation support is normally not given routinely so that the international normalised ratio (INR) can be monitored with regard to prognosis.

CARDIOVASCULAR CONSIDERATIONS

Patients with ALF develop a hyperdynamic circulation with peripheral vasodilation and central volume depletion. Hypotension is common and may initially respond to volume repletion. Assessment of volume responsiveness in the clinical setting may be difficult and pressure measurements are a poor indicator of volume status. Hypotension that does not respond to volume will normally require some form of invasive haemodynamic monitoring and frequently institution of vasopressor agents. Increasingly it is recognised that volume responsiveness, as in general intensive care unit patients, is best determined by dynamic rather than static variables.

The requirement for pressor agents should raise the possibility of adrenal dysfunction. Patients with ALF have been demonstrated to have impaired responses to adrenocorticotropic hormone (ACTH).[20,21] The response at 30 and 60 minutes in terms of cortisol should be examined following 250 μg ACTH in all patients with ALF who are requiring pressor agents. A subnormal response should result in consideration of hydrocortisone replacement therapy, normally given for a period of 10 days. Interestingly, adrenal dysfunction has similarly been reported in acute-on-chronic liver failure and steroid replacement may result in improved outcome.[21,22]

Elevated troponin levels can be observed in patients with liver failure, especially those with cardiovascular failure.[23]

RESPIRATORY CONSIDERATIONS

Ventilatory support is frequently required in patients with ALF, usually because of decreased conscious level rather than hypoxia, at least in the initial stages of disease.

Common respiratory complications are pleural effusions, atelectasis and intrapulmonary shunts. Acute respiratory distress syndrome (ARDS) and acute lung injury may be seen and can be precipitated by extrapulmonary sepsis or inflammation.

Ventilatory strategies are influenced by both the respiratory and the multiorgan involvement that is characteristic of ALF. Thus patients with deep levels of coma and at risk of cerebral oedema will require close attention to CO_2 levels and tailored sedation regimens. Hypercapnia may have to be tolerated in patients progressing to ARDS. This requires balancing against the cerebral needs of these patients as hypercarbia and increased cerebral blood flow will tend to increase ICP. Pleural effusions may require drainage if they are impeding ventilation. Weaning may be facilitated by undertaking tracheostomy during the recovery period of ALF.

RENAL CONSIDERATIONS

Renal failure is common, with an incidence as high as 50%. This is particularly the case with paracetamol-induced liver failure, where the drug may also exert a directly toxic effect on the renal tubule. The aetiology of acute renal dysfunction is frequently multifactorial, with hepatorenal failure being a rare occurrence. Acute tubular necrosis and pre-renal renal failure are common. As such, volume therapy and maintenance of intrathoracic blood volume are essential in the management of such patients, as is the avoidance of nephrotoxins. Intra-abdominal hypertension is frequent and may reduce renal perfusion pressure and contribute to renal dysfunction; the measurement of intra-abdominal pressure may be a valuable component of monitoring.

Established renal failure requires the institution of renal replacement therapy (RRT). In patients with ALF early consideration should be given to RRT to control fluid balance and acid–base disturbances and to avoid rapid changes in osmolarity. It may limit or control elevations of arterial ammonia and retard the development of cerebral complications. The haemodynamic instability and associated cerebral complications of this patient group have resulted in the application of continuous modes of RRT rather than intermittent haemodialysis. Inability of the liver to metabolise and utilise lactate or acetate buffer solutions results in the use of bicarbonate buffers.

A balance needs to be achieved between risk of bleeding and platelet protection across an extracorporeal filter. A prostaglandin such as epoprostenol may be advantageous in terms of decreasing bleeding and prolonging filter life. Alternatively, circuits may be run without anticoagulation, with regional heparin or citrate or low-dose systemic heparin. In patients with thrombocytopenia, consideration should be given to the diagnosis of heparin-induced thrombocytopenia and, if confirmed, heparin should be withdrawn and circuits primed with an alternative agent (e.g. danaparoid).

METABOLISM AND FEEDING

Enteral nutrition should commence as soon as feasible after admission if there are no contraindications. In patients with large aspirates (>200 mL/4 h) a prokinetic agent should be commenced: erythromycin

(250 mg intravenously 6-hourly) appears to be more effective than metoclopramide. Endoscopic placement of a post-pyloric feeding tube should be considered in refractory cases, although this may need to be delayed in patients with or at risk of cerebral oedema. In patients with profound coagulopathy, placement of a nasogastric tube may be associated with nasal/pharyngeal bleeding and oral tube placement may be preferred in ventilated patients. The optimal nature of enteral feed used has not been investigated but metabolic data on these patients demonstrate increased calorific requirements.[24,25] Patients with ALF demonstrate both peripheral and hepatological insulin resistance.[26] Tight glycaemic control would seem reasonable in this population.

Metabolic acidosis is a relatively frequent occurrence that may relate to lactic acidosis, hyperchloraemic acidosis or renal failure.

Hyperlactataemia may be secondary to volume depletion and hence will resolve with appropriate fluid loading or may reflect the inability of the liver to metabolise the lactate produced. A failure of blood lactate to normalise following volume loading is associated with a poor prognosis.[26,27] Metabolic acidosis may be a secondary effect of other drugs ingested as part of an episode of self-harm. Falls in serum phosphate levels are seen in ALF associated with liver regeneration and are associated with a good prognosis in paracetamol-induced ALF.[28] Pancreatitis is a common complication of ALF and should be actively sought.

SPECIFIC TREATMENTS

The management of ALF is largely supportive, providing an optimal environment for either regeneration or stability until a suitable liver becomes available. Once patients develop poor prognostic criteria the chances of effective liver regeneration and thus of spontaneous recovery are low; the prognosis is very poor without liver transplantation. The role of extracorporeal liver support systems remains a hope for the future but at present no system has been shown to have a definitive survival benefit in a controlled trial.

- *N*-acetylcysteine is administered for paracetamol-induced ALF, as mentioned above. Its role in non-paracetamol-induced ALF remains undefined although a US study[29] suggests that it may be of benefit in patients with ALF and grade 1–2 encephalopathy (presumably because transplantation is required to impact on outcome when higher grades of encephalopathy are achieved).
- Chelating agents are not of benefit in patients with established ALF secondary to Wilson's disease but play an important role in chronic presentations. Withdrawal of such treatments, or indeed non-compliance, especially in teenagers, may precipitate ALF.
- Antiviral therapy has a predominant role in preventing re-activation of hepatitis B in patients exposed to chemotherapy and steroids.
- Thrombolytic therapies may be of benefit in patients with early acute Budd–Chiari syndrome, although increasingly the treatment option would be to undertake a transhepatic portosystemic shunt (TIPS) shunt, decompressing the liver with a stent passed either through the hepatic vein (if the clot is soft enough) or via the inferior vena cava and through to the portal vein. Such procedures should be undertaken in units with the facilities to transplant as there is a risk of precipitating ALF. Chemotherapy may be offered to those with lymphoma involving the liver and in these instances tissue is paramount, either of liver or from another diagnostic site.
- Steroid therapy is beneficial in acute autoimmune hepatitis but its role in autoimmune ALF has been less clear. A recent publication from the Paris group suggests that steroids for those with established ALF are potentially detrimental.[30]

PROGNOSIS

Prognostication is important in the management of ALF. It is essential to identify those patients who will not survive without liver transplant but also to identify those who will succumb even if offered such a procedure.[31] Several risk stratification systems are presented in **Box 44.1.2**. The most commonly used are those of

Box 44.1.2 Prognostic criteria for acute liver failure

O'Grady criteria

Paracetamol-related

Acidosis (pH <7.3), *or*

Prothrombin time of >100 seconds (INR >6.5), creatinine >300 mol/L and grade III/IV encephalopathy – all occurring within a 24-hour timeframe

Non-paracetamol-related

Any three of the following in association with encephalopathy:

- Age less than 10 or greater than 40 years
- Bilirubin >300 mol/L
- Time from jaundice to encephalopathy >7 days
- Aetiology: either non-A, non-B (seronegative hepatitis) *or* drug-induced
- Prothrombin time >50 seconds, *or*
- Prothrombin time >100 seconds/INR >6.5

French criteria (Clichy criteria)

The criteria are the presence of encephalopathy (coma or confusion), *and*

Age <20 years with factor V level <20%, *or*

Factor V levels <30% if greater than 30 years of age 59

INR = international normalised ratio.

O'Grady and Clichy. The model for end-stage liver disease (MELD) has also been examined with regard to prognosis in ALF and may be particularly useful in non-paracetamol cases.[32] It is essential that such systems are rigorously applied and in the context of paracetamol are only utilised at least 24 hours post-ingestion and following appropriate volume resuscitation.

Access the complete references list online at http://www.expertconsult.com

5. Bernal W, Hall C, Karvellas CJ, et al. Arterial ammonia and clinical risk factors for encephalopathy and intracranial hypertension in acute liver failure. Hepatology 2007;46:1844–52.
10. Vaquero J, Polson J, Chung C, et al. Infection and the progression of hepatic encephalopathy in acute liver failure. Gastroenterology 2003;125:755–64.
12. Stravitz RT, Kramer AH, Davern T, et al; the Acute Liver Failure Study Group. Intensive care of patients with acute liver failure: recommendations of the U.S. Acute Liver Failure Study Group. Crit Care Med 2007;35(11):2498–508.

44.2 Cirrhosis and acute-on-chronic liver disease

Chronic liver disease is said to be evident when liver dysfunction has been present for a period >6 months. It presents far more commonly to the intensive care unit than does acute liver failure. Acute decompensations in hepatic and extrahepatic organ function in the previously stable cirrhotic are frequently precipitated by infection and bleeding (often variceal), but may also reflect a trajectory of decline in liver function in a patient with end-stage disease. Acute decompensations are termed *acute on chronic liver failure* (ACLF).

AETIOLOGY OF CHRONIC LIVER DISEASE

There are myriad causes of chronic liver disease. Those most frequently encountered are listed in **Box 44.2.1**. It is beyond the scope of this chapter to discuss these in any depth – but we will focus on the management of decompensations, complications and extrahepatic organ failure.

The ICU physician is seldom involved in the management of stable chronic liver disease. Acute on chronic presentations are relatively common, however, and patients with previously unrecognised cirrhosis may decompensate following unrelated medical interventions. Wherever possible, planned interventions in patients with documented cirrhosis should be undertaken in specialist centres with appropriated periprocedural supervision.

Box 44.2.1 Common aetiologies of chronic liver disease

- Chronic infection with hepatitis B and C viruses
- Alcohol
- Primary biliary cirrhosis
- Autoimmune chronic active hepatitis
- Primary sclerosing cholangitis
- Budd–Chiari syndrome
- Veno-occlusive disease
- Amyloidosis
- α_1-antitrypsin deficiency
- Wilson's disease

DECOMPENSATED CHRONIC LIVER DISEASE

ACLF commonly presents with one of the following:

- encephalopathy
- sepsis
- renal failure
- variceal bleeding
- cardiorespiratory failure.

The cause of decompensation should be sought in all cases when it is not clinically apparent. In addition to sepsis and bleeding, alcohol, dehydration, drug therapies (e.g. opiates and sedatives), hepatocellular carcinoma (HCC) and portal vein thrombosis should be considered. Ultrasound should be undertaken in all patients, examining the hepatic veins and portal veins for patency. In patients with ascites a diagnostic tap should always be undertaken for microbiological culture and cell count (a polymorphonuclear count >250/mm^3 is indicative of bacterial peritonitis).

Signs of HCC should be sought on ultrasound, alphafetoprotein and axial imaging techniques. The therapies available for HCC have improved dramatically in recent years and prognosis can be good, especially with the option of cure with liver transplantation.

ENCEPHALOPATHY IN CHRONIC LIVER DISEASE

Hepatic encephalopathy is frequently seen in patients with cirrhosis and a systemic inflammatory response (and so sepsis should be actively sought and treated). Encephalopathy in chronic liver disease has pathophysiological and clinical features that are different from those seen in acute liver failure. Importantly, the cirrhotic cohort does not normally develop intracranial hypertension and as such the management centres on prevention of encephalopathy, the treatment of worsening encephalopathy and control of the airway and prevention of aspiration in those who are deeply encephalopathic.

Ammonia levels are frequently (but not always) elevated in encephalopathy and thus therapy includes bowel cleansing with agents such as lactulose and non-absorbable antibiotics such as rifaximin. There is little evidence-based research to support any particular avenue of treatment. A trial examining the role of albumin dialysis in the management of encephalopathy has been recently completed.[1]

As noted previously, the role of inflammation seems of importance in the development of encephalopathy.[2,3] As many as 70% of patients with bacteraemia demonstrate a 'septic encephalopathy' which manifests as lethargy, confusion, agitation or even coma. There is some evidence that pro-inflammatory mediators mobilised during systemic inflammatory response syndrome (SIRS)/sepsis modulate the action of ammonia on the brain. Shawcross et al in 2004[3] demonstrated that neuropsychological test scores deteriorate when hyperammonaemia is induced in cirrhotics with infection, during the inflammatory state, but not following its resolution. This synergism may be attributed to a number of possible mechanisms:[4]

- Higher levels of inflammatory cytokines such as IL-1, IL-6 and TNFα (see above) may act via activation of vagal afferents in the periphery, via cytokine receptors on the cerebral endothelial cell or have direct action on astrocytes
- The generation of reactive oxygen species and nitric oxide in astrocytes in hyperammonaemia and sepsis[4] with diminished activity of antioxidant enzymes[5]
- Dysregulation of cerebral blood flow, which occurs in cirrhosis, may be exaggerated in sepsis.

The prognosis in cirrhotic patients with sepsis is considerably worse following the onset of encephalopathy.

The role of feeding in the development of encephalopathy has always caused controversy. Recent guidance suggests that protein restriction is not appropriate and a study examining early versus slow introduction of protein into enteral nutrition showed no increase in encephalopathy and indeed appeared beneficial in respect of nitrogen balance.[6,7]

SEPSIS IN CHRONIC LIVER DISEASE

A classical definition of sepsis is SIRS in response to a proven or suspected microbial event. This definition may not be universally applicable, however. The compensated and decompensated cirrhotic may demonstrate components of SIRS under resting conditions. For example, cirrhotics often have an elevated resting heart rate with a hyperdynamic circulation, hyperventilation due to the evolution of hepatic encephalopathy and reduced baseline polymorphonuclear (PMN) count owing to hypersplenism. Indeed, the response of the cirrhotic patient to infection may be characterised only by an exacerbation of circulatory changes already present at baseline or may be distinctly uncharacteristic with, for example, blunting of the elevation in body temperature that is usually seen in sepsis.

The mortality of cirrhotic patients who fulfil SIRS criteria is significantly higher than in those who do not[8] and a majority of those with SIRS have intercurrent infection. It is often unclear whether SIRS acts as a predisposition to or is a consequence of infection in this cohort. In one retrospective analysis of non-transplanted patients with acute on chronic liver failure, bacteraemia was associated with increased illness severity, requirements for organ support, and mortality.[9] The same group found that severity of hepatic encephalopathy and SIRS score >1 were predictive of bacteraemia.[10]

Bacterial infections are more common in cirrhosis than in the general population, and are higher still during episodes of decompensation. Cirrhotic individuals are significantly more likely to die while hospitalised (adjusted risk ratio (RR) 2.7), to have hospitalisations associated with sepsis (adjusted RR 2.6) and to die from sepsis (adjusted RR 2.0).[11]

The increased incidence of sepsis in those with underlying liver disease is multifactorial. Patients are frequently physically debilitated, deconditioned, malnourished and cachectic. Bactericidal and opsonic activity is reduced. Monocyte function is altered and there is depression of the phagocytic activity of the reticuloendothelial system owing to the presence of intra- and extrahepatic shunts through sinusoids without Kupffer cells, and reduced Kupffer cell numbers and function.[12] Serum complement levels are low. Ascites and peripheral oedema are often present. Iatrogenic factors may be contributory. There may be an associated genetic susceptibility to severe infection and sepsis.

The acquisition of a sepsis syndrome is frequently accompanied by encephalopathy, renal failure and worsening coagulopathy. The in-hospital mortality of septic cirrhotics is, accordingly, much higher and has been recently estimated at 70%[13] and infection is responsible for 30–50% of deaths in patients with cirrhosis.[14]

The main sites of infection in cirrhosis are ascites, urinary tract, lungs and blood. The commonest organisms are *Escherichia coli*, followed by *Staphylococcus aureus*, *Enterococcus faecalis*, *Streptococcus pneumoniae*, *Pseudomonas aeruginosa*, and *Staphylococcus epidermidis*. However, resistant Gram-positive organisms and extended spectrum beta lactamase (ESBL)-producing enterobacteria are becoming increasingly common (particularly in nosocomial infection). Cephalosporins therefore fail in a substantial proportion of infections acquired during hospitalisation.

The epidemiology of sepsis in cirrhosis is in a state of flux. Resistant organisms are increasing in prevalence both in nosocomial infection and in patients who require long-term antibacterial prophylaxis. Liver transplantation programmes have given chronic cirrhotics a chance of salvation, and encourage physicians to treat episodes of sepsis more aggressively than ever before. Surveillance and early diagnosis of infection, coupled with adequate and appropriate antibiosis have led to improved outcomes in cirrhotic patients with spontaneous bacterial peritonitis (SBP) and other severe infections.

An enhanced inflammatory response can cause an exaggerated and damaging inflammatory response that may provoke single of multiple organ failures. Organ failure is an important determinant of outcome in patients with cirrhosis, with mortality increasing with the number of organ systems failing. Single-organ failure carries confers a mortality of 33%, double-organ failures a mortality of 73% and three-organ failure a mortality of 97%.[15,16]

Tissue hypoperfusion occurs secondary to systemic hypotension, microvascular dysfunction, shunting, microthrombi formation, vasoplegia, and reduced RBC deformity and tissue oedema. Nitric oxide (NO) synthesis may be responsible for defective mitochondrial respiration. Direct tissue damage is caused by cellular infiltrates, particularly neutrophils releasing lysosomal enzymes and superoxide-derived free radicals.[17]

PATHOPHYSIOLOGY OF SEPSIS IN CIRRHOSIS

ENDOTOXIN SIGNALLING

Lipopolysaccharide (LPS) found on the outer membrane of Gram-negative bacteria and peptidoglycan (PGN) and lipopeptide (LP) from Gram-positive bacteria stimulate Toll-like receptors (TLRs). The interaction of ligand with receptor triggers innate pro-inflammatory signalling cascades[18] with rapid cytokine and chemokine release (**Fig. 44.2.1**).

The Gram-negative flora of the intestine provides a reservoir of LPS. LPS is absorbed and transported in the portal vein where it is rapidly cleared by Kupffer cells. Under normal circumstances the liver does not show signs of excessive inflammation. In addition to its ability to clear LPS, the liver also responds to LPS with the production of cytokines and reactive oxygen intermediates, primarily by Kupffer cells.

In many types of chronic liver disease, levels of endotoxin[19] are elevated and tend to increase progressively as liver function deteriorates. Mortality is higher in patients with significant endotoxaemia than in those without.[20]

Cytokines such as TNFα, IL-6, and IL-1 are essential components of the immune defence mechanism, but may propagate overwhelming septic shock. These may be over-produced and/or up-regulated in chronic liver

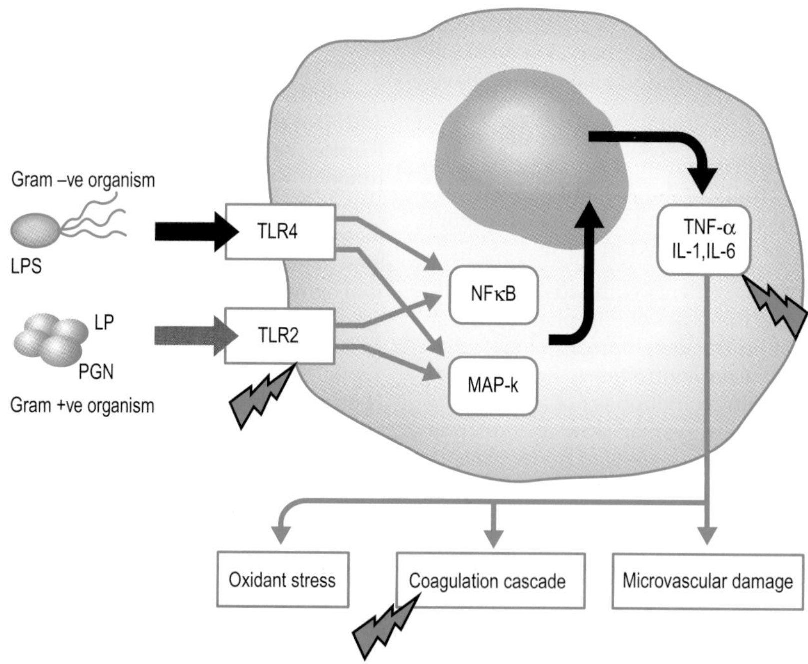

Figure 44.2.1 Endotoxin signalling pathway. The flashpoints represent changes in cirrhosis that make patients more susceptible to infection. LPS=lipopolysaccharide; LP=lipopeptide; PGN=peptidoglycan; TLR=Toll-like receptor; TNF=tumour necrosis factor; IL=interleukin; NFκB=nuclear factor-κB; MAP =membrane-associated protein. *(Reproduced with permission from Wong F, Bernardi M, Balk R, et al; International Ascites Club. Sepsis in cirrhosis: report on the 7th meeting of the International Ascites Club. Gut 2005;54:718–25.)*

disease, although the absolute levels of inflammatory cytokines are extremely variable in cirrhotic cohorts with septic complications. NO production is enhanced in cirrhosis, and is further increased in sepsis, with the induction of nitric oxide synthase (NOS) by LPS.

BACTERIAL TRANSLOCATION

Bacterial translocation is the migration of bacteria or bacterial products from the intestinal lumen to mesenteric lymph nodes or other extraintestinal organs and sites.[21] As mentioned above, elevated levels of endotoxin are a frequent finding in chronic liver disease, and levels tend to increase with disease severity (Child classification). Chromogenic assay in patients undergoing angiographic intervention demonstrates a gradient in terms of endotoxin level between portal and systemic circulations,[22] suggesting that the bowel is the source of the endotoxaemia.

Small bowel hypomotility, alterations in intestinal flora and disruption of mucosal barrier function promote bacterial translocation in the cirrhotic population. It is proposed that bacterial translocation is one of the main causes of spontaneous infection in this cohort and may perpetuate the persistent hyperdynamic state. Portal hypertension, ascites and increased severity of liver dysfunction are risk factors for bacterial translocation in this cohort. The epithelium demonstrates structural changes in cirrhosis, with widening of the intercellular spaces, and there is increased intestinal permeability.[23] Intestinal permeability is increased with portal hypertension (NO may be implicated in disruption of the intestinal epithelium).[24] Permeability is increased further if there is concomitant alcohol intake.

Organisms are usually removed from intestinal tissue by phagocytes. The intestinal immune system is centred on the gut-associated lymphoid tissue (GALT), which is comprised of Peyer's patches, lamina propria lymphocytes, intraepithelial lymphocytes, and mesenteric lymph nodes. The innate immune response is centred on stimulation of TLRs, a cytokine response and bacterial killing by monocytes and lamina propria lymphocytes. Under normal circumstances, any organism breaching the intestinal mucosal barrier is killed. Thus, in order for translocation to become clinically significant, there needs to be an overall failure of local and systemic immune defence.

The currently available therapies are directed towards reducing translocation either by promoting gut motility, decreasing bacterial overgrowth or changing the composition of the gut flora. Selective digestive decontamination has been shown to be effective in preventing infection in patients with gastrointestinal haemorrhage,[25] and in prophylaxis in patients with ascites.

IMMUNE PARESIS

As stated above, there is up-regulation of TLRs and increased levels of circulating cytokines and activation of monocytes in cirrhotics. This does not, however, correspond to increased bacterial killing. Rather, the innate immune system is impaired with decreased phagocytosis and opsonisation.[21] This has been described as a 'sepsis-like immune paralysis'.[26]

GENETIC SUSCEPTIBILITY

It is recognised that a genetic variables may confer a predisposition towards the acquisition of infection in cirrhotic patients.

The management of sepsis in patients with liver failure should proceed along the same lines as in the cohort without liver failure. However, consideration should be given some of the issues outlined below, which are peculiar to this population.

MANAGEMENT OF SEPSIS IN CIRRHOSIS

The principles of early goal-directed therapy in the treatment of sepsis are valid – that is, the early restoration of the circulating volume and maintenance of an adequate cardiac output, but the manner by which adequacy is assessed is complex. The circulation is frequently hyperdynamic in patients with acute or chronic liver failure – with or without infection. The oxygen extraction ratio is not uniform and shunting may occur. As a consequence, central venous oxygen saturations may be artificially high, and not representative of an inadequately resuscitated patient. Early goal-directed therapy titrated to central venous oxygen saturation as outlined by Rivers et al[27] may therefore not be applicable to this cohort. Furthermore, the use of the central venous pressure has been demonstrated to be unreliable[28] as a marker for preload-responsiveness. The authors would therefore advocate the early use of a cardiac output monitor, several of which are in widespread use. These provide markers of preload and preload responsiveness. Stroke volume response to fluid challenge or passive leg raising may be used in the mechanically ventilated or the spontaneously breathing patient.

Lactate levels have been used as markers of the adequacy of fluid resuscitation in sepsis.[29] In sepsis, lactate levels are elevated due to a higher metabolic rate, inhibition of pyruvate dehydrogenase and reflect uptake by the liver. In liver disease, this uptake is markedly diminished and elevated lactate levels may not, therefore, imply anaerobic metabolism. Lactate levels are therefore inadequate markers in this cohort, although elevated levels still unquestionably identify the sicker patients.

In terms of fluid resuscitation, albumin does not confer a mortality benefit over crystalloid in the critically unwell cohort. It does have a specific role in the treatment of patients undergoing large-volume paracentesis and has been demonstrated to preserve haemodynamics and attenuate a tendency towards hepatorenal syndrome.[30,31] A small, unblinded randomised controlled trial suggested that 20% albumin was more effective in terms of improving systemic haemodynamics than a 6% HES solution in spontaneous bacterial peritonitis.[32]

Vasopressor therapy is often required for the maintenance of adequate mean arterial pressure. Norepinephrine (noradrenaline) is the most frequently used pressor agent in the author's unit, with α-agonism attenuating a vasodilated, hyperdynamic systemic circulation and β-agonism augmenting ventricular function (which is frequently impaired in this cohort). Dopamine has no benefit over norepinephrine in the critically unwell and may be associated with a greater number of adverse events.[33] It is also not preferred in the liver failure cohort as it may cause dilatation of the superior mesenteric artery, leading to increased portal pressures. Vasopressin is used in refractory shock and to mitigate very high norepinephrine requirements.

In general terms, ventilatory management should proceed as per management in the general intensive care cohort, with attention paid to protective ventilatory strategies if ARDS is clinically apparent (limiting tidal volumes to ~6 mL/kg and plateau pressure to <30 cmH_2O). Endotracheal intubation is performed for airway protection in advanced (grade III/IV encephalopathy and for the treatment of respiratory failure. It is worth noting that raised intracranial pressure is not normally a feature of chronic liver disease.

Both acute liver failure and chronic cirrhosis are hypermetabolic states with marked catabolism and a net negative nitrogen balance. Assessment of the degree of malnutrition and muscle wasting in the chronic cirrhotic is often difficult owing to the presence of ascites and oedema. Dysphagia and gastroparesis are common in patients with cirrhosis and portal hypertension[34] and the development of encephalopathy of any grade may be associated with a risk of aspiration. In both sepsis and liver failure the potential for both cholestasis and steatosis is significant. In the event of variceal bleeding, it is usual practice at the authors' institution to wait for 48 hours before placement of a nasogastric feeding tube owing to the risk of precipitating further bleeding. Immunonutrition has not been studied in critically unwell patients with liver failure.

The protein load associated with enteral feeding may predispose to hyperammonaemia, which is common in the (decompensated) cirrhotic. Lactulose, L-ornithine L-aspartate (LOLA) and non-absorbable antibiotics such as neomycin, rifaximin, metronidazole, oral vancomycin and oral quinolones have been administered in an effort to decrease the colonic concentration of ammoniagenic bacteria. Branched chain amino acid-enriched formulae may provide protein supplementation in the patient with troublesome hepatic encephalopathy.

Hyperglycaemia is common in sepsis and may be pro-coagulant, induce apoptosis and inhibit neutrophil function. Landmark clinical trials have suggested that the strict maintenance of glycaemic control is beneficial in critically unwell surgical patients.[35] The same group failed to demonstrate a mortality benefit in a medical cohort.[36] Meier el al[37] compared the consequences of intensive glycaemic control (3.5-6.5 mmol/L) with loose glycaemic control (5.0–8.0 mmol/L). The incidences of hypoglycaemia and of bacteraemia were higher in the tight control group, with a trend towards worsened survival at 21 days. There are no RCTs examining the efficacy of tight glycaemic control in the cirrhotic population and there is a high prevalence of hypoglycaemic events in this cohort.

The efficacy of high-volume CVVH in severe sepsis and septic shock has generated a great deal of interest in the critical care community in recent years. It is proposed that the removal of mediators of the inflammatory cascade such as IL-2, IL-6, IL-8, IL-10, TNFα, C3a and C5a may attenuate the inflammatory response, improving haemodynamics and thereby end-organ perfusion and function. Animal studies were initially encouraging. A series of observational, interventional, randomised (but small scale and uncontrolled) studies showed beneficial cardiovascular effects and an improvement in predicted hospital and 28-day mortality.[38] However, a recent large randomised study demonstrated that intensive renal support in critically ill patients with acute kidney injury did not decrease mortality, improve recovery of kidney function, or reduce the rate of non-renal organ failure as compared with less-intensive therapy.[39] There is consequently a lack of consensus on the optimal timing for the commencement of renal replacement therapy, the appropriate dose or the type of membrane (pore size, surface area) for critically ill patients. Data for the septic/cirrhotic cohort are lacking.

SPONTANEOUS BACTERIAL PERITONITIS

Spontaneous bacterial peritonitis (SBP) is infection of cirrhosis-related ascites. It may cause a florid sepsis syndrome with shock and renal failure, or have an onset that is insidious and detected only at paracentesis. Pyrexia, changes in mental state and abdominal tenderness are common. Routine paracentesis demonstrates an incidence of SBP of up to 27% at the time of hospital admission.[40] Mortality rates for patients surviving their first hospital admission are 70% at 1 year, and 80% at 2 years. Prolonged bacteraemia, immune paresis and intrahepatic shunting probably play a role in the aetiology of SBP.

The bacterial concentration in ascitic fluid tends to be comparatively low and so 10–20 mL of ascitic fluid are introduced into blood culture bottles at the bedside to increase the diagnostic yield.

It is extremely important, in terms of management, to differentiate SBP from secondary peritonitis. The mortality rate of SBP approaches 100% if appropriate surgical intervention is omitted. However, the mortality rate is about 80% if a patient with SBP receives an

Box 44.2.2 Diagnostic criteria for HRS

- Cirrhosis with ascites
- Creatinine >1.5 mg/dL
- No improvement in serum creatinine (>1.5) after 2 days of diuretic withdrawal and volume expansion with albumin (1 g/kg/day up to 100 g/day)
- Absence of shock
- No nephrotoxins
- Absence of parenchymal kidney disease (proteinuria >500 mg/day, microhaematuria >50 red blood cells per high-power field) and/or abnormal renal ultrasound

unnecessary exploratory laparotomy.[41] Culture in SBP tends to reveal a single responsible pathogen.

There has been an emergence of enterobacteria strains harbouring ESBLs or beta lactamases which are able to hydrolyse cephalosporins and broad-spectrum penicillins and other resistant bacteria, such as *Pseudomonas aeruginosa*, methicillin-resistant *Staphylococcus aureus* (MRSA) and *Enterococcus faecium*. Predispositions for the acquisition of multi-resistant organisms include hospitalisation, antibiotic exposure and norfloxacin prophylaxis. Authors have suggested that quinolones should be avoided in the treatment of SBP or any other infection in patients on long-term norfloxacin prophylaxis.[42]

RENAL FAILURE IN CHRONIC LIVER DISEASE

Renal failure occurs in 27% of septic cirrhotics in the absence of SBP and in 33% with SBP.[43] Hepatorenal syndrome (HRS) is a prerenal failure that does not respond to fluid therapy. The diagnostic criteria are listed in **Box 44.2.2**.[44]

There is an association with renal/splanchnic insufficiency. Infections, bleeding and large-volume paracentesis without adequate volume replacement are common precipitating factors. Type 1 HRS progresses rapidly, and often occurs in the setting of haemodynamic compromise. Type 2 HRS is said to be characterised by a slowly progressive deterioration in renal indices and is frequently associated with ascites. HRS is associated with a diminished survival probability (**Fig. 44.2.2**).

Ischaemic acute tubular necrosis (ATN) is common in patients with acute or chronic liver failure who develop SIRS/sepsis. The administration of 20% albumin was associated with a reduction in the incidence of renal failure and of mortality.[45] Terlipressin may also have a role in the treatment of hepatorenal syndrome.[46,47] More recent data suggests that norepinephrine may be equally applied.[48-51]

Ascitic drainage should be undertaken with appropriate albumin loading if large-volume drainage is undertaken or in patients at risk of central volume depletion.[52]

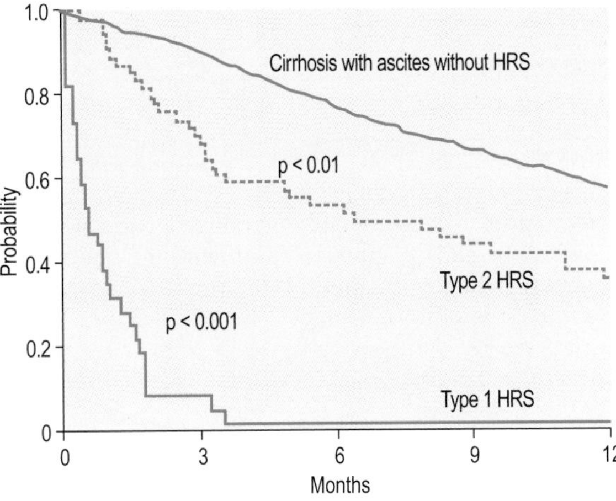

Figure 44.2.2 Actuarial survival probability in cirrhotic patients with HRS. *(From: Salerno F, Gerbes A, Gines P, et al. Diagnosis, prevention and treatment of hepatorenal syndrome in cirrhosis. Gut 2007;56:1310–8, with permission.)*[44]

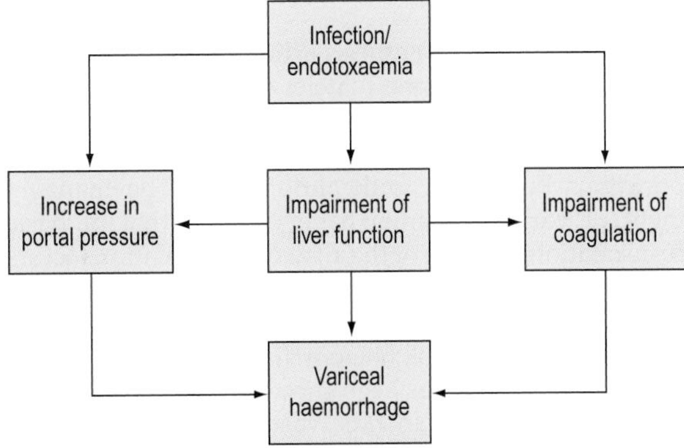

Figure 44.2.3 Pathophysiology of variceal bleeding in ACLF. *(From Thalheimer U, Triantos CK, Samonakis DN, et al. Gut 2005;54:556–63, with permission.)*[12]

VARICEAL BLEEDING IN CHRONIC LIVER DISEASE

The development of infection in cirrhosis is associated with a failure to control variceal bleeding and with early variceal re-bleeding. The incidence of sepsis is also higher in patients with uncontrolled bleeding (**Fig. 44.2.3**).

Propanolol, which is used to lower portal pressures following variceal haemorrhage, was shown to lower incidence of infection from 42% to 15% in a cohort of 73 cirrhotics.[53] It is not clear whether this effect is attributable to increased gut motility, and thus reduced bacterial translocation.

Infection may predispose to variceal bleeding because of an elevation in sinusoidal pressure – and hence portal pressure – and a worsening of

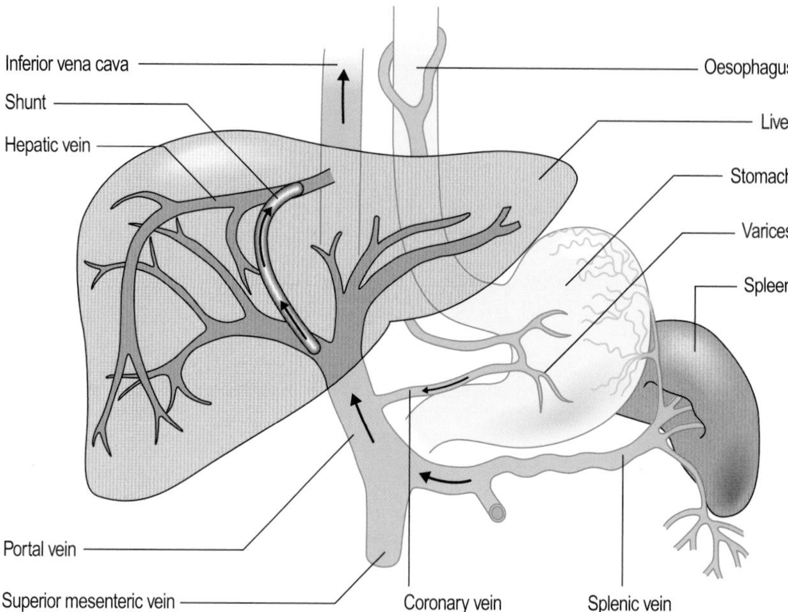

Figure 44.2.4 Transjugular intrahepatic portal systemic shunt.

coagulopathy. NO synthesis (the circulating form is *S*-nitrosothiol) attenuates platelet aggregation and heparinoid synthesis by endothelial cells increases.

It is recommended that patients with bleeding complications be treated with antibiotics.[54] The management of variceal haemorrhage remains that of basic resuscitation and care of the airway. Coagulation factors require appropriate supplementation along with other blood products. Cultures should be taken and all patients with variceal haemorrhage should be given antibiotics and this has been shown to decrease the risk of rebleeding.[55,56] Splanchnic vasoconstrictors, such as terlipressin, are beneficial in controlling oesophageal haemorrhage but their role in gastric variceal haemorrhage per se has not been examined.[48,57] Banding ligation therapy remains the treatment of choice for oesophageal haemorrhage, with tissue adhesives being utilised in gastric varices.

Failure to control variceal bleeding after two endoscopic sessions should result in consideration of TIPS insertion.[58,59] In patients in whom TIPS (**Fig. 44.2.4**) might be considered to be of benefit in controlling variceal bleeding, consideration needs to be given to the severity of the underlying liver disease that may in its own right make TIPS ill-advised.[60]

CARDIORESPIRATORY FAILURE

Cirrhotics display altered haemodynamics at baseline, with a hyperkinetic, vasodilated circulation. Patients tend to be tachycardic and hypotensive, with high cardiac output and low peripheral vascular resistance. Despite this, cirrhotic patients may have markedly abnormal tissue oxygenation, with arteriovenous O_2 content difference and O_2 uptake.[61] These changes become more profound with the onset of the septic state. Fluid resuscitation is complex, and probably best guided by the use of a cardiac output monitor. Patients may not respond to vasopressors as vigorously as the non-cirrhotic septic cohort. Left ventricular dilatation and dysfunction may be apparent on echocardiography.

Respiratory failure is common in the cirrhotic cohort. Intubation is often required for airway protection in encephalopathy. Ventilator-associated pneumonia is common. Alveolar macrophage activity may be diminished.

Tense ascites inhibits diaphragmatic descent and predisposes to basal atelectasis/collapse. There may be an accumulation of fluid owing to increased capillary membrane permeability and exacerbated by attempts to resuscitate a relatively vasoplegic circulation.

There is a relatively high incidence of ARDS in cirrhosis. Mortality rates in ventilated cirrhotics are high.

DECOMPENSATIONS IN LIVER FUNCTION DURING THE SEPTIC EPISODE

Sepsis has the potential to worsen liver function, particularly in chronic cirrhotics. Acute on chronic liver failure has been defined as 'a syndrome characterised by the acute deterioration of liver function in a patient with compensated or decompensated, but hitherto stable cirrhosis. It is commonly precipitated by an acute event/precipitating factor and associated with failure in the function of extra-hepatic organs' (European Association for the Study of Liver failure, EASL). The mechanisms underlying decrements in liver function are likely to be multifactorial.

As outlined above, levels of pro-inflammatory cytokines are increased in many forms of chronic liver

Box 44.2.3 The Child-Pugh classification is a means of assessing the severity of liver cirrhosis

Score	Bilirubin (micromol/l)	Albumin (g/l)	PT (s prolonged)	Encephalopathy	Ascites
1	<34	>35	<4	None	None
2	34–50	28–35	4–6	Mild	Mild
3	>50	<28	>6	Marked	Marked

If there is primary biliary cirrhosis or sclerosing cholangitis then bilirubin is classified as <68=1; 68–170=2; >170=3.
The individual scores are summed and then grouped as:

- <7 = A
- 7–9 = B
- >9 = C

disease. It is now believed that Kupffer cell induction by bacterial cell wall products may mediate hepatic inflammation. Hepatic stellate cells (HSCs), the main fibrogenic cells in the liver, are also mediators of inflammation, regulating leucocyte trafficking and activation.[62] Activation of HSCs by LPS has been proposed as a potential direct link between inflammation and hepatic fibrosis. Activation of the stellate cell to a myofibroblast-like phenotype allows the production of fibrillar collagens and other matrix proteins that characterise the fibrotic response.[63]

There is a large body of evidence to support the role of endotoxin and LPS derived from Gram-negative bacteria in the development of hepatic inflammation. Alcohol exposure (acute and chronic) increases gut permeability to LPS, resulting in increased LPS serum levels.[62] Injury to the liver may be attenuated by selective digestive decontamination and by colectomy whereas the addition of LPS may augment liver injury caused by alcohol.[64]

What is, perhaps, unclear are the relative roles that Gram-negative and Gram-positive bacteria play in the pathogenesis of sepsis-related liver injury. There may be synergy between the TLR-2 and TLR-4 mediated pathways.[63]

COAGULOPATHY

The liver is responsible for the synthesis of the zymogens of both pro- and anti-coagulant factors. Cirrhosis is associated with a relative deficiency of the procoagulant factors II, V VII and X and anticoagulant factors protein C, protein S and antithrombin. Cirrhotic patients with severe sepsis have relatively lower levels of zymogen forms of clotting factors when compared with cirrhotic patients with infection (but not severe sepsis) and uninfected cirrhotics. Decreased zymogen levels are independently correlated with an elevated Child–Pugh score (Box 44.2.3) and are associated with significant increases in the relative risk ratios of in-hospital death.[65] Thrombocytopenia is secondary to hypersplenism and becomes more profound in sepsis.

ACUTE ALCOHOLIC HEPATITIS

Alcoholic hepatitis is a frequent cause of decompensation and requires aggressive treatment. The severity can be assessed using the Glasgow score or Madrey score and in high-risk patients steroid therapy may be considered.[66,67] Response to steroids over the first 7 days is associated with improved outcome.[68] The role of antioxidants has been examined but no benefit was seen.[69,70] Another approach has been to look at the value of enteral feeding, which was comparable with steroid treatment over a 4-week period, albeit in a small study.[71] The use of pentoxifylline has been reported in a single-centre study to decrease the risk of developing hepatorenal failure and hence impacting on outcome.[72]

Access the complete references list online at http://www.expertconsult.com

3. Shawcross DL, Davies NA, Williams R, et al. Systemic inflammatory response exacerbates the neuropsychological effects of induced hyperammonemia in cirrhosis. J Hepatol 2004;40:247–54.
9. Karvellas CJ, Pink F, McPhail M, et al. Bacteremia, acute physiology and chronic health evaluation II and modified end stage liver disease are independent predictors of mortality in critically ill nontransplanted patients with acute on chronic liver failure. Crit Care Med 2010;38(1):121–6.
13. Gustot T, Durand F, Lebrec D, et al. Severe sepsis in cirrhosis. Hepatology 2009;50(6):2022–33. Erratum in: Hepatology 2010; 51(2):725.
14. Wong F, Bernardi M, Balk R, et al; International Ascites Club. Sepsis in cirrhosis: report on the 7th meeting of the International Ascites Club. Gut 2005;54:718–25.
21. Wiest R, Garcia-Tsao G. Bacterial translocation (BT) in cirrhosis. Hepatology 2005;41(3):422–33.
44. Salerno F, Gerbes A, Gines P, et al. Diagnosis, prevention and treatment of hepatorenal syndrome in cirrhosis. Gut 2007;56:1310–18.
46. Triantos CK, Samonakis D, Thalheimer U, et al. Terlipressin therapy for renal failure in cirrhosis. Eur J Gastroenterol Hepatol 2010;22(4):481–6.

45

Abdominal surgical catastrophes

Stephen J Streat

Intra-abdominal surgical catastrophes are common in intensive care units,[1] typically occurring in older patients with co-morbidity and reduced physiological reserve.[2] They are often associated with sepsis (primarily or secondarily), multiple organ failure, multiple surgical procedures and prolonged intensive care stay. Mortality is high[2,3] both within ICUs and afterwards, post-ICU hospital length of stay is often very long and there is both increased post-hospital mortality and reduced functional status[4,5] particularly if severe co-morbidity and functional impairment were previously present.

These factors necessitate treating clinicians to reconsider carefully and frequently the costs and benefits[6,7] of treatment during an illness that often has the character of a tragic saga.[8] The clinical issues alone are complex and decisions must often be made without the benefit of controlled trials of various strategic approaches. These difficulties create the potential for conflict to arise between intensivists and other involved clinicians, particularly surgeons whose relationship with the patient may reflect a different 'moral economy'[8] and who may have different views of what constitutes realistic goals and reasonable strategies[9] for patients who are often near the end of life.[10,11] It is in the care of these patients that the particular day-to-day work skills of the intensivist[12,13] ('seeing the big picture', providing meticulous bedside care, negotiating and maintaining consensus, facilitating communication and cooperation between clinicians and the family) are tested to the limits. Vascular catastrophes, intra-abdominal sepsis and a few serious abdominal complications are discussed in this chapter; gastrointestinal bleeding and pancreatitis are covered elsewhere (Chs 42 and 43).

VASCULAR CATASTROPHES

ABDOMINAL AORTIC ANEURYSM

Abdominal aortic aneurysm (AAA) is a disease of the elderly, and up to six times more common in men than women.[14] Rupture of an abdominal aortic aneurysm is the most common vascular catastrophe seen in ICUs and accounts for 2% of all deaths in men over 60 years of age.[15] The prevalence of AAA, defined as infrarenal aortic diameter of 30 mm or more, as detected by screening in men, rises from less than 1% at age 50 to around 4% at aged 60, 5–10% at age 70 and around 10% at age 80. Ultrasound screening of elderly men for AAA reduces mortality and is probably cost-effective,[16] but in the Western world as smoking declines this may not remain the case.[17]

Aortic diameter is the strongest predictor of the risk of rupture, which is below 1% per year with aortic diameter <5 cm and about 17% per year with aortic diameter of 6 cm or more.[15] The risk of rupture is higher in women (who have faster aneurysm growth rates than men[18]) and is increased by current smoking and hypertension. Aortic aneurysm expansion is around 0.3 cm per year for aneurysms smaller than 5 cm and around 0.5 cm per year for those larger than 5 cm and this rate may be able to be reduced by a short course of macrolide or by stopping smoking. Perioperative mortality for open elective aneurysm repair has fallen to ~3%[19] (higher when there is significant preoperative respiratory or renal dysfunction[20]) and endovascular repair has rapidly overtaken open repair[21] because of lower perioperative mortality (0.5%[19]). A slight mortality benefit for endovascular repair persists for 2–3 years, but after this there is a 'catch-up' in mortality and other complications including rupture after endovascular treatment with associated increase in cost.[22] Endovascular repair does not improve survival in patients judged medically unfit for open repair.[23,24] Operative mortality is increased to around 15% in urgently repaired (non-ruptured) aneurysms[25] and around 40% in ruptured aneurysms repaired as an emergency.[26] Endovascular repair of ruptured aneurysms is associated with lower perioperative mortality (e.g. 24% vs 44% in a non-randomised study[27]).

Ruptured aneurysm may lead to death before hospital admission in around 30% of cases,[28] is almost always lethal without repair[29] and not all patients are offered repair. These results have led to recommendations for population screening by ultrasound at age 65, continued surveillance for small aneurysms[30] and elective repair in patients without severe co-morbidity when aneurysm diameter exceeds 5 or 6 cm.[31,32]

RUPTURE OF AN ABDOMINAL AORTIC (OR ILIAC ARTERY) ANEURYSM

The clinical features of rupture include the sudden onset of shock and back pain or abdominal pain or tenderness in a patient typically over the age of 70. Most ruptures are, at least initially, retroperitoneal with intraperitoneal rupture resulting in greater physiological disturbance and much higher subsequent operative mortality.[33] The correct clinical diagnosis is often not made by the first attending doctor[34] as a pulsatile abdominal mass is commonly not detectable[33] and many patients do not have shock when first seen. Although immediate bedside ultrasound may sometimes be able to confirm the clinical diagnosis without increasing delay, others have found that this investigation commonly delayed vascular surgical referral and subsequent operation without diagnostic benefit.[35] The diagnosis of ruptured aneurysm is confirmed (by CT angiography) in only half of the patients in whom it is suspected,[36] but CT comes with risk of sudden deterioration outside the operating room. It is sometimes inappropriate to proceed to repair (very severe co-morbidity, poor quality of life) and this decision should be very carefully considered.[37] Lack of physiological reserve (often associated with advanced age) predicts high operative mortality and long periods of intensive care and hospitalisation in survivors. Open repair is commonly offered, but endovascular repair is increasingly advocated[38] although randomised trial evidence of superiority is not yet available.[36,39,40] A very small number of patients with aortic aneurysm have infection of the aneurysm, usually with *Staphylococcus* or *Salmonella*, which is often diagnosed at rupture.[41]

A period of intensive care after aneurysm repair is appropriate for most patients. During this time, common physiological abnormalities (e.g. hypothermia, dilutional coagulopathy, minor bleeding, circulatory shock, renal tubular dysfunction) can be corrected and serious complications can be sought and if possible treated (e.g. major bleeding, renal failure, myocardial infarction, acute lung injury, peripheral ischaemia, stroke, pulmonary embolism, persistent ileus, mesenteric ischaemia, pancreatitis, acalculous cholecystitis, increased intra-abdominal pressure). Rapid ventilator weaning and extubation is recommended, perhaps with thoracic epidural anaesthesia[42] if coagulation allows. Abdominal decompression in these particular patients may not be helpful.[43] Finally, an assessment of overall progress should be made after 24–48 hours. Severe or progressive multiple organ failure[44] or major visceral or limb infarction should lead to a reappraisal of the appropriateness of continued intensive therapies. Persistent renal failure occurs more commonly after acute renal failure in this context than in other intensive care patients. Massive upper gastrointestinal haemorrhage (usually aorto-duodenal) is a rare complication usually resulting from infection of a previous aortic repair and less commonly from primary infection in an aortic aneurysm. Some of these patients can be rescued surgically.

ACUTE AORTIC OCCLUSION

This is an uncommon syndrome and is usually due to thrombotic occlusion (of a stenotic or aneurysmal aorta) or to saddle embolism that presents with painful lower limb paraparesis or paraplegia and absent distal circulation. Minimising delay to emergency revascularisation is of the essence, but mortality and multi-system morbidity remain high.[45,46]

MESENTERIC INFARCTION

This uncommon syndrome presents with an acute abdomen, may develop in critically patients and is commonly due to non-occlusive arterial ischaemia, arterial embolism or atherosclerotic arterial thrombosis and less often to venous occlusion, low-flow or hypercoagulable states.[47] Recently reported outcomes have improved[48] with a coordinated multidisciplinary approach including endovascular revascularisation,[49,50] surgery (often including gut resection) and intensive care.

AORTIC DISSECTION

Aortic dissection[51] has an incidence of 5–30 per million per year. The typical patient is elderly, has a history of hypertension[52] and presents with pain in a distribution corresponding to the site of dissection. Cases have been reported in young people and after circumstances suggesting acute situational hypertension. Pericardial tamponade, haemothorax, myocardial infarction, stroke, paraplegia due to spinal cord ischaemia, anuria or an acute abdomen may be present. Most aortic dissections originate in the ascending thoracic aorta. Some dissections extend to involve the abdominal aorta, but spontaneous dissection of the abdominal aorta alone is rare. Mortality remains high but is falling in association with earlier diagnosis and treatment,[51] which now most commonly involves endovascular repair for uncomplicated abdominal aortic dissection.[53–55]

SPONTANEOUS RETROPERITONEAL HAEMORRHAGE

Spontaneous retroperitoneal haemorrhage (excluding aortic aneurysm rupture) is uncommon and usually associated with anticoagulant therapy, including warfarin, unfractionated heparin, low-molecular-weight heparin and antiplatelet agents,[56] or with vascular or malignant disease of the kidney or adrenal gland and less commonly with spontaneous rupture of the retroperitoneal veins. The presentation is most often with acute abdominal pain, shock and a palpable abdominal or groin mass, and CT will confirm the diagnosis.[57] Transfusion, correction of coagulopathy and interventional radiological embolisation may control some situations but surgery may be required in others, either to stop bleeding or to relieve associated intra-abdominal hypertension.

INTRA-ABDOMINAL SEPSIS

Intra-abdominal sepsis is very common in the ICU. In our own experience the abdomen (including CAPD peritonitis) was the most common septic site in patients admitted to ICU with severe sepsis and accounted for 404 (35.9%) of the 1131 such admissions over the 9 years 2000–2008.[58] Only 11% of these patients with intra-abdominal sepsis died in ICU but higher mortality is commonly reported for such patients, depending on the extent of co-morbidity[59] and the severity of the acute illness.

The general principles of the treatment of severe sepsis are to support oxygen transport with ventilator support, fluid therapy and inotropic support, to diagnose and if possible remove the septic source[60,61] and to give appropriate antimicrobial therapy.[62] Sepsis should be thought of as a time-critical condition[62] wherein delay in the execution of these principles is likely to worsen outcome. A clear role for other therapies is not yet established.[62] The issue of severe sepsis in general is covered in Chapter 69. In the critically ill patient with intra-abdominal sepsis, effective source control usually involves surgery although occasionally interventional procedures may suffice. Laparotomy is recommended (without delay or further investigation) for most patients presenting acutely with shock and clinical evidence of peritonitis. Diagnostic peritoneal aspiration or lavage, ultrasonography, CT scanning or laparoscopy may have limited applicability in some circumstances.

Common syndromes[63] include:

- faecal peritonitis
- primarily – diverticular disease or colonic malignancy
- secondarily – after prior anterior resection
- perforated upper abdominal viscus (usually of a gastric or duodenal ulcer)
- biliary obstruction (sometimes with perforation)
- intestinal infarction without perforation (usually adhesive, less commonly ischaemic)
- appendicitis (often perforated in older patients).

Less common syndromes include localised intra-abdominal abscess, acalculous cholecystitis, toxic megacolon, perforation of a fallopian tube abscess, spontaneous bacterial peritonitis (in end-stage liver disease or nephrotic syndrome) and CAPD-associated peritonitis (some of which is surgical).

SURGICAL SOURCE CONTROL

Surgical source control should remove the septic focus at the first ('damage control') operation, but definitive surgery may not be feasible or desirable at this time. Initial surgery[60] involves:

- removal of all peritoneal contamination (both macroscopically and by generous lavage)
- drainage of abscesses
- resection of devitalised tissue
- defunctioning of the gut (diverting the enteric stream) to prevent ongoing contamination.

The abdomen may be left open (with a temporary fascial closure) if required for intra-abdominal hypertension or to facilitate repeat laparotomy. Successful primary colonic anastomosis (even left-sided) after resection in the presence of sepsis is supported by evidence from case series[60,64] and a recent small randomised controlled trial.[65]

Failure of the sepsis syndrome to settle ('failure to thrive') after apparently definitive surgical source control should suggest ongoing contamination or ischaemia or the development of abscess. Repeat laparotomy on clinical grounds is recommended when early postoperative progress is unsatisfactory,[3] as CT performs poorly in this situation,[66] whereas CT scanning followed by either directed laparotomy[67] or interventional radiological drainage is a more successful strategy for late abscess formation.

INTESTINAL-SOURCE PERITONITIS

Peritonitis secondary to contamination by intestinal contents usually results in mixed aerobic and anaerobic infection. Recommended antibiotic regimens[58,61,68] are based on a paucity of randomised controlled trial evidence and usually involve either monotherapy with a carbapenem (or piperacillin–tazobactam) or combination therapy with a third- or fourth-generation cephalosporin and metronidazole. An aminoglycoside is often recommended in addition where the risk of resistant Gram-negative bacteria is particularly high.[61] Similar antibiotic regimens are appropriate in sepsis following intestinal infarction without perforation. An agent active against *Staphylococcus aureus*[69] should be considered in patients with peritonitis following gastric or duodenal perforation.

BILIARY SEPSIS

Biliary ultrasound followed by endoscopic sphincteromy and stone removal is recommended for critically ill patients with cholangitis. Antibiotic regimens should cover enterococci and aerobic Gram-negative bacilli.

ACALCULOUS CHOLECYSTITIS

Acalculous cholecystitis is a rare but serious condition in intensive care units. A small number of patients with the syndrome of acute cholecystitis will have acalculous cholecystitis, but these patients have low mortality and do not present to intensive care units. Of greater concern are the perhaps half of all cases of acalculous cholecystitis that develop insidiously in intensive care patients already critically ill for another reason (e.g. recent trauma or surgery) and can therefore go unrecognised until gangrene, perforation or abscess develop. The gallbladder histology in such patients usually includes prominent ischaemia and arteriosclerosis and low cardiac output may predispose to the condition. There should be a high index of suspicion in an intensive care patient who develops new abdominal pain or clinical signs of sepsis. Although a variety of investigations including scintigraphy, CT scanning, ultrasound and laparoscopy[70] have been used to help establish the diagnosis, none perform reliably[71] and many surgeons advocate a low threshold to exploratory laparotomy on clinical grounds where suspicion exists. Percutaneous cholecystostomy[60] has been used successfully, whereas early cholecystectomy is advocated by others[72] as infarction or perforation of the gallbladder is commonly found at laparotomy.

TOXIC MEGACOLON

Toxic megacolon[73] is now a rare indication for intensive care admission. It is characterised by systemic toxicity accompanying a dilated, inflamed colon and is usually due to inflammatory bowel disease. Infection by *Clostridium difficile*, cytomegalovirus (in patients with HIV disease or immunosuppression) or rarely other organisms may also precipitate toxic megacolon. The diagnosis should be considered in patients with diarrhoea and abdominal distension. Limited colonoscopy (despite the risk of perforation) and biopsy may both yield important microbiological information and help in the decision to operate. Supportive therapy in an intensive care unit is usually recommended and includes both antibiotics as for colonic perforation and steroids (equivalent of ~300 mg/day of hydrocortisone). Other immunosuppression (with calcineurin inhibitors or anti-TNF monoclonal antibody) has also been used. Frequent surgical reassessment and abdominal X-rays are used to monitor progress. Intravenous nutrition may help to reduce the activity of Crohn's disease but does not reduce hospital stay or the need for surgery in ulcerative colitis. A period of several days of careful observation may be reasonable to assess the response to medical treatment but urgent surgery (subtotal colectomy with end-ileostomy) is indicated for increasing colonic dilatation, perforation, bleeding or progressive systemic toxicity.[74] Parenteral metronidazole may be effective in severe pseudomembranous colitis without megacolon (but early surgery is often recommended if megacolon develops).

RUPTURE OF A TUBO-OVARIAN ABSCESS

Rupture of a tubo-ovarian abscess is a rare cause of peritonitis presenting to intensive care units and is best treated with surgical extirpation. Antibiotic therapy should including activity against anaerobic organisms.

SPONTANEOUS BACTERIAL PERITONITIS

Spontaneous bacterial peritonitis (SBP) is usually a monomicrobial infection (usually with *Escherichia coli*, *Klebsiella pneumoniae*, pneumococci or enterococci and rarely with anaerobes).[58] The development of SBP in patients with end-stage liver disease is often followed by hepatic decompensation and multiple organ failure (see Ch. 44). Those who recover are at high risk of death without liver transplantation. Early albumin supplementation has been shown to reduce both renal failure and mortality in SBP associated with end-stage liver disease.[75] Treatment with a broad-spectrum beta-lactam antibiotic should be followed by secondary oral antibiotic prophylaxis.

CAPD-ASSOCIATED PERITONITIS

Peritonitis in CAPD patients rarely necessitates intensive care admission and such patients should be assessed for abscess formation, the presence of unusual organisms including fungi or an unrecognised gastrointestinal septic source.[76]

TERTIARY PERITONITIS

Tertiary peritonitis ('peritonitis in the critically ill patient that persists or recurs at least 48 hours after the apparently adequate management of primary or secondary peritonitis'[77]) occurs occasionally in severely ill patients with prior laparotomy. It is commonly due to *Pseudomonas aeruginosa*, *Staphylococcus epidermidis*, *Enterococcus* spp., *Enterobacter* spp., resistant *Bacteroides* or *Candida* spp.[58,61,77] and antimicrobial treatment should reflect these organisms until guided by cultures. When infection is due to *Candida* spp. other antimicrobial agents should be discontinued, any foreign bodies removed if possible, and treatment with amphotericin B given for at least 4 weeks.[78]

COMPLICATIONS

INTRA-ABDOMINAL HYPERTENSION AND THE ABDOMINAL COMPARTMENT SYNDROME

These phenomena occur uncommonly in critically ill patients, particularly after laparotomy for trauma or sepsis and in association with obesity[79] and excessive fluid administration. Intra-abdominal hypertension has been defined as intra-abdominal pressure (IAP) >12 mmHg (1.6 kPa) and abdominal compartment syndrome as IAP>20 mmHg (2.66 kPa) with associated organ dysfunction.[80] Intra-abdominal pressure (IAP) can be conveniently and easily measured via intravesical pressure,[43,80] is normally 5–7 mmHg (0.66–0.93 kPa) in critically ill adults and is increased in patients with increased body mass index. Physiological impairment (including cardiorespiratory, renal, splanchnic, and neurological) can occur with acute increases in IAP to levels above 12 mmHg. However, in the absence of evidence from randomised controlled trials, expert opinion[81] suggests that the development of the abdominal compartment syndrome (IAP>20 mmHg with associated organ dysfunction) should prompt a search for decompressive measures. Traditionally this has involved urgent decompressive laparotomy and temporary fascial closure; however, other measures (avoidance of the prone position, gastric and colonic decompression, neostigmine or other prokinetic agents, neuromuscular blockade, diuresis or ultrafiltration, percutaneous drainage of intraperitoneal fluid or gas) may be effective in some patients and should also be considered.[81] Mortality for such patients is probably falling with early use of decompression but remains high (~25%).[82]

THE OPEN ABDOMEN AND STAGED ABDOMINAL REPAIR

The use of synthetic materials to provide temporary fascial closure or of a negative-pressure wound technique over porous materials (sponge or towels) has facilitated the care of the patient with an open abdomen and allowed repeat laparotomy and staged abdominal repair to proceed in a timely and unhurried manner.[83] Our own practice[43] used to involve the use of polypropylene mesh for fascial closure if the abdomen was to be open for a short time (less than a week) to remove it before significant adhesion occurred. Alternatively a negative-pressure wound dressing[84] over a porous material (sponge or towels) can also achieve the necessary objectives of decompression, ascites removal and prevention of evisceration. Care should be taken to prevent adherence of any material placed over the abdominal contents to minimise the risk of gut perforation and fistula during removal of the material and eventual wound closure. The management of fistulation in the open abdomen remains problematic as proximal defunctioning is often impossible and better control of wound contamination is probably achieved with a negative-pressure wound care system rather than with soft-catheter intubation of the small bowel via the fistulous tract.

ENTEROCUTANEOUS FISTULAS – INTESTINAL, BILIARY AND PANCREATIC

These are rare complications in intensive care patients but they usually present formidable problems because of their common associations with serious gastrointestinal co-morbidity (e.g. inflammatory bowel disease, intestinal malignancy, pancreatitis) and concurrent severe sepsis. In addition, fistulation through an open abdomen, complex fistulation with multiple collections, inability to proximally defunction or distal intestinal obstruction are commonly present. A standard approach to fistula management should apply[85] including attention to drainage of sepsis, control of the fistula by drainage or if necessary by proximal defunctioning, protection of the skin from the deleterious effects of the fistula fluid, nutritional support and replacement of fluid and electrolyte losses.

Somatostatin analogues have been shown to reduce high-output small bowel fistula losses, probably enhance fistula closure[86] and may reduce the incidence of pancreatic fistula when used prophylactically in pancreatic surgery.[87] Parenteral nutrition is usually recommended for proximal small bowel fistulas but more distal intestinal, biliary or pancreatic fistulas can probably be safely treated with a trial of enteral nutrition. Treatment with an anti-TNF antibody has been shown to be effective in chronic enterocutaneous fistulas in (non-ICU) patients with Crohn's disease.[88,89] Persistent high-output fistula should lead to investigation of possible causes including complete disruption of the gut lumen, distal obstruction or persistent intra-abdominal sepsis. Definitive operative treatment for fistulas that do not close should await clinical recovery and if possible nutritional repletion.

COLONIC PSEUDO-OBSTRUCTION

Colonic pseudo-obstruction (Ogilvie's syndrome, a severe form of colonic ileus) is not uncommon in critically ill patients. The syndrome may contribute to ventilatory difficulty, intra-abdominal hypertension and failure of enteral feeding and carries a small risk of spontaneous perforation with high resultant mortality. Conventional conservative treatment includes nasogastric drainage, intravenous fluid replacement and avoidance of opioids and anticholinergic agents. Treatment with neostigmine has been found to be highly effective[90] but may cause symptomatic bradycardia and even cardiac arrest.[91]

Colonoscopy or surgery may be required if these measures fail.[92,93]

Access the complete references list online at http://www.expertconsult.com

9. Cassell J, Buchman TG, Streat S, et al. Surgeons, intensivists, and the covenant of care: administrative models and values affecting care at the end of life – updated. Crit Care Med 2003;31(5):1551–7.
40. Dillon M, Cardwell C, Blair PH, et al. Endovascular treatment for ruptured abdominal aortic aneurysm. Cochrane Database Syst Rev 2007;1:CD005261.
60. Marshall JC, Maier RV, Jimenez M, et al. Source control in the management of severe sepsis and septic shock: an evidence-based review. Crit Care Med 2004;32(Suppl. 11):S513–26.
61. Chow AW, Evans GA, Nathens AB, et al. Canadian practice guidelines for surgical intra-abdominal infections. Can J Infect Dis Med Microbiol 2010; 21(1):11–37.
62. Dellinger RP, Levy MM, Rhodes A, et al. Surviving Sepsis Campaign Guidelines Committee including the Pediatric Subgroup. Surviving sepsis campaign:

international guidelines for management of severe sepsis and septic shock: 2012. Crit Care Med 2013; 41(2):580–637.
68. Wong PF, Gilliam AD, Kumar S, et al. Antibiotic regimens for secondary peritonitis of gastrointestinal origin in adults. Cochrane Database Syst Rev 2005; 2:CD004539.
81. Cheatham ML, Malbrain ML, Kirkpatrick A et al. Results from the International Conference of Experts on Intra-abdominal Hypertension and Abdominal Compartment Syndrome. II. Recommendations. Intensive Care Med 2007;33(6):951–62.
83. Open Abdomen Advisory Panel, Campbell A, Chang M, et al. Management of the open abdomen: from initial operation to definitive closure. Am Surg 2009;75(Suppl. 11):S1–22.
86. Rahbour G, Siddiqui MR, Ullah MR, et al. A meta-analysis of outcomes following use of somatostatin and its analogues for the management of enterocutaneous fistulas. Ann Surg 2012;256(6):946–54.

46

Solid tumours and their implications in the ICU

Timothy Wigmore and Pascale Gruber

The term 'solid tumour' refers to masses of tissue not containing cysts or liquid. There are over 200 types and they are classified according to the tissue of origin. Most arise from epithelial tissues and are termed carcinomas. They are further differentiated into squamous cell (which include tumours of skin, oropharynx, oesophagus, cervix and lung) and adeno- (which include those originating in lung, colon, breast, pancreas and stomach). Rarer tumours originate from connective tissue (sarcomas), the neuroectoderm (gliomas, glioblastomas, neuroblastomas, medulloblastomas) or germ cells (teratomas, seminomas and choriocarcinomas).

There were 12.7 million new cancer cases worldwide in 2008 and this number is expected to reach 26 million by 2030.[1] This increase is attributable to an ageing population and lifestyle changes, with diet, lack of physical activity and obesity all playing a role. The most common cancers worldwide are lung (12.7% of the total), breast (10.9%) and colorectal cancers (9.7%) whilst the commonest causes of cancer deaths are lung (18.2% of the total), stomach (9.7%) and liver cancer (9.2%).

This case-load presents a substantial challenge to intensive care physicians. In the SOAP (Sepsis Occurrence in Acutely Ill Patients) study[2] cancer patients accounted for 15% of all ICU admissions, 85% of which were solid tumours. The Intensive Care National Audit and Research Centre case-mix review of 128 adult general ICUs in the United Kingdom demonstrated that bowel and oesophageal tumours accounted for the fourth and eighth most common reasons for ICU admission respectively.[3]

Patients with solid cancers present to ICU either postoperatively, with complications of cancer treatment, as a result of the underlying cancer itself or with other co-morbidities unrelated to the cancer.

CANCER TREATMENTS

Cancer treatments fall broadly into the three main categories: chemotherapy, radiotherapy and surgery. Many patients have a combination of all three, and it is increasingly common for patients to receive neoadjuvant chemotherapy prior to surgery to facilitate surgical resection. Chemotherapeutic agents affect DNA synthesis, structure or repair and are usually unselective in that they affect all rapidly dividing cells. They may therefore also affect cells in the gut (with resulting mucositis and diarrhoea), bone marrow (leading to thrombocytopenia, anaemia and immunosuppression) and hair (causing alopecia). Additionally, many chemotherapeutic drugs have agent-specific side-effects that may have implications for ICU (see Table 46.1), for example anthracyclines- or trastuzumab-related cardiomyopathy, bleomycin-related lung injury or ifosfamide-induced encephalopathy.

Agents commonly used in combinations are represented by acronyms. Confusingly, the same agent may be represented by different letters depending on whether the generic or brand name has been used, and equally multiple agents may be represented by the same letter (**Table 46.1**).

SPECIFIC CHEMOTHERAPY-INDUCED TOXICITIES

BLEOMYCIN-RELATED LUNG INJURY

Bleomycin is an antibiotic derived from *Streptomyces* spp. that causes DNA scission through the generation of oxygen superoxide radicals. It is used for the treatment of head and neck squamous cell carcinomas, cancers of the cervix and germ cell tumours. It causes pneumonitis in up to 40% of patients, with subsequent mortality in up to 2%.[4] Toxicity is caused by the generation of oxygen free radicals with subsequent alveolitis and fibrosis. This is exacerbated by high oxygen concentrations.

IFOSFAMIDE NEUROTOXICITY

Ifosfamide is an alkylating agent used in the treatment of head and neck, cervical, ovarian, breast and lung cancers. It causes encephalopathy in between 10 and 30% of patients, with a severity ranging from mild confusion to coma. The diagnosis is essentially one of exclusion with normal brain imaging and an EEG demonstrating metabolic encephalopathy. The aetiology is thought to be related to direct toxicity from metabolites of ifosfamide, notably chloracetaldehyde or dicarboxylic acid. The incidence is greater in those with pre-existing low albumin, raised creatinine or with cisplatin pretreatment.[5] The natural history of the

Table 46.1 Examples of commonly used chemotherapy regimens

AC	Breast cancer	Adriamycin® (doxorubicin), cyclophosphamide
BEP	Germ cell tumours	Bleomycin, etoposide, cisplatin
CAV	Lung cancer	Cyclophosphamide, Adriamycin®(doxorubicin), vincristine
CEF	Breast cancer	Cyclophosphamide, epirubicin, fluorouracil,
FOLFOX	Colorectal tumours	Fluorouracil, folinic acid (leucovorin), oxaliplatin
FOLFIRI	Colorectal tumours	Fluorouracil, folinic acid (leucovorin), irinotecan
PCV	Brain tumours	Procarbazine, CCNU (lomustine), vincristine
VIP	Germ cell tumours	Ifosfamide, cisplatin, etoposide

encephalopathy is to regress over a period of days to weeks after cessation of ifosfamide. Methylene blue (50 mg 4-hourly intravenously) has been shown to ameliorate or even terminate symptoms.[6] (Proposed mechanism is inhibition of the conversion of chloroethylamine to toxic chloroacetaldehyde probably by inhibiting several different amine oxidases.)

ANTHRACYCLINE CARDIOMYOPATHY

Anthracylines, such as daunorubicin, doxorubicin and epirubucin, are widely used anticancer agents. Anthracyclines can cause both acute and chronic cardiac dysfunction. Acutely, 5% of patients suffer from arrhythmias or acute cardiac failure that resolves with standard treatment. Chronically, anthracyclines cause a dose-dependent cardiomyopathy that becomes apparent anywhere between 3 months and several years after treatment and can result in severe myocardial dysfunction. Initial treatment is with ACE inhibition, but the full range of medical therapies for heart failure may be required, including cardiac resynchronisation.[7]

TRASTUZUMAB (HERCEPTIN®) CARDIOTOXICITY

Trastumuzab may cause a non-dose-related, reversible myocardial dysfunction. This appears to involve an element of myocardial stunning rather than myocyte destruction. It is often asymptomatic but can cause symptoms of cardiac failure. Its occurrence does not preclude future dosing provided cardiac function has recovered prior to further use[8] (**Table 46.2**).

RADIOTHERAPY

Radiotherapy causes damage to cells through the production of oxygen free radicals by the ionisation of water molecules. These in turn cause damage to cellular DNA. Damage to healthy surrounding tissue is minimised by targeting the radiation beam through multiple planes that intersect within the tumour. Despite this, radiation commonly causes acute inflammation and subsequent fibrosis in the tissues through which it passes. Common examples are pericarditis, pericardial, myocardial and lung fibrosis. This can cause organ dysfunction, particularly when combined with a chemotherapeutic agent known to have toxicities associated with that same organ.

DISEASE-RELATED ADMISSIONS

A number of oncological emergencies can occur that require admission to ICU.

TUMOUR LYSIS SYNDROME (TLS)

Tumour lysis occasionally follows treatment for bulky solid tumours, particularly small-cell lung tumours, neuroblastomas and breast carcinomas.[9,10] The syndrome results from the rapid death of large numbers of tumour cells. This may occur spontaneously but usually follows chemotherapy, radiotherapy and occasionally surgery, with a consequent release of a high concentration of intracellular contents. This results in a constellation of metabolic abnormalities, specifically hyperuricaemia (and subsequent nephropathy due to deposition of uric acid crystals in the distal tubules), hyperkalaemia, hyperphosphataemia and hypocalcaemia (due to the precipitation of calcium phosphate). The priority with TLS is prevention, and patients with high- or intermediate-risk tumours should receive intravenous hydration and rasburicase (recombinant urate oxidase) as prophylaxis.[11] Rasburicase has generally replaced allopurinol as the agent of choice. Rasburicase catalyses the formation of water-soluble allantoin from uric acid, resulting in a rapid reduction in uric acid levels. In contrast, allopurinol prevents uric acid formation through the inhibition of xanthine oxidase, which results in a slower decrease in uric acid concentration and increases the concentrations of xanthine, which can result in xanthinuria - in itself a cause of renal failure.[12] Urinary alkinisation reduces the risk of uric acid precipitation by rendering it more water-soluble, but simultaneously increases the risk of calcium phosphate precipitation in the kidneys and other organs. Hyperkalaemia and hyperphosphataemia sometimes require renal replacement therapy.

SPINAL CORD COMPRESSION

Breast, prostate, lung and kidney cancers have a predilection for bony metastasis. High spinal cord

Table 46.2 Characteristic toxicities of commonly used chemotherapeutic agents

DRUG NAME OR GROUP	SOLID TUMOURS FOR WHICH TYPICALLY USED	MODE OF ACTION	CHARACTERISTIC TOXICITIES
Anthracyclines – doxorubicin, idarubicin	Breast, bladder, stomach, lung, ovary, thyroid	Intercalates DNA	Cardiotoxicity, 'hand-foot syndrome'
Alkylating agents – cyclophosphamide, ifosfamide	Many	Inhibits DNA replication	Immunosuppression, haemorrhagic cystitis, LV dysfunction, hyponatraemia
– ifosfamide	Ovarian, breast, lung, testicular		Neurotoxicity
– melphalan	Multiple myeloma, ovarian		Myelosuppression, interstitial pneumonitis
Bleomycin	Squamous cell, testicular	Induces DNA strand breaks	Pulmonary fibrosis
Cyproterone	Prostate	Inhibit tumour 'flare'	Hepatotoxicity
Fluorouracil	Colorectal, pancreatic	Thymidylate synthase inhibitor	Cardiotoxicity, neurodegeneration
Methotrexate	Choricarcinoma	Inhibits folic acid metabolism	Mucositis, pulmonary fibrosis, hepatitis, immunosuppression
Platinum analogues, e.g. carboplatin, cisplatin, oxaliplatin	Lymphoma, sarcoma, ovarian, small-cell lung	Selective inhibition of tumour DNA synthesis	Myelosuppression, nephro/oto/neurotoxicity, hypomagnesaemia with cisplatin
Procarbazine	Glioblastoma multiforme	Causes free radical formation	Myelosuppression, hypersensitivity rash
Monoclonal antibodies			
– Bevacizumab (Avastin®)	Colon, non-small-cell lung	Inhibits VEGF, inhibiting cell growth	Mucocutaneous bleeding, GI perforation
– Cetuximab	Colorectal, squamous cell, head and neck	Binds to EGFR, inhibits cell division	Severe hypersensitivity reactions
Trastuzumab (Herceptin®)	Breast	Binds HER2 receptor, inhibits cell division	Cardiotoxicity, hypersensitivity
Tamoxifen	Breast	Oestrogen receptor antagonist	Thrombosis, endometrial Ca, strokes
Taxanes, e.g. docetaxel, paclitaxel	Breast, prostate, non-small-cell lung	Impair mitosis	Cardiac conduction defects, peripheral neuropathy, hypersensitivity
Topoismerase inhibitors, e.g. irinotecan, topotecan	Colon	Inhibits DNA replication	Acute cholinergic syndrome
Vinca alkaloids – vincristine, vinblastine	Nephroblastoma	Inhibits assembly of microtubules arresting mitosis	Neuropathic ileus, peripheral neuropathy, hyponatraemia

VEGF=vascular endothelial growth factor; EGFR=epidermal growth factor receptor; HER2=human epidermal growth factor 2.

compression may require semi-urgent invasive mechanical ventilation. Treatment usually takes the form of steroids followed either by surgery or radiotherapy.

CARDIAC TAMPONADE

Pericardial effusions due to epicardial metastasis or mediastinal lymph drainage obstruction are relatively common with advanced lung and breast cancers.[13] Cardiac tamponade is less frequent and may develop with pericardial effusions as small as 200 mL if accumulated rapidly. On echocardiography, cardiac tamponade classically demonstrates right atrial or ventricular diastolic collapse, increase in right ventricular size or failure of inferior vena cava collapse on inspiration. The management of cardiac tamponade in the acute setting is pericardiocentesis with subsequent pericardial window formation. For some tumours, treatment of the underlying cancer with chemotherapy and/or radiotherapy will result in longer-term resolution.

ELECTROLYTE DISORDERS

Rapid and life-threatening changes in electrolyte concentrations may result from paraneoplastic disorders, losses from treatment-induced diarrhoea or renal dysfunction. Paraneoplastic disorders result from the secretion of hormones or hormone-like substances from tumours. Syndrome of inappropriate antidiuretic hormone secretion (SIADH) typically occurs in the setting of small-cell lung carcinomas, which account for 80% of the total incidences of SIADH. SIADH also occurs with pancreatic, colonic, prostate, duodenal and head and neck tumours. It can be seen with cisplatin, ifosfamide, vincristine, vinblastine and cyclophosphamide use. Hyponatraemia is particularly marked when secondary to cyclophosphamide due to concurrent fluid loading to reduce the risk of haemorrhagic cystitis.[14] Chronic mild hyponatraemia ($Na+>125$ mmol/L) rarely requires intervention, whereas severe hyponatraemia ($Na+<125$ mmol/L) should be cautiously corrected to avoid osmotic demyelination.

Hypercalcaemia represents the most common metabolic consequence of solid tumours and occurs in 10–20% of patients.[15] The release of parathyroid-hormone-related peptides from lung, head and neck, kidney and pancreatic cancers, together with osteolytic calcium release from tumours with bony metastases (e.g. breast and prostate), can result in life-threatening hypercalcaemia. Treatment of hypercalcaemia is with a combination of saline rehydration, calcitonin and bisphosphonates (e.g. pamidronic acid (pamidronate)). Saline corrects hypercalcaemia-induced dehydration, calcitonin reduces resorption from bone by blocking osteoclast maturation and increasing renal calcium excretion, and bisphosphonates cause osteoclasts to apoptose.[16] The response to furosemide is variable and often requires the use of high doses resulting in electrolyte abnormalities, and is therefore not recommended.[17] The effect of bisphosphonates may be poor in those with parathyroid hormone related protein (PTHrP)-induced hypercalcaemia, although zoledronic acid may be useful.[18,19]

Hypokalaemia requiring admission to ICU is often the result of diarrhoea due to chemotherapy or radiotherapy. Hypokalaemia may also be caused by ACTH-producing lung tumours or from tumours that produce insulin.

Electrolyte disorders may be of sufficient severity to be life-threatening requiring immediate correction with intravenous replacement. They are also often accompanied by a normal anion gap hyperchloraemic metabolic acidosis caused by concomitant bicarbonate loss. This can result in marked acidaemia with consequent respiratory compensation that can lead to exhaustion in an already debilitated patient. It is best managed with bicarbonate replacement, although care needs to be taken to avoid worsening hypokalaemia.

SUPERIOR MEDIASTINAL SYNDROME

Patients with anterior mediastinal compression typically present to ICU either postoperatively or as an emergency with airway obstruction, cardiac compression or superior vena cava obstruction. The aetiology in adults is most commonly a thymoma, although lymphomas, germ cell tumours and sarcomas can also be responsible.[20] Airway obstruction may occur owing to compression of the trachea or bronchi. In an emergency there is often little time for formal assessment. Imaging may be available in the form of CT or MRI demonstrating the level and degree of compression. A decrease in cross-sectional area of 50% is predictive of airway complications.[21,22] If available, and symptoms permit, a CT scan can be conducted with the patient at 20–30 degrees of head-up, or in lateral or prone position to minimise airway compromise. Flow volume loops can demonstrate intrathoracic or extrathoracic airway obstruction although correlation with subsequent airway obstruction is variable.

Induction of anaesthesia may result in catastrophic airway obstruction due to a reduction in intrathoracic volume, increased size of (often very vascular) tumours with increased central blood volume, and increased compressibility of airways with reduction in smooth muscle tone. Equally, cardiovascular collapse may occur due to compression of the pulmonary arteries or superior vena cava. Should it be necessary to intubate the patient with superior mediastinal syndrome there are a number of key points that need to be considered.[23,24]

1. Establish venous access in the lower half of the body in case of superior vena caval obstruction, which would result in significantly slowed transit of administered drugs and fluids.
2. Have intravenous fluid administration established to minimise the effect of vascular obstruction.
3. In high-risk cases, establishment of femoral veno-venous bypass under local anaesthesia prior to induction offers a route out in the event of complete airway obstruction. Having bypass on 'standby' is unlikely to be adequate due to the time required to establish it in the event of emergency.
4. Employ gaseous induction with preservation of spontaneous respiration or, if circumstances permit, an awake fibreoptic intubation to assess the degree of airway obstruction is advisable.
5. Neuromuscular blockade is best avoided. Subsequent positive-pressure ventilation (in concert with smooth muscle relaxation) may cause worsened bronchiolar obstruction leading to atelectasis and ventilation/perfusion mismatch. It will also increase

the pressure of the mass on mediastinal structures such as the superior vena cava, heart and pulmonary arteries with consequent potential cardiovascular collapse. If blockade is absolutely necessary, a trial of short-acting paralysis (e.g. with suxamethonium chloride (succinylcholine)) should be undertaken first. Should airway obstruction or cardiovascular collapse occur following intubation, repositioning the patient either sitting up, laterally or prone may be effective by reducing the mass effect. If this is ineffective and venovenous bypass is not possible, then emergency thoracotomy with manual displacement of the mass can be considered.

SUPERIOR VENA CAVA (SVC) COMPRESSION

SVC compression may be part of superior mediastinal syndrome but often occurs in isolation. When caused by tumour, the aetiology is normally lung cancer, lymphoma or a germ cell tumour.[25] The clinical presentation depends on the time period during which the compression has evolved as collaterals involving the azygos, internal mammary or oesophageal vessels develop over time and relieve the pressure. Patients typically present with facial and arm swelling, dyspnoea, cough and dysphagia. Those presenting to ICU are likely to have more immediately life-threatening features of either airway obstruction or cerebral oedema, in which case they may have stridor and a headache or a decreased level of consciousness.[26] In the absence of these features, SVC obstruction does not represent a true emergency and management should await histological diagnosis if one has yet to be made.[27] Endovascular stenting results in rapid resolution of symptoms in the vast majority of cases[28] and can be undertaken even in cases of complete obstruction. Radiotherapy is also effective in reducing tumour burden and achieving disease control in those cancers that are radiosensitive (which includes the majority responsible for SVC obstruction), but takes up to 4 weeks to take effect and can make subsequent histological diagnosis impossible. Steroids such as dexamethasone have a role in cases where the tumour is known to be steroid-sensitive (e.g. with lymphomas or thymomas) but are otherwise not indicated.[29]

NEUTROPENIA

Neutropenia is a common occurrence following the administration of chemotherapy and obviously predisposes the patient to infection. Care of the neutropenic patient in the intensive care setting is detailed in Chapter 99.

USE OF CHEMOTHERAPY IN THE ICU SETTING

There are little published data on the administration of chemotherapy for solid tumours in the ICU. Chemotherapy in ICU should be considered if its administration results in amelioration of life-threatening symptoms or a significant chance of improved patient outcome.[30] Prognostic indicators following chemotherapy administration appear to be similar to those for the general critically ill patient with cancer.[31]

THE EFFECT OF CRITICAL CARE ON CANCER

There has been little work looking into the effect of an ICU stay on tumour progression, but much of what happens to a patient during this period (be it disease- or treatment-mediated) has an impact on the function of the immune system and a potential consequent effect on tumour growth and metastases. The systemic inflammatory response syndrome associated with critical illness has been shown to decrease 5-year survival in patients with lung cancer.[32] Studies conducted in animals have shown that surgery in itself promotes metastasis. This is probably due to a combination of production of pro-inflammatory stimulators of tumour growth, the release of tumour cells directly into the circulation and the stress response. The stress response is mediated through the effect of catecholamines. Epinephrine (adrenaline) acts via β_2-receptors to decrease the number and activity of cytotoxic T and natural killer (NK) cells, both of which are known to destroy cancer cells. Norepinephrine (noradrenaline) has a similar effect, and has been found to induce the production of metastases in a rat model.[33,34] Interestingly, this effect was abolished by the administration of beta blockers. Tumours such as breast, colon and prostate seem to express β-receptors, which up-regulate growth when stimulated.

Hypoxia is tumour-simulating. Hypoxia leads to the production of cellular proliferative and angiogenic growth factors (notably vascular endothelial growth factor) via the generation of hypoxia-inducible factors 1α and 2α. The invasive mechanical ventilation that is commonly a response to hypoxia may similarly have a role to play; it results in the generation of immunomodulatory cytokines that add to the complex interplay of pro- and anti-inflammatory pathways.[35]

Blood transfusion can also increase the risk of tumour progression, particularly in the case of colorectal tumours. This is again thought to be related to immunosuppression. However, leucodepletion appears to make no difference to the impact on cancer recurrence after transfusion, and animal studies have suggested that transfusion of older blood may be implicated.[36]

Sedatives, induction agents and analgesics are also known to impact on cancer progression. Thiopentone, ketamine and propofol all decrease NK activity and numbers, with propofol having the least effect.[35] Morphine and fentanyl both decrease NK activity, and morphine has also been reported to promote angiogenesis and increase breast tumour cell growth in mice.[37]

In summary, admission to ICU for a patient with cancer carries a significant potential risk of promoting tumour growth and metastasis.

OUTCOMES FOR PATIENTS ADMITTED TO ICU WITH SOLID TUMOURS

The traditional view of the outcome for the critically ill cancer patient has been almost universally poor. However, for those with solid tumours, recent evidence has challenged and indeed overturned this view. Survival figures for those admitted to ICU have steadily improved over the past 15 years and approach those of patients admitted with non-oncological diagnoses in the most recent publications.[38,39,40] That said, the concept of considering all patients with solid tumours as a homogeneous group is probably flawed. A substantial proportion of the patients that present to ICU with an underlying diagnosis of solid tumour will be there for postoperative management. They have a similar mortality to patients admitted following any other major operative procedure. At the other extreme, patients with lung cancer admitted with a complication of disease or treatment have a completely different risk profile (and have an average medical ICU mortality of 36%).[41]

However, once in the ICU, prognostic indicators have, contrary to expectations, not shown disease progression, neutropenia or recent treatment with chemotherapy to be important. Instead, they are more related to the degree of acute physiological disturbance present at the time of presentation to ICU[39] and to the continued progression of organ dysfunction over the succeeding 72 hours after ICU admission. In this, the patients differ little from patients admitted to the ICU with a non-oncological diagnosis.

The reason for the improvements in reported survival of critically ill cancer patients are probably based around general improvements in ICU care including non-invasive ventilation and early goal-directed therapy, the existence of novel antitumour agents that are less cytotoxic and more efficacious, novel antifungal agents for the treatment of the neutropenic patient with fungal infection and better understanding of the management of oncological emergencies. Perhaps more importantly, there has been a change in attitude of intensive care physicians with more of us willing to admit and support critically ill cancer patients on the ICU.

Access the complete references list online at http://www.expertconsult.com

2. Taccone FS, Artigas AA, Sprung CL, et al. Characteristics and outcomes of cancer patients in European ICUs. Crit Care 2009;13:R15.
11. Coiffier B, Altman A, Pui CH, et al. Guidelines for the management of pediatric and adult tumor lysis syndrome: an evidence-based review. J Clin Oncol 2008;26(16):2767–678.
23. Erdos G, Tzanova I. Perioperative management of mediastinal mass in adults. Eur J Anaesthesiol 2009;26:627–32.
24. Slinger P, Karsli C. Management of the patient with a large anterior mediastinal mass: recurring myths. Curr Opin Anaesthesiol 2007;20(1):1–3.
35. Kelly P. Focus on oncology. The cancer critical care paradox. Curr Anaesth Crit Care 2008;19:96–104.
39. Azoulay E, Moreau D, Alberti C. Predictors of short-term mortality in critically ill patients with solid malignancies. Intensive Care Med 2000;26(12):1817–23.

Part Six

Acute Renal Failure

47

Acute kidney injury

Rinaldo Bellomo

Acute kidney injury (AKI), formerly referred to as acute renal failure (ARF), is the new international consensus term for a condition that remains a major complication of critical illness and a therapeutic challenge for the intensivist. The term AKI has been introduced to emphasise a gradation of dysfunction and abnormality that begins long before 'failure' occurs.[1] In the ICU, AKI describes a syndrome characterised by a rapid (hours to days) decrease in the kidney's ability to eliminate waste products such as urea and creatinine. Other typical clinical manifestations include decreased urine output, metabolic acidosis and hyperkalaemia.

AKI can now be defined and classified using changes in serum creatinine and urine output using the so-called RIFLE criteria.[2] This classification uses the acronym of RIFLE, to divide AKI into the categories of Risk, Injury, Failure, Loss and ESKD (**Fig. 47.1**). Using this classification, the incidence of some degree of renal dysfunction has reported to be up to 67% in a recent study of >5000 ICU patients.[3] In a study of patients admitted to Australian and New Zealand (ANZ) ICU on day one, 36% of patients had a degree of AKI.[4] In hospital patients, the development of Failure (RIFLE classification) increases the odds ratio of death 10 times.[5] Later on another consensus definition was proposed by the AKIN (Acute Kidney Injury Network) group,[5] with minor modifications and, more recently, by the KDIGO consensus group.[6] Whatever the system of classification, however, the incidence of AKI appears to be increasing in ANZ ICUs (**Fig. 47.2**).

ASSESSMENT OF RENAL FUNCTION

Renal function is complex but, in the clinical context, monitoring of renal function is reduced to the indirect assessment of GFR by the measurement of urea and creatinine in blood. These waste products of nitrogen metabolism are insensitive markers of GFR and are heavily modified by many factors and by the administration of intravenous fluids.[7] Furthermore, they start becoming abnormal only after more than 50% of GFR is lost and do not reflect dynamic changes in GFR. The use of creatinine clearance (2- or 4-hour collections) or of calculated clearance by means of formulae rarely changes clinical management. The use of more sophisticated radionuclide-based tests is useful only for research purposes.

DIAGNOSIS AND CLINICAL CLASSIFICATION

The most practically useful approach to the aetiological diagnosis of AKI is to divide its causes according to the probable source of renal injury: prerenal, renal (parenchymal or intrinsic) or postrenal.

PRERENAL RENAL FAILURE

This form of AKI is by far the most common in ICU and is considered, at least in its initial phases, to be *functional* in nature. The term indicates that the kidney malfunctions predominantly because of systemic factors that decrease glomerular filtration rate (GFR) (i.e. decreased cardiac output, hypotension, sepsis and the like). If the systemic cause of AKI is rapidly removed or corrected, renal function improves and relatively rapidly returns to near normal levels. However, if intervention is delayed or unsuccessful, renal injury becomes established (*structural*) and several days or weeks are then necessary for recovery. Several urine tests (measurement of urinary sodium, fractional excretion of sodium and other derived indices) have been promoted to help clinicians identify the development of such 'established' AKI; unfortunately, their accuracy is doubtful.[8] Their clinical utility is low. Furthermore, prerenal ARF and established ARF are part of a continuum, and their separation has limited clinical implications.[9]

PARENCHYMAL (INTRINSIC) RENAL FAILURE

This term is used to define a syndrome where the principal source of damage is within the kidney and where *structural* changes can be seen on microscopy. Disorders that affect the glomeruli or tubules can be responsible (**Box 47.1**).

Among these, nephrotoxins are particularly important, especially in hospital patients. The most common nephrotoxic drugs affecting ICU patients are listed in **Box 47.2**. Many cases of drug-induced AKI rapidly improve upon removal of the offending agent. Accordingly, a careful history of drug administration is *mandatory* in all patients with ARF. In some cases of parenchymal AKI, a correct working diagnosis can be obtained from history, physical examination and radiological and laboratory investigations. In such

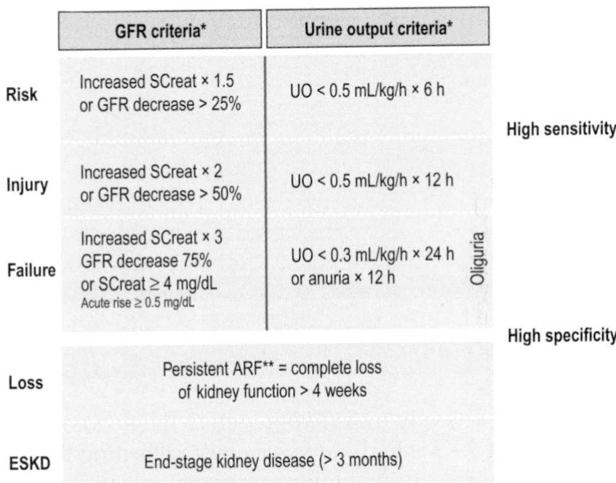

GFR criteria*
Urine output criteria*
Risk
Increased SCreat × 1.5 or GFR decrease > 25%
UO < 0.5 mL/kg/h × 6 h
High sensitivity
Injury
Increased SCreat × 2 or GFR decrease > 50%
UO < 0.5 mL/kg/h × 12 h
Failure
Increased SCreat × 3 GFR decrease 75% or SCreat ≥ 4 mg/dL Acute rise ≥ 0.5 mg/dL
UO < 0.3 mL/kg/h × 24 h or anuria × 12 h
Oliguria
High specificity
Loss
Persistent ARF** = complete loss of kidney function > 4 weeks
ESKD
End-stage kidney disease (> 3 months)

Figure 47.1 RIFLE (Risk Injury Failure Loss End stage) classification scheme for acute kidney injury. The classification system includes separate criteria for creatinine and urine output. The criteria, which lead to the worst possible classification should be used. Note that RIFLE-F (F=failure) is present even if the increase in serum creatinine concentration (S_{Creat}) is < threefold so long as the new S_{Creat}>4.0 mg/dL (350 μmol/L) in the setting of an acute increase of at least 0.5 mg/dL (44 μmol/L). The designation RIFLE-F_C should be used in this case to denote 'acute-on-chronic' disease. Similarly when RIFLE-F classification is reached by urine output criteria only, a designation of RIFLE-F_O should be used to denote oliguria. The shape of the figure denotes the fact that more patients (high sensitivity) will be included in the mild category, including some without actually having 'renal failure' (less specificity). In contrast, at the bottom, the criteria are strict and therefore specific, but some patients with renal dysfunction might be missed. GFR=glomerular filtration rate; ARF=acute renal failure; UO=urine output.

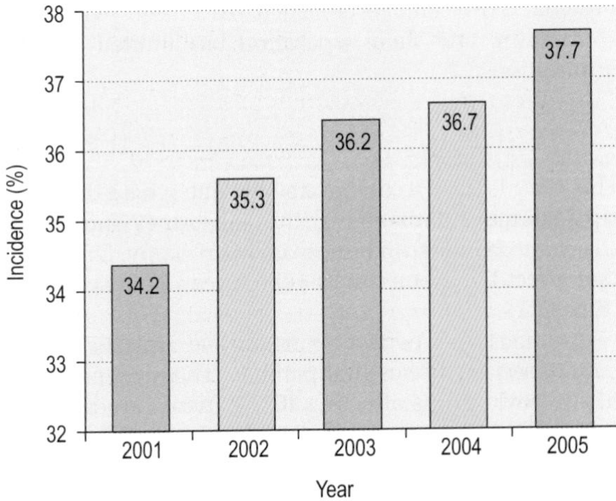

Figure 47.2 Graphic representation of the change in the incidence of AKI on day one after ICU admission in ICUs contributing to the adult patient database in Australia and New Zealand.

Box 47.1 Causes of intrinsic (parenchymal) AKI

- Glomerulonephritis
- Vasculitis
- Interstitial nephritis
- Malignant hypertension
- Pyelonephritis
- Bilateral cortical necrosis
- Amyloidosis
- Malignancy
- Nephrotoxins
- Cholesterol embolism

Box 47.2 Drugs that may contribute to AKI in the ICU

Radiocontrast agents
Aminoglycosides
Amphotericin
Non-steroidal anti-inflammatory drugs
β-lactam antibiotics (interstitial nephropathy)
Sulfonamides
Aciclovir (acyclovir)
Methotrexate
Cisplatin
Cyclosporin A
Tacrolimus
Sirolimus (rapamycin)
Starch solutions

patients one can proceed to a therapeutic trial without the need to resort to renal biopsy. However, if immunosuppressive therapy is considered, renal biopsy is recommended.

More than a third of patients who develop AKI in ICU have chronic renal dysfunction due to factors such as age-related changes, long-standing hypertension, diabetes or atheromatous disease of the renal vessels. Such chronic renal dysfunction may be manifest by a raised serum creatinine. However, this is not always the case. Often, what may seem to the clinician to be a relatively trivial insult that does not fully explain the onset of AKI in a normal patient is sufficient to unmask lack of renal functional reserve in another patient.

Beyond all the above considerations, however, the most common type of so-called intrinsic AKI falls under the traditional name of acute tubular necrosis (ATN). In classic teaching, ATN is used to describe a form of 'intrinsic' AKI that follows from severe and persistent prerenal AKI. It is assumed that tubular necrosis results from such continued hypoperfusion. This approach is widely accepted and used by textbooks and clinicians, but raises serious concerns.[10]

The first concern with the term ATN is that it conflates a histological diagnosis (tubular necrosis) that is rarely confirmed by biopsy (and is therefore not scientifically verifiable or falsifiable) with a complex clinical syndrome (typically AKI of >72 hours). Such a syndrome, in many cases, has *not* been convincingly linked with the specific histopathological appearance of ATN in both animal experiments and human disease.[10]

The second concern is that ATN is believed to represent the consequence of sustained or severe prerenal azotaemia, which, unlike ATN, is believed not to be associated with histopathological changes (and is therefore not classified as intrinsic AKI). Such prerenal azotaemia can be expected to resolve over 2–3 days. Unfortunately, the term 'prerenal azotaemia' is, like ATN, conceptually flawed[11–12] because it implies that clinicians can know with a sufficient degree of certainty, by taking a history, examining the patient and performing urine and blood tests, that there is no histopathological injury to the tubules.

The third concern is that such concepts are biologically flawed because they imply that AKI does not represent (like all other known diseases) a continuum of injury but rather a yes-or-no phenomenon in terms of histological damage. For these reasons, terms like prerenal azotaemia and ATN are increasingly being challenged.[9,12]

HEPATORENAL SYNDROME (HRS)

This condition is a form of ARF that occurs in the setting of severe liver dysfunction in the absence of other known causes of ARF.[13] Typically, it presents as progressive oliguria with a very low urinary sodium concentration (<10 mmol/L). Its pathogenesis is not well understood. New consensus definitions, however, now define HRS as any development of AKI in the setting of advanced liver disease that is not due to intrinsic causes. Thus, sepsis, paracentesis-induced hypovolaemia, raised intra-abdominal pressure due to tense ascites, diuretic-induced hypovolaemia, lactulose-induced hypovolaemia, and any combination of these, which in the past were used to exclude HRS, are now acknowledged triggers of this condition.[14] The avoidance of hypovolaemia by albumin administration in patients with spontaneous bacterial peritonitis has been shown to decrease the incidence of AKI.[15] More importantly, multiple observational studies, several controlled trials and growing clinical experience have led to the acceptance and widespread use of terlipressin to improve GFR in this condition.[16]

RHABDOMYOLYSIS-ASSOCIATED ARF

This condition accounts for close to 5–10%[17] of cases of ARF in ICU depending on the setting. Its pathogenesis involves prerenal, renal and postrenal factors. It is now typically seen following major trauma, drug overdose with narcotics, vascular embolism, and in response to a variety of agents that can induce major muscle injury. The principles of treatment are based on retrospective data. They include prompt and aggressive fluid resuscitation, elimination of causative agents, correction of compartment syndromes, the alkalinisation of urine (pH>6.5) and the maintenance of polyuria (>300 ml/h). The role of mannitol is controversial.

POSTRENAL RENAL FAILURE

Obstruction to urine outflow is the most common cause of functional renal impairment in the community,[18] but is uncommon in the ICU. The clinical presentation of obstruction may be acute or acute-on-chronic in patients with long-standing renal calculi. It may not always be associated with oliguria. If obstruction is suspected, ultrasonography can be easily performed at the bedside. However, not all cases of acute obstruction have an abnormal ultrasound and, in many cases, obstruction occurs in conjunction with other renal insults (e.g. staghorn calculi and severe sepsis of renal origin). Assessment of the role of each factor and overall management should be conducted in conjunction with a urologist. Finally, the sudden and unexpected development of anuria in an ICU patient should always suggest obstruction of the urinary catheter as the cause. Appropriate flushing or changing of the catheter should be implemented in this setting.

PATHOGENESIS OF ACUTE KIDNEY INJURY

The pathogenesis of obstructive AKI involves several humoral responses as well as mechanical factors. The pathogenesis of parenchymal renal failure as seen with glomerulonephritis is typically immunological. It varies from vasculitis to interstitial nephropathy and involves an extraordinary complexity of immunological mechanisms. The pathogenesis of prerenal AKI is of greater direct relevance to the intensivist.

The overwhelming majority of our conceptions of the pathophysiology of prerenal AKI are derived from animal models[19,20] using ischaemia by the acute and complete occlusion of the arterial vascular supply to the kidney.

Unfortunately, the clinical relevance of such models is limited, maybe even negligible to conditions like sepsis,[21,22] now the most common triggers of AKI in hospital and ICU patients. However, models of septic AKI that fully resemble the human phenotype are difficult to develop. When a hyperdynamic sepsis phenotype with AKI is produced in large animals, renal blood flow actually increases to supranormal levels and renal histopathology is essentially normal.[23, 24] If experimental septic AKI can occur in the setting of increased renal blood flow, it is impossible to know for sure that this does not also happen in humans. Histopathological assessment in humans remains confined to rapid postmortem assessment, and assessment of renal blood flow is similarly extremely difficult and confined to invasive techniques.

Despite all of the above observations, activation of the renin–angiotensin system (RAS), activation of the renal sympathetic system,[25] and activation of the tubule-glomerular feedback (TGF) system seem to play a role.[26] However, it remains unclear which particular pathway of injury has *primacy* in terms of *importance or timing* or *both*. Finally, it remains unknown whether intrarenal shunting contributes to decreased GFR and ischaemia of the renal medulla. Such shunting may also be coupled with changes in the microcirculation, suggesting that, even if one could measure global renal blood flow with reasonable accuracy, unless the microcirculation is also assessed our understanding of AKI will remain poor.

THE CLINICAL PICTURE

The most common clinical picture seen in ICU is that of a patient who has sustained/is experiencing a major systemic insult (trauma, sepsis, myocardial infarction, severe haemorrhage, cardiogenic shock, major surgery and the like). When the patient arrives in the ICU, resuscitation is typically well under way or surgery may have just been completed. Despite such efforts, the patient is already anuric or oliguric, the serum creatinine is rising and a metabolic acidosis may be developing. Potassium and phosphate levels may be rising as well. Mechanical ventilation and the need for vasoactive drugs are common. Fluid resuscitation is typically undertaken in the ICU under the guidance of invasive haemodynamic monitoring. Vasoactive drugs are often used to restore MAP to 'acceptable' levels (typically >65–70 mmHg). The patient may improve over time and urine output may return with or without the assistance of diuretic agents. If urine output does not return, however, renal replacement therapy (RRT) needs to be considered. Once the cause of AKI has been removed and the patient has become physiologically stable, slow (days to weeks) recovery will typically occur. If the cause of AKI has not been adequately remedied, the patient remains gravely ill, the kidneys do not recover and death from multi-organ failure may occur.

PREVENTING ACUTE KIDNEY INJURY

The fundamental principle of AKI prevention is to treat its cause. If prerenal factors contribute, these must be identified, and haemodynamic resuscitation quickly instituted.

RESUSCITATION

Intravascular volume must be maintained or rapidly restored, and this is often best done using invasive haemodynamic monitoring (central venous catheter, arterial cannula, and pulmonary artery catheter or pulse contour cardiac output catheters in some cases). Oxygenation must be maintained. An adequate haemoglobin concentration (at least >70 g/L) must be maintained or immediately restored. Once intravascular volume has been restored, some patients remain hypotensive (mean arterial pressure (MAP) <70 mmHg). In these patients, autoregulation of renal blood flow may be lost. Restoration of MAP to near-normal levels may increase GFR. Such elevations in MAP, however, require the addition of vasopressor drugs.[27] The nephroprotective role of additional fluid therapy in a patient with a normal or increased cardiac output and blood pressure is questionable. Despite these resuscitation measures, AKI may still develop if cardiac output is inadequate. This may require a variety of interventions from the use of inotropic drugs to the application of ventricular assist devices.

NEPHROPROTECTIVE DRUGS

Following haemodynamic resuscitation and removal of nephrotoxins, it is unclear whether the use of additional pharmacological measures is of further benefit to the kidneys. A phase III trial in critically ill patients showed that low-dose dopamine is only as effective as placebo in the prevention of renal dysfunction in ICU patients.[28] The use of loop diuretics is controversial and not supported by high-quality evidence. Other agents such as theophylline, urodilatin, anaritide (a synthetic atrial natriuretic factor) and fenoldopam have failed to show consistent benefits.

In patients receiving radiocontrast saline, infusion to maintain intravascular fluid expansion is helpful in attenuating kidney injury. The relevance of such treatment in critically ill patients, however, remains unclear. The benefits of *n*-acetylcysteine and bicarbonate infusion as protective strategies in this context also remain controversial.

DIAGNOSTIC INVESTIGATIONS

An aetiological diagnosis of AKI must always be established. Such diagnosis may be obvious on clinical grounds. In other cases, investigations including the examination of urinary sediment and exclusion of a urinary tract infection (most if not all patients), the exclusion of obstruction when appropriate (some patients) and the careful exclusion of nephrotoxins (all patients) may be needed.

In specific situations, other investigations are necessary to establish the diagnosis, such as creatine kinase and free myoglobin for possible rhabdomyolysis. A chest radiograph, a blood film, the measurement of non-specific inflammatory markers, and the measurement of specific antibodies (anti-GBM, antineutrophil cytoplasm, anti-DNA, anti-smooth muscle, etc.) may help diagnose vasculitis or of certain types of collagen disease or glomerulonephritis. If thrombotic–thrombocytopenic purpura is suspected, the additional measurement of lactic dehydrogenase, haptoglobin, unconjugated bilirubin and free haemoglobin are needed. In some patients, specific findings (cryoglobulins, Bence–Jones proteins) are almost diagnostic. In a few rare patients, a renal biopsy might become necessary.

NOVEL BIOMARKERS OF AKI

Using new search techniques based on proteomics investigators have identified novel biomarkers of AKI.[29] The identification of these biomarkers may change our classification and treatment of this condition in the near future. These biomarkers appear to change significantly earlier than changes in serum creatinine.[30] They appear to reflect different aspects of renal injury. For example, cystatin C appears to reflects changes in glomerular filtration rate, while neutrophil gelatinase-associated lipocalin (NGAL) appears to reflect tubular stress/injury. They also appear to dynamically change with treatment or recovery, which suggests that they can be used to monitor interventions. They may identify subpopulations of patients who do not have AKI according to creatinine-based criteria, but actually have a degree of kidney stress/injury that can be detected by biomarkers and is associated with worse outcomes.[30] Finally, by identifying possible mechanisms of injury they may increase our understanding of the pathogenesis of AKI. Their therapeutic implications however, remain unclear.

MANAGEMENT OF ESTABLISHED ACUTE KIDNEY INJURY

The principles of management of established AKI are the treatment or removal of its cause, the avoidance of nephrotoxins and the maintenance of physiological homeostasis while recovery takes place. Complications such as encephalopathy, pericarditis, myopathy, neuropathy, electrolyte disturbances or other major electrolyte, fluid or metabolic derangement should never occur in a modern ICU. Their prevention may include several measures that vary in complexity, from fluid restriction to the initiation of extracorporeal renal replacement therapy.

Nutritional support should be started early and should contain adequate calories (20–30 kcal/kg/day) as a mixture of carbohydrates and lipids. Adequate protein (1–2 g/kg/day) should be administered. There is no evidence that specific renal nutritional solutions are useful. Vitamins and trace elements should be administered at least according to their recommended daily allowance. The role of newer immunonutritional solution remains controversial. The enteral route is preferred to the use of parenteral nutrition.

Hyperkalaemia (>6 mmol/L) must be promptly treated either with insulin and dextrose administration, the infusion of bicarbonate if acidosis is present, the administration of nebulised salbutamol, or all of the above together. If the 'true' serum potassium is >7 mmol/L or electrocardiographic signs of hyperkalaemia appear, calcium gluconate (10 mL of 10% solution i.v.) should also be administered. The above measures are temporising actions, while renal replacement therapy is being set up. The presence of hyperkalaemia is a major indication for the immediate institution of renal replacement therapy.

Metabolic acidosis is almost always present but rarely requires treatment per se. Anaemia requires correction to maintain a haemoglobin of at least >70 g/L. More aggressive transfusion needs individual patient assessment. Drug therapy must be adjusted to take into account the effect of the decreased clearances associated with loss of renal function. Stress ulcer prophylaxis is advisable. Assiduous attention should be paid to the prevention of infection.

Fluid overload can be prevented by the use of loop diuretics in polyuric patients. However, if the patient is oliguric, the only way to avoid fluid overload is to institute renal replacement therapy (RRT) at an early stage (see Ch. 48). Marked azotaemia ([urea]>40 mmol/L or [creatinine] >400 µmol/L) is undesirable and should probably be treated with RRT unless recovery is imminent or already under way and a return toward normal values is expected within 24–48 hours. It is recognised, however, that no RCTs exist to define the ideal time for intervention with artificial renal support.

PROGNOSIS

The mortality of critically ill patients with ARF remains high (40–50% depending on case-mix). It is frequently stated that patients die with renal failure rather than of renal failure. However, much indirect evidence supports a careful and proactive approach to the treatment of patients with ARF, which is based on the prevention of uncontrolled uraemia and the maintenance of low urea levels throughout the patient's illness. Finally ICU patients with AKI typically recover to baseline or near-baseline function even when suffering from severe AKI and long-term dialysis is an uncommon complication.

Access the complete references list online at http://www.expertconsult.com

1. Kellum JA, Bellomo R, Ronco C. Kidney attack. JAMA 2012;307:2265–6.
2. Bellomo R, Ronco C, Kellum JA, et al. and the ADQI workgroup. Acute renal failure – definition, outcome measures, animal models, fluid therapy and information technology needs: the Second International Consensus Conference of the Acute Dialysis Quality Initiative (ADQI) Group. Crit Care 2004;8:R204–10.
7. Liu K, Thomson T, Ancukiewics M, et al. Acute kidney injury with acute lung injury: impact of fluid accumulation on classification of acute kidney injury and associated outcomes. Crit Care Med 2011;39: 2665–71.
17. Uchino S, Kellum J, Bellomo R, et al. Acute renal failure in critically ill patients – A multinational, multicenter study. JAMA 2005;294:813–18.
29. Devarajan P, Krawczeski CD, Nguyen MT, et al. Proteomic identification of early biomarkers of acute kidney injury after cardiac surgery in children. Am J Kidney Dis 2010;56:632–42.

48

Renal replacement therapy

Rinaldo Bellomo

When acute kidney injury (AKI) is severe, resolution can take several days or weeks. During this time, the kidneys cannot maintain homeostasis of fluid, potassium, metabolic acid and waste products. Life-threatening complications frequently develop. In these patients, extracorporeal techniques of blood purification must be applied to prevent such complications. Such techniques, broadly named renal replacement therapy (RRT), include continuous haemofiltration and its technical variations, intermittent haemodialysis and peritoneal dialysis, each with its technical variations. All of these techniques rely on the principle of removing unwanted solutes and water through a semipermeable membrane. Such membrane is either biological (peritoneum) or artificial (haemodialysis or haemofiltration membranes) and each offers several advantages, disadvantages and limitations.

PRINCIPLES

The principles of RRT have been extensively studied and described.[1–3] This is a summary of some aspects that are relevant to the critical care physician.

WATER REMOVAL

The removal of unwanted solvent (water) is therapeutically probably as important as the removal of unwanted solute (acid, uraemic toxins, potassium and the like). During RRT, water is removed through a process called *ultrafiltration*. This process is essentially the same as that performed by the glomerulus. It requires a driving pressure to move fluid across a semipermeable membrane because such fluid would normally be kept within the circulation due to oncotic pressure (colloid osmotic pressure). This pressure is achieved by:

1. Generating a *transmembrane pressure* though pumped blood flow (as in haemofiltration or during intermittent haemodialysis) that is greater than oncotic pressure
2. Increasing osmolarity of the dialysate (as in peritoneal dialysis).

SOLUTE REMOVAL

The removal of unwanted solute can be achieved by:

1. Creating an electrochemical gradient across the membrane using a flow-past system with toxin-free dialysate (*diffusion*) as in intermittent haemodialysis (IHD) and peritoneal dialysis (PD)
2. Creating a transmembrane-pressure-driven 'solvent drag', where solutes move together with solvent (*convection*) across a porous membrane, are discarded together with the solvent and then replaced with toxin-free replacement fluid as in haemofiltration (HF).

The rate of diffusion of a given solute depends on its molecular weight, the porosity of the membrane, the blood flow rate, the dialysate flow rate, the degree of protein binding, and its concentration gradient across the membrane. If standard, low-flux, cellulose-based membranes are used, middle molecules of >500 Daltons (D) molecular weight (MW) cannot be removed. If synthetic high-flux membranes are used (cut-off at 10–20 kiloDaltons (kD) in MW), larger molecules can be removed. With these membranes, convection is superior to diffusion in achieving the clearance of middle molecules.

INDICATIONS FOR RENAL REPLACEMENT THERAPY

In the critically ill patient, RRT should be initiated early, prior to the development of complications. Fear of early RRT stems from historical experience with the adverse effects of conventional intermittent haemodialysis (IHD) with cuprophane membranes, especially haemodynamic instability, and from the risks and limitations of continuous or intermittent PD.[4–5] However, continuous renal replacement therapy (CRRT)[6,7] or slow extended daily dialysis (SLEDD)[8] minimise these effects. The criteria for the initiation of RRT in patients with chronic renal failure are probably inappropriate in the critically ill.[9,10] A set of modern criteria for the initiation of RRT in the ICU is presented in **Box 48.1**.

With IHD or CRRT or SLEDD, there are limited data on what is 'adequate' intensity of dialysis. However, the concept of dialytic adequacy should include maintenance of homeostasis at all levels[10] and better uraemic control may translate into better survival.[11,12] An appropriate target urea might be 15–25 mmol/L, with a

Box 48.1 Modern criteria for the initiation of RRT in the ICU*

1. Oliguria (urine output <200 mL/12 hours)
2. Anuria (urine output: 0–50 mL/12 hours)
3. [Urea]>35 mmol/L
4. [Creatinine]>400 μmol/L
5. $[K^+]$>6.5 mmol/L or rapidly rising†
6. Pulmonary oedema unresponsive to diuretics
7. Uncompensated metabolic acidosis (pH<7.1)
8. $[Na^+]$<110 and >160 mmol/L
9. Temperature >40°C
10. Uraemic complications (encephalopathy/myopathy/neuropathy/pericarditis)
11. Overdose with a dialysable toxin (e.g. lithium)

*If one criterion is present, RRT should be considered. If two criteria are simultaneously present, RRT is strongly recommended.
†Please be aware of differences between plasma vs serum measurement in your laboratory.

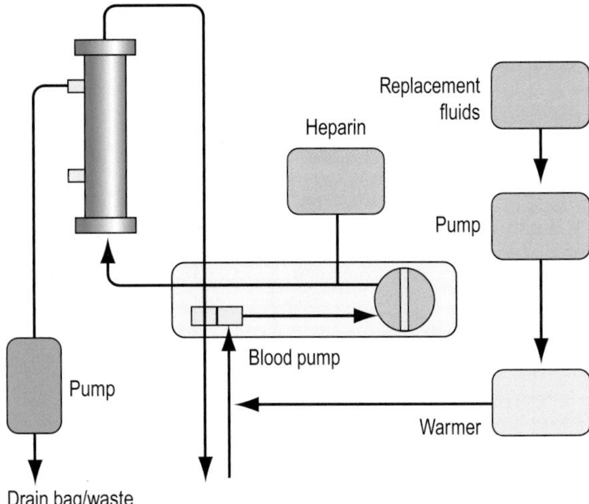

Figure 48.1 A continuous veno-venous haemofiltration (CVVH) circuit.

protein intake around 1.5 g/kg/day. This can be easily achieved using CRRT at urea clearances of 20–25 mL/kg/h depending on catabolic rate. If intermittent therapy is used, daily and extended treatment as described with SLEDD may be desirable in the ICU.[13]

MODALITY OF RENAL REPLACEMENT THERAPY

There is a great deal of controversy as to which modality of RRT is 'best' in the ICU, due to the lack of randomised controlled trials comparing different modalities (IHD or CRRT). In their absence, modalities of RRT may be judged on the basis of the following criteria:

1. Haemodynamic side-effects
2. Ability to control fluid status
3. Biocompatibility
4. Risk of infection
5. Uraemic control
6. Avoidance of cerebral oedema
7. Ability to allow full nutritional support
8. Ability to control acidosis
9. Absence of specific side-effects
10. Cost.

In relation to the above criteria, CRRT and slow low-efficiency daily dialysis (SLEDD) offer many advantages over PD and conventional IHD (3–4 hours/day, 3–4 times/week)[13] and, while CRRT or SLEDD are almost exclusively used in Australia and New Zealand,[14] only a percentage of American ICU patients receive CRRT. Irrespective of the choice of modality, some salient aspects of CRRT, IHD and PD require discussion.

CONTINUOUS RENAL REPLACEMENT THERAPY

First described in 1977, CRRT has undergone several technical modifications. It is now performed using double-lumen catheters and peristaltic blood pumps with control of ultrafiltration rate. If no dialysate is used and effluent is replaced with replacement solutions, the technique is called continuous veno-venous haemofiltration (CVVH). During CVVH, ultrafiltration rates of 2 L/h yield urea clearances of approximately 25 mL/kg/h in the average 80-kg patient. Diagrams illustrating typical haemofiltration circuits are presented in **Figures 48.1–48.3**.

In a veno-venous system, dialysate can also be delivered countercurrent to blood flow (continuous veno-venous haemodialysis/haemodiafiltration) to achieve either almost pure diffusive clearance or a mixture of diffusive and convective clearance.

No matter what technique is used, the following outcomes are predictable:

1. Continuous control of fluid status
2. Haemodynamic stability
3. Control of acid–base status
4. Ability to provide protein-rich nutrition while achieving uraemic control
5. Control of electrolyte balance, including phosphate and calcium balance
6. Prevention of swings in intracerebral water
7. Minimal risk of infection
8. High level of biocompatibility.

However, CRRT mandates the presence of specifically trained nursing and medical staff 24 hours a day and the issues of continuous circuit anticoagulation or the potential risk of bleeding have been of concern.

CIRCUIT ANTICOAGULATION

The flow of blood through an extracorporeal circuit causes activation of the coagulation cascade and promotes clotting of the filter and circuit itself. In order to delay such clotting and achieve acceptable operational lives (approximately 24 hours) for the circuit,

Dialysate
Pump
Warmer
Replacement fluids
Heparin
Pump
Blood pump
Pump
Drain bag/waste

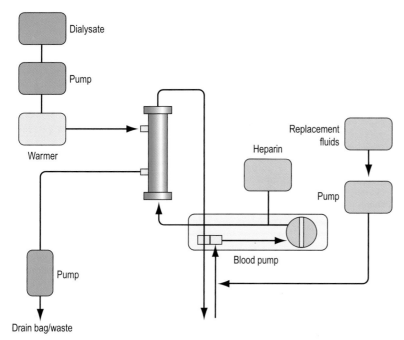

Figure 48.2 A continuous veno-venous haemodiafiltration (CVVHDF) circuit.

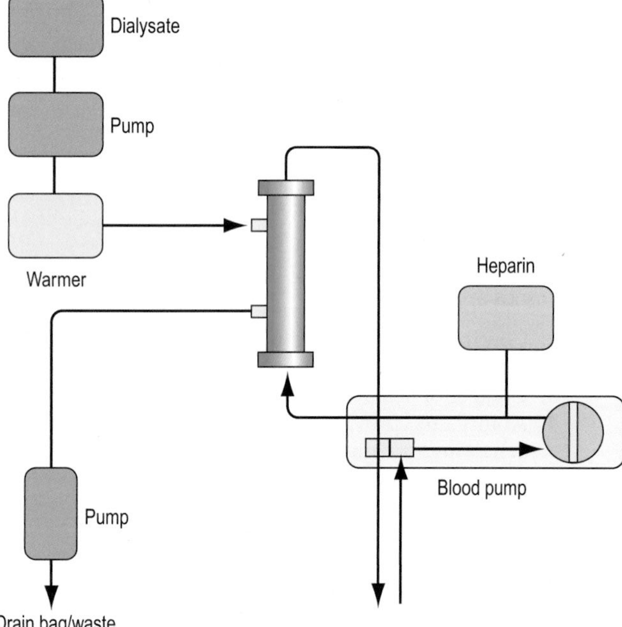

Figure 48.3 A continuous veno-venous hemodialysis (CVVHD) circuit.

anticoagulants are frequently used.[15] However, circuit anticoagulation increases the risk of bleeding. Therefore, the risks and benefits of more or less intense anticoagulation and alternative strategies (**Box 48.2**) must be considered.

In the vast majority of patients, low-dose heparin (<500 IU/h) is sufficient to achieve adequate (approximately 24 hours) circuit life, is easy and cheap to administer and has almost no effect on the patient's coagulation tests. In some patients, a higher dose is necessary. In others (pulmonary embolism, myocardial ischaemia) full heparinisation may actually be concomitantly indicated.

Regional citrate anticoagulation is very effective but requires a special dialysate or replacement fluid.[16] Nevertheless, it is safe and effective in patients who do not have liver failure. In patients with liver failure, citrate may accumulate and induce a coagulopathy. The

Box 48.2 Strategies for circuit anticoagulation during CRRT

1. No anticoagulation
2. Low-dose pre-filter heparin (<500 IU/h)
3. Medium-dose pre-filter heparin (500–1000 IU/h)
4. Full heparinisation
5. Regional anticoagulation (pre-filter heparin and post-filter protamine usually at a 100 IU: IU 1 mg ratio) (1500 IU/h of heparin pre-filter and 15 mg/h of protamine post-filter)
6. Regional citrate anticoagulation (pre-filter citrate and post-filter calcium and magnesium – special calcium-free dialysate needed or citrate-containing replacement fluid delivered pre-filter)
7. Low-molecular-weight heparin
8. Prostacyclin
9. Heparinoids

biochemical signs of citrate accumulation are an increasing base deficit, an increasing requirement for calcium administration to maintain the target level of calcaemia and widening of the total calcium to ionised calcium ratio. Magnesium supplementation is also needed. Due to development of commercially available dialysate and replacement fluids to facilitate citrate anticoagulation, and due to new CRRT machine technology to enable such anticoagulation to be performed with minimal risk, the use of citrate anticoagulation is rapidly expanding.[17]

Regional heparin/protamine anticoagulation is also somewhat complex, but simpler than citrate anticoagulation, and may be useful if frequent filter clotting occurs and further anticoagulation of the patient is considered dangerous. Low-molecular-weight heparin is also easy to administer, but more expensive. If enoxaparin is used, its dose should be adjusted for the loss of renal function. Heparinoids and prostacyclin may be useful if the patient has developed heparin-induced thrombocytopenia and thrombosis. Finally, in perhaps 10–20% of patients anticoagulation of any kind is best avoided because of endogenous coagulopathy or recent surgery or inability to metabolise citrate. In such patients, adequate filter life can be achieved provided that blood flow is kept at about 200 mL/min and vascular access is reliable.[18]

Many circuits clot for *mechanical reasons* (e.g. inadequate access, unreliable blood flow from double-lumen catheter depending on patient position, kinking of catheter). Responding to frequent filter clotting by simply increasing anticoagulation without making the correct aetiological diagnosis (e.g. checking catheter flow and position, taking a history surrounding the episode of clotting, identifying the site of clotting) is often futile and exposes the patient to unnecessary risk. Particular attention needs to be paid to the adequacy/ease of flow through the double-lumen catheter. Smaller (11.5 Fr) catheters in the subclavian position are a particular problem. Larger catheters (13.5 Fr) in the femoral position or internal jugular position appear to perform more reliably.[19]

CRRT TECHNOLOGY

The increasing use of veno-venous CRRT has led to the development of a field of CRRT technology, which offers different kinds of machines to facilitate its performance.[20] Some understanding of these devices is important to the successful implementation of CRRT in any ICU. These machines are safer and have much more sophisticated pump control systems, alarms and graphic displays. They are much more user-friendly, especially with respect to the set-up procedure. They provide information on outflow pressure (the suction pressure applied to the outflow lumen of the dialysis catheter and a marker of its performance), the transmembrane pressure (a marker of membrane fouling and clotting) and inflow pressure (a marker of resistance to inflow). Such pressures are often useful is assessing catheter function and the aetiology of circuit loss.

The choice of membrane is also a matter of controversy. There are no controlled studies to show that one of them confers a clinical advantage over the others. The AN 69 is the most commonly used CRRT membrane in Australia. The issue of membrane size is also controversial as no controlled studies have compared different membrane surface sizes. If high-volume haemofiltration is planned, however, the membrane surface needs to be in the 1.6–2 m^2 range.

INTENSITY OF CRRT

The optimal dose (expressed at effective effluent/kg/h) of CRRT has been the subject of controversy for almost a decade. Several studies had initially suggested that higher dose may translate into better outcome.[21–23] However, such studies had been single centre in nature and were considered to require confirmation in multicentre randomised controlled trials. Two such trials were completed in 2008[24] and 2009.[25] Both showed no difference with increasing the intensity of RRT indicating that, in current practice, the prescribed dose of RRT should be equivalent to 25–30 mL/kg/h to take into account the impact of 'down-time' on delivered dose. Moreover, essentially all AKI patients on vasopressor support received CRRT in the ATN and RENAL trial. Thus, by practice consensus, CRRT has now become the de facto standard of care in haemodynamically unstable patients. Renal recovery was much greater in the RENAL trial (with essentially exclusive use of CRRT) than in the ATN trial (with substantial use of IHD) suggesting that the use of CRRT might facilitate renal recovery.

INTERMITTENT HAEMODIALYSIS

Vascular access is typically by double-lumen catheter as in continuous haemofiltration. The circuit is also the same. Countercurrent dialysate flow is used as in CVVHD. The major differences are that standard IHD uses high dialysate flows (300–400 mL/min), generates dialysate by mixing purified water and concentrate and treatment is applied for short periods of time (3–4 hours), usually every second day. These differences have important implications. Firstly, volume has to be removed over a short period of time and this may cause hypotension. Repeated hypotensive episodes may delay renal recovery.[4] Secondly, solute removal is episodic. This translates into inferior uraemic control[26] and acid–base control. Limited fluid and uraemic control imposes unnecessary limitations on nutritional support. Furthermore, rapid solute shifts increase brain water content and raise intracranial pressure.[27] Finally, much controversy has surrounded the issue of membrane bioincompatibility. Standard low-flux dialysing membranes made of cuprophane are known to trigger the activation of several inflammatory pathways, compared with high-flux synthetic membranes (also used for continuous haemofiltration). It is possible that such pro-inflammatory effect contributes to further renal damage and delays recovery or even affects mortality. Given the minimal difference in cost between biocompatible and bioincompatible low-flux membranes, biocompatible (polysulfone) membranes are now preferred.

The limitations of applying 'standard' IHD to the treatment of ARF[9] have led to the development of new approaches (so-called 'hybrid techniques') such as SLEDD.[13] These techniques seek to adapt IHD to the clinical circumstances and thereby increase its tolerance and its clearances.

PERITONEAL DIALYSIS

This technique is now uncommonly used in the treatment of adult ARF in developed countries.[23] However, it may be an adequate technique in developing countries or in children where the peritoneal membrane has a greater relative surface or alternatives are considered too expensive, too invasive, or are not available. Typically access is by the insertion of an intraperitoneal catheter. Glucose-rich dialysate is then inserted into the peritoneal cavity and acts as the 'dialysate'. After a given 'dwell time' it is removed and discarded with the extra fluid and toxins that have moved from the blood vessels of the peritoneum to the dialysate fluid. Machines are also available that deliver and remove dialysate at higher flows providing intermittent treatment or higher solute clearances. Several major shortcomings make PD relatively unsuited to the treatment of adult ARF:

1. Limited and sometimes inadequate solute clearance
2. High risk of peritonitis
3. Unpredictable hyperglycemia
4. Fluid leaks
5. Protein loss
6. Interference with diaphragm function.

There have not been any reports of the sole use of PD for the treatment of adult patients with ARF in the last 15 years. A randomised trial comparing PD with CVVH found that PD was associated with increased mortality.[28]

OTHER BLOOD PURIFICATION TECHNIQUES

HAEMOPERFUSION

During haemoperfusion, blood is circulated through a circuit similar to one used for CVVH. However, a charcoal cartridge is perfused with blood instead of a dialysis membrane. In some cases an ion exchange resin (Amberlite) has been used. Charcoal microcapsules effectively remove molecules of 300–500 D in molecular weight; including some lipid-soluble and protein-bound substances. Heparinisation is necessary to prevent clotting. Attention must also be paid to changes in intravascular volume at the start of therapy because of the large priming volume of the cartridge (260 mL). Glucose absorption is significant and monitoring of blood glucose is necessary to avoid hypoglycaemia. Also thrombocytopenia is common, and can be marked. The role of haemoperfusion is controversial, as no controlled trials have ever shown it to confer clinically significant advantages. It may be useful, however, in patients with life-threatening theophylline overdose because it removes the agent effectively.

PLASMAPHERESIS OR PLASMA EXCHANGE

With this technique, plasma is removed from the patient and exchanged with fresh frozen plasma (FFP) and a mixture of colloid and crystalloid solutions. This technique can also be performed in an ICU familiar with CRRT techniques. A plasmafilter (a filter that allows the passage of molecules up to 500 kD) instead of a haemofilter is inserted in the CVVH circuit, and the filtrate (plasma) discarded. Plasmapheresis can also be performed with special machines using the principles of centrifugation. The differences, if any, between centrifugation and filtration technology are unclear. Replacement (post-filter) will occur as in CVVH using, for example, a 50/50 combination of FFP and albumin. Plasmapheresis has been shown to be effective treatment for thrombotic thrombocytopenic purpura (TTP) and for several diseases mediated by abnormal antibodies (Guillain–Barré syndrome, cryoglobulinaemia, myasthenia gravis, Goodpasture syndrome, etc.) in which antibody removal appears desirable. Its role in the treatment of sepsis remains uncertain.[29]

BLOOD PURIFICATION TECHNOLOGY OUTSIDE OF ARF

There is growing interest in the possibility that blood purification may provide a clinically significant benefit in patients with severe sepsis/septic shock by removing circulating 'mediators'. A variety of techniques including plasmapheresis, high-volume haemofiltration, very-high-volume haemofiltration, and coupled plasma filtration adsorption and large-pore haemofiltration[29-31] are being studied in animals and in phase I/II studies in humans. Initial experiments support the need to continue exploring this therapeutic option. However, no suitably powered randomised controlled trials have yet been reported. Also, blood purification technology in combination with bioreactors containing either human or porcine liver cells is under active investigation as a form of artificial liver support for patients with fulminant liver failure or for patients with acute-on-chronic liver failure. Albumin-based dialysis has been developed to deal with protein-bound toxins in patients with liver failure. This system, known as MARS (molecular adsorption recirculating system), has shown benefits in patients with elevated intracranial pressure and/or acute-on-chronic liver failure, but not in patients with fulminant liver failure.[32]

DRUG PRESCRIPTION DURING DIALYTIC THERAPY

Acute renal failure and RRT profoundly affect drug clearance. A comprehensive description of changes in drug dosage according to the technique of RRT, residual creatinine clearance and other determinants of pharmacodynamics is beyond the scope of this chapter and can be found in specialist texts.[33] **Table 48.1** provides general guidelines for the prescription of drugs commonly used in the ICU.

Table 48.1 Drug dosage during dialytic therapy*

DRUG	CRRT	IHD
Aminoglycosides	Normal dose q. 36 h	50% normal dose q. 48 h–2/3 re-dose after IHD
Cefotaxime or Ceftazidime	1g q. 8–12 h	1g q. 12–24 h after IHD
Imipenem	500 mg q. 8 h	250 mg q. 8 h and after IHD
Meropenem	500 mg q. 8 h	250 mg q. 8 h and after IHD
Metronidazole	500 mg q. 8 h	250 mg q. 8 h and after IHD
Co-trimoxazole	Normal dose q 18 h	Normal dose q 24 h after IHD
Amoxicillin	500 mg q. 8 h	500 mg daily and after IHD
Vancomycin	1 g q. 24 h	1 g q. 96–120 h
Piperacillin	3–4 g q. 6 h	3–4 g q. 8 h and after IHD
Ticarcillin	1–2 g q. 8 h	1–2 g q. 12 h and after IHD
Ciprofloxacin	200 mg q. 12 h	200 mg q. 24 h and after IHD
Fluconazole	200 mg q. 24 h	200 mg q. 48 h and after IHD
Aciclovir (acyclovir)	3.5 mg/kg q. 24 h	2.5 mg/kg/d and after IHD
Ganciclovir	5mg/kg/d	5mg/kg/48 h and after IHD
Amphotericin B	Normal dose	Normal dose
Liposomal amphotericin	Normal dose	Normal dose
Ceftriaxone	Normal dose	Normal dose
Erythomycin	Normal dose	Normal dose
Milrinone	Titrate to effect	Titrate to effect
Amrinone	Titrate to effect	Titrate to effect
Catecholamines	Titrate to effect	Titrate to effect
Ampicillin	500 mg q 8 hourly	500 mg daily and after IHD

*The above values represent approximations and should be used as a general guide only. Critically ill patients have markedly abnormal volumes of distribution for these agents, which will affect dosage. CRRT is conducted at variable levels of intensity in different units, also requiring adjustment. The values reported here relate to CVVH at 2 L/h of ultrafiltration. Vancomycin is poorly removed by CVVHD. IHD may also differ from unit to unit. The values reported here relate to standard IHD with low-flux membranes for 3–4 hours every second day. D=day; q=frequency; h=hours.

SUMMARY

The field of renal replacement therapy has undergone remarkable changes over the last 10 years and is continuing to evolve rapidly. Technology is being improved to facilitate clinical application and new areas of research are developing. CRRT is now firmly established throughout the world as perhaps the most commonly used form of RRT. Conventional dialysis, however, which was slowly losing ground, is reappearing in the form of extended, slow-efficiency treatment, especially in the USA. Two large-phase III trials (>1000 patients) have been completed in the USA and in Australia/New Zealand to define the optimal dose of RRT in ICU patients and the results indicate that a dose of 25/kg/h of effluent generation provides appropriate therapy in this setting. In the meanwhile the use of novel membranes, sorbents and different intensities of treatment are being explored in the area of sepsis management and liver support. Intensivists need to keep abreast of this rapid evolution if they are to offer their patients the best of care.

Access the complete references list online at http://www.expertconsult.com

10. Bellomo R, Ronco C. Adequacy of dialysis in the acute renal failure of the critically ill: the case for continuous therapies. Int J Artif Organs 1996;19:129–42.
15. Mehta R, Dobos GJ, Ward DM. Anticoagulation procedures in continuous renal replacement. Seminars Dial 1992;5:61–8.
19. Parienti JJ, Thirion M, Fischer MO, et al. Catheter dysfunction and dialysis performance according to vascular access among 736 critically ill adults requiring renal replacement therapy: a randomized controlled trial. Crit Care Med 2010;38:1118–25.
24. Palevsky PM, Zhang JH, O'Connor TZ, et al. Intensity of renal support in critically ill patients with acute kidney injury. N Engl J Med 2008;359:7–20.
25. The RENAL Replacement Therapy Study Investigators. Intensity of continuous renal replacement therapy in critically ill patients. New Engl J Med 2009;361:1627–38.

Part Seven

Neurological Disorders

49

Disorders of consciousness

Balasubramanian Venkatesh

NEUROANATOMY AND PHYSIOLOGY OF WAKEFULNESS

A normal level of consciousness depends on the interaction between the cerebral hemispheres and the rostral reticular activating system (RAS) located in the upper brainstem. Although the RAS is a diffuse projection, the areas of RAS of particular importance to the maintenance of consciousness are those located between the rostral pons and the diencephalon. In contrast, however, consciousness is not focally represented in any of the cerebral hemispheres and is in many ways related to the mass of functioning cortex. Thus anatomical bilateral hemispheric lesions or brainstem lesions may result in an altered conscious state.[1] Large unilateral hemispheric lesions may produce impairment of consciousness by compression of the upper brainstem. In addition metabolic processes may also result in coma from interruption of energy substrate delivery or alteration of neuronal excitability. Disorders of consciousness are characterised either by an alteration in the level or by content of consciousness (**Box 49.1**). These are also illustrated in **Figure 49.1**.

The last three conditions described in Box 49.1 are a frequent source of confusion and require further discussion (**Table 49.1**). These neurological states are seen more frequently in modern day clinical practice partly because of the advances in therapy of severe brain injury and intensive care, which have led to the survival of many patients who would have otherwise died.

DIFFERENTIAL DIAGNOSIS OF COMA

Although the aetiology of coma is invariably multifactorial, the differential diagnosis of coma can be broadly grouped into three classes:

- diseases that produce focal or lateralising signs
- coma without focal or lateralising signs, but with signs of meningeal irritation
- coma without focal or lateralising signs or signs of meningeal irritation.

These are considered in greater detail in **Table 49.2**.

CLINICAL EXAMINATION OF THE COMATOSE PATIENT

The neurological examination of the comatose patient is of crucial importance to assess the depth of coma and to locate the site of lesion. Although the detailed neurological examination that can be carried out in a conscious patient is not possible in a comatose individual, useful information can be obtained by performing a thorough general examination and a neurological examination, particularly evaluating the level of consciousness, brainstem signs and motor responses in coma.

GENERAL EXAMINATION

General examination of the patient may point to the aetiology of coma. Skin changes may be seen in carbon monoxide poisoning (cherry-red discolouration of skin), alcoholic liver disease (telangiectasia, clubbing), hypothyroidism (puffy facies) and hypopituitarism (sallow complexion). The presence of cutaneous petechiae or ecchymoses may point to meningococcaemia, rickettsial infection or endocarditis as possible causes of coma. Needle puncture marks may suggest substance abuse. Bullous skin lesions are a feature of barbiturate overdose. An excessively dry skin may indicate diabetic ketoacidosis or anticholinergic overdose.

Periorbital haematomas (raccoon eyes) indicate an anterior basal skull fracture, particularly if there is associated cerebrospinal fluid rhinorrhoea. The other signs of a basal skull fracture include Battle's sign and cerebrospinal fluid otorrhoea. Nuchal rigidity may be seen in meningoencephalitis and subarachnoid haemorrhage, although this sign may not be present in the elderly and in patients in deep coma.

The presence of hepatomegaly or stigmata of chronic liver disease may suggest hepatic encephalopathy. Bilateral enlarged kidneys may indicate polycystic kidney disease and should prompt one to consider subarachnoid haemorrhage as a possible aetiology of coma. The breath may smell of alcohol or other poisons (organophosphates). The smell of ketones in the breath is an unreliable sign and hepatic and uraemic foetor are rare.

Box 49.1 Disorders of consciousness

Consciousness	An awake individual demonstrates full awareness of self and environment
Confusion	Inability to think with customary speed and clarity, associated with inattentiveness, reduced awareness and disorientation
Delirium	Confusion with agitation and hallucination
Stupor	Unresponsiveness with arousal only by deep and repeated stimuli
Coma	Unarousable unresponsiveness
Locked-in syndrome	Total paralysis below third cranial nerve nuclei; normal or impaired mental function
Persistent vegetative state	Prolonged coma >1 month, some preservation of brainstem and motor reflexes
Akinetic mutism	Prolonged coma with apparent alertness and flaccid motor tone
Minimally conscious state	Preserved wakefulness, awareness and brainstem reflexes, but poorly responsive

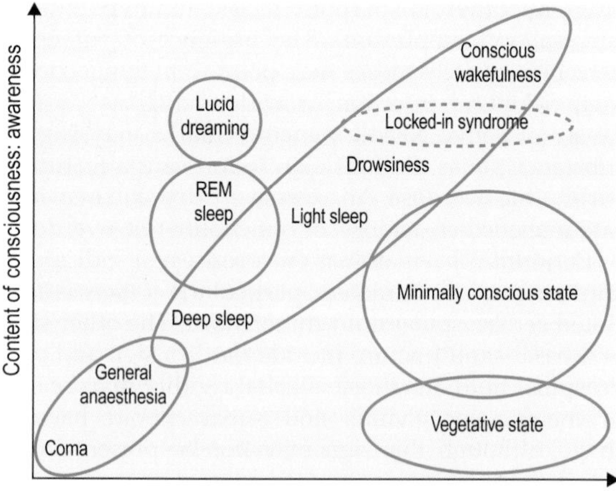

Figure 49.1 Disorders of consciousness are characterised by an alteration in either the level or content of consciousness. *(From Gosseries et al. Disorders of Consciousness: Coma, Vegetative and Minimally Conscious States. In: Cvetkovic D, Cosic I, editors. States of Consciousness: Experimental Insights into Meditation, Waking, Sleep and Dreams. Berlin: Springer; 2011, with permission.)*

LEVEL OF CONSCIOUSNESS

This is assessed by the Glasgow Coma Scale (GCS),[2] which takes into account the patient's response to command and physical stimuli. The GCS (**Table 49.3**), which was originally developed to grade the severity of head injury and prognosticate outcome, has now been extended for all causes of impaired consciousness and coma. Although it is a simple clinical score easily performed by both medical and nursing staff by the bedside, there are a number of caveats:

1. The GCS should always be determined prior to administration of sedative drugs or endotracheal intubation.
2. It should also be defined with regard to patient's vital signs, namely blood pressure, heart rate and temperature.
3. The GCS must be interpreted in light of previous or concomitant drug therapy.
4. The presence of alcohol in the breath or in the serum should always be documented.
5. Because of the considerable inter-observer variation in scoring, it is important to define the responses in descriptive terms rather than emphasising the numerical score associated with each response.
6. The measurement of awareness by the GCS is limited. Subtle changes in brainstem reflexes are not adequately assessed by the GCS.

To overcome the limitations of the GCS in assessing brain stem activity, the FOUR (Full Outline of UnResponsiveness) score was proposed by Wijdicks et al.[3,4] The components of the FOUR score include eye movements, motor score, brainstem reflexes and respiration. Each subscomponent is scored out of a maximum of four and therefore the maximum score is 16. It does not include verbal response and may be more suitable in the intubated patient.

PUPILLARY RESPONSES IN COMA[5]

The presence of normal pupils (2–5 mm and equal in size and demonstrate both direct and consensual light reflexes) confirms the integrity of the pupillary pathway (retina, optic nerve, optic chiasma and tracts, midbrain and third cranial nerve nuclei and nerves). The size of the pupil is a balance between the opposing influences of both sympathetic (causing dilatation) and parasympathetic (causing constriction) systems. Pupillary abnormalities have localising and diagnostic value in clinical neurology (**Table 49.4**). When the pupils are miosed, the light reaction is difficult to appreciate and may require a magnifying glass.

OPHTHALMOSCOPY IN COMA

The pupils *should never be dilated pharmacologically* without prior documentation of the pupillary size and the light reflex. The presence of papilloedema suggests

Table 49.1 Coma-like syndromes and related states

SYNDROME	FEATURES	SITE OF LESION	EEG	METABOLISM (% OF NORMAL)[49]	COMMENTS
Locked-in syndrome[50] (de-efferented state)	Alert and aware, vertical eye movements present, and able to blink Quadriplegic, lower cranial nerve palsies, no speech, facial or pharyngeal movements	Bilateral anterior pontine lesion which transects all descending motor pathways, but spares ascending sensory and RAS systems	Normal	90–100%	Similar state seen with severe polyneuropathies, myasthenia gravis and neuromuscular blocking agents
Persistent vegetative state (PVS)[51] (apallic syndrome, neocortical death)	Previously comatose, who now appear to be awake. Spontaneous limb movements, eye movements and yawning seen. However, patient inattentive, no speech, no awareness of environment and total inability to respond to commands	Extensive damage to both cerebral hemispheres with relative preservation of the brainstem	Polymorphic delta or theta waves, sometimes alpha	40–60%	When vegetative state lasts longer than 4 weeks, it is termed persistent. PVS lasting for longer than 2 weeks implies a poor prognosis
Akinetic mutism[52] (coma vigile)	Partially or fully awake patient, immobile and silent	Lesion in bilateral frontal lobes or hydrocephalus or third ventricular masses	Diffuse slowing	40–80%	Abulia is the term applied to milder forms of akinetic mutism
Catatonia	Awake patients, sometimes a fixed posture, muteness with decreased motor activity	Usually of psychiatric origin	Non-specific EEG patterns associated with medical conditions	Variable metabolic changes in prefrontal cortex	May be mimicked by frontal lobe disease and drugs
Minimally conscious state[49]	Globally impaired responsiveness, limited but discernible evidence of self and environment	Global neuronal damage	Theta and alpha waves	40–60%	Differs from PVS in that patients diagnosed with minimally conscious state have some level of awareness

the presence of intracranial hypertension, but is frequently absent when the lesion is acute. Subhyaloid and vitreous haemorrhages are seen in patients with subarachnoid haemorrhage.[6]

EYE MOVEMENTS IN COMA[7]

Horizontal eye movements to the contralateral side are initiated in the ipsilateral frontal lobe and closely coordinated with the corresponding centre in the contralateral pons. To facilitate conjugate eye movements, yoking of the 3rd, 4th and 6th nerve nuclei is achieved by the medial longitudinal fasciculus.

To look to the left, the movement originates in the right frontal lobe and is coordinated by the left pontine region and vice versa. In contrast to horizontal gaze, vertical eye movements are under bilateral control of the cortex and upper midbrain.

The position and movements of the eyes are observed at rest. The presence of spontaneous roving eye movements excludes brainstem pathology as a cause of coma. In a paralytic frontal lobe pathology the eyes will deviate towards the side of the lesion, whereas in pontine pathologies the eyes will deviate away from the side of the lesion. Ocular bobbing, an intermittent downward jerking eye movement, is seen in pontine lesions owing to loss of horizontal gaze and unopposed midbrain-controlled vertical gaze activity[8]. Skew deviation (vertical separation of the ocular axes) occurs with pontine and cerebellar disorders[9].

Table 49.2 Differential diagnosis of coma

CATEGORY	SPECIFIC DISORDER	FEATURES IN HISTORY AND EXAMINATION	INVESTIGATIONS	COMMENTS
Coma with focal signs	*Trauma* – extradural, subdural and parenchymal haemorrhage, concussions	History of trauma, findings of fracture base of skull, scalp haematoma, other associated body injuries	Usually an abnormal CT	Exclude coexisting drug or alcohol ingestion
	Vascular –intracerebral haemorrhage	Sudden onset, history of headaches or hypertension, neck stiffness may be present	Abnormal CT scan	Consider causes of secondary hypertension in young hypertensives
	Vascular – thromboembolic	Sudden onset, atrial fibrillation, vascular bruits, endocarditis	An abnormal CT after a few days	Consider echocardiography to diagnose cardiac sources of emboli
	Brain abscess	Subacute onset, look for ENT and dental sources of infection	Abnormal CT and CSF	Consider infective endocarditis and suppurative lung disease as sources of sepsis
Coma without focal signs, but with meningeal irritation	Infection Meningitis, encephalitis	Onset of illness over a few hours to days, neck stiffness, rash of meningococcaemia	Abnormal CSF	Consider underlying immunosuppressive states
	Subarachnoid haemorrhage	Onset usually sudden, subhyaloid haemorrhages on fundoscopy	Abnormal CT and CSF	Consider polycystic kidney disease in subarachnoid haemorrhage
Coma without focal signs and no meningeal irritation	Metabolic causes Hyponatraemia Hypoglycaemia, hyperglycaemia Hypoxia Hypercapnia Hypo- and hyperthermia Hyper- and hypo-osmolar states	History might point to the cause of metabolic disturbance, asterixis a feature of hypercapnia-induced coma	Abnormal blood results	Rapid correction of hyponatraemia and osmolality should be avoided
	Endocrine causes Myxoedema Adrenal insufficiency Hypopituitarism	Puffy facies, may be hypothermic	Abnormal electrolyte profile, hypoglycaemia	Multiple disorders may be present in the same patient
	Seizure disorders	History typical	Abnormal EEG, check anticonvulsant levels	CT scan to exclude an underlying space-occupying lesion
	Organ failure Hepatic Renal	History of jaundice, chronic alcohol ingestion, stigmata of liver disease, asterixis	Abnormal hepatic and renal functions	Presence of A–V fistula may be a pointer to chronic renal failure
	Toxic/drug Sedatives Narcotics Alcohol Psychotropic Carbon monoxide Poisons	History, may be hypothermic at presentation except in psychotropic drug overdose	Metabolic screen is usually normal	Rapid improvement in conscious states with antidotes
	Behavioural Sleep deprivation Pseudocoma	No typical features	No specific diagnostic tests	Diagnosis of exclusion

Table 49.3 Glasgow Coma Scale

EYE OPENING	POINTS
Spontaneous	4
To speech	3
To pain	2
Nil	1
BEST VERBAL RESPONSE	
Oriented	5
Confused	4
Inappropriate	3
Incomprehensible	2
Nil	1
Intubated	T
BEST MOTOR RESPONSE	
Obeys commands	6
Localises to pain	5
Withdraws to pain	4
Abnormal flexion	3
Extensor response	2
Nil	1

The presence of full and conjugate eye movements in response to oculocephalic and oculovestibular stimuli demonstrates the functional integrity of a large segment of the brainstem. Corneal reflexes are preserved until late in coma. Upward rolling of the eyes after corneal stimulation (Bell's phenomenon) implies intact midbrain and pontine function.

LIMB MOVEMENTS AND POSTURAL CHANGES IN COMA

Restlessness, crossing of legs and spontaneous coughing, yawning, swallowing and localising movements suggest only a mild depression of the conscious state. Choreoathetotic or ballistic movements suggest a basal ganglion lesion. Myoclonic movements indicate a metabolic disorder usually of post-anoxic origin. Asterixis is seen with metabolic encephalopathies. Hiccup is a nonspecific sign and does not have any localising value.

Decerebrate rigidity is characterised by stiff extension of the limbs, internal rotation of the arms and plantar flexion of the ankles. With severe rigidity, opisthotonos and jaw clenching may be observed. These movements may be unilateral or bilateral, and spontaneous or in response to a noxious stimulus. Whereas animal studies suggest that the lesion is usually in the midbrain or caudal diencephalon (leading to exaggeration of antigravity reflexes), in humans such posturing may be seen in a variety of disease states: midbrain lesion, certain metabolic disorders such as

Table 49.4 Pupillary abnormalities in coma

ABNORMALITY	CAUSE	NEUROANATOMICAL BASIS
MIOSIS (<2 MM IN SIZE)		
Unilateral	Horner's syndrome Local pathology	Sympathetic paralysis Trauma to sympathetics
Bilateral	Pontine lesions Thalamic haemorrhage Metabolic encephalopathy Drug ingestion Organophosphate Barbiturate Narcotics	Sympathetic paralysis Cholinesterase inhibition Central effect
MYDRIASIS (>5 MM IN SIZE)		
Unilateral fixed pupil	Midbrain lesion Uncal herniation	3rd nerve damage Stretch of 3rd nerve against the petroclinoid ligament
Bilateral fixed pupils	Massive midbrain haemorrhage Hypoxic cerebral injury *DRUGS* Atropine Tricyclics Sympathomimetics	Bilateral 3rd nerve damage Mesencephalic damage Paralysis of parasympathetics Prevent local reuptake of catecholamines by nerve endings Stimulation of sympathetics

Table 49.5 Disorders of respiratory rate and pattern in coma

ABNORMALITY	SIGNIFICANCE
Bradypnoea	Drug-induced coma, hypothyroid coma
Tachypnoea	Central neurogenic hyperventilation (mid brain lesion), metabolic encephalopathy
Cheyne–Stokes respiration	Deep cerebral lesions, metabolic encephalopathy (hyperpnoea alternating regularly with apnoea)
Apneustic breathing (an inspiratory pause)	Pontine lesions
Ataxic breathing (ataxic breathing normally progresses to agonal gasps and terminal apnoea)	Medullary lesions

hypoglycaemia, anoxia, hepatic coma and in drug intoxication. Decorticate posturing is characterised by flexion of elbows and wrists and extension of the lower limbs. The lesion is usually above the midbrain in the cerebral white matter.

RESPIRATORY SYSTEM[10]

Abnormal respiratory rate and patterns have been described in coma, but their precise localising value is uncertain. As a general rule, at lighter levels of impaired consciousness tachypnoea predominates, whereas respiratory depression increases with the depth of coma. Some of the commonly observed respiratory abnormalities are summarised in **Table 49.5**. Respiratory failure in comatose patients may result from hypoventilation, aspiration pneumonia and neurogenic pulmonary oedema, a sympathetic nervous system mediated syndrome seen in acute brain injury.

BODY TEMPERATURE IN COMA

The presence of altered core body temperature is a useful aid in the diagnosis of coma. Hypothermia (<35°C) is frequently observed with alcohol or barbiturate intoxication, sepsis with shock, drowning, hypoglycaemia, myxoedema coma and exposure to cold. Severe hyperthermia may be seen in pontine haemorrhage, intracranial infections, heat stroke and anticholinergic drug toxicity.

RECOGNITION OF BRAIN HERNIATION[11-13]

When patients with an impaired level of consciousness deteriorate, it is important to consider brain herniation as a possible cause of the worsening. Several herniation syndromes have been described Subfalcine herniation usually results from the lateral displacement of the brain and is identified by the horizontal shift of the pineal gland. Ischaemia of the medial aspect of the cerebral hemispheres can result from compression of the pericallosal and the marginal arteries. Transtentorial herniation results from the downward displacement of the upper brainstem (central herniation) with or without involvement of the uncus (lateral herniation). The clinical signs of a central herniation are progressive obtundation, Cheyne–Stokes respiration, small pupils followed by extensor posturing and medium-sized fixed dilated pupils. Uncal herniation differs from central herniation in that pupillary dilatation occurs early in the process because of third-nerve compression. The traditional Cushing's response of hypertension and bradycardia is not always a feature of herniation and any heart rhythm may be present. Tonsillar herniation is the protrusion of the cerebellar tonsils through the foramen magnum, resulting in caudal medullary compression and obstruction of the fourth ventricle.

DIFFERENTIATING TRUE COMA FROM PSEUDOCOMA

Patients feigning coma resist passive eye opening and may even hold their eyes tightly closed. They may blink in response to a threat and do not demonstrate spontaneous roving eye movements. In contrast, they move the eyes concomitantly with head rotation and with cold caloric testing they may wake up or demonstrate preservation of the fast component of nystagmus. They also demonstrate avoidance of 'self-injury'. In addition, the pattern of clinical 'abnormalities' does not fit any specific neurological syndromes.

MANAGEMENT OF THE COMATOSE PATIENT

EMERGENT THERAPEUTIC MEASURES

Irrespective of the aetiology of coma, certain emergent therapeutic measures apply to the care of all patients. These take precedence over any diagnostic investigation.

1. Ensure adequate airway and oxygenation.
2. Secure intravenous access and maintain circulation.
3. Administer 50% dextrose after drawing a sample of blood for serum glucose levels. Although there are theoretical concerns about augmentation of brain lactic acid production[14,15] in anoxic coma, the relatively good prognosis for hypoglycaemic coma when treated expeditiously far outweighs any potential risks of glucose administration.
4. Thiamine must always be administered in conjunction with dextrose to prevent precipitation of Wernicke's encephalopathy.

5. Consideration should be given to administering naloxone, when there is a suspicion of narcotic overdose with impending respiratory arrest.
6. If hypertension, bradycardia and fixed dilated pupils are present at the time of the initial presentation, suggestive of marked intracranial hypertension and tentorial herniation, 20% mannitol at a dose 0.5–1 g/kg body weight should be administered. Consideration should be given to the emergency placement of an external ventricular drain.
7. Treat suspected meningitis with antibiotics even if CSF results are not available. A combination of penicillin and ceftriaxone is usually recommended for a community-acquired bacterial meningitis.
8. Control of seizures must be achieved as outlined in the chapter on status epilepticus.
9. Treat extreme body temperatures.
10. Stabilisation of the cervical spine if trauma is suspected.

INVESTIGATIONS

The order of investigation depends on the clinical circumstance. In the majority of cases, history and examination will provide enough information to be able to perform specific cause-related investigation. In general, the investigations can be grouped as follows.

ROUTINE INVESTIGATIONS

Measurements of serum glucose, electrolytes, arterial blood gases, liver and renal function tests, osmolality, and blood count and blood film are part of the routine investigations. When drug overdose is suspected a toxicology screen for alcohol, paracetamol, salicylates, benodiazepines and tricyclic antidepressants should be performed. A sample of serum should be stored for later analysis for uncommon drug ingestions.

NEUROIMAGING

CT SCAN

The most commonly used radiological investigation for evaluation of the comatose patient is computerised tomography (CT) scan of the brain. This is useful for diagnosing CNS trauma, subarachnoid (SAH) and intracerebral haemorrhage, haemorrhagic and non-haemorrhagic strokes, cerebral oedema, hydrocephalus and the presence of a space-occupying lesion (SOL). Frequently a CT is performed prior to a lumbar puncture to exclude rather than confirm the presence of severe cerebral oedema or a SOL. Its other advantages include lower cost, easy availability, short examination time and safety in the presence of pacemakers, surgical clips and other ferromagnetic substances. The advent of helical CT whereby multiple images are possible has reduced scanning times and is suitable for the uncooperative patient. The limitations of a CT scan include:

- the need to transfer the patient to a site where resuscitation and monitoring facilities are limited
- the need to sedate and possibly endotracheally intubate patients who are agitated
- its low sensitivity to demonstrate an abnormality in the acute phase of a stroke
- its low sensitivity for detecting brainstem lesions
- the need to administer i.v. contrast agents: the two major side-effects of i.v. contrast include anaphylaxis (with an approximate death rate of 1 in 40000) and renal failure. The use of *N*-acetylcysteine, sodium bicarbonate and haemodialysis has been reported to reduce the incidence of contrast-induced nephropathy, although data in critically ill patients are minimal[16]. There are a series of CT images (Figs 42.1 to 42.12) available at Excon site under 'Ancillary' tab. 

MAGNETIC RESONANCE IMAGING (MRI)

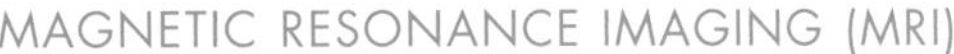

MRI scans provide superior contrast and resolution of the grey and white matter compared with CT scans, thus facilitating easy identification of the deep nuclear structures within the brain. MRI is more sensitive than CT for the detection of acute ischaemia, diffuse axonal injury, and cerebral oedema, tumour and abscess. Brainstem and posterior fossa structures are better visualised. The other advantage of MRI is the use of non-ionising energy. The use of gadolinium, a paramagnetic agent, as a contrast agent permits sharp definition of lesions. MR coupled with angiography (MRA) may enable diagnosis of vascular lesions. MRI is, however, limited by:

- the need for special equipment
- long imaging times
- the need to transfer the patient to a site where resuscitation and monitoring facilities are limited
- the need to sedate and possibly endotracheally intubate patients who are agitated
- risk of dislodgement of metal clips on blood vessels and resetting of pacemakers. MRI images are better for the detection of ischaemia, cerebral oedema, diffuse axonal injury and abscess. They can also be used to see vasculature. Examples can be seen on Figures 42.11 to 42.13 available at Excon site under 'Ancillary' tab.

PET AND SPECT SCANS

Newer nuclear medicine scans such as SPECT (single photon emission with computerised tomography) and PET (positron emission tomography) are useful for the assessment of cerebral blood flow and oxygenation and in the prognostication of neurotrauma, but have little role to play in the management of acute disorders of consciousness. In PET scans, positron-emitting isotopes such as ^{11}C, ^{18}F and ^{15}O are incorporated into biologically active compounds such as deoxyglucose or fluoro-deoxyglucose, which are metabolised in the body. By determining the concentration of the various tracers in the brain and constructing tomographic images, cerebral blood flow and metabolism can be measured by PET scanning.

SPECT scans use iodine-containing isotopes incorporated into biologically active compounds and, like PET scans, their cranial distribution is determined after a dose of tracer. Information on cerebral blood flow and metabolism can be obtained from SPECT scans. The advantage of a PET scan is that it does not require a cyclotron for the generation of isotopes. Despite their many advantages, both these technologies continue to be research tools and are not routinely available in many medical centres.

LUMBAR PUNCTURE (LP)[17]

Cerebrospinal fluid is most commonly obtained by means of a lumbar puncture. This should be performed after ensuring that raised intracranial pressure has been excluded clinically or radiologically. The major use of a lumbar puncture is to diagnose an intracranial infection and to detect abnormal cytology in cases of suspected malignant meningeal infiltration. The advent of CT scans has diminished the role of LP in the diagnosis of SAH. Some of the commonly reported complications post lumbar puncture include post-puncture headache (12–39%) and traumatic tap (15–20%). Brain herniation is a rare potential complication seen with conditions associated with raised intracranial pressure due to a space-occupying lesion.

EEG IN COMA[18–20]

The usefulness of EEG in coma is summarised in **Box 49.2**. Continuous EEG monitoring in the ICU has been reported to be useful in the identification of acute cerebral ischaemia and non-convulsive seizures and for monitoring therapy used in induced coma, such as thiopentone infusion for refractory status, and to assess level of sedation.

Box 49.2 Usefulness of EEG in coma

Identification of non-convulsive status epilepticus
Diagnosis of hepatic encephalopathy
- presence of paroxysmal triphasic waves

Assessing severity of hypoxic encephalopathy
- presence of theta activity
- diffuse slowing
- burst suppression (seen with more severe forms)
- alpha coma (seen with more severe forms)

Herpes encephalitis
- periodic sharp spikes

Monitoring of therapy (e.g. thiopentone infusion for status epilepticus)

EVOKED POTENTIALS

Visual, brainstem and somatosensory evoked potentials test the integrity of neuroanatomical pathways within the brain and the spinal cord. They may be used in the diagnosis of blindness in comatose patients and in the assessment of locked-in states. There are data to suggest that they have better prognostic value than clinical judgement in patients with anoxic coma.[21–22]

BIOCHEMICAL ABNORMALITIES[23–26]

A number of biomarkers of brain injury have been evaluated as predictors of severity of brain injury and to assess progression of injury severity from traumatic and non-traumatic aetiologies. These include neuron-specific enolase (cytoplasm of neurons), S-100B protein (astroglial cells), CK-BB fraction (astrocytes), glial fibrillary acidic protein (glial origin), calpain and caspase. Although early studies showed S-100B as a reliable marker of traumatic brain injury, concerns remain about their sensitivity and specificity for assessment of severity and prediction of outcome.

CARE OF THE COMATOSE PATIENT

AIRWAY

As mentioned before, assessment of airway adequacy should take precedence over any diagnostic investigation in comatose patients. This is best done by assessing the patient's response to command and physical stimulation, and whether a gag reflex is present. Securing the airway will depend on the level of consciousness. This may entail simple manoeuvres such as jaw thrust, chin lift, use of oropharyngeal airways or, in the comatose patient, mandate endotracheal intubation. All of these patients are at risk of pulmonary aspiration and there must be a low threshold for establishing a definitive airway.

As a general rule, patients presenting with medical causes of coma may be nursed on their side (coma position) if the airway is adequate. However, all traumatised patients should be assumed to have a potential cervical spine injury and must be nursed with the cervical spine in the neutral position and/or with a rigid collar until an injury is excluded by definitive radiological views. All patients with disordered consciousness must receive supplemental oxygen.

VENTILATION

It is important to ensure optimal gas exchange and avoid hypoxia and hypercapnia. Generally a Pa_{O_2} of >80 torr (10.66 kPa) and P_{CO_2} of 35–40 torr (4.66–5.33 kPa) is desirable. If spontaneous ventilatory efforts are not adequate to achieve these levels of arterial blood gases, mechanical ventilatory support may be necessary.

CIRCULATION

Adequacy of circulation should be assessed by conventional clinical end-points. The goals of circulatory therapy in coma include prompt restoration of appropriate mean arterial blood pressure, correction of dehydration and hypovolaemia and urgent attention to life-threatening causes of shock.

SPECIFIC TREATMENT

This will depend on the underlying aetiology of the coma and is discussed in the relevant chapters. Avoidance of secondary insults is of paramount importance in the management of these patients.[27,28]

NURSING CARE

Meticulous eye and mouth care, regular changes in limb position, limb physiotherapy, bronchial toilet and psychological support are mandatory. Nosocomial infections and iatrogenic complications are associated with an increased mortality and morbidity in these patients and must be promptly diagnosed and treated. The rational use of daily investigations, invasive procedures and antibiotic prescription is essential.

OTHER THERAPY

Stress ulcer and deep vein thrombosis prophylaxis should be instituted. Early establishment of enteral feeding via a nasoenteric tube is preferable. It is important to exclude a basal skull fracture before insertion of a nasoenteric tube.

ANOXIC COMA/ENCEPHALOPATHY

Cardiac arrest is the third leading cause of coma resulting in ICU admission after trauma and drug overdose. The symptomatology and clinical outcome of patients with anoxic brain damage depend on the severity and duration of oxygen deprivation to the brain. A number of criteria have been developed to prognosticate outcome in anoxic coma. Although a number of laboratory and imaging criteria contribute to the prognostic assessment, clinical signs still have major prognostic impact. The important clinical predictors of outcome are listed in **Table 49.6**. However, there are data to suggest that electrophysiological studies using evoked potentials have far greater prognostic accuracy compared with clinical assessment.[29] It is important to note that the clinical criteria of poor prognosis were developed in the pre-hypothermia era. The optimal time for prognostication following hypothermia is unclear.[30]

Table 49.6 Clinical and laboratory predictors of unfavourable prognosis in anoxic coma[21,29,53]

CLINICAL PREDICTOR	UNFAVOURABLE PROGNOSIS
Duration of anoxia (time interval between collapse and initiation of CPR)	8–10 min
Duration of CPR (time interval between initiation of CPR and ROSC)	>30 min
Duration of postanoxic coma	>72 hours
Pupillary reaction	Absent on day 3
Motor response to pain (absent=a motor response worse than withdrawal)	Absent on day 3
Roving spontaneous eye movements	Absent on day 1
Elevated neuron-specific enolase	>33 µg/L
SSEP recording	Absent N20

Box 49.3 Aetiology of metabolic/toxic encephalopathy[54–56]

Hepatic failure
Renal failure
Respiratory failure
Sepsis
Electrolyte abnormalities: hyponatraemia, hypernatraemia, hypercalcaemia
Hypoglycaemia and hyperglycaemia
Acute pancreatitis
Endocrine – Addisonian crisis, myxoedema coma, thyroid storm
Drug withdrawal – benzodiazepine, opiates
Hyperthermia
Toxins: alcohols, glycols, tricyclic antidepressants
ICU syndrome
D-lactic acidosis

THE CONFUSED/ENCEPHALOPATHIC PATIENT IN THE ICU

Encephalopathy is a term used to describe the alteration in the level or content of consciousness due to a process extrinsic to the brain. Metabolic encephalopathy, particularly of septic aetiology, is the most common cause of altered mental status in the ICU setting.[31,32] A number of processes can lead to metabolic encephalopathy (**Box 49.3**). A number of features in the history and examination help to differentiate metabolic from structural causes of altered conscious states (**Table 49.7**).

Owing to their increased frequency in and exclusiveness to the critical care setting, two types of encephalopathy will be considered in detail: septic encephalopathy and ICU syndrome.

Table 49.7 Distinguishing features of structural and metabolic encephalopathy[56]

FEATURE	STRUCTURAL	METABOLIC
State of consciousness	Usually fixed level of depressed conscious state, may deteriorate progressively	Milder alteration of conscious state, waxing and waning of altered sensorium
Fundoscopy	May be abnormal	Usually normal
Pupils	May be abnormal, either in size or response to light	Usually preserved light response (although pupil shape and reactivity affected in certain overdoses – see above)
Eye movements	May be affected	Usually preserved
Motor findings	Asymmetrical involvement	Abnormalities usually symmetrical
Involuntary movements	Not common	Asterixis, tremor, myoclonus frequently seen

Sepsis-associated encephalopathy (SAE) has been reported to occur in 8–80% of patients with sepsis.[33] The criteria to diagnose SAE include presence of impaired mental function, evidence of an extracranial infection and absence of other obvious aetiologies for the altered conscious state. Although the precise mechanism of damage to the brain has not been delineated, the pathogenesis of the encephalopathy is thought to be multifactorial: alteration in cerebral blood flow induced by mediators of inflammation, generation of free radicals by activated leucocytes resulting in erythrocyte sludging in the microcirculation, breakdown of the blood–brain barrier resulting in cerebral oedema, reduced brain oxygen consumption induced by endotoxin and cytokines, neuronal degeneration and increased neuronal apoptosis, increases in aromatic amino acids resulting in altered neurotransmitter function and increased GABA-mediated neurotransmission leading to general inhibition of the CNS. Hypotension may contribute to the encephalopathy.[34,35] The asterixis, tremor and myoclonus - features of other metabolic encephalopathies - are uncommon in sepsis. The presence of lateralising signs is extremely rare in SAE and warrants exclusion of other causes such as stroke. The mortality of patients with SAE is higher than in those with sepsis without encephalopathy.[36] Therapy is largely directed at the underlying septic process.

ICU ENCEPHALOPATHY OR ICU SYNDROME[37,38]

This is a term used to describe behavioural disorders that develop in patients 5–7 days after admission to intensive care. Clinically this may present as agitation, restlessness and frank delirium. The causes are multifactorial: prolonged ventilation, sleep deprivation,[39,40] distortion of perception with loss of day–night cycles, immobilisation, noisy environment and monotony. These coupled with administration of multiple sedatives and neurological consequences of the underlying disease can precipitate psychotic behaviour in the ICU. It is important to bear in mind that *this is a diagnosis of exclusion and that all other reversible causes are looked for (see Box 49.2)* before this diagnostic label is applied. Tools to assess delirium such as the CAM-ICU have been developed and validated for the critical care setting.[41]

Abnormal behaviour can increase patient morbidity (self-extubation, ripping of catheters, soft tissue damage, etc.). Episodes of delirium in the ICU are also associated with increased mortality.[42] Postoperative delirium after cardiac surgery has also been associated with a significant decline in cognitive ability during the first year after cardiac surgery.[43] It is important to identify the underlying cause of the abnormal behaviour to institute appropriate therapy. Management of this condition may require the use of restraints, sedation and major tranquillisers. Improvement of sleep quality (minimising interruption of nocturnal sleep, adjusting lighting in the ICU), reducing patient boredom by the use of television and music and better communication with the patient may reduce the incidence and severity of this syndrome. Dexmedetomidine has been advocated as an agent to minimise delirium in the critically ill patient.[44]

PROGNOSIS IN COMA

Drug-induced comas usually have a good prognosis unless hypoxia and hypotension have resulted in severe secondary insults. Coma following head injury has a statistically better outcome compared with non-traumatic coma (coma occurring during the course of a medical illness). In non-traumatic coma lasting for 6 hours or greater, only 15% of the patients make a meaningful recovery to be able to return to their pre-morbid state of health.[45] The prognosis following anoxic coma has been described in a separate section. Within the non-traumatic coma category, coma resulting from infection, metabolic causes and multiple organ dysfunction syndrome have better outcome compared with anoxic coma.[46] A number of outcome scales have been developed to assess neurological recovery following brain injury.[47] These include the Barthel Index, Rankin Scale and the Glasgow Outcome Scale (GOS). The GOS is widely used to assess recovery after traumatic brain injury. It has five broad categories: 1=good recovery, 2=moderate disability, 3=severe disability, 4=persistent vegetative state and 5=death. It is simple, easy to administer and has been reported to have good inter-rater agreement.

TREATMENT OPTIONS IN DISORDERS OF CONSCIOUSNESS[48]

No effective standardised treatment exists for these patients. Currently evaluated interventions can be divided into pharmacological and non-pharmacological measures. Pharmacological measures include the use of levodopa and amantadine. Initiial trials reported some recovery response in terms of reduction in spasticity and improved cognitive behaviour and communication such as following simple commands. Zolpidem has also been trialled in patients with traumatic and anoxic aetiologies of reduced consciousness and results have been variable. Although some investigators report enhanced verbal, motor and cognitive functions, these have not been reproduced in other small trials. Moreover, the duration of effect of zolpidem is short. Bromocriptine and intrathecal baclofen have also been tried, but no large-scale studies have been reported.

Non-pharmacological measures include deep brain stimulation, extradural cortical stimulation, spinal cord stimulation and median nerve stimulation. Although reports of improved responsiveness have been published, the evidence is largely anecdotal and data from large studies are lacking.

Access the complete references list online at http://www.expertconsult.com

3. Wijdicks EF, Bamlet WR, Maramattom BV, et al. Validation of a new coma scale: The FOUR score. Ann Neurol 2005;58:585–93.
4. Wijdicks EF, Rabinstein AA, Bamlet WR, et al. FOUR score and Glasgow Coma Scale in predicting outcome of comatose patients: a pooled analysis. Neurology 2011;77:84–5.
22. Guerit JM, Amantini A, Amodio P, et al. Consensus on the use of neurophysiological tests in the intensive care unit (ICU): electroencephalogram (EEG), evoked potentials (EP), and electroneuromyography (ENMG). Neurophysiol Clin 2009;39:71–83.
27. White H, Venkatesh B. Cerebral perfusion pressure in neurotrauma: a review. Anesth Analg 2008;107:979–88.
29. Young GB. Clinical practice. Neurologic prognosis after cardiac arrest. N Engl J Med 2009;361:605–11.
32. Stevens RD, Nyquist PA. Types of brain dysfunction in critical illness. Neurol Clin 2008;26:469–86, ix.
37. Jones SF, Pisani MA. ICU delirium: an update. Curr Opin Crit Care 2012;18:146–51.
44. Riker RR, Shehabi Y, Bokesch PM, et al. Dexmedetomidine vs midazolam for sedation of critically ill patients: a randomized trial. JAMA 2009;301:489–99.
48. Georgiopoulos M, Katsakiori P, Kefalopoulou Z, et al. Vegetative state and minimally conscious state: a review of the therapeutic interventions. Stereotact Funct Neurosurg 2010;88:199–207.

50

Status epilepticus

Helen I Opdam

Status epilepticus (SE) is a medical emergency requiring prompt intervention to prevent the development of irreversible brain damage.

DEFINITION AND CLASSIFICATION

The duration of seizure activity required to define SE has not been universally agreed upon. Most authors have defined SE as more than 30 minutes duration of either a single seizure, or intermittent seizures with no regaining of consciousness between seizures.[1-4] This definition is most useful for epidemiological research[5] and is based on experimental studies that show irreversible neuronal damage occurs after 30 minutes of seizure activity.[6]

There is general acceptance of an operational definition of SE as 5 minutes of continuous seizure activity, or two or more discrete seizures with no intervening recovery of consciousness. It has arisen from the need to rapidly initiate treatment for SE and the observation that seizures persisting beyond this duration are unlikely to remit spontaneously.[7] Promulgation of this definition and resultant earlier treatment may be responsible for a decline in the incidence of SE.[5]

Refractory SE is defined as failure of initial therapy, such as benzodiazepines and phenytoin, usually necessitating treatment with agents that induce general anaesthesia.[8-10] Refractory SE develops in about one in five patients presenting with an SE episode and is associated with a worse prognosis.[9,11]

Continuation or recurrence of SE beyond 24 hours of anaesthetic therapy has been termed 'super-refractory SE'.[12]

SE is commonly separated into two categories:

- *Generalised convulsive SE (GCSE):* seizures are primary or secondarily generalised and the patient has generalised tonic and/or clonic convulsive movements with loss of consciousness.
- *Non-convulsive SE (NCSE):* there is altered consciousness and electroencephalography (EEG) evidence of seizures without convulsive movements. NCSE is a heterogeneous disorder with multiple subtypes. NCSE may evolve from GCSE when electrical seizure activity continues with loss of motor manifestations.

The incidence of SE is U-shaped, being greatest under 1 year and over 60 years of age.[5]

PATHOPHYSIOLOGY

Ongoing or recurrent seizures result from failure of normal seizure terminating mechanisms and predominance of excitation causing seizure activity to persist. The major inhibitory mechanism in the brain is γ-aminobutyric acid A ($GABA_A$) receptor-mediated inhibition. With ongoing seizure activity $GABA_A$ receptors undergo cellular internalisation and subsequent degradation, leading to loss of endogenous inhibition and sustainability of seizures. This reduction in synaptic $GABA_A$ receptors explains the progressive pharmacoresistance to GABAergic anticonvulsants such as benzodiazepines.[13]

Excitatory mechanisms are predominantly via glutamine acting on *N*-methyl-D-aspartate (NMDA) receptors. NMDA receptors increase on synapses during ongoing epileptic activity, facilitating neuronal excitability and persistence of seizures. This in contrast explains the efficacy of NMDA antagonists, even late in the course of SE.

The pathophysiological effects of seizures on the brain are thought to result from both direct excitotoxic neuronal injury and secondary injury due to systemic complications such as hypotension, hypoxia and hyperthermia. Ongoing excitation leads to neuronal injury and death, predominantly through mitochondrial dysfunction. Experimental models and anecdotal human evidence suggest also that SE is epileptogenic, although the mechanisms of this are not well understood.[13]

AETIOLOGY

Status epilepticus may occur de novo (approximately 60% of presentations) or less commonly in a previously diagnosed epileptic.[5] In the situation where refractory SE does not have a clear cause, more unusual conditions should be considered as their diagnosis may lead to a specific therapy. These include autoimmune conditions, mitochondrial diseases and unusual infections.[14] The aetiologies of SE are given in **Box 50.1**.[2,5,14,15]

Box 50.1 Causes of status epilepticus in adults[2,4,14,15]

Low antiepileptic drug levels – poor compliance, recent dose reduction or discontinuation (most common cause in patients with epilepsy)
Stroke – vascular occlusion or haemorrhage
Metabolic disturbances – electrolyte abnormalities (hyponatraemia, hypocalcaemia, hypomagnesaemia, hypophosphataemia), hyperglycaemia, hypoglycaemia
Organ failure – uraemia, hepatic encephalopathy
CNS infection – bacterial meningitis, viral encephalitis, cerebral toxoplasmosis, tuberculosis, other
Cerebral hypoxia/anoxia
Alcohol – withdrawal or intoxication
Head trauma
Drug toxicity – cephalosporins, isoniazid, tranexamic acid, tacrolimus, cyclosporine, tricyclic antidepressants, olanzapine, phenothiazines, theophylline, cocaine, amphetamine, antiepileptic drugs, other
CNS tumours – primary or secondary
Temporally remote causes (previous CNS injury) – stroke, trauma, tumour, meningitis
Hypertensive encephalopathy, eclampsia
Immunological disorders – paraneoplastic syndromes, Hashimoto's encephalopathy, anti-NMDA receptor encephalitis (may have associated ovarian tumour), cerebral lupus, thrombotic thrombocytopenic purpura, other
Mitochondrial diseases

GENERALISED CONVULSIVE STATUS EPILEPTICUS (GCSE)

GCSE is the most common and most dangerous type of SE and accounts for approximately 75%.[2] It encompasses a broad spectrum of clinical presentations, from overt generalised tonic–clonic seizures to subtle convulsive movements in a profoundly comatose patient.[16]

CLINICAL

Typically, early in the evolution of seizures, patients are unresponsive with obvious tonic (sustained contractions) and/or clonic (rhythmic jerking) movements (overt GCSE). Motor manifestations may be symmetrical or asymmetrical.

With time, the clinical manifestations may become subtle, and patients have only small-amplitude twitching movements of the face, hands, or feet, or nystagmoid jerking of the eyes (late or subtle GCSE).[16]

Later still some patients will have no observable repetitive motor activity and the detection of ongoing seizures requires EEG (electrical GCSE). Most authors classify this as a form of NCSE.[7,17] Such patients are still at risk of CNS injury and require prompt treatment.

EEG CHANGES

Just as there is a progression from overt to increasingly subtle motor manifestations, there is also a predictable sequence of EEG changes during untreated GCSE. Initially, discrete electrographic seizures merge to a waxing and waning pattern of seizure activity, followed by continuous monomorphic discharges, which become interspersed with increasing periods of electrographic silence and, eventually, periodic epileptiform discharges on a relatively flat background.[16] The presence of any of these EEG patterns should suggest the diagnosis of GCSE.

Box 50.2 Physiological changes in generalised convulsive status epilepticus[18]

Hypoxia
Respiratory acidosis
Lactic acidosis
Hyperpyrexia
Hypertension (early)/hypotension (late)
Hyperglycaemia (early)/hypoglycaemia (late)
Tachycardia
Cardiac arrhythmias
Blood leucocytosis
CSF pleocytosis, increased CSF protein
Intracranial hypertension
Neurogenic pulmonary oedema
Aspiration pneumonitis
Rhabdomyolysis

ENDOCRINE AND METABOLIC EFFECTS

Early in GCSE there is a marked increase in plasma catecholamines, producing systemic physiological changes that resolve if SE is stopped early (**Box 50.2**). However, if seizures continue, many of these early physiological changes reverse and the resultant hypotension and hypoglycaemia may exacerbate neurological injury.[18]

Hyperthermia is due to both muscle activity and central sympathetic drive, and thus may still occur when paralysing agents prevent motor activity. In early SE, both cerebral metabolic activity and cerebral blood flow (CBF) are increased. In late SE, although cerebral metabolic activity remains high, CBF may fall owing to hypotension and loss of cerebral autoregulation leading to cerebral ischaemia.

PSEUDOSEIZURES

An important differential diagnosis of generalised convulsive epilepsy is pseudoseizures.[19] These can occur in patients with or without a history of epilepsy. Clinical features suggestive of pseudoseizures are listed in **Box 50.3**. "Distinction between the two may be extremely difficult, and can be made with complete certainty only using EEG monitoring." Pseudostatus, misdiagnosed as true SE, is often refractory to initial therapy and can lead to patients receiving general anaesthesia and mechanical ventilation.

Box 50.3 Features suggestive of pseudoseizures

Lack of stereotyped seizures, with behavioural manifestations varying from event to event
Lack of sustained convulsive activity – 'on–off' appearance
Increase in movement if restraint is applied
Abolition of motor movements with reassurance or suggestion
Resistance to eye opening and gaze aversion
Poor response to treatment, refractory status epilepticus
Absence of pupillary dilatation
Normal tendon reflexes and plantar responses immediately after convulsion
Lack of metabolic consequences despite some hours of apparent fitting

Box 50.4 Investigations in status epilepticus

Initial studies
Blood glucose, electrolytes (sodium, potassium, calcium, magnesium), urea
Arterial blood gases
Anticonvulsant drug levels
Full blood count
Urinalysis
Further investigations after stabilisation
Liver function tests, lactate, creatine kinase
Toxicology screen
Lumbar puncture
Electroencephalogram
Brain imaging with computed tomography or magnetic resonance imaging

NON-CONVULSIVE STATUS EPILEPTICUS (NCSE)

This accounts for approximately 25% of SE, though its incidence is probably underestimated because of failure to recognise and diagnose the condition.

The diagnosis of NCSE generally requires a change in behaviour and/or responsiveness from baseline for at least 30 minutes, no overt seizure activity and an EEG with epileptiform discharges.[20] A response to intravenous antiepileptic drugs (e.g. benzodiazepines), with clinical improvement and resolution or improvement in EEG epileptic activity, is helpful in confirming the diagnosis.[21]

The diagnosis of NCSE should be considered in any patient with an unexplained altered conscious state, particularly those with CNS injury, metabolic disturbance, hepatic encephalopathy or sepsis. Series where EEG has been performed in critically ill patients with an unexplained depressed conscious state have found a high incidence of NCSE (8–18%).[22–24] EEG monitoring is required in patients with GCSE who do not recover consciousness after resolution of overt convulsive activity; in one study more than 14% of such patients had NCSE.[17]

NCSE is a heterogeneous disorder with multiple subtypes and published reports often describe diverse cohorts of patients. Although attempts have been made to define and classify this disorder, there is yet no universally accepted definition or classification.[20,25]

Traditionally NCSE is divided into absence status epilepticus (ASE) and complex partial status epilepticus (CPSE).[21] ASE is associated with bilateral diffuse synchronous seizures and may be 'typical' as characterised by generalised 3 Hz spike-wave EEG activity during periods of altered behaviour, or responsiveness that occurs in children with idiopathic generalised epilepsy who are otherwise normal.[21] Atypical ASE is a heterogeneous syndrome occurring in patients with mental retardation and epilepsy with multiple seizure types.

CPSE may present with a wide variety of clinical features and a variable degree of impairment of consciousness, which includes confusion, agitation, bizarre or aggressive behaviour and coma.[20] More recently other possible classification systems have been proposed.[20,25–27]

The most important factor in determining outcome in NCSE is the underlying cause.[4,20,21]

NCSE is often mistaken for other conditions, resulting in a delay in diagnosis and treatment. A high index of suspicion must therefore be present to trigger investigation with an EEG.

The differential diagnosis of NCSE includes:

- metabolic encephalopathy
- drug intoxication
- cerebrovascular disease
- psychiatric syndromes (dissociative reactions, acute psychosis)
- post-ictal confusion.

EPILEPTIFORM ENCEPHALOPATHIES

In many advanced coma stages, the EEG exhibits continuous or periodic EEG abnormalities, but in such situations it is unclear whether the abnormal discharges are responsible for, or contribute to, the altered consciousness or are merely a reflection of a severe cerebral insult.[27]

Some consider myoclonic SE that follows an anoxic insult as part of this category, rather than as a form of NCSE.[27]

INVESTIGATIONS

Not all of the investigations listed in **Box 50.4** need to be performed in every patient. The selection of tests depends on both the patient's history and the presentation.

NEUROIMAGING

Most patients with SE should have a computed tomography (CT) scan of the brain performed, although this may not always be necessary if another episode of SE occurs in a patient with established epilepsy who has previously been thoroughly evaluated. Magnetic resonance imaging (MRI) may occasionally reveal abnormalities not visualised on CT scans and should be considered for non-emergency imaging. Imaging should be performed only after control of SE and patient stabilisation.[28]

LUMBAR PUNCTURE

In any patient, especially in young children with fever and SE, CNS infection and lumbar puncture along with blood cultures should be considered.[29] Meningitis is an uncommon cause of SE in adults and, unless the suspicion of CNS infection is high, brain imaging should be performed before a lumbar puncture. Contraindications to lumbar puncture include intracranial hypertension, mass lesion and hydrocephalus. If meningitis is suspected and a lumbar puncture cannot be performed expediently, antibiotics should be administered immediately rather than delayed. Approximately 20% of patients have a modest CSF white cell count pleocytosis after SE and such patients should be treated for suspected meningitis until the diagnosis is excluded.[1]

MANAGEMENT

GENERALISED CONVULSIVE STATUS EPILEPTICUS (GCSE)

An accurate history should be obtained, with particular emphasis on eye-witness accounts of the onset and nature of the seizures, and a full physical examination performed. However, neither should delay initial emergency management. Rapid control of seizures is crucial to prevent brain injury and the development of refractory SE. There is evidence that the longer SE goes untreated the harder it is to control with drugs.[8,9,30,31]

Management of SE involves termination of seizures, treating precipitating causes and underlying conditions, and prevention of complications and recurrence of seizures.

Few controlled data are available to support the use of any particular agents. One of the few randomised, double-blind clinical trials for treatment of GCSE found that lorazepam, phenobarbital or diazepam followed by phenytoin are all acceptable as initial treatment, but that phenytoin alone was not as effective as lorazepam.[31] Another randomised controlled trial in the pre-hospital setting found intravenous lorazepam and diazepam to be equally effective and superior to placebo in terminating GCSE.[32]

There are few data to guide the treatment of refractory SE, for which anaesthetising agents such as thiopental, propofol or midazolam infusions are commonly used. A randomised controlled trial of propofol versus barbiturates was terminated after 3 years with only 24 of the required 150 patients recruited.[33]

The EEG goal of treatment for refractory SE remains controversial, with some advocating EEG background suppression (isoelectric) and others suppression of seizures regardless of the EEG background activity.[7,9,10,34]

Various protocols for SE management have been suggested.[1,7,9,34] One approach is outlined in **Box 50.5**.

NON-CONVULSIVE STATUS EPILEPTICUS (NCSE)

Patients with NCSE are a heterogeneous group and as such there is a variable response to treatment.[25] Prognosis is most closely related to the underlying aetiology.[20,21]

Clinical response to intravenous benzodiazepine is predictive of a good outcome.[35]

There is considerable debate as to whether NCSE presents the same degree of risk of neurological injury as GCSE.[36] Prompt treatment is generally recommended and the use of additional non-anaesthetising anticonvulsants, such as levetiracetam, phenobarbital and valproate, has been suggested prior to embarking upon general anaesthesia.[7,21,37]

The potential side-effects of aggressive treatment (hypotension, immunosuppression) need to be balanced against the potential neurological morbidity of NCSE.[38] Particularly in elderly patients, aggressive treatment and anaesthesia may be associated with more risk than benefit and result in a worse outcome.[20,38,39]

DRUGS FOR STATUS EPILEPTICUS

BENZODIAZEPINES

Benzodiazepines are fast-acting antiseizure drugs and are therefore preferred as initial therapy. They act mainly by enhancing the neuroinhibitory effects of γ-aminobutyric $acid_A$ ($GABA_A$). The efficacy of benzodiazepines diminishes with duration of SE as a result of a reduction in synaptic $GABA_A$ receptors with prolonged seizures.[13]

Diazepam is a highly lipid-soluble drug with rapid CNS penetration, but then redistribution resulting in a short duration of action. It can be administered either intravenously or by the rectal route. Rectal administration can be achieved using a specially formulated rectal gel, or the intravenous preparation can be diluted with an equal amount of saline and flushed into the rectum. Rectal administration should be considered when vascular access is delayed and may be particularly useful in the pre-hospital setting.

Lorazepam has a longer duration of action and has a lower incidence of seizure recurrence when used as a single agent.[31] A double-blind, randomised comparison of intravenous diazepam, lorazepam and placebo in SE in the pre-hospital setting found both benzodiazepines to be associated with greater cessation of seizures and lower requirement for intubation than placebo. There

Box 50.5 Protocol for management of SE

1. Assess A, B, C, GCS
2. Give O_2 and consider need for intubation/ventilation
3. Monitor blood pressure, ECG, pulse oximetry
4. Obtain i.v. access and draw blood for investigations
5. If patient is hypoglycaemic, or if blood glucose estimation is not available, give glucose:
   adults: give thiamine 100 mg i.v. and 50 mL of 50% glucose i.v.
   children: give 2 mL/kg of 25% glucose i.v.
6. Seizure control:
   A. Give benzodiazepine,* for example:
      diazepam: 0.2 mg/kg i.v. at 5 mg/min up to total dose of 20 mg;
      lorazepam: 0.1 mg/kg i.v. at 2 mg/min up to total dose of 10 mg;
      clonazepam: 0.01–0.02 mg/kg i.v. at 0.5 mg/min up to total dose of 4 mg.
      If diazepam stops the seizures, phenytoin should be given next to prevent recurrence.
      Repeat dose every 2–5 min if required. Note: risk of respiratory depression with cumulative doses.
   B. If seizures persist, give phenytoin:
      phenytoin: 15–20 mg/kg (adults ≤50 mg/min; children ≤1 mg/kg/min) or fosphenytoin 15–20 phenytoin equivalents (PE) mg/kg i.v. (adults ≤150 mg/min; children ≤3 mg/kg per min).
      Additional doses of 5 mg/kg i.v., to a maximum dose of 30 mg/kg can be given for persistent seizures.
      Monitor blood pressure and the ECG during infusion. If hypotension or arrhythmias develop, stop or slow the rate of the infusion.
   C. If seizures persist (refractory SE), intubate and ventilate patient. Give either:
      thiopental: slow bolus 3–5 mg/kg i.v., followed by infusion 1–5 mg/kg per h, *or*
      propofol: slow bolus 1–2 mg/kg i.v., followed by infusion 2–5 mg/kg per h,† *or*
      midazolam: slow bolus 0.1–0.2 mg/kg, followed by infusion 0.1–1.0 mg/kg per h.
      Titrate doses based on clinical and electrographic evidence of seizures, targeting electrographic suppression of seizures or EEG background suppression (isoelectric).
      Monitor BP and maintain normotension by reducing infusion rate and/or giving fluids/pressor agents.
   D. Insert nasogastric tube and administer usual anticonvulsant medications if patient is receiving treatment for pre-existing epilepsy.
   E. Beware of ongoing unrecognised seizures.
      Use EEG monitoring until seizures are controlled and then for 1–2 hours after seizures stop. Continue to monitor the EEG continuously, or for periods of more than 30 minutes every 2 hours, during the maintenance phase.
      Avoid muscle relaxants (use continuous EEG if giving repeated doses of muscle relaxants).
   F. Discontinue midazolam or thiopental, or start reducing propofol, approximately 12 hours after resolution of seizures. Use continuous EEG monitoring and observe for further clinical and/or electrographic seizure activity. If seizures recur, reinstate the infusion and repeat this step at 12–24-hour intervals or longer if the patient's seizures remain refractory.
   In addition:
   Look for and treat cause and precipitant.††
   Look for and treat complications: hypotension, hyperthermia, and rhabdomyolysis.

*If i.v. access is not obtainable, consider rectal diazepam, buccal/sublingual or intranasal or i.m. midazolam, i.m. fosphenytoin.
†High infusion rates for prolonged periods require caution.
††In refractory SE, consider giving pyridoxine for children <18 months or if isoniazid toxicity is suspected in adults.

was a trend toward lorazepam being more efficacious than diazepam.[32]

Midazolam has a short duration of action and, unlike other benzodiazepines, can be administered via intramuscular, buccal and intranasal routes. These alternative routes of administration may be more convenient, acceptable and efficacious than diazepam administered by the rectal route.[40,41] A recent study found that intramuscular midazolam was as safe and efficacious as intravenous lorazepam and resulted in faster and more reliable administration in the pre-hospital setting.[42]

Midazolam administered by intravenous bolus and infusion may terminate seizures when other agents have failed. It may also have fewer side effects than alternative agents available for the treatment of refractory SE.[43] A limiting factor in its use is tachyphylaxis, which may necessitate a several-fold increase in the dose to maintain seizure control.[34] There is a wide variation in recommended infusion rates, from 0.05–0.4 mg/kg per hour[7] to 0.2–2.9 mg/kg per hour.[10]

Clonazepam has a longer duration of action than diazepam and is given by intravenous bolus. Early reports suggested that it has better efficacy and fewer side-effects than diazepam, though there are no published comparisons.

PHENYTOIN

Phenytoin is useful for maintaining a prolonged anti-seizure effect after rapid termination of seizures with a benzodiazepine, or when benzodiazepines fail. When used alone as initial therapy phenytoin is not as efficacious as benzodiazepines for terminating seizures.[31]

The recommended intravenous loading dose is 20 mg/kg. The common practice of giving a standard loading dose of 1000 mg of phenytoin may provide inadequate therapy for some adults.

When phenytoin is infused at the maximal adult recommended rate of 50 mg/min, hypotension occurs in up to 50% of patients and cardiac rhythm disturbance occurs in 2%. These adverse effects are more common in older patients and those with cardiac disease and are due to the phenytoin itself as well as the propylene glycol diluent. Blood pressure and the ECG should be monitored during infusion of phenytoin and the infusion slowed or stopped if cardiovascular complications occur.

Intramuscular administration of phenytoin is not recommended as absorption is erratic and it can cause local tissue reactions.

Fosphenytoin, a new water-soluble prodrug of phenytoin, is converted to phenytoin by endogenous phosphatases.[44] Doses of fosphenytoin are expressed as phenytoin equivalents (PE). Fosphenytoin can be administered at rates of up to 150 PE mg/min, since it is not formulated with propylene glycol, allowing therapeutic serum concentrations of fosphenytoin to be attained within 10 minutes. However, this may not necessarily result in more rapid CNS penetration and onset of action.[45]

Systemic side-effects are similar for phenytoin and fosphenytoin, although reactions at the infusion site are less common with fosphenytoin.[44]

Fosphenytoin can also be administered intramuscularly, although absorption is slower than with intravenous administration, and this route should be used only when intravenous access is not possible.

SODIUM VALPROATE

There are reports of intravenous valproate being used to treat both GCSE and NCSE in adults and children. It is non-sedating and it appears to be well tolerated with few reports of hypotension or respiratory depression.[46]

It may be particularly useful as a second- or third-line drug in situations where it is not possible, or it is preferable to avoid the use of sedating anaesthetic agents and the associated requirement for intubation.[47]

An initial dose of 10 mg/kg followed by continuous infusion or divided doses up to 20-40 mg/kg daily is recommended.[7,48]

LEVETIRACETAM

Although the data are mostly uncontrolled and retrospective, there is some evidence for the use of levetiracetam as second- or third-line therapy and in situations where it is desirable to avoid intubation, such as in NCSE and treatment of the elderly.[8,37,47,49] Levetiracetam may have particular utility in controlling seizures after hypoxic brain injury.[8]

Levetiracetam may be given intravenously in bolus doses of between 1000 and 3000 mg.

BARBITURATES

Phenobarbital is a potent anticonvulsant with a long duration of action. The usual dose is 15–20 mg/kg intravenously. It has equal efficacy to benzodiazepines and phenytoin when used first-line, but may cause greater depression of respiration, blood pressure and consciousness and therefore is often used only if these agents fail. However, many would advocate alternative and more aggressive measures for treatment of refractory SE at this point as the likelihood of phenobarbital controlling seizures when these other agents have failed is small.[10]

Thiopental is an intravenous anaesthetic agent used for refractory SE. A dose of 3–5 mg/kg is usually given for intubation, followed by repeated doses of 0.5–1 mg/kg until seizures are controlled. Following bolus intravenous administration, the drug is rapidly redistributed into peripheral fat stores and an infusion of 1–5 mg/kg per hour is required for ongoing suppression of seizures. Once lipid stores are saturated the duration of action is prolonged and recovery may take hours to days. Prolonged therapy requires the use of EEG monitoring to ensure that the seizures remain suppressed and to allow titration to the lowest dose that achieves the EEG target of seizure and/or EEG background suppression. Side-effects include hypotension, myocardial depression and immunosuppression with increased risk of infection.

Pentobarbital (the first metabolite of thiopental) is available in the USA as the alternative to thiopental.

Compared with other agents used in refractory SE (midazolam and propofol), barbiturates may result in a lower frequency of short-term treatment failure and breakthrough seizures, but result in more hypotension and slower recovery from anaesthesia.[50]

PROPOFOL

Propofol (2,6-diisopropylphenol) is an anaesthetic agent that has become increasingly popular for the treatment of refractory SE. It is administered as an intravenous bolus followed by infusion and intubation and ventilation are required.

Compared with high-dose barbiturates (pentobarbital) in adult patients with refractory SE, propofol has been found to control seizures more quickly and, because of its shorter duration of action, allows earlier re-emergence from anaesthesia.[51] However, seizures tend to recur with sudden discontinuation of propofol, necessitating recommencement of the infusion and a more gradual tapering of the dose, such that both drugs ultimately may result in a similar duration of ventilation and ICU stay.[51]

There is concern that prolonged high-dose propofol use (e.g. >5 mg/kg per hour) may result in myocardial failure, hypoxia, metabolic acidosis, lipaemia, rhabdomyolysis and death (propofol infusion syndrome).[52] Early reports were in children and later adults and its use requires caution. There are series, however, of prolonged high-dose propofol use in adults with SE without major adverse effects.[53]

NEUROMUSCULAR-BLOCKING AGENTS

Paralysis is indicated if uncontrolled fitting causes difficulty with providing adequate ventilation or severe lactic acidosis. Neuromuscular blockade should be used only if continuous EEG monitoring is available, as the clinical expression of seizure activity is abolished.

OTHER AGENTS OF POTENTIAL USE IN REFRACTORY SE

Ketamine acts as an antagonist at the NMDA receptor and may have a role in the treatment of prolonged refractory SE.[12]

Intravenous lacosamide is a new anticonvulsant drug available in intravenous and oral formulations that may be an option for treatment of established SE after failure of standard therapy, or when standard agents are considered unsuitable. Evidence exists mainly in the form of limited case series.[54]

Pregabalin appears to be an interesting option as add-on treatment in refractory NCSE and may lessen the requirement for ICU treatment.[55]

Magnesium is the drug of choice in eclamptic seizures and also is effective in seizures due to hypomagnesaemia, but there is little evidence to support its use in other forms of SE.[12]

SURGERY

Surgery has occasionally been used in refractory SE with procedures based on standard epilepsy surgery techniques. Some success has been reported with focal resections, subpial transection, corpus callosotomy, hemispherectomy and vagus nerve stimulation.[12,56]

INTENSIVE CARE MONITORING

Monitoring using ECG, intra-arterial and central venous catheters, capnography and pulse oximetry should be considered in patients with, or at risk of, cardiorespiratory compromise. Indications for EEG monitoring are listed in **Box 50.6.**[17] Cerebral function monitors are useful in titrating doses of anaesthetic agents to EEG background suppression, but may not have sufficient sensitivity to detect seizure activity. Intracranial pressure monitoring should be considered if elevated intracranial pressure is present owing to the underlying brain pathology.

Box 50.6 Indications for EEG monitoring[17]

- Refractory SE, to aid the titration of anticonvulsant anaesthetic drugs (minimizing dose and toxicity) and ensure suppression of seizure activity*
- Patients receiving neuromuscular blockade*
- Patients who continue to have a poor conscious state after apparent cessation of seizures
- Suspected non-convulsive status epilepticus in a patient with an altered conscious state
- Suspected pseudoseizures

*Continuous or regular intermittent EEG monitoring recommended.

OUTCOME

The prognosis of patients with SE is related to age, aetiology, degree of impairment of consciousness at presentation, and duration of SE.[15,57] Refractory SE is associated with a worse prognosis and very prolonged 'super-refractory' SE an even higher mortality. However, where no underlying irreversible brain damage is present, good recovery is possible even after weeks of SE.[9,12]

Children have a much lower mortality of 3%[58] whereas those aged over 65 years have a mortality rate of 30%.[3,4]

SE that is precipitated by low antiepileptic drug levels, alcohol abuse or systemic infection has a very low mortality, whereas SE secondary to an acute CNS insult such as stroke or infection has a higher mortality.[3,5] SE associated with hypoxic brain injury is most often fatal.[59] NCSE detected in comatose critically ill patients, despite recognition and treatment, has a poor outcome.[24,39]

Consequences of SE include brain damage resulting in permanent neurological deficits and also the development of focal epilepsy (epileptogenesis). Multiorgan failure and death can result from uncontrolled seizures, the underlying illness or complications of treatment.

STATUS EPILEPTICUS IN CHILDREN[58–61]

Most paediatric cases of SE occur in young children, with 80% occurring in those below 4 years of age.[58] The vast majority of cases are convulsive and generalised.[28]

The distribution of causes is highly age-dependent, with febrile SE and that due to acute neurological disease (e.g. CNS infection) being more common in children under 4 years. Remote symptomatic causes and SE in a child with previously diagnosed epilepsy are more common in older children.[58] The most frequent aetiologies of SE in children are listed in **Box 50.7.**[28,29,58]

The likelihood of bacterial meningitis is much higher in febrile children presenting with a first-ever episode of SE (12%) as opposed to a brief seizure (1%) and a high index of suspicion is required to investigate and treat for meningitis.[58]

Treatment of SE in children is essentially the same as in adults.[60]

Box 50.7 Causes of status epilepticus in children[28,29,58]

Febrile – previously neurologically normal, temp. >38°C, CNS infection excluded
Acute symptomatic – meningitis, encephalitis, cerebrovascular disease, trauma, metabolic derangement, hypoxia, sepsis, drug-related
Remote symptomatic causes – previous traumatic brain injury or insult, CNS malformation, cerebral palsy
Progressive neurological conditions – tumours, degenerative, autoimmune diseases
Cryptogenic

The underlying cause is the main determinant of mortality, which is negligible for prolonged febrile seizures and 12–16% for acute symptomatic causes.[61] Similarly, the risk of subsequent epilepsy is low in neurologically normal children but higher than 50% in those with acute or remote symptomatic causes.[61]

Access the complete references list online at http://www.expertconsult.com

7. Meierkord H, Boon P, Engelsen B, et al. EFNS guideline on the management of status epilepticus in adults. Eur J Neurol 2010;17(3):348–55.
8. Holtkamp M. Treatment strategies for refractory status epilepticus. Curr Opin Crit Care 2011;17(2): 94–100.
9. Rossetti AO, Lowenstein DH. Management of refractory status epilepticus in adults: still more questions than answers. Lancet Neurol 2011;10(10):922–30.
12. Shorvon S, Ferlisi M. The treatment of super-refractory status epilepticus: a critical review of available therapies and a clinical treatment protocol. Brain 2011;134(Pt 10):2802–18.
13. Chen JW, Wasterlain CG. Status epilepticus: pathophysiology and management in adults. Lancet Neurol 2006;5(3):246–56.
14. Tan RY, Neligan A, Shorvon SD. The uncommon causes of status epilepticus: a systematic review. Epilepsy Res 2010;91(2-3):111–22.
20. Meierkord H, Holtkamp M. Non-convulsive status epilepticus in adults: clinical forms and treatment. Lancet Neurol 2007;6(4):329–39.
60. Abend NS, Gutierrez-Colina AM, Dlugos DJ. Medical treatment of pediatric status epilepticus. Semin Pediatr Neurol 2010;17(3):169–75.

51

Acute cerebrovascular complications

Bernard Riley and Thearina de Beer

Cerebrovascular disease is common and its acute manifestation, stroke, produces considerable morbidity and mortality. Stroke is defined as an acute focal neurological deficit caused by cerebrovascular disease, which lasts for more than 24 hours or causes death before 24 hours. Transient ischaemic attack (TIA) also causes focal neurology, but this resolves within 24 hours. In the UK, stroke is responsible for 9% of all deaths accounting for around 53 000 deaths per year and is the most common cause of physical disability in adults. The incidence in most developed countries is about 1–2/1000 population per year with a 42% reduction in high-income countries but a 100% increase in low- to middle-income countries in the past four decades.[1] The main causes of stroke are cerebral infarction as a consequence of thromboembolism and spontaneous intracranial haemorrhage (either intracerebral or subarachnoid haemorrhage (SAH)), causing about 85% and 15% of strokes, respectively. The main risk factors are increasing age, hypertension, ischaemic heart disease, atrial fibrillation, smoking, diabetes, obesity, some oral contraceptives and raised cholesterol or haematocrit. The manifestations of stroke are cerebral infarction (thrombosis, embolism) and intracranial haemorrhage (intracerebral haemorrhage, SAH).

PROGNOSIS IN ACUTE CEREBROVASCULAR DISEASE

Mortality after stroke averages 30% within a month, with more patients dying after SAH or intracerebral haemorrhage than after cerebral infarction, although survival to 1 year is slightly better in the haemorrhagic group. In all types of stroke about 30% of survivors remain disabled to the point of being dependent on others. Risk of stroke increases with age and very old age is an independent predictor of death.[2] Thus stroke is often accompanied by significant age-related medical co-morbidity. In the past this may have been partially responsible for a relatively non-aggressive approach to the treatment of stroke patients, so that the gloomy prognosis of stroke becomes a self-fulfilling prophecy. The challenge for intensivists is to identify those patients who are most likely to survive and not to offer aggressive therapy to those who are not. Stroke should be regarded as a medical emergency. Patients should initially be treated in a stroke unit as there is good evidence of reduction in both mortality and dependency compared with those treated in a general ward. The UK National Institute for Health and Clinical Excellence (NICE) has published guidelines aimed at ensuring early diagnosis and aggressive therapy.[3,4]

CEREBRAL INFARCTION

Infarction of cerebral tissue (ischaemic stroke) occurs as a result of inadequate perfusion from occlusion of cerebral blood vessels in association with inadequate collateral circulation. It may occur due to cerebral thrombosis or embolism.

AETIOLOGY AND PATHOLOGY

CEREBRAL THROMBOSIS

Atherosclerosis is the major cause of major arterial occlusion and most often produces symptoms if it occurs at the bifurcation of the carotid artery or the carotid syphon. Progressive plaque formation causes narrowing and forms a nidus for platelet aggregation and thrombus formation. Ulceration and rupture of the plaque exposes its thrombogenic lipid core, activating the clotting cascade. Hypertension and diabetes mellitus are common causes of smaller arterial thrombosis. Rarer causes of thrombosis include any disease resulting in vasculitis, vertebral or carotid artery dissection (either spontaneous or posttraumatic) or carotid occlusion by strangulation or systemic hypotension after cardiac arrest. Cerebral venous thrombosis, responsible for less than 1% of strokes, may occur in hypercoagulable states such as dehydration, polycythaemia, thrombocythaemia, some oral contraceptive pills, protein C or S deficiency or antithrombin III deficiency, or vessel occlusion by tumour or abscess. Cerebral infarction may also result from sustained systemic hypotension from any cause, particularly if associated with hypoxaemia.

CEREBRAL EMBOLISM

Embolism commonly occurs from thrombus or platelet aggregations overlying arterial atherosclerotic plaques, but 30% of cerebral emboli will arise from thrombus in the left atrium or ventricle of the heart. This is very likely in the presence of atrial fibrillation, left-sided valvular disease, recent myocardial infarction, chronic atrial enlargement or ventricular aneurysm. The presence of a patent foramen ovale or septal defects allows paradoxical embolism to occur. Iatrogenic air embolism may occur during cardiopulmonary bypass, cardiac catheterisation or cerebral angiography. Embolisation may also occur as a complication of attempted coil embolisation of cerebral aneurysms or arteriovenous malformations (AVMs) after SAH.

CLINICAL PRESENTATION

In cerebral thrombosis, there is initially no loss of consciousness or headache and the initial neurological deficit develops over several hours. Cerebral embolism may be characterised by sudden onset and rapid development of complete neurological deficit. No single clinical sign or symptom can reliably distinguish a thrombotic from an embolic event.

Where infarction occurs in a limited arterial territory the clinical signs are often characteristic. The commonest site involves the middle cerebral artery, which classically produces acute contralateral brachiofacial hemiparesis with sensory or motor deficits, depending on the precise area of infarction. Infarction of the middle cerebral territory leads to a dense contralateral hemiplegia, contralateral facial paralysis, contralateral hemianopia and ipsilateral eye deviation. Dominant left-hemisphere lesions result in language difficulties from aphasia, dysphasia, dysgraphia and dyscalculia. Non-dominant right hemispheric lesions cause the patient to neglect the left side, and failure to communicate with anyone approaching from that side. In strokes involving the posterior fossa the precise pattern of symptoms depends on the arterial territories involved and the presence or absence of collaterals. The onset of symptoms such as gait disturbance, headache, nausea, vomiting and loss of consciousness may be very rapid. Venous thrombosis may occur particularly in the cerebral veins, sagittal or transverse dural sinuses, causing headache, seizures, focal neurology and loss of consciousness. Other cognitive effects of stroke include memory impairment, anxiety, depression, emotional lability, aprosody and spatial impairment. Bilateral brainstem infarction after basilar artery thrombosis may produce deep coma and tetraparesis. Pontine stroke may produce the 'locked-in' syndrome. The precise clinical presentation depends on the size of the infarcted area and its position in the brain. Vascular lesions such as carotid dissection can present with ipsilateral Horner's syndrome with facial pain, a painful Horner's from local stellate ganglion damage or if there is significant ischaemia from impaired flow or emboli, then with contralateral signs consistent with infarction.[5]

INVESTIGATIONS

A full history and examination of the patient will produce a differential diagnosis that will require specific investigations. The aim is to make the diagnosis, establish the nature, size and position of the pathology, so that correct treatment can target the effects of the primary injury, and prevent extension of the lesion or complications occurring.

BLOOD TESTS

A full blood count should be taken to look for polycythaemia, infection or thrombocythaemia. A raised erythrocyte sedimentation rate or C-reactive protein level may indicate vasculitis, infection or carcinoma, warranting further appropriate investigations. Coagulation screen should also be taken together with serum cholesterol, triglyceride and syphilis serology. Specific investigation for thrombophilia due to protein C, protein S, Leiden factor V and antithrombin III abnormalities should be undertaken in patients with venous thrombosis or patients with otherwise unexplained cerebral infarction or TIA.

ELECTROCARDIOGRAPHY

This may demonstrate atrial fibrillation or other arrhythmia, or recent myocardial infarct.

ECHOCARDIOGRAPHY

Either transthoracic or transoesophageal echocardiography (TOE) may demonstrate mural or atrial appendage thrombus as a source of embolism. TOE is more effective in detecting patent foramen ovale, aortic arteriosclerosis or dissection.

COMPUTED TOMOGRAPHY (CT) OR MAGNETIC RESONANCE IMAGING (MRI) SCANNING

These techniques are used to distinguish infarction from haemorrhage. Tumour, abscess or subdural haematoma may also produce the symptoms and signs of stroke. Ideally, the scans should be undertaken as soon as possible to exclude conditions that are treatable by neurosurgery. Early scanning is vital if interventional treatment such as thrombolysis, anticoagulation, antiplatelet therapy or surgery is planned.

The CT scan may be normal or show only minor loss of grey/white matter differentiation in the first 24 hours after ischaemic stroke, but haemorrhage is seen as areas of increased attenuation within minutes. After a couple of weeks the CT appearances of an infarct or haemorrhage become very similar and it may be impossible to distinguish them if CT is delayed beyond this time. CT angiography will often demonstrate vascular abnormalities and vasospasm but multimodal MRI, a combination of diffusion and perfusion-weighted MRI and magnetic resonance angiography (MRA), is much more sensitive in demonstrating small areas of ischaemia and targeting those patients most suitable for thrombolysis.[6] Where cerebral infarction has occurred as a result of venous thrombosis, the best imaging technique is MRA. Other imaging techniques are appropriate to identify the source of stroke in specific areas. Any patient with a stroke or TIA in the internal carotid artery territory should have duplex Doppler ultrasonography, which may demonstrate stenosis, occlusion or dissection of the internal carotid. Where trauma is an aetiological factor reconstruction CT bone window views are required to demonstrate any site of fracture-associated vascular injury. MRA (magnetic resonance angiography) is increasingly useful for rapid diagnosis of vascular problems as can be seen in Figure 51.1.

MANAGEMENT

The UK national sentinel stroke audit in 2008 suggested that if 80% rather than 68% of the 2000 patients with ischaemic stroke studied had been managed on a stroke unit the number dead or dependent could be reduced

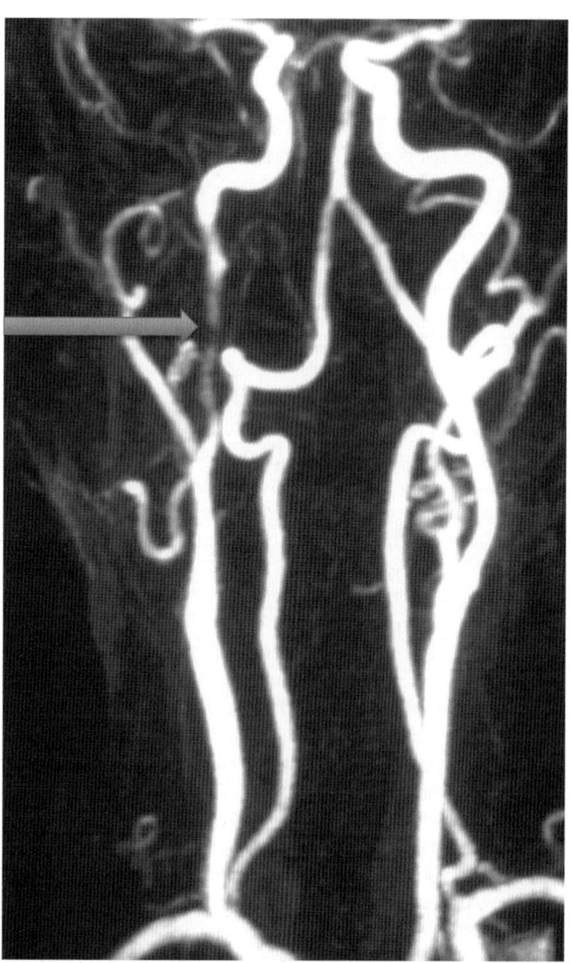

Figure 51.1 MRA. Internal carotid dissection associated with exercise, skiing the bumps. Presentation painful Horner's.

by 69, equating to 5% of all 1300 new cases of death and dependency in a population of 1 million.[7] In general, only those patients with a compromised airway due to depressed level of consciousness or life-threatening cardiorespiratory disturbances require admission to medical or neurosurgical ICUs. In either case, attention to basic resuscitation, involving stabilisation of airway, breathing and circulation, is self-evident.

AIRWAY AND BREATHING

Patients with Glasgow Coma Scores (GCS) of 8 or less, or those with absent gag or defects of swallowing (both of which may occur at higher GCS), will require intubation to preserve their airway and prevent aspiration. Where this requirement is likely to be prolonged, early tracheostomy should be considered. Adequate oxygenation and ventilation should be confirmed by arterial blood gas analysis, and supplemental oxygen prescribed if there is any evidence of hypoxia. If hypercarbia occurs then ventilatory support to achieve normocarbia is necessary to prevent exacerbation of cerebral oedema. Mortality and poor functional outcome can be poor in patients over 65 who require mechanical ventilation with only 40% surviving for 6 months, but 25% of survivors may recover to good functional outcome and reasonable quality of life.[8] There is currently no evidence to suggest that early tracheostomy in ventilated stroke patients is of any benefit, although a randomised prospective trial of early tracheostomy versus prolonged intubation has been mooted.[9]

CIRCULATORY SUPPORT

A large number of stroke patients will have raised blood pressure on admission, presumably as an attempt by the vasomotor centre to improve cerebral perfusion. Hypertensive patients may have impaired autoregulation and regional cerebral perfusion may be very dependent on blood pressure. The patient's clinical condition and neurological status should determine treatment rather than an arbitrary level of blood pressure. Current recommendations are that emergency administration of antihypertensive agents should be withheld unless the systolic pressure is >220 mmHg (29 kPa) or the diastolic pressure is >120 mmHg (16 kPa). Aggressive lowering of blood pressure is not without risk and may result in progression of ischaemic stroke, so reduction should be monitored closely.[10] It would seem reasonable on physiological grounds to avoid drugs that cause cerebral vasodilatation in that they may aggravate cerebral oedema, although there is no hard evidence for this. Animal experiments suggested that haemodilution could improve blood flow by reducing whole-blood viscosity but a multicentre study failed to identify any clinical benefit and euvolaemia remains the ideal end-point.[11] Cardiac output should be maintained and any underlying cardiac pathology such as failure, infarction and atrial fibrillation treated appropriately.

METABOLIC SUPPORT

Both hypo- and hyperglycaemia have been shown to worsen prognosis after acute stroke, therefore blood sugar levels should be maintained in the normal range.[12] In the long term, nutritional support must not be neglected and early enteral feeding instituted by nasogastric intubation. In the longer term, particularly where bulbar function is reduced, percutaneous endoscopic gastrostomy is necessary.

ANTICOAGULATION

In theory, the use of anticoagulation reduces the propagation of thrombus and should prevent further embolism. In practice, the reduction in risk of further thromboembolic stroke is offset by a similar number of patients dying from cerebral or systemic haemorrhage as a result of anticoagulation.[13,14] Anticoagulation can only be recommended in individuals where there is a high risk of recurrence, such as in those patients with prosthetic heart valves, atrial fibrillation with thrombus or those with thrombophilic disorders. A CT scan must be obtained prior to commencing therapy to exclude haemorrhage, and careful monitoring used. In patients with large infarcts there is always the risk of haemorrhage (haemorrhagic conversion) into the infarct and early heparinisation is best avoided.

THROMBOLYSIS

Thrombolysis with intravenous recombinant tissue plasminogen activator (rtPA alteplase) is now an established treatment for acute ischaemic stroke.[15] There are specific inclusion and exclusion criteria. Inclusion criteria are a diagnosis of ischaemic stroke causing measurable neurological deficit, age over 18 and less than 80 with an onset of symptoms to treatment time of less than 3 hours. Patients should be excluded if there is a history of head trauma or stroke (ischaemic or haemorrhagic) in the previous 3 months, evidence of subarachnoid or intracranial haemorrhage, arterial puncture in a non-compressible site in the past 7 days, any active bleeding or bleeding diathesis including platelet count less than 100 000/mm^3, heparin within 48 hours, current anticoagulant therapy, hypoglycaemia or multilobar infarction (more than one-third of a cerebral hemisphere) on CT scan. Relative contraindications include minor or rapidly improving stroke symptoms, seizure at time of stroke with residual post-ictal signs, major trauma in the past 14 days, GI or urinary tract bleeding in the past 21 days or myocardial infarction within the past 3 months.

There is some evidence for improved clinical outcome after rtPA use between 3 and 4.5 hours after symptom onset, although the degree of clinical benefit is less.[16] Patients must be in an environment where they can be monitored for potential complications, the most serious of which is intracranial haemorrhage. This risk is reduced where there is strict adherence to the inclusion and exclusion criteria and the appropriate dose used.

ENDOVASCULAR THERAPY

Selective catheterisation of the occluded cerebral arteries is possible and there have been some reports of direct intra-arterial infusion of thrombolytic drugs such as urokinase for middle cerebral artery strokes.[17] Mechanical disruption or displacement of the thrombus causing acute ischaemic stroke has been reported using several kinds of neuroembolectomy catheters placed on selective angiography allowing for fragmentation and suction of the clot.[18] Intravascular placement of self-expanding stents is also under investigation.[19] All of these methods are available only in specialist neuroradiology departments and have yet to be the subject of large-scale randomised trials.

CEREBRAL PROTECTION

Various agents such as free-radical scavengers, calcium antagonists, magnesium, amino-3-hydroxy-5-methyl-4-isoxazolepropionate (AMPA) antagonists, glutamate antagonists and γ-aminobutyric acid antagonists have been used in attempts to limit the deleterious effects of the biochemical changes that occur intracellularly following ischaemia. No agent has been shown to be effective in placebo-controlled phase III trials.[20]

DECOMPRESSIVE CRANIECTOMY

Some patients with malignant middle cerebral artery infarction syndrome (MMCAS) may benefit from decompressive craniectomy, especially patients with large middle cerebral artery territory infarcts aged <60 years. Decompressive craniectomy must be done within 48 hours of symptom onset. The NNT for survival is 2 and for severe disability is 6. Untreated, MMCAS has a mortality of 80% and it is suggested craniectomy can reduce mortality to around 30%, but with residual neurological deficit. This procedure is limited to specialist centres. MMCAS development is predicted by MCA territory stroke of >50%, a perfusion deficit of >66% on CT, an infarct volume of >145 mL within 14 hours and >82 mL within 6 hours of onset. EEG and tissue cerebral tissue oxygenation have been used to predict cerebral oedema, ICP monitoring has not been proven to change outcome. Craniectomy has to be large enough to extend past the margins of the infarct. This seems to be well tolerated even after thrombolysis. There is no difference in outcome whether dominant or non-dominant hemispheres are involved. The patients who survive after craniectomy have moderate to severe disability and may have a high incidence of psychological complications. Whether this is acceptable to patients has not been studied.[21]

Other forms of surgical intervention proven to be effective in making more intracranial space and reducing intracranial pressure are drainage of secondary hydrocephalus by extraventricular drain (EVD) insertion or evacuation of haemorrhage into infarcted areas, resulting in new compressive symptoms. This is especially useful in the posterior fossa where the room for expansion of mass lesions is limited by its anatomy.

COMPLICATIONS

Local complications include cerebral oedema, haemorrhage into infarcted areas or secondary hydrocephalus. General complications include bronchopneumonia, aspiration pneumonia, deep-vein thrombosis, urinary tract infections, pressure sores, contractures and depression. Stroke patients who are ventilated seem particularly susceptible to ventilator-acquired pneumonia.[22] A team approach of specialist nursing, physiotherapists, occupational and speech and language therapists is best able to avoid these complications.

SPONTANEOUS INTRACRANIAL HAEMORRHAGE

Spontaneous intracranial haemorrhage (ICH) producing stroke may occur from either intracerebral haemorrhage (10%) or SAH (5%).

INTRACEREBRAL HAEMORRHAGE

The incidence of intracerebral haemorrhage is about 9/100 000 of the population, mostly in the age range of 40–70 years, with an equal incidence in males and females.

AETIOLOGY AND PATHOLOGY

The commonest cause is the effect of chronic systemic hypertension. This results in degeneration of the walls of vessels or microaneurysms, by the process of lipohyalinosis, and these microaneurysms then suddenly rupture. This may also occur in malignant tumour neovasculature, vasculitis, mycotic aneurysms, amyloidosis, sarcoidosis, malignant hypertension, primary haemorrhagic disorders and over-anticoagulation.

Occasionally, cerebral aneurysms or AVMs may cause intracerebral haemorrhage without SAH. Where intracerebral haemorrhage occurs in young patients the most likely cause is an underlying vascular abnormality. In some areas this is also associated with the abuse of drugs with sympathomimetic activity such as cocaine. The rupture of microaneurysms tends to occur at the bifurcation of small perforating arteries. Common sites of haemorrhage are the putamen (55%), cerebral cortex (15%), thalamus (10%), pons (10%) and cerebellum (10%). Haemorrhage is usually due to rupture of a single vessel, and the size of the haemorrhage is influenced by the anatomical resistance of the site into which it occurs. The effect of the haemorrhage is determined by the area of brain tissue that it destroys. Cortical haemorrhages tend to be larger than pontine bleeds, but the latter are much more destructive owing to the anatomical density of neural tracts and nuclei.

CLINICAL PRESENTATION

Usually, there are no prodromal symptoms and a sudden onset of focal neurology or depressed level of consciousness occurs. Headache and neck stiffness will occur in conscious patients if there is subarachnoid extension by haemorrhage into the ventricles. Where intraventricular extension occurs there may be a progressive fall in GCS as secondary hydrocephalus occurs, and this may be accompanied by ocular palsies, resulting in 'sunset eyes'. Early deterioration is common in the first few hours after haemorrhagic stroke and more than 20% of patients will drop their GCS by two or more points between initial onset of symptoms and arrival in the emergency department.[23] As with ischaemic stroke, focal neurology is determined by which area of the brain is involved. The only way to differentiate absolutely between ischaemic, intracerebral or SAH is by appropriate imaging. The symptoms relate to tissue destruction, compression and raised intracranial pressure, which if progressive will result in brainstem ischaemia and death.

INVESTIGATIONS

The general investigations are essentially those listed previously for ischaemic stroke, since it is difficult to distinguish between the two in the early stages. Patients undergoing treatment with oral anticoagulants, particularly warfarin in atrial fibrillation, mean that anticoagulant-associated ICH is increasing in frequency and a full coagulation screen is essential.[24] CT and/or MRI should be performed at the earliest opportunity. The early deterioration seen in ICH relates to active bleeding and repeat imaging after 3 hours of symptom onset often shows significant enlargement of the initial haematoma. CT angiography/MR angiography or venography is very important to determine the cause of the haemorrhage such as arteriovenous malformations (AVM), aneurysm or tumour neovasculature (**Figs 51.2** and **51.3**). Lumbar puncture may be performed to exclude infection if mycotic aneurysm is suspected, but only after CT has excluded raised intracranial pressure or non-communicating hydrocephalus.

MANAGEMENT

The general management principles are identical to those for ischaemic stroke. There is, of course, no place for anticoagulation or thrombolysis, and reversal of any coagulation defect either primary or secondary to therapeutic anticoagulation must be undertaken as a matter of urgency. A full coagulation screen must be performed and the administration of vitamin K, fresh

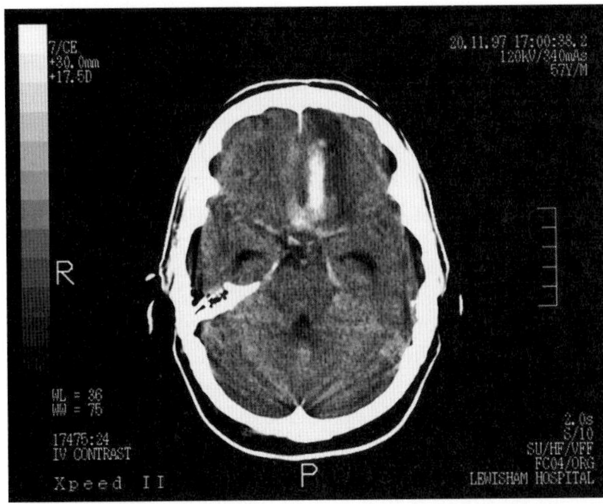

Figure 51.2 Left frontal intraparenchymal bleed with local oedema.

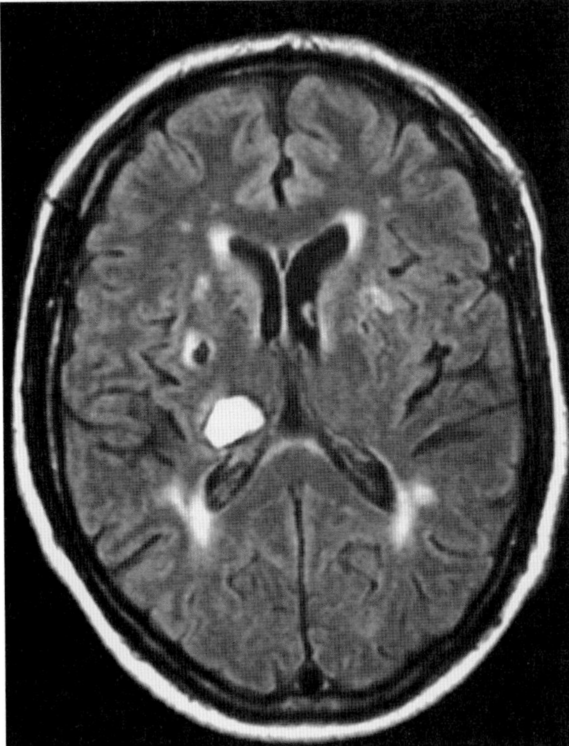

Figure 51.3 Magnetic resonance imaging: thalamic bleed.

frozen plasma, cryoprecipitate, etc., directed by the results. Where emergency decompressive surgery is indicated, warfarin-induced coagulopathy should be corrected using prothrombin complex concentrate (Beriplex or Octaplex). Intraventricular extension occurs in around 45% of cases and the insertion of an extraventricular drain (EVD) may increase conscious level, particularly in the presence of secondary hydrocephalus. The EVD level should be set such that the cerebrospinal fluid (CSF) drains at around 10 mmHg (1.33 kPa). The normal production of CSF should produce an hourly output and a sudden fall in output to zero should alert staff to the possibility that the drain has blocked. This is particularly likely if the CSF is heavily blood-stained. The meniscus of the CSF within the drain tubing should be examined for transmitted vascular pulsation or the level of the drain temporally lowered by a few centimetres to see if drainage occurs. If the drain is blocked, secondary hydrocephalus will recur. Because of the risk of introducing infection and causing a ventriculitis, the drain must be unblocked in a sterile manner by the neurosurgeons. Blood in the CSF acts as a pyrogen, but the patient's high temperature should never be ascribed to this alone and regular blood cultures and CSF samples are required as part of sepsis surveillance. Operative decompression of the haematoma should be undertaken only in neurosurgical centres and safe transfer must be assured if this is considered. The administration of mannitol prior to transfer should be discussed with the neurosurgical unit. There is some evidence that patients with supratentorial intracerebral haemorrhage less than 1 cm from the cortical surface benefitted from surgery within 96 hours, although this finding did not reach statistical significance.[25] Patients presenting with a GCS of less than 8/15 had an almost universally poor outcome. Not all intracerebral haematomata are amenable to surgery, and the CT scans should be reviewed by the neurosurgical unit, preferably prior to transfer by digital image link. In patients with a cerebellar ICH larger than 3 cm in diameter, or those with brainstem compression or secondary hydrocephalus, surgical decompression gives better results than those managed medically and despite the lack of randomised trials the current recommendation is to remove the clot surgically.[26]

The management of hypertension following spontaneous intracerebral haemorrhage may be difficult as too high a blood pressure (BP) may provoke further bleeding, whereas too low a BP may result in ischaemia. Current recommendations of the American Heart Association/American Stroke Association are to lower BP if the systolic BP is >200 mmHg (26.6 kPa) (MAP>150) with monitoring every 5 minutes. If the SBP is >180 mmHg (23.9 kPa) or MAP is >130 mmHg (17.3 kPa) and a high ICP is suspected then ICP and CCP should be measured while the BP is reduced keeping CPP above 60 mmHg (8 kPa). If SBP is >180 mmHg (23.9 kPa) or MAP is >130 mmHg (17.3 kPa) but no evidence of increased ICP then the MAP should be reduced to 110 mmHg or a target BP of 160/90.[26] These guidelines are not evidence based. The INTERACT2 trial on acute targeted blood pressure control after spontaneous intracerebral haemorrhage has shown that a systolic target of 140 mmHg was safe. It did not result in a significant reduction in death or major disability although there was a trend towards improved functional outcome.[44] The adoption of these guidelines may have significant resource indications regarding access to ICU beds to provide the required levels of monitoring. There is no place for steroids, and hyperventilation to Pa_{CO_2} of 30 mmHg (4 kPa) or less to control raised intracranial pressure will have detrimental effects on cerebral blood flow in other areas of the brain.

SUBARACHNOID HAEMORRHAGE

SAH refers to bleeding that occurs principally into the subarachnoid space and not into the brain parenchyma. The incidence of SAH is around 6/100 000; the apparent decrease, compared with earlier studies, is due to more frequent use of CT scanning, which allows exclusion of other types of haemorrhage. Risk factors are the same as for stroke, but SAH patients are usually younger, peaking in the sixth decade, with a female-to-male ratio of 1.24:1. People of Afro-Caribbean ancestry have twice the risk for SAH as whites. Between 5 and 20% of patients with SAH have a positive family history, with first-degree relatives having a three- to sevenfold risk, whereas second-degree relatives have the same degree of risk as the general population. Specific inheritable disorders are rare and account for only a minority of all patients with SAH.[23] The only modifiable risk factors for SAH are smoking, heavy drinking, the use of sympathomimetics (e.g. cocaine) and hypertension, which increase the risk odds ratio by 2 or 3. Overall mortality is 50%, of which 15% die before reaching hospital, with up to 30% of survivors having residual deficit producing dependency. High-volume centres (>60 cases per year) have shown a much-improved outcome over that of low-volume centres (<20 cases per year).[27]

AETIOLOGY AND PATHOLOGY

The majority of cases of SAH are caused by ruptured saccular (berry) aneurysms (85%), the remainder being caused by non-aneurysmal perimesencephalic haemorrhage (10%) and rarer causes such as arterial dissection, cerebral or dural AVMs, mycotic aneurysm, pituitary apoplexy, vascular lesions at the top of the spinal cord and cocaine abuse. Saccular aneurysms are not congenital, almost never occur in neonates and young children and develop during later life. It is not known why some adults develop aneurysms at arterial bifurcations in the circle of Willis and some do not. It was thought that there was a congenital weakness in the tunica media, but gaps in the arterial muscle wall are equally as common in patients with or without aneurysms and, once the aneurysm is formed, the weakness is found in the wall of the sac and not at its neck.[28] The association with smoking, hypertension and heavy drinking would suggest that degenerative processes are involved. Sudden hypertension plays a role in causing rupture, as shown by SAH in patients taking crack cocaine or, rarely, high doses of decongestants such as pseudoephedrine.

CLINICAL PRESENTATION

Classically, there is a 'thunderclap' headache developing in seconds, with half of patients describing its onset as instantaneous. This is followed by a period of depressed consciousness for less than an hour in 50% of patients, with focal neurology in about 30% of patients. About a fifth of patients recall similar headaches and these may have been due to sentinel bleeds; this increases the chances of early rebleed 10-fold. The degree of depression of consciousness depends upon the site and extent of the haemorrhage. Meningism – neck stiffness, photophobia, vomiting and a positive Kernig's sign – is common in those patients with higher GCS. A high index of suspicion is needed for patients presenting with the classical headache; a non-contrast CT is recommended and, if negative, a lumbar puncture should be done. If that is also negative, consider computed tomographic angiography (CTA).

The clinical severity of SAH is often described by a grade, the most widely used being that described by the World Federation of Neurological Surgeons (WFNS),[29] which is summarised in **Table 51.1**. This grading, together with the extent of the haemorrhage and the age of the patient, gives some indication of the prognosis, in that the worse the grade the bigger is the bleed, and the older the patient the less likely a good prognosis. Other poor prognostic signs are pre-existing severe medical illness, clinically symptomatic vasospasm, delayed multiple cerebral infarction, hyperglycaemia, fever, anaemia and medical complications such as

Table 51.1 Clinical neurological classification of subarachnoid haemorrhage

GRADE	SIGNS
I	Conscious patient with or without meningism
II	Drowsy patient with no significant neurological deficit
III	Drowsy patient with neurological deficit – probably intracerebral clot
IV	Deteriorating patient with major neurological deficit (because of large intracerebral clot)
V	Moribund patient with extensor rigidity and failing vital centres

WFNS GRADE	*GCS*	*MOTOR DEFICIT*
I	15	Absent
II	14–13	Absent
III	14–13	Present
IV	12–7	Present or absent
V	3–6	Present or absent

WFNS = World Federation of Neurological Surgeons; GCS = Glasgow Coma Score.

pneumonia and sepsis. Anatomical risk factors may increase periprocedural risk of complications. On the other hand better outcomes seem to be associated with treatment in a high-volume centre.

In a recently published study on the natural history of cerebral aneurysms, the annual rupture rate was 0.95%. Risk factors that made it more likely to rupture were the location, MCA more likely than posterior communicating (PCOM) or anterior communicating (ACOM), size (the larger the more likely to rupture) and if the aneurysm has an irregular shape.[30]

COMPLICATIONS

The clinical status of the patient may be complicated by factors other than the physical effect of initial bleed, and factors such as acute hydrocephalus, early rebleeding, cerebral vasospasm, parenchymal haematoma, seizures and medical complications must be considered.

REBLEEDING

This may occur within the first few hours after admission and 15% of patients may deteriorate from their admission status. They may require urgent intubation and resuscitation, but not all rebleeds are unsurvivable and such deterioration should be treated. The chance of rebleeding is dependent on the site of the aneurysm, presence of clot, degree of vasospasm, age and sex of the patient. Although most studies quote an incidence for rebleeding of 4% in the first 24 hours, more recent studies suggest an incidence of 9–17% with most cases occurring within 6 hours. A few small studies have shown that antifibrinolytics such as tranexamic acid can be used, early, short term (<72 hours) in patients who do not have a pre-existing high risk for thrombotic events, for the prevention of rebleeding while awaiting securing of the aneurysm. It is an off-licence use of antifibrinolytics.[31]

ACUTE HYDROCEPHALUS

This may occur within the first 24 hours post ictus and is often characterised by a drop in the GCS, sluggish pupillary responses and bilateral downward deviation of the eyes ('sunset eyes'). If these signs occur, CT scan should be repeated and, if hydrocephalus is confirmed or there is a large amount of intraventricular blood, then a ventricular drain may be inserted. This is not without risk as it may provoke more bleeding and introduce infection. Only observational studies exist and these are contradictory so no firm recommendation can be made (**Fig. 51.4**).

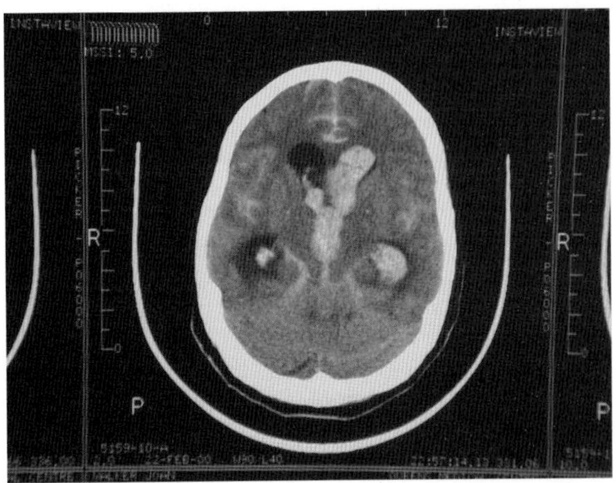

Figure 51.4 Spontaneous subarachnoid haemorrhage and secondary hydrocephalus.

DELAYED CEREBRAL ISCHAEMIA (DCI)

Vasospasm is the term used to describe narrowing of the cerebral blood vessels in response to SAH seen on angiography. It occurs in up to 70% of patients, but not all of these patients will have symptoms. Delayed cerebral ischaemia refers to the onset of focal neurological deficit, drop in GCS by 2 or more points, and/or cerebral infarction that occurs typically 4–12 days post SAH unrelated to aneurysm treatment or other causes of neurological deficit such as hydrocephalus, cerebral oedema or metabolic disorder.[32] Use of transcranial Doppler (TCD) to estimate middle cerebral artery blood velocity has shown that a velocity of more than 120 cm/s correlates with angiographic evidence of vasospasm. This technology allows diagnosis in the ICU and provides a means of monitoring the success of treatment to reduce DCI, which is undertaken to reduce the severity of delayed neurological deficit secondary to vasospasm. The problem is that not all patients who have angiographic vasospasm or high Doppler velocities have symptoms. If there is evidence of a depressed level of consciousness in the absence of rebleeding, hydrocephalus or metabolic disturbances, but there is evidence of DCI clinically, on TCD or angiogram, then it would seem appropriate to initiate treatment. If vasospasm occurs at the time of angiography or coiling, then intravascular vasodilators such as papaverine or nimodipine have been used. CTA is the imaging modality of choice unless intracerebral therapy is planned, then DSA is recommended as first-line imaging.

PARENCHYMAL HAEMATOMA

This may occur in up to 30% of SAH following aneurysm rupture and has a much worse prognosis than SAH alone. If there is mass effect with compressive symptoms then evacuation of haematoma and simultaneous clipping of the aneurysm may improve outcome.

MEDICAL COMPLICATIONS

During the placebo-controlled study of nicardipine in WFNS grade I and II SAH patients, there was a 40% incidence of at least one life-threatening medical complication in the placebo group.[33] The mortality due to medical complications was almost the same as that due to the combined effects of the initial bleed, rebleeds and

Table 51.2 Types of medical complication seen in patients with subarachnoid haemorrhage

MEDICAL COMPLICATION	INCIDENCE (%)
Arrhythmias	35
Liver dysfunction	24
Neurogenic pulmonary oedema	23
Pneumonia	22
ARDS and atelectasis	20
Renal dysfunction	5

ARDS=acute respiratory distress syndrome.

delayed cerebral ischaemia. The types of medical complication seen are shown in **Table 51.2**.

INVESTIGATIONS

The general investigations for stroke should be performed and early CT imaging is mandatory. Blood appears characteristically hyperdense on CT and the pattern of haemorrhage may enable localisation of the arterial territory involved. Very rarely, a false-positive diagnosis may be made if there is severe generalised oedema resulting in venous congestion in the subarachnoid space. Small amounts of blood may not be detected and the incidence of false-negative reports is around 2%.[34] It may be difficult to distinguish between post-traumatic SAH and primary aneurysmal SAH, which precipitates a fall in the level of consciousness that provokes an accident or fall. MR scanning is particularly effective for localising the bleed after 48 hours when extravasated blood is denatured, and provides a good signal on MRI.[34]

Lumbar puncture is still necessary in those patients where the suspicion of SAH is high despite a negative CT, or there is a need to exclude infection. There must be no raised intracranial pressure and at least 6 hours should have passed to give time for the blood in the CSF to lyse, enabling xanthochromia to develop.

Angiography via arterial catheterisation is still the most commonly used investigation for localising the aneurysm or other vascular abnormality prior to surgery. It is generally performed on patients who remain, or become, conscious after SAH. It is not without risk and aneurysms may rupture during the procedure and a meta-analysis has shown a complication rate of 1.8%. Other methods under investigation include CT angiography and MR angiography. Digital subtraction angiography (DSA) is the diagnostic tool of choice in cases where CTA is still inconclusive.[35]

Intracranial pressure monitoring is of limited use in SAH patients except in those where hydrocephalus or parenchymal haematoma is present and early detection of pressure increases may be the trigger for drainage or decompressive surgery.

Transcranial Doppler studies may be useful in detecting vasospasm or those patients in whom autoregulation is impaired.[36] The technique is dependent on there being a 'window' of thin temporal bone allowing insonation of the Doppler signal along the middle cerebral artery. It is very user-dependent and 15% of patients do not have an adequate bone window.

MANAGEMENT

The initial management of SAH is influenced by the grading, medical co-morbidity or complications, and the timing or need for surgery. Patients with decreased GCS may need early intubation and ventilation, simply for airway protection, whereas those with less severe symptoms require regular neurological observation, analgesia for headache and bed rest prior to investigation and surgery. Other management options are: stress ulcer prophylaxis, deep-vein thrombosis prophylaxis using compression stockings or boots, and seizure control with phenytoin or barbiturates. If the patient is sedated and ventilated, the use of an analysing cerebral function monitor should be considered to detect subclinical seizure activity.

Hyponatraemia is a common finding and adequate fluid therapy with normal saline is required with electrolyte levels maintained in the normal range. Occasionally, as in other types of brain injury, excessive natriuresis occurs and may result in hyponatraemic dehydration – cerebral salt-wasting syndrome (CSWS).[37] Its aetiology is not known, but some suggest increased levels of atrial natriuretic peptide. It usually occurs within the first week after insult and resolves spontaneously in 2–4 weeks. Failure to distinguish CSWS from the syndrome of inappropriate secretion of antidiuretic hormone (SIADH) could lead to inappropriate treatment by fluid restriction, which would have adverse effects on cerebral perfusion. Urine sodium concentrations are usually elevated in both SIADH and CSWS (>40 mmol/L) but urinary sodium excretion, urine sodium concentration [Na mmol/L]×urine volume [L/24 hours] is high in CSWS and normal in SIADH. If CSWS does not respond to fluid replacement with saline or is not self-limiting then fludrocortisone therapy may be useful.

BLOOD PRESSURE CONTROL

Elevation of blood pressure is commonly seen after SAH and there are no precise data on what constitutes an unacceptably high pressure that is likely to cause rebleeding. Equally, there are no precise data on a minimum level of pressure below which infarction is likely to occur, since this will depend on the patient's normal pressure, degree of cerebral oedema and the presence or absence of intact autoregulation. One observational study has demonstrated reduced rebleeding, but higher rates of infarction, in newly treated compared with untreated post-SAH hypertensive patients. Although there are no precise data on specific blood pressure controls, the AHA guidelines recommend that systolic blood pressure is kept <160 mmHg (21.3 kPa) or mean arterial pressure of <110 mmHg (14.6 kPa) in a person with an unsecured aneurysmal SAH.[38] Beta-adrenergic blockers or calcium antagonists are the most widely used agents, since drugs producing cerebral vasodilation may increase intracranial pressure. The choice is less important than the titratability of the drug, as the balance between increase of rebleed and cerebral perfusion needs to be maintained. If nimodipine causes severe hypotension, timing and dose need to be changed too (i.e. 30 mg 2-hourly instead of 60 mg 4-hourly). If nimodipine still remains a problem, consider omitting doses until more cardiovascularly stable.

DELAYED CEREBRAL ISCHAEMIA (DCI)

Angiographic demonstration of vasospasm may be seen in about 70% of SAH patients, but only about 30% develop cerebral symptoms related to vasospasm, hence the change of nomenclature. Transcranial Doppler-derived flow velocities in the middle cerebral arteries of more than 120 cm/s are accurate in predicting ischaemia. Symptoms tend to occur between 4 and 14 days post bleed, which is the period when cerebral blood flow is decreased after SAH.

PREVENTION

One method of pre-empting vasospasm is the prescription of oral nimodipine at 60 mg given 4-hourly for 21 days, which has been shown to achieve a reduction in the risk of ischaemic stroke of 34%.[39] Intravenous nimodipine should be used in the patients who are not absorbing, but it must be titrated against blood pressure to avoid hypotension. Other calcium antagonists, notably nicardipine and the experimental drug AT877, reduce vasospasm but do not improve outcome.

There have been some studies looking at statins to prevent DCI. These have been small trials but have shown promising results. A large randomised control trial (STASH) is under way to give us definitive answers on statins. Statins should at least be considered in the prevention of DCI and definitely continued if they were prescribed pre-event.[38]

Routine hypermagnesaemia for the prevention of DCI is not recommended, but hypomagnesaemia should be prevented. The 2012 MASH 2 trial showed no improvement in clinical outcome following routine administration of intravenous magnesium.

TREATMENT

Low cerebral blood flow is known to worsen outcome and this resulted in the development of prophylactic hypertensive hypervolaemic haemodilution – so-called triple-H therapy.[40] As originally described, the therapy involved the use of fluid loading to achieve haemodilution and vasopressor therapy to increase cerebral blood flow, and was combined with surgery within 24 hours if possible. The therapy was continued for 21 days and all patients remained neurologically stable or improved as a result, apparently, of the absence of vasospasm. Very few centres use the strict protocol as originally described, but fluid loading rather than fluid restriction is the norm and inotropes or vasopressors are used subsequently if neurological function decreases. Despite its widespread use, there remains no prospective randomised trial that demonstrates its utility. The focus now is on normovolaemia and, if indicated and blood pressure not already raised, hypertension is induced with vasopressors. This needs to be done in a stepwise fashion with assessment of neurological function at each step.[38] Cerebral angioplasty or direct intracerebral vasodilators should be considered if induced hypertension is not reversing the DCI symptoms.[38] Where symptoms develop it is important to exclude other causes such as rebleeding, hydrocephalus or metabolic disorder. Poor-grade SAH patients who are sedated or have low GCS are clinically difficult to assess; multimodal monitoring is recommended to look for deterioration.[38]

SEIZURES

Seizure occurs in up to 26% of SAH sufferers. The evidence for prophylactic use of anticonvulsants is poor and not recommended. Some prognostic indicators for the development of seizures have been identified: increased intracerebral blood, poor-grade SAH, rebleeding infarction and MCA aneurysm. Patients should be observed for seizure activity and treated appropriately. A patient with poor-grade SAH who is not improving or is deteriorating neurologically, from an unknown cause, should have continuous EEG monitoring.[38]

SURGERY

Clipping of the aneurysm is the surgical treatment of choice, with wrapping, proximal ligation or bypass grafting being used if the aneurysm is inaccessible to Yasargil clipping. The timing of surgery remains debatable. Early surgery, within 3 days of the bleed, has the advantage of fewer deaths occurring from rebleeding but is technically difficult owing to the friability of associated tissues. Delayed surgery, around 10–12 days post bleed, gives better operating conditions but allows some patients to suffer a rebleed. Recommendations by the AHA are to secure the aneurysm as early as is possible. Large intracerebral haematomas associated with the SAH and middle cerebral artery aneurysms should be strongly considered for surgery. There is no good level one evidence for the use of induced hypertension or hypothermia during clipping, but in certain patients it could be considered. What is clear is that hypotension and hyperglycaemia should be avoided.[38]

ENDOVASCULAR COILING

The development of detachable microcoils made of platinum by Guglielmi in 1992 has resulted in endovascular embolisation of aneurysms or AVMs by interventional radiology.[41] A microcatheter is passed from the femoral artery to the cerebral aneurysm and the coils positioned sequentially in the lumen of saccular aneurysms to occlude it. Rupture of the aneurysm or adjacent vessel occlusion, causing ischaemia, is the most frequent complication. The International Subarachnoid Aneurysm Trial (ISAT) of neurosurgical clipping versus endovascular coiling in 2143 patients with ruptured intracranial aneurysms – a randomised comparison of effects on survival, dependency, seizures, rebleeding, subgroups and aneurysm occlusion – has come down in favour of coiling rather than open surgical technique at 1-year follow-up. In patients with ruptured intracranial aneurysms suitable for both treatments, endovascular coiling is more likely to result in independent survival at 1 year than neurosurgical clipping; the survival benefit continues for at least 7 years. The risk of late rebleeding is low, but is more common after endovascular coiling than after neurosurgical clipping.[42] Additional complications of coiling include rupture during catheter placement in the aneurysm, coil embolisation and vasospasm. Not all aneurysms, particularly those with wide necks, multiple filling vessels or giant aneurysms, are suitable for coiling. Aneurysms that are amenable to either surgery or coiling should be coiled; if patients are elderly (>70 years) or have poor-grade SAH then coiling is preferred. Stenting of acute SAH carries a worse prognosis.[38]

NEUROPROTECTIVE THERAPY

There has been a great deal of research on the cellular and biochemical responses to brain injury and several drugs have been investigated to try to reduce mortality in SAH. The 21-amino steroid tirilazad, nicaraven and ebselen, all free-radical scavengers, have been the most widely investigated. None has been shown to improve outcome consistently in all types of patient with SAH.

THERAPY OF MEDICAL COMPLICATIONS

This is obviously specific to the type of complication. Pneumonia may require continuous positive-airways pressure or ventilatory support together with directed antimicrobial therapy, acute respiratory distress syndrome requires lung-protective/recruitment ventilatory strategies, and renal failure necessitates an appropriate means of renal replacement therapy. Arrhythmias require correction of trigger factors such as hypovolaemia and electrolyte or acid–base disturbances prior to the appropriate antiarrhythmic drug or DC cardioversion. Cardiac function should be evaluated in patients with cardiovascular deterioration, by means of serial enzymes and echocardiography. Cardiac output monitoring should be considered. Neurogenic pulmonary oedema may be associated with severe cardiogenic shock, which may require inotropic support or even temporary intra-aortic balloon counterpulsation. The cardiogenic shock is reversible and patients can make a good recovery despite the need for aggressive support.[43]

Hyper- and hyponatraemia are frequently seen, with hyponatraemia occurring in up to 30% of cases and implicated in the development of DCI. The aim is for normovolaemia; if it cannot be achieved because of a persistent negative fluid balance as a result of cerebral salt-wasting syndrome, then fludrocortisone should be considered. Hyponatraemia should be corrected by no more than 0.5 mmol/L per hour with a maximum of 8 mmol/L per day (if it is chronic, i.e. of more than 48 hours' duration) during which 4-hourly sodium levels should be taken. This may be achieved by using intravenous fluid that has more sodium than the serum concentration of the patient. In patients who are resistant to vasopressors, hypothalamic dysfunction should be considered and hydrocortisone should be administered, but no more than 300 mg per day.

Blood glucose should be kept at 4.4–11.1 mmol/L (80–200 mg/dL), as higher and lower levels of blood glucose has been shown to be detrimental to outcome.

Fever should be controlled by antipyretics as first line, especially when DCI is suspected. Cooling devices should be considered if first-line antipyretics have failed, but care should be taken to monitor for pressure ulcers and venous thrombotic events. Shivering needs to be addressed, as this will be counterproductive to therapy by increasing oxygen consumption.

Deep-vein thrombosis prophylaxis should be instituted as soon as possible in the form of graduated compression devices; heparin (unfractionated or low-molecular weight) should be started 24 hours after securing of the aneurysm.

Anaemia should be minimised by limiting the amount of blood taken for blood test. A transfusion trigger of 8–10 g/dL has been recommended.

 Access the complete references list online at http://www.expertconsult.com

5. Redekop GJ. Extracranial carotid and vertebral artery dissection: a review. Can J Neurol Sci 2008;35(2):146–52.
9. Bosel J, Schller P, Hacke W, et al. Benefits of early tracheostomy in ventilated stroke patients? Current evidence and study protocol of the randomised pilot trial SETPOINT (Stroke-related Early Tracheostomy vs. Prolonged Orotracheal Intubation in Neurocritical care Trial). Int J Stroke 2012;7:173–82.
18. Kawanishi M, Kawai N, Tamiya T. Mechanical thrombectomy for the acute ischaemic stroke using the Penumbra system. Proceedings of the 2012

International Conference on Complex Medica Engineering 2012;388–91. Online. Available: http://ieeexplore.ieee.org/xpl/.

21. Wartenberg KE. Malignant middle cerebral artery infarction. Curr Opin Crit Care 2012;18:152–63.
26. Morgenstern LB, Hemphill JC, Anderson C, et al. Guidelines for the management of spontaneous intracerebral hemorrhage: a guideline for healthcare professionals from the American Heart Association/American Stroke Association. Stroke 2012;41:2108–29.
27. Diringer MN, Bleck TP, Hemphill JC, et al. Critical care management of patients following aneurysmal subarachnoid hemorrhage: recommendations from the Neurocritical Care Society's Multidisciplinary Consensus Conference. Neurocritical Care 2011;15:211–40.
32. Washington CW, Zipfel GJ. Detection and monitoring of vasospasm and delayed cerebral ischaemia: a review and assessment of the literature. Neurocrit Care 2011;15:312–17.
38. Connolly Jr ES, Rabinstein AA, Ricardo Carhuapoma J, et al. Guidelines for the management of aneurysmal subarachnoid hemorrhage. A guideline for healthcare professionals from the American Heart Association/American Stroke Association. Stroke 2012;43:1711–37.
44. Anderson CS, Heeley E, Huang Y, et al. Rapid blood-pressure lowering in patients with acute intracerebral hemorrhage. N Engl J Med 2013. DOI: 10.1056/NEJMoa1214609.

52

Cerebral protection

Victoria Heaviside and Michelle Hayes

The cerebral circulation is arguably the most important and most vulnerable in the body. Circulatory impairment or arrest for only a few minutes can cause neuronal death. Cerebral protection is the application of therapeutic interventions following a primary brain injury, in the hope of preventing secondary injury and improving neurological outcome. It has been incorporated into the prophylaxis, treatment and management of brain injury irrespective of aetiology. A complete review is beyond the scope of this chapter, but an understanding of the current approaches to cerebral protection is certainly helpful in the management of cerebral insults.

NORMAL BRAIN PHYSIOLOGY

The brain has high energy requirements, utilising approximately 3–5 mL O_2/min per 100 g tissue (45–75 mL O_2/min per 1500 g brain) and 5 mg glucose/min per 100 g tissue (75 mg glucose/min per 1500 g brain). It has little ability to store precursors of metabolism and thus depends on a constant supply of nutrients from the blood.

With a cerebral blood flow (CBF) of 50 mL/min per 100 g tissue (750 mL/min per 1500 g brain) and a normal oxygen content of 20 mL O_2/100 mL blood, the brain receives approximately 150 mL O_2/min per 1500 g brain, or 2–3 times the amount needed for normal brain activity.

At the same CBF of 50 mL/min per 100 g tissue and a blood glucose concentration of 5.5 mmol/l (100 mg/100 mL blood), there is 50 mg/min per 100 g tissue (750 mg/min per 1500 g brain) delivery of glucose. Glucose extraction by the brain, at 5 mg/min per 100 g brain tissue, is a tenth of that delivered; minimal compared with oxygen.

Although cerebral injury has many aetiologies, the mechanisms of injury are thought to be few. The most common is lack of the essential nutrients, oxygen and glucose, either separately with preserved blood flow (i.e. hypoxia or hypoglycaemia), or together, because of reduced or absent perfusion (i.e. ischaemia or infarction). A reduction in these energy precursors is a major contributor in the mechanism of brain injury.

NATURAL PROTECTIVE MECHANISMS

The importance of the brain is highlighted by the presence of integral protective mechanisms that aim to prevent cerebral ischaemia.

COLLATERAL BLOOD SUPPLY

An elaborate vascular architecture is designed to ensure adequate CBF. The anterior cerebral circulation is provided by bilateral internal carotid arteries as they each divide into anterior and middle cerebral arteries. They provide approximately 70% of the cerebral circulation and supply the anterior cerebrum (frontal, parietal and temporal lobes) and anterior diencephalon (basal ganglia and hypothalamus). The remaining 30% of the cerebral circulation is provided posteriorly by the vertebrobasilar system, which runs the length of the posterior fossa, supplying the brainstem, cerebellum, posterior portion of the cerebrum (occipital lobes) and diencephalon (thalamus). These two circulations are joined by communicating arteries, ultimately forming the circle of Willis (**Fig. 52.1**). This joining of the anterior and posterior circulations at the base of the brain is the major component of cerebral vasculature in humans. Between these arterial distributions are watershed zones fed by leptomeningeal connections. In addition, persistent fetal arteries can infrequently provide collateral routes between the anterior and posterior arterial systems in the brain.

CEREBRAL BLOOD FLOW

CEREBRAL PERFUSION PRESSURE

The amount of blood delivered to the brain is highly regulated and is determined by several factors. CBF is determined in part by the perfusion pressure across the brain, called cerebral perfusion pressure (CPP). CPP is the difference between the arterial pressure in the feeding arteries as they enter the subarachnoid space and the pressure in the draining veins before they enter the major dural sinuses. These pressures are difficult to measure, thus CPP is derived from the difference between the systemic mean arterial pressure (MAP)

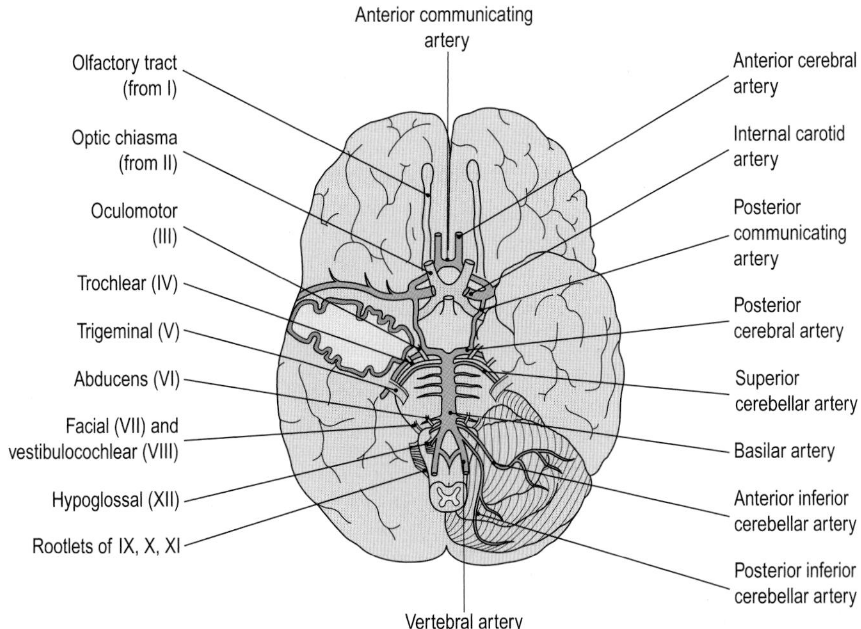

Figure 52.1 Circle of Willis.

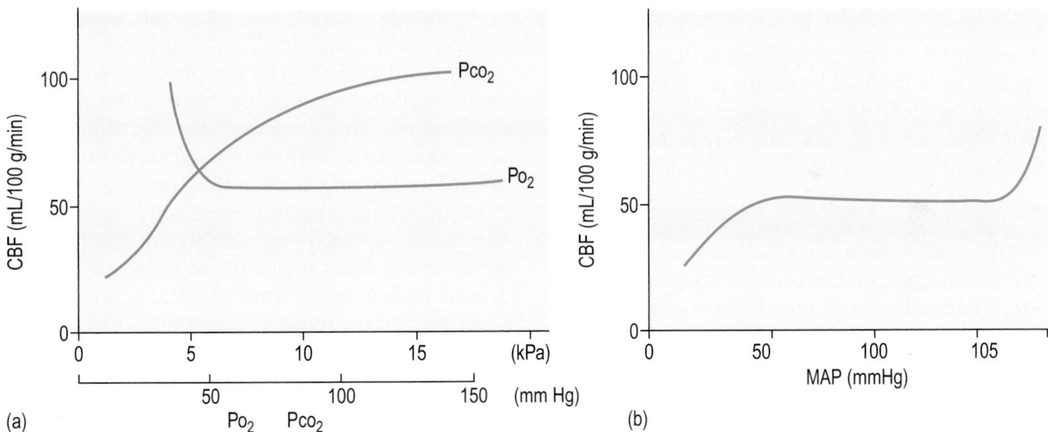

Figure 52.2 (a) The relationship between the partial pressure of oxygen (P_{O_2}) and carbon dioxide (P_{CO_2}) and cerebral blood flow (CBF). (b) The relationship between mean arterial pressure (MAP) and cerebral blood flow under normal circumstances, illustrating the range of autoregulation.

and the intracranial pressure (ICP) (an estimate of tissue pressure).

The cerebral vessels change diameter inversely with changing perfusion pressure. As CPP rises, the vessels constrict and as CPP falls the vessels dilate, such that blood flow is kept constant over a wide range of CPP (**Fig. 52.2a**). This 'autoregulated' pressure is thought to be controlled by local myogenic responses of the vessel wall to changes in intra-arterial pressure. At pressures above and below this range of 6.7–20 kPa (50–150 mmHg), cerebral perfusion becomes pressure-passive and increases or decreases in direct proportion to changes in CPP. The autoregulatory range varies with age, being shifted to the left in newborns and to the right in those with chronic hypertension. The latter is important to remember to avoid overtreating systolic blood pressure in such patients and thus incur the risk of cerebral ischaemia at the lower limits of autoregulation. Alternatively, cerebral perfusion above normal can be caused by acute hypertension overcoming the upper limits of autoregulation. This may lead to cerebral oedema secondary to increased hydrostatic pressures (hypertensive encephalopathy) and potentially lead to seizures or cerebral haemorrhage.

Pa_{O_2} AND Pa_{CO_2} EFFECTS

Oxygen and carbon dioxide manipulate CBF through an influence on the local metabolic milieu. The arterial content or partial pressure of oxygen in the normal or hyperoxic range causes very little change in CBF. This changes with the onset of hypoxaemia (Pa_{O_2} 60 mmHg or 8 kPa), where there is a prompt increase in CBF proportional to the decrease in blood oxygen content, in order to maintain oxygen delivery constant (Fig. 52.2b).

There is also a direct relationship between CBF and Pa_{CO_2}, such that CBF increases with increasing Pa_{CO_2} (Fig. 52.2b). This probably represents the need of the brain to maintain a homeostatic pH by removing metabolic breakdown products more efficiently through increased blood flow. Unlike the response to oxygen, the CBF response to changes in Pa_{CO_2} is dramatic in the physiological range, such that for every 0.13 kPa (1.0 mmHg) change in Pa_{CO_2} there is a 1–2 mL/min per 100 g tissue change in CBF. Therefore, an increase in Pa_{CO_2} to 10.6 kPa (80 mmHg) will increase CBF to approximately 100 mL/min per 100 g and a decrease in Pa_{CO_2} to 2.7 kPa (20 mmHg) will decrease CBF to 25 mL/min per 100 g. Thus:

- doubling Pa_{CO_2} doubles CBF
- halving Pa_{CO_2} halves CBF within this range.

Understanding this basic physiology will make treatment logical (see below), as increases in CBF often lead to increases in cerebral blood volume, which in turn can increase ICP, a common cause of cerebral ischaemia and a significant predictor in patient outcome.

CEREBRAL INJURY

Vascular insufficiency or disruption, trauma, tumour, infection, inflammation and metabolic and nutritional derangement can all cause damage. Whatever the cause, the mechanism of injury is usually hypoxic and/or ischaemic injury. Therefore, it is possible to have high flow but no oxygen or, alternatively, no flow but plenty of oxygen. At the cellular level the consequence is the same.

The protective mechanisms that are in place to increase CBF with the generous oversupply of nutrients under normal conditions, allow for sufficient blood flow, oxygen delivery and supply of nutrients in milder injurious cases. However, in situations of trauma and developing pathology such as cerebrovascular disease restricting perfusion, or intracranial masses causing oedema, alterations in blood flow, hypoxia and or ischaemic injury will occur. This in turn can disturb systemic circulatory homeostasis, cause hypotension and worsen the ischaemic injury further. Thus hypoxic and ischaemic injury may be considered synonymous, be there aetiological differences between them. A more important distinction to be made is that between global and focal hypoxic or ischaemic insults.

GLOBAL HYPOXIC/ISCHAEMIC INSULTS

These types of insult are caused by hypoxaemia and cardiovascular insufficiency or arrest, respectively. These are usually sudden, short and severe. If there is to be recovery, prompt return of oxygen delivery and spontaneous circulation are necessary. The recovery may be variable, depending on the severity and duration of the insult and the selective vulnerability of the cell types involved. Different mechanisms are responsible for reversible loss of cellular function and for irreversible cell death and there are also differences between the mechanisms that cause death of neurons, glia and endothelial cells. After 4–6 minutes of complete global ischaemia, there are signs of permanent histological damage in selective neuronal populations and the beginnings of neurological deficits in survivors. Outcome worsens significantly after 15 minutes of global ischaemia.[1]

FOCAL HYPOXIC/ISCHAEMIC INSULTS

These insults often occur suddenly but are usually of more prolonged duration. Only a subtotal of the brain is affected and the injury may be less severe if the surrounding brain is preserved by collateral blood supply.

The area of the focal ischaemia supplied by end-arteries will result in cell death unless reperfusion is established rapidly. The periphery of an infarcted area is the ischaemic penumbra. Here, CBF is greater than at the infarcted core, but less than in the normal tissue around it. Animal studies suggest that the time course for infarction and irreversible damage to brain from a focal hypoxic/ischaemic event is around 30–60 minutes. The focus of therapeutic intervention is the penumbral area, on the basis that if blood flow can be normalised in this region, or pharmacological agents can be delivered despite the reduced blood flow, there is a potential for recovery. Conversely, failure to maintain this area will result in a coalescing of the penumbra into the infarcted area, as the ischaemic stimulus continues.

It is likely that the ongoing ischaemic penumbral areas of a focal insult and transient whole-brain ischaemia (e.g. during early cardiac arrest, low-flow cardiopulmonary resuscitation (CPR) or elevated ICP states) are subject to similar pathophysiological processes. As pretreatment is usually impossible, prevention and treatment of the secondary insult is the focus in neuroprotection and tissue salvage strategies.

BRAIN ISCHAEMIC AND INFARCTION PROCESSES

Changes in normal physiology begin to occur when blood flow is reduced.

- At CBF below 50 mL/min per 100 g neurological function is impaired and there is slowing of the electroencephalogram (EEG).

- A CBF of 15–25 mL/min per 100 g results in loss of electrical activity.
- A CBF between 10 and 15 mL/min per 100 g can maintain adenosine triphosphate (ATP) levels sufficiently to support ionic pump function for a time, despite the lack of electrical activity and normal neurological function.
- At a CBF of 10 mL/min per 100 g membrane failure occurs, due to a critical loss of ATP, which causes ionic imbalance between the cell and the extracellular milieu. If prolonged or worsened, CBF at this level will lead to permanent neurological impairment as a result of cell death.

EFFECTS OF ISCHAEMIA

In the non-fasting state, glucose is metabolised to ATP via oxidative phosphorylation. ATP is needed for homeostasis and cellular activities such as mitochondrial expression, protein synthesis, ionic gradient maintenance, cell membrane stability and CO_2 elimination. Ischaemia results in reduced availability of oxygen and glucose to support aerobic production of ATP. Levels of ATP are depleted within 2–3 minutes of complete ischaemia (animal studies). There is little brain storage of either glucose or oxygen, and ATP production during ischaemia relies on anaerobic glycolysis for as long as stores last. This results in continued ATP use, but suboptimal production of ATP to fuel aerobic metabolism, so a lactic acidosis develops.

Loss of ATP causes failure of membrane ionic pump function, the beginnings of cytotoxic oedema and a cascade of events, which result in eventual cell death:

- potassium efflux with cell membrane depolarisation, ion channel opening and the release of excitatory amino acid (EAA) neurotransmitters (glutamate, aspartate and others)
- EAA damage by further depolarisation of neighbouring and distal unaffected cells
- sodium and chloride influx via kainate (K) and quisqualate (Q) receptors (with worsening intracellular oedema)
- sodium and calcium influx via *N*-methyl-D-aspartate (NMDA) receptors
- conversion of phosphorylases, uncoupling of oxidative phosphorylation, activation of proteases, degradation of cystosolic protein and stimulation of lipases. Lipases liberate arachidonic acid and other free fatty acids that cause tissue damage via production of oxygen radicals and prostaglandins.

Other effects within the cell influence DNA and RNA production, hence inhibiting protein production. This may explain why cellular and clinical recovery is partial, even with restoration of ionic equilibrium and near-normal ATP levels after successful reperfusion. Necrosis is thought to occur in the core of the cerebral infarct following acute vascular occlusion, with further neurodegeneration occurring more slowly in the penumbra, by apoptosis or release of various immunological mediators.[2]

EXTRACELLULAR EFFECTS

Leucocytes are thought to be major contributors to reperfusion injury in that:

- they may plug up small capillaries under conditions of low blood flow and prevent reflow in certain areas, thus hindering restoration of perfusion
- they may enhance production of oxygen radicals and begin a cascade of inflammatory mediators, which may potentiate cell destruction in injured tissue.

These mechanisms result in tissue oedema, which may affect the core lesion by narrowing blood vessels and worsening chances of reperfusion. Local mechanical compression of tissue or its blood supply can cause deterioration in neighbouring tissue. The alteration in volume is of extreme importance in the adult brain because the cranial vault is non-distensible, preventing accommodation to an expanding lesion. This will impede CBF both locally and globally.

Hypoxic/ischaemic insults are rarely predictable, so that the process is usually well established when clinicians intervene. It is therefore highly likely that the injury will be only partially remediable.

MANAGEMENT

In neurological injury, the initial aims are to provide basic support. Assessment of the airway and respiration are the first priority, closely followed by optimisation of the circulation.

In cases of head trauma, it is very important to prevent secondary brain injury. Reviews of intensive care practice have resulted in recommendations for treatment in this group of patients.[3] These involve:

- institution of systemic and neurological monitoring
- early treatment of hypoxia, hypotension, hyperthermia, hyperglycaemia and intracranial hypertension
- maintenance of CPP.

Following stroke, it is also important to optimise homeostasis and address any extreme hypertension, hyperglycaemia, hyperthermia and intracranial hypertension, as these are independent factors of a poor prognosis.

HYPOXIA

This is defined as O_2 saturation <90% or a P_{O_2} <8 kPa. Irrespective of aetiology, hypoxia occurs when impaired consciousness and loss of airway reflexes cause partial or complete airway obstruction, hypoventilation, aspiration pneumonia or atelectasis.

In mechanically ventilated patients with traumatic brain injury, settings should aim to achieve a $P_{O_2} \geq 10$ kPa and a P_{CO_2} of 4.5–5.0 kPa. It has been suggested that high PEEP≥15 cmH_2O may decrease cerebral venous drainage by increasing intrathoracic pressure, thus increasing cerebral blood volume and intracranial pressure.[3] In the brain-injured patient with ALI/ARDS these requirements pose a ventilatory challenge as they tend against those employed for lung protection.

In patients who have had an acute stroke oxygen saturations should be kept greater than or equal to 92%.[4] In stroke patients who require intubation either for decreased GCS or hypoxia, prognosis is poor with about 50% being dead within 30 days of the clinical event.[5]

There is currently no evidence for the use of hyperbaric oxygen in the treatment of stroke or traumatic brain injury,[6,7] but there is continuing interest in the early application of normobaric hyperoxia treatment in these two conditions as guided by cerebral tissue oxygen monitors.[8]

BLOOD PRESSURE CONTROL

Fluctuating haemodynamics occur in the majority of patients following an acute brain injury. The therapeutic type, timing and extent of intervention to correct this instability are still being debated, but there appears to be growing evidence that the aetiology of the brain injury should be clarified prior to initiating any treatment.

In stroke patients the mechanism and effects of blood pressure elevation are not well understood. Most experts would not advocate antihypertensive treatment in the acute phase unless the blood pressure is particularly high. Currently hypertension (systolic blood pressure >180 mmHg (24 kPa) or diastolic blood pressure >110 mmHg (14.6 kPa)) is a contraindication to thrombolysis, based on the trials involving rtPA in which the blood pressure was lowered prior to treatment.[9,10]

The International Stroke Trial involving patients with ischaemic stroke found that systolic blood pressures >200 mmHg (26.6 kPa) and <120 mmHg (16 kPa) were associated with poor clinical outcome, systolic blood pressures between 140 and 160 mmHg (18.6–21.3 kPa) were associated with the best outcome and reducing the systolic blood pressure of patients who were in this range was associated with a 17.9% increase in mortality for every 10 mmHg below 150 mmHg (20 kPa).[11]

Conversely, in haemorrhagic stroke, The Intensive Blood Pressure Reduction in Acute Intracerebral Haemorrhage Trial (INTERACT) suggested early blood pressure reduction within 6 hours of diagnostic imaging. Patients whose systolic blood pressure was reduced to 140 mmHg (18.6 kPa) compared with a standard group of 180 mmHg (24 kPa) showed a reduction in haematoma growth over the subsequent 72 hours.[12] Phase III of this trial, INTERACT 2 aims to look at the long-term functional benefits of this intervention.

Following traumatic brain injury hypotension (systolic blood pressure <90 mmHg (12 kPa)) is more common and significantly associated with increased mortality.[3] It is often caused by cardiogenic, hypovolaemic or neurogenic shock from other injuries rather than the brain injury itself. Fluid and blood product resuscitation should be employed along with vasopressors if appropriate and guided by systemic invasive monitoring. Hypertension in traumatic brain injury should be treated cautiously. Secondary brain injury hypertension may increase ICP through vasogenic cerebral oedema but it may also be a physiological response to poor cerebral perfusion. Rapid reduction of blood pressure may worsen cerebral ischaemia and treatment of high systolic blood pressure (>180 mmHg (24 kPa)) should not occur until another causes have been excluded and neurospecific monitoring employed.[3]

HYPERGLYCAEMIA

Hyperglycaemia has been associated with increased mortality and reduced functional outcome irrespective of brain injury aetiology or a diabetic history.[13] Proposed explanations for this are:

- potential direct hyperglycaemic toxicity to the ischaemic brain
- decreased levels of insulin and its peripheral uptake thus increasing cerebral glucose availability and potential impairment of endothelial-dependent vasodilatation
- possible dysglycaemia, which is associated with vascular disease and endothelial dysfunction, both of which may exacerbate ischaemic damage at the time of stroke
- increased risk of a hypercoagulable state, with decreased plasma fibrinolytic activity, which may delay reperfusion and increase haemorrhagic infarct conversion in tissue plasminogen activator-treated patients.[14]

For these reasons many studies have investigated the effects of tight glucose control in stroke and traumatic brain injury, unfortunately with disappointing results.

The Cochrane review, 'Insulin for glycaemic control in acute stroke' compared tight and 'standard' glucose control employed within 24 hours of the stroke, in terms of death and dependency. There was no difference between the groups but patients in the intervention group experienced significantly more symptomatic and asymptomatic hypoglycaemic episodes.[15] The INSULINFARCT trial compared intravenous with subcutaneous insulin treatment on post-stroke glycaemic control and MRI-imaged cerebral infarct size. Again there was no difference in functionality, death or serious adverse events between the two groups. There was an association in the intravenous insulin group with increased infarct size.[16] Thus there is no evidence for intensive insulin therapy in hyperacute ischaemic stroke.

There are studies, albeit with small numbers of patients, using cerebral microdialysis to assess cerebral metabolism, which infer that tight glucose control reduces extracellular cerebral glucose availability, causes a cerebral metabolic crisis and is associated with increased mortality.[17,18]

TEMPERATURE CONTROL

An increased temperature increases cerebral metabolism, oxygen requirements, CBF and ICP. Hyperpyrexia following acute stroke adversely influences stroke severity, infarct size, functional outcome and mortality.[19] A raised temperature should, therefore, be treated aggressively using ice packs, cooling blankets, or intravascular cooling systems if available. Any evidence of infection should be identified early and treated with appropriate antibiotics.

Potential mechanisms by which hyperthermia worsens cerebral ischaemia may include:

- neurotransmitter and oxygen free radical production
- blood–brain barrier failure
- damaging depolarisations in the ischaemic penumbra
- impaired recovery of energy metabolism
- cytoskeletal proteolysis.[20]

Hypothermia has been known for years to offer protection. Classically the primary neuroprotective effect of hypothermia has been attributed to reduction in cerebral metabolic rate and hence oxygen consumption with improved glucose utilisation. Animal models have demonstrated the beneficial effects of hypothermia on secondary injury, namely reduced cerebral oedema, reduced ischaemia and reperfusion injuries, decreased infarct size, decreased excitatory neurotransmitters, less acidaemia and preservation of the blood–brain barrier vascular integrity.[21,22] Complications of hypothermia include hypotension, pneumonia, electrolyte derangement, cardiac arrythmias and coagulopathy.

In contrast to preventing hyperthermia, the use of induced hypothermia is more complex. It has been used extensively in cardiac surgery to provide optimal operating conditions and protection against organ ischaemia. Induced hypothermia (28–30°C) for coronary artery bypass is commonplace and deep hypothermia (<20°C) allows prolonged circulatory arrest for complex surgical procedures such as aortic arch repairs.

Two randomised clinical trials of induced hypothermia after witnessed out-of-hospital ventricular fibrillation cardiac arrest demonstrated improved survival and neurological outcome after 12 or 24 hours of hypothermia at 32–34°C (see online Appendix 9).[23,24] This has led to recommendations by the International Liaison Committee on Resuscitation.[25]

The benefits of therapeutic hypothermia in traumatic brain injury and ischaemic stroke are unproven. Therapeutic hypothermia for treatment of TBI was first used in 1943 without success. There have been many studies, meta-analyses and reviews that have looked at the effects of induced moderate hypothermia (above 30°C) on the outcome of patients with TBI in the last 20 years. Although the majority of studies have shown a decrease in ICP with cooling, there haven't been any proven benefits on outcome. The results have been inconclusive because of variations in methodology, patient numbers and demographics, centre cooling experience and adjuvant treatments to name but a few.[26,27] The European Society of Intensive Care Medicine study of therapeutic hypothermia (32–35°C) for ICP reduction after traumatic brain injury (EUROTHERM3235Trial) is currently recruiting. Its primary objective is to look at the effects of hypothermia on patient outcome at 6 months using the extended Glasgow Outcome Score (GOSE) questionnaire.[28]

Although therapeutic hypothermia is well established to improve survival and neurological outcome in global cerebral ischaemia following cardiac arrest, its benefits in focal cerebral ischaemia are not yet established. Clinical trials have studied pharmacological (antipyretic and anti-inflammatory agents) and physical ways of inducing hypothermia. Pharmacological ways of reducing temperature have been disappointing with no clinical benefit. Physical methods involve either surface or intravascular cooling. Surface cooling is often easier to apply but target temperature takes longer to reach (peripheral vasoconstriction) and prevention of shivering may require sedation and paralysis. Intravascular cooling is more effective, allows for surface warming thus reducing shivering but its invasive nature carries risks.[22] The rate of reaching target temperature, the duration of hypothermia and the rate of rewarming have been investigated in several trials. From clinical trials and experimental work done so far, early therapeutic hypothermia for 24–72 hours followed by slow rewarming appears to be the best combination for a promising neurological outcome.[22] EUROHYP-1 is a major phase III clinical trial and will be launched imminently.

REVASCULARISATION

Aims of treatment for focal cerebral ischaemia are:

- Start treatment as early as possible.
- Increase local CBF (fibrinolysis).
- Try to ameliorate ischaemic cascade (neuroprotection).

Ischaemic neuronal degeneration follows the onset of perfusion failure so that interventional therapy must begin immediately. Diagnostic imaging is required before using thrombolytic agents. For acute ischaemic stroke the National Institute of Neurological Disorders and Stroke (NINDS study) suggested efficacy if intravenous thrombolytic therapy is initiated within the first

3 hours of stroke symptoms (using recombinant tissue plasminogen activator).[29] In fact subgroup analysis within the study showed improved outcome the earlier the thrombolysis was given.

Current issues in implementing this treatment include:

- diagnosis, including imaging within this timeframe
- the potential risks of thrombolysis and the need for specialist stroke services for monitoring and reimaging as necessary
- accurately selecting patients eligible for thrombolysis.

'TRIPLE H' THERAPY

Hypervolaemic haemodilution and deliberate hypertension or 'triple H' therapy has been an accepted but controversial intervention to prevent delayed cerebral ischaemia secondary to vasospasm following subarachnoid haemorrhage. Cerebral vasospasm usually develops from about 72 hours after the primary insult and peaks over the subsequent 2 weeks before resolving spontaneously at days 21–28. As the efficacy of 'triple H' therapy is still unproven and is not without its complications there has been a therapeutic shift towards euvolaemia and induced hypertension.[30,31]

INTRACRANIAL PRESSURE

Raised ICP can cause global ischaemia. Treating ICP requires knowledge of the three compartments contributing to ICP within a fixed cranium:

- blood
- relatively non-compliant brain tissue
- cerebrospinal fluid (CSF).

The relationship between ICP and intracranial volume is described by a non-linear pressure–volume curve. At lower intracranial volumes the ICP remains low and reasonably constant. Any increases in intracranial volume are compensated for by decreases in intracerebral blood or CSF volume. If greater intracranial volumes persist, this compensation is lost and ICP rises considerably, despite relatively small increases in intracerebral blood volume. Eventually at high levels of ICP cerebrovascular responses are lost, ICP equals MAP and CPP is very low.

To maintain adequate cerebral perfusion, treatment should be targeted at ensuring an adequate perfusion pressure and a reduction in ICP. MAP should be raised to a level at or above the usual pressure for that patient, within a patient-specific zone of pressure autoregulation. If the majority of the vasculature is autoregulating, raising the blood pressure may decrease vascular diameter and reduce blood volume within the cranium. If the cause of the raised ICP cannot be corrected (e.g. blood clot or brain tumour), then the focus should be to prevent secondary injury around the lesion. An increased ICP can cause further ischaemia, and a reduction in ICP may facilitate adequate perfusion to areas at risk. Whenever possible, the offending compartment should be treated promptly (e.g. tumour removal, blood evacuation, drainage of hydrocephalus and, on occasion, craniectomy). If this is not advisable, reducing the relative volumes of other compartments may improve compliance overall and reduce the ICP.

MONITORING OF ICP (FIG. 52.3)

ICP-monitoring devices have been ranked by the Brain Trauma Foundation[32] on their accuracy, stability and ability to drain CSF. Intraventricular and intraparenchymal catheter tip microtransducer catheters are the most commonly used. Subdural, subarachnoid and epidural devices are now rarely used.

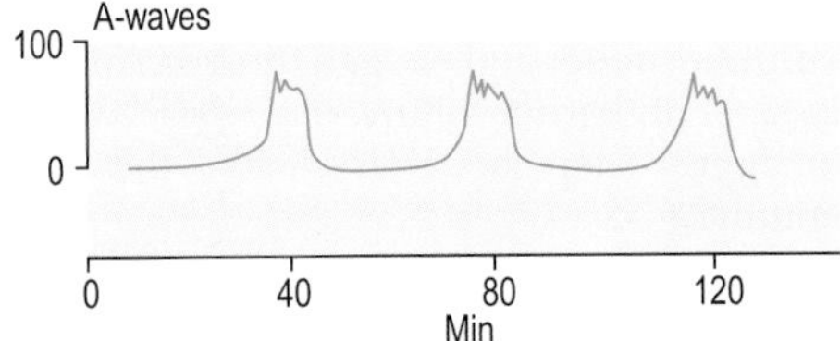

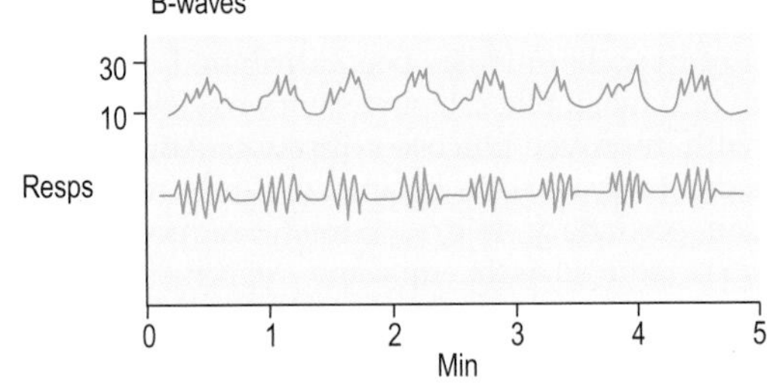

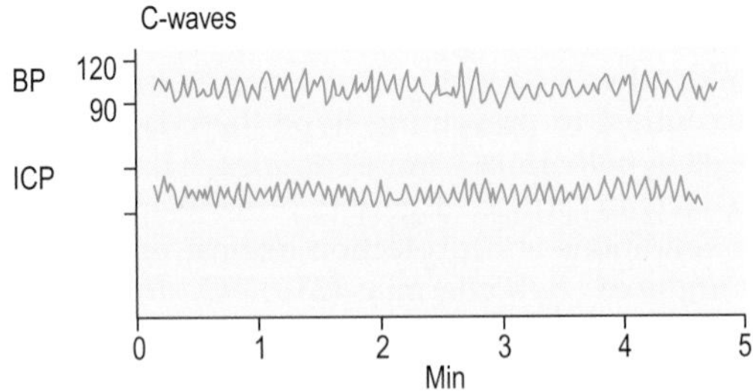

Figure 52.3 Intracranial pressure (ICP) waveforms. A-waves are plateau waves of 50–100 mmHg, sustained for 5–15 minutes, associated with raised ICP and compromised cerebral blood flow. B-waves are small changes in pressure every 0.5–2 minutes, often associated with breathing patterns and possibly due to local variations in the partial pressure of oxygen and carbon dioxide. C-waves are low-amplitude oscillations with a frequency of about 5 per minute, associated with variation in vasomotor tone. Resps=respirations; BP=blood pressure.

INTRAVENTRICULAR DEVICES

This is the gold standard of ICP measurement and is capable of measuring global ICP. The pressure transducers can either be external and attached to a fluid-filled catheter or internal, within the catheter lumen. Insertion is into the lateral ventricle usually via a small right frontal burr hole. The external auditory meatus is used as the reference point.[33] This device allows CSF sampling for culture or therapeutic drainage, the administration of antibiotics and the ability to recalibrate following insertion. The main disadvantage is the high infection rate associated with their use.[32,33] Infection rates increase significantly after 5 days of catheter insertion and with repeated use of the device's flushing system. The use of antibiotic-impregnated catheters may lower the infection rate. Air, blood, tissue debris and ventricular collapse can all adversely affect measurement.

INTRAPARENCHYMAL DEVICES

ICP can be measured by either a miniature strain gauge pressure transducer mounted at the end of a thin catheter or by a fibreoptic cable, which directs light to a miniature mirror at the end of the cable. The catheter can be placed in brain tissue or the subdural space via a skull bolt, burr hole or neurosurgical procedure. These monitors are advantageous when lateral ventricles have collapsed secondary to raised ICP. This system is not dependent on fluid coupling for pressure transduction so waveform damping and artefact are avoided. The infection rates are very low. Its main disadvantages include lack of recalibration in vivo, a tendency for baseline drift requiring transducer replacement, the inability to drain CSF and the ability to measure only localised pressure, which may not be representative of the global ICP.[33,34]

Alternative invasive ICP monitoring includes epidural, subarachnoid and subdural devices, although these are not as accurate. All invasive ICP-monitoring devices are associated with a risk of infection and parenchymal damage with the potential for parenchymal and subdural bleeding. Less-invasive methods of measuring ICP are being investigated. These include infrared spectroscopy, visual evoked potentials, transcranial Doppler and with perhaps the most promising correlation to invasive measurements, optic nerve sheath diameter ultrasound. When it is not possible to insert or interpret an ICP-monitoring device clarification should be sought by computed tomographic (CT) or MRI scanning.

REGULATION OF INTRACRANIAL PRESSURE

BRAIN COMPARTMENT

Reduction in the parenchymal compartment depends on removal of either free water or the lesion causing the raised ICP.

Free water must be moved across an intact blood-brain barrier. Mannitol is recommended as first-line osmotic agent for elevated ICP, although this is controversial. Two meta-analyses have indicated that hypertonic saline is more effective than mannitol for the treatment of raised ICP caused by differing pathologies.[35,36] Choice of agent may be influenced by their individual properties: whereas hypertonic saline improves volume status, cardiac output, regional blood flow and CSF absorption, mannitol may improve microvascular cerebral blood flow, reduce blood viscosity, reduce CSF production and inhibit apoptosis. Further evaluation is required.

Removal of tumour or blood clot, drainage of abscesses and extirpation of infarcted brain are all therapies aimed at improving compliance. Mounting evidence now suggests that there is a penumbra of functionally impaired but potentially reversible neuronal injury surrounding a haematoma. Indications for clot removal, despite numerous studies performed over the last four decades, has been controversial. The Surgical Trial in Intracerebral Haemorrhage (STICH) compared early surgical evacuation (within 24 hours) of haematoma with initial conservative treatment, but found no significant difference in outcomes between the two treatments. However, a subgroup analysis indicated that patients with superficial haematomas and without an associated intraventricular haemorrhage may do better with early surgical removal.[37] For these reasons STICH II is underway recruiting a more select group of patients with superficial lobar haematomas to compare conservative versus surgical treatment.[38]

The rationale for removing part of the skull is to decompress the brain, prevent cerebral herniation and thus reduce ICP, a significant predictor of patient outcome. The benefits of craniectomy versus medical treatment for refractory raised ICP in TBI remain uncertain. The Decompressive Craniectomy in Diffuse Traumatic Injury Trial (DECRA) compared bifronto-temporoparietal decompressive craniectomy with standard medical treatment for the effects on patients with refractory raised ICP and their functional outcome. The patients in the surgical group had fewer days with a raised ICP, required fewer interventions to control their ICP and had a shorter length of ICU stay. Unfortunately the 6-month outcome in the surgical group was unfavourable as measured by the Extended Glasgow Outcome Scale and hypotheses for this included axonal stretch and injury, changes in cerebral blood flow and metabolism and differing surgical techniques.[39] The Randomised Evaluation of Surgery with Craniectomy for Uncontrollable Elevation of raised Intra-Cranial Pressure trial (RESCUEicp) is still recruiting to evaluate whether decompressive craniectomy improves outcome in those patients whose raised ICP is refractory to treatment at a higher ICP.[40]

The outcome of craniectomy for ischaemic stroke is much more favourable. Massive middle cerebral artery stroke, 'malignant' stroke, has a very high mortality due to the very extensive cerebral oedema, raised ICP and resultant herniation. Surgical intervention succeeds where medical treatment fails, reducing mortality from 80% to 20%.[40] Three European trials, Decompressive Craniectomy in Malignant Middle cerebral Artery Infarction (DECIMAL),[41] Decompressive Surgery for the Treatment of Malignant Infarction of the Middle Cerebral Artery (DESTINY)[42] and Hemicraniectomy After Middle Cerebral Artery infarction with Life-threatening Edema Trial (HAMLET),[43] indicated that surgery is not just life-saving but if done early (within 48 hours) has benefits on the severity of functional disability.[40]

The role of decompressive craniectomy in subarachnoid haemorrhage is still uncertain. Loss of cerebral perfusion is mainly due to vasospasm, a physiological response unlikely to be reversed by expanding intracranial space.[44]

BLOOD COMPARTMENT

Although a small component of intracranial volume, the blood compartment is the most compliant. Reduction in blood volume is useful in the treatment of raised ICP, especially in the acute setting. Hypoxia and hypercarbia can lead to hyperaemia and an increase in cerebral blood volume, potentially worsening ICP. Induced hypocarbia is accompanied by a fall in global CBF, which may result in critical ischaemia and a worsened outcome particularly if applied within the first 24 hours. The Brain Trauma Foundation's recommendation is that hyperventilation should be used only as a temporising measure to reduce raised ICP and that ideally some form of neurospecific oxygen monitoring should be employed. Secondary treatment for raised ICP should be instituted as soon as possible.

CEREBROSPINAL FLUID COMPARTMENT

CSF drainage can be used to reduce ICP but is only possible if there is a ventricular catheter in place. Care is taken regarding the route and rate of CSF drainage to avoid herniation of a mass lesion, either towards the other side of the brain or through the tentorium. Less-invasive methods of measuring ICP are being employed. However, the Brain Trauma Foundation guidelines for the management of severe head injury provide some evidence supporting the increased use of CSF drainage for ICP control.[45]

ANAESTHETIC AGENTS

Barbiturates have been used for decades for controlling raised ICP. Barbiturate-mediated neuroprotection was initially attributed to suppression of cerebral metabolic rate, but more recently to coupling of CBF to regional metabolic demands, the blockade of glutamate receptors and sodium channels, inhibition of free radical formation and potentiation of GABAergic activity.[46,47] Barbiturates are now less commonly used in head-injured patients but can play a role in those patients who have intractable intracranial hypertension.

Propofol has been shown to be neuroprotective in vivo, in focal and global models of cerebral ischaemia. It decreases cerebral metabolic rate and hence CBF. It has been shown to have antioxidant properties, potentiate $GABA_A$-mediated inhibition of synaptic transmission and inhibit glutamate release. It delays neuronal death by being a free radical scavenger, preventing lipid peroxidation and modulating apoptosis-regulating proteins.[46,48] Its side-effects include hypotension with a reducing CPP and hyperlipidaemia when an infusion of 200 μg/kg per min is used to produce burst suppression.[48] This latter problem has been lessened by the introduction of a more concentrated formulation.

Inhalational agents have significant neuroprotective effects but the precise mechanism by which they reduce cerebral injury is unclear.[48] It is possible that isoflurane may attenuate excitotoxicity by inhibiting glutamate release and its postsynaptic responses at both anaesthetic and EEG burst suppression concentrations. The neuroprotection provided by volatile agents may also be attributable to their effect at $GABA_A$ receptors and ability to reduce the sympathetic vascular response to ischaemia. Certainly their effect on reducing cerebral metabolic rate is not sufficient to explain their neuroprotective properties.[46,47] These potential benefits in adults are offset by recent studies which have suggested that in neonatal animal studies there may be disturbing increases in cerebral apoptosis, although this has yet to be confirmed.

Nitrous oxide exhibits the neuroprotective and neurotoxic features of an NMDA antagonist. Studies, however, have shown that, when combined with an opioid (e.g. fentanyl), its neuroprotective effect during incomplete cerebral ischaemia is still inferior compared with volatile agents.[47]

Midazolam reduces the cerebral metabolic rate for oxygen, CBF and volume. It does not produce burst suppression or an isoelectric EEG, even in large doses.

Neuromuscular blockade is often used in head-injured patients to prevent any coughing on the tracheal tube and subsequent rise in ICP. Their use is not associated with better outcome despite the improvements in ICP control.

CALCIUM ANTAGONISTS

The influx of calcium from the extracellular space and from intracellular organelles has been implicated as the common mediator of cell death from a variety of causes. Calcium antagonists were among the first neuroprotective agents studied to prevent cerebral ischaemia. Despite the effects seen in animal models, human studies in both global and focal ischaemia have been disappointing. Two large trials of intravenous nimodipine in patients with acute ischaemic stroke were terminated early as neurological and functional outcome were significantly poorer in the nimodipine group.[49,50] A close relationship was found between a reduction in diastolic and mean blood pressure in the group treated with nimodipine and an unfavourable neurological outcome. A review of 29 randomised acute stroke trials involving calcium antagonists concluded that the use of calcium antagonists could not be justified in patients with ischaemic stroke and that, although the published trials showed no overall effect on death and dependency, unpublished trials were associated with a statistically significant worse outcome.[51] Nimodipine, however, has become the standard prophylactic treatment for cerebral vasospasm after subarachnoid haemorrhage, with a consequent decrease in cerebral infarction and better patient outcome.[52] Benefits appear to be due to an effect on smaller penetrating vessels not seen by angiography, or a neuroprotective effect at the cellular level, rather than cerebral vasodilatation identifiable by angiography.

Nimodipine was shown to be neuroprotective in head-injured patients with traumatic subarachnoid haemorrhage.[53] Regrettably, further studies to test the neuroprotective effect of nimodipine in severely head-injured patients with traumatic subarachnoid haemorrhage (including the multicentre study, HIT 4) failed to confirm the beneficial effects of nimodipine. A small group of patients with a Glasgow Coma Score <9 did appear to be a have a better outcome in the nimodipine-treated group.[54] However, a recent systematic review concluded that there was no beneficial effect on outcome.[55] Its use therefore remains contentious.

STEROIDS

Glucocorticoids were used for over 30 years in the treatment of raised ICP from head injury despite the fact that randomised trials had failed to demonstrate their effectiveness reliably. They were thought to decrease cerebral oedema associated with breakdown of the blood–brain barrier (i.e. vasogenic oedema), decrease CSF production, attenuate free radical production and show improvement in central nervous system function in patients with brain tumours and abscesses.[56,57]

The Corticosteroid Randomisation After Significant Head injury (CRASH) trial[58] investigated the effects of a 48-hour infusion of methylprednisolone on death within 14 days or disability at 6 months in 10008 adults with clinically significant head injury. The trial was stopped early as, at interim analysis, the steroid-treated subjects had significantly higher all-cause 2-week mortality (21.1% versus 17.9%, $p=0.0001$). The 6-month mortality was also higher in steroid-treated subjects (25.7% versus 22.3%, $p=0.0001$), with a trend toward increases in the combined end-point of death or severe disability (38.1% versus 36.3%, $p=0.08$). In neither report did the results differ by injury severity or time since injury.[58] The cause for the increased mortality is unclear.

In subarachnoid and primary intracerebral haemorrhage, corticosteroids have also been commonly used. In 2005, a Cochrane Review concluded that there was no evidence to support the use of mineralocorticoids or glucocorticoids in subarachnoid haemorrhage or to support the use of glucocorticoids in primary intracerebral haemorrhage. Corticosteroid use may also be associated with adverse events.[59]

TRANEXAMIC ACID

Tranexamic acid has been shown to safely reduce patient blood loss during elective surgery. The Clinical Randomisation of an Antifibrinolytic in Significant Haemorrhage study (CRASH II) compared the effects of an early short course of tranexamic acid versus placebo on mortality in trauma patients who were at risk of significant blood loss. Cause of death was categorised into bleeding, vascular occlusive events (myocardial infarction, stroke and pulmonary embolism), multiorgan failure, head injury and other. All-cause mortality was significantly reduced with tranexamic acid, but particularly in the bleeding category.[60] CRASH III aims to quantify the effects of tranexamic acid versus placebo on death and disability in trauma patients who have suffered intracranial bleeding.

Optimal cerebral management of patients suffering an acute brain injury remains controversial. Certainly it appears that early clarification of the cause of the brain injury and access to specialist centres is increasingly important for guiding treatment and improving outcome (e.g. blood pressure control, thrombolysis, pharmaceutical intervention and rehabilitation). Unfortunately both old established and new experimental treatments have still yielded disappointing results or safety concerns when applied on a large scale. There are however some new and amended therapeutic interventions which appear promising and are currently under investigation. Hopefully the outcome of these will add to our knowledge and help to improve the management of patients with cerebral injury.

Access the complete references list online at http://www.expertconsult.com

3. Haddah SH, Arabi YM. Critical care management of severe traumatic brain injury in adults. Scand J Trauma Resusc Emerg Med 2012;20:12.
10. Blood Pressure in Acute Stroke Collaboration (BASC). Interventions for deliberately altering blood pressure in acute stroke. Cochrane Database Syst Rev 2001; 3:CD000039.
12. Anderson CS, Huang Y, Arima H, et al. INTERACT Investigators. The Intensive Blood Pressure Reduction in Acute Cerebral Haemorrhage Trial (INTERACT). Stroke 2008;41:307–12.
15. Bellolio MF, Gilmore RM, Stead LG. Insulin for glycaemic control in acute stroke. Cochrane Database Syst Rev 2011;9:CD005346.
18. Vespa P, MacArthur DL, Stein N, et al. Tight glycaemic control increases metabolic distress in traumatic brain injury: A randomized controlled within subjects trial. Crit Care Med 2012;40(6):1923–9.
25. Nolan JP, Morley PT, Vanden Hoek TL, et al. ALS Task Force. Therapeutic hypothermia after cardiac arrest. An advisory statement by the Advanced Life Support Task Force of the International Liaison Committee on Resuscitation. Resuscitation 2003;57:231–5.
44. Hempenstall J, Sadek A-R, Eynon CA. Decompressive craniectomy in acute brain injury- lifting the lid on neurosurgical practice. J Intensive Care Soc 2012;13(3):221–6.
60. CRASH 2 trial collaborators. Effects of tranexamic acid on death, vascular occlusive events, and blood transfusion in trauma patients with significant haemorrhage (CRASH-2): a randomized, placebo-controlled trial. Lancet 2010;376:23–32.

53

Brain death

Martin Smith

The determination of death by neurological criteria, or brain death, has been recognised in many countries for more than 40 years. Brain death describes a state of irreversible loss of brain function, including brainstem function, that provides a professional and legal framework for the withdrawal of therapies, including mechanical ventilation, from an individual who is (brain) dead. A further benefit for society is the availability of organs for transplantation from heart-beating donors.

HISTORICAL PERSPECTIVE

In the 1950s, developments in critical care led to the prospect of somatic function being sustained by mechanical ventilation long after brain function had ceased in patients who did not fulfil the historical criteria for death (i.e. the absence of a heart-beat). This state of unconsciousness, brainstem areflexia and the absence of spontaneous respiration and cortical electrical activity was described in 1959 by Mollaret and Goulon as 'le coma dépasse' – literally a state beyond coma.[1] Although it was agreed that it was futile to maintain treatment in such patients, it was not until the development of heart transplantation, and the associated importance of determining death in heart-beating donors prior to organ retrieval, that the first widely accepted standard for the confirmation of brain death was published by an ad hoc Committee of the Harvard Medical School in 1968.[2] Whilst these initial recommendations defining brain death were temporally associated with advances in transplantation, the concept of brain death was not primarily designed to facilitate donation. Rather it was developed to allow the withdrawal of therapies from an individual who has died and who can no longer conceivably derive benefit from them.[3]

The 'Harvard criteria' defined brain death in terms of the irreversible loss of function of the whole brain and described a clinical picture of lack of responsiveness, absence of brainstem reflexes and apnoea – a definition that remains largely unchanged today. In the following year the committee indicated that brain death could be diagnosed on clinical grounds alone, without the need for a confirmatory electroencephalogram (EEG), so long as certain aetiological preconditions were present.

In the UK in 1976 the Conference of Medical Colleges and their Faculties took a slightly different approach and concluded that permanent functional death of the *brainstem* constitutes brain death and that this could be diagnosed clinically in the context of irremediable structural brain damage after certain specified conditions had been excluded.[4] A set of guidelines and clinical tests for the diagnosis of brainstem death were established and these have become the foundation of modern practice. A subsequent memorandum in 1983 made additional recommendations about the timing of the clinical tests and who should perform them. It also confirmed that there may be circumstances in which it is impossible or inappropriate to carry out every one of the tests and that it is for the doctor at the bedside to determine that the patient is dead.

DEFINITIONS OF BRAIN DEATH

Death is not a single event but a process that leads progressively to the failure of all functions that constitute the life of the human organism. Once a threshold of irreversibility has been reached, and brain death is such a point, it is not necessary to wait for the death of the whole organism for the inevitable consequence of its biological death to be certain.[3] There is widespread acceptance that human death is ultimately death of the brain and that this crucially involves the irreversible loss of the capacity for consciousness combined with the irreversible loss of the capacity to breathe. These elements represent the most basic manner in which human beings interact with their environment.

Two modes of death are described – cardiorespiratory arrest and brain death – but this distinction is artificial because cardiorespiratory arrest results in inevitable death of the whole person only if the period of arrest is long enough to result in irreversible damage to the brain, particularly to the brainstem. The neurons of the brainstem are the most resistant to anoxia so shorter periods of cardiac or respiratory arrest may result in retention of the ability to breathe but survival with differing, and often severe, degrees of cortical damage.

CAUSES OF BRAIN DEATH

Brain death results from massive brain swelling, a sustained rise in intracranial pressure equal to or above systemic arterial pressure causing cessation of cerebral circulation and brainstem herniation. Around 5% to 10% of all comatose patients admitted to intensive care units become brain dead. The principal causes in adults are traumatic and haemorrhagic brain injury, and severe cerebral hypoxia–ischaemia.

After the onset of brain death, brainstem reflexes are lost sequentially in a craniocaudal direction. This process may take several hours to become complete but finally results in apnoea due to failure of the medulla oblongata. Because of the fundamental controlling role of the brainstem, myocardial and other systemic physiological functions deteriorate after the onset of brain death and, without cardiovascular support, brain-dead patients progress to asystolic cardiac arrest within a relatively short time.[5]

WHOLE BRAIN AND BRAINSTEM DEATH

Brain death is confusingly defined in two different ways based on 'whole' brain and 'brainstem' formulations. The Uniform Determination of Death Act states that 'an individual who has sustained irreversible cessation of all functions of the entire brain, including the brainstem, is dead' and gives equivalence to death determined by neurological and cardiovascular criteria.[6] This whole brain formulation is the standard for the determination of death by neurological criteria in many parts of the world, including the USA and most European countries, and requires confirmation of the loss of *all* brain function, including the brainstem.

On the other hand, the diagnosis of brainstem death, such as that used in the UK, does not require confirmation that all brain functions have ceased, but rather that none of those functions that might persist should indicate any form of consciousness.[7] In determining brainstem death, confirmation of the irreversible loss of the capacity for consciousness combined with the irreversible loss of the capacity to breathe relies on the fact that key components of consciousness and respiratory control, the reticular activating system and nuclei for cardiorespiratory regulation, are located in the brainstem.

Early arguments to support the concept of brain death relied on the brain as the central integrator of somatic function, but brain dead patients may exhibit levels of somatic integration that can persist for some time. A 'loss of personhood' was therefore proposed as an alternative rationale because the loss of certain key human functions, such as the ability to be conscious or apply reason, is deemed to be sufficient for the philosophical and ethical justification, as well as the legal determination, of death.[8] In the USA in 2008, the President's Council on Bioethics concluded that it is the 'ability to conduct the vital work of a living organism – the work of self-preservation, achieved through the organism's need-driven commerce with the world' that supports the continued use of brain death as a valid determinant of human death.[9] An individual with irreversible loss of brainstem function who has no drive to breathe, and who can neither perceive nor interact with their environment to meet their basic requirement for oxygen and other nutrients, can no longer be considered to be living. In this way brain death is equivalent to the death of the individual as a whole.

DIAGNOSIS OF BRAIN DEATH

The majority of countries have followed the lead of the USA and the UK in specifying that the clinical diagnosis of brain death is sufficient for the determination of death in adults.

The diagnostic algorithm has three sequential but interdependent steps. Certain preconditions and exclusions must be fulfilled before clinical tests of brainstem function are performed.[7]

PRECONDITIONS

- The patient should be in apnoeic coma (i.e. unresponsive and dependent on mechanical ventilation).
- The cause of coma must be known and due to brain damage that is consistent with the diagnosis of brain death.
- The underlying disorder that has led to this state must be established.

In all cases a cranial computed tomography scan is essential. Establishing the causative diagnosis is relatively straightforward in the case of head injury or intracranial haemorrhage but may take longer in coma arising from hypoxia or other causes.

EXCLUSIONS

Reversible causes of coma must be excluded (**Table 53.1**). The original Harvard criteria specifically required the exclusion of the effects of hypothermia and depressant drugs and, although these are consistently cited in modern recommendations, the thresholds for testing vary considerably between countries.[10]

CLINICAL TESTS

There is no evidence to define a minimum period of observation between the onset of apnoeic coma and clinical examination to ensure irreversibility.[11] Many countries recommend a minimum of 6 hours, whereas in others no minimum period is specified.[12] Most guidelines recommend a longer period of observation, typically 24 hours, in coma related to anoxic brain injury.

The clinical examination is designed to demonstrate the absence of brainstem reflexes and confirm the

Table 53.1 UK recommendations for the exclusion of potentially reversible causes of coma and apnoea

VARIABLE	REQUIREMENTS
Drugs	• Exclude sedative drug effects: – consider specific antagonists, e.g. naloxone, flumazenil – serum drug levels should be measured where assays are available – no consensus regarding the minimal concentration at which brain death can be diagnosed • Exclude residual effects of neuromuscular-blocking drugs: – presence of deep tendon reflexes – train-of-four present on peripheral nerve stimulation
Hypothermia	• Temperature >34°C
Cardiorespiratory	• Mean arterial blood pressure consistently >60 mmHg • Pa_{O_2}>10 kPa • Pa_{CO_2}<6.0 kPa • pH 7.35–7.45
Electrolytes	• Sodium 115–160 mmol/L • Potassium >2.0 mmol/L • Magnesium 0.5–3.0 mmol/L • Phosphate 0.5–3.0 mmol/L
Endocrine	• Hormonal assays if suspicion of myxoedema or Addisonian crisis

Box 53.1 Components of the clinical examination to confirm brain death in the UK

Cranial nerve examination

- Pupils are fixed and do not respond to light
  - no pupillary response to sharp changes in the intensity of incident light
  - the pupils do not need to be maximally dilated, simply unresponsive
- Absent corneal reflexes
- Absent oculo-vestibular reflex
  - no eye movements during or following slow injection of 50 mL ice-cold water over 1 minute into each external auditory meatus
  - clear access to tympanic membrane confirmed by direct inspection prior to testing
  - head at 30° to the horizontal plane unless contraindicated by unstable spine injury
- No motor response within cranial nerve distribution to adequate stimulation of any somatic area
  - supraorbital pressure often used as the stimulus
- Absent cough reflex
  - no response to a suction catheter inserted into the trachea to the carina
- Absent gag reflex
  - no response to stimulation (under direct vision) of the posterior pharynx with a spatula

Apnoea test

- Absence of respiratory effort observed for >5 min
  - Sp_{O_2} must be maintained >95% throughout
  - cardiovascular stability during the test
  - Pa_{CO_2} must rise to >6.5 kPa (>50 mmHg) (pH<7.40) confirmed by arterial blood gas analysis

presence of persistent apnoea, and should be performed only when the preconditions and exclusions have been met.

CRANIAL NERVE EXAMINATION

A rigorous clinical examination of brainstem reflexes must be undertaken to confirm the diagnosis of brain death (**Box 53.1**). The clinical tests are designed to be easy to perform at the bedside, require no special equipment and have unequivocal results.

Confirmation of the absence of the oculo-cephalic reflex ('doll's-eye' movements) is not included in UK criteria but is part of the protocol in some countries. The presence of this reflex confirms that brainstem function persists and that further tests are inappropriate. Facial trauma or obstruction to external ear canals may make assessment of brainstem reflexes difficult, but injury preventing bilateral examination of some reflexes does not invalidate the diagnosis of brain death.

APNOEA TEST

Confirmation of apnoea is required by all guidelines but the end-points are inconsistent.[13] The overall aim is to produce an acidaemic respiratory stimulus (pH<7.4) in the presence of normoxia and ardiovascular stability. This applies even in those with chronic respiratory disease, although the Pa_{CO_2} required to achieve the end-point may be higher. To minimise the risk of further damage to potentially recoverable brain tissue, the apnoea test should only be performed after the absence of brainstem reflex activity has been confirmed. The following method describes a safe method for conducting the apnoea test in the UK.

- Pre-oxygenate with 100% oxygenation – ensure Sp_{O_2}>95%.
- Reduce minute ventilation until E_{TCO_2} 6.0 kPa (45 mmHg) and pH is 7.4.
- Disconnect from the ventilator and maintain apnoeic oxygenation delivering oxygen by bulk flow using a re-breathing circuit and CPAP.
- Sp_{O_2} should remain >95% with cardiovascular stability (MAP>60 mmHg) throughout the procedure.
- Confirm a further rise in Pa_{CO_2} of more than 0.5 kPa (4 mmHg) (Pa_{CO_2}>6.5 kPa (48.8 mmHg)) and pH<7.4 with blood gas analysis. (Pa_{CO_2} rises at about 3 mmHg/min or 0.5 kPa). In some countries, including Australia, the level required is >60 mmHg (8kPa) or >20 mmHg (2.7kPa) above the baseline level in those with chronic hypercapnia.
- Observe for the absence of respiratory activity for >5 minutes.

Following completion of the apnoea test the ventilator should be reconnected and normal minute ventilation resumed to allow return of acid–base variables to their pre-test levels.

TIMING AND REPETITION OF CLINICAL TESTS

More than one set of clinical tests is required in many jurisdictions to minimise the likelihood of errors in diagnosis.[10] However, after more than 30 years of applying clinical criteria for the diagnosis of brain death, there have been no cases of a response during the second examination in a patient who has satisfied the clinical criteria for brain death during the first. Where two sets of tests are required there is often no specified time interval between them. In the original Harvard criteria the two clinical examinations were separated by 24 hours but subsequent US guidance recommends that they may be repeated after 6 hours.[11] In the UK, the second set of tests may be performed as soon as arterial blood gas values have normalised following the first apnoea test.[7] The legal time for certification of death is often that of the initial testing but in some countries, such as Australia, the time of death is the time of the second confirmatory examination.

The number of doctors required to determine brain death varies. In most jurisdictions a single doctor is sufficient, but in the UK, Australia and some states in the USA two medical practitioners are required.[12] There are specific requirements for the base specialty of the doctors in some countries, whereas relevant competencies are defined in others. To avoid any conflict of interest, those diagnosing brain death are usually required to have no involvement with organ transplantation.

CONFIRMATORY TESTS

Clinical tests remain the gold standard for the diagnosis of brain death but confirmatory tests may have a place when the preconditions for clinical testing are unmet or where clinical testing cannot be completed. An alternative view argues that confirmatory tests have no role because the determination of brain death based on a comprehensive clinical examination is robust and, if clinical tests cannot be completed, support should be withdrawn on the grounds of futility.[14] The relevance of confirmatory tests varies between jurisdictions; patients with preserved cortical electrical activity or intracranial blood flow can be considered to be dead in countries that utilise a brainstem approach but not in those that apply a whole brain concept to the diagnosis of brain death.

Confirmatory tests are not specifically required in the UK, Australia or New Zealand but are required by law in some European countries.[7,12] US guidance recommends ancillary tests only where a clinical diagnosis cannot be made, but there is wide variability in their choice and application.[11]

Confirmatory tests fall into two main categories: those that assess cerebral blood flow (CBF) and those that evaluate the brain's electrophysiological activity.[15]

ASSESSMENT OF CEREBRAL BLOOD FLOW

Investigations of CBF are independent of confounding variables such as sedation, metabolic disturbance or hypothermia. The presence of residual CBF does not preclude a diagnosis of brain death and CBF methods of assessment may produce false-negative results, particularly after decompressive craniectomy or in the presence of skull fracture or cerebrospinal fluid drains.

Cerebral angiography

Four-vessel digital subtraction cerebral angiograph (DSA) is the gold-standard confirmatory test for brain death in some jurisdictions.[16] Following injection of contrast into both vertebral and carotid arteries, absence of flow beyond the foramen magnum will be confirmed in the posterior circulation and no flow beyond the petrosal portion of the carotid artery in the anterior circulation. Isolated or minimal filling necessitates repeat examination. DSA is invasive, time-consuming and readily available only in neuroscience units but it is reliable and easy to interpret. Newer imaging modalities, such as spiral CT angiography, are less invasive than DSA and accurately demonstrate the absence of CBF.

Cerebral tissue perfusion

Contrast-enhanced CT cerebral perfusion techniques are now widely available and their application in the diagnosis of brain death is likely to increase. Positron emission tomography is also accurate and unambiguous for the determination of absence of perfusion. Nuclear imaging techniques are also able to confirm absent cerebral perfusion but are not widely used in this context.

Transcranial Doppler ultrasonography

Transcranial Doppler (TCD) is a non-invasive bedside investigation used as a confirmatory test during the diagnosis of brain death.[17] Blood flow through both middle cerebral and vertebral arteries is compared with flow through extracranial vessels. Typical findings after brain death include diastolic reverberating flow and little or no forward systolic flow. There is significant operator dependence, and previous surgery or the presence of a ventricular drain may make waveform interpretation difficult. The absence of an acoustic window in some patients means that an absence of signal should not be taken as diagnostic of absence of blood flow.

ELECTROPHYSIOLOGY

The EEG is widely used as a confirmatory test in the diagnosis of brain death but specialist expertise is required for interpretation.[16] The absence of cortical electrical activity during high-sensitivity recordings from 16 or 18 channels over 30 minutes is usually taken as confirmatory evidence of brain death. However, an isoelectric cortical EEG cannot confirm or exclude brainstem activity or the presence of viable neurons in other deep structures. Conversely, electrical activity in some cortical cells does not mean that the brain as a whole is alive. Confirmatory EEG examination is mandatory in many European countries and strongly recommended in some jurisdictions in the USA where loss of whole brain function must be confirmed. The EEG is affected by hypothermia and sedation and is therefore of limited value in circumstances where prolonged sedation precludes clinical testing.[15]

Evoked potentials (EPs) monitor the integrity of discrete sensory pathways and are thus able to assess components of the brainstem. Somatosensory and brainstem EPs demonstrate successive loss of function of various afferent pathways of the brainstem but, because they rely on the integrity of the whole pathway, a lesion affecting any point of that pathway may result in an absent EP and a false-positive result.[16] Like EEG, EPs are susceptible to sedative drugs and metabolic derangement and, in association with their anatomical limitations, this renders them unreliable as sole confirmatory tests of brain death.

DIAGNOSING BRAIN DEATH IN SPECIAL CIRCUMSTANCES

Although there are no published reports of recovery of neurological function after a diagnosis of brain death using standard criteria,[11] there are numerous case reports highlighting situations or conditions that may mimic brain death and thus lead to erroneous conclusions if unrecognised. These invariably involve failure to consider the preconditions and exclusions prior to clinical testing.

SEDATIVE DRUGS AND HYPOTHERMIA

The effects of high-dose sedative infusions may persist for several days after discontinuation, particularly in critically ill patients. During this time the patient fails to satisfy the preconditions for the clinical confirmation of brain death. This is particularly an issue following infusion of barbiturates, which are increasingly being used to treat intractable intracranial hypertension. As with other sedatives, plasma barbiturate levels may not reflect clinical effect, particularly in the context of brain injury, and there is no consensus regarding a minimal plasma concentration at which brain death can be diagnosed. On the other hand, waiting an arbitrary period of time, usually several days, to allow sedative effects to wear off represents an inefficient use of ICU resources and additional pressures for relatives. Although the effects of high-dose barbiturates can mimic brain death, particularly in the presence of hypothermia, this is rare except in children. Therefore, in the presence of other stigmata of brain death, such as dilated unreactive pupils, characteristic cardiovascular changes and diabetes insipidus, the diagnosis is rarely in doubt.

A case of misdiagnosed 'reversible' brain death has been reported in a 55-year-old man who had been treated with therapeutic hypothermia and propofol and fentanyl infusions following cardiopulmonary arrest and serves to highlight the potential pitfalls.[18] Sixteen hours after re-warming the patient satisfied the clinical criteria for brain death and these findings were confirmed 6 hours later. However, cough and gag reflexes, and spontaneous respiration, returned after a further 24 hours, although this recovery was transient and did not affect the ultimate outcome. The potential confounding effects of a very high cumulative dose of fentanyl in the presence of renal and hepatic impairment, and therapeutic hypothermia, were not given sufficient weight in this case, which illustrates the importance of meticulous attention to exclusion of confounding factors prior to proceeding with clinical examination of the brainstem.

Confirmatory tests may have a role when the diagnosis of brain death using clinical criteria is complicated by the effects of prolonged sedation, particularly in the context of hypothermia. The Australian and New Zealand guidance offers the greatest assistance in this regard, permitting brain death to be determined by demonstration of the absence of intracranial blood flow if any of the preconditions for clinical testing, including the presence of residual sedation, are not met.[19]

INABILITY TO COMPLETE THE APNOEA TEST

In patients with high spinal cord injury the possibility that apnoea might be related to the cord injury itself brings some uncertainty to the diagnosis of brain death. The degree of any spinal cord injury must therefore be quantified clinically, structurally and functionally by meticulous clinical examination, magnetic resonance imaging and electrophysiological tests.[20] In other situations, such as after polytrauma, the apnoea test cannot be attempted, or has to be abandoned, because of haemodynamic instability or poor oxygenation. The majority of guidelines consider the apnoea test to be a fundamental component of the clinical determination of brain death, although in Australia and New Zealand brain death can be confirmed by demonstration of the absence of intracranial blood flow if the apnoea test cannot be completed.

OTHER CONDITIONS

Other brain death mimics, including baclofen and valproic acid overdose, snake bite and some neurological conditions, have been reported. Cranial nerve involvement and respiratory paralysis are features of Guillain-Barré syndrome and may cause diagnostic confusion, although pupil dilatation is rare. Brainstem reflexes may also be absent in brainstem encephalitis but the patient is usually drowsy rather than comatose. The preconditions for the diagnosis of brain death are not met in any of these conditions and meticulous application of the clinical criteria and careful examination will ensure that they cannot be mistaken for brain death.

CHILDREN

Special care is recommended in diagnosing brain death in children younger than 5 years of age.[21] In those over 2 months, the general criteria are the same as for adults but the period of observation should be longer and confirmatory investigations, such as EEG or cerebral angiography, are often conducted. A higher Pa_{CO_2} target is also recommended during the apnoea test. As in adults the tests must be undertaken by two competent clinicians but, in the case of young children, one should be a paediatrician and one not directly involved in the child's care.

Coma may occur for a wide variety of reasons in infants younger than 2 months of age but hypoxic–ischaemic encephalopathy is the most likely cause of devastating brain injury in this age group. Diagnosing brain death can be difficult because it may be impossible to demonstrate structural brain damage and thus the preconditions are rarely met. Associated severe multi-system failure is common at this young age, so it may not be appropriate or necessary to confirm brain death if care can be withdrawn on the grounds of futility.

Apnoea and coma are common in preterm infants (gestational age less than 37 weeks) but the development of brainstem reflexes is variable and therefore their absence difficult to demonstrate. In the UK it has been suggested that the concept of brain death is inappropriate in this age group and decisions to withdraw support should be made on the basis of futility.

SUMMARY

More than 40 years since the concept was first introduced, practice guidelines to determine brain death are available in many countries but there is large international variation in their content and application. There is thus a need for an international consensus on the determination of brain death; this should retain clinical tests at its core and clarify the role of, and indications for, confirmatory investigations. Flexibility should be maintained and, as in other areas of medicine, the clinical findings should be interpreted with common sense by an experienced and humane physician.

Access the complete references list online at http://www.expertconsult.com

3. Smith M. Brain death: time for an international consensus. Br J Anaesth 2012;108(Suppl. 1):i6–9.
8. Zamperetti N, Bellomo R, Defanti CA, et al. Irreversible apnoeic coma 35 years later. Towards a more rigorous definition of brain death? Intensive Care Med 2004;30:1715–22.
10. Baron L, Shemie SD, Teitelbaum J, et al. Brief review: history, concept and controversies in the neurological determination of death. Can J Anaesth 2006;53:602–8.
11. Wijdicks EF, Varelas PN, Gronseth GS, et al. Evidence-based guideline update: determining brain death in adults: report of the Quality Standards Subcommittee of the American Academy of Neurology. Neurology 2010;74:1911–18.
12. Wijdicks EF. Brain death worldwide: accepted fact but no global consensus in diagnostic criteria. Neurology 2002;58:20–5.
14. Wijdicks EF. The case against confirmatory tests for determining brain death in adults. Neurology 2010;75:77–83.
15. Young GB, Shemie SD, Doig CJ, et al. Brief review: the role of ancillary tests in the neurological determination of death. Can J Anaesth 2006;53:620–7.
21. Shemie SD, Pollack MM, Morioka M, et al. Diagnosis of brain death in children. Lancet Neurol 2007;6:87–92.

54

Meningitis and encephalomyelitis

Angus M Kennedy

Infections of the cranial contents can be divided into those that affect the meninges (meningitis) and those that affect the brain parenchyma (encephalitis). Chronic, insidious or rare infections are beyond the scope of this chapter, which will focus on acute bacterial and viral causes of meningitis and encephalomyelitis. The crucial questions to be considered for an individual patient with a neurological infection are to determine why this individual, in this place, has developed this disease, at this time.[1]

Definitions

- *Meningitis:* infection or inflammation of the meninges and subarachnoid space. The infection can be caused by viruses, bacteria, fungi or protozoa. Meningeal inflammation may be caused by subarachnoid haemorrhage, vaccination or be a manifestation of other multi-organ diseases such as systemic lupus erythematosus, sarcoidosis, lymphoma or meningeal micro-metastases from a disseminated carcinoma.
- *Aseptic meningitis:* a generic term for cases of meningitis in which bacteria cannot be isolated from the cerebrospinal fluid. The differential diagnosis includes: (1) viral meningitis, (2) partially treated bacterial meningitis, (3) TB meningitis, (4) fungal meningitis, (5) lymphoma, (6) sarcoidosis, and (7) other collagen vascular diseases. The most common causes of aseptic meningitis are viral infection most often due to an enterovirus or coxsackie infection.
- *Encephalitis:* an infection of the brain parenchyma. The patient may have a history of focal symptoms including preceding seizures together with cognitive or behavioural symptoms.
- *Tuberculous meningitis:* causes subacute lymphocytic meningitis. Patients may have a non-specific prodromal phase, including symptoms such as headache, vomiting and fever.
- *Subdural empyema:* a suppurative process in the space between the pia and dura maters.
- *Brain abscess:* a collection of pus within the brain tissue.

BACTERIAL MENINGITIS

Bacterial meningitis is an inflammatory response to infection of the lepto meninges and subarachnoid space. This is characterised by the clinical syndrome of fever, headache, neck stiffness and cerebrospinal fluid pleocytosis. Despite antibiotic therapy some patients continue to suffer significant morbidity and mortality.

The bacterial organisms are usually not confined to the brain and meninges and frequently cause systemic illness - for example, severe sepsis, shock, acute respiratory distress syndrome, and bleeding disorders such as disseminated intravascular coagulation.[2,3]

A variety of other pathogens cause meningeal inflammation, resulting in very similar clinical presentations. Bacterial infections must be treated urgently and appropriately to limit ongoing central nervous system damage. It is also important to treat the complications of meningitis such as seizures and raised intracranial pressure (ICP).

Where possible, spinal fluid examination following a lumbar puncture is required in order to confirm the diagnosis and establish the pathogenic organism responsible. A cerebrospinal fluid (CSF) examination may be contraindicated if there are signs of raised intracranial pressure including:

- papilloedema
- focal neurological signs
- seizures.

These features raise the possibility of an undiagnosed cerebral mass lesion, which, in turn, could cause cerebral herniation should lumbar puncture be performed. A computed tomography (CT) brain scan is required prior to CSF examination in order to rule out this possibility and lessen, but not obviate, the risk of cerebral herniation. Even if the CT brain scan is normal, intracranial pressure may be raised. The importance of performing a safe CSF examination must be balanced against the need to commence immediate treatment in each individual patient.[4,5]

AETIOLOGY

All three main causes of meningitis (see below) are spread by droplet infection or exchange of saliva. Meningitis may occur when pathogenic organisms colonise the nasopharynx and reach the blood–brain barrier. It can also occur as a consequence of infection in the middle ear, sinus or teeth leading to secondary meningeal infection. Most bacteria obtain entry into the central nervous system via the haematogenous route. As the organisms multiply, exponentially, they release cell wall products and lipopolysaccharide, which can generate a local inflammatory reaction that itself also releases inflammatory mediators. The net result of the release of cytokines, tumour necrosis factor and other factors is associated with a significant inflammatory response. Vasculitis of central nervous system (CNS) vessels, thrombosis, cell damage and exudative material all contribute to vasogenic and cytotoxic oedema, altered blood flow and cerebral perfusion pressure. Later on, infarction and raised intracranial pressure occur.[6]

The inflammatory events seen with infection are summarised in **Figure 54.1**.

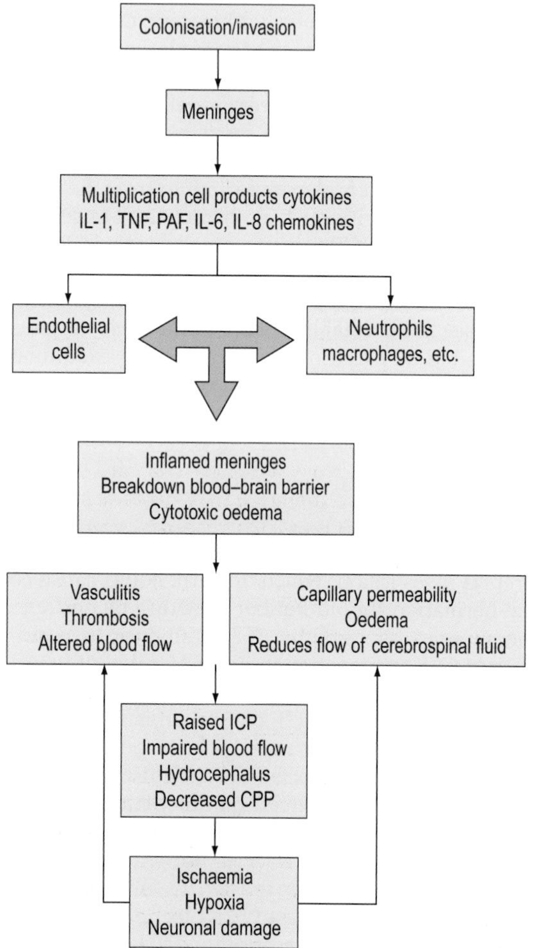

Figure 54.1 Cascade of events in meningitis. IL=interleukin; TNF=tumour necrosis factor; PAF=platelet-activating factor; ICP=intracranial pressure; CPP=cerebral perfusion pressure.

ORGANISMS

Acute bacterial meningitis can be caused by many species of bacteria, although three organisms are commonly reported, including:

- *Haemophilus influenzae*
- *Streptococcus pneumoniae*
- *Neisseria meningitidis* (which account for 70% of cases in the neonatal period).

Until the advent of the meningitis vaccination programme *H. influenzae* type B was the most common cause of bacterial meningitis. Recently *S. pneumoniae* and *N. meningitidis* were considered the main causes, although one study suggested that *Listeria monocytogenes* is the second most common isolate in the adult population. The emergence of pneumococcal strains that are resistant to penicillin has also influenced the epidemiology of meningitis.[7]

NOSOCOMIAL INFECTIONS

Common systemic nosocomial pathogens such as *Escherichia coli, Pseudomonas* spp., *Klebsiella* and *Acinetobacter* spp. account for a high percentage of nosocomial infections of the meninges.

IMMUNOCOMPROMISED HOSTS

In the immunocompromised patient with meningitis (e.g. human immunodeficiency virus, HIV), fungal, viral and cryptococcal meningitis should be considered.[8]

NEUROSURGERY AND TRAUMA

Infections following skull trauma are frequently caused by *Staphylococcus aureus* and *Staphylococcus epidermis*, which should be considered in those with shunts or other intracranial devices.

CLINICAL PRESENTATION

The history may reveal evidence of trauma or infection. Meningitis usually presents with an acute onset of:

- fever
- headache
- neck stiffness
- photophobia
- altered conscious level
- irritability
- seizures (paediatric).

However, in the immunocompromised, elderly or infant patient, non-specific features such as a low-grade fever or mild behavioural change may be all that is apparent. Many of the classic symptoms are late manifestations of meningitis and are preceeded by early symptoms such as leg pain or cold hands, which may not immediately suggest the more serious underlying diagnosis.

If the presenting symptoms are highly suggestive of pyogenic bacterial meningitis, empirical administration

Table 54.1 Cerebrospinal fluid changes in meningitis

	NORMAL	BACTERIAL	VIRAL
Appearance	Clear	Turbid/purulent	Clear/turbid
White cell count	<5 per mm^3 mononuclear	200–10000 per mm^3 predominantly polymorphonuclear	<500 per mm^3 mainly lymphocytes
Protein	0.2–0.4 g/L	0.5–2.0 g/L	0.4–0.8 g/L
Glucose	Blood glucose	≤Blood glucose	Blood glucose pressure is usually raised

Table 54.2 Empirical antibiotics for meningitis

INDICATION	ANTIBIOTIC	DOSE
<50 years	Ceftriaxone *or* cefotaxime	2–4 g q. 24 h, 2 g q. 4 h
>50 years or impaired cell immunity	Ceftriaxone *or* cefotaxime Cefotaxime+ampicillin *or* penicillin G	2–4 g q. 24 h, 2 g q. 4 h 2 g q. 4 h or 3–4 MU q. 4 h
Drug-resistant *Streptococcus pneumoniae*	Ceftriaxone+rifampicin *or* vancomycin	2–4 g q. 8 h, 2 g q. 4 h 0.5 g q. 6 h
Neurosurgery shunts trauma	Ceftazidime+nafcillin *or* vancomycin+aminoglycoside (gentamicin 5–7 mg/kg stat)	2 g q. 8 h, 2 g q.4 h 0.5 g q. 6 h 2 mg/kg q. 8 h

of a third-generation cephalosporin such as cefotaxime or ceftriaxone should be given.

It is important to identify from the history any reports of preceding trauma, upper respiratory tract infection or ear infection. Symptoms may develop over hours or days. Specific infections relate partly to an individual's age.

Neurological signs can be present with meningitis, but signs such as nuchal rigidity, stiffness and a positive Kernig's sign (pain and hamstring spasm resulting from attempts to straighten, e.g. with the hip flexed) are not always present, and a number of studies have shown that the classic triad of signs were present in less than 50% of cases. There may be focal neurological signs. Systemic signs may occur most often in meningococcal disease where a haemorrhagic, petechial or purpuric rash may be observed. Digital gangrene or skin necrosis may occur. Some patients present severely septic with acute respiratory distress syndrome and disseminated intravascular coagulation.

Approximately 25% of patients have a seizure during the course of the illness. Differential diagnosis may include subarachnoid haemorrhage, migraine, encephalitis and tumour.

INVESTIGATIONS

The patient with suspected bacterial meningitis requires immediate blood cultures and should be given empirical i.v. antibiotics if there is likely to be any delay in further assessment (**Table 54.1**).

CSF FINDINGS

A CSF examination is a vitally important investigation that will definitively confirm the diagnosis of bacterial meningitis. Its value should, in this regard, not be dismissed. Concern about the risks of coning following lumbar puncture should be considered in the context of patients' symptoms where the presence of coma, seizures, focal neurological signs and papilloedema may suggest raised intracranial pressure. Neuroimaging may not always predict whether it is safe to lumbar puncture a patient, although it may provide some level of reassurance that it is safe to proceed. A young patient who is alert, orientated, immune competent and without focal signs can safely have a lumbar puncture without prior imaging.

Bacterial meningitis is suggested when there is:

- polymorphic leucocytosis
- low CSF glucose relative to the plasma value
- raised CSF protein concentration.

An urgent Gram stain and microbiological culture are mandatory. The Gram stain is positive in approximately 50–60% of cases. A CSF examination shortly after empirical antibiotics may, but does not necessarily, decrease the diagnostic sensitivity of CSF culture. Polymerase chain reaction (PCR) techniques can now be used to detect the presence of different organisms. A throat swab should be routinely taken. The clinical decision-making process to determine whether a patient does or does not have bacterial meningitis cannot be modelled easily and is reliant on both clinical and laboratory findings as well as observation of the patient over time.

As spread is haematogenous, blood cultures comprise an important investigation in meningitis, and a number of sets of cultures should be sent. It is advisable to routinely check a full blood count clotting profile (to exclude DIC) and biochemistry including blood glucose level. A chest X-ray and blood gases should be performed to identify systemic involvement. Obviously, relevant areas such as infected sinuses or ears should be examined if there is any indication that they are implicated.

MANAGEMENT

Broad-spectrum antibiotics should be started as early as possible and continued until bacterial identification is made (**Table 54.2**). Antibiotic selection is influenced by the clinical situation in conjunction with known allergies or local patterns of antibiotic resistance and the CSF findings. Delay in administering antibiotics is a significant risk factor for a poor prognosis. In the abscence of a known organism, empirical choice for antibiotics has been complicated by the development of resistance. Penicillin G, ampicillin and third-generation cephalosporins are typical first-line agents. Until recently, ampicillin was appropriate for pneumococcal, meningococcal and listerial infections but the emergence of resistant strains significantly influences local antibiotic practice and hence choice. If there is a history of recent head injury, a broad-spectrum cephalosporin may be indicated with vancomycin. Discussions with local microbiology services are recommended. If the CSF examination identifies the organism then specific regimens can be prescribed (**Table 54.3**).

It is more difficult to select an appropriate empirical antibiotic in the immunocompromised patient. When the organism has been identified and sensitivity results are available, it will probably be necessary either to change or to rationalise the antibiotics being given.[9]

In all cases, it is important to monitor the clinical response and antibiotics should be reviewed and appropriately altered once antibiotic sensitivities are known, or if a patient is not improving. A repeat CSF examination should be performed if there is concern about antibiotic sensitivity or selection. In those with penicillin-resistant pneumococcal meningitis, a CSF examination 48 hours after presentation is recommended to ensure bacteriological improvement. Antibiotics should be given for 10–14 days, although a shorter course may be adequate in some circumstances. Intrathecal antibiotics are not recommended.

STEROID ADMINISTRATION

The benefit of steroid administration in adult meningitis has been debated, but clear guidance is now available to support its routine use as the Cochrane Database of 1800 adults and children demonstrated a reduction in mortality, hearing loss and and neurological complications. Concerns still remain, however, that dexamethasone may adversely effect CSF penetration or cause longer-term cognitive problems.[10] An extended and more established literature exists for the use of steroids in bacterial meningitis in children and these studies confirm a benefit for those with *H. influenzae* type B infection with a reduction in the frequency of post-meningitis deafness.

RECOMMENDATIONS IN ADULTS

Dexamethasone is an adjuvant treatment and should be given with the first dose of antibiotics and continued 6-hourly for 4 days (0.6 mg/kg daily).

ANTICONVULSANTS

Focal or generalised seizures should be treated immediately with i.v. benzodiazepines to stop the seizures and the individual then subsequently loaded with i.v.

Table 54.3 General recommendation for known organisms

ORGANISM	ANTIBIOTIC	SECOND LINE OR ALLERGY
Streptococcus pneumoniae (penicillin-resistant)	Ceftriaxone+vancomycin *or* rifampicin	Vancomycin+rifampicin
Streptococcus pneumoniae (penicillin-sensitive)	Penicillin G	Ceftriaxone *or* chloramphenicol
β-Haemolytic *Streptococcus*	Penicillin *or* ampicillin	Cefotaxime *or* chloramphenicol *or* vancomycin
Haemophilus influenzae	Ceftriaxone *or* cefotaxime	Chloramphenicol
Neisseria meningitidis	Penicillin G	Ceftriaxone *or* chloramphenicol
Listeria monocytogenes	Ampicillin+gentamicin	Trimethoprim+sulfamethoxazole
Enterobacteriaceae	Ceftriaxone+gentamicin	Quinolones
Pseudomonas aeruginosa	Ceftazidime+tobramycin	Quinolones

Always check local sensitivity as resistance patterns are variable.

phenytoin or levetiracetam. The possibility of the following should be considered:

- raised intracranial pressure
- cerebritis
- cerebral abscess
- septic venous thrombosis.

The development of seizures may be indicative of a poor prognosis.

INTRACRANIAL PRESSURE

Intracranial hypertension is a common complication of meningitis. Intracranial pressure monitoring may be required and standard measures such as hyperventilation, mannitol infusion or CSF drainage may be considered. Depending upon the particular circumstance, serial lumbar punctures or external ventricular drainage should be implemented.

GENERAL MANAGEMENT CONSIDERATIONS[11]

Intravenous fluid therapy

Normal haemodynamics should be maintained. Currently, there is emphasis on maintaining the cerebral perfusion pressure at around 70 mmHg (9.33 kPa). Inappropriate antidiuretic hormone secretion may occur in meningitis.

Respiratory

It is important to secure the airway and respiratory support may be required for those with severe shock or profound coma. Attention should be paid to management of the unconscious patient with appropriate mouth and eye care. Physiotherapy will be required in order to prevent the onset of pressure sores. Surgical evaluation may be needed for skin necrosis.[12,13]

Public health

Meningitis prophylaxis is recommended for close (kissing contacts) associates and for those medical personnel with close contact. A 2-day course of oral rifampicin 600 mg 12-hourly is recommended. There should be procedures in place for alerting the infectious disease team and public health.

PROGNOSIS

Untreated bacterial meningitis is usually fatal. Appropriate therapy significantly reduces the mortality rate, but recent studies still show that the overall mortality is approximately 18%. Mortality is slightly higher in those who have seizures, when there have been delays introducing treatment, and if the patient is either elderly or very young[13,14] (see Table 54.3).

CRYPTOCOCCAL MENINGITIS

Cryptococcus neoformans is a yeast that can cause a chronic meningitis that is clinically similar to *tuberculous meningitis*. It is most frequently found in those who are immunocompromised, such as with HIV infection. The CSF should be stained with India ink and appropriate antifungal chemotherapy instituted (amphotericin B). Management of the raised intracranial pressure may necessitate daily lumbar punctures or CSF diversion.

VIRAL MENINGITIS

The majority of cases of viral meningitis are benign, usually self-limiting conditions that are often caused by enterovirus or coxsackie infection. Some are caused by arboviruses. The same viruses that produce meningitis can also cause encephalitis. Herpes simplex virus type 1 usually produces encephalitis but rarely causes meningitis. Other viruses causing CNS infections include echoviruses, mumps, polio and HIV. Patients with migrainous headaches often receive a lumbar puncture to rule out viral meningitis, which paradoxically may prolong their hospital stay with a post-lumbar-puncture headache and migraine.

CLINICAL PRESENTATION

Patients usually present with symptoms of meningeal irritation, fever, headache, neck stiffness, retrobulbar pain, photophobia, vertigo, nausea and vomiting that are less severe than those with bacterial meningitis. The presence of intellectual impairment, focal neurological symptoms or seizures suggests that the brain parenchyma is involved often due to meningo-encephalitis. A detailed travel history should be obtained as this may alter the differential diagnosis in terms of the likely organism. True viral meningitis develops over hours to days but rarely lasts longer than 7–10 days. A variety of associated symptoms, such as nausea, vomiting and generalised malaise, may accompany this condition.[15]

INVESTIGATIONS

A CSF examination is important and usually shows:

- a mild to moderate lymphocytic pleocytosis
- a mildly elevated CSF protein concentration
- normal glucose concentration.

Staining for microorganisms, including bacteria, mycobacterium tuberculosis and cryptococcal meningitis, is necessary. Sites for culture include the mucous membranes, throat, skin and rectum.

MANAGEMENT

Acute viral meningitis is usually a self-limiting condition and only supportive therapy is required with analgesia and bedrest. Viral meningitis caused by herpes simplex virus (HSV) 1 or 2 may require i.v. aciclovir. Acute HIV infection causing meningitis may respond to retroviral therapy.

ENCEPHALITIS

Encephalitis is a viral infection of the brain but can be due to either direct infection or by post-infectious, immune-mediated mechanisms. HSV-1, the most common and serious cause of focal encephalitis, usually affects the temporal and frontal lobes. There are a large number of arboviruses that cause epidemics of encephalitis. Encephalitis acts as a sentinel for new and emerging infections, including Japanese encephalitis, Nipah virus, Hendra virus, a variety of bat-associated viruses as well as West Nile and some tick-borne encephalitides such as Murray Valley encephalitis.

West Nile virus is now the most common cause of epidemic viral encephalitis in some countries. Although, on neuroimaging, changes in the basal ganglia may suggest the diagnosis, a CSF pleocytosis may be a more obvious diagnostic finding. Specific CSF antibodies can be sent for West Nile virus. There are also a variety of antibody-mediated encephalitides that target synaptic proteins. These include myeloid cell nuclear differentiation antigen (MNDA) receptor antibodies and voltage-gated K^+ channel antibodies.[16]

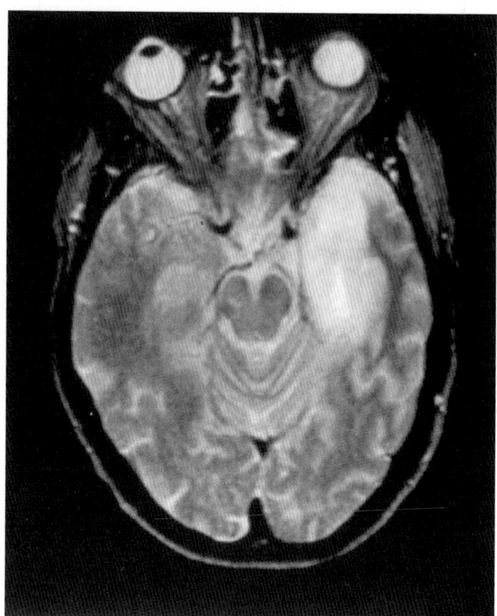

Figure 54.2 Enhanced temporal lobe with herpes simplex encephalitis.

CLINICAL PRESENTATION

The key clinical pointer to encephalitis is the presence of focal neurological symptoms indicating involvement of the brain parenchyma. In particular, the presence of speech disturbance, seizures, altered cognition and disturbance of conscious level suggest this.

Diagnosis can be difficult.

- Abnormalities on cranial imaging such as T2-weighted magnetic resonance imaging (MRI) may support this diagnosis (**Fig. 54.2**).
- Electroencephalogram (EEG) studies may show slow-wave activity or epileptiform discharges in temporal lobe.
- PCR examination of the CSF examination may confirm the virus at a later date.

A systematic approach to the investigation of those with encephalitis has been proposed and national guidelines developed in order to reduce the proportion of unidentified cases.[17]

TREATMENT

Understanding, and if at all possible identifying, the specific aetiological cause of an individual's encephalitis may ultimately have the greatest influence on the successful management of individual patients.[18]

Specific treatment for HSV encephalitis requires i.v. aciclovir at a dose of 30 mg/kg per day for 14 days. If untreated, the mortality of HSV encephalitis is approximately 70% but there is still a 25% mortality in patients treated with optimal therapy, and patients can be left with significant disability in terms of cognitive dysfunction or seizures. Most patients with significant cerebral oedema receive empirical steroids, although there are no clinical trials to support this therapy. Aciclovir can cause renal impairment and the patient should be hydrated intravenously and renal function monitored.[19] Aggressive treatment of seizures is important.

Cytomegalovirus (CMV) infection requires antiviral therapy with ganciclovir or valganciclovir. CMV may cause a ganglionitis and polyradiculitis, which may suggest this diagnosis clinically in an immunocompromised patient.

Most CNS viruses cause neuronal damage but chronic Jakob–Creuzfeldt (JC) virus infection in oligodendrocyes causes the syndrome of progressive multifocal leucoencephalopathy (PML). This condition presents with a subacute onset of confusion, weakness and visual symptoms, usually in an immunosuppressed individual. The MRI scan is usually suggestive but CSF examination with PCR amplification of the JC virus particles may be required. Currently, no specific therapy for PML exists. The survival of HIV patients with associated PML is poor, averaging 6 months in 90% of individuals.

Viral infection with HIV-1, measles and rubella can also cause chronic CNS infection leading to chronic encephalitides. *Mycoplasma* infection can give rise to post-infectious encephalitis.

A number of systemic neurological conditions (e.g. lymphoma, Lyme disease, sarcoidosis and vasculitides such as Behçet disease) may present with aseptic meningitis. It is therefore important to consider these systemic conditions in those presenting with viral meningitis or encephalitis.

TUBERCULOUS MENINGITIS

Tuberculous meningitis has a variable natural history with a range of different clinical presentations. This and the lack of specific and sensitive tests hinder the diagnosis of this condition. Approximately 10% of individuals with tuberculosis develop meningeal involvement. A variety of risk factors such as HIV, diabetes mellitus and the recent use of steroid use may increase the risk of tuberculous meningitis.[20]

CLINICAL FEATURES

Tuberculous meningitis has a very varied clinical presentation. Often, it is heralded by a non-specific prodromal phase, frequently but not necessarily including headache, vomiting and fever. Of one case series that included those admitted to an intensive care unit, only 65% had fever, 52% had focal neurology and 88% had signs of meningism. A variety of cranial nerve palsies can occur, but other presentations include those seen with stroke, hydrocephalus and tuberculoma.

DIAGNOSIS

An investigation of the differential diagnosis of tuberculous meningitis is important. PCR amplification of mycobacterial DNA, which in the case of TB meningitis has not been fully evaluated, usually requires a lumbar puncture examination. Those who are immunosuppressed may have an atypical CSF appearance, but this may include normal CSF examinations in occasional HIV individuals. Tuberculosis culture from CSF is required but may take up to 6 weeks before a positive culture result is available. Imaging studies may show a basal meningitis and hydrocephalus but these features are non-specific.[21]

Current advice suggests that the first 2 months of treatment should comprise quadruple therapy:

- Isoniazid oral/i.v. 10 mg/kg per day up to 300 mg; it is bactericidal and has good CNS penetration
- Pyrazinamide oral/i.v. 25 mg/kg per day up to 2.5 g/day
- Rifampicin high dosage as poor penetration, 10 mg/kg per day up to 600 mg
- Ethambutol i.v. high dosage as it is highly protein bound and therefore has poor penetration.

Streptomycin is used rarely. The toxicity of the agents must be monitored in terms of renal and liver function and the effect on other organs such as the eye.

There is increasing multidrug-resistant tuberculous meningitis, especially in the HIV-positive population, and so sensitivity is important. Some clinical trials suggest that steroids have a beneficial effect in some groups of patients.[22] Patients may require neurosurgical intervention for the treatment of hydrocephalus.

SUBDURAL EMPYEMA

This is a collection of pus between the dural and arachnoid space and usually is a consequence of middle ear or sinus disease. It may follow cranial osteomyelitis related to previous neurosurgery. Head trauma can also be responsible.

Individuals present acutely with headache, fever, neck stiffness, seizures and focal neurological symptoms. Meningeal signs and evidence of hemispheric dysfunction with sinusitis should suggest the diagnosis.

DIAGNOSIS

CT and MRI are both effective in demonstrating a fluid collection.

Surgical intervention, drainage and appropriate antibiotic regimens are required. Both Gram-positive, *Staphylococcus* and *Streptococcus*, and Gram-negative organisms may be implicated. Initial broad-spectrum cover should be narrowed to targeted treatment when the organism or organisms are known.

PROGNOSIS

This condition if left untreated is invariably fatal. With treatment, mortality is in the order of 20% but neurological sequelae are common.

EPIDURAL INFECTION

Cranial and spinal epidural abscess is an infection between skull and dura often as a consequence of osteomyelitis, from an orbital infection or malignancy. There is an occasional incidence following an epidural. It is similar to subdural empyema. The organism involved where a catheter or drain is implicated is often the same as that found at the skin; hence *S. aureus* is frequently responsible.

PRESENTATION

Inflammation is commonly, but not always, present on the back, and is usually generalised to the area of the back involved. There may be local tenderness over the site associated with redness of the catheter insertion site. Fever is common. Initially mild neurological deficit may rapidly progress leading to para/quadriparesis.

Blood cultures may be positive and may indicate the organism.

DIAGNOSIS

CT and MRI are both effective in diagnosis.

Spinal decompression and drainage are urgently required. This is usually a nosocomial infection and therefore resistant organisms are commonly found. Antibiotics should be specific for the organisms involved and may need to be continued for prolonged periods, often weeks, to eradicate the infection.

Where there have been neurological symptoms and signs prior to surgery, residual deficit is common. In one series, the recovery rate for patients with paresis/plegia after lumbar epidural abscess was 50%, whereas no patients with paresis/plegia following a thoracic abscess recovered. The majority of long-term survivors had severe neurological deficits.

CEREBRAL VENOUS AND SAGITTAL SINUS THROMBOSIS

Venous and sinus thrombosis may occur in the context of infection; in particular meningitis, and epidural or subdural abscess. It may also be secondary to facial or dental infection. It may have no septic aetiology but can occur either as an isolated event or in association with prothrombotic problems such as diabetic ketoacidosis, MDMA (ecstasy) abuse, oral contraceptives and hereditary prothrombotic conditions in pregnancy.[23]

Clinical signs at presentation include:

- headache
- focal neurological deficits in particular cranial nerves
- seizures
- papilloedema.

The diagnostic sensitivity of CT, MRI and digital subtract angiography are 59%, 86% and 100%, respectively, but MRI with magnetic resonance angiography reaches 96% (**Fig. 54.3**).

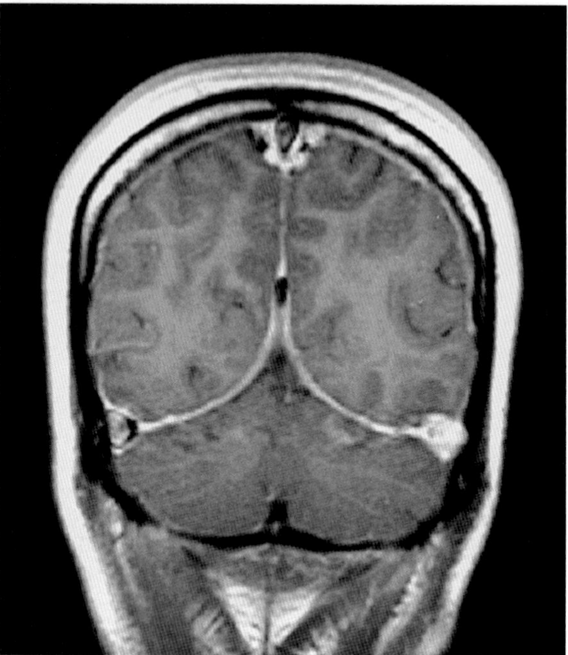

Figure 54.3 Magnetic resonance imaging (MRI) of superior sagittal sinus thrombosis: coronal T1-weighted post-contrast MRI; patient developed a sinus thrombosis following protracted labour and delivery.

TREATMENT

- Treat the primary infection if present.
- Anticoagulants are the mainstay of treatment. Paradoxically there are often areas of intracerebral haemorrhage in patients with sinus thrombosis. The presence of such haemorrhages is not a contraindication to anticoagulation.

BRAIN ABSCESS

AETIOLOGY

Direct spread from bone or dura or may be via haematogenous spread. Predisposition includes cranial trauma, neurosurgery, chronic ear or sinus disease, suppurative lung disease, congenital heart disease and recurrent sepsis. Immunological compromise may predispose to more exotic organisms, but more common organisms include *Staphylococcus* spp. associated with trauma, and *Streptococcus*, *Bacteroides* and Gram-negative bacteria, which are common with lung disease or recurrent sepsis.

PRESENTATION

Severe headache, vomiting, obtundation, seizures and focal neurological signs. Neck stiffness is often absent. Clinical sepsis may not be obvious.

DIAGNOSIS (**FIG. 54.4**)

- An obvious primary source of infection
- Evidence of raised ICP
- Focal cerebral or cerebellar signs.

INVESTIGATIONS

- Lumbar puncture is potentially dangerous and contraindicated
- CT scan – contrast will usually show a ring-enhancing lesion
- MRI
- Assessment of the patient's immune status
- Specific blood tests such as HIV and toxoplasma serology.

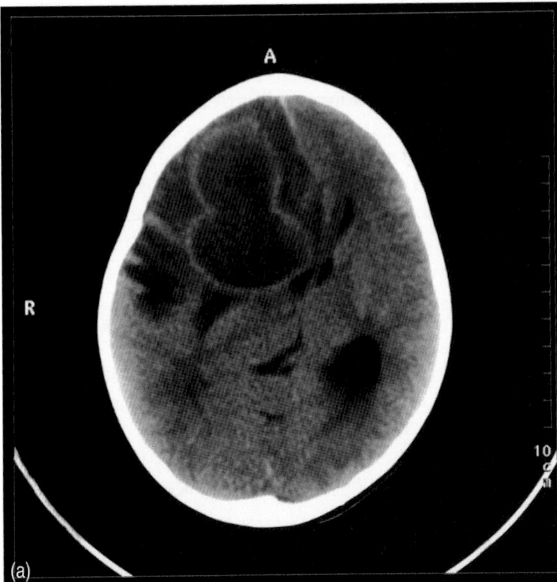

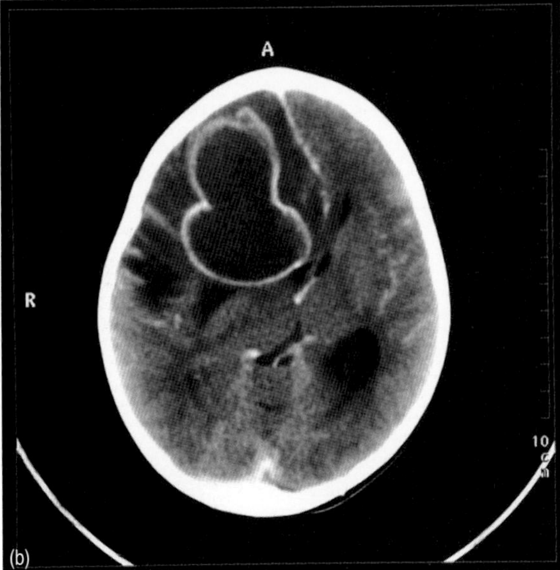

Figure 54.4 Abscess: (a) pre-contrast and (b) post-contrast.

TREATMENT

Indications for surgery include large single lesions, relief of raised ICP and the need for tissue diagnosis.

Antibiotics are the mainstay of therapy. If the organism is known then the treatment should be specific. In the absence of a definitive organism, penicillin plus chloramphenicol (as for meningitis) and metronidazole 500 mg i.v. 8-hourly or 500 mg rectally 12-hourly should be empirical therapy. Administer cefotaxime 1–2 g i.v. 6–8-hourly and metronidazole 500 mg i.v. 8-hourly. If there is a recent history of trauma or neurosurgery, then a regimen that will cover *Staphylococcus* should he used. Antibiotics should be continued for 3–6 weeks.

Supportive therapy limits morbidity, which is nevertheless high. Mortality from cerebral abscesses is still 10–20%.[24]

LYME DISEASE

This is a tick-borne multisystem disease with dermatological, cardiological, rheumatological and neurological effects caused by the spirochaete *Borrelia burgdorferi*.

A history of potential exposure should be sought but is not always found. Usually the disease presents as an acute febrile illness with gastrointestinal upset, but it may present in a variable fashion neurologically including as a cranial neuropathy (commonly a facial palsy) or as meningo-encephalitis or radiculopathy. It may also cause lymphocytic meningitis and may have been diagnosed as 'viral' meningitis in the past. A variety of longer-term neurological sequelae have been described.[25]

INVESTIGATIONS

CSF

White cell count is equivocal but may be raised. Protein is normal or marginally raised and sugar is normal or marginally low. Serology and ELISA may be difficult. PCR may be helpful. It may have characteristic MRI appearances. Vaccination is the only empirically demonstrated method to prevent Lyme disease.

TREATMENT

Beta-lactam antibacterials such as penicillin V, amoxicillin and cefuroxime are effective first-line treatment. The optimal duration of treatment is not known, but 10–21 days is recommended.[26,27] Practice parameters for the treatment of nervous system Lyme disease state that nervous system infection responds favourably to penicillin, ceftrixaone, cefotaxime and doxycycline. Prolonged treatment with antibiotic appears to have no benefit in preventing post-Lyme syndrome.

OTHER DISEASES

There are several other diseases that may have an encephalopathic component. Cerebral malaria is dealt with elsewhere. *Legionella* may lead to subclinical or clinical neurological manifestations, ranging from headache to coma or encephalopathy usually seen in conjunction with pneumonia, in addition to possible renal impairment. Similarly, *Mycoplasma* has been associated with an encephalitic picture characterised by impaired consciousness and seizures, and by normal or non-specific neuroradiological findings. Occasionally, symmetrical lesions in the putamen and its external surrounding areas have been seen.

Septic encephalopathy has been described as a common complication in the critically ill, presenting in a panoply of ways, from the agitated confused state seen in acute sepsis through to profound loss of consciousness. The aetiology is almost certainly multifactorial involving changes in cerebral blood flow, alteration in oxygen extraction, cerebral oedema, disruption of the blood–brain barrier, the presence and effects of diverse inflammatory mediators and abnormal neurotransmitter activity. Deranged liver and renal function contribute. It is a syndrome of exclusion based on observation and circumstantial evidence. The EEG is usually abnormal with decreased fast activity and an increase of slow-wave activity, but the findings are not pathognomonic. There are no specific treatments. In general terms, outcome appears to correlate with the management of the underlying sepsis.[28]

Access the complete references list online at http://www.expertconsult.com

1. Davies N, Thwaites G. Infections of the nervous system. Pract Neurol 2011;11:121–31.
10. Van de Beek D, de Gans J, McIntyre P, et al. Corticosteroids for acute bacterial meningitis. Cochrane Database Syst Rev 2007;1:CD004405.
16. Granerod J, Davies N. Encephalitis: recent advances and challenges ahead. ACNR 2012;12(5):8–11.
17. Solomon T, Michael BD, Smith PE, et al; National Encephalitis Guidelines Development and Stakeholder Groups. Management of suspected viral encephalitis in adults – Association of British Neurologists and British Infection Association national guidelines. J Infection 2012;64(4):347–73.
23. de Bruijn SF, Stam J, Koopman MM, et al. Case-control study of risk of cerebral sinus thrombosis in oral contraceptive users and in carriers of hereditary prothrombotic conditions. The Cerebral Venous Sinus Thrombosis Study Group. BMJ 1998;316:589–92.
27. Halperin JJ, Shapiro D, Logigian E, et al. Practice parameter: treatment of nervous system Lyme disease (an evidence-based review): report of the Quality Standards Subcommittee of the American Academy of Neurology. Neurology 2007;69:91–102.

55

Tetanus

Jeffrey Lipman

Tetanus is a preventable, often Third-World disease frequently requiring expensive First-World technology to treat. It is an acute, often fatal disease caused by exotoxins produced by *Clostridium tetani,* and is characterised by generalised muscle rigidity, autonomic instability and sometimes convulsions.

EPIDEMIOLOGY

Recently, tetanus has become a disease of the elderly and debilitated in developed countries, as younger people are likely to have been immunised.[1] In the USA, its incidence decreased from 0.23 per 100 000 in 1955 to 0.04 per 100 000 in 1975, and remained stable thereafter.[1] It is reported that 1 million people annually are afflicted with tetanus signifying a global incidence about 18 per 100 000 population, with an estimated world mortality of about 500 000 per year. [2] It is geographically prevalent in rural areas with poor hygiene and medical services. Thus, tetanus remains a significant public health problem in the developing world, primarily because of poor access to immunisation programmes. In addition, modern management requires ICU facilities, which are rarely available in the most severely afflicted populations.[3] Therefore, tetanus will continue to afflict developing populations in the foreseeable future.

PATHOGENESIS

C. tetani is an obligate anaerobic, spore-bearing, Gram-positive bacillus. Spores exist ubiquitously in soil and in animal and human faeces. After gaining access to devitalised tissue, spores proliferate in the vegetative form, producing the toxins tetanospasmin and tetanolysin. Tetanospasmin is extremely potent; an estimated 240 g could kill the entire world population,[4] with 0.01 mg being lethal for an average man. Tetanolysin is of little clinical importance.

C. tetani is non-invasive. Hence, tetanus occurs only when the spores gain access to tissues to produce vegetative forms. The usual mode of entry is through a puncture wound or laceration, although tetanus may follow surgery, burns, gangrene, chronic ulcers, dog bites, injections such as with drug users, dental infection, abortion and childbirth. Tetanus neonatorum usually follows infection of the umbilical stump. The injury itself may be trivial, and in 20% of cases there is no history or evidence of a wound.[1] Germination of spores occurs in oxygen-poor media (e.g. in necrotic tissue), with foreign bodies, and with infections. *C. tetani* infection remains localised, but the exotoxin tetanospasmin is distributed widely via the bloodstream, taken up into motor nerve endings, and transported into the nervous system. Here, it affects motor neuron end-plates in skeletal muscle (to decrease release of acetylcholine), the spinal cord (with dysfunction of polysynaptic reflexes) and the brain (with seizures, inhibition of cortical activity and autonomic dysfunction). Tetanus is not communicable from person to person.

The symptoms of tetanus appear only after tetanospasmin has diffused from the cell body through the extracellular space, and gained access to the presynaptic terminals of adjacent neurons.[1] Tetanospasmin spreads to all local neurons, but is preferentially bound by inhibitory interneurons – that is, glycinergic terminals in the spinal cord, and γ-aminobutyric acid (GABA) terminals in the brain.[3] Its principal effect is to block these inhibitory pathways. Hence stimuli to and from the central nervous system (CNS) are not 'damped down'.

ACTIVE IMMUNOPROPHYLAXIS[1,2,4]

Natural immunity to tetanus does not occur. Tetanus may both relapse and recur. Victims of tetanus must be *actively immunised.* Tetanus toxoid is a cheap and effective vaccine that is thermally stable.[4] It is a non-toxic derivative of the toxin that, nevertheless, elicits and reacts with antitoxic antibody. By consensus, an antibody titre of 0.01 U/mL serum is protective.[5] In a damped-down form, tetanus has been reported in a few victims with much higher serum antibody titres.[1]

In adults, a full immunisation course consists of three toxoid doses, given at an optimal interval of 6–12 weeks between the first and second doses, and 6–12 months between the second and third doses. A single dose will offer no immediate protection in the unimmunised, but a full course should never be repeated. Neonates have immunity from maternal antibodies. Children over 3 months should be actively immunised, and need four doses in total. Two or more doses to child-bearing females over 14 years will protect any child produced within the next 5 years. Pregnant females who are not immunised should thus be given two spaced-out doses 2 weeks to 2 months before delivery. Booster doses should be given routinely every 10 years.

Side-effects of tetanus toxoid are uncommon and not life-threatening. They are associated with excessive levels of antibody due to indiscriminate use.[6] Common reactions include urticaria, angio-oedema and diffuse, indurated swelling at the site of injection.

CLINICAL PRESENTATION[1,2,5,7]

The incubation period (i.e. time from injury to onset of symptoms) varies from 2 to 60 days. The period of onset (i.e. from first symptom to first spasm) similarly varies. Nearly all cases (90%), however, present within 15 days of infection.[7] The incubation period and the period of onset are of prognostic importance, with shorter times signifying more severe disease.

Presenting symptoms are pain and stiffness. Stiffness gives way to rigidity, and there is difficulty in mouth opening - trismus or lockjaw. Most (75%) non-neonatal generalised tetanus cases present with trismus.[7] Rigidity becomes generalised, and facial muscles produce a characteristic clenched-teeth expression called risus sardonicus. The disease progresses in a descending fashion. Typical spasms, with flexion and adduction of the arms, extension of the legs and opisthotonos, are very painful and may be so intense that fractures and tendon separations occur.[1] Spasms are caused by external stimuli (e.g. noise and pressure). As the disease worsens, even minimal stimuli produce more intense and longer-lasting spasms. Spasms are life-threatening when they involve the larynx and/or diaphragm.

Neonatal tetanus presents most often on day 7 of life,[5] with a short (1-day) history of failure of the infant to feed. The neonate displays typical spasms that can be easily misdiagnosed as convulsions of another aetiology. In addition, because these infants vomit (as a result of the increased intra-abdominal pressure) and are dehydrated (because of their inability to swallow), meningitis and sepsis are often considered first.

Autonomic dysfunction occurs in severe cases,[7-9] and begins a few days after the muscle spasms. (The toxin has further to diffuse to reach the lateral horns of the spinal cord.) There is increased basal sympathetic tone, manifesting as tachycardia and bladder and bowel dysfunction. Also, episodes of marked sympathetic overactivity involving both α- and β-receptors occur. Vascular resistance, central venous pressure and, usually, cardiac output are increased, manifesting clinically as labile hypertension, pyrexia, sweating, and pallor and cyanosis of the digits.[8] These episodes are usually of short duration and may occur without any provocation. They are caused by reduced inhibition of postsynaptic sympathetic fibres in the intermediolateral cell column, as evidenced by very high circulating norepinephrine (noradrenaline) concentrations.[1,9] Other postulated causes of this variable sympathetic overactivity include loss of inhibition of the adrenal medulla with increased epinephrine (adrenaline) secretion, direct inhibition by tetanospasmin of the release of endogenous opiates, and increased release of thyroid hormone.[1,3]

The role of the parasympathetic nervous system is debatable. Episodes of bradycardia, low peripheral vascular resistance, low central venous pressure and profound hypotension are seen, and are frequently preterminal.[8] Sudden and repeated cardiac arrests occur, particularly in intravenous drug abusers.[9] These events have been attributed to total withdrawal of sympathetic tone, since it is unresponsive to atropine.[10] However, they may be caused by catecholamine-induced myocardial damage[9,11] or direct brainstem damage.[9] Whatever the mechanism, patients afflicted with the autonomic dysfunction of tetanus are at risk of sudden death.

Local tetanus is an uncommon mild form of tetanus with a mortality of 1%. The signs and symptoms are confined to a limb or muscle, and may be the result of immunisation. *Cephalic tetanus* is also rare. It results from head and neck injuries, eye infections and otitis media. The cranial nerves, especially the seventh, are frequently involved and the prognosis is poor. This form may progress to a more generalised form. Tetanus in heroin addicts seems to be severe, with a high mortality, but numbers are small.[9,12]

DIAGNOSIS

The diagnosis is clinical and often straightforward. There are no laboratory tests specific to tetanus. *C. tetani* is cultured from the wound in only a third of cases. The most common differential diagnosis is dystonic reaction to tricyclics. Other differential diagnoses include strychnine poisoning, local temporomandibular disease, local oral disease, convulsions, tetany, intracranial infections or haemorrhage and psychiatric disorders.

MANAGEMENT

Initial objectives of treatment are to neutralise circulating toxin (i.e. passive immunisation) and prevent it from entering peripheral nerves (i.e. wound care), as well as eradicating the source of the toxin (i.e. extensive surgery, hygiene, wound care and antibiotics). Treatment then aims to minimise the effect of toxin already bound in the nervous system, and to provide general supportive care.

PASSIVE IMMUNISATION[1,2,13]

Human antitetanus immunoglobulin (HIG) has now largely replaced antitetanus serum (ATS) of horse origin, as it is less antigenic. HIG will at best neutralise only circulating toxin, but does not affect toxins already fixed in the CNS (i.e. it does not ameliorate symptoms already present).

Current recommendations for HIG in tetanus are 500 IU.[2] It has been suggested that unimmunised patients or those whose immunisation status is unknown should be given HIG on presentation with contaminated wounds. No controlled study has shown this to be more effective than wound toilet and penicillin administration.

Intrathecal administration of antitetanus toxin is still controversial[14,15] with the most recent meta-analysis reporting benefit. [16] Moreover, suitable intrathecal preparations are not widely available. Side-effects of human antitetanus toxin include fever, shivering and chest or back pains. Cardiovascular parameters need to be monitored, and the infusion may need to be stopped temporarily if significant tachycardia and hypotension are present.[1,6,13] If HIG is not available, equine ATS can be used after testing and desensitisation.[1]

ERADICATION OF THE ORGANISM

WOUND CARE

Once HIG has been given, the infected site should be thoroughly cleaned and all necrotic tissue extensively debrided.

ANTIBIOTICS

Tetanus spores are destroyed by antibiotics. The vegetative form (bacillus) is sensitive to antibiotics in vitro. However, in vivo efficacy depends on the antibiotic concentration at the wound site, and large doses may be required, Recommended antibiotic regimens include:

- *metronidazole 500 mg IV 8-hourly for 10 days:* the drug has a spectrum of activity against anaerobes, is able to penetrate necrotic tissue, and has been shown to be more effective than penicillin in this situation[17]
- *penicillin G 1–3 Mu IV 6-hourly for 10 days:* penicillin is a GABA antagonist in the CNS,[18] and may aggravate the spasms; nevertheless, it is still often used in this situation
- *erythromycin:* this has been used, but should not be routinely used.

SUPPRESSION OF EFFECTS OF TETANOSPASMIN

CONTROLLING MUSCLE SPASMS

In the early stages of tetanus, the patient is most at risk from laryngeal and other respiratory muscle spasm. Therefore, if muscle spasms are present, the airway should be urgently secured by endotracheal intubation or tracheostomy. If respiratory muscles are affected, mechanical ventilation should be instituted. In severe tetanus, spasms usually preclude effective ventilation, and muscle relaxants may be required. Any muscle relaxant can be used.[19] Heavy sedation alone may prevent muscle spasms and improve autonomic dysfunction (see below).

MANAGEMENT OF AUTONOMIC DYSFUNCTION

Autonomic dysfunction manifests in increased basal sympathetic activity[20] and episodic massive outpourings of catecholamines.[20–22] During these episodes, norepinephrine and epinephrine may be up to 10 times basal levels.[20,21] The clinical picture is variable.[22] Hypertension, tachycardia and sweating do not always occur concurrently.

Traditionally, a combination of alpha- and beta-adrenergic blockers has been used to treat sympathetic overactivity. Phenoxybenzamine, phentolamine, bethanidine and chlorpromazine have been used as α-receptor blockers. Ganglion blockers and nitroprusside have occasionally been used. Propranolol and labetalol have had limited success.[23–25] However, unopposed beta-adrenergic blockade cannot be advised. Deaths from acute congestive cardiac failure have resulted.[23,24] Removal of beta-mediated vasodilatation in limb muscle causes a rise in systemic vascular resistance, and beta-blocked myocardium may not be able to maintain adequate cardiac output. Also, with beta blockade, hypotension follows when sympathetic overactivity abates. Esmolol, a very short-acting beta-adrenergic blocker given IV, has been reported to be useful.[26] However, although sympathetic crises can be controlled by esmolol, catecholamine levels remain raised.[22] This raises concern because excessive catecholamine secretion is associated with myocardial damage.[11]

From the above, it appears more logical to decrease catecholamine output. This can be done with sedatives. Benzodiazepines and morphine are successfully used.[21] Morphine and diazepam act centrally to minimise the effects of tetanospasmin. Morphine probably acts by replacing deficient endogenous opioids.[1] Benzodiazepines increase the affinity and efficacy of GABA.[1] Very large doses of these agents (e.g. diazepam 3400 mg/day[21] and morphine 235 mg/day [27]) may be required, and are well tolerated.

Magnesium has been used as an adjunct to sedation,[21,28] now confirmed by a large trial.[29] Magnesium sulphate infusions to keep serum concentrations between 2.5 and 4.0 mmol/L have decreased systemic vascular resistance and pulse rate, with a small decrease in cardiac output.[21,28] In animal studies, magnesium inhibits release of epinephrine and norepinephrine, and reduces the sensitivity of receptors to these neurotransmitters. Magnesium also has a marked neuromuscular-blocking effect, and may reduce the intensity of muscle spasms. Nevertheless, it could not be shown to decrease the need for mechanical ventilation.[29] However, magnesium sulphate must be used with sedatives,[21] and calcium supplements may be needed when it is infused. Anecdotally, clonidine, a central α_2-stimulant, has successfully produced sedation with control of autonomic dysfunction.[30] It seems sensible to attempt to make use of the central nervous system effects of an α_2-adrenergic agonist, namely sedation and vasodilatation.[31] Intrathecal baclofen has produced similar beneficial results in a series of cases, but significant respiratory depression occurred in a third.[32] When given intrathecally, baclofen can diminish spasms and spasticity, allowing for a reduction in sedative and paralysis requirements.[33]

SUPPORTIVE TREATMENT

Steps should be taken to prevent contractures, nosocomial pneumonias and deep-vein thrombosis. The patient (including the mother if a neonate is afflicted) must be actively immunised. Where possible, supportive psychotherapy should be offered to both patient and family.

COMPLICATIONS[1,5,7,11,34]

Muscle spasms disappear after 1–3 weeks, but residual stiffness may persist. Although most survivors recover completely by 6 weeks, cardiovascular complications, including cardiac failure, arrhythmias, pulmonary oedema and hypertensive crises, can be fatal. No obvious cause of death can be found at autopsy in up to 20% of deaths. Other complications include those associated with factors shown in **Box 55.1**.

Box 55.1 Factors contributing to death in tetanus

Hypoxia
Complications of mechanical ventilation
Myoglobinuria and its attendant problems
Sepsis, particularly pneumonia
Fluid and electrolyte problems (including inappropriate antidiuretic hormone secretion)
Deep-vein thrombosis and embolic phenomena
Bed sores
Bony fractures

OUTCOME

Recovery from tetanus is thought to be complete. However, in 25 non-neonatal patients followed for up to 11 years,[35] 15 were reported to have one or more abnormal neurological features such as intellectual or emotional changes, fits and myoclonic jerks, sleep disturbance and decreased libido. Of the 10 apparently normal survivors, 6 had electroencephalogram changes. Some of these symptoms resolved within 2 years.

Mortality figures depend on the availability of intensive care. In neonates, the mortality from African countries with no ICU facilities can be up to 80% of cases, but falls to about 10% when artificial ventilation is used. In the USA, mortality in non-neonates relates directly to age, with rates from 0% in patients under 30 years rising to 50% in those 60 years or older. An average of 10% mortality would seem to be reasonable for most ICUs. However, as this disease is easily and completely preventable, loss of life is unacceptable.

Access the complete references list online at http://www.expertconsult.com

1. Bleck TP. Tetanus: Pathophysiology, management and prophylaxis. Dis Mon 1991;37(9):556–603.
2. Afshar M, Raju M, Ansell D, et al. Narrative review: tetanus – a health threat after natural disasters in developing countries. Ann Intern Med 2011; 154:329–35.
8. Kerr JH, Corbett JL, Prys-Roberts C, et al. Involvement of the sympathetic nervous system in tetanus. Lancet 1968;2:236–41.
15. Miranda-Filho Dde B, Ximenes RA, Barone AA, et al. Randomised controlled trial of tetanus treatment with antitetanus immunoglobulin by the intrathecal or intramuscular route. Br Med J 2004;328:615–17.
16. Kabura L, Ilibagiza D, Menten J, et al. Intrathecal vs. intramuscular administration of human antitetanus immunoglobulin or equine tetanus antitoxin in the treatment of tetanus: a meta-analysis. Trop Med Int Health 2006;11:1075–81.
17. Ahmadsyah I, Salim A. Treatment of tetanus: An open study to compare the efficacy of procaine penicillin and metronidazole. Br Med J 1985;291:648–50.
23. Buchanan N, Smit L, Cane RD, et al. Sympathetic overactivity in tetanus: Fatality associated with propanolol. Br Med J 1978;2:254–5.
27. Rocke DA, Wesley AG, Pather M, et al. Morphine in tetanus – the management of sympathetic nervous system overactivity. S Afr Med J 1986;70:666–8.
29. Thwaites CL, Yen LM, Loan HT, et al. Magnesium sulphate for treatment of severe tetanus: a randomised controlled trial. Lancet 2006;368:1436–43.

56

Delirium

Timothy M Alce, Valerie Page and Marcela P Vizcaychipi

Delirium is an acute confusional state common in critically ill patients, particularly those who require ventilation. It is an independent predictor of death and long-term cognitive decline. Prompt identification and treatment of delirium in patients aims to improve patient outcomes reducing morbidity, length of stay in ICU and mortality as well as associated financial costs of intensive care.

DEFINITION

Delirium, as defined by the American Psychiatric Association in the Diagnostic and Statistical Manual of Mental Disorders, 4th edition, text revised (DSM-IV-TR), is a disturbance of consciousness that develops over a short period of time, fluctuates and is associated with perceptual changes such as hallucinations (**Box 56.1**).[1] Consciousness in this context consists of arousal and cognition - awake and aware.

Three clinical subtypes of delirium are recognised: hypoactive, hyperactive and mixed, each distinguishable by psychomotor behaviour and arousal. Hypoactive delirium, which is the most common subtype, is often unrecognised or misdiagnosed as depression or sedation. Patients will appear cooperative and docile but will show signs of inattention and will be unable to organise thoughts. Pure hyperactive delirium, in contrast, is much less common (approximately 5%) but more familiar to the clinician and recognisable. Patients will be obviously agitated and aggressive, being uncooperative and combative. These patients are more likely to have hallucinations. Mixed delirium exists when patients fluctuate between hypoactive and hyperactive subtypes.

Delirium tremens, a state of confusion, agitation and hallucinations specifically relates to delirium following alcohol withdrawal.

HISTORICAL PERSPECTIVE

The first records of delirium are from the 5th century BC by Hippocrates who described delirium in an acutely confused patient using the terms phrenitis (frenzy) and lethargus. Da Medicina, a 1st century BC treatise by Aulus Cornelius Celsus used well into the 15th century as a source of medical wisdom, has the first written entry of delirium to describe the acutely confused state. The word delirium comes from the latin *de* away from + *lira* furrow in a field, hence literally meaning *going away from the ploughed track.* Until relatively recently those ICU patients who were recognised as delirious were described as either having an encephalopathy or ICU psychosis.

ICU INCIDENCE AND RELEVANCE

The highest incidence rates of delirium of all clinical areas in the hospital, including orthopaedic/care of the elderly wards, is the ICU. Delirium can occur in up to 69% of ventilated patients in the UK.[2] Delirium is an independent predictor of mortality.[3] Compared with case-matched critically ill patients without delirium, those with delirium have three times higher 6-month mortality following ICU admission.[3] Delirium is known to be associated with long-term cognitive decline and early dementia and results in a three-fold increase in the risk of discharge to long-term care.[4] Patients with delirium in ICU are nine times more likely to experience some degree of cognitive impairment following discharge compared with non-delirious ICU patients.[3] In specific risk conditions such as Alzheimer disease the development of delirium has been shown to accelerate cognitive decline.

Clearly, delirium has implications for quality of life and independence of patients and their relatives. Patients with delirium have longer ICU and hospital stays. Moreover, there are increased ICU costs (1.4 fold) and increased overall hospital costs (1.3 fold).[5]

PATHOPHYSIOLOGY

The pathophysiology of delirium is ill defined but there are a number of theories regarding the pathological changes in the brain that result in and from delirium. These range from neuroinflammation with TNFα activation of microglia, impaired oxidative metabolism, altered cerebral blood flow, increased blood–brain barrier permeability, thalamic dysfunction and aberrant levels of large neutral amino acids.[6,7]

It is likely that several mechanisms contribute to the development of delirium, which then results in a common pathway of neurotransmitter imbalance and

Box 56.1 DSM-IV-TR definition of delirium

1. Altered consciousness: reduced clarity of awareness of environment with reduced ability to focus, sustain or shift attention
2. Change in cognition: disorientation, memory disturbance, problem-solving impairment, development of perceptual disturbance
3. Rapid onset (hours to days) and tendency to fluctuate during the day
4. Evidence the condition is caused by physiological consequences of a clinical condition or drug withdrawal/ overdose

resultant cholinergic hypoactivity.[8,9] There is then, inevitably, a relative state of dopamine excess, which can also cause deterioration in attention or consciousness. The interlinking role of acetylcholine and dopamine makes it difficult to ascertain which of these imbalances is primarily responsible for delirium.

Other theories relate to the availability of tryptophan, a metabolic precursor of serotonin, which may play a role since both increased and decreased levels of serotonin are seen in delirium. It is also possible that there is a genetic component for developing delirium. Apolipoprotein E4 (ApoE4) genotype, rather than ApoE2 or ApoE3, is a susceptibility factor for Alzheimer disease possibly by being less able to suppress cerebral inflammation than the other isoforms. In all of these mechanisms of the cause of delirium, the data are conflicting.[10,11]

RISK FACTORS

The numerous risk factors for delirium fall in to two main categories: predisposing (non-modifiable) and precipitating (both modifiable and non-modifiable) (**Box 56.2**). It is important to realise that the risk of delirium increases with the number of risk factors to which the patient is exposed,[12] and a frail, elderly patient with many predisposing factors may develop delirium from only a minor precipitating factor.

The PRE-DELIRIC model described by van den Boogaard et al[13] has been developed to help predict the likelihood that a patient admitted to ICU will develop delirium based on risk factors. It uses various parameters readily available during the first 24 hours of admission – for example, the Acute Physiology and Chronic Health Evaluation score (APACHE-II), metabolic acidosis, urea concentration, use of sedatives, etc. Using this model, the risk factors that confer the highest risk of developing delirium in ICU are coma (from any cause), sedatives and infection.

Box 56.2 Risk factors for developing delirium in intensive care

ICU delirium modifiable risk factors		Non-modifiable risk factors
Infection	Hyponatraemia	Age, especially over 65
Anticholinergic drugs	Hypoxia	Cognitive impairment
	Hypercarbia	
Opiates	Acidosis	Dementia
Pain	Polypharmacy	
Immobility	Sleep disturbance	Depression
Dehydration or constipation	Use of physical restraints	Genetic factors
		Institutionalised residence
Sedative drugs	Use of bladder catheter	Liver impairment
Sensory impairment (visual/auditory)		

DIAGNOSIS/SCREENING

Diagnosis of delirium is challenging and difficult. In one study nurses detected daily delirium in only 34.8% of cases, with doctors detecting delirium in only 28%.[14] The key feature to detecting delirium is evidence of inattention. Delirious patients can appear to have normal mental status as they are often able to obey direct commands and will nod randomly to questions.

There are several delirium screening tools available to the clinician to assist in diagnosis of delirium, but few of them have been validated for use in ICU with intubated patients. The most widely used in critical care are the Confusion Assessment Model for ICU (CAM-ICU)[12] (**Fig. 56.1**) and the Intensive Care Delirium Screening Checklist (ICDSC).[15] These tools are designed for clinical use and have been validated for intubated patients. They are non-verbal, simple to use and require minimal training. CAM-ICU is a point-in-time assessment, whereas ICDSC uses information gathered over a nursing shift. These screening tools aim to detect the key features of delirium, which are inattention, disorganised thinking, altered level of arousal with or without hallucinations and altered sleep pattern in the case of ICDSC. Specificity and sensitivity for each of these tools in critically ill patients are 81% and 96% respectively (CAM-ICU)[16] and 99% and 66% respectively (ICDSC).[15] However, a cautionary note was sounded by van Eijk et al. who discovered in a multicentre trial that routine, daily use of CAM-ICU by nursing staff has a specificity of 98% but a sensitivity of only 47%.[17]

MANAGEMENT OF DELIRIUM

GENERAL MANAGEMENT

Initial management should aim at correcting the cause of delirium. If a medical condition has been the trigger or has caused delirium, it is likely that the patient will continue to be delirious, with all the associated neuroinflammation, neurotransmitter imbalance and alterations in cerebral blood flow, until the medical condition has successfully been treated. Reversal of the underlying cause is important and necessary examination and

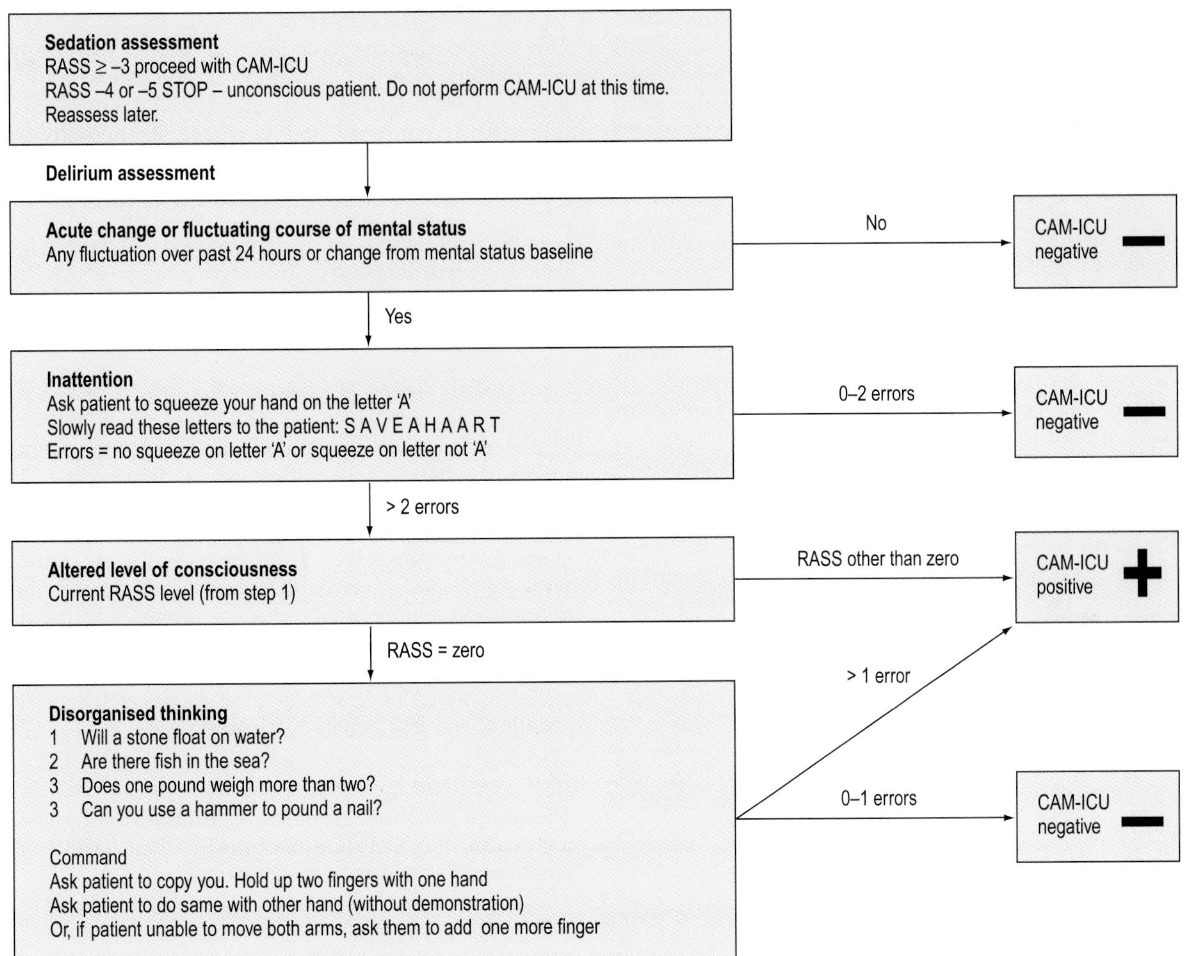

Figure 56.1 Confusion assessment method for ICU (CAM-ICU) flow chart. *(Reproduced with permission from E Wesley Ely, MD MPH.)*

investigations should be undertaken, bearing in mind that there may be more than one precipitating cause.

There are several simple and easy non-pharmacological measures, free from adverse effects, that can be usefully employed with the aim of preventing delirium or reducing its severity.[18] These include clear and firm communication with frequent verbal orientation clues, such as date, time and location. Involvement of relatives assists in giving the patient a sense of familiarity, security and control, and can give the clinician information about the patient's normal mental status before illness. Other environmental factors include keeping noise to a minimum, correcting sensory impairment with hearing aids or spectacles, if worn, and avoiding sleep disturbance by careful timing of treatments and interventions, and by promoting a normal sleep–wake cycle.

Other measures such as correcting electrolytes, restoring oxygenation, controlling febrile episodes, maintaining blood pressure within patient's normal range and treating constipation may be sufficient to treat delirium. Physical restraints, rarely used in the UK, are known to increase the risk of delirium. They should be avoided. Medical restraints, including urinary catheters, ECG leads within other monitoring tools, which will also impact the mobility of patients, should be removed as early as is prudent.

Pain control in critical care is important. Although opioids can be deliriogenic, higher doses of opiates are associated with a significantly lower risk of delirium in intensive care burns patients.[19] It is a difficult balancing act to weigh the risk of opioids precipitating delirium against suffering and possible delirium caused by pain.

Sedation plays a large role in delirium in ICU. All sedative drugs including propofol and fentanyl are likely to precipitate delirium. It is essential to have a sedation protocol with routine sedation scoring, sedation targets and daily sedation holds where appropriate.[20] How the sedatives are used, the type of sedative, the dose and patient susceptibility are all important considerations. Daily wake-ups combined with spontaneous breathing trials, as the patient clinical condition allows, have been shown to decrease mortality.[21] Deep sedation (i.e. RASS -3 (Richmond Agitation Sedation Scale)) in the first 48 hours of sedation and ventilation on intensive care has been associated with increased time to extubation and mortality.[22] Unless there is a clinical reason to keep a patient sedated (e.g. severe asthma) it is suggested that a daily sedation target of RASS 0 to −1 is appropriate.

It is also good practice to stop any unnecessary drugs, in particular benzodiazepines, steroids and drugs with anticholinergic activity including furosemide and digoxin. Early mobilisation of critically ill patients has been demonstrated to decrease delirium and improves outcomes.[23]

Clinical trials have attempted to address the question whether antipsychotics can be used in prevention of delirium.[24,25] Although these have shown positive effects on delirium, reducing either severity or duration, this has not been translated to an improvement in outcome. Thus, there is currently insufficient robust scientific evidence to recommend the use of prophylactic antipsychotics.

PHARMACOLOGICAL MANAGEMENT

Pharmacological treatment primarily involves the use of dopamine antagonists - typical and atypical antipsychotics.

HALOPERIDOL

Haloperidol is a butyrophenone with partial selectivity for dopamine D2 receptors. Its licensing is variable in different countries (i.v. haloperidol is not licensed in the US) but it is commonly used in critically ill patients, in the UK, where enteral absorption may be impaired and close monitoring is available.

Side-effects include sedation, autonomic effects and, more importantly, extrapyramidal symptoms (e.g. excessive salivation, dystonia). Akathisia, an unpleasant sensation of restlessness, may be confused for continuing agitation. Haloperidol should not be given to patients with Parkinson disease or with a family history of dystonia.

More serious side-effects are neuroleptic malignant syndrome and torsades de pointes, both potentially life threatening. Electrocardiogram (ECG) monitoring to check for QTc prolongation, which increases the risk of torsades, should be carried out prior to starting haloperidol and daily while the patient is receiving the drug. Haloperidol can be used cautiously with a QTc greater than 450 ms (or use an alternative drug) but should not be used at all if the QTc is over 500 ms.

Doses of haloperidol used clinically range from 0.5 mg to 10 mg, although 2.5–5 mg is more common. Maximum dose in 24 hours is 18 mg.

OLANZAPINE, QUETIAPINE, RISPERIDONE

Other antipsychotics have lower incidence of extrapyramidal side-effects. Olanzapine can be given both i.v. and intramuscularly. It is as effective as haloperidol in critically ill patients[25] and is a useful alternative if haloperidol is contraindicated.[26] The starting dose is usually 5 mg, up to 20 mg daily (10 mg in renal failure). For patients with dementia who are agitated, quetiapine and risperidone are recommended. Quetiapine has been shown to decrease delirium in a placebo-controlled trial[27] and risperidone was seen to be as effective as olanzapine in managing delirium.[28]

CLONIDINE, DEXMEDETOMIDINE

Alpha-2 agonists have a sedative effect without GABAergic activity, potentially reducing the requirements of sedation, which itself can be deliriogenic.

Clonidine is favoured by some clinicians if a patient is requiring large doses of sedatives due to agitation. A starting dose would be 1 μg/kg enterally or diluted with saline and given slowly intravenously. Dexmedetomidine, a more highly selective alpha-2 agonist but significantly more expensive, has recently been licensed for use in the UK as a sedative infusion. It may be beneficial in terms of length of time at targeted level of sedation, and less agitated delirium.[29]

ANTICHOLINESTERASES

The use of anticholinesterases, including rivastigmine, for treatment of delirium in critically ill patients is not recommended and may be harmful.[30]

BENZODIAZEPINES

Benzodiazepines should be used only for the treatment of delirium tremens resulting from alcohol withdrawal. A Cochrane review of benzodiazepines in delirium treatment concluded that their use is not indicated in non-alcohol-withdrawal agitated delirium.[31] Indeed, a study in critically ill burns patients revealed benzodiazepine exposure to be an independent risk factor with these patients approximately seven times more likely to develop delirium.[19] However, if agitation is severe and is putting the patient at risk, a *stat* dose of a benzodiazepine might be indicated for rapid control of the incident. Up to 2 mg i.v. of lorazepam every 4 hours may be of benefit. It has rapid onset, short duration of action and low risk of accumulation. Use a lower dose when administering to elderly patients and those with hepatic disease.

SUBSYNDROMAL DELIRIUM

Some patients will not present or progress to full-blown delirium but do have altered mental status. For instance, patients may be able to attend to a conversation while obviously hallucinating. Subsyndromal delirium can be

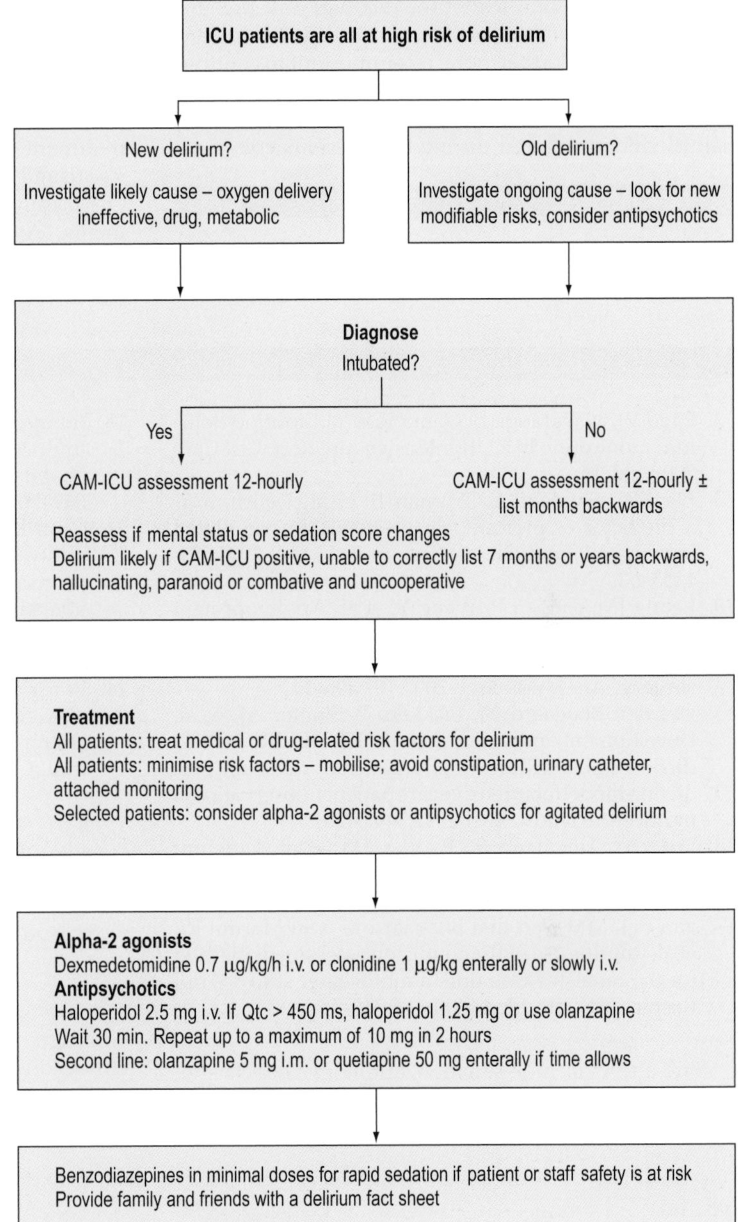

Figure 56.2 Critical care unit guideline for treatment of delirium.

diagnosed using the ICDSC and it has been associated with worse outcomes, although better than those in patients who demonstrate the full clinical syndrome.

PERSISTENT DELIRIUM

Elderly care patients may be left with persistent delirium, lasting beyond 3 months. The use of antipsychotics may be considered in individual cases, although generally care-of-the-elderly physicians avoid antipsychotics in their practice, relying on non-pharmacological interventions.

A possible ICU management protocol is outlined in **Figure 56.2**.

REMEMBER THE RELATIVES

ICU admission is already a distressing time for relatives and friends of patients and this is exacerbated by their witnessing the delirious patient. It is important to make the relatives aware that mental status changes in ICU are common and inform them that, although delirium can lead to cognitive impairment, generally any acute psychosis is transient. It is often useful to provide a delirium information leaflet for relatives and reassure them that clinicians are looking for and addressing any treatable cause. Furthermore, it is important to continue to support the patient after recovery. This may involve them talking about their experience, in particular any hallucinations endured during the delirious episode.

SUMMARY

Delirium is commonly encountered in ICU, particularly in intubated patients. Regular assessment of sedation and cognitive function will identify delirious patients early, facilitating prompt management. Delirium primarily requires correction of likely causes (medical or drug related) and minimising known risks (mobilising, avoiding constipation, etc.). First-line treatment of agitated delirium consists of antipsychotics, usually i.v. haloperidol provided QTc is <500 ms. Olanzapine or quetiapine are useful second-line treatments. Avoid benzodiazepines and anticholinergics. Keep friends and relatives, and, whenever possible, the patient informed.

Access the complete references list online at http://www.expertconsult.com

2. Page VJ, Navarange S, Gama S, et al. Routine delirium monitoring in a UK intensive care unit. Crit Care 2009;13:R16.
3. Ely EW, Shintani A, Truman B, et al. Delirium as a predictor of mortality in mechanically ventilated patients in the intensive care unit. JAMA 2004;291:1753–62.
10. Leung JM, Sands LP, Wang Y, et al. Apolipoprotein E e4 allele increases the risk of early postoperative delirium in older patients undergoing noncardiac surgery. Anesthesiology 2007;107:406–11.
13. van den Boogaard M, Pickkers P, Slooter AJ, et al. Development and validation of PRE-DELIRIC (PREdiction of DELIRium in ICu patients) delirium prediction model for intensive care patients: observational multicentre study. BMJ 2012;344:e420.
16. Luetz A, Heymann A, Radtke FM, et al. Different assessment tools for intensive care unit delirium: which score to use? Crit Care Med 2010;38:409–18.
17. van Eijk MM, van den Boogaard M, van Marum RJ, et al. Routine use of the confusion assessment method for the intensive care unit: a multicenter study. Am J Respir Crit Care Med 2011;184:340–4.
18. Inouye SK, Bogardus ST Jr, Charpentier PA, et al. A multicomponent intervention to prevent delirium in hospitalized older patients. N Engl J Med 1999;340:669–76.
21. Girard TD, Kress JP, Fuchs BD, et al. Efficacy and safety of a paired sedation and ventilator weaning protocol for mechanically ventilated patients in intensive care (Awakening and Breathing Controlled trial): a randomised controlled trial. Lancet 2008;371:126–34.
24. Wang W, Li HL, Wang DX, et al. Haloperidol prophylaxis decreases delirium incidence in elderly patients after noncardiac surgery: a randomized controlled trial. Crit Care Med 2012;40:731–9.

WEBSITES

Hospital Elderly Life Program, http://www.hospitalelderlylifeprogram.org
www.icudelirium.co.uk
www.icudelirium.org

57

Neuromuscular diseases in intensive care

George Skowronski and Manoj K Saxena

A number of disorders producing generalised neuromuscular weakness can require admission to the ICU, or complicate the course of ICU patients. These may involve:

- spinal anterior horn cells: motor neuron (or neurone) disease, poliomyelitis
- peripheral nerve conduction: Guillain–Barré syndrome (GBS) and related disorders
- the neuromuscular junction: myasthenia gravis, botulism
- muscle contraction: myopathies, periodic paralysis
- mixed disorders: intensive care acquired weakness.

Box 57.1 lists a differential diagnosis of muscle weakness in critically ill patients.

GUILLAIN–BARRÉ SYNDROME AND RELATED DISORDERS

In 1834 James Wardrop reported a case of ascending sensory loss and weakness in a 35-year-old man, leading to almost complete quadriparesis over 10 days, and complete recovery over several months.[1] In 1859, Landry described an acute ascending paralysis occurring in 10 patients, 2 of whom died. Guillain, Barré and Strohl in 1916[2] reported two cases of motor weakness, paraesthesiae and muscle tenderness in association with increased protein in the cerebrospinal fluid – lumbar puncture for cerebrospinal fluid (CSF) examination was first described only in the 1890s.

The many variants of this syndrome and the lack of specific diagnostic criteria have previously resulted in confusion in nomenclature. More recently clinical, electrical and laboratory criteria for the predominant variant – acute inflammatory demyelinating polyradiculopathy (AIDP) – are well described,[3] though 10–15% of cases do not fit these criteria. GBS is best regarded as a heterogeneous group of immunologically mediated disorders of peripheral nerve function.

INCIDENCE

Since the incidence of poliomyelitis has markedly declined due to mass immunisation programmes, GBS has become the major cause of rapid-onset flaccid paralysis in previously healthy people, with an incidence of approximately 1.7 per 100 000.[4] Epidemics have occurred in large populations exposed to viral illness or immunisation but immunosuppression and concurrent autoimmune disease may also be predisposing factors.[5–7] The disorder is commoner in males, and up to 4 times commoner in the elderly. No consistent seasonal or racial predilection has been demonstrated.[4]

AETIOLOGY

Most recent evidence supports the proposition that GBS is caused by immunologically mediated nerve injury.[8] Cell-mediated immunity, in particular, probably plays a significant role, and inflammatory cell infiltrates are often seen in association with demyelination, which is generally regarded as the primary pathological process. Antibodies to a number of nervous system components have been demonstrated in GBS patients, with most interest in recent years focusing on anti-ganglioside antibodies.

The precise mechanism of sensitisation is not known, but clinical associations suggest that antecedent infections or immunisations are commonly involved and two-thirds of cases are preceded by symptoms suggestive of respiratory or gastrointestinal infection. Infective agents implicated include influenza A, parainfluenza, varicella-zoster, Epstein–Barr, chickenpox, mumps, human immunodeficiency virus (HIV),[9] measles virus and *Mycoplasma. Campylobacter jejuni* gastroenteritis now appears to be the most common predisposing infection and may be associated with a more severe clinical course; 26–41% of GBS patients show evidence of recent *C. jejuni* infection.[10] Cytomegalovirus infection accounts for a further 10–22% of cases.[11] Immunisations against viral infections, tuberculosis, tetanus[12] and typhoid have all been reported to be associated with the onset of GBS, but most of these reports are anecdotal and of questionable aetiological significance; 65% of patients present within a few weeks of minor respiratory (43%) or gastrointestinal (21%) illness. Surveillance data following the 2009 H1N1 influenza epidemic suggested that the risk of GBS following immunisation was only slightly increased over baseline.[13]

Box 57.1 Differential diagnosis of muscle weakness in critically ill patients

Brainstem
Lower pontine hemorrhage or infarction (locked-in state)
Spinal cord
Transverse myelitis
Compression by tumour, abscess, or haemorrhage
Carcinomatous or lymphomatous meningitis
Peripheral nerve
Intensive care unit acquired neuropathy/neuromyopathy
Phrenic nerve injury during thoracic surgery
Guillain–Barré syndrome
Ingested toxins, including arsenic, thallium, cyanide
Neuromuscular junction
Delayed reversal of neuromuscular blockade
Myasthenia gravis
Lambert–Eaton syndrome
Botulism
Pesticide poisoning
Skeletal muscle
Acute necrotising myopathy
Steroid myopathy
Severe hypokalaemia, hypophosphataemia, and/or hypomagnesaemia
Acute alcoholic myopathy
Polymyositis or dermatomyositis
Toxic myopathy (colchicine, lovastatin, cocaine, bumetanide, amiodarone and others)
Intensive care unit acquired myopathy/neuromyopathy

Adapted with permission from Hansen-Flaschen J. Neuromuscular disorders of critical illness. UpToDate 2006; Ver. 14.3[93]

PATHOGENESIS[8]

The peripheral nerves of patients who have died of GBS show infiltration of the endoneurium by mononuclear cells, in a predominantly perivenular distribution. The inflammatory process may be distributed throughout the length of the nerves, but with more marked focal changes in the nerve roots, spinal nerves and major plexuses. Electron micrographs show macrophages actively stripping myelin from the bodies of Schwann cells and axons. In some cases, Wallerian degeneration of axons is also seen, and failure of regeneration in these cases may correspond with a poor clinical outcome.

The underlying immune response is complex and poorly understood, but serum from GBS patients produces myelin damage in vitro when complement is present.[14] Although antibodies to various glycolipids have been demonstrated in GBS, these are generally in low titre and can occasionally be seen in controls. Patients with recent *C. jejuni* infection have a high incidence of antibodies to the ganglioside GM1.[10] Antibodies to GD1a and GQ1b gangliosides are associated with the rarer AMAN and AMSAN variants (see below).[15] The basis of the effectiveness of plasma exchange and immunoglobulin therapy is likely to be blocking of demyelinating antibodies by several mechanisms.[16]

CLINICAL PRESENTATION

The majority of patients describe a minor illness in the 8 weeks prior to presentation, with a peak incidence 2 weeks beforehand. Approximately half the patients initially experience paraesthesiae, typically beginning in the hands and feet. One-quarter complain of motor weakness, and the remainder have both.[8] Motor weakness proceeds to flaccid paralysis, which becomes the predominant complaint. Objective loss of power and reduction or loss of tendon reflexes usually commence distally and ascend, but a more haphazard spread may occur. Cranial nerves are involved in 45% of cases, most commonly the facial nerve, followed by the glossopharyngeal and vagus nerves. One-third of patients require ventilatory support.

In the Miller–Fisher syndrome, a variant of GBS,[17] cranial nerve abnormalities predominate, with ataxia, areflexia and ophthalmoplegia as the main features. This is strongly associated with recent *C. jejuni* infection and with the presence of GQ1b antibodies.

Another subgroup of patients presents with a primarily axonal neuropathy – acute motor–sensory axonal neuropathy (AMSAN). In these cases motor and sensory axons appear to be the primary targets of immune attack, rather than myelin. These patients have a more fulminant and severe course, and there is again a strong association with *C. jejuni* infection.[18]

In typical GBS, sensory loss is generally mild, with paraesthesiae or loss of vibration and proprioception, but occasionally sensory loss, pain or hyperaesthesia can be prominent features. Autonomic dysfunction is common, and a major contributor to morbidity and mortality in ventilator-dependent cases.[19] Orthostatic or persistent hypotension, paroxysmal hypertension and bradycardia are all described, as are fatal ventricular tachyarrhythmias. Sinus tachycardia is seen in 30% of cases. Paralytic ileus, urinary retention and abnormalities of sweating are also commonly seen.

DIFFERENTIAL DIAGNOSIS

Most of the important alternative diagnoses are listed in **Box 57.2**. In patients with prolonged illness, the possibility of chronic inflammatory demyelinating polyradiculopathy (CIDP) should be considered.[20] In this condition, preceding viral infection is uncommon, the onset is more insidious and the course is one of slow worsening or stepwise relapses. Corticosteroids and plasma exchange are possibly effective in this disorder, but adequate studies of immunosuppressive drugs have not been carried out.

An intermediate *subacute* polyradiculopathy (SIDP) as well as a recurrent form of GBS are also described, and all of these variants may be part of the spectrum of a single condition. However, a purely motor axonal neuropathy (acute motor–axonal neuropathy, AMAN), which causes seasonal childhood epidemics mimicking classical GBS in China and elsewhere,[21] appears to be a distinct entity. Once again, this is strongly associated with *C. jejuni* infection.

Box 57.2 Diagnostic criteria for typical Guillain–Barré syndrome[3]

Features required for diagnosis
Progressive weakness in both arms and both legs
Areflexia
Features strongly supportive of the diagnosis
Progression over days to 4 weeks
Relative symmetry of symptoms
Mild sensory symptoms or signs
Cranial nerve involvement, especially bilateral weakness of facial muscles
Recovery beginning 2–4 weeks after progression ceases
Autonomic dysfunction
Absence of fever at onset
High concentration of protein in cerebrospinal fluid protein, with fewer than 10×10^6 cells/L
Typical electrodiagnostic features
Features excluding diagnosis
Diagnosis of botulism, myasthenia, poliomyelitis or toxic neuropathy
Abnormal porphyrin metabolism
Recent diphtheria
History or evidence of lead intoxication
Purely sensory syndrome, without weakness

INVESTIGATIONS

In over 90% of patients, CSF protein is increased (greater than 0.4 g/L), within 2 weeks of onset of symptoms. The level does not correlate with the clinical findings. A pleocytosis with lymphocytes and monocytes in the CSF may be seen in a small proportion of patients, especially later in the disease. Nerve conduction studies typically demonstrate reduced conduction velocity and prolonged distal latencies,[22] but there is no consensus on precise electrophysiological criteria for the various subtypes.[22] Severely reduced distal motor amplitude and a predominantly axonal pattern are associated with more severe disease and a guarded prognosis.

MANAGEMENT

Although the management of the patient with severe and protracted GBS provides a major challenge, the prognosis is generally good if complications can be treated early or avoided.

SPECIFIC THERAPY

Plasma exchange (plasmapheresis) is of value in GBS and in two trials a reduction in patients requiring mechanical ventilation, reduced duration of mechanical ventilation for those who required it, reduced time to motor recovery and time to walking without assistance were demonstrated.[23,24] Mortality, however, was not altered. Plasma exchange was most effective when carried out within 7 days of onset of symptoms. The currently recommended plasma exchange schedules consist of four exchanges of 1–2 plasma volumes each, over 1–2 weeks.[25] Adverse events are common, and some relate to the disease itself.[26] Fresh frozen plasma is reported to have more side-effects than albumin as the replacement fluid.[26]

Immunoglobulin therapy was as effective as plasmapheresis[27] and previous concerns of higher recurrence rates are probably unfounded. Because of its ease of use, many authorities now advocate immunoglobulin as the treatment of choice.[28] A dose of 2 g/kg body weight intravenously, over 2–5 days, is the current recommendation.[29]

About 10% of patients relapse after initial treatment with either plasmapheresis or immunoglobulin; most respond well to a further course. There appears to be no benefit in combining plasmapheresis and immunoglobulin treatments, or in crossing over from one to the other.[30]

A Cochrane review confirms that low- or high-dose corticosteroids are of no value,[31] and may even slow recovery. The combination of high-dose steroids with immunoglobulin does not affect the long-term outcome.[32]

SUPPORTIVE CARE

RESPIRATORY

In the spontaneously breathing patient, chest physiotherapy and careful monitoring of respiratory function are of paramount importance. Regular measurement of vital capacity is probably the best way to predict respiratory failure, and is more reliable than arterial blood gases.[33] The latter nevertheless remain a useful guide. Any patient with a vital capacity less than 15 mL/kg or 30% of the predicted level, or a rising arterial P_{CO_2} is likely to require mechanical ventilation.

Bulbar involvement should be carefully sought, as there is a significant risk of aspiration of upper airway secretions, gastric contents or ingested food. The cough reflex may be inadequate, and airway protection by tracheal intubation or tracheostomy is then required. Oral feeding should be stopped in any patient in whom bulbar involvement is suspected.

Mechanical ventilation is mandatory if coughing is inadequate, pulmonary collapse or consolidation develop, arterial blood gases are significantly abnormal, vital capacity is less than predicted tidal volume (approximately 10 mL/kg), or the patient is dyspnoeic, tachypnoeic or appears exhausted. Mechanical ventilation, if necessary, will probably be required for several weeks (although there is wide variation), and early tracheostomy should be considered.

CARDIOVASCULAR

Cardiac rhythm and blood pressure should be monitored. Sinus tachycardia is the commonest autonomic manifestation of GBS and usually requires no active treatment. Induction of anaesthesia appears particularly likely to induce serious arrhythmias. Use of suxamethonium may contribute significantly to this[34] and, as with many other neuromuscular disorders, should be avoided. Endotracheal suctioning has also been associated with serious arrhythmias. Cardiovascular instability may also be exacerbated by a number of other drugs (**Box 57.3**). These, likewise, should be avoided or used with great care.

Mild hypotension and bradycardia may require no treatment, particularly if renal and cerebral functions are maintained. However, blood volume expansion or inotropic drugs may be required in some cases. Hypertension is often transient, but occasionally requires appropriate drug therapy. Hypoxia, hypercarbia, pain and visceral distension should be excluded as causes.

FLUIDS, ELECTROLYTES AND NUTRITION

Paralytic ileus is not uncommon, especially immediately following the institution of mechanical ventilation, and a period of parenteral nutrition may be required. However, wherever possible, nasoenteric feeding should be instituted because of its significantly greater safety. Energy and fluid requirements are considerably reduced in these patients.

SEDATION AND ANALGESIA

In non-ventilated patients, sedation should be avoided because of the potential for worsening respiratory and upper airway function. In ventilated patients, sedation becomes less necessary as the patient becomes accustomed to the ventilator, but night sedation may help to preserve diurnal rhythms. Limb pain, particularly with passive movement, is very common and often quite severe. Quinine, minor and non-steroidal analgesics and antidepressant drugs may all be tried, but the pain can be difficult to control and opioids are often required. Methadone, transdermal fentanyl, gabapentin and tramadol have all been advocated.

GENERAL AND NURSING CARE

A comprehensive programme of physiotherapy should be implemented by nurses and physiotherapists, with careful attention to pressure area care, the maintenance of joint mobility and pulmonary function. Nosocomial infection should be actively sought with culture of urine and respiratory secretions at least twice weekly. Sites of vascular access should be inspected frequently, and changed whenever necessary. It may be possible to manage stable long-term patients without venous access. Care should be taken to prevent corneal ulceration and faecal impaction.

Prophylaxis against venous thromboembolism should be given, and enterally administered low-dose warfarin may be preferable to twice-daily heparin injections in long-stay patients. Psychological problems, especially depression, are common, and some patients are helped by antidepressant drugs. Good communication and rapport between the patient and staff, involvement of allied health practitioners, the provision of television, radio and reading aids and, where possible, occasional trips out of the ICU are all of great value.

Box 57.3 Drugs associated with cardiovascular instability in Guillain–Barré syndrome[94]

Exaggerated hypotensive response
Phentolamine
Nitroglycerin
Edrophonium
Thiopentone
Morphine
Furosemide

Exaggerated hypertensive response
Phenylephrine
Ephedrine
Dopamine
Isoprenaline

Arrhythmias
Suxamethonium

Cardiac arrest
General anaesthesia

Modified from Dalos et al,[94] with permission.

PROGNOSIS

The nadir of the disease is reached within 2–4 weeks, and gradual resolution follows over weeks to months. Of those who survive the acute illness, 70% are fully recovered within 1 year, and a further 20% are left with only minor limitation. Poor prognostic features[35] include age over 60 years, rapid progression to quadriparesis in less than 7 days, the need for mechanical ventilation (except for children),[36] and a preceding diarrhoeal illness.[37] Even in patients ventilated for more than 2 months, gradual improvement may continue for 18 months to 2 years.[38] These severely affected patients require a protracted period of rehabilitation.

Death in up to 25% of GBS patients has been reported in those requiring intensive care.[39] Many of these deaths were due to potentially avoidable problems such as respiratory arrest, ventilator malfunction and intercurrent sepsis, and considerably better results have been achieved.[23] A more representative estimate of the overall mortality is 5–8%.[35]

WEAKNESS SYNDROMES COMPLICATING CRITICAL ILLNESS[40,41]

A number of neuromuscular disorders specifically associated with critical illness have been described over the last 30 years. They are probably much more common than previously appreciated and may occur in up to 46% (95% CI 43–49%) of patients who require prolonged mechanical ventilation, have sepsis, or multiorgan failure.[42] These disorders include neuropathies, myopathies and combinations of both. Variations in nomenclature, the lack of a pragmatic, simple diagnostic test, and confusion with other disorders, such as GBS and corticosteroid-induced myopathy, have further complicated this area. There is also considerable overlap among the various subtypes. Sepsis, neuromuscular-blocking agents (NMBA), disuse atrophy, asthma, corticosteroids and the multiple organ dysfunction syndrome (MODS) have all been implicated.

Intensive care unit acquired weakness (ICUAW) is now the preferred term used to encompass this broad group of heterogeneous disorders and is potentially classifiable (based on electrophysiology and tissue biopsy) into the subcategories of critical illness neuropathy, myopathy and neuromyopathy.[43] The diagnosis of ICUAW requires the clinical context of an acute process of high illness severity often requiring prolonged organ support, and is usually associated with a period of protracted immobilisation. Key clinical signs that support a diagnosis of ICUAW include the presence of normal cognition and consciousness, sparing of the cranial nerves, and the presence of symmetrical flaccid weakness. A common feature of ICUAW is the involvement of the respiratory musculature, which results in rapid shallow breathing with reduced clearance of respiratory secretions.

Although two subgroups of ICUAW are outlined below, a number of rarer variants have also been described.

CRITICAL ILLNESS POLYNEUROPATHY

This acute, diffuse, mainly motor neuropathy is probably the commonest of these disorders. It usually presents in the recovery phase of a severe systemic illness with persistent quadriparetic weakness, hyporeflexia and difficulty in weaning from respiratory support. There appears to be a specific association with severe sepsis and MODS. Histological and electrophysiological features are consistent with axonal degeneration. The mortality in this group is high, presumably reflecting that of the underlying condition.

CRITICAL ILLNESS MYOPATHY

This disorder is linked with asthma and with the use of corticosteroids, NMBA and, less convincingly, aminoglycosides and beta-adrenergic agonists. Reflexes are preserved except in severe cases, as is sensation. Elevated blood CPK concentrations are often seen. A few patients have a more severe, fulminant form with very high CPK levels, frank rhabdomyolysis and, rarely, renal failure. Electrophysiological findings are somewhat variable, though muscle necrosis is usually apparent on histology. Although steroidal muscle relaxants (pancuronium or vecuronium)[44] have been particularly implicated, the disorder has also been seen with other types of NMBA.

DIFFERENTIAL DIAGNOSIS (**BOX 57.4**)

The influence of drugs (particularly anxiolytics and analgesics), metabolic abnormalities (electrolyte abnormalities, altered renal and hepatic function) and hypothermia should always be excluded when unexplained neuromuscular weakness appears in an intensive care patient. The possibility of a coincident illness such as the Eaton–Lambert syndrome, myasthenia gravis, vasculitis or GBS must also be carefully considered. Severe catabolism and disuse atrophy are common in many of these patients and can themselves result in significant weakness.

MANAGEMENT

No specific therapies are available, but minimisation of corticosteroids, sedatives and NMBA, with the aim of maintaining an awake, communicative patient, may be beneficial. Patient evaluation ideally should include daily grading of muscle strength. In a cooperative patient this may be performed using the Medical Research Council (MRC) score, which grades strength from 0 to 5 in three functional muscle groups in each limb. This gives a sum score that ranges from 0 (paralysis) to 60 (full strength), with ICUAW defined as a score of less than 48.[43,45]

Ancillary investigations (nerve conduction, electromyogram and tissue biopsy) assist with the classification of ICUAW, but remain primarily research tools because of technical difficulties and the lack of a specific therapeutic intervention.

PROGNOSIS

The prognosis is generally good providing the underlying acute and chronic disorders can be addressed. The influence of these factors is reflected in the variable extent and duration of recovery (from a few weeks to several months, with some symptoms and signs persisting long term). ICUAW has been associated with prolonged weaning from mechanical ventilation, increased duration of intensive care and hospital stay.[46] Long-term associations include increased physical disability and increased mortality,[47] but it remains difficult to

Box 57.4 Clinical features suggesting intensive care unit acquired weakness

- Onset of weakness is after the acute presentation
- Clinical context includes acute, severe illness requiring either prolonged mechanical ventilation, or sepsis and multi-organ support
- Exclude direct effects of sedation or neuromuscular blockade
- Normal cognition presence of flaccid, symmetrical motor weakness (with muscle wasting) affecting limbs and respiratory muscles, but sparing cranial nerves
- Reflexes are absent if a primarily neuropathic pathology, or reduced/absent if primarily a myopathic pathology. Sensation may be affected with primarily neuropathic lesions
- Muscle strength grade (using Medical Research Council sum score – see text) <48/60

distinguish whether these associations are modifiable by intervention or whether they are simply a consequence of the underlying illness.

MYASTHENIA GRAVIS

MG is an autoimmune disorder caused by antibodies directed against acetylcholine (ACh) receptors in skeletal muscle. Despite its relative rarity, it is the most studied and best understood clinical disorder of neuroreceptor function, and arguably the best understood organ-specific autoimmune disease. It is characterised clinically by weakness or exaggerated fatigability on sustained effort. Intensive care is most commonly required because of severe involvement of the bulbar or respiratory muscles, which may be the result of a spontaneous exacerbation of the disease, a complication of drug therapy, intercurrent illness or surgery, or following surgical thymectomy – a definitive treatment for some patients.

INCIDENCE

The incidence of MG is approximately 1 in 20 000 in the USA. There is no racial or geographic predilection. Although MG can occur at any age, it is very rare in the first 2 years of life, and the peak incidence is in young adult females. Overall, females are affected about twice as often as males. This gender predilection decreases with increasing age, and there is a smaller, second incidence peak in elderly males.[48]

AETIOLOGY AND PATHOPHYSIOLOGY

In 75% of cases, there is histological evidence of thymic abnormality. Thymic hyperplasia is present in the majority of patients, but approximately 10% have a thymoma. The latter appears more common in the older age group. The precise role of the thymus is uncertain, but ACh receptors are present in the myoid cells of the normal thymus, and there is evidence that anti-ACh receptor antibody production is mediated by both B and T lymphocytes of thymic origin. Other organ-specific autoimmune disorders, most commonly thyroid disease[49] but also rheumatoid arthritis, lupus erythematosus and pernicious anaemia, are significantly associated with MG, and autoantibodies to other organs may be seen in MG patients without evidence of disease.

Children born to mothers with MG demonstrate transient weakness ('neonatal MG') in about 15% of cases. A number of congenital myasthenic syndromes exist, in which symptoms develop in infancy, without evidence of autoantibody production.[50] A familial tendency is more common in this group, and structural changes at the neuromuscular junction have been demonstrated.

The stimulus to autoantibody production is not known, but these can be detected in about 90% of patients with generalised myastheni a. They may interfere with neuromuscular transmission by competitively blocking receptor sites, by initiating immune-mediated destruction of receptors, or by binding to portions of the receptor molecule that are not part of the ACh receptor site but nevertheless are important in allowing ACh to bind.

CLINICAL PRESENTATION

Ptosis and diplopia are the most common initial symptoms and in 20% of cases the disorder remains confined to the eye muscles (ocular MG).[51] Bulbar muscle weakness is common and may result in nasal regurgitation, dysarthria and dysphagia. Limb and trunk weakness can occur with varying distribution, and is usually asymmetrical. Some patients complain of fatigue rather than weakness, and may be misdiagnosed as having psychiatric problems. However, weakness can be elicited by sustained effort of an involved muscle group (e.g. sustained upward gaze is often worse at the end of the day and improves with rest).

INVESTIGATIONS

Impairment of neuromuscular transmission may be confirmed by a positive edrophonium (Tensilon) test. However, this traditional test has waned in popularity as it has high sensitivity but rather poor specificity.[52] Atropine 0.6 mg is given i.v. to prevent muscarinic side-effects, and this is followed by 1 mg edrophonium. If there is no obvious improvement within 1–2 minutes, a further 5 mg may be given. Some authors recommend the use of a saline placebo injection, and the presence of a second doctor as a 'blinded' observer. Resuscitation facilities should be available as profound weakness may ensue, especially in patients already receiving anticholinesterase drugs. Intramuscular neostigmine, 1–2 mg, may produce a positive response in 5–10% of patients who do not respond to edrophonium.[53]

The presence of autoantibodies against nicotinic ACh receptors (AChR) is quite specific, but false positives may occur in patients with penicillamine-treated rheumatoid disease, other autoimmune diseases and in some first-degree relatives of myasthenic patients.[54] About 20% of patients are seronegative. Some of these may have antibodies to muscle-specific kinase (MuSK), which appears to be associated with more severe, treatment-resistant disease, predominantly in women.

Electromyography shows characteristic changes in 90% of patients with generalised MG, and also in many patients with ocular symptoms only.

A syndrome of myasthenic weakness occurs in association with malignancy and other autoimmune diseases (Eaton–Lambert syndrome). Although fatigability is present, the pelvic and thigh muscles are predominantly affected, whereas ocular and bulbar involvement is rare. Tendon reflexes are reduced or absent, and there are specific electromyographic changes.

MANAGEMENT

1. *Symptomatic treatment* is provided by anticholinesterase drugs, which potentiate the action of ACh at receptor sites. Pyridostigmine (Mestinon) is the most commonly used, and is usually commenced at a dose of 60 mg orally four times daily. Considerable adjustment of dosage may be required.
2. *Corticosteroids* are effective in approximately 70% of patients, and give best results when high doses (e.g. prednisolone 50–100 mg/day) are used initially, and then gradually reduced. However, transient exacerbation upon commencement of steroids is very common,[55] and severely affected patients are often hospitalised for the initiation of therapy with gradually increasing doses. Older patients are more likely to respond, but an average of 4 months' treatment is required to achieve clinical stability and the majority will require continuing treatment indefinitely.[56]
3. *Azathioprine and cyclophosphamide* are both effective adjuncts to corticosteroid therapy. Overall, 80% of patients are improved, but this may be seen only after some months. A few patients may achieve complete remission.[57]
4. *Ciclosporin (cyclosporine),*[58] *mycophenolate and tacrolimus* are all supported by limited evidence in MG and are occasionally used.[59]
5. *Plasma exchange* is effective in producing short-term clinical improvement.[60] It is mainly used in myasthenic crisis or to improve severely affected patients before thymectomy. Its use should be considered, particularly in patients with severe respiratory failure refractory to conventional therapy (see below).[61] Typically, five exchanges of 3–4 litres each are performed over a 2-week period, and this results in improvement within days. However, the benefits are short-lived, lasting only weeks.[62]
6. *Intravenous immunoglobulin* has similar effects to those of plasma exchange. A dose of 400 mg/kg per day is usually given for 5 successive days, and occasional patients derive long-term benefit.[63] Interestingly, immunoglobulin has no consistent effect on ACh receptor antibody concentrations, and its mechanism of action is poorly understood. Clinical trial evidence suggests that immunoglobulin is as effective as plasmapheresis,[64] but some clinical experts continue to favour the latter, claiming the clinical response is more rapid.
7. *Thymectomy* offers the prospect of long-term, drug-free remission and has long been advocated as a mainstay of MG treatment. However, there is a lack of unequivocal clinical trial evidence to support its role.[59] Most experts advocate early thymectomy in younger patients with more than mild disease, regardless of the presence of a thymoma.[65]

   As with non-thymic surgery, preoperative optimisation of neuromuscular function is essential, using anticholinesterase drugs and steroids, supplemented by plasma exchange or immunoglobulin if necessary. Though anticholinesterase requirements are usually reduced in the immediate postoperative period to about three-quarters of the preoperative dose, sustained improvement following thymectomy may not be seen for months or even years. A thoracoscopic approach may achieve equivalent results with less short-term morbidity,[66] but the traditional sternotomy approach continues to be commonly used.[67]

MYASTHENIC AND CHOLINERGIC CRISIS

Patients with known MG may undergo life-threatening episodes of acute deterioration affecting bulbar and respiratory function. These may occur spontaneously, or may follow intercurrent infection, pregnancy, surgery, the administration of various drugs (**Box 57.5**),[68] or attempts to reduce the level of immunosuppression. Such episodes, known as myasthenic crises, usually resolve over several weeks, but occasionally last for months. The incidence of myasthenic crisis increases markedly with age.[69]

Rarely, a patient may deteriorate due to excessive dosage of anticholinesterase drugs ('cholinergic crisis'). Abdominal cramps, diarrhoea, excessive pulmonary secretions, sweating, salivation and bradycardia may be present, but these can also occur in patients with myasthenic crisis on high doses of pyridostigmine. Though the two situations may be difficult to distinguish, myasthenic crisis is far more likely unless extremely large doses of pyridostigmine (at least 120 mg every 3 hours) have been administered.

A Tensilon test is now considered an unreliable method of distinguishing between these two possibilities, may be hazardous, and is generally not recommended.

Patients with myasthenic crisis should be admitted directly to the ICU, as there is a significant risk of pulmonary aspiration due to bulbar involvement, bacterial pneumonia due to stasis, acute respiratory failure or cardiorespiratory arrest. After initial stabilisation and resuscitation, every effort should be made to identify and correct reversible causes, especially respiratory infections and electrolyte disturbances.

Box 57.5 Drugs that may exacerbate myasthenia gravis

Antibiotics	**Local anaesthetics**
Streptomycin	Procaine
Kanamycin	Lidocaine
Tobramycin	**General anaesthetics**
Gentamicin	Ether
Polymyxin group	**Muscle relaxants**
Tetracycline	Curare
Antiarrhythmics	Suxamethonium
Quinidine	**Analgesics**
Quinine	Morphine
Procainamide	Pethidine

Frequent estimations of vital capacity and maximum inspiratory force should be made and recorded. Tracheal intubation and mechanical ventilation should be considered in patients with significant bulbar involvement or clinical evidence of worsening respiratory failure. As with other neuromuscular disorders, deterioration of blood gases may occur late, and is an unreliable sign of progressive respiratory failure.[70] Aggressive chest physiotherapy, urinary drainage and nasogastric feeding may be required. Hypokalaemia, hypocalcaemia and hypermagnesaemia should be avoided, as all may exacerbate muscle weakness.

If the patient's clinical status cannot be rapidly improved by the adjustment of anticholinesterase dosage and aggressive treatment of intercurrent illness, high-dose corticosteroids and plasma exchange or immunoglobulin should be commenced simultaneously, and may produce some benefit within as little as 24 hours.[71]

PERIOPERATIVE MANAGEMENT

MG patients often require intensive care in relation to surgery for intercurrent illness or for thymectomy. Unstable patients should be admitted to hospital some days in advance for stabilisation. In severely affected patients, preoperative high-dose corticosteroids and/or plasma exchange may be used to improve the patient's fitness for surgery. It may be prudent to omit premedication, and an anaesthetic technique that avoids the use of non-depolarising muscle relaxants is usually advocated, though vecuronium and atracurium are probably safe in reduced dosage.[72,73] Suxamethonium can be used safely in normal dosage.[74]

Up to one-third of patients require continuing mechanical ventilation postoperatively following thymectomy. Predictive factors include a long preoperative duration of myasthenia, coexistent chronic respiratory disease, high anticholinesterase requirements (e.g. pyridostigmine >750 mg/day) and a preoperative vital capacity of less than 2.9 litres.[75] In those cases requiring mechanical ventilation, some authors advocate temporary cessation of anticholinesterase drugs to reduce respiratory secretions,[76] but generally they should be continued, though dosage requirements must be reassessed carefully and repeatedly.

MOTOR NEURON DISEASE (AMYOTROPHIC LATERAL SCLEROSIS, LOU GEHRIG'S DISEASE)[77]

Motor neuron disease refers to a group of related disorders (**Box 57.6**), a few of which are clearly genetically determined, while most arise sporadically, are of completely unknown aetiology, and are generally untreatable. The most common variant is the sporadic form known as amyotrophic lateral sclerosis (ALS), a relentlessly progressive degenerative disease which most commonly affects males over 50 years of age.[78] In North America the term ALS is often used more generically, essentially equivalent to the broader term motor neuron disease.

PATHOGENESIS

The disease affects both upper and lower motor neurons. The involvement of either can predominate early on, giving rise to several clinically recognisable subgroups (see Box 57.6). The cerebral cortex as well as the anterior horns of the spinal cord are involved, with shrinkage, degenerative pigmentation and, eventually, disappearance of the affected cells accompanied by gliosis of the lateral columns ('lateral sclerosis'). As muscles are denervated, there is progressive atrophy of muscle fibres ('amyotrophy'), but, remarkably, sensory neurons as well as those concerned with autonomic function, coordination and higher cerebral function are all spared. The precise cause remains unknown. Postulated pathogenetic causes include oxygen free radicals, viral or prion infection, excess excitatory neurotransmitters and growth factors, and immunological abnormalities.[79] Heavy metal exposure has also been implicated. The only established clinical risk factors are age and family history.

CLINICAL PRESENTATION[80]

The earliest symptoms are those of insidiously developing limb weakness, often asymmetrical, accompanied by obvious muscle wasting. This classically affects the small muscles of the hand and may be accompanied by fasciculation. As time passes, the disease becomes more generalised and more symmetrical, with a mixture of upper and lower motor neuron signs (i.e. spasticity and hyperreflexia in addition to gross wasting), eventually involving bulbar and respiratory muscles. Awareness and intellect were previously thought to be preserved, but it is now recognised that up to half the patients have evidence of cognitive dysfunction.[81] Death occurs in 50% of cases within 3–5 years, usually due to

Box 57.6 Degenerative motor neuron disease[95]

Amyotrophic lateral sclerosis
Spinal muscular atrophy
Bulbar palsy
Primary lateral sclerosis
Pseudobulbar palsy
Heritable motor neuron diseases
Autosomal recessive spinal muscular atrophy
Familial amyotrophic lateral sclerosis
Other
Associated with other degenerative disorders

Modified from Beal et al,[95] with permission.

respiratory infection, aspiration or ventilatory failure from profound weakness. However, there is wide variability, and a few patients may survive for many years.

DIAGNOSIS

There are no specific investigations, and the diagnosis must be made on clinical grounds together with electromyogram (EMG) evidence of denervation in at least three limbs. Experienced neurologists correctly diagnose the condition with 95% accuracy.[82] The most important differential diagnosis is multifocal motor neuropathy. The distinction is of clinical importance, as the latter is amenable to treatment. Poliomyelitis can also result in a syndrome of progressive weakness, wasting and fasciculation, beginning many years after the initial illness (the post-polio syndrome), and leading occasionally to respiratory failure and death.[83]

MANAGEMENT

Treatment is essentially symptomatic and supportive. No benefit has been shown with antioxidants, growth factors and immunosuppressants.[79] Current evidence suggests that non-invasive ventilation improves both quality of life and survival in patients who do not have severe bulbar dysfunction,[84] but the evidence favouring enteral tube feeding is much less convincing.[85] The centrally acting glutamate antagonist riluzole has been shown to slow slightly the progression of ALS.[86]

Admission to ICU is sometimes requested when these patients present with an acute deterioration or intercurrent illness. The intensivist may also be asked to assist with ambulatory or home respiratory support for gradually worsening chronic respiratory failure.

Respiratory support may be given by facemask, nasal mask or, rarely, by tracheostomy using simple, compact ventilators. Some patients require only intermittent support, particularly at night or during periods of acute deterioration due to intercurrent illness. Although home-based non-invasive ventilation has become routine, long-term invasive respiratory support outside the ICU is a major undertaking, requiring specific equipment and extensive liaison with the patient, the family and numerous specialised support services.

RARE CAUSES OF ACUTE WEAKNESS IN THE ICU

PERIODIC PARALYSIS[87]

This term describes a group of rare primary disorders, mostly inherited as autosomal dominant traits, producing episodic weakness. They must be distinguished from other causes of intermittent weakness, including electrolyte abnormalities, MG and transient ischaemic attacks. The inherited types are now grouped together with the various forms of myotonia and susceptibility to malignant hyperthermia. All are classified as congenital defects of skeletal muscle ion channels and there is an association with long QT syndrome and other cardiac channelopathies.[88] Symptoms begin early in life (before age 25), and follow rest or sleep rather than exertion. Alertness during attacks is completely preserved, and muscle strength between attacks is normal. Treatment is usually successful in preventing both the attacks and the chronic weakness, which can develop after many years in untreated patients.

The *hypokalaemic* form of periodic paralysis is predominantly inherited, but can also present sporadically in association with thyrotoxicosis. Involvement of bulbar or respiratory muscles occurs rarely. The degree of hypokalaemia during attacks is mild, but patients rapidly respond to potassium administration. Effective prophylaxis is conferred by acetazolamide, with potassium replacement. Many patients eventually develop established myopathy. Depolarising muscle relaxants should be avoided in these patients.

The *hyperkalaemic* form is milder, almost always inherited and rarely requires intensive care. The serum potassium is modestly elevated at the beginning of attacks, but may be normal at other times. CK may be elevated during attacks. Attacks respond to carbohydrate administration, sympathomimetics (which activate the sodium/potassium pump) and acetazolamide. Thiazide diuretics or acetazolamide provide effective prophylaxis. Non-depolarising muscle relaxants should be avoided in these patients.

A *normokalaemic* form and several eponymously named congenital syndromes are also included in this group of disorders.

BOTULISM[89]

Botulism is a widespread but very uncommon potentially lethal disease caused by exotoxins produced by *Clostridium botulinum* – an anaerobic, spore-forming Gram-positive bacillus. The vast majority of botulism is *foodborne* and outbreaks are largely due to home-preserved vegetables (type A toxin), meat (type B) or fish (type E), but high-risk foods also include low-acid fruit and condiments. Signs and symptoms are caused by toxin produced in vitro and then ingested.

The first recorded outbreak occurred in Germany in 1817, from ingestion of improperly preserved blood sausage (*Botulus* (Latin) = 'sausage').

Wound botulism arises rarely, when wounds (typically open fractures) are contaminated by soil containing type A or B organisms. Intravenous drug abusers are an increasing source of this condition through infected injection sites.

Infantile botulism arises in infants under 6 months of age, and is due to the active production of toxin by organisms in the gut rather than the direct ingestion of toxin.

Hidden botulism describes the adult equivalent of infantile botulism, and is a rare complication of various gastrointestinal abnormalities.

Inadvertent botulism is the most recently described form, and occurs as a complication of the medical or cosmetic use of botulinum toxin.

Inhalational botulism is the form that would occur as a result of aerosolised toxin released in the context of bioterrorism. Botulinum toxin (BoNT) is the most potent known neurotoxin, and some authors have estimated that as little as 1 gram of aerosolised BoNT could lead to the death of over 1.5 million people.[90]

In most cases, exogenously produced exotoxin is absorbed (primarily in the upper small intestine), and carried by the bloodstream to cholinergic nerves at the neuromuscular junction, postganglionic parasympathetic nerve endings and autonomic ganglia, to which it irreversibly binds. The toxin enters the nerve endings to interfere with ACh release.

Most patients become ill about 3 days after ingestion of toxin, with gastrointestinal symptoms (nausea, vomiting, abdominal pain, diarrhoea or constipation), dryness of the eyes and mouth, dysphagia and generalised weakness, which progresses in a symmetrical, descending fashion, with ventilatory failure in severe cases. Cranial nerve dysfunction is a prominent early feature, manifested by ptosis and diplopia, facial weakness and impaired upper airway reflexes. The pupils may be fixed and dilated in severe cases. Patients are usually afebrile and have no sensory involvement.

The differential diagnosis includes food poisoning from other causes, MG and GBS. Botulism can be confirmed by the presence of toxin (either in the patient's serum or stool, or in contaminated food) in about two-thirds of cases. Contact tracing, in the case of foodborne botulism, is of great importance.

Treatment is mainly supportive, with airway protection and mechanical ventilation when required. Mean duration of mechanical ventilation, when required, is 7 weeks. Clearance of toxin from the bowel with enemas and cathartics has been advocated. Guanidine hydrochloride, which enhances the release of ACh from nerve terminals, has been reported to improve muscle strength, especially in ocular muscles, and may be useful in milder cases.[91] Antibiotics have not been clearly shown to be useful. Equine antitoxins are available, but side-effects are common and their efficacy is limited. A human-derived antitoxin has been shown to be effective in *infantile botulism*,[92] and the United States Defense Department has a pentavalent antitoxin, which is not available for public use. Antitoxin must be given before the onset of paralysis in order to be effective. In *wound botulism*, antibiotics (penicillin or metronidazole) and aggressive debridement are recommended.

Most patients begin to improve after a week or so, but hospitalisation is usually required for 1–3 months. The mortality is low (5–8%) with good supportive care, including mechanical ventilation. Mild weakness and constipation may persist for many months.

Access the complete references list online at http://www.expertconsult.com

4. Sejvar JJ, Baughman AL, Wise M, et al. Population incidence of Guillain–Barré syndrome: a systematic review and meta-analysis. Neuroepidemiology 2011;36:123–33.
27. Plasma Exchange/Sandoglobulin Guillain–Barré Syndrome Trial Group. Randomised trial of plasma exchange, intravenous immunoglobulin and combined treatments in Guillain–Barré syndrome. Lancet 1997;349:225–30.
28. Patwa HS, Chaudhry V, Katzberg H, et al. Evidence-based guideline: Intravenous immunoglobulin in the treatment of neuromuscular disorders: Report of the Therapeutics and Technology Assessment Subcommittee of the American Academy of Neurology. Neurology 2012;78:1009–15.
35. Rajabally YA, Uncini A. Outcome and its predictors in Guillain–Barré syndrome. J Neurol Neurosurg Psychiatry 2012;83(7):711–18. Epub 2012 May 7.
42. Stevens RD, Dowdy DW, Michaels RK, et al. Neuromuscular dysfunction acquired in critical illness: a systematic review. Intensive Care Med 2007;33: 1876–91.
43. Stevens RD, Marshall SA, Cornblath DR, et al. A framework for diagnosing and classifying intensive care unit-acquired weakness. Crit Care Med 2009;37:S299–308.
46. De Jonghe B, Bastuji-Garin S, Sharshar T, et al. Does ICU-acquired paresis lengthen weaning from mechanical ventilation? Intensive Care Med 2004;30:1117–21.
64. Gajdos P, Chevret S, Clair B, et al; Myasthenia Gravis Clinical Study Group. Clinical trial of plasma exchange and high-dose intravenous immunoglobulin in myasthenia gravis. Ann Neurol 1997;41:789–96.
84. Bourke SC, Tomlinson M, Williams TL, et al. Effects of non-invasive ventilation on survival and quality of life in patients with amyotrophic lateral sclerosis: a randomised controlled trial. Lancet Neurol 2006;5:140–7.
85. Katzberg HD, Benatar M. Enteral tube feeding for amyotrophic lateral sclerosis/motor neuron disease. Cochrane Database Syst Rev 2011;1:CD004030.
89. Zhang JZ, Sun L, Nie QH. Botulism, where are we now? ClinToxicol 2010;48:867–79.

Part Eight

Endocrine Disorders

58

Diabetic emergencies

Richard Keays

Diabetes mellitus is due to an absolute or relative deficiency of insulin. The sustained effect of poor glycaemic control results in a wide array of end-organ damage as a consequence of small- and large-vessel pathology. Mortality and morbidity are related to the progress of this damage but often there are acute metabolic deteriorations that can be life-threatening. Diabetic ketoacidosis (DKA) and hyperosmolar hyperglycaemic state (HHS) are two of the most common acute complications of diabetes, both accompanied by hyperglycaemia. The pathophysiological changes that occur in both disease states represent an extreme example of the super-fasted state. Coma may also result from severe hypoglycaemia due to overtreatment - usually with insulin.

DIABETES MELLITUS

Type I insulin-dependent diabetes mellitus (IDDM) has a peak incidence in the young rising from 9 months to 14 years and declining thereafter. In 25% of patients the presentation is with ketoacidosis, especially in those under 5 years of age. Usually the fasting plasma glucose is >7.8 mmol/L and glucose and ketones may be present in the urine. In the asymptomatic patient with an equivocal fasting plasma glucose, an impaired glucose tolerance test may be demonstrated.

Type II non-insulin-dependent diabetes mellitus (NIDDM) is prevalent in the elderly but can occur at any age. Truncal obesity is a risk factor and there is ethnic variation in susceptibility. Diagnosis is often delayed and may be incidental from blood or urine sugar screening.[1] Increasingly it is recognised that individuals can be in a prediabetic state of impaired glucose regulation for many years, which makes them 5 to 15 times more likely to progress to diabetes. It may present with classical symptoms, as a diabetic emergency, with complications of organ damage or vascular disease.

EPIDEMIOLOGY

The worldwide prevalence of diabetes is estimated to be 366 million people in 2011. Diabetes mellitus affects about 6% of the world's population and is set to rise to 552 million sufferers by 2030.[2] Most of these (97%) will have type II diabetes but the resources required to treat the complications of type I diabetes are such that health care costs are equivalent between the two groups. The annual incidence of DKA is around 14 episodes per thousand patients with diabetes and it has been estimated in the USA that about $1 billion are spent each year in treating DKA. Hospital admissions for DKA have gone up by 30% in the last decade and this is most likely due to the increase in ketosis-prone type II diabetics. HHS represents approximately 1% of primary admissions to hospital with diabetes as compared with DKA. The mortality rate in HHS remains high at 5–20%, whereas the mortality in DKA has been falling dramatically in recent years and is less than 1% but still remains high in the elderly.[3] An interplay of both genetic and environmental factors contribute to disease development. In type I diabetes there is some evidence for genetic susceptibility but environmental factors play a greater part. It varies across race and regions, being highest in northern Europe and the USA and lowest in Asia and Australasia. Genetic factors in type 2 diabetes are evidently crucial, with a concordance between monozygotic twins approaching 100%.

PATHOGENESIS

Normal carbohydrate metabolism depends upon the presence of insulin (**Fig. 58.1**). However, different tissues handle glucose in different ways; for example, red blood cells lack mitochondria and therefore pyruvate dehydrogenase and the enzymes involved in β-oxidation, whereas liver parenchymal cells are able to perform the full range of glucose disposal (**Fig. 58.2**). Both DKA and HHS result from a reduction in the effect of insulin with a concomitant rise in the counterregulatory hormones such as glucagon, catecholamines, cortisol and growth hormone. Hyperglycaemia occurs as a consequence of three processes: increased gluconeogenesis, increased glycogenolysis and reduced peripheral glucose utilisation. The increase in glucose production occurs in both the liver and the kidneys as there is a high availability of gluconeogenic precursors such as amino acids (protein turnover shifts from balanced synthesis and degradation to reduced synthesis and increased degradation). Lactate and glycerol also become available owing to an increase in skeletal muscle glycogenolysis and an increase in adipose tissue

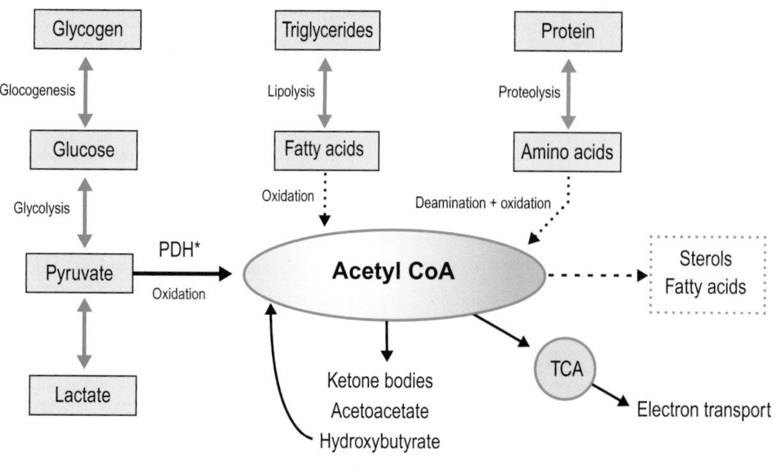

Figure 58.1 Sources and fate of acetyl CoA. *Pyruvate conversion by pyruvate dehydrogenase (PDH) is essentially irreversible, therefore no net conversion of fatty acids to carbohydrates can occur. TCA=tricarboxylic acid.

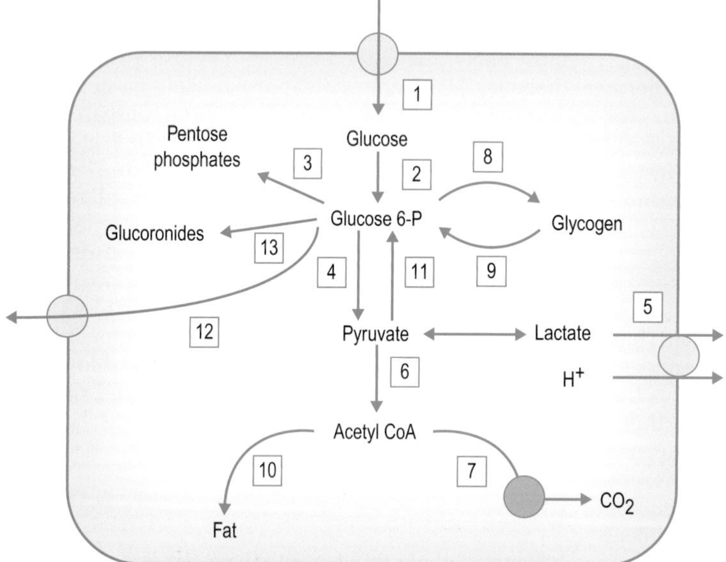

Figure 58.2 Glucose metabolism within hepatocyte: (1) glucose transport GLUT-1; (2) hexokinase phosphorylation; (3) pentose phosphate pathway (hexose monophosphate shunt); (4) glycolysis; (5) lactate transport out of cell; (6) pyruvate decarboxylation; (7) tricarboxylic acid cycle; (8) glycogenesis; (9) glycogenolysis; (10) lipogenesis; (11) gluconeogenesis; (12) glucose-6-phosphate (G 6-P) hydrolysis and release of glucose; (13) glucuronidation.

lipolysis respectively. Lastly, there is an increase in gluconeogenic enzyme activity enhanced further by stress hormones. Although hepatic gluconeogenesis is the main mechanism for producing hyperglycaemia a significant proportion can be produced by the kidneys.[4] What is unclear is the temporal relationship of these changes, although an increase in both catecholamines and the glucagon/insulin ratio are early features.[5]

Decreased insulin and increased epinephrine levels activate adipose tissue lipase causing a breakdown of triglycerides into glycerol and free fatty acids (FFAs). Once again glucagon is implicated as hepatic oxidation of FFAs to ketone bodies is stimulated predominantly by its inhibitory effect on acetyl-CoA carboxylase. The resultant reduced synthesis of malonyl-CoA causes a disinhibition of acyl-carnitine synthesis and subsequent promotion of fatty acid transport into mitochondria where ketone body formation occurs. Both cortisol and growth hormone are capable of increasing FFA and ketone levels and once again the exact contribution of insulin deficiency or stress hormone increase to ketogenesis is undetermined. As ketone bodies are comparatively strong acids, a large hydrogen ion load is produced owing to their dissociation at physiological pH. The need to buffer hydrogen ions depletes the body's alkali reserves and ketone anions accumulate, accounting for the elevated plasma anion gap.

By contrast, HHS does not share the ketogenic features of DKA. Reduced levels of FFAs, glucagon, cortisol and growth hormone have been demonstrated in HHS relative to DKA although this is by no means a consistent observation. However, the presence of higher levels of C-peptide in HHS (with lower levels of growth hormone) relative to DKA suggests there is just enough insulin present in HHS to prevent lipolysis but not enough to promote peripheral glucose utilisation.[6]

Hyperosmolarity, which is a prominent feature of HHS, is caused by the prolonged effect of an osmotic diuresis with impaired ability to take adequate fluids. It has been shown that, even when well, patients who have suffered from HHS have impaired thirst reflexes. However, the hyperosmolarity seen in about one-third of patients with DKA results from a shorter osmotic diuresis and to variable fluid intake due to nausea and vomiting - which is often ascribed to the brainstem effects of ketones.

Interestingly, hyperglycaemia with or without ketoacidosis leads to a significant increase in pro-inflammatory cytokine production, which resolves when insulin therapy is commenced.[7] This has led others to postulate a wider beneficial anti-inflammatory effect attributable to insulin therapy. This pro-inflammatory, pro-thrombotic state may explain the relatively high incidence of thrombotic events associated with diabetic emergencies.

CLINICAL PRESENTATION

DKA and HHS represent the two extremes of presentation due to the absolute or relative deficiency of insulin. However, up to one-third of cases can present with mixed features.[8] DKA develops over a shorter time period whereas HHS appears more insidiously - see **Table 58.1**. Polyuria, polydipsia and weight loss are experienced for a variable period prior to admission and, in patients with DKA, nausea and vomiting are also common symptoms. Abdominal pain is commonly seen in children and occasionally in adults and may mimic an acute abdomen. Dehydration presents with loss of skin turgor, dry mucous membranes, tachycardia and hypotension. Mental obtundation occurs more frequently in HHS than DKA as more patients, by definition, are hyperosmolar and the presence of stupor or coma in patients who are not hyperosmolar requires consideration of other potential causes for altered mental status.[9] However, loss of consciousness is not a common presentation with DKA or HHS (<20%). Most hospitalisations are caused by infection (29%) or non-compliance with medication (17%) in previously diagnosed diabetics; however, in some patients it is the first presentation with undiagnosed diabetes (17%).[10] Given that there is a high likelihood of concurrent infection, most patients have a normal or low temperature and most patients also have a leucocytosis, whether there is infection present or not.

Table 58.1 Comparison of DKA and HHS

PRESENTATION	DKA	HHS
Prodromal illness	Days	Weeks
Coma	++	+++
Blood glucose	++	+++
Ketones	+++	0 or +
Acidaemia	+++	0 or +
Anion gap	++	0 or +
Osmolality	++	+++
TYPICAL DEFICITS		
Total water (litres)	6	9
Water (mL/kg)	100	100–200
Na^+ (mEq/kg/kg)	7–10	5–13
Cl^- (mEq/kg/kg)	3–5	5–15
K^+ (mEq/kg/kg)	3–5	4–6
PO_4^{3-} (mEq/kg/kg)	5–7	3–7
Mg^{2+} (mEq/kg/kg)	1–2	1–2
Ca^{2+} (mEq/kg/kg)	1–2	1–2

DIABETIC KETOACIDOSIS

This tends to occur more often in patients with type I diabetes, although a third of hospitalisations for DKA occurs in patients with type 2 diabetes. The predominant feature is ketoacidosis. Rapid, deep breathing due to the acidosis (Kussmaul breathing) may be present, as may the breath odour that is characteristic of ketones, which is somewhat like nail polish remover. Insulin therapy omission or inadequate dosing is the commonest precipitant of DKA (40%) with underlying infection the next most likely cause (30%).[6] Other causes should be actively sought such as silent myocardial infarction, pancreatitis and drugs that interfere with carbohydrate metabolism. Diagnostic criteria include pH<7.3, HCO_3^- <15 mmol/L and blood glucose >14 mmol/L. Increasing acidaemia, ketonaemia and deteriorating conscious level indicate an increasing severity. Blood glucose per se is not a good determinant of severity and euglycaemic ketoacidosis is possible, depending on the hepatic glycogen stores *prior* to the onset of DKA - a patient who has not been eating well in the recent past may well have a minimally elevated blood glucose. A high amylase is frequently seen and may be extrapancreatic in origin. It should be interpreted cautiously as a sign of pancreatitis.

HYPEROSMOLAR HYPERGLYCAEMIC SYNDROME

HHS is more often seen in patients with type II diabetes and the dominant feature is hyperosmolarity (>320 mOsm/kg). HHS is typically observed in elderly patients with non-insulin-dependent diabetes mellitus, although it may rarely be a complication in younger patients with insulin-dependent diabetes, or those without diabetes following severe burns,[11] parenteral hyperalimentation, peritoneal dialysis, or haemodialysis. Patients receiving certain drugs including diuretics, corticosteroids, β-blockers, phenytoin and diazoxide are at increased risk of developing this syndrome. HHS may be caused by lithium-induced diabetes insipidus.[12] Not only may mental obtundation occur, but also occasionally focal neurological features or seizures are present.

MANAGEMENT

ICU admission is indicated in the management of DKA, HHS and mixed cases in the presence of cardiovascular instability, inability to protect the airway, altered sensoria and the presence of acute abdominal signs or symptoms suggestive of acute gastric dilatation. It is now possible to direct therapy to the underlying metabolic problems of ketogenesis and acidosis rather than the surrogate marker of the blood glucose level. This is increasingly important in euglycaemic DKA. Assessment of response to therapy guided by measurement of ketone concentration is becoming part of best practice.[13]

INITIAL ASSESSMENT

These conditions are medical emergencies and a prompt and thorough history and physical examination should be obtained with special attention paid to airway patency, conscious level, cardiovascular and renal status, possible sources of infection and state of hydration. Some assessment of the severity of DKA is also aided by the degree of acidosis. The majority of patients have a leucocytosis irrespective of whether or not they have a source of sepsis. Attention must also focus on any underlying precipitant. The two major factors involved are inadequate insulin treatment and infection causing a change in insulin responsiveness. The latter must be actively sought in the management of these patients.

FLUID REQUIREMENTS

Dehydration and sodium depletion develop as a result of the osmotic diuresis that accompanies hyperglycaemia in both DKA and HHS. In DKA there is an additional ketoanion excretion, which is approximately half that of glucose. This obligates cation (sodium, potassium and ammonium) excretion and contributes to the electrolyte losses. Despite the dual osmotic load of glucose and ketones in DKA, dehydration is often worse in HHS owing to the more prolonged onset. Insulin itself also promotes salt, water and phosphate reabsorption in the kidney and its lack can contribute further to these losses. The total osmolar load on the kidney in DKA can be as much as 2000 mOsm/day.[14] Fluid resuscitation is initially directed to repleting the intravascular volume, and colloids achieve this more rapidly than crystalloids. Fluids alone will reduce glucose and counterregulatory hormone levels and diminish peripheral insulin resistance. There is individual variation as to how much fluid will be required and simple vital signs such as heart rate, blood pressure and peripheral perfusion should guide the resuscitation. Fluid challenges with assessment of response may be less likely to avoid the problems of fluid overload. The usual urinary sodium concentration is 60–70 mmol/L, which is roughly similar to half-normal saline and this is the logical fluid to use for rehydration.[15] This avoids too great a sodium load and is less likely to produce a hyperchloraemic acidosis, which, if rhabdomyolysis occurs, will further acidify the urine and promote precipitation of myoglobin in the renal tubule. As insulin therapy is commenced extracellular water is driven into the intracellular compartment, exacerbating hypovolaemia, which is why it is most important to commence fluid resuscitation early. This can also lead to a rapid rise in serum sodium concentrations as the true sodium in hyperglycaemia is higher than the measured sodium. Such rapid changes in sodium levels can lead to prolonged neurological dysfunction such as pontine myelinolysis.[16]

Inappropriate fluid replacement can lead to problems. Studies of DKA and cerebral oedema are limited but there is some evidence that overaggressive replacement of water losses can precipitate cerebral and other forms of oedema. Water losses do not need to be corrected rapidly and hyperosmolality should not be corrected more rapidly than 3 mOsm/kg H_2O/h.

General guidelines are given in **Figure 58.3** but it must be remembered that each case needs individual tailoring of treatment. It is mostly agreed that the first litre should be isotonic saline, even in patients with marked hypertonicity. This should be given over the first hour. If there is any evidence of cardiovascular compromise due to hypovolaemia, plasma expansion with colloids should also be given as a matter of urgency. That saline has a pH of 5.5 and a high chloride content is a source of some concern as a resolving ketoacidosis would be compounded by a hyperchloraemic acidosis. A recent study using a balanced electrolyte solution has shown reduced resuscitation-associated hyperchloraemia and an improved serum bicarbonate level.[17] For the next 2 hours 0.45% saline can be given if the serum sodium is normal or high. If the corrected sodium is low then 0.9% saline should be continued. When the blood glucose falls below 15 mmol/L in DKA or HHS then a combination of 5 or 10% dextrose solution with some further saline-containing solution should be commenced (100–250 mL/h) and continued until the ketonaemia has resolved. Assuming cardiovascular stability, the aim should be to correct the remaining fluid deficit gradually over the next 24–48 hours whilst also taking account of ongoing urinary losses.

INSULIN THERAPY

Low-dose, physiological insulin replacement resolves the biochemical abnormalities as quickly as higher

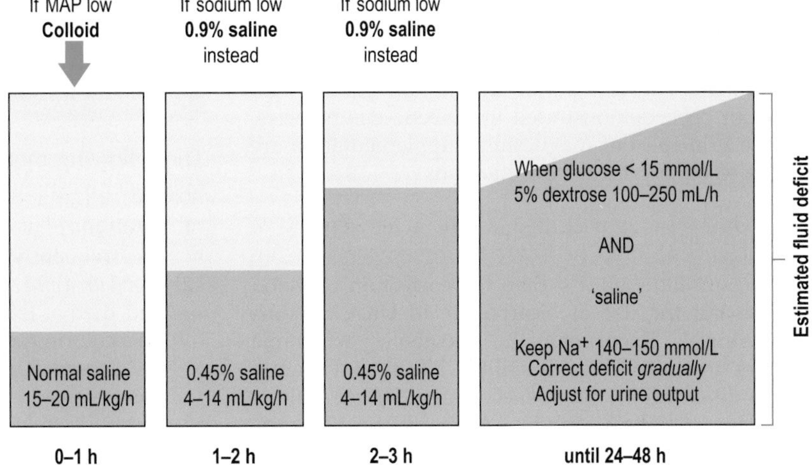

Figure 58.3 Fluid regimen in hyperglycaemic emergencies. No major differences between DKA and HHS. MAP=mean arterial pressure.

doses without running the risk of hypoglycaemia and hypokalaemia, and gradual correction of hyperglycaemia is associated with a lower mortality.[18] A recent study has even questioned the need for an initial insulin bolus dose, contending that commencing the infusion at 0.14 U/kg/h may well be sufficient. A bolus dose (0.14 U/kg) may be required after 1 hour if the blood glucose level has not fallen by at least 10%.[19] Alternatively, a regimen consisting of an initial bolus dose of 0.1 U/kg followed by low dose (0.1 U/kg/h) insulin infusion is similarly acceptable and safe. Weight-based fixed infusion rates are preferable to sliding-scale regimens. Intravenous rather than subcutaneous or intramuscular delivery is preferable as glucose decrement is the same whatever route is chosen, but intravenous insulin reduces ketone body production faster. It is mandatory to use the intravenous route where hypovolaemic shock is present. The aim of treatment is to achieve metabolic targets, specifically: increasing bicarbonate concentration by 3 mmol/L/h, reducing the blood glucose concentration by 3 mmol/L/h and reducing the blood ketone concentration by 0.5 mmol/L/h whilst maintaining normal potassium levels. If the glucose levels fail to reduce appropriately it may indicate insufficient fluid resuscitation. Severe insulin resistance occurs in 10% of cases and will necessitate the use of higher doses. The insulin infusion rate should be reduced to 0.02–0.05 U/kg/h when the glucose level falls to below 12 mmol/L (DKA) or below 15 mmol/L (HHS), and maintained at a level tailored to the patient's need.

ELECTROLYTE THERAPY

POTASSIUM

Hyperosmolarity causes a shift of potassium from within cells to the extracellular space and this potassium is lost as a result of the osmotic diuresis. Renal losses are augmented by secondary hyperaldosteronism and ketoanion excretion as potassium salts. Typical total body deficits are shown in Table 58.1. Serum potassium levels may initially be high and potassium replacement should not commence until this has fallen to <5.5 mmol/L. Potassium can be replaced as a combination of the chloride and phosphate salt as this can avoid hyperchloraemia and hypophosphataemia. Occasionally the presenting potassium level will be low (<3.3 mmol/L), which represents profound potassium depletion (600–800 mmol) and replacement should commence immediately and before insulin therapy is initiated. If the patient is in between these two levels then 20–40 mmol of potassium may be given in the first hour - this should not generally be exceeded. Further decisions regarding potassium replacement need to be adjusted with respect to serum levels and the urine output but usually 20–30 mmol/h are required. ECG monitoring has been recommended where potassium replacement is needed for patients who present with hypokalaemia or cardiac rhythms other than sinus tachycardia.[6]

PHOSPHATE

A total body phosphate deficit of greater than 1 mmol/kg is typical. Once again the shift is from the intracellular compartment with subsequent urinary loss; however, serum levels are typically normal or increased. Insulin causes an intracellular shift of phosphate and, although hypophosphataemia rarely results in adverse complications, muscle weakness, haemolytic anaemia and impaired cardiac systolic performance can occur. Routine phosphate replacement has not been shown to be beneficial in DKA,[20] but correction of severely low levels (<0.4 mmol/L) may be necessary. Excessive phosphate replacement leads to hypocalcaemia and serum calcium should be monitored.

MAGNESIUM

A chronic magnesium deficiency may be present in type I or II diabetes and may be exacerbated by renal impairment. The benefits of magnesium replacement have not been demonstrated in diabetic emergencies, but the principles of magnesium supplementation are similar to other critical care situations.

CORRECTION OF ACIDOSIS

This occurs more slowly than the correction of blood glucose but the use of bicarbonate in DKA remains controversial. Experimentally, metabolic acidaemia impairs myocardial contractility, affects oxyhaemoglobin dissociation and tissue oxygen delivery, alters cellular metabolism, inhibits intracellular enzymes, such as the pH-dependent enzyme phosphofructokinase, and results in organ dysfunction. Not only that, but insulin resistance increases sharply below pH 7.2. Bicarbonate treatment to rapidly correct the acidosis should offer some benefit but, in most studies, the use of sodium bicarbonate fails to provide any benefit. There are no haemodynamic benefits that could not be attributed purely to osmotic load of sodium administered.[21] There is no doubt that blood pH can be improved but at the expense of worsening the intracellular acidosis.[22] Sodium bicarbonate treatment may cause paradoxical cerebrospinal fluid (CSF) acidosis.[23] It is also associated with other side-effects that may overshadow any potential benefits such as: increased CO_2 production, hypokalaemia, rebound alkalosis, volume overload and altered tissue oxygenation. In the context of DKA, sodium bicarbonate also delays the clearance of ketones and may enhance further hepatic production even when insulin and glucose are being delivered.[24] At pH>7.0 insulin will block lipolysis and ketoacid production; however, when the pH is between 6.9 and 7.1 it remains uncertain whether bicarbonate is beneficial or otherwise. Although a recent systematic review of trials in both adult and paediatric populations concluded that there was no obvious benefit with bicarbonate treatment, there were reassuringly few clinically significant complications resulting from its use either.[23] These studies did not include patients with pH<6.85 and recommendations in such patients are difficult. Below pH 6.9 most authorities would recommend the use of bicarbonate to correct the pH partially to the threshold. The threshold for correction is debatable (between pH 6.9 and 7.15) but life-threatening hyperkalaemia is an undisputed indication for bicarbonate therapy.

Sometimes there is a persistent acidosis without ketosis. Regeneration of bicarbonate in DKA once insulin activity has been restored occurs via two mechanisms: renal and hepatic. The latter requires a metabolisable substrate, typically ketones, which are lost to the body especially if the diuresis is substantial. The former is slow and hyperchloraemia may persist, particularly if a high-chloride-containing fluid such as normal saline is used.[25]

MONITORING

The following monitoring parameters are also undertaken as investigations on presentation:

1. *Blood glucose concentration:* initially every hour, then less frequently
2. *Blood urea and creatinine concentrations:* on admission and then at least daily. Creatinine assays that rely on a colorimetric method may be interfered with by the presence of acetoacetate, giving a falsely elevated value
3. *Serum electrolytes:*
   a. *Serum sodium*: on admission and at least daily. It represents the relative water and electrolyte losses and cannot be used to infer a state of hydration. It may be normal (50% of cases), raised or lowered. Each 1.0 mmol/L rise in blood glucose will decrease serum sodium by 0.3 mmol/L, so hypernatraemia represents a profound loss of water
   b. *Serum potassium*: initially every hour, then less frequently (every 2–4 hours). DKA patients have a K^+ deficit of 3–5 mmol/kg. However, serum concentrations are usually normal or raised because of a shift from the intracellular to the extracellular compartment due to acidaemia, insulin deficiency and hypertonicity. Hypokalaemia on admission represents severe potassium depletion (>600–800 mmol) and requires potassium administration before starting insulin therapy
   c. *Serum chloride*: as indicated
   d. *Serum phosphate*: on admission and every 1–2 days. Routine replacement is not of any benefit. Despite evidence that hypophosphataemia leads to a decrease in 2,3-diphosphoglycerate levels, subsequent correction has no impact on the oxyhaemoglobin dissociation curve and dangerous hypocalcaemia may result[20]
   e. *Serum magnesium*: on admission and every 1–2 days. Chronic hypomagnesaemia may be present and may contribute to insulin resistance, carbohydrate intolerance and hypertension. Severe uncontrolled diabetes also results in magnesium depletion. However, the benefits of replacement therapy have not been demonstrated but may be necessary if arrythmias are present
4. *Serum ketones (if available):* on admission. This test relies on the nitroprusside reaction and, because it measures acetoacetate and acetone but not β-hydroxybutyrate, which is the main ketoacid in DKA, it consequently underestimates the degree of ketoacidosis. Near patient testing for β-hydroxybutyrate is now more readily available

5. *Urinary glucose and ketones:* 4-hourly; ketonuria may persist up to 2 days after the correction of acidosis due to the presence of acetone, which is not an acid anion and is highly lipid soluble. The ratio of acetoacetate : β-hydroxybutyrate (approximately 1:3) increases as acidosis improves with treatment; this can lead to the paradoxical impression that ketosis is worsening but is merely an anomaly of the nitroprusside test
6. *Arterial blood gases:* frequently, as indicated
7. *Serum osmolality and anion gap:* initially and as indicated. Serum osmolality can be measured with an osmometer or estimated
8. *Serum lactate:* if acidosis is severe and anion gap is large
9. *Full blood count and coagulation studies:* daily and as indicated. Leucocytosis with left shift may occur in the absence of sepsis
10. *Chest X-ray*
11. *Blood cultures, urine and sputum microscopy and culture and culture of relevant specimens:* as indicated
12. *Pulse oximetry:* continuously
13. *Electrocardiogram:* 12-lead recording and continuous monitoring
14. *Invasive haemodynamic monitoring:* as indicated
15. *Neurological status and observations:* including Glasgow Coma Scale and computed tomography (CT) scans as indicated for persistent coma or worsening neurological state
16. *Other investigations:* as indicated (e.g. liver function tests, serum amylase, cardiac enzymes and creatinine clearance).

COMPLICATIONS

EARLY

The commonest early complications are hypoglycaemia due to overtreatment with insulin, hypokalaemia due to inadequate replacement and hyperglycaemia due to interruption of insulin. A hyperchloraemic acidosis can develop in about 10% of patients with DKA. It can be exaggerated by excessive saline use and is not usually clinically significant except in cases of acute renal failure or extreme oliguria.

Clinically apparent cerebral oedema is a rare (0.5–1%) but extremely serious complication of DKA occurring predominantly in children and the mortality is high (25%), with a quarter of survivors being left with some permanent neurological sequelae. Recent studies have suggested a subclinical incidence approaching 50%.[26] Risk factors for developing cerebral oedema include: degree of hypocapnia and dehydration, the failure of serum sodium to rise with treatment and the use of sodium bicarbonate.[27] It also occurs in young adults and may be associated with rapid deterioration in conscious level with or without seizures. If progressive signs of brainstem herniation are present the mortality is high with only 7–14% likely to make a complete recovery. The risks of brain herniation are related to the degree of acidosis and the volume of initial fluid resuscitation. Oedema formation most likely occurs due to a vasogenic mechanism[28] and cerebral hyperaemia with loss of autoregulation is evident, which can take up to 36 hours to resolve.[29,30] It has been recommended that plasma osmolality is reduced slowly and that glucose must be added to the hydrating fluids when the plasma glucose has fallen below 15 mmol/L in DKA and HHS. Fatal cases of cerebral oedema have been reported in HHS as well and treatment is aimed at maintaining plasma osmolality with intravenous mannitol.

Some degree of brain dysfunction is apparent even in those patients who are not comatose but who have severe DKA as measured by sensory evoked potentials. This reverts to normal with correction of the ketoacidosis.[31]

Hypoxia, non-cardiogenic pulmonary oedema and myocardial infarction can also occur – particularly in the elderly.

INTERMEDIATE

A reversible critical illness motor syndrome has been described in HHS and led to slowness to wake up and reversible tetraplegia.[32] Deep venous thrombosis and pulmonary embolism occur more frequently in DKA and are a significant cause of mortality in HHS.[33,34] Prophylaxis with subcutaneous heparin is advisable. Full anticoagulation may be indicated in HHS.[3]

LATE

Various movement disorders can rarely persist after recovery from HHS.[35] The effects of neuroglycopenia can result in an array of late complications from amnesia to optic atrophy.

PROGNOSIS

In a series of 610 patients with DKA or HHS the overall mortality was 6.2%. HHS is a more serious disease and has an associated mortality 2–3 times higher than DKA; nevertheless DKA is approximately six times commoner. A retrospective analysis of causes of death in this group of patients revealed that pneumonia was the commonest cause of death (37%), followed by myocardial infarction (21%), with mesenteric or iliac thrombosis accounting for 16% of deaths.[36] Rhabdomyolysis has been reported in both DKA and HHS and, when present, increases the mortality.[37] The likelihood of a poorer outcome in HHS was associated with: older age, low blood pressure, low sodium, pH and bicarbonate plasma levels, and high urea plasma levels, of which urea has the strongest association.[38] Mortality is also age-related in DKA. Pregnant women with type I diabetes are more likely to have a worse outcome from DKA than non-pregnant diabetic women who develop DKA. The presence of hypothermia is also a poor prognostic sign.

Survival depends upon establishing a high index of suspicion and a rapid diagnosis.[39]

HYPOGLYCAEMIC COMA

This results from overtreatment with insulin and is the commonest cause of diabetic coma. Clinically, there is confusion, agitation progressing to coma and fitting. Tremor, tachycardia and sweating may be blunted by diabetic autonomic neuropathy. It may be precipitated in known type I diabetic patients (up to 10% of patients per year) by missed meals, exercise and overdose of insulin or oral hypoglycaemic agents. Changing therapy or insulin periods are susceptible periods and there is an increased risk associated with long-acting sulfonylurea agents. Alcoholic ketoacidosis is a syndrome of hypoglycaemia, ketoacidosis and dehydration associated with starvation, vomiting, upper abdominal pain and neurological changes including seizures and coma. Hypoglycaemia may complicate other disease states (e.g. liver and renal failure, or adrenocortical insufficiency).

Severe hypoglycaemia (blood glucose <1 mmol/L) is a medical emergency. Brain metabolism uses half the glucose produced by the liver and neuronal stores of glycogen are depleted within 2 minutes, after which the brain is susceptible to damage. Urgent glucose infusion (50 mL of 50% glucose) is required and leads to rapid resolution of coma. Intramuscular glucagon is an alternative especially suited to out-of-hospital circumstances, but achieves a slower result when compared with intravenous glucose.[40] Hypoglycaemia due to long-acting insulins or oral hypoglycaemic agents will require ongoing glucose infusion.

Access the complete references list online at http://www.expertconsult.com

3. Nyenwe E, Kitabchi A. Evidence-based management of hyperglycemic emergencies in diabetes mellitus. Diabetes Res Clin Pract 2011;94:340–51.
8. Magee MF, Bhatt BA. Management of decompensated diabetes. Diabetic ketoacidosis and hyperglycemic hyperosmolar syndrome. Crit Care Clin 2001; 17(1):75–106.
13. Joint British Diabetes Societies Inpatient Care Group. The management of diabetic ketoacidosis in adults. March 2010. Online. Available: http://www.diabetes.org.uk/Documents/.
18. Wagner A, Risse A, Brill HL, et al. Therapy of severe diabetic ketoacidosis. Zero-mortality under very-low-dose insulin application. Diabetes Care 1999; 22(5):674–7.
19. Kitabchi A, Murphy M, Spencer J, et al. Is a priming dose of insulin necessary in a low-dose insulin protocol for the treatment of diabetic ketoacidosis? Diabetes Care 2008;31:2081–5.
23. Chua H, Schneider A, Bellomo R. Bicarbonate in diabetic ketoacidosis – a systematic review. Ann Intensive Care 2011;1:23.
27. Glaser N, Barnett P, McCaslin I, et al. Risk factors for cerebral edema in children with diabetic ketoacidosis. The Pediatric Emergency Medicine Collaborative Research Committee of the American Academy of Pediatrics. N Engl J Med 2001;344: 264–9.

59

Diabetes insipidus and other polyuric syndromes

Alastair C Carr

Diabetes insipidus (literal translation 'tasteless siphon') refers to a syndrome characterised by pathological polyuria, excessive thirst and polydipsia. Polyuria is arbitrarily defined as a urine loss of >3 litres per day in an adult of normal mass or >2 L/m^2 in children. The urine produced in DI is inappropriately dilute having both low specific gravity and low osmolality in the face of a high or normal plasma osmolality.

Three subtypes of DI are recognised: (i) *nephrogenic DI* – caused by insensitivity of the kidney to antidiuretic hormone (ADH), (ii) *central/hypothalamic/neurogenic DI* – caused by reduced or absent production of ADH, and (iii) *gestational DI* – caused by an increase in the placental production of vasopressinase or as a variant of central or nephrogenic DI developing during pregnancy. A separate disorder is occasionally classified as a fourth form of DI: *primary polydipsia* (also called psychogenic or neurogenic polydipsia or polydipsic DI). This is caused by excessive water ingestion usually due to psychological disturbance but occasionally associated with a lesion of the hypothalamus. In the context of hospital in-patients, a similar iatrogenic condition is created by overenthusiastic administration of intravenous solutions of dextrose 5% or hypotonic saline. Although water overload will reduce plasma osmolality and reduce the ability of the kidney to maximally concentrate urine, the diuresis of hypo-osmolar urine seen with water overload is not pathological but physiological and appropriate. In this instance, plasma osmolality is low or in the low–normal range and the body is attempting to restore plasma osmolality to normality by reducing water reabsorption in the kidneys and inducing a water diuresis.

In critically ill patients, polyuria may be the sole part of the DI syndrome apparent to the clinician. Patients are seldom in control of their own fluid intake and are frequently unable to report thirst. The recognition of DI is important as failure to recognise and treat the syndrome appropriately will result in severe dehydration and hyperosmolality with a significant risk of morbidity and mortality. As there are many causes of polyuria in the critically ill (**Box 59.1**), it is important to adopt a systematic approach to the clinical assessment, investigations, diagnosis and management of such patients.

The classification as a solute or water diuresis is not always absolute; the table provides a convenient structure but a diuresis should be considered in terms of the individual patient and both physical and biochemical assessments. A diuresis may frequently represent the clearance of both an excess of water and solute such as is usually the case following the resolution of septic shock with multi-organ failure.

BACKGROUND PHYSIOLOGY AND ANATOMY

OSMOLALITY

Osmolality is the measure of osmoles (Osm) of solute per kilogram of solvent and includes both permeant (e.g. urea) and impermeant solutes (e.g. sodium). It may change owing to both water movement and the movement of permeant solute. Osmolarity is the measure of osmoles per litre of solute and, unlike osmolality, is temperature dependent. Normal plasma osmolality is in the range of 275–295 mOsm/kg. Plasma osmolality can be estimated from several equations.[1] The formula of Worthley[2] below is both simple and correlates well with measured values.[3]

$$\text{plasma osmolality (mOsm/kg)} = 2\,[\text{Na+}] + [\text{urea}] + [\text{glucose}$$

All units of solute are mmol/L.

Where a patient is markedly uraemic, a value of 8 mmol/L is substituted for the actual urea. Actual osmolality may differ markedly from estimated osmolality in the presence of unmeasured, osmotically active solutes such as mannitol, ethanol, bicarbonate, lactate and amino acids. Whenever concern exists that a patient may be hyper- or hypo-osmolal, osmolality should be measured by assessing the freezing point depression of the plasma or urine. Increasing the osmolality results in depression of the freezing point.

The osmolal gap is the difference between the calculated and measured osmolality in plasma or urine. The normal osmolal gap is <10 mOsm/kg. An increased osmolal gap indicates the presence of an unmeasured osmotically active solute.

TONICITY

Tonicity describes the ability of a solution of impermeant solute (such as sodium) to cause the movement

Box 59.1 Causes of polyuria

Water diuresis

Pathological: Diabetes insipidus – cranial, nephrogenic, gestational

Physiological:

- Psychogenic polydipsia (excess drinking is pathological but the diuresis is not)
- Iatrogenic – excessive administration of hypotonic solutions (e.g. 5% dextrose solution, 0.45% saline, 0.18% saline 4% dextrose solutions)

Solute diuresis

Pathological:

- Hyperglycaemia, azotaemia (uraemia), Fanconi syndrome, renal tubular acidosis, glomerulonephritis, hyperaldosteronism, Addison disease, anorexia nervosa, migraines, paroxysmal tachycardia (via increased ANP release)
- Poisons/drugs – ethanol, methanol, ethylene glycol, mannitol, loop diuretics, thiazide diuretics

Physiological:

- Resolving sepsis (redistribution of fluid into the vascular compartment from the third space)
- Iatrogenic – excessive administration of isotonic or hypertonic solutions e.g. 0.9% saline, hypertonic saline, Hartman's solution, Gelofusin

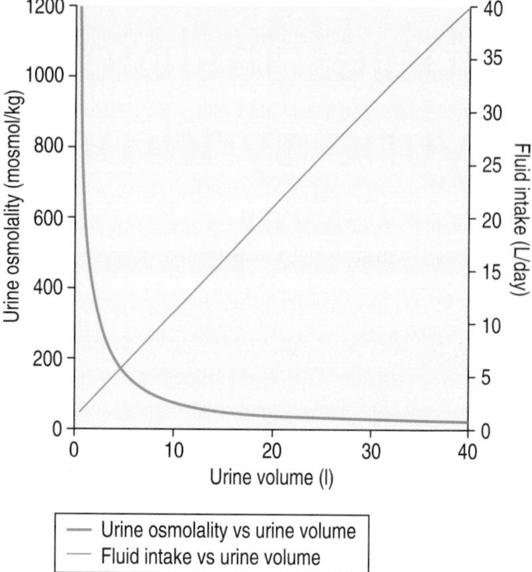

Figure 59.1 Urine output rises and urine osmolality falls in health as a function of increasing water intake. Assuming normal solute ingestion, normal solute excretion (around 800 mmol/day) is preserved between water intakes of 1.5 and 32 litres/day.

of water between itself and another fluid compartment. It may be considered an index of the water concentration rather than the solute concentration as the solute is impermeant. The tonicity of plasma is largely determined by its sodium content; the main solute in extracellular fluid that is not freely permeable to cross into the intracellular space. This characteristic facilitates the control of extracellular fluid volume through the regulation of sodium balance.

It is possible for a solution to be both hypotonic and iso-osmolar. Dextrose solution 5% is an example of this; the solution contains no impermeant solute (assuming no absence of insulin, glucose freely enters the cell) but is iso-osmolar with the intracellular milieu.

SOLUTE AND WATER INTAKE AND LOSSES

Assuming a normal diet, in a 75 kg man there is every day an obligatory loss of around 800 mmol of solute: approximately 300 mmol of urea and 500 mmol of cations and anions. The maximum concentrating ability of the healthy kidney is around 1200 mOsm/kg; consequently, a minimum of 666 mL of urine a day is required to excrete osmotically active solutes. Additionally, insensible losses of water (respiratory water, faecal water and sweat) approximate 10 mL/kg/day and this rises markedly with fever and hot dry climates. Thus, obligatory water losses of around 1.5 litres per day arise owing to insensible losses and obligatory solute excretion.

NORMAL URINARY OSMOLALITY

In health, urinary osmolality is usually maintained between 500 and 700 mOsm/kg. As the obligatory solute load to be excreted is relatively constant in value, urine osmolality will fall in response to an increased intake in free water and rise in response to dehydration or water restriction (**Fig. 59.1**). The minimum osmolality of urine achievable in man is around 25 mOsm/kg. Diuresis refers to the passage of a high volume of urine (>1.5 mL/kg/h) and may be transient or persistent, physiological or pathological. The production of >3 L/day is arbitrarily defined as polyuria. Water diuresis occurs when the total solute in the urine excreted per day is within the normal range but the osmolality of the urine passed is low. An osmotic or solute diuresis occurs when the total solute passed per day is higher than normal; the urine passed is usually iso-osmolar to plasma if the extracellular fluid volume is expanded or hyperosmolar if the patient is hypo- or euvolaemic.

PLASMA OSMOLALITY AND PLASMA VOLUME REGULATION

Changes in plasma osmolality and changes in plasma volume can occur in tandem or independently of one another. Whereas normal plasma osmolality lies in a population range of 275–295 mOsm/kg (270–280 mOsm/kg in pregnancy), individuals tend to vary less than ±1% around their set value. In pregnancy this set value falls but the limited variability around it does not. The body regulates osmolality and volume by separate mechanisms. Water balance and osmolality are maintained via osmoreceptors, which mediate their control via control of thirst and ADH production.

Control of the plasma volume is maintained via volume receptors and sodium receptors, which mediate their actions through the sympathetic nervous system and the renin–angiotensin–aldosterone system. Additionally, the volume receptors have inputs to the hypothalamus via which they too can mediate ADH release and the sensation of thirst. Atrial natriuretic peptide (ANP) and brain natriuretic peptide (BNP), predominantly released from atrial and ventricular myocytes respectively, inhibit the release of renin, aldosterone, vasopressin and endothelin leading to both a natriuresis and a diuresis.[4]

THIRST

In health fluid intake is determined by the sensation of thirst and the subsequent ingestion of fluid. A plasma osmolality of >290 mOsm/kg, elevated angiotensin II (AII) concentrations, sympathetic nervous system activation and circulating volume depletion of 5–10% are all associated with the onset of thirst. Fluid and solute excretion are largely regulated through the kidney, although some solutes such as ethanol and glucose are largely cleared through metabolism rather than excretion.

In the ICU, the patient loses control over intake of fluids and solute and frequently has impaired excretory mechanisms. Thus both volume and solute homeostasis may become heavily dependent upon the skills of attending clinicians.

OSMORECEPTORS AND OTHER INPUTS TO THE SUPRAOPTIC AND PARAVENTRICULAR NUCLEI

Detection of osmolality occurs largely at osmo- (Na^+) receptors sited around the anterior aspect of the third ventricle of the brain. These are sensitive to plasma osmolality and CSF sodium concentration. Hypertonic saline is a more potent stimulus than equi-isotonic equi-ososmolar solutions of other solutes.[5] These osmoreceptors link to the cells of the paraventricular nuclei (PVN) and supraoptic nuclei (SON), the sites of ADH synthesis. The axons of the cells in the PVN and SON form part of the pituitary stalk linking the hypothalamus to the pituitary gland, in which they terminate. A smaller proportion of the axons terminate in the median eminence where they release ADH and oxytocin, which is transported to the anterior lobe of the pituitary by portal vessels. The ADH and oxytocin so released cause release of ACTH and prolactin respectively; the ADH acts synergistically with corticotropin-releasing factor (CRF) but is also believed to have ACTH secretagogue properties in its own right.[6,7]

Direct inputs from the sympathetic nervous system to the PVN and SON can stimulate ADH release via α-adrenoreceptors. Other central osmoreceptors lie outside the blood–brain barrier in the subfornical organ and come into contact with plasma. It is believed that ANP and AII[8] act via these receptors to inhibit or elicit ADH synthesis, ADH release and to modify the sensation of thirst. Additional osmoreceptors in the mouth, stomach, and liver are believed to play a role in the anticipation of an osmolal load following ingestion of food and pre-emptively can stimulate ADH synthesis in the hypothalamus.

As the baroreceptor and osmoreceptor inputs to the PVN and SON are distinct, it is possible to lose the normal ADH response to hyperosmolality but maintain a normal ADH response to hypovolaemia.[9] Additionally, in animal experiments, when hypotension increases the basal plasma ADH concentration, there is a simultaneous resetting of the osmomolality–plasma ADH response curve in an attempt to preserve osmoregulatory function from the new higher baseline.[10] If this did not occur, the ADH response to hypotension would always result in the development of a hypo-osmolal state in addition to causing vasoconstriction.

The normal response of osmoreceptors to changing plasma osmolality in terms of ADH is illustrated in **Figure 59.2**. At plasma osmolalities of <275 mOsm/kg, the osmoreceptors remain hyperpolarised and virtually no ADH release occurs via them. At osmolalities >295 mOsm/kg, the osmoreceptors are maximally depolarised and plasma concentrations of ADH of >5 pg/mL are attained. Other inputs and influences upon ADH release are summarised in **Figure 59.3** and **Box 59.2**.

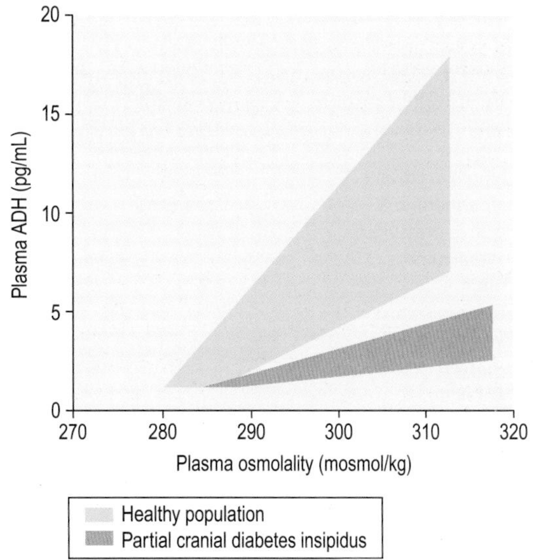

Figure 59.2 Plasma antidiuretic hormone (ADH) and plasma osmolality in health and partial cranial diabetes insipidus.

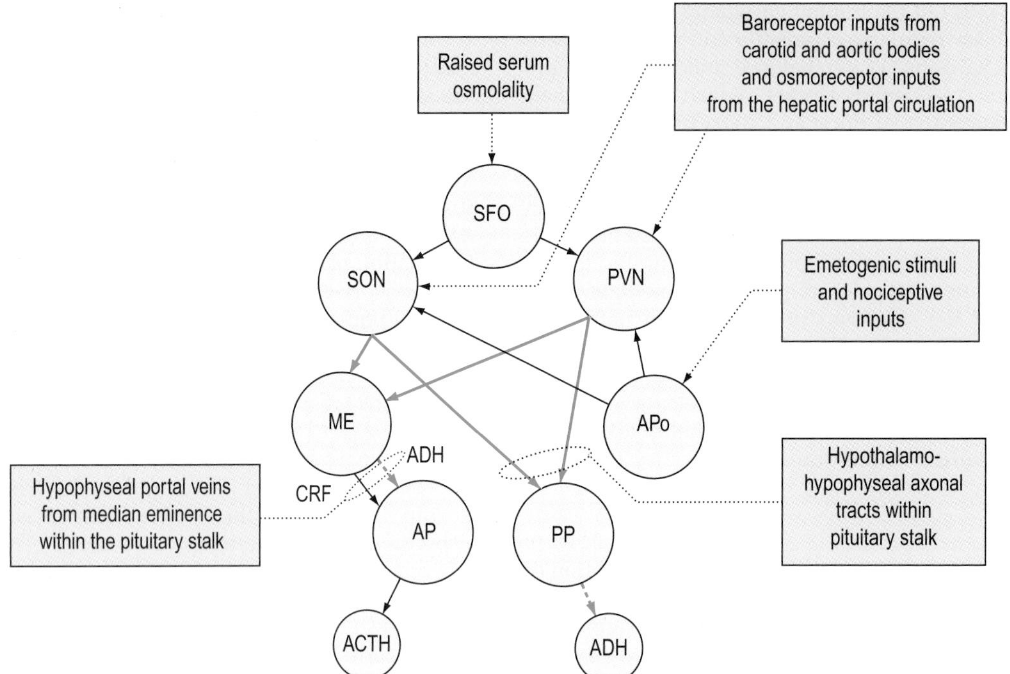

Figure 59.3 A schematic representation of anatomical and physiological connections of the supraoptic and paraventricular nuclei (SON and PVN), the principal sites of antidiuretic hormone (ADH) synthesis within the hypothalamus. Blue arrows represent the transport of ADH or its precursor between anatomically distinct sites. Baroreceptor inputs into these nuclei travel via the vagus nerve to reach the central nervous system. Whereas the majority of ADH produced in the SON and PVN is transported to the posterior pituitary (PP) for storage, some is transported to the median eminence (ME) then onwards to the anterior pituitary (AP), where it acts synergistically as a secretagogue for adrenocorticotropic hormone (ACTH). APo=area postrema; SFO=subfornical organ; CRF=corticotropin-releasing factor.

Box 59.2 Factors influencing ADH release

Increased ADH release with:	Decreased ADH release with:
Hyperosmolality	Elevated ANP, BNP
Hypovolaemia	Hypo-osmolality
Hypotension	Hypervolaemia
Hypoxia	Hypertension
Hypothyroidism	Ethanol
Hyperthermia	Cranial DI
Positive-pressure ventilation	
Pain	
Emotional stress	
Exercise	
Nausea	
Nicotine	
Trauma/surgery	

ANTIDIURETIC HORMONE (ADH)/ARGININE VASOPRESSIN (AVP)

ADH (8-arginine vasopressin) is a nine amino acid peptide that differs from oxytocin at only two residues but shares the disulphide bond between the 1st and 6th ones. This similar structure and conformation results in some cross-reactivity at receptors and in function.[11] It is synthesised in the SON and PVN, bound to neurophysin, transferred through axons to the posterior pituitary gland and stored in granules prior to release. Synthesis to replace any released stores is a rapid process (1–2 hours from synthesis to storage) and patients with damage to the pituitary can achieve near-normal plasma concentrations of ADH, in terms of osmoregulatory function, via release of newly synthesised ADH via the axons terminating in the median eminence. However, the higher plasma concentrations associated with hypovolaemia cannot be achieved. Normal osmoregulatory plasma ADH concentrations are in the range of 1–8 pg/mL but rise as high as 40 pg/mL in hypovolaemic patients under the influence of the sympathetic nervous system, baroreceptor responses and AII.

Once released from the pituitary, ADH has a plasma half-life of around 10–35 minutes.[12] It is metabolised by hepatic, renal and placental vasopressinases and around 10% of the active hormone is excreted unchanged in the urine.

ACTIONS OF ADH

ADH has antidiuretic, vasopressor, haemostatic and ACTH secretagogue actions. Additionally, it has roles in memory, water permeability of the blood–brain barrier, nociception, splenic contraction and thermoregulation. These actions are mediated through V_1, V_2 and V_3 receptors. It also has actions on the uterus and mammary tissue mediated through oxytocin receptors. Cardiac inotropic effects are reported to be mediated through purinergic P_2 receptors, but this remains controversial.[13] Animal studies give conflicting reports of both positive and negative inotropic effects and their receptor mediation.[14]

Antidiuresis

ADH binds to V_2 receptors on the basal membranes of the principal cells of the collecting duct and distal tubule. The activated receptor induces production of cAMP by adenylate cyclase and this in turn activates protein kinases, which effect the integration into the luminal membrane of vesicles containing aquaporin-2 highly selective water channels. The production of prostaglandin E_2 (PGE_2) inhibits cAMP production. PGE_2 synthesis is stimulated by the action of ADH on V_1 receptors on the luminal membrane of the collecting duct.[15] Thus, a form of autoregulatory limitation of the antidiuretic effect of ADH may exist. Hypokalaemia, lithium and hypercalcaemia also antagonise the renal actions of ADH.

ADH also increases the urinary concentrating ability of the kidney by increasing the expression of urea transport proteins in the collecting duct and reducing renal medullary blood flow (V_1 mediated) facilitating an increase in medullary interstitial hypertonicity. This hypertonicity additionally depends upon intact functioning of the ascending loop of Henle where sodium and chloride are reabsorbed without absorption of water at the same time. Interference with this process reduces the osmolal gradient between the collecting duct and the interstitium and reduces water absorption even in the presence of ADH and functioning aquaporin-2.

In low dose, administration of exogenous ADH may paradoxically cause a diuresis in patients with septic shock.[16] This may be due to increased renal perfusion pressure resulting in an increase in GFR.

Vasoconstriction

At higher concentrations (>40 pg/cm), ADH activates not only V_2 receptors but also V_1 receptors through which it causes preferential vasoconstriction in muscle, skin and fat with relative sparing of coronary, cerebral and mesenteric circulations. However, these relative sparing effects are controversial, with some authors reporting relative sparing and others reporting significant vasoconstriction.[17–20] Activation of V_1 receptors activates phospholipase C and increases inositol triphosphate intracellularly. Ultimately this increases intracellular free calcium and leads to smooth muscle constriction in the blood vessel wall.

In brain-dead organ donors, a failure to produce ADH may result in the development of both hypotension and cranial diabetes insipidus with disturbances of osmolality and organ function. Treatment with α-adrenoceptor agonists may restore organ perfusion pressure but also cause ischaemic damage. The use of low-dose ADH infusions at 0.5–3 U/h titrated against urine output reduces the need for catecholamine support and also reduces perturbations in plasma osmolality and fluid balance; 1-deamino-8-*O*-arginine vasopressin (DDAVP) has similar benefits but causes less vasoconstriction. It is preferred for the treatment of cranial diabetes insipidus associated with brainstem death where hypotension is not a concomitant feature.

Coagulation

ADH increases circulating levels of tissue plasminogen activator, factor VIII and von Willebrand factor.[21] These effects may be mediated by V_2 receptors but this remains controversial. At high but physiological concentrations it can act as a platelet -aggregating agent.[22,23] Platelet aggregation is mediated through activation of platelet V_1 receptors.[24] ADH and its synthetic analogue DDAVP are used as first-line treatments in patients with von Willebrand's disease, and may be used in bleeding associated with renal failure and platelet dysfunction.

ACTH secretion

ADH transported via the portal venous system between the median eminence and the anterior pituitary acts upon V_3 receptors in the anterior pituitary to stimulate release of ACTH, which in turn increases plasma cortisol. The ADH both increases the efficacy of CRF in releasing ACTH and also has independent efficacy in stimulating ACTH release itself. In septic shock, it is possible that ADH insufficiency partially accounts for the relative adrenal insufficiency noted in certain patients. The relative importance and potency of ADH compared with CRF in stimulating ACTH release in humans is unclear.

VOLUME RECEPTORS

Volume homeostasis takes precedence over sodium homeostasis and so rises and falls in sodium will occur in order to preserve the circulating volume. In euvolaemic patients, sodium homeostasis is maintained. Sodium concentration is detected by both the osmoreceptors of the SFO outside the blood–brain barrier and the juxtaglomerular apparatus, which secretes renin in response to reduced GFR and a lower sodium load in the tubule.[25] The predominant determinants of sodium balance, however, are the high-pressure baroreceptors in the pulmonary veins, left atrium, carotid sinus and aortic arch.[26] Reduced stretch of these receptors increases sympathetic nervous system activity and activation of the renin–angiotensin–aldosterone system, resulting in reduced sodium excretion (via reduced GFR) and increased reabsorption of sodium in the proximal and distal convoluted tubules. Additionally, release of ADH can be stimulated resulting in concomitant water retention. Conversely, stretch of the baroreceptors will result in a fall in sodium retention through reduced activity of the sympathetic nervous and renin–angiotensin–aldosterone systems. Stretch additionally results in the release of ANP/BNP and a natriuresis through reduced sodium reabsorption in the distal convoluted tubule and collecting duct. ADH release is reduced by the fall in sympathetic nervous tone from the baroreceptors. ADH secretion may also be inhibited by the action of ANP on cerebral osmoreceptors lying outside the blood–brain barrier.[27]

The role of low-pressure baroreceptors in the systemic venous circulation and right atrium is less clearly defined. When venodilatation occurs, as is seen in sepsis or when there is a reduction in cardiac output, reduced baroreceptor signalling in the high-pressure system will result in both sodium and water retention as outlined previously. This will expand the extracellular fluid compartment and potentially cause tissue oedema. As sepsis resolves, venous tone is restored, capillary leak reduces, an increase in the loading of the high-pressure baroreceptors results and a natriuresis takes place. Patients may become transiently polyuric as they clear the excess salt and water accumulated whilst shocked. During this physiological diuresis, plasma osmolality remains tightly within the normal range provided that renal concentrating mechanisms have not been injured during the septic episode or by drug administration.

CRANIAL DIABETES INSIPIDUS (CDI)

CONGENTIAL CDI

Congenital CDI is rare and usually inherited as an autosomal dominant characteristic that results from mutations of the gene encoding an ADH precursor – preprovasopressin neurophysin II.[28] The onset of the disease may occur anywhere between 1 year of age and middle adult life and is associated with the final destruction of the ADH-producing cells due to an accumulation of the abnormal ADH precursor.[29] Until the destruction of the SON and PVN cells occurs, ADH secretion (facilitated by expression of the normal gene) and regulation of plasma osmolality are often unaffected.

ACQUIRED CDI

Acquired CDI may be transient or permanent and can arise from an absolute (complete) or relative (incomplete) lack of ADH. Complete central DI is usually associated with lesions above the level of the median eminence, in the supraoptic or paraventricular nuclei or of the neurohypophyseal stalk whereby the production of ADH in the hypothalamus is terminated.[30] Permanent central DI tends to be associated with transecting, obliterating or chronic inflammatory lesions, whereas transient DI is more likely to be associated with acute inflammatory or oedematous lesions with some recovery of ADH secretion occurring as the inflammation or oedema resolves. An exception to this is the transient DI seen following excision or destruction of the posterior pituitary; ADH produced in the hypothalamus can still be released into the systemic circulation from capillaries in the median eminence. In the past the majority of acquired non-traumatic CDI was categorised as idiopathic but it has become apparent that the majority of these cases are associated with abnormality of the inferior hypophyseal arterial system[31] or autoimmune reactivity against ADH-producing cells.[32] However, association does not necessitate causality.

When the normal release of ADH into the circulation in response to rising plasma osmolality is reduced or absent, inappropriately high urine volumes are passed and the urine osmolality becomes inappropriately low for the state of water depletion being suffered by the patient. Where ADH is entirely absent from the circulation, over 20 litres of very dilute urine (25–200 mOsm/kg) per day may be produced. If the patient is unable to drink freely (most ICU patients), or the thirst mechanisms are impaired, profound dehydration will result very rapidly unless appropriate interventions are made by the physician. Where ADH deficiency is relative rather than absolute, it is possible for the patient to partially concentrate the urine and values of 500–800 mOsm/kg would not be atypical. However, these osmolalities are inappropriately low relative to the plasma osmolality. In partial ADH deficiency, volumes of urine as low as 3 litres per day may be evidenced. These are still inappropriately high when assessed in terms of the solute excretion of the patient, but are more difficult to recognise as being due to DI as there are many other causes of diureses of this magnitude. Additionally, extrinsic stimulants of ADH release (see Box 59.2) may have an antidiuretic effect further complicating the diagnosis.

The plasma osmolality measured in central DI is usually in the higher regions of the normal range or very slightly supranormal. It is remarkably constant in those with free access to water and intact thirst mechanisms as they will drink huge quantities of water to regulate and maintain their water balance. Hyperosmolality or hypernatraemia suggests impaired sensation of thirst or inability to access water (see water deprivation test later) and can also be seen if patients are administered large quantities of isotonic saline or Hartman's solution to replace their hypotonic urine losses. If unrecognised and untreated, hyperosmolality and hypernatraemia may result in death.

Cranial diabetes insipidus is usually associated with reduced production of ADH or damage to the normal release mechanisms of ADH. However, there can be dysfunction of the osmolality sensing mechanism at receptor or intracellular signalling levels whilst actual

Box 59.3 Causes of cranial DI

Acquired:
Idiopathic
Autoimmune
Tumours (especially suprasellar, lung, breast, lymphoma and leukaemia)
Surgery (especially trans-sphenoidal surgery)
Traumatic head injury (strongly associated with base of skull fracture[82])
Hypoxic brain injury
Brainstem death
Electrolyte disturbance – profound hyponatraemia
Radiotherapy
Drugs – amiodarone, lithium (Li more likely to cause nephrogenic DI)
Inflammatory/infectious diseases – sickle cell disease, tuberculosis, abscesses, encephalitis, meningitis, sarcoidosis (may also cause nephrogenic DI), Wegner's granulomatosis, histiocytosis X
Vascular disease – ischaemic or haemorrhagic strokes, aneurysmal bleeds (especially anterior communicating artery SAH), Sheehan syndrome, pituitary apoplexy

Congenital (1–2% of all cases)
Autosomal dominant mutations of ADH expression (despite the dominant expression of the gene, the onset of clinical DI may take up to 30 years to develop)[34]
Wolfram syndrome – autosomal recessive condition characterised by DI, diabetes mellitus, optic atrophy and deafness

ADH production and storage are normal. It is possible to have a normal release of ADH in response to baroreceptor detection of hypotension but subnormal release in response to hyperosmolality. This has been described in association with chronic hypernatraemia.[33]

The main recognised causes of central DI are listed in **Box 59.3**. A particularly common cause of DI seen in the ICU is traumatic or post-surgical brain injury. Trans-sphenoidal surgery for treatment of suprasellar tumours can result in DI in between 10 and 70% of patients; the frequency parallels the magnitude of the tumour being removed. Additionally, transcranial surgery may cause the development of DI in the absence of a fall in plasma ADH. This is postulated to be due to the release of a hypothalamic ADH precursor that acts as a competitive antagonist of both ADH and synthetic analogues. The presence of a competitive antagonist effectively creates an endocrinological picture similar to nephrogenic DI with normal or high plasma ADH levels but an inappropriate diuresis of dilute urine.

Following surgery or traumatic brain injury, several different patterns of polyuria can be seen. Immediate polyuria is common and may be transient or permanent. Occasionally it is preceded by a period of oliguria due to an initial surge of ADH release. Additionally, a classical triphasic pattern of urine output may be observed with: (i) transient polyuria due to transient impairment of the release of ADH (0–5 days in duration), then (ii) a phase of normal or reduced urine output – the ADH previously stored in the pituitary gland is gradually released into the circulation as the cells storing it involute (3–6 days in duration), and finally (iii) persistent polyuria as the pituitary stores exhaust and no replacement hormone from the hypothalamus is produced. During the second phase of this pattern, administration of fluids may result in volume overload and hyponatraemia as the ADH release is not under feedback control from osmoreceptors but occurs in an uncontrolled manner as a result of pituitary degeneration. Effectively, there is a transient syndrome of inappropriate ADH (SIADH) secretion. The triphasic pattern is usually associated with sudden severe damage to the hypothalamus or pituitary from trauma, surgery or intracranial bleed, and careful, regular clinical and biochemical assessment is essential to ensure normal water balance and osmolality during this transition from DI to SIADH and back to DI again.

The exact nature of the urinary pattern seen in DI is relatively unimportant and gradual resolution may occur over several months in those with transient DI. Imaging the hypothalamus and pituitary with T1 MRI may provide prognostic information as to whether recovery is likely or not; hypothalamic lesions have a poorer prognosis than pituitary ones.[35] What is essential is that meticulous assessments of the patient and their plasma and urinary biochemistry as well as fluid inputs and outputs are made to prevent the development of unnecessary fluid and solute imbalances that could lead to worsening morbidity or mortality. It is important to maintain a high level of suspicion for the development of DI in anyone who is suffering from pituitary disease or who has suffered a pituitary injury as the symptoms may have gradual onset. Anterior pituitary failure can lessen the impact of central DI because of the deficiency of ACTH and cortisol, which reduces GFR and free water loss. Additionally, the loss of feedback inhibition may stimulate increased release of ADH from the median eminence. Thus, in Sheehan's syndrome and pituitary apoplexy, the presenting symptoms tend not to be those of DI with polyuria. However, once corticosteroid therapy is commenced then polyuria indicating DI may become apparent or exacerbated. Conversely, patients with persistent DI of idiopathic origin should have long-term endocrine follow-up as a number will go on to develop tumours of the pituitary several years after the diagnosis of DI.[36,37]

TREATMENT OF CDI

Four separate problems have to be addressed when treating CDI:

1. Associated anterior pituitary dysfunction should be considered and managed when present.
2. Hypernatraemia must be recognised and treated with painstaking care.

3. Any deficit of total body water must be recognised and addressed (this may be urgent if the patient is shocked).
4. The underlying deficiency of ADH causing the polyuria must be addressed.

In all ICU patients with DI, hourly urine measurements, hourly fluid losses and fluid inputs and at least twice-daily urine and plasma osmolalities are recommended. In shocked patients and those with hypernatraemia, hourly monitoring of plasma sodium is recommended to prevent worsening of hyperosmolality or over-rapid correction of hypernatraemia.

ANTERIOR PITUITARY DYSFUNCTION

If this is present, it requires recognition and treatment. In the emergent situation with a shocked patient, hydrocortisone 100 mg can be administered as an i.v. bolus, and steroid replacement continued if needed. Steroid administration may worsen the diuresis but will improve cardiovascular stability in patients with pituitary ablation.

HYPERNATRAEMIA

If the patient with CDI and ongoing water diuresis has had restricted access to fluids and developed hyperosmolality/hypertonicity, or has developed hypertonicity through replacement of dilute urine with equal volumes of isotonic (to plasma) intravenous fluids, then sudden reduction in plasma tonicity may result in cerebral oedema, pontine myelonecrosis and permanent neurological damage as a result of water moving into brain cells down an osmotic gradient (see below). In order to counteract cellular dehydration in chronic (>24 hours) hypernatraemic states, the brain accumulates intracellular organic osmolytes such as amino acids, taurine and sorbitol.[38–40]

When a euvolaemic state is present, arginine vasopressin or DDAVP may be administered to reduce urine output (see below). At the same time, fluid restriction should be imposed and replacement of the previous hour's urine output undertaken with an appropriate fluid to avoid a fall in concentration of sodium by more than 0.5 mmol/h.[41] Absolute safety data are not available to determine the ideal rate of reduction of plasma sodium. However, when a patient has been hypernatraemic for more than 48 hours, a fall of more than 8 mmol/L in any 24-hour period should be avoided.[42] Several formulae exist to guide fluid replacement regimens controlling the rate of fall of plasma sodium concentrations; reliance on these is not recommended and extremely close monitoring with hourly review of plasma sodium is less likely to result in sudden unexpected changes in tonicity.[43]

DEHYDRATION AND HYPOVOLAEMIA

If associated with shock, hypovolaemia requires rapid resuscitation. If hypovolaemia is also associated with hypernatraemia, extreme caution is required in the resuscitation, which should take place with isotonic saline solution and frequent reassessments of plasma sodium and cardiovascular and neurological status. Where the hypernatraemia is very marked (>155 mmol/L), consideration of a combination of isotonic (0.9%) and hypertonic saline should be given to reduce the rate of sodium reduction. In the face of hypertonicity of the plasma, cells reduce their chloride and potassium conductance in addition to synthesising intracellular osmolytes. If 0.9% saline (effective osmolality 290 mOsm/kg when diluted by plasma proteins) is infused rapidly into hypertonic plasma with a sodium of 160 mmol/L, an effective osmolality of 330 mOsm/kg, a rapid drop in plasma osmolality may cause cerebral and other organ oedema, seizures and death. By reducing the tonicity of the plasma gradually, the cells have time to down-regulate their synthesis of intracellular osmolytes and increase potassium and chloride conductance to reduce swelling as plasma tonicity falls.

CORRECTION OF POLYURIA AND ADH DEFICIENCY

At mild levels of polyuria (2–3 mL/kg/h) where there is an expectation that the condition may resolve, it may be appropriate to merely replace the previous hours' urine output with an appropriate fluid (usually 5% dextrose or 0.18% saline/4% dextrose) whilst undertaking regular measurements of plasma and urine osmolality and electrolytes. Care must be taken not to give so much dextrose as to result in hyperglycaemia, hyperosmolality and osmotic diuresis.

Where polyuria is expected to be persistent or is excessive, either ADH/AVP or DDAVP may be administered. DDAVP is a selective V_2 receptor agonist and thus is less likely to cause hypertension. It is also longer acting, resisting breakdown by vasopressinases, and is usually administered once or twice daily. The usual daily dose rate, when administered intravenously, intramuscularly or subcutaneously is 1–4 μg daily. ADH may be administered subcutaneously or by intravenous infusion and DDAVP may be presented intranasally, subcutaneously, intravenously or orally. In the acute situation, an ADH infusion (0.1–3 U/h) can be conveniently titrated against urine output. The use of the infusion ensures 100% bioavailability and facilitates re-establishment of the hypertonic renal medullary interstitium before changing the patient to the longer acting DDAVP. The dose of ADH or DDAVP is often higher during the acute onset phase of CDI – this may be due to the loss of hypertonicity in the medullary interstitium or due to biologically inactive ADH precursors released from the damaged hypothalamic–pituitary tract, which act as competitive antagonists at the V_2 renal receptors. The dose of ADH or DDAVP used is the minimum dose required to control urine output to an acceptable rate. Excessive administration can result in water retention and the development of hypo-osmolal syndromes.

Other drugs may also be used to reduce the polyuria of CDI. Provided there is some residual ADH synthesis, chlorpropamide, clofibrate and carbamazepine are all reported to enhance ADH release and also increase the renal responsiveness to ADH. Thiazide diuretics may also be effective. Although these agents all reduce urine output, there is little place for them in the modern management of CDI in the ICU where DDAVP and ADH have excellent safety profiles and are more easily titrated to effect. These alternative drugs are discussed later in the treatment of nephrogenic DI.

NEPHROGENIC DIABETES INSIPIDUS

Nephrogenic diabetes insipidus (NDI) may be congenital or acquired (**Box 59.4**). As the majority of congenital cases present in the first week of life, the majority of cases seen in the adult ICU are acquired. The commonest of these are lithium toxicity due to long-term drug treatment, hypercalcaemia and post-obstructive uropathy following relief of ureteric or urethral obstruction.

CONGENITAL NDI

Some 80–90% of patients with congenital NDI have an X-linked recessive abnormality of the $AVPR_2$ gene coding for the V_2-receptor.[28,44] Different mutations of the gene are described but the majority result in trapping of the V_2-receptor intracellularly, and unable to integrate into the membrane of the collecting duct cell. Drugs have been developed that can facilitate receptor integration into the membrane, restoring some of the urine-concentrating abilities of ADH.[45] The sex linkage results in the vast majority of affected patients being male. However, female children can also present less severe polyuria and polydipsia due to expression of the abnormal gene. Non-sex-linked genetic abnormalities can also cause NDI. Approximately 10% of cases of congenital NDI have mutations of the AQP_2 (aquaporin 2) gene, which codes for the AQP_2 channel. Over 40 mutations, both autosomal dominant and recessive, have been described to date.

The remainder of cases of congenital NDI arises from a variety of pathophysiologies that result in failure to generate a hypertonic renal medulla, with inability to reabsorb water even if the V_2 receptor and acquaporin$_2$ channels are normal. A lack of the Kidd antigen (a blood group antigen) results in an inability to concentrate urine to more than 800 mOsm/kg even with water deprivation and exogenous ADH administration.[46] This is because the antigen is also expressed in the collecting duct epithelium where it functions as a urea transporter (urea transport B protein) and facilitates movement of urea from urine into the medullary interstitium maintaining some of the gradients required to facilitate water reabsorption. Similarly, patients with mutations in chloride channel genes, potassium channel genes or the sodium–potassium–chloride co-transporter gene resulting in the Bartter syndrome are unable to generate a hypertonic medullary interstitium. However, in these patients the defect is more marked and urine can rarely be concentrated above 350 mOsm/kg.[47]

With congenital NDI, early diagnosis and management are essential as avoidance of hypernatraemia and dehydration facilitate the achievement of normal developmental milestones and avoid the cerebral damage once commonly accepted as an inevitable association of NDI.

Box 59.4 Causes of nephrogenic DI

Acquired	Congenital
Lithium toxicity	X-linked recessive: $AVPR_2$ gene mutations
Postobstructive diuresis	Autosomal recessive or dominant: AQP_2 gene mutations
Hypercalcaemia	Bartter syndrome
Hypokalaemia	Gitelman syndrome
Hypoproteinaemia	Urea transport protein B (Kidd Ag) deficiency/absence
Sjögren's syndrome	
Amyloid	
Multiple myeloma	
Sickle cell disease	
Polycystic kidney disease	
Pyelonephritis	
Renal transplantation	
Other drugs: amiodarone, amphotericin B, clozapine, colchicine, demeclocycline, foscarnet, gentamicin, loop diuretics, rifampicin	

ACQUIRED NDI

Lithium-associated nephrotoxicity remains the commonest form of acquired NDI with more than 20% of patients on chronic lithium therapy developing polyuria. Lithium is taken up into the principal cells of the collecting duct via sodium channels and inhibits intracellular adenylate cyclase, antagonising the effects of ADH. Additionally, it reduces the medullary interstitial hypertonicity possibly through reducing expression of urea transport protein B. If patients with early lithium-related NDI are prescribed amiloride, some reversal of both the polyuria and lithium mediated toxicity is possible. Amiloride's natriuretic action is achieved through closure of the luminal sodium channels in the collecting duct, the sodium channels through which lithium enters the cells.[48] Indomethacin increases intracellular cAMP and counteracts the diminution of this and AQP_2 caused by lithium, resulting in a marked and immediate drop in urine output. However, care is required as NSAIDs may worsen renal failure, reducing GFR and lithium excretion thereby worsening toxicity.

Hypercalcaemia, hypokalaemia, release of ureteric or urethral obstruction and hypoproteinaemia are also recognised as causing NDI and are associated with reduced expression of AQP_2 channels, urea transport proteins and a loss of interstitial hypertonicity. These defects normally cause milder polyuria than that associated with lithium toxicity. Finally, the attritions of ageing lead to loss of urinary concentrating ability. It is suggested that this is due to a combination of pathophysiological changes characteristic of both NDI and CDI with relative reductions of both AQP_2 and AVP production.[49]

TREATMENT OF NDI

The treatment of NDI aims to minimise the occurrence of hypernatraemia and hypovolaemia and wherever possible to remove the underlying cause.

1. *Correct reversible causes:* stop any drugs suspected in the aetiology; then correct hypokalaemia, hypercalcaemia and hypoproteinaemia.
2. *Reduce solute load:* as urine output is determined by the solute load to be excreted, reducing the solute intake will reduce the urine volume accordingly; if maximum urine concentration is 250 mOsm/kg, a solute intake of 750 mOsm day requires production of at least 3 litres of urine to clear the solute, whereas if intake is reduced to 500 mmol then 2 litres of urine will suffice. In ICU, the reduction of solute can be difficult as many drugs and diluents have a high solute load. Additionally, patients may be catabolic and have a high protein requirement. It may be more appropriate not to aim to restrict solute intake for certain patients but to monitor fluid balance closely and ensure adequate appropriate replacement:
   a. Restrict salt intake (aiming at <100 mmol/day)
   b. Reduce protein intake aiming to provide the minimum daily requirement including essential amino acids. This should be done with specialist dietetic advice and requires careful follow-up to avoid protein malnutrition. It is not appropriate to protein-restrict children where it may adversely affect normal growth and development)
3. *Diuretics – thiazides and amiloride:*
   a. Thiazides – whereas DI loses water in excess to solute rendering the plasma hyperosmolal, resulting in intracellular dehydration to maintain the intravascular volume, thiazide diuretics cause solute loss in excess of water and lead to a drop in intravascular volume. This causes activation of the sympathetic nervous system and the renin–angiotensin–aldosterone system and a fall in glomerular filtration and ANP. Additionally, thiazides are associated with an increased expression of AQP_2 channels in the collecting duct.[50] These neuroendocrine changes lead to an increase in proximal tubular reabsorption of sodium and water and an increase in ADH release. Less ultrafiltrate reaches the collecting duct and urine volume can fall by as much as 30%. Combined with a solute-reduced diet, the fall in urine production can be as high as 50%.
   b. Amiloride is a useful adjunct to thiazide diuretics in NDI where it causes a further slight reduction in urine output and combats the hypokalaemia associated with the thiazides. It may have benefit in its own right in lithium-associated nephrotoxicity where it blocks the sodium channels through which lithium enters the principal cells. If administered before lithium damage becomes irreversible, it can both reduce the damage to the cells themselves and reverse the antagonism of lithium on the effects of ADH.

   Loop diuretics are not effective in reducing the diuresis of NDI as, whilst they reduce intravascular volume and stimulate the sympathetic nervous system in a similar manner to thiazides, they also reduce interstitial medullary sodium concentrations and hypertonicity thus reducing water reabsorption by the collecting duct rather than enhancing it.
4. *ADH:* where NDI is not absolute (most cases of acquired NDI), supplementing endogenous ADH to create supraphysiological concentrations in the plasma can result in a fall of urine production by up to 25%. This may occur by antagonism of the effects of any V_2 receptor antagonists present or through greater receptor occupation. Care is required with long-term use as hypertension and its associated complications may result.
5. *NSAIDs:* PGE_2 increases GFR and urine flow and decreases intracellular cAMP and thus aquaporin expression. NSAIDs reduce the formation of renal PGE_2 and when used alone may reduce urine output by up to 50%.[51] Combination with low-solute diet and a thiazide diuretic may provide additional antidiuretic benefit.[52] However, the use of NSAIDs has to be weighed against their long-term complications. This is particularly true in the ICU population who are at increased risk of both renal impairment and gastric erosions. Indomethacin is cited to have greater treatment benefit than other NSAIDs in NDI.[53] It is also more likely to produce unwanted adverse effects.
6. *Chlorpropamide:* this oral hypoglycaemic agent enhances both ADH release and the sensitivity of the kidney to it. It is suggested to act via increasing the hypertonicity of the renal medulla. Doses of 250 mg o.d. or b.d. are prescribed, but are likely to cause hypoglycaemia.[54] Its use is therefore reserved for severe refractory cases of partial NDI.
7. *Clofibrate:* this oral lipid-lowering agent is reported to enhance ADH release and increase the renal sensitivity to ADH.[55] Its use in CDI has largely been superseded by the introduction of safer, more efficacious DDAVP therapy. Its use in treatment of DI has been associated with myopathy.[56] If considered for

treatment of partial NDI, biochemical markers of myopathy should be measured regularly.

8. *Carbamazepine:* carbamazepine can also be tried as a treatment in partial NDI although it is more effective in treating partial CDI. It increases the renal responsiveness to ADH, but requires a dose rate three times higher than that effective as an antiepileptic. This high dose rate limits its usefulness in therapy.
9. *Molecular chaperones:* novel drugs described as 'molecular chaperones' are being developed to treat NDI where the V_2 receptor is functional and intact but confined to the intracellular space, unable to integrate into the basolateral membrane of the principal cell.[57] The drugs are membrane-permeable V_2 receptor antagonists and are believed to cause refolding of the receptor in a form that allows normal processing of the receptor into the membrane.[58] These are showing some success in animal models of congenital NDI and with human V_2R mutations associated with NDI in testing in vitro. Early studies in humans report some success.[59] Unfortunately, a recent study with Relcovaptan (SR49059), whilst showing very promising clinical results, had to be discontinued owing to possible interference in the cytochrome P450 pathway. Nevertheless, other chaperone molecules are currently being explored for human testing.[60]

GESTATIONAL DI (GDI) (BOX 59.5)

In pregnancy the normal range of plasma osmolalities falls to 265–285 mOsm/kg and the plasma sodium is <140 mmol/L. The reduction in osmolality is attributed to a resetting of the central osmostat[61,62] with the onset of development of thirst at an osmolality around 10 mOsm/kg lower than in the non-pregnant state. This has been attributed to increases in the plasma concentration of human chorionic gonadotropin (hCG).[63] The retention of water and sodium is mediated by reduced baroreceptor stimulation.[64]

During pregnancy, the placenta produces vasopressinases (cysteine-aminopeptidases) that increase ADH metabolism up to fourfold[65] and relaxin, which contributes to the 50% increase in GFR and venodilatation.[66] Aldosterone concentrations rise up to fivefold. Solute elimination also increases; a small reduction in urine-concentrating ability may have a more marked effect. The volume of urine passed per day increases as a result of passage of an increased solute load (including urinary proteins, glucose and amino acids), increased drinking and a raised GFR. A diagnosis of DI therefore requires careful differentiation from a physiological polyuria or potentially pathological polyuria of separate aetiology (e.g. gestational diabetes) in pregnancy.

GDI occurs in around 1:300 000 pregnancies and can result from:

1. Increased destruction of ADH by excessive production of placental vasopressinases[67] (especially gemellar pregnancies) or reduced deactivation of vasopressinases (e.g. in acute fatty liver of pregnancy,[68] pre-eclampsia or HELLP syndrome) – this may be unresponsive to exogenous ADH administration as it too is rapidly metabolised. DDAVP can be used instead as it is resistant to degradation by placental vasopressinase.
2. Permanently deficient reserve of ADH secretion, which in the non-pregnant state is asymptomatic but in the pregnant state is unmasked by the higher vasopressinase activity that cannot be compensated for by increased secretion.[69] This condition responds to treatment with ADH/DDAVP and is indicative of latent, subclinical DI that predated pregnancy. Investigation and follow-up following pregnancy is warranted as a proportion of patients in this category will develop later hypothalamo–pituitary axis pathologies such as tumours or autoimmune hypophysitis.
3. Central DI associated with Sheehan syndrome and pituitary apoplexy – Sheehan syndrome is commonest, and is usually preceded by major bleeding or hypotension at the time of delivery. Pituitary apoplexy has been described antenatally too.[70]
4. Gestational nephrogenic DI of unknown aetiology that is resistant to both ADH and DDAVP, with resolution in the postnatal period.[71]

The treatment of GDI varies depending on the underlying cause. In all cases, it is important not to allow the patient to become hypernatraemic and hyperosmolal as this is likely to have adverse effects on both mother and child. Where hypernatraemia and hyperosmolality do occur, careful correction is required in a closely monitored, very gradual, stepwise fashion. A lowering of sodium by as little as 10 mmol/L per day has been associated with pontine myelinolysis.[72]

The associations between acute fatty liver of pregnancy, HELLP and pre-eclampsia and DI are well recognised, if not fully understood. It has been suggested that liver dysfunction results in reduced clearance of the vasopressinases released by the placenta and thus increased clearance of maternal ADH.[73,74] It is important to bear these associations in mind as the polyuria of

Box 59.5 Causes of gestational DI

Sheehan syndrome Pituitary apoplexy Hepatic dysfunction: acute fatty liver of pregnancy, pre-eclampsia, HELLP syndrome	Vasopressinase release by placenta Idiopathic gestational NDI (resolves post-partum)

DI may mask the hypertension and fluid overload of pre-eclampsia and HELLP leading to later diagnosis, delayed management and poorer outcome.[75]

POLYDIPSIA (PSYCHOGENIC/ NEUROGENIC/PRIMARY)

Polydipsia may result from: (i) a psychiatric disorder or disturbance,[76] (ii) drugs that give the sensation of dry mouth[77] or airways to the patient (e.g. oxygen therapy, phenothiazines, anticholinergics), or (iii) hypothalamic lesions that directly disturb the thirst centre[78] (e.g. sarcoidosis). In all three of the above causes of polydipsia, excessive drinking is associated with the production of large quantities of urine of appropriate osmolality. If the fluid ingested is largely hypotonic, the urine will be hypo-osmolal and result from a fall in ADH secretion. If the fluid ingested is hypertonic, the urine will have high osmolality but remain of high volume because of the combination of low ADH production and high ANP production causing a solute diuresis.

Polydipsia may also result from the appropriate detection by osmoreceptors of a raised plasma osmolality due to raised glucose, alcohol or sodium. The glycosuria itself will cause an osmotic diuresis and plasma osmolality may be normal or raised depending on the severity of the hyperglycaemia and any accompanying ketoacidosis and dehydration.

Excessive drinking of hypotonic fluids leads to hyponatraemia and may progress to water intoxication with cerebral oedema, confusion, impaired consciousness, seizures and death. It has also been postulated that long-term polydipsia may lead to the development of dysregulation of ADH secretion and cranial DI.[79] These are important considerations in patients presenting with reduced consciousness and polyuria; water intoxication, more usually associated with SIADH, and DI may coexist.

SOLUTE DIURESIS

Just as failure to reabsorb water can result in polyuria, failure to reabsorb solute can result in an osmotic load in the tubule that opposes water absorption in the convoluted tubules and collecting duct. The commonest cause of this in the general patient population is glycosuria. In the ICU setting, a solute diuresis may also be associated with the administration of diuretic drugs, high-protein feeds (increased urea load), supranormal quantities of sodium and other solutes through fluids, feeds and drugs, recovery from acute renal failure with tubular inability to reabsorb solute, and drug-induced tubular damage.

To differentiate a solute diuresis from a water diuresis it is advisable to measure the 24-hour excretion of solute in the urine. Normally, between 600 and 900 mOsm/day of solute are excreted in the urine. Values higher than this indicate a solute diuresis. A spot urine osmolality may be measured; osmolality higher than 300 mOsm/kg, is suggestive of a solute diuresis. It would not be uncommon in the critically ill patient to encounter simultaneous impairment of both water reabsorption and impaired solute elimination. In this instance, 24-hour solute excretion will be increased but the urine may be hypo-osmolal.

THE DIAGNOSIS OF POLYURIC SYNDROMES

MEASURE AND CALCULATE PLASMA OSMOLALITY AND URINE OSMOLALITY

A high urine osmolality in the presence of a high plasma osmolality is appropriate and if the plasma osmolality is higher than 295 mOsm/L, urine osmolality should reach 1000–1200 mOsm/kg. Urine osmolalities of less than this imply that there is a urine-concentrating defect and lead to consideration of the causes of diabetes insipidus or medications that might reduce renal interstitial hypertonicity such as loop diuretics. Urine osmolalities of <150 mOsm/kg in this circumstance are sufficient to make the diagnosis of DI provided there is not obvious gross fluid and solute overload of the patient.

Where the patient is polyuric with a high plasma osmolality and maximum urine osmolalities are being achieved, an osmotic diuresis is implied. The diuresis may be inappropriate in as much as it is leading to dehydration, but appropriate in that the kidneys are retaining as much water as they can for the large solute load being excreted. If there is a normal *osmolal gap* (the difference between measured and calculated plasma osmolality, normal <10 mOsm/kg), hyperglycaemia, hypernatraemia or hyperkalaemia are implied. If the osmolal gap is greater than 10 mOsm/kg, investigation should be undertaken to look for an unmeasured solute such as ethanol, mannitol, ethylene glycol, sorbitol or methanol. If plasma osmolality is less than 280 mOsm/kg, urine osmolality would also be expected to be lower than this to clear free water. This picture implies water overload, which may be iatrogenic or patient mediated. Low plasma osmolality with high urine osmolality implies SIADH and would not normally be associated with polyuria.

WATER DEPRIVATION AND ADH TESTS

In health, being deprived of water rapidly results in an increase in plasma osmolality, which causes ADH release and an increase in urine osmolality to 1000–1200 mOsm/kg in order to preserve water and reduce plasma osmolality back towards its normal value. When the cause of polyuria is unclear and the patient is not already clinically dehydrated, a water deprivation test may be useful to determine the cause of the diuresis. In patients with severe polyuria, the test is potentially dangerous as dehydration and hyperosmolality may develop very rapidly resulting in permanent cerebral damage and cardiovascular collapse. It is therefore necessary to undertake the test under very close supervision during daylight hours.

The limitations of the test should also be appreciated:

1. In acute CDI, release of ADH precursors from injured brain tissue may render interpretation of ADH tests unreliable through cross-reactions with ADH measurement assays.
2. At high concentrations of ADH, the urine concentrations achieved in partial NDI and primary polydipsia may be similar.
3. Patients with partial CDI may occasionally become hypersensitive to relatively small rises in ADH, which may be induced by the rise in osmolality associated with water deprivation and thus maximally concentrate urine once osmolality is raised leading to an erroneous diagnosis of primary polydipsia.[80]
4. In patients with chronic hypernatraemia and CDI secondary to osmoreceptor dysfunction, hypovolaemia with water deprivation may cause sufficient baroreceptor stimulus to release ADH and suggest normal urine concentrating abilities.[81]

Step 1: plasma and urine osmolalities, plasma ADH and patient body weight are measured at time zero and access to i.v./oral fluids is denied.

Step 2: plasma and urine osmolalities and patient body weight are measured hourly until either three consecutive urine osmolalities are within 30 mOsm/kg of one another or plasma osmolality is >295 mOsm/kg, or the patient loses more than 5% of the body weight from baseline. At this time, plasma ADH is measured again.

Step 3: if plasma osmolality is >295 mOsm/kg and urine osmolality is <800 mOsm/kg, ADH (5 units AVP s.c. or 4 μg DDAVP s.c.) is administered to the patient and plasma and urine osmolalities are measured hourly for 3 hours (this time is necessary to allow time for at least partial recovery of the medullary interstitial hypertonic gradient in patients with primary polydipsia). DDAVP is preferred to AVP as it avoids misinterpretation of results in the presence of vasopressinases, which would rapidly metabolise AVP and suggest a diagnosis of NDI rather than CDI. Although neither is the correct diagnosis if vasopressinases are present, the treatment is as for CDI (i.e. the administration of DDAVP).

Step 4: urine osmolality is then plotted against plasma osmolality (**Fig. 59.4**).

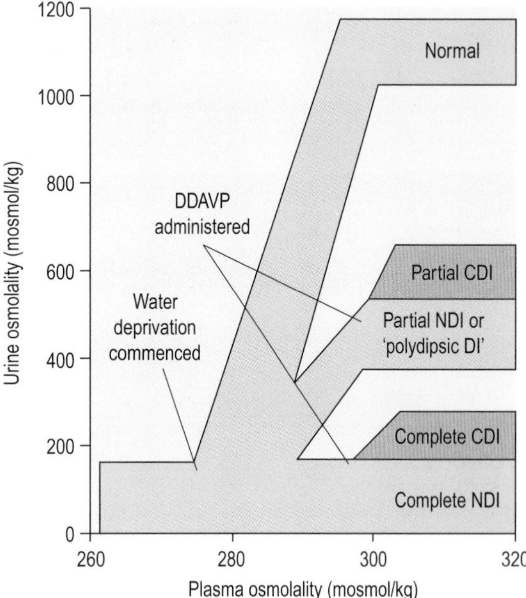

Figure 59.4 Urine versus plasma osmolality during water deprivation testing. DDAVP = 1-deamino-8-O-arginine vasopressin; CDI = cranial diabetes insipidus; NDI = nephrogenic diabetes insipidus. *(Adapted from Sands JM, Bichet DG. Nephrogenic diabetes insipidus. Ann Intern Med 2006;144:186–94.[49])*

Step 5: plasma and urine osmolalities are plotted against plasma ADH concentrations (**Fig. 59.5**).

INTERPRETATION OF THE TESTS (SEE FIGS 59.4 AND 59.5)

In complete DI, plasma osmolality will rise but urine osmolality will not rise above 300 mOsm/kg. Upon administration of ADH, patients with complete CDI will raise their urine osmolality to 500 mOsm/kg or higher, whereas there will be no rise in urine osmolality in complete NDI. In complete CDI the original plasma ADH measurement will be zero, whereas in complete NDI the initial ADH measurement will be normal or high depending upon the corresponding plasma osmolality at the time of measurement. In partial DI, plasma osmolality will rise and urine osmolality will also increase but usually plateaus between 400 and 800 mOsm/kg. In partial CDI the ADH will initially be normal or low and will rise with increasing plasma osmolality but is unlikely to rise above 4–5 pg/mL. In partial NDI, the ADH will initially be normal or high and will increase with plasma osmolality to >8 pg/mL but without achieving a correspondingly appropriate rise in urine concentration.

Following administration of ADH or DDAVP, urine osmolality is expected to at least double in complete

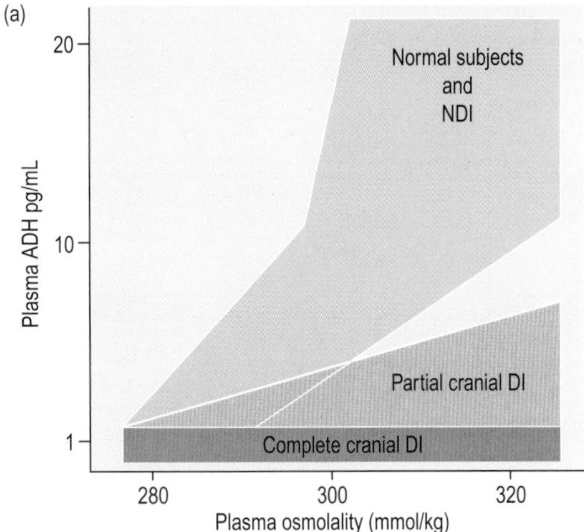

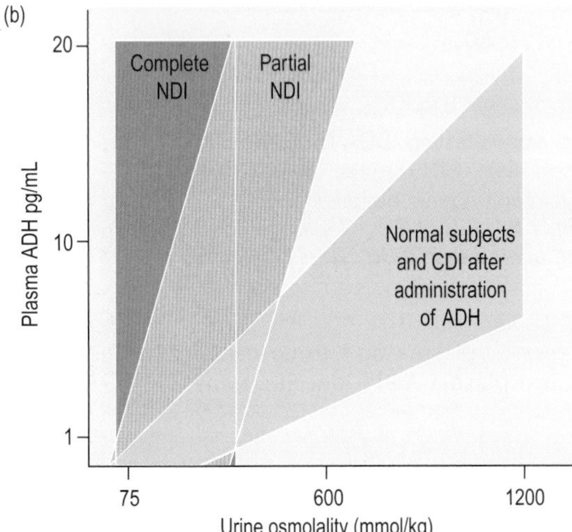

Figure 59.5 (a) As plasma osmolality increases as a result of water deprivation or hypertonic saline infusion, the measured concentration of antidiuretic hormone (ADH) should rise. Failure to do so suggests cranial diabetes insipidus. (b) At a given value of plasma ADH, whether endogenous or exogenous in origin, urine osmolality is expected to lie within a corresponding range of osmolality. However, the range of expected osmolalities is high as osmoreceptors adjust regulation around the basal level of ADH, which is also partly determined by volume receptors. In nephrogenic diabetes insipidus (NDI), the urine osmolality remains low even when high plasma ADH concentrations are measured.

CDI and rise by 10–50% in partial CDI or NDI. In complete NDI, there will be no rise in urine osmolality. Partial CDI may be inferentially differentiated from partial NDI on the basis of urine osmolality alone; in the former, urine osmolality rises above plasma osmolality whereas in partial NDI it tends to remain hypo-osmolal or iso-osmolal to plasma following ADH/DDAVP administration. However, this generalisation is indicative only and for greater certainty it is preferred to have measured sequential ADH concentrations to assess hypothalamic–pituitary function independently of the renal concentrating ability.

Water deprivation tests should not be conducted in infants, patients with pre-existing hypovolaemia or hyperosmolality. In the latter two categories, treatment of the fluid deficit and/or solute excess should precede further investigations. In infants and in adults with equivocal water deprivation test results, an infusion of hypertonic saline should be considered.

HYPERTONIC SALINE INFUSION TEST

In patients with equivocal results from a water deprivation test and in those at high risk of dehydration and hypovolaemia from water deprivation, a hypertonic saline infusion test may be undertaken to establish the cause of a water diuresis. Interpretation of the test is as for the water deprivation test, but there is a clearer demarcation between partial CDI and primary polydipsia (the latter having a normal rise in ADH in response to increasing plasma osmolality, whereas the former will have no rise or an obtunded one) and the risk of missing a diagnosis of CDI secondary to osmoreceptor dysfunction is reduced.[82]

Hypertonic saline is available in multiple different concentrations. Care is required in calculating the appropriate infusion rate to use for the test as this varies with the concentration of the hypertonic preparation stocked. 0.0425 mmol/kg/min of hypertonic sodium chloride solution is infused for up to 3 hours or until a plasma osmolality of 300 mOsm/kg is achieved.

Blood samples are taken 30 minutes before and at 30-minute intervals throughout the duration of the test and plasma sodium, osmolality and ADH are measured. Urine samples are collected before and where possible at 60-minute intervals throughout the test period and measurements of osmolality and sodium performed. Thirst and blood pressure are recorded at 30-minute intervals.

MRI-T-1-WEIGHTED IMAGING OF THE NEUROHYPOPHYSEAL TRACT

Imaging may be helpful in differentiating partial CDI from psychogenic polydipsia where results of a water deprivation test and the history make the differentiation uncertain. In CDI, the normal bright spot (stored ADH[34]) seen in the posterior pituitary is usually reduced or absent, whereas in psychogenic polydipsia it is usually well preserved or even enhanced (**Fig. 59.6**).

Although rapid and less labour intensive than a hypertonic saline infusion test, the results of MRI are not yet held to be entirely specific or sensitive. It is reported that the signal is often reduced in nephrogenic

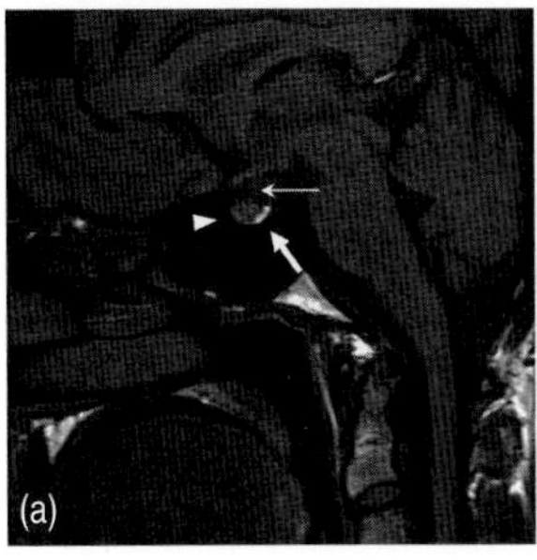

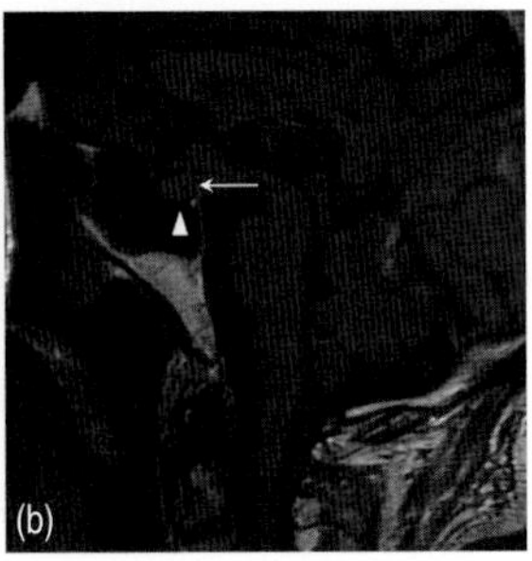

Figure 59.6 Sagittal T1-weighted magnetic resonance imaging scans of the hypothalamic-pituitary region in a patient with PP (a) and a patient with CDI (b). (a) A normal anterior pituitary (arrowhead) and pituitary stalk (thin *white arrow)* and hyperintensity of the posterior pituitary (thick *white arrow)*. (b) Sagittal T1-weighted scan obtained in a patient with CDI due to lymphoma shows a massively thickened pituitary stalk (thin *white arrow)* and an absent hyperintense signal in the posterior pituitary gland (arrowhead). *(Reproduced with permission from Journal of Clinical Endocrinology and Metabolism 2012;97:3426–37, Wiebke Fenske and Bruno Allolio. Clinical Review: Current State and Future Perspectives in the Diagnosis of Diabetes Insipidus.)*

diabetes (possibly due to ADH store depletion secondary to over-secretion)[28] and in up to 30% of elderly subjects without any clinical symptoms of DI.[83] Additionally, the signal intensity may change bi-directionally over time, even in young subjects.[84] Given these findings, MRI-derived diagnostic information should probably be considered indicative rather than conclusive.

OTHER TESTS

Other tests have been explored to investigate polyuric syndromes in patients believed to have DI. Non-osmotic stimuli of ADH release such as nicotine, nausea and hypotension are not considered sufficiently reliable or consistent to be of practical use. More promisingly, it appears that the biochemically stable C-terminal glycoprotein cleaved from the ADH pro-hormone at the time of pro-hormone activation is relatively easy to measure and correlates well with plasma ADH concentrations. This 'plasma copeptin' may offer a future alternative to ADH for measurement during standard water deprivation and hypertonic saline tests.[85]

Access the complete references list online at http://www.expertconsult.com

5. McKinely MJ, Denton DA, Weisinger RS. Sensors for antidiuresis and thirst - osmoreceptors or CSF sodium detectors? Brain Res 1978;141:89–103.
11. Antunes-Rodrigues J, de Castro M, Elias LLK, et al. Neuroendocrine control of body fluid metabolism. Physiol Rev 2004;84:169–208.
26. Schrier RW. Water and sodium retention in edematous disorders: role of vasopressin and aldosterone. Am J Med 2006;119(7A):S47–53.
31. Maghnie M, Altobelli M, di Iorgi N, et al. Idiopathic central diabetes insipidus is associated with abnormal blood supply to the posterior pituitary gland caused by vascular impairment of the inferior hypophyseal artery system. J Endocrinol Metab 2004;89: 1891–6.
35. Makaryus AN, McFarlane SI. Diabetes insipidus: diagnosis and treatment of a complex disease. Clev Clin J Med 2006;73(1):65–71.
49. Sands JM, Bichet DG. Nephrogenic diabetes insipidus. Ann Intern Med 2006;144:186–94.
59. Bernier V, Morello JP, Zarruk A, et al. Pharmacologic chaperones as a potential treatment for x-linked nephrogenic diabetes insipidus. J Am Soc Nephrol 2006;17:232–43.
75. Aleksandrov N, Audibert F, Bedard MJ, et al. Gestational diabetes insipidus: a review of an underdiagnosed condition. J Obstet Gynaecol Can 2010;32(3): 225–31.

60

Thyroid emergencies

Jonathan M Handy and Alexander M Man Ying Li

Thyroid emergencies are a rare cause for admission to critical care. However, mortality is high unless specific treatment is provided in an expeditious manner. Abnormal thyroid function tests are commonly encountered during critical illness; numerous factors must be considered before interpreting these findings as indicating thyroid disease.

BASIC PHYSIOLOGY

Thyroid hormones affect the function of virtually every organ system and must be constantly available for these functions to continue. The two biologically active hormones are tetraiodothyronine (thyroxine or T_4) and tri-iodothyronine (T_3). These are synthesised by incorporating iodine into tyrosine residues, a process which occurs in thyroglobulin contained within the lumena of the thyroid gland (**Fig. 60.1**). Stimulation of hormone release by thyroid-stimulating hormone (TSH) results in endocytosis of thyroglobulin from the lumen into the follicular cells, followed by hydrolysis to form T_4 and T_3, which are released into the circulation.[1]

Both T_4 and T_3 contain two iodine atoms on their inner (tyrosine) ring. They differ in that T_4 contains two further iodine atoms on its outer (phenol) ring whereas T_3 contains only one, resulting in a comparatively longer plasma half-life for T_4 of 5–7 days compared with that of 10 hours for T_3. T_4 is produced solely by the thyroid gland whereas the majority of T_3 is synthesised peripherally by the removal of one iodine atom (deiodination) from the outer ring of T_4. If deiodination of an inner ring iodine atom occurs, the metabolically inert reverse-T_3 (rT_3) is formed. This is produced in preference to T_3 during starvation and many non-thyroidal illnesses, and the ratio of inactive (rT_3) to active T_3 synthesis appears to play an important role in the control of metabolism.[2] Numerous factors can affect the peripheral deiodination process (**Box 60.1**). Both T_4 and T_3 are highly protein bound in the serum, predominantly to thyroid-binding globulin (TBG), but to a lesser extent to albumin and pre-albumin. Changes in concentration of these serum-binding proteins have a large effect on total T_4 and T_3 serum concentrations. Such protein changes do not, however, effect the concentration of free hormone or their rates of metabolism. The serum-binding proteins act as both a store and a buffer to allow an immediate supply of the metabolically active free-T_4 (fT_4) and free-T_3 (fT_3). In addition, protein binding reduces the glomerular filtration and renal excretion of the hormones.

On reaching the target organs, fT_4 and fT_3 enter the cells predominantly by diffusion. Here, microsomal enzymes deiodinate the fT_4 to form fT_3. This varies in differing tissues, the majority occurring in the liver, kidney and muscle. The fT_3 subsequently diffuses into the nucleus where it binds nuclear receptors and exerts its affect through stimulation of messenger RNA (mRNA) with subsequent synthesis of polypeptides including hormones and enzymes. The role of thyroid hormones in development and homeostasis is widespread and profound; the most obvious effects are to stimulate basal metabolic rate and sensitivity of the cardiovascular and nervous systems to catecholamines.

The regulation of thyroid function is predominantly determined by three main mechanisms, the latter two providing physiological control. First, availability of iodine is crucial for the synthesis of the thyroid hormones. Dietary iodide is absorbed and rapidly distributed in the extracellular fluid, which also contains iodide released from the thyroid gland and from peripheral deiodination processes. This becomes trapped within thyroid follicular cells, from which it is actively transported into the lumen to be oxidised into iodine and subsequently combined with tyrosine.[3] Other ions such as perchlorate and pertechnetate share this follicular cell active transport mechanism and thus act as competitive inhibitors for the process.

Secondly, thyroid hormone release is controlled by a close feedback loop with the anterior pituitary. Diminished levels of circulating hormones trigger secretion of TSH, which acts on the follicular cells of the thyroid gland causing them to release thyroglobulin-rich colloid from the lumena. This thyroglobulin is hydrolysed to form T_4 and T_3 for systemic release. Increased levels of T_4 and T_3 cause diminished TSH secretion, resulting in the follicular cells becoming flat and allowing increased capacity for colloid storage. As a result, less thyroglobulin is mobilised and hydrolysed with less T_4 and T_3 release. The degree to which TSH is secreted in response to changes in circulating thyroid hormones is

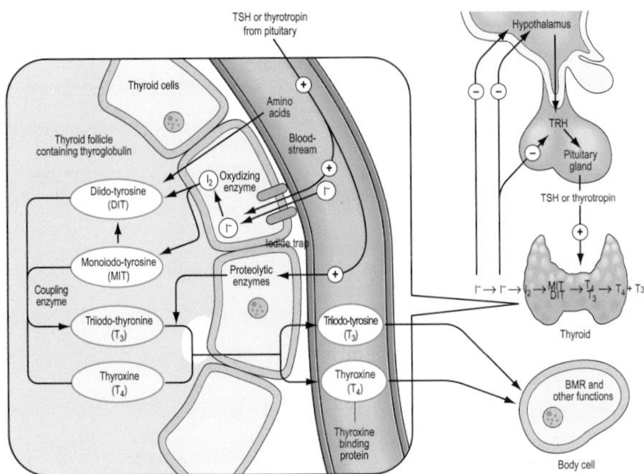

Figure 60.1 Synthesis of tetraiodothyronine (T_4) and tri-iodothyronine (T_3). Stimulation of hormone release by thyroid-stimulating hormone (TSH) produced in the pituitary gland results in endocytosis of thyroglobulin from the lumen into the follicular cells, followed by hydrolysis to form T_4 and T_3, which is released into the circulation.

Box 60.1 States associated with decreased deiodination of T_4 to T_3

- Systemic illness
- Fasting
- Malnutrition
- Postoperative state
- Trauma
- Drugs: propylthiouracil, glucocorticoids, propanolol, amiodarone
- Radiographic contrast agents (ipodate, ipanoate)

dependent on the hypothalamic hormone thyrotropin-releasing hormone (TRH), which is itself modulated by feedback from the thyroid hormones (see Fig. 60.1). TRH secretion is inhibited by dopamine, glucocorticoids and somatostatin.

Lastly, further regulation occurs during the enzyme-dependent peripheral conversion of fT_4 to fT_3. It is this latter stage that provides the rapid and fine control of local fT_3 availability. All of these mechanisms may be altered by drugs and in pathological states.

THYROID CRISIS (THYROID STORM)

Thyrotoxic storm is arguably the most serious complication of hyperthyroidism, with reported mortality ranging from 10 to 75% in hospitalised patients.[4,5] Crisis most commonly occurs as a result of unrecognised or poorly controlled Grave's disease; however, other underlying diseases may be the cause.[6,7] Females outnumber males. Laboratory findings are inconsistent owing to acute disruption of the normal steady state of the circulating hormones and there is no definitive value that separates thyrotoxicosis from thyroid storm. The latter is a clinical diagnosis, and a scoring system has been proposed to guide the likelihood of the diagnosis (**Table 60.1**).[8] Precipitating factors are not always present, though many have been identified (**Box 60.2**).

CLINICAL PRESENTATION (Box 60.3)

The classic signs of thyroid crisis include fever, tachycardia, tremor, diarrhoea, nausea and vomiting.[9] However, presentation is extremely variable and may range from apathetic hyperthyroidism (apathy, depression, hyporeflexia and myopathy)[10] to multiple organ

Table 60.1 Severity assessment in thyroid crisis*

TEMP (°C)	PULSE	CARDIAC FAILURE	CNS EFFECTS	GI SYMPTOMS	SCORE
Normal	<99	Absent	Normal	Normal	0
37.2–37.7	99–109	Pedal oedema	–	–	5
37.8–38.2	110–119	Bibasal crepitations, atrial fibrillation	Agitation	Diarrhoea, nausea, vomiting, abdominal pain	10
38.3–38.8	120–129	Pulmonary oedema	–	–	15
38.9–39.3	130–139	–	Delirium	Unexplained jaundice	20
39.4–39.9	>140	–	–	–	25
>40	–	–	Seizure, coma	–	30

*Adapted from Tietgens ST, Leinung MC. Thyroid storm. Medical Clinics of North America, 1995;79:169–184.
Calculations:
1. Add the scores for each of the five clinically observed parameters.
2. Add a further *10 points* if *atrial fibrillation* is present.
3. Add a further *10 points* if an identifiable *precipitating factor* is present.
4. Total score of *45* or greater is highly suggestive of thyroid storm. Total score of *25–44* supports impending crisis. Total score of less than *25* makes thyroid storm unlikely.
CNS=central nervous system; GI=gastrointestinal.

Box 60.2 Factors associated with precipitating thyroid storm

- Infection; sepsis
- Withdrawal of antithyroid treatment
- Surgery; trauma
- Parturition
- Diabetic ketoacidosis
- Radioactive iodine therapy
- Iodinated contrast dyes
- Hypoglycaemia
- Excessive palpation of the thyroid gland
- Emotional stress
- Burn injury
- Pulmonary thromboembolism
- Cerebrovascular accident; seizure disorder (including eclampsia)
- Thyroid hormone overdose

dysfunction.[11,12] Differential diagnosis includes sepsis and other causes of hyperpyrexia such as adrenergic and anticholinergic syndromes.

FEVER

This is the most characteristic feature. Temperature may rise above 41°C. There have been suggestions that pyrexia is present in all cases of thyroid storm,[13] though normothermia has also been reported.[11] Pyrexia is rare in uncomplicated thyrotoxicosis and should always raise suspicion of thyroid storm. It is not clear whether this febrile response is due to alteration of central thermoregulation or elevation of basal metabolic thermogenesis beyond the body's ability to lose heat.

CARDIOVASCULAR FEATURES

Fluid requirements may be substantial in some patients, whereas diuresis may be required in those with severe heart failure. Cardiac decompensation can occur in young patients with no known antecedent cardiac disease. Systolic hypertension with widened pulse pressure is common initially; however, hypotension supervenes later. Shock with vascular collapse is a pre-terminal sign.[14]

NEUROMUSCULAR FEATURES

Tremor is a common early sign, but as 'storm' progresses central nervous dysfunction evolves with progression from agitation and anxiety to encephalopathy or even coma.[15] Thyroid storm has been reported in association with status epilepticus and cerebrovascular accident.[16] Weakness may be a feature, particularly with apathetic thyrotoxicosis.[11] Thyrotoxic myopathy and rhabdomyolysis may be present,[11,17] the latter being differentiated from the former by its association with markedly elevated creatine phosphokinase levels. A number of other syndromes of neuromuscular weakness have been described including hypokalaemic periodic paralysis[18,19] and myasthenia gravis.[20]

Box 60.3 Clinical features of hyperthyroidism/thyroid crisis

- Fever
- Cardiovascular:
  - Tachycardia, atrial fibrillation, ventricular arrhythmias
  - Heart failure
  - Hypertension (early), hypotension (late)
- Neuromuscular:
  - Tremor
  - Encephalopathy, coma
  - Weakness
- Gastrointestinal:
  - Diarrhoea, nausea and vomiting
- Respiratory:
  - Dyspnoea
  - Increased oxygen consumption and carbon dioxide production
- Goitre (possible airway compromise)
- Laboratory abnormalities

GASTROINTESTINAL FEATURES

Diarrhoea, nausea and vomiting are common, though the patient may present with symptoms of an acute abdomen.[21] Severe abdominal tenderness should raise the possibility of an abdominal emergency. Liver function tests may be abnormal due to congestion or necrosis and tenderness over the hepatic area may be present. Hepatosplenomegaly may be present. The presence of jaundice is a poor prognostic sign.[14]

RESPIRATORY CONSIDERATIONS

Dyspnoea at rest or on exertion may be present for a number of reasons. Oxygen consumption and carbon dioxide production are increased with subsequent increase in the respiratory burden. This may be exacerbated by pulmonary oedema, respiratory muscle weakness and tracheal obstruction from enlarged goitre (rare).

LABORATORY FINDINGS

Numerous abnormalities may be found:

- fT_4 and fT_3 are usually increased, though this does not correlate with clinical severity; TSH is undetectable
- hyperglycemia in non-diabetics
- leucocytosis with a left shift, even in the absence of infection (leucopenia may be present in patients with Graves' disease)
- abnormal liver function tests and hyperbilirubinaemia
- hypercalcemia due to haemoconcentration and the effect of thyroid hormones on bone resorption
- hypokalaemia and hypomagnesaemia (particularly in apathetic thyrotoxicosis)

- serum cortisol should be elevated – if low values are found, adrenal insufficiency should be considered and treated; adrenal reserve in thyrotoxic patients is often exceeded in the absence of absolute adrenal insufficiency.

MANAGEMENT

Treatment is aimed at:

- control and relief of adrenergic symptoms
- correction of thyroid hormone abnormalities
- the precipitating cause
- investigation and treatment of the underlying thyroid disease
- supportive measures.

BETA-ADRENERGIC BLOCKADE

This is the mainstay of controlling adrenergic symptoms.[22] Intravenous propranolol titrated in 0.5–1mg increments while monitoring cardiovascular response diminishes the systemic hypersensitivity to catecholamines. In addition it inhibits peripheral conversion of T_4 to T_3.[23] Concurrent administration of enteral propranolol is the norm, with doses as high as 60–120 mg 4–6-hourly often being necessary owing to enhanced elimination during thyroid crisis.[24] An alternative regimen uses intravenous esmolol with a loading dose of 250–500 μg/kg followed by infusion at 50–100 μg/kg/min. This allows rapid titration of beta blockade while minimising adverse reactions.[25] Patients with contraindications to beta blockade or who exhibit resistance to this treatment may be successfully treated with reserpine or guanethidine, though their onset of action is slow and side-effects may be significant.

DIGOXIN

Control of heart rate and rhythm may result in significant improvement in cardiac performance. Electrolyte imbalance, particularly hypokalaemia and hypomagnesaemia, should be corrected prior to drug therapy. Relative resistance to digoxin may occur due to increased renal clearance[26] and increased Na/K ATPase units in cardiac muscle.[27] Arterial thromboembolic phenomena are common (10–40%) in thyrotoxicosis-related atrial fibrillation. This may be due to a procoagulant state or an increased incidence of mitral valve prolapse. Anticoagulation is controversial given the increased sensitivity to warfarin and potential for bleeding; however, it should be considered in the management of these patients.

AMIODARONE

Amiodarone has theoretical benefits in thyrotoxicosis as it inhibits peripheral conversion of T_4 to T_3 and reduces the concentration of T_3-induced adrenoceptors in cardiac myocytes.[28] It does, however, cause profound (and sometimes physiologically irrelevant) changes to thyroid function tests and should not therefore be used as the first-line agent.

THIONAMIDES

These drugs block de novo synthesis of thyroid hormones within 1–2 hours of administration, but have no effect on the release of preformed glandular stores of thyroid hormones. Transient leucopenia is common (20%) and agranulocytosis can rarely occur with carbimazole use.

Propylthiouracil

This is usually considered the drug of choice in thyroid storm owing to its ability to partially block peripheral conversion of T_4 to T_3. Its main mechanism of action is to block the iodination of tyrosine. Only enteral preparations are available and absorption may be unpredictable during thyroid crisis. Rectal administration has been reported. The loading dose is 100 mg followed by 100 mg every 2 hours.

Methimazole

Methimazole lacks peripheral effects, but has a long duration of action making administration easier and more reliable. It may be used in combination with drugs that block peripheral T_4-to-T_3 conversion (such as iopanoate or ipodate). Only enteral preparations are available, though rectal administration has been reported. Loading dose is 100 mg followed by 20 mg every 8 hours.

Carbimazole

This is metabolised to methimazole and is rarely associated with agranulocytosis. Only enteral preparations are available.

IODINE

The release of preformed glandular thyroid hormones is inhibited by administering either inorganic iodine or lithium. Enterally administered iodides include Lugol's solution and sodium or potassium iodide. Intravenous infusion of sterile sodium iodide may be used at a dose of 1 g 12-hourly; however, this is not always available commercially. If not, it may be prepared by the hospital pharmacy. Iodine therapy should not commence without prior thionamide administration. Used alone, it will enrich hormone stores within the thyroid gland and exacerbate thyrotoxicosis.

Iodine-containing contrast media (e.g. ipodate and iopanoate) may be used instead of the simple iodides, the former blocking T_4-to-T_3 conversion and inhibiting the cardiac effects of thyroxine. Ipodate is administered orally as a loading dose of 3 g followed by 1 g daily. As with the iodides, treatment should always be preceded by thionamide administration.

LITHIUM

Lithium carbonate has a similar, though weaker, action to iodine and can be used in patients with iodine allergy. An initial dose regimen of 300 mg 6-hourly has been used with subsequent dosage adjusted to maintain serum drug levels at about 1 mmol/L.[29] Renal and neurological toxicity tend to limit its use.

STEROIDS

Glucocorticoids reduce T_4-to-T_3 conversion and may modulate any autoimmune process underlying the thyroid crisis (e.g. Graves' disease). In addition, relative glucocorticoid deficiency may be a feature of the crisis. An ACTH stimulation test is desirable prior to administration of hydrocortisone (100 mg 6- to 8-hourly); alternatively dexamethasone (4 mg 6-hourly) can be administered until the test has been performed. Combination therapy with iodides can produce rapid results. Glucocorticoids are the most effective treatment for type-2 amiodarone-induced thyrotoxicosis.[30]

OTHER THERAPIES

Plasmapheresis, charcoal haemoperfusion and dantrolene have all been used as novel therapies in thyroid storm; however, their use is not established or proven.

SUPPORTIVE THERAPY

Fluid management

Fluid management may be extremely difficult in patients suffering from thyroid storm, particularly the elderly. Fluid losses may be profound due to diarrhoea, vomiting, pyrexia and reduced intake. However, congestive cardiac failure may also develop as a result of the high cardiac demand. Echocardiography and cardiac output monitoring may be invaluable in guiding therapy for such patients.

Nutrition

Thyrotoxic patients have high energy expenditure and may present with a significant energy, vitamin and nitrogen deficit. Nutritional requirements should take account of any deficit and the ongoing hypercatabolic state. Thiamine is usually supplemented.

Drug therapy

Consideration should be given to the enhanced metabolism and elimination of drugs that occurs in thyrotoxic patients. Salicylates and furosemide should be avoided as both displace thyroid hormones from their binding proteins and can rapidly exacerbate systemic symptoms.

Precipitating factors

Both the precipitating factors and the disease process underlying the thyroid crisis should be sought and treated aggressively. Infection is the leading precipitant of crisis; thus early microbiological cultures and antibiotic therapy should be considered.

MYXOEDEMA COMA

Myxoedema coma is the extreme manifestation of hypothyroidism, which, although rare, carries a mortality ranging from 30 to 60%. The term is a misnomer in that the majority of patients present with neither the non-pitting oedema known as myxeodema nor coma.[31]

Box 60.4 Factors precipitating myxoedema coma

- Infection
- Cold environmental temperatures/hypothermia
- Burns
- Stroke
- Surgery
- Trauma
- Chronic heart failure
- Carbon dioxide retention
- Gastrointestinal haemorrhage
- Hypoglycaemia
- Carbon dioxide retention
- Gastrointestinal haemorrhage
- Hypoglycaemia
- Medications:
  - Amiodarone
  - Anaesthetic agents
  - Analgesics/narcotics
  - Beta blockers
  - Diuretics
  - Lithium
  - Phenytoin
  - Rifampicin
  - Sedatives/tranquilisers

The condition should be considered in any patient presenting with a reduced level of consciousness and hypothermia. The crisis occurs most commonly in elderly women with long-standing undiagnosed or undertreated hypothyroidism in whom an additional significant stress is experienced. Numerous precipitating factors have been identified (**Box 60.4**).

CLINICAL PRESENTATION (Box 60.5)

Myxoedema coma can be defined when decreased mental status, hypothermia and clinical features of hypothyroidism are present (Box 60.5). When these features are present, diagnosis is straightforward; however, asymptomatic or atypical presentation (e.g. decreased mobility) may occur.[32] The presence of hypotension and bradycardia at presentation, a need for mechanical ventilation, hypothermia unresponsive to treatment, sepsis, intake of sedative drugs, lower GCS, high APACHE II score, and high SOFA score have been associated with an increased predicted mortality.[33]

NEUROMUSCULAR

Alteration of conscious or mental state is present in all patients. This can range from personality changes to coma, with about 25% of patients experiencing seizures prior to the onset of coma. Electroencephalogram usually reveals non-specific changes. Weakness is common and skeletal muscle dysfunction may develop secondary to increased membrane permeability. The latter can lead to a rise in creatine phosphokinase. Hyponatraemia is present in up to 50% of patients and

Box 60.5 Clinical features of myxoedema coma

- Neuromuscular
  - Abnormal conscious level
  - Psychiatric alterations
  - Weakness
  - Slow relaxing reflexes
  - Fatigue
- Hypothermia
- Cardiovascular
  - Diastolic hypertension
  - Bradycardia
  - Low cardiac output
  - Pericardial effusions
  - ECG alterations
- Respiratory
  - Diminished central response to hypoxia and hypercapnia
  - Respiratory alkalosis
  - Respiratory muscle weakness
  - Increased sensitivity to sedative drugs
  - Pleural effusions
  - Sleep apnoea
- Airway
  - Deep voice, goitre, vocal cord oedema, macroglossia
- Gastrointestinal
  - Gastric atony, distension, paralytic ileus, faecal impaction and megacolon (late)
  - Weight gain
  - Malabsorption
  - Ascites (rare)
- Bladder distension, urinary retention
- Cold intolerance
- Coarse hair
- Dry, pale, cool skin
- Laboratory abnormalities

may contribute to alterations in conscious level (see below). Lumbar puncture often reveals elevated protein levels and a high opening pressure.

HYPOTHERMIA

Hypothermia represents the decrease in thermogenesis that accompanies reduced metabolism and is exacerbated by low ambient temperatures. Mortality is proportional to the degree of hypothermia. A low-reading thermometer should be used during assessment.

CARDIOVASCULAR FEATURES

Diastolic hypertension is due to increased systemic vascular resistance and blood volume reduction.[34] However, myxoedema is associated with bradycardia and impaired myocardial contractility, with reduced cardiac output and hypotension a common feature. Although pericardial effusions may occur, tamponade is uncommon. Creatine phosphokinase may be elevated, though this more commonly originates from skeletal than from cardiac muscle. Acute coronary syndrome must nevertheless be excluded as a precipitant of the crisis. ECG changes include bradycardia, decreased voltage, non-specific ST and T changes, varying types of block and prolonged QT interval. All of the cardiovascular abnormalities are reversible with thyroid hormone treatment.[35]

RESPIRATORY FEATURES

Hypothyroidism causes numerous respiratory alterations (see Box 60.5). There is a propensity to respiratory alkalosis, particularly during artificial ventilation. This is due to low metabolic rate which may be compounded by iatrogenic hyperventilation.[36] Diaphragmatic weakness may occur owing to abnormalities of the phrenic nerve; as a result, exercise tolerance may be significantly reduced. These abnormalities improve with thyroid hormone replacement, though full recovery can take several months.

LABORATORY FINDINGS

Thyroid function tests will reveal low T_4 and T_3; TSH is raised in primary and low in secondary and tertiary hypothyroidism.

Hyponatraemia is common and usually develops owing to free water retention resulting from excess vasopressin secretion or impaired renal function.[37] It may be severe and can contribute to diminished mental function. Although total body water is increased, intravascular volume is usually decreased.

Hypoglycaemia may result from hypothyroidism alone, or as a result of concurrent adrenal insufficiency (Schmidt's syndrome). The mechanism is probably reduced gluconeogenesis, but infection and starvation may contribute.

Azotaemia and hypophosphataemia are common; renal function may be severely abnormal owing to low cardiac output and vasoconstriction. Mild leucopenia and normocytic anaemia are frequently present, though macrocytic and pernicious anaemia due to autoimmune dysfunction may occur.

Arterial blood gases often reveal respiratory acidosis, hypoxia and hypercapnia.

MANAGEMENT

The mainstay of therapy consists of thyroid hormone replacement, steroid replacement and supportive measures. Once clinical diagnosis has been made or is suspected, blood should be collected for thyroid function and plasma cortisol tests. This should be followed by thyroid hormone treatment, which should not be delayed to await laboratory results. Consideration should be given to identifying and treating precipitating factors and complications of the crisis.

THYROID HORMONE THERAPY

All patients with suspected myxedema coma should receive presumptive treatment with thyroid hormone.

The optimum speed, type, route and dose of thyroid hormone replacement in myxoedema coma are unknown owing to the rarity of the condition and paucity of trials. The severity of clinical presentation does not correlate with the doses of replacement hormone that are required. Rapid replacement can result in life-threatening myocardial ischaemia or arrhythmias; delayed therapy exposes patients to prolonged risk of complications from the crisis. Both scenarios are associated with increased mortality.

Some experts favour administration of T_3 as it is biologically more active; has more rapid onset of action, and bypasses the impaired deiodination of T_4 to T_3 that occurs in hypothyroidism and non-thyroidal illness. High serum T_3 concentration has, however, been associated with increased mortality[38] and T_3 is expensive and may be difficult to obtain. T_3 may be administered orally or intravenously and has been combined with T_4 therapy.[39,40] In one study of 23 successive patients suffering from myxoedema coma, those who received oral L-thyroxine had no difference in outcome from those receiving i.v. thyroxine.[33]

Most authorities recommend use of T_4 alone[38,40,41] as the delayed conversion to T_3 allows more gradual replacement of the deficient hormone. Bioavailability of orally administered T_4 is unpredictable given the high incidence of gastrointestinal dysfunction; therefore intravenous administration is more frequently used. A loading dose of intravenous levothyroxine 100–500 μg is recommended[40] as this saturates the binding proteins. This should be followed by 50–100 μg daily until conversion to the bioequivalent oral formulation is possible. The doses must be adjusted to allow for patient age, weight and their cardiovascular risk factors; the lower doses should be administered to patients who are elderly, frail or have co-morbidities (particularly cardiovascular disease).

CORTICOSTEROIDS

Corticosteroids are an important part of treatment as relative or absolute hypoadrenalism may occur concurrently with hypothyroid disease. A random serum cortisol level should be collected prior to commencing hydrocortisone therapy at 100 mg 8-hourly. If ACTH stimulation test is warranted, dexamethasone 4 mg 6-hourly should be commenced with conversion to hydrocortisone or cessation of treatment once the results are known. If random serum cortisol levels return at normal levels, steroid treatment can be discontinued.

SUPPORTIVE THERAPY

Hypothermia should be treated by passive rewarming where possible, but active measures may be required. Appropriate cardiovascular, temperature gradient, electrolyte and acid–base monitoring should be provided during the rewarming phase in order to prevent haemodynamic and metabolic compromise.

Numerous alterations in respiratory physiology occur, including hypoventilation and altered response to arterial oxygen and carbon dioxide tensions. In addition, anatomical changes to the airway, delayed gastric emptying and increased sensitivity to sedative drugs may be present. These changes should be considered when mechanical ventilation is required; particularly during intubation and the weaning process.[36]

Patients usually present with intravascular fluid depletion despite peripheral oedema. Cardiac output monitoring may help guide fluid resuscitation and therapy. Echocardiography is useful in identifying cardiac dysfunction, pericardial effusions and assisting in assessment of intravascular volume status. Cardiac monitoring should be used to alert to the presence of arrhythmias. Inotropes and vasopressors should be avoided where possible owing to their potential to precipitate cardiac arrhythmias. Where inotropes are required, increased dosage may be necessary as reduction in β-adrenoceptors is common; α-adrenoceptor function is usually preserved.

Hyponatraemia is reversible with thyroid hormone treatment, but severe abnormalities contributing to neurological dysfunction may require more expeditious correction. Free water intake should be restricted and hypertonic saline solutions may be required. Hypotonic fluid therapy should be avoided. If glucose therapy is required, hypertonic solutions (20–50%) should be infused via a central venous catheter.

Precipitating factors must be considered. As with all critically ill patients, microbial cultures should be collected and antibiotic therapy commenced unless cultures are negative. Prophylaxis against venous thromboembolism and peptic ulceration should be considered. Enteral feeding should be attempted, but may be unsuccessful if gastrointestinal dysfunction and stasis is present.

NON-THYROIDAL ILLNESS

Non-thyroidal illness describes the phenomenon of starved or systemically unwell patients with abnormal serum thyroid function tests but with no apparent thyroidal illness. Low T_3, T_4 and TSH are commonly found, the degree of abnormality correlating with the severity of illness. Variants of these hormone levels are well described. Low serum T_3 is a frequent finding and occurs due to down-regulation of the monodeiodinase enzyme that converts T_4 to T_3, while rT_3 may increase owing to increased activity of the T_4-to-T_3 monodeiodinase.[42]

Serum T_4 is also commonly low in the critically ill. This is due to a decrease in the concentration of thyroid hormone-binding proteins and the presence of inhibitors that reduce T_4 binding to these proteins. There is also suggestion that T_4 entry into cells may be impaired.[43] Free T_4 levels should be normal in less severe illness; however, in severe illness the level may be low owing to inadequate correction during the fT_4 assay.[44]

Low serum TSH levels were previously thought to be associated with the euthyroid state; however, more recent work suggests that acquired transient central hypothyroidism is present in these patients.[45] Cytokines such as tumour necrosis factor-α are known to inhibit TSH secretion. Such phenomena are probably evolutionary adaptations to conserve protein and energy during severe illness. Elevated TSH may also occur in non-thyroidal illness, but few of these patients prove to have hypothyroidism following recovery from their acute illness.

Changes in thyroid function test (TFT) are well described during starvation, sepsis, bone marrow transplantation, surgery, myocardial infarction, coronary artery bypass surgery, and probably any critical illness. However, replacement of thyroid hormone in these patients is of no benefit and may be harmful;[46] hence thyroid function should not be assessed in critically ill patients unless there is a strong clinical indication to do so. A number of specific non-thyroidal illnesses are associated with abnormal TFTs. These include: some psychiatric illnesses, hepatic disease, nephritic syndrome, acromegaly, acute intermittent porphyria and Cushing's syndrome. Where assays are performed, TSH should not be interpreted in isolation as low values will not discriminate between true thyroid versus non-thyroidal disease. If low T_4 is also present, non-thyroidal illness is likely. If T_4 is elevated then hyperthyroidism is the likely diagnosis, though elevated T_4 has been documented in non-thyroidal illness.

Given the alterations in these hormones and difficulties with their assay during critical illness, thyroid hormone replacement should not be undertaken on the strength of TFT results alone. Additional laboratory and clinical indications must also be present (**Table 60.2**).

Table 60.2 Changes in thyroid hormone concentrations

	fT_4	T_3	TSH
Euthyroid	N	N	N
Hyperthyroid	↑	↑	↓
Hypothyroid	↓	↓ N	↑
Non-thyroidal illness	↑ N ↓	↓	N ↓

fT_4=free tetraiodothyronine; T_3=tri-iodothyronine; TSH=thyroid-stimulating hormone; N=normal; ↑=increased; ↓=decreased.

Access the complete references list online at http://www.expertconsult.com

1. Kopp P. Thyroid hormone synthesis. In: Braverman LE, Utiger RD, editors. The Thyroid: Fundamental and Clinical Text. 9th ed. Philadelphia: Lippincott Williams & Wilkins; 2005. p. 52.
2. Marshall W, Bangert S. The thyroid gland. In: Marshall W, Bangert S, editors. Clinical Chemistry. 5th ed. Mosby: Elsevier; 2004. p. 161–75.
14. Wartofsky L. Thyroid storm. In: Wass JAH, Shalet SM, Gale E, et al., editors. Oxford Textbook of Endocrinology and Diabetes. Oxford: Oxford University Press; 2002. p. 481–5.
43. De Groot LJ. Dangerous dogmas in medicine: the nonthyroidal illness syndrome. J Clin Endocrinol Metab 1999;84(1):151–264.
45. Chopra IJ. Clinical review 86: Euthyroid sick syndrome: is it a misnomer? J Clin Endocrinol Metab 1997;82(2):329–34.
46. Utiger RD. Altered thyroid function in nonthyroidal illness and surgery. To treat or not to treat? N Engl J Med 1995;333(23):1562–3.

61

Adrenocortical insufficiency in critical illness

Balasubramanian Venkatesh and Jeremy Cohen

The adrenal glands form an essential part of the organism's response to stress. Hence, in intensive care, an adequate adrenal response is considered to be of prime importance. Although primary adrenal insufficiency is a well-recognised but rare condition in intensive care, secondary, or relative, adrenal insufficiency is thought to be more prevalent. Adrenocortical insufficiency may present as an insidious, occult disorder, unmasked by conditions of stress, or as a catastrophic syndrome that may result in death.

PHYSIOLOGY

The adrenal glands are functionally divided into medulla and cortex; the latter is responsible for the secretion of three major classes of hormones: glucocorticoids, mineralocorticoids and sex hormones. The major pathogenic effects of disease result from cortisol and aldosterone deficiency.

Cortisol, the major glucocorticoid (GC) synthesised by the adrenal cortex, plays a pivotal role in normal metabolism. It is necessary for the synthesis of adrenergic receptors, normal immune function, wound healing and vascular tone. These actions are mediated by the glucocorticoid receptor, a member of the nuclear hormone receptor superfamily. The activated receptor migrates to the nucleus and binds to specific recognition sequences within target genes, but also interacts with numerous transcription factors and cytosolic proteins. Numerous isoforms of the glucocorticoids receptor have now been described; the alpha subtype, a 777-amino-acid polypeptide chain, was initially felt to be the primary mediator of glucocorticoid action. In contrast the beta isoform, a 742-amino-acid chain, was felt to have no physiological activity. More recently it appears that the beta subtype has a negative effect on alpha-mediated gene transactivation, the physiological relevance of which remains controversial. Furthermore, additional isoforms have now been described, suggesting that glucocorticoid receptor diversity may be an important factor in understanding the complex effects of corticosteroid action.[1]

Under normal circumstances, cortisol is secreted in pulses, and in a diurnal pattern.[2] The normal basal output of cortisol is estimated to be 15–30 mg/day, producing a peak plasma cortisol concentration of 110–520 nmol/L (4–19 μg/dL) at 8–9 a.m., and a minimal cortisol level of <140 nmol/L (<5 μg/dL) after midnight. The daily output of aldosterone is estimated to be 100–150 μg/day.

Secretion is under the control of the hypothalamic-pituitary axis. There are a variety of stimuli to secretion, including stress, tissue damage, cytokine release, hypoxia, hypotension and hypoglycaemia. These factors act upon the hypothalamus to favour the release of corticotrophin-releasing hormone (CRH) and vasopressin. CRH is synthesised in the hypothalamus and carried to the anterior pituitary in portal blood, where it stimulates the secretion of adrenocorticotrophic hormone (ACTH), which in turn stimulates the release of cortisol, mineralocorticoids (principally aldosterone) and androgens from the adrenal cortex. CRH is the major (but not the only) regulator of ACTH release and is secreted in response to a normal hypothalamic circadian regulation and various forms of 'stress'. Vasopressin, oxytocin, angiotensin II and beta-adrenergic agents also stimulate ACTH release, whereas somatostatin, beta endorphin and enkephalin reduce it. Cortisol has a negative feedback on the hypothalamus and pituitary, inhibiting hypothalamic CRH release induced by stress and pituitary ACTH release induced by CRH. During periods of stress, trauma or infection, there is an increase in CRH and ACTH secretion and a reduction in the negative-feedback effect, resulting in increased cortisol levels in amounts roughly proportional to the severity of the illness.[3–5]

Cortisol is transported in the blood to the tissues in three fractions: approximately 80% is closely bound to corticosteroid-binding globulin (CBG), 10–15% is loosely bound to albumin, and 5–8% is a free fraction. At normal levels of total plasma cortisol (e.g. 375 nmol/L or 13.5 μg/dL) less than 5% exists as free cortisol in the plasma; however, it is this free fraction that is biologically active. Circulating CBG concentrations are approximately 700 nmol/L. In normal subjects CBG can bind approximately 700 nmol/L (i.e. 25 μg/dL).[6] At levels greater than this, the increase in plasma cortisol is largely in the unbound fraction. The affinity of CBG for synthetic corticosteroids, with the exception of prednisolone, is negligible. CBG is a substrate for elastase, a polymorphonuclear enzyme that cleaves CBG, markedly decreasing its affinity for cortisol.[7] This enzymatic cleavage results in the liberation of free cortisol at sites of inflammation. CBG levels have been documented to fall during critical illness,[8–10] and these changes are postulated to increase the amount of circulating free cortisol.

Cortisol is lipophilic and diffuses into the cell freely. However, once inside the cell the concentrations of cortisol are profoundly affected by the activity of the 11β-hydroxysteroid dehydrogenase 1 and 2 (11β-HSD1 and 2) enzyme system.[11–14] 11β-HSD1 acts in vivo primarily as a reductase, generating active cortisol from inactive cortisone. By contrast, 11β-HSD2 has dehydrogenase action, inactivating cortisol by conversion to cortisone. 11β-HSD2 is found primarily in mineralocorticoid target tissues such as kidney, sweat glands and colonic mucosa, where it prevents illicit activation of the mineralocorticoid receptor by cortisol. 11β-HSD1 has a wide distribution including liver, adipose and vascular tissues and, although its primary action is reductase, there is some evidence its directionality may be tissue specific.[15] The system is able to regulate intracellular GC concentration irrespective of circulation concentration, thus rendering circulating levels highly problematic as indicators of tissue GC activity. Altered HSD status has been reported in critical illness.[16,17]

Cortisol has a half-life of 70–120 minutes. It is eliminated primarily by hepatic metabolism and glomerular filtration. The excretion of free cortisol through the kidney represents 1% of the total secretion rate. Currently, available routine assays measure only total cortisol levels: bound and free.

The metabolic effects of cortisol are complex and varied. In the liver, cortisol stimulates glycogen deposition by increasing glycogen synthase and inhibiting the glycogen-mobilising enzyme glycogen phosphorylase.[18] Hepatic gluconeogenesis is stimulated, leading to increased blood glucose levels. Concurrently, glucose uptake by peripheral tissues is inhibited.[19] Free fatty acid release into the circulation is increased, and triglyceride levels rise.

In the circulatory system, cortisol increases blood pressure both by direct actions upon smooth muscle and via renal mechanisms. The actions of pressor agents such as catecholamines are potentiated, whereas nitric-oxide-mediated vasodilation is reduced.[20,21] Renal effects include both an increase in glomerular filtration rate and sodium transport in the proximal tubule and sodium retention and potassium loss in the distal tubule.[22]

The primary effects of cortisol upon the immune system are anti-inflammatory and immunosuppressive. Lymphocyte cell counts decrease, whereas neutrophil counts rise.[22] Accumulation of immunologically active cells at inflammatory sites is decreased. The production of cytokines is inhibited, an effect that is mediated via nuclear factor κB (NF-κB). This occurs by induction of NF-κB inhibitor or by direct binding of cortisol to NF-κB, thus preventing its translocation to the nucleus.

Although the well-defined effects of cortisol upon the immune system are primarily inhibitory, it is also suggested that normal host defence function requires some cortisol secretion. Cortisol has been described to have a positive effect upon immunoglobulin synthesis, potentiation of the acute phase response, wound healing, and opsonisation.[23]

CLASSIFICATION

Adrenal insufficiency (AI) may be considered to be primary, secondary or relative. Primary AI, otherwise known as Addison's disease, results from hypofunction of the adrenal cortex. Secondary AI occurs when there is suppression or absence of ACTH secretion from the anterior pituitary. Relative AI describes a situation of inadequate cortisol response to stress in the setting of critical illness.

PRIMARY ADRENAL INSUFFICIENCY

Primary adrenal insufficiency or Addison's disease is a rare disorder. In the Western world its estimated prevalence is 120 per million.[24] In adulthood, the commonest cause is autoimmune, but in the intensive care setting consideration should be given to other causes of adrenal gland destruction (**Box 61.1**). These include infection, haemorrhage and infiltration. Tuberculosis is the commonest infective cause worldwide, but rarer infections such as histoplasmosis, coccidiomycosis and cytomegalovirus (CMV), especially in patients with HIV, have also been implicated. Haemorrhage into the glands is associated with septicaemias, particularly meningococcal (Waterhouse–Fredrickson syndrome). Asplenia and the antiphospholipid syndrome may also be associated with adrenal haemorrhage. Adrenal gland destruction

Box 61.1 Causes of primary adrenal insufficiency

Infections
Tuberculosis
Histoplasmosis
Coccidiomycosis
Cytomegalovirus
Autoimmune mediated
Haemorrhagic
Sepsis (especially meningococcal)
Antiphospholipid syndrome
Trauma
Surgery
Coagulation disorders
Infiltrative
Tumour
Amyloid
Sarcoidosis
Haemochromatosis
Drug related
Etomidate
Fluconazole
Ketoconazole
Metyrapone
Suramin
Rifampicin
Phenytoin
Congenital
Adrenal dysgenesis
Adrenoleucodystrophy
Impaired steroidogenesis
Cytokine mediated

may also be secondary to infiltration with tumour, or amyloid.

Drugs may impair adrenal function either by inhibiting cortisol synthesis (etomidate, ketoconazole) or by inducing hepatic cortisol metabolism (rifampicin, phenytoin). High levels of circulating cytokines are also reported to have a suppressive effect upon ACTH release.[25]

PRESENTATION (BOX 61.2)

The disease is often unrecognised in its early stages as the presenting features are ill defined. Symptoms include tiredness and fatigue, vomiting, weight loss, anorexia and postural hypotension. Hyperpigmentation is seen in non-exposed areas (such as palmar skin creases) and is due to the hypersecretion of melatonin, a breakdown product from the ACTH precursor pro-opiomelanocortin (POMC).

Presentation to an intensive care physician is likely to be in the form of adrenal crisis. This may be precipitated by concurrent illness or surgery, or by failure to take replacement medication. Adrenal crisis will present classically as refractory shock with a poor response to inotropic or pressor agents. Abdominal or flank pain is often present and may lead to an erroneous diagnosis of an acute surgical abdomen.

Treatment should consist of immediate supportive measures, fluid resuscitation and high-dose intravenous glucocorticoid therapy. *A standard dose would be 100 mg of hydrocortisone 6-hourly, or as an infusion.* At these doses, separate mineralocorticoid replacement is not required.[26]

Adrenal crisis should be suspected in cases of undifferentiated shock not responding to standard management. Suggestive features would include a history of symptomatology consistent with the diagnosis, hyperpigmentation on examination, and demonstration of hyponatraemia, hyperkalaemia and peripheral blood eosinophilia. A random plasma total cortisol taken during a crisis will be low (below 80 nmol/L) and in the acute phase ACTH stimulation testing is not required.

Box 61.2 Clinical features of Addison disease

Symptoms	Signs
Muscular weakness	Hyperpigmentation – skin creases, buccal mucosa
Fatigue	Postural hypotension
Abdominal pain	Associated vitiligo
Vomiting	Decreased axillary and pubic hair
Diarrhoea	Auricular calcification
Salt craving	Vasodilated shock (in crisis)
Weight loss	
Arthralgia and myalgia	
Mood change	
Headache	
Sweating	
Syncope	

SECONDARY ADRENAL INSUFFICIENCY

The commonest cause of ACTH deficiency is sudden cessation of exogenous glucocorticoid treatment. Patients who have been taking more than 30 mg/day of hydrocortisone or the equivalent for more than 3 weeks are at risk of adrenal suppression.[22] Other causes include pituitary surgery, pituitary infarction (Sheehan syndrome) and pituitary tumour.

Presentation is similar to that of primary AI. The major distinguishing characteristics are a lack of hyperpigmentation and the absence of mineralocorticoid deficiency; hence hyperkalaemia is not a feature of secondary AI, although hyponatraemia may still be present owing to increased vasopressin levels.

INVESTIGATION OF ADRENAL INSUFFICIENCY

In a stable patient, suspected adrenal insufficiency is routinely investigated by an ACTH stimulation test. The test is performed by administering 250 μg of a synthetic ACTH molecule comprising the first 24 amino acids: tetracosactrin (Synacthen). Plasma total cortisol is measured at 0 and 30 minutes after administration, and a normal response is defined as a peak cortisol measurement over 525 nmol/L.[27] However, it should be noted that current immunoassays exhibit a significant degree of variability, and thus local laboratory reference ranges should be used.[28] The test cannot be performed if the patient is currently being prescribed hydrocortisone as this will cross-react with the assays; *an alternative replacement therapy such as dexamethasone should be used in these cases.*

Secondary AI may be differentiated from primary by a prolonged ACTH test. This is performed by the use of a depot preparation or an intravenous infusion of tetracosactrin for 24–48 hours. Patients with secondary hypoadrenalism show a greater plasma cortisol response at 24 hours than at 4 hours; alternatively, measurement of a baseline ACTH level may be used. In patients with primary AI this will be elevated.

Other biochemical tests that may be used in investigation of AI include the insulin hypoglycaemia test, the overnight metyrapone test and the CRH stimulation test. These investigations are not normally necessary in uncomplicated cases. In addition the use of the low-dose ACTH stimulation test has been advocated, in which only 1 μg of tetracosactrin is used. This approach has not yet gained widespread acceptance.

RELATIVE ADRENAL INSUFFICIENCY

The term *relative adrenal insufficiency* (RAI) was coined to describe a syndrome where the adrenal gland partially responds to stress but the magnitude of response is not commensurate.

Annane et al prospectively studied 189 patients with septic shock and detailed a three-level classification system based upon the basal cortisol level and response to ACTH.[29] Mortality was found to be highest in those patients with a basal cortisol level above 34 μg/dL (938 nmol/L) and response to ACTH of less than 9 μg/dL (248 nmol/L). Patients with a basal cortisol above 34 μg/dL but a cortisol response greater than 9 μg/dL did better, although the best prognosis was seen in the group with a lower basal cortisol level and high response to ACTH. This pattern of a high basal cortisol and blunted response to ACTH[30–33] is associated with increasing mortality. Although the term 'relative adrenal insufficiency' is often applied to a cortisol response to ACTH of less than 9 μg/dL (248 nmol/L), the changes in glucocorticoid secretion and responsiveness, protein binding, and activity in critical illness have also been described by the terms 'critical-illness-related corticosteroid insufficiency' (CIRCI).[34] The significance of this observation is not clear, however. It has been suggested either to represent a partially suppressed adrenal axis, implying a role for cortisol replacement therapy, or to indicate an 'overstressed' axis, in which case steroid treatment would be inappropriate. Treatment of septic patients fulfilling RAI criteria with hydrocortisone has been shown to improve outcome in only one study,[35] but these results have not been widely accepted (see below). Alternative diagnostic criteria relying on baseline plasma cortisol levels without ACTH stimulation have been proposed,[36] but the lack of a consistently observed relationship between cortisol levels and mortality means that the optimal diagnostic criteria for RAI remain controversial (**Box 61.3**). Possible explanations for the difficulties in assessing adrenal function in this patient group include spontaneous fluctuations in the measured cortisol values,[37] increased variability of assays[28] and changes in CBG levels affecting free cortisol values.[10,38] Measurement of the free cortisol fraction, representing the bioavailable active hormone, has been the focus of recent research interest, with some evidence suggesting it may give a more accurate representation of adrenal function.[10,38] However, the superiority of free cortisol estimations is by no means clear[16,39] and the limited availability of the assay means the test is not in general clinical use.

An alternative hypothesis put forward to explain the constellation of adrenocortical changes in critical illness is a sick euadrenal syndrome analogous of the sick euthyroid state,[40] in which changes in the free cortisol fraction, intracellular cortisol:cortisone interconversion, glucocorticoid receptor density and gene transcription may all act to affect adrenal function at a tissue level. The complexity of this system suggests that simple measurement of total plasma cortisol levels may give only a partial insight into the true functioning of the 'stress response' in the critically ill.

STEROID THERAPY IN CRITICAL ILLNESS

Steroids have an established role in the management of a number of critical illnesses as outlined in **Box 61.4**.

Box 61.3 Controversies in the diagnosis of adrenal insufficiency in the critically ill

1. Limitations of a random cortisol
   a. In the critically ill there is a marked fluctuation in plasma cortisol concentration limiting the utility of a random cortisol[37]
   b. The 'normal' range of cortisol in critical illness is not defined
   c. There is no consensus 'cut-off' value below which adrenal insufficiency is present
2. Limitations of total cortisol
   a. Free cortisol is the bioactive fraction of cortisol
   b. There is large variation in total cortisol assay results when the same specimen is tested in different laboratories and using different assays[28]
   c. Peripheral tissue-specific glucocorticoid resistance is not tested
3. Limitations of the conventional Synacthen test
   a. The HDSST results in plasma Synacthen concentrations that are supraphysiological
   b. Published data may have overestimated the incidence of adrenal insufficiency as many studies have not excluded patients who received etomidate.
   c. The low-dose SST may be a better predictor of outcome

HDSST=high-dose short Synacthen test; SST=short Synacthen test.

Box 61.4 Proven role for steroids in critical illness

1. Addisonian crisis
2. Anaphylaxis
3. Asthma
4. Bacterial meningitis
5. COPD with acute respiratory failure
6. Croup
7. Hypercalcaemia
8. Fulminant vasculitis
9. Idiopathic thrombocytopenic purpura
10. Myasthenic crisis
11. Myxoedema coma
12. Organ transplantation
13. *Pneumocystis carinii* pneumonia
14. Thyroid storm

However, their use in other conditions has not been without controversy.

SPINAL INJURY

Following the publication of the NASCIS II and III trials, high-dose methylprednisolone has been advocated in the management of patients with spinal cord injury. The major criticism of these studies is the lack of a demonstrable improvement in the primary outcome measures. For a more detailed review of the use of steroids in spinal cord injury, the reader is referred to Chapter 78.

HEAD INJURY

The role of steroids in the management of cerebral oedema secondary to tumours is well documented and accepted. However, their role in the management of head injury has been the subject of intense debate. Several prospective studies have not been able to prove any benefit with steroids in head trauma. However, these studies were not adequately powered to detect a difference. The recent CRASH trial with nearly 10 000 patients clearly demonstrated the lack of any benefit with steroids in head injury.[41]

However, a more recent study of multiple trauma suggested that patients fulfilling criteria for CIRCI had a lower rate of development of ventilator-associated pneumonia when treated with hydrocortisone,[42] and these findings were more marked in patients with head injury. This study is awaiting replication.

ACUTE RESPIRATORY DISTRESS SYNDROME (ARDS)

The ARDS clinical trial network published the results of its multicentre study where corticosteroids were administered to patients with ARDS persisting beyond 7 days. Although steroid use was associated with earlier ventilatory wean, improved arterial oxygenation and increased respiratory compliance, there was a higher rate of return to assisted ventilation and neuromuscular weakness.[43] No overall mortality difference was demonstrable between steroid and placebo groups. Commencement of steroids more than 2 weeks after onset of ARDS led to almost a fourfold increase in mortality compared with the placebo group. Consequently, steroids cannot be routinely recommended for persistent ARDS and may be harmful in late-stage ARDS. Although one randomised controlled trial demonstrated some benefit in early ARDS, trial design issues preclude widespread application of these results.[44] Steroids were also not found to be of benefit in ARDS associated with severe H1N1 pneumonia.[45]

SEPTIC SHOCK

Since the first reported use of steroids in sepsis in 1951, therapy with this drug has undergone several transformations, from 'steroid success' in sepsis and malaria in the 70s and early 80s, to 'steroid excess' (30 mg/kg methylprednisolone) in severe sepsis in the mid to late 80s, to total abandonment in the early 90s, and finally a resurgence of its use in the new millennium. The results of the only prospective randomised trial of steroids in septic shock, by Annane et al,[35] which found a beneficial effect, have not been widely accepted owing to problems of randomisation, change of protocol and the use of etomidate (an adrenal suppressant drug) in the study. A European multicentre randomised trial of steroids in septic shock (CORTICUS),[46] did not demonstrate a mortality difference between steroids and placebo. Neither the CORTICUS trial (n=499) nor the French study[35] (n=299) had adequate statistical power to demonstrate a clinically significant reduction in mortality. A recent meta-analysis[47] of 17 trials with 2138 patients reported reduced mortality in patients with septic shock treated with hydrocortisone. These conflicting data mean that the role of glucocorticoid treatment in the management of septic shock is still uncertain, and the Surviving Sepsis Campaign Guidelines of 2008 have downgraded their support for the use of low-dose hydrocortisone in septic shock (weak, low-grade recommendation) in the most recent revision.[48] Currently an ANZICS CTG-driven large multicentre randomised controlled trial (ADRENAL) of hydrocortisone in septic shock is under way (clinical trials.gov NCT01448109).

The role of fludrocortisone in septic shock also remains controversial. The study by Annane at al, quoted above, included a dose of 50 µg of fludrocortisone administered orally.[35] It has been argued, however, that doses of cortisol above 50 mg a day provide sufficient mineralocorticoid cover, and thus separate supplementation is unnecessary.[26]

Furthermore, the oral route of administration is unreliable in critically ill patients. A study comparing fludrocortisone plus hydrocortisone with hydrocortisone alone in septic patients failed to demonstrate a difference in outcome.[49]

PNEUMONIA

Adjunctive treatment with glucocorticoids has been advocated in the management of pneumonia as a strategy to reduce systemic effects of locally produced pulmonary cytokines, although results from these studies have been conflicting. A pilot study reported an improvement in oxygenation and mortality in patients with severe pneumonia treated with 7 days of hydrocortisone.[50] A larger trial in community-acquired pneumonia reported a reduced length of stay in patients receiving a 4-day course of dexamethasone; however, only 5% of these patients required ICU care.[51] Conversely, a trial of 7 days of prednisolone treatment in patients with community-acquired pneumonia showed no evidence of efficacy in either cure rate or length of stay,[52] and a recent observational study of 316 patients with ICU-acquired pneumonia suggested that systemic steroid treatment was associated with an increase in mortality.[53] At present, glucocorticoid treatment is not routinely recommended for critically ill patients with pneumonia; an exception would be for the case of *Pneumocystis jirovecii* infection in patients suffering from human immunodeficiency virus (HIV).[54]

MENINGITIS

Randomised controlled trials have demonstrated the benefit of early steroid therapy in paediatric meningitis, particularly with *H. influenzae* infections. There is also

Box 61.5 Side-effects of corticosteroid therapy

Adrenal suppression	Hypertension
Hypokalaemia	Osteoporosis
Glucose intolerance	Peptic ulcer disease
Truncal obesity	Glaucoma
Myopathy	Hyperlipidaemia
Mood alterations including psychosis	Aseptic necrosis of femoral/humeral head

evidence of benefit in adult patients with meningitis, particularly with pneumococcal infections. (For more detail refer to Ch. 54.)

SIDE-EFFECTS OF STEROID THERAPY

Steroid therapy is associated with numerous side-effects. Those that would be of particular relevance to intensive care are (a full list is given in **Box 61.5**):

- *suppression of the adrenal axis (discussed above):* patients who have been receiving steroid treatment for less than a week are unlikely to be affected
- *hyperglycaemia:* this may be associated with adverse outcomes in critically ill patients[55]
- *myopathy:* steroid therapy is known to be associated with muscle weakness and also shown to be an independent risk factor for developing ICU-acquired muscle paresis; this has significant clinical implications for weaning patients from mechanical ventilation
- *hypokalaemia*
- *leucocytosis:* corticosteroids increase the neutrophil count by a shift from the marginating to the circulating pool; this effect may lead to concerns that the patient has developed an occult infection
- *poor wound healing*
- *immunosupression*
- *pancreatitis.*

Access the complete references list online at http://www.expertconsult.com

1. Yudt MR, Cidlowski JA. The glucocorticoid receptor: coding a diversity of proteins and responses through a single gene. Mol Endocrinol 2002;16:1719–26.
16. Cohen J, Smith ML, Deans RV, et al. Serial changes in plasma total cortisol, plasma free cortisol, and tissue cortisol activity in patients with septic shock: an observational study. Shock 2012;37:28–33.
29. Annane D, Sebille V, Troche G, et al. A 3-level prognostic classification in septic shock based on cortisol levels and cortisol response to corticotropin. JAMA 2000;283:1038–45.
35. Annane D, Sebille V, Charpentier C, et al. Effect of treatment with low doses of hydrocortisone and fludrocortisone on mortality in patients with septic shock. JAMA 2002;288:862–71.
36. Cooper MS, Stewart PM. Corticosteroid insufficiency in acutely ill patients. N Engl J Med 2003;348:727–34.
40. Venkatesh B, Cohen J. Adrenocortical (dys)function in septic shock – a sick euadrenal state. Best Pract Res Clin Endocrinol Metab 2011;25:719–33.
42. Roquilly A, Mahe PJ, Seguin P, et al. Hydrocortisone therapy for patients with multiple trauma: the randomized controlled HYPOLYTE study. JAMA 2011;305:1201–9.
46. Sprung CL, Annane D, Keh D, et al. Hydrocortisone therapy for patients with septic shock. N Engl J Med 2008;358:111–24.

62

Acute calcium disorders

Balasubramanian Venkatesh

Calcium is an important cation and the principal electrolyte of the body. A total of 1–2 kg is present in the average adult, of which 99% is found in the bone. Of the remaining 1%, nine-tenths are present in the cells and only a tenth in the extracellular fluid. In the plasma, 50% of the calcium is ionised, 40% bound to plasma proteins, mainly to albumin, and the remaining 10% is chelated to anions such as citrate, bicarbonate, lactate, sulphate phosphate and ketones. The chelated fraction is usually of little clinical importance, but is increased in conditions where some of these anionic concentrations might be elevated, as in renal failure. Whereas most calcium inside the cell is in the form of insoluble complexes, the concentration of intracellular ionised calcium is about 0.1 µmol/L, creating a gradient of 10 000 : 1 between plasma and intracellular fluid (ICF) levels of ionised calcium.[1] A schematic illustration of calcium distribution within the various body compartments is shown in **Figure 62.1**.

Because ionised calcium is the biologically active component of ECF calcium with respect to physiological functions (**Box 62.1**) and is also the reference variable for endocrine regulation of calcium homeostasis, its measurement is recognised as being one of prime importance in the management of disorders of calcium homeostasis.

HORMONAL REGULATION OF CALCIUM HOMEOSTASIS[2,3]

The concentration of ionised calcium in the plasma is subject to tight hormonal control, particularly parathyroid hormone (PTH). A G-protein coupled calcium receptor plays a significant role in the maintenance of calcium homeostasis. This receptor, responsible for sensing extracellular calcium concentration, is present on the cell membrane of the chief cells of the parathyroid and in bone, gut and the kidney. In response to ionised hypocalcaemia, PTH secretion is stimulated, which in turn serves to restore serum calcium levels back to normal by increasing osteoclastic activity in the bone and renal reabsorption of calcium and stimulating renal synthesis of $1,25(OH)D_3$ (calcitriol – the active metabolite of vitamin D), which increases gut absorption of calcium.

Calcitriol production is stimulated by hypocalcaemia, and vice versa. Calcitriol increases serum calcium by largely promoting gut reabsorption, and to a lesser extent renal reabsorption of calcium.

Calcitonin, a hypocalcaemic peptide hormone, produced by the thyroid, acts as a physiological antagonist to PTH. Although calcitonin has been shown to reduce serum calcium levels in animals by increasing renal clearance of calcium and inhibiting bone resorption, its role in humans is less clear. Despite extreme variations in calcitonin levels, for example total lack in patients who have undergone total thyroidectomy, or excess plasma levels, as seen in patients with medullary carcinoma of the thyroid gland, no significant changes in calcium and phosphate metabolism are seen. Calcitonin is useful as a pharmacological agent in the management of hypercalcaemia.

METABOLIC FACTORS INFLUENCING CALCIUM HOMEOSTASIS

Alterations in serum protein, pH, serum phosphate and magnesium closely impact on serum calcium concentrations. Total plasma calcium levels vary with alterations in plasma protein concentration. Several equations have been put forward for the adjustment of serum calcium in the face of alterations in serum protein concentrations. The validity of these equations is dependent upon the patient population, the methodology used for assessment of serum calcium and the reference intervals.[4] Clinicians often use simple rules of thumb – a correction is made for hypoalbuminaemia by adding 0.2 mmol/L to the measured serum calcium concentration for every 10 g/L decrease in serum albumin concentration below normal (40 g/L). The corresponding correction factor for globulins is –0.04 mmol/L of serum calcium for every 10 g/L rise in serum globulin.

Changes in pH alter protein binding of calcium. As the relationship between ionised calcium (iCa) and changes in pH is well defined, iCa concentrations can be predicted for a given pH using the following formula:

$$\text{corrected iCa at pH 7.4} = \text{measured iCa} \times [1 - (0.53 \times (7.40 - \text{measured pH}))]^4$$

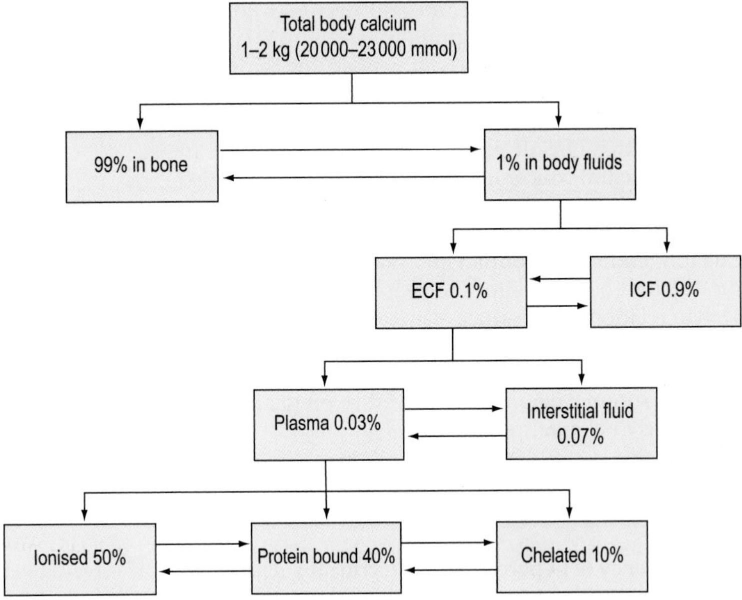

Figure 62.1 Distribution of body calcium. ECF=extracellular fluid; ICF=intracellular fluid.

Box 62.1 Functions of calcium[1,15]

- Excitation – contraction coupling in cardiac, skeletal and smooth muscle
- Cardiac action potentials and pacemaker activity
- Release of neurotransmitters
- Coagulation of blood
- Bone formation and metabolism
- Hormone release
- Ciliary motility
- Catecholamine responsiveness at the receptor site[7]
- Strong cation
- Regulation of cell growth and apoptosis

Table 62.1 Daily calcium balance

GASTROINTESTINAL TRACT	
Diet	600–1200 mg/day
Absorbed	200–400 mg/day
Secreted	150–800 mg/day
RENAL	
Filtered	11000 mg/day
Reabsorbed (97% in the proximal convoluted tubule)	10800 mg/day
Urinary calcium	200 mg/day
BONE	
Turnover	600–800 mg/day

Another rule of thumb is that an increase in pH by 0.1 pH units results in a decrease in ionised calcium by approximately 0.1 mmol/L.[5]

Calcium and phosphate are closely linked by the following reaction in the extracellular fluid. $HPO_4^{2-}+Ca^{2+}=CaHPO_4$. Increases in serum phosphate shift the reaction to the right. When the calcium phosphate solubility product exceeds the critical value of 5 mmol/L, calcium deposition occurs in the tissues, resulting in a fall in serum calcium concentration and a secondary increase in PTH secretion. Reductions in phosphate concentration lead to corresponding changes in the opposite direction.

As magnesium is required for PTH secretion and end-organ responsiveness, alterations in serum magnesium have an impact on serum calcium concentration.

Turnover of calcium in the bone is predominantly under the control of PTH and calcitriol, although prostaglandins and some of the cytokines also play a role in it. Bone resorption is mediated by osteoclasts, whereas osteoblasts are involved in bone formation. The daily calcium balance is summarised in **Table 62.1**.

MEASUREMENT OF SERUM CALCIUM

Most hospital laboratories measure total serum calcium. The normal plasma concentration is 2.2–2.6 mmol/L. However, the ionised form (1.1–1.3 mmol/L) is the active fraction and its measurement is not routine in many laboratories, although most state-of-the-art blood gas analysers can measure serum ionised calcium concentrations. Estimation of ionised calcium from total serum calcium concentration using mathematical algorithms is unreliable in critically ill patients.[6–8] Heparin forms complexes with calcium and decreases ionised calcium.[9] A heparin concentration of <15 units/mL of whole blood is therefore recommended for the measurement of ionised calcium.[10] Anaerobic collection of the specimen is recommended as CO_2 loss from the specimen may result in alkalosis and reduction in ionised calcium concentration. Calcium levels are also reduced by a concomitant lactic acidosis owing to chelation by lactate ion.[11] Free fatty acids (FFAs) increase calcium binding to albumin and may form a portion of the calcium-binding site.[12] Increases in FFAs may be seen in relation to stress, use of steroids, catecholamines and heparin. The impact of pH on calcium measurements has been described above. The normal reference levels of serum calcium are reduced in pregnancy and in the early neonatal period.[13]

HYPERCALCAEMIA IN CRITICALLY ILL PATIENTS

The frequency of hypercalcaemia in critically ill patients is not well established, although it is not as common as hypocalcaemia. Depending on the patient population, the reported incidence ranges from 3–5% to as high as 32%.[14,15] Admission to the ICU with a primary diagnosis of a hypercalcaemic crisis is uncommon. Although a number of aetiologies have been described (**Box 62.2**), in the critical care setting, hypercalcaemic crisis is usually due to malignancy-related hypercalcaemia, renal failure or posthypocalcaemic hypercalcaemia.[16] Before undertaking a work-up for hypercalcaemia, it is important to exclude false-positive measurements. This is usually the result of inadvertent haemoconcentration during venepuncture and elevation in serum protein, although ionised calcium levels are not reported to be affected by haemoconcentration.[17] *Pseudohypercalcaemia* has also been described in the setting of essential thrombocythaemia. The erroneous result is thought to be due to in vitro release of calcium from platelets, analogous to the pseudohyperkalaemia seen in the same condition.[18]

From a pathophysiological standpoint, hypercalcaemia may be due to an elevation in PTH, in which case the homeostatic regulatory and feedback mechanisms are preserved, and this is termed *equilibrium hypercalcaemia*. Alternatively, it could be a non-parathyroid-mediated hypercalcaemia with associated breakdown of homeostatic mechanisms, and this situation is termed *disequilibrium hypercalcaemia*.

MECHANISMS OF HYPERCALCAEMIA

Malignancy-related hypercalcaemia might arise from bony metastases or humoral hypercalcaemia of malignancy. In the latter (seen with bronchogenic carcinoma and hypernephroma), tumour osteolysis of bone resulting from the release of PTH-like substances (which cross-react with PTH in the radioimmunoassay, but are not identical to PTH), calcitriol, osteoclast-activating factor and prostaglandins are thought to be the major underlying mechanisms. Aggravating factors include dehydration, immobilisation and renal failure.

Posthypocalcaemic hypercalcaemia is a transient phenomenon seen in patients following a period of hypocalcaemia.[16] This has been attributed to a parathyroid hyperplasia that develops during the period of hypocalcaemia, which results in a rebound hypercalcaemia following resolution of the underlying hypocalcaemic disorder.

Immobilisation hypercalcaemia results from an alteration in balance between bone formation and resorption.[19–22] This leads to loss of bone minerals, hypercalcaemia, hypercalciuria and increased risk of renal failure. In patients with normal bone turnover, immobilisation rarely causes significant hypercalcaemia. However, in patients with rapid turnover of bone (children, post-fracture patients, hyperparathyroidism, Paget's disease, spinal injuries and Guillain–Barré syndrome), this may result in severe hypercalcaemia.

Intravascular volume depletion reduces renal calcium excretion by a combination of reduced glomerular filtration and increased tubular reabsorption

Box 62.2 Causes of hypercalcaemia

Common causes of hypercalcaemia in the critically ill patient

Complication of malignancy:
- bony metastases
- humoral hypercalcaemia of malignancy

Posthypocalcaemic hypercalcaemia:
- recovery from pancreatitis[15]
- recovery from acute renal failure following rhabdomyolysis[37–41]

Primary hyperparathyroidism
Adrenal insufficiency[23,24]
Prolonged immobilisation[18–21]
Disorders of magnesium metabolism
Use of TPN[42]
Hypovolaemia
Iatrogenic calcium administration

Less common causes of hypercalcaemia in the critically ill patient

Granulomatous diseases – sarcoidosis, tuberculosis, berylliosis
Vitamin A and D intoxication
Multiple myeloma
Endocrine:
- thyrotoxicosis
- acromegaly
- phaeochromocytoma

Lithium – chronic therapy
Tamoxifen
Rare association between drugs and hypercalcaemia
Theophylline, omeprazole and growth hormone therapy

of calcium. Hypercalcaemia further compounds this problem by causing a concentrating defect in the renal tubules, thus creating a polyuria and further aggravating the hypovolaemia. Extrarenal production of calcitriol by lymphocytes in granulomata is thought to be the predominant mechanism of hypercalcaemia in granulomatous diseases.[23,24] Only 10–20% of patients with adrenal insufficiency develop hypercalcaemia.[25,26] The aetiology of this is thought to be multifactorial: intravascular volume depletion, haemoconcentration of plasma proteins and the loss of anti-vitamin D effects of glucocorticoids. Hypercalcaemia can be associated with the use of certain medications – vitamin D toxicity, loop diuretics, thiazide diuretics and lithium. For rarer causes of hypercalcaemia, the reader is referred to the reviews by Kallas et al and Jacobs & Bilezikian.[23,27]

MANIFESTATIONS OF HYPERCALCAEMIA

The clinical manifestations of hypercalcaemia (commonly encountered when total serum calcium exceeds 3 mmol/L) are outlined in **Box 62.3**. *Hypercalcaemic crisis* is defined as severe hypercalcaemia (total serum Ca >3.5 mmol/L) associated with acute symptoms and signs.

INVESTIGATIONS

A detailed diagnostic algorithm is outside of the scope of this chapter. The basic work-up should include serum calcium, phosphorus and alkaline phosphatase estimation, PTH assay, renal function assessment and a skeletal survey.

Box 62.3 Clinical manifestations of hypercalcaemia*

Cardiovascular
Hypertension
Arrhythmias
Digitalis sensitivity
Catecholamine resistance
Urinary system
Nephrocalcinosis
Nephrolithiasis
Tubular dysfunction
Renal failure
Gastrointestinal
Anorexia/nausea/vomiting
Constipation
Peptic ulcer
Pancreatitis
Neuromuscular
Weakness
Neuropsychiatric
Depression
Disorientation
Psychosis
Coma
Seizures

*Ectopic calcification is usually seen with chronic hypercalcaemia.

THERAPY OF HYPERCALCAEMIA AND HYPERCALCAEMIC CRISIS

Mild asymptomatic hypercalcaemia does not require emergent treatment. Therapy is usually directed at the underlying cause. The management of hypercalcaemic crisis consists of two principal components:

1. Increasing urinary excretion of calcium
2. Reducing bone resorption.

INCREASING URINARY EXCRETION OF CALCIUM

As almost all patients with hypercalcaemia are volume-depleted, the initial therapy consists of rehydration with normal saline, followed by diuresis with furosemide. Rehydration with normal saline improves intravascular volume, reducing serum calcium by extracellular dilution, and saliuresis promotes calcium loss in the urine. Volume expansion should be titrated to clinical end-points and CVP monitoring. A urine output of 4–5 L should be aimed for in these patients to promote calciuresis. In many patients, these measures would achieve a reduction in serum calcium by about 0.4–0.5 mmol/L. Hypokalaemia, hypomagnesaemia and calcium stone formation in the urine are potential side-effects of this mode of treatment.

In patients with established renal failure, in whom forced diuresis cannot be instituted, dialysis against a dialysate with zero or low calcium concentrations should be the treatment of choice.

REDUCTION OF BONE RESORPTION

Measures to increase urinary excretion of calcium should be followed up with administration of agents that minimise bone resorption. A number of agents are available and these are listed in **Table 62.2**. Disodium EDTA at a dose of 15–50 mg/kg i.v. rapidly lowers serum calcium. However, its propensity to reduce serum calcium rapidly coupled with its nephrotoxic effects limits its usefulness to life-threatening hypercalcaemia. Other therapeutic modalities include the use of NSAIDs and parathyroidectomy. Calcimimetics are agents that increase the activation of the calcium receptor thus reducing serum PTH concentrations. Cinacalcet is a first-generation calcimimetic, which has shown promise in early randomised trials for the management of hypercalcaemia; it has also been shown to be effective in the management of primary hyperparathyroidism across a wide spectrum of disease severity.[28] However, its role in the management of acute hypercalcaemia[29] is limited.

At the present time, several newer and more potent bisphosphonates are under development. Their efficacy combined with a relative lack of side-effects

Table 62.2 Therapeutic agents for reducing bone resorption

THERAPY	INDICATIONS	DOSE	ONSET TIME/ DURATION	LIMITATIONS	MECHANISM OF ACTION	COMMENTS
Bi-Phosponates* Etidronate (first-generation)	Malignancy-related hypercalcaemia	5 mg/kg per day	1–2 days, lasts 5–7 days	Hyperphosphataemia, short duration of action	Inhibit osteoclast activity, may have some effect on osteoblasts	High-potency group. Pamidronate lowers Ca levels more rapidly than etidronate
Pamidronate (second-generation)		90 mg as an infusion every 4 weeks	1–2 days, lasts 10–14 days	Hypophosphataemia, fever and hypomagnesaemia		
Calcitonin	Hypercalcaemia, Paget's disease	Initial IV dose 3–4 U/kg followed by 4 U/kg s.c. 12-hourly	Hours, lasts 2–3 days	Nausea, abdominal pain, flushing, tachyphylaxis, limited efficacy	Inhibit osteoclast activity, reduces renal tubular reabsorption of calcium	Tachyphylaxis minimised by concomitant steroid therapy
Glucocorticoids	Vitamin D toxicity, myeloma, lymphoma, granulomata	i.v. hydrocortisone 200–400 mg/day	Days, lasts days to weeks	Glucocorticoid side-effects	Inhibit inflammatory cell production of calcitriol, reduce gut absorption of calcium	Improve the efficacy of calcitonin
Gallium nitrate	Malignancy-related hypercalcaemia	100–200 mg/m^2 per day for 5–7 days	5–6 days, lasts 7–10 days	Nephrotoxic	Inhibits bone resorption and alters bone crystal structure	Recent phase II data suggest equivalent efficacy with pamidronate[45]
Plicamycin	Malignancy-related hypercalcaemia	25 µg/kg i.v.	Rapid onset, lasts for a few days	Hepatotoxic, nephrotoxic and thrombocytopoenia	Inhibits cellular RNA synthesis	Side-effect profile limits the use of this drug
Intravenous phosphates	Limited clinical role	10–15 mmol as an infusion repeated at regular intervals	Hours, lasts 24–48 hours after cessation	Ectopic calcification, severe hypocalcaemia	Ectopic calcification, reduce gut absorption, inhibition of bone resorption	Use superseded by the other modalities described

*Other biphosphonates include ibandronate, risedronate and zoledronate. As compared to pamidronate, zoledronate has the advantage of simplicity of administration and better control of hypercalcemia.
i.v., intravenous; s.c., subcutaneous.

make them the agents of choice for the treatment of malignancy-related hypercalcaemia. Other drugs that have been used in the management of hypercalcaemia include prostaglandin inhibitors for cancer-related hypercalcaemia, ketoconazole and chloroquine (for sarcoid-induced hypercalcaemia).[24]

ADJUNCTIVE MEASURES IN THE MANAGEMENT OF HYPERCALCAEMIA

Monitoring of cardiorespiratory function and biochemical status is mandatory during therapy of hypercalcaemia. Thiazide diuretics, vitamin D and absorbable antacids should be avoided. Hypercalcaemia potentiates digitalis effect and dosage should be adjusted accordingly. Endocrinologists should be consulted for further management.

HYPOCALCAEMIA

Hypocalcaemia is more common than hypercalcaemia in critically ill patients, with an estimated incidence of around 70–90%.[16] As the ionised calcium is the biologically active moiety, it is important to look at ionised hypocalcaemia. The frequency of this is far more varied, ranging from 15 to 70%.[16,30,31] *Spurious hypocalcaemia* is seen with poor storage of specimens prior to analysis, resulting in CO_2 loss from the specimen, use of EDTA or large doses of heparin as anticoagulants in the syringe. Gadodiamide used in association with MRI as a contrast medium can interfere with the colorimetric assay and cause spurious hypocalcaemia.[32]

AETIOLOGIES

The aetiology of ionised hypocalcaemia based on the predominant pathophysiological mechanism is listed in **Box 62.4**. The other contributory mechanisms of hypocalcaemia in each of the conditions are shown in brackets.

Although a long list of causes exists for hypocalcaemia, calcium chelation and hypoparathyroidism constitute the common mechanisms of ionised hypocalcaemia in intensive care. The increasing prevalence of citrate anticoagulation used for renal replacement therapy, if not accompanied by appropriate metabolic monitoring, could emerge as another cause of hypocalcaemia in critically ill patients. Frequently, hypocalcaemia is accompanied by a number of other biochemical abnormalities, thus a pattern recognition approach towards the cause of hypocalcaemia will point to its aetiology and save a considerable amount of investigations for the patient. Common diagnostic patterns are listed below in **Table 62.3**.

Although alkalosis is frequently associated with ionised hypocalcaemia, the presence of a metabolic acidosis in the face of low serum ionised calcium narrows the differential diagnosis even further (**Box 62.5**).

Box 62.4 Aetiology of ionised hypocalcaemia

Calcium chelation
- Alkalosis (increased binding of calcium by albumin)
- Citrate toxicity (calcium chelation)
- Hyperphosphataemia (calcium chelation, ectopic calcification, reduced vitamin D3 activity)
- Pancreatitis (calcium soap formation, reduced parathyroid secretion)
- Tumour lysis syndrome (hyperphosphataemia)
- Rhabdomyolysis (hyperphosphataemia and reduced levels of calcitriol)

Hypoparathyroidism
- Hypo- and hypermagnesaemia
- Sepsis (decrease PTH secretion, calcitriol resistance, intracellular shift of calcium)
- Burns (decrease in PTH secretion)
- Neck surgery (removal of parathyroid gland, calcitonin release during thyroid surgery and hungry bone syndrome post-parathyroidectomy)

Hypovitaminosis D
- Inadequate intake
- Malabsorption
- Liver disease (impaired 25-hydroxylation of cholecalciferol)
- Renal failure (impaired 1-hydroxylation of cholecalciferol, hyperphosphataemia)

Reduced bone turnover
- Osteoporosis
- Elderly
- Cachexia

Drug induced
- Phenytoin (accelerated metabolism of vitamin D3)
- Diphosphonates (see under hypercalcaemia)
- Propofol
- EDTA (calcium chelation)
- Ethylene glycol (formation of calcium oxalate crystals in the urine
- Cis-platinum (renal tubular damage leading to hypermagnesuria)
- Protamine
- Gentamicin (hypermagnesuria leading to hypomagnesaemia and therefore hypocalcaemia)

CLINICAL MANIFESTATIONS OF HYPOCALCAEMIA

Mild degrees of hypocalcaemia are usually asymptomatic. Ionised calcium levels less than 0.8 mmol/L may cause neuromuscular irritability and result in clinical symptoms. The clinical manifestations of hypocalcaemia are summarised in **Box 62.6**. The manifestations listed in Box 62.6 are by no means a comprehensive list of all the clinical features, but include the ones most commonly seen in the critical care setting.

When eliciting tetany, Trousseau's sign (carpopedal spasm) is more specific for hypocalcaemia than is Chvostek's sign (facial twitch in response to facial nerve stimulus, which is present in 10–30% of the normal population). ECG changes do not correlate well with

Table 62.3 Pattern recognition in the diagnosis of common causes of hypocalcaemia

AETIOLOGY OF HYPOCALCAEMIA	CLINICAL/BIOCHEMICAL PATTERNS
Low serum albumin	Reduced total calcium, normal ionised calcium
Alkalosis	Normal total calcium, reduced ionised calcium
Hypomagnesaemia	Reduced ionised calcium and hypokalaemia
Pancreatitis	Hypocalcaemia, elevated serum lipase and glucose
Renal failure	Elevated blood urea nitrogen, elevated phosphate
Rhabdomyolysis	Hypocalcaemia, elevated phosphate, creatine kinase and urinary myoglobin
Tumour lysis syndrome	Hypocalcaemia, elevated phosphate, potassium and urate

Box 62.5 Hypocalcaemia with metabolic acidosis

Acute renal failure
Tumour lysis
Rhabdomyolysis
Pancreatitis
Ethylene glycol poisoning
Hydrofluoric acid intoxication

Box 62.6 Clinical manifestations of hypocalcaemia

Central nervous system
Circumoral and peripheral paraesthesia
Muscle cramps
Tetany
Seizures
Extrapyramidal manifestations: tremor, ataxia, dystonia
Proximal myopathy
Depression, anxiety, psychosis
Cardiovascular
Arrhythmias
Hypotension, inotrope unresponsiveness
Prolonged QT intervals, T-wave inversion
Loss of digitalis effect
Respiratory
Apnoea
Laryngospasm
Bronchospasm

Table 62.4 Commonly used i.v. calcium preparations

PREPARATION	DOSAGE (ML)	ELEMENTAL CALCIUM/GRAM
Calcium gluconate	10	93 mg (2.3 mmol)
Calcium chloride	10	272 mg (6.8 mmol)
Calcium acetate	10	253 mg (6.35 mmol)

the degree of hypocalcaemia. The symptoms of hypocalcaemia are exacerbated by a coexisting hypokalaemia and a hypomagnesaemia.

The laboratory work-up should include serum calcium, phosphorus, magnesium and alkaline phosphatase, PTH and vitamin D assays and renal function assessment.

APPROACH TO THE TREATMENT OF ASYMPTOMATIC AND SYMPTOMATIC HYPOCALCAEMIA

ARGUMENTS FOR AND AGAINST CORRECTION OF ASYMPTOMATIC HYPOCALCAEMIA

As stated before, it is not clear if asymptomatic hypocalcaemia needs correction. Based on published data which suggest that critical care hypocalcaemia is associated with a higher mortality and increased length of stay in intensive care,[33–35] it is advocated that ionised hypocalcaemia be corrected routinely irrespective of the level. However, arguments exist against the routine correction of asymptomatic ionised hypocalcaemia. Increases in cytosolic calcium lead to disruption of intracellular processes, activation of proteases and can lead to ischaemia and reperfusion injury.[36] Also, there are data suggesting that ionised calcium is an important participant in the pathogenesis of coronary and cerebral vasospasm.[37] In rodent models of endotoxic shock, there are also data demonstrating an increased mortality when these rats were administered intravenous calcium.[38] Most clinicians agree that an ionised calcium level of <0.8 mmol/L needs correction even if asymptomatic.

MANAGEMENT OF ACUTE SYMPTOMATIC HYPOCALCAEMIA

Acute symptomatic hypocalcaemia is a medical emergency that requires immediate therapy. In addition to treatment of underlying cause and support of airway, breathing and circulation, the definitive treatment includes administration of intravenous calcium. Intravenous calcium is available as a calcium salt of chloride or gluconate or acetate. The main difference between these formulations is the amount of elemental calcium available at equivalent volumes of drug (**Table 62.4**). The dose of calcium required should be based on the elemental calcium.[39] Intravenous calcium can be administered as a bolus or as an infusion. Rapid administration of calcium may cause nausea, flushing, headache

Box 62.7 Indications for calcium administration

Absolute
Symptomatic hypocalcaemia
Ionised Ca <0.8 mmol/L
Hyperkalaemia
Ca channel blocker overdose
Relative
β-blocker overdose
Hypermagnesaemia
Hypocalcaemia in the face of high inotrope requirement
Massive blood transfusion post cardiopulmonary bypass to augment cardiac contractility

and arrhythmias. Digitalis toxicity may be precipitated. Extravasation of calcium may lead to tissue irritation, particularly with the chloride salt. Calcium chloride may be better than calcium gluconate for the management of hypocalcaemia, if there is concomitant alkalosis. Following an initial bolus, an infusion may be commenced at a rate of 1–2 mg/kg/h of elemental calcium to maintain target levels of ionised calcium. With correction of the underlying disorder and restoration of calcium to normal levels, the infusion can be tapered and stopped. Adequacy of calcium therapy can be monitored clinically and by performing serial determinations of ionised calcium. Failure of ionised calcium to increase after commencement of i.v. calcium may indicate an underlying magnesium deficiency. This can be corrected by administration of 10 mmol of intravenous magnesium over 20 minutes.

Administration of calcium in the setting of hyperphosphataemia may result in calcium precipitation in the tissues. In these situations, a phosphate binder may be administered. Calcium salts should not be administered with bicarbonate since the two precipitate. The other indications for calcium administration are listed in **Box 62.7**. Other therapy for hypocalcaemia consists of oral calcium supplements and calcitriol administration, although these are usually used in the management of chronic hypocalcaemia.

ASSOCIATION BETWEEN IONISED CALCIUM CONCENTRATION AND OUTCOME IN CRITICAL ILLNESS

A recent retrospective study examined the association between serum ionised calcium (iCa) and mortality in a heterogeneous cohort of critically ill patients.[40] Data from >7000 patients generating >175 000 iCa measurements were analysed. The investigators concluded that, within a broad range of values, ionised calcium concentration has no independent association with hospital or intensive care unit mortality. However, from multivariate logistic regression analysis, an ionised calcium <0.8 mmol/L or an ionised calcium >1.4 mmol/L was independently associated with intensive care unit and hospital mortality. In patients requiring massive blood transfusion, another study reported a concentration-dependent effect of hypocalcaemia on mortality.[41]

VITAMIN D AND CRITICAL ILLNESS

The traditional role of vitamin D has been thought to be the maintenance of adequate serum calcium and phosphate levels, for bone mineralisation and optimal cardiac and skeletal muscle function. Over the past decade, data from biochemical and molecular genetic studies indicate that vitamin D has a much wider range of effects than this traditional role. These non-skeletal effects, termed pleiotropic, include potentiation of antimicrobial action, modification of inflammation, cardioprotective effects and immunomodulatory effects. Several large observational studies have demonstrated an association between increased morbidity and mortality and lower vitamin D levels as measured by serum $25(OH)D_3$ in critically ill patients. On the other hand there are data to suggest that a single measurement of vitamin D may not be reflective of the 24-hour profile in critically ill patients owing to the marked variability.[42,43] Moreover there are also data to suggest that $1,25(OH)D_3$ levels may be increased during the inflammatory response. Currently, the existing data are insufficient to make an evidence-based recommendation regarding its potential benefit in the ICU.[44] Results from large prospective randomised controlled trials are lacking.

Access the complete references list online at http://www.expertconsult.com

4. Baird GS. Ionized calcium. Clin Chim Acta 2011; 412:696–701.
22. Sam R, Vaseemuddin M, Siddique A, et al. Hypercalcemia in patients in the burn intensive care unit. J Burn Care Res 2007;28:742–6.
27. Jacobs TP, Bilezikian JP. Clinical review: Rare causes of hypercalcemia. J Clin Endocrinol Metab 2005;90: 6316–22.
28. Peacock M, Bilezikian JP, Bolognese MA, et al. Cinacalcet HCl reduces hypercalcemia in primary hyperparathyroidism across a wide spectrum of disease severity. J Clin Endocrinol Metab 2011;96: E9–18.
29. Steddon SJ, Cunningham J. Calcimimetics and calcilytics – fooling the calcium receptor. Lancet 2005;365: 2237–9.
40. Egi M, Kim I, Nichol A, et al. Ionized calcium concentration and outcome in critical illness. Crit Care Med 2011;39:314–21.
42. Venkatesh B, Davidson B, Robinson K, et al. Do random estimations of vitamin D3 and parathyroid hormone reflect the 24-h profile in the critically ill? Intensive Care Med 2012;38:177–9.
44. Amrein K, Venkatesh B. Vitamin D and the critically ill patient. Curr Opin Clin Nutr Metab Care 2012; 15:188–93.

Part Nine

Obstetric Emergencies

63

Preeclampsia and eclampsia

Wai Ka Ming and Tony Gin

Pre-eclampsia is a syndrome specific to pregnancy. Although diagnostic criteria have varied among countries and over time, it is generally defined as new onset of hypertension and proteinuria after 20 weeks' gestation (**Table 63.1**). In Australian practice, pre-eclampsia is defined as new-onset hypertension after 20 weeks' gestation with organ involvement; proteinuria is not mandatory for establishing the clinical diagnosis.[1] Many organisations have issued extensive national guidelines for the prevention, diagnosis and treatment of pre-eclampsia and other hypertensive disorders in pregnancy.[1-5] Eclampsia describes the occurrence in a pre-eclamptic woman of seizures not attributable to other causes.

Pre-eclampsia complicates 2–10% of pregnancies worldwide.[6] In the United Kingdom, the maternal mortality attributed to pre-eclampsia in 2006–2008 was 0.83 per 100 000 deliveries.[7] In developed countries, eclampsia complicates 2–3 cases per 10 000 deliveries with mortality less than 1%.[8] Despite the decline of maternal mortality from pre-eclampsia and related complications in developed countries over the past two decades, hypertensive disorders remain one of the three leading cause of maternal death. The incidence of eclampsia and maternal mortality are higher in developing countries.[9] This may be related to poor antenatal care services, and lack of expertise and health care resources.[10]

Factors associated with increased maternal risk include:[11,12]

- onset at or less than 32 weeks' gestation
- greater maternal age and parity
- pre-existing hypertension or medical complications
- Afro-Caribbean descent
- nausea and vomiting and epigastric pain
- abnormal laboratory tests, including raised liver enzymes, increased serum creatinine and increased serum uric acid.

Patients may be referred to the intensive care unit (ICU) for poorly controlled hypertension, convulsions, postoperative care, or following complications such as pulmonary oedema, renal failure, haemorrhage, coagulopathy and stroke.

AETIOLOGY

The cause of pre-eclampsia is unknown, and there is no satisfactory single unifying hypothesis. Pre-eclampsia is more common in primigravidae, multiple gestation, obesity, African–American race, molar pregnancy, pre-existing hypertension, underlying disease (e.g. autoimmune disease, renal disease, diabetes and thrombophilia) and previous or family history of pre-eclampsia.[13] Although there is a genetic predisposition, no particular gene or mode of inheritance has been strongly implicated. Pre-eclampsia may be a result of cumulative effects of variants at multiple genes, both fetal and maternal.[14-15] Genetic factors could influence not only the aetiology of pre-eclampsia, but also the development of the disease and response to treatment. Some investigators differentiate early-onset (before 34 weeks' gestation) and late-onset pre-eclampsia (at or after 34 weeks) because of differences in outcomes, biochemical markers and clinical features.[16]

PATHOGENESIS

Pre-eclampsia is a systemic disease that affects most organ systems. Many theories of pathogenesis have been proposed, but a common concept is that of a two-stage disease with an initial stage of abnormal placentation and placental ischaemia, followed by a second stage of clinical disease. Initially, there is inadequate endovascular invasion of fetal trophoblast into the spiral arteries with reduced dilatation of uterine spiral arteries and placental hypoxia. This acts as a precipitating factor that leads to an imbalance of angiogenic and antiangiogenic factors and a generalised inflammatory response. The exact link between placental triggering and the systemic response is unknown, but there is placental release of circulating antiangiogenic factors such as soluble Fms-like tyrosine kinase-1 (sFlt1) and soluble endoglin, and inflammatory cytokines. There are reduced concentrations of angiogenic factors such as vascular endothelial growth factor and placental growth factor.[17] All this leads to diffuse endothelial dysfunction with an increase in sensitivity to vasoactive

Table 63.1 Basic diagnostic criteria for pre-eclampsia

Hypertension *and*	Systolic arterial pressure >140 mmHg (18.6 kPa) *or* Diastolic arterial pressure* >90 mmHg (12 kPa)
Proteinuria	>/=300 mg protein in a 24-hour collection** *or* Random urine protein/ creatinine >/=30 mg/mmol

*Korotkoff phase V.
A rise in blood pressure above baseline and oedema are now not usually included.
**A positive dipstick test for proteinuria should be confirmed by 24-hour urine collection.

substances and activation of a key vasoconstrictor endothelin-1,[18] a decrease in endothelial synthesis of vasodilator substances such as prostaglandin and nitric oxide, activation of platelets and coagulation, and an increase in capillary permeability. This then causes widespread vasoconstriction, fluid extravasation, proteinuria, decreased intravascular volume, haemoconcentration and decreased organ perfusion.

Table 63.2 Clinical features suggestive of severe pre-eclampsia

Blood pressure	Systolic arterial pressure >160 mmHg (21.3 kPa) Diastolic arterial pressure >110 mmHg (14.6 kPa)
Renal	Proteinuria ≥2 g/24 h Oliguria <500 mL/24 h Serum creatinine >0.09 mmol/L
Hepatic	Epigastric or right-upper-quadrant pain Elevated bilirubin and/or transaminases
Neurological	Persistent headaches Visual disturbances, papilloedema, clonus Convulsions (eclampsia)
Haematological	Thrombocytopenia Deranged coagulation tests Haemolysis
Cardiac/ respiratory	Pulmonary oedema Cyanosis

CLINICAL PRESENTATION

Pre-eclampsia is a syndrome with a spectrum of presentations. Although hypertension is the cardinal sign, some women present with convulsions, abdominal pain or general malaise and some complications may be life-threatening without a marked increase in blood pressure. Features typical of severe disease are listed in **Table 63.2**. Rarely, cocaine intoxication and phaeochromocytoma may be confused with pre-eclampsia.

Haemodynamic changes of pre-eclampsia consist of hypertension, increased systemic vascular resistance and decreased intravascular volume. Cardiac output is often decreased, usually secondary to changes in preload and afterload rather than contractility.[19] Sympathetic activation occurs, and this may account for observations of increased cardiac output in the early stage.[20] However early-onset and late-onset pre-eclampsia appear to have different patterns of cardiovascular change.[21]

Pulmonary oedema may occur because of iatrogenic fluid overload, decreased left ventricular function, increased capillary permeability and narrowing of the colloid osmotic–pulmonary capillary wedge pressure gradient; this is more likely to occur after delivery. Sudden ventricular tachycardia may occur during hypertensive crises.

Neurological complications include eclamptic convulsions, cerebral oedema and stroke. Intracranial haemorrhage is an important cause of death. In recent decades, posterior reversible encephalopathy syndrome has been recognised as a primary event in eclampsia.[22]

Renal changes include reduced glomerular filtration rate due to reduced renal plasma flow and filtration coefficient. These features, together with proteinuria, are associated with the characteristic lesion of glomeruloendotheliosis. Hyperuricaemia is associated with increased prenatal risk, particularly if serum uric acid concentration rises rapidly.

Haemostatic abnormalities include thrombocytopenia, which may be associated with decreased platelet function. Associated coagulation abnormalities may occur but are unlikely unless the platelet count is $<100\,000\times10^9/L$.[23,24]

Hepatic complications include liver oedema, hepatocellular necrosis, periportal and subcapsular haemorrhage, hepatic infarcts and rupture. Patients with HELLP syndrome (see below) are particularly at risk.

The leading causes of maternal death in pre-eclampsia/eclampsia are intracranial haemorrhage, pulmonary oedema and hepatic complications. Fetal morbidity results from placental insufficiency, prematurity and abruptio placentae.

MANAGEMENT

The principles of management include:

- timely delivery of the placenta and fetus
- supportive care before delivery, and during the immediate postpartum period, focusing on:
  - control of blood pressure
  - prevention of seizures with magnesium sulphate
  - maintenance of placental perfusion
  - prevention of complications
  - monitoring of fetal well-being.

Table 63.3 Management in severe pre-eclampsia

General measures	Keep patient in lateral position Stress ulcer prophylaxis DVT prophylaxis
Maternal monitoring	Intra-arterial blood pressure monitoring in severe cases Sp_{O_2}, urine output, intake–output chart Consider central venous catheter or pulmonary artery catheter
Investigations	Complete blood count, renal function and electrolytes Urate Liver function test Clotting profile Blood group matching Urinalysis
Fetal monitoring	Continuous fetal heart monitoring Other options as assessed by obstetricians: ultrasound, amniotic fluid index (AFI), umbilical artery Doppler
Magnesium sulphate prophylaxis and treatment of eclampsia For recurrent eclampsia	Intravenous regimen: loading dose 4 g over 10–15 min Maintenance 1–2 g/h Intramuscular regimen: 4 g every 4 h A further i.v. loading dose of 2–4 g over 10 min May increase maintenance up to 2 g/h
Antihypertensive therapy	Acute treatment indicated if SBP>160 mmHg (21.3 kPa) *or* DBP>110 mmHg (14.6 kPa) Control of blood pressure should be gradual and sustained while preserving maternal organ perfusion and placental perfusion
Liaison with obstetricians regarding timing of delivery	Antenatal steroid if gestation <34 weeks

The management for severe pre-eclampsia is summarised in **Table 63.3**.

If complications are avoided, the disease normally resolves completely after delivery. Transfer of the mother to a tertiary centre before delivery should be considered if a level III neonatal unit is not available (see Ch. 1). Admission into an ICU before delivery may be appropriate in severe cases, or when the labour ward lacks the expertise or equipment for intensive monitoring. Because prematurity is a major cause of neonatal morbidity, expectant management of select patients with severe pre-eclampsia <34 weeks' gestation to prolong pregnancy may improve outcomes.[25] This requires collaboration with obstetricians and careful balancing of the maternal and perinatal risks. In all cases, the maternal benefit should always outweigh the benefit of the fetus. Consulting a neonatologist for prenatal counselling is preferable if time is available. After delivery, severe cases should preferably be managed in an ICU for 24–72 hours.

ANTIHYPERTENSIVE THERAPY

The aim of antihypertensive therapy is to prevent maternal complications (intracerebral haemorrhage, cardiac failure and abruptio placentae) while maintaining placental blood flow. It is important to appreciate that hypertension is a marker and not a causal factor in pre-eclampsia. Therefore, although controlling hypertension reduces the risk of complications, it does not ameliorate the underlying pathological process. Acute treatment is indicated when blood pressure is greater than 160 mmHg (21.3 kPa) systolic or 105–110 mmHg (14–14.6 kPa) diastolic. Reduction of systolic pressure is particularly important for the prevention of stroke.[26] Initially, systolic blood pressure should only be reduced by about 20–30 mmHg (2.66–4 kPa) and diastolic pressure by 10–15 mmHg (1.33–2 kPa) while monitoring the fetus. Concomitant plasma expansion reduces the risk of sudden hypotension when vasodilators are used. Recommended antihypertensive drugs for acute treatment are summarised in **Table 63.4**.[1,2,5,27] The most commonly used drugs are labetalol, hydralazine and nifedipine; insufficient data are available to show which of these is superior.[28,29]

OTHER AGENTS

These agents are not routinely used and indicated only when hypertension is refractory to conventional treatment. *Sodium nitroprusside* (initial dose 0.25 μg/kg per min, maximum dose 5 μg/kg per min) can be used to reduce blood pressure rapidly in a hypertensive emergency but care should be taken in patients with depleted

Table 63.4 Drug treatment of hypertension in severe pre-eclampsia

DRUG	DOSAGE GUIDE	MECHANISM OF ACTION	NOTES
Labetalol	Bolus 20–40 mg i.v. every 10–15 min to maximum dose of 300 mg Infusion 1–2 mg/min, reducing to 0.5 mg/min or less after blood pressure is controlled	Non-selective beta-adrenergic receptor block with alpha$_1$-blocking effect	Reduces blood pressure without decrease in uteroplacental flow[29] Crosses placenta, but neonatal hypoglycaemia and bradycardia are rarely seen Need fetal heart monitoring Should not be given to patients with asthma or myocardial dysfunction
Hydralazine	Bolus 5 mg i.v. followed with 5–10 mg every 20 min to maximum of 20 mg	Direct arteriolar vasodilator	Slow onset of action of 10–20 min but may cause sudden hypotension Consider concomitant fluid bolus (<250 mL) Adverse effects include headache, tachycardia, tremor, nausea, rarely neonatal thrombocytopenia
Nifedipine	Oral route is preferred, 10 mg, repeat after 30 min as required (sublingual route may cause sudden hypotension)	Calcium channel blocker	Cause uterine muscle relaxation that may increase risk of postpartum haemorrhage Potentiation of neuromuscular block in patient receiving magnesium sulphate

intravascular volume and duration should be limited to <4 hours to avoid fetal cyanide poisoning. *Nitroglycerin* infusion (initial dose 5 μg/min, maximum dose 100 μg/min) may be useful in cases complicated by pulmonary oedema.

Methyldopa has been used for mild cases, but its slow onset time makes it unsuitable for acute treatment. *Diazoxide, ketanserin, nimodipine* and *magnesium* are not recommended as first-line agents. *Beta blockers* other than labetalol may cause decreased uteroplacental perfusion, fetal bradycardia and decreased fetal tolerance to hypoxia. *Angiotensin-converting enzyme inhibitors* and *angiotensin antagonists* should not be used before delivery because of adverse fetal effects. *Diuretics* should generally be avoided because pre-eclamptic patients have reduced plasma volume.

ANTICONVULSANT THERAPY

Anticonvulsants are used to prevent recurrent convulsions in eclampsia or to prevent initial convulsions in pre-eclampsia. Magnesium sulphate should be used as first-line treatment for prophylaxis and treatment of eclamptic seizures, and for prophylaxis of seizures in severe pre-eclampsia. The Magpie trial conducted in 33 countries showed that women in the magnesium group had a 58% (95% CI 40–71%) lower risk of eclampsia and probably lower maternal mortality.[30] Magnesium was more cost-effective in developing countries where pre-eclampsia is a more significant problem.[31] However, the benefits of using magnesium in mild pre-eclampsia are uncertain, especially in developed countries. Adverse maternal events are increased, and there is no reduction in maternal or perinatal morbidity.[32]

The mechanism of action of magnesium for preventing eclamptic seizures is unknown. Although abnormal electroencephalograms are frequent in pre-eclampsia and eclampsia, they are not altered by magnesium sulphate. Part of magnesium's action may be reduction of cerebral vasospasm via antagonism of calcium at membrane channels or intracellular sites. However, the cerebral vasodilator nimodipine was ineffective for preventing seizures.[33] Magnesium amplifies release of prostacyclin by vascular endothelium, and this may inhibit platelet aggregation and vasoconstriction. Doppler ultrasonography suggests that magnesium vasodilates smaller-diameter intracranial blood vessels, and some of its effects may be from relieving cerebral ischaemia. Part of the anticonvulsant activity of magnesium may be mediated by blockade or suppression of *N*-methyl-D-aspartate (NMDA) receptors. Magnesium has tocolytic effects and mild general vasodilator and antihypertensive actions, and increases renal and uterine blood flow.

Guidelines for administration of magnesium sulphate are summarised in Table 63.3. The kidney rapidly excretes magnesium. The half-life in patients with normal renal function is 4 hours and 90% of the dose is excreted by 24 hours after the infusion.[34] When there is renal impairment or oliguria the dose should be reduced and serum concentration should be monitored. Suggested target serum concentration for severe pre-eclampsia is 2–3.5 mmol/L (4–7 mEq/L or 4.8–8.4 mg/dL). Magnesium toxicity is associated with muscle weakness and may lead to respiratory paralysis (>7.5 mmol/L). Increased conduction time with increased PR and QT intervals and QRS duration can lead to sinoatrial and atrioventricular block

(>7.5 mmol/L) and cardiac arrest in diastole (>12.5 mmol/L). Toxicity is unlikely when deep tendon reflexes are present (the upper limb should be used during epidural analgesia). Magnesium toxicity can be treated with small intravenous doses of calcium and enhanced clearance with renal replacement therapy when it is associated with renal failure. Other reported adverse effects of magnesium include death from overdose, increased bleeding, slowed cervical dilatation and increased risk of pulmonary oedema. Magnesium crosses the placenta and can cause neonatal flaccidity and respiratory depression.

ECLAMPSIA

With modern obstetric care, eclampsia may present without marked preceding hypertension or proteinuria, and up to 40% of cases occur postpartum, often more than 48 hours after delivery.[35,36] Priorities in the management of eclamptic seizures are airway protection, oxygenation, and termination and prevention of seizures. Delivery of the fetus should be considered after maternal stabilisation. Patients should be placed in the left-lateral position and given oxygen. Magnesium should be given if not already started. A further 2 g loading dose of $MgSO_4$ can be given if the patient is already on magnesium therapy (see Table 63.3). Approximately 10% of eclamptic patients will have a recurrent seizure despite receiving magnesium. Prolonged seizures can be terminated by diazepam 5–10 mg intravenously. If seizures are refractory, thiopental and suxamethonium should be given and the airway secured.

It is important to appreciate that eclampsia is not the only cause of seizure during pregnancy. Recurrent convulsions or prolonged unconsciousness may indicate additional cerebral pathology (e.g. cerebral oedema, intracerebral haemorrhage, venous thrombosis) and an urgent computed tomographic (CT) scan should be done whenever possible.

OTHER ANTICONVULSANTS

If repeated seizures occur despite therapeutic levels of magnesium, conventional anticonvulsants can be considered, but it is important to exclude other causes of convulsions. Although diazepam and phenytoin are inferior to magnesium for preventing eclamptic seizures, these agents may be considered when magnesium sulphate is contraindicated (e.g. renal failure, muscle weakness, allergy).

Diazepam as a bolus dose could be considered for immediate treatment of convulsions while preparing for magnesium therapy. Intravenous infusion of diazepam has been used (40 mg diazepam in 500 mL normal saline titrated to keep patients sedated but rousable) as prophylaxis when magnesium therapy is contraindicated.

Phenytoin is given as an initial intravenous loading dose of 10 mg/kg followed 2 hours later by 5 mg/kg. Doses are diluted in normal saline and given no faster than 50 mg/min. Electrocardiogram and arterial pressure should be monitored. Maintenance doses of 200 mg orally or intravenously are started 12 hours after the second bolus and given 8-hourly. However, there is no consensus on the optimal dosing regimen. Monitoring of phenytoin level is necessary to avoid toxicity.

FLUID BALANCE

Fluid management in pre-eclampsia is controversial. Pre-eclamptic patients usually have reduced circulating intravascular volume. There may also be a significant decrease in blood pressure upon initiation of antihypertensive therapy, particularly with hydralazine. However, the effectiveness of fluid loading is uncertain,[37] and there is a risk of pulmonary oedema. Oliguria is common in patients with pre-eclampsia, but this does not necessarily imply volume depletion. Hence fluid challenge should be considered for treatment of oliguria only when there are other signs of hypovolaemia. Renal failure in pre-eclampsia is uncommon. Some patients with persistent oliguria and a rising serum creatinine concentration may require a period of continuous renal replacement therapy, but the majority of cases recover. However, the risk of irreversible renal damage is greater when there is associated abruptio placentae, disseminated intravascular coagulation (DIC), hypotensive shock, or sepsis.

Low-dose dopamine (3 μg/kg per min) infusions have been used after correction of hypovolaemia to improve urine output, but they have not been shown to improve renal outcome and are no longer recommended.[38]

Furosemide could be considered if pulmonary oedema develops. Furosemide should not be used to treat oliguria without pulmonary oedema because this may exacerbate the fluid-depleted state.

There is controversy over the effectiveness of CVP and pulmonary capillary wedge pressure (PCWP) for assisting fluid management in pre-eclamptic patients. CVP and PCWP have poor correlation, especially when CVP is greater than 6 mmHg (0.8 kPa).[39] Optimal CVP and PCWP values are unknown, but the measured response to fluid challenge may be informative and useful. Pulmonary artery catheterisation placement carries inherent risks and should be considered only when there are clear indications (e.g. refractory hypertension, pulmonary oedema, severe cardiac disease and refractory oliguria), and the obtained data will be used to guide decision making.[39] Should pulmonary oedema develop, it is managed with oxygen therapy, positive end-expiratory pressure with or without ventilation, inotropes, vasodilators, morphine or diuretics as indicated. The echocardiogram can be used for assessment of cardiac function and guiding further therapy.[40]

POSTPARTUM CARE

Patients are frequently referred to an ICU for postpartum care, particularly after caesarean delivery. Pre-eclampsia may persist or even develop post partum.[41] The risk of pulmonary oedema is greatest after delivery. After delivery, there is often an initial improvement with a relapse in the first 24 hours. Magnesium should be continued for 24 hours after delivery or the last seizure. Ongoing monitoring for signs of severe pre-eclampsia should be continued in the postpartum period. Antihypertensive drugs may be reduced according to the blood pressure. Some patients may require a change to oral medication that may need to be continued for several weeks. Psychological support is important, especially if there has been an adverse neonatal outcome. Full recovery from the organ dysfunction of pre-eclampsia is normally expected within 6 weeks. However, patients are more likely to develop pre-eclampsia in subsequent pregnancies, and have double the risk of early cardiovascular disease and mortality.[42]

HELLP SYNDROME AND HEPATIC COMPLICATIONS

HELLP syndrome is a particularly high-risk form of pre-eclampsia characterised by more pronounced hepatic rather than cerebral or renal involvement. Diagnosis is based on laboratory findings showing *h*aemolysis (microangiopathic haemolytic anaemia), *e*levated *l*iver enzymes and *l*ow *p*latelets, although exact criteria vary.[43,44] The pathogenesis of HELPP is similar to that of early-onset pre-eclampsia, but biomarker derangements are more severe.[45] Clinical presentation is variable. Many patients have non-specific signs such as right-upper-quadrant or epigastric pain, nausea, malaise or headache. Although most patients will have hypertension and proteinuria, these can be mild or absent. Important differential diagnoses include idiopathic thrombocytopenic purpura, systemic lupus erythematosus, thrombotic thrombocytopenic purpura, haemolytic–uraemic syndrome and acute fatty liver of pregnancy. Typically, HELLP syndrome presents at early gestational ages and is more common in white and multiparous women. In about 30% of cases, it first presents in the postpartum period, sometimes with no evidence of pre-eclampsia before delivery. After delivery, patients usually show a continuing deterioration in platelet count and liver enzymes, with a peak in severity 24–48 hours after delivery followed by gradual resolution and complete recovery if complications are avoided. Complications of HELLP syndrome include DIC, abruptio placentae, acute renal failure, pulmonary oedema, severe ascites, pleural effusion, liver haemorrhage or failure, acute respiratory distress syndrome (ARDS), sepsis and stroke.

Patients with HELLP should be managed aggressively, similarly to pre-eclampsia, with an emphasis on stabilisation and delivery.[46] Expectant management of patients with gestation less than 34 weeks has been described but the relative benefits and risks of this are controversial.[44]

Corticosteroids are given to promote fetal lung maturation before premature delivery, but there is controversy concerning the use of high-dose corticosteroids for maternal benefit. The anti-inflammatory actions of corticosteroids are postulated to be beneficial for the disease, and the platelet count is increased. Although corticosteroids are part of a standardised protocol at one hospital,[47] a recent Cochrane review of 11 trials concluded that there is no difference in maternal or perinatal death, and no evidence of significant maternal benefit.[48] Plasma exchange with fresh frozen plasma has been described for postpartum patients with delayed resolution of HELLP, with variable response.[49]

Life-threatening hepatic complications may occur in pre-eclampsia, particularly in patients with HELLP syndrome. These include segmental hepatic infarction, parenchymal haemorrhage and subcapsular haemotoma with or without rupture. If suspected, patients should have an urgent CT scan. Hepatic rupture is a surgical emergency. Hepatic haemorrhage without rupture has been managed conservatively.

ANAESTHESIA AND ANALGESIA

Platelet count and coagulation tests should be checked before regional anaesthesia. Epidural analgesia in labour reduces fluctuations in arterial pressure and improves placental blood flow.[50] For caesarean delivery, the use of epidural or spinal anaesthesia avoids the risks of aspiration, difficult intubation from airway oedema, exaggerated hypertensive response to intubation and magnesium-induced sensitivity to muscle relaxants associated with general anaesthesia.

If general anaesthesia is required, smaller-size endotracheal tubes may be required. The hypertensive response to intubation should be attenuated with drugs such as fentanyl (2.5 μg/kg), alfentanil (10 μg/kg), magnesium sulphate (40 mg/kg), a combination of alfentanil (7.5 μg/kg) with magnesium sulphate (30 mg/kg), or remifentanil (1 μg/kg). Occasionally, awake intubation under topical anaesthesia may be necessary when there is airway obstruction.

 Access the complete references list online at http://www.expertconsult.com

1. Society of Obstetric Medicine of Australia and New Zealand. Guidelines for the management of hypertensive disorders of pregnancy. 2008. Online. Available: http://www.somanz.org.
2. National Collaborating Centre for Women's and Children's Health (UK). Hypertension in Pregnancy: The Management of Hypertensive Disorders during Pregnancy. National Institute for Health and Clinical Excellence (NICE) clinical guideline 107. 2010 Aug, updated 2011 Jan. Online. Available: http://guidance.nice.org.uk/CG107/NICEGuidance/pdf/English.
7. Centre for Maternal and Child Enquiries (CMACE). Saving Mothers' Lives: reviewing maternal deaths to make motherhood safer: 2006–2008. The Eighth Report of the Confidential Enquiries into Maternal Deaths in the United Kingdom. BJOG 2011;118(Suppl. 1):1–203.
17. Eiland E, Nzerue C, Faulkner M. Preeclampsia 2012. J Pregnancy 2012;2012:586578.
22. Zeeman GG. Neurologic complications of pre-eclampsia. Semin Perinatol 2009;33:166–72.
27. American College of Obstetricians and Gynecologists. Committee Opinion No. 514. Emergent therapy for acute-onset, severe hypertension with preeclampsia or eclampsia. Obstet Gynecol 2011;118:1465–8.
45. Abildgaard U, Heimdal K. Pathogenesis of the syndrome of hemolysis, elevated liver enzymes, and low platelet count (HELLP): a review. Eur J Obstet Gynecol Reprod Biol 2012;PII:S0301-2115(12)00449-6.

64

General obstetric emergencies

Winnie TP Wan and Tony Gin

The intensive care unit (ICU) will receive obstetric patients with the usual range of medical and surgical emergencies, and also provide supportive care for patients who suffer specific obstetric complications. The pattern of admission varies widely among countries with different standards of obstetric care. A recent prospective cohort study in the Netherlands reported the incidence of ICU admission to be 2.4 per 1000 deliveries. The most common reasons for ICU admission were major obstetric haemorrhage, hypertensive disorder of pregnancy and sepsis.[1] Data from the Centre for Maternal and Child Enquiries (CMACE) in the United Kingdom showed that the overall maternal mortality rate for the triennium 2006–2008 was 11.39 per 100 000 maternities, with the commonest cause of direct death now being sepsis (1.13 per 100 000 maternities).[2] Over half of the mothers that die will spend some time in an ICU, and many die there. This latest report highlighted the need for early consultation by obstetricians to intensivists, and discussed in more detail the management of sepsis and haemorrhage.

PATHOPHYSIOLOGY

Two important points to recognise in treating obstetric patients are:

1. During pregnancy, the normal ranges for physiological variables change (**Table 64.1**).[3] This may modify the presentation of the problem, variables used to guide treatment, and the response to treatment. The majority of physiological changes revert to normal several days after delivery.
2. Both mother and fetus are affected by the pathology and subsequent treatment.

AIRWAY AND VENTILATION

Several factors may complicate tracheal intubation in pregnancy:

- altered anatomy in pregnancy predisposes to a potentially difficult airway
- oedematous tissues
- delayed gastric emptying
- increased oxygen consumption.

Intensivists must be familiar with the difficult airway algorithm and the use of the laryngeal mask airway.[4,5] Avoidance of intubation and the use of non-invasive ventilation may, in selected cases, be a good option.

CIRCULATION

Tachycardia, low blood pressure, increased cardiac output and warm peripheries are normal in late pregnancy. After 20 weeks' gestation, aortocaval compression by the gravid uterus can decrease uterine perfusion and venous return to the heart. This is best prevented by using the full left-lateral position, but a left-lateral tilt or manual displacement of the uterus may be more practicable.

Haemodynamic support should generally start with good hydration, and assessment should take into account the altered cardiovascular variables in pregnancy. Non-invasive cardiac output monitoring is inaccurate and invasive monitoring with pulmonary artery catheters may be helpful in severe pre-eclampsia, pulmonary oedema and cardiac disease.[6] The uterine vascular bed is considered maximally dilated but still responsive to stimuli that cause vasoconstriction, such as circulating catecholamines. Ephedrine has traditionally been the vasoconstrictor used in obstetrics because it was thought to preserve uterine blood flow better than pure alpha agonists. However, alpha agonists such as phenylephrine are more effective and not associated with fetal acidosis when used to manage hypotension during caesarean delivery.[7] There is no evidence favouring any particular inotrope.

COAGULATION

Pregnancy is associated with a fivefold increase in thromboembolism, and patients should be given thromboembolic prophylaxis, typically with unfractionated heparin or low-molecular-weight heparin (LMWH) and elastic compression stockings.

MOTHER AND FETUS

In the critically ill it is important to monitor the fetus because of the problems associated with:

Table 64.1 Changes in physiological variables during pregnancy

PARAMETER	NON-PREGNANT	FIRST TRIMESTER	SECOND TRIMESTER	THIRD TRIMESTER
CARDIOVASCULAR				
SBP (mmHg)	110 (14.63 kPa)		100 (–8%)	105 (–5)
MAP (mmHg)	90 (11.97 kPa)			85 (–5)
DAP (mmHg)	60 (7.98 kPa)		50 (–12%)	50 (–12)
CVP (mmHg)	4 (0.53 kPa)			4 (no change)
PCWP (mmHg)	6 (0.8 kPa)			6 (no change)
HR (b.p.m.)	75	82 (+10%)	82 (+10%)	90 (+25%)
SV (mL)	65	80 (+20%)	85 (+30%)	82 (25%)
CO (L)	5	6.5 (+30%)	7 (+50%)	7 (+50%)
SVR (dyn cm/s^{-5})	1530			1210 (–20%)
PVR (dyn cm/s^{-5})	119			78 (–30%)
Total blood vol (L)	3.2	3.5 (+10%)	4.1 (+30%)	4.6 (+45%)
Haematocrit				–33%
Plasma albumin (g/L)	35			30
Oncotic pressure (mmHg)	28 (3.72 kPa)			25 (–3–0.4 kPa)
RESPIRATORY				
pH	7.40	7.44	7.44	7.44
Pa_{CO_2} (mmHg)	40 (5.32 kPa)	30	30	30
Pa_{O_2} (mmHg)	100 (13.3 kPa)	107	105	103
HCO_3 (mmol/L)	24	21	20	20
TV (mL)	500			700 (+40%)
RR (breath/min)	15			17 (+15%)
MV (mL/min)	7500			10500 (+40%)
FRC (mL)	2800			2300 (–20%)
VC (mL)	3500			3500 (no change)
IC (mL)	2200			2500 (+15%)
ERV (mL)	1300			1100 (–20%)
RV (mL)	1500			1200 (–20%)
TLC (mL)	5000			4800 (–5%)
O2 consumption (mL/min)	250			300 (+20%)

SBP=systolic arterial pressure; MAP=mean arterial pressure; DBP=diastolic arterial pressure; CVP=central venous pressure; PCWP=pulmonary capillary wedge pressure; HR=heart rate; SV=stroke volume; CO=cardiac output; SVR=systemic vascular resistance; PVR=pulmonary vascular resistance; TV=tidal volume; RR=respiratory rate; MV=minute volume; FRC=functional residual capacity; VC=vital capacity; IC=inspiratory capacity; ERV=expiratory reserve volume; RV=residual volume; TLC=total lung capacity.

- premature labour
- the placental transfer of drugs
- maintenance of placental perfusion and oxygenation.

An obstetric opinion should be sought as soon as possible regarding cardiotocography, ultrasound examination and timing of delivery. Nutrition is also very important for the fetus and adequate maternal feeding should be started as soon as possible. Neither perineal nor breast nursing care should be neglected.

CARDIOPULMONARY RESUSCITATION[8,9]

Despite being younger than the more usual cardiac arrest patients, pregnant patients have a poor survival rate.[10,11] The obstetrician and neonatologist should be notified when the cardiac arrest call is activated, and preparations be made for perimortem caesarean delivery.

MODIFICATION OF CPR

The 2010 International Liaison Committee on Resuscitation (ILCOR) guideline emphasises the importance of good-quality chest compression, and suggests rescuers may consider starting CPR with chest compression rather than ventilations (the sequence changes from 'ABC' to 'CAB').

After about 20 weeks' gestation, the gravid uterus can compress the inferior vena cava and impede venous return and cardiac output from CPR. Positioning for obstetric CPR should aim at relieving aortocaval compression and optimising the quality of chest compression. It can be done by manual left uterine displacement in the supine position first, either at the patient's left side with a two-handed technique, or at the patient's right side with a one-handed technique. The mother can also be placed in left-lateral tilt of 27–30° using a firm wedge to support the pelvis and thorax. Chest compression should be performed with a slightly higher hand position (slightly above the centre of the sternum). Airway management in pregnant patients is generally more difficult. Bag-mask ventilation with high-flow oxygen before intubation is especially important. Early tracheal intubation after cricoid pressure will facilitate ventilation and decrease the risk of acid aspiration. During advanced life support (ALS), drugs are given and defibrillation performed according to the normal protocols. Apical placement of the paddle may be difficult because of position and breast enlargement, and adhesive defibrillation pads are preferred. Fetal or uterine monitors should be removed before defibrillation.

Case reports at advanced gestation indicate that both maternal and fetal survival from cardiac arrest may depend on prompt caesarean delivery to relieve the effects of aortocaval compression. The ILCOR advisory statement suggests that the resuscitation team leaders should activate the protocol for an emergency caesarean delivery as soon as cardiac arrest is identified in a pregnant woman with an obviously gravid uterus. Emergency caesarean section may be considered at 4 minutes after onset of maternal cardiac arrest if there is no return of spontaneous circulation.

POST-RESUSCITATION CARE

Therapeutic hypothermia has been shown to improve outcome in post-arrest adult patients. There is one case report of hypothermia in early pregnancy without emergency caesarean section, but not in patients after perimortem caesarean section. The ILCOR 2010 guideline suggests hypothermia may be considered on an individual basis in comatose pregnant patients.

TRAUMA[12,13]

More than 10% of pregnancy-related traumas are associated with the use of illicit drugs or alcohol. Most injuries occur as the result of motor vehicle accidents, and other common causes are suicide (usually postpartum), falls and assaults.

Special considerations of trauma in obstetric patients include the potential for miscarriage, preterm rupture of membrane, placenta abruptio, inadequate uteroplacental blood flow, preterm labour, and fetal distress and demise. The gravid uterus displaces the bowel cephalad so visceral injuries are less common after lower abdominal injuries. The dilated pelvic vasculature increases the risk of retroperitoneal hemorrhage following pelvic injuries. Head injuries and haemorrhagic shock account for most maternal deaths, whereas placental abruption and maternal death are the most frequent causes of fetal death.[14]

PRIMARY AND SECONDARY SURVEY

Initial resuscitation should follow the normal plan of attention to airway, breathing and circulation.[15] Unless a spinal injury is suspected, the pregnant patient should be transported and examined in the left-lateral tilt position or with manual left uterine displacement. Blood volume is increased during pregnancy and hypotension may not be evident until 35% or more of total blood volume is lost. Uterine blood flow is not autoregulated and may be decreased despite normal maternal haemodynamics, so that slight overhydration may be preferred to underhydration. Excessive resuscitation with crystalloids or non-blood colloids may increase the mortality from severe haemorrhage. Drug treatment of modest hypotension can be started with ephedrine, but more potent vasopressors should be used if necessary. Continuous fetal heart rate monitoring should be used.

In trauma assessment the increased significance of pelvic fractures in terms of uterine injury and retroperitoneal haemorrhage should be considered.

- Ultrasound is the investigation of choice.
- Diagnostic peritoneal lavage, if performed, should be through an open surgical incision above the fundus.
- Chest drains are placed slightly higher than normal, in the third or fourth intercostal space.
- It is important to exclude herniation of abdominal contents through a ruptured diaphragm.
- Vaginal examination to look for either leak of amniotic fluid and/or vaginal bleeding is vital.

Necessary radiological investigations should be performed as indicated as the radiation hazard to the fetus is very small, except in the early first trimester when exposure to more than 50–100 mGy is a cause for concern. A chest X-ray delivers less than 5 mGy to the lungs and very little to the shielded abdomen. The fetal radiation dose from abdominal examinations can range from 1 mGy for a plain film up to 20–50 mGy for an abdominal pelvic computed tomography (CT) with fluoroscopy.[16]

DEFINITIVE CARE

Cardiotocographic monitoring is considered essential, but there is wide variation in practice and recommended duration of monitoring. Premature labour and placental abruption may not be diagnosed unless regular monitoring is continued for at least 6 hours and even 24 hours if indicated.[17] Rh immune globulin 300 μg should be considered for all Rh D-negative within 72 hours of injury to prevent future Rh alloimmunisation of the newborn. The Kleihauer–Betke test can be used to detect fetal blood in the maternal circulation and give an estimate of the volume of feto-maternal haemorrhage.

BURNS

Approximately 7% of women of reproductive age are seen for treatment for major burns.[18] Although the women are usually young and healthy, pregnancy is already a hypermetabolic state and the fetus is at great risk from many complications.[19] Factors influencing morbidity and mortality include the depth and size of burn wound, the underlying health and age of the pregnant women, the estimated gestational age of the fetus, associated inhalational injury, and significant secondary complications. Preterm labour and stillbirth are more likely in the first few days after the burn injury. The presumed pathogenesis is due to the high levels of prostaglandins and maternal acidosis.[20]

SPECIAL CONSIDERATIONS IN PREGNANT BURN PATIENTS[20]

FLUID RESUSCITATION

Replacement of fluid loss from burns must keep in mind the normally increased circulating volume of pregnancy. Pregnant burn patients usually require significantly more fluid to maintain haemodynamic stability. Pregnancy affects the total body surface area (TBSA) as the abdomen increases in size. The Lund–Browder chart is still the commonly used method for burn area estimation.

DEFINITIVE BURN CARE

Continuous enteral feeding should be initiated as soon as possible and can be within the first 24 hours of burn. Canadian Clinical Practice Guidelines suggest enteral glutamine should be considered in burn patients, but its role in pregnant burn patients is unclear.[21] Topical povidone-iodine solution should be avoided because the iodine may be absorbed and affect fetal thyroid function. Inhalational injuries with hypoxia and carbon monoxide are especially detrimental to the fetus, because carbon monoxide has a greater affinity and longer half-life when it is bound to fetal haemoglobulin.

SEVERE OBSTETRIC HAEMORRHAGE

Obstetric haemorrhage accounts for 25–30% of all maternal mortality.[22] The aim of management is rapid restoration of circulating volume, correct coagulopathy and remedy the underlying cause of haemorrhage.

Antepartum haemorrhage is defined as bleeding from the genital tract after 24 weeks of gestation. Its incidence is 2–5% of all pregnancies.[23] The common causes are placenta praevia and placental abruption; both are ultimately managed by delivery. In placenta praevia, the placenta implants in advance of the presenting part and classically presents as painless bleeding during the second or third trimester. Placenta praevia is relatively common (1 in 200 pregnancies) but severe haemorrhage is relatively rare. In placental abruption, a normally implanted placenta separates from the uterine wall. The incidence of placental abruption is low (0.5–2%) but perinatal mortality may be as high as 50%. In concealed abruption, vaginal bleeding can be absent and several litres of blood may be concealed in the uterus.

Postpartum haemorrhage is most commonly due to uterine atony and abnormal placentation, with retained tissues, trauma to the genital tract and coagulopathy as other causes. In an emergency, the aorta can be compressed against the vertebral column by a fist pressed on the abdomen above the umbilicus.

Uterine atony is managed initially with bimanual compression, uterine massage and drugs that include:[24]

- *oxytocin:* 5 units slow intravenous injection, or infusion (40 units in 500 mL Ringer's lactate solution at 125 mL/h)
- *ergonovine (ergometrine):* 0.5 mg slow intravenous or intramuscular injection (contraindicated in patients with hypertension)
- *carboprost:* 250 μg intramuscular injection, repeated at intervals of not less than 15 minutes to a maximum of 8 doses (contraindicated in patients with asthma) or 500 μg direct intramyometrial injection
- *misoprostol:* 1000 μg rectally.

If bleeding persists, tamponade techniques using gauze packs or balloons can be useful. Otherwise, specific invasive management such as angiographic arterial embolisation, laparotomy for uterine haemostatic suturing techniques such as B-lynch and multiple square sutures, surgical bilateral uterine artery ligation, or definitive hysterectomy may be required. Recombinant factor VIIa has also been used; the recommended initial dose is 90 μg/kg, and a second dose can be given 20–60 minutes after the first dose if there is no response.

For patients with known and suspected risk factors for postpartum haemorrhage, prophylactic interventional radiology can be employed. Balloons are placed in the internal iliac or uterine arteries before delivery. The balloons then can be inflated to occlude the vessels in the event of postpartum haemorrhage.[25]

With massive bleeding and transfusion, there should be no need to wait for a coagulation profile before giving coagulation factors. Disseminated intravascular coagulation still develops in 10–30% of cases, partly because tissue thromboplastin is released during abruption.

SEPSIS AND SEPTIC SHOCK[26]

Maternal sepsis and septic shock are relatively uncommon. However, sepsis should always be carefully considered because the underlying physiological changes in pregnancy and the response to labour can confound the presentation of sepsis and make its diagnosis difficult. The most common sources of infection are chorioamnionitis, postpartum endometritis, urinary tract infections, pyelonephritis and septic abortion. Animal studies suggest that pregnancy increases the susceptibility to endotoxin, and that metabolic acidosis and cardiovascular collapse occur earlier.

Management of septic shock follows the same guidelines as for non-pregnant population, with initial resuscitation, source control and prompt antibiotics. Gram-negative organisms are the frequent causative organisms, but streptococci and *Bacteroides* may also be present. Antimicrobial therapy is dependent on hospital prevalence and susceptibility patterns; empirical broad-spectrum therapy should be started early. Typical combinations are ampicillin, gentamicin and clindamycin, or carbapenem and vancomycin. Tetracyclines and quinolones should not be used in pregnancy.

Other treatment modalities, including insulin therapy, corticosteroids and activated protein C were never evaluated in pregnancy.

VENOUS THROMBOEMBOLISM[27]

The incidence of venous thromboembolism (VTE) ranges from 0.6 to 1.3 episodes per 1000 deliveries, which is a fivefold to tenfold increase in risk compared with those reported in non-pregnant women of comparable age. Pulmonary thromboembolism is a common cause of maternal death, accounting for 15–25% of maternal mortality. Pregnancy is associated with increased risk of VTE because of:

- venous stasis
- hypercoagulable state
- vascular injury associated with delivery.

Accurate diagnosis of venous thromboembolism is crucial because of the long-term implications for therapy. Symptoms of dyspnoea or pain in the leg or chest require accurate diagnosis, especially in the immediate postpartum period. Although contrast venography is the gold-standard test for diagnosing deep-vein thrombosis, the radiation exposure and invasive nature of the test mean that duplex Doppler ultrasonography is the usual first choice. D-dimer testing may also be useful but a positive test must be interpreted carefully because D-dimer values normally increase throughout pregnancy. Venography, perfusion lung scanning, pulmonary angiography and helical CT scan should not be avoided if indicated.

TREATMENT OF VTE DURING PREGNANCY[28]

Treatment is either subcutaneous LMWH or intravenous unfractionated heparin. LMWH has gradually replaced unfractionated heparin, based on the results of large trials in non-pregnant patients showing that LMWHs are at least as safe and effective as unfractionated heparin. In addition, the risk of heparin-induced thrombocytopenia and osteoporosis appears lower with LMWH than unfractionated heparin. The need for dose adjustments in proportion to change in weight over the course of pregnancy remains controversial. Full-dose anticoagulation should be continued during pregnancy. Subcutaneous LMWH can be discontinued 24–36 hours, and intravenous unfractionated heparin 4–6 hours, before elective induction of labour or caesarean section. A temporary retrievable venous filter can be inserted and removed postpartum. LMWH or unfractionated heparin should be restarted in the postpartum patient for at least 6–12 weeks. Neuraxial anaesthesia should not be used on patients with full anticoagulation.

With life-threatening massive pulmonary embolus, surgical treatment or thrombolysis must be considered. Thrombolysis was thought to be relatively contraindicated during pregnancy because of the risk of maternal and fetal haemorrhagic complications. No controlled trials are feasible and outcome data must be extracted from case reports. A review found that thrombolytic therapy was associated with a low maternal mortality rate of 1%, with a 6% rate of fetal loss and 6% rate of premature delivery.[29] The fetal risks appear to be lower than that obtained with surgical intervention in pregnant patients, and maternal risks lower than reported risks for surgery, thrombolysis or transvenous filters in non-pregnant patients. Although heparin remains the treatment of choice, thrombolysis appears to be a viable option except during the immediate postpartum period.

AMNIOTIC FLUID EMBOLISM (AFE)[30]

The incidence of AFE has been reported as 1 in 13 000 deliveries in the United States, and 1 in 50 000 deliveries in the UK.[31,32] The maternal mortality rate in developed countries ranges from 13% to 61%.

PATHOPHYSIOLOGY

The pathophysiology of AFE remains uncertain. Traditionally, it is thought that amniotic fluid and fetal debris enter the maternal circulation by forceful uterine contraction. However, recent studies show that fetal cells are commonly found in the maternal circulation. AFE has more in common with anaphylaxis and septic shock than other embolic diseases. The exact trigger is unknown. There is an abnormal maternal immune response to fetal antigen exposure, and inflammatory mediators cause pulmonary vasoconstriction, complement activation and coagulopathy. Recently, the term 'anaphylactoid syndrome of pregnancy' has been proposed.

CLINICAL PRESENTATION

AFE is a clinical diagnosis. Classically, patients present with severe dyspnoea, cyanosis, sudden cardiovascular collapse, and coma or convulsions during labour, but AFE may occur earlier during pregnancy, during delivery or in the early puerperium. Some patients may present with bleeding and most patients eventually develop a coagulopathy.

Animal studies indicate that AFE causes a biphasic haemodynamic response. The early phase probably lasts less than half an hour and is characterised by severe hypoxia and right heart failure as a result of pulmonary hypertension from vasoconstriction or vessel damage. Patients who survive this first phase develop left ventricular failure with return of normal right ventricular function. Left ventricular failure may be a result of the initial hypoxia or the depressant effects of mediators. Disseminated intravascular coagulation is present in most patients. It could be caused by a specific activator of factor X, tissue factor or other substances, such as trophoblasts, in the amniotic fluid.

TREATMENT

Treatment is supportive. Assessment of central venous pressure may be misleading, and early pulmonary artery catheterisation has been advocated in a series reporting 100% survival in 5 patients by treating left ventricular failure aggressively.[33] The differential diagnoses must be evaluated quickly. Survivors of AFE regain normal cardiorespiratory function but may have neurological sequelae.

ACUTE RESPIRATORY FAILURE

Pregnant women should receive medication for optimal asthma control. There is no evidence that appropriate use of inhaled glucocorticosteroids, beta agonists and leukotriene modifiers is associated with increased incidence of fetal abnormalities. In contrast, there is a substantial risk of preterm delivery posed by poorly controlled maternal asthma.[34] Acute exacerbation should also be treated aggressively with systemic glucocorticosteroids when necessary.

Pulmonary oedema is more likely in the pregnant patient (1:1000 pregnancies) because of the increased cardiac output and blood volume, and the decreased plasma oncotic pressure. The principles of treatment are relatively straightforward in terms of determining the cause of the oedema and improving oxygenation, although it can be difficult to distinguish between hydrostatic and permeability oedema.

The prevalence of acute respiratory distress syndrome during pregnancy has been estimated at 16–70 cases per 100 000 pregnancies, with mortality rates from 23 to 50%.[35] Important causes of ARDS in pregnancy are sepsis, aspiration and pre-eclampsia. Non-invasive positive pressure ventilation has not been evaluated for treatment of hypoxaemic respiratory failure in pregnancy. Clinical criteria for intubation are similar to those in non-pregnant patients, but arterial blood gases must be interpreted carefully because of the underlying respiratory alkalosis in pregnancy. The ARDS Network lung protective strategy can be adopted in pregnant patients by using the non-pregnant predicted body weight and gestational age-appropriate blood gas targets. Permissive hypercapnia may cause fetal respiratory acidosis that will reduce the ability of fetal haemoglobin to bind oxygen. Furthermore, transfer of CO_2 across the placenta requires a gradient of 10 mmHg (1.33 kPa). Therefore, $Pa\text{CO}_2$ should probably be kept below 45 mmHg (6.0 kPa) and $Pa\text{O}_2$ above 70 mmHg (9.3 kPa). If conventional ventilation fails, the effectiveness of alternative strategies is unknown.[35] There are case reports of the use of extracorporeal membrane oxygenation (ECMO) in pregnant patients with severe ARDS.[36]

ACID ASPIRATION (MENDELSON'S SYNDROME)

Obstetric patients are at increased risk of acid aspiration because of decreased gastric emptying, increased gastric acidity and volume and increased intra-abdominal pressure. Aspiration of acidic material will cause acute lung injury, the severity being related to the amount, content and acidity of the aspirate.

The initial presentation is hypoxaemia and bronchospasm. Chemical pneumonitis and increased permeability pulmonary oedema develop over several hours.

Treatment includes standard respiratory support. Rigid bronchoscopy may be required to remove large food particles. Bronchoalveolar lavage and steroids are not useful and antibiotics should only be given for proven infection.

PERIPARTUM CARDIOMYOPATHY (PPCM)[37]

Peripartum cardiomyopathy is characterised by new onset of heart failure between 1 month before and 5 months after delivery in previously healthy women. Diagnosis requires echocardiographic evidence of left ventricular dysfunction (ejection fraction <45%). The incidence varies from 1:100 to 1:10000 pregnancies. PPCM often presents as acute heart failure. The echocardiogram usually shows features of dilated cardiomyopathy.

The exact aetiology of PPCM remains controversial. A number of mechanisms have been proposed, including genetic factors, volume overload, viral illness, autoimmune, and hormonal imbalance. Treatment is largely supportive with diuretics, inotropes and non-invasive positive-pressure ventilation (NIPPV). Intra-aortic balloon pump and left ventricular assist device may be used in severe case. Recently, 16 kDa prolactin has been shown to have detrimental effects on the maternal heart. A small-scale randomised study showed that addition of bromocriptine to standard heart failure therapy can improve left ventricular ejection fraction.[38]

TOCOLYTIC THERAPY AND PULMONARY OEDEMA[39]

Pulmonary oedema is an uncommon (1 in 400 pregnancies) but serious complication of tocolytic therapy with beta-adrenergic agonists. The underlying mechanism for pulmonary oedema is unclear, but it is probably related to fluid overload and the cardiovascular effects of beta-adrenergic agonists leading to increased pulmonary capillary hydrostatic pressure. The initial management of pulmonary oedema is discontinuation of the beta-adrenergic agonist and oxygen therapy, with further monitoring, diuretics and respiratory support as necessary. This problem should disappear as alternative tocolytics such as nifedipine and atosiban are used.

COCAINE TOXICITY[40]

Cocaine abuse during pregnancy has become a significant problem in the USA, affecting more than 30 million people, with 90% of the women of child-bearing age. Cocaine has local anaesthetic and sympathomimetic actions and can cause:

- hypertension, dysrhythmias, myocardial ischaemia and infarction
- tachycardia and increased cardiac output, but decreased uterine blood flow
- increased uterine contractility.

Patients commonly present with chest pain, cardiovascular complications, or placental abruption and fetal distress. Acute toxicity may also mimic pre-eclampsia by presenting with cerebral haemorrhage or convulsions.

For the treatment of hypertension, the drug of choice is controversial. Although hydralazine is often used in obstetrics to treat maternal hypertension, labetalol is also widely used. However, concerns about beta blockers allowing unopposed alpha-adrenergic stimulation may also apply to a lesser extent with labetalol, and calcium channel antagonists and nitroglycerin have also been advocated. Nitroglycerin and benzodiazepines have been recommended for the treatment of cocaine-related myocardial ischaemia and infarction.

OVARIAN HYPERSTIMULATION SYNDROME[41]

Ovarian hyperstimulation syndrome (OHSS) is a rare iatrogenic complication of ovarian stimulation usually occurring during the luteal phase or early part of pregnancy. The prevalence of severe OHSS is low, at 0.5–5% of stimulated ovarian cycles. However, it is becoming more recognised owing to the increasing number of women undergoing assisted reproductive technique.

The exact aetiology and pathogenesis of OHSS remain uncertain. It appears that exogenous or endogenous human chorionic gonadotropin (hCG) is the central triggering factor. OHSS usually occurs a few days after follicular rupture or follicular aspiration, after follicular growth has been medically stimulated or induced with either gonadotropins or clomiphene citrate. The stimulated ovaries become markedly enlarged with overproduction of ovarian hormones and vasoactive substances, including cytokines, angiotensin and vascular endothelial growth factor (VEGF). As a result, the capillary permeability increases leading to hypovolaemia with haemoconcentration, oedema and accumulation of fluid in the abdomen and pleural spaces.

OHSS can be classified as mild, moderate, severe or life threatening. For the life-threatening form, patients could have oliguria, renal failure, tense ascites, hydrothorax, thromboembolism, pericardial effusion, liver derangement, ovarian torsion, cerebral oedema and ARDS.

The treatment of OHSS is supportive until the condition resolves. In most cases, the syndrome follows a self-limiting course that parallels the decline in serum hCG level. Invasive haemodynamic monitoring is necessary to assist fluid management. Abdominal and pleural tapping is needed to release the accumulated fluid. Albumin can be used as a plasma expander. Prophylaxis for thromboembolism with anticoagulant should be given, and surgical intervention may be necessary for ovarian torsion.

Access the complete references list online at http://www.expertconsult.com

2. Centre for Maternal and Child Enquiries (CMACE). Saving Mothers' Lives: reviewing maternal deaths to make motherhood safer: 2006–08. The Eighth Report on Confidential Enquiries into Maternal Deaths in the United Kingdom. BJOG 2011;118(Suppl. 1):1–203.
8. Vanden Hoek TL, Morrison LJ, Shuster M, et al. Part 12: cardiac arrest in special situations: 2010 American Heart Association Guideline for Cardiopulmonary Resuscitation and Emergency Cardiovascular Care. Circulation 2010;122(18 Suppl. 3):S829–61.
9. Hazinski MF, Nolan JP, Billi JE, et al. Part 1: Executive Summary: 2010 International Consensus on Cardiopulmonary Resuscitation and Emergency Cardiovascular Care Science With Treatment Recommendation. Circulation 2010;122(16 Suppl. 2): S250–75.
12. Barraco RD, Chiu WC, Clancy TV, et al. Practice management guidelines for the diagnosis and management of injury in the pregnant patient: the EAST Practice Management Guidelines Work Group. J Trauma 2010;69(1):211–14.
24. Royal College of Obstetricians and Gynaecologists. Green-top Guideline No. 52. Prevention and Management of Postpartum Haemorrhage. 2009. Online. Available: http://www.rcog.org.uk.
26. Barton JR, Sibai BM. Severe sepsis and septic shock in pregnancy. Obstet Gynecol 2012;120:689–706.
28. Bates SM, Greer IA, Pabinger I, et al. Venous thromboembolism, thrombophilia, antithrombotic therapy, and pregnancy: American College of Chest Physicians Evidence-Based Clinical Practice Guidelines, 8th edn. Chest 2008;133:S844–86.

65

Severe pre-existing disease in pregnancy

Jeremy P Campbell and Steve M Yentis

The two main sources of information about pre-existing conditions that result in severe morbidity in pregnancy are local or national registries/databases (e.g. UK Obstetric Surveillance System (UKOSS)) and published case series of admissions to intensive care, high-dependency or obstetric units. Information about mortality comes from registries of maternal death such as the Report of the Confidential Enquiries into Maternal Deaths in the United Kingdom, or from individual case series.

The most important pre-existing conditions likely to lead to intensive care unit (ICU) admission and/or death are cardiac disease, respiratory disease, neurological disease, psychiatric disease (including drug addiction) and haematological, connective tissue and metabolic diseases.

With increasingly successful medical care during childhood and early adulthood, the number of women with severe disease who survive to childbearing age has increased. Part of such women's desire to lead a normal life includes a wish to have children, and this places increasing demands on obstetric, anaesthetic and ICU services, as well as on women's physiological reserves.

CARDIAC DISEASE

In the UK, cardiac disease is the commonest cause of maternal death, killing more women than pre-eclampsia/eclampsia, thromboembolism and haemorrhage combined.[1] Over the last 40 years, there has been a shift away from acquired cardiac disease (mainly rheumatic heart disease) towards congenital heart disease as modern techniques of cardiac surgery in early life enable female babies with previously fatal conditions to reach maturity.[2] More recently, there has been an increase in the prevalence of ischaemic heart disease resulting from increased obesity, maternal age and smoking.

Mortality varies from less than 1% in uncomplicated conditions to over 40% in Eisenmenger's syndrome, even with modern methods of medical management.[3]

PHYSIOLOGY AND PATHOPHYSIOLOGY

The physiological changes of pregnancy most important to cardiac disease are:

- aortocaval compression
- reduction in systemic vascular resistance
- increased cardiac output (40–50% by the 20th week of gestation, with a further increase of up to 50% during labour).

In patients whose cardiac function is already impaired, inability to increase their cardiac output may result in cardiac failure. If there is a large right-to-left shunt, the fall in systemic vascular resistance results in blood bypassing the lungs. This, together with increasing maternal and fetal oxygen requirements and decreased maternal pulmonary reserve, may lead to severe exacerbation of hypoxaemia.

ANTEPARTUM MANAGEMENT

It is important that women with severe cardiac disease are appropriately counselled before pregnancy since the risks both to them and to their fetuses may be considerable. This early counselling should include anaesthetic input.

Women with cardiac disease must be assessed regularly throughout pregnancy. Electrocardiography, chest X-ray and echocardiography are the most useful investigations. For patients with valve lesions, echocardiographic measurement of valve areas provides a consistent measure of severity since flow gradients across stenosed valves usually increase in pregnancy because of the increase in cardiac output that occurs. Pulse oximetry is a simple, non-invasive tool for monitoring the degree of right-to-left shunt and can easily be repeated during pregnancy. Measures may be taken to reduced cardiac workload, for example by reducing activity and treating arrhythmias and/or cardiac failure. Prophylaxis against thromboembolism should be considered since patients with cardiac disease are more at risk, especially if confined to prolonged bed rest.[4] Low-molecular-weight heparins are now standard for prophylaxis. Heparin requirements increase with body weight, so it is vital to ensure that heparin dosing is adequate.

An obstetric and anaesthetic delivery plan should be prepared, taking into account different scenarios such as vaginal delivery and caesarean section, and the intensivists informed of the anticipated delivery date.

PERIPARTUM MANAGEMENT

The overall aim of peripartum management of the patient with cardiac disease is to minimise stress on the maternal heart and to maintain cardiac output and placental and fetal circulations. In the past, elective caesarean section (traditionally under general anaesthesia) was advocated, but the stresses and complications of surgery are now felt to exceed those of a well-controlled vaginal delivery. Therefore, over the last decade there has been a move towards vaginal delivery unless caesarean section is indicated for obstetric reasons.

Low-dose epidural analgesia regimens using weak solutions of local anaesthetic (e.g. 0.1% bupivacaine or less) with opioids such as fentanyl have been found to be effective and cardiostable.[5] Combined spinal-epidural analgesia using similar low concentrations is also suitable, and continuous spinal analgesia has also been described. In patients with marked exercise intolerance, instrumental delivery using forceps or ventouse is usually indicated to limit pushing during the second stage of labour. If a caesarean section is required, either regional or general anaesthesia has been advocated[6,7] so long as due care is taken.

Peripartum complications may be tolerated poorly by patients with limited reserves. Common peripartum complications are listed in **Box 65.1**.

The cardiovascular effects of oxytocin analogues (e.g. Syntocinon®) include a decrease in mean arterial pressure due to a fall in systemic vascular resistance and an increase in heart rate, stroke volume and cardiac output.[8] Although these are usually tolerated in healthy patients, they may cause profound hypotension in patients with limited cardiac reserves, with a worsening of shunt in susceptible individuals. If oxytocin is required, it should be diluted and given very slowly (e.g. 5 units infused over 10–20 minutes). In patients with fixed cardiac outputs and no pulmonary hypertension, ergometrine may be preferable. Withholding oxytocin altogether may be problematic because such patients may also be sensitive to the effects of acute blood loss. At caesarean section, mechanical compression of the uterus with a 'brace' suture may be used to reduce or avoid the need for oxytocics.[9]

Box 65.1 Common peripartum problems in patients with pre-existing cardiac disease

- Arrhythmias
- Cardiac failure/pulmonary oedema
- Pulmonary embolism
- Bacterial endocarditis
- Increased susceptibility to the effects of haemorrhage
- Increased risk of cardiovascular collapse in response to iatrogenic reductions in systemic vascular resistance (e.g. regional anaesthesia, intravenous bolus of oxytocin)
- Myocardial ischaemia (certain lesions)
- Increased risk from air embolism (certain lesions)

Monitoring ranges from simple non-invasive methods to peripheral arterial, central venous and pulmonary arterial cannulation, depending on the severity of the underlying disease. Central venous cannulation is often difficult because of the increased soft tissues and fluid retention of pregnancy, and the inability to lie flat, let alone head-down. Meticulous attention must be paid to avoiding intravascular air in patients with right-to-left shunts because of the risk of systemic embolism.

The principles of haemodynamic support are generally the same as in non-pregnant patients. The physiological changes of pregnancy should be remembered, especially tachycardia and increased cardiac output. Aortocaval compression must be avoided at all times, with the woman placed in the lateral or supine wedged position. The propensity for pregnant women to acute pulmonary oedema if overloaded with fluid should also be borne in mind. Exacerbation of right-to-left shunt is manifested by worsening hypoxaemia and may be improved by vasoconstrictors such as phenylephrine. If a pregnant woman requires intensive care before the baby is born, there may be a conflict between the maternal need for vasopressors and/or inotropes and the adverse effects of these drugs on uteroplacental blood flow. Similarly, attempts to prolong pregnancy with steroids and β_2-adrenergic agonists such as terbutaline or salbutamol may cause adverse cardiovascular effects (primarily pulmonary oedema) in the mother.

POSTPARTUM MANAGEMENT

Women continue to be at risk from bleeding, arrhythmias and cardiac failure postpartum. Monitoring in an area able to provide high-dependency care is vital.[10] Several problems need to be considered:

- Postoperative analgesia must be adequate.
- If oxytocin has been withheld, postpartum haemorrhage may become a problem.
- Thromboembolic prophylaxis should be (re)started.
- Prophylactic antibiotics against endocarditis should be considered (typically amoxicillin and gentamicin, or vancomycin if the woman is allergic to penicillin). Although recent guidelines suggest these are not necessary for routine use in women with cardiac disease,[11] many clinicians caring for such women give them, after weighing up the individual risks and benefits.
- There should be a high index of suspicion and aggressive early management of infection (especially of the chest, wound and genital tract).

The duration of postpartum observation will depend on the underlying disease. In Eisenmenger's syndrome, sudden death typically occurs 1–2 weeks after delivery from pulmonary embolism and/or pulmonary haemorrhage.[12]

RESPIRATORY DISEASE

The most common pre-existing respiratory diseases that cause mothers to present to ICUs are asthma and cystic fibrosis.

Asthma is very common but rarely causes serious morbidity in its own right, although there is a higher risk of several complications of pregnancy and neonatal morbidity.[13]

Cystic fibrosis is comparatively rare, but recent advances in its management have resulted in many young women achieving successful pregnancies with excellent maternal and fetal outcomes.[14] Pregnancy per se does not appear to confer an increased risk of maternal mortality or accelerate decline in lung function. Risk factors are the same as in non-pregnant patients: pre-pregnancy forced expiratory volume in 1 second (FEV_1) <60% of predicted, colonisation with *Burkholderia cepacia*, pancreatic insufficiency, and diabetes mellitus. Successful pregnancy following lung transplantation may be possible. Pre-pregnancy counselling and psychological support are important considerations since the decision to have a child, with the risk of passing on the cystic fibrosis gene, is one that imposes a great deal of stress on the mother, her partner and their relatives.

PHYSIOLOGY AND PATHOPHYSIOLOGY

If respiratory function is already impaired, the physiological effects of pregnancy add an additional burden on the respiratory system that may precipitate respiratory failure. These include:

- reduced functional residual capacity
- increased oxygen demand
- increased minute ventilation ($PaCO_2$ in late pregnancy is typically 27–32 mmHg (3.6–4.3 kPa) compared with 40 mmHg (5.3 kPa) in the non-pregnant state.

In addition, chronic hypoxaemia may lead to pulmonary vasoconstriction, pulmonary hypertension and cor pulmonale. In cystic fibrosis, an additional stress is the increased nutritional demand in a patient who may already be malnourished because of malabsorption. The increased minute ventilation in late pregnancy should be borne in mind when interpreting arterial blood gases: an arterial partial pressure of carbon dioxide of 45 mmHg (6 kPa) represents a much greater deviation from the normal value in pregnancy than in non-pregnant patients.

GENERAL MANAGEMENT AND COMPLICATIONS

Antepartum management comprises regular assessment and adjustment of medical treatment if required. Patients may be taking a variety of drugs, including steroids. Chronic use of steroids may be associated with impaired glucose tolerance in pregnant patients.

Regional analgesia is indicated in patients with moderate or severe functional limitation in order to reduce the demands of labour. If caesarean section is required, regional anaesthesia is thought to reduce the risk of pulmonary complications, although women with severe respiratory disease may be unable to lie flat. Care must be taken to ensure that the regional anaesthetic block does not extend too high as this may impair the woman's ability to breathe and cough.

In cystic fibrosis, the principles of intensive care are generally the same as in non-pregnant patients. The mainstay of treatment is regular physiotherapy and antibiotic therapy. It is important to know whether the patient has been previously colonised with unusual and/or resistant organisms (e.g. *Burkholderia cepacia*). The biggest single hazard for the mother is an acute infective exacerbation in the second or third trimester provoking respiratory failure. Infection must be treated early and aggressively. Respiratory failure has been managed with non-invasive ventilatory techniques with some success. Delivery of the fetus usually results in an immediate improvement in maternal oxygenation, although pain following caesarean section may limit deep inspiration and the ability to cough, encouraging basal atelectasis and retained secretions. Continuing respiratory support postpartum therefore remains essential.

NEUROLOGICAL DISEASE

Epilepsy is the most frequent pre-existing neurological disorder in pregnancy and remains an important cause of maternal death, often related to poor seizure control as a result of altered pharmacodynamics and pharmacokinetics of anticonvulsant drugs in pregnancy.[1] Neurological conditions that potentially affect respiratory function (e.g. myasthenia gravis, multiple sclerosis, high spinal cord lesions) can be expected to cause particular problems in pregnancy.

GENERAL MANAGEMENT

Traditionally, regional analgesia and anaesthesia were avoided in most neurological diseases for fear of exacerbating the condition, or being blamed for an exacerbation should it occur. Nowadays, most authorities encourage regional analgesia for labour in parturients at risk of respiratory insufficiency secondary to their neurological condition since it reduces the physiological demands of labour. Similarly, regional anaesthesia for caesarean section avoids the problems of postoperative sedation, and whether or how to use neuromuscular-blocking drugs. Initial fears about an increased relapse rate in multiple sclerosis following regional anaesthesia have fortunately not been borne out by a large prospective series.[15]

If there is raised intracranial pressure, the use of regional techniques is more controversial. Although

Table 65.1 Guide to converting oral to systemic medication in mothers with myasthenia gravis*

DRUG	ORAL DOSE (MG)	INTRAMUSCULAR DOSE (MG)	INTRAVENOUS DOSE (MG)
Neostigmine	15	0.7–1.0	0.5
Pyridostigmine	60	3–4	2

*Approximate conversion doses are given.

labour and vaginal delivery without effective analgesia can result in marked increases in intracranial pressure, accidental dural puncture is potentially disastrous. Even if successfully placed, rapid epidural injection may be associated with increases in intracranial pressure.[16]

Management of conditions in which there are spinal abnormalities is also controversial. Spinal bifida and other spinal cord lesions have been successfully managed using regional techniques, although a careful balance between risk and benefit must be achieved in each case. These patients are unlikely to present to intensivists unless they are associated with respiratory impairment.

Myasthenia gravis poses a particular problem because of the need for regular medication throughout labour and after delivery. Gastric emptying may be decreased during labour, especially if the mother has been given systemic opioids. It is therefore important to consider parenteral administration of anticholinesterase therapy during this period. A useful guide is given in **Table 65.1**. Epidural analgesia can be helpful in limiting maternal fatigue during labour. The mother should be observed for signs of increasing weakness for up to 10 days postpartum.

PSYCHIATRIC DISEASE (INCLUDING DRUG ADDICTION)

Psychiatric disorders are common in pregnancy and after delivery, and recent maternal mortality reports have highlighted suicide and the complications of drug addiction as relatively common causes of maternal death.[1] Patients with psychiatric disease may be more vulnerable to becoming pregnant, and pregnant women are more likely to suffer from psychiatric disease during and/or after pregnancy.

Abuse of drugs poses similar problems to those in the non-pregnant population, with the additional effects of fetal addiction and growth retardation. In particular, cocaine abuse has been implicated in causing placental abruption and maternal convulsions, hypertension and tachycardia, with increasing morbidity and mortality for both mother and fetus.[17] Unplanned operative intervention is more likely, and these patients may require admission to ICU postoperatively.

Intensive care management is usually similar to that in non-pregnant patients. If antepartum, the effects of drugs (both those taken in overdose and their antidotes) on the fetus should be considered.

HAEMATOLOGICAL, CONNECTIVE TISSUE AND METABOLIC DISEASES

Several haematological conditions may predispose to critical illness in pregnancy, the commonest being sickle cell disease. In general, ICU management of patients with haematological disease is as for non-pregnant patients.

Connective tissue disease rarely presents to the intensivist unless there is systemic involvement resulting in cardiac and respiratory insufficiency. These may be exacerbated by the physiological demands of pregnancy. Such patients are also at increased risk of obstetric complications such as haemorrhage.

Diabetes mellitus is the most important pre-existing metabolic disease in pregnancy and is well known to increase both maternal and fetal morbidity. It usually presents in the ICU as diabetic ketoacidosis, or as a contributory factor to other conditions (e.g. sepsis). Anecdotal reports suggest that diabetic ketoacidosis in pregnancy may be particularly difficult to treat and stability of blood glucose may be achieved only after delivery of the fetus.

Access the complete references list online at http://www.expertconsult.com

1. Lewis G (ed.) Saving mothers' lives: reviewing maternal deaths to make motherhood safer - 2006–8. The Eighth Report of the Confidential Enquiries into Maternal Deaths in the United Kingdom. London: CMACE; 2011.
3. Naguib MA, Dob DP, Gatzoulis MA. A functional understanding of moderate to complex congenital heart disease and the impact of pregnancy. Part II: Tetralogy of Fallot, Eisenmenger's syndrome and the Fontan operation. Int J Obstet Anesth 2010;19:306–12.
5. Suntharalingam G, Dob D, Yentis SM. Obstetric epidural analgesia in aortic stenosis: a low-dose technique for labour and instrumental delivery. Int J Obstet Anesth 2001;10:129–34.
13. Schatz M, Dombrowski MP. Asthma in pregnancy. N Engl J Med 2009;360:1862–9.
17. Ludlow JP, Evans SF, Hulse G. Obstetric and perinatal outcomes in pregnancies associated with illicit substance abuse. Aust NZ J Obstet Gynaecol 2004;44:302–6.

Part Ten

Infections and Immune Disorders

66

Anaphylaxis

Malcolm M Fisher

Anaphylaxis is a symptom complex accompanying the acute reaction to a chemical recognised as hostile. In the classical reaction the patient has been previously sensitised (immediate hypersensitivity or type 1 hypersensitivity), although the sensitising agent may be unknown. The term 'anaphylactoid reaction' is used to describe reactions clinically indistinguishable from anaphylaxis, in which the mechanism is non-immunological, or has not been determined. Recent consensus meetings have suggested the use of the term 'anaphylactoid' be discontinued and 'anaphylaxis' used to describe the symptom complex which may be either 'non-immune' or 'immune',[1] but the 'new' terminology has not been generally accepted. The clinical signs of anaphylaxis may be produced by direct drug effects, physical factors or exercise, and a causative agent cannot always be determined. The mediators involved are the same as those in other acute inflammatory responses such as sepsis, but the rate of release is more rapid and of shorter duration.

AETIOLOGY

Clinical anaphylaxis in hospital commonly follows injection of drugs, blood products, plasma substitutes, contrast media, or exposure to latex products or chlorhexidine. Outside hospital, ingestion of foods or food additives (especially peanut products) or insect stings may be more common causes than drugs.

Neugut et al[2] estimated 1400–1500 deaths per year in the USA and between 3.3 and 40.9 million patients at risk. They estimated radiocontrast media and penicillin to be the greatest causes of death, with food and stings the next groups. In contrast a postmortem study of 56 deaths in the UK[3] attributed 19 deaths to venoms, 16 to foods and 19 to drugs and radiocontrast media.

In anaphylaxis, sensitisation occurs following exposure to an allergenic substance, which either alone, or by combination with a protein or hapten, stimulates the synthesis of immunoglobulin E (IgE). Some IgE binds to the surface of mast cells and basophils. Later, re-exposure to antigen produces an antigen–cell surface IgE antibody interaction where two IgE molecules are bridged. This results in mast cell degranulation, and the release of histamine and other mediators, including interleukin, prostaglandins and platelet-activating factor. Histamine is responsible for the early signs and symptoms, but is rapidly cleared from plasma. The overall effects of the mediators are to produce vasodilatation, smooth-muscle contraction, increased glandular secretion and increased capillary permeability. The mediators act both locally and upon distant target organs.

Anaphylactoid reactions may be due to a direct histamine-releasing effect of drugs or other triggers on basophils and mast cells. The symptom complex may also be produced by other mechanisms. Some intravenous drugs and X-ray contrast media may activate the complement system. Plasma protein and human serum albumin reactions may be induced by either albumin aggregates or stabilising agent-modified albumin molecules. Other reactions, including those to dextrans and gelatin preparations, may be activated by non-IgE antibody already present in the plasma or osmotic factors (dextrose, mannitol).

The direct histamine-releasing effects of some drugs may produce reactions due to the effect of histamine alone, and such reactions are related to volume, rate and amount of infusion. Recent work suggests that the site of release of histamine may be important in its clinical effects. Drugs such as morphine and Haemaccel release histamine from skin alone,[4] and are unlikely to produce symptoms such as bronchospasm, whereas drugs which produce release from lung mast cells (e.g. atracurium, vecuronium and propofol) may be more likely to produce bronchospasm.[5] Direct histamine release is usually a transient phenomenon, but in some patients severe manifestations may occur, particularly with Haemaccel and vancomycin.

Anaphylactic reactions are usually seen in fit and well patients. It is likely that the adrenal response to stress 'pretreats' sick patients, and blocks the release and effects of anaphylactic mediators. The exception to this appears to be patients with asthma, in whom reactions to the additives in steroid and aminophylline preparations may occur, and this may be related to the reduced catecholamine response in asthma.[6] Patients on beta blockers and with epidural blockade may be more likely to develop adverse responses due to histamine release, and this may also be related to reduced catecholamine responsiveness. Reactions occurring in these groups are more difficult to treat.

CLINICAL PRESENTATION

The latent period between exposure and development of symptoms is variable, but usually occurs within 5 minutes if the provoking agent is given parenterally. Reactions may be transient or protracted (lasting days), and may vary in severity from mild to fatal. Recurrent anaphylaxis is described. Cutaneous, cardiovascular, respiratory or gastrointestinal manifestations may occur singly or in combination.

Cutaneous features include piloerection, erythematous flush, generalised or localised urticaria, angioneurotic oedema, conjunctival injection, pallor and cyanosis. Awake patients may experience an aura, warning of an impending reaction. Cardiovascular system involvement occurs most commonly and may occur as a sole clinical manifestation.[7] It is characterised by initial bradycardia then sinus tachycardia, hypotension and the development of shock.

In patients reacting due to venom desensitisation, bradycardia may be severe and require treatment.[8] Respiratory manifestations include rhinitis, bronchospasm and laryngeal obstruction. Gastrointestinal symptoms of nausea, vomiting, abdominal cramps and diarrhoea may be present. Other features include apprehension, metallic taste, choking sensation, coughing, paraesthesiae, arthralgia, convulsions, clotting abnormalities and loss of consciousness. Pulmonary oedema is a rare sign. Rarely, some women develop a profuse, watery, vaginal discharge 3–5 days after anaphylaxis. It is self-limiting.

Anaphylaxis is rare in the intensive care unit (ICU), probably because of the protective effects of the adrenal response to stress. However, use of the mast cell tryptase assay (see below) may detect anaphylaxis as an unsuspected cause of shock in intensive care.

PATHOPHYSIOLOGY OF CARDIOVASCULAR CHANGES

The traditional concept of the cardiovascular changes in clinical anaphylaxis is that of an initial vasodilatation, followed by capillary leak of plasma, which produces endogenous hypovolaemia, reduced venous return and lowered cardiac output.

Whether or not cardiac function is impaired has been controversial. Although most anaphylactic mediators adversely affect myocardial function in vitro, most case reports of anaphylaxis in which invasive cardiovascular monitoring has been used suggest minimal impairment of cardiac function. Patients with normal cardiac function before the reaction rarely show evidence of cardiac failure or arrhythmias other than supraventricular tachycardia, but the incidence of serious arrhythmias and cardiac failure increases in those with prior cardiac disease.[7] Echocardiography in anaphylaxis usually shows an 'empty', normally contracting heart. Troponins are elevated after anaphylaxis, but these elevations do not normally predict coronary artery disease requiring intervention. A recent study of patients with anaphylaxis during venom desensitisation showed that bradycardia requiring treatment was a common finding.[8] Two reactions in patients with no previous cardiac disease, where the major manifestation was prolonged global myocardial dysfunction, and the use of a balloon counterpulsator was life-saving, have been reported.[9]

TREATMENT

There are no randomised controlled trials of treatment in anaphylaxis, and the unexpected onset, rapid course and usual rapid response to treatment preclude performing such trials. Treatment recommendations are based on historical practice, case reports, series of cases and animal models.

OXYGEN

Oxygen is given by facemask. Endotracheal intubation may be required to facilitate ventilation, especially if angioedema or laryngeal oedema is present. Oedema of the upper airway is more common when anaphylaxis is due to foods than to drugs.[3] Mechanical ventilation is indicated for severe bronchospasm, apnoea or cardiac arrest.

EPINEPHRINE (ADRENALINE)

Epinephrine is universally recommended as the drug of choice for severe reactions. In the community epinephrine may be given intramuscularly in a dose of 0.3–1.0 mg early in anaphylaxis. Intramuscular epinephrine produces higher levels earlier in stable allergic patients than subcutaneous epinephrine.[10] In severe shock or in patients in whom muscle blood flow is thought to be compromised by shock, intravenous injection of 3–5 ml of 1:10 000 epinephrine is given. A second dose is necessary in 35%[11] and an infusion in 10%.

Epinephrine, by increasing intracellular levels of cyclic adenosine monophosphate (cAMP) in leukocytes and mast cells, inhibits further release of histamine. It has beneficial effects on myocardial contractility, peripheral vascular tone and bronchial smooth muscle, and stabilises mast cells. A common management error is not to institute external cardiac massage (ECM) as the arrhythmia is 'benign'. If the patient is pulseless, ECM should be instituted irrespective of rhythm, although there are no data to support its efficacy.

There has been controversy regarding the best route of administration of epinephrine outside hospital. Both case reports and patients self-injecting show efficacy for intramuscular epinephrine when given early. Intravenous epinephrine may rarely cause arrhythmias and myocardial infarction, particularly in unmonitored patients. In our series it seems to be more hazardous when the diagnosis of anaphylaxis is incorrect. Recent recommendations endorse the use of intramuscular epinephrine.[12]

OTHER SYMPATHOMIMETIC AMINES

Other sympathomimetic drugs may reverse the symptoms, but appear (albeit in the absence of any randomised trials) to be less effective than epinephrine. Norepinephrine by infusion may be life saving in the absence of a response to fluid loading and epinephrine. Methoxamine and phenylephrine have been used to treat anaphylactic hypotension successfully as first-line treatment and in 'rescue' therapy when epinephrine appears ineffective. More recently, case reports have shown vasopressin and methylene blue to be effective in refractory cases of hypotension.

COLLOIDS

Plasma expanders are given rapidly to correct the hypovolaemia consequent to acute vasodilatation and leakage of fluid from the intravascular space.[13] The author favours plasma protein solution or gelatin preparations rather than crystalloids, as they remain in the vascular compartment earlier and for longer. There are, however, no data showing improved outcomes from colloid over crystalloid, and there are many patients who have been successfully resuscitated with crystalloid alone. Greater volumes of crystalloid are necessary and on occasions very large volumes of fluid may be required; central venous pressure monitoring and measurement of haematocrit are helpful.

BRONCHOSPASM

Epinephrine should be given. Nebulised salbutamol should be given for severe asthma. Aminophylline 5–6 mg / kg intravenously may be given over 30 minutes, if bronchospasm is unresponsive to epinephrine alone. Aminophylline increases intracellular cAMP by phosphodiesterase inhibition, and its effect on inhibiting histamine and interleukin release is theoretically additive to that of epinephrine. Adverse responses have not been observed in our series but a recent comprehensive review[14] suggested safer agents with proven efficacy should be preferred. Volatile anaesthesia, ketamine and magnesium sulphate may produce improvement in some patients with severe asthma.

CORTICOSTEROIDS

Steroids have no proven benefit, particularly early, and should be reserved for refractory bronchospasm. Conversely, steroids are often given and there is no evidence of harm.

ANTIHISTAMINES

Antihistamines are the treatment of choice in localised non-severe reactions. In severe reactions they are only indicated in protracted cases or in those with angioneurotic oedema, which may recur. The data on antihistamines are not conclusive, but in protracted anaphylaxis, improvement is often reported with H_2-blockers.

A comprehensive review of the evidence for efficacy and recommendations from the evidence has recently been produced by the World Allergy Organisation.[15]

DIAGNOSIS

The most important advance in the diagnosis of anaphylaxis has been the introduction of an assay for mast cell tryptase. The mast cell enzyme is elevated 1 hour after a reaction begins, and the elevation may persist for up to 4 hours. It can also be helpful in the diagnosis of anaphylaxis from postmortem specimens.[16] The assay is highly specific and sensitive for anaphylaxis, although elevated levels are found with direct histamine release, and at postmortem in some patients with myocardial infarction. A negative mast cell tryptase assay does not exclude anaphylaxis as the diagnosis. Mast cell tryptase has been used to diagnose anaphylaxis postmortem.

FOLLOW-UP

Following successful acute management, the drug or agent responsible should be determined by in vitro or in vivo testing if possible. Hyposensitisation should be considered for food, pollen and bee venom allergy. A medic alert bracelet should be worn and the patient should be given a letter stating the nature of the reaction to the particular causative agent.

If re-exposure to the allergen is likely at home, patients or their relatives should be instructed in the use of epinephrine, salbutamol inhalation and antihistamines. Clinical anaphylaxis may be modified by pretreatment with disodium cromoglycate, corticosteroids, antihistamines, salbutamol and isoprenaline.

In patients with recurrent anaphylaxis in whom no cause can be found corticosteroids on alternate days reduce the incidence and severity of attacks.

Access the complete references list online at http://www.expertconsult.com

1. Sampson HA, Munoz-Furlong A, Campbell RL, et al. Second symposium on the definition and management of anaphylaxis: summary report. Second National Institute of Allergy and Infectious Disease / Food Allergy and Anaphylaxis Network symposium. J Allerg Clin Immunol 2006;117:391–7.
3. Pumphrey RS, Roberts IS. Postmortem findings after fatal anaphylactic reactions. J Clin Pathol 2000;53: 273–6.
7. Fisher MM. Clinical observations on the pathophysiology and treatment of anaphylactic cardiovascular collapse. Anaesth Intensive Care 1986;14:17–21.
8. Brown SG, Blackman KE, Stenlake V, et al. Insect sting anaphylaxis; prospective evaluation of treatment with intravenous adrenaline and volume resuscitation. Emerg Med J 2004;21:149–54.
9. Raper RF, Fisher MM. Profound reversible myocardial depression following human anaphylaxis. Lancet 1988;8582:386–8.
15. Simons FE, Ardusso LR, Bilò MB, et al. World Allergy Organisation Guidelines for the treatment of anaphylaxis. World Allergy Organ J 2011;4(2):13–37.

67

Host defence mechanisms and immunodeficiency disorders

Steven McGloughlin and Alexander A Padiglione

The outcome of an infection is determined by the balance between our ability to eliminate an invading microorganism and that microorganism's virulence. Diverse host defence mechanisms protect the different anatomical compartments of the body from a great variety of microorganisms. In particular there is a coordinated immunological response to infection, involving both cellular and humoral components. The immune system can be defective in many ways, leading to an increased propensity to infections. The response also needs to be controlled to avoid inappropriate and excessive activation, such as when excessive systemic activation results in disseminated intravascular coagulation (DIC).

INNATE IMMUNE RESPONSES

Innate immune responses provide a first line of defence against many microorganisms, capable of reacting without prior exposure to antigens from those microorganisms. This innate immune system consists of plasma proteins, including alternative-pathway components of the complement system and mannose-binding lectin (MBL), some lymphocytes with cytotoxic activity (natural killer or NK cells) and some macrophage functions.

ACUTE-PHASE REACTION

The acute-phase reaction is a response of the haematopoietic and hepatic systems, involving many plasma proteins and the cellular components of the blood. It occurs within hours of acute physical stress or infection. Most of the proteins are inflammatory mediators or inhibitors of transport proteins. Fibrinogen, the bulk protein of the coagulation system, is one of the plasma proteins to show the greatest rise in the acute-phase reaction, and is responsible for the elevation in the erythrocyte sedimentation rate. Decreases in haemoglobin, serum iron and albumin are all normal in the acute-phase reaction. The fall in albumin is due to redistribution and decreased synthesis and generally does not require supplementation. The function of many acute-phase proteins remains unclear, but may be beneficial to the patient.

THE ADAPTIVE IMMUNE SYSTEM

Adaptive immune responses exhibit specificity, memory, amplification and diversity. This specificity (immune response against a particular antigen) and memory (prompt response on subsequent exposures) is mediated by antigen receptors on the surface of lymphocytes. Amplification and diversity of immune responses are regulated by cytokines, which are secreted by lymphocytes and other cells, and through the effects of various lymphocyte surface molecules, including adhesion molecules and co-stimulatory molecules. Cytokines have various activities, the most important of which are cell activation (e.g. interferon gamma (IFN-γ)), regulation of immune responses (e.g. interleukin (IL)-10) and pro-inflammatory effects (e.g. tumour necrosis factor (TNF)) and lymphotoxins).

ANTIGEN PRESENTATION AND THE ROLE OF T AND B LYMPHOCYTES

An adaptive immune response is initiated by the processing and presentation of fragments of a microorganism in a form that makes them antigenic to lymphocytes. Major histocompatibility complex (MHC) class I (human leucocyte antigen (HLA)-A, B, C) and class II (HLA-DR, DP, DQ) molecules are the major cell-surface antigen presentation molecules, and determine the nature of the subsequent response against the antigen.

Class I MHC molecules are present on most nucleated cells, and present processed *endogenous* peptides (such as fragments of viruses) to the T-cell receptor (TcR) of CD8+ (cytotoxic) T lymphocytes. Activated CD8+ T cells have a cytotoxic effect on the presenting cell, resulting in the death of the cell and inhibition of viral replication.

Class II MHC molecules are found on macrophages and monocytes (where they present fragments of phagocytosed microorganisms to TcRs on CD4+ (helper) T cells) and B cells (where antigen is bound to specific surface immunoglobulins, the B-cell antigen receptor).

Activation of CD4+ T cells by these *exogenous* antigens results in the expression of cell-surface molecules and secretion of cytokines with immunoregulatory effects. These immunoregulatory molecules augment the functions of many other cells, including B cells, T cells and macrophages (T-cell help). CD4+ T-cell activation may also elicit macrophage activation (critically dependent on the production of IFN-γ) to assist in killing of the microorganism.

Proliferating B cells differentiate into plasma cells, which secrete immunoglobulins with antibody activity against the initiating antigen, or into memory B cells, which live for a long time and rapidly respond on re-exposure to an antigen.

IMMUNOGLOBULINS AND ANTIBODIES

Nine isotypes of immunoglobulin can be produced, each of which has a different function. Immunoglobulin M (IgM) is a large pentamer that has its major effect within the circulation early in the immune response, and works as a bacterial agglutinator and complement activator. IgA_1 and IgA_2 are produced at secretory surfaces, such as the mucosa of the gut and respiratory tract, and also in the breast, where IgA is a major constituent of colostrum and provides secretory antibody to the gut of the neonate. IgE is also produced at mucosal surfaces and is an important part of the immune response against parasitic infections. IgD acts mainly as a B-cell receptor. IgG occurs in four subclasses, and is the only antibody able to cross the placenta: IgG_1 and IgG_3 are particularly effective at activating complement and binding to Fc receptors on phagocytic cells; IgG_2 are mainly active against polysaccharide antigens, such as those present in bacterial cell walls; the functions of IgG_4 antibodies are unclear.

SECONDARY ANTIBODY FUNCTION

Antibodies must act through one of several secondary effector mechanisms to eliminate a micro-organism. Antibodies complexed with antigens can activate the complement system through the classical pathway. The complement system may also be activated directly by components of microorganisms through the alternative (or MBL) pathway. Activation of the complement system results in the generation of biologically active molecules, such as C3b, which is an important opsonin, and the activation of the membrane attack complex (MAC), which lyses bacterial cell walls. Like C3b, antibodies of the IgM, IgG_1 and IgG_3 isotypes are also important opsonins. These molecules, when bound to the surface of a microorganism, facilitate their opsonisation and phagocytosis. These effects of complement and antibody are mediated through complement receptors (CRs) and receptors for the Fc portion of the immunoglobulin molecules (Fc receptors) on the surface of phagocytic cells such as neutrophils and macrophages.

DIVERSITY OF IMMUNE RESPONSES

The type of immune response produced against a microorganism varies according to the nature of the infecting organism. Thus virus-infected cells elicit a cytotoxic CD8+ T-cell response; intracellular pathogens such as mycobacteria and protozoa elicit a CD4+ T-cell response, which results in macrophage activation; encapsulated bacteria elicit an opsonising antibody response; other bacteria such as *Neisseria* spp. elicit a complement-activating antibody response, which lyses the cell wall of the bacterium. The nature of the immune response is regulated by cytokines, which provide T-cell help (Th) in the course of an immune response. Thus IL-2, IL-12 and IFN-γ production induces a predominantly cellular immune response (Th1), whereas the production of IL-4 and IL-13 induces a predominantly antibody-mediated immune response (Th2).

IMMUNODEFICIENCY DISORDERS

Immunodeficiency disorders can generally be classified functionally into five groups: antibody deficiency, complement deficiency, cellular immunodeficiency, phagocyte dysfunction and combined immunodeficiency (T cells, B cells and NK cells).

Immunodeficiency disorders may also be classified aetiologically as either primary or acquired.

Primary immunodeficiency disorders are the result of a developmental anomaly or a genetically determined defect of the immune system. Primary immunodeficiency due to an absent or non-functional gene product critical for the normal immune function is more severe, so it tends to present early in life. Primary immunodeficiency due to aberrant regulation of lymphocyte differentiation, which is probably determined by the products of several genes and may be influenced by environmental factors, tends to be less severe so it presents later. Our understanding of the genetic basis of many of these conditions is improving, including a number of specific gene defects that lead to selective susceptibility to single pathogens.

Acquired immunodeficiency disorders are more common than primary immunodeficiency disorders and may present at any time after early childhood. Most result from an immune defect that is a consequence of a disease process, infection or complication of a therapeutic procedure such as splenectomy, immunosuppressant therapy or haemopoietic stem cell transplantation (HSCT).

An immunodeficiency disorder may be considered in an adult patient with an unexplained abnormal propensity to infections, such as recurrent or multiple serious infections (e.g. deep abscess, meningitis, osteomyelitis, sepsis, pneumonia), persistent thrush, opportunistic infections or poor response to antimicrobial therapy, and requires the demonstration of a specific immune defect (**Table 67.1**).

Table 67.1 Tests of immunocompetence

IMMUNE DEFICIENCY SYNDROME	CLINICAL MANIFESTATION	TESTS
Antibody-mediated	Recurrent bacterial infection, especially with encapsulated bacteria, e.g.: *Streptococcus pneumoniae* *Neisseria meningitides* *Haemophilus influenzae*	Immunoglobulin G, A and M levels IgG subclasses Peripheral blood B-cell count (CD 19) *Consider:* Immunisation response to: Polysaccharide antigens (e.g. pneumococcal, pre and post vaccination) Protein antigens (e.g. tetanus and diptheria antibodies)
Cell-mediated immunity	Predominantly intracellular pathogens: Viruses Herpes simplex viruses Cytomegalovirus Varicella-zoster virus Epstein–Barr virus Molluscum contagiosum virus JC virus (cause of progressive multifocal leucoencephalopathy) Mycobacteria *Mycobacterium tuberculosis* Non-tuberculous mycobacteria Bacterial *Salmonella* spp. *Shigella* spp. *Listeria monocytogenes* Fungi and yeasts *Candida* spp. (mucosal infections) Cryptococci *Aspergillus* spp. Protozoa *Toxoplasma gondii* Cryptosporidia *Pneumocystis jiroveci*	Peripheral blood T-cell subsets (CD3+, CD4+ and CD8+) Serology for HIV (+/– HTLV) *Consider:* T-cell response to antigens Cytokine assays Delayed-type hypersensitivity (DTH) skin test responses to antigens (rarely done now)
Phagocyte function	Recurrent severe bacterial infection, esp. *Neisseria meningitides*	Neutrophil count *Consider:* Tests of oxidative killing mechanisms, e.g. nitroblue tetrazolium reduction test (NBT) or dihydrorhodamine oxidation Neutrophil migration assays Bacteria or *Candida* killing assays
Complement system	*Streptococcus pneumoniae* *Neisseria meningitides* *Moraxella* spp. *Acinetobacter* spp.	Immunochemical quantitation of C3 and C4 Functional assay of the classical pathway (CH50) *Consider:* Functional assay of the alternative pathway (AH50) Immunochemical quantification of other individual components

ANTIBODY DEFICIENCY

A poor systemic antibody response most commonly results in a lack of opsonising antibody, and a propensity to infections with encapsulated bacteria such as *Streptococcus pneumoniae* or *Haemophilus influenzae*, most often manifesting as recurrent respiratory tract infections including sinusitis. Chronic echovirus infections of the nervous system and infection with some mycoplasmas may also occur in patients with severe primary immunoglobulin deficiency (agammaglobulinaemia).

PRIMARY ANTIBODY DEFICIENCY DISORDERS

Failure of B-cell production or differentiation is the cause of most primary antibody deficiency disorders.[1] B cells are absent from blood and secondary lymphoid tissues in patients with X-linked agammaglobulinaemia (XLA) because mutations of the *Btk* gene on the X-chromosome result in the absence of a B-cell tyrosine kinase necessary for the maturation of pre-B cells to B cells in the bone marrow. In the hyper-IgM immunodeficiency syndrome, B cells are able to differentiate into plasma cells secreting IgM, but not IgG or IgA.

Common variable immunodeficiency (CVID) is a group of disorders that appear to be the consequence of immunoregulatory defects that result in impaired B-cell differentiation, leading to hypogammaglobulinaemia.

IgA deficiency also results from impaired B-cell differentiation. Deficient secretory antibody responses are common in patients with IgA deficiency, but most affected individuals are able to produce compensatory secretory IgM or IgG antibody responses and do not suffer from infections. Some may also have a defect of systemic antibody responses, such as an IgG subclass deficiency and/or impairment of antibody responses to polysaccharide antigens, and hence may suffer from recurrent infections.[2]

The immunoregulatory defect underlying CVID and IgA deficiency sometimes results in an increased propensity to autoimmunity. This can include the production of anti-IgA antibodies, which may result in anaphylactoid reactions to blood products containing IgA.

ACQUIRED ANTIBODY DEFICIENCY DISORDERS

B-cell chronic lymphocytic leukaemia or lymphoma and myeloma are commonly associated with reduced synthesis of normal immunoglobulins, which may result in bacterial infections.[3] A thymoma is a rare cause of immunoglobulin and antibody deficiency, and should be considered in a patient presenting with primary immunoglobulin deficiency after the age of 40.[4] Asplenic patients have impaired production of antibodies against polysaccharide antigens leading to infection with encapsulated bacteria, such as pneumococci and meningococci, particularly in patients who have haematological malignancy.[5]

Drugs occasionally affect B-cell differentiation and cause immunoglobulin deficiency, particularly IgA deficiency. The most common offender is phenytoin. Most patients do not have antibody deficiency severe enough to cause infections. Intensive plasmapheresis may also cause severe immunoglobulin deficiency if immunoglobulin replacement is not used.

TREATMENT OF ANTIBODY DEFICIENCY DISORDERS

Infections can be prevented by regular infusions of intravenous immunoglobulin (IVIg) in patients with primary or acquired antibody deficiency. The usual dose is 0.4 g/kg given monthly. Acute infections should be treated with appropriate antibiotics. The routine use of IVIg as an adjunct in the management of sepsis in adults cannot be recommended, as higher-quality studies have failed to confirm earlier suggestions of benefit.

CELLULAR IMMUNODEFICIENCY

Impairment of cell-mediated immune responses leads to an increased propensity to infections normally controlled by cellular immune responses (see Table 67.1). These microorganisms are often pathogens that replicate intracellularly and cause persistent (latent) infections that reactivate when the cellular immune response against them becomes ineffective.

PRIMARY CELLULAR IMMUNODEFICIENCY

Children with the Di George syndrome have a complete or partial absence of the thymus, resulting in depletion of T cells from blood and lymphoid tissue.[6] A less severe defect of cellular immunity occurs in patients with chronic mucocutaneous candidiasis. This is usually seen in patients with the autoimmune polyendocrinopathy–candidiasis–ectodermal dystrophy (APECED) syndrome, which results from a disorder of T-cell processing in the thymus.[7]

ACQUIRED CELLULAR IMMUNODEFICIENCY

Acquired defects of cellular immunity are by far the most common cause of cellular immunodeficiency, with human immunodeficiency virus (HIV) infection the most common (see Ch. 68). Less commonly, Hodgkin's disease, T-cell lymphomas and sarcoidosis may also be complicated by opportunistic infections occurring as a consequence of cellular immunodeficiency. A thymoma is a rare cause of chronic mucocutaneous candidiasis that, like thymoma and immunoglobulin deficiency, occurs later in life.[4]

Suppression of cellular immune responses is an intended effect of many immunosuppressant drugs used to treat allograft rejection, graft-versus-host disease (GvHD), autoimmune diseases and vasculitis. Opportunistic infections may complicate this type of immunodeficiency.

TREATMENT OF CELLULAR IMMUNODEFICIENCY DISORDERS

Most infections complicating cellular immunodeficiency are re-activated latent infections, so prevention by the use of prophylactic antimicrobial drugs is important, and is best defined in HIV-induced immunodeficiency.[8] The risk and type of infection are determined by the degree and duration of cellular immunodeficiency, allowing for appropriate decisions to be made regarding investigations, treatment and prophylaxis.

Acquired cellular immunodeficiency may be corrected, at least temporarily, by removing its cause (e.g. by suppressing HIV infection or ceasing immunosuppressive therapy). Thymus transplantation may be effective in children with thymus aplasia.

COMPLEMENT COMPONENT DEFICIENCY

Deficiency of complement components is an uncommon but often overlooked cause of recurrent bacterial infections. Complement-mediated lysis of bacterial cell walls is a critical defence against certain bacteria, especially *Neisseria* spp. and related bacteria such as *Moraxella* spp. and *Acinetobacter* spp. Deficiency of classical pathway components may also result in impaired antibody responses.

PRIMARY COMPLEMENT DEFICIENCY

Congenital deficiency of C3 is extremely rare. C3b is an important opsonin and C3 deficiency will often impair phagocytosis of bacteria, causing a propensity to severe pyogenic infections. Deficiency of MAC components is more common, and should be considered in patients with recurrent meningococcal infections.[9] Deficiency of classical pathway components (C1, C2, C4) may also result in an increased propensity to infection with meningococci and some other bacteria, but most affected individuals do not experience recurrent infections.

ACQUIRED COMPLEMENT DEFICIENCY

Disease processes that cause persistent activation of the complement system may cause depletion of complement components, particularly classical pathway components. This can result in infections with *Neisseria* spp. or related bacteria, and sometimes overwhelming septicaemia when the complement deficiency is severe. Systemic lupus erythematosus, myeloma and chronic atrioventricular shunt infections are rare causes of complement component deficiency.

MANAGEMENT OF PATIENTS WITH COMPLEMENT DEFICIENCY

An awareness of the possibility of complement deficiency is the most important aspect of management. Replacement therapy is not available. If a complement component deficiency is identified, screening of family members should be considered.

PHAGOCYTE DISORDERS

Phagocytosis of a bacterium or fungus by a neutrophil, leucocyte or macrophage is dependent on chemotaxis (attraction of phagocytes to the site of infection), adhesion (to endothelial cells via molecules such as integrins), binding (to opsonins on the microorganism), ingestion and intracellular killing (which involves both oxidative and non-oxidative mechanisms).

Depletion or functional impairment of phagocytes results in an increased propensity to bacterial and fungal infections, particularly infection with *Staphylococcus aureus*, Gram-negative enteric bacteria, *Candida* spp. and *Aspergillus* spp. Primary or acquired defects of phagocytes may result in localised pyogenic infections or pneumonia. In patients with severe neutropenia, however, localised infections may show little inflammatory reaction and overwhelming systemic infections, in particular systemic fungal and yeast infections, are common.

PRIMARY DISORDERS OF PHAGOCYTOSIS

Congenital neutropenias are rare. Defects of phagocyte function usually affect chemotaxis, adhesion or intracellular killing, either alone or in combination. The best-characterised defect of phagocyte adherence results from a congenital absence of the β-subunit of CD18 integrins in patients with leucocyte adhesion deficiency syndrome type 1.[10] Defects of intracellular killing are usually caused by a deficiency of microbicidal enzymes. Chronic granulomatous disease (CGD) results from a deficiency of a phagosome enzyme (NADPH oxidase) leading to ineffective oxidative killing.[11] CGD usually presents in childhood but may present in adults, even as late as the seventh decade. It should be considered in patients with recurrent abscesses or suppurative lymphadenitis, and in patients with pneumonia caused by *S. aureus* or *Aspergillus* spp. infection.

ACQUIRED DISORDERS OF PHAGOCYTOSIS

Severe neutropenia may be complicated by bacterial or fungal infections. There are many causes of neutropenia, including autoimmune neutropenia, drug therapy and haematological diseases such as cyclic neutropenia, myelodysplastic syndromes and aplastic anaemia. Cytotoxic chemotherapy, used to treat various malignancies, commonly causes neutropenia, which is often complicated by severe bacterial and fungal infections.

MANAGEMENT OF PHAGOCYTE DISORDERS

Acquired neutropenia may be corrected by removing the underlying cause and/or use of granulocyte colony-stimulating factor (G-CSF). Febrile neutropenia requires investigation for the source of sepsis and empirical antibiotics. If fever persists then antifungals should be added. IFN-γ therapy may be effective in patients with CGD.

COMBINED IMMUNODEFICIENCY DISORDERS

Several immunodeficiency disorders result from a combination of immune defects. Some combinations of congenital immune defects are so severe that death is a common occurrence, unless the defect can be corrected. Such conditions are classified as severe combined immune deficiency (SCID) syndromes.

PRIMARY COMBINED IMMUNODEFICIENCY

There are many primary combined immunodeficiency syndromes, which present in early childhood.[12] Specific molecular defects have now been demonstrated for many of them. For example, defective expression of MHC class II molecules, adenosine deaminase (ADA) deficiency, and deficiency of the common γ-chain of the receptor for several interleukins (IL-2, 4, 7, 9, 15, 21) all result in a deficiency and/or functional impairment of B cells, T cells and sometimes NK cells. Deficiency of the interleukin receptor common γ-chain results from mutations of its gene on the X-chromosome and is the underlying defect of X-linked SCID.

Treatment of primary combined immunodeficiency

HSCT is the main treatment for many types of primary SCID, though enzyme replacement therapy can be effective in ADA deficiency and gene replacement therapy has been used to treat X-linked SCID. Antibody replacement with IVIg therapy and prophylaxis for opportunistic infections are also important in primary SCID.

ACQUIRED COMBINED IMMUNODEFICIENCY

Combined immune defects are a characteristic of several acquired immunodeficiency disorders.

Haemopoietic stem cell transplantation

Combined immune defects may result in severe infections in patients who have received HSCT.[13] Following transplantation, the recipient's immune system is reconstituted with donor cells. A degree of immunocompetence is passively transferred from the donor to recipient by antigen-specific lymphocytes, but as this and any residual immunocompetence of the recipient declines an immunodeficient state exists until the donor immune system is established. Consequently, both antibody-mediated and cell-mediated immunity are deficient in the first 3–4 months after transplantation and may remain deficient for a longer period of time in patients with GvHD. This combined immune defect is often compounded by neutropenia and/or the effects of corticosteroid or immunosuppressant therapy for GvHD. Defective antibody responses may persist for several years after transplantation, particularly antibody responses against polysaccharide antigens.

Critical illness

Many patients who are critically ill as a result of surgery, trauma, thermal injury or overwhelming sepsis also have acquired immune defects. These defects include abnormalities of cellular immunity, immunoglobulin deficiency and impaired neutrophil function and appear to be associated with an increased propensity to infections. Impairment of cell-mediated immune responses usually manifests as decreased T-cell proliferation and impaired delayed-type hypersensitivity responses, and probably results from a combination of factors, including the effects of anaesthetic drugs, blood transfusion, negative nitrogen balance and serum suppressor factors, including cytokines such as TNF. Phagocyte defects are mostly due to impairment of neutrophil chemotaxis by serum factors, and impaired intracellular killing. Deficiency of serum immunoglobulins also occurs, especially IgG deficiency, and may be associated with antibody deficiency. Serum leakage is a factor in patients with thermal injuries, and reduced synthesis and increased catabolism of immunoglobulins occur in many critically ill patients.

The correction of immune defects in critically ill patients has been intensely investigated, but no effective treatment regimen has been defined. General measures such as adequate nutrition, achieving a positive nitrogen balance and excision of thermally injured tissue appear helpful. Biological response modifiers, cytokine and mediator inhibitors, and IVIg therapy have all been evaluated. The number of acute infections, particularly pneumonia, can be reduced by the use of IVIg therapy, but patient survival is not increased. G-CSF levels are increased during critical illnesses and correlate with the severity of illness. Although administration of G-CSF has been shown to be safe in intensive care patients, there is no current evidence that the administration of G-CSF improves outcome and cannot be routinely recommended in the treatment of critically ill intensive care unit patients.

Asplenia and hyposplenism

The spleen is an important part of the immune system's response to infections, particularly bloodstream infections. Splenic macrophages remove opsonised microorganisms from the blood, and IgM memory B cells (also known as mantle-zone B cells) produce an early antibody response to the polysaccharide antigens of encapsulated bacteria. The risk of overwhelming post-splenectomy infection (OPSI) is around 1 in 500 per annum, with 50% mortality. OPSI is most commonly caused by encapsulated bacteria, such as *Pneumococcus, Meningococcus* and *Haemophilus influenzae*, for which vaccines are available. Other bacteria that are sometimes important include group A *Streptococcus, Capnocytophaga canimorsus* (following dog bites), *Salmonella, Enterococcus* and *Bacteroides*.

Asplenic/hyposplenic patients require education, vaccination and appropriate use of antibiotics. Pneumococcal, meningococcal and *H. influenzae* vaccines, including regular boosters, and annual influenza vaccine are recommended, preferably 14 days before removal of the spleen if performed electively, or 14 days after if not.[14] Chemoprophylaxis with antibiotics (with a penicillin, or if allergic macrolides) should be given in accordance with national guidelines; our practice is to offer them for at least 2 years post splenectomy in adults. Enrolment of patients in spleen registries, where available, can offer ongoing patient education, vaccination reminders and access to updated recommendations.

Biological immune response modulators

Anti-TNF agents such as infliximab have been associated with increased rates of bacterial infection,[15] tuberculosis and some opportunistic infection.

Antibodies targeting various B- and T-cell antigens are increasingly used for rheumatological and haematological diseases. Not unexpectedly, these agents have been increasingly associated with infectious complications. For example, the anti-CD20 antibody rituximab specifically targets B cells for its therapeutic action, but has also been associated with infectious complications such as recurrent bacterial infection, reactivation of hepatitis B, CMV and PML.

Access the complete references list online at http://www.expertconsult.com

1. Buckley RH. Primary immunodeficiency diseases due to defects in lymphocytes. N Engl J Med 2000; 343:1313–24.
8. Kovacs JA, Masur H. Prophylaxis against opportunistic infections in patients with human immunodeficiency virus infection. N Engl J Med 2000;342:1416–29.
9. Fijen CA, Kuijper EJ, te Bulte MT, et al. Assessment of complement deficiency in patients with meningococcal disease in The Netherlands. Clin Infect Dis 1999;28:98–105.
12. Buckley RH. Advances in the understanding and treatment of human severe combined immunodeficiency. Immunol Res 2001;22:237–51.
13. Ninin E, Milpied N, Moreau P, et al. Longitudinal study of bacterial, viral, and fungal infections in adult recipients of bone marrow transplants. Clin Infect Dis 2001;33:41–7.
14. Shatz DV, Schinsky MF, Pais LB, et al. Immune responses of splenectomized trauma patients to the 23-valent pneumococcal polysaccharide vaccine at 1 versus 7 versus 14 days after splenectomy. J Trauma 1998;44(5):760.
15. Curtis JR, Patkar N, Xie A, et al. Risk of serious bacterial infections among rheumatoid arthritis patients exposed to tumor necrosis factor α antagonists. Arthritis Rheum 2007;56(4):1125–33.

68

HIV and acquired immunodeficiency syndrome

Alexander A Padiglione and Steve McGloughlin

HIV/AIDS AND THE INTENSIVE CARE UNIT (ICU)

Modern antiretroviral therapy (ART) is so effective at controlling HIV replication that the mortality of patients with HIV is now similar to that for the general population. Correspondingly, the mortality risk for patients with HIV in ICU is now more closely related to their acute illness severity than to their degree of immunosuppression.[1] The proportion of HIV patients being admitted to intensive care with illnesses unrelated to their immune suppression, such as major surgery, self-poisoning and trauma, is increasing.[2]

Patients with HIV may be admitted to intensive care because of:

- *direct complications of the immune deficiency induced by HIV:* classically infections such as *Pneumocystis jiroveci* pneumonia (PJP) or cryptococcal meningitis, and occasionally tumours, especially lymphoma
- *indirect complications of HIV or its treatment not due to immune deficiency:* examples include sepsis or myocardial infarction, or drug side-effects including chemotherapy for HIV-associated cancers
- *problems unrelated to HIV infection:* such as major surgery or trauma.

The most common cause overall for admission to intensive care remains respiratory failure. Previously the predominant cause for this was PJP, but bacterial pneumonia and non-HIV-related respiratory illnesses such as chronic obstructive pulmonary disease (COPD) and asthma are increasing in prevalence. Immune reconstitution disease related to PJP, tuberculosis and other mycobacterial diseases can also cause respiratory failure in patients recently commenced on ART.

Sepsis is an important cause of admission to intensive care units amongst HIV patients, and is an independent predictor of mortality in HIV patients admitted to ICU. Bloodstream and lower respiratory tract infections are the most common. Early recognition of bacterial sepsis as a cause for an acute illness in HIV patients is vital. HIV patients in ICU also appear to be at an increased risk of developing severe nosocomial infections.[1]

HIV REPLICATION

Human immunodeficiency viruses 1 and 2 are retroviruses that exhibit tropism for cells of the immune system with subsequent immune disturbance, especially immunodeficiency. The major cell surface receptor for HIV is the CD4 molecule, but one of the chemokine receptors CCR5 or CXCR4 acts as a co-receptor. Inside the cell, the viral RNA is reverse-transcribed into DNA by a viral reverse transcriptase enzyme. This proviral DNA is integrated into the host DNA by a viral integrase enzyme. The proviral DNA remains in the nucleus until the cell is activated, when it is transcribed into RNA, which provides the template for assembly of new HIVs under the control of viral enzymes such as proteases. Budding of new virus from the cell is followed by infection of new cells and a repeat of the replication cycle.

PRIMARY HIV INFECTION

Primary HIV infection ('seroconversion illness') occurs in 50–75% of infected patients, typically 1–4 weeks after exposure to HIV. This infectious mononucleosis-like syndrome is characterised by fever, lymphadenopathy, headache, photophobia, fatigue and myalgia. However, mucocutaneous lesions, neurological disease and even transient immunodeficiency with secondary infections may occur.[3]

CHRONIC HIV INFECTION

The viraemia associated with primary HIV infection is controlled by cellular and antibody-mediated immune responses, which correspond with resolution of symptoms. However, HIV replication continues to take place even though most patients are asymptomatic. This results in activation of the immune system and immune dysregulation, but especially cellular immunodeficiency and in particular depletion of CD4+ T cells. These abnormalities develop at different rates in different individuals, depending on both host and viral factors. In untreated patients the median time to develop the acquired immunodeficiency syndrome

(AIDS) after acquiring HIV infection is around 9 years. However, about 5% of HIV-infected individuals have no abnormalities or evidence of CD4 loss even after 15 or more years and are referred to as long-term non-progressors.

There is a persistent immune response against the virus, but this usually slowly fails owing to CD4 cell depletion, immune dysregulation and viral mutation; viral replication increases and the other cells become infected, including macrophages and microglial cells of the nervous system.

Chronic HIV infection may cause weight loss, fevers, lymphadenopathy and diarrhoea, though such symptoms are more likely to be caused by an opportunistic infection in immunodeficient patients. Worsening HIV infection leads to a T-cell immunodeficiency syndrome manifesting in the development of opportunistic infections and tumours. These are classically PJP, Kaposi's sarcoma and T-cell lymphoma. Neurological disease may also develop, and is a consequence of HIV infection of macrophages and microglial cells in the central and peripheral nervous system. At very severe T-cell deficiency (<100 cells/mL) diseases such as cryptococcal meningitis, disseminated *Mycobacterium avium* complex (MAC) and cerebral toxoplasmosis can also occur. Globally tuberculosis (TB) is the most common consequence of HIV immunodeficiency, presenting classically as pulmonary disease at higher CD4 counts, with more unusual extrapulmonary manifestations including meningitis and miliary disease increasingly likely at lower CD4 counts.

DIAGNOSIS

A definitive diagnosis of HIV infection can be made by demonstrating anti-HIV antibodies in the patient's serum. It may take a number of weeks for HIV antibody to become positive during seroconversion. Most current testing is with combination antigen/antibody tests, which dramatically reduce any window period.[4] Laboratories have generally confirmed a positive antibody result with an HIV-specific Western blot immunoassay (though this may take time to become positive in acute HIV infection), best done on a repeat blood draw.

Most patients who develop HIV will have positive antibodies by 3 months after their exposure to the virus; after this time, absence of HIV antibodies excludes HIV infection in almost all cases.

HIV VIRAL LOAD MONITORING/GENOTYPE TESTING

Polymerase chain reaction (PCR) testing allows the quantification of viral nucleic acid in body fluids. The HIV viral load is useful in prognostication and monitoring response to treatment[5] so in stable patients it is usually tested every 3–4 months. Specific mutations in the viral RNA confer resistance to specific antiretroviral drugs. These mutations can be detected by PCR and sequencing of complementary DNA (cDNA); this genotyping is normally done at first diagnosis, or when a treatment regimen is failing, to guide subsequent therapy.[6]

IMMUNOLOGICAL MONITORING

Immunodeficiency and neurological disease caused by HIV infection usually develop gradually over years. The blood CD4+ T-cell count or percentage is the best indicator of the severity of HIV-induced immunodeficiency, and therefore of the patient's susceptibility to opportunistic infections, and may be a useful guide to starting therapy. Significant AIDS-related illnesses tend to occur at a CD4+ count of less than 200, but there is clear benefit at starting therapy in any patient with a subnormal CD4+ count.[7]

MANAGEMENT OF THE HIV-INFECTED PATIENT[8]

The impact of combination antiretroviral therapy on the morbidity and mortality associated with HIV infection has been dramatic, and patients currently on effective treatment can expect a near-normal lifespan. Six classes of antiretroviral drugs are currently in use and function at various points in the HIV replication cycle (**Table 68.1**).

Antiretroviral drugs should not be used individually but triple combination therapy against a sensitive virus usually leads to sustained virological control without the development of resistance. Adherence to antiretroviral therapy is critical to the success of treatment. The choice of drug therapy should be based on national guidelines and individualised for patient characteristics and genotyping results.

DRUG TOXICITY

Improvements in antiretroviral therapy have seen reductions in serious adverse events due to HIV medications. Older nucleoside analogue reverse transcriptase inhibitors (NRTIs) previously associated with lipodystrophy, lactic acidosis and peripheral neuropathy and pancreatitis are now rarely used in the developed world.[9] Severe allergic reactions to abacavir have been significantly reduced by HLAB5701 testing of patients to exclude those with a predisposition.

Long-term toxicities including liver, kidney and bone disease are now more significant concerns. In some cases a combination of viral, treatment and other factors may play a synergistic or additive role in generating these toxicities; for example co-infection with hepatitis C virus is a significant risk factor for hepatotoxicity and at least some cases are probably a type of immune restoration syndrome.[10]

Table 68.1 Antiretroviral drugs used to treat human immunodeficiency virus (HIV) infection

ANTIRETROVIRAL CLASS AND EXAMPLES	MECHANISM
FUSION INHIBITORS	Block binding/fusion of the virus with the cell membrane
Enfuvirtide (T20) Maraviroc	
NUCLEOSIDE/NUCLEOTIDE ANALOGUE REVERSE TRANSCRIPTASE INHIBITORS	Substitute natural nucleoside or nucleotide analogues during HIV replication, thereby inhibiting DNA chain elongation and the effects of the reverse transcriptase enzyme
NUCLEOSIDE ANALOGUES	
Abacavir (ABV) Didanosine (ddl) Emtricitabine (FTC) Lamivudine (3TC) Stavudine (d4T) Zidovudine (AZT)	
NUCLEOTIDE ANALOGUES	
Tenofovir (TDF)	
NON-NUCLEOSIDE REVERSE TRANSCRIPTASE INHIBITORS	Inhibit the reverse transcriptase enzyme preventing the formation of HIV DNA
Etravirine (ETR) Rilpivirine Efavirenz Nevirapine	
INTEGRASE INHIBITORS	Block integration of viral DNA into host DNA
Raltegravir Elvitegravir Dolutegravir	
PROTEASE INHIBITORS	Inhibit the viral protease
Atazanavir Darunavir Fosamprenavir Indinavir Lopinivir Nelfinavir Saquinavir Tipranavir Ritonavir*	

*Administered with other PIs to increase serum levels.

IMMUNE RECONSTITUTION INFLAMMATORY SYNDROME (IRIS)

IRIS is a complication related to the commencement of antiretroviral therapy and the subsequent reconstitution of the immune system. The syndrome can lead to a worsening of treated opportunistic infections or even unmask untreated infections. IRIS is more common in those patients with a history of cytomegalovirus retinitis, cryptococcal meningitis and tuberculosis, and in those with low CD4 counts. However, it can occur with virtually any opportunistic infection. ART is usually continued if mild IRIS develops. Corticosteroids, other immunosuppressive agents and even cessation of ART may be considered for the management of severe IRIS.[11–13]

HIV TREATMENT IN ICU

ART is a lifelong therapy that should be commenced in consultation with an HIV specialist. Patients already on ART should continue their therapy during an acute ICU admission, if possible. Maintenance of adequate drug delivery and absorption of ART is a particular challenge in the ICU. Options include syrup formulations, crushing tablets and the use of intravenous preparations, and drug levels of some medications can be monitored. This complex area should be managed in consultation with a pharmacist with specialist HIV knowledge.

ART also has the potential for serious drug interactions, particularly when ART includes protease inhibitors or efavirenz (metabolised via the P450 hepatic enzyme system). For example, protease inhibitors can significantly potentiate the effect of midazolam. Web-based tools are very useful (e.g. www.HIV-druginteractions.org) when prescribing antimicrobials, antiemetics and lipid-lowering drugs. The presence of renal or hepatic failure will also potentially affect the dosing of ART.

In patients who are not on ART admitted to ICU for a problem unrelated to immunosuppression, the commencement of ART can usually be delayed until after they recover. In patients admitted for an AIDS-related illness, the timing of therapy is somewhat more controversial. The potential earlier improvements in immune function need to be balanced against potential side-effects from the introduction of new drugs and increased risk of complications from immune reconstitution. Overall there is evidence in most opportunistic infections that early ART therapy is associated with improved survival.[14] Our specific practice is to initiate ART within 2–4 weeks after diagnosis of most AIDS-related infections as by this time the patient's clinical status has often stabilised, and tolerability of treatment for the infection has been established. Specific exceptions to early treatment are cryptococcal meningitis and probably TB meningitis, where early therapy is associated with a poor outcome mainly because IRIS reactions can be very severe, but also in part because drug interactions and side-effects are problematic. In these conditions, ART should not be commenced for at least 4–6 weeks.

HIV-INDUCED IMMUNODEFICIENCY

There is a strong relationship between the degree of immunodeficiency (as indicated by CD4+ count/percentage) and susceptibility to opportunistic infections. It can also guide the need for prophylactic

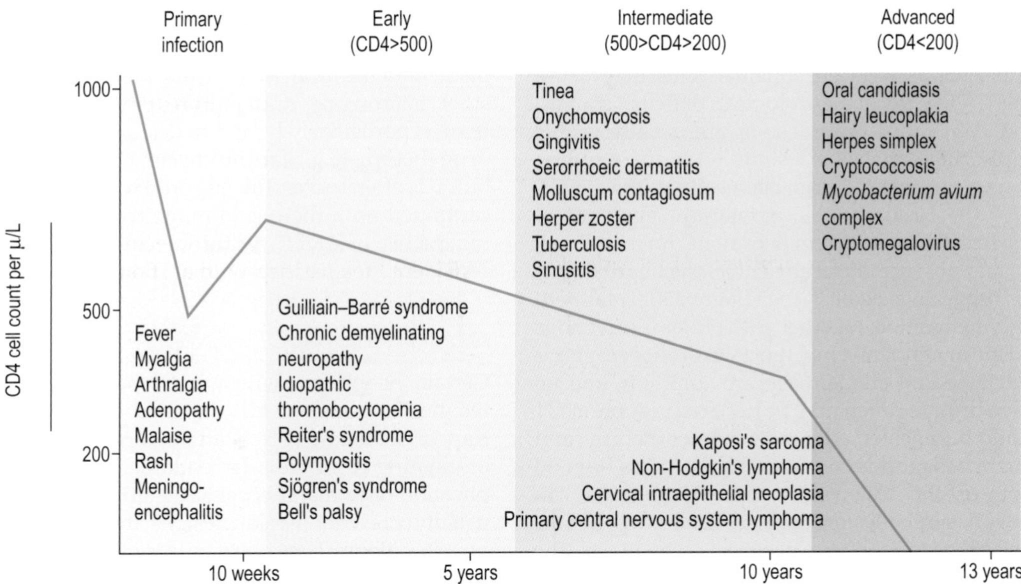

Figure 68.1 Chronological framework for understanding human immunodeficiency virus (HIV) disease and its management.

antimicrobials (**Fig. 68.1**). In addition, some patients have impaired antibody responses and phagocyte dysfunction, which predisposes them to bacterial sepsis.

MAJOR OPPORTUNISTIC INFECTIONS

PNEUMOCYSTIS JIROVECI *PNEUMONITIS*

Interstitial pneumonitis due to *Pneumocystis jiroveci* presents as subacute progressive dyspnoea, non-productive cough and fever. Respiratory examination reveals fever and tachypnoea; however, focal signs are uncommon. The critical finding is that of hypoxia. The chest X-ray or CT scan classically demonstrates interstitial 'ground glass' infiltrates but can be normal. A definitive diagnosis is made by demonstrating *Pneumocystis* cysts in an induced sputum specimen, bronchoalveolar lavage fluid or a transbronchial biopsy.

Severe PJP is best treated with high-dose intravenous co-trimoxazole (trimethoprim-sulfamethoxazole). Many patients develop a hypersensitivity reaction to co-trimoxazole; only severe reactions necessitate changing to intravenous pentamidine. Steroid therapy must be used if the Pa_{O_2} is <70 mmHg (9.3 kPa)[15] with an Fi_{O_2} of 0.21 or if the A-a gradient is >35 mmHg. These patients are also at high risk of a pneumothorax; this needs to be considered if there is a sudden deterioration in respiratory status. Non-invasive ventilation can be effective for severe hypoxaemia; however, if mechanical ventilation is required then lung protective strategies such as low tidal volumes and plateau pressures must be implemented.

Patients with a CD4 T-cell count of <200/mL should receive PJP prophylaxis; most effective is co-trimoxazole, which has added benefit in protecting against other bacterial infections and cerebral toxoplasmosis.[16]

OESOPHAGEAL CANDIDIASIS

Candida infection of the oesophageal mucosa presents with odynophagia and dysphagia. The occurrence of such symptoms in association with oral candidiasis is usually sufficient to start treatment, most commonly with fluconazole. Endoscopy is required for a definitive diagnosis. Patients with severe immunodeficiency and prior azole exposure may have azole resistance and require intravenous amphotericin or an echinocandin.

CRYPTOCOCCAL MENINGITIS

Meningitis is the most common manifestation of infection with *Cryptococcus neoformans* in patients with AIDS. It usually presents with subacute headache and fever, but sometimes confusion or behavioural abnormalities are the predominant abnormalities. Neck stiffness is often minimal or absent, as the immune response responsible for producing this sign is minimal. Cerebrospinal fluid examination (performed after CT imaging has excluded a space-occupying lesion) may also reveal little evidence of inflammation, particularly in the most severe cases. Cryptococcal antigen is virtually always present in both serum and cerebrospinal fluid, and cultures for cryptococci are positive.[17] Intravenous amphotericin is the treatment of choice, usually given in combination with flucytosine; it must be followed by suppressive therapy with oral fluconazole until immune reconstitution is achieved with antiretroviral therapy to prevent relapses.[18]

TOXOPLASMA *ENCEPHALITIS*

Reactivation of *Toxoplasma gondii* infection most commonly presents as focal encephalitis. This may cause headaches, fever, focal neurological deficits, convulsions and even coma. Brain lesions are usually visible as multiple ring-enhancing lesions with surrounding oedema on a contrast CT scan, classically with a predilection for the basal ganglia. Serological evidence of previous *Toxoplasma* infection is present in virtually all patients, and absence of serum *Toxoplasma* antibody is strongly suggestive against the diagnosis. Treatment is oral pyrimethamine, together with either intravenous sulfadiazine or clindamycin. Hypersensitivity reactions to sulfadiazine and clindamycin are common, and an alternative drug regimen may be necessary. A brain CT scan should be repeated after 2–3 weeks of therapy, and an alternative diagnosis considered if there has been no resolution of the lesions. Cerebral lymphoma can produce very similar lesions to *Toxoplasma* encephalitis. A brain biopsy is often necessary to make the diagnosis.[19]

CYTOMEGALOVIRUS (CMV) DISEASE

CMV disease most often occurs in patients with very severe immunodeficiency (CD4 T-cell count <50/mL). The most common site for reactivation of CMV infection is the retina. CMV retinitis usually presents with unilateral blurred vision, visual field loss or 'floaters'. Diagnosis is by fundoscopy and should be confirmed by an ophthalmologist. Treatment is usually with oral valganciclovir; intravenous ganciclovir or foscarnet are alternatives, and rarely intravitreal treatment is given. Induction is followed by suppressive therapy to prevent relapses until there is immune reconstitution following the use of ART.

CMV infection less commonly presents with disease of other organs, particularly the oesophagus, bile ducts or colon. Biopsy of affected tissue is necessary to make a definitive diagnosis. High or increasing CMV viral load in blood should prompt a search for end-organ CMV disease. CMV PCR can be used to monitor the response to therapy and detect antiviral resistance.

CRYPTOSPORIDIOSIS

Infection of the gastrointestinal tract by *Cryptosporidium parvum* causes a severe and intractable secretory diarrhoea, which is often associated with a malabsorption syndrome. It can also cause cholangitis. Diagnosis is by demonstrating *Cryptosporidium* oocysts in faeces and/or a rectal or duodenal biopsy. Antiretroviral therapy to raise the CD4 count is the best treatment.

MYCOBACTERIUM AVIUM *COMPLEX (MAC) INFECTION*

Infection with MAC is usually disseminated and affects blood leukocytes, liver, spleen and lymph nodes, and the gastrointestinal tract. Active infection often results in non-specific symptoms such as weight loss, fatigue, fevers, anaemia and diarrhoea. The diagnosis is usually made by culturing MAC from blood, but sometimes stool microscopy and culture or biopsy of affected tissues, particularly lymph nodes, are necessary. Multidrug therapy (e.g. clarithromycin, rifabutin and ethambutol) is often successful. Suppressive therapy should be continued until there is immune reconstitution following the use of ART.[20] Azithromycin prophylaxis can be considered for patients with a CD4 count less than 50.

AIDS-RELATED NEOPLASMS

Certain neoplasms with a viral pathogenesis characteristically occur in HIV-induced immunodeficiency. Kaposi's sarcoma (KS) is an angioproliferative tumour originating from vascular endothelium, and is a complication of human herpesvirus-8 (HHV-8) infection. It usually presents as skin lesions that have a reddish-purple colour. They vary in extent from one or two small papules to numerous bulbous lesions. The gastrointestinal tract, lymph nodes and internal organs may also be involved in the severely immunosuppressed. A clinical diagnosis of KS can be confirmed by biopsy of a lesion. KS may present at any degree of immunodeficiency but occurs most often, and is more severe, in patients with moderate to severe immunodeficiency. New antimitotic agents plus antiretroviral therapy have resulted in KS essentially disappearing as a clinical problem in treated individuals.

Lymphomas can also complicate HIV-induced immunodeficiency. The great majority are B-cell lymphomas (non-Hodgkin's), and reactivation of Epstein–Barr virus infection is implicated in the pathogenesis of most cases. Primary cerebral lymphoma or extracerebral lymphoma, which often has extranodal involvement, is common in patients with severe immunodeficiency. These lymphomas are usually high grade. Treatment consists of whole brain radiation, steroids and antiretroviral therapy.[21]

Cervical intraepithelial neoplasia and cancer are more common and aggressive in women with HIV infection, as are anal neoplasia and cancer in males.

HIV-RELATED NEUROLOGICAL DISEASE

HIV infection of macrophages and microglial cells in the nervous system often results in neurological disease by incompletely understood mechanisms. Encephalopathy, myelopathy and peripheral neuropathy are all possible. In a small number of patients, the neurological disease is more problematic than the immunodeficiency. The encephalopathy usually develops insidiously in individuals with advanced immunodeficiency and eventually results in cognitive, motor and behavioural abnormalities. Myelopathy, which is now rare, results in an ataxic spastic paraparesis.[22]

Investigation of HIV patients with space-occupying cerebral lesions requires analysis of serology, cerebrospinal fluid and neuroimaging investigations. Analysis of cerebrospinal fluid includes polymerase chain reaction (PCR) for Epstein–Barr virus (indicative of lymphoma), herpes simplex virus, CMV, varicella–zoster virus (viral encephalitis), JC virus (indicative of progressive multifocal leucoencephalopathy), toxoplasmosis and *Mycobacterium tuberculosis*.[23]

NEEDLE-STICK INJURIES AND POSTEXPOSURE PROPHYLAXIS

Patients with unrecognised HIV infection or AIDS may also be admitted to an ICU with the first manifestation of HIV disease. Known patients with HIV in the ICU may be outnumbered by undiagnosed patients with HIV; it is therefore important for all ICU staff to practice stringent infection control procedures at all times, and this will also protect them against other bloodborne viruses.

HIV transmission from needle sticks occurs at a rate of approximately 0.3%, and from mucosal exposure at a rate of approximately 0.009%. There have been no reported seroconversions after skin exposure. The major risk factors for infection after a needle-stick injury are: (1) deep injury; (2) visible blood on device; (3) needle placement in a vein or artery; and (4) a source patient with late-stage HIV/AIDS (high viral load).

Antiretroviral prophylaxis reduces transmission rates.[24] A protocol for dealing with blood and body fluid exposure should therefore be developed for every health care institution.

Access the complete references list online at http://www.expertconsult.com

1. Greenberg JA, Lennox JL, Martin GS. Outcomes for critically ill patients with HIV and severe sepsis in the era of highly active antiretroviral therapy. J Crit Care 2012;27(1):51–7.
2. Masur H. Caring for AIDS patients in the ICU: expanding horizons. Chest 2009;135(1):1–2.
11. Müller M, Wandel S, Colebunders R, et al; IeDEA Southern and Central Africa. Immune reconstitution inflammatory syndrome in patients starting antiretroviral therapy for HIV infection: a systematic review and meta-analysis. Lancet Infect Dis 2010;10(4):251–61.
12. French MA, Lenzo N, John M, et al. Immune restoration disease after the treatment of immunodeficient HIV-infected patients with highly active antiretroviral therapy. HIV Med 2000;1:107–15.
14. Zolopa AR, Andersen J, Komarow L, et al. Early antiretroviral therapy reduces AIDS progression/death in individuals with acute opportunistic infections: a multicenter randomized strategy trial. PloS one, 2009;4(5):5575–e5575.
23. Antinori A, Ammassari A, De Luca A, et al. Diagnosis of AIDS-related focal brain lesions: a decision-making analysis based on clinical and neuroradiologic characteristics combined with polymerase chain reaction assays in CSF. Neurology 1997;48:687–94.
24. Young TN, Arens FJ, Kennedy GE , et al. Antiretroviral post-exposure prophylaxis (PEP) for occupational HIV exposure. Cochrane Database Syst Rev 2007;1:CD002835.

69

Severe sepsis

A Raffaele De Gaudio

Sepsis remains a common problem in critically ill patients, and is strongly related to morbidity, mortality and costs. The incidence of severe sepsis has been increasing steadily over the last three decades, in part due to the ageing of Western populations. Nearly 15% of patients in intensive care units present with severe sepsis, and two-thirds of them have septic shock. Despite intense research, only a few new therapies have been developed, and the mainstay of treatment remains non-specific advanced life support.[1–3] The failure to develop new therapies suggests that our knowledge of the pathological process of sepsis in humans is inadequate.[4]

DEFINITION

The internationally accepted definition of severe sepsis was outlined during a conference held in 2001 and 2003 and requires a specific set of physiological and laboratory indices associated with a clinical suspicion of a new onset of an infection as the source of the abnormalities[5,6] (**Box 69.1**).

Sepsis is defined as an infection associated with a systemically activated inflammation response syndrome (SIRS) and has a mortality rate of 10–15%. To further differentiate illness severity, severe sepsis is defined as sepsis with multi-organ dysfunction (mortality rate 17–20%), and septic shock is defined as severe sepsis with haemodynamic instability despite fluids and vasoactive drugs (mortality rate 43–54%) (**Fig. 69.1**). The compensatory anti-inflammatory response syndrome (CARS) following SIRS is indicative of immunosuppression that may last for a long period of time. These definitions delineate gradations of mortality risk, but they do not adequately stratify patients into homogeneous groups with respect to the underlying pathophysiology or their potential response to therapy. That is, they define concepts but do not identify patients with a single disease. To resolve this problem, a staging system (PIRO) was proposed that includes domains for **p**redisposition (premorbid illness), **i**nsult/infection (site, microbiology of infection and severity of other insults, such as trauma), **r**esponse (hypotension) and **o**rgan dysfunction (sequential organ failure assessment, SOFA).[5–7]

PATHOGENESIS

Severe sepsis represents an uncontrolled immune response (SIRS) to exposure to different types of micro-organisms and microbial products (**Table 69.1**). Gram-negative bacilli (mainly *Escherichia coli*, *Klebsiella* spp. and *Pseudomonas aeruginosa*) and Gram-positive cocci (mainly staphylococci) are the pathogens most commonly associated with the development of the syndrome. Fungi, mostly *Candida albicans*, account for 17% of all cases of severe sepsis.[8]

The innate immune system describes a network of immune cells and their surface receptors designed to recognise and react to either dead tissue or pathogens. When either of these elements encounters certain lymphocytes or monocytes, it binds to pre-existing receptors and causes the activation of lymphocytes, or is ingested and then presented to cell surface receptors to activate monocytes. The expansion and activation of several immune cell lines, such as polymorphonucleocytes (PMNs) and B lymphocytes stimulated by the pro-inflammatory cytokines, then follows.

The pathophysiology of bacterial sepsis is initiated by the outer membrane components of Gram-negative organisms (lipopolysaccharide, lipid A, flagellin and peptidoglycan), Gram-positive organisms (teichoic acid, lipoteichoic acid and peptidoglycan) and fungi (mannan-proteins). These outer-membrane components and products of tissue destruction are able to bind to the CD14 receptor, a protein anchored in the outer leaflet of the surface of monocytes. Microorganism components also interact with co-receptors called Toll-like receptors (TLR), which show a degree of specificity for pathogenic microbes and tissue products (e.g. TLR2 for teichoic and lipoteichoic acid or TLR4 for lipopolysaccharide) (**Fig. 69.2**).[9–11]

The binding of TLR activates intracellular signalling pathways that trigger transcription factors, such as nuclear factor-κB, which in turn control the expression of immune response genes, resulting in the release of cytokines (**Fig. 69.3**). The appearance of a 'cytokine storm' expands beyond a restricted local microenvironment and spreads to the systemic circulation (such as through bacteraemia).[12] Immune cells secrete cytokines with inflammatory properties (TNF-α, IL-1, IL-2 and

Box 69.1 Diagnosis of sepsis

SIRS criteria
Heart rate >90 beats/min
Temperature <36.0 or >38.3°C
Blood glucose >7.7 mmol/L (in the absence of diabetes)
Respiratory rate >20/min
White cell count <4 or >12×10⁹/L
Acutely altered mental state

Sites responsible for infection
Cough/sputum/chest pain
Abdominal pain/distension/diarrhoea
Line infection
Endocarditis
Dysuria
Headache with neck stiffness
Cellulitis/wound/joint infection

Evidence of organ dysfunction
Blood pressure systolic <90/mean <65 mmHg (12/8.66 kPa) (after initial fluid challenge)
Lactate >2 mmol/L after initial fluids
INR >1.5 or a PTT >60 s
Bilirubin >34 μmol/L
Urine output <0.5 mL/kg/h for 2 h
Creatinine >177 μmol/L
Platelets <100×10⁹/L
Sp_{O_2} >90% unless O_2 given

From Daniels.[6]

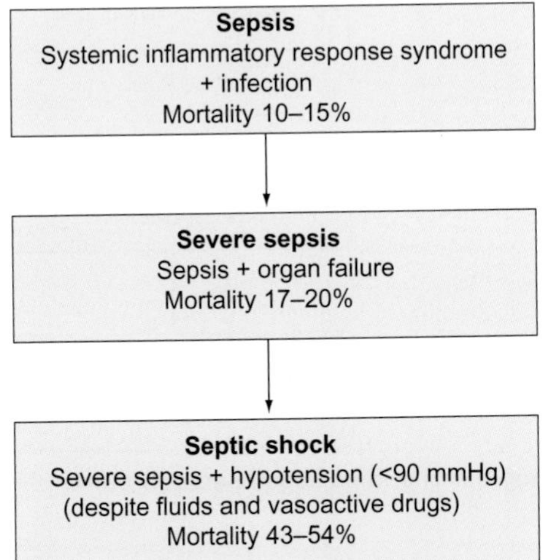

Figure 69.1 Sepsis definitions: despite significant advances, sepsis continues to be associated with high morbidity and mortality.

Table 69.1 Types of microorganisms in culture-positive infected patients in critically ill septic patients

ORGANISM	(%)
Gram-positive (%)	46.8
Staphylococcus aureus	20.5
MRSA	10.2
S. epidermis	10.8
Streptococcus pneumoniae	4.1
VSE	7.1
VRE	3.8
Other	6.4
Gram-negative (%)	62.2
Escherichia coli	16.0
Enterobacter	7.0
Klebsiella species	12.7
Pseudomonas species	19.9
Acinetobacter species	8.8
Other	17.0
ESBL-producing	1.9
Anaerobes	4.5
Other bacteria	1.5
Fungi (%)	
Candida	17
Aspergillus	1.4
Other	1
Parasites	0.7
Other organisms	3.9

From Vincent et al.[8]

IL-6) and activated leucocytes, promote leucocyte-vascular endothelium adhesion and induce endothelial damage.[7] This endothelial damage, in turn, leads to tissue factor expression and activation of the tissue-factor-dependent clotting cascade with subsequent formation of thrombin such that microaggregates of fibrin, platelets, neutrophils and red blood cells impair capillary blood flow, thereby decreasing the delivery of oxygen and nutrients.[7,9]

Early inflammatory cytokines increase the expression of enzyme-inducible nitric oxide synthase (iNOS) in endothelial cells, and increased synthesis of the potent vasodilator nitric oxide leads to a decrease in systemic vascular resistance characteristic of septic shock. Cytokines and other inflammatory mediators induce gaps between endothelial cells by disassembling intercellular junctions, by altering the cellular cytoskeletal structure or by directly damaging the cell monolayer. The creation of these gaps can result in microvascular leaking and tissue oedema, both of which are characteristic of sepsis.[13]

IL-6 alters hepatocyte protein synthesis, inducing the synthesis of acute-phase reactants and promoting

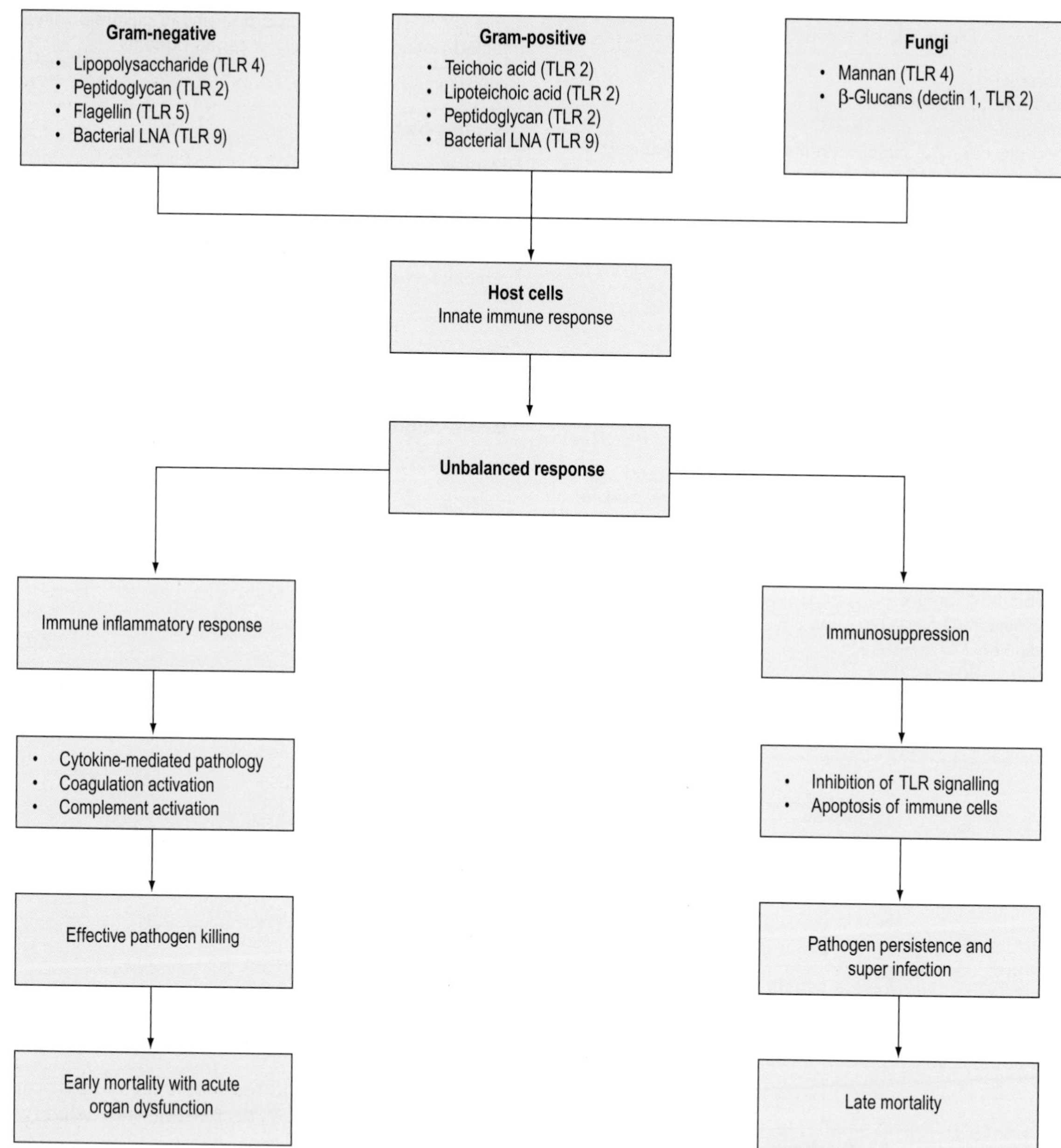

Figure 69.2 Sepsis pathogenesis and progression from effective pathogen killing to pathogen persistence and superinfection.

anaemia. The acute-phase response also results in the down-regulation of albumin production and anticoagulant proteins, such as protein C.[14]

Microcirculatory dysfunction plays a key role in the development of organ failure in severely septic patients.[15] As a result of the vicious cycle of inflammation and coagulation, cardiovascular insufficiency (due to the myocardial-depressant effect of TNF, vasodilation and capillary leaking) and multiple-organ failure occur, often leading to death.[14]

The production of anti-inflammatory cytokines (IL-4 and IL-10) during SIRS results in the expression of CARS, which is considered to be a compensatory response by the immune system in an attempt to reduce the systemic activated inflammatory immune responses responsible for tissue injury and organ failure.[16,17] This anti-inflammatory response indicates that sepsis can be associated with a state of immunosuppression that may last for extended periods of time (weeks, months and/or years) following the initial onset of SIRS.[12,16,17]

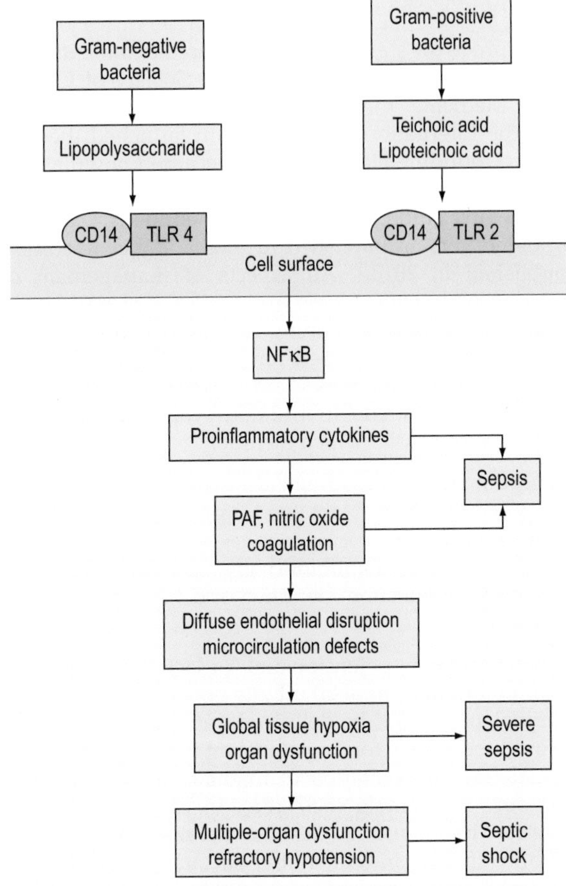

Figure 69.3 Pathogenesis of bacterial sepsis.

In many cases of sepsis, the immune system fails to eradicate the infectious pathogens, and a prolonged phase of sepsis-induced immunosuppression begins, characterised by a failure to eradicate the primary infection and by the development of secondary nosocomial infections. This immunosuppression is mediated by multiple mechanisms, including massive apoptosis of lymphocytes (see Fig. 69.2).[17]

DIAGNOSIS

The initial presentation of severe sepsis and septic shock is often non-specific and 'cryptic'. The diagnosis requires a presumed or known site of infection, evidence of SIRS and acute sepsis-associated organ dysfunction (Table 69.1).

CARDIOVASCULAR FAILURE

Adequately resuscitated patients with severe sepsis display hyperdynamic circulation with warm peripheries, low systemic vascular resistance and high cardiac output (CO). However, despite the increase in CO and normal stroke volume, many patients suffer from intrinsic myocardial dysfunction with a reduction in ejection fraction. Septic cardiomyopathy is characterised by biventricular impairment of intrinsic myocardial contractility with a subsequent reduction in left ventricular (LV) ejection fraction and LV stroke work index.[18] Bedside echocardiography is critical in the evaluation of ventricular size and function.

PULMONARY DYSFUNCTION

Detection of sepsis is facilitated by the nearly universal presence of tachypnoea and hypoxaemia. The lung can be one of the targets of the overwhelming acute systemic inflammatory response triggered in other organs. Mild, moderate or severe[19] acute respiratory distress syndrome (ARDS) can be caused by direct (pulmonary) injury, such as pneumonia, or by an indirect (extrapulmonary) insult to the lung in the case of sepsis and septic shock.[20]

SEPSIS AND ACUTE KIDNEY INJURY

According to the RIFLE (**r**isk, **i**njury, **f**ailure, **l**oss, **e**nd-stage renal disease) criteria, acute kidney injury (AKI) can be diagnosed by small changes in serum creatinine or acute reductions in urine output.[20] The development of AKI during sepsis increases patient morbidity, predicts higher mortality and has a significant effect on multiple organ functions.[21]

Until recently, it was generally believed that, like other causes of shock (hypovolaemic or cardiogenic), sepsis-induced AKI was mainly due to kidney hypoperfusion. If true, this would imply that hypoperfusion improvement and renal blood flow should be the primary targets of renoprotection in sepsis.[22]

LIVER DYSFUNCTION

The liver is a mechanical and immunological filter for portal blood and may be a major source of cytokines. An increase in aminotransferase and bilirubin levels is common, but hepatic failure is rare. Recently, subclinical liver injury has been identified in critically ill patients.

Microcirculatory changes in the liver sinusoids, neutrophil sequestration, and platelet activation and adhesion have been proposed as the main contributors to known hepatic dysfunction parameters. Cholestasis, steatosis, hepatocellular injury, impaired cellular regeneration and impaired hepatic mitochondrial respiration are factors implicated in the clinical septic hepatic dysfunction.[23]

COAGULATION ABNORMALITIES

Subclinical coagulopathy, with a mild elevation of the prothrombin or partial thromboplastin time, a moderate reduction in platelet count or an increase in plasma fibrinogen degradation and D-dimer levels, may occur. Coagulopathy is caused by deficiencies of the coagulation system proteins antithrombin III, protein C, the tissue factor pathway and the kinin system. Simultaneous activation of coagulation by inflammatory cytokines and reduced production of anticoagulant proteins contribute to disseminated intravascular coagulation.[23]

SEPSIS-ASSOCIATED ENCEPHALOPATHY

Diffuse cerebral dysfunction is often present in sepsis and may ensue even before signs of other organ failure. It is better defined as 'sepsis-associated encephalopathy' (SAE) to stress the absence of direct infection of the central nervous system. The main sign of SAE is altered mental status. Electroencephalography is the most sensitive diagnostic test and allows the grading of the severity of cerebral dysfunction that is related to outcome. SAE is potentially reversible but always worsens the prognosis. The pathophysiology of SAE is still not completely understood, and it is most likely multifactorial. Indeed, brain dysfunction in sepsis may be related to microorganism toxin activity, the effects of inflammatory mediators, metabolic alterations and to abnormalities in cerebral circulation. Experimental studies have shown that microcirculatory dysfunction, a consequence of endothelial activation, is an early pathogenic step.[24–26]

BIOMARKERS

More than 80 biological markers of sepsis have been proposed for diagnosis and prognosis, including C-reactive protein, IL-6 and procalcitonin (PCT). PCT has emerged as the most specific biomarker for bacterial infections. A multitude of observational studies have reported on its diagnostic potential in distinct types of infections. However, PCT measurements may decrease antibiotic use without compromising clinical outcome.[27]

Several polymorphisms of genes broadly involved in inflammation, immunity and coagulation have been linked with outcome in sepsis. Since management of severe sepsis suffers from the lack of effective biomarkers and largely empirical predictions of disease progression and therapeutic responses, the availability of genetic biomarkers for predicting therapeutic responses would be very useful.[28]

TREATMENT

Timely and proper care of the patient with severe sepsis is essential. There has been considerable debate around treatment guidelines, particularly those relating to invasive management. The most widely discussed guidelines are those from the Surviving Sepsis Campaign.[6]

SURVIVING SEPSIS CAMPAIGN (SSC)

To improve the standard of care offered to patients with severe sepsis and septic shock, the Society of Critical Care Medicine, the European Intensive Care Society and the International Sepsis Forum launched the SSC with a founding statement that became known as the 'Barcelona declaration'.

The first guidelines were published in 2004, with an updated version published in 2008 and a new edition published in 2013.[29] All aspects of management of patients with severe sepsis were covered; recommendations or bundles, depending on the available level of evidence, were developed for each category. A set of the following recommendations has to be completed for all patients within the first 12 hours following the onset of severe sepsis,[29,30] which include:

- serum lactate measurements
- blood cultures obtained prior to antibiotic administration
- broad-spectrum antibiotics given within 3 hours
- source of infection identified and treated within 12 hours.

When there is hypotension and/or lactate >4 mmol/L, an initial minimum of 30 mL/kg crystalloid (or colloid equivalent) should be delivered and vasoactive drugs should be given for hypotension not responding to initial fluid resuscitation to maintain a mean arterial pressure ≥65 mmHg (8.67 kPa). In case of persistent arterial hypotension, despite volume resuscitation (septic shock) and/or initial lactate >4 mmol/L, a central venous pressure of ≥8 mmHg (1.07 kPa) should be maintained and a central venous (superior vena cava) oxygen saturation of ≥70% should be achieved.

These guidelines have been endorsed by many professional organisations worldwide and are regarded as the standard of care for the management of patients with severe sepsis.[6,29,31] However, at the moment, there is no evidence of additional beneficial effects.[6,31]

SOURCE CONTROL OF INFECTION

Adequate source control of infection is as important as appropriate antimicrobial therapy. All patients presenting with the clinical suspicion of sepsis should be evaluated for the possible presence of a focus of infection amenable to treatment by source control measures. A source of infection should be rapidly sought through integration of the clinical history, physical examination and the results of focused diagnostic tests and imaging examinations. Advances in diagnostic or interventional radiology and surgical procedures have revolutionised the management of human infections. Source control includes removal of infected foreign bodies (such as intravascular catheters and vascular draft) incision and drainage (open or percutaneous) of abscesses or fluid collections and the debridement of infected necrotic tissue; the restoration of anatomy and physiological function is often the goal of surgical intervention. For patients with necrotising fasciitis, mortality and extent of tissue loss are directly related to the rapidity of surgical intervention.[7]

ANTIMICROBIAL THERAPY

The site of infection and causative organisms are often unknown. Broad-spectrum antimicrobial therapy must be administered empirically in these cases, guided by knowledge of the most common site of infection and the most common infecting organisms. Specimens for culture and sensitivity testing should be obtained before empirical antibiotic therapy is started. Observational studies suggest a significant reduction in mortality when antibiotics are administered within 4–8 hours of hospital admission. Current SSC recommendations consider administration of antibiotics within 3 hours of sepsis diagnosis. Despite the absence of strong evidence, antibiotic de-escalation has been recommended.[32,33] Specific antibiotic strategies may be found in Chapters 36, 54 and 70–73.

EARLY HAEMODYNAMIC RESUSCITATION (FIRST 6 HOURS)

Haemodynamic resuscitation to normal physiological parameters has been defined as early goal-directed therapy (EGDT). EGDT aims to restore the balance between oxygen supply and demand within the first 6 hours from diagnosis, leading to a significant reduction of mortality[30] and optimising the intravascular volume. A low central venous saturation ($Scv_{O_2} \leq 70\%$) coupled with an elevated lactate level suggests a mismatch between systemic oxygen delivery and oxygen consumption in the tissues. When low Scv_{O_2} is identified, therapies to increase the components of oxygen delivery are recommended to restore the balance between systemic oxygen delivery and consumption (oxygen-carrying capacity, arterial oxygen saturation and cardiac output). Despite the fact that early and vigorous fluid replacement is widely recognised as good clinical practice, EGDT has faced significant criticisms: the protocol is complex and should be implemented very early, some of the steps (use of packed red blood cells and inotropes) are not universally accepted and there is a great deal of controversy over the use of Scv_{O_2} as a surrogate of tissue hypoxia.[34] In addition, central venous pressure neither reflects intravascular volume nor predicts fluid responsiveness and has no place in the resuscitation of patients with sepsis.[31]

FLUID THERAPY

Recent advances in the pathophysiology of sepsis-related multiorgan dysfunction and on restoring tissue perfusion have provided the basis for protocols using physiology-based approaches to guide fluid therapy.[34] Initial resuscitation efforts should incorporate intravenous fluid therapy. The first goal of volume therapy of sepsis is repletion of the patient's intravascular volume deficit. The selection of crystalloid versus colloid solutions has been vigorously debated. Recently in a multicentre randomised clinical trial it was demonstrated that patients with severe sepsis assigned to fluid resuscitation with HES 130/0.4 had an increased risk of death at day 90 and were more likely to require renal replacement therapy, compared with those receiving Ringer's acetate.[35] A large volume of crystalloids is usually required, and more oedema will result. However, it is not likely that peripheral oedema carries significant clinical risk.[6] Intravenous fluid therapy should begin with 30 mL/kg of crystalloids.[29]

VASOPRESSORS

The initial goal for septic shock resuscitation includes the administration of intravenous fluid followed by vasopressor if organ perfusion cannot be maintained with fluids alone. Vasoactive agents should be administered when hypotension is persistent or mean arterial blood pressure is less than 65 mmHg (8.67 kPa). However, no evidence clearly supports the superiority of one vasopressor over another (among norepinephrine, epinephrine and vasopressin). Norepinephrine is considered as the first-line agent, followed by dobutamine or epinephrine, in patients with poor left ventricular (LV) function.[31] Dopamine has a number of theoretical disadvantages in patients with sepsis. It tends to increase heart rate and myocardial oxygen demand, and it is associated with splanchnic mucosal ischaemia.[31] Dopamine appears to increase the risk for arrhythmia if administered at high-level doses, even if there is no difference in mortality between norepinephrine and dopamine treatment.[36] The SSC recommends vasopressin infusion for refractory shock and in limited doses with the intent of raising MAP to target or decreasing norepinephrine dosage.[29] The choice of a specific vasopressor may be individualised and left to the discretion of the treating physicians.[36]

ADMINISTRATION OF ERYTHROCYTES

The patient's oxygen-carrying capacity may be augmented by the administration of packed erythrocytes to achieve a haematocrit above 30%, with a more restrictive transfusion strategy in the convalescent phase of the disease.[29,37] Although the intent of blood transfusions is to increase tissue oxygenation, this intervention may have unexpected effects. Poorly deformable transfused red blood cells may alter microvascular flow. Furthermore, the P50 of stored red cells may be as low as 6 mmHg (0.8 kPa), with the red blood cells being able to unload less than 6% of the carried oxygen; stored cells may thereby increase the Scv_{O_2} (by binding oxygen) but compound the tissue oxygen debt by decreasing oxygen unloading.[31]

ADDITIONAL GENERAL TREATMENT COMPONENTS

Additional components in the care of severe sepsis include:

- strategies to minimise oxygen demand and the fatigue of breathing (non-invasive and invasive ventilation)
- sedation with daily awakening
- adequate early enteral nutrition
- deep-vein thrombus prevention
- gastric ulcer prophylaxis
- selective antimicrobial decontamination of the gastrointestinal tract.

ADJUVANT THERAPIES

Several additional therapies initiated early after the identification of severe sepsis have been proposed to improve patient outcome. Currently, there is no consensus regarding these issues.

STEROIDS

Corticosteroid therapy has been used in various doses for more than 50 years with no clear benefit in mortality.[38] Therefore, steroid administration in severe sepsis and septic shock remains controversial. The SSC recommends the use of intravenous corticosteroids in patients with septic shock who, despite adequate fluid replacement, require vasopressor therapy to maintain blood pressure.[29] The administration of hydrocortisone in a dose of 50 mg every 6 hours or 10 mg/h[31] can be considered.

BLOOD GLUCOSE CONTROL

The prevalence of hyperglycaemia is estimated to be higher than 40% among critically ill septic patients. It is considered to be associated with increased adverse outcomes, such as poor immune response, increased cardiovascular events, thrombosis, delayed wound healing, infection and mortality. Intensive insulin therapy (IIT) is defined as the maintenance of blood glucose between 80 and 110 mg/dL (4.4 to 6.1 mmol/L). This intervention has generated a great deal of controversy. There is no evidence that IIT reduces mortality, infection rates, length of stay or the need for renal replacement therapy. Additionally there is an increased risk of severe hypoglycaemia. Currently, a target blood glucose level of 140–200 mg/dL is recommended (7.8–11.1 mmol/L).[39]

EXTRACORPOREAL BLOOD PURIFICATION TECHNIQUES[40,41]

Multiple applications of blood purification techniques in critically ill patients have made possible the evolution of management of such patients using a new therapeutic strategy called 'multiple organ support therapy'.

As in severe sepsis, the strategy is to overtake renal support and to modulate systemic inflammation, and high-volume haemofiltration (HVHF) appears to be a promising option. Although there are still no large, multicentre, randomised, controlled trials showing beneficial effects on mortality with HVHF, preliminary studies in humans and preclinical animal data support this intervention. Other extracorporeal blood purification therapies are currently available: coupled plasma filtration adsorption, polymyxin-B haemoperfusion and the use of high cut-off membranes have been proposed as adjuvant treatments for sepsis. However, it is not currently possible to determine which technique is the most effective because they have not been compared with one another. Nevertheless, an additional hybrid technique can synergistically combine HVHF and haemoadsorption in a technique called 'high adsorptive haemofiltration.'[41]

PROTECTIVE LUNG STRATEGIES, ECCO2R AND ECMO[42,43]

Low-tidal-volume ventilation (6 mL/kg with plateau pressure maintained at <30 cmH_2O) is generally well tolerated and may confer some protection against ventilator-associated lung injury. This intervention has not been associated with clinically important adverse outcomes except for hypercapnic respiratory acidosis. When lung-protective strategies are unsuccessful, various technologies, such as extracorporeal CO_2 removal (ECCO2R) and veno-venous extracorporeal membrane oxygenation (ECMO), can produce significant temporary improvement. Benefits in patient outcome have been shown with the use of these techniques in H1N1 septic patients, but this improvement does not seem to affect the outcome of other patients.[43]

ACTIVATED PROTEIN C (APC)

The use of recombinant human APC to treat severe sepsis was believed to have unique effects on the immune-coagulatory pathways; in 2001, it became the only pharmaceutical aid on the market designed specifically to treat sepsis. This intervention has generated a great deal of controversy since its introduction and in 2011, after negative preliminary results of the PROWESS-SHOCK trial, its market withdrawal was announced.[39,44]

CONCLUSIONS

The past two decades have seen a remarkable growth in our understanding of the complex interconnection of multiple biological pathways involved in the sepsis pathogenesis. However, the overall mortality rate for patients is still high. The early source control, the administration of appropriate antibiotics and the haemodynamic resuscitation remain the cornerstone of the management of patients with severe sepsis.

Access the complete references list online at http://www.expertconsult.com

6. Daniels R. Surviving the first hours in sepsis: getting the basics rights (an intensivist 's perspective). J Antimicrob Chemother 2011;66(Suppl 2):ii11–23.
12. Carson WF, Cavassani K, Dou Y. Epigenetic regulation of immune cell functions during post-septic immunosuppression. Epigenetics 2011;6:273–83.
16. Ward PA. Immunosuppression in sepsis. JAMA 2011;306:2618–19.
22. Zarjou A, Agarwall A. Sepsis and acute kidney injury. J Am Soc Nephrol 2011;22:999–1006.
27. Kopterides P, Tsangaris I. Procalcitonin and sepsis: recent data on diagnostic utility, prognosticpotential and therapeutic implications in critically ill patients. Minerva Anestesiol 2012;78(7):823–35. Epub 2012 May 4.
29. Dellinger RP, Levy M, Rhodes A, et al. Surviving Sepsis campaign: international guidelines for management of severe sepsis and septic shock: 2013. Critical Care Med 2013;41:580–637.
43. Gattinoni L, Carlesso E, Langer T. Towards ultraprotective mechanical ventilation. Curr Op Anaesthesiol 2012;25:14–17.

70

Nosocomial infections

James Hatcher and Rishi H-P Dhillon

Nosocomial or health-care-associated infections (HCAI) are a major problem in hospitals, affecting up to 9% of inpatients at any one time. Intensive care units (ICUs) represent 2–10% of hospital beds, but are responsible for 25% of all nosocomial bloodstream and pulmonary infections. In the European Prevalence of Infection in Intensive Care (EPIC) and EPIC II studies' snapshot of prevalence showed the infection rate in ICU was 44.8% and 51% respectively, with ICU-associated infection 20.6% in the EPIC study.[1,2] Nosocomial infection is, at least in theory, a preventable cause of morbidity and mortality (**Box 70.1**).

EPIDEMIOLOGY

The prevalence of nosocomial infection is reported as being between 3 and 12% in most institutions but varies considerably between different sites within each institution.[3] The vulnerability of the patient population, the nature of interventions and cross-infection are but three of many factors. This is seen clearly if one compares the range between ophthalmology and critical care: 0–23%.[4]

The site of infection varies with location so that, whereas the urinary tract and the chest are common throughout the hospital, within the ICU surgical wound infection, pneumonia and bloodstream infection are far more common (8–12%).

The impact of nosocomial infection is impressive. Ventilator-associated pneumonia (VAP) is common, has significant morbidity with increased length of stay, associated costs and a twofold increase in mortality.[5] It has been suggested that bloodstream infections, surgical wound infections and nosocomial pneumonia result in 14, 12 and 13 attributable extra hospital days respectively.[6] Catheter-related bloodstream infection (CR-BSI) was also associated with major morbidity although, curiously, not necessarily mortality.[7] The mortality rates directly due to these infections are hard to separate from the mortality attributed to the presenting severity of illness, which in its own right may have predisposed to infection. What is clear is that nosocomial infection is associated with increased mortality, and huge financial and resource costs.[2]

INTERACTION BETWEEN PATIENT, ORGANISM AND ENVIRONMENT

A number of factors come together to enable nosocomial infection to occur. Some may be risk factors in their own right, whereas others may simply represent an identifier of a sicker and therefore more vulnerable population (**Box 70.2**).

The host usually lives in synergistic or symbiotic tranquillity with a huge range of organisms (**Table 70.1**). Antibiotics suppress many normal organisms and allow the emergence and overgrowth of a usually insignificant organism or a resistant organism of the same type. For example, an intrinsic organism such as *Candida* will flourish in the presence of broad-spectrum antibiotics and this overgrowth may result in symptomatic or even invasive candidiasis; cephalosporin use may encourage the intrinsically resistant but quiescent enterococci to emerge as a problematic organism.

Extrinsic organisms may be introduced from the environment, from other patients, from staff or from surfaces. These may be organisms that are thriving in that environment because of local pressures (e.g. antibiotics), or from poor hygiene. Examples include *Acinetobacter baumanii* and, of course, meticillin (methicillin)-resistant *Staphylococcus aureus* (MRSA). On admission, patients will be carrying a range of organisms that have the potential to cause problems, but during their stay they are likely to acquire a new ecology from their surroundings. In a hospital that ecology may be quite hostile, with multiresistance being common.

The great debate remains as to interpretation of microbiology results in the context of a non-septic patient; is this infection or colonisation? This can be challenging to decipher and highlights the importance of reviewing the patient clinically whilst making a judgement on any positive microbiology result. No results should be acted on in isolation, and best care is often enacted through multidisciplinary efforts.

A vast range of organisms can cause nosocomial infection (**Box 70.3**). It must be emphasised that each hospital and each ICU will have its own local ecology and knowing this information is important. Regional, national and international surveys give indications of

Box 70.1 Principles of diagnosis of nosocomial infections

- Diagnosis of infection usually requires the combination of both clinical findings and the results of diagnostic tests
- Clinical diagnosis of infection from direct observation at surgery, endoscopy or other diagnostic procedure is an acceptable criterion for an infection
- It must be hospital-acquired. There must be no evidence that the infection was present or incubating at the time of hospital admission. Infection acquired in hospital, but only evident after hospital discharge, also fulfils the criteria
- Usually no specific time during or after hospitalisation is given to determine whether an infection is nosocomial or community-acquired. Each infection is examined for evidence that links it to hospitalisation (this is a matter of controversy)

Box 70.2 Risk factors for nosocomial infection

Patient
Severity of illness
Underlying diseases
Nutritional state
Immunosuppression
Open wounds
Invasive devices
Multiple procedures
Prolonged stay
Ventilation
Multiple or prolonged antibiotics
Blood transfusion
Environment
Changes in procedures or protocols
Multiple changes in staff; new staff
Poor aseptic practice – poor hand washing
Patient-to-patient – busy, crowded unit, staff shortages
The organism
Resistance
Resilience in terms of survival
Formation of slime or ability to adhere
Pathogenicity
Prevalence

general trends, but this does not supplant local knowledge.

The individual characteristics of the organism are important. These include their resilience in the local environment, the ease of transmission and the individual pathogenicity. This clearly interacts with the vulnerability of the host, as some usually innocuous organisms such as *Candida* spp. or *Serratia marcescens* will cause problems only in vulnerable hosts, whereas others such as some strains of *S. aureus, Pseudomonas aeruginosa* or *Clostridium difficile* may be intrinsically more virulent.

Box 70.3 Organisms responsible for the majority of nosocomial infections

Meticillin-resistant *Staphylococcus aureus* (MRSA)
Coagulase-negative *Staphylococcus* (CNS)
Enterococcus spp. (*E. faecalis, E. faecium*)
Pseudomonas aeruginosa
Acinetobacter baumanii
Stenotrophomonas maltophilia
Enterobacter spp.
Klebsiella spp.
Escherichia coli
Serratia marcescens
Proteus spp.
Candida spp. (*C. albicans, C. glabrata, C. krusei*)

Other organisms may be a problem in the severely immunocompromised, such as those with acquired immunodeficiency syndrome (AIDS; see Ch. 68).

Table 70.1 Common commensals that may cause infection in a vulnerable host

SITE	COMMON COMMENSAL ORGANISMS
Skin	*Staphylococcus epidermidis*, streptococci, *Corynebacterium* (diphtheroids), *Candida* spp.
Throat	*Viridans group streptococci*, diphtheroids
Mouth	*Viridans group streptococci*, *Moraxella catarrhalis*, *Actinomyces*, spirochaetes
Respiratory tract	*Viridans group streptococci*, *Moraxella*, diphtheroids, micrococci
Vagina	Lactobacilli, diphtheroids, streptococci, yeast
Intestines	*Bacteroides* spp., anaerobic streptococci, *Clostridium perfringens*, *Escherichia coli*, *Klebsiella* spp., *Proteus* spp., enterococci

Nosocomial infection is dynamic in that it is influenced by many environmental factors, the type of patient, type of surgery or illness, the antibiotic usage profile and many other variables. This dynamism is illustrated by the Gram-positive infections of the 1950s and 1960s giving way to the Gram-negative infections of the 1970s and, although the multiresistant Gram-positive organisms are a major anxiety currently, they are already being superseded by superresistant Gram-negative organisms such as extended-spectrum β-lactamase (ESBL)-producing *Enterobacteriaceae*, MDR *Pseudomonas aeruginosa*, *Stenotrophomonas maltophila* and *Acinetobacter baumanii*. The ease of transmission or development of resistance is a key factor in the current explosion in multiresistance.

The combination of sick patients and widespread use of potent antibiotics selects out problematic organisms and, as this epitomises intensive care practice, it is in ICU where multiresistance is common.

RESISTANT ORGANISMS

Many of the organisms that cause nosocomial infection are characterised by multiresistance. There are several mechanisms involved in resistance and in its spread. Generally speaking, there are four main mechanisms of antibiotic resistance:[8]

1. Enzymatic inactivation of drug
2. Altered drug-binding site
3. Decreased uptake of drug, either by decreased penetration or up-regulated efflux pumps
4. Bypass pathways.

Resistance is acquired in a variety of ways. Mutation of any gene occurs at a rate of one cell in 10^7 and, if this cell is then presented with antibiotics that it can survive, it will become a dominant cell, reproducing at a rate of 10^9 overnight. An example of this might be the development of AmpC β-lactamase in *Enterobacter* spp., when patients are treated with third-generation cephalosporins. A similar example is the loss of porin OprD in *P. aeruginosa* in the presence of imipenem.

Enzymes such as the β-lactamases render a large array of antibiotics useless. Class 1 β-lactamase is effective against some β-lactam-containing antibiotics but ESBLs, which incorporate enzymes such as TEM-24, will produce cross-resistance to multiple classes of antibiotics, including fluoroquinolones and aminoglycosides.[9–12]

The Ambler classification categorised all β-lactamases into four classes A–D, based upon molecular structure, and ESBLs are Class A enzymes. The major ESBL types are TEM, SHV and CTX-M, the latter being the predominant genotype globally.

AMPc enzymes are Class C, and differ chiefly in the fact they are not inhibited by clavulanate in vitro. *Enterobacter*, *Serratia* and *Citrobacter* can all produce AMPc β-lactamases. This fact is mainly of use in the diagnostic laboratory, where different markers aid in helping define potential therapeutic options. For example, β-lactamase inhibitor combinations such as co-amoxiclav and piperacillin-tazobactam may be considered in ESBL producers with mild infection, but not in AMPc producers. However, this is rarely appropriate in the ICU setting.

Resistance may be produced by a combination of mechanisms, such as in *P. aeruginosa* where the resistance is due to a combination of protein efflux systems, cephalosporinases and derepression of AmpC enzyme.

Carbapenemases were first described in the 1980s but have become prominent over the last 10 years, especially with the rise of metallo β-lactamases (MBLs). In particular the New Delhi MBL (NDM-1), which was characterised in 2008, is of growing concern as the plasmid carrying the enzyme also carries other resistance mechanisms, rendering such infections extremely drug resistant.[13]

The big problem particularly with ESBLs is that they can spread by plasmid transmission, which is very rapid. The enzyme production is encoded chromosomally within an organism, and can then be transferred between bacteria by plasmids. Transposons transfer genes between plasmids.

The phenomenon of induction is also seen. This is the process whereby the presence of an antibiotic appears to 'induce' or switch on the production of the relevant enzyme so that the organism becomes resistant. For example, staphylococcal resistance to meticillin occurs due to an altered penicillin-binding protein that has low affinity for all β-lactam agents. It is linked to a *MecA* gene, which is usually expressed only when stressed by antibiotic pressure. This gene does not develop readily and spread of meticillin resistance is by vector transmission, not de novo production of resistance[9] (**Table 70.2**).

Table 70.2 The influence of extended-spectrum β-lactamases (ESBL) on resistance in *Klebsiella*

ANTIBIOTICS	ESBL-NEGATIVE (% RESISTANT)	ESBL-POSITIVE (% RESISTANT)
Gentamicin	8	76
Amikacin	3	52
Ciprofloxacin	3	31
All the above	0	5

(Reproduced from Livermore DM, Yuan M. Antibiotic resistance and production of extended-spectrum beta-lactamases amongst *Klebsiella* spp. from intensive care units in Europe. J Antimicrob Chemother 1996;38:409–24.)

PROBLEM ORGANISMS

See Box 70.3 for organisms responsible for the majority of nosocomial infections.

These infections are likely to be associated with an increase in morbidity and mortality, primarily due to delayed recognition (no quick, reliable test currently exists that can rapidly identify such enzyme-producing strains), an association with other resistant mechanisms (ESBLs are often aminoglycoside and quinolone resistant too) and a lack of therapeutic options.[11]

An indication of their perceived importance is that, in 2010, the Infectious Diseases Society of America gave testimony before the House Committee on Energy and Commerce Subcommittee on Health on the need for antibiotic stewardship and the dire need for research and development into newer therapies. The epidemiological evidence shows that the prevalence of such infections is increasing worldwide.[12]

ESBL-PRODUCING ENTEROBACTERIACEAE

Enterobactericeae encompasses a large family of enteric, oxidase-negative, Gram-negative bacilli. In terms of nosocomial infection, *E. coli* and *Klebsiella* spp. are the most frequently seen but *Enterobacter*,

Citrobacter spp., *Serratia* spp. and *Proteus* spp. (amongst others) are also commonly implicated.

Of these *E. coli* and *Klebsiella* are particularly able to produce ESBLs, which may be defined as transferable plasmid-mediated enzymes that hydrolyse oxyimino-cephalosporins but are inhibited in vitro by clavulanate.[10]

PSEUDOMONAS

Pseudomonas spp. are versatile opportunistic pathogens common in the critically ill; they may colonise patients with chronic lung disease. *P. aeruginosa* is one of the commonest pathogens associated with hospital-acquired pneumonia. Resistance is able to develop in a range of ways and produces a very broad spectrum of resistance, making it potentially very difficult to treat and resulting in the increased popularity of combination therapy.[14] It is associated with an adverse outcome in the critically ill[15] and, like the ESBL producers, multidrug-resistant (MDR) pseudomonal strains are growing in number.[16]

STENOTROPHOMONAS MALTOPHILIA

This is an increasingly common and troublesome environmental organism. It is often resistant to β-lactam antibiotics, quinolones and to aminoglycosides. Co-trimoxazole is the only reliably effective antibiotic agent. It also produces a carbapenamase, which makes it intrinsically resistant to carbapenems. Indeed the use of carbapenems predisposes to *Stenotrophomonas* selection.

ACINETOBACTER BAUMANII

Acinetobacter baumanii is an increasing and major problem. It survives even in dry environments and, despite its name, spreads and cross-infects readily (*a cineto*: without movement). It is multiresistant and, although generally sensitive to carbapenems, it is increasingly resistant even to these agents. It becomes rapidly resistant and the profile of resistance is unpredictable but can be extremely broad, with some organisms sensitive only to colistin. [17]

It has the potential to cause significant outbreaks, and MDR strains have also been implicated in military personnel returning from Iraq and Afghanistan.[18]

COAGULASE-NEGATIVE STAPHYLOCOCCI (CoNS)

CoNS are low-virulence organisms and common skin contaminants, but are increasingly causing nosocomial infection. Their resilience may be in part due to the production of biofilm, when associated with catheter-related or bone and joint infections. Frequently meticillin resistant, they are also resistant to multiple classes of antibiotics, but are usually sensitive to glycopeptides. As glycopeptide resistance patterns alter, newer agents such as linezolid and tigecycline will have a role.

METICILLIN-RESISTANT STAPHYLOCOCCUS AUREUS *(MRSA)*

Staphylococcus aureus is a virulent pathogen causing a wide range of infections. It has a plethora of virulence factors but it is the toxins that produce most of the clinical syndromes such as invasive skin and soft tissue infections, food poisoning and necrotising pneumonia.

Meticillin resistance was first noted in the early 1960s and, although rates between countries and ICUs vary considerably, there has been an inexorable rise in its prevalence in most countries. Glycopeptides are currently commonly used to treat invasive MRSA infections but, as ever, source control is of paramount importance. Newer anti-MRSA agents include linezolid, tigecycline and daptomycin. Anti-MRSA cephalosporins have also been developed. MRSA has been a model of the failure of some infection control methods and is a well-publicised marker of quality in a health-care setting.

CLOSTRIDIUM DIFFICILE

This originally emerged as an organism that became a problem after administration of certain antibiotics, including clindamycin. It is now clear that in the critically ill it often emerges after using almost any broad-spectrum antibiotics. The organism produces toxins that can cause pseudomembranous colitis, a potentially catastrophic disease. Although it usually settles on metronidazole or vancomycin orally, recurrence is common and it can also progress to a severe colitis that necessitates radical surgery such as colectomy.[19] A newer therapeutic agent fidaxomicin shows promise against recurrent disease.[20] Surgery carries a high mortality rate, quoted at 11% for total colectomy, and very high mortality for less aggressive surgery such as hemicolectomy in the presence of toxic megacolon.[21] Almost as important is the observation of case clusters, indicating that cross-infection is important.

CANDIDA *SEPSIS*

Candida sepsis is almost always a nosocomial problem, probably endogenous in origin, and related to overgrowth secondary to antibiotic pressures. It is the fourth commonest bloodstream infection in the USA and the sixth commonest in Europe.[22]

The prevalence of species is defined by each unit, but *C. albicans* is most common. There is some evidence to suggest that the widespread use of azoles may have influenced the relative increase in *C. glabrata* and *C. krusei* species. Definitive diagnosis is by blood culture, but presumptive diagnosis is suggested by the triad of clinical infection, a high-risk patient and *Candida* at more than two sites (**Fig. 70.1**). Antifungal treatment should depend on the sensitivity of the species involved.

SITES OF INFECTION

The main sites of nosocomial infection are the respiratory system, surgical site wounds and intravenous

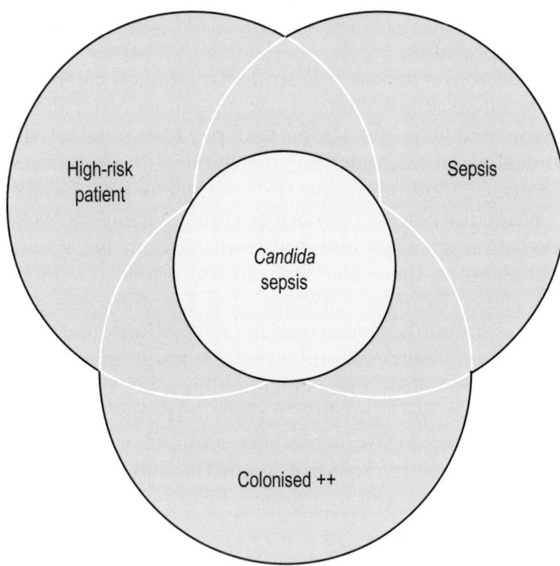

Figure 70.1 Diagnostic triad of *Candida* sepsis.

lines. Urinary tract infection appears to be relatively uncommon compared with non-critical care environments, with only 14% point prevalence in the EPIC II study compared with 64% of respiratory-related infections.

NOSOCOMIAL PNEUMONIA

Nosocomial pneumonia is a common problem in the critically ill, particularly in ventilated patients, with an incidence of 15–30%.[23-25]

AETIOLOGY

There are several possible mechanisms, including aspiration from the nasopharynx, local spread and haematogenous spread of infection. Some 45% of healthy adults aspirate in their sleep. In the sick the nasopharynx colonises rapidly with a wide range of organisms, usually Gram-negatives, and aspiration is encouraged by the unconscious state, the presence of a nasogastric tube or endotracheal intubation. Pneumonia will develop in up to 25% of colonised patients, compared with a 3% incidence in non-colonised patients. It may also be related to the colonisation of the upper gastrointestinal tract, which may in turn colonise the nasopharynx.

Factors that are likely to encourage colonisation of the pharyngeal areas with organisms include antibiotics and nasogastric tubes. Also implicated are alterations in the host defences in the pharynx, changes in the local pH, the amount of surface mucin and impairment of other local immune defence mechanisms.

Patient factors predisposing to nosocomial pneumonia include acute severity of illness, chronic illness, especially chronic lung disease, diabetes, immunosuppression, advanced age, recent surgery to thorax or abdomen, intubation, and bronchoscopy. Environmental factors include broad-spectrum and prolonged use of antibiotics, potential pathogens in the vicinity, bacterial properties such as ability to adhere to surfaces, cross-infection, 24-hour ventilator tubing changes, and foreign bodies such as nasogastric tubes. Intubated and ventilated patients have a higher rate of nosocomial infection than patients receiving non-invasive ventilation. However, this may be due to different patient populations with different underlying problems and background morbidity.[26] The role of neutralisation by H_2 antagonists and proton pump inhibitors is still debated.[27-29]

Box 70.4 Principles for the diagnosis of nosocomial pneumonia

Crackles on auscultation or dullness to percussion on physical examination of the chest and any of the following:

- New onset of purulent sputum
- Organism isolated from blood cultures
- Isolation of pathogen from specimen obtained by transtracheal aspirate, bronchial brushing or biopsy
- Chest radiography examination shows new or progressive infiltration, consolidation, cavitation or pleural effusion
- Isolation of virus or detection of virus antigen in respiratory secretions
- Diagnostic single antibody titre (IgM) or fourfold increase in paired serum samples (IgG) for pathogen
- Histopathological evidence of pneumonia

IgM = immunoglobulin M.

DIAGNOSIS

The general criteria for diagnosis are general signs of infection, clinical signs of a chest infection, purulent sputum, rising inflammatory markers, radiological evidence such as new pulmonary infiltrates, and positive cultures from sputum or blood.[23,25,30,31] These criteria are non-specific, and obtaining deep respiratory samples with quantitiative analysis remains the stated gold standard method of diagnosis. This can be achieved with protected brush specimens (PBS) bronchoalveolar lavage (BAL) and protected BAL. These are difficult and time consuming and it appears that non-bronchoscopic techniques such as blind tracheal aspirates through the endotracheal tube are both practical and reasonably effective from a clinical – if not a research – viewpoint.[25,32] A recent Cochrane review showed there was no evidence that quantitative cultures (compared with qualitative analysis) reduced mortality, length of stay, time on mechanical ventilation or antibiotic change[33] (**Box 70.4**).

THE ORGANISMS

The majority of VAP is due to aerobic Gram-negative organisms such as *Klebsiella* spp., *Escherichia coli* and *Pseudomonas* spp. but early-onset VAP, between 48 hours and 5 days, may be due to community pathogens, such as meticillin-sensitive *Staphylococcus aureus, Streptococcus pneumoniae* and *Haemophilus infiuenzae*. This has been described as early endogenous infection.

In late-onset VAP (after 5–7 days), multidrug-resistant organisms such as MRSA, *P. aeruginosa, Acinetobacter baumannii* and *Stenotrophomonas maltophilia* occur more commonly than in non-ICU patients.[34–36] This has been called secondary endogenous and exogenous infection.

PREVENTION

Prevention is by methods that reduce aspiration, cross-infection and contamination of respiratory devices.[31] Recommended methods include:

- hand washing
- limiting antibiotic use
- changing ventilator circuits at longer intervals – 1 week
- orotracheal, rather than nasotracheal intubation
- removing nasogastric tubes
- semirecumbent position – this reduces aspiration
- avoiding muscle relaxants
- avoiding re-intubation
- using non-invasive ventilation, where possible.

Other more controversial methods include:

- antibiotic prophylaxis after intubation
- continuous suctioning of subglottic secretions
- early enteral nutrition benefits of the colonisation of the gastrointestinal tract might be offset by problems with nasogastric tubes and nasopharyngeal colonisation
- the use of heat moisture exchangers
- closed suctioning – there is some limited evidence that it reduces VAP.

TREATMENT

The use of inappropriate or inadequate antibiotics leads to an increased mortality, so current trends are towards initial broad-spectrum antibiotics followed by reassessment and de-escalation.[37,38] As the spectrum of resistance grows it is highly likely that it will be increasingly difficult to apply this broad-spectrum empirical treatment, especially with late-onset VAP. Surveillance of current colonisation, awareness of an individual ICU's ecology and targeted treatment will replace empiric regimens. Most guidelines, including those of the Infectious Diseases Society of America, advocate the initial use of combination therapy, usually an antipseudomonal β-lactam with an aminoglycoside, especially in late-onset VAP.[25,37,39–41] The evidence is not conclusive, however, and many studies have shown good results with monotherapy.[42,43]

Duration of treatment has always been widely debated. Shorter courses are increasingly being advocated, with an 8-day course shown to be effective.[32,44] Pseudomonal or MRSA pneumonia may require longer courses, of 14 and 21 days respectively, depending on severity.[45] Linezolid appears to be a better choice than vancomycin for treatment of MRSA pneumonia.[46,47]

The attributable mortality with nosocomial pneumonia is difficult to determine because patients requiring ventilation often have a high intrinsic mortality. Rates of 30% have been quoted; pneumonia accounts for 60% of deaths from nosocomial infections. In addition, nosocomial pneumonia increases length of stay by 12–23 days.[5,48,49]

SURGICAL SITE INFECTIONS

Surgical site infections (SSI) are common and represent 20% of all nosocomial infections. The organisms involved may be those introduced at the time or from later contamination.

RISK FACTORS

- The procedure itself and the level of contamination prior to or during surgery. In clean elective surgery the incidence should be less than 10%, but where contamination may occur (e.g. bowel surgery) it may be as high as 15%. In contaminated procedures, the rate rises to around 20%, and where infection already exists it may be 40% or higher
- The surgeon's technical ability[50]
- Host factors: see Box 70.2
- The use of antibiotic prophylaxis
- Duration of stay in ICU.

PREVENTION

Clean theatres, good operating technique and thorough asepsis, both in the theatre and postoperatively, are important.

ANTIBIOTIC PROPHYLAXIS

Efficacy of antibiotic prophylaxis has clearly been demonstrated, but the unnecessary use of broad-spectrum antibiotics should be avoided. If there is no risk of infection with a clean procedure there is no place for antibiotics. If contamination is either seen or likely to occur, the use of antibiotics is to provide cover for the spillage. Effective prophylaxis requires an antibiotic:

- that covers the most likely organisms
- to be given prior to contamination (0–2 hours preoperatively)[51]
- at peak dosage at the time of contamination.

A single dose should suffice, although a second dose is recommended if the procedure extends beyond 4 hours or a significant amount of blood loss occurs. Prolonged administration:

- increases the chance of antibiotic resistance
- unnecessarily exposes the patient to adverse effects from the drugs
- encourages colonisation with resistant organisms
- ensures that if a late infection occurs it will be with an organism resistant to the prophylaxis.

Table 70.3 Surgical prophylaxis

TYPE OF SURGERY	
Abdominal wall	Insertion of mesh. Staphylococcal or streptococcal cover. In the groin, Gram-negative cover may be needed
Cardiac	Protection of valves and grafts. Staphylococci may be resistant
Vascular	Protection of grafts. Staphylococci are a major consideration. If the groin is involved, it may require Gram-negative cover
Orthopaedic	Prostheses. Staphylococci are an increasing problem
Biliary upper GI	Usually Gram-negative and anaerobic cover, with an awareness of resistant enterococci
Colorectal	Protection against faecal flora. Cephalosporins and metronidazole have been popular but predispose to developing enterococci such as *Enterococcus faecalis* or *E. faecium*, which may be multiresistant
Gynaecological	Conventionally broad-spectrum involving cephalosporins or, currently, co-amoxiclav. Metronidazole is also favoured
Urological	Protection from instrumentation of the urinary tract, Gram-negative cover. Awareness of any existing infection

GI=gastrointestinal.

In many circumstances the evidence supporting prophylaxis is minimal, and frequently the antibiotics used are inappropriate to the perceived risk. Most hospitals will have specific guidance on appropriate antibiotic prophylaxis tailored to the procedure, taking into account local microbial resistance data. With grafts, mesh or prostheses the morbidity from infection is so great as to justify using prophylaxis even if the evidence is marginal (**Table 70.3**).

LINE SEPSIS

The use of intravascular devices in hospital practice is ubiquitous. There is both a significant morbidity, resulting in prolongation of hospital stay, and an attributable mortality due to infection associated with their use.[52-54] The catheter type influences the rate of infection. A systematic review[55] showed the following rates per 1000 catheter days:

- peripheral intravenous catheters – 0.5 (95% CI 0.2–0.7)
- non-cuffed central venous catheters
  - non-medicated and nontunneled – 2.7 (95% CI 2.6–2.9)
  - non-medicated and tunneled – 1.7 (95% CI 1.2–2.3)
- cuffed and tunnelled central venous catheters – 1.6 (95% CI 1.5–1.7)
- arterial catheters for haemodynamic monitoring – 1.7 (95% CI 1.2–2.3)
- pulmonary artery catheters – 3.7 (95% CI 2.4–5.0)
- peripherally inserted central catheters – 1.1 (95% CI 0.9–1.3)
- peripherally inserted midline catheters – 0.2 (0.0–0.5).

Box 70.5 Risk factors for catheter infection

Host risk factors
Site: subclavian is a lower risk than internal jugular and femoral
Catheter material: antibacterial catheters may reduce infection; antiseptic catheters reduce colonisation
Number of lumens: multilumen catheters increase the infection risk[30]
Number of administrations through the lines
Dressing type: frequency of changes
Skin preparation
Experience of technique of personnel
Occurrence of bacteraemia
Tunnelling: often used for long-term access but the data are contentious[31]

Central venous catheters common in the ICU have a higher rate of infection, but it is important to note that all indwelling lines pose an infection risk. Many other factors influence development of infection, such as conditions of insertion, catheter care and duration of catheter. Peripheral catheters should be changed every 72 hours; however, there is no indication for routine CVC line changing based on catheter days (**Box 70.5**).

CENTRAL VENOUS CATHETERS

Colonisation of catheters is common and it is likely that this is a precursor of infection. Colonisation rates are in the order of 5–40%, determined in part by the risk factors involved (see below). Infection rates are approximately 10% of the colonised catheters.[56]

DEFINITIONS

1. *Colonised catheter:* growth of >15 colony-forming units (semiquantitative) or 10^3 (quantitative) from a proximal or distal catheter segment in the absence of accompanying clinical symptoms and signs.
2. *CR-BSI:* isolation of the same organism from the catheter segment (see above) as from a peripheral blood culture in a patient with signs of infection and in the absence of another source. In the absence of laboratory corroboration of infection, effervescence of infection after removal of the catheter may be taken as circumstantial evidence.

Extrinsic mechanisms associated with developing catheter sepsis include infection from the skin and insertion site, contamination from the hub and then internally spread, and contamination of drugs or fluids administered through the catheter. Bacteraemia seeding to the catheter is an intrinsic mechanism.

THE ORGANISMS

The organisms involved in catheter sepsis are influenced predominantly by the patient's endogenous flora. There is a 25% incidence of CoNS, which are increasingly recognised as pathogens due to their ability to form biofilms on prosthetic material. A biofilm is a three-dimensional matrix of extracellular polymeric material (slime) that allows bacteria to live in communities. These are important owing to the increased resistance to antimicrobials and strong adherence to prosthetic material.[57] *Staphylococcus aureus* (meticillin susceptible and resistant) and *Candida* spp. can cause significant bacteraemia, and seeding to other organs such as the eyes and heart valves must be ruled out. Gram-negative pathogens predominate in patients with haematological malignancies, and *Pseudomonas* is frequent in burns patients.

TREATMENT OF CATHETER INFECTION

The most important aspect of treatment is a high index of suspicion that leads to removal of the device if infection is present either locally or systemically.[53] Antibiotics after line removal are recommended. Duration of treatment varies: 5–7 days for CoNS, and 10–14 days for *S. aureus*, Gram-negative organisms and *Candida* spp.[53] If bacteraemia is present it is best to avoid replacing the central venous catheter if possible for a few days. In situations where it is uncertain whether the line is implicated in infection, some advocate replacing a new line over a wire. If the removed catheter is subsequently shown to be infected then it must be removed.

Due to biofilm production, all lines should be considered for removal, but some long-term lines such as Hickman catheters may not be appropriate to remove, and salvage therapy instigated instead. This high-risk strategy is not routinely recommended, especially if the organism is highly virulent, but 14 days' antibiotics via the line would be minimum.

PREVENTION

Important issues include adequate hand washing, adequate skin disinfection, insertion under aseptic conditions, intravenous team to insert and manage lines, anchoring of lines to prevent excessive movement, closed systems with limited interruptions to the lines, application of sterile dressings to the insertion site, and daily inspection of catheter site. Replacement of intravenous administration sets at 72 hours is optimal. Stopcocks may be essential, but are portals of infection. Local antiseptics are advocated for site care, but there is little difference between gauze and transparent dressings, although efforts to reduce local humidity at the site may be important.[58–60]

Techniques of unproven benefit include antiseptic cream at insertion site, routine changes of dressings at frequent intervals, antibiotic lock therapy, occlusive antimicrobial dressings, in-line filters, tunnelling of central venous catheters, and routine flushing of long-term central venous catheters.

METHODS OF INFECTION CONTROL

Each hospital has an infection control team that can employ techniques to reduce infection (**Box 70.6**). Prevention of nosocomial infection, thus reducing length of stay, will decrease antibiotic utilisation and therefore generation of multidrug resistance.

The most important aspects of preventing nosocomial infection and facilitating infection control are simple hygiene, such as hand washing, and being aware that the problem exists. There are several ways in which the issue of nosocomial infection can be addressed. These include surveillance, screening, isolation and strategic planning.[61]

SURVEILLANCE AND SCREENING

Routine culture surveillance of both patients and environment provides information on the organisms currently prevalent, and is a useful tool in guiding management when infection occurs. Molecular typing of specific pathogens allows identification of cross-infection, and gives the clinician the ability to track the organism during an outbreak.

Screening of patients allows identification of multidrug resistance organisms and therefore barrier precautions to be implemented. MRSA, VRE and *Acinetobacter baumanii* are organisms targeted during screening.

ISOLATION

Although physical barriers undoubtedly reduce cross-contamination, isolation may be hazardous as it often indicates lower-intensity care. The relative risks need to be addressed.

STRATEGIC PLANNING

There are two elements. One is enforcing hygienic practice, which is simple, cheap and very effective. The other is looking towards means of reducing both

Box 70.6 Roles of infection control teams

Surveillance and investigation of infection outbreaks
Education of staff
Review of antibiotic utilisation
Review of antibiotic resistance patterns
Review of infection control procedures and policies

nosocomial infection and the emergence of resistance by good antimicrobial stewardship.

On an individual basis the approach to management must change. In the past, empirical treatment on the basis of likely organisms led to the use of very-broad-spectrum antibiotics. Narrow-spectrum targeted treatment will cease to be an option and will become a necessity. Prolonged broad-spectrum antibiotic management aimed at dealing with any eventuality will be replaced by short-duration specific and effective regimens.

SELECTIVE DECONTAMINATION OF THE DIGESTIVE TRACT

SDD is based on the idea that elimination of colonising organisms in the gut will reduce nosocomial infection as the majority of infections arise from endogenous flora. Administration of oral non-absorbable antibiotics, such as polymyxin and nystatin, are applied to the oropharynx and stomach in conjunction with a parenteral cephalosporin. The uptake of this technique has been limited owing to concerns over antibiotic resistance generation, but it is associated with a higher survival at day 28, lower incidence of bacteraemia, and reduced VAP.[34,62–64] It is likely to be most effective in ICUs with low levels of antibiotic resistance.[65]

USEFUL WEBSITES

http://www.cdc.gov/ncidod/dhqp/pdf/nnis/NosInfDefinitions.pdfhttp://www.cdc.gov/ncidod/dhqp/pdf/nnis/NosInfDefinitions.pdf.

http://www.ecdc.europa.eu/en/activities/surveillance/EARS-Net/Pages/index.aspx.

Access the complete references list online at http://www.expertconsult.com

1. Vincent JL, Bihari DJ, Suter PM, et al. The prevalence of nosocomial infection in intensive care units in Europe. Results of the European Prevalence of Infection in Intensive Care (EPIC) Study. EPIC International Advisory Committee. JAMA 1995;274:639–44.
8. Hawkey P. The origins and molecular basis of antibiotic resistance. BMJ 1998;317:657.
10. Paterson DL, Bonomo RA. Extended-spectrum beta-lactamases: a clinical update. Clin Microbiol Rev 2005;18:657–86.
20. Louie TJ, Miller MA, Mullane KM, et al. Fidaxomicin versus vancomycin for *Clostridium difficile* infection. N Engl J Med 2011;364:422–31.
22. Pfaller MA, Diekema DJ, Jones RN, et al. International surveillance of bloodstream infections due to Candida species: frequency of occurrence and in vitro susceptibilities to fluconazole, ravuconazole, and voriconazole of isolates collected from 1997 through 1999 in the SENTRY antimicrobial surveillance program. J Clin Microbiol 2001;39(9):3254–9.
36. American Thoracic Society. Guidelines for the management of adults with hospital-acquired, ventilator-associated, and healthcare-associated pneumonia. Am J Respir Crit Care Med 2005;171(4):388–416.
45. Liu C, Bayer A, Cosgrove SE, et al. Clinical practice guidelines by the infectious diseases society of america for the treatment of methicillin-resistant *Staphylococcus aureus* infections in adults and children: executive summary. Clin Infect Dis 2011;52(3):285–92.

71

Severe soft-tissue infections

Ilker Uçkay, Hugo Sax, Pierre Hoffmeyer, Daniel Lew and Didier Pittet

PATHOGENESIS

The skin is the largest organ and acts as an excellent barrier against infection. It consists of the epidermis and dermis and resides on fibrous connective tissue, the superficial and deep fasciae. The fascial cleft, with nerves, arteries, veins, lymphatic and adipose tissue, lies between these fascial planes. Microorganisms cause skin and soft-tissue infections if there is a break in the skin because of traumatic lesion or maceration; soft tissues are ischaemic; particularly virulent bacteria such as community-acquired meticillin-resistant *Staphylococcus aureus* (CA-MRSA),[1] surgical site infections,[2] or in severely immune-compromised patients.[2–4] Skin lesions can on occasion be manifestations of systemic infection; examples are bacteraemia due to meningococci, staphylococci, and endocarditis. This issue is not specifically addressed here.

MICROBIOLOGY

Normal human skin flora includes coagulase-negative staphylococci, *Corynebacterium* spp., *Micrococcus* spp. and *S. aureus* for roughly 20–30% of all humans. Colonisation by Gram-negative bacteria usually occurs in hospital patients or transiently in arid areas by *Acinetobacter* spp. However, substantial skin infections due to human skin flora are exceptions. The classical pathogens of deep-layer soft-tissue infections are beta-haemolytic streptococci, notably *Staphylococcus pyogenes*, and *S. aureus* in iatrogenic cases. Of note, the virulent *S. pyogenes* can equally cause nosocomial infections (including necrotising fasciitis[5]) following needle stick injury from patient to surgeon[6] or from patient to nurse,[7] or cause invasive disease among elderly home patients.[8] This microbiology of severe soft-tissue infections has not changed significantly over recent decades[9] with three main exceptional trends: CA-MRSA is an emerging severe tissue infection in certain parts of the world,[1,10] there is awareness of severe *Acinetobacter* infections following war trauma and natural disasters in arid regions of northern Africa and the Middle East,[11,12] and earthquakes (with associated tsunamis) all over the world have highlighted the potential of atypical microorganisms (mycobacteria, *Scedosporium* spp., *Aeromonas* spp., *Vibrio* spp., *Pseudomonas* spp.) as causes of soft-tissue infections.[11,13]

DIAGNOSIS

Diagnosis of skin and soft-tissue infections is essentially clinical. Chemistry confirms inflammation and measures its severity for the follow-up of patients. Microbiological confirmation (blood cultures, abscesses) is necessary for a targeted antibiotic therapy by avoiding empirical broad-spectrum antimicrobial therapy. Growth of microorganisms per se in superficial or deep necrotic swabs is not evidence of infection, as the differential diagnoses of skin and soft-tissue infections (ischaemia, necrosis, allergy, pyoderma gangrenosum) may equally interrupt the cutaneous barrier with consequent colonisation with all kind of bacteria. Additionally, a positive skin carriage for MRSA correlates only poorly with the pathogen of subsequent cutaneous infection[14] and patients who were pretreated with antibiotics before hospital admission may reveal negative results. Serology is of inferior importance. Practically, only the serum antistreptolysin-O antibody titres may diagnose infection by beta-haemolytic streptococci of groups A, C and G.[15] Histology may help to confirm clinical suspicion, especially for necrotising fasciitis,[16] whereas radiology detects abscesses or confirms fasciitis,[17] guiding the surgeon for appropriate debridement.

CLASSIFICATION

The classification of skin and soft-tissue infections based upon pathogenesis or microbiology can be confusing, because almost every pathogen can reveal every clinical picture. For example, *S. pyogenes* can be responsible for erysipelas infecting only superficial skin layers, or can spread into deeper tissues to cause fasciitis with or without associated myositis. The exact reason why some infections remain superficial and others turn bacteraemic or penetrate to deeper structures is largely unknown (besides surgical site or trauma-related infections). Many clinicians' experience is that *S. aureus* tends to form localised abscesses or evolves to bacteraemic diseases without local spread, whereas streptococci, and especially *S. pyogenes*, tend to spread within collagenous tissue and fascias owing specialised virulence factors such as hyaluronidase. However, this distinction can be arbitrary. In the following text, we will summarise some key elements of possible clinical presentations.

CLINICAL PRESENTATIONS

SUPERFICIAL SKIN INFECTIONS

Most of this group will never progress to a severe sepsis necessitating intensive care. Impetigo, more common in children, is a superficial skin infection characterised by yellow pigmentation and caused by *S. aureus*, or *S. pyogenes*. Mild infections are managed with topical antibiotics; more severe ones need a first-generation cephalosporin or a penicillinase-resistant penicillin.[18] Resistance in streptococci and staphylococci might prohibit macrolides or clindamycin, which are alternatives in penicillin-allergic patients. For CA-MRSA, oral co-trimoxazole or clindamycin is the usual choice.[1,10] Folliculitis with subsequent abscesses arises spontaneously in hair follicles and apocrine glands. Classically, *S. aureus* is the causative organism. When confluent, folliculitis can evolve to furunculosis and may need surgical drainage. Topical or systemic antibiotics may be required to prevent recurrence in selected cases. Repeated folliculitis raises the possibility of diabetes mellitus or chronic granulomatous disease, an inherited immunodeficiency syndrome based on granulocyte malfunction.[19]

Erysipelas is the most severe form of a skin infection, which can lead to bacteraemia in roughly 2% of cases. This dermal infection is largely caused by group beta-haemolytic streptococci and by *S. aureus*.[3,4] The prominent lymphatic blockade results in a painful bright red patch with a raised sharp border, which clearly demarcates infection from surrounding skin. Predisposing conditions include interdigital mycoses, foot abrasions, chronic ulcers, lymphoedema, venous stasis, and diabetes. (Amino) penicillins, cephalosporins or amoxicillin/clavulanate are the drugs of choice. Often clinicians empirically administer antibiotic agents with a broader spectrum, especially for pretreated patients or those in intensive care. However, cases not covered by cephalosporins or amoxicillin/clavulanate are rare (with the exceptions of CA-MRSA). It is rather a hallmark of clinical disease that severe erysipelas does not respond immediately to (correct) antibiotic administration. Often, it takes courage to wait several days and to retain, giving escalation of anti-infective therapy to a broader spectrum. When there is a poor response, collections and abscesses amenable for drainage need to be searched for. In patients with lymphoedema and recurrent erysipelas, secondary prophylactic therapy with (benzathyl)-penicillin may help to prevent further episodes.[18]

DEEP SKIN AND SOFT-TISSUE INFECTIONS

Cellulitis[4,5,18] is an acute spreading infection with tissue necrosis and eventual collections, but does not involve the fascias. There is less lymphatic involvement so the borders of the infection are often not well defined and differentiation between cellulitis and erysipelas is sometimes difficult. Fever, malaise and rigors are common. Cellulitis is most commonly due to streptococci, but other Gram-positive and -negative organisms can also cause this condition.[4,18] External facial cellulitis may involve the venous system draining into the sinus venosus and thus lead to thrombosis. Periocular cellulitis is a medical emergency. Clinical signs for the latter include visual disturbance because of optic nerve involvement. The orbital entity includes a wider range of bacteria: *S. pneumoniae, Haemophilus influenzae, Moraxella catarrhalis, S. aureus, S. pyogenes* and anaerobes. Another severe form of cellulitis with hemorrhagic bullous lesions can be caused by marine bacteria such as *Vibrio* spp., mostly in cases with a history of contact with seawater.[11]

TOXIN DISEASE

S. aureus and streptococci may cause sepsis not only by local inflammatory damage, but also by superantigens and toxin production. These cases are called staphylococcal or streptococcal '(toxin) shock syndromes' and are marked with signs of septic shock with absence of locally spreading infection. Sometimes, a fine macular rash on the patient's skin indicates the toxin. Regarding staphylococcal shock syndrome, a forgotten female vaginal absorption tissue (tampon), has been identified as a possible origin.[13]

NECROTISING FASCIITIS AND MYOSITIS

Necrotising fasciitis and myositis are the most feared soft-tissue infections that can affect even the healthiest young individual with very rapid onset and rapid progression to death.[18,20,21] Fatality rates range between 20–30% all over the world,[22–24] although a lower incidence of 17% is also reported.[25,26] Involvement of genitalia is called Fournier's gangrene.[24] Unsurprisingly, many papers have been published on necrotising fasciitis (e.g. a PubMed search at the end of 2011 reveals 2848 citations for 'necrotising fasciitis'). Patients with immune suppression such as diabetes mellitus appear to be particularly at risk.[27] Formally, two types are described, depending on causative organisms.[20] Type I comprises mixed infections (in immune-suppressed individuals). Type II infections are by definition caused by *S. pyogenes* and are very rapidly progressive (in otherwise healthy patients). However, this distinction is academic. There is no difference in morbidity, mortality or initial management between the two types of infection.

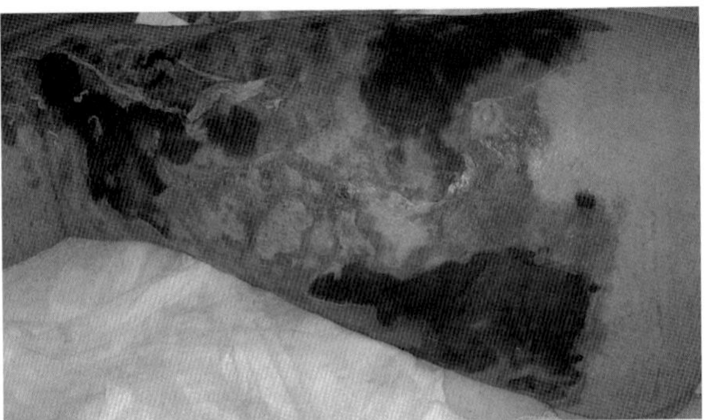

Figure 71.1 Necrosis on the calf due to progressive underlying necrotising fasciitis.

Clinically, necrotising fasciitis begins as cellulitis or erysipelas that fails to improve on antibiotics and quickly spreads along fascial planes, accompanied by destructive bacterial enzymes and toxins that cause necrosis and liquefaction of the surrounding tissue.[27] From the outside, there is often a disproportion between the character of the visible injury or erythema and the intensity of pain. Fever and crepitus on admission may be rare.[28] Microthrombi[16] and impaired blood supply lead to deep gangrene. Spontaneous drainage of debris and pus does not occur. Bullae may form and late lesions may resemble deep burns (**Fig. 71.1**) that may become pain-free because of nerve fibre necrosis. In untreated cases, there is a rapid spread to surrounding tissues and bacteraemia, with onset of multiorgan failure and death.

Often, the fasciitis also involves musculature. Thus, anatomically speaking, most necrotising fasciitis cases are musculofascitiis, or fasciomyositis, although separate myositis cases may occur. Increases in serum creatine phosphokinase may suggest muscle involvement. The bacterial infection of muscles by *Clostridium perfringens* or *C. septicum* is called 'gas gangrene', as crepitus may occur (**Fig. 71.2**), but is rare nowadays. Predisposing causes for gas gangrene are contaminated anaerobic wounds (e.g. in war or septic abortions).

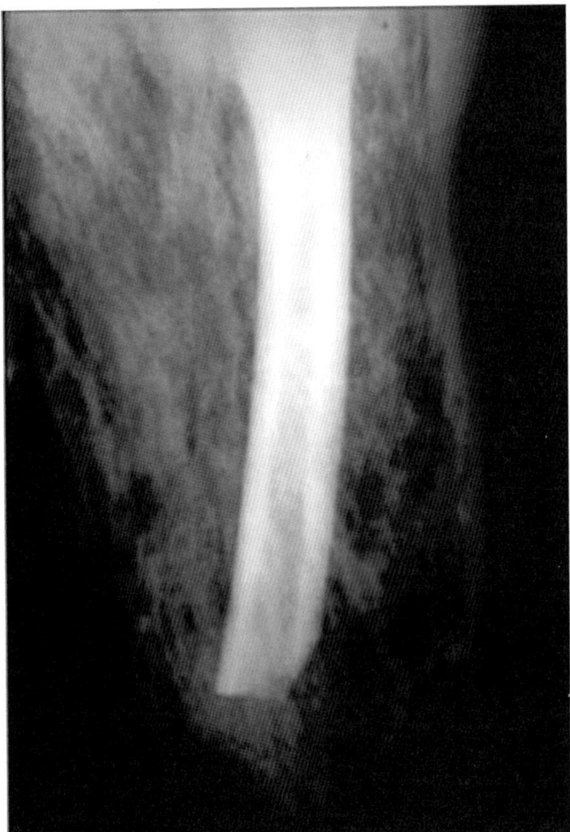

Figure 71.2 Gaseous cellulitis in a standard X-ray.

TREATMENT

Superficial skin infections, erysipelas and cellulitis are treated by antibiotics alone, whereas abscesses, fasciitis, or myositis require a combined surgical and medical treatment (**Table 71.1**). Only in selected cases of deep severe soft-tissue infections and absence of sepsis or collections can a purely conservative medical approach lead to success.[22,29]

SURGICAL TREATMENT

A surgeon experienced in the treatment of necrotising fasciitis should be involved as early as possible, even if there is no immediate surgery performed. The decision for surgical intervention and timing should be taken together. Often, experienced surgeons may delay and avoid intervention if the patient is stable and the clinical diagnosis is unclear. When the decision for intervention is made, an extensive surgical removal of damaged tissues is essential.[30,31] During intervention, the surgeons may see greyish necrotic fascia, a lack of resistance of normally adherent muscular fascia to blunt finger dissection, lack of bleeding from the fascia or dishwater pus. All involved tissue that can easily be elevated off the fascia with gentle pressure or finger spreading is debrided[27] (**Fig. 71.3**). Numerous studies have shown the importance of the extent of the first debridement.[27] A planned second look at 24-hour intervals to debride necrotic tissue is usual. In extreme cases, if only the extremities are involved, amputation may be life-saving.

When infection is stopped and all necrotic tissues debrided, wound closure may become a major problem. Besides healing by secondary intention or meshing, musculocutaneous flaps or vacuum-assisted closure therapy[32] are modern approaches of reconstructive surgery.

Table 71.1 Pathogens and presumptive antibiotic therapy in severe soft-tissue infections*

DISEASE	MAIN PATHOGENS	ANTIBIOTIC CHOICE*	REMARKS**
Erysipelas	Beta-haemolytic streptococci (rarely, *S. aureus*)	Penicillin G or amoxicillin/ clavulanate or first-generation cephalosporin	
Cellulitis	Beta-haemolytic streptococci, *S. aureus*; rarely, various other organisms	First-generation cephalosporin, amoxicillin/clavulanate clindamycin (for severe penicillin allergy)	Clindamycin resistance in *S. pyogenes* and *S. aureus* exists. Vancomycin when high suspicion of MRSA
Necrotising fasciitis	Type I: mixed. Anaerobic species together, streptococci and Enterobacteriaceae Type II: *S. pyogenes*	Empirically, high-dose amoxicillin/clavulanate IV, plus clindamycin IV	Surgical debridement essential Add vancomycin if MRSA likely Immunoglobulin in severe life-threatening sepsis
Myositis	*S. aureus*, beta-haemolytic streptococci, rarely *C. perfringens*	Empirically, high-dose amoxicillin/clavulanate IV, plus clindamycin IV	Surgical debridement essential Add vancomycin if MRSA likely Immunoglobulin in severe life-threatening sepsis

*Once causative pathogens have been identified, antibiotic choice can be modified and its spectrum narrowed.
**Be aware of local endemicity of community- or hospital-acquired meticillin-resistant *S. aureus* (MRSA). Co-trimoxazole or clindamycin are the choice in most community-acquired low-grade infections, for all other cases vancomycin.

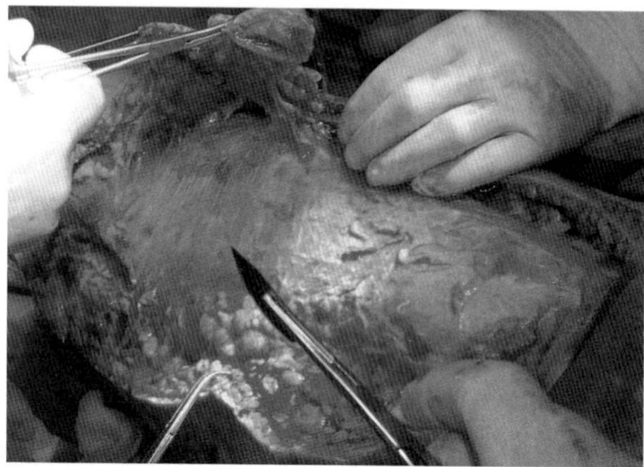

Figure 71.3 Debridement of fascia. All infected tissue is elevated off.

MEDICAL TREATMENT

Besides supportive intensive care, which is discussed in other chapters, appropriate antimicrobial agents are central to medical management of necrotising fasciitis, myositis, cellulitis and erysipelas. The role of immunoglobulins or hyperbaric oxygen is supportive at best.

Initial empirical antibiotic therapy often includes a carbapenem or other broad-spectrum antibiotic (plus vancomycin in many cases) while awaiting culture results. This broad-spectrum choice is due to fear of a potentially lethal evolution rather than supported by microbiological data. Indeed, beta-haemolytic streptococci and *C. perfringens* are susceptible to penicillin. *S. aureus* is usually susceptible to first- and second-generation cephalosporins or amoxicillin/clavulanate. Hence, even in polymicrobial infection, these most damaging pathogens are still largely covered by cephalosporins or amoxicillin/clavulanate. Besides eventual allergies or nosocomial infection, there is no need to cover larger. According to the published literature[5,20] and personal experience, almost all retrospective assessment of community-acquired fasciitis cases confirms that initial broad-spectrum coverage was excessive and antibiotic therapy could have been restricted to penicillins.

The duration of antibiotic therapy for patients with septic shock depends on the presence of secondary haematogenous seeding and the patient's evolution.[33] As for non-bacteraemic severe skin and soft-tissue infections, there is no convincing evidence regarding the ideal duration of antibiotic therapy. Often, the clinical evolution, the presence of undrained microabscesses and the experience of the physician should decide the duration, which might nevertheless be excessive in many cases. For erysipelas, the authors of this chapter performed a single-centre retrospective study highlighting that, after case-mix adjustment, less than 12 days of treatment yielded the same outcome as a prolonged treatment for more than 21 days.[14] Another randomised study among 121 cellulitis patients showed the clinical equivalence of a 5-day levofloxacin therapy compared with 10 days of levofloxacin.[34]

For (myo)fasciitis, and shock syndromes due to superantigens and toxin production, clindamycin 600 mg intravenously 6-hourly (or 900 mg t.i.d) is often added for 3–5 days,[35] even if the pathogen is clindamycin-resistant. The rationale lies in the inhibition of toxin production.[35] This is mostly supported by in vitro data. In vivo, to the best of our knowledge, only one observational study investigated the clinical benefit of supplementary clindamycin and found a positive result with a large confidence interval (univariate analysis, non-adjusted odds ratio 4.7, 95%CI 1.0–25).[36] Likewise, limiting the duration of clindamycin administration to 3–5 days or the absence of other superantigen-blocking agents relies on expert opinion.

Intravenous immunoglobulins are regularly debated as supportive therapy to antimicrobial agents. Today, their rationale lies in the activation of complement, promotion of antibody-dependent cytotoxicity, reduction of interleukin-6 and TNF-alpha production,[36] and in the inhibition of superantigens.[37] Their clinical evidence stems from several in vitro and at least five in vivo articles published in one scientific journal[29,35–39] by the same group of researchers. This group published the best available evidence in 2003 with a European randomised double-blind placebo-controlled trial among patients with toxic shock syndrome (not all patients had necrotising fasciitis). The primary end-point was mortality after 28 days. There was a non-significant trend to lower mortality in the group treated with immunoglobulins compared with placebo (2/10 vs 4/11).[39] Adjustment for case-mix could not be performed owing to the small study population of only 21 patients. The authors concluded from their dataset that immunoglobulins are very probably beneficial. The recommended doses of immunoglobulins vary according to different authors and time. The literature suggests either single doses of 2 g/kg[36] or a 3-day course beginning with 1 g/kg the first day, followed by 0.5 g/kg the two other days.[39] Taken together, these studies provide some promise, however, additional studies are urgently needed before a strong recommendation can be made regarding use of expensive and potentially harmful immunoglobulins in necrotising fasciitis. Of note, different formulations of pooled polyspecific immunoglobulins seem to have different potency against streptococcal and staphylococcal superantigens,[38] of which the clinical significance remains unclear.

Hyperbaric oxygen therapy is costly, labour-intensive, and not without risk, but can be delivered safely also to critically ill patients.[40] The rationale for soft-tissue infections is based on logical concepts (e.g. for anaerobic gas gangrene) and on personal experience. To the best of our knowledge, no randomised trials and no case–control studies exist. Nevertheless, good outcomes in individual cases allow the Center for Medicare and Medicaid Services in the USA to reimburse its use in necrotising fasciitis and gas gangrene. The situation is similar in many European countries. Hyperbaric oxygen therapy harbours today a grade C evidence level and a grade IIb class of recommendation.[40] Its importance remains behind surgical and antibiotic treatment. Importantly, hyperbaric oxygen therapy should never delay surgical intervention, including for gas gangrene.[27]

FUTURE ASPECTS

The future will hopefully show strong prospective-randomised data about the optimal management of severe soft-tissue infections. Due to their low incidence and the large and heterogeneous case-mix of these infections, multidisciplinary and multicentre trials are needed regarding all aspects of care - from the post-debridement surgical approach to the role and dosing of clindamycin and immunoglobulins in the early management of these infections. Finally, the benefit of the available 26-valent vaccine against *S. pyogenes* and related invasive infections has to be better shown, and potentially implemented on a large scale.[23]

Acknowledgements

We are indebted to Mrs Rosemary Sudan for editorial assistance. We thank our colleagues from the Orthopedic Surgery Service, University Hospitals of Geneva, for support.

Access the complete references list online at http://www.expertconsult.com

2. Uçkay I, Harbarth S, Peter R, et al. Preventing surgical site infections. Expert Rev Anti Infect Ther 2010; 8:657–70.
3. Vinh DC, Embil JM. Rapidly progressive soft tissue infections. Lancet Infect Dis 2005;5:501–13.
6. Corti G, Bartoloni A, von Hunolstein C, et al. Invasive *Streptococcus pyogenes* infection in a surgeon after an occupational exposure. Clin Microbiol Inf 2000;6: 170–1.
11. Uçkay I, Sax H, Harbarth S, et al. Multi-resistant infections in repatriated patients after natural disasters: lessons learned from the 2004 tsunami for hospital infection control. J Hosp Infect 2008;68:1–8.
16. Stamenkovic I, Lew PD. Early recognition of potentially fatal necrotising fasciitis: use of frozen-section biopsy. N Engl J Med 1984;310:1689–93.
39. Darenberg J, Ihendyane N, Sjölin J, et al. Intravenous immunoglobulin G therapy in streptococcal toxic shock syndrome: a European randomized, double-blind, placebo-controlled trial. Clin Infect Dis 2003; 37:333–40.

72

Principles of antibiotic use

Jeffrey Lipman

The intensive care unit is always the area of any hospital associated with the greatest use of antibiotics. Much of this high usage is unavoidable, but the clinician working in the ICU must realise that there is an essential consequence of this use. Antibiotic use, which should eliminate susceptible organisms, promotes (over)growth of other non-susceptible organisms, especially fungi. As far as bacteria are concerned, antibiotics confer enormous selective advantage to resistant strains, and therefore these strains will congregate where their advantage is greatest – in the ICU. Resistance (and fungal overgrowth) is a direct consequence of usage, and every course of inappropriate antibiotics should be avoided to help reduce the burden of resistance.

Antibiotic stewardship[1,2] has been suggested as a new strategy to help limit resistance. This involves selecting an appropriate drug and optimising its dose and duration to cure an infection while minimising toxicity and conditions for selection of resistant bacterial strains. Inadequate doses of even the 'correct' antibiotic may lead to survival of initially susceptible organisms.[3,4] For the optimal use of antibiotics not only should antibiotic pharmacokinetics be understood but also there should be clear and rational principles on which each specific antibiotic prescription in the ICU is based. In addition, it is probably better to have portions of the ICU population receive different classes of antibiotics at the same time.[5]

Although this chapter will provide basic principles for most of the antibiotic classes commonly used in ICUs, some important antimicrobial agents will not be specifically addressed here, namely macrolides, clindamycin and the antifungal agents.

GENERAL PRINCIPLES[6,7]

1. All appropriate microbiological specimens, including blood cultures, should be obtained before commencing antibiotic therapy. An immediate Gram-stained report may indicate the appropriate antibiotic to use, otherwise a 'best guess' choice is made depending on the clinical situation. This important and common clinical phenomenon involves trying to predict the infecting organism(s).
2. Blood cultures should be taken from a venepuncture site, after adequate skin antisepsis, and not from an intravenous or arterial catheter. Two *separate* sets of 20 mL (for adults) should be taken, the timing of which is less important.[8] Depending on what system is used, probably 10 mL should be placed into two different blood culture bottles.
3. Once a decision is made to administer antibiotics, they should be administered *without delay*.[9]
4. The decision for empirical therapy (i.e. cover for the most 'likely' organisms causing any specific infection) must include various factors such as: the site of the infecting organism (respiratory tract pathogens differ from those of abdominal infections), community- versus hospital-associated infection, recent previous antibiotic prescription, ward-versus ICU-acquired infection, and knowledge of the organisms commonly grown in patients in any specific area. This latter point is where ward/unit surveillance becomes important.[10,11]
5. Although there should be an attempt to use a narrow-spectrum antibiotic whenever practicable, appropriate therapy particularly for empirical choice for nosocomial sepsis mandates starting off with broad-spectrum antibiotics, even a combination, until culture results are back[12,13] – at which time de-escalation should be embarked upon (see below).[7] Inappropriate[14] and/or delayed correct[9] antibiotic use in the ICU has been shown to impact on morbidity and mortality (**Table 72.1**).[7]
6. Monotherapy with a single agent effective against the expected organisms aims to decrease the risk of drug antagonism, reaction or toxicity.[15]

Table 72.1 New paradigm of treatment for nosocomial sepsis

OLD	NEW
Start with penicillin	Get it right 1st time (broad spectrum)
Cost-efficient low dose	Hit hard up front
Low doses = fewer side effects	Low dose → resistance
Long courses ≥ 2 weeks	Seldom longer than 7 days

From Lipman J, Boots R. A new paradigm for treating infections: "go hard and go home". Crit Care Resusc 2009;11:276–81.

Monotherapy often costs less than multiple antibiotic usage.

7. The clinical response to treatment already given should always be considered when bacteriological results suggest reduced susceptibility.
8. A standard 2-week course of antibiotics is unnecessary and probably harmful. There is a move to use shorter courses for pneumonias[16,17] (see Table 72.1).
9. In consultation with infectious disease specialists, additional tests such as antibiotic minimum inhibitory concentration (MIC), antibiotic assay, serum bactericidal activity and synergy tests of antibiotic combinations may be useful in serious infections (e.g. endocarditis and infections in immunocompromised patients). Susceptibility tests should be interpreted carefully. In vitro sensitivity does not equate with clinical effectiveness; in vitro resistance is a better negative predictor.
10. Consultations with the laboratory staff and infectious diseases/clinical microbiology specialists are always useful and should be mandatory in serious infections (e.g. meningococcal sepsis, meticillin-resistant staphylococci, and multiresistant Enterobacteriaceae).
11. The pharmacokinetics and pharmacodynamics (e.g. penetration into relevant tissues) as well as the spectrum of activity of the antibiotic must be considered. Antibiotic pharmacokinetic principles should determine the dosage and frequency of antibiotic regimens (see below).[18]
12. Adequate drug doses should be given. The intravenous route is preferable in critically ill patients, but other routes should be considered when appropriate.
13. Serum levels of potentially toxic antibiotics should be monitored, especially if hepatic or renal dysfunction is present.
14. Prophylactic use of antibiotics should be limited to certain situations, should cover organisms that potentially can cause infections in that specific group of patients (e.g. organisms causing skin and soft-tissue infections differ from those implicated in intra-abdominal infections) and should be given at the appropriate timing (see below).
15. General signs of infection are signs of systemic inflammation. Although bacterial infection is likely, non-bacterial infection and non-infective causes should also be considered. High procalcitonin and C-reactive protein levels may be discriminatory for infection, but have limitations.[19,20]
16. Antibiotic guidelines are only one aspect of infection control.[21-23] Hand washing and hand hygiene in general are vital and the fundamental aspect of infection control.[21] Identification and elimination of reservoirs of infection,[22,23] blocking transmission of infection,[23] barrier nursing, as well as terminal cleaning of high-touch areas are imperative controls that need to be in place in every ICU.[22,23]

COMMON ERRORS WHEN USING ANTIBIOTICS

1. Administration of antibiotics before microbiological specimens are obtained.
2. Quantity and quality of blood cultures.
3. Extended use of antibiotics after eradication of infection (e.g. a 2-week course for ventilation-associated pneumonia).[16]
4. Antibiotic 'surfing' (i.e. switching from one combination to another) when the patient is not improving without delving into the cause of persistent inflammatory response.
5. Inadequate and delayed therapy and/or incorrect dosing of antibiotics.
6. Failure to adequately predict 'resident' microbial flora and therefore inability to correctly choose empiric antibiotics for nosocomial infections, i.e. no adequate surveillance data.
7. Failure to recognise toxic effects of antibiotics, particularly when polypharmacy is used.
8. Use of combination therapy, irrespective of infection.

SPECIFIC ISSUES

PHARMACOKINETIC PRINCIPLES

The goal of antimicrobial prescription is to achieve effective active drug concentrations (a combination of dose and duration) at the site of infection whilst avoiding, or at least minimising, toxicity.

The various antibiotic classes have different 'kill characteristics' and therefore should be dosed differently[18,24] (**Table 72.2**).

Table 72.2 Pharmacodynamic properties of selected antibiotics

ANTIBIOTICS	Aminoglycosides	Fluoroquinolones Glycopeptides	β-lactams Carbapenems Glycopeptides
PD KILL CHARACTERISTICS	Concentration dependent	Concentration dependent with time dependence	Time dependent
OPTIMAL PK PARAMETER	C_{max} : MIC	AUC : MIC	*T*>MIC

PD=pharmacodynamics; PK=pharmacokinetic; C_{max}=peak serum concentration; MIC=minimum inhibitory concentration; AUC=area under concentration–time curve; *T*>MIC=time above MIC.
From Roberts JA, Lipman J. Pharmacokinetic issues for antibiotics in the critically ill patient. Crit Care Med 2009;37:840–51.

β-LACTAMS (ALL PENICILLINS AND CEPHALOSPORINS, MONOBACTAMS)[18,24]

1. Studies of β-lactam antibiotics on Gram-negative bacilli show a bactericidal activity that is relatively slow, time-dependent and maximal at relatively low concentrations. Bacterial killing is almost entirely related to the time that levels in tissue and plasma exceed a certain threshold. The maximum time that plasma β-lactam levels should be allowed to fall below minimum inhibitory concentration (MIC) is 40% of the dosing interval.
2. β-lactam antibiotics lack a significant post-antibiotic effect particularly against Gram-negative organisms, and it is not necessary to achieve very high peak plasma concentrations. Post-antibiotic effect (PAE) is the continued suppression of bacterial growth despite zero serum concentration of antibiotic. It is suggested that concentrations of any β-lactam should be maintained at about 4–5 times MIC for long periods, as maximum killing of bacteria in vitro occurs at this level. If antibiotic concentrations fall below this threshold in the in vitro models, bacterial growth is immediately resumed.[3,4,18,24]
3. Thus, it is important for the efficacy of β-lactams that the dosing regimen maintains adequate plasma levels for as long as possible during the dosing interval. A recent meta-analysis demonstrated that lower doses could be used with continuous infusions for the same outcomes.[25] There is currently one randomised controlled trial that formally addresses the place of continuous infusions of β-lactams.[26]

CARBAPENEMS

1. Similar to β-lactams, the carbapenems also have time-dependent kill characteristics but have some PAE.
2. Prolonged infusions (over 3 hours) have been utilised to improve time above MIC.[27]
3. In vitro data suggest that low concentrations may predispose to development of resistant organisms.[3]

AMINOGLYCOSIDES[18,24]

1. The agents above contrast with the kill characteristic of the aminoglycosides, which is concentration-dependent. Experimentally, a high peak concentration of an aminoglycoside antibiotic provides a better, faster killing effect on standard bacterial inocula.
2. All aminoglycosides exhibit a significant PAE. The duration of this effect is variable, but the higher the previous peak the longer is the PAE. This phenomenon allows drug concentration to fall significantly below MIC of the pathogen without allowing regrowth of bacteria.
3. These principles allow for single daily doses of aminoglycosides (also termed extended interval dosing). Combining various meta-analyses involving thousands of patients, once-daily administration was found to be more efficacious with reduced toxicity, higher peak/MIC ratios, further prolonged PAE and reduced administration costs.
4. With renal dysfunction[28] the dose should be altered according to creatinine clearance. If ≥60 mL/min give 5–7 mg/kg/daily; if 59–40 mL/min, give the same dose at an interval of 36 hours; 39–20 mL/min increases the dosing interval to 48 hours.

QUINOLONES[18,24]

1. Ciprofloxacin, in contrast, has a combination of both of the above characteristics (i.e. concentration-dependent and time-dependent effects), as well as some PAE.
2. Although one suggested 'target' parameter for a good clinical bactericidal effect is a high peak, the most validated parameter is the area under the inhibitor curve (AUIC) – that is, AUC/MIC>125.
3. There is general concern about the emergence of resistance related to inappropriately low doses of ciprofloxacin (see Table 72.1).

GLYCOPEPTIDES[18,29]

1. Vancomycin induces a PAE and a post-antibiotic sub-MIC effect. These combined effects suggest that bacterial regrowth will not occur for prolonged periods following a fall in drug concentrations to levels below the MIC.
2. Continuous infusions of vancomycin may have some advantages.

Aminoglycosides and glycopeptides distribute well into fluids of the extravascular, extracellular space, and less well into tissues. This has two important implications. First, these agents should not be first-line agents, or monotherapy, for solid organ infections (lung, kidney, liver, etc.). Secondly, in situations where extravascular fluid shifts are significant (such as in situations of 'third-space losses' of abdominal sepsis, in severe burns, etc.), the volume of distribution of these drugs is significantly affected. Hence for any serum level required a larger than usual dose may have to be administered.[29] The volume of distribution of the quinolones (very large) suggests penetration is excellent into most tissues and hence these drugs are good for solid organ infections. Similarly, β-lactams as a group (including carbapenems) all have reasonable tissue penetration.

ANTIBIOTIC PROPHYLAXIS[6,30]

The main indications for prophylaxis are:

- when surgery involves incision through an area of colonisation or normal commensal flora and a resultant potential infection has morbidity or mortality
- when a procedure (e.g. catheterisation, instrumentation, intubation, dental work) potentially produces a bacteraemia in the presence of an immunocompromised patient, or when the potential

bacteraemia occurs in the presence of an abnormal heart valve or a prosthesis.

Basic principles of choice of prophylactic regimen should include the following:

1. The organisms colonising the area through which the incision is made should be covered (Gram-positives if skin is breached, Gram-negatives and anaerobes if bowel is opened).
2. A similar case should be made for colonising organisms through the area breached by catheterisation or instrumentation, etc. (Gram-negatives for bladder catheterisation, Gram-positives and anaerobes for dental procedures).
3. If prevalence of a resistant organism in a specific area is high (e.g. *Pseudomonas* in burns units) then those organisms should be covered by the prophylactic regimen.

TIMING AND DURATION OF PROPHYLAXIS

1. Optimal blood levels of antibiotic(s) are needed when the occurrence of the potential bacteraemia occurs (i.e. for surgery optimal timing of the antibiotic should be at, or just prior to, induction of anaesthesia and skin incision).[30]
2. For prolonged procedures where bacteraemias are still a potential occurrence, a second dose of antibiotic(s) may be considered.
3. There is no extra benefit to postoperative antibiotic prophylaxis.

DOSES[18,29,31]

Comments on dosing regimens are provided below. Doses suggested below are intravenous, for a 70-kg adult with *normal* renal function. All these drugs accumulate with renal dysfunction and modified doses should be used accordingly. It should be noted that some patients with 'normal' renal function may have increased renal clearance of antibiotics and hence need a higher than usual dose.[31]

1. Doses for β-lactams vary with each different drug, *but* recent emphasis supports lower boluses with more frequent administration (i.e. 4-hourly versus 8-hourly, or b.d. versus daily).[31] Continuous infusions may become standard practice.[26]
2. *Aminoglycosides:* give tobramycin and gentamicin at 7 mg/kg as a loading dose on the first day, followed by 5 mg/kg/day. Amikacin 25 mg/kg as the loading dose followed by 15 mg/kg/day. These doses are the same for adults and children, neonates excluded.
3. *Quinolones:* the ciprofloxacin dose is *at least* 400 mg b.d. (up to t.d.s.).
4. *Glycopeptides:* the vancomycin[29] dose is at least 30 mg/kg loading and similar/day either as continuous infusion or in divided doses (40 mg/kg/day for children).
5. *Carbapenems:* give meropenem or imipenem at 3 g/day in at least three divided doses.

SURVEILLANCE

Some type of simple laboratory-oriented surveillance, which primarily collects data and resistance patterns of microbiological isolates, is important. Each unit should have access to its own such data as there is an increasing prevalence of resistant organisms in intensive care units. This is complicated even further by different units having differing resistance patterns.[10] Empirical antibiotic therapy must take these factors into account. Some form of surveillance that provides units with their own microbiological data, updateable quarterly or biannually, is therefore beneficial in helping choose empirical and prophylactic regimens that are applicable to any specific unit.[10]

MULTIRESISTANT ORGANISMS

Although this chapter is on antibiotics, the point must be made that without good, efficient and effective infection control policies in all areas treating critically ill patients the spread of multiresistant organisms would be rampant and their control useless.[21–23] Part of these policies should involve attention to good hand hygiene and the use of antiseptic soaps and alcohol-based hand rubs.[21] Hands are still the most documented and incriminated mode of transmission of infection. In this regard a decrement in nursing numbers has also been incriminated in outbreaks of infections possibly due to the time it takes to adequately wash between procedures.[21] High-touch areas are important areas to address with terminal cleaning procedures.[22,23]

1. Multiresistant streptococci and vancomycin-resistant enterococci (VRE), although not common in all countries, are an increasing worldwide problem, as is community-acquired MRSA.
2. New agents are available for treatment of resistant Gram-positive infections.[32]
3. Antibiotic resistance is agent-specific. Often resistance is claimed to be against third-generation cephalosporins, but this is largely to ceftazidime (particularly the extended-spectrum β-lactamases of *Klebsiella pneumoniae, E. coli* and some Enterobacteriaceae).
4. Worrying Gram-negative organisms are *K. pneumoniae, Pseudomonas aeruginosa, Acinetobacter baumanii* spp. *and Stenotrophomonas maltophilia* (the latter specifically, for which trimethoprim may need to be used). A common feature of these organisms is intrinsic resistance to multiple antibiotics. *P. aeruginosa* and *Acinetobacter* complex (also named *A. baumanii*) have become particular problems. Sulbactam and polymyxin B or colistin have been used for these problem organisms.
5. Although the antibiotic pipeline is drying up, there are some new agents on the horizon.[33]

MONO- VERSUS COMBINATION THERAPY[12,13,15]

1. Much of the work in this area was performed before the clinical introduction of the carbapenems, penicillin/β-lactamase combinations and fourth-generation cephalosporins. It seems that newer single agents are adequate, apart possibly from resistant pseudomonal infections.[15]
2. There is no clear evidence supporting the claim that combination antimicrobial therapy prevents emergence of resistance.[15]
3. However, combination therapy is often suggested for endocarditis and some pseudomonal infections.[13] When combination therapy is used, preference should be given to the combination therapy of two different classes of antibiotics that act synergistically. The combination of two β-lactam antibiotics should not be used.

BROAD-SPECTRUM INITIAL COVER WITH DE-ESCALATION[7,13,14]

In view of the morbidity and mortality of delayed appropriate therapy for nosocomial sepsis,[9,14] patients with risk factors for infection with resistant pathogens should initially receive broad-spectrum antibiotics, possibly even combination therapy,[7,13,14] then, as soon as the pathogen and the susceptibilities are available, treatment should be simplified to a more targeted one – so-called 'de-escalation' therapy (see Table 72.1).[7] In the limited studies to date, de-escalation has led to less antibiotic usage, shorter durations of therapy, fewer episodes of secondary pneumonia and reduced mortality, without increasing the frequency of antibiotic resistance.

TIME TO ANTIBIOTICS AS A QUALITY INDICATOR

Recent data suggest that, particularly in septic shock, a delay of even hours of appropriate antibiotic administration increases morbidity and mortality.[9] A delay in antibiotic administration has therefore become an important negative factor in patient outcomes. Similar to the concept of 'time to lysis', antibiotic administration from the time of recognition of infection may in future become a quality indicator of infection management.

Access the complete references list online at http://www.expertconsult.com

7. Lipman J, Boots R. A new paradigm for treating infections: 'go hard and go home'. Crit Care Resusc 2009;11:276–81.
13. Traugott KA, Echevarria K, Maxwell P, et al. Monotherapy or combination therapy? The *Pseudomonas aeruginosa* conundrum. Pharmacotherapy 2011;31:598–608.
15. Safar N, Handelsman J, Maki DG. Does combination antimicrobial therapy reduce mortality in Gram-negative bacteraemia? A meta-analysis. Lancet Infect Dis 2004;4:519–27.
16. Chastre J, Wolff M, Fagon JY, et al. Comparison of 8 vs 15 days of antibiotic therapy for ventilator-associated pneumonia in adults: a randomized trial. JAMA 2003;290:2588–98.
18. Roberts JA, Lipman J. Pharmacokinetic issues for antibiotics in the critically ill patient. Crit Care Med 2009;37:840–51.
19. Hayashi Y, Paterson DL. Strategies for reduction in duration of antibiotic use in hospitalized patients. Clin Infect Dis 2011;52:1232–40.
31. Udy AA, Roberts JA, Boots RJ, et al. ARC – Augmented renal clearance: implications for antibiotic dosing in the critically ill. Clin Pharmacokinet 2010;49:1–16.

73

Tropical diseases

Ramachandran Sivakumar and Michael E Pelly

Once an exotic and esoteric topic, modern travel and the quest for unusual holidays has the potential to bring tropical diseases to every ICU. This chapter covers some important diseases, which are common in the tropical belt.

MALARIA

EPIDEMIOLOGY AND PATHOGENESIS

It is estimated that four species of *Plasmodium* (*vivax, malariae, ovale* and *falciparum*) cause 200 to 300 million infections per year. Most of the 600–700 000 deaths per year due to malaria are caused by *P. falciparum* and the majority of deaths are in children under 5 years of age in sub-Saharan Africa. Malaria is also widely prevalent in the Indian subcontinent and South-East Asia. It is transmitted from human to human by the bite of infected female *Anopheles* mosquitoes. After development in the liver, there is invasion of red cells by parasites, which is followed by their multiplication, and rupture of the red cells. The cycle is then repeated in red cells. In *vivax* and *ovale* infections, development to dormant forms can occur in the liver, which may lead to relapse.

CLINICAL FEATURES

UNCOMPLICATED MALARIA

Initial symptoms of malaria are non-specific and similar to a viral illness. Classic symptoms of fever, aches and headache are usually, but not always, present. Other features such as diarrhoea, vomiting, cough and abdominal pain may confuse the unwary. Unusual presentations are more common in children and may be missed. Classical rigors or fevers occurring on specific days (tertian or quartan) are usually absent in early *falciparum* infection. Clinical signs may be unhelpful, although hepatosplenomegaly may be present fairly early.

SEVERE MALARIA

Risk factors for severe malaria[1]

- Children under 5 years in endemic regions
- Adults and children in areas of low endemicity
- Non-immune travellers to endemic areas.

Definition

Clinical features include:

- impaired consciousness or unrousable coma
- prostration (i.e. generalised weakness so that the patient is unable walk or sit up without assistance)
- failure to feed
- multiple convulsions – more than two episodes in 24 hours
- deep breathing, respiratory distress (acidotic breathing)
- circulatory collapse or shock, systolic blood pressure <70 mmHg (9.31 kPa) in adults and <50 mmHg (6.65 kPa) in children
- clinical jaundice plus evidence of other vital organ dysfunction
- haemoglobinuria
- abnormal spontaneous bleeding
- pulmonary oedema (radiological).

Laboratory findings include:

- hypoglycaemia (blood glucose <2.2 mmol/L or <40 mg/dL)
- metabolic acidosis (plasma bicarbonate <15 mmol/L)
- severe normocytic anaemia (Hb <5 g/dL, packed cell volume <15%)
- haemoglobinuria
- hyperparasitaemia (>2%/100 000/µL in low-intensity transmission areas or >5% or 250 000/µL in areas of high stable malaria transmission intensity)
- hyperlactataemia (lactate >5 mmol/L)
- renal impairment (serum creatinine >265 µmol/L).

The incubation period is 7 days (usual range 9–14 days), but this may be prolonged. Several of the above coexist or may develop in rapid succession. Cough, convulsions and hypoglycemia are more common in children. Jaundice is common, but hepatic failure is uncommon. The acidosis of malaria is multifactorial and probably very similar to other forms of sepsis involving tissue hypoxia, liver dysfunction and impaired renal handling of bicarbonate.

The differential diagnosis of malaria includes:

- meningitis, typhoid fever, septicaemia
- severe influenza, dengue and other arboviral infections
- haemorrhagic fevers

- hepatitis, leptospirosis
- rickettsial diseases (e.g. scrub typhus)
- relapsing fever (*Borrelia recurrentis*)
- febrile convulsions in children.

Pregnancy increases the risk of development of severe malaria. During pregnancy both maternal and fetal morbidity and mortality are increased.

Poor prognostic indicators include age under 3 years, cerebral malaria, circulatory collapse and organ dysfunction. Laboratory evidence of poor prognosis includes hyperparasitaemia (>250 000/μL or >5%), peripheral schizontaemia, severe anaemia (PCV<15% or Hb<50 g/L), raised blood urea >60 mg/dL and serum creatinine >265 μmol/L (>3.0 mg/dL), raised venous lactate (>5 mmol/L), raised CSF lactate (>6 mmol/L), low CSF glucose and a very high concentration of TNF-α.

Cerebral malaria

Cerebral malaria may be the most common non-traumatic encephalopathy worldwide. The term is restricted to the syndrome in which altered consciousness due to malaria could not be attributed to convulsions, sedatives, hypoglycaemia or to a non-malarial cause.

Clinical, histopathological and laboratory studies have suggested two potential mechanisms:

- *mechanical hypothesis:* cytoadherence of parasitised erythrocytes
- *cytotoxic hypothesis:* neuronal injury by malarial toxin and excessive cytokine production.

Cerebral malaria has few specific features, but there are differences in clinical presentation between African children and non-immune adults.[2]

Clinical findings include:

- coma
- convulsions
- raised intracranial pressure
- hypoglycaemia
- acidosis
- abnormalities of tone and posture (the commonest being symmetrical pyramidal signs)
- retinopathy – retinal haemorrhages, cotton wool spots, papilloedema, retinal whitening and retinal vessel abnormalities – all of which are more common in children.

DIAGNOSIS

- Microscopy of thick and thin films remains the gold standard for both the diagnosis, and to follow the efficacy of treatment. In the non-immune patient there is a close association between parasite levels and complications; however, severe complications can occur in patients with low counts.
- Rapid diagnostic tests (RDT) that detect specific antigens (proteins) produced by malaria parasites are useful in diagnosis. Current tests are based on the detection of histidine-rich protein 2 (HRP2) (which is specific for *P. falciparum*), pan-specific or species-specific parasite lactate dehydrogenase (pLDH) or other pan-specific antigens such as aldolase. Many commercial assays are available. Some tests detect only one species (*P. falciparum*), whereas others detect one or more of the other three species. RDTs do not give information about the parasite load and their sensitivity and specificity decrease at low parasitaemia. Hence, it is important to seek microbiological advice regarding the RDT tests used locally.
- PCR tests based on detecting malarial DNA are more sensitive than microscopy but are expensive and do not give estimates of parasite load.
- In areas where two or more species of malaria parasites are common, only microscopy will permit a species diagnosis. Where mono-infection with *P. vivax* is common and microscopy is not available, it is recommended that a combination RDT, which contains a pan-malarial antigen, is used. Where *P. vivax, P. malariae* or *P. ovale* occur, almost always as a co-infection with *P. falciparum*, an RDT detecting *P. falciparum* alone may be sufficient; the treatment for non-*falciparum* malaria is given only to cases with a negative test result and where no other obvious cause of illness is present. Treatment solely on the basis of clinical suspicion should only be considered when a parasitological diagnosis is not accessible.

TREATMENT OF MALARIA[3]

WHO has recently issued new guidelines for the treatment of malaria.

FALCIPARUM MALARIA (Box 73.1)

To counter the threat of resistance of *P. falciparum* to monotherapies, and to improve treatment outcome, combinations of antimalarials are now recommended by WHO for the treatment of falciparum malaria. Antimalarial combination therapy is the simultaneous use of two or more blood schizontocidal drugs with independent modes of action. Artemisinin-based combination therapy (ACT) is recommended treatment for uncomplicated falciparum malaria. The choice of ACT in a country or region will be based on the level of resistance of the partner medicine in the combination.

Severe falciparum malaria (Box 73.2)

Two classes of drugs are currently available for the parenteral treatment of severe malaria: the cinchona alkaloids (quinine and quinidine) and the artemisinin derivatives (artesunate, artemether and artemotil). Recent evidence[4,5] suggests superior efficacy of artesunate over quinine in adults. The dosage of artemisinin

Box 73.1 WHO recommendations for treatment of uncomplicated *P. falciparum* malaria

Artesunate + amodiaquine
4 mg/kg of artesunate and 10 mg base/kg of amodiaquine given once a day for 3 days
Artesunate + sulfadoxine–pyrimethamine
4 mg/kg of artesunate given once a day for 3 days and a single administration of sulfadoxinepyrimethamine (25/1.25 mg base/kg bw) on day 1
Artesunate + mefloquine
4 mg/kg of artesunate given once a day for 3 days and 25 mg base/kg of mefloquine usually split over 2 or 3 days
Artemether–lumefantrine
They are available as co-formulated tablets containing 20 mg of artemether and 120 mg of lumefantrine; the recommended treatment for persons weighing more than 34 kg is 4 tablets twice a day for 3 days
Dihydroartemisinin plus piperaquine
4 mg/kg/day dihydroartemisinin and 18 mg/kg/day piperaquine once a day for 3 days
Second-line antimalarial treatment
Artesunate (2 mg/kg once a day) plus doxycycline (3.5 mg/kg once a day) or clindamycin (10 mg/kg twice a day) for 7 days
Quinine plus doxycycline or clindamycin for 7 days

Box 73.2 WHO recommendations for treatment of severe falciparum malaria

Artesunate
2.4 mg/kg i.v. or i.m. given on admission (time = 0), then at 12 hours and 24 hours, then once a day
Artemether, or quinine, is an acceptable alternative if parenteral artesunate is not available: artemether 3.2 mg/kg BW i.m. given on admission, then 1.6 mg/kg BW per day; or quinine 20 mg salt/kg BW on admission (i.v. infusion or divided i.m. injection), then 10 mg/kg BW every 8 hours; infusion rate should not exceed 5 mg salt/kg BW per hour
Give parenteral antimalarials in the treatment of severe malaria for a minimum of 24 hours, once started (irrespective of the patient's ability to tolerate oral medication earlier) and, thereafter, complete treatment by giving a complete course of one of the regimens listed in Box 73.1 except artesunate + mefloquine regimen

derivatives does not need adjustment in vital organ dysfunction.

In patients with features of severe malaria, a mixed infection with *P. falciparum* should be assumed even if only a benign species is identified in the film. Occasionally, severe malaria can occur with *P. vivax* species. If clinical suspicion is high, a therapeutic trial of antimalarial treatment is justified even if the film is negative.

Box 73.3 WHO recommendations for treatment of *P. vivax, ovale* and *malariae* malaria

Uncomplicated *P. vivax* malaria
Chloroquine 25 mg base/kg divided over 3 days, combined with primaquine 0.25 mg base/kg, taken with food once daily for 14 days is the treatment of choice for chloroquine-sensitive infections; in Oceania and South-East Asia the dose of primaquine should be 0.5 mg/kg
For chloroquine-resistant *vivax* malaria, ACTs combined with primaquine except artesunate plus sulfadoxine–pyrimethamine as this is not effective against *P. vivax* in many places
Complicated *P. vivax* malaria
Treatment is the same as severe *P. falciparum* malaria
P. ovale and *malariae* malaria
Treatment is the same as uncomplicated *P. vivax* malaria but without primaquine for *P. malariae*

Severe malaria leads to severe septic shock, and the principles of management are the same, including resuscitation and provision of supportive treatment. These patients are at risk of acute lung injury but do need adequate fluid resuscitation. Convulsions must be actively treated. Complications should be managed as they present. The threshold for dialysis should be low. Pneumonia and bacterial septicaemia are also common, and should be recognised and treated.

Exchange blood transfusion (EBT) has been used in severe malaria. However, recent WHO guidelines[3] do not make any recommendation and note the lack of consensus on indications, benefits and dangers involved, or on practical details such as the volume of blood that should be exchanged. Traditional indications for EBT if pathogen-free compatible blood is available are:

- parasitaemia >30% even in the absence of clinical complications
- parasitaemia >10% in the presence of severe disease, especially cerebral malaria, acute renal failure, ARDS, jaundice and severe anaemia and/or poor prognostic factors (e.g. elderly patient, late-stage parasites (schizonts) in the peripheral blood)
- parasitaemia >10 % and failure to respond to optimal chemotherapy after 12–24 hours.

OTHER FORMS OF MALARIA (Box 73.3)

PROGNOSIS

Data are largely derived from endemic areas where presentation with convulsions, acidosis or hypoglycaemia is associated with a poorer outcome. Mortality in artesunate-treated severe *falciparum* malaria group in one trial[5] was still high (15% vs 22% in quinine-treated patients). In cerebral malaria, mortality is around 20%. The prognosis of cerebral malaria is frequently determined by the management of other complications such as renal failure and acidosis, but neurological sequelae are increasingly recognised.

TUBERCULOSIS

EPIDEMIOLOGY

Tuberculosis continues to be a devastating disease worldwide, with an estimated 9 million new cases and 1.5 million deaths annually. Medical conditions that predispose to tuberculosis include HIV infection, silicosis, diabetes, chronic renal failure/haemodialysis, malnutrition, solid organ transplant, gastrectomy, jejunoileal bypass, injection and inhalational drug abuse, alcoholism, chronic pulmonary disease, and prolonged steroid use. Social factors such as institutional living conditions (nursing homes, homeless shelters, prisons), urban dwelling and poverty are associated with an increased risk of tuberculosis.

PATHOGENESIS

Tuberculosis is usually caused by *Mycobacterium tuberculosis* and four other species (*M. bovis*, *M. africanum*, *M. microti* and *M. canetti*) grouped in the *Mycobacterium* complex. The genus *Mycobacterium* consists of many different species, all of which appear similar on acid-fast staining.

Inhalation of tubercle bacilli leads to one of four possible outcomes: immediate clearance of the organism, primary or progressive primary disease, chronic or latent infection, and reactivation disease. Latent infection refers to the presence of tuberculous infection (positive tuberculin reaction) without the disease.

The majority of primary TB infections are asymptomatic; clinical pneumonia occurs in 5–10% of adults, with a higher incidence in children and those suffering HIV infection. *M tuberculosis* microfoci that have remained dormant after primary infection may undergo reactivation resulting in secondary TB, often referred to as reactivation disease. This is responsible for 90% of TB in patients not infected with HIV.

CLINICAL SPECTRUM

The manifestations of TB are protean and TB should be considered in the differential diagnosis of all patients with fever of unknown origin, night sweats or unexplained weight loss. Besides the lungs, it can also involve the central nervous system, peritoneum, pericardium, gastrointestinal and genitourinary tract, bone and joints, lymph nodes and skin. Occasionally it can be disseminated in the form of miliary tuberculosis.

PULMONARY TUBERCULOSIS

Typically reactivation disease starts in the apex of one or both lungs leading to chronic inflammation and fibrosis. Pulmonary TB is often asymptomatic initially, though cough, dyspnoea and haemoptysis are useful clues. Hilar lymphadenopathy is the most common pulmonary presentation in children. It may occasionally present very late as extensive disease in both lungs with severe lung damage including cavitation and pneumothoraces.

Sputum, induced sputum, bronchial washings and transbronchial biopsy of infiltrates should be performed to isolate the organism. Computed tomography (CT) is more sensitive than chest radiography for detection of infiltrates, cavities, lymphadenopathy, miliary disease, bronchiectasis, bronchial stenosis, bronchopleural fistula and pleural effusion.

Tuberculous pleural effusion

Pleural TB may result in pleural effusion, or pleural empyema with or without bronchopleural fistula. Thoracentesis and pleural biopsy should be performed. The pleural fluid should be examined for total protein and glucose content, WBC count and differential, and fluid pH.

Positive cultures are found in less than 25% of cases. Pleural biopsy shows granulomatous inflammation in approximately 60% of patients. However, when culture of three biopsy specimens is combined with histological examination, the diagnosis can be made in up to 90% of cases. Pleuroscopy-guided biopsies increase the yield in pleural sampling. Conventional diagnostic tests have limitations.[6] Raised adenosine deaminase (ADA) levels have been found to be useful in the diagnosis with levels more than 70 U/L in pleural fluid strongly favouring tuberculous aetiology and levels less than 40 U/L making it less likely; ADA also has a good negative predictive value. However ADA assay should not be considered as an alternative to biopsy and culture.[7] Raised γ-interferon has also been found to be useful. Nucleic acid amplification tests have high specificity but low and variable sensitivity. Hence these tests are useful in confirming the disease, but not useful in excluding the disease.

TUBERCULOUS MENINGITIS

Tuberculous meningitis[8] remains the most serious relevant manifestation of TB to the intensive care physician. Tuberculous meningitis results from haematogenous spread. There is a thick gelatinous exudate around the sylvian fissures, basal cisterns, brainstem and cerebellum.

The majority of patients with TB meningitis have had recent contact with TB, followed by a prodrome of vague ill-health lasting 2–8 weeks. Later, signs and symptoms of meningeal irritation appear. Cranial nerve palsies occur in 20–25% of patients and papilloedema may be present. Choroidal tubercles are rare but almost pathognomonic. Visual loss due to optic nerve involvement may occasionally be the presenting feature. There may be focal neurological deficit such as hemiplegia; extrapyramidal movements and seizures are other manifestations. As the disease progresses, cerebral dysfunction sets in and the mortality approaches 50%.

Diagnostic algorithms have been suggested but they are unlikely to provide sufficient assurance to confidently exclude other diagnoses.[9,10] The key is a high degree of clinical suspicion, especially in the critically ill. In one study, TB meningitis was considered as a diagnosis in only 36% of cases and only 6% received immediate treatment.[11]

Definitive diagnosis of TB meningitis depends upon the detection of the organism in CSF, either by smear examination or by bacterial culture. The yield from smear is variable, but generally low. Culture of the CSF for the organisms is not invariably positive. Raised adenosine deaminase level is not specific. Various molecular-based methods including nucleic acid amplification (NAA) assays have emerged as a promising new method for the diagnosis of CNS tuberculosis because of its rapidity, sensitivity and specificity. In particular, nested PCR assay technique may improve the diagnosis of CNS tuberculosis.[12]

Computed tomography (CT) or magnetic resonance imaging (MRI) of the brain, both of which are sensitive but not specific, may reveal thickening and intense enhancement of meninges especially in basilar regions. Hydrocephalus and tuberculomas may also be present. Infarcts due to either vasculitis or mechanical strangulation of the vessels by the surrounding exudates are detected in up to 40%. The radiological differential diagnosis includes cryptococcal meningitis, CMV encephalitis, sarcoidosis, meningeal metastases and lymphoma.

TUBERCULOUS EMERGENCIES

- Massive haemoptysis
- Respiratory failure
- Pericardial tamponade
- Small intestinal obstruction
- Tuberculous meningitis
- Status epilepsy due to tuberculomas.

DIAGNOSIS OF TUBERCULOSIS

Once considered, isolate the patient and sample all potential sites for acid-fast staining and culture. Pleural, peritoneal, pericardial and other fluids must be cultured and analysed for differential cell count, protein, glucose and adenosine deaminase.

Histological examination for granulomatous infection is useful in bronchial tissue, pleural, peritoneal and skeletal tissues. Peritoneal biopsies are best obtained via laparoscopy. Newer culture media have reduced the time for culture to 2 weeks.

Nucleic acid amplification (NAA) tests amplify target nucleic acid regions that uniquely identify the *M. tuberculosis* complex, and are available as commercial kits or in-house assays. They can be applied to clinical specimens within hours. Based on current evidence, NAA tests cannot entirely replace conventional diagnostic approaches using microscopy and culture. A sensitive and specific fully automated and commercially available NAA Xpert MTB/RIF assay (Cepheid, Sunnyvale, CA, USA) can produce results in less than 2 hours, permitting a specific tuberculosis diagnosis and rapid detection of rifampicin resistance.[13]

The current status of NAA tests is summarised below:

- NAA tests, in general, have high specificity and positive predictive value; they are useful in ruling in rather than ruling out TB.
- A positive NAA test in smear-positive patients can differentiate *M. tuberculosis* from non-tuberculous *Mycobacteria* (NTM); treatment can then be started.
- The interpretation of smear-positive but negative-NAA test is controversial.
- In smear-negative and NAA-positive patients with a high clinical suspicion, treatment can be started particularly when prompt treatment is imperative.
- If clinical suspicion is high, TB is not excluded by both a negative smear and NAA.
- NAA results may remain positive for months. This method should be used only for initial diagnosis and not for follow-up.

Serodiagnosis of tuberculosis, despite remaining as a poor confirmatory tool, may be useful in exclusion of disease in areas of low incidence. The tuberculin skin test is useful in the diagnosis of latent infection with tuberculosis, but it cannot reliably distinguish individuals infected with *M. tuberculosis* from individuals sensitised to other mycobacteria including BCG. Interferon-γ release assays (IGRAs) are at least as sensitive and more specific than the tuberculin skin test. These IGRAs show high sensitivities but low specificities and hence can be used as rule out, but not rule in, tests for diagnosis of active tuberculosis.[14] Drug susceptibility tests should be performed on initial isolates from all patients in order to identify an effective antituberculous regimen, and may have to be repeated if the patient remains culture positive after 3 months.

TREATMENT OF TUBERCULOSIS[15]

Local guidelines are of paramount importance and advice should be sought. The commonest regimen used is isoniazid (5 mg/kg; max. 300 mg daily), and rifampicin (10 mg/kg; max. 600 mg daily) for 6 months with the addition of pyrazinamide (25 mg/kg) and ethambutol (15 mg/kg) for the first 2 months. It has been suggested that, instead of ethambutol, streptomycin is preferable as a fourth drug in tuberculous meningitis. Steroids are generally recommended in tuberculous meningitis and pericardial tuberculosis.

DRUG-RESISTANT TUBERCULOSIS

This is an increasing problem. Multidrug-resistant tuberculosis (defined as resistance to two or more of the first-line antituberculous drugs, usually INH and rifampicin) can be primary (no prior antituberculous therapy) or secondary (development of resistance during or after chemotherapy). Extensively drug-resistant (XDR) tuberculosis, defined by additional resistance to two second-line drug classes, is more difficult to treat and may be incurable.

Diagnosis depends upon collection of adequate specimens for culture prior to the initiation of antituberculous therapy. In critically ill patients, rapid diagnosis of drug resistance is of paramount importance. With the improvements in the culture methods and the availability of newer techniques, rapid identification of resistance is possible.[13] When resistance is present to two or more first-line agents, parenteral aminoglycoside (streptomycin, amikacin, etc.) and fluoroquinolones are generally added. Specialist microbiological advice should be sought.

TYPHOID FEVER

Typhoid fever is caused by *S. typhi* and less commonly by paratyphi A, B and C. Even non-typhoidal salmonellae have occasionally been isolated.[16] Typhoid fever, common in South and South-East Asia, is almost exclusively caused by fecal–oral spread. In the developed world, cases are either seen in international travellers or occasionally caused by infected food.

CLINICAL FEATURES

The incubation period is 5–21 days. Typhoid presents non-specifically with fever, chills, abdominal pain and constitutional symptoms. Constipation may be more frequent than diarrhoea. Hepatosplenomegaly, erythematous macular rash (30%) and relative bradycardia may be present. Relative bradycardia is not specific for enteric fever, but is a useful clue.[17]

COMPLICATIONS

- Shock
- Intestinal perforation
- Gastrointestinal haemorrhage
- Jaundice and encephalopathy[18]
- Neuropsychiatric manifestations
- Septic arthritis, pericarditis, etc.
- Obstetric complications in pregnant women.

DIAGNOSIS[19]

Anaemia, leucopenia/leucocytosis and deranged liver function are common. Blood cultures are positive in up to 80% of cases, and are the investigation of choice; 10–15 mL yields higher success than smaller volumes.[20] Though culturing urine, stool, rose spots and duodenal contents are useful, bone marrow culture is the most sensitive, and its yield remains unchanged up to 5 days after commencement of treatment.[21]

Serodiagnosis using Widal tests has limited clinical value. Commercial serological tests such as Typhidot-M® and Tubex®, which detect IgM antibodies against different *S typhi* antigens, have a higher sensitivity and specificity.[22] Nested PCR is very promising in the diagnosis of typhoid fever.

TREATMENT[23]

In both uncomplicated and complicated typhoid fever, the treatment of choice is fluoroquinolones (ciprofloxacin or ofloxacin for 5–7 days in uncomplicated and 10–14 days in complicated infections). In fluoroquinolone-resistant cases, azithromycin, cefixime or ceftriaxone can be used. There is some concern in using fluoroquinolones in children as they have been shown to cause cartilage toxicity in immature animals, but this appears largely unfounded in clinical trials.[24] A recent Cochrane review reported that, when compared with fluoroquinolones, azithromycin significantly reduced clinical failure.[25]

Dexamethasone reduces mortality in severe typhoid fever: delirium, obtundation, stupor, coma or shock. [26] Ileal perforation, which may occur late, classically in the third week of febrile illness, requires prompt surgical intervention, and segmental resection has been recommended as the procedure of choice. [27,28]

CHOLERA

Cholera is caused by enterotoxin-producing *Vibrio cholera*.[29] The incubation period varies from 12 hours to several days. The clinical case:infection ratio is about 1:10. It starts abruptly with painless watery diarrhoea associated with vomiting and painful muscle cramps. Vomiting may be the first symptom before diarrhoea.

Stool examination shows neither leucocytes nor erythrocytes. Dark-field microscopy examination may reveal rapidly motile comma-shaped bacilli in fresh stool. Commercial assays detecting O antigen in stool samples, which take less than 5 minutes, are now available and are as sensitive and specific as stool culture. Aggressive rehydration is the mainstay of treatment; very large quantities of fluid may be needed. Adjunctive antimicrobial therapy is effective in shortening the duration of diarrhoea. Single-dose doxycycline (300 mg) or single-dose ciprofloxacin (1 g) is very effective, but azithromycin has recently been shown to be superior.[30]

LEPTOSPIROSIS

This is caused by *Leptospira interrogans*. It occurs due to exposure to contaminated water. The disease has an incubation period of 7–10 days with a range of 2–20 days. It has two phases: septicaemic phase and immune phase. Clinical features include conjunctival suffusion or haemorrhages (useful diagnostic clue), uveitis, severe muscle tenderness, non-oliguric renal failure, hypokalaemia, hepatic dysfunction, pulmonary haemorrhage, ARDS, myocarditis, rhabdomyolysis, thrombocytopenia, DIC, haemorrhage into the skin and internal organs, and digital gangrene. Weil's syndrome is characterised by hepatorenal dysfunction, bleeding diathesis and pulmonary involvement.

Diagnosis is made with isolation of the organism by culture (blood, urine, CSF) or serology using the gold standard microscopic agglutination test (MAT). Alternative serology tests including ELISA tests are available. Both culture and serology should be attempted if available, and local microbiological advice should be sought. Treatment is with penicillin G or ceftriaxone. In penicillin-allergic patients, doxycycline can be used.

DENGUE FEVER

EPIDEMIOLOGY AND PATHOGENESIS

It is estimated that 50 million cases of dengue fever occur worldwide annually and half a million people suffering from DHF require hospitalisation each year, a very large proportion of whom (approximately 90%) are children less than 5 years old.[31] The causative agent is a flavivirus with four distinct serogroups, and it is transmitted by the bite of *Aedes* mosquitoes. Two patterns of transmission have been recognised, epidemic due to isolated introduction of dengue to a region, usually due to a single serotype, and hyperendemic referring to the continuous circulation of multiple dengue virus serotypes.

Following a mosquito bite, viraemia begins and usually lasts up to 7 days. Infection with one of the four serotypes (primary infection) provides life-long immunity against that serotype, but not against the other serotypes (secondary infection). Epidemiological studies have suggested that the risk of severe disease (DHF/DSS) is significantly higher in secondary infection than in primary infection.

CLINICAL FEATURES

The clinical presentation varies from mild febrile illness to severe haemorrhagic fever. Most infections are asymptomatic. WHO classifies dengue infection as undifferentiated fever, dengue fever (DF), and dengue haemorrhagic fever (DHF)/dengue shock syndrome (DSS).[31]

Dengue fever has an incubation period of 3–14 days and is characterised by the sudden onset of fever, severe headache, retro-orbital pain on moving the eyes, and fatigue. It is often associated with severe myalgia and arthralgia (breakbone fever). Maculopapular rash, flushed facies and injected conjunctiva are common. Haemorrhagic manifestations can occur in DF and should not be confused with DHF.

Dengue haemorrhagic fever occurs primarily in children <10 years and is characterised by plasma leakage syndrome and haemoconcentration (20% or greater rise in haematocrit), pleural effusion or ascites. The diagnosis is made if the following symptoms and signs are present: bleeding, a platelet count of less than 100 000 per cubic millimetre, and plasma leakage. Haemorrhagic manifestations without evidence of plasma leakage do not constitute DHF. The mechanism underlying the profound capillary leak in DHF but not in DF is poorly understood. It is important to watch for the onset of DHF, which typically occurs 4–7 days after the onset of the disease, approximately at the time of defervescence. Decrease in platelet count and rise in haematocrit are useful clues.[32]

Dengue shock syndrome is characterised by profound hypotension and shock.

DIAGNOSIS

Dengue should be suspected in all febrile patients who live in, or have returned from, endemic areas in the preceding 2 weeks. Leucopenia, thrombocytopenia with a positive tourniquet test and raised AST are frequently seen; the former two tests have the highest sensitivity (about 90%) for the diagnosis of early dengue.[32] A positive tourniquet test alone cannot differentiate DHF from DF.

IgM immunoassay allows rapid confirmation of the diagnosis. If it is negative, particularly in the first 6 days of the illness, the diagnosis should not be ruled out. Acute and convalescent sera should be analysed by haemagglutination assay or IgG immunoassay for a fourfold rise in titre. Virus isolation, viral nucleic acid detection by techniques such as reverse transcriptase PCR, and viral antigen detection are available.[31]

TREATMENT

Supportive therapy for shock, especially appropriate and prompt fluid replacement can reduce mortality. Fluid management is complex and WHO guidelines on fluid management are available.[31] In DSS, steroids have not been shown to be useful.[33] Once capillary leakage abates, fluid overload and pulmonary oedema can become problematic.

HANTAVIRUS

Hantaviruses are rodent viruses distributed worldwide, with over 150 000 cases being registered annually. There are two major clinical syndromes: haemorrhagic fever with renal syndrome (HFRS) and hantavirus cardiopulmonary syndrome (HCPS). Both are acquired by exposure to aerosols of rodent excreta.

HANTAVIRUS CARDIOPULMONARY SYNDROME

The incubation period is about 3 weeks. There are two phases: the prodromal phase is characterised by a relatively mild febrile illness, typically lasting 3–5 days, and the cardiopulmonary phase is characterised by severe, rapidly progressive respiratory failure. In the latter phase, acute pulmonary oedema due to increased capillary permeability occurs. The progress from the prodromal phase to cardiopulmonary phase is dramatic. In severe cases, significant myocardial depression also occurs, resulting in low cardiac output and hypotension. Acute renal failure can occur. The combination of thrombocytopenia, myelocytosis, haemoconcentration, lack of significant toxic granulation in neutrophils, and more than 10% of lymphocytes with immunoblastic morphological features is highly sensitive and specific. ELISA for IgM and IgG antibodies is useful in the diagnosis. Hantavirus can also be detected by tissue RT-PCR. Immunohistochemical staining of tissue reveals hantaviral antigen. Treatment is mainly supportive with intravenous fluids, inotropes, mechanical ventilation, extracorporeal membrane oxygenation and blood products. Intravenous ribavirin is probably ineffective in the treatment of HCPS in the cardiopulmonary stage.[34]

HAEMORRHAGIC FEVER WITH RENAL SYNDROME

This is characterised by fever, renal failure and haemorrhagic manifestations. The disease has five progressive stages: febrile, hypotensive, oliguric, diuretic and convalescent. Non-specific constitutional symptoms are followed by shock, oliguria, disseminated intravascular coagulation (DIC) and haemorrhagic manifestations. Diagnosis is made using ELISA for IgG and IGM antibodies. Treatment is supportive, including renal support. Ribavirin has been found to be useful.[35]

ARBOVIRAL ENCEPHALITIS

Viruses transmitted to human beings by the bites of arthropods (especially mosquitoes and ticks) are major causes of encephalitis worldwide. Although different viruses can cause encephalitis, an antigenically related group of flaviviruses[36] accounts for a major proportion of cases worldwide. These include mosquito-borne diseases such as Japanese encephalitis, West Nile virus encephalitis, St Louis encephalitis, Murray Valley encephalitis[37] and tick-borne encephalitis.[38] Viral encephalitis is characterised by a triad of fever, headache and altered level of consciousness. Other common clinical findings include disorientation, behavioural and speech disturbances, and focal or diffuse neurological signs such as hemiparesis or seizures. The incubation period is usually 5–15 days. Other manifestations include recurrent seizures, including status epilepticus, a flaccid paralysis resembling that of poliomyelitis, and Parkinsonian-type movement disorders. Flavivirus encephalitis is diagnosed usually by the IgM capture enzyme-linked immunosorbent assay (ELISA). Treatment is supportive. Interferon-α, ribavirin and intravenous immunoglobulin have all been tried with mixed success.

VIRAL HAEMORRHAGIC FEVERS (VHF)

Viral haemorrhagic fever is a general term for a severe illness, sometimes associated with bleeding, caused by a number of viruses.

EPIDEMIOLOGY

Lassa virus, Rift Valley fever, Crimean–Congo HF, haemorrhagic fever with renal syndrome (HFRS-hantavirus), Marburg and Ebola virus, yellow fever and dengue haemorrhagic fever are some of the most important viral haemorrhagic fevers. Haemorrhagic fever viruses have an affinity for the vascular system and increased vascular permeability is the primary defect. Petechial haemorrhages are usually associated with fever and myalgias. Later, frank mucous membrane haemorrhage may occur, with accompanying hypotension, shock and circulatory collapse. Multisystem organ failure can occur. There is a wide variation in the relative severity of the clinical presentation.

The sources of infection are rodents for Lassa virus and hantavirus, mosquitoes for Rift Valley fever, yellow fever and dengue haemorrhagic fever, and ticks for Congo–Crimean haemorrhagic fever virus. At least four of the haemorrhagic fevers - Lassa fever (LF), Ebola virus, Marburg virus and CCHF - are capable of person-to-person transmission through close contact with infected blood and other body secretions. Epidemiological studies of VHF in humans indicate that although possible, the airborne route does not readily transmit infection from person to person.

CLINICAL FEATURES

The patient will have either been in an endemic area or been in contact with someone from an endemic area.

Viral haemorrhagic fevers[39] generally have an abrupt onset with an incubation period <10 days. The incubation period can be up to 21 days. They present as acute febrile illnesses with a prodrome that often includes severe headache, dizziness, flushing, conjunctival injection, myalgia, lumbar pain and prostration. Gastrointestinal symptoms with nausea, vomiting, abdominal pain and diarrhoea may occur.

Leucopenia or leucocytosis, thrombocytopenia and elevated serum aminotransferases may be evident early in the disease; a petechial rash may appear on days 3–10. Coagulation profiles become progressively more abnormal, and overt haemorrhagic features of the disease (ecchymoses, epistaxis, gingival bleeding, malaena, haematuria, etc.) may supervene from day 5 onward, or sometimes even earlier. Multiple organ failure supervenes and death may ensue. Clinical improvement becomes apparent toward the end of the second week of illness in patients who survive.

DIAGNOSIS

A high index of suspicion is needed and VHF should be suspected in the following circumstances:

- unexplained fever in patients who have visited areas where VHF are endemic, within 3 weeks of becoming ill; the likelihood is greater if they have camped in the bush, slept on the ground or in rural farms, or had any bites or contact with sick animals
- febrile medical and nursing staff in the endemic areas and laboratory workers who handle VHF viruses
- febrile contacts.

Tests on samples present an extreme biohazard risk. The diagnosis may be made by isolating virus from blood or body fluids, by positive IgM antibody or by showing a fourfold rise in antibody titre. Early diagnosis is mainly based on direct detection of viral antigens or RNA.[40] Diagnosis can be confirmed by visualisation of characteristic viral particles by electron microscopy.

TREATMENT

Therapy is essentially supportive for a severe shock state. Haemorrhage is managed by replacement of blood, platelets and clotting factors as indicated. Ribavirin is useful in treating LF, Rift Valley fever and CCHF.[40] Ribavirin may reduce mortality by tenfold if treatment is begun within 6 days of onset. A 30 mg/kg i.v. loading dose is followed by 15 mg/kg q 6 h for 4 days and then 7.5 mg/kg q 8 h for another 6 days. Other treatment options are post-exposure vaccination.

PRECAUTIONS

In most countries these diseases must be notified immediately. In addition to universal blood and body fluid precautions, airborne isolation, including use of goggles, high-efficiency masks, a negative-pressure room with no air circulation, and positive-pressure filtered air respirators have all been recommended, as is surveillance of contacts. If applicable, to prevent further mosquito transmission, patients should be isolated in well-screened rooms sprayed with residual insecticides. Guidelines on infection control in the management of highly pathogenic infectious diseases have been published.[41]

Access the complete references list online at http://www.expertconsult.com

3. WHO. Guidelines for the treatment of malaria. 2nd ed. Geneva: WHO; 2010. Online. Available: http://whqlibdoc.who.int/publications/2010/9789241547925_eng.pdf.
15. WHO. Treatment of Tuberculosis Guidelines. 4th ed. Geneva: WHO; 2010. Online. Available: http://whqlibdoc.who.int/publications/2010/9789241547833_eng.pdf. (Accessed 17/06/2012.).
20. Bhan MK, Bahl R, Bhatnagar S. Typhoid and paratyphoid fever. Lancet 2005;366:749–62.
31. WHO. Comprehensive Guidelines for Prevention and Control of Dengue and Dengue Haemorrhagic Fever Dengue. 2011. Online. Available: http://www.searo.who.int/LinkFiles/Dengue_DHF_prevention&control_guidelines_rev.pdf. (Accessed 20 June 2012.).
32. Wilder-Smith A, Schwartz E. Dengue in travelers. N Engl J Med 2005;353(9):924–32.
36. Gould EA, Solomon T. Pathogenic flaviviruses. Lancet 2008;371(9611):500–9.
38. Lindquist L, Vapalahti O. Tick-borne encephalitis. Lancet 2008;371(9627):1861–71.

Part Eleven

Severe and Multiple Trauma

74

Severe and multiple trauma

James A Judson and Li C Hsee

Trauma can be defined as physical injury from mechanical energy. It is usually categorised as blunt or penetrating. In Western countries, severe blunt trauma is common, caused by road crashes, falls and, less frequently, blows and assault. Severe penetrating trauma, usually from stabbings and gunshots, is less common except in larger cities of the USA,[1,2] South Africa and war zones. Blunt trauma is often more difficult to treat than penetrating trauma. Assessment is more difficult, because injuries are frequently internal, multiple and not obvious initially. The risk of missing serious injuries can only be lessened by a systematic approach and repeated assessments.[3-5]

ASSESSMENT AND PRIORITIES

TRIAGE

An important first step is triage – sorting patients with acute life-threatening injuries and complications from those whose lives are not in danger. Depending on the complexity of injury, it is important to ensure resources are available for treatment. If institutional capacity is lacking, consider transferring the patient to an advanced trauma unit. The severity of total body injury is related to the number of separate injuries present, and to the severity of individual injuries. Assessment can be made either at the scene of injury or on arrival at hospital. As in any emergency, assessment, diagnosis and treatment need to be concurrent. There is limited time for detailed histories, examinations, investigations or well-considered diagnoses before starting emergency care.

RECOGNITION OF SEVERITY

Most patients with severe injury can be distinguished early by the following:

- *Depressed consciousness:* in the trauma patient, depressed consciousness can be related to brain injury, hypoxaemia, shock, alcohol or other ingested drugs, or precipitating neurological or cardiac events. Frequently, a combination of factors is present, and the precise extent of physical brain injury is not known initially. Initial treatment is in any case determined by the level of consciousness rather than its exact cause.
- *Breathing difficulty:* this is common in patients with trauma to the head, face, neck and chest. If rapid or distressed breathing is present then airway obstruction, laryngeal injury, pulmonary aspiration and lung or chest wall injury (especially pneumothorax and lung contusion) must be considered.
- *Signs of shock:* shock is almost always hypovolaemic from blood loss, but other types of shock occasionally occur in trauma (see below).

PRIORITIES

A trauma patient often has multiple problems requiring attention. Determining priorities is not always easy. In general, the priorities are to:

- *support life*: the patient is kept alive with resuscitative techniques, while the various injuries and complications are attended to
- *locate and control bleeding*, which may be varied (see below)
- *prevent brainstem compression* and spinal cord damage
- *diagnose and treat* all other injuries and complications.

BASIC TREATMENT PRINCIPLES

A systematic approach to managing severe and multiple trauma is important. Effective programmes developed by the American College of Surgeons are now well established.[6] A number of basic treatment principles apply to all severe trauma patients.

EMERGENCY ASSESSMENT (PRIMARY SURVEY)

The following must be recognised and treated before anything else:

- A – *Airway obstruction*: is suggested by noisy (or silent) breathing, with paradoxical chest movements and breathing distress, and inadequate airway protection from impaired gag reflexes in patients with depressed consciousness. Airway obstruction should be managed with cervical spine protection.

- *B – Breathing difficulty*: is suggested by tachypnoea, abnormal pattern of breathing, cyanosis or mental confusion.
- *C – Circulatory shock*: is manifested by cold peripheries with delayed capillary refill, rapid weak pulse or low blood pressure (see below).
- *D – Disability:* neurological status needs to be evaluated by checking the pupils and GCS. A decreased level of consciousness can be caused by poor cerebral perfusion, direct cerebral injuries, alcohol, recreational drugs and opiates.[6]
- *E – Exposure:* the patient needs to be exposed for examination, but at the same time hypothermia must be prevented and dignity preserved.[6]

OXYGEN AND VENTILATORY THERAPY

High-flow oxygen by mask is given to all trauma patients. Patients with severe trauma frequently require ventilatory support. A restless uncooperative patient should be anaesthetised and intubated under a rapid sequence induction to facilitate resuscitation.

BLOOD CROSSMATCH AND TESTS

Six units of red cells should be crossmatched urgently, but it is impossible to predict the amount of blood that will be required. Blood is concurrently sent for baseline haematological and biochemical tests, including blood ethanol level. Blood ethanol level is clinically useful in assessing individual patients with depressed consciousness, quite apart from epidemiological and preventive medicine,[7] and legal considerations.

FLUID RESUSCITATION

Resuscitation fluids are given (see below). If necessary, two or three large 14- or 16-gauge i.v. cannulae are inserted in upper limb, external jugular or femoral veins.

ANALGESIA

Analgesia is easily overlooked. Opioid agents should be titrated i.v., and not given i.m. or subcutaneously. Large doses may be needed.

URINE OUTPUT

A urinary catheter is inserted unless a ruptured urethra is suspected (because of blood at the urinary meatus, severe fractured pelvis or abnormal prostate position on rectal examination), in which case a urethrogram is indicated before catheterisation. Urine output monitoring is an important guide to resuscitation.

CLINICAL EVALUATION OF INJURIES (SECONDARY SURVEY)

Injuries are easily missed in an emergency, especially when one injury is obvious. A secondary, and even a tertiary, survey should be performed.[5] The back and the front of the patient should be examined. Special attention is paid to regions with external lacerations, contusions and abrasions. All body regions are examined systematically.

HEAD

Neurological observations are made. The ears and nose are inspected for cerebrospinal fluid and blood, and the scalp is examined thoroughly.

FACE

Bleeding into the airway should be excluded, and the face and jaws tested for abnormal mobility.

SPINE

A cervical spine fracture or dislocation is assumed in all patients with depressed consciousness until proved otherwise. Signs of spinal cord injury should be sought (e.g. warm dilated peripheries from loss of vasomotor tone, diaphragmatic breathing, paralysis, priapism and loss of anal tone). The thoracic and lumbar spine should be inspected and palpated.

THORAX

Fractured ribs in themselves are not usually life threatening, but haemothorax, pneumothorax, lung contusion and chest wall instability (flail chest) will require attention if present. Tension pneumothorax is a life-threatening emergency that needs to be detected and treated early. Less common but very serious injuries can occur to the heart and great vessels (see Ch. 77).

ABDOMEN

The spleen, liver and mesenteries are often damaged. Retroperitoneal haemorrhage is common. Injuries to the pancreas, duodenum and other hollow viscera are less frequent, and may be missed until signs of peritonitis occur. Renal injury with retroperitoneal haemorrhage is suggested by haematuria and loin pain (see Ch. 79).

PELVIS

Pelvic fractures may be difficult to detect clinically, especially in the unconscious patient. Blood loss may be massive, particularly with posterior fractures involving sacroiliac dislocation. Ruptured bladder and ruptured urethra may occur with anterior fractures.

EXTREMITIES

A litre or more of blood may be lost into a fractured femur. Long-bone fractures are more serious when they are open, comminuted or displaced, or if associated with nerve or arterial damage.

EXTERNAL

Contusions may be extensive and serious, especially in falls from heights, and may be overlooked if the victim's back is not examined. Road crash victims may sustain serious burns or abrasions.

SHOCK IN THE TRAUMA PATIENT

The earliest, most constant and reliable signs of shock are seen in the peripheral circulation. A patient with cold, pale peripheries has shock until proved otherwise. Tachycardia is not always present and hypotension is a late sign of shock. The commonest form of shock in trauma is hypovolaemic shock.

HYPOVOLAEMIC SHOCK

If the neck veins are empty, hypovolaemic shock should be inferred. Possible sites of blood loss causing shock are:

- *external loss*, which is obvious clinically from blood-soaked clothing and pooled blood
- *major fractures*, which are obvious clinically by deformity, swelling, crepitus, pain and tenderness (e.g. femurs) or seen on a plain X-ray (e.g. pelvis)
- *pleural cavity*, detected on urgent chest X-ray. Intrapleural drains will reveal the amount and rate of blood loss
- *peritoneal cavity*, detected by laparotomy, diagnostic peritoneal lavage, computed tomography (CT) scan or ultrasound. Clinical examination of the abdomen can be misleading when the patient is intoxicated, has depressed consciousness or has multiple injuries. A single clinical examination is of limited value; changes over time are more important
- *retroperitoneum*, detected at laparotomy or by CT scan, or inferred when all the above are negative, especially in the presence of pelvic or lumbar spine fracture.

CARDIOGENIC SHOCK

If the trauma patient with shock has distended neck veins, possible causes are tension pneumothorax, concurrent myocardial infarction, cardiac tamponade or myocardial contusion.

NEUROLOGICAL SHOCK

Patients with paraplegia or tetraplegia from spinal cord injury may have low blood pressure with warm dilated peripheries accompanied by lax anal tone and by priapism in the male (see Ch. 78). This is a diagnosis of exclusion and all causes of hypovolaemic shock (see above) must be sought.

SEPTIC SHOCK

Occasionally, patients with pulmonary aspiration may develop septic shock. This is unlikely to confuse the initial trauma assessment soon after injury, but may require consideration some hours or a day or two later.

ABDOMINAL ULTRASOUND

The non-invasive nature and increasing availability of FAST (focused assessment with sonography for trauma) scanning in emergency departments has made this modality attractive in trauma to detect haemoperitoneum and haemopericardium.

However:[8]

- it is operator dependent and needs to be performed by trained personnel
- it may have an unacceptably high false-negative rate
- there is a small but important false-positive rate for intra-abdominal bleeding
- it is unable to diagnose ruptured bowel
- it is not good for bleeding in the pelvis.

Its main usefulness is in the shocked patient, where a positive FAST indicates the need for immediate laparotomy without further investigation.[6,9,10]

DIAGNOSTIC PERITONEAL LAVAGE

Diagnostic peritoneal lavage (DPL) is indicated to diagnose intra-abdominal bleeding and sometimes bowel injury.

This is an invasive procedure that may make subsequent clinical abdominal examination difficult.[6,11]

Caution is needed with pregnancy, previous abdominal surgery or massive pelvic injury. Isotonic saline 1 L (or 10 mL/kg) is instilled into the peritoneal cavity, after drainage of the stomach and bladder. The presence of more than 10 mL frank blood on catheter aspiration necessitates immediate laparotomy; otherwise a lavage fluid specimen should be examined for red and white cell counts and amylase concentration. A red cell count over 100 000 per mm^3, white cell count over 500 per mm^3, or an increased amylase concentration suggests bleeding or viscus injury, and laparotomy should be undertaken immediately. These absolute figures are debatable, however, and lower values are accepted in penetrating trauma.[6,12,13]

CT ABDOMEN

Improved availability, reduced scanning times and better definition are increasingly favouring CT abdomen over DPL in patients who are sufficiently stable to tolerate the procedure safely. It needs to be performed quickly and safely, with gastric and i.v. contrast, and interpreted by radiologists experienced in trauma. Visualisation of abdominal and pelvic organs and haemorrhage is excellent.[14,15] Diaphragm, pancreas and hollow viscus injuries may be difficult to visualise on CT, but the presence of free fluid in the absence of solid organ injury raises suspicion of hollow viscus injury.[16]

FLUID RESUSCITATION

TYPES OF FLUIDS

Almost all patients who are hypotensive or noticeably vasoconstricted will need blood transfusion but, in general, transfusion of large quantities of blood is wasteful while bleeding is uncontrolled. Isotonic saline or a balanced salt solution should be the first fluid infused. Shocked patients may need 2–3 L in the first few minutes. One-litre bags or bottles and giving sets with in-line pumps should be used on all i.v. lines. If fluid resuscitation is likely to be extensive, warmed fluids and rapid infusion devices should be used. Albumin solutions (and probably other colloid resuscitation fluids) are contraindicated in trauma patients as the SAFE study conducted in ICU patients showed higher mortality in patients given albumin, in the predetermined trauma subgroup, particularly in those with traumatic brain injury.[17] By 20–30 minutes cross-matched red cells should be available. Uncrossmatched group O Rh-negative blood is occasionally indicated in the exsanguinating patient.

All resuscitation fluids have a high sodium concentration, similar to that of extracellular fluid. Glucose 5% and glucose–saline solutions are not effective resuscitation fluids. Few trauma patients actually require them in the first day.

THE EXSANGUINATING PATIENT

With exsanguination secondary to penetrating thoracic injury, there is a place for emergency room thoracotomy, but this approach has little place in blunt trauma.[18] The exsanguinating blunt trauma patient needs rapid intubation, volume resuscitation, bilateral intrapleural drains, chest and pelvic X-ray, and a rapid trip to the operating room if it seems likely that the bleeding is in the thorax or abdomen.

MASSIVE TRANSFUSION PROTOCOL

Coagulopathy is common in patients with haemorrhagic shock and can be made worse by fluid resuscitation. Many institutions will have a massive transfusion protocol (MTP) for exsanguinating patients. The principle of MTP is to increase plasma to platelet to red blood cells ratios during the resuscitation phase.[19] MTP is shown to improve outcome. Haemostatic agents such as tranexamic acid and factor VIIa are increasingly used as a part of MTP.[20,21]

PERMISSIVE HYPOTENSION

In penetrating trauma, there is some evidence that extensive fluid resuscitation prior to haemostasis may be detrimental, presumably because of higher blood pressure, displacement of blood clot and dilution of coagulation factors.[22,23]

In blunt trauma, there is no such evidence. Furthermore, it is not appropriate to generalise the evidence from penetrating trauma to blunt trauma because these two types of trauma are quite different. In penetrating trauma, the bleeding is often from single arteries without extensive tissue injury, and complete haemostasis can often be easily achieved. In contrast, in blunt trauma, the bleeding is often venous as well as arterial, with capillary oozing into the soft tissues, which may continue for hours. It can often not be completely controlled by operative surgery, interventional radiology or reduction and fixation of fractures. Accordingly, fluid resuscitation is an important part of the treatment of circulatory shock in blunt trauma (see section on Inadequate resuscitation). Nevertheless, fluid resuscitation must not be used as an excuse for delaying haemostasis in blunt trauma.

Furthermore, traumatic brain injury is often present in blunt trauma, which frequently involves several body regions. Hypotension is disastrous to an already injured brain, and must not be prolonged by under-resuscitation (see Ch. 75, section on Traumatic brain injury – emergency treatment).[24–26]

DAMAGE CONTROL RESUSCITATION (DCR)

Damage control surgery was described some years ago as abbreviated surgery to stop bleeding and contamination, followed by a period of ICU care before further surgery, to try to arrest the lethal triad of acidosis, hypothermia and coagulopathy.[27] US military experience with combat patients is extending this concept to fluid resuscitation as well, with a tendency to give no (or only small amounts of) resuscitation fluids before haemostatic surgery. As such, DCR is seen to integrate permissive hypotension, haemostatic resuscitation, and damage control surgery.[28] Some enthusiasts are now injudiciously extending DCR to other types of trauma.[29] As mentioned above under permissive hypotension, great caution should be exercised before extending this concept to non-exsanguinating blunt trauma, particularly if a traumatic brain injury is present,[26] or if remote from a trauma centre.

URINE OUTPUT

Hourly urine output is a useful guide to resuscitation from shock. Minimal acceptable urine output is 0.5 mL/kg per hour, but 1–2 mL/kg per hour is more adequate. Furosemide has no place in initial resuscitation. Apart from adequate resuscitation, diuresis can be due to ethanol, mannitol, dopamine, nephrogenic or neurogenic diabetes insipidus, or non-oliguric renal failure. Polyuria may mask early recognition of acute renal failure.

INADEQUATE RESUSCITATION

Patients in shock have depleted interstitial fluid as well as circulating blood volume, and need trauma resuscitation fluid volumes greater than the actual volume of blood lost. With blunt injury, volume losses often continue for 24–48 hours. Prolonged shock from delayed and inadequate resuscitation leads to renal failure, acute respiratory distress syndrome (ARDS), sepsis, disseminated intravascular coagulation (DIC) and multiple organ dysfunction.[30,31]

PULMONARY OEDEMA

Pulmonary oedema during resuscitation may be related to fluid overload, direct lung trauma, aspiration of gastric contents, pulmonary responses to non-thoracic trauma and reactions to resuscitation fluids. They can all cause leaky capillaries and produce non-cardiogenic pulmonary oedema.

RADIOLOGY FOR TRAUMA PATIENTS

Patients with depressed consciousness, breathing difficulties or unstable circulation should be X-rayed in the emergency department, and not sent to a radiology department remote from skilled resuscitation facilities. Conversely, extensive imaging examinations of shocked patients in the emergency department are unacceptable. Only three examinations should ever be requested in the emergency department.

CHEST

This is the only X-ray ever justified in an unresuscitated patient. A supine film is usually sufficient. An erect film is better for showing intrapleural air or fluid, ruptured diaphragm, free abdominal gas and for defining an abnormal mediastinum, but is often impractical in shock or suspected spinal injury. It can be done later if feasible. Tension pneumothorax is a clinical diagnosis and does not require a chest X-ray before insertion of an intercostal drain.

LATERAL CERVICAL SPINE

Lateral cervical spine X-ray in the severely injured patient is now largely replaced by CT. It is only an initial screening examination for cervical spine fractures and does not 'clear' the spine. With head or facial injuries, a cervical fracture should be assumed initially and a cervical collar applied.

PELVIS

Unexplained blood loss can be due to a missed pelvic fracture. A dislocated hip can be missed in multiple injuries. A pelvic X-ray is not needed in awake patients with no pelvic abnormalities.

OTHER RADIOLOGICAL INVESTIGATIONS

Other X-rays should be performed after adequate resuscitation in the radiology department, operating room or intensive care unit (ICU):

- *Skull*: plain skull X-rays are not useful and do not guide immediate treatment. An urgent CT scan of the brain is a more useful investigation.
- *Extremities*: X-rays of the extremities to assess bony injuries are not urgent unless there is vascular injury. Therefore, these films should not be taken in the emergency department, unless the patient is going directly to the operating room for fracture fixation.
- *Spine*: X-rays of thoracic or lumbosacral spine are seldom indicated in the emergency department.
- *Abdomen*: a plain abdominal X-ray is of limited value in the initial evaluation of trauma. It may be helpful in high-velocity penetrating injuries, such as gunshot wounds, to help determine trajectory.
- *CT abdomen*: this can be valuable to evaluate a patient who is haemodynamically sufficiently stable to tolerate the procedure safely (see above).
- *CT head*: this is vital in the treatment of traumatic brain injuries.
- *CT neck*: the most reliable way to exclude or delineate cervical spine injuries is by a CT neck scan,[4,32] which can conveniently be done when the patient is going to the CT scanner for other examinations.
- *CT thorax*: apart from diagnosis of aortic injury, CT thorax is of limited value in the trauma patient. Visualisation of thoracic structures is excellent, but it seldom discovers important undiagnosed injuries that affect patient treatment.[33] If aortic injury is suspected, multislice CT is the current definitive diagnostic test. The use of aortic stent grafts for this injury, in locations where this technology is available, means that CT is not only the best diagnostic test but also necessary for preoperative planning.[34] Aortography is no longer the definitive diagnostic test for traumatic aortic rupture.
- *Urethrography:* this is used when urethral injury is suspected. Properly done CT abdomen may well demonstrate bladder injury; otherwise *cystography* is used.
- *Interventional radiology*: percutaneous transcatheter embolisation is therapeutic rather than diagnostic. It can provide life-saving haemostasis in massive retroperitoneal haemorrhage associated with pelvic fracture.[35] The logistics of managing such haemodynamically unstable patients in the radiology department are formidable.

TRAUMATIC BRAIN INJURY (SEE CH. 75)

Injuries to the head region are common, but those requiring urgent cranial operations are less so. Traumatic brain injury may initially be obvious amongst multiple injuries, but may not be the most important injury. Conversely, traumatic brain injury may seem initially unimportant. Traumatic brain injury is a major determinant of outcome in critically injured patients.

EMERGENCY TREATMENT

Resuscitation measures, as in the emergency assessment (primary survey) section above, are undertaken. Victims with one or both dilated unreactive pupils, or a rapidly deteriorating level of consciousness not due to hypoxia or shock, should be given mannitol 1 g/kg i.v. to relieve brainstem compression until definitive diagnosis and treatment can be arranged. However, mannitol should be given only if the patient has been adequately volume-resuscitated as it may add to hypovolaemia. In the ICU, concentrated salt is often preferred to mannitol because it is readily available and does not produce hypovolaemia.[36,37]

Shocked trauma patients with or without traumatic brain injuries require the same crystalloid resuscitation fluids. Treatment of shock and maintenance of cerebral perfusion are vital, as hypotension is disastrous to an already damaged brain.[24-26] Contrary to common belief, sodium-containing fluids are not inherently dangerous in traumatic brain injury. However, after adequate resuscitation further sodium administration is usually not indicated. Excessive (free) water is potentially dangerous, however, as it can lead to hypo-osmolar brain swelling.[38]

NEUROLOGICAL EVALUATION

Factors such as hypoxaemia, shock, alcohol, analgesics, anaesthetic agents, muscle relaxants and other drugs confound neurological signs. Clinical neurological evaluation includes the Glasgow Coma Scale (GCS)[39,40] and a search for lateralising signs.

CT scanning is indicated in all patients who will not obey verbal commands, especially if they are rendered neurologically inaccessible by sedative and relaxant agents. Lateralising motor or pupillary signs with a deteriorating level of consciousness are indications for immediate CT scanning (or, if unavailable, emergency burr holes). In an unstable patient, a laparotomy for intra-abdominal haemorrhage should take priority over a head CT scan.[41]

SEVERITY AND MORBIDITY OF TRAUMA

Severity of injury is measured by the Abbreviated Injury Scale (AIS), updated over the years, most recently in 2008.[42–44] AIS divides the body into six regions: head and neck, face, thorax, abdomen, pelvis and extremities, and external. Specific injuries in each body region are coded on a scale of 1 (minor), 2 (moderate), 3 (serious, not life threatening), 4 (severe, life threatening, survival probable), 5 (critical, survival uncertain) and 6 (unsurvivable). The AIS was designed for motor vehicle injuries, but has been validated for blunt and penetrating trauma. It can provide a basis for research, education, audit and allocation of resources.

Severity of trauma is related not just to the severity of individual injuries, but also to the combined effects of multiple injuries. Multiple injuries are graded by the Injury Severity Score (ISS), which is an empirical system based on the AIS grades for the three worst body regions.[45,46] ISS gives a score between 0 and 75 for total body injury; 16 or more indicates major trauma. Death with an ISS below 24 should be rare. Above an ISS of 25, there is a stepwise increase in mortality, with very high rates over 50.[47,48]

The AIS and ISS study mostly the anatomy of injury. Other factors influence trauma mortality and morbidity, including age, pre-existing health, degree of physiological derangement, standard of prehospital and early hospital care, and complications. Degree of physiological derangement can be measured by the Revised Trauma Score (RTS),[49] which is computed from the coded values of the GCS, systolic blood pressure and respiratory rate, usually at admission to the emergency department. The Trauma Score – Injury Severity Score (TRISS) is based on the RTS, ISS and patient age.[50] It correlates well with outcome, and has been used to compile survival norms for blunt and penetrating trauma.[47,48] Physiological scoring systems such as APACHE (Acute Physiology and Chronic Health Evaluation) do not work well for trauma patients (see Ch. 3).[51,52] Pre-injury illness (co-morbidity) has a profound effect on trauma outcome.[53]

Shock influences trauma mortality and morbidity. Complications of shock include renal failure, ARDS, sepsis, liver failure and multi-organ dysfunction.[30,31,54] Acute oliguric renal failure on the first day after trauma is now rare, but non-oliguric renal failure is often seen 2–4 days later, caused by the shock and delayed or inadequate resuscitation. It is often heralded by polyuria, which is misinterpreted as a sign of adequate resuscitation.

EPIDEMIOLOGY OF INJURIES

Only a minority of victims of severe trauma reach hospital alive.[55,56] The majority of deaths are immediate (within minutes) at the scene of injury. Some deaths are early (within hours) in the emergency department or the operating room, and a few are late (after days or weeks) and occur in the ICU or ward.[57] Those in the ICU are mostly from severe head injury within a few days and, less commonly, multi-organ dysfunction later.

Of trauma admissions to hospital, only a minority have severe or multiple trauma.[58] In order of frequency, life-threatening injuries involve the head, abdomen and chest (**Table 74.1**), and are often multiple. The hospital services that this small number of severely injured patients use out of proportion to their numbers are major surgery, intensive care, radiography and CT scanning.[58] Major trauma outcome studies in the USA,[47] the UK[48] and Australasia[59,60] offer valuable epidemiological data. The USA study found that the mortality of direct admissions is strongly related to serious head injury.

ORGANISATION OF TRAUMA CARE

Many of the problems of trauma care are organisational. Problems faced by health authorities are the

Table 74.1 Percentage of ICU trauma patients with grades of injury in different body regions

	AIS≥4	AIS 3	AIS 1 OR 2	AIS 0
Head and neck	63	9	9	19
Face	2	11	8	79
Thorax	10	17	7	66
Abdomen	17	6	2	75
Extremities	1	31	11	57
External	0	<1	63	37

Data on 5031 trauma patients (excluding burns) in the Department of Critical Care Medicine, Auckland City Hospital, 1988–2011. Abbreviated injury scale (AIS-80) codes: 0= no injury; 1=minor; 2=moderate; 3=serious; not life threatening; 4=severe; life threatening, survival probable; 5=critical; survival uncertain; 6=unsurvivable. In tertiary referral centres (like Auckland City Hospital) these figures will vary with the mix of local and referred patients.[60]

provision of advanced care at the scene of injury, rapid transportation to hospital, policies on which hospitals should receive trauma patients, systems for rapid evaluation and decision making in hospitals, and rapid, safe patient transfer between hospitals. If survival from major trauma is to be maximised then prehospital and hospital care must be coordinated.

Regionalisation of trauma care has become an accepted concept.[2,61] Trauma centres are designated hospitals that meet certain requirements. The main prerequisites are rapidly available experienced surgeons, anaesthetists and neurosurgeons, and a minimum number of patients seen annually for staff expertise. Regionalisation involves the concept of ambulances bypassing non-designated hospitals.[2] Helicopters are used increasingly to speed patient transportation.[62] Trauma teams are teams of surgeons and intensivists or anaesthetists who immediately attend the trauma victim on arrival at hospital.[2-4,54]

Trauma registries and databases are important tools in organising and improving trauma care. The UK major trauma outcome study[48] showed that the doctors in charge of resuscitation were often junior, delays in performing urgent operations were common, and the number of preventable deaths was significant. A hospital may not see enough trauma patients to justify a trauma team or supply adequate experience for its staff, and may not have all the facilities required by trauma patients. Transfer to a trauma hospital may be desirable, but geography and limited transport facilities may make such transfers hazardous.

In Western countries, trauma is a leading cause of death and disability under the age of 38 years.[47] Reduction of mortality and morbidity depends on public education, new legislations, on-site advanced care, rapid evacuation (see Ch. 4), hospital trauma expertise and coordination of services.[63,64]

Access the complete references list online at http://www.expertconsult.com

6. Committee on Trauma, American College of Surgeons. Advanced Trauma Life Support (ATLS) Program for Doctors: Student Course Manual. 8th ed. Chicago: American College of Surgeons; 2008.
19. Holcomb JB, Wade CE, Michalek JE, et al. Increased plasma and platelet to red blood cell ratios improves outcome in 466 massively transfused civilian trauma patients. Ann Surg 2008;248:447–58.
21. CRASH 2 Trial Collaborators. Effect of tranexamic acid on death, vascular occlusive events, and blood transfusion in trauma patients with significant hemorrhage (CRASH-2): a randomised placebo-controlled trial, Lancet 2011;376:23–32.
22. Morrison CA, Carrick MM, Norman MA, et al. Hypotensive resuscitation strategy reduces transfusion requirements and severe post operative coagulopathy in trauma patients with hemorrhagic shock: preliminary results of a randomized controlled trial. J Trauma 2011, 70:652–63.
26. Brain Trauma Foundation. Guidelines for the Management of Severe Traumatic Brain Injury. 3rd ed. New York: Brain Trauma Foundation; 2007. Online. Available: http://www.braintrauma.org/ (accessed 28 June 2012).
43. Committee on Injury Scaling. The Abbreviated Injury Scale – 1980 revision. Morton Grove, IL: American Association for Automotive Medicine; 1980.
60. Data updated from that published in Gardiner JP, Judson JA, Smith GS, et al. A decade of ICU trauma admissions in Auckland, New Zealand. N Z Med J 2000;113:326–7.

75

Severe head injuries

John A Myburgh and Manoj K Saxena

Despite improvements in resuscitation and vital organ support, the management of patients with traumatic brain injury in the intensive care unit (ICU) presents a challenge to all members of the critical care team.

EPIDEMIOLOGY

Traumatic brain injury has been termed a 'silent global epidemic'. It accounts for up to 30% of all trauma-related deaths and is the leading cause of death in young males in developed countries. The impact of mechanisation in low- and middle-income countries has resulted in a substantial increase in the incidence and mortality from vehicular trauma.

In addition to this high mortality, the cost of survivors in these societies in emotional, social and financial terms is substantial as the effects of the original injury may persist for many years.

AETIOLOGY

Vehicular trauma, industrial accidents, falls and assaults account for the majority of head injury, with marked variations in patterns of injury across the world. In high-income countries such as Australia, the incidence of head injury due to vehicular trauma has significantly decreased due to technical improvements in vehicle design and safety and public health initiatives such as restraint devices, speed control and drink-driving legislation.[1]

DEMOGRAPHICS

The numbers of patients with traumatic brain injury presenting to hospitals vary widely in accordance with hospital admission policies and capabilities. Typical figures of all-cause head injury admissions in high-income countries range from 200 to 300 per 100 000 patients, with the majority of these managed in dedicated trauma centres.

Age- and gender-specific data typically show two peaks: one in the second and third decades, with a male : female ratio of 2 : 1, and the latter in the seventh to ninth decades with a more equal gender ratio.

PATTERNS OF INJURY

Traumatic brain injury represents a range of injury from mild head injury that may fully recover to severe injury associated with high mortality or high levels of disability.

Injury may be either blunt or penetrating, with the latter associated with a higher mortality.

Although the majority of head injuries (70–80%) are minor, a significant proportion of these patients have poor functional outcomes due to secondary brain insults and co-morbidities. Of the 20–30% who constitute moderate to severe head injury, approximately 10% of these are dead on admission whereas the remainder will usually require admission to the ICU for management in the first 7–10 days.

PATHOPHYSIOLOGY

Brain injury is a heterogeneous pathophysiological process.[2] It encompasses a spectrum of injury that includes the degree of brain damage at the time of injury (primary injury) in addition to insults that occur during the post-injury phase (secondary injury). These processes are depicted in **Figure 75.1.**

PRIMARY BRAIN INJURY

The severity of primary injury is determined by the degree of neuronal damage or death at the time of impact. This is the major determinant of outcome from traumatic brain injury.

Primary brain injuries include all types of injury to the brain parenchyma and vasculature. Primary injuries that are associated with adverse outcome include traumatic subarachnoid haemorrhage and non-evacuable mass lesions, particularly in critical parts of the brain such as the posterior fossa.

SECONDARY BRAIN INJURY

Secondary brain insults are characterised by a reduction in cerebral substrate availability and utilisation[3] (**Box 75.1**). Of these, hypotension (defined as a systolic blood pressure of <90 mmHg (11.97 kPa)), hypoxia (oxygen saturation <90% or Pa_{O_2} <50 mmHg (6.65 kPa)), hypoglycaemia, hyperpyrexia (temperature

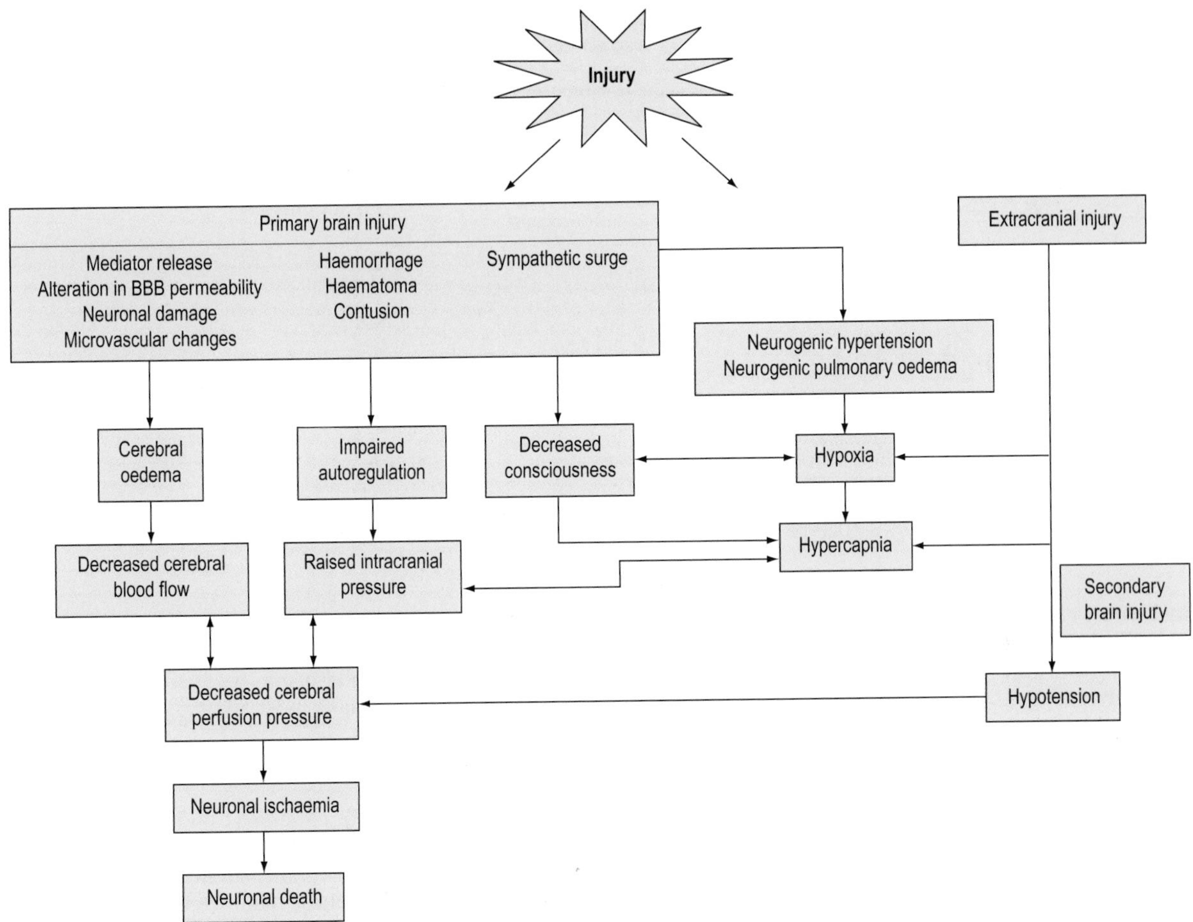

Figure 75.1 Pathophysiology of traumatic brain injury. BBB=blood brain barrier.

Box 75.1 Secondary brain insults following traumatic brain injury that are associated with increased morbidity and mortality

Systemic	Intracranial
Hypoxia	Seizure
Hypotension	Delayed haematoma
Hypocapnia	Subarachnoid haemorrhage
Hypercapnia	Vasospasm
Hyperthermia	Hydrocephalus
Hypoglycaemia	Neuroinfection
Hyperglycaemia	
Hyponatraemia	
Hypernatraemia	
Hyperosmolality	
Infection	

>39°C) and prolonged hypocapnia (Pa_{CO_2}<30 mmHg (3.99 kPa)) have been shown to independently worsen survival following traumatic brain injury.

Secondary insults may occur during initial resuscitation, transport both between and within hospitals, during anaesthesia and surgery, and in the ICU. These insults may initiate or propagate pathophysiological processes that may damage neurons already rendered susceptible by the primary injury.

INTRACRANIAL INFLAMMATION

As the brain is enclosed within the rigid skull and dura, small increases in intracranial volume result in sharp increases in intracranial pressure (Monroe–Kelly doctrine). Consequently, the brain is a poorly elastant organ with a limited capacity to accommodate pathological increases in intracranial pressure.

Traumatic brain injury invokes an inflammatory response characterised by the release of pro- and anti-inflammatory mediators. The consequence of this response is disruption and alteration in the permeability of the blood–brain barrier, glial swelling and alterations in regional and global cerebral blood flow. The extent of this inflammatory process is an important determinant of intracranial pressure that may persist for some time following injury. Furthermore, alteration

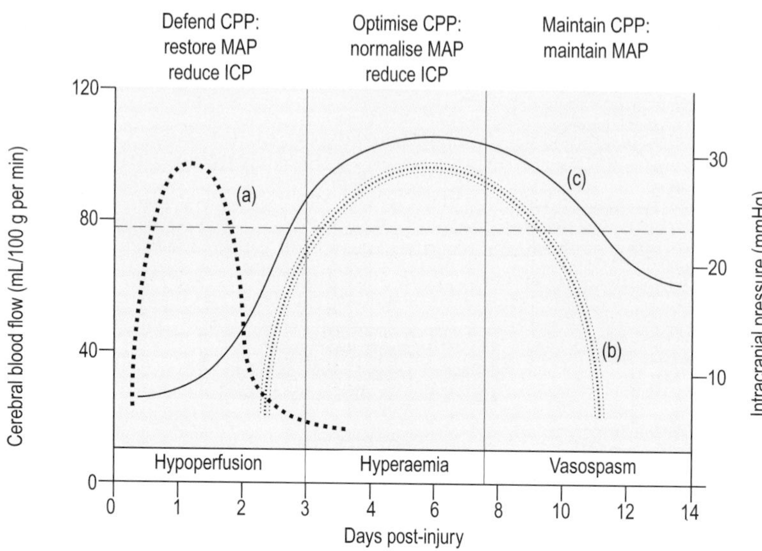

Figure 75.2 Conceptual changes in cerebral blood flow and intracranial pressure (ICP) over time following traumatic brain injury: (a) cytotoxic oedema; (b) vasogenic oedema; (c) cerebral blood flow. CPP=cerebral perfusion pressure, MAP=mean arterial pressure.

in blood–brain permeability may change the normal physiology of the cerebral circulation and alter the response to intravenous fluids, osmotic diuretics and vasoactive drugs.

CEREBRAL BLOOD FLOW AND AUTOREGULATION

Normally, cerebral blood flow is maintained at a constant rate in the presence of changing perfusion pressures by regional myogenic and metabolic autoregulation. These homeostatic mechanisms are impaired following head injury due to neuronal damage and intracranial inflammation. Distinct patterns of cerebral blood flow have been described following head injuries that have direct clinical relevance with regard to management[4] (**Fig. 75.2**).

THE HYPOPERFUSION PHASE

Cerebral blood flow is reduced by extrinsic and intrinsic mechanisms in the first 72 hours following injury, with resultant global and regional ischaemia. Because autoregulation is impaired during this period, cerebral blood flow is largely dependent on systemic blood pressure. Resultant neuronal ischaemia may result in 'cytotoxic' cerebral oedema and increased intracranial pressure.

THE HYPERAEMIC PHASE

Following the initial hypoperfusion phase, autoregulatory mechanisms may start to recover with improved cerebral blood flow.

During this phase, intracranial inflammation and/or effects of medical therapies directed at maintaining adequate cerebral perfusion pressure may result in cerebral hyperaemia and increased intracranial pressure. The consequences of hyperaemia, inflammation and altered blood–brain permeability may result in 'vasogenic' cerebral oedema.

This hyperaemic phase may persist for a variable period, up to 7–10 days post injury, and occurs in 25–30% patients.

THE VASOSPASTIC PHASE

In a small proportion of patients (10–15%), particularly those with severe primary and secondary injuries or those with significant traumatic subarachnoid haemorrhage, a vasospastic phase characterised by typical cerebral blood flow patterns may occur. This phase represents a complex of cerebral hypoperfusion due to arterial vasospasm, post-traumatic hypometabolism and impaired autoregulation.

RESUSCITATION

INITIAL ASSESSMENT

The resuscitation of head-injured patients should follow the principles outlined in the Advanced Trauma Life Support (ATLS®) guidelines for the early management of severe trauma.[5]

The initial emphasis is directed at assessing and controlling the airway, ensuring adequate oxygenation and ventilation, establishing adequate intravenous access and correcting hypotension. Neurological assessment and brain-specific treatment should follow only after cardiorespiratory stability has been established.

AIRWAY

All patients with severe head injury (traumatic coma), marked agitation or significant extracranial trauma require early oral endotracheal intubation.

Depending on the skill of the operator and available facilities, this should be performed using a rapid sequence induction of anaesthesia with cricoid pressure and in-line immobilisation of the cervical spine.

All head-injured patients should be assumed to have a potential cervical spine injury, and should be immobilised in a rigid collar until that possibility is definitively excluded.

BREATHING (=VENTILATION)

Patients should be ventilated with 100% oxygen using 6–10 mL/kg tidal volumes until blood gas analysis is available.

Oxygenation should be maintained at least 80–100 mmHg (13 kPa) and the ventilator adjusted to achieve a normal arterial carbon dioxide tension (35–40 mmHg; 4.5–5.0 kPa).

Non-depolarising muscle relaxants and narcotics such as fentanyl may facilitate ventilation in the immediate post-intubation period in combative patients.

Empirical hyperventilation during initial resuscitation is not indicated.

CIRCULATION (=CONTROL OF SHOCK)

Prompt restoration of circulating blood volume and restoration of a euvolaemia is critical.

Early arterial monitoring for accurate measurement of mean arterial pressure and central venous catheter placement for providing a guide to volume replacement and administration of blood and drugs is essential. The placement of these lines must not delay volume resuscitation.

Blood transfusion should be commenced as soon as possible in actively bleeding patients with early administration of coagulation factors where appropriate.

Crystalloid, specifically normal saline, is recommended for fluid resuscitation of patients with traumatic brain injury.[6] Hypertonic saline may have a role as a small-volume resuscitation fluid in patients with traumatic brain injury, although there is no evidence of reduced mortality when used in the pre-hospital period.[7]

Vasoactive drugs such as epinephrine (adrenaline) or norepinephrine (noradrenaline) may be used to defend blood pressure once correction of hypovolaemia is under way. This may be necessary if sedatives or narcotics are co-administered.

DISABILITY (=NEUROLOGICAL ASSESSMENT)

Assessment of neurological function following injury is important to quantify the severity of traumatic brain injury and to provide prognostic information. This may be influenced by associated injuries, hypoxia, hypotension and/or drug or alcohol intoxication.

Recording the mechanism of injury is important, as high-velocity injuries are associated with a greater degree of neuronal damage. It is important to review ambulance and emergency personnel and records in order to obtain the most accurate information.

Level of consciousness

The ATLS® recommends an initial assessment during initial resuscitation based on the response to stimulation: Awake, Verbal, Pain, Unresponsive (AVPU). This provides a rapid and practical grading of function with severe head injuries defined as those who respond to pain only or who are unresponsive.

The Glasgow Coma Scale (GCS) has an established place in the management of traumatic brain injury and is the most widely accepted and understood scale.[8] Although originally described as a prognostic index, it provides an overall assessment of neurological function, derived from three parameters: eye opening, verbal response and motor response (**Table 75.1**).

The best responses in the GCS components should be recorded following cardiorespiratory resuscitation prior to surgical intervention. A GCS of 14–15 indicates a mild injury, 9–13 a moderate injury and 3–8 is classified as severe (traumatic coma). In severely injured patients or those who are intubated or with ocular or facial trauma, the motor response is the most useful.

Pupillary responses

Pupil size and reactivity are important when consciousness is impaired. Whilst not part of the GCS, pupillary function should always be assessed and recorded at the same time as the GCS, particularly prior to the administration of narcotics, sedatives or muscle relaxants.

Table 75.1 The Glasgow Coma Score[8] – the best response following non-surgical resuscitation is scored

BEST EYES OPEN SCORE		BEST VERBAL RESPONSE		BEST MOTOR RESPONSE	
Spontaneously	4	Orientated, adequate	5	Obeys spoken command	6
On spoken command	3	Disorientated, confused	4	Localised pain	5
To pain	2	Inappropriate words	3	Flexion withdrawal	4
No response	1	Incomprehensible	2	Abnormal flexion	3
		No response	1	Extension	2
		INTUBATED PATIENTS:		No response	1
		Appears able to converse	5		
		Questionable ability to converse	3		
		Unresponsive	1		

In the absence of traumatic mydriasis, abnormalities of pupil size and reactivity may indicate compression of the third cranial nerve, suggesting raised intracranial pressure or impending herniation, particularly when associated with lateralising motor signs and depressed consciousness.

Papilloedema is uncommon in the acute phase of head injuries.

Motor function

In addition to the motor response of the GCS, decerebrate or decorticate posturing, hemiparesis or lateralising signs, paraparesis and quadriparesis (given the high association with spinal injuries with traumatic brain injury) should be documented concurrently with the GCS and pupillary responses.

SECONDARY SURVEY

Once the initial assessment is complete and resuscitation under way, a thorough secondary survey adopting a 'top-to-toe' approach, as outlined in the ATLS®, is mandatory.

The principles outlined in the initial assessment form the basis for prioritising interventions in the secondary survey. Extracranial causes of hypoxia such as pulmonary contusion or haemo/pneumothorax must be excluded and promptly treated. Haemorrhage - both externally from fractures or lacerations and internally from major vascular disruption or visceral injuries - must be aggressively treated until circulatory stability is achieved. There is no place for 'permissive hypotension' in head-injured patients as has been advocated in selected cases of penetrating trauma.

Target mean arterial pressure should be estimated in the context of the patient's premorbid blood pressure. Higher pressures may be necessary in hypertensive or elderly patients. The early use of vasoactive drugs such as epinephrine or norepinephrine may be necessary to achieve this.

An approach of 'damage-control surgery' is recommended in patients with traumatic brain injury to minimise secondary insults.[9] In the initial 24–48 hours following injury, only life- or limb-threatening injuries should be addressed, following which patients should be transferred to the ICU for stabilisation and monitoring. Thereafter, semiurgent surgery such as fixation of closed fractures or delayed plastic repairs may be done.[10] Patients with severe traumatic brain injury undergoing prolonged emergency surgery should have intracranial pressure monitoring placed as soon as possible.

BRAIN-SPECIFIC RESUSCITATION

The place of interventions and therapies specifically directed at reducing intracranial pressure has been extensively reviewed in evidence-based guidelines for the management of severe head injury.[11]

HYPERVENTILATION

Ventilation-induced reductions in Pa_{CO_2} result in marked reductions in cerebral blood flow and consequently in intracranial pressure. However, as cerebral blood flow may be reduced during the initial period following injury, further reductions in cerebral perfusion will result if hyperventilation is used during this phase. Consequently, empirical hyperventilation is not indicated during initial resuscitation.

In the resuscitated head-injured patient with unequivocal clinical signs of raised intracranial pressure or impending tentorial herniation (pupillary dilatation, lateralising signs or a witnessed neurological deterioration), temporary hyperventilation is an option. Reductions of Pa_{CO_2} to levels ≤30 mmHg (4 kPa) may be considered prior to urgent imaging or surgery for evacuation of a mass lesion.[12]

OSMOTHERAPY

Osmotically active agents, such as mannitol, are administered to increase plasma osmolality in order to cause net efflux of fluid from areas of oedematous brain, with resultant reduction in intracranial pressure. An intact blood–brain barrier is necessary for this to occur. Following intravenous administration of mannitol, an immediate plasma-expanding effect that reduces haematocrit and viscosity ensues, which temporarily increases cerebral blood flow. Subsequent reductions in intracranial pressure probably result from restoration in cerebral perfusion pressure and rheological changes in cerebral blood flow rather than specific cerebral dehydration.

Osmotherapy is associated with a number of potentially adverse effects. Mannitol exerts an osmotic effect over a narrow range of plasma osmolality (290–330 mosm/L), above which theoretically beneficial effects may be negated, and induces an osmolal gap between measured and calculated osmolality. This gap may be increased by alcohol, which is frequently present in the acute period. Mannitol will enter the brain where the blood–brain barrier is damaged, thereby potentially increasing cerebral oedema by increasing brain osmolality. It is a potent osmotic diuretic that may compromise haemodynamic stability by inducing an inappropriate diuresis in a hypovolaemic patient.

Given the high risk with minimal benefit during resuscitation, the routine use of mannitol is not recommended in the absence of raised intracranial pressure.[13]

Similarly to hyperventilation, mannitol is considered as an option only in resuscitated patients with unequivocal signs of raised intracranial pressure prior to imaging or evacuation of a mass lesion. Although doses are frequently quoted as 0.25–1.0 g/kg, lower doses are equally as effective as higher doses in terms of improving cerebral perfusion and are associated with a lower incidence of side-effects.

Hypertonic saline (3% solution) exerts similar osmotic plasma-expanding effects to mannitol. These solutions do not exert an osmolal gap so serum sodium reflects serum osmolality allowing easier titration.[14]

EMERGENCY SURGICAL DECOMPRESSION ('BURR HOLES')

The advent of advanced in-field resuscitation, medical retrieval, imaging, teleradiology and telemedicine in high-income countries has largely superseded the need to perform urgent, undirected craniotomy in patients with traumatic brain injury. In most instances, patients are resuscitated, stabilised and imaged with CT scans prior to any surgical intervention. This usually involves transfer to a specialised trauma centre.

In remote communities or in low- and middle-income countries without immediate access to CT scanning, surgical evacuation may be life-saving in selected patients with a strong clinical probability of an expanding mass lesion such as an extradural or subdural haematoma. These include patients with low-velocity injuries to the temporal region with an associated skull fracture and developing lateralising neurological signs.

IMAGING

X-RAYS

Routine 'trauma series' of X-rays, namely chest, pelvis, skull and cervical spine, have been superseded by high-resolution, multislice computerised tomography (CT). In areas without immediate access to CT, X-rays should focus on identifying injuries or confirmation of placement of lines and tubes post resuscitation.

COMPUTED TOMOGRAPHY (CT) SCAN

CT scanning is now standard in all patients following traumatic brain injury. As CT scanning requires moving the patient to a radiological suite, this must be done only when initial assessment and resuscitation are complete and the patient is stable enough to be transported by appropriately trained and equipped personnel.

The following patients should undergo CT head scan following traumatic brain injury:

- all patients with a history of loss of consciousness or traumatic coma (GCS<8)
- combative patients where clinical assessment is masked by associated alcohol, drugs or extracranial injuries; these patients may require endotracheal intubation, sedation and ventilation to facilitate completion of CT scanning
- to exclude a cervical spine injury.[15]

The most important role of CT scanning is prompt detection of intracranial mass lesions such as extradural or subdural haematomas. Thereafter, the degree of brain injury may be quantified by radiological criteria (**Table 75.2** and **Fig. 75.3a**).[16,17]

Table 75.2 Classification of CT scan appearance following traumatic brain injury[16]*

CATEGORY	DEFINITION
DI I (diffuse injury)	No visible intracranial pathology seen on CT scan
DI II (diffuse injury)	Cisterns are present with midline shift 0–5 mm and/or: Lesion densities present No high- or mixed-density lesion >25 mm May include bony fragments and foreign bodies
DI III (swelling)	Cisterns are compressed or absent with midline shift 0–5 mm *No* high- or mixed-density lesion >25 mm
DI IV (shift)	Midline shift >5 mm *No* high- or mixed-density lesion >25 mm
Evacuated mass lesion	Any lesion surgically evacuated
Non-evacuated mass lesion	High- or mixed-density lesion >25 mm, not surgically evacuated

*An example is shown in Figure 75.3a.

These criteria are important for providing an index of injury severity, providing criteria for intracranial pressure monitoring, comparing the progression of injuries with subsequent scans and providing an index for prognosis. Examples of typical injuries appear in **Figure 75.3**.

The presence of traumatic subarachnoid haemorrhage should be recorded. This is an important index of severity of injury and is relevant for prognostication.[18]

MAGNETIC RESONANCE IMAGING (MRI)

Magnetic resonance imaging provides accurate details of parenchymal damage, specifically small collections and non-haemorrhagic contusions. The information provided is not significantly better than that obtained from CT scanning to warrant routine use of MRI in the acute phase of injury.

In patients when a major intracranial vascular injury is suspected, such as carotid artery dissection where the patient's clinical condition is not consistent with the CT findings (e.g. a dense hemiparesis in the absence of a mass lesion), magnetic resonance angiography (MRA) or direct cerebral angiography is indicated.

MRI has an emerging role in prognostication at a later stage in management.[19]

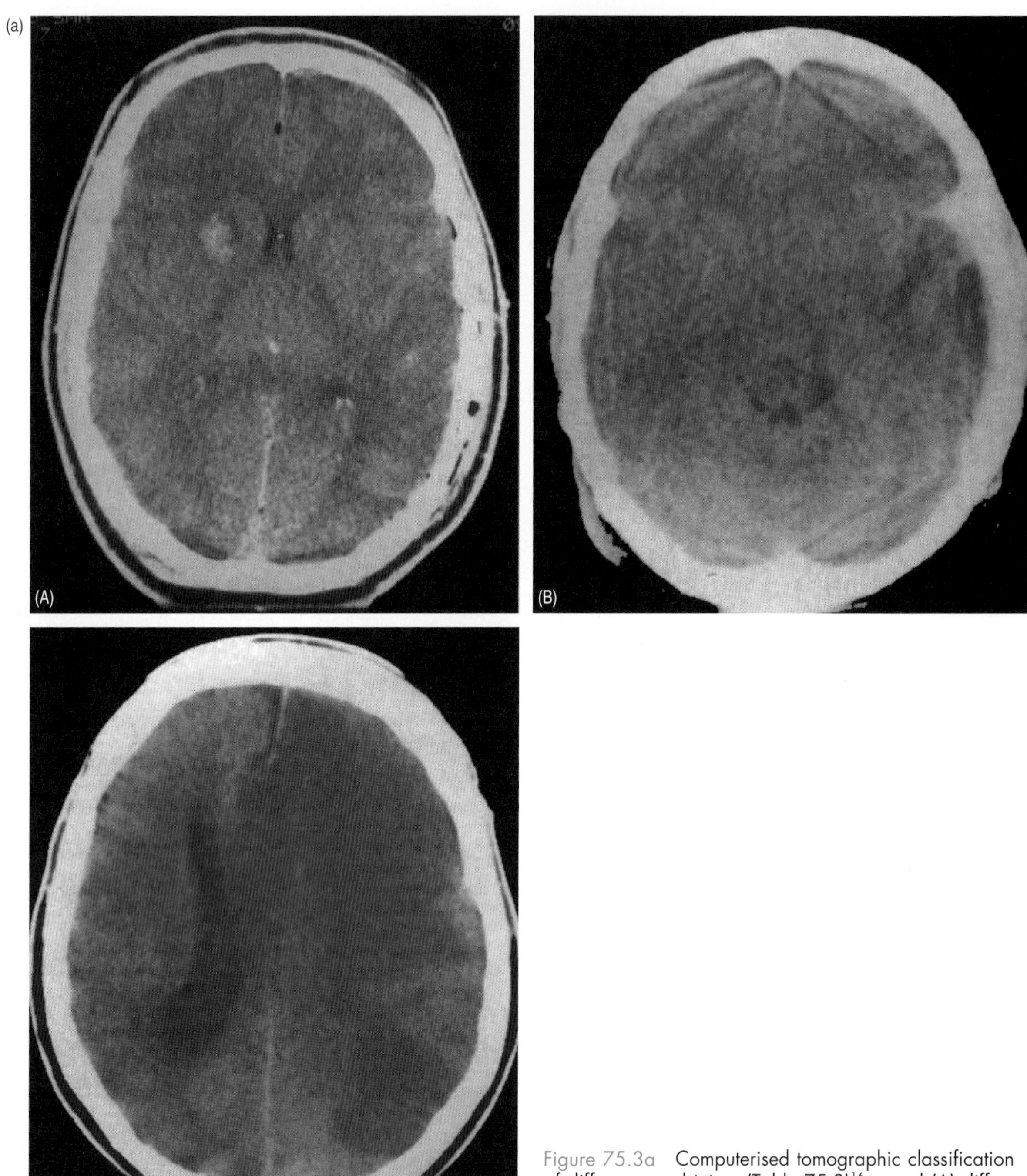

Figure 75.3a Computerised tomographic classification of diffuse axonal injury (Table 75.2)[16]: panel (A) diffuse injury II; panel (B) diffuse injury III; panel (C) diffuse injury IV.

INTER-HOSPITAL TRANSFER

All severely head-injured patients should be managed at a specialised neurotrauma centre in close collaboration with intensive care physicians and neurosurgeons. This may involve intra- or inter-hospital transportation. Appropriately skilled and equipped personnel should do this only once resuscitation, stabilisation and initial imaging are completed.

A full primary and secondary survey and review of all documentation and investigation is required following transfer to a secondary or tertiary centre.

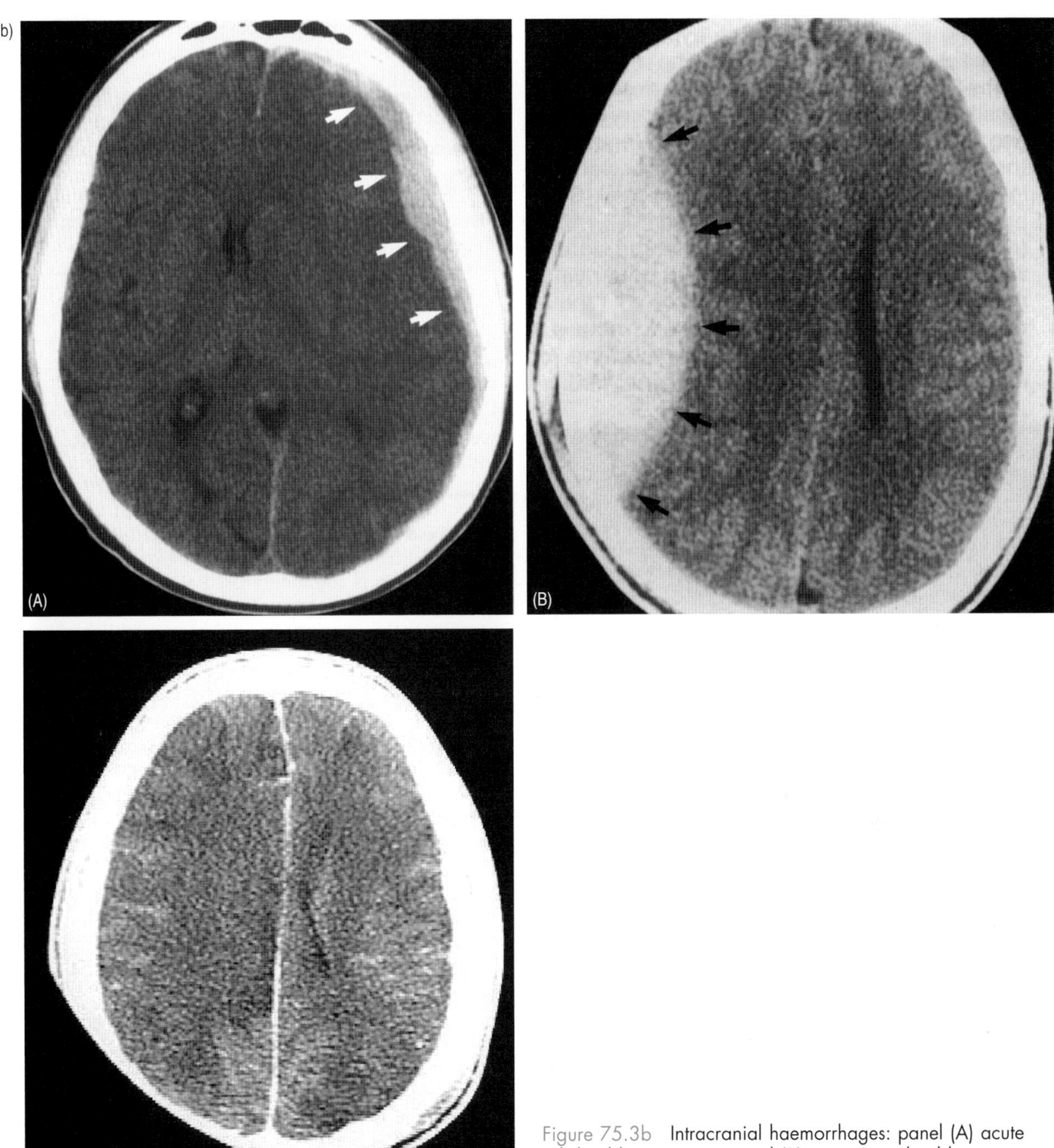

Figure 75.3b Intracranial haemorrhages: panel (A) acute subdural haematoma; panel (B) acute extradural haematoma; panel (C) acute traumatic subarachnoid haemorrhage.

INTENSIVE CARE MANAGEMENT

There is no standard or uniform method of managing traumatic brain injury in the ICU. Most practices are determined by local preferences and experience, caseload and resources. The Brain Trauma Foundation of the American Association of Neurological Surgeons has published evidence-based management guidelines for the management of severe brain injury.[11]

Following initial resuscitation, good intensive care management forms the basis of head injury management and is regarded as a continuum of care. This takes priority over brain-specific therapies, which to date remain inconclusive in their efficacy.

HAEMODYNAMIC MANAGEMENT

Monitoring

Accurate measurement of systemic blood pressure is essential and should be measured via an arterial catheter referenced to the aortic root. A large artery such as the femoral artery should be considered in haemodynamically unstable patients as radial or dorsalis pedis arterial catheters may underestimate systemic pressure in shocked patients. Given the importance of maintaining adequate systemic blood pressure, non-invasive measurement of blood pressure is not recommended during the acute phase of monitoring.

Therapy should be titrated to mean arterial pressure in accordance with the patient's premorbid blood pressure – i.e. in older patients, higher mean arterial pressure (e.g. 70–80 mmHg; 9.31–10.64 kPa) may be necessary.[3]

Volume status should be assessed using clinical criteria including pulse rate, right atrial and mean arterial pressure, urine output serum sodium and osmolality, urea and creatinine.

Pulmonary artery catheterisation for the measurement of cardiac output and pulmonary artery pressures is rarely indicated in head-injured patients and is not recommended.

Fluid management

The attainment of euvolaemia is essential throughout intensive care management; both dehydration and fluid overload should be avoided.

Normal saline is the resuscitation fluid of choice for patients with traumatic brain injury. The use of albumin is associated with increased mortality due to increased intracranial pressure; whether this applies to other colloids is unknown but, on current evidence, resuscitation with colloids should be avoided.[6] Equally, hypotonic crystalloids such as compounded sodium lactate (Ringer's lactate or Hartmann's solution) should be avoided.

Maintenance fluids should be restricted to a minimum and directed at maintaining normal serum sodium (140–145 mmol/L) and osmolality (290–310 mosmol/L). As a general principle, glucose-containing solutions are not recommended; however, these may be required if patients become hyperosmolal (>320 mosm/L).

Vasoactive therapy

Catecholamines such as epinephrine, norepinephrine or dopamine are frequently used to augment mean arterial pressure to attain an adequate cerebral perfusion pressure. These should be commenced once volume resuscitation is actively under way. The early use of vasoactive drugs is increasingly being advocated during resuscitation as an important strategy during the hypoperfusion phase.[20]

There are no conclusive trials to recommend one vasoactive drug over another or combination of drugs. Epinephrine, norepinephrine and dopamine are equally effective in augmenting cerebral perfusion pressure.[21] The degree by which these agents directly affect the cerebral circulation following head injury is unknown, although there is some evidence suggesting that dopamine has both direct cerebrovascular and adverse neuroendocrine effects.[21]

Norepinephrine is currently regarded as the initial agent of choice for patients with traumatic brain injury in doses titrated to achieve a target mean arterial or cerebral perfusion pressure. Epinephrine is widely used, particularly in low-income countries, but may be associated with transient metabolic side-effects such as hyperlactataemia and hyperglycaemia, which may confound assessment of the adequacy of circulatory and metabolic resuscitation.[22]

Doses may range widely between and within patients to attain a target cerebral perfusion pressure. However, excessive doses of catecholamines (i.e. >40 μg/min) should be avoided, particularly after 72 hours after injury when lower cerebral perfusion pressure targets (i.e. 40–60 mmHg) may be appropriate. At all times, other causes of hypotension such as dehydration, sedatives, bleeding and sepsis must to be excluded.

Vasopressin is commonly used as a catecholamine-sparing agent or as a primary vasopressor, but its role in traumatic brain injury has not been established and is not recommended.

Neurogenic hypertension

Neurogenic hypertension is common in the latter phases following injury (>5 days) and is usually centrally mediated. It may be associated with ECG changes and/or supraventricular arrhythmias. It is usually self-limiting and correlates with the severity of injury, although a proportion may require long-term therapy. Treatment depends on the severity of the problem: beta blockers or centrally acting agents such as clonidine are usually effective; vasodilators are contraindicated.

RESPIRATORY THERAPY

Monitoring

Continuous measurement of arterial oxygen saturation is essential.

Continuous measurement of end-tidal carbon dioxide is frequently performed in ventilated patients, although the reliability is questionable and should be intermittently checked with arterial blood gases to maintain normocapnia.

Monitoring of ventilatory parameters should be consistent with standard approaches and includes measurement of tidal volumes, respiratory rates, and inspiratory and expiratory airway pressures.

Ventilation

The majority of patients with severe head injury will require mechanical ventilation to ensure adequate oxygenation and to maintain normocapnia (36–40 mmHg; 4.8–5.3 kPa).

The principles of optimal ventilation, humidification and weaning are addressed elsewhere. Strategies such as 'permissive hypercapnia' that are advocated for selected patients with acute lung injury or acute respiratory distress syndrome do not have a role in head-injured patients owing to the requirement to maintain normocapnia.

Positive end-expiratory pressure (PEEP) is recommended at low levels (5–10 cmH_2O) to maintain functional residual capacity and oxygenation. Higher levels may compromise systemic blood pressure, particularly in hypovolaemic patients, and should be used with caution. High levels of PEEP (>15 cmH_2O) may compromise cerebral venous return but adverse effects on intracranial pressure are uncommon.

Weaning from ventilation should commence once intracranial pathology has stabilised – that is, resolution of cerebral oedema on CT scan and control of intracranial hypertension.

Trials of extubation should be carefully considered so that subsequent hypoxic episodes do not occur, as these are potent secondary insults.

Patients with slow recovery of adequate consciousness should be considered for early tracheostomy, either percutaneously or surgically.

Neurogenic pulmonary oedema

This is a dramatic clinical syndrome that occurs in some patients with severe head injury and correlates with severity of injury. The underlying pathophysiological process is complex, but is primarily related to centrally mediated sympathetic overactivity. It is characterised by sudden onset of clinical pulmonary oedema, hypoxia, low filling pressures, poor lung compliance and bilateral lung infiltrates, usually within 2–8 hours following injury.

The process is usually self-limiting and treatment is primarily supportive, aimed at ensuring adequate oxygenation and ventilation. This usually requires endotracheal intubation and mechanical ventilation with the administration of PEEP. Ablation of sympathetic overactivity is effectively done with adequate sedation; beta blockade is usually unnecessary. Diuretics are effective, particularly if patients have received substantive fluid resuscitation, and must be titrated against the volume status of the patient.

The development of pulmonary oedema in patients with cardiac disease should be regarded as cardiogenic until proven otherwise.

Nosocomial pneumonia

Head-injured patients who require prolonged ventilation are at increased risk of nosocomial pneumonia. Risk factors include barbiturate and hypothermia therapy. Diagnosis and treatment are discussed elsewhere.

SEDATION, ANALGESIA AND MUSCLE RELAXANTS

There are no standards for sedation and analgesia in head-injured patients – protocols will depend on local preferences and resources. The level of sedation and analgesia required for head-injured patients depends on the degree of traumatic coma, haemodynamic stability, intracranial pressure and systemic effects of the head injury itself.[23]

During the initial resuscitation phase, sedation should be titrated to cause the least effect on systemic blood pressure. During this period, short-acting narcotics such as fentanyl are useful particularly if patients have associated extracranial injuries. These agents have relatively little adverse effect on haemodynamics and have the additional benefit of tempering the systemic sympathetic surges that frequently occur after injury. As narcotics affect pupillary responses, these must be documented before administration. Short-term muscle relaxants such as vecuronium are useful to control combative patients following intubation, ventilation and sedation.

During the intensive care phase, the requirements for sedation are different. Sedation should be titrated to have the patient sedated as lightly as possible to allow clinical assessment of neurological function and to facilitate mechanical ventilation. The level of sedation will depend on haemodynamic stability and the degree of intracranial pressure. Infusions of narcotics and benzodiazepines (e.g. morphine and midazolam) are useful in providing moderate to deep levels of sedation and are effective in controlling surges of intracranial pressure. However, these agents may accumulate, resulting in a delay in return of consciousness or, if used for prolonged periods, may be associated with an emergent delirium state.

The use of propofol as a sole sedating agent has become popular. It provides deep levels of sedation, which is effective in controlling systemic sympathetic swings and rises in intracranial pressure. It is rapidly reversible on cessation allowing prompt assessment of neurological status and does not accumulate. In addition, pupillary responses are not directly affected. Propofol should be used with caution in haemodynamically unstable patients, however, as it is a potent negative inotrope. The prolonged use of propofol is associated with tachyphylaxis and significant caloric loading from the lipid vector. Concerns have been raised about myocardial depression and sudden cardiac death, particularly if large doses are administered.[24]

The routine use of muscle relaxants is not recommended either to facilitate sedation or to control raised intracranial pressure. The prolonged use of these agents is associated with adverse outcome in traumatic brain injury and prolonged use of non-depolarising muscle relaxants is associated with polyneuromyopathies.

BODY POSITION AND PHYSIOTHERAPY

Patients should be nursed at 30–45° head elevation to facilitate ventilation, improve oxygenation and reduce the risk of aspiration. The head should be kept in a neutral position.

Physiotherapy has an important role in the removal of lung secretions, prevention of contractures and venous thrombosis. Patients with raised intracranial pressure may require boluses of sedation before chest physiotherapy to prevent acute rises in intracranial pressure.

METABOLIC MANAGEMENT

Routine measurement of biochemistry is essential with the aim of keeping all parameters within normal limits, in particular serum sodium levels.

Hyperglycaemia is common following severe head injury and is usually centrally mediated and transient. Blood sugar levels should be maintained within normal limits with insulin infusions, between 8.0–10.0 mmol/L; hypoglycaemia should be avoided.

Core temperature should be routinely monitored as hyperthermia has been identified as a cause of secondary injury. Normothermia (core temperature at 37°C) is recommended.

NUTRITION

The caloric needs of head-injured patients must be addressed as soon as possible following resuscitation. Early enteral feeding is recommended.[25]

Placement of a nasogastric and/or enteral feeding tubes in head-injured patients is usually via the oral route until an anterior cranial fossa (fractured cribriform plate) is excluded.

STRESS ULCER PROPHYLAXIS

The incidence of gastric erosions and 'stress ulceration' has markedly decreased with better resuscitation and early enteral feeding. Head-injured patients are at no more risk than other critically ill patients for developing stress ulceration.

H_2 antagonists or proton pump inhibitors should be used in ventilated patients until enteral feeding is established, following which they may be ceased.

Patients with a previous history of peptic ulceration should remain on proton pump inhibitors for the duration of the intensive care stay.

THROMBOPROPHYLAXIS

Head-injured patients, particularly those requiring prolonged ventilation and sedation or with extracranial injuries, are at increased risk for developing thromboembolism. The use of anticoagulants such as fractionated or low-molecular-weight heparins is contraindicated in patients with clinically significant intracranial haemorrhage. Consequently, the role of thromboprophylactic agents in head injury is difficult and there are no standards for their use.[26]

As a general rule, anticoagulants should not be used in head-injured patients with any evidence of destructive intracranial pathology or haemorrhage until there is resolution of these processes on CT scan.

Non-pharmacological methods of thromboprophylaxis such as elastic stockings or pneumatic calf compressors are of unproven effectiveness, but provide a reasonable alternative. Frequent surveillance using Doppler ultrasound of the iliofemoral veins in high-risk patients, such as those with pelvic fractures, should be considered. Patients who develop deep-vein thromboses and who cannot be anticoagulated should be considered for inferior vena caval filters. The use of anticoagulants in head-injured patients with proven pulmonary embolism will depend on the relative risk to the patient's life.

ANTIBIOTICS

These should be used sparingly and in accordance with accepted microbiological principles. Prophylactic antibiotics should be prescribed only to cover insertion of intracranial pressure monitors and are not recommended for basal skull fractures. Frequent cultures of leaking or draining cerebrospinal fluid should be taken and infection treated specifically.[27]

BRAIN-SPECIFIC MONITORING

The most accurate assessment of brain function following traumatic brain injury is a full clinical neurological examination in the absence of drugs or sedatives. However, this is often not possible for the majority of head-injured patients managed in the ICU.

Ideally, neuromonitoring should provide accurate and integrated information about intracranial pressure, patterns and adequacy of cerebral perfusion, and an assessment of cerebral function. No such monitor exists, although each of these parameters may be monitored in various ways with variable levels of accuracy and clinical utility.

CLINICAL ASSESSMENT

Regular assessments of GCS, pupillary signs and motor responses should be made and recorded in the ICU flow chart. Concomitant sedation may influence the level of consciousness and this should be recorded. Initially, these assessments are recorded hourly, but this may change as patients become more stable.

A witnessed deterioration in GCS, especially the motor response, or the development of new lateralising signs should be regarded as life-threatening intracranial hypertension or tentorial herniation until proven otherwise.

INTRACRANIAL PRESSURE MONITORING

The recognition that raised intracranial pressure is associated with adverse outcome led to the measurement of this parameter in order to quantify the degree of injury and to assess the response to treatments directed at reducing intracranial pressure.

Indications

The Brain Trauma Foundation guidelines[28] recommend intracranial pressure monitoring in patients with traumatic coma (severe head injury: GCS=8 following non-surgical resuscitation) with any of the following:

- abnormal CT scan
- diffuse injury II–IV (see Table 75.2) or
- high- or mixed-density lesions >25 mm^3
- normal CT scan with two or more of the following features:
  - age >40 years
  - unilateral or bilateral motor posturing
  - significant extracranial trauma with systolic hypotension (<90 mmHg (11.97 kPa)).

Coagulopathy is a relative contraindication to intracranial pressure monitoring.

Methods

Measurement of intracranial pressure[29] with an intraventricular catheter is the most accurate and clinically useful method. It has the advantages of zero calibration and drainage of cerebrospinal fluid drainage. Disadvantages include technical difficulty with insertion, particularly in patients with cerebral oedema and compression of the lateral ventricles, and an increased incidence of infection.

Solid-state systems such as fibreoptic (e.g. Camino®) or strain gauge tipped catheters (e.g. Codman®) may be placed intraparenchymally or intraventricularly. These systems transduce intracranial pressure to provide high-fidelity waveforms. They are small calibre and, although requiring a small craniotomy (burr hole) for insertion, may be inserted at the bedside. Disadvantages include inability to perform zero calibration after insertion and baseline drift that may be significant after 5 days.

Fluid-filled subdural catheters have been used for many years. However, these are no longer recommended owing to the development of more accurate solid-state systems. Subdural pressures do not accurately reflect global intracranial pressure, particularly in the presence of a craniectomy. Pressure readings may also be affected by local clot formation within the catheter.

Thresholds

Measurements are used to calculate cerebral perfusion pressure: mean arterial pressure minus intracranial pressure. For this calculation, both measurements should be referenced to the external auditory meatus (equivalent to the circle of Willis).

Intracranial pressure monitoring should be continued until the patient can be assessed clinically and intracranial pressure has stabilised (<20–25 cmH_2O). This occurs in the majority of patients within 7 days. Patients with refractory intracranial hypertension may require monitoring for longer periods, although this may be complicated by drift (with solid-state systems), infection (with intraventricular catheters) or occlusion (subdural catheters). In this situation, intracranial pressure monitors may need to be replaced or removed and patients assessed by serial CT scan or clinically.[30]

CEREBRAL BLOOD FLOW MONITORING

Currently, there is no method of routinely measuring cerebral blood flow at the bedside. Technological advances such as mapping with labelled xenon under computed tomography and laser Doppler flowmetry provide useful imaging of regional and cerebral blood flow. However, these techniques are intermittent, labour-intensive and limited to research-based units.

A number of qualitative measurement techniques are available that provide an indirect assessment of cerebral blood flow and have a limited and undefined role in routine management.

Jugular bulb oximetry

Measurement of oxygen saturation in the jugular bulb by the retrograde placement of a fibreoptic catheter provides an indirect assessment of cerebral perfusion. Low jugular venous saturations (<55%) may be indicative of cerebral hypoperfusion whereas high levels of jugular venous saturation (>85%) may be indicative of cerebral hyperaemia or inadequate neuronal metabolism, such as occurs during the hyperaemic phase or during the evolution of brain death. Both low and high jugular venous saturations are associated with adverse outcomes.[31]

There are insufficient data to provide evidence-based indications for the routine use of jugular bulb oximetry. Its use is limited to experienced units when an index of cerebral blood flow may be required during adjunctive therapies in patients with intracranial hypertension – for example, augmentation with catecholamines, barbiturate coma, hyperventilation or hypothermia.[32]

Transcranial Doppler

Transcranial Doppler ultrasonography with a 2-MHz pulsed Doppler probe allows non-invasive, intermittent or continuous assessment of the velocity of blood flow through large cerebral vessels. Insonation through a naturally occurring acoustic window such as the transtemporal approach allows insonation of the anterior, middle and posterior cerebral arteries, terminal internal carotid artery and anterior and posterior communicating arteries. However, the technique is operator-dependent and there may be significant variations in velocity patterns during the course of the injury. Measured indices of flow include systolic, mean and diastolic flow velocities.

Distinct patterns associated with normal, hyperaemic, vasospastic and absent flow are recognised. Derived indices such as the Gosling pulsatility index (systolic/diastolic difference divided by the mean velocity) and Lindegaard ratio (between middle cerebral artery to extracranial internal carotid artery) may assist in differentiating these flow patterns.

Despite an increasing use of transcranial Doppler to diagnose post-traumatic hyperaemia and vasospasm, there are insufficient data to provide evidence-based indications for its routine use.[33]

CEREBRAL FUNCTION AND METABOLISM

Electroencephalography

Electroencephalography has been used for many years to assess seizure activity that may be masked by sedatives or muscle relaxants and to provide an objective estimate of the degree of electrical neuronal depression with barbiturate therapy. Although seizures may not be clinically apparent in a proportion of patients, and may constitute an important secondary insult, the accuracy and reliability of electroencephalography in ICU is questionable owing to outside electrical interference from monitors and ventilators.[34]

The development of bispectral index (BIS monitoring) as a measurement of depth of anaesthesia has led to the suggestion that this may be an alternative to the use of electroencephalography with barbiturate or sedative therapy in traumatic brain injury. Nevertheless, bispectral index has not been validated in this context and cannot be recommended as a titration end-point.[35]

Evoked potentials

Measurement of evoked potentials, assessing the integrity of sensory and motor pathways, may provide diagnostic and prognostic information; however, because of the complexity of the technique it is not recommended for general use. The reliance on one variable, such as evoked potentials, to predict outcome from traumatic brain injury is not recommended.[36]

Neuronal function

Research developments in microprobe technology have resulted in specific electrodes that may be placed into the brain parenchyma to measure brain oxygen, pH, lactate and carbon dioxide tensions. These may be individual electrodes or combined with other sensors such as pressure monitors to form multimodal tissue monitors.[32]

Cerebral microdialysis is a technique that measures brain extracellular fluid metabolites. Dialysate is obtained through a microdialysis catheter inserted through the same burr hole as an intracranial pressure monitor to measure concentration and fluxes of markers of intracranial inflammation (e.g. lactate, pyruvate and purines).

Although these systems provide highly specific information about the biochemical milieu of focal areas of brain tissue, their clinical utility is limited to research centres.

BRAIN INJURY SURVEILLANCE

Serial assessment of the anatomical injury is an important part of monitoring head injury. This is done by serial CT scanning at frequent intervals depending on the neurological status of the patient.

Any patient who develops an unexplained neurological deterioration or significant validated deviation of monitored parameters should have a CT scan so that new or delayed intracranial mass lesions are identified.

CT scans should be assessed and scored according to the classification outlined in Table 75.2. The progression or resolution of axonal injury, cerebral oedema, contusion and haemorrhages should be recorded. However, as CT scanning requires transport of the patient to a radiology suite, this should be done only by experienced personnel, when the patient is stable.

BRAIN-SPECIFIC THERAPY

Treatment options directed at ameliorating brain injury are limited. Despite intensive research into defining the pathobiological processes in primary injury, studies analysing therapies designed to modulate intracranial inflammation have not been successful. These include aminosteroids, calcium channel blockade and *N*-methyl-D-aspartic acid antagonists.

Brain-specific or 'targeted' therapy is directed at maintaining cerebral perfusion pressure and minimising intracranial pressure. Although there is an inherent relationship between these two principles, priorities are different depending on the time course of the underlying injury. This is important as strategies directed at one may have adverse effects on the other (see Fig. 75.2).

DEFENCE OF CEREBRAL PERFUSION PRESSURE

The Brain Trauma Foundation guidelines recommend a range of cerebral perfusion pressure of 60 mmHg (7.98 kPa).[37]

This requires a change from a 'set and forget' philosophy to one of 'titration against time' in order to prescribe desirable therapeutic targets.

Hypoperfusion phase (0–72 hours)

Cerebral hypoperfusion is present in the majority of patients with severe head injury (GCS=8). During this phase, there is an imperative to maintain cerebral perfusion pressure by supporting systemic haemodynamic function.

During this period, a cerebral perfusion pressure of at least 60 mmHg (7.98 kPa) is recommended. In addition to reduced cerebral blood flow, intracranial pressure may be increased by mass lesions or 'cytotoxic' cerebral oedema.

During this phase, medical therapies directed at raised intracranial pressure such as osmotherapy or hyperventilation should be used only if cerebral perfusion pressure is maintained at an appropriate level and the patient is adequately monitored.

Assessment of adequacy of the response to augmentation of cerebral perfusion pressure is made by intracranial pressure trends, CT scan appearance and, where possible, neurological assessment. If patients appear to have stabilised, sedation may be reduced with the aim of extubation.

Hyperaemic phase (3–7 days)

Approximately 25–30% of patients will develop clinical signs of cerebral hyperaemia, characterised by increased intracranial pressure and persistent cerebral oedema on CT scan. This may occur due to vasogenic cerebral oedema caused by intracranial inflammation or in patients who require increasing doses of catecholamines (e.g. >40 μg/min of epinephrine or norepinephrine) to attain a target cerebral perfusion pressure.

In this context, a target cerebral perfusion pressure target of 40–60 mmHg (5.32–7.98 kPa) is recommended.

If patients continue to have raised intracranial pressure, strategies directed at reducing intracranial pressure should be considered.

REDUCTION OF INTRACRANIAL PRESSURE

In the absence of intracranial mass lesions, raised intracranial pressure is usually an indicator of severity of the underlying injury and represents exhausted intracranial elastance.

The most effective methods of reducing raised intracranial pressure are mechanical interventions such as removal of mass lesions, drainage of cerebrospinal fluid or decompressive craniectomy.

A number of medical strategies directed at reducing intracranial pressure have been used for many years. Despite widespread use and firmly held beliefs, there is little evidence to support the routine use of these therapies.[38]

Intracranial pressure should be maintained at <20–25 cmH_2O. Trends of intracranial pressure are equally as important and should be assessed within the context of cerebral perfusion pressure and the methods used to defend it.[30]

Surgical evacuation of mass lesions

The prompt detection and evacuation of mass lesions causing raised intracranial pressure is the most effective method of relieving intracranial hypertension. Although the majority of these lesions will be present immediately after injury and will be treated during the resuscitative phase, approximately 10% of patients will develop delayed intracranial haematomas. These are detected by sudden unexplained rises in intracranial pressure or by CT scan surveillance.

Cerebrospinal fluid drainage

Drainage of cerebrospinal fluid through an intraventricular catheter is an effective method of reducing intracranial pressure. If present, these catheters should be placed 5–10 cm above the head and opened for drainage every 1–4 hours.

Decompressive craniectomy

Wide, bilateral, frontoparietal craniectomies are highly effective in reducing intracranial pressure and have mainly been used in patients with refractory intracranial hypertension without evacuable mass lesions.

However, a large randomised-controlled trial of early decompressive craniectomy in patients with diffuse traumatic brain injury and early intracranial hypertension demonstrated an increase in unfavourable neurological outcome in survivors.[39] The role of decompressive craniectomy is now questioned in these patients.

Osmotherapy

The rationale and role of osmotherapy using mannitol or hypertonic solution are addressed above (in the section 'Brain-specific resuscitation'). These same principles also apply during intensive care management.

Mannitol or hypertonic saline should be used only in patients with validated intracranial hypertension who are euvolaemic, haemodynamically stable, with a serum osmolality <320 mosm/L.

There is no evidence that osmotherapy or induced dehydration improves outcome or is more effective in cytotoxic than vasogenic cerebral oedema.[13]

Hyperventilation

The role of hyperventilation during intensive care management is limited to the indications outlined in the section 'Brain-specific resuscitation'.

The routine prolonged use of hyperventilation in head-injured patients is associated with a worse outcome than patients ventilated to normocapnia. This is probably due to reduction of cerebral blood flow and secondary brain ischaemia.

Current evidence-based guidelines do not recommend the use of routine hyperventilation.[12]

Hypothermia

Induced hypothermia has been used for many years to reduce cerebral metabolism and thereby raised intracranial pressure. A theoretical benefit exists in experimental models where hypothermia is induced immediately following injury with prompt reduction in raised intracranial pressure. However, these benefits have not translated into improved outcomes in a number of clinical trials.[40]

Induced hypothermia (to temperatures of 30–33°C) is associated with prolonged ventilation and increased susceptibility to nosocomial infection, and may also be associated with increased morbidity and mortality in head-injured patients.

Currently, hypothermia is regarded as a 'second tier' option in patients with refractory intracranial hypertension but, on current evidence, cannot be recommended.[41]

Barbiturate coma

The role of barbiturates in traumatic brain injury is similar to hypothermia. Despite experimental evidence that barbiturates reduce cerebral metabolism and reduce intracranial pressure, no definitive studies have shown a benefit in clinical trials. Barbiturates have invariably been used in patients with refractory intracranial hypertension where a positive outcome was unlikely, making interpretation of these trials difficult.

Barbiturates may cause hypotension and reduce cerebral blood flow, potentially exacerbating secondary insults in patients with cerebral oligaemia. Prolonged use of barbiturates will delay awakening and predispose the patient to nosocomial infection.

Barbiturates are a 'second-tier' option in patients with refractory intracranial hypertension and are not recommended on current evidence.[23]

Steroids

Steroids have been advocated for many years to ameliorate intracranial inflammation, thereby reducing intracranial pressure. A large international study has provided conclusive evidence that high doses of steroids are associated with adverse outcomes in traumatic brain injury, and therefore have no place in management.[42,43]

CEREBRAL VASOSPASM

Post-traumatic cerebral vasospasm occurs in approximately 10–15% of patients. It is associated with a high morbidity and mortality. It is frequently present in patients with traumatic subarachnoid haemorrhage and is a marker of severity of injury, although the true incidence of clinically significant vasospasm is uncertain.

Treatment options remain limited. Calcium antagonists, such as nimodipine, have not been shown to be effective in traumatic subarachnoid haemorrhage. Strategies that have been used in aneurysmal subarachnoid haemorrhage such as 'triple H' therapy (induced hypertension, hypervolaemia and haemodilution) or chemical angioplasty have not been evaluated in traumatic subarachnoid haemorrhage and are not recommended.

SEIZURE PROPHYLAXIS

Seizures are infrequent following traumatic brain injury and usually present at the time of injury. These should be treated with anticonvulsants (e.g. diazepam, midazolam) when they occur. Subsequent prophylaxis with phenytoin is recommended only in patients with destructive parenchymal lesions on CT scan and should be continued for 10 days following injury. Short-term seizure prophylaxis does not prevent late-onset post-traumatic epilepsy.[44]

OUTCOME AND PROGNOSIS

Patient factors that determine outcome from traumatic brain injury include severity of primary and secondary injuries, traumatic coma (GCS<8), age >60 years and co-morbidities. Prediction of outcome is difficult as significant functional improvements, particularly in young patients, may occur over time.

There are patients in whom the prognosis is clearly very poor or hopeless. A proportion of these patients will become brain dead and may be considered for organ donation. In other patients, it may be appropriate to withdraw active treatment. This increasingly complex process requires time, careful consideration and consensus with all members of the healthcare team and relatives.

Outcomes from traumatic brain injury are difficult to quantify. Although mortality is an easy end-point to measure, functional outcome is an equally important measurement as the effects of traumatic brain injury on psychosocial recovery and duration of rehabilitation often take extended periods of time.

Access the complete references list online at http://www.expertconsult.com

9. Curry N, Davis PW. What's new in resuscitation strategies for the patient with multiple trauma? Injury 2012;43:1021–8.
17. BTF Guidelines. Brain Trauma Foundation. American Association of Neurological Surgeons. Computed tomography scan features. J Neurotrauma 2000;17:597–627.
28. Bratton SL, Chestnut RM, Ghajar J, et al. Guidelines for the management of severe traumatic brain injury. VI. Indications for intracranial pressure monitoring. J Neurotrauma 2007;24(Suppl 1):S37–44.
30. Bratton SL, Chestnut RM, Ghajar J, et al. Guidelines for the management of severe traumatic brain injury. VIII. Intracranial pressure thresholds. J Neurotrauma 2007;24(Suppl 1):S55–8.
37. Bratton SL, Chestnut RM, Ghajar J, et al. Guidelines for the management of severe traumatic brain injury. IX. Cerebral perfusion thresholds. J Neurotrauma 2007;24(Suppl 1):S59–64.
39. Cooper DJ, Rosenfeld JV, Murray L, et al. Decompressive craniectomy in diffuse traumatic brain injury. N Engl J Med 2011;364:1493–502.
42. Edwards P, Arango M, Balica L, et al. Final results of MRC CRASH, a randomised placebo-controlled trial of intravenous corticosteroid in adults with head injury-outcomes at 6 months. Lancet 2005; 365:1957–9.

76

Faciomaxillary and upper-airway injuries

Cyrus Edibam and Hayley Robinson

MAXILLOFACIAL INJURIES

Blunt or penetrating faciomaxillary injuries may be isolated or part of multisystem trauma. Life-threatening associated injuries occur in 6.2% of patients with facial injuries and commonly include head, cervical spine and chest injury.[1] Life-threatening airway haemorrhage and airway obstruction are challenging issues and require skilled airway management to prevent adverse outcomes. This chapter outlines the basic anatomy, pathology, complications and common pitfalls in the emergency management of maxillofacial and upper-airway trauma.

EPIDEMIOLOGY

Maxillofacial trauma occurs most frequently in the 20–25-years age group and occurs three to five times more often in males than in females. Blunt injury mechanisms account for nearly 98% of all maxillofacial injuries.[2] Motor vehicle trauma accounts for nearly three-quarters of blunt injuries, the remainder being due to falls, physical assault, contact sports and industrial accidents. In some areas, legislative changes and preventative measures involving drink–driving, seat-belt and airbag use have seen a reduction in the incidence of motor-vehicle-related maxillofacial injury.[3] However, others have seen a large increase owing to alcohol and interpersonal violence.[4] In multiple trauma patients with an Injury Severity Score (ISS) > 15, maxillofacial injury occurs in up to 16%, with a corresponding mortality rate of 10.5%.[2]

ANATOMICAL ASPECTS

Fractures, haemorrhage, soft-tissue damage and oedema are the commonest manifestations of blunt facial trauma. The severity of facial injury is directly related to the velocity of force applied. Common maxillofacial fractures involve the midface (71.5%), mandible (24.3%) and frontal bone (4.2%).[5]

MANDIBULAR FRACTURES

The mandible is a unique horseshoe-shaped bone that is tubular and weakest where the cortices are thinnest. Most fractures occur at vulnerable points, regardless of the point of impact.[6] Common sites of weakness include the condylar area, followed by the symphyseal and parasymphyseal area, and then the angle. Multiple fractures are common (64%),[6] with body of mandible fractures often being accompanied by fractures of the opposite angle or neck due to transmitted forces. Mandibular fragments are often distracted owing to the action of the lower jaw muscles. Respiratory obstruction may occur after bilateral mandibular angle or body fractures due to the posterior displacement of the tongue – the 'Andy Gump' fracture.[7]

MIDFACIAL FRACTURES

The bones of the middle third of the face are relatively thin and poorly reinforced. Fracture dislocations occur through the bones and suture lines and the facial skeleton acts as a compressible energy-absorbing mass that gives on impact. The series of compartments (nasal cavity, paranasal sinuses and orbits) within the bony framework collapse progressively, absorbing energy and protecting the brain, spinal cord and other vital structures.[8] Multiple complex facial fractures usually result and isolated facial bone fractures are rare. Le Fort described three great lines of weakness in the facial skeleton and subsequently derived the Le Fort fracture classification[9] **(Fig. 76.1)**. Le Fort fractures are perpendicular to the three main vertical buttresses of the facial skeleton – the nasomaxillary, zygomaticomaxillary and pterygomaxillary 'pillars'. Such fractures usually occur with mixed patterns as impact to the face is rarely centred (e.g. right hemifacial Le Fort I and left hemifacial Le Fort II). Airway obstruction may occur from posterior movement of the soft palate against the tongue and the posterior pharyngeal wall. Oral secretions, blood, bone and tooth debris and pharyngeal wall haematomas may worsen airway compromise.

LE FORT I (ALSO KNOWN AS GUERIN'S FRACTURE)

This fracture involves only the maxilla at the level of the nasal fossa. It follows a horizontal plane at the level of the nose. The fracture separates the palate from the remainder of the facial skeleton (i.e. palate–facial disjunction) and is usually caused by direct low-maxillary blows or by a lateral blow to the maxilla.

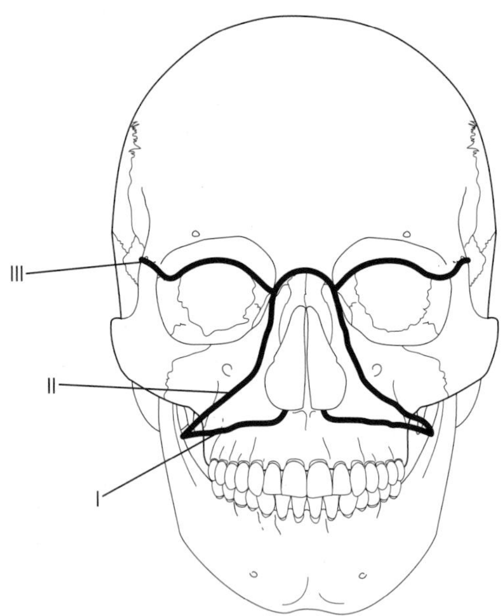

Figure 76.1 Le Fort classification of facial fractures.

LE FORT II

This is the most common midface fracture. The maxilla, nasal bones and medial aspect of the orbit are involved, which results in a freely mobile, pyramidal-shaped portion of the maxilla (i.e. pyramidal disjunction). The fracture line extends from the lower nasal bridge through the medial wall of the orbit, and crosses the zygomaticomaxillary process. It is caused by direct blows to the mid-alveolar area, or by lateral impacts and inferior blows to the mandible when the mouth is closed.

LE FORT III

This is known as craniofacial disjunction because the fracture line runs parallel to the base of the skull, separating the midfacial skeleton from the cranium. The fracture extends through the upper nasal bridge and most of the orbit and across the zygomatic arch. It involves the ethmoid bone, and thus may transect the cribriform plate at the base of the skull.[10,11] These fractures result from superiorly directed blows to the nasal bones.[11]

TEMPOROMANDIBULAR JOINT (TMJ)

Mechanical TMJ impairment may result from condylar or zygomatic arch fractures and can prevent jaw opening even after muscle relaxants have been administered.

ZYGOMATIC, ORBITAL AND NASAL FRACTURES

Zygomatic fractures account for 20% of all facial bone fractures. Its attachments to the maxilla, frontal and temporal bones are vulnerable and may be disrupted. When the zygoma is displaced, disruption of the lateral wall and floor of the orbit may ensue. Orbital injury is commonly associated with midface trauma. The severity of injury in the orbital region varies from oedema and ecchymosis of the periosteal soft tissue to subconjunctival haemorrhage[12] and loss of visual acuity or ocular rupture. Facial fractures are associated with visual loss and blinding in 0.7–10% of patients.[13-15] The blinding mechanism is usually associated with globe perforation rather than optic nerve injury. Orbital blowout fractures occur when pressure that is directly applied to the eye is hydraulically transmitted via the globe to the interior bony structures. The weaker inferior orbital wall usually fractures, causing enophthalmos, diplopia, impaired eye movement and infraorbital hypoaesthesia. Nasal fractures are common, with epistaxis and septal haematoma being the prime concerns.

SOFT-TISSUE INJURIES

Abrasions, contusions, lacerations to the tongue, palate, pharynx, cheek, eyelids, nasolacrimal duct, ear, parotid gland and facial nerve can occur. Oedema evolving over 24–48 hours can be massive and cause gross distortion of soft-tissue structures. Patency of an initially unobstructed airway may become compromised during this period.

HAEMORRHAGE

Haemorrhage following blunt maxillofacial injury is extremely common. Life-threatening bleeding is rare. Various series have reported the incidence to be between 1.25 and 11%.[12-14] Most severe haemorrhage is associated with midfacial fractures, although soft-tissue lacerations alone can cause significant blood loss. Swallowing of large quantities of blood may conceal haemorrhage and predispose to vomiting and aspiration.[15]

The origin of bleeding in facial trauma is complicated, as the vascular supply is derived from both the internal and external carotid arteries, with anastomoses occurring between them as well as between both halves of the face. The internal maxillary artery, especially the intraosseous branches, is the main source of bleeding in facial injury because the artery passes within the common Le Fort fracture borders.[16] The comminuted nature of maxillary fractures makes the detection of an exact site of vessel damage nearly impossible.[16] Branches of the internal carotid artery such as the lacrimal and zygomatic branches, as well as the anterior and posterior ethmoidal arteries, may contribute to bleeding.

ASSOCIATED INJURIES

More than half of all patients with maxillofacial injuries will have other injuries and these are listed below.

BASILAR SKULL FRACTURE

The anterior cranial fossa is often involved in craniofacial injuries. Fractures involving the frontal bone, frontal sinus, nasoethmoid complex, or fronto-orbital complex result in bone defects in the skull base and can cause dural tears with resultant leakage of cerebrospinal fluid (CSF). CSF fistulae occur in 10–30% of basilar skull fractures.[17] The clinical finding of CSF rhinorrhoea represents only the site of exiting CSF and is not diagnostic for anterior cranial fossa lesions. The origin may be from a temporal bone fracture, because CSF from the middle ear discharges into the nose via the Eustachian tube. A middle cranial fossa defect can produce rhinorrhoea through the sphenoid sinus. The vast majority of fistulae present within 1 week of injury. Meningitis in patients with midface fractures is uncommon, despite the fact that approximately 25% develop CSF leaks.[18]

Pulsating exophthalmos and the presence of an orbital bruit may lead to the diagnosis of a carotido-cavernous fistula, which may develop following fractures involving the skull base and orbit.

HEAD AND CERVICAL SPINE INJURY

The incidence of head injury in those with maxillofacial trauma has been variably reported to be from 15% for severe head injury, increasing to 80% if all grades of head injuries are included.[14,19,20] Cervical spine injury has been reported in up to 11% of patients. The prevalence of cervical spine fracture with mandibular injury is 6.5%[21] and is attributed to forces exerted directly or indirectly from the facial skeleton to the neck. C1/C2 and C5–C7 are at particular risk.

The association between maxillofacial and cervical spine injury depends on the mechanism of injury. Falls and motor vehicle accident victims are more likely to have cervical injury than are sporting or personal assault victims.

OTHER INJURIES

Thoracic trauma (9–40%), abdominal trauma (5–40%) and limb fractures (30%) are other common coexistent injuries.[19,22] Traumatic injury of the internal carotid artery following maxillofacial trauma occurs in less than 0.5% of patients presenting with blunt maxillofacial injury.[23] It is often associated with mandible fractures or laterally displaced midface fractures (LeFort II and III[24]) and is recognised when a patient develops an unexplained neurological deficit, most often hemiplegia, subsequent to trauma or surgery of the head, face or neck. Assessment of the carotid circulation by CT angiography is a useful investigation if carotid injury is suspected.

ASSESSMENT OF INJURY

The obvious priorities are airway management and control of haemorrhage and identification of other life-threatening injuries. These are discussed later in detail. Once the patient is stable, formal assessment of the facial injuries can proceed.

HISTORY

Evaluation of facial fractures begins with a history of the injury. The mechanism of injury is important in order to assess the likelihood of other injuries.

EXAMINATION

Physical examination includes inspection of the deformity, presence of enophthalmos, asymmetry, dental malocclusion, nasal septal deviation or haematoma, CSF rhinorrhoea and the extent of jaw opening. Other signs associated with basal skull fracture should also be noted (haemotympanum, Battle's sign, raccoon eyes). Tenderness and mobility on bimanual palpation of the alveolar process and the infraorbital rim or frontozygomatic suture indicates the presence of a complex midfacial fracture. Naso-orbito-ethmoid instability can also be established by bimanual palpation. Visual acuity (in the conscious patient), corneal integrity and pupillary reflexes as well as eye movements (failure of upward movements in orbital blowout fracture) should be assessed early and thoroughly. Facial nerve function should also be assessed if possible. The presence of a bruit over the orbit may indicate a carotido-cavernous fistula.

INVESTIGATION

CT scanning, especially with three-dimensional reconstruction, is the preferred and most accurate method of imaging.[25] In addition to bony distortion, fluid in the paranasal sinuses, optic nerve integrity and soft-tissue distortion, the brain, upper cervical spine and other body areas can be visualised concurrently. Other investigations such as colour Doppler ultrasound studies, CT angiography or standard angiography of the great vessels in the neck may be required in cases of possible carotid dissection or carotid-cavernous fistulae. Nasal discharge should be tested for β_2-transferrin to confirm the presence of a CSF fistula.[26]

AIRWAY MANAGEMENT

Airway management in maxillofacial injury is potentially complex owing to multiple concurrent compromising factors **(Table 76.1)**.

IMMEDIATE PRIORITIES

- Assess and monitor for signs of airway obstruction whilst maintaining cervical spine precautions
- Clear airway, assist respiration
- Definitive airway intervention.

An initially unobstructed airway may become compromised as swelling and oedema can progress in the initial hours after injury. Careful close monitoring in an intensive care unit (ICU) or high-dependency unit (HDU) is essential. Maintaining the head-up position and the use of humidified oxygen may lessen the likelihood of later airway compromise. Sudden obstruction may occur

Table 76.1 Airway problems in maxillofacial trauma

GENERAL PROBLEMS	MANAGEMENT
Haemorrhage/debris Impaired laryngoscopy Aspiration risk from blood swallowing Clot inhalation/obstruction Teeth, bone fragments	Suction, volume replacement Head down Definitive control of haemorrhage (see text)
Oedema soft-tissue haemotomas Increases over 48 hours Mask fit can be poor	Monitor airway closely Head up 30° Maintain spontaneous ventilation during airway Manipulation; laryngeal mask ventilation
SPECIFIC PROBLEMS	
Bilateral mandibular body/angle fractures Posterior displacement of tongue	Anterior traction on tongue or jaw, towel clip or suture through tongue and elevate
TMJ impairment from mandibular condyle and or zygomatic arch fracture Mouth opening limited	Nasotracheal intubation (blind/fibreoptic) or surgical airway may be required (see text)
Midfacial fracture Mask seal poor Soft palate collapses against pharynx	Anterior traction on mobile segment
Basilar skull Nasotracheal intubation contraindicated Pneumocephalus from mask ventilation	Avoid nasal intubation
Cervical spine injury	Orotracheal intubation with in-line stabilisation; fibreoptic intubation; surgical airway

with clot dislodgement and inhalation. Signs of partial obstruction include noisy breathing, stridor, intercostal or supraclavicular recession and restlessness.

Occasionally, patients may assume positions that lessen airway obstruction (e.g. sitting forward or even prone). Simple measures such as suction and clearing the airway and insertion of an oropharyngeal airway may suffice.

In midfacial injuries, anterior digital traction on the mobile mid-segment may relieve obstruction. In bilateral mandibular fractures of the angle or body, a towel clip or suture through the tongue may allow anterior traction on the unsupported tongue and relieve obstruction.

Bag and mask ventilation may be difficult owing to distorted anatomy, and this should be borne in mind when a decision to intubate is made. Failure of these simple manoeuvres necessitates definitive airway management

TECHNIQUES (FIG. 76.2)

Facilities to perform a surgical airway must be available prior to elective intubation. The chosen technique for securing the airway depends on the presence of airway obstruction and the likelihood of difficult direct laryngoscopy (extent of jaw opening, gross anatomical distortion and swelling, operator experience). In a combative patient, or if urgent intubation is necessary, a rapid sequence induction can be used if difficulty in direct laryngoscopy is not anticipated. If direct laryngoscopy is likely to be difficult or impossible, spontaneous respiration must be maintained and intubation carried out under local anaesthesia.

Analgesia can be achieved with a combination of sprayed or nebulised lignocaine (4%) to the posterior pharynx as well as a transcricoid injection of 2–4 mL lignocaine (2%). Adjunctive superior laryngeal and glossopharyngeal nerve blocks can be used.[27, 28] The orotracheal route for intubation is the route of choice in the presence of basal skull fracture.

If cervical spine injury is present or suspected, in-line stabilisation is mandatory. A variety of intubation techniques can be used – for example, direct laryngoscopy, awake fibreoptic-guided laryngoscopy, video laryngoscopy as well as retrograde intubation techniques.[29] The operator should use the technique with which he/she is most comfortable. Excessive bleeding or debris may render fibreoptic techniques difficult.

Failure to intubate and ventilate in the presence of airway obstruction necessitates the passage of an appropriate-sized laryngeal mask. If ventilation is not possible with a laryngeal mask in situ then emergency cricothyroidotomy should be performed. Formal tracheostomy may be required in those likely to need prolonged ventilatory support (e.g. multiple facial fractures combined with a head injury) and is best

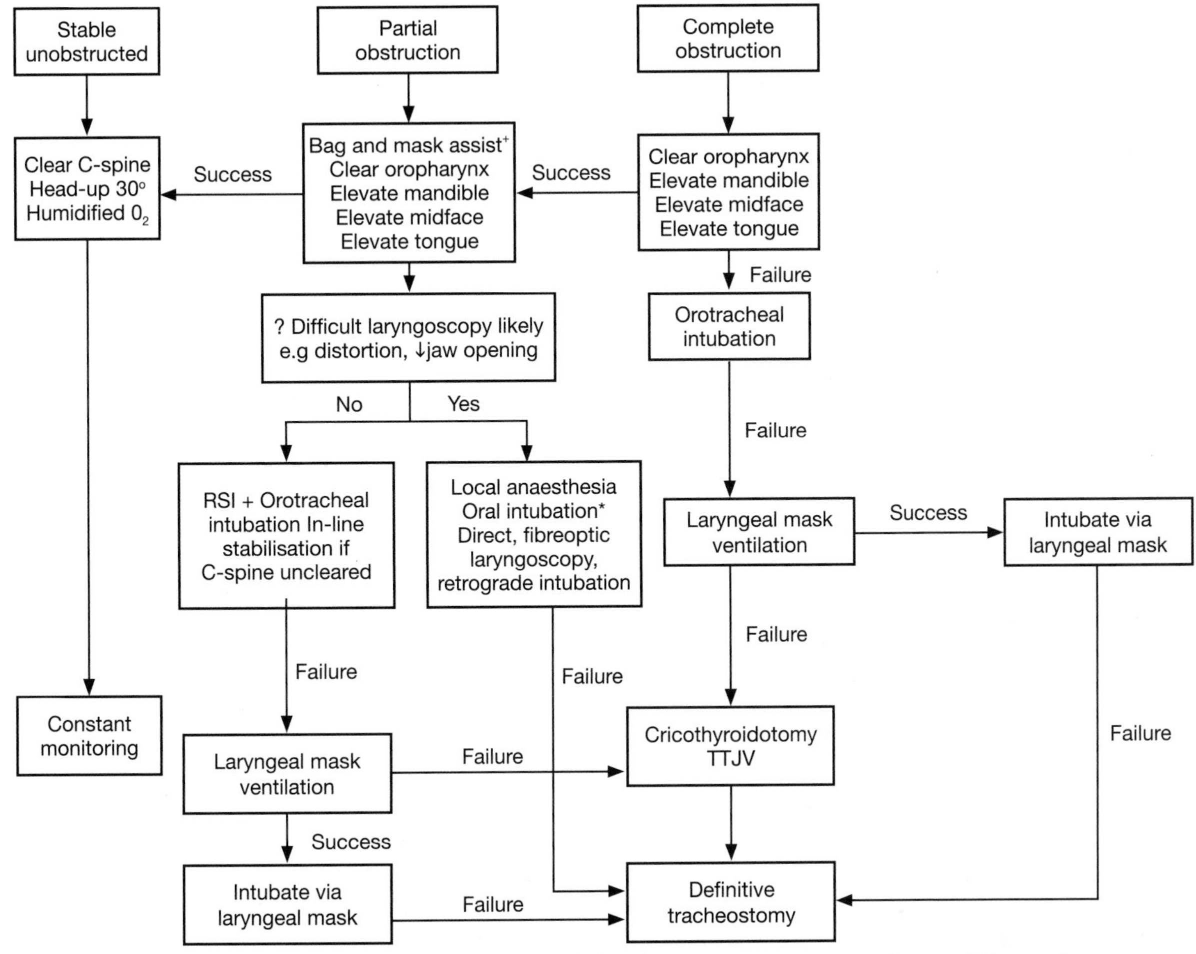

Figure 76.2 An airway management algorithm for maxillofacial trauma. C-spine=cervical spine; RSI=rapid sequence induction; TTJV=transtracheal jet ventilation. +Mask seal may be poor. *Nasotracheal route contraindicated in basilar skull fracture.

performed as a semi-elective procedure in the operating room.[16]

MANAGEMENT OF HAEMORRHAGE

Topical vasoconstrictors may not be effective with ongoing nasal haemorrhage. Anterior or posterior nasopharyngeal packs are sometimes effective at reducing blood loss. Foley catheters passed into the posterior nasopharynx with the balloons filled with air may stem blood loss, especially if anterior traction is applied in mild to moderate haemorrhage.[30] Angiographic embolisation has an increasing role as first-line approach for life-threatening intractable bleeding for blunt and penetrating trauma, with a success rate of greater than 85%.[30] Plastic or maxillofacial surgical opinion should always be sought early on regarding the appropriateness of angiographic versus operative intervention for persistent haemorrhage. Operative intervention includes reduction and stabilisation of fractures and direct ligation of bleeding vessels. External carotid ligation has failed to show consistent efficacy.

DEFINITIVE MANAGEMENT

Definitive surgery is generally delayed 4–10 days to allow swelling to subside. The timing of surgery may be further delayed if a severe head injury coexists. Early surgery may be warranted if orbital injury with optic nerve compromise is present. The use of high-dose steroids in optic nerve compression is controversial and no good data exist regarding its efficacy.[16] Irrigation and debridement of open wounds, closure of facial lacerations and removal of foreign bodies must be undertaken as soon as is practicable, preferably within 24 hours.

The use of prophylactic antibiotics for CSF leak is debateable and local protocols should be followed. The timing of operative intervention is still under discussion but the recent trend is for conservative management due to high rate of spontaneous closure, with lumbar drain insertion for leakage lasting longer than 5- 7 days and endoscopic or surgical closure for those that persist.[31] Appropriate tetanus prophylaxis must be given.

The use of modern internal fixation techniques has reduced the need for intermaxillary fixation following elective facial fracture repair, with only unstable comminuted fractures requiring this form of fixation. Submental intubation during fracture repair is now being used as an alternative to tracheostomy in some centres.[32]

INJURIES TO THE LARYNX AND TRACHEA

Direct trauma to the airway is rare, accounting for less than 1% of traumatic injury seen in most major centres.[33,34] The bony protection afforded to the airway by the sternum and mandible and death from asphyxia at the accident scene account for the rarity of the injury. Laryngotracheal injury can be classified as blunt or penetrating. Failure to recognise these injuries, their complications and specific pitfalls in airway management can lead to death.[35]

MECHANISM OF INJURY

BLUNT INJURY

Common causes include motor vehicle accidents where the extended neck impacts with the steering wheel or dashboard. The 'clothes-line injury' occurs when a cyclist or horse rider collides with a cable or wire causing direct injury to the upper airway. Assaults and strangulation account for the remainder of blunt injuries. Direct blows are more likely to injure the cartilages of the larynx whereas flexion/extension injuries are most commonly associated with tracheal tears and laryngotracheal transection.[36] The larynx above the cricoid cartilage is injured in 35%, manifesting as oedema, contusions, haematomas, lacerations, avulsion and fracture dislocation, most commonly of the thyroid and arytenoid cartilages.

The cricoid cartilage itself is injured in 15%, which may cause recurrent laryngeal nerve dysfunction.[37] The cervical trachea is injured in 45%.[38] Tracheal transection most often occurs at the junction between the cricoid cartilage and trachea.[39] Oedema fluid and air dissecting within submucosal layers of the larynx and trachea may cause airway obstruction. Air in the soft tissues can cause epiglottic emphysema and narrowing of the supraglottic airway.[40] Straining, talking and coughing may worsen the oedema.

Common associations with blunt laryngotracheal injury include thoracic spine injury (15.5%), closed head injury (8.5%) and vascular injuries (11.3%).[33] Up to 96% of patients with laryngotracheal trauma also have maxillofacial injuries.[34]

PENETRATING INJURY

Penetrating injuries usually result from stab or gunshot wounds. The anterior triangle of the neck is the most common site of entry. The cervical trachea is most commonly involved in stab wounds. The larynx is injured in about one-third of those with upper-airway injuries.[38] Of patients with penetrating laryngotracheal trauma, 19% also had cervicothoracic vascular injury, 15% had oesophageal injury and 34% had chest trauma.[33]

ASSESSMENT OF INJURY

Definitive investigation and management depend on the airway status and presence of associated injury. The degree of injury is not readily assessable on the basis of any one clinical symptom or sign **(Box 76.1)** and delayed diagnosis is common. The emphasis has moved towards CT scanning in the first instance in stable patients with laryngeal tenderness, endolaryngeal oedema and small haematomas. CT demonstrates fractures of cartilages, haematomas and other injuries. Further investigation with fibreoptic laryngotracheoscopy under local anaesthesia can be used to demonstrate vocal cord dysfunction, integrity of the cartilaginous framework and laryngeal mucosa. Rigid laryngoscopy can be used when adequate visualisation is not achieved with the former. Pharyngo-oesophagoscopy, contrast studies, open exploration and angiography may be required to exclude aerodigestive tract and major vascular injuries.

AIRWAY MANAGEMENT

Up to three-quarters of patients with laryngotracheal injury require intubation.[34] The safest mode of intubation is via tracheostomy under local anaesthesia

Box 76.1 Clinical features in laryngotracheal injury

- Symptoms
  - Respiratory distress, stridor, noisy breathing
  - Neck tenderness or oedema
  - Hoarseness
  - Dysphonia
  - Cough
  - Dysphagia
- Signs
  - Abnormal laryngeal contour
  - Subcutaneous emphysema
  - Cervical ecchymosis
  - Haemoptysis
- Investigations
  - Plain radiography
    - Air in soft tissues
    - Pneumomediastinum
    - Pneumothorax
    - Cervical spine fracture
  - CT scan
    - Cartilage and soft-tissue injury
    - Altered airway patency
  - Laryngoscopy
    - Vocal paralysis
    - Mucosal or cartilage disruption
    - Haematoma
    - Laceration

Figure 76.3 Airway assessment and management algorithm for suspected laryngotracheal trauma. CT=computed tomography.

(Fig. 76.3). Blind intubation can lead to complete airway obstruction owing to creation of false passages and mucosal disruption.[35] Cricoid pressure can lead to laryngotracheal separation and is contraindicated. Positive-pressure ventilation can rapidly worsen air leaks and wherever possible the patient should maintain spontaneous respiration until a tube has been placed distal to the site of injury. Cricothyroidotomy is not recommended as it may compound laryngeal injury. In an emergency, gaping airway wounds (e.g. with tracheal transection) can be intubated under direct vision pending subsequent surgery.

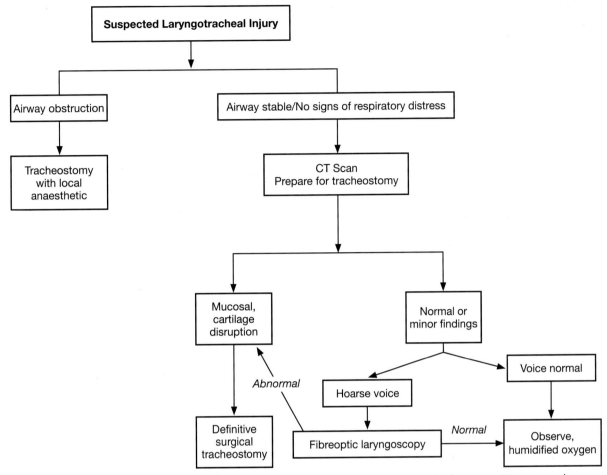
Access the complete references list online at http://www.expertconsult.com

1. Tung TC, Tseng WS, Chen CT, et al. Acute life-threatening injuries in facial fracture patients: a review of 1,025 patients. J Trauma 2000;49(3):420–4.
21. Mulligan RP, Mahabir RC. The prevalence of cervical spine injury, head injury, or both with isolated and multiple craniomaxillofacial fractures. Plast Reconstr Surg 2010;126(5):1647–51.
29. Kellman RM, Losquadro WD. Comprehensive airway management of patients with maxillofacial trauma. Craniomaxillofac Trauma Reconstr 2008;1(1):39–47.
30. Cogbill TH, Cothren CC, Ahearn MK, et al. Management of maxillofacial injuries with severe oronasal hemorrhage: a multicenter perspective. J Trauma 2008;65(5):994–9.
34. Verschueren DS, Bell RB, Bagheri SC, et al. Management of laryngo-tracheal injuries associated with craniomaxillofacial trauma. J Oral Maxillofac Surg 2006;64(2):203–14.

77

Chest injuries

Ubbo F Wiersema

Chest injuries account for a quarter of all trauma deaths. Immediate death from severe blunt trauma is usually due to blunt rupture of the thoracic aorta, heart or major vessel. Patients who survive to hospital presentation may still have life-threatening chest injuries that require immediate intervention. The majority can be managed with simple measures such as intercostal tube thoracostomy, oxygen therapy, analgesia and mechanical ventilation.[1-3] Tension pneumothorax, open pneumothorax or massive haemothorax require immediate intercostal tube drainage. Urgent thoracotomy is indicated for pericardial tamponade, diaphragmatic rupture and massive haemothorax with ongoing bleeding.[2] Following the resuscitation phase, extensive pulmonary contusions with respiratory failure may require prolonged ventilatory support. Chest injuries that are initially missed may also significantly prolong intensive care stay.

IMMEDIATE MANAGEMENT

Identification of chest injuries forms a core component of the initial assessment of a patient with major trauma – both because immediate intervention can be life saving, and because restoration of respiratory and circulatory stability minimises secondary injury to extrathoracic organs, particularly traumatic brain injury.[1] A history of the mechanism and force of injury should be sought as this will guide the likelihood of different injuries and determine the need for more extensive investigation.

During the primary survey the airway patency is ensured, oxygen administered by face mask and ventilation assessed. The degree of circulatory compromise is determined and obvious external bleeding is controlled. Two large-bore intravenous cannulae are sited, blood samples taken and intravenous fluids commenced. Intravenous opioid analgesia is given as repeated small boluses, titrated to effect. Complete exposure is important to facilitate examination of the chest and facilitate intercostal tube insertion, if required. With penetrating trauma all surface wounds must be located so that the pathway of potential injuries can be determined.[2] There are four life-threatening chest injuries that require immediate intervention:

- tension pneumothorax
- open (sucking) pneumothorax
- massive haemothorax
- pericardial tamponade.

In addition, the clinical features of flail chest should be sought, as these will no longer be apparent if positive-pressure ventilation is instituted (see below). Interventions required during initial management are outlined in **Box 77.1**. A chest radiograph is integral to the initial assessment and should be performed promptly. However, the severity of physiological derangement will dictate the time available for confirmatory imaging, and a patient with clinical signs of tension pneumothorax should undergo immediate intercostal tube thoracostomy before the chest radiograph (see below). If there is no physiological improvement after unilateral tube thoracostomy, a second drain should be inserted in the contralateral chest.

Lung ultrasound can be completed faster than a chest radiograph, and has significantly higher diagnostic accuracy for pneumothorax and haemothorax when performed by experienced operators.[4] However, clinicians not experienced with lung ultrasound should avoid decision-making based on this technique. Subcostal ultrasonography of the heart to look for pericardial fluid forms part of the focused assessment with sonography for trauma (FAST) and should be performed with penetrating chest trauma, or if there is haemodynamic instability with blunt trauma.[2,4,5] An electrocardiogram (ECG) is important in the assessment for blunt cardiac injury.[2,6]

Endotracheal intubation and mechanical ventilation are indicated for the patient with a compromised airway, severe head injury, or gross hypoventilation and/or hypoxaemia not attributable to pneumothorax. Haemodynamic instability should be anticipated (**Box 77.2**). Rarely, emergency cricothyroidotomy or tracheostomy is required when an airway obstruction cannot be bypassed by translaryngeal intubation. A nasogastric or orogastric tube (if facial injuries are suspected) should be inserted to decompress the stomach after endotracheal intubation.

PNEUMOTHORAX

Pneumothorax visible on the initial chest radiograph should be treated with insertion of an intercostal tube connected to an underwater seal drainage system

Box 77.1 Immediate management of chest trauma

Indications for intercostal drain insertion
- Pneumothorax
- Haemothorax

Indications for urgent thoracotomy
- Pericardial tamponade
- Diaphragmatic rupture
- Massive haemothorax with ongoing bleeding

Indications for emergency thoracotomy
- Witnessed loss of vital signs after penetrating trauma

Indications for intubation and positive pressure ventilation
- Airway compromise
- Gross hypoventilation and/or hypoxaemia (not attributable to pneumothorax)
- Severe head injury

Box 77.2 Causes of cardiovascular collapse on induction of anaesthesia and positive-pressure ventilation in chest-injured patients

- Excessive anaesthetic agent
- Hypovolaemia
- Oesophageal intubation with hypoxaemia
- Tension pneumothorax
- Pericardial tamponade
- Anaphylaxis
- Systemic air embolism
- Severe blunt cardiac injury

(**Fig. 77.1**). A single bottle drainage system without suction is usually adequate. Low-pressure suction (20 cmH_2O) is applied if the pneumothorax fails to fully resolve, or if there is associated haemothorax (**Fig. 77.2**). A three-bottle system (or a commercially available three-in-one system) allows more accurate control of suction (**Fig. 77.3**). Use of antibiotics (to prevent empyema) is controversial, but contamination during intercostal tube insertion is common and a 24-hour course of a first-generation cephalosporin may be appropriate.[7,8]

Tension pneumothorax results from progressive accumulation of air in the pleural space, positive intrapleural pressure and cardiorespiratory decompensation.[9] In awake patients, slow development of positive intrapleural pressure leads to progressive hypoxaemia and respiratory distress. Tachycardia is common, but preserved venous return maintains cardiac function and blood pressure. In sedated patients on positive-pressure ventilation, the positive intrapleural pressure throughout the respiratory cycle can lead to the rapid development of hypoxaemia. Cardiac output is compromised by obstructed venous return; hypotension is prominent and may progress to cardiac arrest. In both awake and ventilated patients, chest signs (hyperexpansion, decreased breath sounds and tracheal deviation) are not reliably present.[9]

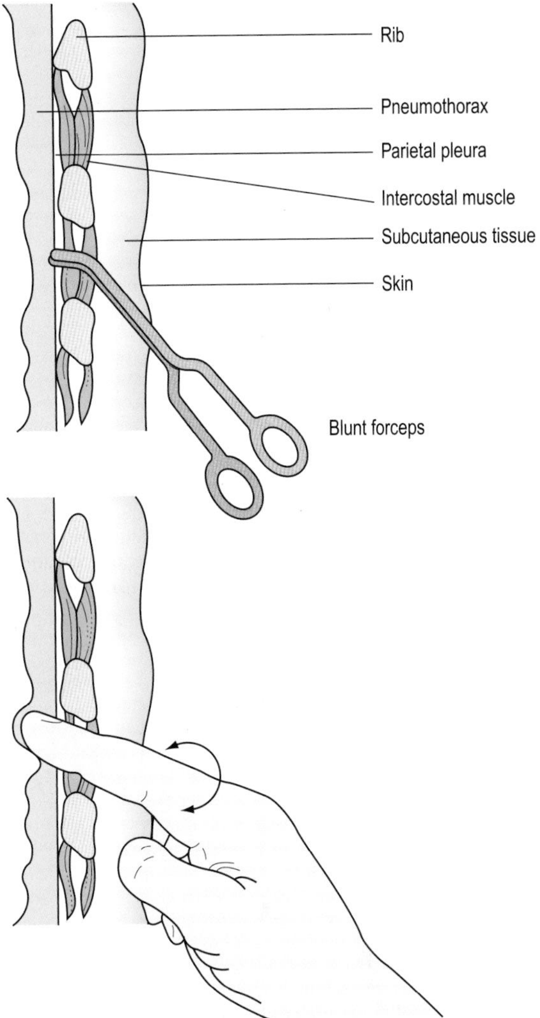

Figure 77.1 Intercostal tube insertion. After sterile preparation and drape 1% lidocaine is infiltrated in the midaxillary line at the level of the nipple. A 2–3 cm transverse skin incision is made. Dissection is performed by blunt forceps down to the pleura passing just superior to the rib surface to avoid injury to neurovascular structures. A gloved finger is used to confirm separation of lung from chest wall. A large-bore (28–32 Fr) intercostal tube is inserted without a trocar and advanced in a postero-superior direction. Curved forceps clamped to the distal side hole of the tube can be used to guide the tube through the chest wall. The tube is immediately connected to an underwater seal drainage system (see Figs 77.2 and 77.3) and checked for satisfactory drainage and tidal rise and fall in fluid level with respiration. Non-absorbable sutures are used to seal the skin incision around the tube and secure the tube. The intrathoracic position of the tube is checked with a chest radiograph.

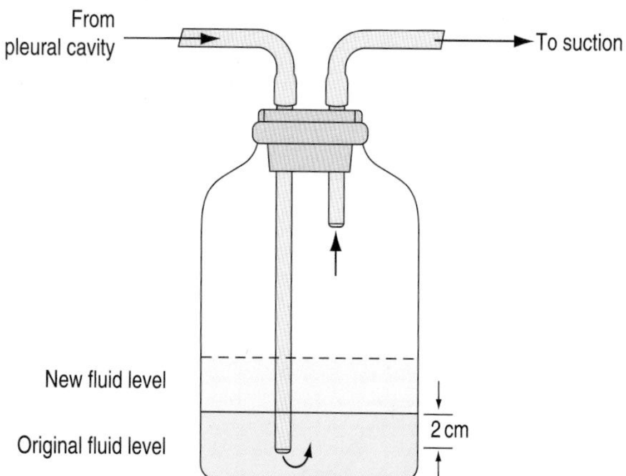

Figure 77.2 Single-bottle drainage system for haemopneumothorax. Air drainage will become more difficult if there is also fluid drainage, raising the fluid level in the bottle (dashed line) and increasing the depth of immersion of the hollow rod. This can be overcome by applying low-pressure suction (20 cmH_2O). Arrows indicate direction of air flow.

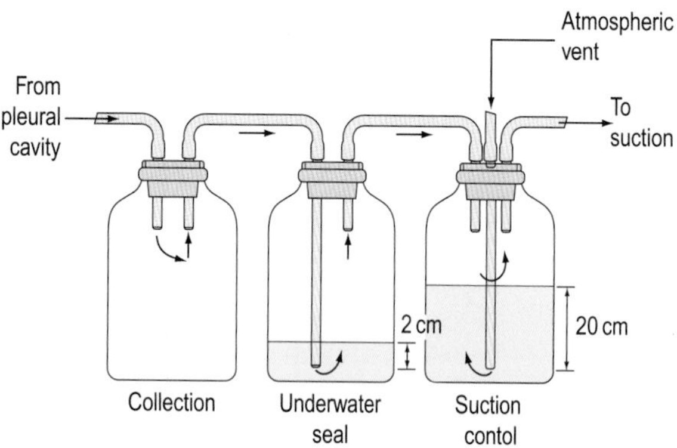

Figure 77.3 Three-bottle chest drainage system. The first bottle (connected to the intercostal tube) is a fluid collection chamber, the second functions as a one-way valve (underwater seal), and the third (connected to wall suction) limits the amount of suction applied. The level of suction is set by adjusting the depth of the atmospheric vent whilst ensuring that it bubbles continuously. Commercially available drainage systems function on the same principles as the three-bottle system. Arrows indicate direction of air flow.

If tension pneumothorax is suspected clinically, an intercostal tube should be inserted immediately, prior to the chest radiograph. Blunt dissection and insertion of a gloved finger into the pleural space allow rapid decompression of tension, prior to intercostal tube insertion.[7] Needle thoracostomy with a large-bore cannula inserted into the second intercostal space in the midclavicular line may be used to drain air more rapidly for patients in extremis. However, this is rarely necessary and may puncture the lung, or a blood vessel, fail to reach the pleural space, or kink when the needle is removed from within the cannula.[7] Furthermore the landmarks for needle thoracostomy are often identified incorrectly, increasing the risk of adverse outcome. Whether successful or not, needle thoracostomy must be followed by intercostal tube drainage.

Open pneumothorax occurs when a chest wall defect allows direct communication of a pneumothorax with the exterior, usually after penetrating trauma. Tension can develop if air can enter but not exit through the defect. Treatment involves application of an occlusive, non-adherent, square dressing sealed along three edges over the wound after sterile skin preparation. This allows air to escape but not enter through the wound, but should be followed by intercostal tube insertion at a site not immediately adjacent to the wound.

Simple pneumothorax may develop tension at any stage, especially with positive-pressure ventilation (see Box 77.2). A small pneumothorax may be missed on the initial chest radiograph. In the supine position pleural air collects antero-inferiorly and is demonstrated radiologically by a deep sulcus sign or increased radioluscency of one side of the chest compared with the other (**Fig. 77.4**).[10]

Occult pneumothorax is defined as visible on chest CT (or upper slices of an abdominal CT) but not plain radiograph. Drainage is not usually required, but should be considered if prolonged surgery is anticipated, there is significant cardiorespiratory compromise, or interhospital transport is necessary. With a conservative approach the patient should be carefully monitored for deterioration from expansion of the pneumothorax.[11,12]

Subcutaneous emphysema over the chest wall in a patient with blunt chest trauma is almost always associated with pneumothorax, but should raise suspicion of other injuries (**Box 77.3**). The pneumothorax may not be visible on chest radiograph, either because it is obscured by the emphysema, or because it has largely decompressed into subcutaneous tissues. An intercostal tube should be inserted.

If there is no associated fluid collection, the intercostal tube can be removed once the pneumothorax is no longer visible on chest radiograph and there has been no air drained for at least 24 hours. Persistent air leak and incomplete drainage of a pneumothorax after intercostal tube insertion should prompt investigation for tracheobronchial injury. However, the depth of the tube within the pleural space and tubing connections should be checked to ensure that air is not being inadvertently entrained from outside the chest. Incomplete drainage with no air leak is usually due to tube malplacement.

HAEMOTHORAX

Haemothorax visible on chest radiograph should be drained as completely as possible (Fig. 77.1). The tube can be removed once radiographic clearance is achieved,

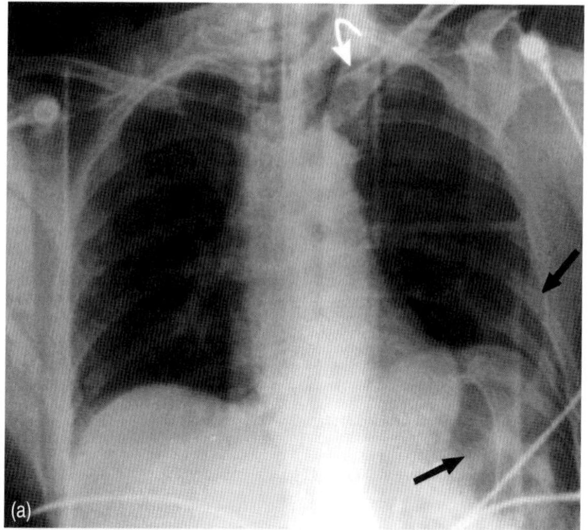
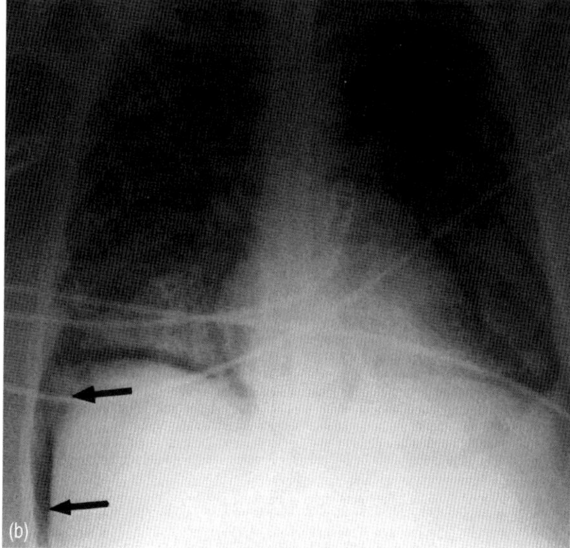

Figure 77.4 (a) Moderate-sized left pneumothorax on supine chest radiograph. The visceral pleura is visible at the lung apex (curved arrows). Hyperlucency is visible in the left lower chest (straight arrows), (b) Supine chest radiograph of right-sided deep sulcus sign (arrows). *(From Miller LA. Chest wall, lung, and pleural space trauma. Radiol Clin North Am 2006; 44(2):213–24, viii.)*

Box 77.3 Causes of pneumothorax, subcutaneous emphysema and/or pneumomediastinum

- Lung puncture
- Tracheobronchial injury
- Oesophageal injury
- Facial or pharyngeal injury
- Abdominal or retroperitoneal injury (air tracking up)

with <100 mL per 24 hours drainage. A small haemothorax (<300 mL) (visible on ultrasound or CT) may initially be managed conservatively, but should be drained if it enlarges. Persistent opacity on chest radiograph after tube placement should be investigated with CT or ultrasound to determine whether there is significant undrained fluid (see retained haemothorax below).

Massive haemothorax, defined as >1500 mL, causes life-threatening circulatory compromise from hypovolaemia and vena caval compression, as well as hypoxaemia. This requires immediate tube drainage and consideration of surgical exploration.[12] If the amount of ongoing bleeding following initial drainage is low, the patient remains haemodynamically stable after initial resuscitation and the blood is venous in appearance, the patient can be managed with close observation. Ongoing bleeding of >200 mL per hour, or >600 mL over 6 hours (massive haemothorax equivalent), is an indication for thoracotomy.

PERICARDIAL TAMPONADE

Pericardial tamponade should be suspected in any patient with a gunshot wound to the chest, or stab wound to the precordium. It occurs rarely with blunt trauma, but should be suspected if there is hypotension out of proportion to blood loss, and distended neck veins. Pulsus paradoxus may be detected in the spontaneously breathing patient. The differential diagnosis includes tension pneumothorax (most likely), cardiogenic shock from severe blunt cardiac injury, or inadequate resuscitation. Pericardial fluid can be detected with ultrasound via a subcostal view (as part of the FAST scan).[4] Echocardiography, or operative subxiphoid window, can be used if diagnostic uncertainty remains.

Haemodynamically unstable patients should undergo thoracotomy.[13] Subxiphoid pericardiotomy can be performed in selected stable patients, but may require conversion to open thoracotomy. Needle pericardiocentesis is rarely effective in the acute setting, but may have a role in the drainage of delayed pericardial effusions following stab wounds.[13]

CARDIAC ARREST AND EMERGENCY THORACOTOMY

External cardiac massage is invariably unsuccessful in the trauma setting, and may cause further injury to intrathoracic structures, and obstruct access to the patient for more potentially useful interventions such as bilateral pleural decompression. For patients with witnessed loss of vital signs after penetrating chest trauma, emergency thoracotomy should be considered if suitably experienced medical personnel are available.[13] This is rarely successful for blunt trauma. The standard approach is a left-sided antero-lateral thoracotomy. Access to the thoracic cavity facilitates specific interventions:[8]

- release of pericardial tamponade
- control of intrathoracic bleeding
- control of massive air embolism, or bronchopleural fistula
- cross-clamping of the descending aorta
- internal cardiac massage.

These temporising (damage control) measures are followed by transfer to the operating room for completion of surgery:[14]

- definitive repair of cardiac injury
- pulmonary tractotomy, wedge resection, or lobectomy/pneumonectomy for lung injury
- Repair or grafting of vascular injury.

Postoperatively the patient is admitted to ICU for rewarming, correction of coagulopathy and resuscitation.

SPECIFIC INJURIES

After addressing initial management issues, a secondary survey and further imaging are performed to identify all injuries. Extrathoracic injuries causing haemodynamic instability should be addressed (e.g. laparotomy) before completion of thoracic imaging; unstable patients should not be transferred to an imaging department away from resuscitation facilities. With the widespread availability of multislice helical CT, chest CT angiography has become the primary imaging modality for the diagnosis of specific chest injuries. This is usually performed as part of a whole body 'pan scan' (CT head, neck, chest, abdomen and pelvis) with injection of intravenous contrast timed to provide aortic angiography. Endotracheal intubation and mechanical ventilation may be required to facilitate CT (e.g. the combative trauma patient with ethanol intoxication). Exposure to high doses of radiation has raised concern about the liberal use of the pan scan.[15] Chest CT is unlikely to identify additional significant injuries if the chest radiograph is normal and the mechanism of injury was low risk.[16]

BLUNT AORTIC INJURY

Blunt aortic injury usually occurs as a result of severe deceleration injury causing a tear at the junction between the fixed descending aorta and the mobile aortic arch, just distal to the origin of the left subclavian artery.[5] Less frequently the ascending aorta (or arch vessels) is injured by direct trauma. Most patients with blunt aortic injury die at the scene from complete aortic wall transection, or associated injuries. Of those that reach hospital, 90% will have a significant aortic injury and up to 50% of these will die before repair.[5] Blunt aortic injuries may be divided into:[17–19]

- *significant aortic injury*, with disruption of the intima and full thickness of the media; there is a high risk of rupture
- *minimal aortic injury*, with laceration limited to the intima and inner media – radiologically this manifests as an intimal flap or pseudoaneurysm <1 cm in length, with minimal or no periaortic haematoma; there is a low risk of rupture.

Aortic injury should be suspected if the mechanism of injury is suggestive of rapid deceleration, such as high-speed (greater than 50 km/h) motor vehicle or motorcycle crash, pedestrian hit by a vehicle, or fall from a height greater than 3 metres.[5,20] Clinical signs of significant aortic injury include unequal upper limb pulses, pseudocoarctation or interscapular murmur, but these are often absent.

Historically chest radiography has been the screening test (to detect mediastinal haematoma), and aortic angiography the diagnostic test for blunt aortic injury.[18] Helical CT chest angiography is now the diagnostic test of choice, although transoesophageal echocardiography may be more appropriate in certain circumstances:[19–21]

- *Chest radiograph* features of blunt aortic injury are caused by distortion of normal mediastinal contour by periaortic haemorrhage. A widened mediastinum (greater than 8 cm at the level of the aortic knuckle) is the principal finding (**Box 77.4**).[22] A supine chest radiograph accentuates mediastinal width and in the acute trauma setting is often of suboptimal quality. Measurement of left mediastinal width (>6 cm), or left mediastinal width to mediastinal width ratio (>0.6), may improve specificity.[22]
- *Multislice helical (multiple row detector) chest CT angiography* (with more than 16 detectors) provides sufficient resolution in multiple planes for CT to be used as the sole diagnostic test, and has largely superseded other imaging modalities for diagnosis of aortic injury.[19]
- *Single-slice helical chest CT* may demonstrate direct signs of aortic injury. However, more commonly aortic injury manifests indirectly with periaortic haematoma, and a further diagnostic test is required.[19] Nevertheless by differentiating periaortic

Box 77.4 Chest radiograph signs of blunt aortic injury

Signs of periaortic haematoma	Indirect signs
Widened mediastinum (>8 cm)	Left haemothorax
Obscured aortic knuckle	Left pleural cap
Opacification of aortopulmonary window	Fractured first or second ribs
Deviation of trachea, left main bronchus or nasogastric tube	
Thickened paratracheal stripe	

haematoma from other types of mediastinal haematoma, and excluding other causes of an abnormal mediastinal contour, single-slice helical CT provides a useful screening test[19] where multislice CT is not available.

- *Transoesophageal echocardiography* is rapid and portable, making it suitable for examination of the unstable patient (e.g. in the operating room). It provides high diagnostic accuracy for aortic injury and also allows examination for blunt cardiac injury.[21] However, imaging of the distal ascending aorta, proximal arch and major branches is limited. Thus if signs of mediastinal haematoma are detected, but an aortic injury is not identified, further diagnostic imaging is warranted.[19] It is contraindicated if an upper airway or oesophageal injury is suspected.
- *Aortic angiography* is relatively time consuming and requires transfer of the patient to the angiography room, making it potentially hazardous for the unstable patient. However, it is the preferred diagnostic test if branch vessel injury is suspected (**Box 77.5**), or if uncertainty remains after other diagnostic imaging.[19] It is also necessary for endovascular aortic repair, and may be required for operative planning.

Significant aortic injury requires prompt surgical or thoracic endovascular aortic repair (TEVAR).[5,18,23] However, this should not take priority over other life-saving interventions (e.g. control of external or pelvic bleeding, laparotomy, or craniotomy for intracranial haemorrhage). Open surgical repair requires a left postero-lateral thoracotomy and selective right-lung ventilation. Operative techniques include direct repair (clamp and sew), or techniques that maintain distal aortic perfusion (bypass). [5,18,23] The latter reduce the risk of postoperative paraplegia from spinal cord ischaemia, but often require systemic heparinisation, which may exacerbate bleeding from other injuries. Sometimes a lumbar drain for cerebrospinal fluid (CSF) drainage is placed perioperatively to improve spinal cord perfusion and potentially reduce the incidence of paraplegia. Postoperatively CSF is drained freely to maintain a CSF pressure less than 10 mmHg. The drain is removed after 3 days if there are no neurological complications. Surgery should be deferred, sometimes indefinitely, if severe associated injuries or co-morbidities make the operative risk unacceptably high. In such cases TEVAR may still be feasible and in many institutions has become the primary method of aortic repair.[5,18,23] The procedure involves isolation of the injured section of aorta by deployment of endoluminal stents, usually via cannulation of the iliac or femoral artery. Although less invasive and less time consuming than open repair, long-term outcome data are lacking and complications may occur.[5,18,23] Endoleaks can arise from incomplete exclusion of the site of injury, or inadequate apposition along the lesser curve of the aorta. Lesions immediately adjacent to the left subclavian artery may require stent coverage of the artery to fully exclude the site of injury. This may result in endoleak due to retrograde blood flow from the left subclavian artery, or ischaemia of the left upper limb or vertebral artery territory requiring left subclavian to left carotid artery grafting. Device collapse causing catastrophic aortic occlusion can occur if the endograft is oversized. Serial follow-up imaging is recommended after TEVAR[5,18]

In patients unfit for immediate intervention, beta blocker +/− vasodilator therapy is given as tolerated to decrease aortic wall shear forces, aiming for a systolic blood pressure <100–120 mmHg and heart rate <100 beats per minute. Minimal aortic injury, with no associated periaortic haematoma or pseudoaneurysm on initial CT can be managed expectantly, with serial imaging.[17] Development of pseudoaneurysm, or periaortic haematoma should prompt consideration for TEVAR.[18]

Box 77.5 Signs of aortic branch vessel injury

Supraclavicular haematoma
Pulse discrepancy in arms
Brachial plexus palsy or stroke
Widened upper mediastinum on chest radiograph

BLUNT CARDIAC INJURY

Blunt cardiac injury results from compression of the heart between the sternum and the spine, abrupt pressure changes within cardiac chambers, or deceleration shear injury. A wide spectrum of injuries has been described, but may be classified according to the clinical sequelae and need for intervention:[6]

- *Minor ECG and cardiac enzyme abnormalities:* sinus tachycardia and premature beats are common, but usually resolve within 24 hours without intervention.
- *Complex arrhythmias:* these may cause heart failure, or persistent hypotension, and may warrant antiarrhythmic therapy.
- *Free wall rupture:* this is usually fatal, but atrial rupture may present with haemopericardium +/− tamponade. Immediate drainage and repair is required.
- *Heart failure:* this may develop from gross myocardial injury, septal rupture (causing left to right shunt), or valvular injury (causing regurgitation). The latter may not manifest until weeks later. Septal rupture and severe valvular injury require surgery. Myocardial dysfunction may require inotropic support.
- *Coronary artery injury:* this is very rare and ST elevation on ECG is more likely to be due to a primary myocardial infarction.

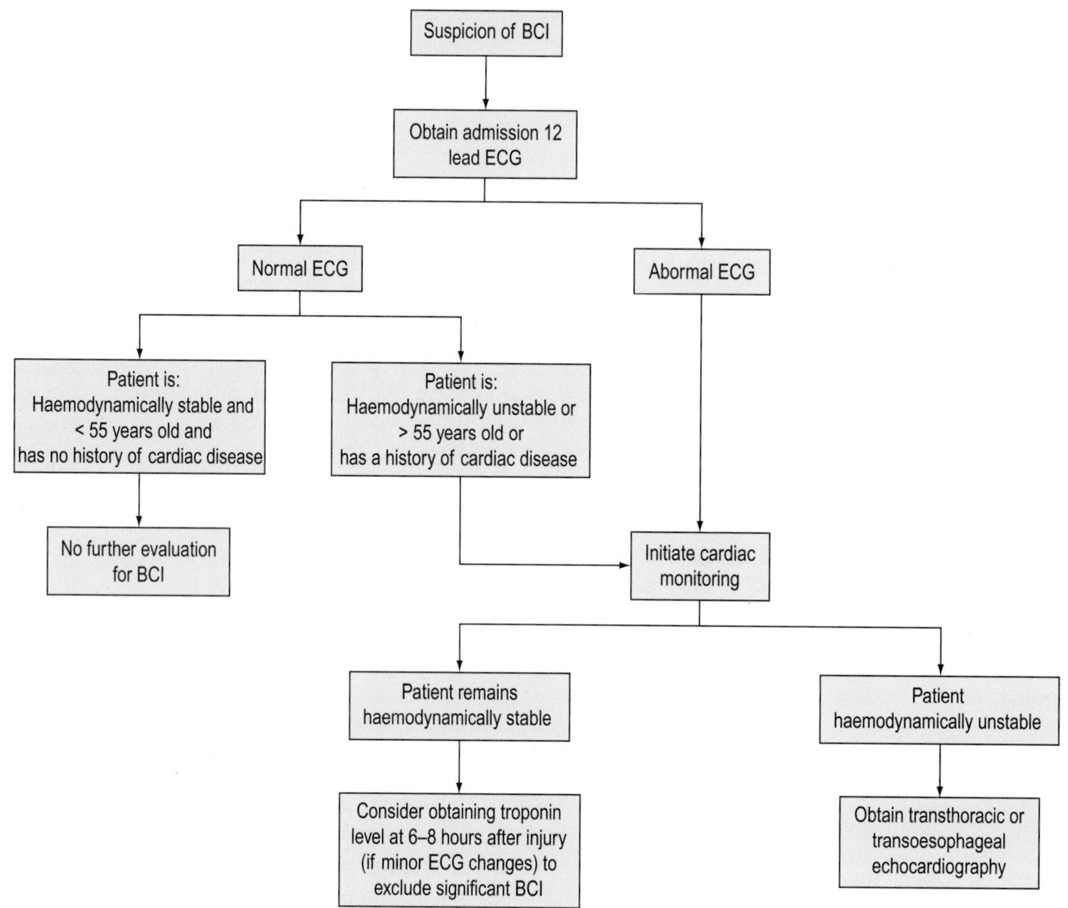

Figure 77.5 Algorithm for evaluation of patients suspected of having blunt cardiac injury (BCI). *(Modified from Schultz JM, Trunkey DD. Blunt cardiac injury. Crit Care Clin 2004;20:57–70.)*

All patients should have an ECG on admission (**Fig. 77.5**). If this is normal and the patient is young, haemodynamically stable and has no history of cardiac disease, the risk of significant injury is very low and no further cardiac evaluation is required. Other patients should be monitored for late sequelae of significant cardiac injury (arrhythmia or heart failure).[6] Patients who remain haemodynamically stable with only minor ECG changes, and who have a normal troponin level at 6–8 hours post injury, have a low risk of cardiac complications.[24]

Echocardiography is indicated for patients with hypotension unexplained by other injuries, heart failure, or persistent arrhythmias.[2] Undisplaced sternal fracture does not of itself warrant cardiac evaluation.[25]

TRACHEOBRONCHIAL INJURY

Blunt rupture of the trachea or bronchi results from crush injury or rapid deceleration with shearing of the airway between a fixed trachea and mobile lungs. The proximal right main bronchus is the most common site of injury.[2,26] Large injuries present with respiratory distress, subcutaneous emphysema and haemoptysis (Box 77.3).[27] The chest radiograph demonstrates pneumothorax and mediastinal emphysema. Dramatic deterioration may follow the institution of positive-pressure ventilation (Box 77.2). With smaller injuries, initial findings are often overshadowed by associated injuries with delay in diagnosis. Persistent pneumothorax with a large air leak, or recurrent pneumothoraces and pulmonary collapse, should prompt further investigation. Flexible bronchoscopy confirms the diagnosis and identifies the level of injury. Treatment is usually primary repair, although non-operative management has been described.[28] Late complications of either approach include post obstructive pneumonia, empyema or bronchiectasis.[26]

With penetrating trauma the cervical trachea is most commonly injured. Immediate management involves tracheal intubation (preferably with flexible bronchoscopy) with the cuff positioned distal to the tear to ablate the air leak. With a large neck wound the endotracheal tube can be passed directly through the wound in emergency situations.

DIAPHRAGMATIC RUPTURE AND DIAPHRAGMATIC PARESIS

The usual mechanism of diaphragmatic rupture is gross abdominal compression from direct vehicular intrusion. The risk of rupture is higher with lateral impact collisions, but not seat belt use.[29] Associated injuries are very common.[29] Rupture of the left hemidiaphragm is more common because the right hemidiaphragm is congenitally stronger and protected by the liver.

Symptoms (dyspnoea and chest pain) are nonspecific. Rarely bowel sounds are audible on chest auscultation. Diagnostic chest radiograph findings are herniation of bowel into the thoracic cavity and nasogastric tube above the left hemidiaphragm. Indirect signs include an elevated or distorted diaphragmatic outline, or pleural effusion, but these may be obscured by adjacent pulmonary pathology, phrenic nerve injury, or by positive-pressure ventilation.[30] The low diagnostic accuracy of chest radiography often results in delayed diagnosis unless further imaging is performed. Multislice helical CT has high diagnostic accuracy, but magnetic resonance imaging, or video-assisted thoracscopy (VATS) may be required if uncertainty persists.[30,31] Prompt operative repair is important to prevent bowel incarceration or perforation. The choice of surgical approach (laparotomy or thoracotomy) is dictated by associated injuries.

Traumatic phrenic nerve palsy, or postoperative diaphragmatic dysfunction, may go unrecognised whilst the patient is on mandatory positive-pressure ventilation. With the transition to spontaneous ventilation, paradoxical abdominal and chest wall movement, reduced vital capacity and difficulty weaning from ventilatory support become evident.

OESOPHAGEAL INJURY

Rupture of the oesophagus from blunt trauma is rare. Penetrating trauma usually causes injury to the cervical portion of the oesophagus. Oesophageal injury may also result from attempted endotracheal intubation or gastric tube insertion during resuscitation of the trauma patient.[32] Clinical features include chest pain, dysphagia, pain on swallowing and subcutaneous emphysema (Box 77.3). Chest radiograph findings include pneumothorax and/or hydrothorax, mediastinal emphysema, or widened mediastinum.[27] Prompt diagnosis by oesophagoscopy or gastrograffin swallow is important. Treatment is immediate surgical repair.[32] Delayed recognition or repair (more than 12 hours post injury) leads to septic shock from mediastinal contamination. Extensive irrigation and drainage is then required, but postoperative complications are common.[32]

PULMONARY INJURY

Pulmonary contusion is characterised by interstitial haemorrhage and oedema, with a secondary inflammatory reaction. Clinically there are signs of increased work of breathing, associated with impaired gas exchange and sometimes haemoptysis. The chest radiograph demonstrates patchy interstitial infiltrates, or consolidation not confined to anatomical segments. Gas exchange and radiographic findings may initially be unremarkable, with deterioration over the first 24–48 hours.[3,10] CT and lung ultrasound are more sensitive at detecting contusion, and quantification of lung volume affected predicts risk of ARDS.[33,34] In the absence of complications (ARDS, pneumonia, or aspiration) clinical and radiological recovery can be expected within 3–5 days.[10]

Treatment is supportive with humidified oxygen therapy, and encouragement of deep breathing and coughing in the spontaneously breathing patient. Noninvasive ventilation can be used in selected patients if gas exchange is poor. Intubation and mechanical ventilation is indicated for refractory hypoxaemia, or if intubation is required for non-pulmonary reasons. Routine corticosteroids are not indicated. Antibiotics should be reserved for superimposed pneumonia.[3]

Pulmonary laceration occurs when disruption of lung architecture, with formation of an air or blood-filled cavity, occurs after blunt or penetrating trauma. On chest radiography, lacerations are often initially obscured by adjacent contusion, but typically take many weeks to resolve and may be complicated by abscess formation or bronchopleural fistula.[10]

BONY INJURIES

Half of all rib fractures are missed on plain chest radiography, but should be suspected if there is localised tenderness over the chest wall. Good analgesia to prevent pulmonary complications from sputum retention is essential.[35] This risk may not be clinically apparent initially, but deterioration in respiratory status over the next few days should be anticipated, especially in the elderly, smokers, or patients with pre-existing pulmonary disease. First- and second-rib fractures, scapula fracture and sternoclavicular dislocation are markers of high-energy trauma.[3]

Most sternal fractures occur in restrained occupants involved in frontal impact vehicular crashes. Associated thoracolumbar spine fractures are common.[25] Blunt cardiac injury should be suspected with displaced sternal fractures.[25]

FLAIL CHEST

Fracture of at least four consecutive ribs in two or more places results in a flail segment with paradoxical movement of the chest wall during tidal breathing (**Fig. 77.6**).[3] Associated pulmonary contusion is often present. Younger patients with no other major injuries, no

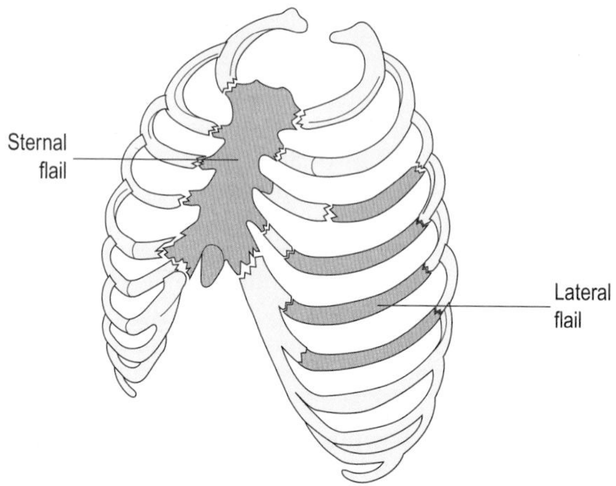

Figure 77.6 Types of flail chest. *(Modified from Wanek S, Mayberry JC. Blunt thoracic trauma: flail chest, pulmonary contusion, and blast injury. Crit Care Clin 2004;20:71–81.)*

pulmonary comorbidities and good analgesia can often be managed with non-invasive ventilation or oxygen therapy alone.[36] Deteriorating gas exchange and sputum retention are indications for intubation and mechanical ventilation. Prolonged ventilatory support is often not necessary in patients whose associated injuries and co-morbidities are not severe. Surgical stabilisation has been advocated for severe flail to reduce duration of ventilation.[37]

EXTRAPLEURAL HAEMATOMA

Traumatic extrapleural haemorrhage arises when chest wall bleeding does not enter the pleural space.[38] Chest radiography shows a parietal shadow that does not cause blunting of the costophrenic angle or shift with gravity. A large haematoma should be evacuated with an intercostal tube or by thoracotomy.

SYSTEMIC AIR EMBOLISM

This is more frequent with penetrating injuries and is immediately life threatening. The typical presentation is circulatory collapse after institution of positive-pressure ventilation, when the pulmonary air-space pressure exceeds pulmonary venous pressure (Box 77.2). Focal neurological changes in the absence of head injury also suggest the diagnosis. Characteristic head CT findings have been described.[39]

When suspected, maintenance of spontaneous ventilation is preferred. If positive-pressure ventilation is necessary, an Fi_{O_2} of 1.0 should be used, with ventilatory pressures and volumes reduced to a minimum. Selective lung ventilation, using a double-lumen endotracheal tube or bronchial blocker, and/or high-frequency ventilation, should be considered.[39] However, urgent thoracotomy, with hilar clampling or lung isolation, is usually indicated.[13] Hyperbaric oxygen therapy has been used to treat cerebral air embolism, but is often impractical.[39]

COMPLICATIONS AND ICU MANAGEMENT

On admission to ICU, rewarming, correction of coagulopathy and ongoing fluid resuscitation are often required. Pericardial tamponade and persistent air leak should be anticipated in post-thoracotomy patients.[14] A restrictive approach to fluid therapy is indicated for patients who have undergone lung surgery. However, care should be taken to ensure adequate fluid resuscitation. A judicious transfusion policy should be employed with all patients.[40]

As with other critically ill or injured patients, prophylactic measures against thromboembolism[41] and upper gastrointestinal stress ulceration should be used. Adequate nutrition is important to ameliorate the hypermetabolic and catabolic metabolic changes, reduce the incidence of sepsis and improve outcome. Nutrition should be instituted early, preferably via the enteral route.

ACUTE RESPIRATORY FAILURE AND MECHANICAL VENTILATION

Respiratory complications are common. When acute lung injury occurs early after trauma, common causes are pulmonary contusion, aspiration, massive transfusion and prolonged shock or delayed resuscitation with severe systemic inflammatory response. Aspiration with persistent lobar collapse is an indication for bronchoscopy to exclude bronchial obstruction from particulate obstruction. When lung injury develops several days later, sepsis of either pulmonary or non-pulmonary origin is a more likely cause.

The approach to mechanical ventilation for intubated patients follows the same principles as with other critically ill patients.

- Patients with acute lung injury/ARDS should be ventilated with a lung-protective strategy. However, high PEEP and permissive hypercapnia are contraindicated if there is associated head injury.
- Patients with pneumothorax or tracheobronchial injury should be managed with low PEEP, low peak airway pressures, and early transition to spontaneous ventilation if possible.
- Patients with flail chest may benefit from the splinting effect of moderate levels of PEEP.
- Failure to wean from mechanical ventilation should raise suspicion of fluid overload, diaphragmatic injury, cardiac dysfunction or flail.

Select patients with hypoxaemia refractory to optimal mechanical ventilation may be supported with veno-venous extracorporeal membrane oxygenation.

SPUTUM RETENTION

Sputum retention leads to progressive pulmonary collapse, with impaired gas exchange, increased work of breathing and increased risk of infection. Smokers, or patients with pre-existing respiratory disease, are particularly at risk. In the spontaneously breathing patient, good analgesia and incentive spirometry facilitate coughing and deep breathing. In the intubated/ventilated patient, humidification, tracheal suctioning and regular position changes are important.

ANALGESIA

Adequate analgesia is essential for deep breathing and effective coughing, which, if achieved, will reduce the likelihood that endotracheal intubation will be needed for less severely injured patients. Analgesia also facilitates chest physiotherapy and early mobilisation, reducing pulmonary morbidity. The choice of analgesia depends on the severity of illness and may vary over time. Options include the following:[35]

- *Intravenous morphine or fentanyl by frequent small boluses or continuous infusion:* this is the mainstay of analgesia for severely injured patients who are intubated and ventilated. Patient-controlled analgesia (PCA) can be used for cooperative unintubated patients.
- *Thoracic epidural infusion of combined opioid and local anaesthetic agent (e.g. fentanyl 2 µg/mL+bupivicaine 0.125% at 5–15 mL/h):* this may be the preferred option for unintubated patients, particularly the elderly, if four or more ribs are fractured, or if there are cardiopulmonary co-morbidities. It may also be used to facilitate successful extubation of ventilated patients who still have significant analgesia requirements.
- *Intercostal nerve block:* this can be used if only a few lower ribs are fractured. Either a single bolus (20 mL of 0.5% bupivicaine) can be injected into one intercostal space, or smaller amounts can be injected at multiple levels. Repeated injections may be required.
- *Paravertebral block:* this is rarely used unless thoracic surgery is performed.
- *Non-steroidal anti-inflammatory agents:* these should be used only in fully resuscitated patients with normal renal function and no other contraindications.
- *Paracetamol:* this is given regularly except in the presence of hepatic dysfunction.

PNEUMONIA

Sepsis is the principal cause of late death after major trauma. Breach of the skin surface barrier, devitalised tissues and the presence of invasive drains and catheters make the trauma patient especially prone to bacterial invasion. In the chest-injured patient, pulmonary contusion, emergency intubation, shock, blood transfusion and the presence of extrathoracic injuries increase the risk of nosocomial pneumonia.

Early-onset pneumonia (within the first few days of hospitalisation) may result from aspiration at the time of injury, particularly after head injury. Common pathogens are *Haemophilus influenzae, Pneumococcus* and anaerobes. Later-onset nosocomial pneumonia is more likely to be due to aerobic Gram-negative bacilli and *Staphylococcus aureus.*

The diagnosis of pneumonia is suspected if there are new or progressive infiltrates on the chest radiograph and deterioration in respiratory status. However, new infiltrates may also be caused by pulmonary contusion, pleural fluid collections, atelectasis, aspiration and pulmonary oedema. Infection is supported by the presence of purulent sputum, new fever and leucocytosis. Confirmation depends on culture of tracheal aspirate, or bronchoscopic samples.[42]

Antibiotic therapy should be targeted at causative organisms. Prompt empirical antibiotics should be started in unstable patients, with re-evaluation at 48–72 hours.

Preventative measures include careful hand cleansing, reduced duration of intubation and ventilation, semirecumbent position, enteral nutrition, avoidance of excessive sedation or hyperglycaemia, and avoidance of prolonged prophylactic antibiotics.[42]

RETAINED HAEMOTHORAX AND EMPYEMA

Haemothorax that is not adequately drained within a few days becomes clotted and unable to drain via intercostal tube. The clot becomes organised and fibrosed with progressive pleural thickening (fibrothorax). This results in loss of lung volume, impaired pulmonary compliance and increased risk of empyema formation. Patients with persistent opacity on chest radiograph after intercostal tube placement should undergo ultrasound or CT imaging to determine whether a significant retained haemothorax is present.[12] Small haemothoraces (<300 mL) in clinically stable patients where the pleural cavity has not been breached may be observed. However, in the presence of respiratory compromise, suspected empyema, or retained haemothorax over 300 mL, further intervention is required. Several management options are available, but complete drainage should be achieved within 3–7 days, before the development of fibrothorax or empyema.

If the initial intercostal tube is poorly positioned, or blocked, a second tube may be placed through a different skin incision, preferably under ultrasound or CT guidance. In other circumstances a second intercostal tube should be avoided because of increased risk of empyema formation and high failure rate.[12,43] If the initial intercostal tube remains patent, evacuation of retained haemothorax can be attempted with intrapleural administration of thrombolytic agent, after exclusion of a bleeding diathesis or intrathoracic organ injury.[12,44] Thrombolysis is most likely to be successful if attempted within 3 days of initial haemothorax. Streptokinase 250 000 units, or urokinase 100 000 units, in 100 mL saline is instilled into the intercostal tube for 4 hours each day until resolution of haemothorax with minimal further drain losses.[12,44] However, video-assisted thoracoscopic surgery (VATS) is the recommended approach in haemodynamically stable patients who can tolerate single-lung ventilation.[12,31,43] Failure of these techniques, or empyema formation, requires formal thoracotomy +/− decortication. VATS and thoracotomy allow direct inspection for a missed pulmonary, diaphragmatic or oesophageal injury.[31]

Patients who did not require initial intercostal tube drainage, but who subsequently develop respiratory compromise or opacification on chest radiograph, should be imaged with ultrasound or CT to look for delayed haemothorax. This should also prompt reconsideration of an occult injury to the diaphragm or an intrathoracic organ.[44]

FAT EMBOLISM SYNDROME

Fat embolism is very common in patients with long-bone fractures[45] and frequently causes oxygen desaturation, which may be severe and prolonged in patients with parenchymal lung injury.[46] However, fat embolism *syndrome*, with pulmonary, neurological and cutaneous sequelae, is rare. Treatment of fat embolism is supportive, but early resuscitation and fracture stabilisation are important preventative measures.[45] Early (<24 hours) intramedullary nailing is the fixation method of choice, resulting in fewer orthopaedic complications than other fixation methods, and fewer pulmonary complications than delayed surgery.[47] However, internal fixation may provoke further fat embolism, require a longer operative time and result in more blood loss than external fixation.[47] Thus in severely chest-injured patients, temporary stabilisation using external fixation with intramedullary nailing several days later is preferred.[47]

PROGNOSIS

Risk of death and length of intensive care stay depend on severity of chest injury, extent of extrathoracic injuries and pre-existing co-morbidities.[1,48] Initial physiological markers that predict adverse outcome are low Glasgow Coma Scale score, hypotension and high respiratory rate. In patients with severe blunt trauma the mortality is significantly higher with bilateral than with unilateral chest injuries, and depends more on the extent of parenchymal lung injury than the extent of chest wall injury.[49] Older age correlates strongly with worse outcome, even though the elderly are more likely to suffer rib fractures than parenchymal lung injury.[48,49] In the elderly the risk of death or pneumonia increases with each additional rib fractured.

Access the complete references list online at http://www.expertconsult.com

4. Kirkpatrick AW. Clinician-performed focused sonography for the resuscitation of trauma. Crit Care Med 2007;35: S162–72.
7. Fitzgerald M, Mackenzie CF, Marasco S, et al. Pleural decompression and drainage during trauma reception and resuscitation. Injury 2008;39:9–20.
9. Leigh-Smith S, Harris T. Tension pneumothorax-time for a re-think? Emerg Med J 2005;22:8–16.
12. Mowery NT, Gunter OL, Collier BR, et al. Practice management guidelines for management of hemothorax and occult pneumothorax. J Trauma 2011;70:510–18.
13. Hunt PA, Greaves I, Owens WA. Emergency thoracotomy in thoracic trauma – a review. Injury 2006; 37(1):1–19.
35. Simon BJ, Cushman J, Barraco R, et al. Pain management guidelines for blunt thoracic trauma. J Trauma 2005;59(5):1256–67.

78

Spinal injuries

Sumesh Arora and Oliver J Flower

Spinal cord injury (SCI) has immense consequences for patients, their families, healthcare resources and society. Initial management of SCI and prevention of secondary injury may make substantial differences to long-term functional outcome. SCI is best managed in specialised spinal injury units, with specialist medical, nursing and allied health expertise.[1,2] The prognosis for SCI has improved tremendously in the last 50 years and, despite their disability, survivors often report high levels of life satisfaction years after their injury.[3] Non-traumatic spinal cord injury, from a broad range of aetiologies, has an equal incidence to traumatic SCI and shares many clinical, pathological and management features with traumatic SCI. However, the specific differences in managing non-traumatic SCI are beyond the scope of this chapter, which will focus on traumatic SCI.

EPIDEMIOLOGY

Approximately 5% of trauma victims have spinal fractures, and 20% of these have SCI.[4] The incidence of traumatic SCI ranges from 2.3 to 83 cases per million population per year, with a prevalence ranging from 236 to 1800 per million population in developed countries.[5] Approximately 80% of SCI are male, usually in the 15–35 age group. Motor vehicle accidents are the commonest cause, followed by falls and sports-related injuries. The proportion of injuries relating to falls, especially in the over 60s, is increasing.[4,6] Pre-existing spinal pathology such as spinal canal stenosis or ankylosing spondylitis increases the risk of SCI from relatively minor trauma. Improved availability and quality of pre-hospital treatment has increased early survival and prevalence of SCI. The epidemiology of neurological level of injury varies dramatically depending on location. In developed countries, more than 50% of patients have cervical SCI, but developing countries report lower rates. This may be due to fewer of these patients surviving to hospital, as well as aetiological, geographical and economic global variation.[5] Approximately one-third of patients are tetraplegic and half have complete injuries, with both of these factors increasing in prevalence in recent years.[7]

PATHOGENESIS

APPLIED ANATOMY AND PHYSIOLOGY

The spinal cord extends from foramen magnum to approximately L1–L2 level. The conical lower end of the spinal cord is called the conus medullaris, from which a filament of connective tissue, known as filum terminale, continues inferiorly. The cauda equina refers to the bundle of spinal nerves for the lumbo-sacral segments that continue below the spinal cord. At the C1 level, the spinal cord occupies one-third of the spinal canal, whereas in the lower cervical and thoracic region it occupies 50% of the space. Compared with the spinal cord in the cervical and thoracic regions, the cauda equina is less susceptible to injury owing to a relatively larger canal size in the lumbar region. Corresponding to each intervertebral level, dorsal and ventral roots exit the spinal cord and join within the dural sac to form the spinal nerve. The spinal nerves run caudally within the spinal column until reaching the corresponding spinal levels, exiting through the spinal foramen. The sympathetic nerve supply originates from the intermediolateral column of segments T1–L2. The parasympathetic outflow originates from S2–S4 level and supplies the pelvic viscera. A cross-section of the spinal cord is shown in **Figure 78.1**.

SPINAL CORD INJURY

The pathophysiology of SCI is described as biphasic, consisting of primary and secondary phases.

PRIMARY INJURY

Direct mechanical injury may produce focal compression, laceration or traction injury to the cord. Actual transection is unusual. Ischaemic injury may result from interference to the segmental spinal arterial supply. Initial pathological changes include the traumatic severing of axons, blood vessels and cell membranes.[8,9]

SECONDARY INJURY

Local hypoperfusion and ischaemia begin at the site of injury, extending progressively over hours from the site

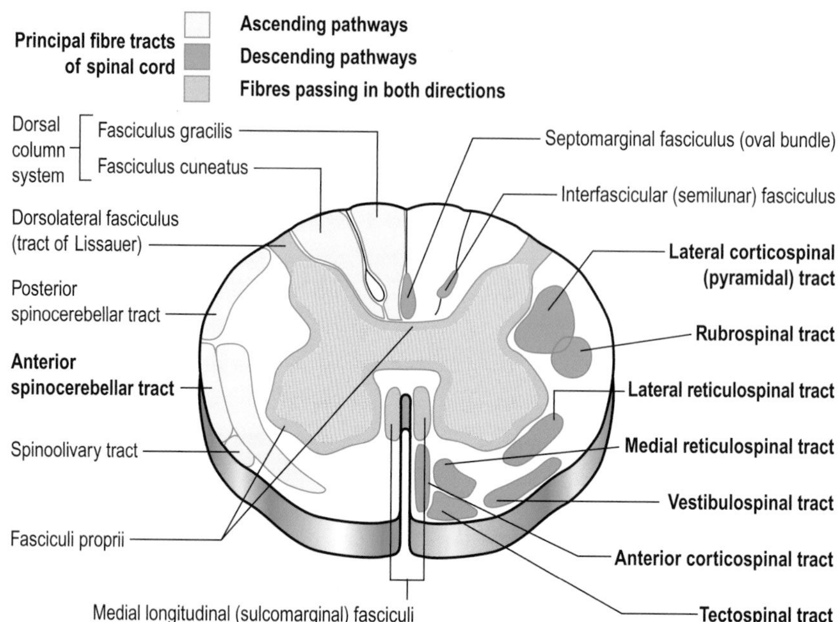

Figure 78.1 Cross-section of the spinal cord. *(From Principal Tracts of Spinal Cord, Image ID: 60477, published in Netter's Concise Neuroanatomy, Author: Michael Rubin, and Joseph E. Safdieh, Chapter: Gross Anatomy of the Brain and Spinal Cord, p 49, 2007.)*

of injury in both directions. There is loss of spinal cord autoregulation, often complicated by arterial hypotension in high SCI. Apart from ischaemia, other mechanisms may contribute to the secondary injury, including release of free radicals, reactive oxygen species, eicosanoids, calcium, proteases, phospholipases and excitotoxic neurotransmitters (e.g. glutamate).[8,9]

Petechial haemorrhages begin in the grey matter, progress over hours and may result in significant haemorrhage into the cord. There is oedema, cellular chromatolysis and vacuolation, and ultimately neuronal necrosis. Apoptosis, especially of oligodendrocytes, also occurs.[8] In the white matter vasogenic oedema, axonal degeneration and demyelination follow. Infiltration of polymorphs occurs in the haemorrhagic areas. Late coagulative necrosis and cavitation subsequently take place.[10]

INITIAL ASSESSMENT AND MANAGEMENT

The main principles in the early management of a spinal injury relate to the prevention of secondary injury and the provision of optimum conditions for neurological recovery. This includes prevention of secondary cord injury with immobilisation, prevention of hypoxia, defending blood pressure and avoiding metabolic abnormalities.

The general principles of managing severe trauma are outlined in Chapter 74. Resuscitation must occur synchronously with evaluation, initial investigations and management. The specific considerations in the acute setting are outlined in **Table 78.1**.

IMMOBILISATION

If a cervical SCI is suspected, the patient may have to be extricated from the scene of the accident. Manual stabilisation of the head in a neutral position is used with four people lifting and one controlling the head and neck. The neck is immobilised in a rigid, hard collar that should be applied without neck movement. The patient is placed supine on a rigid spine board with straps and occipital padding. Sandbags should be placed on either side of the head, and the head secured with the application of broad tape across the forehead. With a suspected thoracolumbar spinal injury, the patient is again lifted as a single unit or log rolled as necessary. Rigid collars and hard spinal boards cause rapid development of pressure areas. This risk can be minimised by transferring the patient off a hard board as soon as possible, safely rolling the patient every 2 hours, and by changing the hard collar if there could be any delay in cervical spine clearance. Of the collars available, evidence suggests the Miami J and Philadelphia collars restrict cervical range of movement more than Aspen or Miami J/Occian Back, and the Miami J and Miami J/Occian Back have the lowest levels of mandibular and occipital pressure.[11]

Complications of prolonged immobilisation and spinal precautions include cutaneous pressure

Table 78.1 Acute issues following SCI

ISSUE	PATHOPHYSIOLOGY RELEVANT TO SCI	MANAGEMENT
Need for intubation	Paralysis of muscles of respiration below NLOI Increased secretions and bronchospasm from loss of sympathetic innervation	Consider: • respiratory failure • decreased level of consciousness • transport with an unstable patient • need for surgery
Intubation	Excessive movement of neck in unstable cervical injury may cause further spinal cord damage	If intubation is urgent, rapid sequence induction and intubation with manual in-line stabilisation Minimise neck movement Video laryngoscopy improves view and minimises movement Consider awake fibreoptic intubation if time and expertise available
Hypotension	Loss of vasomotor tone below NLOI Bradycardia for NLOI above T_1 Traumatic abdominal or long-bone haemorrhage presents differently in patients insensate below the NLOI	Must exclude hypovolaemia/haemorrhagic shock Usually vasoplegia and bradycardia from SCI causing neurogenic distributive shock Give fluids initially Have low threshold for inserting central line and using norepinephrine (noradrenaline) Consider targeting a MAP of 85 mmHg (11.3 kPa) to maintain spinal cord perfusion
Bradycardia	Loss of cardiac sympathetic innervation (T_1–T_4)	May require anticholinergics (e.g. atropine), chronotropics (e.g. isoprenaline) or pacing
Neurological examination	NLOI and ASIA grade may be difficult to assess once patient is intubated	Obtain NLOI and ASIA grade if patient alert before sedation or intubation
Medications	Sedation may prevent accurate assessment of neurological status	Use short-acting sedatives and analgesics to permit ongoing neurological assessment Avoid paralytic agents if possible
Pressure area care	Loss of sensation and paralysis predisposes to early decubitus ulcers	Transfer off hard board Change collar to Miami J as soon as possible Roll every 2 hours
Hypothermia	Vasoplegia Loss of thermoregulatory control Exposure during resuscitation Pre-hospital environmental factors	External passive and active warming often required
Urinary retention	Paralysis of detrusor Loss of bladder sensation	Indwelling bladder catheter
Gastroparesis	Loss of gastrointestinal sympathetic innervation Ileus Gastroparesis	Nasogastric insertion
Refer and transfer	Better outcome in specialist spinal care centres	Early liaison and transfer to SCI specialist unit

NLOI = neurological level of injury.

ulceration, difficulties with the airway and intubation, potential venous obstruction affecting intracranial pressure, less options for central venous access, higher risk of VTE, and a higher risk of respiratory infections due to restricted physiotherapy, gastrostasis and an inability to provide optimal oral care.[12]

NEUROLOGICAL ASSESSMENT

TERMINOLOGY

The terminology for SCI has now been standardised:[13]

Tetraplegia: Greek nomenclature, preferred to quadriplegia, which is a mixture of Latin and Greek, is defined as motor and/or sensory deficits affecting both upper and lower limbs, due to cervical SCI.

Paraplegia: motor and/or sensory deficits affecting only lower limbs due to SCI below the cervical levels.

Neurological level of injury (NLOI): the most caudal cord segment with normal motor and sensory function bilaterally. As differences often exist, it is preferred to describe the individual motor and sensory levels on each side (as the most caudal segments with normal motor and sensory function, respectively). In this context, normal motor function refers to a motor grade of 3, with all cephalad motor levels being grade 5. This is distinct from the skeletal or radiological level of injury.

Complete SCI: absence of both motor and sensory function in the lowest sacral segments (i.e. no anal tone and no sensation).

Zone of partial preservation: only used in describing complete (ASIA A) SCI. This refers to the spinal segments that have any motor or sensory function below the NLOI.

Spinal shock: the period of flaccid paresis and areflexia following a spinal injury, lasting from 48 hours to weeks, and ending with return of reflexes such as the bulbocavernosus reflex.[14]

Neurogenic shock: a form of distributive (cardiovascular) shock following SCI due to loss of sympathetic tone in peripheral vasculature.

A thorough neurological examination should be performed as early as feasible after presentation, prior to administration of any sedative or paralytic agents. The American Spinal Injury Association (ASIA) impairment scale[13] is the most validated instrument for diagnosing and classifying SCI. It is currently the only standardised neurological examination available that allows prognostication, and has sufficient inter-rater reliability for local and international data collection and comparison. A bilateral sensory and motor exam, including digital rectal examination, determines a single neurological level of injury (NLOI); completeness of injury and the ASIA grade (**Fig. 78.2**, **Box 78.1**) describes the grades of the ASIA impairment scale.[13] The physical exam should also include palpation of the spine for steps or gaps.

With conscious, alert patients, SCI may be obvious, with limb weakness, hypoaesthesia and absence of reflexes below the NLOI, vasodilatation, priapism, urinary retention and paralytic ileus. When assessing sensation, it should be remembered that the C4 dermatome can extend as low as the nipple line, misleading the examiner to believing the T_4 dermatome has sensation. An initial ASIA classification may reliably predict long-term motor outcome.[15] However, head or other injuries, pain, alcohol or the administration of analgesic or other drugs may make initial assessment impossible. Signs of SCI in unconscious or uncooperative patients include:

- response to pain above, but not below, a suspected level
- flaccid areflexia in the arms and/or legs
- elbow flexion with the inability to extend suggestive of cervical SCI
- paradoxical pattern of breathing with in-drawing of upper chest on inspiration (in the absence of upper respiratory tract obstruction or chest injury)
- inappropriate vasodilatation (in association with hypothermia, or in the legs but not the arms with thoracolumbar SCI)
- unexplained bradycardia, hypotension
- priapism
- loss of anal tone and reflexes.

Box 78.1 American Spinal Injury Association (ASIA) impairment scale

A	*Complete:* no sensory or motor function is preserved in the sacral segments S4–S5
B	*Incomplete:* sensory but not motor function is preserved below the neurological level and includes the sacral segments S4–S5
C	*Incomplete:* motor function is preserved below the neurological level, and more than half of key muscles below the neurological level have a muscle grade less than 3
D	*Incomplete:* motor function is preserved below the neurological level, and at least half of key muscles below the neurological level have a muscle grade greater than or equal to 3
E	*Normal:* sensory and motor function is normal

INCOMPLETE SCI

Incomplete SCI tends to occur in characteristic syndromes.[13] (See Fig. 78.1.)

SYNDROMES

- *Central cord:* weakness and sensory loss, greater in the arms than the legs – it typically follows a hyperextension injury with pre-existing canal stenosis, such as an elderly man falling onto his chin. Ischaemia or haematoma in the centre of the cord affects the cervical segments more due to the pattern of lamination of the corticospinal and spinothalamic tracts.
- *Anterior cord:* loss of motor function and pain and temperature sensation below the NLOI, with preservation of fine touch and proprioception – it is less common, typically following interruption of the blood supply to the anterior spinal cord.
- *Brown-Séquard:* ipsilateral loss of motor, proprioception and fine touch, with contralateral loss of pain and temperature sensation below the NLOI – it usually follows a penetrating SCI damaging only one-half of the spinal cord.
- *Conus medullaris:* sudden onset, symmetrical paraplegia with mixed upper and lower motor neuron findings, caused by injury at T12/L1.

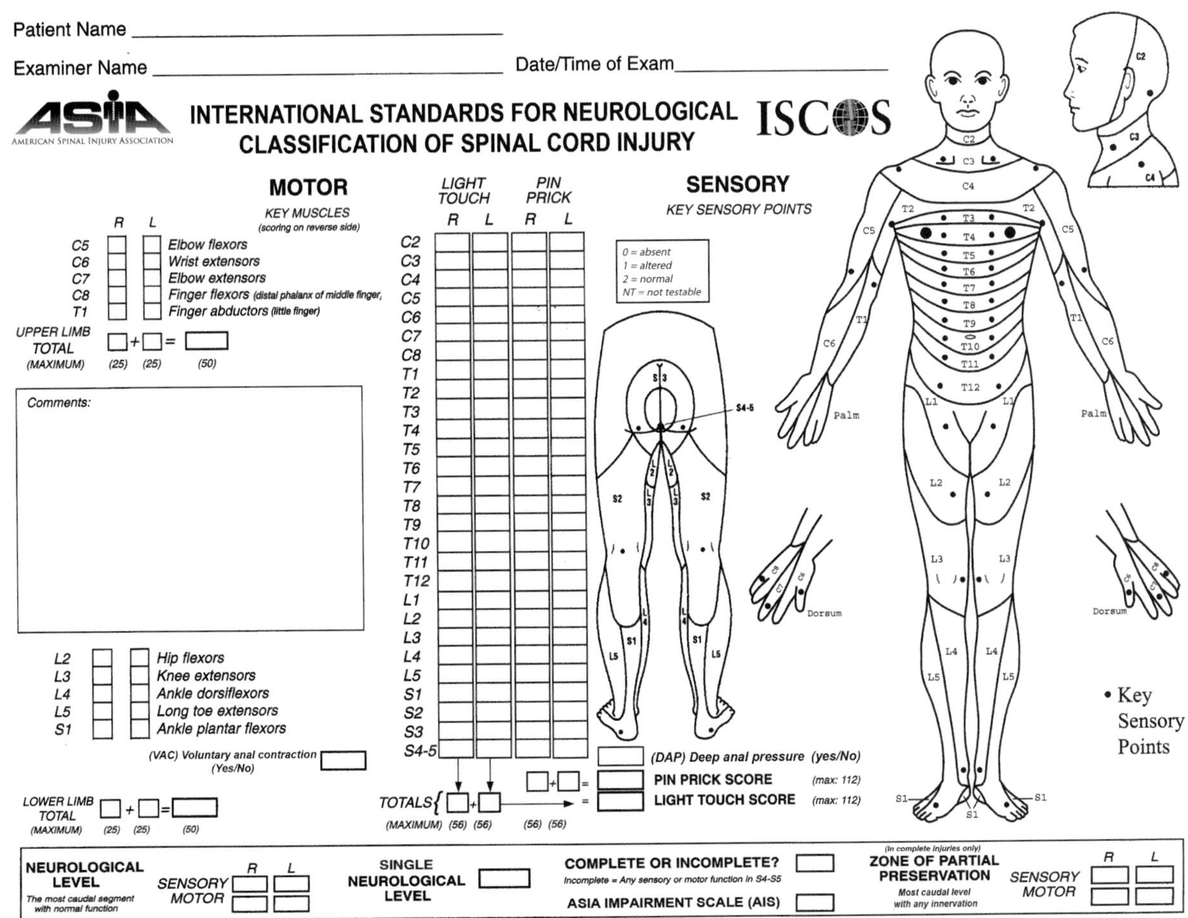

Patient Name ______________________

Examiner Name ______________________ Date/Time of Exam ______________________

ASIA — AMERICAN SPINAL INJURY ASSOCIATION

INTERNATIONAL STANDARDS FOR NEUROLOGICAL CLASSIFICATION OF SPINAL CORD INJURY

ISCoS

MOTOR

KEY MUSCLES (scoring on reverse side)

	R	L	
C5			Elbow flexors
C6			Wrist extensors
C7			Elbow extensors
C8			Finger flexors (distal phalanx of middle finger)
T1			Finger abductors (little finger)

UPPER LIMB TOTAL (MAXIMUM) ☐ + ☐ = ☐ (25) (25) (50)

Comments:

	R	L	
L2			Hip flexors
L3			Knee extensors
L4			Ankle dorsiflexors
L5			Long toe extensors
S1			Ankle plantar flexors

(VAC) Voluntary anal contraction (Yes/No) ☐

LOWER LIMB TOTAL (MAXIMUM) ☐ + ☐ = ☐ (25) (25) (50)

	LIGHT TOUCH R	LIGHT TOUCH L	PIN PRICK R	PIN PRICK L
C2				
C3				
C4				
C5				
C6				
C7				
C8				
T1				
T2				
T3				
T4				
T5				
T6				
T7				
T8				
T9				
T10				
T11				
T12				
L1				
L2				
L3				
L4				
L5				
S1				
S2				
S3				
S4-5				

TOTALS { ☐ + ☐ ☐ + ☐ = (MAXIMUM) (56) (56) (56) (56)

SENSORY

KEY SENSORY POINTS

0 = absent
1 = altered
2 = normal
NT = not testable

(DAP) Deep anal pressure (yes/No) ☐

PIN PRICK SCORE (max: 112) ☐

LIGHT TOUCH SCORE (max: 112) ☐

NEUROLOGICAL LEVEL (The most caudal segment with normal function)		R	L
	SENSORY		
	MOTOR		

SINGLE NEUROLOGICAL LEVEL ☐

COMPLETE OR INCOMPLETE? ☐ Incomplete = Any sensory or motor function in S4-S5

ASIA IMPAIRMENT SCALE (AIS) ☐

ZONE OF PARTIAL PRESERVATION (In complete injuries only) Most caudal level with any innervation		R	L
	SENSORY		
	MOTOR		

This form may be copied freely but should not be altered without permission from the American Spinal Injury Association.

REV 04/11

Figure 78.2 American Spinal Injury Association: International Standards for Neurological Classification of Spinal Cord Injury, revised 2011. *(From American Spinal Injury Association. International Standards for Neurological Classification of Spinal Cord Injury, revised 2011.)*

- *Cauda equina:* often asymmetrical, lower motor neuron lower limb weakness with saddle area hypoaesthesia or paraesthesia, with bladder and bowel areflexia – it is caused by injuries below L1 damaging the lumbosacral nerve roots.

ASSOCIATED INJURIES

Cervical spine injury/tetraplegia

Overall with major trauma the incidence of cervical spine injury (CSI) is 1–3%. However, 2–10% of patients with head injuries have a CSI. The more severe the head injury, the more likely CSI is to be present. Patients with head injuries should be assumed to have a CSI until proved otherwise. Of patients with a cervical SCI, 25% have some degree of head injury, with 2–3% having a severe injury.[8]

Thoracolumbar spine injury/paraplegia

Chest injuries are often present and are difficult to assess with the inability to take an erect chest X-ray, and the presence of a mediastinal haematoma associated with the vertebral injury. Computerised tomography (CT) of the chest may be used to assess other chest injuries, with contrast to exclude aortic injuries. There should be a high index of suspicion of abdominal injuries, as the lack of sensation, hypotension and bradycardia from the SCI may mask the usual presentation. Abdominal ultrasound and CT are usually required to delineate these injuries.

IMAGING

IS IMAGING REQUIRED?

Some trauma patients may not require cervical spinal imaging and the inherent risks that this entails. Two clinical decision tools are used in this context: The National Emergency X-Radiography Utilization Study (NEXUS) criteria and the Canadian C-Spine rules. NEXUS suggests cervical spine imaging is

Muscle Function Grading

0 = total paralysis

1 = palpable or visible contraction

2 = active movement, full range of motion (ROM) with gravity eliminated

3 = active movement, full ROM against gravity

4 = active movement, full ROM against gravity and moderate resistance in a muscle specific position.

5 = (normal) active movement, full ROM against gravity and full resistance in a muscle specific position expected from an otherwise unimpaired peson.

5* = (normal) active movement, full ROM against gravity and sufficient resistance to be considered normal if identified inhibiting factors (i.e. pain, disuse) were not present.

NT = not testable (i.e. due to immobilization, severe pain such that the patient cannot be graded, amputation of limb, or contracture of >50% of the range of motion).

ASIA Impairment (AIS) Scale

☐ **A = Complete.** No sensory or motor function is preserved in the sacral segments S4-S5.

☐ **B = Sensory Incomplete.** Sensory but not motor function is preserved below the neurological level and includes the sacral segments S4-S5 (light touch, pin prick at S4-S5: or deep anal pressure (DAP)), AND no motor function is preserved more than three levels below the motor level on either side of the body.

☐ **C = Motor Incomplete.** Motor function is preserved below the neurological level**, and more than half of key muscle functions below the single neurological level of injury (NLI) have a muscle grade less than 3 (Grades 0-2).

☐ **D = Motor Incomplete.** Motor function is preserved below the neurological level**, and at least half (half or more) of key muscle functions below the NLI have a muscle grade ≥ 3.

☐ **E = Normal.** If sensation and motor function as tested with the ISNCSCI are graded as normal in all segments, and the patient had prior deficits, then the AIS grade is E. Someone without an initial SCI does not receive an AIS grade.

**For an individual to receive a grade of C or D, i.e. motor incomplete status, they must have either (1) voluntary anal sphincter contraction or (2) sacral sensory sparing with sparing of motor function more than three levels below the motor level for that side of the body. The Standards at this time allows even non-key muscle function more than 3 levels below the motor level to be used in determining motor incomplete status (AIS B versus C).

NOTE: When assessing the extent of motor sparing below the level for distinguishing between AIS B and C, the ***motor level*** on each side is used; whereas to differentiate between AIS C and D (based on proportion of key muscle functions with strength grade 3 or greater) the ***single neurological level*** is used.

Steps in Classification

The following order is recommended in determining the classification of individuals with SCI.

1. Determine sensory levels for right and left sides.
2. Determine motor levels for right and left sides.
   Note: in regions where there is no myotome to test, the motor level is presumed to be the same as the sensory level, if testable motor function above that level is also normal.
3. Determine the single neurological level.
   This is the lowest segment where motor and sensory function is normal on both sides, and is the most cephalad of the sensory and motor levels determined in steps 1 and 2.
4. Determine whether the injury is Complete or Incomplete.
   (i.e. absence or presence of sacral sparing)
   If voluntary anal contraction = **No** *AND all S4-5 sensory scores =* **0** *AND deep anal pressure =* **No,** *then injury is COMPLETE. Otherwise, injury is incomplete.*
5. Determine ASIA Impairment Scale (AIS) Grade:
   Is injury Complete? If **YES,** AIS=A and can record ZPP (lowest dermatome or myotome on each side with some preservation)

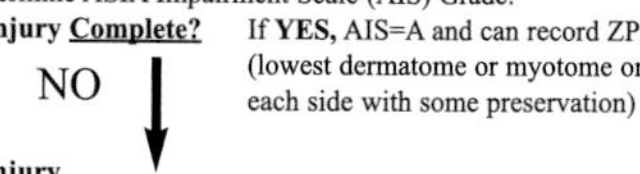

Is injury motor Incomplete? If **NO,** AIS=B (Yes=voluntary anal contraction OR motor function more than three levels below the motor level on a given side, if the patient has sensory incomplete classification)

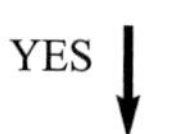

Are at least half of the key muscles below the single neurological level graded 3 or better?

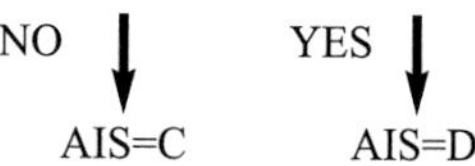

AIS=C AIS=D

If sensation and motor function is normal in all segments, AIS=E
Note: AIS E is used in follow-up testing when an individual with a documented SCI has recovered normal function. If at initial testing no deficits are found, the individual is neurologically intact; the ASIA Impairment Scale does not apply.

Figure 78.2, cont'd

indicated for patients with trauma unless they meet all of the following criteria:[16]

- no posterior midline cervical spine tenderness
- no evidence of intoxication
- a normal level of alertness
- no focal neurological deficit
- no painful distracting injuries.

NEXUS criteria have a very high sensitivity (99.6% for significant injuries) if used as initially intended, although the specificity is only 12.9%. They require there to be no evidence of any intoxication (including even an odour of alcohol), an alert level of consciousness sufficient to allow *three-object recall at 5 minutes*, no focal neurological deficits and there should be no painful distracting injuries. This subjective component includes any long-bone fractures, de-gloving injuries, deep lacerations, visceral injuries, crush injuries, large burns or any injury that causes any acute functional impairment. The Canadian C-Spine rules have a higher degree of sensitivity (100%) and specificity (45%) but were based on a smaller cohort of patients than NEXUS.[16] Again, they define only which patients may be clinically cleared without imaging.

IMAGING MODALITIES

PLAIN RADIOGRAPHS

Adequate, three-view combination plain radiography misses injuries of the spinal column in both alert and obtunded patients, with a pooled sensitivity of detecting significant injuries of 52%.[17] Despite reducing thyroid radiation exposure in comparison to CT, plain radiography has no role in this context, unless other modalities are not available.[18]

DYNAMIC STUDIES (e.g. DYNAMIC FLUOROSCOPY OR FLEXION/EXTENSION RADIOGRAPHY)

This imaging modality visualises the relevant anatomy poorly[19] and has a low sensitivity to detect injury.[20] It is labour- and resource-intensive[21] and has now been superseded by CT and MRI.

COMPUTERISED TOMOGRAPHY

CT technology has improved considerably in recent years, with multi-detector row CT (MDCT) offering sensitivity of detecting spinal injuries, including ligamentous injury, close to 100%.[22] MDCT is readily available, easily performed as part of a polytrauma evaluation and is more time- and cost-effective than plain radiography. However, MDCT may miss some significant and unstable injuries (subsequently detectable by MRI) in approximately 4%, with 0.29% requiring surgical stabilisation. Other disadvantages include significant thyroid radiation exposure and transport of a trauma patient to CT.[12]

MAGNETIC RESONANCE IMAGING (MRI)

For investigating suspected myelopathy and cord injury, MRI provides superior imaging to any other modality.[23] It is the most sensitive screening test available to detect soft-tissue and ligamentous injuries that could contribute to instability of the cervical spine[24] and MR angiography may detect associated vertebral artery injury. However, MRI has a rate of false positives as high as 40%,[25] which may result in unnecessary and detrimental immobilisation, transfers and imaging in patients who have no injury. Complications of prolonged immobilisation are a significant cause of morbidity and mortality. Timing of MRI is another contentious issue as, with time, the MR signal may change due to a decrease in ligamentous oedema. The Eastern Association for the Surgery of Trauma guidelines recommend that MRI should be performed within 72 hours.[26] However, there is only limited evidence that delay between injury and imaging results in a false-negative MRI.[27]

AN APPROACH TO IMAGING

There is currently no universal consensus. Following trauma, if there is evidence of any new neurological deficit attributable to a spinal injury then an urgent MRI should be performed. If there is no neurological deficit but the other conditions of the CCCR or NEXUS rules are not met, then high-resolution MDCT of the entire spine is indicated. For the obtunded blunt trauma patient who is likely to be unassessable for a prolonged period, an MRI may follow the MDCT.

Policy for the use of MRI in this context should be discussed at an institutional level, with the knowledge that a policy with MDCT alone may miss a small percentage of injuries that would otherwise have required intervention, but the false-positive rate of MRI results in significant morbidity to patients with no injuries who are kept immobilised.[12]

INTENSIVE CARE MANAGEMENT OF SCI

PREVENTION OF SECONDARY NEUROLOGICAL INJURY AFTER SCI

Spinal cord compression may occur owing to misalignment of spine, oedema or haemorrhage. Incomplete injury with spinal cord compression should be urgently decompressed. Stability is the ability of the spine, under physiological loads, to limit patterns of displacement, which would result in neurological injury, pain, or deformity.[28] It is affected by fracture morphology and osteo-ligamentous integrity. Most unstable spinal injuries require operative intervention. Where indicated, early surgery within 24 hours of injury is safe, may improve neurological outcome, reduces length of stay in acute care, permits early mobilisation and commencement of DVT prophylaxis and lowers hospital cost.[29] Most spinal surgeons prefer to operate as early as possible in patients with incomplete or cervical spinal cord injury.

Many pharmacological agents have been investigated in secondary injury to aid recovery of damaged neurons; however, none of these have proven successful. NASCIS 2[30] and NASCIS 3[31] were the largest trials that investigated the effects of corticosteroids in SCI. They both were negative studies, showing no significant difference in motor score between treatment groups at any time points. Post-hoc subgroup analysis of these data suggesting neurological outcome benefit was fundamentally flawed. The lack of evidence of efficacy and the adverse effects of steroids such as sepsis (particularly pneumonia), detrimental effects on concomitant head injury, risk of gastrointestinal bleeding and pancreatitis, has seen steroid use fall out of favour in recent years. Other agents that have been investigated with no evidence of benefit include GM-1 ganglioside, tirilazad, naloxone and nimodipine.

There is weak evidence that a mean arterial pressure (MAP) >85 mmHg (11.3 kPa) should be maintained for up to 7 days following injury,[32] theoretically improving cord perfusion pressure and preventing secondary injury. After initial fluid resuscitation vasopressors such as norepinephrine (noradrenaline) are commonly required to meet this target. Induced hypothermia has been reported to be beneficial in case reports, but there is not enough evidence to recommend this intervention currently.[33] Fever may worsen outcome and normothermia should be maintained.

RESPIRATORY DYSFUNCTION

Respiratory dysfunction is a major cause of morbidity after SCI, especially after cervical SCI. The diaphragm, external intercostals, scalene and sternocleidomastoid are the key muscles of inspiration. Quiet expiration is passive, but forceful expiration and cough require the abdominal muscles, the interosseous part of the internal intercostals, lattisimus dorsi, serratus posterior and inferior, triangularis sterni and quadratus lumborum. The effect of SCI on respiratory function depends upon the NLOI. Various effects of cervical SCI on respiratory function are listed in **Table 78.2**. The diaphragm is innervated by C3–5. If the NLOI is above C5, the sternocleidomastoid (innervated by cranial nerve XI and anterior rami of C2, 3) and scalenus medius and posterior (innervated by C3–4) become important muscles of inspiration. The abdominal wall muscles are innervated by T_7–L1, and if the NLOI is above this the cough is generated only by the muscles of the upper chest, particularly the pectoralis major.[34]

Table 78.2 Effect of cervical SCI on respiratory function

Decreased vital capacity	Paralysis of diaphragm and intercostal muscles Distortion of rib cage in inspiration due to paralysed diaphragm
Reduced compliance of lungs and chest wall	Spasticity of intercostal muscles Altered articulation of ribs to sternum and vertebrae Low functional residual capacity Atelectasis Possible alteration of surfactant
Increased abdominal compliance	Paralysis of abdominal muscles
Increased bronchial tone and secretions	Sympathetic denervation
Poor cough	Reduced vital capacity Abdominal muscle paralysis
Sleep disordered breathing (develops within 6 months)	Unknown cause Increased adipose tissue around neck Anti-spasticity drugs

RESPIRATORY MANAGEMENT AFTER CERVICAL SPINAL CORD INJURY

Intubation may be required for respiratory failure, secretion clearance, imminent surgery, decreased level of consciousness or because of other injuries. Almost 75% of patients with cervical SCI will require intubation and mechanical ventilation.[35]

The cervical spine should be immobilised during endotracheal intubation. If time and expertise are available, awake fibreoptic intubation minimises the movement of the neck. Video laryngoscopes may improve glottic view when the neck is immobilised. Direct laryngoscopy with manual inline stabilisation does not eliminate all movement at the cervical spine, but there is no evidence that it is associated with neurological outcomes that are worse than other intubation techniques.

In the initial period after cervical SCI, ventilator settings are dictated by associated injuries and other co-morbidities. For example, in patients with severe traumatic brain injury, normocapnia should be maintained. Once acute issues have resolved, mechanical ventilation should be tailored to SCI. Baseline spirometry should be obtained to allow monitoring of progress.

Tidal volumes (V_T) in excess of 10 mL/kg are often used in patients with cervical SCI. The rationale for high V_T ventilation is to prevent atelectasis and the common sensation of 'air hunger' experienced following SCI. This avoids the need for high-level PEEP that may lower the position of diaphragm to one of mechanical disadvantage. In many spinal centres, V_T of 10–20 mL/kg is used routinely.[36] With high V_T, dead space must be incorporated into the circuit to avoid hypocapnoea. Another approach is to use more conventional V_T and higher PEEP to prevent atelectasis. Until better-quality evidence is available, an individualised approach to ventilator settings should be used.

Box 78.2 Checklist prior to extubation

1. No further procedure or imaging outside ICU anticipated in next 24 hours
2. No significant hypoxia or reversible respiratory pathology
3. Ability to tolerate non-invasive ventilation
4. No contraindication for the assist cough or chest physiotherapy (e.g. rib fractures, major laparotomy)
5. Minimal respiratory secretions
6. Negative inspiratory force >20 cmH_2O
7. Vital capacity >10 mL/kg
8. Presence of cuff leak (particularly after spinal fixation by anterior approach)
9. Airway plan and equipment ready for re-intubation

Extubation after mechanical ventilation in patients with cervical SCI requires careful consideration of several factors (**Box 78.2**), with failure likely to necessitate a tracheostomy. Extubation failure is commonly due to retained, excessive secretions, inadequate cough and sputum plugs. Patients may benefit from extubation to non-invasive ventilation directly, which may be required for several days post extubation. A variety of non-invasive ventilation interface devices should be available and nasal skin should be protected from developing pressure ulcers. Aggressive chest physiotherapy and assisted coughing are required to clear secretions.

The tracheostomy rate after cervical SCI varies between 20 and 60%. Complete injuries above C5 usually require tracheostomy.[37] A high NLOI, complete SCI, associated facial fractures, thoracic trauma and emergency intubation are associated with need for tracheostomy. Percutaneous tracheostomy is as safe as surgical tracheostomy.[38] Early tracheostomy may reduce the duration of mechanical ventilation and ICU length of stay and it does not increase the risk of wound or implant infection even after anterior spinal fixation.[39]

Weaning from MV after cervical SCI may take considerable time. In some centres, high-level tetraplegics are cared for in chronic respiratory care facilities rather than ICUs. It is important that a long-term weaning strategy is agreed upon and adhered to by all members of the multidisciplinary team. Accurate neurological assessment, progressive ventilator-free breathing guided by vital capacity, adequate rest periods with controlled ventilation, and secretion control with aggressive physiotherapy are associated with successful weaning.[40] Inspiratory muscle training uses an inspiratory resistor to increase the strength of inspiratory muscles. Although more studies are needed to delineate clearly the role of inspiratory muscle training in weaning of patients with cervical SCI, its use makes physiological sense and is being used increasingly.[41] It should be remembered that most patients with cervical SCI ventilate more easily when supine compared with being upright, as their abdominal contents can push the diaphragm up into a position of better mechanical advantage in supine position. An abdominal binder may be used in the sitting position, which also helps in this regard.

Inhaled anticholinergics and β_2-agonists reduce airway resistance but have not been shown to improve success of weaning. Anabolic steroids like oxandrolone do not lead to significant improvement in respiratory function and may cause hepatotoxicity and dyslipidaemia. Phrenic nerve or direct diaphragmatic-pacing systems are occasionally used for respiratory support in high-level tetraplegics.

The NLOI is the strongest predictor of successful weaning.[42] Patients with complete injuries at or above C3 are likely to need permanent ventilation. Early identification of patients who cannot be weaned helps reduce their ICU length of stay and expedites the arrangements for equipment and care personnel required for home ventilation or transfer to a chronic respiratory care facility. Overall, approximately 2% of patients with SCI, mostly with complete injuries at C1–C4, require lifelong ventilation.[43]

CARDIOVASCULAR DYSFUNCTION AFTER SCI

The heart receives its sympathetic innervation from the upper thoracic segments via the superior, middle and inferior cervical ganglions. Vasomotor tone of the peripheral vasculature is also controlled by segmental sympathetic innervation. The heart's parasympathetic innervation comes from the vagus, and therefore is not affected by SCI. Following SCI, loss of sympathetic supply and unopposed vagal activity may cause profound vasoplegia combined with bradycardia, resulting in hypotension and neurogenic shock. This occurs in 19% of patients with cervical and 7% of thoracic SCI.[44] Other causes of hypotension, particularly hypovolaemic shock, must be excluded before a diagnosis of neurogenic shock is made. Bradycardia and even asystole may occur during routine ICU procedures like endotracheal suction or repositioning in bed in patients with a cervical NLOI. This phenomenon occurs most commonly in the first week and generally resolves within 2–6 weeks after injury.[45]

CARDIOVASCULAR COMPLICATIONS

AUTONOMIC DYSREFLEXIA

Autonomic dysreflexia (AD) is a medical emergency characterised by acute hypertension due to severe sympathetic stimulation in patients with injuries above T6. It occurs following the resolution of spinal shock (once reflexes have returned) and is a frequent cause for admission to ICU. AD occurs due to dysregulated sympathetic activation leading to intense vasoconstriction below the level of lesion. Compensatory parasympathetic activation leads to bradycardia, vasodilatation and sweating above the NLOI. Other symptoms include headache, blurred vision, nausea and nasal congestion. The precipitants, investigations and treatments of precipitating factors are outlined in **Table 78.3**.

Initial management includes primarily detecting and treating the precipitant, sitting the patient up (to induce an orthostatic hypotensive response), loosening tight clothing and antihypertensives. Sublingual or transdermal glyceryl trinitrate is used initially. Sublingual captopril or oral prazocin may be used in unresponsive patients before intravenous agents such as sodium nitroprusside or glyceryl trinitrate infusions are used. Invasive BP monitoring is required if infusion of intravenous agents is used. Some patients may develop chronic, severe AD requiring multiple classes of antihypertensive. It must be remembered that, in the setting of chronic hypotension following SCI, systolic blood pressure of >150 mmHg (≈20 kPa) is life-threatening,[46] and may lead to intracerebral or retinal haemorrhage or myocardial ischaemia.

VENOUS THROMBOEMBOLISM

If inadequate or no prophylaxis is used, venous thromboembolism (VTE) following SCI has a very high incidence of up to 100%.[47] With prophylaxis, this incidence has reduced; however, 5% of patients with SCI will still develop VTE,[48] and pulmonary embolism (PE) remains a leading cause of death. The use of low-molecular-weight heparin (LMWH) or unfractionated heparin in combination with mechanical measures for thromboprophylaxis is recommended. LMWH is superior to subcutaneous heparin in decreasing the incidence of deep-vein thrombosis, but not PE, and carries less bleeding complications. Commencement of adequate VTE prophylaxis is easier if all planned surgical procedures can occur as soon as practicable. The risk of venous thromboembolism increases significantly if prophylaxis is started more than 72 hours after the injury.[49] If pharmacological VTE prophylaxis is contraindicated, a retrievable inferior vena cava filter should be considered.[50]

Table 78.3 Precipitants, investigations and treatment of autonomic dysreflexia[56]

PRECIPITANT	INVESTIGATION AND TREATMENT
Bladder distension (cause in 75–85%)	Insert or change bladder catheter
Faecal impaction (cause in 13–19%)	Digital examination Laxatives Enema Manual disimpaction
Urinary tract calculi	CT of urinary tract Cystoscopy or surgery to remove calculi
Urinary tract infection	Urinary microscopy and culture Appropriate antibiotics
Haemorrhoids or anal fissure	Laxatives Dietary management
Decubitus ulcers, with or without infection	Rule out underlying osteomyelitis Pressure care Consider plastic surgery Consider antibiotics
Foot disease including ingrown toenails	Nail care
Procedures (e.g. suprapubic catheter insertion, cystoscopy, urodynamic studies)	Spinal anaesthesia may prevent AD
Heterotopic ossification	Bone scintigraphy Measure C-reactive protein and creatine kinase Physiotherapy Surgery
Pelvic stimulation (sexual activity, menstruation, labour)	Education Be prepared in peripartum period
Skeletal fractures	High index of suspicion below NLOI

NLOI = neurological level of injury.

MUSCULOSKELETAL COMPLICATIONS

Muscle spasticity is a common but late issue. It develops after resolution of spinal shock and is characterised by increased muscle tone, hyperreflexia and muscle spasms below the NLOI. The initial treatment is enteral baclofen, the side-effects of which include sedation, fatigue and confusion that may interfere with weaning from mechanical ventilation or participation in a rehabilitation programme. Intrathecal baclofen, gabapentin, pregabalin and benzodiazepines may also be used for severe spasticity.[46] Physiotherapy measures are needed to preserve a full range of movement in paralysed joints and to prevent contractures. Special attention should be given to hand and shoulder physiotherapy after cervical SCI to preserve maximum functionality.

CHRONIC PAIN

Chronic pain is a frequent complication after SCI that occurs in up to two-thirds of patients. Pain after SCI may be classified as nociceptive pain from stimulation of nociceptors, or neuropathic pain from damage to the sensory system itself. Most patients will report onset of chronic pain within 6 months after the injury, and frequently whilst still in ICU. Gabapentinoids (gabapentin and pregabalin) for neuropathic pain have the strongest evidence to support their efficacy.[51] Tricyclic antidepressants such as amitriptyline are effective for neuropathic pain in patients who also have depression. Infusions of opiates, ketamine and lidocaine are effective for neuropathic pain in the short term.[51] Behavioural therapy may be useful in addition to pharmacological treatment. Consultation with a pain specialist should be sought in patients with severe, refractory pain.

GASTROINTESTINAL

Paralytic ileus and acute gastric dilatation are common initially following SCI. The upper motor neuron bowel syndrome is seen following lesions above the cauda equina; it is characterised by increased colonic wall and anal tone with loss of external anal sphincter control, which results in constipation and faecal retention. Defaecation may be induced by a reflex activity caused by a rectal stimulus such as an irritant suppository or digital stimulation. Other components of bowel management programmes include adequate fluid intake, diet, laxatives and, rarely, surgery or electrical stimulation. Daily suppositories are commonly required, with polyethylene glycol-based suppositories having advantages over hydrogenated vegetable-oil-based bisacodyl suppositories. Opioids and other constipating medications should be avoided where possible.[52]

In lower motor neuron bowel syndrome, seen in cauda equina injuries, the external anal sphincter is lax but colonic peristalsis is inhibited leading to both constipation and overflow incontinence.

Unopposed parasympathetic activity results in stomach hyperacidity, necessitating a proton pump inhibitor for ulcer prophylaxis.

URINARY TRACT

Most patients with a NLOI above L1 experience detrusor overactivity associated with sphincter dysynergia.

This results from the upper motor neuron lesion causing overactivity of both detrusor and bladder sphincters. As a result, the detrusor contracts against a closed sphincter, leading to high intravesical pressure, vesico-uretheral reflux, high residual volume, incontinence, bladder spasm and an increased risk of urinary tract infections. Most patients with complete cervical SCI will require a suprapubic cystostomy, whereas thoraco-lumbar injuries may be managed by intermittent self-catheterisation. Bladder spasticity is common and anticholinergic agents like oxybutynin, tolterodine or trospium should be commenced early in the admission to prevent a contracted, low-volume bladder. The anti-cholinergic side-effects of these agents may be significant. Most patients require a combination of two anticholinergic medications.

Following SCI, there is a marked alteration in calcium homeostasis, with potential hypercalcaemia, hypercalciuria and a significant risk of calcium oxalate nephrolithiasis. A baseline CT of the renal tract should be obtained a couple of months after SCI, and renal calculi and urinary tract infections should be suspected as precipitants of autonomic dysreflexia.

SKIN CARE

Pressure ulcers are common due to immobility and lack of sensation; 10–30% of patients with SCI develop pressure ulcers.[53] They are a source of significant morbidity and are associated with increased hospital length of stay, life-threatening infections, chronic refractory osteomyelitis and autonomic dysreflexia. Skin healing in denervated skin is significantly delayed, so prevention is vital. The incidence of pressure areas may be reduced by:

- daily skin inspection to detect early pressure areas
- prevention of accumulation of moisture
- good bowel and bladder care
- pressure-relieving mattresses
- protocol-based frequent patient repositioning
- optimal nutrition
- patient participation in their skin care programme.

PSYCHOLOGICAL

Prolonged supportive care is necessary for both patients and their families to help them accept and adapt to neurological disability. Depression is common after SCI. Major depression should be differentiated from depressed mood. Healthcare workers may have the tendency to overdiagnose depression and, conversely, depressive symptoms may be misinterpreted as somatic symptoms (e.g. fatigue) following SCI. Since many patients require antidepressants for pain and are also on drugs with anticholinergic effects (e.g. tolterodine, oxybutynin), management of depression is complex and specialist psychiatric consultation should be sought.

RE-ADMISSION TO ICU

Common causes for re-admission to ICU for patients with pre-existing SCI are infections (urinary tract infections, pneumonia), AD, VTE and surgery (commonly after urinary tract procedure for renal stones). Meticulous attention should be given to skin care. All usual medications should be continued if possible. Abrupt withdrawal of baclofen may lower the seizure threshold. The use of succinylcholine may lead to severe hyperkalaemia.

OUTCOMES FOLLOWING SCI

Hospital survival after SCI is now more than 90%, with long-term survival substantially better than 40 years ago. Factors predictive of higher mortality include higher NLOI, complete SCI, older age and presence of co-morbidities.[54] Depending on the individual circumstances, it may be appropriate to have limitations on treatment for elderly patients with complete and high NLOI. Most deaths are now due to respiratory and cardiovascular disease, with a decreasing proportion due to urinary complications.

The neurological outcome post SCI is best prognosticated with an accurate neurological assessment using the AIS. Even during the first 24 hours, a reliable exam is highly predictive of outcome. Complete (ASIA A) injuries have the least potential for recovery, with only 7% converting to ASIA B by 1 year and none becoming motor incomplete. However 54% of ASIA B patients convert to ASIA C or D by 1 year with much better functional outcomes, and nearly all ASIA C under 50 years of age and all ASIA D patients are expected to be ambulatory on discharge from rehabilitation.[15] In the absence of a clinical exam, an MRI may be used to prognosticate but is far less reliable. Most patients improve by one NLOI, with the majority of improvement seen in the first 6 months, but clinically significant strength gains can occur for up to 2 years after injury. Despite significant disability requiring considerable care, functional ability may be surprising to those who manage only the acute phase of SCI. For example, someone with a C5 ASIA A SCI may be able to mobilise with a power wheelchair with hand controls, drive a modified vehicle, and have a family and a rewarding career.

Access the complete references list online at http://www.expertconsult.com

6. Devivo MJ. Epidemiology of traumatic spinal cord injury: trends and future implications. Spinal Cord 2012;50(5):365–72.
16. Stiell IG, Clement CM, McKnight RD, et al. The Canadian C-spine rule versus the NEXUS low-risk criteria in patients with trauma. New England J Med 2003;349(26):2510–18.
29. Furlan JC, Noonan V, Cadotte DW, et al. Timing of decompressive surgery of spinal cord after traumatic spinal cord injury: an evidence-based examination of pre-clinical and clinical studies. J Neurotrauma 2011;28(8):1371–99.
30. Bracken MB, Shepard MJ, Collins WF, et al. A randomized, controlled trial of methylprednisolone or naloxone in the treatment of acute spinal-cord injury. Results of the Second National Acute Spinal Cord Injury Study. New Engl J Med 1990;322(20):1405–11.
32. Casha S, Christie S. A systematic review of intensive cardiopulmonary management after spinal cord injury. J Neurotrauma 2011;28(8):1479–95.
36. Peterson WP, Barbalata L, Brooks CA, et al. The effect of tidal volumes on the time to wean persons with high tetraplegia from ventilators. Spinal Cord 1999;37(4):284–8.
37. Berney SC, Gordon IR, Opdam HI, et al. A classification and regression tree to assist clinical decision making in airway management for patients with cervical spinal cord injury. Spinal Cord 2011;49(2): 244–50.
39. Arora S, Flower O, Murray NP, et al. Respiratory care of patients with cervical spinal cord injury: a review. Crit Care Resusc 2012;14(1):73.
51. Teasell RW, Mehta S, Aubut JAL, et al. A systematic review of pharmacological treatments of pain following spinal cord injury. Arch Phys Med Rehabil 2010;91(5):816–31.
55. American Spinal Injury Association. International Standards for Neurological Classification of Spinal Cord Injury. Atlanta, GA, 2011.

79

Abdominal and pelvic injuries

Colin McArthur and Pieter HW Lubbert

Although important abdominal injuries are present in only about 20% of hospital trauma admissions,[1] haemorrhage from abdominal and pelvic injuries is the most common cause of preventable trauma death.[2] Most abdominal and pelvic injuries are caused by blunt trauma; penetrating aetiologies can account for up to a quarter of cases, depending on the society concerned.[3] Important considerations with abdominal and pelvic injuries are:

- potential for severe haemorrhage
- difficulties in diagnosing visceral injury
- severity of associated injuries (e.g. chest and head)
- complications, especially sepsis.

MECHANISMS OF INJURY

BLUNT INJURIES

Road crashes account for most abdominal and pelvic blunt injuries. Injuries may also result from falls, assaults and industrial accidents.[3] Associated injuries are frequent, involving the thorax (most common), head and extremities. Seat belts and airbags reduce mortality in motor vehicle crashes (mainly by limiting brain injury), but are associated with more lower body injuries including decelerating trauma to cardiovascular structures such as thoracic aorta.

PENETRATING INJURIES

Stab and gunshot wounds account for most penetrating injuries to the abdomen.

STAB AND LACERATION WOUNDS

Entry sites do not accurately predict the nature of deeper injury. Penetration of the thoracic cavity should be suspected with upper abdominal wounds; conversely, lower chest wounds may involve abdominal structures. Selective management of haemodynamically stable patients using investigation and observation algorithms that accurately predict intra-abdominal injury have superseded mandatory laparotomy in high-volume centres.[4]

GUNSHOT WOUNDS

Injuries depend on missile calibre, and its velocity and trajectory. Intra-abdominal, thoracic and multiple organ injuries and mortality are substantially greater than with stab wounds. Laparotomy should be performed in all cases with haemodynamic instability, peritonitis or a clinically un-evaluable abdomen. A non-operative approach for selected low-risk patients remains controversial.[5]

INITIAL TREATMENT AND INVESTIGATIONS

RESUSCITATION

Ensuring adequacy of airway, ventilation and oxygenation are immediate priorities. However, circulatory resuscitation should not delay surgery for uncontrolled haemorrhage.[6] If rapid surgical haemostasis is provided in penetrating trauma, delaying or limiting fluid resuscitation before surgery improves outcome.[7] 'Damage control resuscitation'[8] combining permissive hypovolaemia/hypotension with a haemostatic fluid regimen may limit bleeding and transfusion, but is controversial in blunt injury (see Haemorrhage and Coagulopathy section below). Pneumatic anti-shock garments provide no benefit.[9]

CLINICAL ASSESSMENT

A full clinical examination (including the back) by experienced clinicians is most important. The mechanism of injury may direct attention to particular anatomical areas.

- Contusions, external wounds and their relationship to underlying viscera are noted.
- Abdominal distension, tenderness and peritonism are sought but auscultation for bowel sounds is not useful.
- The rectum is examined for prostatic position, anal tone, blood or other evidence of injury.
- Gastric aspirate and urine are inspected for blood.

Isolated penetrating injuries present few diagnostic problems, but the decision to explore the abdomen can be difficult. Blunt abdominal trauma is often part of multiple injuries, and is more difficult to diagnose clinically, except when abdominal signs are obvious. Nevertheless, in conscious patients, serial assessments can accurately identify those with significant intra-abdominal pathology. In the presence of impaired consciousness, intellectual disability or spinal, chest or pelvic injury, clinical assessment is unreliable. Other more visually spectacular injuries may also divert attention from the abdomen. Laparotomy is indicated on clinical grounds when there is evisceration, peritonism, or signs of shock with free abdominal fluid.

In all other situations where clinical examination is inadequate, further investigations must be undertaken.[10]

PLAIN X-RAYS

A chest X-ray (preferably erect) is essential. It may demonstrate free intraperitoneal gas, herniation of abdominal contents through a ruptured diaphragm, or an alternative focus of bleeding. Plain films of the abdomen are of no benefit in blunt injuries; however, they may show presence of foreign bodies in penetrating injuries. An anteroposterior pelvic X-ray (or computed tomography (CT) scan) is indicated for all victims of blunt trauma, except conscious patients with normal pelvis on examination.[11]

INVESTIGATIONS FOR OCCULT ABDOMINAL INJURY

ULTRASONOGRAPHY

Focused abdominal sonography for trauma (FAST) can be performed rapidly in the resuscitation room without compromising ongoing treatment. It requires significant training to achieve acceptable accuracy[12] and, although highly specific, its sensitivity of around 85%[13] is less than that of peritoneal lavage or CT in detecting free intra-abdominal fluid following either blunt[14,15] or penetrating[16] trauma. FAST cannot identify hollow viscus injury or the nature of solid organ injury. FAST may reduce the need for other investigations,[17] but the small but important false-negative rate must be considered in determining its role in abdominal assessment algorithms. A limited transthoracic echocardiogram (LTTE) can assess IVC size (an index of volume status) and ventricular contractility, and detect pericardial fluid.[18]

PERITONEAL LAVAGE

Diagnostic peritoneal lavage (DPL)[19] is indicated to exclude intra-abdominal injuries when other methods of investigation (FAST, CT scan) are not available. DPL detects intraperitoneal injury with up to 98% accuracy,[19] but its high sensitivity can result in a significant non-therapeutic laparotomy rate.

DPL is unjustified when an indication for laparotomy already exists. It is relatively contraindicated in pregnancy, significant obesity and previous abdominal surgery.

Generally accepted criteria for a positive DPL are shown in **Table 79.1**.

Table 79.1 Criteria for positive diagnostic peritoneal lavage

CLINICAL		
Initial aspiration of >10 mL frank blood		
Egress of lavage fluid via chest tube or urinary catheter		
Bile or vegetable material in lavage fluid		
LABORATORY		
	BLUNT INJURY	PENETRATING INJURY
Red cells		
Definite	$>100\times10^9$/L	$>20\times10^9$/L
Indeterminate	$50–100\times10^9$/L	$5–20\times10^9$/L
White cells	$>0.5\times10^9$/L	0.5×10^9/L
Amylase	>20 IU/L	>20 IU/L
Alkaline phosphatase	>10 IU/L	>10 IU/L

COMPUTED TOMOGRAPHY

CT requires a still patient, a high-resolution scanner and experienced interpretation to match the sensitivity of peritoneal lavage. Imaging from the top of the diaphragm to the symphysis pubis following i.v. contrast is required to fully assess the abdominal cavity. The safety of undertaking CT in acute trauma depends on the degree of cardiorespiratory stability relative to the speed of scanning and access to resuscitation support. CT is particularly indicated for assessing the retroperitoneum and pelvic fractures, and delineating the nature of abdominal injury (thus guiding non-operative management of some solid organ injuries). It may not detect all hollow viscus traumas, but multidetector CT is more specific and sensitive for bowel injury.[20] Enteric contrast may not improve accuracy.[21] Magnetic resonance imaging offers no advantage over CT in evaluating acute abdominal trauma, and poses significant logistical problems.

CHOICE OF INVESTIGATION

- FAST is non-invasive, rapid, and reasonably accurate when used by trained staff. It can screen for haemoperitoneum, but negative studies should be followed by another investigation.[15,16]
- CT is non-invasive, time-consuming, accurate and has a primary role in defining the location and magnitude of intra-abdominal injuries in stable patients with blunt trauma or penetrating trauma to the flank or back.

FAST and CT are complementary and ideally both should be available. If CT is unavailable, a negative FAST should be followed by either a DPL or a delayed repeat FAST[22] in the patient with blunt trauma in whom clinical examination is inadequate.

LAPAROSCOPY

Diagnostic laparoscopy may be useful in the haemodynamically stable patient. It is good at visualising the diaphragm and identifying a need for laparotomy, but may miss specific organ injuries in blunt abdominal injuries, particularly of the bowel. Laparoscopy appears best suited for the evaluation of equivocal penetrating wounds.[5]

ANGIOGRAPHY

Selective angiography and embolisation are valuable in detecting and treating the source of major haemorrhage from surgically difficult-to-access pelvic and retroperitoneal structures. In selected patients embolisation can also treat haemorrhage from liver and splenic injuries. Angiography in unstable patients is best undertaken in a hybrid operating room.

LAPAROTOMY

Laparotomy can be regarded as both therapeutic and diagnostic. Intra-abdominal injury may be detected by means discussed above, but often only laparotomy can accurately diagnose specific injuries. In severe and multiple trauma, the morbidity of a negative laparotomy is insignificant compared with the dire consequences of not diagnosing and treating a serious injury.

Operative treatment of more severe injuries with difficult haemostasis can cause a lethal triad of hypothermia, acidosis and coagulopathy. A 'damage control' laparotomy[23] with control of haemorrhage and contamination, intraperitoneal packing, elective re-exploration and removal of packs 24–48 hours later should be performed.

- Angiography should be considered and may be required for inaccessible arterial bleeding.
- Temporary prosthetic closure may be required to avoid elevated intra-abdominal pressure.
- Survival is better when the decision to terminate the initial procedure is made earlier.

SPECIFIC INJURIES

SPLEEN

The spleen is the organ most frequently injured by blunt trauma. Injuries vary from a small subcapsular haematoma to hilar devascularisation or shattered spleen, but are rarely fatal with good medical care.[24] Diagnosis may be delayed in mild trauma. Fractures of the lower left ribs are a common association. When associated chest or neurological injuries are severe, minor splenic injury may not initially be detected unless further investigation is undertaken. Minor trauma may cause splenic injury when the spleen is enlarged (e.g. from malaria, lymphoma and haemolytic anaemia).

Immediate splenectomy is indicated in patients with splenic avulsion, fragmentation or rupture, extensive hilar injuries, failure of haemostasis, associated peritoneal contamination from gastrointestinal injury or rupture of diseased spleen. However, overwhelming post-splenectomy infection (OPSI) by encapsulated organisms, such as *Pneumococcus,* can occur early or late (even years) after splenectomy in 0–2% of individuals. It is a particular risk following splenectomy in children and young adults. Polyvalent pneumococcal vaccine should be administered following splenectomy together with vaccination for *Meningococcus* and *Haemophilus influenzae*.[25]

If associated abdominal injuries have been excluded, a non-operative approach can give splenic salvage rates of over 80%. Arterial embolisation can further reduce the need for laparotomy. Failure rates are higher with more severe injuries.[26]

Other treatment alternatives include operative procedures to conserve splenic tissue (e.g. topical haemostatic agents, suture repair, absorbable mesh, partial splenectomy and splenic artery ligation). Benefits of splenectomy with autotransplantation of splenic tissue are unproven.

LIVER

The liver is the second most commonly injured organ after blunt abdominal trauma, and has been the most frequently missed injury in deaths from trauma.[2] Diagnosis is made by laparotomy in unstable patients, or CT in stable patients. Injuries range from small subcapsular haematomas to major parenchymal disruption and laceration of hepatic veins or even hepatic avulsion.

CT assessment enables most patients to be managed without operation. Patients should be haemodynamically stable, have associated major abdominal injuries excluded, and be assessed repeatedly. Follow-up CT scans can show the resolution of injury, which typically takes 2–3 months. CT-guided percutaneous drainage, ERCP and angioembolisation can treat the complications of a non-operative approach such as bile leak, haemobilia, necrosis, abscess and delayed haemorrhage.

If surgery is required, early determination of indications for a damage control approach is important. Perihepatic packing gives best haemostasis. Angiography may identify and treat uncontrolled arterial bleeding. Early complications of liver injury relate to the effects of hypoperfusion or massive blood transfusion. Late complications are usually associated with sepsis.[27]

GASTROINTESTINAL TRACT (GIT)

Injury to the GIT is more common following penetrating than blunt trauma. The very high likelihood of bowel injury in abdominal gunshot wounds should mandate laparotomy. Laparoscopy can be used to identify those with stab wounds for laparotomy when peritoneal violation cannot be excluded. Posterior stab wounds may damage retroperitoneal structures. CT examination with contrast enema may identify colonic injury better than clinical assessment.[5]

Blunt abdominal injuries include perforation or devascularisation of stomach, duodenum, small intestine, colon and their mesenteries, all of which are difficult to evaluate. Physical signs may be absent initially. FAST may provide a general indication for laparotomy, but is insensitive to bowel injury. CT is a sensitive indicator of free intraperitoneal air, but signs of duodenal perforation or haematoma are subtle even with multidetector CT or enteral contrast. Consequently, duodenal injury may be missed. A high index of suspicion should be maintained in patients with persistent abdominal pain and tenderness.[28]

Bleeding from mesenteric vessels is often self-limiting and may not require surgical control. However, vessel damage can cause ischaemia and infarction, and may require resection of affected bowel. Uncomplicated blunt or penetrating bowel injury can usually be managed by primary repair and anastomosis rather than colostomy.[29] A faecal diversion procedure with delayed repair is indicated in significant peritoneal contamination or severe perineal injury.

PANCREAS

Blunt injuries to the pancreas require considerable force with compression of abdominal contents against the spinal column and are often associated with duodenal, liver and splenic trauma. CT is the most useful initial investigation; however, pancreatic duct injury might be better visualised by MRCP or ERCP. Acute hyperamylasaemia does not predict pancreatic or hollow viscus injury.[30]

Minor injuries require simple drainage and haemostasis. Severe injuries to the body and tail of the pancreas are best managed by distal pancreatectomy. Severe injuries involving the proximal pancreas and duodenum with intact ampulla and common bile duct can be treated by drainage alone if associated duodenal injury is simple to repair. Acute pancreaticoduodenectomy is rarely required; however, it should be considered if there is disruption of the ampullary–biliary–pancreatic union or major devitalisation. Complications such as pancreatitis, fistula, abscess and pseudocyst are common.[31]

KIDNEY AND URINARY TRACT

Blunt injury to the urinary tract is more common than penetrating injury. Identification and treatment of other major injuries often take precedence. Gross haematuria should be investigated; CT is the examination of choice for haemorrhage. Urinary extravasation may be identified only on a repeat scan 10–20 minutes after contrast injection or on a formal retrograde (CT) cystogram. Unless there is unexplained shock, microscopic haematuria does not require further investigation. Renovascular pedicle or ureteric injuries may not cause any haematuria. Most renal injuries resolve with expectant management. Lacerations involving the collecting system or injury to the renal pedicle usually require operative intervention, although restoration of renal function following long warm ischaemic times is unusual. If major renal injury is discovered at emergency laparotomy, intraoperative i.v. urography is an option to ensure contralateral function and identify urinary extravasation. Angio-embolisation may be useful for controlling renal haemorrhage.[32]

Bladder rupture is commonly associated with pelvic fractures. Blunt injury to patients with a distended bladder can cause isolated intraperitoneal bladder rupture. Over 95% of patients have macroscopic haematuria. Retrograde cystography is the investigation of choice because plain abdominal CT has a high false-negative rate. Intraperitoneal bladder rupture requires operative repair and urinary drainage. Patients with sterile urine and extraperitoneal rupture can be managed with catheter drainage alone.[33]

Urethral trauma is caused by direct blunt injury, or occurs in association with pelvic injury. It should be suspected if there is blood at the urinary meatus, perineal injury or abnormal position of the prostate on rectal examination in the male. In the absence of these findings, cautious urethral catheterisation is appropriate. Treatment of urethral trauma is suprapubic drainage and subsequent definitive repair.

DIAPHRAGM

Diaphragmatic injury occurs in fewer than 5% of cases of blunt injury, is left-sided in 80% of cases, and is commonly associated with injuries to abdominal organs. It should also be suspected in penetrating trauma below the fifth rib. Diagnosis can be difficult, especially in the presence of positive-pressure ventilation, and may become evident only after ventilatory support is discontinued. Chest X-rays are commonly abnormal but often with non-specific findings. Laparoscopy and thoracoscopy provide good views of the diaphragm.

Spontaneous healing does not occur, and all defects over 1 cm should be repaired. The risk of associated injuries in acute cases mandates an abdominal approach.[34]

BONY PELVIS AND PERINEUM

Pelvic fractures are primarily caused by vehicular trauma or falls. Associated injuries to the bladder, urethra and intra-abdominal organs are common. Injuries may be life-threatening, initially from major haemorrhage, and later from sepsis. Significant morbidity can result from damage to pelvic nerves, urethra or the structural integrity of the pelvis. Pelvic injury is suggested by pain on movement, structural instability, gross haematuria or peripelvic ecchymosis. Rectal examination is mandatory to identify rectal injury and prostatic position.

Radiography can confirm bony injury, but CT is usually required to identify associated intra-abdominal injuries (in the haemodynamically stable) and can assist in planning operative stabilisation.

Patients with haemodynamic instability and pelvic fractures must have intra-abdominal haemorrhage excluded. Early FAST is the investigation of choice but has a significant false-negative rate with major pelvic fractures. If grossly positive, laparotomy should precede pelvic interventions. If FAST negative, the risk of life-threatening intra-abdominal haemorrhage is relatively low, and achieving haemostasis for pelvic bleeding becomes the priority; CT and/or laparotomy should follow if the patient is still unstable.[35]

- Temporary pelvic binding (and avoidance of external rotation of the legs) is the preferred emergency measure to improve tamponade by reducing pelvic volume.
- Angiography and selective embolisation is effective in controlling arterial bleeding.[36]
- Retroperitoneal (preperitoneal) packing may reduce the need for angiography.[37]
- External fixation of the pelvis may reduce bleeding near fracture sites and reduce the volume of an open pelvis, but reduced blood loss and improved outcomes are unproven.[35]
- Bleeding from large vessels such as the aorta, common and external iliac arteries, and common femoral artery requires surgical control.

Pelvic fractures range from simple fractures of individual bones requiring bed rest alone to complex fractures. Early operative stabilisation of complex pelvic fractures is preferred in the intensive care unit (ICU), as it facilitates respiratory care, pain control and early mobilisation. Compound pelvic fractures involving the perineum, rectum or vagina require aggressive surgery (which may include diversion of the faecal stream) to avoid high mortality.

RETROPERITONEAL HAEMATOMA

Retroperitoneal haematoma is frequent following blunt trauma, and is commonly caused by injury to the lumbar spine, bony pelvis, bladder or kidney or, less commonly, to the pancreas, duodenum or major vascular structures. Diagnosis may be inferred by excluding other sites of major blood loss, or presumed by signs of underlying organ injury. CT is the most useful investigation in the stable patient.

A central haematoma should be explored with proximal vascular control because of the risk of pancreatic, duodenal or major vascular injury. A lateral or pelvic haematoma should not be explored, unless there is evidence of major arterial injury, intraperitoneal bladder rupture or colonic injury.[38]

TRAUMA IN PREGNANCY

Women injured during pregnancy pose problems of altered physiology, risk to the gravid uterus and fetus, and potential conflict of priorities between mother and fetus, In general, however, the best treatment for the fetus is to treat the mother optimally.

High-flow oxygen must be given until maternal hypoxaemia, hypovolaemia and fetal distress have been excluded:

- Reduced respiratory reserve demands earlier intervention.
- Maternal compensation for blood loss is at the expense of uteroplacental blood flow.
- Pregnant women should be positioned to avoid aortocaval compression.
- Secondary survey must include a vaginal examination and obstetric consultation.
- Upper limbs are preferred for intravenous access.
- Transfusions should be Rhesus compatible.
- All Rhesus-negative mothers should receive immune globulin, because of the immunological risk of even minor fetomaternal haemorrhage.[39]

Only X-rays and CT scans that may significantly alter therapy should be taken (with appropriate shielding), especially in those under 20 weeks' gestation, although examination of body regions outside the abdomen/pelvis offers minimal fetal risk. Ultrasound is the preferred investigation as it is safe and can accurately detect free intra-abdominal fluid, confirm gestation and fetal well-being, and identify placental abnormalities.[40]

CT may miss injuries owing to abdominal crowding. Retroperitoneal haemorrhage is more common in pregnant patients. Placental abruption may conceal significant blood loss. Treatment may be expectant or by caesarean section, depending on the condition of the mother and fetus. Uterine rupture is unusual and will often require hysterectomy. Perimortem caesarean section must commence within 4 minutes of maternal cardiac arrest for best fetal outcome.[40]

Placental abruption, fetal distress and fetal loss are rare following blunt injury, but premature uterine contractions are common. Continuous cardiotocography (indicated at viable gestations) for 6 hours is the most sensitive test to detect obstetric complications.[40] Kleihauer–Betke tests to identify fetomaternal haemorrhage can predict preterm labour[41] and guide additional Rh immune globulin doses.

COMPLICATIONS

HAEMORRHAGE AND COAGULOPATHY

Haemorrhage from abdominal and pelvic injuries is the most common cause of preventable trauma death.[2] Direct tissue injury plus the hypoperfusion of shock causes early acute coagulopathy and hyperfibrinolysis, exacerbated by subsequent haemodilution of clotting factors, hypothermia and acidosis.[42] Disseminated intravascular coagulation occurs infrequently in trauma. Damage control surgery can limit progression to the 'lethal triad' (coagulopathy, hypothermia, acidosis).[23] Low-volume resuscitation ('permissive hypovolaemia/hypotension') for short periods prior to haemostatic intervention is established for penetrating trauma,[7,43] but controversial for blunt injuries due to limited evidence and potential risks to patients with long transport times, cardiovascular disease or central nervous system injury.[44,45] In the absence of such factors, a target systolic pressure of 80–100 mmHg (11–13 kPa) prior to haemostatic intervention may be adequate.[6] Early initiation of a 'massive transfusion protocol', with a high ratio of plasma to packed red cells (typically 1 plasma unit per 1–2 red cells, and often including regular platelets and cryoprecipitate), limits the dilution of asanguineous resuscitation and is effective in minimising acute coagulopathy, and may improve outcome in both blunt and penetrating trauma.[46–48] The combination of limited resuscitation volumes and target blood pressure with a haemostatic transfusion strategy is termed 'damage control resuscitation'.[8] Patient-specific treatment for acute coagulopathy in trauma, including fibrinolysis, may be better guided by point-of-care viscoelastic haemostatic testing (e.g. thromboelastography) than standard laboratory assays.[49,50] The prophylactic administration of the antifibrinolytic tranexamic acid within 3 hours of injury reduced death from bleeding without increasing vascular occlusive events in a large study of patients treated in diverse hospital settings.[51] Its use in advanced trauma care may be best in the pre-hospital environment. Empirical use of recombinant activated factor VII based on number of transfused red cell units is not effective,[52] but still may benefit individual patients with resistant coagulopathy if not significantly hypothermic or acidaemic and if they have adequate fibrinogen.

SEPSIS

Intra-abdominal sepsis remains an important preventable cause of death after trauma. Predisposing factors include:

- peritoneal contamination from GIT injury
- external wounds
- invasive procedures
- delayed diagnosis of hollow viscus injuries
- splenectomy
- devitalised tissue.

Early diagnosis and effective lavage and drainage procedures may reduce the incidence *of* intra-abdominal sepsis. Prophylactic antibiotics for 24 hours are satisfactory for penetrating injuries.[53] Intra-abdominal sepsis should be excluded if unexplained fever and/or neutrophil leucytosis, or multiple organ failure develops. Septic shock may represent a second shock insult to the trauma patient, leading to multiorgan dysfunction. Selective decontamination of the digestive tract may reduce infections in multiple trauma,[54] but its use remains controversial.

GASTROINTESTINAL FAILURE

GIT failure in various forms, ranging from stress ulceration and delayed gastric emptying to paralytic ileus, is a frequent occurrence. Prophylaxis against stress ulceration is indicated in ventilated patients not tolerating gastric feeding.[55] Enteral nutrition is associated with a lower incidence of complications following abdominal trauma.[56] Feeding through a jejunostomy tube placed during surgery or radiologically in the ICU is usually feasible. Parenteral nutrition may be necessary in patients with severe bowel or retroperitoneal injuries.

RAISED INTRA-ABDOMINAL PRESSURE

Although less common than in the past, abdominal distension with raised intra-abdominal pressure may be seen in the critically injured as a consequence of haemorrhage, bowel oedema, ileus or surgical packs. This can have severe adverse effects on respiratory, cardiovascular and renal function.[57] Alleviation is by abdominal decompression and temporary closure,[58] with or without visceral packing. The abdomen is subsequently closed by staged repair as the distension resolves.

VENOUS THROMBOEMBOLISM

Pelvic trauma, postoperative status, higher Injury Severity Score (ISS – see Ch. 3) and underlying medical risk factors increase the risk of venous thromboembolism 1.5 to 3 times greater than trauma patients without such factors.[59] Early initiation of mechanical prophylaxis is usually feasible, and chemoprophylaxis when the risk of injury-associated bleeding has reduced.

Access the complete references list online at http://www.expertconsult.com

5. Como J, Bokhari F, Chiu W, et al. Practice management guidelines for selective nonoperative management of penetrating abdominal trauma. J Trauma 2010;68:721–33.
6. Rossaint R, Bouillon B, Cerny V, et al. Management of bleeding following major trauma: an updated European guideline. Critical Care 2010;14:R52.
8. Harris T, Thomas R, Brohi K. Early fluid resuscitation in severe trauma. BMJ 2012;345:e5752.
23. Shapiro MB, Jenkins DH, Schwab CW, et al. Damage control: collective review. J Trauma 2000;49:969–78.
35. Cullinane D, Schiller H, Zielinski M, et al. Eastern Association for the Surgery of Trauma practice management guidelines for hemorrhage in pelvic fracture – update and systematic review. J Trauma 2011;71:1850–68.
40. Barraco R, Chiu W, Clancy T, et al. Practice management guidelines for the diagnosis and management of injury in the pregnant patient: The EAST practice management guidelines work group. J Trauma 2010; 69:211–14.
51. CRASH-2 trial collaborators, Shakur H, Roberts I, et al. Effects of tranexamic acid on death, vascular occlusive events, and blood transfusion in trauma patients with significant haemorrhage (CRASH-2): a randomised, placebo-controlled trial. Lancet 2010; 376:23–32.

Part Twelve

Environmental Injuries

80

Submersion

Cyrus Edibam and Tim Bowles

DEFINITIONS

Drowning has been defined by the World Health Organization in 2002 as follows: 'Drowning is the process of experiencing respiratory impairment from submersion/immersion in liquid'.[1] If the victim dies as a result, the event should be referred to as 'fatal drowning', if the drowning process is interrupted, it should be referred to as 'non-fatal drowning'. The Utstein template can be adopted to provide consistent reporting of drowning events and allow accurate categorisation.[2]

EPIDEMIOLOGY

Drowning causes an estimated 400 000 deaths worldwide per year.[3] Of these, 4000 are reported from the USA (approximately 1.5 deaths per 100 000 population) and 290 (1.4 deaths/100 000 population) from Australia.[4,5] Ninety-six per cent of fatal drownings occur in low- or middle-income countries and, worldwide, drowning is the third most common cause of unintentional injury death.[3] In the USA, twice as many non-fatal drownings as fatal ones were recorded in 2009.[4] In Australia, drowning is the leading cause of unintentional injury death in children aged 1 to 3 years.[6] Males predominate, with peaks at 5 and 20 years of age. Private swimming pools and natural water bodies close to home present the greatest risk to young children.[7] Other sites include bath tubs, fish tanks, buckets, toilets and washing machines. Adolescent drowning tends to occur in rivers, lakes, canals and beaches.[8] Lack of adult supervision is almost always to blame for toddler accidents; however, child abuse must also be considered. Alcohol and drug intoxication are associated with up to 40% of adolescent drowning.[9] Other risk factors include epilepsy (18%), trauma (16%) and cardiopulmonary disease (14%).[10] Hyperventilation prior to underwater swimming suppresses the physiological response to rising carbon dioxide tension, allowing hypoxia to ensue with consequent loss of consciousness and water breathing.[11]

PATHOPHYSIOLOGY

Voluntary apnoea and reflex responses occur upon submersion. The *diving response* is characterised by apnoea, marked generalised vasoconstriction and bradycardia in response to cold-water stimulus of the ophthalmic division of the trigeminal nerve. Blood is thus shunted preferentially to the brain and heart. In infants the response may be marked,[12] but only 15% of fully clothed adults show a significant response. Although the diving reflex appears to play a powerful role in oxygen conservation in animals, its role in humans is unknown but may be protective.[13]

After airway immersion, breath holding followed by laryngospasm occurs. This causes progressive hypoxia and hypercarbia, eventually resulting in relaxation of airway reflexes and water aspiration.[11] Up to 22 mL/kg of water has been estimated to be the maximal survivable inhaled water volume.[14] This is followed by a phase of secondary apnoea and loss of consciousness. Hypoxaemic death ensues if the person is not retrieved and resuscitated; acute respiratory distress syndrome (ARDS) occurs in up to 72% of symptomatic survivors.[15] Multiple organ dysfunction and cerebral damage may become evident in those who survive to hospital.

SALT- VERSUS FRESH-WATER ASPIRATION

The differences between salt- and fresh-water drowning have traditionally been emphasised. This is largely on the basis of animal data. In canine models, after aspiration of massive volumes of salt water, it was possible to recover by suction or mechanical drainage greater volumes than were initially instilled.[16] The hypertonic salt water was drawing fluid into the pulmonary interstitial space, which was thought to result in hypovolaemia, hypernatraemia and haemoconcentration as well as pulmonary oedema.

Conversely, after fresh-water aspiration in dogs minimal volumes of fluid were retrievable from the lungs.[17] The hypotonic water was absorbed into the circulation. The pulmonary oedema seen was thought to be secondary to removal of surfactant, and hypervolaemia, dilutional hyponatraemia and haemolysis were expected.

More recent animal data and human case series have demonstrated that the tonicity of the fluid aspirated is not clinically relevant.[18] No clinically detectable difference in the patterns of lung injury is seen between salt- and fresh-water drowning; both types reduce pulmonary surfactant quantity and function, causing pulmonary oedema and hypoxia by collapse, atelectasis and shunting. Differences in electrolyte disturbance are not generally clinically significant.[14]

WATER CONTAMINANTS

The incidence of pneumonia complicating submersion injury may be greater than 15% in those who survive long enough.[15] Rivers, lakes and coastal waters are greater reservoirs for microbes than well-kept swimming pools. In fresh water, Gram-negative bacteria predominate along with anaerobes and *Staphylococcus* spp., fungi, algal and protozoan species. *Aeromonas* spp. are ubiquitous water-borne bacteria and can be responsible for severe pneumonia.[19] Infection with oral commensals is common, as is infection with multiple organisms. Although prophylactic antibiotic treatment is not recommended in general, if infection is suspected then broad-spectrum antibiotics with antipseudomonal cover is required.[20]

Chemicals in polluted water such as kerosene,[21] chlorine[22] and particulate matter like sand[23] can cause severe pulmonary dysfunction.

TEMPERATURE

Victims of submersion may develop primary or secondary hypothermia. If submersion occurs in icy water (<5°C) hypothermia may develop rapidly and provide some protection against hypoxia. Surface cooling is unlikely to produce adequate protective hypothermia before hypoxia ensues.[13] Most reports of survival after prolonged submersion involve small children in icy water and it has been postulated that protective core cooling occurs rapidly due to cold-water aspiration, ingestion and absorption, though the mechanisms remain controversial.[24]

Of more importance in cold-water submersion are the detrimental 'cold-shock' responses.[25] These responses include a 'gasp' followed by uncontrollable hyperventilation and reduction in maximal breath-hold times, vasoconstriction, tachycardia, hypertension and increased myocardial oxygen consumption. These responses may lead to motor dyscoordination and swimming failure as well as cardiac arrhythmia; hence even strong swimmers may drown quickly in icy waters.

MANAGEMENT

BASIC LIFE SUPPORT

Prompt retrieval from the water is essential, as is immediate on-site resuscitation. As any cardiac arrest is normally secondary to hypoxaemia, five rescue breaths should be administered first, followed by standard basic life support. Compression-only CPR is inappropriate in this case. Rescue breathing can be performed effectively in the water; chest compressions cannot.[18]

The risk of cervical spine injury is small (<0.5%), and attempted cervical spine immobilisation can compromise effective rescue and resuscitation in the water. Therefore, spinal immobilisation is indicated only in the presence of severe injury or consistent history.[18] The Heimlich manoeuvre is no longer recommended in the management of submersion injury as the volume of aspirated water removed at the time of attempt is small and the risk of gastric aspiration is great.[18]

Rewarming should be commenced immediately with the use of blankets and further heat loss should be avoided. When experienced personnel arrive, bag and mask ventilation and advanced cardiac life support are initiated.

INITIAL HOSPITAL MANAGEMENT

Resuscitation continues on arrival to hospital. Endotracheal intubation and mechanical ventilation are instituted if hypoxaemia is severe despite high-flow oxygen or assisted bag and mask respiration. Ventilatory failure, characterised by increasing respiratory distress and rising carbon dioxide levels, and the presence of an impaired conscious level or severe agitation may also necessitate intubation. The stomach should be decompressed by insertion of a nasogastric tube if possible but this may be difficult in a hypoxic agitated patient. Early active rewarming is indicated for severe hypothermia, but hyperthermia should be meticulously avoided.[18]

ASSESSMENT

HISTORY

Attempts should be made to elucidate the time and the duration of submersion, the presence of polluted water and likely contaminants, delay in resuscitation attempts and the likelihood of alcohol ingestion, drug use, pre-existing medical conditions (particularly seizure disorders) and coexisting trauma. If collateral history is available, any symptoms of illness prior to the submersion event should be elicited to rule out or in a medical cause for the drowning that may require treatment.

EXAMINATION

A thorough secondary survey is carried out, concentrating on cardiorespiratory examination in particular, looking for signs of respiratory distress, wheeze, crepitations and peripheral circulatory insufficiency. Neurological status should also be assessed. Clinical deterioration in those with minor symptoms and signs can occur and the patient should be reassessed at frequent intervals.

INVESTIGATIONS

These depend on the clinical circumstances and could include:

- *arterial blood gases/lactate level*
- *plasma biochemistry/serum osmolality:* electrolyte abnormalities are unlikely in sea- or fresh-water drowning. CK should be measured as rhabdomyolysis has been reported[26]
- *haematology:* tests for haemolysis, e.g. total haemoglobin (tHb), free Hb and myoglobin concentrations in the plasma and urine
- *toxicological assays:* for drug and alcohol levels should be considered
- *chest X-ray, 12-lead ECG*
- *microbiology:* tracheal aspirates or sputum for Gram stain, microscopy and culture
- *trauma imaging:* cervical and/or thoracolumbar spine views; CT head and cervical spine if head and neck injury is suspected or the patient is comatose. Imaging of other body areas is dependent upon the clinical likelihood of injury.

ADMISSION CRITERIA

Asymptomatic patients with no clinical findings on cardiorespiratory examination and a normal chest radiograph and blood gas are unlikely to develop ARDS and pneumonia and thus do not require hospital admission.[15,27] All other patients should be admitted to a high-dependency area or intensive care unit for continuous monitoring and rewarming.

RESPIRATORY SUPPORT

Severe agitation or coma mandates intubation and mechanical ventilation; otherwise oxygenation is initially maintained with high-flow oxygen or continuous positive airway pressure (CPAP) by tight-fitting facemask. Superimposed ventilatory failure may be managed with non-invasive bilevel positive airway pressure assistance (BIPAP). The use of bronchodilators may reduce air-flow resistance and the work of breathing if evidence of bronchospasm is present. Given the high frequency of ARDS after drowning, lung-protective strategies should be employed if mechanical ventilation is required. Selective pulmonary vasodilators such as inhaled nitric oxide or inhaled prostacyclin may be useful in severe refractory hypoxaemia. In severe cases, extracorporeal membrane oxygenation has been used in some centres.[28]

CARDIOVASCULAR SUPPORT

Patients with ARDS are often hypovolaemic regardless of the type of water ingestion. Cautious volume expansion and the use of catecholamine infusion may improve cardiac output and blood pressure. Fluid replacement with isotonic fluids is aimed at restoring adequate end-organ perfusion without compromising respiratory function. The use of a central venous or pulmonary artery catheter may be necessary to achieve these goals. In cases where severe circulatory insufficiency or cardiac arrest is associated with severe hypothermia, cardiopulmonary bypass has been used successfully.[29]

CEREBRAL PROTECTION

Better neurological outcome has been demonstrated with induced hypothermia (32–34°C) after cardiac arrest due to ventricular fibrillation.[30] Although no specific data for the cerebral protective effects of hypothermia exist for patients suffering hypoxic brain injury associated with submersion, the data suggest that comatose drowning victims should not be actively rewarmed above 34°C.[18]

No other specific cerebral protective measures have proven efficacy in post anoxic encephalopathy associated with drowning.[31] Maintenance of an adequate cerebral perfusion pressure (mean arterial pressure >90 mmHg (11.97 kPa) in adults, 60–70 mmHg (7.98–9.31 kPa) in children) is the most important goal of therapy. Prevention of cerebral venous and thus intracranial hypertension can be achieved by neutral neck positioning, avoiding occlusive endotracheal tube ties and head-up positioning. Avoiding hypocapnia (Pa_{CO_2} <30 mmHg (3.99 kPa)), reducing cerebral metabolic rate with sedation, preventing hypoglycaemia and hyperthermia, and the use of anticonvulsants in those with documented seizures are simple measures to prevent secondary cerebral injury.

OTHER THERAPIES

There is no role for prophylactic corticosteroid therapy in the prevention of acute lung injury after submersion.[11] Prophylactic antibiotic therapy is unproven and the decision to commence therapy is made on the degree of water contamination, need for mechanical ventilation and severity of respiratory failure in each case.[15] Baseline microbiological studies should be sent prior to commencement of therapy.

PROGNOSIS

Mortality rate for those surviving more than 24 hours was 24% in a large series,[15] with three-quarters succumbing in the early stages after injury. Moderate to severe brain damage is reported in 33% of survivors.[7] The outcome in children is similar, with 30% having selective deficits and 3% with persistent vegetative state.[32] No difference in mortality between fresh- and salt-water submersion has been documented.[10] Lower core temperatures appear to be associated with a better prognosis, except if this occurs after rescue. However, hypothermia in warm-water immersion and severe hypothermia (<30°C) in cold-water immersion is indicative of prolonged immersion and poor outcome.[26] **Box 80.1** lists some factors associated with death or severe neurological impairment. None of these predictors is infallible and survival with normal cerebral function has been noted despite the presence of some or all of these factors.[33]

Box 80.1 Predictors of death or severe neurological impairment after submersion

At site of immersion
Immersion duration >5 minutes[34]
Delay in commencement of CPR >10 minutes[7]

In the emergency department
Glasgow Coma Score 3[35]
Fixed dilated pupils[36]

In the ICU
Glasgow Coma Scale <6 on arrival in ICU[37]
Arterial pH <7.0 on arrival in ICU[36]
No spontaneous, purposeful movements and abnormal brainstem function 48 hours after immersion[35]
Abnormal CT scan within 36 hours of submersion

Access the complete references list online at http://www.expertconsult.com

1. van Beeck EF, Branche CM, Szpilman D, et al. A new definition of drowning: towards documentation and prevention of a global public health problem. Bull World Health Organ 2005;83:853–6.
15. van Berkel M, Bierens JJL, Lie RLK, et al. Pulmonary oedema, pneumonia and mortality in submersion victims: a retrospective study in 125 patients. Int Care Med 1996;22:101–7.
18. Soar J, Perkins G, Abbas G, et al. European Resuscitation Council Guidelines for Resuscitation 2010 Section 8, Cardiac arrest in special circumstances: Electrolyte abnormalities, poisoning, drowning, accidental hypothermia, hyperthermia, asthma, anaphylaxis, cardiac surgery, trauma, pregnancy, electrocution. Resuscitation 2010;81:1400–33.
20. Tadie JM, Heming N, Serve E, et al. Drowning associated pneumonia: A descriptive cohort. Resuscitation 2012;83:399–401.
33. Layton AJ, Modell JH. Drowning update. Anesthesiology 2009;110:1390–401.

81

Burns

David P Mackie and Jacqueline EHM Vet

The last half of the twentieth century witnessed a sustained improvement in the survival of patients suffering thermal injury. Arguably, the single most important development has been the establishment of centralised burn care, which made possible advances in fluid resuscitation, life support techniques and the prevention of infection. With optimal care, children and young adults with burns of more than 80% of total body surface area (TBSA) now stand a reasonable chance of survival.[1]

Improvements in survival have gradually led to a shift of emphasis in burn care towards qualitative aspects, such as rehabilitation and quality of life. The complexity of care has led to the concept of the multidisciplinary burn team, in which all aspects of care are coordinated in an integrated approach to clinical management.[1]

PATHOPHYSIOLOGY

LOCAL EFFECTS

Thermal injury produces complex local and systemic responses. The local inflammatory response results in vasodilatation and an increase in vascular permeability. The changes are immediate and combine to produce extravasation of fluid and plasma protein at the site of injury. In extensive burns, oedema becomes generalised. The greatest rate of oedema formation occurs in the first few hours, but further extravasation occurs up to 24 hours post burn.[2] The total amount of oedema formed depends on the extent of injury and the volume and rate of fluid administration. Without fluid replacement, hypovolaemic shock occurs, limiting the extent of extravasation. On the other hand, excessive fluid administration will produce excessive oedema. By 24 hours post burn, oedema formation is largely complete and vascular integrity restored.

The process of deepening of the burn wound beyond the area of heat necrosis following injury is at least partly due to microvascular stasis. Events occurring within minutes and hours of injury include microthrombus formation, neutrophil adherence, fibrin deposition and endothelial swelling. Diverse agents, including antioxidants and anti-inflammatory drugs, have been shown to attenuate this process in experimental settings, but none is yet established in clinical practice. Empirically, it is assumed that maintenance of good tissue oxygenation, avoidance of over-resuscitation and prevention of wound dehydration all contribute to wound healing by preventing undue extension of necrosis in the wound bed. Inotropic drugs are largely ineffective and should be avoided.

CIRCULATORY EFFECTS

Circulatory effects of burn injury become significant in burns of over 15% TBSA. Changes are rapid and the magnitude is roughly proportional to the extent of burn injury. Cardiac output is reduced immediately following injury. Secretion of epinephrine (adrenaline), norepinephrine (noradrenaline), vasopressin and angiotensin cause an increase in systemic and pulmonary vascular resistance. Circulating levels of agents with myocardial depressant properties, such as interleukin-1 (IL-1) and tumour necrosis factor alpha (TNF-α), are increased following burn injury, but developing hypovolaemia and increased blood viscosity may be equally important.[3]

Cardiac output recovers gradually during the second post-burn day, reaching supranormal levels by day 3 as the hypermetabolic response to burn injury becomes manifest. Circulatory dynamics are complicated by resorption of oedema fluid and by continuing evaporative fluid loss from the wounds. Prolonged elevation of renin/angiotensin and antidiuretic hormone (ADH) has been well documented and circulating blood volume may remain subnormal into the second week post burn.[4]

METABOLIC EFFECTS

The hypermetabolic state, which ensues from around the third post-burn day until the wounds are substantially healed, is a manifestation of the systemic inflammatory response syndrome. The state is partly sustained by evaporative and radiant heat loss through the wounds, and energy expenditure can be reduced by increasing the ambient temperature[5] and by the use of occlusive dressings.[6] Other factors known to influence the metabolic rate include pain, fear and anxiety. There is also a suggestion that bacterial colonisation may aggravate hypermetabolism.[7,8] Burn patients often develop moderate pyrexia and leucocytosis, even when all microbial cultures are negative.

PHARMACOLOGICAL EFFECTS

The pharmacokinetics and pharmacodynamics of many drugs are altered in burn patients. During the first 24 hours, when the cardiac output is depressed, absorption and distribution of administered drugs are delayed. Thereafter, increased cardiac output leads to accelerated drug absorption and distribution, while oedema fluid acts as an ill-defined third space. At the same time, renal blood flow is increased, particularly in younger patients. Drugs excreted via this route, such as the quinolone and aminoglycoside antibiotics, may therefore fail to reach effective levels at conventional dosages.[9] On the other hand, toxic levels may ensue if renal failure supervenes. If possible, therefore, antibiotic administration should be guided by measurement of plasma concentrations.

Serum albumin levels are low in burn patients, and drugs bound to this protein, including some benzodiazepines, will show increased bioavailability. On the other hand, α_1-glycoprotein levels, which bind fentanyl, are increased. Detoxification via redox pathways such as cytochrome P-450 is depressed, lengthening the half-life of drugs such as diazepam.[10] Accumulation of benzodiazepine derivatives may be increased.

The pharmacodynamics of muscle relaxants are significantly altered owing to an increase in peri-junctional acetylcholine receptors.[11] Patients become relatively insensitive to non-depolarising agents, whereas administration of succinylcholine may give rise to excessive release of potassium, and cardiac arrest.

The burn wound is a significant route of drug absorption as well as drug loss. For example, the topical sulfonamide agent, mafenide, may cause metabolic acidosis through inhibition of renal carbonic anhydrase; deafness has been reported following the topical use of gentamicin.

CLINICAL MANAGEMENT

FIRST AID

Immediate aid comprises stopping the burn process, followed by the removal of clothing and cooling the wound, preferably with tepid, running water, for 10–20 minutes. This provides pain relief and may prevent deepening of the wound.[12] Hypothermia should be avoided. Oxygen should be given, if available, and patients with burns to head and neck should be kept in a semi-upright position. Burn injury can be assessed properly only in hospital conditions, and priority should be given to early evacuation of the victim.

GENERAL MANAGEMENT: 0–24 HOURS

On admission, a careful history should be taken of the circumstances of the injury, and to elucidate past medical history. The patient should be undressed, weighed and carefully examined to exclude additional traumatic injury. The extent and depth of injury are assessed with the aid of printed Lund and Browder charts, or by using the 'rule of nines' (**Fig. 81.1**). The rule of nines is modified for children (**Fig. 81.2**). A nasogastric tube and urinary catheter should be inserted in patients requiring resuscitation therapy. Escharotomies may be required for circular burns of the neck, trunk and limbs.

FLUID THERAPY: 0–24 HOURS

Fluid therapy is required for injuries exceeding 15% of body surface area (10% in children and the elderly), preferably via two wide-bore peripheral i.v. cannulas (preferably not in a burned area). The aim is to maintain moderate hypovolaemia by providing sufficient salt and water to preserve normal organ function while minimising oedema formation. Excessive fluid administration increases the risk of circulatory overload in the days following the resuscitation period. Potentially fatal complications of excessive fluid administration include the abdominal compartment syndrome in adults[13] and cerebral oedema in children.[14] An increasing tendency in recent years to over-resuscitate burn patients has been signalled.[15,16] In contrast to other

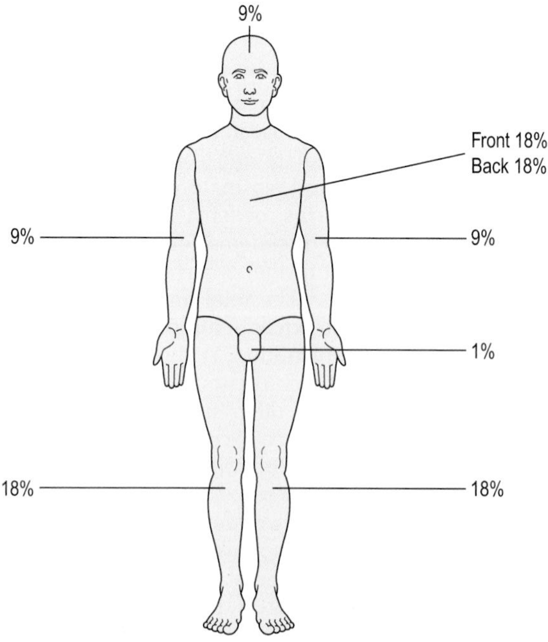

Figure 81.1 'Rule of nine' to estimate body surface area burns in adults.

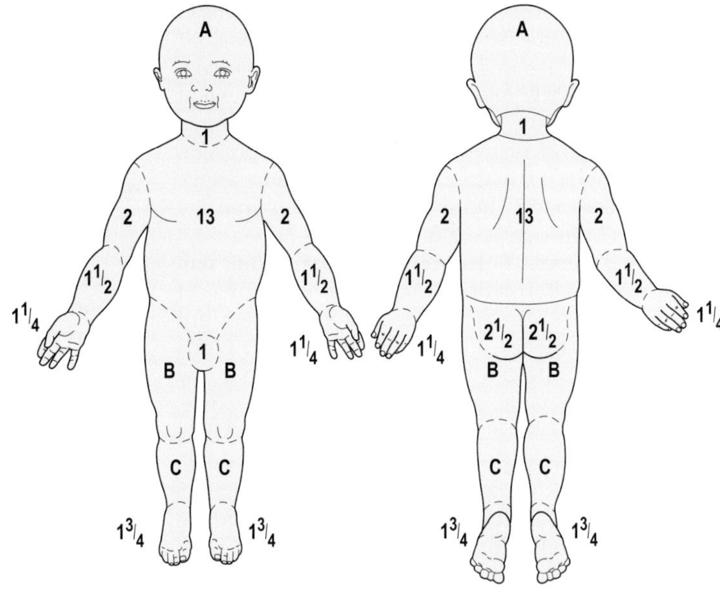

Figure 81.2 Surface area percentages by age.

Age	<1 year	1 year	5 years	10 years	15 years	Adult
Area A = 1/2 of head (%)	9.5	8.5	6.5	5.5	4.5	3.5
Area B = 1/2 of one thigh (%)	2.75	3.25	4.0	4.25	4.5	4.75
Area C = 1/2 of one leg (%)	2.5	2.5	2.75	3.0	3.25	3.5

traumatic injuries, burn hypovolaemia is gradual, obligatory and predictable. Aggressive fluid administration will not restore the circulating volume[17] and, in the absence of frank shock, bolus fluids should not be given.

Various resuscitation formulae have been published in the past to guide initial fluid therapy. These formulae are entirely experience based and many are of historical interest only, but all comprise a fluid intake of 2–4 mL/kg body weight per % burn in 24 hours, and a sodium intake of approximately 0.5 mmol/kg per % burn.[18] These findings have led some to employ resuscitation regimens based on the administration of hypertonic sodium solutions, which require a smaller volume of fluid. However, the solute load may be excessive, requiring extra water administration in subsequent days, with an increased risk of fluid overload. The use of isotonic saline solutions is therefore preferred by those without experience of burns resuscitation.

The most widely used resuscitation formula for adults is based on the Parkland Formula, which has been adopted by major training programmes such as the Advanced Trauma Life Support and the Emergency Medicine for Severe Burns:

> *4 mL Ringer-Lactate solution × kg body weight × % TBSA burn in the first 24 hours; of which half should to be given in the first 8 hours* post burn *and the other half in the next 16 hours.*

The formula thus incorporates a faster rate of administration if initial treatment has been delayed.

Children require extra fluid to compensate for basal needs. For children under 30 kg, the resuscitation formula of Carvajal[19] is useful:

$$\text{fluid requirement (mL): 0–24 hours post burn} \\ = (2000 \times \text{TBSA}) + (5000 \times \text{TBSAB}) \tag{81.1}$$

where TBSA is the total body surface area (m^2) and TBSAB is total body surface area burned (m^2). Again half of the calculated amount is given in the first 8 hours. For children under 1 year of age, one-quarter of the administered fluid should be glucose 5%.

These formulae are to be regarded as guidelines only. The actual amount of fluid given depends on the clinical condition and the actual amount of fluid administered can vary widely from that predicted. Adequacy of resuscitation is monitored by vital signs and a targeted urine output of 0.5–1 mL/kg per hour in adults and 1–2 mL/kg per hour in children. Other indicators include warm extremities and return of gut peristalsis. Fluid intake may be adjusted to maintain urine output at the desired range. Requirements are increased in the presence of mechanical ventilation, additional traumatic injury and dehydration (e.g. firefighters, intoxication).

Invasive monitoring is not essential in uncomplicated burns and the results may be misleading, as central pressures are invariably low. Hypoalbuminaemia develops rapidly and may be extreme. The extent to which burn patients will tolerate hypoalbuminaemia remains the subject of debate. In our unit at present, albumin is given to maintain serum albumin above 15 g/L, commencing 12 hours post burn when capillary integrity has been largely restored.

Thirst is common, but unrestricted oral fluids will increase oedema formation. Controlled quantities of nutritional liquids are recommended to protect gut integrity.[20] In patients with extensive injuries, tube feeding at a low rate can be commenced within a few hours of injury.

FLUID THERAPY AFTER 24 HOURS

During the second 24 hours, enteral nutritional intake is increased, while the total rate of fluid administration is gradually reduced. At the end of the second day, fluid intake should allow for generous urine production, while compensating for evaporative losses through the wounds.

The actual fluid loss through wounds varies widely, and depends on the type of burn and topical wound treatment. A useful formula to obtain a rough estimate for insensible fluid loss is:

$$(25 + \%\ \text{body surface burn}) \times \text{m}^2\ \text{body surface area} = \text{evaporative fluid loss (mL/h)} \quad (81.2)$$

Electrolyte disturbance is common following burn injury and requires treatment. Hypernatraemia is often a sign of dehydration, confirmed if serum urea is elevated. The condition is perilous, especially in the first week post burn, as oliguria and renal failure may develop unexpectedly. The amount of free water given should be increased gradually, particularly in the elderly, to avoid fluid overload. Patients who are in fluid balance may require sodium supplementation to compensate for solute loss in wound exudates.

HAEMOGLOBINUREA/MYOGLOBINUREA

Tissue injury from deep burns, particularly electrical injury, causes the release of myoglobin and haemoglobin from damaged cells. Diagnosis is made on observing discoloration of the urine, from faint pink in mild cases to almost black. Fluid administration should be increased; additional measures such as mannitol (12.5 g/L resuscitation fluid) to encourage diuresis and bicarbonate to alkalinise the urine may be considered, but the value of urine output as a guide to resuscitation is then lost.

PAIN THERAPY

During the first 24 hours, pain management is best achieved by incremental doses of i.v. morphine, or an equivalent opiate. Thereafter, the pain suffered by burn patients may be divided into background pain, which is continuous, and procedural pain caused by interventions.[21] The recurring ordeal of dressing changes, physiotherapy exercises and surgical procedures generates apprehension and anxiety, which compound distress.

Regular pain therapy is required to counter background pain, topped up by extra analgesics prior to procedures. In recent years, the advent of slow-release oral opiate medication has greatly improved the administration of analgesia. Procedural pain is best treated with continuous i.v. morphine or fentanyl, with titrated incremental boluses as required. Patient-controlled analgesia is effective, although modification of the control button may be necessary for those with bandaged hands. Ketamine in subanaesthetic doses is extremely useful for procedural pain in children. The influence of anxiety and depression on pain perception suggests additional avenues of therapy.[22] Non-pharmacological interventions, such as hypnosis and other distraction techniques, are an effective adjunct in susceptible patients.[23] Many burn patients may develop post-traumatic distress syndrome, and the emergence of symptoms may require additional support. Above all, an attitude of reassurance and understanding by all carers is indispensable.

NUTRITION

The hypermetabolic response is roughly proportional to the extent of injury. In young adults and children with extensive burns, energy expenditure may be doubled. In addition, protein and substantial amounts of trace elements, such as zinc, copper and selenium, are lost in wound exudate.[24]

There is no doubt that burn patients require additional calories and proteins, but traditional formulae for calculating requirements produce overestimates in the context of current burn care.[25] In the absence of direct metabolic measurements we currently use an empirical formula for estimating caloric intake:

$$\text{caloric requirement} = \text{REE} + (\text{REE} \times \%\ \text{TBSA burn}/100) \quad (81.3)$$

where REE is the resting energy expenditure calculated from the Harris and Benedict equation.

Patients with extensive burns will require tube feeds, which are generally well tolerated. If gastric emptying is problematic, a post-pyloric tube is usually effective. PEG tubes are useful when facial burns are present. A high-protein proprietary feed is usually adequate, but should be supplemented by extra trace elements and vitamins. The possible benefit of glutamine supplements in burns has recently been reviewed.[26] Adequacy of feeding is best assessed by monitoring body weight.

Adjunctive therapy aimed at promoting anabolism includes the use of insulin to maintain normoglycaemia, the administration of oxandrolone (10 mg twice daily for adults),[27] and the use of propanolol to control tachycardia and extensive catabolism.[28]

WOUND HEALING

Treatment of extensive, full-thickness burn wounds by early excision and grafting has been firmly linked to survival.[29] Wound excision should be completed within the first week, before bacterial colonisation and neovascular infiltration of the wound bed develop. These operations are therefore urgent. Successfully grafted wounds will heal within 5 weeks, reducing the time available for bacterial infection to develop, and shortening the period of physiological disturbance. Wounds covered with widely meshed autografts lose large amounts of fluid unless protected by a semipermeable layer, such as allograft skin. Autograft donor sites are a further source of fluid loss.

For wounds treated conservatively, the main effort is devoted to the prevention of infection. Topical antimicrobial agents are commonly used, but may have potential side-effects (**Table 81.1**). These compounds change the appearance of the wound and should never be applied until expert wound inspection is complete. A number of biosynthetic materials are currently available, which are designed to improve cosmetic and functional outcome. Despite the use of antiseptic dressings or biosynthetic coverings, there is still a risk of microbial infection developing and unexplained signs of sepsis may necessitate urgent wound revision.

PREVENTION OF WOUND INFECTION

Bacterial infection is still the most common cause of death in burns. Depression of the immune system is well documented.[30] At the same time, the burn wound presents a favourable medium for bacterial growth.

BACTERIOLOGICAL SURVEILLANCE

Routine bacteriological surveillance of burn patients (at least twice weekly) is essential. The growth of pathogens from wound swabs may reflect growing resistance to topical wound therapy, indicating a need for change. When infection is suspected, the choice of an appropriate antibiotic will be governed by prior knowledge of the colonising micro-organisms and their antibiograms. In addition, the effectiveness of prophylactic measures can be assessed only by regular monitoring of the microflora present within the burns unit.

PATIENT ISOLATION

In an effort to reduce wound colonisation and contamination from cross-infection, barrier nursing of patients with extensive injuries is mandatory. The importance of isolation measures has been stressed,[31] but a significant proportion of patients still become colonised by micro-organisms from endogenous reservoirs, which cannot be controlled by barrier nursing alone.[32,33]

Table 81.1 Commonly used topical antimicrobial agents

AGENT	COMMENTS
Silver sulfadiazine (SSD)	The most widely used agent with broad-spectrum cover. Hypersensitivity (rarely) and transient leucopenia have been reported
Cerium nitrate 0.5%	Often added to SSD, and forms a stable eschar. It is reported to bind 'burn toxins'. Methaemoglobinaemia has been reported
Silver nitrate 0.5%	Applied as a soak, and is especially effective against *Pseudomonas*. However, it may increase sodium loss, and potentially can cause methaemoglobinaemia
Mafenide acetate 5–10%	Effective but short-lived antimicrobial, requiring repeated application. It has good penetration, and its side-effects (pain and metabolic acidosis) are less evident with 5% solution
Chlorhexidine	Aqueous solution (0.2%) or 1% gel provides broad-spectrum cover, but is rapidly inactivated, and may cause local pain, and rarely causes hypersensitivity
Nitrofurazone	In polyethylene glycol (PEG) solution it is effective against *S. aureus*, but resistance develops early. Side-effects include hypersensitivity (common), hyperosmolarity, and renal failure due to PEG absorption has been reported
Povidone iodine	In PEG solution provides broad-spectrum cover, but is rapidly inactivated. It prevents wound maceration. Side-effects include occasional hypersensitivity, renal dysfunction due to excessive PEG, metabolic acidosis and rarely dysfunction
Antibiotics	Have been used in solutions, creams, gels and sprays, but selection and development of resistant strains is inevitable, with a risk of systemic toxicity through absorption. Their usage is generally discouraged

Positive experiences have been reported with selective decontamination of the digestive tract,[8,34] but large-scale prospective trials have not been performed.

THE GASTROINTESTINAL TRACT

Loss of gut integrity following burn injury has been well demonstrated.[35] In addition to reactive damage following reperfusion of the ischaemic gut, mediators derived from the burn wound itself may also be involved.[36] Clinical strategies aimed at protecting the gastrointestinal tract include optimal fluid therapy during the first hours following injury to prevent mesenteric hypoperfusion, and the institution of early enteral nutrition, which can be safely commenced within a few hours of injury.[20] Diets enriched with glutamine may contribute to the maintenance of gut integrity.[26,37] Whatever the merits of each approach, all are secondary to the maintenance of effective hygienic policies in all aspects of patient care.

WOUND SEPSIS

Local effects include disruption of wound healing and deepening of the injury.

Systemic effects are often insidious. Prodromal signs are common and may include gastrointestinal stasis, increasing positive fluid balance, increasing insulin resistance and increasing pyrexia. As sepsis progresses, clinical deterioration becomes manifest: tachypnoea, circulatory instability, thrombocytopenia and oliguria may herald the onset of multiorgan failure. Leucocyte counts and C-reactive protein levels are affected by the systemic inflammatory response syndrome (SIRS) and are unreliable indicators in the absence of clinical signs and symptoms. Procalcitonin levels seem to be more reliable. Blood cultures are indicated if sepsis is suspected.

ANTIBIOTIC THERAPY

This is chosen on the basis of bacteriological surveillance data, and should be given early if possible. Evaporative fluid loss may increase if the wound surface degenerates. Supportive therapy for (multi-)organ failure should be implemented as indicated.

The causes of sepsis will persist until wound coverage is achieved, and operative wound treatment should not be postponed. Although mortality is appreciable, experience has repeatedly shown that the prognosis is by no means hopeless.

INHALATION INJURY

The term inhalation injury includes three distinct types of injury, which often, but not always, occur together. The presence of inhalation injury may increase resuscitation fluid requirements in patients with extensive cutaneous burns.

HEAT INJURY TO THE UPPER AIRWAY

Burns due to the inhalation of hot gases (steam excepted) rarely extend beyond the larynx. The development of mucosal and facial oedema can cause respiratory obstruction, particularly in children.

DIAGNOSIS

Facial burn, singed nasal hairs, visible burn to oropharynx and hoarseness are typical features.

TREATMENT

If the condition is suspected, early endotracheal intubation is safest, before the procedure is rendered hazardous by oedema formation. However, as mechanical ventilation may aggravate oedema formation, unnecessary intubation should be avoided.

EFFECTS OF SMOKE ON THE RESPIRATORY SYSTEM

Many of the chemicals that are contained in smoke are highly reactive and produce damage to the tracheobronchial tree. Detachment of epithelial cells and the development of tracheobronchial oedema cause airway narrowing and cast formation. Small-airway closure leads to hypoxaemia and respiratory failure. Later, bronchorrhoea and mucosal sloughing may cause atelectasis and provide a focus for infection. In the absence of a cutaneous injury the clinical course is usually benign. However, the presence of an extensive skin burn increases the likelihood of acute respiratory distress syndrome (ARDS); respiratory infection may follow.

DIAGNOSIS

There is a history of exposure in a confined space, cough, breathlessness, wheeze, stridor, hypoxaemia, and soot particles in the pharynx. Diagnosis is confirmed by bronchoscopy, which may reveal soot in the bronchial tree, mucosal injury and tracheobronchial oedema.

TREATMENT

Treatment is essentially symptomatic. Mild cases may be treated by high-flow oxygen administration by mask. In severe cases intubation and ventilatory support are necessary, with positive end-expiratory pressure (PEEP) to maintain small-airway patency. Regular bronchial toilet by bronchoscopy is recommended to clear debris and to prevent respiratory infection. Endotracheal tubes may become blocked with detritus. As small-airway obstruction is common, ventilation pressures may be adversely affected. Various strategies,

Table 81.2 Common inhaled toxic gases

GAS	SOURCE	EFFECT
Carbon monoxide	Organic matter	Tissue hypoxia, lipid peroxidation
Carbon dioxide	Organic matter	Narcosis, tachycardia, hypertension
Nitrogen dioxide	Wallpaper, wood	Bronchial irritation, dizziness, pulmonary oedema
Hydrogen chloride	Plastics	Severe mucosal irritation
Hydrogen cyanide	Wood, silk, nylons, polyurethane	Headache, coma, acidosis
Benzene	Petrol, plastics	Mucosal irritation, coma
Ammonia	Nylon	Mucosal damage, extensive lung injury
Aldehyde	Wood, cotton, paper	Mucosal irritation

such as high-frequency ventilation, have been advocated to minimise the risks of barotrauma.

Prolonged respiratory assistance may be necessary. The added respiratory requirements of the hypermetabolic state combined with inevitable loss of muscle mass frequently frustrate early weaning efforts.

INHALATION OF TOXIC GASES

Of the many toxic compounds[38] in smoke (**Table 81.2**), carbon monoxide (CO) deserves special mention. The affinity of CO for haemoglobin is 240 times that of oxygen. The loss of oxygen transport capacity is dependent on the concentration of inhaled CO and the duration of exposure. In addition, CO binds to cytochrome systems, inhibiting cellular oxidative processes. The half-life of COHb is 4 hours when breathing air, compared with 45 minutes when breathing 100% oxygen.

DIAGNOSIS

Carbon monoxide poisoning should be suspected in all cases of exposure to combustion products in a closed space. The classic cherry-red appearance of the CO victim is seldom evident; early signs may be mistaken for inebriation. Symptoms range from a throbbing headache in mild exposure (10–25% COHb) to weakness, dizziness, confusion and nausea (25–40% COHb), progressing to collapse, unconsciousness and convulsions (40–60% COHb). Death is increasingly likely at COHb concentrations of >60%. Patients exposed to high levels of CO may exhibit signs of cardiac instability. Signs of cerebral irritability may persist for days or weeks following apparent recovery.

TREATMENT

Administer the highest concentration of oxygen available, as soon as possible after exposure. Loss of consciousness is an indication for oxygen delivery via an endotracheal tube. The use of hyperbaric oxygen, if immediately available, seems logical, but additional benefit has not been proven.

HYDROGEN CYANIDE TOXICITY

Hydrogen cyanide (HCN) toxicity frequently occurs in conjunction with CO inhalation. Inhaled concentrations of 200 p.p.m. are rapidly fatal and HCN may account for many deaths at fire accident scenes.[39] Conventional treatment is as for CO intoxication. Removal by chelating agents, such as hydroxycobalamin, or by the administration of sodium thiosulphate, is also possible, but treatment would have to be immediate, based on a presumptive diagnosis and is therefore not generally recommended.

FUTURE PROSPECTS

The outlook for young patients with extensive burn injuries, treated under optimal conditions, is now such that little further progress may be expected in terms of survival alone. Mortality among the elderly does, however, remain high. The major thrust of research is currently directed at improving functional and cosmetic outcome following burns. Although the most visible efforts concern the development of techniques and materials to improve the quality of wound healing, advances in the field of intensive care are also relevant: strategies aimed at preventing ventilator-associated morbidity are equally applicable to burn patients, who often require prolonged ventilatory support; new insights into the inflammatory responses may improve the general condition of burn patients, increasing resistance to infection and improving tissue repair. There is growing interest in the psychological effects of thermal trauma, which includes new approaches to the management of pain and mental distress.

In the past, the establishment of burn centres has been largely opportunistic, often depending on the dedication of individual specialists. As the provision of medical services undergoes increasing scrutiny, the organisation of burn care in many countries may be subject to reorganisation. It is of the utmost importance that specialists involved in the field of burn care become actively engaged in this process, in order to guarantee continued quality of care for their population.

Access the complete references list online at http://www.expertconsult.com

1. Herndon DN, Blakeney PE. Teamwork for total burn care: achievements, directions and hopes. In: Herndon DN, editor. Total Burn Care. 2nd ed. London: WB Saunders; 2002. p. 11–15.
4. Cioffi WG, Vaughan GM, Heironimus JD. Disassociation of blood volume and flow in regulation of salt and water balance in burn patients. Ann Surg 1991;214:213–19.
11. Martyn JAJ, Fukushima Y, Chon JY, et al. Muscle relaxants in burns, trauma, and critical illness. Int Anesthesiol Clin 2006;44:123–43.
15. Pruitt Jr BA. Protection from excessive resuscitation: 'pushing the pendulum back'. J Trauma 2000;49: 567–8.
17. Holm C, Mayr M, Tegeler J. A clinical randomised study on the effects of invasive monitoring on burn shock resuscitation. Burns 2004;30:798–807.
18. Settle JAD. Principles of replacement fluid therapy. In: Settle JAD, editor. Principles and Practice of Burns Management. London: Churchill Livingstone; 1996. p. 217–22.
21. Choinière M, Melzak R, Rondeau J. The pain of burns: characteristics and correlates. J Trauma 1989;29:1531–9.
28. Pereira CT, Murphy KD, Herndon DN. Altering metabolism. J Burn Care Rehabil 2005;26:194–9.
29. Muller MJ, Ralston D, Herndon DN. Operative wound management. In: Herndon DN, editor. Total Burn Care. 2nd ed. London: WB Saunders; 2002. p. 170–82.
35. Deitch EA. Intestinal permeability is increased in burn patients shortly after injury. Surgery 1990; 107:411–16.

82

Thermal disorders

Stephen W Lam and Richard Strickland

NORMAL TEMPERATURE REGULATION

Humans are endotherms and maintain a remarkably constant core body temperature (T_c) across an ambient range that may exceed 100°C. In order to do so, humans produce heat via oxidisation of food substrates or use of stored energy. At equilibrium:

$$\text{energy input} = \text{external work} + \text{stored energy} + \text{heat} \quad (82.1)$$

Broadly speaking, heat production may be obligatory or facultative. Obligatory production is continuous and arises from processes essential for cell survival. The major components are the basal metabolic rate and the specific dynamic action of food. Facultative production is intermittent and arises from non-shivering thermogenesis in small amounts of brown adipose tissue, from shivering thermogenesis in skeletal muscle and as a by-product of physical activity. If the environmental temperature exceeds the mean skin temperature then heat will be gained from the environment; this generally occurs when the ambient temperature exceeds 35°C. Heat is lost by radiation, conduction, convection, and vaporisation of water from sweat and the respiratory tract. These mechanisms are limited by high ambient temperature or humidity. A very small amount of heat is lost in urine and stool.

The body may be visualised as having two thermal compartments: an outer shell comprising the skin and subcutaneous fat, and an inner core. The shell acts to protect the core and provide 'feed-forward' signals that allow the body to respond to potential thermal loads.[1] Current models of thermoregulation suggest T_c is maintained in an interthreshold zone or balance point by a series of relatively autonomous thermoeffector loops dependent on a common variable, T_c.[1,2] Although there is evidence for central reciprocal cross-inhibition of thermoeffector loops, the concept of a centrally regulated set point has now been replaced.

Temperature sensing occurs in skin, tissues of the deep core and centrally, providing afferent input to thermoeffector loops. In the dermis and epidermis, temperature-activated transient receptor potential (thermo-TRP) ion channels are found on free ending axons of dorsal root ganglia. Over 30 thermo-TRP channels exist and may be cold (predominant) or heat activated at differing thresholds.[3] Inputs from these channels travel the dorsal root ganglion to ascend via multiple pathways, including lamina one of the spinal cord and spinothalamic tract to the brainstem, where fibres for discriminative sensation and homeostatic control diverge.[1] Fibres for homeostatic control project to warm sensitive neurons in the preoptic anterior hypothalamus and cold-sensitive neurons in the posterior hypothalamus. Similar afferent inputs are derived from deep thoraco-abdominal musculature, large vessels and many organs. In addition, thermosensitive neurons in the preoptic anterior hypothalamus, circumventricular organs, the midbrain and spinal cord provide central sensory input.

When thermoafferent input reaches a threshold one or more thermoeffector loops are stimulated, with a resultant heat loss or heat gain response mediated via behavioural, autonomic or endocrine changes. Behavioural responses, which appear to be driven predominantly by peripheral input, are generally more energy-efficient, afford the greatest degree of thermoregulation and often pre-empt significant changes in T_c. If behavioural responses are inadequate or unavailable, as in many ICU patients, there is recruitment of autonomic regulation.

Autonomic responses are characterised by a threshold, gain and maximal response. An increase in T_c above 37°C results in a heat loss response comprising cutaneous vasodilatation and sweating mediated via predominantly cholinergic sympathetic nerves. When accompanied by an appropriate increase in cardiac output (≈3 L/min/°C), vasodilatation results in core to cutaneous heat transfer and increased heat loss. Skin blood flow may increase from a basal rate of 0.2 L/min up to 8 L/min at $T_c \approx 39.0$°C. Reflexes maintaining blood volume and pressure take precedence over thermoregulation. An inability to increase cardiac output or dehydration will reduce both the gain and maximal response of the vasodilator and sweating thermoeffector loops respectively.[2,4]

A decrease in T_c initiates heat-preserving responses. At a threshold of 36.8°C, sympathetic adrenergic vasoconstriction occurs, and then non-shivering thermogenesis commences in small amounts of brown adipose tissue. This is of more importance in infants and enables heat production by uncoupling proton movement from ATP production across the mitochondrial inner membrane.[5] If T_c continues to fall toward 35.5°C then shivering thermogenesis begins, although the threshold and gain are reduced if the substrates for this process are inadequate – as may occur in hypoxaemia or hypoglycaemia.[2] Endocrine response includes increased secretion of cortisol and adrenaline.

The net effect of these mechanisms is maintenance of T_c around 36.9±0.4°C, with circadian variation of 0.5–1.0°C, peaking in the evening and being lowest around 6 a.m. T_c is less precisely regulated in young children who may exhibit greater diurnal variation. Whereas T_c is normally maintained in a narrow interthreshold zone, skin temperature may vary widely depending on ambient temperature and regional cutaneous blood flow. Temperature may vary amongst core organs by as much as 1.5°C during periods of rapid heat loss or gain, as in induction of therapeutic hypothermia or rewarming from cardiopulmonary bypass. The significance of this is uncertain, although it is worth noting that although the balance point at which T_c is normally maintained is close to the upper limit of survival, it is distant from the lower limit.

The ability to regulate temperature diminishes with age. In a thermoneutral environment T_c does not change in healthy older adults. When exposed to cold stress, peripheral vasoconstriction and thermogenesis are diminished both in threshold and in maximal response.[6,7] When exposed to heat stress, the elderly exhibit reduced sweat gland output and skin blood flow compared with younger controls.[6] When able, the elderly compensate for diminished autonomic thermoregulation with behavioural thermoregulation; however, this may be impaired when unwell, rendering the elderly prone to thermal insult.[6]

Patients in ICU are likely to have disturbances of both heat production and heat loss. Anaesthetic agents and opiates significantly reduce the threshold for heat loss response in a dose-dependent manner. Threshold for cutaneous vasoconstriction may fall to 34°C under general anaesthesia. Maximal response is also reduced by some agents although gain is unaltered.[8,9] In ICU sedation, cool ambient temperature, exposure, use of adrenergic, cholinergic and neuromuscular-blocking agents, ambient temperature fluid infusion, extracorporeal flow, impairment of neurological or cardiovascular function, or deficiencies of substrate for thermogenesis all alter the body's ability to maintain thermal homeostasis.

FEVER AND HYPERTHERMIA

Fever generally results from a cytokine-mediated change in threshold of thermoeffector loops resulting in regulated thermogenesis and transient elevation in T_c by 1–4°C. Hyperthermia results from failure of thermoeffector mechanisms to regulate temperature in the face of uncontrolled endogenous or exogenous heat gain. The primary event is not cytokine-mediated and T_c is usually well in excess of 40.0°C.

Various definitions of fever exist and are acceptable depending on the desired sensitivity of fever as an indicator of disease. Recognising differences in measurement technique, fever is often defined as a T_c>38.3°C.[10] Fever is common in the ICU and has many potential aetiologies (**Box 82.1**). Most are mediated by production of the pro-inflammatory cytokines IL-1, IL-6 and TNFα, which bind to receptors on circumventricular organs and up-regulate phospholipase A_2 resulting in production of prostaglandin E_2 via cyclo-oxygenase. This in turn stimulates warm-sensitive neurons in the preoptic anterior hypothalamus, shifting the threshold of cold-sensitive thermoeffectors by as much as 2°C, so inducing vasoconstriction and thermogenesis.[1,11] As pyrogen

Box 82.1 Potential causes of fever in ICU

Infection (50%)
Inflammatory
- Trauma/burns/surgery
- Pancreatitis
- Pneumonitis/VILI/ARDS
- Autoimmune disorders:
  - hypersensitivity reactions (including transplant rejection)
  - connective tissue disorders
  - inflammatory bowel disease
  - hepatitis
  - myocarditis
  - vasculitis
  - neuropathies (GBS)/myopathies
- Gout
- Acalculous cholecystitis
- Granulomatous disease

Infarction
- Myocardial
- Cerebral
- Gastrointestinal tract (GIT)
- Pulmonary
- Other

Haemorrhage
- Subarachnoid (SAH)/GIT/other
- Haematoma reabsorption

Haematological/oncological
- Blood product transfusion
- Malignancy/tumour lysis
- Radiotherapy

Endocrine
- Thyrotoxicosis
- Phaeochromocytoma
- Adrenocorticoid insufficiency

Seizures
Drugs
- Adverse reactions
- Overdose/withdrawal

levels fall, thermoeffector thresholds return to normal and T_c falls.

Mild to moderate fever is a phylogenetically preserved response and may provide survival benefit.[11] There is little evidence to suggest benefit from routine treatment of mild–moderate fever outside the setting of acute brain injury, cardiogenic shock or profound hypoxaemia.[12] As T_c progresses above 40.0°C, however, deleterious effects may occur and measures to control T_c should be considered whilst the underlying disorder is treated. In the case of fever, antipyretics may be adequate. Hyperthermias require active measures.

At a subcellular level hyperthermia has widespread effects that depend on both maximal T_c and duration of exposure. These include alteration of enzymatic function and protein folding that disrupts many cellular systems including ion channels, surface receptors, mitochondrial electron transport and cytoskeletal elements. Different individuals and cell lines exhibit different resistance to thermal injury. In general, short-term elevation in T_c to 40°C is tolerated without harm and may provide transient protection from further thermal injury via up-regulation of heat shock proteins.[13,14] Beyond this cellular and organ system dysfunction occur. These changes represent a spectrum of disease evolution with progressive damage as T_c or exposure duration increases. A T_c greater than 43°C is immediately life-threatening. Major organ system effects as core temperature rises are summarised in **Table 82.1**.

HYPERTHERMIAS

HEAT STROKE

Heat stroke represents the severest form of the spectrum of heat-related illness. It is characterised by T_c>40°C and neurological dysfunction ranging from restlessness to delirium, seizures and coma.[15] Heat stroke may be classified as either classic (passive) or exertional (active). Classic heat stroke occurs following exposure to high ambient temperatures in those at the extremes of age or with co-morbid disease or medications that affect thermoregulation (**Box 82.2**). Exertional heat stroke occurs in healthy individuals who undertake strenuous activity in environments with high ambient temperature and humidity, reducing the efficiency of radiative and evaporative heat loss. Although the incidence of certain organ dysfunction varies slightly between the two forms, management is the same and they will be discussed together.

The pathogenesis of organ dysfunction in heat stroke has been the subject of much research and our understanding remains incomplete. Elevations in T_c alter cellular and organ function as detailed above. The role of the cytokine response is unclear. In humans levels of TNFα and IL-6 have been correlated directly with severity of heat stroke.[15] In murine models pro- and anti-inflammatory cytokines were suppressed during onset of hyperthermia, rising 2–4 hours after maximal T_c was reached, and TNFα and IL-6 double-knockout mice exhibited increased heat stroke mortality.[16,17] It appears likely that components of the cytokine response serve a protective function.

Heat stroke is far more amenable to prevention rather than treatment. Most patients present with a delirium or coma, although focal neurology may occur. T_c is usually >40.5°C and patients are vasodilated with evolving distributive shock and multi-organ dysfunction. Sweating is not always present. Disorders that may present in a similar fashion require exclusion (**Box 82.3**). Management is essentially supportive; principles include the following:

- *Resuscitation:*
  - recognise the need for alveolar hyperventilation
  - restore circulating volume with cold 0.9% saline.
- *Cooling:*
  - accurately monitor core temperature (see section Core temperature measurement)
  - aggressively cool to return and maintain T_c<39°C **(Table 82.2)**
  - non-invasive measures that minimise cutaneous vasoconstriction and shivering are usually adequate.
- *Organ support:*
  - assess and support cardiorespiratory, renal, hepatic, haematological, endocrine and neurological function
  - hypotension usually responds to adequate cooling and volume replacement
  - seizures are probably best treated with benzodiazepines
  - prophylactic antibiotics are not recommended; however, endotoxaemia is a common complication and if clinically suspected appropriate cultures and Gram-negative cover are indicated
  - insulin receptor expression is down-regulated during hyperthermia, so there is a risk of hypoglycaemia after cooling with large initial doses of insulin.
- *Identify and manage precipitants (see Box 82.2):*
  - withhold agents impairing thermoregulation
  - treat underlying infection, dehydration or endocrine disorders.

The use of dantrolene has been reported in case series; however, it has been found to be ineffective.[18] Use of antipyretics is common although benefit has not been established and there is an association between the use of paracetamol and incidence of hepatic dysfunction.[15] The normal response to recovery from hyperthermia in mammals is biphasic, with initial hypothermia and then mild hyperthermia prior to restoration of thermal homeostasis. Traditional teaching has been to avoid hypothermia during recovery. In murine models prevention of hypothermia during recovery was associated with greater hypotension and mortality.[17] It is

Table 82.1 Organ system effects of change in T_c

20°C 28°C	30°C 32°C	34°C 35°C≈T_C	ORGAN SYSTEM	T_C≈38.3 → 40.0°C	42.0°C INCREASING TIME	44.0°C →
Cerebral metabolism falls by around 8%/°C Confusion progresses to coma, hyporeflexia, unreactive pupils Cerebral electrical activity is absent below 20°C			CNS	Increased CMRO and $CMR_{glucose}$ Reduced cerebral blood flow as Pa_{CO_2} falls	Agitation/Delirium Blood–brain barrier injury ↑ CSF protein/ lymphocytes	Coma, seizures Cerebral oedema Cortical infarction – especially cerebellum
Cardiac output halved at 28°C ↓ Contractility AF with slow ventricular rate at <30°C, VF at <28°C, Asystole at <20°C	Increasing PR, QRS and QT_c intervals (slowed K^+ flux) Osborne J wave below 33°C (height increasing with severity of hypothermia)	Initial increase in heart rate, then progressive fall (HR=45–55 at 33°C) ↑ Contractility±mild diastolic dysfunction V_{O_2} falls 8%/°C	CVS	Tachycardia, vasodilatation ↑ Stroke volume ↓ CVP/SVR Small decrease MAP Increase in V_{O_2}≈10%/°C	Progressive tachycardia Reduced stroke volume and MAP Reduced D_{O_2} if acidaemic	Hypotension/shock Myocardial infarction
Pulmonary oedema Apnoea	Respiratory depression ↓ Cough reflex ↑ Bronchial secretions ↓ Mucociliary clearance	↑ Respiratory rate and minute ventilation	Respiratory	Increased minute ventilation – mild respiratory alkalosis	Marked respiratory alkalosis±metabolic acidosis	Intravascular thrombosis Hypoxaemia ARDS
Fluid compartment shifting, haemoconcentration, blood viscosity increases ≈2%/°C Reduced platelet aggregation and adhesion at <35°C (decreased TxA_2 and glycoprotein Ib-IX) Reduced coagulation factors and platelet adhesion inhibitor (PAI) function at <33°C Non-linear reduction in both tPA and plasminogen activator inhibitor-1 activity; net result is unpredictable Hypercoagulability and DIC may also result			Haematological	Increased haematocrit if fluid intake inadequate	Direct activation of endothelium and platelets (increased vWF) Increased fibrinolysis Increased endothelial permeability	↑ Circulating tissue factor Microvascular thrombosis DIC Widespread haemorrhage Endothelial apoptosis

Hepatic and splenic sequestration causing thrombocytopenia and leucopenia Immune dysfunction (including white blood cells, reduced lymphocyte activation, natural killer cells, cytokines, complement)			Immunological	Leucocytosis Increased T- and B-cell activation, neutrophil/ macrophage diapedesis and cytotoxicity ↓ Serum iron	Leucopenia Reduced cell-mediated cytotoxicity Lymphoid apoptosis and necrosis	
Acute tubular dysfunction	↓ ADH tubular ADH resistance	ANP release and diuresis Increased K^+, Mg^{2+}, Pa_4^{3-} excretion	Renal	↓ Renal blood flow	Tubular necrosis Glomerular microthrombus and haemorrhage	
Pancreatitis Lactic and ketoacidosis		↓ GI motility	Gastrointestinal	↓ Splanchnic blood flow	Enterocyte exfoliation – increased mucosal permeability	Bacterial translocation – endotoxaemia Intestinal infarction Pancreatic infarction
Reduced drug metabolism			Hepatic		Hepatocyte oedema and fatty infiltration	Haemorrhagic and coagulative necrosis, hepatic failure
↓ Catecholamine and cortisol secretion		↓ Insulin secretion and insulin resistance Glycogenolysis ↑ Catecholamine and cortisol secretion	Endocrine/ metabolic	↑ Cortisol/glucagon secretion ↑ Metabolic rate	Insulin resistance Hyperglycaemia Hypokalaemia	Hypoglycaemia Hyperkalaemia Adrenal haemorrhage
Loss of shivering, rhabdomyolysis		Shivering	Musculoskeletal		Rhabdomyolysis	
Vasoconstriction			Skin	Vasodilatation (cutaneous blood flow ↑ up to 8 L/min) Sweat production	Vasodilatation Diminishing sweat production	Reduced cutaneous blood flow if cardiac output falls, anhydrosis

Box 82.2 Risk factors for heat stroke

Age
- Extremes of age

Environmental
- High ambient temperature and humidity
- Poor ventilation/lack of air conditioning

Behavioural
- Immobility
- Lack of acclimatisation
- Salt and water deprivation
- Obesity

Underlying conditions
- Cardiovascular disease
- Respiratory disease
- Infection/fever
- Diabetes
- Malnutrition
- Alcoholism
- Hyperthyroidism
- Impaired sweat production

Drugs
- Antihypertensives (angiotensin-converting enzyme inhibitors (ACEIs), beta blockers, diuretics)
- Butyrophenones and phenothiazines
- Anticholinergics
- Antiparkinsonians
- Antihistamines
- Tricyclics
- Sympathomimetics

Box 82.3 Differential diagnosis of hyperthermia

Environmental hyperthermias	CNS disease
Heat stroke	Status epilepticus Hypothalamic stroke Granulomatous disease
Drug-induced hyperthermia	**Infectious**
Malignant hyperpyrexia Neuroleptic malignant syndrome Serotonin syndrome Anticholinergic toxicity Sympathomimetic toxicity Salicylate toxicity MAOI toxicity Withdrawal (alcohol, benzodiazepines, baclofen)	Sepsis Encephalitis Meningitis Cerebral abscess Tetanus Malaria Typhoid
Endocrine disorders	**Psychiatric disease**
Thyrotoxicosis Phaeochromocytoma	Lethal catatonia

uncertain whether mild hypothermia should be allowed in humans during treatment for heat stroke.

Heat stroke mortality remains high with an in-hospital mortality of 65% being reported in a large, prospective observational study of classic heat stroke.[19] Those factors strongly associated with death included immobility, psychiatric or cardiovascular disease, T_c and number of organ failures at admission. Survivors often have significant long-term morbidity, predominantly secondary to neurological impairment.

MALIGNANT HYPERTHERMIA

Malignant hyperthermia (MH) is a rare, autosomal dominant, pharmacogenetic myopathy with variable penetrance. It is characterised by a hypermetabolic state and skeletal muscle rigidity manifested when a susceptible individual is exposed to volatile anaesthetics or depolarising muscle relaxants. The disorder results from abnormal sarcoplasmic calcium flux and in 70% of cases is linked to a mutation in the ryanodine receptor RYR1. However, 30% of individuals with MH do not have RYR1 mutations, and other candidate proteins include calsequestrin-1 and the dihydropyridine receptor.[20] Upon triggering the abnormal RYR1 receptor is thought to release excessive calcium into the cytosol resulting in sustained excitation–contraction coupling. Sustained contraction and increased Ca^{2+}–ATPase activity result in increased aerobic glycolysis; however, muscle blood flow is reduced and eventually metabolism becomes anaerobic, with onset of metabolic acidosis.

Almost all cases are associated with use of a volatile anaesthetic±succinylcholine.[21] The earliest clinical sign is that of masseter spasm; however, this is neither specific nor sensitive. Hypercarbia disproportional to minute ventilation, sinus tachycardia and a rapidly rising temperature are the cardinal features, associated with generalised muscular rigidity in 40%.[21] These usually occur within 2 hours of exposure. In the ICU early diagnosis may be difficult as hypercarbia and tachycardia are common, although if out of keeping with the clinical situation or associated with other features such as muscular rigidity the diagnosis of MH should be considered. Fortunately the incidence of MH is extremely low if volatiles are avoided. Less common signs include tachypnoea, cyanosis, diaphoresis, cola-coloured urine, bleeding and ventricular dysrhythmias.

Triggering agents should be avoided in those with a history or family history of MH. If MH is suspected immediate management includes the following:

- Cease triggering agents. If using an anaesthetic circuit, flush the circuit. Increase minute ventilation.
- Give intravenous dantrolene 2.5 mg/kg rapidly. Repeat every 5–10 minutes until hypercarbia and temperature respond. Maximal initial dose 10 mg/kg (median required 6 mg/kg).[21]
- Treat hyperkalaemia/metabolic acidosis with bicarbonate.
- Cool the patient to T_c 36–38°C.

Table 82.2 Methods of temperature manipulation

CLASSIFICATION		METHOD	RATE OF CHANGE (°C/H)
Passive	Warming	Warm (>24°C) environment Insulating blanket	0.5–1
	Cooling	Cool environment Exposure (removal blankets/clothes)	
Active external	Warming	Warm forced-air blankets Water circulating heating control blanket Radiant heaters Temperature control pads (e.g. Arctic Sun, Medivance Inc., Louisville, CO)	1 1 1–2 1.5–3
	Cooling	Wet towels/ice packs Water circulating cooling control blanket Evaporative cooling (fan+tepid mist) Temperature control pads	1 1 1–2 1.5–3
Active internal	Warming	Humidified warm inspired gases Intravascular temperature control catheter (e.g. Alsius Coolgard, Irvine, CA; Celsius Control System, Innercool Therapies Inc., San Diego, CA) Body cavity lavage isotonic saline (gastric, right pleural 200 mL, peritoneal 10 mL/kg, bladder) Extracorporeal: renal replacement circuit cardiopulmonary bypass	0.5–1 2–4 2–3 5 10
	Cooling	Cool intravenous fluids (4°C: 30–40 mL/kg) Intravascular temperature control catheter Body cavity lavage isotonic saline (gastric, right pleural 200 mL, peritoneal 10 mL/kg, bladder) Extracorporeal: renal replacement circuit cardiopulmonary bypass	2–3 2–4 3 5 10

- Identify and treat complications:
  - cardiac arrhythmias:
    - usually respond to correction of hyperkalaemia and acidosis
    - avoid calcium antagonists, which may cause severe hyperkalaemia and cardiac arrest with high-dose dantrolene
  - rhabdomyolysis
  - disseminated intravascular coagulation (DIC).

All cases should be appropriately monitored until resolution. Dantrolene should be continued at 1 mg/kg 4–6-hourly for 24–48 hours. Failure to respond should prompt a search for an alternative diagnosis. Suspected cases should be referred to a MH screening centre. Testing usually includes a caffeine/halothane contracture test and genetic screening of relatives of confirmed cases for RYR1 mutations. Outcome of MH is good with mortality less than 10%. Additional resources are available from the Malignant Hyperthermia Association of the United States (http://www.mhaus.org/).

NEUROLEPTIC MALIGNANT SYNDROME

Neuroleptic malignant syndrome (NMS) is an idiosyncratic reaction characterised by hyperthermia, muscle rigidity, mental state change and autonomic dysfunction. It typically occurs within a month of introduction, or dose increment of an antipsychotic agent (including atypical antipsychotics). Other drugs that antagonise central dopamine transmission or rapid cessation of central dopamine agonist may also precipitate NMS.[22]

NMS is thought to occur as a result of central dopamine antagonism, predominantly at the D2 receptor. In the hypothalamus this results in hyperthermia, whilst mesocortical and nigrostriatal blockade result in mental state change and extrapyramidal symptoms respectively. It is postulated that a loss of central integration gives rise to autonomic instability.[22,23]

The clinical presentation is one of hyperthermia (usually <42°C), 'lead-pipe' rigidity, tachycardia, labile hypertension and delirium or coma. This may be accompanied by hypoventilation, diaphoresis, tremor, incontinence or mutism. Onset is usually over hours to days and the diagnosis requires exclusion of other conditions that may mimic NMS (see Box 82.3). A peripheral leucocytosis is common, and creatine kinase is usually above 1000 IU/L; however, it may be much higher. Acute kidney injury and DIC complicate severe cases. Neuroimaging studies and CSF analysis are normal in 95% and EEG shows generalised slowing.[23]

Differentiation from other hyperthermias relies predominantly on drug and environmental history, the presence of hypertonia rather than hypotonia (heat stroke) and absence of serotonergic features. If there is clinical suspicion of infection then appropriate cultures including CSF should be performed after neuroimaging. If seizures are suspected an EEG is required.

Usually only severe NMS requires ICU support. Therapy includes:

- resuscitation - sedation±neuromuscular blockade may reduce severity of hyperthermia, rhabdomyolysis and other complications
- cessation of any potentially causative agent or re-introduction of acutely withdrawn dopamine agonist
- cooling to maintain T_c<39°C
- supportive care and management of complications:
  - respiratory failure (hypoventilation or aspiration)
  - rhabdomyolysis
  - AKI
  - DIC
  - arrhythmias
- potential adjunctive therapies including:
  - benzodiazepines or central alpha agonist for agitation
  - benzodiazepines for seizures or catatonia
  - bromocriptine 2.5–5 mg entrally 8-hourly
    - case series suggest reduced extrapyramidal symptoms and mortality
    - may worsen hypotension or psychosis
  - ECT - case series suggest ECT is safe and effective if NMS is prolonged or psychotic symptoms persist, although most patients were not in ICU.[24]

Dantrolene has been used in severe cases; however, there is no RYR1 abnormality in NMS and recent meta-analysis of published cases suggest no benefit.[23] Drug withdrawal and supportive measures are usually adequate and mortality is <10%. Psychiatric advice should be sought prior to re-introduction of antipsychotics.

SEROTONIN SYNDROME

A wide range of drugs are associated with the syndrome of serotoninergic toxicity. These include selective serotonin reuptake inhibitors (SSRIs), serotonin and norepinephrine reuptake inhibitors (SNRIs), monoamine oxidase inhibitors (MAOIs) (including linezolid and methylene blue), lithium, amphetamines, pethidine, fentanyl, tramadol, triptans and St John's wort. Severe serotonin toxicity occurs only after concurrent use of two or more serotoninergic agents, usually a SSRI and MAOI, and is thought to be mediated predominantly via the $5HT_{2A}$ receptor.[25]

Severe serotonin toxicity presents with altered mental state (agitation, delirium, coma), autonomic stimulation (tachycardia, hyperthermia, diaphoresis, tremor) and neuromuscular excitation (clonus, hyperreflexia, rigidity). Features with greater specificity for serotonin toxicity include hyperreflexia, lower limb or ocular clonus and myoclonus. Rigidity tends to be predominantly lower limb.[25]

Management of severe toxicity involves resuscitation, withdrawal of offending agents, cooling and supportive care. Complications are similar to those observed in the other hyperthermias. Adjunctive therapies are of less importance. These include the $5HT_{2A}$ agonist cyproheptadine, 4–8 mg enterally 6-hourly or chlorpromazine if enteral administration is not possible.

SYMPATHOMIMETIC TOXICITY

Hyperthermia may be precipitated by all centrally acting sympathomimetics by increasing release, inhibiting metabolism or preventing re-uptake of norepinephrine (noradrenaline), serotonin and dopamine, usually in a dose-dependent fashion. This results in increased muscle thermogenesis and impairs heat loss. In severe cases the clinical picture is that of a rapidly progressive hyperthermia with marked delirium or coma, rhabdomyolysis, DIC and multi-organ dysfunction. As with other severe hyperthermias, early and aggressive supportive care is indicated. Intubation, neuromuscular blockade and aggressive cooling are often required. Plasma potassium may rise very rapidly and require dialysis. There are no specific therapies and although dantrolene has been advocated there is insufficient evidence to support routine use.

ANTIMUSCARINIC TOXICITY

A wide variety of antimuscarinic agents exist. Peripheral toxicity causes tachycardia, cutaneous vasodilatation, mydriasis, urinary retention and impaired sweating. Central toxicity gives rise to tremor, delirium and occasionally seizures. Severe hyperthermia with rhabdomyolysis and DIC may occur; however, this is unusual and most antimuscarinic toxidromes are adequately managed with drug withdrawal, titrated benzodiazepine and passive cooling.

HYPOTHERMIA

DEFINITION AND CLASSIFICATION

Hypothermia is defined as core temperature less than 35°C, and it may develop due to abnormal

Box 82.4 Important causes and contributors of hypothermia

Increased heat loss
- Surface conduction, convection, radiation, or evaporation
- Vasodilatation, dermatological disruption
- Extremes of age

Reduced heat production
- Endocrine (e.g. diabetic ketoacidosis, hypopituitarism, hypoadrenalism, hypothyroidism)
- Reduced energy reserve or substrate (e.g. hypoglycaemia, malnutrition, hypoxaemia)
- Immobility and reduced neuromuscular activity
- Extremes of age

Impaired or abnormal central thermoregulation
- Central nervous system disorders
- Pharmacological and toxicological (e.g. alcohol, CNS depressants, psychotropics)
- Uraemia
- Sepsis
- Malignancy

thermoregulation or heat loss overwhelming thermoregulatory capacity. Important causes and contributing factors are summarised in **Box 82.4**.

Severity is somewhat arbitrarily classified as:

- mild (32–35°C)
- moderate (28–32 °C)
- severe (T_c<28 °C).

Hypothermia may be unintentional (often referred to as 'accidental'), or intentional (therapeutic hypothermia, TH). This can be further divided into:

- primary (intact thermoregulation)
- secondary (abnormal thermoregulation)
- tertiary hypothermia (induced for therapeutic purpose, as in TH).

PHYSIOLOGICAL EFFECTS OF HYPOTHERMIA

Hypothermia alters a wide range of molecular and cellular functions, some of which may be exploited for therapeutic purpose. However, prolonged or severe hypothermia causes progressive deterioration in organ function.

Manifestations of the normal thermoregulatory response predominate in patients with cold exposure or very mild primary or tertiary hypothermia (generally with T_c above 34°C). Patients with abnormal thermoregulatory capacity (especially those with dysautonomia) may lack some of these features and are more prone to developing secondary hypothermia. There is an increase in catecholamine and cortisol secretion, and sympathetic activation is evident with:

- increase in respiratory rate
- increase in heart rate and contractility
- mild diastolic cardiac dysfunction
- vasoconstriction with reduced tissue perfusion
- increase in muscle tone and shivering. This can increase heat production and oxygen consumption several-fold, but largely settles at temperatures below 34°C. Application of surface warming and the use of alfentanil, fentanyl, pethidine, propofol, dexmedetomidine, clonidine, or magnesium are often effective in reducing shivering.

The Swiss staging system describes five clinical stages of severity in primary hypothermia:[26]

- *stage I:* clearly conscious and shivering
- *stage II:* impaired consciousness without shivering
- *stage III:* unconscious
- *stage IV:* no breathing, no signs of life
- *stage V:* death due to irreversible hypothermia.

Table 82.1 provides a summary of the physiological effects of hypothermia.

MANAGEMENT OF PATIENTS WITH ABNORMAL CORE TEMPERATURE

This section provides a summary of some important clinical considerations in the management of patients with abnormal core temperature.

CORE TEMPERATURE MEASUREMENT

The temperature of blood perfusing the hypothalamus is considered the reference point for T_c. The pulmonary artery catheter is the most accurate means for temperature measurement.

Compared with pulmonary artery catheters, the most accurate means of temperature measurement are oesophageal probe in the lower quarter of the oesophagus (0.11±0.3°C) and urinary bladder catheter (−0.2±0.2°C). Less accurate are rectal, inguinal and axillary measurements.[27–29]

Urinary bladder temperature measurement is less reliable in oliguria. The accuracy of tympanic measurements is somewhat variable and may be inaccurate in significant hypothermia, while oesophageal temperature measurement may be influenced by gas temperature in the trachea.[29,30]

There may also be differences of around 1.5°C between regions of the body and brain, particularly during rapid temperature change, and cerebral thermopooling (regions of increased brain temperature) can occur.[31,32]

PHARMACOLOGICAL EFFECTS OF ALTERED BODY TEMPERATURE

Much work in this area has been performed on animal models and understanding of drug pharmacology in humans during hypothermia or hyperthermia is limited. Although each drug requires characterisation across temperatures, some principles provide guidance.

Febrile patients with SIRS may have high cardiac output with resultant increase in renal and hepatic blood flow. Augmented renal clearance of a number of antimicrobials has been well described in subgroups of ICU patients.[33] Although hepatic blood flow may increase, the acute phase response suppresses expression of many cytokines and the net effect of fever on hepatic clearance in humans is uncertain. In severe hyperthermia organ dysfunction is likely to result in markedly altered pharmacokinetics.

In hypothermia, absorption of orally administered drugs is significantly slowed. Bioavailability, depending upon hepatic extraction, varies between drugs. Effect on volume of distribution (*Vd*) is variable as tissue blood flow, protein binding and ionisation change. For example, the *Vd* of midazolam increases 83% at 33°C, whilst the *Vd* of pancuronium decreases.[34] Altered ionisation is of significance in drugs with a pKa between 7–8 and narrow therapeutic window (e.g. lidocaine). In this setting pH-stat ventilation may be wise.[34] Hypothermia reduces hepatic blood flow and slows enzyme kinetics resulting in reduced hepatic and extrahepatic clearance. Renal flow, glomerular filtration rate (GFR) and tubular secretion are also reduced.[35] In moderate hypothermia clearance of propofol, morphine and vecuronium are reduced by 10–25%.[34] Pro-drugs therefore have a slower onset, whereas active drugs and those with active metabolites have prolonged duration of action and increased risk of toxicity.

Pharmacodynamic changes with hypothermia are variable and poorly characterised. Rewarming brings about further kinetic and dynamic alterations. In patients with significant alterations in T_c it seems wise to dose parenterally, avoid pro-drugs and agents with multiple active metabolites, and when possible titrate to a clinical end-point or undertake temperature-corrected therapeutic drug monitoring.

ACID–BASE AND BLOOD GAS INTERPRETATION

Blood gas analysers heat or cool samples to 37°C at which they are calibrated to perform measurements. Deviation in body temperature from 37°C therefore results in a difference between the patient's true values and those derived from the blood gas analyser, which may be clinically significant.

The solubility of a gas is inversely related to the temperature of the solution. Therefore, a hypothermic patient will actually have lower Pa_{O_2} and Pa_{CO_2} than values derived from blood gas analysis performed at 37°C, whereas the opposite is true in fever and hyperthermia (Henry's law). The relationship between temperature and gas solubility is non-linear and correction factors are required to estimate true blood gas values in the patient.[36]

Because cerebrovascular reactivity to Pa_{CO_2} is preserved, calculation of the patient's true Pa_{CO_2} may be relevant in patients with raised intracranial pressure. Maternal acid–base status may also be particularly relevant to the fetus during pregnancy.[37,38]

VENTILATION STRATEGIES

Data on ventilatory strategies are mostly derived from patients undergoing hypothermic cardiopulmonary bypass and therapeutic hypothermia following central nervous system injury. It is uncertain whether mechanical ventilation should be adjusted to achieve Pa_{CO_2} and pH targets according to the arterial blood gas values measured at 37°C (alpha-stat method), or corrected to the patient's body temperature (pH-stat method).[39–41]

Regardless of ventilation strategy, it should always be noted that measured Pa_{O_2} is not the true patient value if T_c is significantly greater or less than 37°C.

ALPHA-STAT STRATEGY

This strategy is based on the theory that maintaining the pH of neutrality (pN) is important for cellular enzyme function and metabolism. The imidazole group of histadine is an important component of protein acid–base buffering, and has a pN that changes with temperature. Imidazole ionisation fraction (denoted as alpha) remains constant as body temperature changes (if CO_2 content also remains constant) thereby maintaining constant net charge of proteins and maximal ionisation of intracellular metabolic intermediates. When applying alpha-stat theory, measures are taken to adjust Pa_{CO_2} to meet its target value at 37°C, without being corrected for actual patient temperature.

PH-STAT STRATEGY

This strategy is based on the theory that pH should be kept at its target value throughout the range of patient temperatures, and that cerebral blood flow autoregulation continues to react to Pa_{CO_2}. There is no reference range for temperatures other than 37°C, and the pH-stat approach assumes that values appropriate for 37°C remain so for all temperatures. This may be particularly relevant in patients with narrower Pa_{CO_2} and/or pH targets, such as those with raised intracranial pressure and in pregnancy.

Use of pH-stat in hypothermic patients requires an increase in CO_2 content, and therefore results in cerebral vasodilatation above the brain's metabolic demand, which may worsen pre-existing intracranial hypertension. It does, however, counteract the leftward shift in the oxyhaemoglobin dissociation curve caused by hypothermia.

TRANSCUTANEOUS PULSE OXIMETRY RESPONSE TIMES IN HYPOTHERMIA

In hypothermic patients the detection of changes in haemoglobin oxygen saturation by transcutaneous pulse oximetry may be significantly slower using finger probes compared with forehead sensors.[42]

HAEMOSTATIC ASSESSMENT

In the same manner as blood gas analysis, common tests of haemostasis such as the thromboelastograph (TE), activated partial-thromboplastin time (aPTT), and prothrombin and thrombin times are measured with blood samples at 37°C. Hypothermic effects on platelet and coagulation enzyme function are reversible with rewarming, and hence laboratory values may be misleading when considering the patient's haemostatic capacity.[30,43] Measurements can be performed at other temperatures with prior calibration of equipment.

MANAGEMENT OF CARDIAC ARREST

No recommendations for modification of standard cardiopulmonary resuscitation have been made for fever or hyperthemia.

Severe hypothermia can produce a clinical state that mimics prolonged circulatory arrest and poor prognosis with apnoea, asystole, unreactive pupils and areflexia. However, good outcomes have been achieved with prolonged resuscitation in such patients and efforts should be continued in conjunction with aggressive rewarming until return of spontaneous circulation or T_c of 35°C is achieved.[44] Rewarming is important in restoring perfusing cardiac rhythm in patients with VF or VT and may also resolve atrial arrhythmias, atrioventricular block and bradycardia.

The optimal dose and timing of defibrillation and drugs in hypothermic cardiac arrest patients have not been established.[45] Recommendations for reducing or withholding drugs and defibrillation in hypothermic cardiac arrest patients are based on mostly theoretical concerns over cardiac unresponsiveness to drugs and defibrillation, and reduced drug metabolism that might result in drug toxicity with repeated dosing.[44]

The suggested modification for cardiopulmonary resuscitation of hypothermic patients involves:[46]

- withholding drugs until temperature is >30°C, then doubling usual drug intervals until temperature is >35°C
- delivery of up to three shocks using maximum energy for VT or VF, and thereafter withholding further shocks until temperature is >30°C. Rhythms other than VF may revert spontaneously with rewarming.

The optimal timing and dose of cardiac arrest drugs is not known for normothermic or hypothermic patients. Animal studies have found vasoactive drugs and defibrillation to be effective in the setting of hypothermia, and success in humans has been reported.[44,47] Currently, there is inadequate evidence to make strong recommendations on how to modify standard cardiopulmonary resuscitation algorithms in the setting of hypothermia.[44]

TEMPERATURE MANAGEMENT AND CONTROL

CONTROLLING FEVER AND HYPERTHERMIA

In the patient with severe hyperthermia, early aggressive pharmacological and physical measures are indicated to reduce or avoid the adverse consequences of elevated T_c. Sedation, intubation and neuromuscular blockade may be required in severe cases. Physical methods that are rapidly available and achieve high cooling rate should be employed (see Table 82.2).

In the case of fever, and especially sepsis, the concept of manipulating T_c is somewhat more controversial. Although controlling fever may reduce metabolic workload (unless uncontrolled shivering occurs) and appears to reduce vasopressor requirement in septic shock, its net effect on immune function, development of acute lung injury and survival are unknown.[48–51] Similarly, whilst fever and hyperthermia cause secondary neurological injury, benefit from controlled normothermia is yet to be conclusively demonstrated.[52]

Where temperature is pyrogen-mediated the use of an antipyretic such as paracetamol seems logical, although this has been questioned by some animal studies.[53] Paracetamol acts predominantly by central inhibition of cyclo-oxygenase and results in temperature reduction of 0.3–0.4°C, without inducing a counter-regulatory response.[54] Other agents that suppress thresholds for thermogenesis and may be appropriate in the non-ventilated patient include magnesium, opiates, benzodiazepines, clonidine and tramadol.[39]

Control of fever or maintenance of normothermia in the non-sedated, non-intubated patient can be challenging if thermoregulation is intact, with the balance point for T_c often being elevated by endogenous pyrogens or direct hypothalamic insult. The application of physical modes of cooling without pharmacological measures to alter thermoeffector response results in shivering and increased cardiorespiratory workload. In such cases, the risks associated with need for sedation and even intubation and paralysis in order to achieve additional cooling must be weighed against potential benefit of temperature control.

CORRECTING HYPOTHERMIA

The various methods of increasing core temperature are summarised in Table 82.2.

In general, it is considered that:

- for patients with intact autoregulatory thermogenesis and temperature >34°C, passive rewarming alone may be adequate
- patients with spontaneous circulation and temperature <34°C often require addition of active external warming
- patients with temperature <30°C usually require active internal warming; extracorporeal techniques

are the most effective and are generally required in the setting of cardiac arrest.

Warming of intravenous fluid (generally to around 40°C) prior to administration is important in limiting further hypothermia, but is an inefficient means of rewarming. Gastric and bladder irrigation also have limited effectiveness.

During rewarming, care should be taken to avoid precipitation of cardiac arrhythmias by sudden movement and invasive intervention; however, this concern should not influence the performance of life-supportive manoeuvres such as intubation and central venous catheterisation, and it is very rare at temperatures above 30°C.[39,44,46] Hyperkalaemia may develop due to extracellular shifting, and the return of insulin sensitivity may result in potentially detrimental hypoglycaemia and high blood glucose variation.[55,56] Rapid rewarming causes cerebral vasodilatation and impairs cerebral blood flow autoregulation, and hence any intracranial hypertension would be expected to worsen. Vasodilatation often results in the need for intravenous fluid administration; however, the potassium (and perhaps lactate) content in lactated Ringer's solution may be problematic in hypothermic patients being rewarmed.

In patients who have become hypothermic due to surface heat loss, the temperature of the peripheral compartment may be lower than the core compartment. Active surface rewarming in these patients may cause peripheral vasodilatation with blood circulating to the cooler peripheral compartment returning to the core compartment at a lower temperature. This 'core temperature afterdrop' may be mitigated by using active internal rewarming prior to or concurrent with surface rewarming.

RATE OF REWARMING

Concerns in addition to the hazards of sudden physiological change during rewarming have been raised more recently, mostly in the literature on patients undergoing cardiopulmonary bypass or TH. These include:

- that rapid rewarming exacerbates neurological injury and compromises cerebral blood flow autoregulation[57,58]
- a possible association with seizures on rewarming[59,60]
- discrepancy between cerebral and core temperatures during rewarming[30–32,61,62]
- findings of better neurocognitive and renal function following slow rather than fast rewarming from cardiopulmonary bypass.[63,64]

THERAPEUTIC HYPOTHERMIA AND TARGETED TEMPERATURE MANAGEMENT

Hypothermia is potentially beneficial in a variety of circumstances and is the subject of intense laboratory and clinical research interest. The combination of biological plausibility of benefit, positive animal data and some positive human trial data has resulted in its introduction as a therapeutic modality in some circumstances.

POTENTIAL MECHANISMS

Most mechanisms of potential benefit with TH relate to the modification of temperature-sensitive consequences of cellular injury, with particular focus at present on tissues of the central nervous system in the setting of ischaemia or reperfusion. Traumatic or ischaemia/reperfusion injury results in a cascade of destructive processes ranging from subcellular to systemic levels that can continue for several days and perhaps even weeks.[52] A wide range of these processes are temperature-sensitive; however, their duration of such varies following an insult. The clinical implications of this variability such as on optimal timing and duration of TH has not been fully elucidated.[62] **Box 82.5** lists some of the effects of hypothermia with potential benefit for the central nervous system.

Potential benefit may also be derived from its physiological effects such as those on vascular tone and the immune function (in patients with sepsis and septic shock), and reduction of intracranial pressure.

INDICATIONS FOR THERAPEUTIC HYPOTHERMIA

Current consensus amongst resuscitation councils and critical care societies is that:[45,58,65–68]

- therapeutic hypothermia is strongly recommended on the basis of a moderate to strong level of evidence

Box 82.5 Mechanisms of neuronal benefit with hypothermia[52,62]

Early mechanisms
- Reduction in cerebral metabolism (≈8% reduction per 1°C fall) and thermopooling
- Reduction in mitochondrial dysfunction
- Decreased production of nitric oxide and free radicals
- Decrease in excitatory neurotransmitters and calcium influx

Late mechanisms
- Suppression of ischaemia-induced inflammation
- Mitigation of reperfusion-related DNA injury, lipid peroxidation and leukotriene production
- Reduced cell membrane leakage and cytotoxic oedema, blood–brain barrier stabilising effect
- Suppression of seizures
- Reduction in apoptosis (inhibition of caspase activation)

Adapted from: Polderman KH. Mechanisms of action, physiological effects, and complications of hypothermia. Crit Care Med 2009;37(7):S186–202.

for use in adult survivors of out-of-hospital cardiac arrest of cardiac cause with initial rhythm ventricular fibrillation (VF) or ventricular tachycardia (VT), who do not demonstrate meaningful response to voice following return of spontaneous circulation, ROSC (target temperature 32–34°C, maintained for 12–24 hours, rewarmed at a maximum rate of 0.5°C/h)
- therapeutic hypothermia *may* be beneficial and *should* be considered on the basis of extrapolation and weaker levels of evidence for use in:
  - adult survivors of in-hospital cardiac arrest and cardiac arrest of non-shockable rhythm or non-cardiac cause
  - neonates born at ≥36 weeks' gestational age with evolving moderate to severe hypoxic ischaemic encephalopathy (target 33.5–34.5°C, commenced within 6 hours of birth, maintained for 72 hours, rewarmed over at least 4 hours).

Other conditions for which therapeutic hypothermia is being investigated include traumatic brain injury, spinal cord injury, neurosurgery, ischaemic and hemorrhagic cerebrovascular accident, myocardial infarction, cardiogenic shock and liver failure.[52,58]

METHOD

It is currently recommended that TH be provided using similar temperature profiles to those used in human trials, which demonstrated positive outcomes; however, the optimal timing and method of TH are still uncertain.

The risks of TH are most likely to be outweighed by potential benefit in high-level intensive care units with a practice guideline specific for the institution. In addition, it is recommended that a tightly controlled temperature profile over discrete stages of induction, maintenance, reversion and post TH be prescribed. This is referred to as targeted temperature management (TTM); the use of imprecise temperature targets and methods of temperature measurement and control is potentially hazardous.[58]

Induction of TH is generally carried out as quickly as possible, aiming to achieve target temperature within 8 hours of return of spontaneous circulation in the case of post-cardiac-arrest care. In addition to targeting destructive processes that are temperature-sensitive for only a few hours following insult, rapid induction also limits shivering, diuresis and electrolyte loss, fluid compartment shifting and haemodynamic fluctuation, all of which tend to settle once the temperature falls below 33.5°C.[39] Current recommended timeframes for achieving target temperature are derived only from some animal and trial data, and the true therapeutic window is presently unknown.[66,69]

Methods of rapidly inducing TH include (see Table 82.2):

- 4°C intravenous crystalloid fluid bolus of up to 30 mL/kg over 30 minutes
- surface ice packs or cold-air blankets
- temperature control devices with external pads (e.g. Arctic Sun) or intravascular catheters (e.g. Alsius Coolgard, Celsius Control System)
- intranasal evaporative coolant delivery (e.g. Rhinochill, BeneChill, San Diego, CA)
- cooling helmet.

Cold intravenous fluids have been used in pre-hospital initiation of TH and can rapidly lower temperature by around 1.5°C.[66] Numerous studies found no convincing increase in complications (including pulmonary oedema); however, cold fluids alone are not sufficient to maintain hypothermia.[68]

The optimal duration of TH is unknown and may vary between individual cases depending on circumstance and the nature of illness or injury.[62] Current recommendations of 12–24 hours in adults and 72 hours in neonates are based on the methods used in clinical trials with outcome benefit in favour of TH.

Rewarming is recommended to be tightly controlled at a rate of 0.25–0.5°C/h. Although the optimal rate of rewarming is not known, the prevention of rapid rewarming and rebound hyperthermia is thought to be important and often requires active temperature modulation through the use of a temperature control device.[62]

Hyperthermia is common following cardiac arrest and is thought to be an important mechanism of secondary neurological damage. It is recommended that normothermia be maintained beyond the period of TH; however, there is no evidence at present that this improves patient outcome.[66]

Temperature control devices use continuous temperature feedback from patient monitoring (such as oesophageal and bladder catheters) or intermittent intravascular temperature measurements (Celsius Control System) to adjust closed-loop fluid or catheter temperature. These devices do not involve administration of extra fluid, and use conductive cold or heat between device and skin (surface devices) or blood (intravascular devices). They can achieve cooling rates of up to 4.5°C/h and are the most precise methods of controlling temperature through all stages of TTM.[39,70–72]

CLINICAL CONSIDERATIONS DURING TH

All of the physiological effects of hypothermia as discussed earlier in this chapter and their implications on patient management should be borne in mind when applying TH. Of particular importance are:

- its effects on potassium and glucose levels
- interpretation of arterial blood gases and acid–base status
- potential masking of fever due to sepsis
- effects on pharmacokinetics and pharmacodynamics
- the use of anticoagulation and thrombolysis
- safety with percutaneous coronary intervention (PCI)

- potential for worsening of cardiac output and arrhythmias
- its implications in pregnant patients
- potential need to control shivering with sedation and paralysis
- neurological prognostication following anoxic brain injury.

ANTICOAGULATION AND THROMBOLYSIS DURING TTM

There is very little published data on the effect of TH on patients receiving anticoagulation and/or thrombolytic therapy. In the two major trials with outcomes in favour of TH following cardiac arrest, anticoagulation and thrombolytics were used as required; however, only one patient in one study and 27 patients in the other received both TH and thrombolysis.[69,73]

Hypothermia can reduce both tPA and plasminogen activator inhibitor-1 (PAI-1) activity; however, these effects appear non-linear and the net result is unpredictable. No clear change in incidence of intracranial haemorrhage was found in a preliminary study of TH commenced 30–180 minutes following thrombolysis in patients with ischaemic stroke.[74]

TTM AND PERCUTANEOUS CORONARY INTERVENTION (PCI)

Coronary arterial dilatation can occur in response to cold skin contact and mild hypothermia, however vasoconstriction can occur in diseased coronary arteries.[75] Results are somewhat mixed in the very limited data available on the impact of TH on outcomes in patients receiving PCI. The introduction of protocolised TH to patients undergoing PCI may be associated with a higher incidence of infection and need for blood transfusion compared with historical controls.[76,77] In patients treated with TH, those undergoing PCI may not have a higher rate of complication compared with patients not undergoing PCI.[78] It is currently considered safe to provide patients with both TH and PCI.[68]

TTM IN PATIENTS WITH CARDIOGENIC SHOCK

The use of hypothermia in cardiogenic shock may improve haemodynamic stability with an increase in both systemic vascular resistance and stroke volume; however, it may also increase oxygen consumption and demand if shivering is not controlled.[79,80]

There is limited published evidence on the use of TH in patients with cardiogenic shock,[81,82] and importantly there has not been a direct comparison of outcomes between patients with cardiogenic shock treated with TH and patients with cardiogenic shock not treated with TH.

Patients with significant shock (defined as systolic blood pressure less than 60 mmHg (7.98 kPa) despite epinephrine infusion, or mean arterial pressure less than 60 mmHg (7.98 kPa) for greater than 30 minutes) were excluded from the two major trials on cardiac arrest patients.[69,73]

There are some data to suggest that the incidence of ventricular arrhythmias, bleeding, and infection may not be higher when TH is used in patients with cardiogenic shock compared with patients without cardiogenic shock.[82]

THERAPEUTIC HYPOTHERMIA IN PREGNANCY

There are published cases of therapeutic hypothermia in pregnancy; however, there is a lack of trial data and pregnant patients were excluded in the clinical trials that demonstrated benefit with TH. Good maternal outcome with subsequent delivery of an apparently normal neonate has been reported following the use of TH at 13 weeks' gestation,[83] although fetal demise has also been reported during, but not necessarily as a result of, TH.[84]

Given the weight of evidence supporting improved outcomes for a subset of adult survivors of cardiac arrest, it is reasonable to consider the use of TTM in a pregnant woman.

The following should be noted when considering or applying TTM during pregnancy:

- evidence is lacking on the safety of TH for the fetus
- both hypothermia and rewarming can increase uterine tone and contractions, which reduce placental blood flow[85,86]
- hypothermia shifts the maternal haemoglobin-oxygen dissociation curve to the left, reducing placental gas exchange
- maternal acid–base disturbances can further compromise the fetus, and temperature should be taken into consideration in the interpretation of arterial blood gases
- hypothermic cardiopulmonary bypass (CPB) may be associated with higher fetal mortality than normothermic CPB.[87]

Fetal bradycardia may be associated with fetal distress or hypothermia.[88] Increasing maternal Pa_{O_2} may attenuate fetal bradycardia; however, hyperoxia post cardiac arrest has been found to be associated with increased mortality, possibly due to increased reactive oxygen species in the context of ischaemia–reperfusion injury.[89]

Fetal bradycardia with heart rates around 90–100 beats per minute were reported in the case of successful TH in pregnancy.[83]

Maternal hypothermia and alkalaemia decrease fetal Pa_{O_2}.[90] Maternal Pa_{CO_2} and pH should ideally be maintained at values normal for gestation. By 12 weeks' gestation, maternal Pa_{CO_2} is normally around 32 mmHg (4.25 kPa) with pH 7.44. Fetal pH is normally around 0.1 less than maternal. In the TH range of 32–34°C, corrected values can be estimated by the subtraction of 5 mmHg (0.66 kPa) per 1°C below 37°C for Pa_{O_2}, subtraction of 2 mmHg (0.27 kPa) per 1°C below 37°C for Pa_{CO_2}, and addition of 0.012 per 1°C below 37 °C for pH.[36,39] Although an alpha-stat approach is generally recommended during hypothermic cardiopulmonary bypass in pregnancy, the best approach is uncertain.[86,91]

SEDATION, PARALYSIS AND SEIZURES

Seizures occur in around 36% of patients after ROSC, mostly within the first 24 hours (and therefore coinciding with the period of TH[92,93]) and can result in further brain injury in as little as 30 minutes.[92–95]

The use of paralysis to control shivering during TH may mask seizure activity, and electroencephalographic (EEG) monitoring should be considered in paralysed patients.[96] However, it is not known whether the treatment of seizures impacts patient outcome post cardiac arrest and therefore a strong recommendation for EEG monitoring and aggressive attempts to control seizure activity cannot be made at this stage.[97]

NEUROLOGICAL OUTCOME AND PROGNOSTICATION FOLLOWING TH

There is considerable uncertainty about the effect of TH on the reliability of clinical signs as predictors of poor neurological outcome following cardiac arrest. New data suggest that the 2006 American Academy of Neurology (AAN) guidelines for neurological prognostication following cardiac arrest do not have the same degree of accuracy in patients treated with TH.[45,98,99]

The current level of evidence is considered inadequate to support a specific method of determining poor neurological prognosis with certainty.[45]

Access the complete references list online at http://www.expertconsult.com

1. Romanovsky AA. Thermoregulation: some concepts have changed. Functional architecture of the thermoregulatory system. Am J Physiology Integr Comp Physiol 2007;292:R37–46.
11. Marik PE. Fever in the ICU. Chest 2000;117:855–69.
15. Bouchama A, Knochel JP. Heat stroke. N Engl J Med 2002;346:1978–88.
30. Danzl DF, Pozos RS. Accidental hypothermia. N Engl J Med 1994;331:1756–60.
39. Polderman KH, Ingeborg H. Therapeutic hypothermia and controlled normothermia in the intensive care unit: Practical considerations, side effects, and cooling methods. Crit Care Med 2009;37: 1101–20.
58. Nunnally ME, Jaeschke R, Bellingan GJ, et al. Targeted temperature management in critical care: A report and recommendations from five professional societies. Crit Care Med 2011;39:1113–25.
62. Polderman KH. Mechanisms of action, physiological effects, and complications of hypothermia. Crit Care Med 2009;37(7):S186–202.

83

Electrical Safety and Injuries

Lester AH Critchley

Patients suffering from the consequences of electrocution and associated burns occasionally require ICU management. Patterns of presentation include post cardiopulmonary arrest, coma, blunt trauma and severe burns - either direct or indirect from electrical arcs, flashes or fires. An understanding of the physical concepts behind electrical power supplies and how electrocution occurs helps in determining the extent of these injuries.

Patients and staff in the ICU are at risk of electrocution from faulty electrical equipment. The necessity of direct patient contact with electrical equipment increases this risk, and when therapy involves an invasive contact close to the heart, microshock is an additional hazard. Thus, strict adherence to internationally accepted electrical safety standards is desirable. Faulty electrical equipment can also result in power failures, fires and explosions. The use of mobile phones and related devices near patient equipment can lead to malfunctioning.

PHYSICAL CONCEPTS

Electricity is produced by the movement of negatively charged electrons. A *potential difference* or voltage, measured in volts (V), exists between two points if the number or density of electrons is greater at one point. When these points are connected by a conductor, the potential difference will cause electrons or an *electric current* (I), measured in amperes (A), to flow. *Resistance* (R), measured in ohms (Ω), opposes this flow of electrons. Resistance is low in a conductor, because electrons can move freely from atom to atom. However, resistance is high in an insulator as electrons are unable to move freely. Voltage, current and resistance are related by Ohm's law:

$$V = I \times R \quad (83.1)$$

If an electric current flows through a resistance, it dissipates energy as heat. The heating effect per second, or *power*, is measured in joules (J)/s or watts (W):

$$\text{power} = V \times I = I^2 \times R \quad (83.2)$$

A current that flows in one direction, such as produced by a battery, is called a *direct current*. Electricity to homes, hospitals, and factories is supplied as an *alternating current*, which flows back and forth at a *frequency* (i.e. cycles per second or hertz (Hz)). Voltage and frequency specifications vary worldwide. This may cause problems when electrical equipment designed to be used in one region is used elsewhere. Voltage specifications range from 100 V (i.e. Japan) to 240 V (i.e. Australia) with 220 V being most commonly supplied (i.e. Britain, most of Europe and Asia). The frequency most commonly supplied is 50 Hz. North America is a notable exception, where the specification is 110–120 V and 60 Hz.

For efficiency, electricity is distributed from the power station using ultra-high voltages. Main power-grids carry >1 million volts, which is stepped down by transformers to >10 000 V to supply local power-lines, that are further stepped down to 120 to 220 V for domestic, commercial and factory use. Accidental contact with these high-voltage supply lines can be fatal if the current returns to ground with the person in its path. High-voltage currents can also flow via ionised air. This is known as electrical arcing and causes surface or flash burns. If an electrical fault occurs in domestic or hospital equipment, the flow of electricity can be re-routed to ground though a bystander who makes contact, resulting in electrocution.

A current flowing in a circuit produces electric and magnetic fields, which induce currents to flow in neighbouring circuits. When this results in a current flowing between the two circuits, it is called coupling. With *capacitive coupling*, high-frequency currents are most easily passed, and the size of the current is greatest when the circuits are in close proximity. *Inductive coupling* can result from the strong magnetic fields produced by heavy-duty electrical equipment such as transformers, electric motors, and magnetic resonance imaging (MRI) machines. The most common problem associated with coupling is electrical interference or 'noise'. Monitoring equipment is designed to 'filter' out this noise. However, in certain circumstances, such as the use of high-frequency surgical diathermy and magnetic resonance, sufficient amperage can be induced to cause microshock and burns.[1,2] Smaller electromagnetic fields emitted by hand-held devices, such as mobile phones, can affect the programming of microprocessors. Cases of patient equipment malfunctions have been reported.[3]

Static electricity has no free flow of electrons. Insulated objects can become highly charged, usually by repeated rubbing. The charge is dissipated by electrons jumping onto another neighbouring object of a different potential. 'Jumping' electrons ionise and heat the air through which they pass, causing a spark, which may ignite an inflammable liquid or gas. Lightning is a type of static electrical discharge. Direct currents of 12000–200000 A and voltages in the millions are involved; however, flow lasts for only a fraction of a second.[4]

ELECTROPHYSIOLOGICAL CONSIDERATIONS

For a current to flow through the body, the body must complete a circuit. Usually this involves the current flowing from its source to ground through the body, often hand to hand or hand to feet. The pathophysiological effects depend on the size and duration of the current, and this depends on the voltage and electrical resistance of the body. The main pathophysiological effects of current passing through the body are: (i) ventricular fibrillation or asystole, (ii) sustained muscle contraction or tetany causing the 'cannot let go' phenomenon and asphyxiation, and (iii) dissipation of electrical energy as heat causing burns, often to deep-seated structures as well as skin. Muscle, blood vessels and nerves act as the main conduits for currents flowing through the body, and offer a very low resistance 500–1000 Ω.[9] Most of the resistance to passage of the current, and thus burning effect, occurs at the skin contact, which can vary enormously. Dry skin has a resistance in excess of 100000 Ω.[5] However, skin resistance is markedly reduced (to 1000 Ω)[6] if the skin is wet, or if a conductive jelly has been applied. Hence, from Ohm's law, dry skin in contact with 240 V mains supply will result in a harmless 0.24 mA current flowing through the body, whereas moist or wet skin will result in a potentially lethal 240 mA current.

ELECTROCUTION

EPIDEMIOLOGY

Most cases of electrocution occur either in the workplace (about 60%) or at home (about 30%).[6] Most data on the incidence of electrocution come from North America, though significant regional differences exist worldwide. Children under 6 years are most at risk from domestic electrocution, but with greater electrical safety awareness and the use of ground fault circuit interrupters (GFCIs), the oral burns once seen from chewing power cords are much less common.[7] Young adult Caucasian men are the most likely victims of electrocution in the workplace. Power-lines and electrified railway tracks are the most common causes of high-voltage injuries.

CAUSES AND PATTERNS

There are a number of causes of electrocution and each has its own pattern of injuries:

1. *Low-voltage alternating current (AC) with or without loss of consciousness or arrest:* these injuries usually involve exposure to <1000 V in the home or office setting
2. *High-voltage AC with or without loss of consciousness or arrest:* these injuries can cause extensive thermal burns and usually are occupation related
3. *Direct current (DC) injury:* these injuries often involve trauma due to the victim being thrown due to violent muscle contraction
4. *Conducted electrical weapons (CEWs) such as Tazers used by the police:* CEWs deliver high-voltage currents, either AC or pulses of DC in the order of 50,000 V. Injuries are due mainly to trauma secondary to the Tazer shock[8]
5. *Lightening strike:* this is discussed later.

PATHOPHYSIOLOGY

Pathophysiological processes involved in electrical injuries from an electrical engineer's perspective are well described in a short review article by Bernstein.[9] The extent of injury depends on: (i) the amount of current that passes through the body, (ii) the duration of the current, and (iii) the tissues traversed by the current (**Table 83.1**). The extent of injury is most directly related to amperage. However, usually only the voltage involved is known. In general, lower voltages cause less

Table 83.1 Origin and pathophysiological effects of different levels of electrical injury

CURRENT (A)	SOURCE	EFFECTS ON VICTIM
10–100 μA	Earth leakage	Microshock (ventricular fibrillation)
300–400 μA	Faulty equipment	Tingling (harmless)
>1 mA	Faulty equipment	Pain (withdraw)
>10 mA	Faulty equipment	Tetany (cannot let go)
>100 mA	Faulty equipment	Macroshock (ventricular fibrillation)
>1 A	Faulty equipment	Burns and tissue damage
>1000 A	High-tension injury	Severe burns and loss of limbs
>12000 A	Lightning	Coma, severe burns and loss of limbs

injury, although voltages as low as 50 V have caused fatalities.

TISSUE HEAT INJURY

Currents in excess of 1 A generate sufficient heat energy to cause burns to the skin at entrance and grounding points and occult thermal injury to internal tissues and organs. Small blood vessels and nervous tissue appear to be particularly susceptible.[6]

DEPOLARISATION OF MUSCLE CELLS

An alternating current of 30–200 mA will cause ventricular fibrillation.[10] Domestic frequencies of 50–60 Hz are most dangerous, being three times more likely to stop the heart than direct or high-frequency current sources. Currents in excess of 5 A cause sustained cardiac asystole, which is the principle used in defibrillation. Apart from ventricular fibrillation, other arrhythmias may occur. Myocardial damage is common and may result in ST and T-wave changes. Global left ventricular dysfunction may occur hours or days later, despite initial minimal ECG changes.[11,12] Myocardial infarction has also been reported.[13] Specific markers of myocardial injury, such as cardiac troponin, should be checked in all suspected cases of electrical injury to the heart.[14]

Tetanic contractions of skeletal muscle occur with currents in excess of 15–20 mA. The threshold is particularly low with alternating currents at the household frequency of 50–60 Hz. Tetanic contraction will prevent voluntary release of the source of electrocution, the 'cannot let go' phenomenon, and violent muscle contractions may cause fractures of long bones and spinal vertebrae.[6]

VASCULAR INJURIES

Blood vessels may become thrombosed and occluded as a result of the thermal injury. Small vessels are at greater risk as the blood flow in larger vessels dissipates the heat. Compartment syndromes are seen secondary to tissue oedema, causing tissue ischaemia and necrosis. Affected limbs may require fasciotomy and amputation.[15]

NEUROLOGICAL INJURIES

Neurological injuries may be central or peripheral, and immediate or late in onset. Unconsciousness following electrocution may result from cardiorespiratory arrest, trauma to the head or the direct effect of current passing through the brain. This may be one of the main reasons for admission to ICU. Monoparesis may occur in affected limbs, and the median nerve is particularly vulnerable.[6,16] Monoparesis may be due to the direct effect of electricity passing through the body or delayed effect due to scar formation. Electrocution to the head may result in unconsciousness, paralysis of the respiratory centre, and late complications such as epilepsy, encephalopathy and Parkinsonism.[6,16] Spinal cord damage resulting in para- or tetraplegia can result from a current traversing both arms and the spine.[6,16] Autonomic dysfunction may also occur causing acute vasospasm or a late sympathetic dystrophy.[6]

RENAL FAILURE

Direct electrical injury to the kidneys is unusual. However, acute renal failure may result from the myoglobinuria and toxins produced by extensive muscle necrosis.[16]

EXTERNAL BURNS

Victims of high-voltage electrocution can incur extensive superficial or deep external burns from electrical arcs passing over the skin surface, fires especially from clothes catching fire and heated metal objects such as jewellery. Arc formation requires voltages in excess of 350 V and tracks over the body surface. They can generate extremely high temperatures of up to 5000°C that mainly cause skin burns.[9] Victims can also be burnt by the intense flash caused by the electrical discharge.

OTHER INJURIES

High-voltage and direct current electrocution can cause the victim to fall or be thrown, which may result in traumatic blunt injuries. Thus, it is important to get a reliable witness report of the incidence so that the nature of the patients' injuries is properly understood and nothing is missed, like a fractured cervical spine. All unconscious electrocuted patients should be initially treated with neck and spinal protection. High-voltage injuries can commonly rupture the eardrum and affect hearing.[17] Cataracts may later develop.[18]

MACRO- AND MICROSHOCK

The above domestic/workplace electrocution is known as *macroshock*, and occurs when current flows through the intact skin and body.

In the ICU and other high-level patient care areas, the potential for *microshock* electrocution also exists. Microshock occurs when there is a direct current path to the heart muscle that bypasses the protective electrical resistance of the skin surface. Such a pathway may be provided by saline-filled arterial or venous-pressure-monitoring catheters or transvenous pacemaker wires. The current required to produce ventricular fibrillation in microshock settings is extremely small, in the order of 60 μA.[15] Currents of 1–2 mA are barely perceptible and produce tingling of the skin (see Table 83.1). Hence a lethal microshock may be transmitted to a patient via

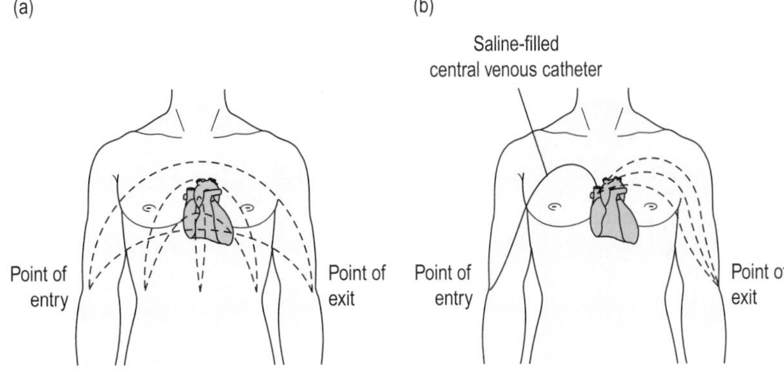

Figure 83.1 Microshock: (a) low current density at the heart; (b) high current density at the heart if there is a conducting pathway, such as a saline-filled catheter.

a staff member who is unaware of the conducted current. Microshock can result from direct contact with faulty electrical equipment, or stray currents from capacitive coupling, or earth leakage. Such small currents are potentially lethal because a high current density is produced at the heart (**Fig. 83.1**). Patients at risk of microshock require higher levels of electrical safety protection.

HIGH-TENSION AND LIGHTNING STRIKE INJURIES

High-tension electricity (>1000 V) involves voltage much greater than domestic supply, usually many thousands of volts. Sources include power-lines, electrified railway tracks and equipment requiring high internal voltages produced by step-up transformers, such as televisions. Tissue damage is mainly due to the generation of heat, as high-amperage currents are involved. Not only does the current pass through the victim, but electrical arcing may also be involved. Witnesses have described tissues actually exploding.[19]

Lightning injury is a type of high-tension injury. Its incidence depends upon geographical location. Generation of lightning is surprisingly complex and involves a number of steps. The victim of a lightning strike may be hit directly, injured by the side-flash from a nearby object, or electrocuted by ground currents which re-route through the victim's legs.[9]

Victims can be thrown several feet as a result of violent muscular contractions. Electrical arcing of the air causes intense heat, resulting in superficial burns and the clothes igniting. Characteristic entrance and exit site burns are seen, which have a spider-like appearance with redness and blistering. Victims are usually unconscious in the initial phase. However, many victims survive (80–90%),[4] and good recovery has been reported despite initial hopeless neurological responsiveness (e.g. fixed dilated pupils).[20] Immediate death usually results from cardiorespiratory arrest; asystole is more common than ventricular fibrillation.[4]

MANAGEMENT OF ELECTRICAL INJURIES

Treatment of electrical injuries is mainly supportive. It includes the following.

FIRST AID AND RESUSCITATION

It is imperative to make the immediate environment safe for rescuers. Power sources should be switched off and wet areas avoided where possible. Instinctive attempts to grab the electrocuted victim must be avoided until it is safe to do so. Cardiopulmonary resuscitation is carried out when indicated, and continued even if the prognosis seems hopeless. The neck and spine should be protected because of possible fractures.

INVESTIGATIONS

Investigations are indicated to detect damaged organs. They include electrocardiogram (ECG), echocardiography, computed tomography (CT) of the head, EEG, X-rays of the spine and long bones, haemoglobin, serum electrolytes, creatinine kinase and urine myoglobin to assess muscle damage, and nerve conduction studies. Arteriograms may help in the decision to amputate a limb.[15]

HOSPITAL AND ICU MANAGEMENT

Management is directed towards treatment of burns, ischaemic and necrotic tissue, and injured organs. The principle of treating electrical burns is complete excision because of the risks of acute renal failure and sepsis. Fasciotomies and amputations may be necessary. Tetanus toxoid and antibiotics, especially penicillin, are given if indicated.

ELECTRICAL HAZARDS IN THE ICU

The ICU has the potential to inflict both macroshock and microshock injuries to staff and patients. Potential sources of these electrical hazards are:

MAJOR ELECTRICAL FAULTS

The casing and insulated wiring of electrical equipment protect against electric shock. Faulty wiring or components, and deterioration of internal insulation, can result in the casing becoming 'live'. Contact with live casing or wires can result in an electric current flowing through the victim to ground. The outcome largely depends on the resistance offered by the body to the current. If it is low, such as in a wet environment, sufficient current can flow to cause death, which is usually due to ventricular fibrillation/asystole or asphyxia from tetanic contraction of respiratory muscles.

MICROSHOCK CURRENTS

EARTH LEAKAGE CURRENTS

Within all pieces of electrical equipment, stray low-amperage electrical currents exist that usually flow to earth, called earth leakage currents. They originate from current leaks across imperfect insulation of wires, capacitive and inductive coupling within the equipment, and coupling from electric and magnetic fields that exist in the working environment, such as the 50–60 Hz mains supply. Normally these currents are small and harmless, but they have the potential to cause microshock.

PACING WIRES AND CENTRAL VENOUS LINES

In certain circumstances, sufficient current to cause microshock can be passed by capacitive and inductive coupling to intracardiac pacing wires and central venous lines. Ventricular fibrillation has been reported from capacitive coupling with thermistor wires in a pulmonary artery catheter.[1]

DIFFERENT EARTH POTENTIALS

Inadequate or faulty earthing can result in separate earthing points being at different resting potentials. If contact is made between the two earthing points, sufficient current can flow to cause microshock.

STAFF–PATIENT CONTACT

Small currents capable of causing microshock can be transmitted unknowingly to a patient by a staff member who simultaneously touches faulty electrical equipment and the patient. If this current returns to earth via an intracardiac connection, a high current density will pass through the heart, resulting in microshock.

INDUCTIVE CURRENTS

Inductive coupling from the strong magnetic fields produced by MRI can cause overheating of wires and equipment. Severe burns have resulted from the use of pulse oximetry during magnetic resonance imaging, and specially designed wiring and probes are recommended.[2] Similar problems can exist with any intravascular device containing wires, such as a pulmonary artery catheter. More recently problems have arisen from the interference caused by personal computers, mobile phones and related devices with patient equipment. Many hospitals have banned the use of such devices in areas where patients are treated.

OTHER RELATED HAZARDS

Electrical equipment has the potential to cause other hazards such as thermal injury, fire and power failures. Preliminary critical incident reports suggest that power failures are the most commonly encountered incidents involving electricity in the ICU. Power failures can be disastrous, as many patients' lives depend on electrically driven 'life support' equipment. As the intensivist frequently works outside the ICU, they should also be aware of potential electrical hazards outside ICU.

MEASURES TO PROTECT STAFF AND PATIENTS[21,22]

EARTHING, FUSES AND CIRCUIT BREAKERS

Earthing reduces the risk of macroshock. The casing in most electrical equipment is connected to ground by a very-low-resistance wire called the earth, which uses the third pin of the electrical socket. If a fault arises, the earth wire offers a low-resistance path to ground. The high-amperage current that results will blow the main fuse or circuit breaker, thus providing protection and warning that a fault is present. However, fuses and circuit breaker do not guarantee patient protection from macroshock and other more sensitive protection strategies are required in patient care locations (see below). Additional protection can be achieved by connecting all the earthing points in a patient care area together by a very-low-resistance wire. This reduces the risk of microshock occurring from earthing points at different potentials, and is commonly used in cardiac protected areas.

ISOLATED POWER SYSTEMS (IPS)

MAINS ISOLATION

The power supply is isolated from earth using a mains isolation transformer. If contact is made with live faulty circuitry, the risk of electric shock is reduced because stray currents no longer preferentially flow through patient or staff member to earth. Presence of stray earth leakage currents can be detected by using a line isolation monitor. This type of system is particularly useful in wet locations where the body may offer a very low resistance to earth.

INTERNAL ISOLATION

In medical equipment the mains power supply is usually isolated from the patient connection by using internal transformers and photoelectric diodes. The casing is still earthed to protect against faulty circuitry.

This method of protection is commonly used in ICU equipment, including most monitoring and patient information systems. Electrical power isolation may limit the use of networks that link patient monitors to printers and information technology systems.

GROUND FAULT CIRCUIT INTERRUPTERS (GFCIs)

Ground fault circuit interrupters are devices that switch off the electrical supply if small currents are detected flowing to earth. GFCIs are designed to protect against electrocution from faulty electrical equipment. They are commonly incorporated into electrical sockets and require activation. When contact is made with the faulty equipment an increased current will flow to earth, which trips the system. GFCIs also protect against microshock. A major concern with using GFCIs in critical patient management areas, however, is that power supply to essential life-supporting equipment such as heart–lung machines can be permanently switched off by small-leakage currents.

ELECTRICAL SAFETY STANDARDS

Most First-World nations have standards of electrical safety that apply to both the design of medical equipment and their use in healthcare locations. A number of well-recognised standards exist that can be easily found and uploaded from the internet. The US follows the National Electric Code, which has a section on Health Care Locations and was most recently updated in 2011. Europe and Great Britain follow the International Electrotechnical Commission Code IEC 60601, first published in 1997 and regularly updated, most recently in 2011. IEC 60601-1 is widely accepted as the benchmark for medical equipment and has become the de facto requirement for medical equipment worldwide. Australia and New Zealand follow similar standards (AS/NZS 3003:2011 and AS/NZS 3200:2010). Hospitals worldwide should establish their own committees to ensure that these standards are applied.

Patient care areas differ in their safety requirements and commonly used classifications are listed below. The ICU should conform to 1(b) and preferably 1(c), as follows:

1. **a.** Unprotected areas, where only routine electrical safety standards are applied
   b. Body-protected areas, where the level of electrical safety is sufficient to minimise the risk of macroshock when the patient is in direct contact with electrical equipment and the skin impedance is reduced or bypassed
   c. Cardiac-protected areas, where the level of electrical safety is sufficient to minimise the risk of direct microshock to the heart
2. Wet locations, where spillage of water and physiological solutions, such as saline and blood, frequently occurs; the US Department of Defense until recently defined wet areas as those used for cystoscopy, arthroscopy and labour/delivery[23]
3. In the past, standards existed for the safe use of inflammable anaesthetic agents.

Currently, the US only requires GFCIs in wet areas that do not include ICUs and most operating theatres. Other countries, such as Australia, New Zealand and Great Britain require IPSs in operating rooms and ICUs. If cost is not an issue, ideally both internal isolation and GFCIs should be used in 1(a) and 1(b) and wet locations. More stringent controls to protect against microshock are required in 1(c) cardiac-protected locations.

EQUIPMENT CHECKS

The purchase of new equipment should be strictly controlled, and circuit diagrams should be provided. All new equipment should be checked that it adheres to the appropriate electrical safety standards, functions properly and for current leaks before it is used in the ICU or other high-risk patient areas. Preventative maintenance of equipment should be done regularly. Dated stickers should be used to show when the equipment was last checked. All faulty equipment must be removed from service, labelled appropriately and recommissioned only after thorough checking.

RESERVE POWER SUPPLIES AND ALARMS

All essential equipment should have a reserve power supply (usually a battery), and alarms that warn of power failure. All hospitals should provide an emergency backup power supply in case of power cuts. Protocol should be in place, or developed, to ensure continuation of ventilation, sedation and other essential life-sustaining therapies in case of complete electrical power failure, or the need to evacuate patients because of fire.

PERSONNEL EDUCATION

Staff should be taught correct ways to handle electrical equipment. Equipment with frayed wires should never be used, plugs should never be tugged, trolleys should never be wheeled over power cords, and two pieces of equipment should never be handled simultaneously. Staff should also respond appropriately to alarms. The increasing use of patient monitoring and information technology systems means that an increasing number of electrical devices are being used at any one time at the patient's bedside, with increasing need for power cords and sockets. Care should be taken when using multiple socket power cables to ensure that their use does not violate electrical safety standards.

Access the complete references list online at http://www.expertconsult.com

4. Apfelberg DB, Masters FW, Robinson DW. Pathophysiology and treatment of lightning injuries. J Trauma 1974;14:453–60.
5. Bruner JMR. Hazards of electrical apparatus. Anesthesiology 1976;28:396–3424.
9. Bernstein T. Electrical injury: electrical engineer's perspective and an historical review. Ann NY Acad Sci 1994;720:1–10.
16. Solem L, Fischer RP, Strate RG. The natural history of electrical injury. J Trauma 1977;17:487–92.
21. Litt L, Ehrenwerth J. Electrical safety in the operating room: Important old wine, disguised new bottles. Anesth Analg 1994;78:417–19.

84

Envenomation

James Tibballs

Envenomation by snakes, spiders, ticks, bees, ants, wasps, jellyfish, octopuses or cone shell snails may threaten life, while envenomation by other creatures may cause serious illness.[1] Although this chapter focuses on management of envenomation in Australia, the principles of management are widely applicable in other countries. Immediate advice on management may be obtained from the Australian Venom Research Unit (AVRU) advisory service on its 24-hour telephone number within Australia on 1300760451, from overseas on +61 3 8344 7753 or from their website at http://www.avru.org.

SNAKES

EPIDEMIOLOGY

Australia is habitat to a large number of venomous terrestrial and marine snakes (Families Elapidae and Hydrophiidae). The genera responsible for the majority of serious illness are Brown Snakes (*Pseudonaja*), Tiger Snakes (*Notechis*), Taipans (*Oxyuranus*), Black Snakes (*Pseudechis*) and Death Adders (*Acanthophis*). Each genus comprises several or many species.

The mean snake bite death rate in Australia from 1982 to 2011 was 2.1 per year (~0.01/100 000) (Ken Winkel, personnal communication), usually occurring because of massive envenomation, snake bite in remote locations, rapid collapse, or delayed or inadequate antivenom therapy. However, as many as 2000 people are bitten each year and, of these, at least 300 require antivenom treatment. This morbidity and mortality is far less than that observed in India, South-East Asia and Africa. Death and critical illness is due to (1) progressive paralysis leading to respiratory failure, (2) haemorrhage, or (3) renal failure or combinations. Renal failure occurs as a consequence of rhabdomyolysis, disseminated intravascular coagulation (DIC), haemorrhage, haemolysis or to their combinations.

Snake bite is often 'accidental' when a snake is trodden upon or suddenly disturbed. However, many bites occur when humans deliberately interfere with snakes or handle them. At special risk are herpetologists and snake collectors who not only invariably sustain bites in the course of their work[2] or hobby, but also develop allergy to venoms and to the antivenoms used in their treatment. Contact with exotic snakes has additional problems.

SNAKE VENOMS

Venoms are complex mixtures of toxins, usually proteins, which kill the snake's prey and aid its digestion. Many toxins are phospholipases. The main toxins cause paralysis, coagulopathy, rhabdomyolysis and haemolysis (**Box 84.1**). Coagulopathy is due either to the procoagulant effect of prothrombin activators (factor Xa-like enzymes), with consumption of clotting factors and possible thrombotic sequelae such as thrombotic microangiopathic renal failure,[3] or to a direct anticoagulant effect. Platelets may be consumed and fibrinolysis may occur as a secondary phenomenon resembling the findings in disseminated intravascular coagulation (DIC) caused by other conditions. When circulating venom has been neutralised by antivenom, it may be 4–6 hours or longer before hepatic manufacture of clotting factors can normalise coagulation tests.

SNAKE BITE AND ENVENOMATION

Although a bite may be observed, envenomation may not occur because no venom or a small amount of venom is injected. Bites by Australian snakes are relatively painless and may be unnoticed. This is in marked contrast to bites of many overseas crotalid and viperid snakes, where massive local reaction and necrosis are caused by proteolytic enzymes. In general, Australian snake venoms do not cause extensive damage to local tissues and are usually confined to mild swelling and bruising, and continued slight bleeding from the bite site. After Australian snake bite, paired fang marks are often visible but sometimes only scratches or single puncture wounds exist.

SYMPTOMS AND SIGNS OF ENVENOMATION

Classical symptoms and signs are given in **Box 84.2**. Sometimes, not all possible symptoms and signs occur. In some cases one symptom or sign may dominate the clinical picture, and in other cases they may wax and wane. These phenomena may be explained by

Box 84.1 Main components of Australian snake venoms

Neurotoxins
Presynaptic and postsynaptic neuromuscular blockers present in all dangerous venomous snakes. Cause paralysis
Postsynaptic blockers readily reversed by antivenom
Presynaptic blockers are more difficult to reverse, particularly if treatment is delayed
Some presynaptic blockers are also rhabdomyolysins

Prothrombin activators
Present in many important species
Cause consumption coagulopathy and possibly thrombotic microangiopathy (disseminated intravascular coagulation)
Intrinsic fibrin(ogen)lysis generates fibrin(ogen) degradation products
Significant risk of haemorrhage

Anticoagulants
Present in a relatively small number of dangerous species
Prevent blood clotting without consumption of clotting factors

Rhabdomyolysins
Some presynaptic neurotoxins also cause lysis of skeletal and cardiac muscle
Apart from loss muscle of mass, may cause myoglobinuria and renal failure

Haemolysins
Present in a few species
Rarely a serious clinical effect

Box 84.2 Progressive onset of major systemic symptoms and signs of untreated envenomation*

<1 hour after bite
Headache
Nausea, vomiting, abdominal pain
Transient hypotension associated with confusion or loss of consciousness
Coagulopathy (laboratory testing)
Regional lymphadenitis

1–3 hours after bite
Paresis/paralysis of cranial nerves (e.g. ptosis, double vision, external ophthalmoplegia, dysphonia, dysphagia, myopathic facies)
Haemorrhage from mucosal surfaces and needle punctures
Tachycardia, hypotension
Tachypnoea, shallow tidal volume

>3 hours after bite
Paresis/paralysis of truncal and limb muscles
Paresis/paralysis of respiratory muscles (respiratory failure)
Peripheral circulatory failure (shock), hypoxaemia, cyanosis
Rhabdomyolysis
Dark urine (due to myoglobinuria or haemoglobin)
Renal failure

*In massive envenomation or in a child, a critical illness may develop in minutes rather than hours.

variations in toxin content of venoms of the same species in different geographical areas, and by variable absorption of different toxins.

The cause of transient or prolonged hypotension soon after envenomation is obscure but it may be related to intravascular coagulation with myocardial ischaemia and pulmonary hypertension culminating in systemic hypotension.[4,5] Prothrombin activators gain access to the circulation within a number of minutes after subcutaneous injection. Tachycardia and relatively minor ECG abnormalities are common. Other causes of hypotension such as direct cardiac toxicity are possible.

Tender or even painful regional lymph nodes are moderately common but are not per se an indication for antivenom therapy. Lymphadenitis also occurs with bites by mildly venomous snakes that do not cause serious systemic illness.

Occasionally intracranial haemorrhage occurs. In the case of untreated or massive envenomation, rhabdomyolysis may occur. This usually involves all skeletal musculature and sometimes cardiac muscle. The resultant myoglobinuria may cause renal failure.

A high intake of alcohol by adults before snake bite is common, and may confound the cluster of symptoms and signs. Pre-existing treatment with anticoagulant (e.g. warfarin) or disease (e.g. gastrointestinal tract ulceration) may complicate management of coagulopathy.

SNAKE BITE IN CHILDREN

Snake bite in young children presents additional problems. Envenomation is difficult to diagnose when a bite has not been observed. The symptoms of early envenomation may pass unsuspected and the signs, particularly cranial nerve effects, are difficult to elicit. Bite marks may be difficult to distinguish from the effects of everyday minor trauma. Lastly, the onset of the syndrome of envenomation is likely to be more rapid and severe because of the relatively higher ratio of venom to body mass. Presentation may be cardiorespiratory failure.

IDENTIFICATION OF THE SNAKE

Identification of the snake is helpful but not essential since a venom detection kit test is available for snakes of Australia and Papua New Guinea. If the snake cannot be identified, a specific monovalent antivenom, or a combination of monovalent antivenoms or polyvalent antivenom should be administered on a geographical basis. Nevertheless, identification guides selection of the appropriate antivenom, and provides an insight into the expected syndrome. Administration of the wrong antivenom may endanger a victim's life because a generic monovalent antivenom (e.g. Brown Snake antivenom) does not neutralise venoms of other genera (e.g. Tiger Snakes, Taipans).

Identification by venom detection kit test

The venom detection kit (VDK) is an in vitro test for detection and identification of snake venom at the bite site, in urine, blood or other tissue in cases of snake bite. It can be performed at the bedside or in the laboratory. It is an enzyme immunoassay using rabbit antibodies and chromogen and peroxide solutions. A positive result will indicate the type of antivenom to be administered. It detects venom from a range of snake genera including Tiger, Brown, Black, Death Adder and Taipan. Individual species of snake cannot be identified by the test and several genera may yield a positive result in a specified well. The test is very sensitive, able to detect venom in concentrations as low as 10 ng/mL, and can yield a visual qualitative result in test wells in approximately 25 minutes. The incidences of false-positive and false-negative tests of the kit are low. On occasions, venom may be detected but the patient is asymptomatic and has no signs of envenomation. A decision to administer antivenom should be made on clinical grounds. A very high concentration of venom in a sample may overwhelm the test and yield a spuriously negative result (Hook effect). If that possibility exists, a diluted sample should be retested.

Identification by physical characteristics

This can be misleading. Not all brown-coloured snakes are Brown Snakes, not all black-coloured snakes are Black Snakes and not all banded snakes are Tiger Snakes. Moreover, Brown Snakes may have bands and Tiger Snakes may lack characteristic bands. Non-herpetologists should consult an identification guide[1] with reference to scale patterns to identify a specimen correctly if antivenom therapy is to be based on morphological characteristics alone.

Identification by clinical effects

The appearance of a bite site cannot be used to reliably identify a snake. The constellation of symptoms and signs may be useful to a limited degree. For example, paralysis associated with procoagulopathy may be caused by a Tiger, Taipan, Brown, or Rough-scaled Snake, *Hoplocephalus* spp. or Red-bellied Black Snake, but if rhabdomyolysis also occurs a bite by a Brown Snake is improbable. Paralysis associated with anticoagulation may be caused by a Black Snake (other than a Red-bellied Black Snake), Copperhead or Death Adder, but if rhabdomyolysis occurs a bite by a Death Adder is improbable. Paralysis with neither coagulopathy nor rhabdomyolysis may be caused by a Death Adder bite.

This information is obviously of limited practical importance. It is essential to administer antivenom at the first opportunity when indicated, rather than wait until the full syndrome becomes apparent, to enable an 'educated clinical guess' in selection of the appropriate antivenom.

MANAGEMENT OF SNAKE ENVENOMATION

The essentials of management are:

- resuscitation – mechanical ventilation and restoration of blood pressure with intravenous fluids, inotropic and vasoactive agents as needed
- application of a pressure-immobilisation first-aid bandage
- administration of antivenom
- performance of investigations.

From a practical point of view, one of three clinical situations arises after snake bite. A plan of management for each of these is summarised in **Figure 84.1**:

- victim presents with a critical illness
- victim is envenomated but not critically ill
- victim is bitten but does not appear envenomated.

When the envenomated victim is not critically ill, time is available to identify the snake by investigations and to administer specific monovalent antivenom. A pressure-immobilisation bandage should be applied if not already in place, and not removed until antivenom has been administered.

When the victim has been bitten but not apparently envenomated, admission to hospital is advisable with observation and examination hourly for at least 12 hours in the case of a child but less time for an adult. The syndrome of envenomation may be very slow in onset over numerous hours with an initial period free of symptoms. A test of coagulation should always be performed. If a coagulopathy is present, specific monovalent antivenom should be administered after identification of the species or as indicated by a VDK test. If only a mild coagulopathy is present it may be acceptable to withhold antivenom in the anticipation of spontaneous resolution, but coagulation should be checked at intervals and the victim maintained under surveillance until coagulation is normal.

THE PRESSURE-IMMOBILISATION TECHNIQUE OF FIRST AID

Since at least 95% of snake bites occur on the arms or legs,[1] Sutherland's first-aid pressure-immobilisation technique[6] is applicable in the majority of cases. With this technique, a crêpe (or crêpe-like) bandage, but preferably elasticised, is applied from the fingers or toes up the limb as far as possible, encompassing the bite site. It should be as firm as required for a sprained ankle. Additional immobilisation is applied to the entire limb by a rigid splint, with the aim of immobilising the joints either side of the bite site.

Venom is usually deposited subcutaneously. The systemic spread of venom is largely dependent on its absorption by way of the lymphatics[7] or the small blood

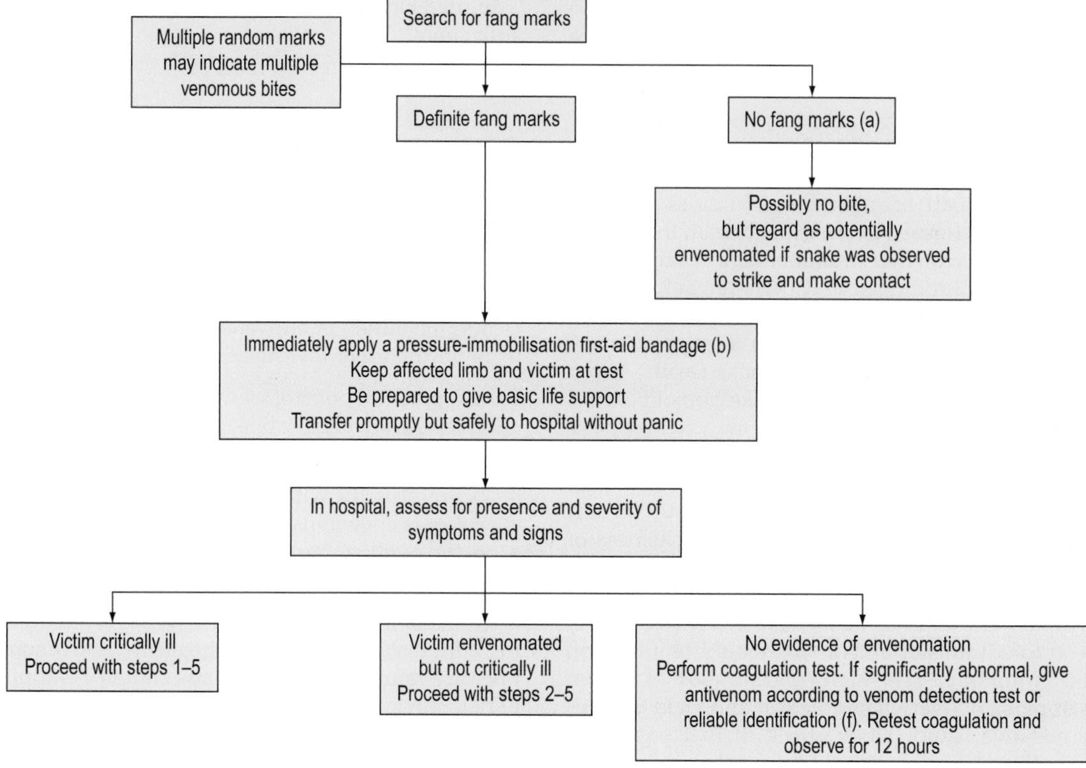

1. Resuscitate (treat hypoxaemia and shock)
   Be prepared to intubate and mechanically ventilate. Admit to intensive care.
2. Apply pressure-immobilisation bandage. Do not remove if already applied [b]
3. Give antivenom intravenously [c,d,e,f,g]
   - Give monovalent if species reliably known or appropriate antivenom indicated by venom detection test.
   - In critically ill victim, don't wait for venom detection test result or if species cannot be determined; give according to geographic location:
     Victoria – Brown and Tiger Snake
     Tasmania – Tiger Snake
     Other states and territories – polyvalent
   - Titrate antivenom against clinical and coagulation status (NOTE: Death Adders don't cause significant coagulopathy).
4. Perform investigations
   - Bite swab for venom detection. (First-aid bandage may be cut to expose bite site, and then reinforced)
   - Blood for venom detection, coagulation, type and cross-match blood (if bleeding), fibrin degradation products, full blood examination, enzymes, electrolytes, urea, creatinine
   - Urine for venom detection, red blood cells, haemoglobin, myoglobin.
5. Examine frequently to detect slow onset of paralysis [h], coagulopathy, rhabdomyolysis and renal failure.

Dangers and mistakes in management

a. Fang marks not visible to naked eye.
b. Premature release of bandage may result in sudden systemic envenomation. Leave in situ until victim reaches full medical facilities. If clinically envenomated, remove only after antivenom given.
c. Erroneous identification of snake may cause wrong antivenom to be given. If in any doubt treat as unidentified.
d. Antivenom without premedication. Anaphylaxis is not rare and may not respond to treatment.
e. Insufficient antivenom. Titrate dose against clinical and coagulation status.
f. Blood and coagulation factors (fresh frozen plasma, cryoprecipitate) not preceded by antivenom will worsen coagulopathy.
g. Antivenom given without clinical or laboratory evidence of envenomation.
h. Delayed onset of paralysis may be missed. Victim must be examined at least hourly.

Figure 84.1 Management of snake bite.

vessels. Application of a pressure less than arterial to the bitten area when combined with immobilisation of the limb effectively delays the movement of venom to the central circulation.[6] Although it is a first-aid technique designed for use in the field, it should be part of initial management in hospital since it halts further absorption of venom. Some experimental and anecdotal evidence with Death Adder bites suggests that the technique inactivates some venom at the bite site,[1] but prolonged application has not been subjected to a controlled study.

Removal of the pressure-immobilisation bandage

Removal in the case of envenomation may precipitate a sudden elevation in blood concentration of venom and collapse of the victim. On the other hand, first aid has not been proven to inactivate venom in humans. Its removal therefore should be dictated by the circumstance. When an asymptomatic snake-bite victim reaches hospital with the recommended first-aid measures in place, these should not be disturbed until antivenom, appropriate staff and equipment have been assembled. If the victim is symptomatic and antivenom is indicated, the first-aid measures should not be removed until after antivenom has been administered, and reapplied if the victim's condition deteriorates. A swab of the bite site may be obtained by removing the splint temporarily and then cutting a window in the bandage. Thereafter the bandage should be made good and the splint reapplied.

ANTIVENOM

CSL Ltd (Parkville, Australia, +61 393891204) produces highly purified equine monovalent antivenoms against the venoms of the main terrestrial snakes, including Tiger Snake, Brown Snake, Black Snake, Death Adder and Taipan. A polyvalent antivenom – a mixture of aliquots of all of these – is also available. A sea-snake antivenom is also produced from horses immunised with Beaked Sea-Snake (*Enhydrina schistosa*) and Tiger Snake venom.

Antivenom should be administered according to the identity of the snake or if unknown or doubtful, according to the result of a VDK test (**Table 84.1**). If neither of these criteria can be fulfilled, and if the situation warrants immediate antivenom therapy, the geographical location may be used a guide, since the distribution of many species is known (**Table 84.2**). Polyvalent antivenom should not be used when a monovalent antivenom could be used appropriately. For bites by uncommon snakes, when antivenom is indicated, polyvalent antivenom or a monovalent antivenom as indicated by a VDK test should be chosen.

Table 84.1 Antivenom and initial dosages when snake identified

SNAKE	ANTIVENOM	DOSE (UNITS)
Common Brown Snake	Brown Snake	4000
Chappell Island Tiger Snake	Tiger Snake	12000
Copperheads	Tiger Snake	3000–6000
Death Adders	Death Adder	6000
Dugite	Brown Snake	4000
Gwardar	Brown Snake	4000
Mulga (King Brown) Snake	Black Snake	18000
Papuan Black Snake	Black Snake	18000
Red-bellied Black Snake	Tiger Snake *or* Black Snake*	3000 18000
Rough-scaled (Clarence River) Snake	Tiger Snake	3000
Sea-Snakes	Sea-Snake *or* Tiger Snake	1000 3000
Small-scaled (Fierce) Snake	Taipan	12000
Taipans	Taipan	12000
Tasmanian Tiger Snake	Tiger Snake	6000
Tiger Snake	Tiger Snake	3000

*Smaller protein mass Tiger Snake antivenom preferable.
Antivenom units per vial: Brown Snake 1000; Tiger Snake 3000; Black Snake 18000; Taipan 12000; Death Adder 6000; polyvalent 40000. Note: (1) If the victim on presentation is critically ill, 2–3 times these amounts should be given initially; (2) additional antivenom may be required in the course of management since absorption of venom may be delayed.

Dose

One vial of specific antivenom neutralises in vitro the average yield on 'milking'– a process whereby venom is harvested by inducing the snake to bite through a latex membrane. If the amount of venom injected at a bite is greater than the average yield on milking, one vial of antivenom will not be adequate therapy. In severe cases of envenomation, a number of vials of antivenom will need to be administered. Absorption of venom from a bite site(s) is a continuing process.

The initial doses of antivenom are given in Tables 84.1 and 84.2. The need for subsequent doses should be guided by the clinical response. After bites by species with coagulopathic effects the victim's coagulation status is a useful but not definitive guide to whether more antivenom is required. In the absence of a rapid measurement of exogenous venom procoagulant in blood, it is difficult to determine whether continued coagulopathy after antivenom administration is due to unneutralised venom or to the fact that hepatic

Table 84.2 Antivenom and initial dosages when identity of snake uncertain

STATE	ANTIVENOM	DOSE (UNITS)
Tasmania	Tiger Snake	6000
Victoria	Tiger Snake *and* Brown Snake	3000 4000
New South Wales and ACT; Queensland; South Australia; Western Australia; Northern Territory	Polyvalent	40 000
Papua New Guinea	Polyvalent	40 000

Note: (1) If the victim on presentation is critically ill, 2–3 times these amounts should be given initially; (2) additional antivenom may be required in the course of management since absorption of venom may be delayed.

manufacture of consumed coagulation factors requires at least 6 hours.

The dose of antivenom required varies because the amount of venom injected cannot be determined, and snakes may bite multiple times. Moreover, victims may present late after envenomation when toxins have already become bound to target tissues and cannot be easily neutralised. Some victims in this circumstance have required mechanical ventilation for many weeks despite large amounts of appropriate antivenom. A child may require more antivenom than an adult envenomated by the same amount of venom, and a victim in poor general health will likewise require more. Finally, antivenoms are manufactured against specific species and may have less neutralising ability against different species of the same genus or against unrelated species, even when the antivenom chosen is nevertheless appropriate.

Administration

The decision to administer antivenom must be based on clinical criteria of envenomation, and not restricted to the result of a VDK test. A positive VDK test of a biological sample establishes the diagnosis of envenomation and the choice of antivenom, but does not imply that antivenom should or should not be given.

If the victim is significantly envenomated, antivenom must be administered as there is no other effective treatment. Antivenom may be withheld if envenomation is so mild that spontaneous recovery may occur or the consequences of antivenom administration are likely to outweigh the benefit to be gained (e.g. in a herpetologist who is mildly envenomated and known to have allergy to antivenom).

Snake antivenoms must be given by the intravenous route, or in dire circumstances if a vein cannot be cannulated then by the intraosseous route. The large volume of fluid and slow absorption render the intramuscular route useless in emergencies.

A test dose of antivenom to determine allergy should not be done. It is unreliable and a waste of precious time.

Premedication

Antivenom should be preceded by premedication with subcutaneous epinephrine (adrenaline), approximately 0.25 mg for an adult and 0.005–0.01 mg/kg for a child, at least 5–10 minutes before commencement of infusion. In the moribund or critically ill victim when it is essential to administer antivenom quickly, the epinephrine may be given intramuscularly or even intravenously in smaller doses. However, in general epinephrine is not recommended by either of those routes because of the risk of intracerebral haemorrhage due to the combination of possible epinephrine-induced hypertension and venom-induced coagulopathy. Although intracerebral haemorrhage has been recorded in the past in association with premedication, all such cases occurred after intravenous epinephrine, and none with subcutaneous epinephrine. On the other hand, the incidence of adverse reactions (8–13%) and occasional death after antivenom are sufficient to warrant premedication with epinephrine, which is the only medication proven effective in reducing the incidence of antivenom-induced reactions and their severity.[8]

It is not prudent to forgo premedication on the assumption that if anaphylaxis occurs it will be treatable. Iatrogenic anaphylaxis has a high mortality despite vigorous and expert resuscitation.[9] If an adverse reaction to the first vial of antivenom has not occurred, subsequent vials do not need to be preceded by epinephrine. The reaction rate to polyvalent antivenom is higher than to monovalent antivenoms and should not be used when a monovalent antivenom or combinations will suffice.

The antihistamine promethazine is ineffective in this setting[10] and contraindicated because it may cause obtundation and hypotension, both of which may exacerbate and confound a state of envenomation. Other drugs such as steroids and aminophylline are also not useful in preventing anaphylaxis because their actions, apart from being unproven, are too slow in onset, but steroids are useful for preventing serum sickness.

Infusion

The antivenom may be injected slowly into a running intravenous line or diluted in Hartmann's or other crystalloid solution in approximately 1 in 10 volumes in a burette and administered over 15–30 minutes if the situation is not critical. This method reduces the risk of an anaphylactoid reaction resulting from its binding with complement. For small children, if multiple vials are required, the dilution may be less to prevent excessive fluid administration. In emergencies the antivenom may be infused quickly in high concentration.

Adverse reactions

Antivenom infusion should be administered in a location equipped and staffed by personnel capable of managing anaphylaxis, which is discussed in detail in Chapter 66. Intramuscular epinephrine is the key treatment in a dose of approximately 0.25–1.00 mg for adults and 10 μg/kg for children. Antivenom therapy should be discontinued temporarily and restarted when the victim's condition is stable.

Lesser degrees of immediate adverse reaction restricted to headache, chest discomfort, fine rash, arthralgia, myalgia, nausea, abdominal pain, vomiting, and pyrexia may be managed by temporary cessation of infusion and administration of steroids and antihistamine before recommencement.

A delayed hypersensitivity reaction, serum sickness, should be anticipated and patients warned of the symptoms and signs, which usually appear several days to 2 weeks after antivenom administration. Severity may range from a faint rash and pyrexia to serious multisystem disease including lymphadenitis, polyarthralgia, urticaria, nephritis, neuropathy and vasculitis. The incidence of serum sickness appears to be greater with the use of multiple doses of monovalent antivenom and with polyvalent antivenom. Prophylactic treatment is a course of steroids (e.g. prednisolone 1 mg/kg per day for 5 days).

INVESTIGATIONS AND MONITORING

Tests should be performed regularly, interpreted quickly and treated promptly to counter venom effects and its complications. Serial coagulation tests and tests of renal function are especially important. Absorption of venom from the bite site is a continuing process that should be anticipated. Apart from regular monitoring of vital signs and oxygenation, the following are specifically needed.

Bite site

A swab for venom testing should be done. It has the highest likelihood of detecting venom provided the site has not been washed. The bite site may be squeezed to yield venom if it has been washed. A positive result identifies venom but does not prove envenomation.

Urine

Test the urine for venom that may be present when venom in blood has been bound by antivenom and is therefore undetectable. Urine should also be tested for blood and protein. If the urine is pigmented a distinction should be made between haemoglobinuria and myoglobinuria, which is impossible with simple ward tests. Urine output should be recorded.

Blood

- Coagulation tests should include prothrombin time, activated thromboplastin time, serum fibrinogen and fibrin degradation products.
- A full-blood examination and blood film for haemoglobin level, evidence of haemolysis and platelet count. A mild elevation in white cell count is expected.
- Electrolytes, urea, creatinine and creatine phosphokinase (isoenzymes and troponin are useful) to monitor rhabdomyolysis and possible renal compromise.

Electrocardiogram

Sinus tachycardia, ventricular ectopy and ST segment and T-wave changes are not uncommon. These effects may be the direct result of venom toxins or from electrolyte disturbances caused by rhabdomyolysis or renal failure.

SECONDARY MANAGEMENT

Coagulation factor and blood transfusion

Although coagulopathy often resolves after several doses of antivenom it does not restore coagulation per se – it permits newly released or manufactured coagulation factors to act unopposed by venom. If haemorrhage is occurring, or if coagulation is not restored after several doses of antivenom over several hours, it is prudent to administer fresh frozen plasma and to remeasure coagulation at intervals. Because regeneration of coagulation factors takes many hours, treatment of isolated coagulopathy entirely with antivenom while waiting for their regeneration exposes the patient to serious haemorrhage. Administration of coagulation factors, such as in the form of fresh frozen plasma, should be preceded by antivenom to neutralise venom prothrombin activator as otherwise consumption coagulopathy may worsen.[11] Platelets may be required but whole blood is rarely needed.

Intravenous fluids, rhabdomyolysis and renal protection

After acute resuscitation, administer intravenous fluids in sufficient volume to maintain urine output at about 40 mL/kg per day in an adult and 1–2 mL/kg per hour in a child to prevent tubular necrosis as a consequence of rhabdomyolysis. Life-threatening hyperkalaemia and hypocalcaemia may develop with rhabdomyolysis. Haemofiltration or dialysis may be required.

Heparin

Although this anticoagulant has prevented the action of prothrombin activators in animal models of envenomation, it does not improve established consumption coagulopathy. It is not recommended. Emphasis instead should be on treating the cause by neutralising venom with antivenom.

Analgesia and sedation

Australian snake bite does not cause severe pain. However, sedation is required for the mechanically ventilated venom-paralysed victim and analgesia for rhabdomyolysis.

Care of the bite site

Usually no specific care is required. Occasionally the site may blister, bruise, ulcerate or necrose, particularly when a first-aid bandage has been in place for a considerable time or when the bite was by a member of the Black Snake genus, such as a Mulga Snake or Red-bellied Black Snake.

Other drugs

Antibiotics are not routinely required but should be considered as for any potentially contaminated wound. Sea-snake bites may cause Gram-negative infections. Tetanus prophylaxis should be reviewed.

SEA-SNAKE BITE

Some sea-snake venoms cause widespread damage to skeletal muscle with consequent myoglobinuria, neuromuscular paralysis or direct renal damage. Many have not been researched. The principles of treatment are essentially the same as for envenomation by terrestrial snakes. The venoms of significant species are neutralised with CSL Ltd Beaked Sea-Snake (*Enhydrina schistosa*) antivenom. If that preparation is not available, Tiger Snake or polyvalent antivenom should be used. Sea-snake bites are uncommon in Australia and no deaths have been recorded.

UNCOMMON AND EXOTIC SNAKE BITE

Zoo personnel, herpetologists and amateur collectors who catch, maintain or breed species of uncommon Australian snakes or who import or breed exotic (overseas) snakes are at risk, as are personnel in the Australian Quarantine and Inspection Service (AQIS) who encounter exotic species. Specific antivenoms to the venoms of uncommon Australian snakes do not exist, but neutralisation is provided by polyvalent antivenom or by monovalent antivenom, as indicated by the VDK.

Exotic snake antivenoms are maintained by Royal Melbourne Hospital (tel: +61 3 9342 7000), Royal Adelaide Hospital (tel: +61 8 8222 4000), Ballarat Hospital (tel: +61 3 5320 4316), Venom Supplies Ltd, Tanunda, South Australia (tel: +61 8 8563 0001), Australian Reptile Park (Tel: +61 2 4340 1022), Taronga Zoo (Mosman, tel: +61 2 9978 4757) and the Australian Venom Research Unit (AVRU) (tel: +61 3 8344 7753). The locations and stocks of antivenoms in Australia for treatment of bites by specific exotic snakes are maintained by AVRU at http://www.avru.org/reference/reference_avhold.html.

LONG-TERM EFFECTS OF SNAKE BITE

After appropriate treatment, recovery is expected but it may be slow, taking many weeks or months, particularly from a critical illness or after delayed presentation involving neurotoxicity and rhabdomyolysis. Isolated neurological or ophthalmic signs may persist. Long-term loss of taste or smell occurs occasionally.

SPIDERS

Although several thousand species of spiders exist in Australia, only Funnel-web Spiders (genera *Atrax* and *Hadronyche*) and the Red-back Spider (*Latrodectus hasselti*) have caused death or significant systemic illness. All spiders have venom and a few, particularly the White-tailed Spider (*Lampona cylindrata*) and the Common Black House Spider (*Badumna insignis*), have caused severe local injury, although this occurs rarely.[1,12,13] Causes for ulcerated skin lesions other than spider bites should be sought.

FUNNEL-WEB SPIDERS

Many species of the Funnel-web genera *Atrax* and *Hadronyche* inhabit Queensland, New South Wales, Victoria, Tasmania and South Australia, but only spiders from New South Wales and southern Queensland have caused significant illness and death. These are large dark-coloured aggressive spiders. A systematic review involving 138 cases identified 77 cases of severe envenomation with 13 deaths, but none occurred after introduction of antivenom in 1981 and the vast majority (97%) responded to antivenom therapy.[14] All deaths were attributed to the Sydney Funnel-web Spider (*A. robustus*)[1] which inhabits an area within an approximate 160 km radius of Sydney. It roams after rainfall, may enter houses and seeks shelter among clothes or bedding, giving a painful bite when disturbed.

Severe envenomation is also caused by the Southern Tree (*H. cerberea*), Northern Tree (*H. formidabilis*), Port Macquarie (*H.* sp. 14), Toowoomba or Darling Downs (*H. infensa*) and Blue Mountains (*H. versuta*) species. In contrast to other spiders, male Funnel-web Spiders have more potent venom than female spiders.

Bites do not always result in envenomation, but envenomation may be rapidly fatal. The early features of the envenomation syndrome include nausea, vomiting, profuse sweating, salivation and abdominal pain. Life-threatening features are usually heralded by the appearance of muscle fasciculation at the bite site, which quickly involves distant muscle groups. Hypertension, tachyarrhythmias, vasoconstriction, hypersalivation and bronchorrhoea occur. The victim may lapse into coma, develop central hypoventilation and have difficulty maintaining an airway free of secretions. Finally, respiratory failure, pulmonary oedema and severe hypotension culminate in death. The syndrome may develop within several hours but it may be more rapid. Several children have died within 90 minutes of envenomation, and one died within 15 minutes.[1] An active component in the venom is a polypeptide that stimulates the release of acetylcholine at neuromuscular junctions and within the autonomic nervous system, and the release of catecholamines.

Treatment consists of the application of a pressure-immobilisation bandage, intravenous administration of antivenom and support of vital functions, which may include airway support, mechanical ventilation and intensive cardiovascular support.

RED-BACK SPIDER

This spider is distributed throughout Australia and is found outdoors in household gardens in suburban and rural areas. Related species and similar effects of envenomation ('latrodectism') occur in many parts of the world. Red-back Spider bite is the most common cause for antivenom administration in Australia, at 300–400 per annum. The adult female is identified easily. Its body is about 1 cm in size and has a distinct red or orange dorsal stripe over its abdomen. When disturbed, it gives a pinprick-like bite. The bite site becomes inflamed and, during the following minutes to several hours, severe pain exacerbated by movement commences locally and may extend up the limb or radiate elsewhere. The pain may be accompanied by profuse sweating, headache, nausea, vomiting, abdominal pain, fever, hypertension, paraesthesiae and rashes. In a small percentage of cases when treatment is delayed, progressive muscle paralysis may occur over many hours, requiring mechanical ventilation. If untreated, muscle weakness, spasm and arthralgia may persist for months after the bite.

If the effects of a bite are trivial and confined to the bite site, antivenom may be withheld; otherwise antivenom should be given intramuscularly or intravenously. The antivenom may be given intravenously in cases of refractory pain but the risk of anaphylaxis may be higher than by the intramuscular route, which is very low (<0.5%). A premedication with promethazine is recommended and epinephrine should be at hand. In contrast to a bite from a snake or Funnel-web Spider, a bite from a Red-back Spider is not immediately life-threatening. There is no proven effective first aid, but application of a cold pack or iced water may help relieve pain. Bites by *Steatoda* spp. (cupboard spiders) may cause a similar syndrome and can be treated effectively with Red-back Spider antivenom.[15]

BOX JELLYFISH

This creature, *Chironex fleckeri,* is probably the most venomous in the world. It has caused approximately 70 deaths in the waters off northern Australia. It has a cuboid bell up to 30 cm in diameter. Numerous tentacles arise from the corners of the bell and trail several metres. It is semitransparent and difficult to see by anyone wading or swimming in shallow water. The tentacles are lined with millions of nematocysts that, on contact with skin, discharge a threaded barb that pierces subcutaneous tissue, including small blood vessels. Contact with the tentacles causes severe pain and envenomation, from which death may occur within minutes. Death is probably due to both neurotoxic effects causing apnoea and direct cardiotoxicity, although the precise mode of action of the venom is unknown. In mechanically ventilated animals, fatal hypotension occurs rapidly on envenomation.[16] The skin that sustains the injury may heal with disfiguring scars.

First aid, which must be administered on the beach, consists of dousing the skin with acetic acid (vinegar), which inactivates undischarged nematocysts. Adherent tentacles can then be removed. Cardiopulmonary resuscitation may be required on the beach and continued en route to hospital where extracorporeal life support could be considered. An ovine antivenom is available but efficacy is doubtful in established critical illness. Prevention is of paramount importance: water must not be entered when this jellyfish is known to be close inshore. Wet suits, clothing and 'stinger suits' offer protection.

IRUKANDJI

Stings by the Irukandji, *Carukia barnesi* (Barnes' jellyfish), and by other Carybdeid jellyfish may cause a syndrome known as Irukandji syndrome.[17] *C. barnesi* is a small cubozoan jellyfish with a squarish bell a little more than 1 cm in diameter. Single tentacles trail from its four corners. When submerged it is virtually impossible to see.

Its sting is mild and marked only by a small area of erythema. However, severe general illness may follow with abdominal cramps, hypertension, back pain, nausea and vomiting, limb cramps, chest tightness and marked distress. Occasionally, cardiogenic pulmonary oedema has necessitated mechanical ventilation and inotropic therapy, while hypertension has caused two deaths by stroke. The mechanism is uncertain, but experimental studies in animals have shown that Irukandji extracts cause a hyperadrenergic syndrome secondary to massive release of catecholamines,[18] which may explain at least in part the cause of heart failure. Pain relief is the most important feature of management in mild to moderate cases. In a series of 10 victims with 'Irukandji syndrome', intravenous magnesium salts provided pain relief and a reduction in blood pressure,[19] but these observations are not supported by a randomised trial showing that magnesium salts did not influence the required amount of analgesia.[20] Antihypertensive therapy with phentolamine or a 'titratable' nitrate may be required in the initial phase of management.

AUSTRALIAN PARALYSIS TICK

This tick (*Ixodes holocyclus*) injects a toxin that causes flaccid paralysis after some 3–5 days of feeding on humans. The onset of illness resembles that of Guillain–Barré syndrome. Prompt, careful and entire removal of tick(s) is necessary, followed by a period of observation to ensure that late-onset paralysis does not occur. No antitoxin is available.

BEES, WASPS AND ANTS

Anaphylactic reactions to bee and wasp stings cause approximately the same number of deaths in Australia each year as do snake bites, at an average of 2.3 per annum.[21] The common European Honey Bee (*Apis mellifera*) is largely responsible. Jumper and Bull Ants (*Myrmecia* spp.) may also cause anaphylaxis. Persons who develop reactions to bites should seek immunotherapy and always carry injectable epinephrine.

BLUE-RINGED OCTOPUSES

Several species of *Hapalochlaena* inhabit the Australian coastline. When handled, these octopuses bite and inject tetrodotoxin – a neurotoxin found in many different species of marine animals. It causes rapid onset of flaccid paralysis. Approximately a dozen deaths have been recorded. The required treatment is mechanical ventilation until spontaneous recovery occurs.

STINGING FISH

Numerous marine and fresh-water fish carry venom in glands attached to stinging spines. The most dangerous is the Stonefish (*Synanceia* spp.). When trodden upon, venom is injected. The immediate effect is extreme pain. Several deaths have been recorded, which are presumably due to the known depressive effects of the toxins on cardiovascular and neuromuscular function, and myotoxicity. An antivenom (CSL Ltd) is available. Local or regional nerve blockade may be required for pain relief. Other stinging fish, such as the fresh-water Bullrout (*Notesthes robusta*) also cause excruciating pain when their spines are contacted. Immersion of the affected limb in warm-to-hot water provides pain relief.

VENOMOUS CONE SHELLS

Many gastropod molluscs rapidly eject a venom-laden harpoon to almost instantaneously immobilise and kill prey. The numerous conotoxins, which are short proteins, stimulate or block neuronal and neuromuscular receptors, causing rapid death. A handful of human deaths have been recorded when shells have been carelessly or unwittingly handled. There is no antivenom. Mechanical ventilation would be required until spontaneous recovery occurs.

Access the complete references list online at http://www.expertconsult.com

1. Sutherland SK, Tibballs J. Australian Animal Toxins. Melbourne: Oxford University Press; 2001.
3. Isbister GK, Scorgie FE, O'Leary MA, et al. Factor deficiencies in venom-induced consumption coagulopathy resulting from Australian elapid envenomation: Australian Snakebite Project (ASP-10). J Thromb Haemostasis 2010;8:2504–13.
6. Sutherland SK, Coulter AR, Harris RD. Rationalization of first-aid measures for elapid snakebite. Lancet 1979;1:183–6.
8. Premawardhena AP, de Silva CE, Fonseka M, et al. Low dose subcutaneous adrenaline to prevent acute adverse reactions to antivenom serum in people bitten by snakes: randomised, placebo controlled trial. BMJ 1999;318:1041–3.
10. Fan HW, Marcopito LF, Cardoso JL, et al. A sequential randomised and double blind trial of promethazine prophylaxis against early anaphylactic reactions to antivenom for *Bothrops* snake bites. BMJ 1999; 318:1451–3.
11. Tibballs J. Fresh frozen plasma after Brown snake bite – helpful or harmful? Anaesth Intens Care 2005; 33:13–15.
12. Isbister GK, Gray MR. White-tail spider bite: a prospective study of 130 definite bites by *Lampona* species. Med J Aust 2003;179:199–202.
14. Isbister GK, Gray MR, Balit CR, et al. Funnel-web spider bite: a systematic review of recorded clinical cases. Med J Aust 2005;182:407–11.
17. Tibballs J, Li R, Gershwin LA, et al. Review: Australian carybdeid jellyfish causing "irukandji syndrome". Toxicon 2012;59:617–25.
18. Winkel KD, Tibballs J, Molenaar P, et al. Cardiovascular actions of the venom from the Irukandji (*Carukia barnesi*) jellyfish: effects in human, rat and guinea-pig tissues in vitro and in pigs in vivo. Clin Exp Pharmacol Physiol 2005;32:777–88.

85

Ballistic injury

Michael C Reade and Peter D (Toby) Thomas

'Ballistics' is the study of projectiles. Strictly, this does not include the effect of blast, but as blast often wounds by accelerating projectiles, this chapter refers to both mechanisms of injury.

Patients with ballistic injury are uncommon in most parts of the developed world. However, understanding ballistic trauma is essential, as failing to do so can result in treatment (e.g. needless extensive debridement) worse than the injury itself. This chapter will hopefully remain a skimmed-over curiosity in an otherwise intensely studied book. For the minority who need to read it in detail, perhaps unexpectedly, we hope it can provide useful advice.

EPIDEMIOLOGY OF BALLISTIC TRAUMA

Military conflicts result in variable wound patterns, summarised in **Table 85.1**.[1–3]

The trend towards a higher proportion of head and neck wounds in recent conflicts (**Table 85.2**)[2–4] has been attributed to better protection from body armour.

CAUSES AND TIMING OF DEATH IN BALLISTIC INJURY

Seventy percent of deaths due to ballistic trauma occur due to brain injury or exsanguination within 5 minutes of wounding,[2] and almost none are survivable regardless of treatment. However, most ballistic wounds are not fatal. Of patients who died in the Vietnam War,[4] 25% had potentially correctable surgical causes, and 12% died of infections and other complications. While most preventable deaths occur in the first 1–2 'golden' hours after wounding, treatment in the 'platinum 10 minutes'[5] is frequently most important. Of preventable deaths, 60% are due to haemorrhage from extremities, 33% from tension pneumothorax, and 6% from airway obstruction.[6] Interventions to address these three mechanisms are central to the training of military personnel.[7]

RATIO OF KILLED TO WOUNDED

The ratio of killed to wounded depends on weapon systems employed, context, protective equipment and medical support. The mortality associated with different weapons systems in combat is shown in **Table 85.3**.[2,8]

The context of wounding is critically important. In modern war the wounded : killed ratio ranges from 1.9 : 1 to 13.0 : 1,[9] with an average over time of around 4 : 1.[2,4] Body armour and better medical care were advanced as possible explanations for the higher survival (ratio 10 : 1) of US casualties in Iraq,[10] although the higher proportion of blast casualties probably also contributed. Weapons used in a civilian context are more lethal, ranging from 0 : 1 to 1 : 3.14,[9] probably because civilian shootings occur at close range with unarmed victims who cannot escape. Higher than expected mortality in war suggests executions rather than combat deaths, and has been used as evidence of war crimes.[9]

BLAST TRAUMA

An explosion occurs when a substance rapidly undergoes a chemical or nuclear reaction, releasing energy in the form of a pressure wave, (usually) gas and heat. *High explosive* produces a supersonic pressure wave; slower burning (*conflagration*) produces a subsonic wave. The first force felt by an affected body is the static pressure wave, depicted in **Figure 85.1**. There is no mass movement of gas; rather pressure rapidly increases then becomes sub atmospheric. Hard surfaces reflect pressure waves, increasing the force in enclosed spaces.[11] The second force felt by a body in air is the mass movement of gases liberated by the exploding substance: the 'blast wind'.

MECHANISMS OF BLAST INJURY

The classification of blast injury is shown in **Table 85.4** and **Figure 85.2**.

PATHOPHYSIOLOGY OF PRIMARY BLAST INJURY

Primary blast injury is a common cause of death due to blast,[12] but (except in confined environments) is uncommon in survivors. For example, only 7% of US personnel wounded by blast surviving to hospital care had primary blast injury.[13] If the casualty is close enough to suffer a primary blast injury, secondary and tertiary effects are usually fatal. The immediate response to

Table 85.1 Historical variation in combat trauma

CONFLICT	BULLETS (%)	BLAST/FRAGMENTATION (%)	OTHER INCL. LAND MINES (%)
World War 1[1]	39	61	–
World War 2[1]	10	85	5
Korean War[1]	7	92	1
Vietnam War[1]	52	44	4
Falkland Islands[1]	31.8	55.8	12.4
Yugoslavia 1991–1992[2]	41	2	52
Iraq and Afghanistan[3]	19	77	4

Table 85.2 Historical anatomical wound patterns

CONFLICT	HEAD/NECK (%)	THORAX (%)	ABDOMEN (%)	LIMBS (%)	OTHER/MULTIPLE (%)
World War 1[2,4]	17	4	2	70	7
World War 2[2,4]	4	8	4	75	9
Korean War[2,4]	17	7	7	67	2
Vietnam War[2,4]	14	7	5	74	–
Falkland Islands[2,4]	16	15	10	59	–
Yugoslavia 1991–1992[2]	21	9	8	62	23 (also incl. in individual %)
Iraq and Afghanistan[3] (3)	30	6	9	55	–

Table 85.3 Mortality associated with different weapons systems employed in combat[2,8]

Military rifle bullet	30–40%
Blast	22%
Blast fragmentation – randomly formed fragments	20% artillery shells; 10% grenades
Blast fragmentation – military preformed fragments	15% artillery shells; 5% grenades

blast to the chest is vagal-mediated hypotension, bradycardia and apnoea. Alternating overpressure and under pressure causes injury at the interfaces of tissues of different densities. This especially affects gas-containing organs (i.e. ears, lungs and gastrointestinal tract). The ear is the most sensitive. The eardrum can be ruptured (generally inferiorly in the pars tensa) by overpressures of approximately 35 kPa, and above 100 kPa rupture is nearly universal. There may be haemorrhage into the membrane without rupture. Rupture of the tympanic membrane may cause tinnitus, pain, hearing loss, and abnormal vestibular function. One-third of casualties experiencing rupture of the tympanic membrane will have permanent hearing loss.

The sensitivity of the tympanic membrane to blast led to recommendations to use this as an effective screen for blast injury to other organs. Unfortunately, this is not supported by clinical experience. Tympanic membrane disruption was present in only 50% of patients with other significant blast injury in one recent study.[13]

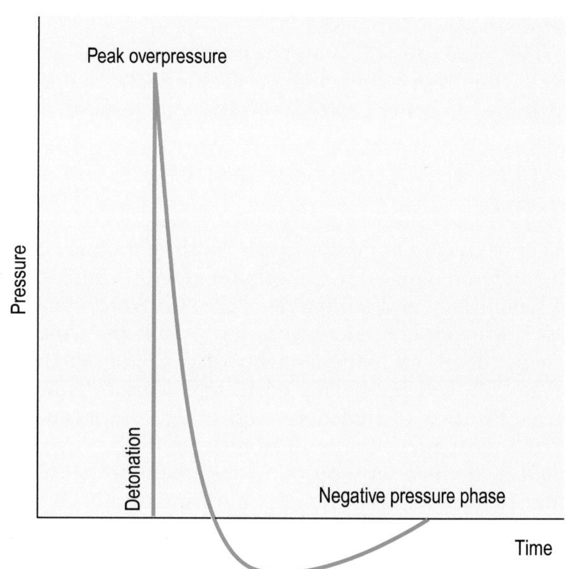

Figure 85.1 The blast static pressure wave in air.

Blast lung injury, with shearing of the alveolar-capillary barrier, can cause air emboli, pneumothorax,

Table 85.4 Mechanisms of blast injury

TYPE OF BLAST INJURY	MECHANISM	EFFECTS
Primary	Static pressure wave, causing barotrauma due to overpressurisation and underpressurisation	Affects mainly air-filled organs: Tympanic membrane rupture 'Blast lung' Hollow viscera rupture (colon) Mild traumatic brain injury (mTBI) Eye injury (globe rupture, hyphaema, serous retinitis)
Secondary	Effects of projectiles propelled by the explosion	Penetrating injury Soft tissue trauma Traumatic amputation
Tertiary	Effects due to mass movement of air ('blast wind'), either directly or by interaction with the surroundings, including collapse of buildings	Blunt and penetrating injury Bone fracture Traumatic amputation Open or closed TBI Crush injury; entrapment
Quaternary	All other effects of blast, including burns, oxygen depletion, creation of dust	Surface and airway burns Inhalation of toxic gases (CO, cyanide) Exposure to radiation Asphyxiation

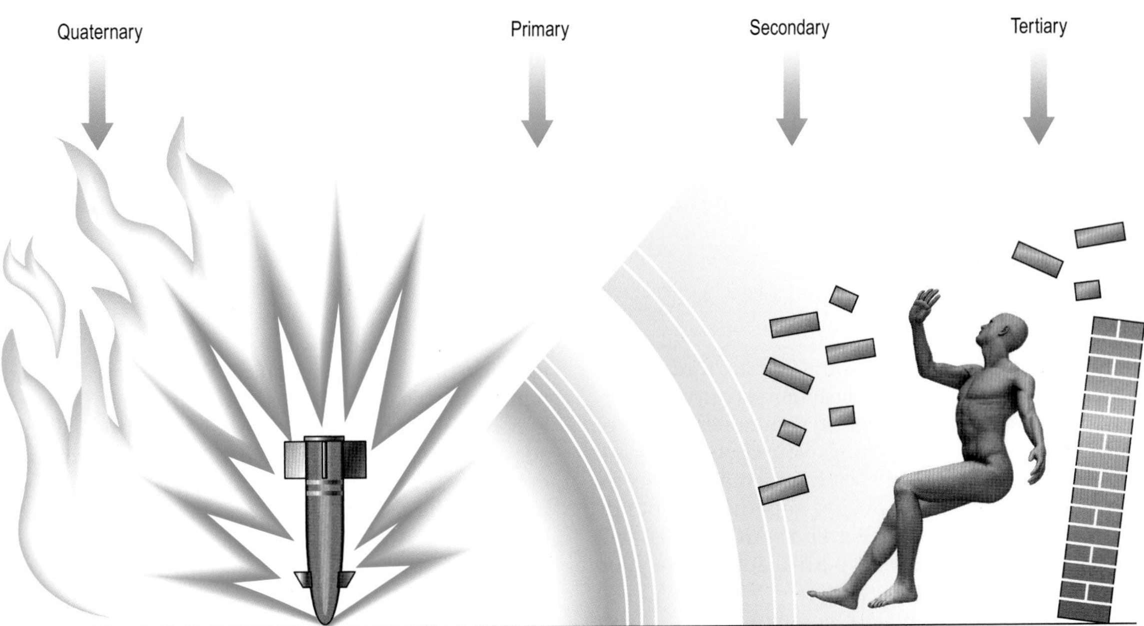

Figure 85.2 Mechanisms of blast injury. *(Courtesy of Major Anthony Chambers FRACS.)*

lung contusion, haemothorax, alveolar haemorrhage, mediastinal air, and subcutaneous emphysema.[14] As alveoli become flooded with fluid and cellular debris, the result is 'blast lung' (**Fig. 85.3**), with hypoxaemia secondary to ventilation–perfusion mismatch. The effect can appear similar to pulmonary contusion from blunt chest trauma. Arterial air emboli from alveolar–pulmonary venous communications cause most early deaths. Signs of air emboli include cerebral dysfunction such as altered affect, confusion, or focal neurological signs. When such findings are noted after an explosion, other closed head injuries must be excluded. Emboli to the coronary arteries may cause arrhythmias or ischaemia.

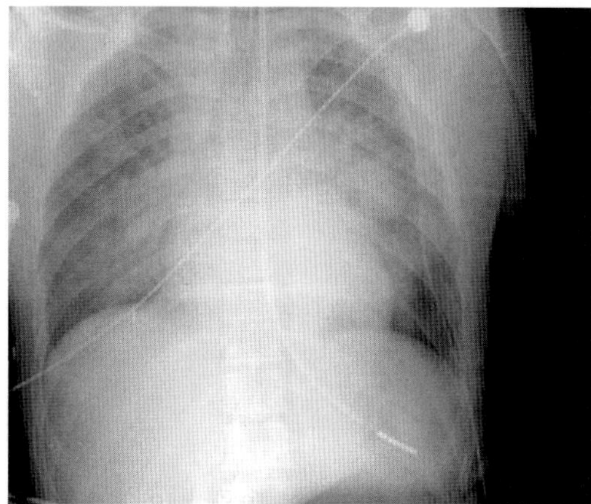

Figure 85.3 Blast lung, showing characteristic perihilar infiltrates. CT is a more sensitive modality than plain radiography. *(Courtesy of Australian Defence Force, Iraq, 2006.)*

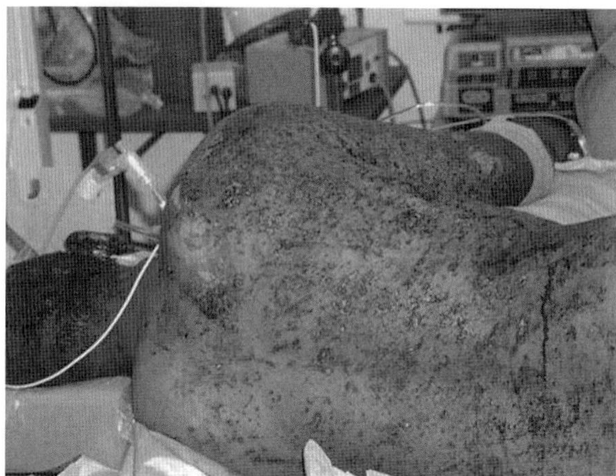

Figure 85.4 'Peppering' or 'battle acne' wounds characteristic of secondary blast injury. *(Courtesy of Australian Defence Force, Iraq, 2006.)*

Primary abdominal blast injury is uncommon, but occurs more frequently in enclosed spaces and under water. It frequently presents late with signs of peritonism and absent bowel sounds indicating visceral rupture. The colon is most commonly affected. Rarely, rupture of the liver or spleen may occur.

The role of primary blast injury in mild traumatic brain injury (mTBI) is unclear. mTBI can be associated with persistent and debilitating symptoms, many of which are shared with post-traumatic stress disorder (PTSD).[15] Diffusion tensor imaging MRI shows abnormalities in mTBI, but these appear to correlate poorly with clinical signs.[16]

PATHOPHYSIOLOGY OF SECONDARY AND TERTIARY BLAST INJURIES

Secondary blast injuries were more than three times more common than primary blast injuries during Operation Iraqi Freedom[17] and are the commonest cause of death, mainly from penetrating wounds to the head, neck or chest. Survivors of blast fragmentation injuries often have many low-velocity superficial wounds ('peppering' or 'battle acne': **Fig. 85.4**). Around 10% will have significant eye injuries,[18] particularly due to glass fragments in urban environments.

Traumatic limb amputation is only partly an effect of the blast wind. Primary blast injury fractures long bones, and the blast wind then detaches the distal portion. This is thought to explain why such amputations are typically not through joints.[19]

MANAGEMENT OF BLAST INJURY

Explosions often cause 'mass casualty' events. Depending on the circumstances, triage should be well away from the incident, as placement of further explosive devices is a common tactic targeting medical personnel.

EAR INJURIES

Tympanic membrane rupture is treated conservatively, as most heal spontaneously. About 25% will require delayed surgical closure.

BLAST LUNG

Blast lung typically develops over 24–48 hours and takes 7–10 days to resolve. Presentation ranges from a slight decrease in oxygen saturation to frothy sputum, profound hypoxaemia, and subcutaneous emphysema. A chest radiograph will distinguish pneumothorax, haemothorax, or pulmonary parenchymal failure from blast or other causes (e.g. inhalation of toxic gases). Recommendations for blast lung are mostly extrapolated from those for other causes of acute respiratory distress syndrome (ARDS), despite the known differences in pathogenic mechanisms. The risk of systematic air embolism increases with mechanical ventilation, suggesting minimising peak inspiratory pressures and permissive hypercapnia may be particularly useful. Excessive fluid administration should be avoided to minimise contusion. Pumpless arteriovenous extracorporeal oxygenation has been used successfully to transport profoundly hypoxaemic casualties from field hospitals to definitive care.

ABDOMINAL INJURIES

CT or focused assessment sonography for trauma (FAST) scanning will guide early management, but clinical suspicion in the days after the injury is even more useful given the likelihood of delayed presentation. Primary anastomosis for colorectal injuries associated with blast is thought unwise because of the high incidence of leak (30%), and most patients require colonic diversion.[20]

TRAUMATIC BRAIN INJURY

The most severe CNS blast effects are diffuse axonal injury, contusion and traumatic subdural haematoma, all of which are managed according to conventional guidelines.[21] A patient with brief loss of consciousness after blast should have brain CT or MRI if there is persistent headache, vomiting, localising neurological signs or a Glasgow Coma Score less than 15.[22]

PENETRATING BALLISTIC TRAUMA

Penetrating ballistic trauma can be caused by fragments energised by explosive devices, or by projectiles from firearms.

BLAST FRAGMENTATION

Casing fragmentation multiplies many times the range and effect of smaller blast weapons such as grenades, mines and mortar bombs, producing fragments with predictable properties that optimise range, kinetic energy and probability of hitting a target. Larger blast weapons (bombs) rely on their greater energy to create effective fragments from surrounding rocks or debris.

BULLETS FROM FIREARMS

A *bullet* is a single projectile shot from a firearm. Modern bullets are attached to *cartridge cases* containing the *percussion cap* or *primer* and *propellant*; the entire structure forms a *round* of *ammunition*. Firearms firing bullets include *rifles* (with a long barrel that is 'rifled' with spiralling grooves inside that make the bullet rotate, increasing gyroscopic stability), *revolvers* (handguns with chambers that rotate to present each round to the barrel) and *pistols* (with short barrels but no rotating chambers). A *shotgun* with a smooth-bored barrel usually fires *shot* (round metal balls) rather than a single formed projectile.

PROJECTILE BALLISTICS

Rapidly expanding propellant gas accelerates the projectile through the firearm barrel. Projectile flight is determined by gravity, air friction and pressure resistance, wind, contact with solid objects (causing *ricochets*), and stability in flight. An aerodynamically shaped bullet tends to *yaw* to the side; this is opposed by gyroscopic stability, leading to a composite movement of *spin* (rotation around the long axis), *precession* (rotation of the rotational axis) and *nutation* (swaying of the rotational axis as it precesses). During flight, yaw progressively reduces. A bullet is therefore more likely to hit point-on after 100 metres of flight than after 3 metres (**Fig. 85.5**).[23,24]

WOUND BALLISTICS

Wound ballistics describes the interaction between a projectile and the biological tissue it hits. The amount of energy that is transferred is determined by the:

- *kinetic energy (KE) of the projectile:* KE = mass × velocity^2/2 × g. The kinetic energy *transferred* to the tissue is mass × (impact velocity − exit velocity)^2/2 × g

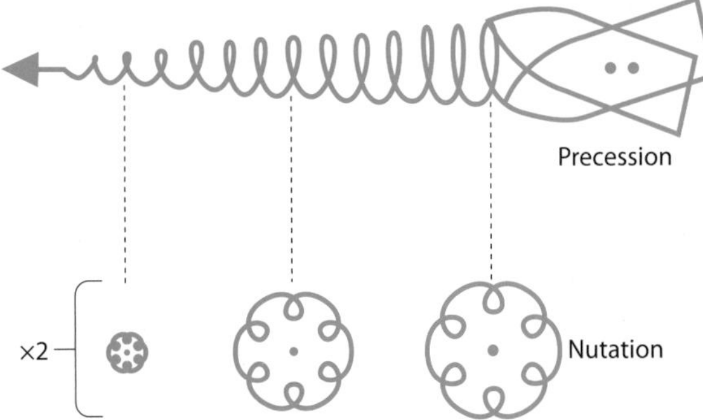

Figure 85.5 Precession and nutation. Both decrease as distance from the barrel increases. *(From Volgas DA, Stannard JP, Alonso JE. Ballistics: a primer for the surgeon. Injury 2005;36(3):373–9.)*

- *rotational energy of the projectile in flight:* usually negligible
- *shape and impact angle of the projectile:* an aerodynamically shaped bullet will impart more energy if it hits side-on; the degree to which this occurs is determined by its properties in flight, including the distance travelled and whether it has hit anything during flight
- *projectile deformability*
- *degree to which the projectile 'tumbles':* a rapid end-over-end motion does not occur; rather, if it remains intact, the bullet typically tumbles through 180 degrees and comes to lie base-first. Tumbling is the main reason why full metal jacket exit wounds are often larger than entry wounds
- *specific gravity of the tissue hit.*[25]

The terms 'high' and 'low' velocity are not as useful as 'power', incorporating projectile mass, and even less useful than the concept of energy transfer. Although most rifles are 'high-powered' and most pistols/revolvers 'low-powered', projectile energy is only one determinant of wound magnitude. A 'high-powered' rifle bullet may cause less trauma if it misses ribs and traverses a short path through the chest than a 'low-powered' pistol bullet that fragments after hitting a rib. Having said this, the kinetic energy of a rifle bullet is many times that from a pistol. Hitting bone, a pistol bullet frequently causes a simple fracture, whereas a rifle bullet causes fragmentation and extensive bone loss.[26] Most wounds caused by blast fragmentation (when the patient survives the explosion) are low-energy transfer.

Further determinants of the effect of the projectile are:

- the function of the tissue affected (e.g. the eye is damaged by minimal energy transfer)
- the ability of the affected tissue to tamponade haemorrhage (e.g. liver bleeds more than muscle).

BULLET DEFORMABILITY

Bullets are typically made of lead or lead–antimony, as high density preserves kinetic energy in flight. Pure lead bullets melt at velocities of greater than 2000 ft/s (≈600 m/s),[25] necessitating at least partial 'jacketing' in a more resilient substance (e.g. aluminium, brass, or steel). Military bullets (according to Third Hague Convention of 1899) must be completely encased in a 'full metal jacket' (a misnomer, as the base of the bullet may have no covering), which reduces deformation in tissues and so causes less 'unnecessary suffering'. By increasing the chance of non-lethal injury, an unintended consequence is to increase combat effect: a wounded enemy soldier consumes more resources than one who is dead. In contrast, hunting rifle bullets have a soft lead or polymer tip, increasing the chance of killing quickly and so reducing suffering. Bullets with hollowed-out points have greater air drag and shorter range, but deform so extensively that exiting the target is unlikely. This is beneficial for police wishing to reduce the chance of harming bystanders.

Doctors are sometimes asked by people concerned with compliance with the laws of armed conflict to classify the type of bullet found in a patient. *Any* bullet can deform and fragment, so finding no intact fully jacketed bullets does not allow this question to be answered (**Fig. 85.6**).[27]

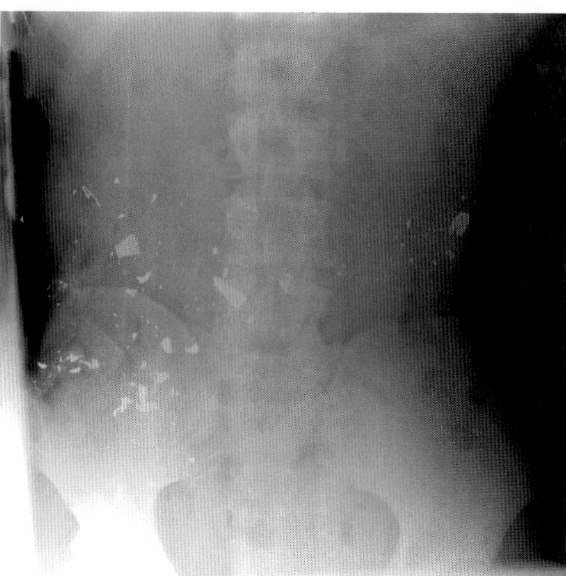

Figure 85.6 Three fully jacketed bullets have entered the right thigh. Two have fragmented after contacting bone, while the third remains intact. *(Courtesy of Australian Defence Force, Afghanistan, 2009.)*

MECHANISMS OF TISSUE DAMAGE

Bullets cause crushing/laceration, shock waves and cavitation. Crushing and laceration are caused by the direct force of the bullet, and are the principal mechanisms of injury due to 'low-powered' firearms. Serious injury generally results only if vital structures are damaged. Shock waves are caused when a 'high-powered' bullet compresses tissues. They cause little damage to most tissues[28] but can rupture gas-filled organs[25] and possibly cause neurological injury.[29] Cavitation results from the inertia imparted by a high-powered bullet to the tissues. As the tissues continue to move away from the bullet track, subatmospheric pressure sucks in debris. The *temporary cavitation* disrupts cells and their microcirculation, producing dead tissue around the wound track *up to* 30–40× the diameter of the bullet.[25] Cavitation is dependent on tissue elasticity; for example, liver is more affected than muscle. Inelastic gelatin blocks overemphasise the implications of temporary cavitation in many tissues.[30,31] The temporary cavity collapses to a much smaller permanent cavity, but the size of the permanent cavity is not an indicator of the extent of devitalised tissue.

MANAGEMENT OF PENETRATING BALLISTIC TRAUMA: BASIC PRINCIPLES

The International Committee of the Red Cross (ICRC) recommends as basic principles: early and thorough wound excision and irrigation, no unnecessary dressing changes, delayed primary closure, antibiotics as an adjuvant, antitetanus vaccine and immunoglobulin if necessary, no internal bone fixation, and early physiotherapy.[2]

DAMAGE CONTROL SURGERY

Damage control surgery aims to stop haemorrhage, restore blood flow and control wound contamination.[32] Wounds are left packed if necessary, and temporarily closed. Restoration of bowel continuity, definitive debridement and wound closure are all deferred until physiology is optimised. This concept fits well with the ICRC basic principles and, as it requires general rather than specialist surgical expertise, can be performed in small hospitals close to the wounded.

DEFINITIVE MANAGEMENT

In general, re-inspection within 24–48 hours will be required for major wounds, with further debridement if required. This process continues every 48 hours until the wound can be closed. Even apparently clean wounds should not be closed before 4–5 days. Of 16172 patients in the ICRC database, 41% required two operations, 14% three and 20% four or more.[2] Serial debridement in this manner is demanding; in mass casualties or resource-poor environments, the ICRC recognises this approach may be impossible and advises wider initial excisions.[2]

There are exceptions to the 'no primary closure' rule. The head, neck and genitals have such good blood supply that primary closure is possible in all but the most contaminated wounds. Oral mucosa should always be closed primarily if possible. In penetrating brain injury the dura should also be closed, if necessary with a patch of pericranium or muscle aponeurosis.[2] Blood vessels that have been repaired should be covered by viable muscle if possible, with the skin left open.

MANAGEMENT OF SPECIFIC TYPES OF PENETRATING BALLISTIC WOUND

EXTREMITY WOUNDS: WOUNDS THAT DO NOT REQUIRE DEBRIDEMENT

Military[33] and civilian[2] consensus guidelines agree that not all bullet wounds require debridement. Extremities with entry and exit wounds <1 cm and no swelling or signs of injury to vital structures can have narrow skin margins excised and the channel irrigated. Wounds that do not penetrate deep fascia require only scrubbing, irrigation, dressings and antibiotics.

EXTREMITY WOUNDS: HOW MUCH TISSUE TO DEBRIDE?

Many published accounts[1,30,34] and the authors' own experience suggest that surgeons sometimes perform extensive debridement around high-powered bullet tracks in the belief that microvascular tissue damage is more extensive than can be seen. This approach, although once advocated in military texts,[35] ignores empirical studies[34] and the distinction between projectile energy and energy transfer.

In penetrating ballistic trauma, muscle viability was historically assessed using the 'four C's'[8] – *capillary* bleeding when cut, *contracts* when pinched, *colour* of red meat, and *consistency* firm. However, apparently dead muscle is often later found to be viable.[30,31,36] Along with substantial consensus,[8,28,30,37] we advocate initial debridement of only tissue and bone that is clearly ischaemic or not attached, with re-inspection and reassessment after 2–3 days. Drawing on experience in Afghanistan and Iraq, detailed consensus recommendations for extremity war wound debridement have recently been published.[33]

SUPERFICIAL BLAST FRAGMENTATION

There is debate about the optimal management of blast fragmentation penetrating trauma. Historically, military teaching was that all wounds should be surgically debrided, as most fragments carry bacteria. However, few open wounds develop infection,[38] implying at least some can be managed non-operatively. The foot wound in **Figure 85.7** was extensively contaminated and contained devitalised tissue, necessitating debridement. Conversely, the superficial wounds in Figure 85.4 were cleaned with a surgical scrub brush; no infection developed and the resultant scars were smaller than if each perforation had been explored. Published indications for surgical debridement of blast fragmentation wounds derived from case series are listed in **Table 85.5**.[39,40]

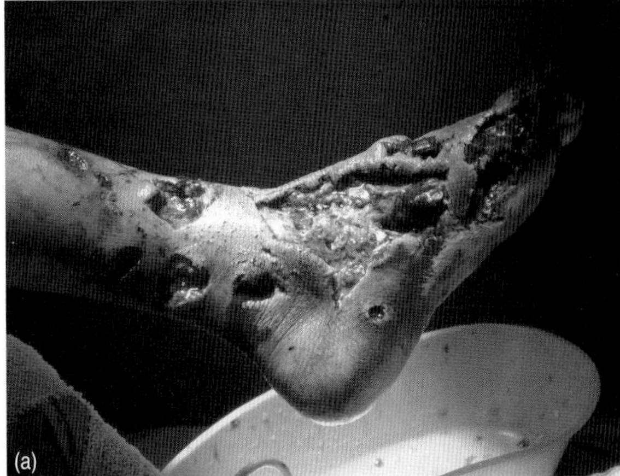

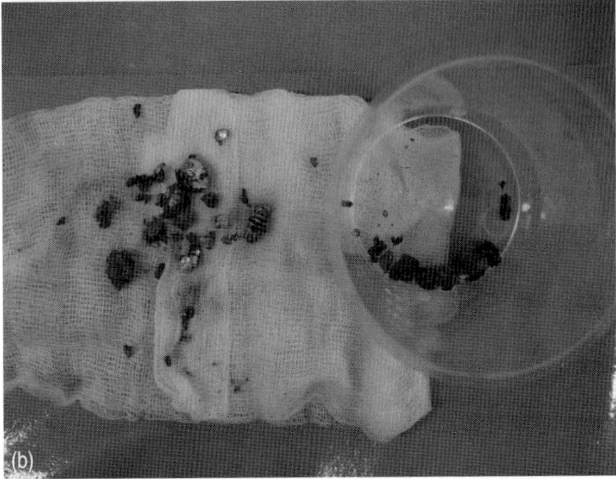

Figure 85.7 Extensive wound contamination and tissue loss due to blast fragmentation from a military explosive device. *(Courtesy of Australian Defence Force, Afghanistan, 2009.)*

BALLISTIC FRACTURE MANAGEMENT

Bone fragments without any soft tissue attachments should be removed.[26] However, *any* soft tissue attachment makes assessment of viability difficult, and at primary surgery such fragments should be retained. High-energy transfer fractures and fractures of the proximal tibia and fibula[41] often require deep fasciotomy to prevent compartment syndrome. Infection risk argues strongly for plaster, external fixation or traction rather than internal fixation of ballistic fractures.[26,42,43]

ABDOMINAL PENETRATING WOUNDS

Low-kinetic-energy bullets and blast fragmentation tend to produce discrete injury to abdominal organs. Up to 30% of civilian anterior abdominal and 67% of lower back gunshot wounds can be managed safely without surgery. This approach is increasing in US civilian practice,[44] probably associated with better and more widespread CT imaging; however, it fails in 21% of cases, and failure is associated with increased

Table 85.5 Indications for surgical debridement of blast fragmentation wounds

ORDOG ET AL 1993[39]	BOWYER 1997[40]
Presentation >24 h after wounding, without basic cleansing before presentation	Involvement of bone, pleura, peritoneum, or major vessels
Wound size >1–2 cm	Wound entry or exit >1–2 cm
Failure to comply with wound care instructions	Evidence of wound cavitation
Fractures	Obvious signs of infection Wounds due to buried mines

mortality.[44] High-energy transfer, haemodynamic instability, peritonitis, or lack of reassuring imaging all indicate laparotomy. In the military context, definitive surgery can avert a more prolonged admission for observation. Without comprehensive imaging, it is our practice and that of others[38] to explore all penetrating abdominal wounds (**Fig. 85.8**). If CT imaging is available, in the light of observational studies,[45] UK military guidelines allow for a selective non-operative approach in the minority of casualties with no peritonitis or haemodynamic instability who can be intensively monitored.[46]

THORAX

Penetrating thoracic injury is either rapidly fatal (e.g. 93% of patients with aortic injuries die before reaching hospital[47]), or managed with simple measures. Eighty-five percent of penetrating thoracic trauma patients who reach medical care can be successfully managed with intercostal catheter (ICC) drainage alone.[48] An ICC should always be placed through a new incision rather than the wound to prevent further haemorrhage. On placement of the ICC, Early Management of Severe Trauma[49] teaching is that >1500 mL initial haemorrhage or >200 mL/h ongoing loss for >2–4 hours necessitates operative thoracotomy. Emergency anterolateral thoracotomy should be considered in patients with penetrating thoracic injuries who arrive pulseless but with ECG activity within the last 6–10 minutes, with the intention of releasing cardiac tamponade, controlling haemorrhage (by cross-clamping the aorta or pulmonary hilum) and allowing internal cardiac massage to 'buy time' for aggressive fluid resuscitation. Thoracic penetrating injury below the level of the nipple, a positive FAST scan or abdominal signs suggests the projectile has traversed the diaphragm.

RETAINED FOREIGN BODIES

Easily accessible projectiles should be surgically removed. However, projectiles buried in healthy tissue *unequivocally do not need to be removed,* with some exceptions:

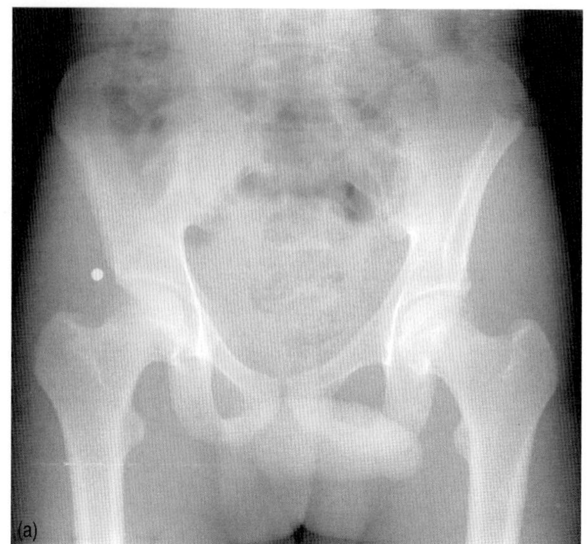

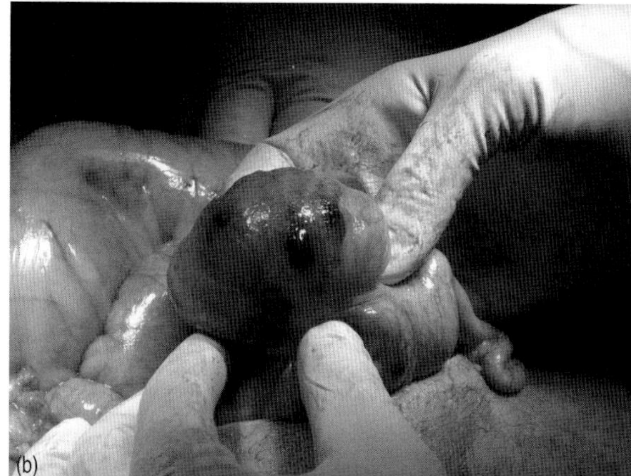

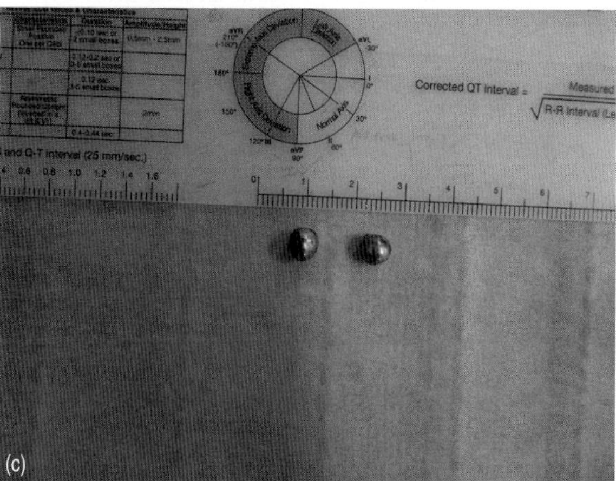

Figure 85.8 Localised bowel damage due to blast fragmentation. *(Courtesy of Australian Defence Force, Afghanistan, 2009.)*

- those lodged in joints or the subarachnoid space, in order to prevent lead arthropathy and systemic toxicity, joint destruction or neural damage
- those that appear to become the source of systemic infection
- those lying next to an internal organ (e.g. bronchus, heart), with the risk of subsequent erosion[31]
- those causing persistent pain, with the caveat that the psychological effects of a retained projectile are often profound, and this can influence pain perception.

Blood lead levels from projectiles retained in muscle peak at 1 month and in synovial fluid at 6 months.[50] If lead toxicity is the sole indication for projectile removal, the threshold serum levels are 10 µg/dL in children and 40 µg/dL in adults. Projectile removal should be attempted only after chelation with EDTA, dimercaprol, D-penicillamine or dimercaptosuccinic acid.[2]

HELPFUL INVESTIGATIONS

Pre- and intraoperative physical examination is the best single method of evaluating ballistic wounds.[34] However, projectiles often follow unpredictable paths. Radiology can be useful in triage, operative planning, and selection of cases for non-operative management. Experience in Iraq and Afghanistan led to a policy of all patients with substantial ballistic trauma having whole-body multidetector computed tomography (MDCT) scanning if this was available, unless operative intervention was immediately required to save life. Wound paths can be plotted using MDCT-derived data, allowing surgical planning.[51]

ICRC WOUND CLASSIFICATION

The ICRC wound classification system[2] categorises disease severity by measuring the size of the entry wound, exit wound and wound cavity, and involvement of fractures, vital structures and metallic foreign bodies. The result is a grade and type of wound. Unable to capture all aspects of anatomy and physiology and not accounting for multiple wounds, the ICRC system is not a predictor of outcome, but is nevertheless useful for quantifying the effects of weapon systems.

SPECIAL CASES OF BALLISTIC TRAUMA

LANDMINES AND IMPROVISED EXPLOSIVE DEVICES

Antipersonnel landmines wound by a combination of blast and fragmentation from their casing and from rocks and soil. Buried mines explode upwards through the leg, commonly resulting in traumatic amputation through the midfoot or distal tibia, with debris driven up fascial planes. Wound severity depends on the quantity of explosive, point of foot contact, debris near the mine, and footwear.[35] Bounding mines contain two charges: a small explosion propels a tethered casing upwards to 1–2 metres, which then explodes propelling fragments 50–100 metres. Horizontal spray mines also cause most of their effect by blast fragmentation. Air-dropped 'butterfly' mines rely on primary blast effect to maim when handled. Improvised explosive devices often mimic the effects of mines, but, being made from anything from artillery shells to household chemicals, their effects are more difficult to predict. All the principles articulated above apply to mine wounds, with particular emphasis on the need to remove soil. Topical negative-pressure dressings are perceived to be particularly useful,[52] but this approach is not yet supported by trial evidence.

INCENDIARY DEVICES (NAPALM, WHITE PHOSPHOROUS)

Military forces use white phosphorus and napalm as incendiaries, and white phosphorus is also used to create smokescreens. Both are also effective psychological weapons due to their capacity to inflict severe wounds. Napalm produces a burning gel that adheres to skin, invariably producing full-thickness burns involving muscle. A 10% burn typically causes rhabdomyolysis and renal failure.[2] Napalm commonly undergoes incomplete combustion, so carbon monoxide poisoning is common. White phosphorus fragments on explosion and ignites on air contact. Debridement requires keeping the wound moist. Dilute (1%) copper sulphate turns phosphorus black, which is safer and easier to remove. Alternatively, phosphorus particles glow in low light. Systemically absorbed white phosphorus causes hypocalcaemia and hyperphosphataemia, requiring intravenous calcium.[53]

BEHIND ARMOUR BLUNT TRAUMA (BABT)

Body armour, consisting of woven textiles with or without ceramic plate supplementation, effectively reduces the lethality of ballistic trauma.[54–56] However, larger rifle bullets can still kill by transmission of a force wave.[55] The immediate effects of BABT are vagally mediated apnoea and hypotension,[57] commonly accompanied by pulmonary and myocardial contusion, rib fractures, haemo- and pneumothorax. The commonest military bullet calibre, 5.56 mm, has negligible BABT potential, but larger calibres (eg. 7.62 mm and 50-cal.) carry substantial risk.[55]

INFECTION IN BALLISTIC INJURY

The two requirements for serious wound infection – a deep inoculum of bacteria and dead tissue, – are frequently present in ballistic trauma. This is particularly true of military wounds, with typically 3–6 different bacterial species isolated compared with only one in infected civilian wounds.[26] Bacteria are mainly

Box 85.1 Infectious Diseases Society of America and Surgical Infection Society guidelines for the prevention of infections associated with combat-related injuries[59]

I.v. antibiotic prophylaxis is indicated as soon as possible (ideally <3 h) after wounding.

Cefazolin 2 g i.v. every 6–8 hours (+metronidazole 500 mg i.v. q8–12 h for oesophageal, abdominal organ, CNS) is appropriate for all wounds except penetrating eye injury, for which levofloxacin 500 mg i.v./p.o. once daily is recommended.

Alternate agents depend on site of wounding:

- *extremity*: thoracic (excl. oesophageal); maxillofacial: clindamycin (300–450 mg p.o. t.i.d. or 600 mg i.v. q8 h)
- *oesophageal:* abdominal: single doses of ertapenem 1 g i.v. or moxifloxacin 400 mg i.v.
- *CNS:* ceftriaxone 2 g i.v. q24 h. Consider adding metronidazole 500 mg i.v. q8–12 h if gross contamination with organic debris. For penicillin-allergic patients, vancomycin 1 g i.v. q12 h plus ciprofloxacin 400 mg i.v. q8–12 h.

Duration of therapy in the absence of signs of infection: extremity; thoracic – 1–3 days; abdominal – 1 day after definitive washout; maxillofacial – 1 day; CNS: 5 days or until CSF leak is closed, whichever is longer.

Tetanus toxoid and immune globulin should be used as appropriate to immunisation status.

Enhanced Gram-negative coverage with aminoglycoside or fluoroquinolone is not recommended.

Addition of penicillin to prevent clostridial gangrene or streptococcal infection is not recommended.

Redose antimicrobials in the setting of large-volume blood produce resuscitation.

Use only topical antimicrobials for burns.

introduced into gunshot wounds by cavitation, but the bullet is not sterilised by firing and can also lead to infection.[25] Historically, the major causative organisms have been beta-haemolytic streptococci and clostridia. Although 'the best antibiotic is good surgery',[2] infection with both organisms is effectively prevented by prophylactic penicillin. Antibiotics alone may be sufficient for wounds left open with sufficient drainage.[58] US consensus guidelines for antimicrobial prophylaxis of combat-related wounds, drawing on experience of modern conflict, were recently published.[59] Essential points are summarised in **Box 85.1**.

Other organisations make different recommendations – for example, the ICRC recommends penicillin for all wounds except those involving hollow abdominal organs (requiring ampicillin+metronidazole +/− gentamicin) and thorax (requiring ampicillin), with the addition of metronidazole to maxillofacial or heavily contaminated soft tissue wounds and chloramphenicol for penetrating head trauma.[2]

Soil potentiates the ability of contamination to cause infection.[31] Wounds contaminated with soil should be thoroughly cleaned, potentially requiring more wound excision than otherwise. Infection is also particularly likely in haematomas,[31] which should be drained. If a wound requires debridement, earlier surgery is associated with less infection. For example, the 10% infection rate in wounds debrided in less than 6 hours after wounding rose to 25% in wounds debrided later.[60]

CONCLUSION

Medical planning and training in the management of ballistic trauma require balancing modern evidence-based medicine with the study of lessons acquired over centuries of conflict. Belligerents may be compelled to repeat the mistakes of the past; doctors should not.

Acknowledgements

The work of Stephen Brett in earlier editions of this book was invaluable in the preparation of this chapter. Major Anthony Chambers FRACS, Major Brett Courtenay FRACS FAOrthA and Commander Paul Luckin FANZCA kindly provided many of the photographs.

Access the complete references list online at http://www.expertconsult.com

2. Giannou G, Baldan M. War surgery: working with limited resources in armed conflict and other situations of violence. Geneva: International Committee of the Red Cross; 2012.
6. Bellamy RF. The causes of death in conventional land warfare: implications for combat casualty care research. Mil Med 1984;149(2):55–62.
7. Tactical Combat Casualty Care. Fort Leavenworth, KS, USA: Center for Army Lessons Learned; 2010. Online. Available: http://publicintelligence.net/ufouo-u-s-army-tactical-combat-casualty-care-handbook/.
13. Harrison CD, Bebarta VS, Grant GA. Tympanic membrane perforation after combat blast exposure in Iraq: a poor biomarker of primary blast injury. J Trauma 2009;67(1):210–11.
33. Guthrie HC, Clasper JC, Kay AR, et al. Initial extremity war wound debridement: a multidisciplinary consensus. J R Army Med Corps 2011;157(2):170–5.
34. Fackler ML. Ballistic injury. Ann Emerg Med 1986; 15(12):1451–5.
59. Hospenthal DR, Murray CK, Andersen RC, et al. Guidelines for the prevention of infections associated with combat-related injuries: 2011 update: endorsed by the Infectious Diseases Society of America and the Surgical Infection Society. J Trauma 2011;71(2 Suppl 2):S210–34.

86

Background information on 'biochemical terrorism'

Munita Grover and Michael Pelly

Biochemical terrorism is defined as the use of biological or chemical agents to intimidate, incapacitate, or eradicate crops, livestock, civilian and military personnel.[1] It is well suited for attack by poorer nations against the rich, and is known as a poor man's atom bomb, or asymmetric method of attack. The large-scale use of mustard and nerve gases in the Iran/Iraq war,[2] the dissemination of nerve gas sarin on the Tokyo underground,[3] and the discovery by UN inspectors in Iraq of SCUD missiles, rockets and aerial bombs primed with *Botulinum* and aflatoxins[4,5] have highlighted that the threat remains real (**Box 86.1**).

CHARACTERISTICS OF BIOLOGICAL WEAPONS

Intended target effects are either due to infection with disease-causing micro-organisms or other replicative entities, including viruses, fungi, and prions, or due to the toxins they elaborate. Their effects depend on the ability to multiply in the person, animal, or plant attacked.[6] Sequelae depend on host factors (state of nutrition, immunocompetence) and environment (sanitation, temperature, humidity, water quality, population density).[7]

CLASSIFICATION

Although classification of biological weapons can be taxonomy-based, for example, bacterial/viral/fungal, it is also useful to examine particular features such as:

- *infectivity:* proportion of persons exposed to a given dose who become infected.; reflects capability of agent to enter, survive and replicate
- *virulence:* ratio of the number of clinical cases to the number of infected hosts; this may differ for strains of the same pathogen
- *lethality:* ability of agent to cause death in an infected population
- *pathogenicity:* ratio of number of clinical cases to the number of exposed persons; reflects capability of agent to cause disease
- *incubation period:* time elapsing between exposure to the agent and first signs and symptoms of disease
- *contagiousness:* number of secondary cases following exposure to a primary case in relation to the total number exposed
- *stability:* ability of an agent to survive the environment.

Another useful classification system available is that from the CDC Atlanta:

CATEGORY A

High-priority agents include organisms that pose a risk to national security because they can be easily disseminated or transmitted from person to person, result in high mortality rates and have the potential for major public health impact, might cause public panic and social disruption, and require special action for public health preparedness. Examples include anthrax, botulism, plague, smallpox, tularaemia and viral haemorrrhagic fevers.

CATEGORY B

Agents of second highest priority include those that are moderately easy to disseminate, result in moderate morbidity rates and low mortality rates, and require specific enhancements of CDC's diagnostic capacity and enhanced disease surveillance. Examples include brucellosis, *Salmonella*, glanders, melioidosis, psittacosis, Q fever, ricin toxin, typhus, staphylococcal eneterotoxin B and viral encephalitis (**Box 86.2**).

ROUTES OF DISSEMINATION

- *Inhalational exposure using sprays or aerosols:* the optimal particle size for alveolar deposition is 0.6–5 μm. Those larger than this are filtered by the nose and smaller ones are exhaled. This can be achieved using aerosol generators mounted on stationary objects or primed onto trucks, cars, boats, cruise missiles and planes. Environmental factors such as wind velocity, cloud cover, rainfall and humidity affect the efficiency of dissemination[7]
- *Cutaneous:* via wounds and mucous membranes
- *Ingestion via food and water:* hand-to-mouth contact is a suitable vehicle (e.g. the Rajneeshee cult successfully disseminated *Salmonella* via salads, infecting 750 people in 1984)

Box 86.1 Potential weapons

Biological diseases	Chemical agents
Bacillus anthracis (anthrax)	*Blisters/vesicants*
Clostridium botulinum toxin (botulism)	Distilled mustard (HD)
Yersinia pestis (plague)	Lewisite (L)
Variola major (smallpox)	Mustard gas (H)
Francisella tularensis (tularaemia)	Nitrogen mustard (HN-2)
Viral haemorrhagic fever	Phosgene oxime (CX)
Coxiella burnetii (Q fever)	*Blood*
Brucella melitensis (brucellosis)	Arsine (SA)
Burkholderia mallei (glanders)	Cyanogen chloride (CK)
Ricin toxin (*Ricinus communis* – castor beans)	Hydrogen chloride
Staphylococcus enterotoxin B	Hydrogen cyanide (AC)
Nipah virus	*Choking/pulmonary damage*
Hantaviruses	Chlorine (CL)
	Nitrogen oxide (NO)
	Phosgene (CG)
	Nerve
	Sarin (GF)
	Soman (GD)
	Tabun (GA)
	VX
	Incapacitating
	LSD
	Cannabinoids

Box 86.2 Criteria for a successful biological weapon[6]

Assailant
Has methods to treat own forces and population

Target population
Non-immune
Little or no access to immunisation or treatment

Bioweapon
Consistently produces disease/death
Highly contagious or infective in low doses
Short and predictable incubation period
Difficult to identify in target population
Suitable for mass production, storage and weaponisation
Stable during dissemination
Low persistence after delivery

DETECTION OF A BIOTERRORIST EVENT

This may be obvious if large numbers of military personnel become ill with similar syndromes, but any release is likely to be a covert event. Furthermore, genetic engineering may result in altered pathogenicity, incubation periods, clinical effects and response to treatment or immunisation (**Box 86.3**).

SPECIFIC BIOLOGICAL AGENTS

ANTHRAX

Anthrax[8] is an acute infectious zoonosis caused by *Bacillus anthracis*, a Gram-positive spore-forming bacillus. The infective dose is 8000–50 000 spores and routes of transmission include inhalation, ingestion and skin contact. Person-to-person transmission does not occur for the pulmonary form but secondary cutaneous lesions may occur after direct exposure to vesicle secretions. Spraying by aircraft is a potential threat to a large city; hence pulmonary exposure is the most likely route in a mass casualty situation.

Box 86.3 Epidemiological evidence of an attack

Increasing incidence of disease in a normally healthy population
Higher incidence in subgroups, e.g. outdoor workers/shared ventilation
Increasing numbers seeking help with similar symptoms
Rise in endemic disease at an uncharacteristic time
Large numbers of rapidly fatal cases
Any patient with an uncommon disease that has bioterrorist potential
Large numbers of dying animals or fish, and unusual swarms of insects

CLINICAL FEATURES

Pulmonary exposure[9,10]

The incubation period is 2–60 days. The prodrome has flu-like symptoms. There may be interim improvement followed by respiratory failure and cardiovascular collapse. A widened mediastinum is seen on CXR, owing to haemorrhagic mediastinitis and lymphadenopathy. Gram-positive bacilli are found on blood cultures.

Cutaneous exposure

The incubation period is 1–7 days. Mostly the head, hands and forearms are affected, with pruritis, erythema, oedema and maculopapular lesions progressing to depressed black eschars within 2–6 days. Eschars fall off without scarring.

Gastrointestinal exposure

The incubation period is 1–7 days, usually following ingestion of infected meat. It presents with abdominal pain, cramps, haematemesis and bloody diarrhoea followed by toxaemia and cardiovascular collapse. There are Gram-positive blood cultures.

Post-exposure management[11]

There should be universal precautions for medical personnel, including warning the laboratory and coroner's personnel regarding pathology specimens. Contact the infection control team.

Handle fomites minimally. Thoroughly decontaminate with soap and water, and disinfect surfaces with 0.5% hypochlorite solution.

TREATMENT

Most strains used for bioterrorism will produce beta lactamases, and cephalosporinases were produced by the latest cases in the USA. Appropriate antibiotics include:

- *ciprofloxacin:* adults 500 mg b.d. for 8 weeks; children 20–30 mg/kg per day
- *doxycycline:* adults 100 mg b.d. for 8 weeks; children 5 mg/kg per day
- *amoxicillin:* in children and pregnant patients 40 mg/kg per day (max 500 mg t.d.s.) is appropriate if the organism is penicillin-sensitive.

Immunisation with anthrax vaccine consists of 3 doses at 0, 2 and 4 weeks. Prophylaxis of contacts should continue for 8 weeks and include immunisation if exposure is confirmed. Preventative immunisation using an inactivated cell-free vaccine is available but presently only administered to military personnel.

BOTULISM

Botulism[5] is caused by *Clostridium botulinum*, an anaerobic Gram-positive bacillus that produces a neurotoxin. Seven forms of the toxin have been identified from A to G, but human botulism is due mainly to strains A, B, or E. The neurotoxin contains a zinc protease that acts at the presynaptic terminal of the neuromuscular junction to prevent the fusion of vesicles of acetylcholine with the presynaptic membrane, therefore preventing release of acetylcholine leading to a flaccid paralysis. The LD_{50} for type A is 0.001 μg/kg. Routes of exposure are either inhalation or ingestion, and there is an incubation period of 12–36 hours. Person-to-person transmission does not occur.

CLINICAL FEATURES

Clinical features include a responsive patient with no fever. There is a symmetric descending flaccid paralysis in a proximal-to-distal pattern without a sensory deficit. Cranial neuropathies (mainly bulbar) lead to diplopia, dysphagia, dysphonia and dysarthria. Respiratory dysfunction may occur owing to upper airway obstruction or muscle paralysis. The diagnosis is clinical, and confirmation is with the mouse bioassay in which mice are pretreated with antitoxin and exposed to the patient's serum. A pentavalent toxoid vaccine is available for prevention, but routine immunisation is not recommended.

TREATMENT

Patients should be monitored with frequent assessment of gag, cough reflexes, inspiratory force and vital capacity. Mechanical ventilation may be protracted, and may be punctuated by nosocomial infections requiring antibiotics.

Aminoglycosides and clindamycin are contraindicated because of their ability to increase blockade.[12] Administration of the trivalent (A, B, E) antitoxin should not be delayed while awaiting confirmation of the diagnosis. This horse serum has <9% hypersensitivity reactions and <2% incidence of anaphylaxis. Skin testing is advisable.[13] A heptavalent antitoxin is under investigation. Passive administration of neutralising antibody minimises further damage.[14]

Treatment of children, pregnant women and immunocompromised patients should be no different; all have received equine antitoxin without short-term sequelae. Prophylaxis of contacts involves close observation and, at the first sign of illness, treatment with antitoxin, neutralising antibody and administration of the pentavalent toxoid vaccine.

SMALLPOX

Smallpox[15] is an acute viral illness caused by variola virus (orthopoxvirus). The last documented case was in Somalia in 1977. It is transmitted from person to person via the airborne route, and its release into a non-immune population would be catastrophic.[16] The infective dose is 10–100 virions, with an incubation period of 7–17 days. In a non-immune society, the impact would be devastating as the human–human spread would be difficult to check, and many countries have very poor health structures with overcrowding in the cities. Also, the impact of global travel would change the epidemic and allow it to move rapidly from continent to continent. There are two other major factors that may change the profile of a predicted epidemic: the potential use of new antiviral agents against smallpox and the HIV epidemic. Predictions are difficult.

CLINICAL FEATURES[17]

There is a flu-like prodrome with malaise, fever, and headache. There is also a synchronously evolving maculopapular rash forming pustules over the head and extremities, and the mouth and pharynx may also be affected. Multi-organ failure commonly complicates smallpox. Diagnosis is clinical with confirmation by identification of brick-shaped virions from vesicular fluid using electron microscopy.

PREVENTION

Routine vaccination with vaccinia virus stopped in 1972. The immune status of vaccinated individuals is unclear, but if a single-dose vaccine was administered it is assumed the subject is non-immune. A preventative vaccination programme is currently under review.

TREATMENT

Vaccinate within 4 days of exposure.[18] However, complications include: post-vaccinial encephalitis, vaccinia gangrenosa, eczema vaccinatum, generalised vaccinia and inadvertant inoculation. Five groups are considered high risk for these. They are: pregnancy, HIV infection, chemotherapy, eczema and immune disorders.[19] In these cases, vaccinia immune globulin should be given simultaneously. Other treatments include:

- supportive care with isolation
- antibiotics for secondary bacterial infections

- cidofovir, a nucleoside DNA polymerase inhibitor, which is under investigation but needs to be given i.v. and causes renal toxicity.[20]

PLAGUE

Plague[21] is an acute bacterial disease caused by the Gram-negative *Yersinia pestis*, from the *Enterobacter* species.[22] Although usually transmitted by fleas causing bubonic and septicaemic plague, a bioterrorist event is likely to be airborne resulting in pneumonic plague. The infective dose is <100 organisms, and has an incubation period of 2–3 days. It is unlikely that spread would be person to person.

CLINICAL FEATURES

Plague presents with fever, haemoptysis, chest pain and dyspnoea. Gram-negative rods are found in mucopurulent sputum, and on Wright's, Giemsa or Wayson stain appear as bipolar rods with a safety-pin appearance. The diagnosis can be confirmed on blood culture and with fluorescent antibody testing. There is radiographic evidence of bronchopneumonia, and multi-organ failure soon develops. Until 72 hours of antibiotic therapy have been completed, plague is communicable.

PREVENTION

A formalin-killed vaccine exists but is ineffective and unavailable. Post-exposure immunisation has no benefit.

TREATMENT[21]

Once the diagnosis is considered, isolation and universal precautions should be instituted. Historically streptomycin (1 g b.d. i.m.) reduced mortality to 5%, and gentamicin (5 mg/kg per day) has also been used successfully. Tetracycline and doxycycline (100 mg b.d.), have been used, but in Madagascar 13% of strains are resistant to doxycycline. Animal studies have demonstrated efficacy of fluoroquinolones including ciprofloxacin (400 mg b.d.), ofloxacin and levofloxacin. No human trials exist so far. Chloramphenicol (25 mg/kg q.i.d.) is recommended for plague meningitis.

CHARACTERISTICS OF CHEMICAL AGENTS

The North Atlantic Treaty Organization definition of a chemical agent is a 'chemical substance which is intended for use in military operations to kill, seriously injure, or incapacitate people because of its physiological effects'.[2] In addition to physiological effects these agents promote psychological warfare.[23]

POSSIBLE ROUTES OF DISSEMINATION

The principal hazard is inhalation of liquid, vapour, or droplets (0.6–5 μm). Delivery may be by artillery shells, missiles or aerial bombing. In the Tokyo subway attack in 1995, terrorists left plastic bags on the subway filled with Sarin after piercing them with umbrella tips. There were 3796 casualties and 12 deaths.[3]

Toxicity depends on the concentration and time of exposure, and is measured in units of concentration and time (mg/min m^3), known as the Haber product.[7] Most chemical agents are designed to penetrate the skin, respiratory epithelium and cornea, unlike biological agents. Penetration is promoted by thinner, more vascular, moister, hairy skin, and by high humidity, spills and aerosols.

RICIN

Ricin is one of the most toxic biological agents known – a Category B bioterrorism agent and a Schedule number 1 chemical warfare agent. Ricin toxin can be extracted from castor beans, purified and treated to form a pellet, a white powder, or dissolved in water or weak acid to be released as a liquid. It is stable under ambient conditions. Particles of <5 μm have been used for aerosol dispersion in animal studies. Ricin particles can remain suspended in undisturbed air for several hours and finally resuspension of settled ricin from disturbed surfaces also may occur.

TRANSMISSION

Ricin is transmitted through skin contact, or by the airborne route through release of ricin in the form of a powder, or a mist, or reaerosolisation of ricin into the air from disturbed surfaces. Ricin would need to be dispersed in particles smaller than 5 μm to be used as an effective weapon by the airborne route. It is very difficult to prepare particles of this size. Routes of exposure include inhalation, parenteral (injection), ingestion, dermal contact (exposure risk is low; absorption through non-intact skin or via a solvent carrier), or ocular contact. Although ricin may adhere to skin, person-to-person transmission through casual contact has not been reported. Despite the fact that ricin may adhere to clothing or be present on surfaces, there is low potential for transmission via contact with contaminated clothing or contaminated surfaces.

RISK GROUPS

There is worldwide distribution of castor plants. Ricin is produced when castor oil is made from castor beans, but the general public is not considered at risk for exposure. Those at particular risk include: (i) persons in or around castor-oil-processing plants (however, it would take a deliberate act to make ricin and use it as a poison); (ii) persons in the dispersal area of a ricin aerosol release if ricin is used as an agent of terrorism; (iii) persons who are victims of parenteral injection with ricin; (iv) persons who ingest castor beans, or food or water contaminated with ricin. It is not known whether certain populations are more vulnerable to the health effects of ricin exposure (e.g. children, pregnant women, the elderly, those with immunosuppression, or underlying respiratory or gastrointestinal tract disease); however, persons with pre-existing tissue irritation or damage who are exposed to ricin may sustain further injury and greater absorption of ricin toxin.

PATHOGENESIS

Ricin is a toxalbumin, a biological toxin whose mechanism of action is inhibition of protein synthesis in eukaryotic cells; cell death results from the absence of proteins. The effects of ricin poisoning depend upon the amount of ricin exposure, the route of exposure and the person's premorbid condition. Ingestion and mastication of three to six castor beans is the estimated fatal dose in adults. The fatal dose in children is not known, but is probably less. Most cases of castor bean ingestion do not result in poisoning, because it is difficult for ricin to be released from ingested castor beans, ricin release requires mastication, and the degree of mastication is likely to be important in determining the extent of poisoning. Ricin is not as well absorbed through the gastrointestinal tract compared with injection or inhalation. Inhalation or injection of ricin would be expected to lead to a more rapid onset of symptoms of ricin poisoning and to a more rapid progression of poisoning compared to ingestion, given the same exposure amount.

Data on inhalational exposure to ricin in humans are extremely limited, and systemic toxicity has not been described. Animal studies suggest that inhalation is one of the most lethal forms of ricin poisoning. Following severe ricin poisoning, damage to vital organs may be permanent or have lasting effects. No long-term effects are known to exist from ricin exposure that did not result in symptoms.

LABORATORY DIAGNOSIS AND TESTS

Non-specific laboratory findings in ricin poisoning include:

- metabolic acidosis
- increased liver function tests
- increased renal function tests
- haematuria
- leucocytosis (two- to five-fold higher than normal value).

There are no specific clinically validated assays for detection of ricin that can be performed by the hospital/health care facility clinical laboratory. Tests for ricinine, an alkaloidal component of the castor bean plant, are being developed. The potential uses of tests for either ricin or ricinine in human biological samples would primarily be for purposes of confirming exposure or assessing the prevalence of exposure rather than diagnostic use as the results would most likely not be immediately available. Laboratory criterion for diagnosis include detection of ricin in environmental samples. Laboratory tests performed on ricin-suspicious samples include:

- time-resolved fluorescence immunoassay: antibody binds to ricin
- polymerase chain reaction for the ricin protein.

TREATMENT

Because no antidote exists for ricin, the most important factor is avoiding ricin exposure in the first place. If exposure cannot be avoided, then rapid elimination and supportive care targeted at the route of exposure are required. This might include respiratory support, intravenous fluids and management of shock, prevention of seizures, enteral charcoal and ophthalmic irrigation.

SARIN

Sarin ($C_4H_{10}FO_2P$, isopropylmethylphosphofluoridate) is a colourless, odourless liquid at room temperature. It is volatile and incompatible with metals or concrete, which lead to production of hydrogen gas. Hydrolysis of Sarin forms acid. It is thermally stable <49°C, but clings to clothing and releases slowly for 30 minutes. Toxicity is through inhibition of the enzyme acetylcholinesterase (**Table 86.1**).

The route of exposure determines which clinical features appear first.[24] Post inhalation respiratory and eye symptoms appear, whereas post cutaneous exposure diaphoresis and muscle fasciculation occur. Immediate first aid is to remove the patient from the area of danger to a well-ventilated area before removal of clothing, and decontamination of the skin. This can be achieved using mists of water, or dilute sodium hypochlorite. Eyes are irrigated with water or normal saline.

Assessment follows airway, breathing and circulation principles. Patients with compromised airways due either to direct effects or secondary to reduced level of consciousness require intubation and positive-pressure ventilation. Aggressive suctioning may be needed for the bronchial secretions.

TREATMENT

- *Anticholinergics:* to antagonise the muscarinic effects, usually i.v. atropine in 2 mg doses, every 3–5 min until the patient is atropinised; atropine may need to be continued for 24 h at 2 mg/h[2]

Table 86.1 Sarin toxicity

MILD	Rhinitis, dyspnoea, miosis, blurred vision
MODERATE	Diaphoresis, drooling, bronchospasm, nausea, vomiting, cramps, weakness, twitching, headache, confusion
SEVERE	Involuntary defaecation/urination, convulsions, respiratory arrest, coma, death

Table 86.2 Features of mustard gas toxicity

EYES	Lacrimation, conjunctivitis, photophobia
SKIN	Erythema, blistering, partial- to full-thickness burns
RESPIRATORY TRACT	Rhinorrhoea, tracheobronchitis, bronchopneumonia
SYSTEMIC	Nausea, vomiting, diarrhoea, bradycardia, hypotension

- *Oximes:* to reactivate the anticholinesterase enzyme at nicotinic sites (e.g. pralidoxime mesilate 30 mg/kg by slow i.v. injection, up to 2–4 g); this should be prompt, as dealkylation of the inhibited enzyme renders it resistant to reactivation
- *Prophylactic anticonvulsants:* to prevent seizures, diazepam 5 mg by any route has been shown to reduce morbidity in animal studies.

MUSTARD GAS

Mustard gas ($C_4H_8Cl_2S$, bis-(2-chloroethyl) sulphide) is a yellow oily liquid at room temperature. It has a faint garlic odour and evaporates to form a vapour that penetrates clothing. There is a low mortality, but it tends to incapacitate. It is a bi-functional alkylating agent that is carcinogenic (oral cavity, larynx, bronchus), and irritates skin and mucosa. Mustard gas is also myelotoxic (pancytopenia) and teratogenic. Assessment is similar to that of Sarin (**Table 86.2**).[25]

TREATMENT

Patients with large burns are resuscitated as any other burn injuries; however, fluid losses are transudates so protein losses are less.[26] Pain control is important and frequently requires analgesics, such as morphine. Tense blisters are dressed with silver sulfadiazine. Mustard burns take at least 12 weeks to heal, but early excision and grafting do not reduce healing time.[27,28] Eye lesions usually heal in 2 weeks, and are aided by topical antibiotics and saline irrigation. Oxygen, antibiotics for secondary pneumonia, physiotherapy and ventilation are the mainstays of treatment for respiratory effects.

ACUTE RADIATION SYNDROME

Acute radiation syndrome (ARS) can also be termed radiation poisoning, radiation sickness or radiation toxicity. It is a collection of symptoms and signs that present within 24 hours of exposure to high amounts of ionising radiation. It can last for months but acute radiation syndrome really refers to the acute medical problems rather than ones that develop after a prolonged period of time. There is a dose–response relationship to both the onset and type of symptoms, with smaller doses resulting in gastrointestinal effects such as nausea and vomiting, and symptoms related to fall in blood count such as infection and bleeding, whereas relatively larger doses tend to produce neurological effects and rapid death. Treatment is largely supportive with blood transfusions and antibiotics.

TYPES OF RADIATION

Alpha and beta radiation have low penetrating power and are unlikely to affect internal organs from outside the body. Any type of ionising radiation can cause burns but alpha and beta radiation do so only if fallout actually causes contamination of individuals' clothing. Gamma and neutron radiation can travel much further distances and penetrate the body easily, so whole-body irradiation generally causes ARS before skin effects are evident. Local gamma irradiation can cause skin effects without any sickness.

PATHOPHYSIOLOGY

One of the predictors of the radiation symptoms is whole-body absorbed dose of radiation. Other equivalent measurements include effective dose and committed dose, which are used to gauge long-term biological effects such as cancer incidence, but they are not designed to evaluate ARS. Absorbed dose is measured in units of gray (Gy) or rad.

Diagnosis is made on history of significant exposure to radiation and absolute lymphocyte count can give a rough estimate of radiation exposure. Time from exposure to vomiting can also give estimates of exposure levels if they are less than 1000 rad.

SIGNS AND SYMPTOMS

The three main systems affected tend to be haematopoietic, gastrointestinal and neurological. These symptoms can be preceded by a prodrome and the speed of onset of symptoms related to the radiation exposure, with greater doses resulting in a shorter delay in symptom onset.

Any prodrome tends to have symptoms and signs common to other illnesses and by itself do not indicate ARS. Nausea, vomiting, headaches and fever with a short period of skin reddening can occur, but these resolve very quickly and therefore the diagnosis of ARS can be overlooked.

SKIN

Cutaneous radiation syndrome refers to the constellation of skin effects after exposure. It usually happens within a few hours after irradiation, consisting of redness, associated itching, followed by a latent period that can last from a day to weeks, during which there is intense reddening, blistering and ulceration of the irradiated site. Very large doses can cause permanent hair loss, damaged sebaceous and sweat glands, atrophy, fibrosis and increased skin pigmentation together with ulceration or necrosis of the exposed tissue, such as seen at Chernobyl and during the Litvinenko exposure in 2006.

HAEMATOPOIETIC

Aplastic anaemia leads to increased risk of infections due to leucopenia, bleeding tendencies due to thrombocytopenia and anaemia due to reduced red cell counts.

GASTROINTESTINAL

The main symptoms encountered include nausea, vomiting, loss of appetite, and abdominal pain. Vomiting is a marker for high exposure doses and therefore heralds a likely fatality. Death is common without bone marrow transplantation.

NEUROVASCULAR

This syndrome occurs at doses greater than 30 Gy, but can occur below 10 Gy. It presents with symptoms of dizziness, headache and decreased levels of consciousness occurring within minutes to a few hours, and with an absence of vomiting. It is invariably fatal.

PREVENTION

1. *Exposure:* increasing the distance from the radiation source reduces the dose according to the inverse-square law for a point source. Distance can sometimes be effectively increased by means of a simple handling source.
2. *Time:* minimise exposure duration.
3. *Shielding:* matter will attenuate radiation, so placing any mass, dirt, sandbags, vehicles between humans and the source will reduce the radiation dose. A gas mask, dust mask, or good hygiene practices may offer protection, depending on the nature of the contaminant. Potassium iodide tablets can reduce the risk of cancer in some situations.
4. *Fractionation of dose:* if a dose is broken up into a number of smaller doses then the total dose causes less cell deaths.

MANAGEMENT

Treatment is supportive with the use of antibiotics for infection in neutropenic patients, blood products to support the haematopoietic system, colony-stimulating factors to boost bone marrow production and eventually cell stem transplant as clinically indicated. Symptomatic measures in order to decrease nausea and vomiting and dressings for skin lesions may further help management.

Access the complete references list online at http://www.expertconsult.com

1. Spencer R, Wilcox M. Agents of biological warfare. Rev Med Microbiol 1993;4:138–43.
2. Evison D, Hinsley D, Rice P. Chemical weapons. BMJ 2002;324:332–5.
5. Arnon SS, Schechter R, Inglesby TV, et al. Botulinum toxin as a biological weapon. Medical and Public Health Management. JAMA 2001;285:1059–70.
8. Inglesby TV, Henderson DA, Bartlett JG, et al. Anthrax as a biological weapon. Consensus statement. JAMA 1999;281:1735–45.
15. Breman J, Henderson D. Poxvirus dilemmas: monkeypox, smallpox and biological terrorism. N Engl J Med 1998;339:556–9.
17. Henderson DA, Inglesby TV, Bartlett JG, et al. Smallpox as a biological weapon: medical and public health management. JAMA 1999;281:2127–30.
21. Inglesby TV, Dennis DT, Henderson DA, et al. Plague as a biological weapon: medical and public health management. JAMA 2000;285:2763–73.

Part Thirteen

Pharmacologic Considerations

87

Pharmacokinetics, pharmacodynamics and drug monitoring in critical illness

Christine Chung

Pharmacokinetics (PK) describes a drug's journey through the body and is quantified by the measurement of plasma levels. The four parameters usually studied are absorption, distribution, metabolism and excretion. Pharmacodynamics (PD) examines the effects of the drug on the body during its time course. The relationship between the two can be used to individualise dosing regimens by predicting how a drug will behave in a given patient.

Most PK–PD studies are performed in patients outside of the intensive care setting, so the results are not always applicable to this patient group. Data from ICU studies may be more accurate at predicting outcome but, due to labile PK–PD of the critically ill, optimisation of treatment still remains a therapeutic challenge. As a patient improves or deteriorates clinically, dosing may need adjustment depending on the drug in question.

The aim of this chapter is to provide the reader with the basic principles of pharmacokinetics and pharmacodynamics and to aid in the understanding of drug dosing in the ICU patient.

PHARMACOKINETICS

The basic terms used in pharmacokinetics include bioavailability (F), target (desired) plasma concentration (C_p), volume of distribution (V_d), clearance (Cl) and half-life ($t_{1/2}$).

Bioavailability is the fraction of administered dose that reaches the systemic circulation[1] and is dependent on many variables including absorption (see below). The value of F for the intravenous (i.v.) route is usually 1 unless the drug in question is a prodrug (i.e. requires metabolism to its active form). For an oral dosage form, F would also be less than 1 in the majority of cases as a certain percentage of the drug can be lost at each stage of the journey from the gastrointestinal tract to its site of metabolism. For example, bioavailability of digoxin tablets is 0.63 and the liquid 0.75.[2] Therefore, strictly speaking, converting from an oral to an i.v. dose requires a 20–30% reduction to provide an equivalent amount of drug. In practice, it is recommended that the dose is reduced by 25%. C_p is the desired plasma concentration.[1]

ABSORPTION

In order for a drug molecule to be absorbed, it is required to cross a membrane. Membranes are comprised of a phospholipid bilayer, with a hydrophilic exterior and a hydrophobic core. Fat-soluble drugs use passive diffusion to cross the membrane barrier. Extremely small water-soluble molecules gain entry through narrow aqueous membrane channels. The majority of water-soluble drugs travel by other mechanisms (e.g. via an active transport process facilitated by an energy source, i.e. ATP).[3]

Unionised molecules pass freely through membranes; ionised molecules do not.

Therefore, lipid-soluble drugs such as phenytoin can be easily absorbed from the gastrointestinal tract whereas large, water-soluble and polar drugs such as gentamicin cannot (**Fig. 87.1**).

Oral

The majority of drugs used in critical care are administered via the intravenous route. There are occasions, however, where an essential drug exists only in the oral form. How much is absorbed via the enteral route is governed by many factors such as:

- whether the pH of the stomach is optimal (e.g. bioavailability of atazanavir is significantly reduced by agents used for stress ulcer prophylaxis. Proton pump inhibitors reduce atazanavir's solubility by raising the pH of the stomach.[4] Weak basic drugs such as atazanavir require a low pH for absorption.)
- presence of enteral feed that may significantly reduce the efficacy of certain drugs (e.g. phenytoin is best administered in the middle of a 4-hour rest period from enteral feed[5])
- presence of other drugs that may bind and reduce bioavailability if administered at the same time, e.g. ciprofloxacin and ferrous fumarate[6]
- formulation of drug administered (e.g. liquid versus tablet)
- gut transit time (e.g. profuse diarrhoea may lead to reduced time for absorption and potentially therapeutic failure)
- gut integrity and perfusion (often reduced in the critically ill)

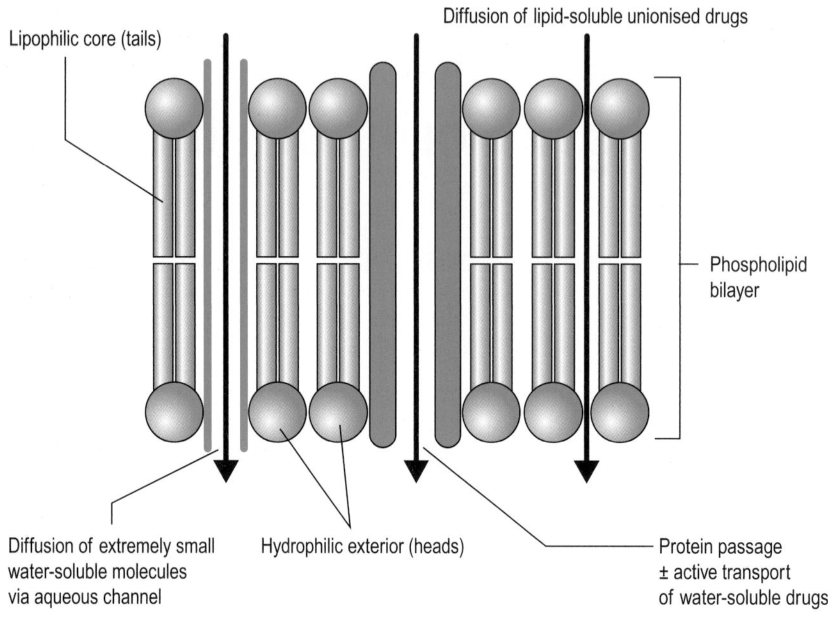

Figure 87.1 Diagram of a membrane.

- extent of first-pass metabolism (see metabolism), which can significantly reduce the amount of drug reaching the systemic circulation or lead to drug toxicity if the liver is failing.[7]

Intramuscular (i.m.) and subcutaneous (s.c.)

The effects via i.m. or s.c. can be erratic and unpredictable depending on local blood flow to tissues, adipose and muscle mass. Muscle perfusion is often significantly reduced in patients with haemorrhagic shock making it an undesirable route of administration if rapid systemic effects are required. Also, patients with a coagulopathy may be at increased risk of bleeding from the i.m. injection site.

Intravenous (i.v.)

The most common form of drug administration in ICU as it usually guarantees 100% bioavailability. However, several factors can still affect drug efficacy:

- drug–drug incompatibility when drugs of very different pHs are administered via the same i.v. line, e.g. propofol (near neutral pH) and atracurium (acidic pH)[8]
- drug–diluent incompatibility when a very acidic drug (e.g. amiodarone) is diluted with sodium chloride 0.9% (near neutral pH)[9] or a very basic drug (e.g. furosemide) is diluted with dextrose 5% (weakly acidic).[10]

The resultant salt-formed precipitates can lead to line occlusion, loss of drug efficacy and possible danger of systemic embolisation.

- Temperature and light can lead to degradation of, e.g., parenteral nutrition,[11] or sodium nitroprusside to cyanide ions,[12] which explains the need for an opaque covering.
- Too much diluent (e.g. amiodarone diluted beyond 0.6 mg/L comes out of solution, leading to loss of efficacy).[9]

DISTRIBUTION

Volume of distribution (V_d) is the theoretical volume of fluid into which the total drug administered would have to be diluted to produce the concentration in plasma. It is unrelated to volume of the body or its fluid compartments but rather its distribution.[13] V_d is increased by factors decreasing plasma drug concentration:[1]

- reduced protein binding (increased drug available for tissue binding)
- increased tissue binding
- increased lipid solubility (for fat-soluble drugs)
- oedema, ascites, effusion fluid (for water-soluble drugs)
- sepsis (endothelial damage and increased capillary permeability where fluid leaks into the interstitial space)
- mechanical ventilation (for water-soluble drugs),

and vice versa.

$$V_d = \frac{A}{C} \tag{87.1}$$

where V_d = apparent volume of distribution (L), A = total amount of drug in organ (mg), C = plasma concentration of drug (mg/L).

For example, gentamicin, a hydrophilic drug with minimal protein binding, has a low V_d similar to the extracellular fluid volume (0.25 L/kg).[14] In a septic, mechanically ventilated patient, the V_d of gentamicin increases as the effective extracellular volume increases, and a larger dose is required to obtain therapeutic levels.[15,16]

Phenytoin, a lipophilic drug, is 90% protein bound with a V_d similar to total body volume (0.65 L/kg).[1] Hypoalbuminaemia in critical illness increases the free, pharmacologically active fraction of phenytoin. This should be taken into account when interpreting phenytoin levels. The latter is normally reported as total serum concentrations that assume normal protein binding.

Morphine extensively binds to tissue and has a high V_d (4 L/kg).[17] Uraemia displaces drugs such as morphine from their tissue-binding sites, thereby increasing their plasma concentration whilst reducing the V_d, and this can lead to toxicity.

A drug with a high V_d will take considerable time to reach organ equilibration (approximately four to five times the half-life):[1]

$$t_{1/2} = 0.693 \times V_d / Q \quad (87.2)$$

where Q=organ blood flow.

V_d is used to calculate the *loading dose* (L_d), that is, the dose required to rapidly achieve a desired therapeutic concentration (C_p) of drug:

$$L_d = \frac{V_d \times C_{pss}}{S \times F} \quad (87.3)$$

where C_{pss}=desired plasma concentration at steady state, S=salt factor of drug, F=bioavailability as a fraction.

For example, the L_d of phenytoin sodium for a 70-kg patient via the i.v. route would be:

$$L_d = \frac{0.65\ \text{L/kg} \times 70\ \text{kg} \times 15\ \text{mg/L}}{0.92 \times 1}$$
$$= 741.8\ \text{mg}$$

The dose is usually rounded to the nearest easily measurable value (i.e. 750 mg in this case). (**NB** This differs considerably from the standard 15 mg/kg dose often used in emergency practice where other prior antiepileptic medicines may have been given.)

Critically ill patients sometimes demonstrate subtherapeutic levels of phenytoin despite accounting for the unbound fraction due to hypoalbuminaemia. A possible explanation is that, as there is more of the free fraction available, more is available for metabolism and excretion. Alternatively, reduced hepatic function may lead to accumulation.[18]

Blood–brain barrier (BBB)

A combination of narrow junctions between the endothelial capillary cells and inherent resistance to the penetration of polar substances allows only the passage of lipophilic drugs via the transcellular route. Proteins, and therefore protein-bound drugs, are too large to cross. Conversely, drugs with low protein binding are able to penetrate the BBB.

In some cases active transporters prevent certain drugs from crossing the BBB. For example, loperamide is an opioid with no central effect at therapeutic doses as P-glycoprotein (an acute phase protein) excludes it from the brain. Conversely, in hepatic encephalopathy, damage to the BBB allows penetration of higher than normal amounts of opioids and, therefore, the patient's sensitivity to the drug's effects increases.

METABOLISM

Metabolism can occur using either or both of the following:[19]

- *Phase I reactions:* these involve addition or exposure of a polar group, for example -OH. Oxidation or reduction reactions in liver microsomes are catalysed by cytochrome P-450 (CYP) enzymes and hydrolysis of esters to alcohol and carboxylic acid by esterases.
- *Phase II reactions:* these increase a drug's hydrophilicity, promoting its renal or biliary excretion. Conjugation or synthesis takes place in the liver or the lung (e.g. glucuronidation, sulphation, acetylation, methylation). The kidney can excrete the drug metabolite by both filtration, and potentially, also by active secretion, into the urine. Usually metabolites are less active than their parent compound, more polar and more readily excreted in bile or urine.

Extensive first-pass metabolism refers to a drug that is significantly metabolised by the liver prior to becoming available to the systemic circulation.

ELIMINATION

CLEARANCE IN AN ORGAN

The liver and the kidney are the main organs involved in drug removal from the body. The liver can either transport a drug from the blood into the bile or metabolise it into another chemical entity (metabolite).

The rate (R) that the liver or kidney can remove drug from the body is usually proportional to the concentration of drug in the blood (C) (first-order kinetics). This proportionality constant is known as the drug's clearance (Cl) (**Fig. 87.2**).

Clearance is related to the half-life ($t_{1/2}$) of the drug. Half-life is the time taken for the plasma drug concentration to fall by 50% and is dependent on V_d:

$$t_{1/2} = \frac{0.693 \times V_d}{Cl} \quad (87.4)$$

(Note: alpha $t_{1/2}$ refers to the distribution $t_{1/2}$; beta $t_{1/2}$ refers to the terminal elimination $t_{1/2}$.)

Figure 87.3 shows the graph of alpha and beta $t_{1/2}$.

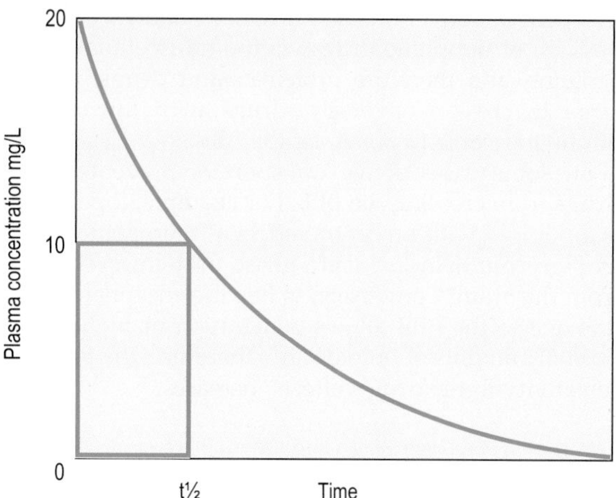

Figure 87.2 First-order elimination graph (plasma drug concentration versus time).

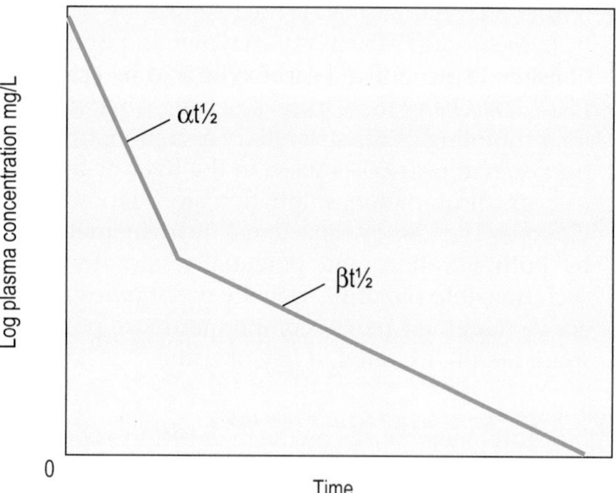

Figure 87.3 Graph of α $t_{1/2}$ and β $t_{1/2}$.

Any process that reduces V_d without affecting clearance will shorten $t_{1/2}$ and vice versa.

$t_{1/2}$ can also be expressed as an equation involving the elimination rate constant (fraction of total drug removed per unit time):

$$k = \frac{Cl}{V_d} \qquad (87.5)$$

This assumes the drug follows first-order kinetics (i.e. Cl and V_d do not change with dose or concentration).

Caution must be taken with interpreting half-lives with respect to a drug's duration of action. Simply using terminal elimination $t_{1/2}$ to predict the length of drug effect may not be accurate. For example, lipophilic fentanyl exhibits a three-compartment pharmacokinetic model post an i.v. bolus:[20]

1. *Short-distribution phase:* high concentrations are achieved rapidly in well-perfused organs (brain, kidneys, lungs)
2. *Slower redistribution phase:* in other tissues, skeletal muscle, fat
3. *Elimination phase.*

The terminal $t_{1/2}$ is 3.7 hours, but the duration of action of fentanyl may vary due to 80% protein binding (see effects of hypoalbuminaemia above) and redistribution into body compartments. Hepatic impairment prolongs $t_{1/2}$.

Steady state

$t_{1/2}$ can be used to predict the time for a drug to reach 'steady state' (i.e. when the rate of drug administered equals the rate it is eliminated). Usually this is reached within 4 or 5 half-lives. Similarly, the time taken for a drug to be eliminated from the body would also be 4 to 5 half-lives. A drug that is 90% dependent on metabolic clearance compared with 10% renal will, in hepatic failure, be eliminated primarily by the renal route, but total clearance will still remain at 10% so accumulation will occur.

Hepatic drug clearance

Hepatic drug clearance is affected by blood flow to the liver and the fraction of drug removed as it passes through – that is, the extraction ratio (ER):[19]

$$\mathrm{ER} = C_{in} - C_{out} / C_{in} \qquad (87.6)$$

where C_{in}=concentration in; C_{out}=concentration out.

- *High-extraction drugs (>0.7) e.g. morphine:* have significant first-pass metabolism and low oral bioavailability: There is a relative excess of the enzymes that metabolise a drug (i.e. a high intrinsic clearance) and a high proportion of the drug is removed by the liver before reaching the systemic circulation. The rate-limiting step is supply of the drug to the liver. Hepatic clearance therefore depends on hepatic blood flow, which is proportional to cardiac output,[21] and is unaffected by changes in the amount of active enzyme (and therefore enzyme inhibition or enzyme induction) and changes in free fraction of the drug. In advanced sepsis the hepatic blood flow is reduced, but in hyperdynamic sepsis the hepatic perfusion may be spared as blood is diverted to vital organs.

  Conversely, in cirrhosis, functional hepatocytes are bypassed when intrinsic clearance falls or portosystemic shunts form, both of which increase drug bioavailability.
- *Intermediate-extraction drugs pharmacokinetics (0.3–0.7) e.g. midazolam:* are more complex to predict. Drugs that fall into this category include those that are normally in the high ER group but alter in this respect when used in patients with hepatic dysfunction. Hepatic dysfunction and reduced metabolism lead to accumulation of active drug. This is further enhanced if drug metabolites are also active.
- *Low-extraction drugs (<0.3) e.g. lorazepam:* have negligible first-pass metabolism and high oral bioavailability: There is a relative deficit of enzymes that

Box 87.1 High and low extraction ratio (ER) drugs

High ER	Low ER
Propranolol	Lorazepam
Morphine	Theophylline
Fentanyl	Chlordiazepoxide
Amitriptyline	Phenytoin

metabolise the drug (i.e. a low intrinsic clearance) and the rate-limiting step is enzymatic activity. Hepatic clearance is independent of hepatic blood flow but is influenced by enzyme inhibition or enzyme induction, other competing drugs and changes in free fraction of the drug (the form accessible to the enzyme). Reduced liver perfusion and a fall in ER do not significantly affect drug bioavailability.

- Hepatic dysfunction can reduce the effects of pro-drugs that require metabolism to become active.

Box 87.1 lists high and low hepatic extraction drugs.

Zero-order metabolism Most drugs follow first-order pharmacokinetics (i.e. rate of metabolism correlates proportionally with plasma concentration). However, drugs such as phenytoin follow zero-order pharmacokinetics. In this situation metabolism reaches its peak as the enzyme system is saturated and relative clearance falls as plasma concentrations rise. The process is concentration-independent and so an increase in dose will produce a disproportionate rise in plasma levels. The rate of metabolism is constant regardless of the amount of drug present (**Fig. 87.4**).

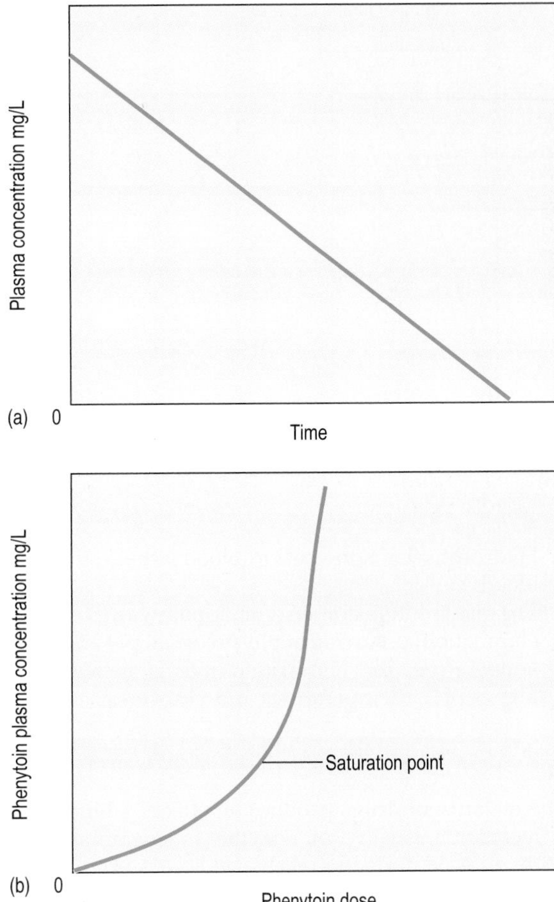

Figure 87.4 (a) Zero-order elimination. (b) Saturation point phenytoin pharmacokinetics.

Renal drug clearance[22]

Renal clearance of a drug or metabolite is influenced by glomerular filtration, tubular secretion and tubular reabsorption.

Glomerular filtration usually allows the passage of the free but not protein-bound drug into the renal tubules. Drugs that are not subject to tubular secretion or reabsorption therefore have a renal clearance that equals the glomerular filtration rate. For a healthy 70-kg 20-year-old man this is normally 0.1 L/min (i.e. a relatively low clearance rate is achieved). Conversely, drugs that undergo active tubular secretion can have higher renal clearances up to a theoretical maximum of renal blood flow (1.2 L/min). Such drugs are usually charged and can have a high affinity for transporter sites, which allows the passage of even protein-bound drugs. Tubular secretion normally occurs in the proximal tubule and is assumed if clearance rate exceeds calculated filtration rate.

Tubular reabsorption involves the passive diffusion of drugs back across the tubule into the systemic circulation. Such drugs are usually lipophilic and uncharged. The extent of reabsorption is determined by degree of ionisation and concentration gradient determined by urine pH and flow rate respectively. Reabsorption is assumed if clearance rate is less than calculated filtration rate (e.g. fluconazole reabsorption is considerable in normal renal function but reduced in acute kidney injury, therefore, dose reduction is not necessary or even an increase may be warranted).

Biliary clearance[1,3]

Large molecules can be actively transported by hepatocytes and excreted in the bile either unchanged or conjugated. Conjugated molecules can undergo enterohepatic recirculation (i.e. be hydrolysed by gut bacteria, secreted into the ileum, reabsorbed into the systemic circulation and transported back to the liver via the portal vein). Phenytoin and loperamide are examples of drugs that undergo significant enterohepatic circulation. Biliary obstruction will increase levels of active drug and metabolites excreted via this route.

Other drug clearance routes

Atracurium is an example of a drug that is independent of hepatic or renal clearance and is eliminated via two non-oxidative routes to inactive metabolites:[23]

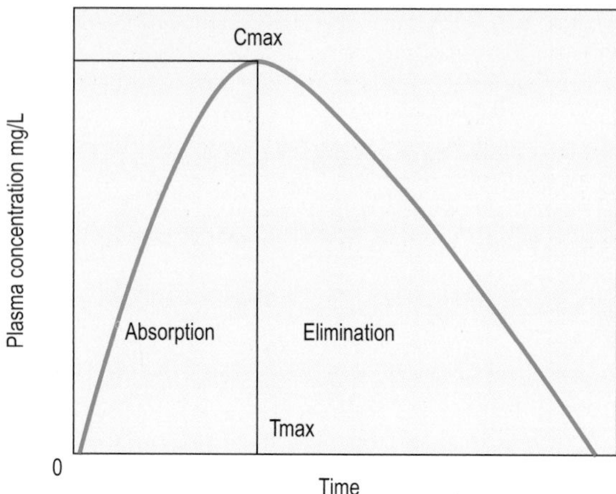

Figure 87.5 Areas under the curve (AUC).

1. Hydrolysis by non-specific blood esterases in the blood
2. The main route, a non-enzymatic pathway (Hofmann elimination) occurring at physiological pH and body temperature; the elimination rate is increased at higher pH or temperatures and vice versa.

DOSE–RESPONSE RELATIONSHIPS

The majority of drugs produce an effect by binding to a receptor,[1] usually an enzyme or membrane ion channel. A conformational change occurs producing a direct physiological response, the extent of which is dependent on the:

- number of receptors present
- affinity of drug for the receptor
- presence of agonists/antagonists competing for the receptor-binding site
- concentration of the free (unbound) drug within the vicinity of the receptor.

Drugs achieve a maximum effect as there are only a finite number of receptors upon which to act. A graph of plasma concentration of drug versus time is shown in **Figure 87.5**.

- C_{max} is the maximum plasma concentration achieved during the time course of the drug.
- T_{max} is the time taken to achieve C_{max}.
- $t_{1/2}$ is the time taken for the plasma level to fall by 50%.
- k is the elimination rate constant.

PHARMACOKINETIC MODELS[3]

The ability to predict the effects of dose changes on concentration and outcome requires a mathematical representation or model of the behaviour of the drug. A model is defined by a set of equations (representing the basic structure) and a set of parameter values for those equations (representing the behaviour of a specific drug).

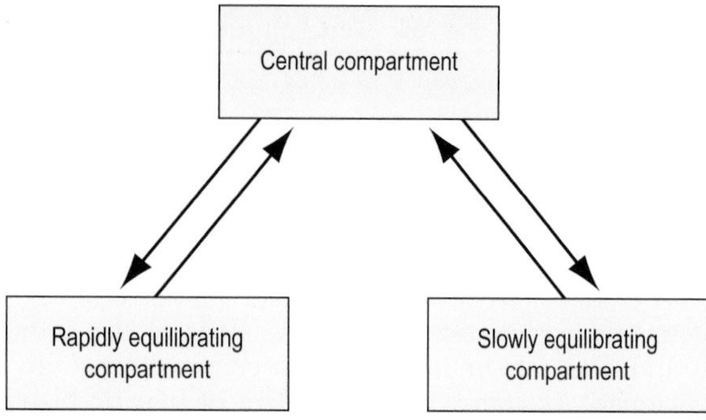

Figure 87.6 Compartment models.

There are three basic forms of pharmacokinetic models:

- *Compartmental models* are the most commonly utilised. The body is represented by a central compartment plus one or more peripheral compartments. Drugs used in anaesthesia usually follow a three-compartment model: one compartment that is central, one that is slowly equilibrating and the other that is rapidly equilibrating (**Fig. 87.6**). As blood flow is not taken into account, compartment models have limited use in the critically ill where patient physiology is variable.
- *Physiological models* represent the major body organs. Drug supply to and from organs is influenced by vascular anatomy and organ perfusion. Animal models tend to be used as they are far easier to develop than human models (with some notable exceptions[24]). They are able to predict the consequences of changes in both dose regimen and physiological status.
- *Recirculatory models* are an intermediate between compartment and physiological models. They can provide a simple conceptual framework for the important relationship between cardiac output, bolus injection rate and initial drug concentrations[25] that is lacking in compartmental models.

More recently, population modelling aims to take into account patient variability with respect to physiology and pharmacological response to a given drug.[26]

TITRATION

The majority of drugs used in intensive care are relatively rapid in onset with a direct measurable effect. The dose can, therefore, be titrated to desired therapeutic outcome. Although titration can be empirical, optimal titration strategies are guided by an understanding of drug kinetics and dynamics. Important points to consider include:

- time required for the drug to achieve peak effect after an i.v. bolus; multiple doses within this time period may result in 'overshooting' the desired outcome
- potential dose range for titration
- time to offset of effect
- influence of evolving pathophysiology and tolerance on drug effect
- potential kinetic and dynamic interactions with co-administered drugs.

PRACTICAL APPLICATIONS

BOLUS INJECTION RATE

The rate of injection is often important to avoid toxic effects. Ranitidine can cause asystole and bradycardia if administered too fast – that is, greater than 25 mg/min.[27] Conversely, an 'i.v. push' refers to a rapid i.v. bolus; for example, adenosine is administered over 2 seconds due to its short half-life (less than 10 seconds).[28] If the time over which an i.v. bolus dose is not specified, it would be prudent to assume the drug should be administered over at least 3 minutes (i.e. as a slow i.v. bolus).

REPEAT BOLUS OR INFUSION

Drugs with relatively long half-lives and wide therapeutic indices can be administered by repeat bolus administration (e.g. ceftazidime); those with short half-lives and narrow therapeutic indices (e.g. catecholamines) should be administered in a more predictable and titratable manner by continuous infusion.

MAINTENANCE DOSE

ALTERING INFUSION RATES

The consequence of altering drug infusion rates is dependent on the half-life of the drug. If the half-life is relatively long (e.g. midazolam and morphine), an increase in dose requirements should be met by titrating small boluses to achieve the desired goal, and then increasing the infusion rate by the appropriate amount. Decreases in requirements can be met by stopping the infusion and recommencing at a lower rate after the new desired state has been reached. If severe illness causes the volume of distribution of a drug to be doubled then its half-life will also be doubled. Severe illness may also decrease clearance of a drug; halving clearance will cause a similar doubling of half-life. Should both effects occur together, half-life will be increased fourfold, having a significant effect on the duration of action of a drug.

OFFSET TIMES

The half-life for some drugs depends on the duration of the infusion (e.g. fentanyl's half-life increases with duration of continuous infusion). This is particularly evident for drugs with high distribution volumes and with bolus kinetics governed significantly by redistribution rather than clearance. For short infusions, the plasma half-life after the infusion will be less than the terminal elimination half-life. However, as the duration of infusion becomes sufficient to achieve steady state, the half-life upon stopping the infusion will increase until it equals the terminal elimination half-life.[29]

PK–PD CHANGES IN CRITICAL ILLNESS

Multi-organ failure significantly alters drug kinetics and dynamics making prediction of effects a therapeutic challenge.

CIRCULATORY FAILURE

Circulatory failure diverts blood flow to essential organs such as the heart and brain at the expense of the peripheral tissues. This results in:

- increased levels of drug in the heart and brain
- decreased levels of drug in the peripheries
- reduced renal blood flow and shunting of blood from cortical to juxtamedullary nephrons; glomerular filtration rate and tubular excretion fall, decreasing extraction of drugs and renally excreted metabolites
- reduced hepatic blood flow; liver function may be impaired, decreasing clearance of both highly extracted drugs (reduced delivery to the liver) and of poorly extracted drugs (reduced cellular metabolism).

Mechanical ventilation may cause further decline in hepatic perfusion by increasing intrathoracic pressure and therefore decreasing venous return.

The initial effect is a large decrease in distribution volumes and clearance of drugs. The effects are more profound on drugs that are usually rapidly distributed such as sedatives. Fluid and inotropic therapy may alter these effects over brief periods of time. With volume overload, there may be an increase in initial distribution volume (of water-soluble drugs) but with a more prolonged distribution half-life.

HEPATIC FAILURE

Drug dosing in hepatic failure is more difficult to predict compared with renal failure. Derangements in liver function tests do not usually serve as a strict guide for the extent of dose reduction compared with trends in creatinine clearance and other parameters used to estimate renal function.

Liver failure significantly affects the pharmacokinetics of drugs.

Absorption

Bioavailability of lipid-soluble drugs is reduced in cholestasis where bile salts are used to enhance their absorption.

Distribution
Patients with ascites may require larger loading doses of water-soluble drugs due to increased V_d.

Hypoalbuminaemia as a result of catabolism, sepsis, reduced protein intake and synthesis leads to an increase in free fraction of highly albumin-bound drug (e.g. phenytoin). Total serum concentration may appear low or within range but lead to toxic effects if the pharmacologically active free fraction is unaccounted for. Conversely, increased concentrations of α_1-acid glycoprotein (an acute-phase glycoprotein often raised in sepsis), to which phenytoin is 20% bound, can decrease the free fraction.[18] Phenytoin, therefore, exhibits complex and sometimes unpredictable pharmacokinetics in the critically ill.

Metabolism
(See extraction ratio (ER).)

Elimination
Cholestasis can reduce elimination of active drug or their metabolites that undergo biliary excretion and enterohepatic circulation. Concomitant renal dysfunction as in hepatorenal syndrome may require a dose reduction of renally excreted drugs.

RENAL FAILURE

Absorption[16]
Uraemia has been linked to reduced gut integrity in animal studies.

Certain drugs used in, for example, chronic renal failure, such as phosphate binders, can reduce the enteral absorption of certain drugs (e.g. ciprofloxacin).

Distribution[16]
Significant fluid retention due to volume resuscitation or reduced diuresis increases the V_d and, therefore, distribution $t_{1/2}$ of water-soluble drugs (e.g. gentamicin and beta lactams).

Reduced plasma protein binding of acidic drugs (e.g. amiodarone) can occur. Possible explanations include the displacement of acidic drugs from their albumin-binding sites by endogenous substances that accumulate in renal failure and compete for a position (see Metabolism below).

Plasma protein binding for basic drugs (e.g. epoprostenol) is not usually affected; however, certain interventions such as haemodialysis can raise levels of α_1-glycoprotein, an acute-phase protein to which basic drugs usually bind.[21]

If the unbound fraction of a drug increases and intrinsic clearance remains constant, plasma clearance will increase proportionally. Total plasma concentration will fall but the unbound plasma concentration will not be affected (e.g. phenytoin).

Reduced tissue binding can occur in end-stage renal failure (ESRF) causing a decrease in V_d.

Metabolism
Certain drugs that are mainly or completely eliminated from the body by non-renal mechanisms can still accumulate in renal dysfunction. This implies that their metabolism is impaired by renal failure. Possible explanations for this include reduced activity of metabolic enzymes.[22]

Accumulation of metabolic products can reduce protein binding of drugs. For example, uraemia displaces penicillins, sulphonamides and cephalosporins from their binding sites. The reduced affinity of plasma proteins for phenytoin increases the drug's free fraction. Therefore, a non-uraemic patient with a normal free fraction of phenytoin of 0.1 and a total phenytoin level of 7 mg/L will have the same free phenytoin concentration as a uraemic patient with a free fraction of 0.2 and a total phenytoin level of 14 mg/L:[1]

$$C_{\text{paj}} = \frac{\text{total phenytoin level (mg/L)}}{0.9 \times (\text{albumin level}/\text{normal albumin level}) + 0.1} \quad (87.7)$$

where C_{padj}=adjusted phenytoin level (free phenytoin concentration), and normal albumin=40 g/dL.

Elimination
Reduced renal clearance prolongs the terminal elimination $t_{1/2}$.

Renal failure can lead to toxicity if dose adjustments are not made to account for accumulation of drugs and their active metabolites cleared primarily by the kidneys. Dose can either be reduced, for instance vancomycin (time-dependent bacterial kill) or their dosing intervals increased, for instance gentamicin (concentration-dependent kill). Renal failure usually affects glomerular function more than tubular function so excretion of aminoglycosides, which depend more on glomerular filtration, is affected more than that of penicillins, which are dependent on tubular function.

Serum creatinine is usually a poor guide to renal function in the critically ill because creatinine is:

- a by-product of muscle often reduced in critical illness, the elderly or low-weight patients
- influenced by diet (recent protein intake, which can often be insufficient due to variable absorption if administered via the gastrointestinal tract)
- increased or reduced by drugs or disease states without necessarily influencing GFR (e.g. trimethoprim inhibits the renal secretion of creatinine without reducing renal clearance)
- used to calculate C_rCl based on a normal population data of healthy individuals
- usually fluctuating in the critically ill
- a very late marker of renal dysfunction – the GFR has to fall by at least 50% before a significant rise in creatinine is seen; it is better to monitor levels for accumulation of renally cleared drugs (e.g. vancomycin) or electrolytes (e.g. potassium).

Renal replacement therapy drastically alters volumes and clearances of drugs. Effects vary with the mode of dialysis, the filter life, the type of membrane in use and the drugs in question.

RESPIRATORY FAILURE

Insufficient gaseous exchange can disrupt the normal acid–base balance and consequently affect protein binding and V_d. Mechanical ventilation increases intrathoracic pressure, reducing cardiac output, hepatic and renal perfusion. Therefore, drugs with a high extraction ratio or those that are predominantly renally cleared may be at risk of accumulation. The V_d of water-soluble drugs (e.g. aminoglycosides) and the risk of a stress ulcer are also increased by mechanical ventilation.

SYSTEMIC INFLAMMATORY RESPONSE SYNDROME

In sepsis and multi-organ failure, an increase in capillary permeability and a tendency towards increased total body water occurs, associated with hypoalbuminaemia. Larger loading doses are required to achieve the desired therapeutic response due to the consequent increased V_d of many drugs. Similar changes occur in patients with major burns. The volume of distribution may also change over short periods of time. When patients start to recover, serum concentrations may increase because of the decreasing volume of distribution of the drug (e.g. vancomycin[30]) as well as decrease because of resumption of normal metabolism and clearance (e.g. midazolam[31]). Circulatory, hepatic and renal failure may also add the characteristic changes already described, of decreased clearance or metabolism and accumulation of active metabolites.

The consequence of hypoalbuminaemia on highly protein-bound antibiotics

Hypoalbuminaemia increases V_d by increasing the free fraction of drug in the extracellular compartment. Unbound drug leaves the systemic circulation to distribute to tissues and total drug concentrations fall in the intravascular compartment; that is, there is a fall in total effective serum concentrations over time (area under the curve). The consequences of this include:

- reduced time above the MIC for time-dependent antibiotics
- reduced C_{max}/MIC for concentration-dependent antibiotics.

Continuous vancomycin infusions are often used in ICU. This is a more convenient method of administration for the time-dependent antibiotic as levels can be taken at any time post steady state (see 'sampling time for drug levels'). In contrast, once-daily dosing of relatively larger doses of gentamicin (as opposed to smaller doses administered more frequently) are used to optimise its concentration-dependent kill whilst minimising accumulation risk. Therapeutic drug monitoring (TDM) guides dosing (see TDM), but for other antibiotics with wider therapeutic indices, such as caspofungin, TDM is not routinely performed. Dosing should ideally be at the maximum dose possible whilst avoiding accumulation (usually manifested as an accentuation of the drug's usual side-effects). Extended infusion times of beta lactam antibiotics beyond the manufacturer's licensed duration (e.g. meropenem) have been shown to achieve better pharmacodynamics targets against less susceptible microorganisms such as *P. aeruginosa* and *Acinetobacter*[15,32] (**Box 87.2**).

Box 87.2 Highly protein-bound and minimally protein-bound antibiotics

Highly protein bound	Minimally protein bound
Amphotericin B 90%	Gentamicin <30%
Caspofungin 97%	Vancomycin 10–50%
Ceftriaxone 85–95%	Meropenem 2%
Teicoplanin 90–95%	Imipenem <30%

An increased $t_{1/2}$ is caused by redistribution of drug from the tissues to blood. This is beneficial in both time- and concentration-dependent antibiotics with high susceptibility (i.e. it increases the time above the MIC).

CHANGES IN RECEPTORS IN ACUTE ILLNESS

Catecholamines demonstrate increased receptor numbers in response to a lack of agonist (up-regulation) and reduced receptor numbers in the presence of excess agonist (down-regulation). Drug affinity for receptors is also influenced by pH. Acidosis decreases the affinity of catecholamines for their receptors, and becomes a clinically significant problem when there is a pH<7.1. Body temperature also affects pharmacodynamics – hypothermia decreases drug affinity for receptors.

Proliferation of extrajunctional acetylcholine receptors on muscle after acute injuries such as burns and denervation can lead to hyperkalaemia following the use of suxamethonium.

THERAPEUTIC DRUG MONITORING (TDM)

TDM is used to guide dosing of drugs with a narrow therapeutic range (i.e. a small therapeutic to toxic window) – for example gentamicin, phenytoin and theophylline. Toxicity may be associated with peak drug concentrations (e.g. seizures and arrhythmias from theophylline) or with mean concentrations (e.g. ototoxicity from aminoglycosides). **Table 87.1** displays examples of drugs with a narrow therapeutic window.[33-35] Hospital laboratories measure total plasma drug concentration. However, it is the unbound drug fraction that is pharmacologically active (see phenytoin).

Regardless of measured concentration, evidence of clinical efficacy or toxicity must be monitored regularly (e.g. altering the maintenance dose of digoxin in a patient with a subtherapeutic level is unnecessary if ventricular rate is adequately controlled). Conversely,

Table 87.1 Therapeutic drug monitoring in the critically ill

DRUG	THERAPEUTIC CONCENTRATION	TOXIC EFFECTS
Digoxin	1–2 μg/L	CNS and visual disturbances, dizziness, nausea and vomiting[1]
Gentamicin	<1 mg/L (trough)	Nephrotoxicity, ototoxicity[14]
Amikacin	<5 mg/L (trough)	Nephrotoxicity, ototoxicity[33]
Vancomycin	20–25 mg/L (continuous infusion)	Nephrotoxicity, ototoxicity, reversible neutropenia[34]
Phenytoin	10–20 mg/L	Nystagmus, ataxia, dysarthria, cardiovascular collapse[5] Correct for hypoalbuminaemia Caution in uraemia
Theophylline	10–20 mg/L	Arrhythmias, nausea, vomiting[35]

it would be prudent to reload a previously stable epileptic patient presenting with seizures if the phenytoin level is subtherapeutic. If the phenytoin level is therapeutic and the patient's convulsions persist, a neurology review is required. This usually results in addition of, or change to, another agent.

SAMPLING TIME FOR DRUG LEVELS

The ideal sampling time for a drug level is either just prior to the next due dose or once distribution into the tissue is known to be complete. If taken prior to distribution, the levels will be falsely interpreted as higher than expected for the dose administered. For example, an i.v. loading dose of phenytoin takes at least 2 hours for distribution.[1] A level taken prior to this time would not be a true reflection of the dose administered and subsequent dosing based on the result will be incorrect.

The majority of drug levels are obtained as a 'trough' – that is, a pre-dose level as suggested in the case of phenytoin. Usually, levels should not be taken prior to steady state being reached; for example, it would take approximately 10 days following a formulation change for phenytoin to reach steady state. However, if the patient's pharmacokinetics is suspected not to follow the normal population, as in the case of the critically ill, and if there is a risk of accumulation or underdosing before this time, it would be prudent to sample much sooner so the dose can be promptly optimised.

THE EFFECT OF DRUG INTERACTIONS ON PHARMACODYNAMICS

Multiple drug therapy in the critically ill increases their vulnerability to the effects of drug interactions. It could also be argued that ICU patients are monitored more closely than their counterparts on general wards so any adverse effects are likely to be identified sooner. Nevertheless, if a patient does not demonstrate a normal response to a drug treatment, it may be due to a drug interaction.

The consequence of drug interactions is naturally dependent on the drugs in question. **Table 87.2** provides a few examples of interactions involving commonly used drugs in ICU. Certain drugs (e.g. warfarin) are usually avoided altogether in the critically ill due to their numerous drug interactions, long $t_{1/2}$ and potentially catastrophic effects on coagulation in an already vulnerable patient with variable physiology.

SUMMARY

The relationship between PK and PD can be used to predict a dosing regimen for a patient. However, wide inter-patient variability and the labile nature of the critically ill means careful consideration needs to be applied when formulating an appropriate dose. Best clinical judgement is required. Treatment may need to be individualised and titrated, especially when the outcome does not follow the normal expected clinical response. Levels should be taken to guide dosing in drugs with narrow therapeutic windows but caution must be taken with interpretation, especially when the clinical symptoms do not correlate with apparently therapeutic readings. For drugs with 'silent' pharmacodynamics, other markers of therapeutic effect should be sought – for example, a reduction in temperature, C-reactive protein (CRP) and white cell count (WCC) in anti-infectives with a wide therapeutic index. At the same time, optimising dosage in ICU should take into account the adverse effects of accumulation if higher doses are used beyond what is normally recommended.

In line with non-drug therapies in the ICU, drug kinetic and dynamics are never simple or straightforward and rarely does one dosage regimen fit all. For further advice, please consult your pharmacist.

Acknowledgements

Updated and modified from the chapter in the previous edition by R N Upton, J A Myburgh and R G Morris. Dose regimens are for illustration only and local guidelines should be consulted.

Many thanks to Vanessa Marvin, PharmD for reviewing this chapter prior to submission.

Table 87.2 Examples of drug–drug interactions in ICU patients

DRUG A	DRUG B	INTERACTION	COMMENT
Norepinephrine (noradrenaline)	Amitriptyline	Amitriptyline and related antidepressants block norepinephrine uptake into adrenergic neurons thereby potentiating its effect	Results in ↑ blood pressure and heart rate beyond what is usually expected
Midazolam	Amiodarone	Amiodarone is an inhibitor of cytochrome P450 isoenzyme by which midazolam is metabolised	Results in ↑ levels of midazolam
Midazolam	Fluconazole	Fluconazole is an inhibitor of cytochrome P450 isoenzyme by which midazolam is metabolised	Results in ↑ levels of midazolam
Haloperidol	Amiodarone	Both drugs prolong QT interval	Results in ↑ risk of ventricular arrhythmias
Phenytoin	Hydrocortisone	Phenytoin is a potent enzyme inducer	↑ Hydrocortisone metabolism, ↓Therapeutic and adrenal suppressant effects
Amiodarone	Simvastatin	Amiodarone is an inhibitor of cytochrome P450 isoenzyme by which simvastatin is metabolised	↑ Risk of myopathy

Access the complete references list online at http://www.expertconsult.com

1. Winter ME. Basic Clinical Pharmacokinetics. 5th revised ed. London: Pharmaceutical Press; 2009.
15. Varghese JM, Roberts JA, Lipman J. Pharmacokinetics and pharmacodynamics in critically ill patients. Curr Opin Anaesthesiol 2010;23:472–8.
18. Von Wincklelmann SL, Spriet I, Willems L. Therapeutic drug monitoring of phenytoin in critically ill. Pharmacotherapy 2008;28(11):1391–400.
19. North-Lewis P, editor. Drugs and the Liver: A Guide to Drug Handling in Liver Dysfunction. 1st ed. London: Pharmaceutical Press; 2008.
22. Verbeeck RK, Flora TM. Pharmacokinetics and dosage adjustment in patients with renal dysfunction. Eur J Clin Pharmacol 2009;65:757–73.
32. Sutep J, Thanya L, Jullangkoon M, et al. Pharmacodynamics of meropenem in critically ill patients with febrile neutropenia and bacteraemia. Int J Antimicrob Agents 2011;38:231–6.

FURTHER READING

Cook DJ, Fuller HD, Guyatt GH, et al. Risk factors for gastrointestinal bleeding in critically ill patients. New Engl J Med 1994;330:377–81.

Crandon JL, Ariano RE, Zelenitsky SA, et al. Optimisation of meropenem dosage in the critically ill population based on renal function. Intensive Care Med 2011;37:632–8.

Dryden MS. Linezolid pharmacokinetics and pharmacodynamics in clinical treatment. J Antimicrob Chemther 2011;66(Suppl 4):iv7–15.

Jean-Marle C, Bernard G, Stephanie R, et al. Tobramycin disposition in ICU patients receiving once daily regimens: population approach and dosage simulations. Br J Clin Pharmacol 2010;71(1):61–71.

Robert JA, Lipman J. Pharmacokinetic issues for antibiotics in the critically ill patient. Crit Care Med 2009;37(3):840–51.

Roberts JA, Joynt GM, Choi GYS, et al. How to optimize antimicrobial prescriptions in the Intensive Care Unit: principles of individualized dosing using pharmacokinetics and pharmacodynamics. Int J Antimicrob Agents 2012;39:187–92.

Taccone FS, Laterre PF, Dugernier T, et al. Insufficient β-lactam concentrations in the early phase of severe sepsis and septic shock. Crit Care 2010;14:R126.

88

Management of acute poisoning

David M Wood and Duncan LA Wyncoll

Acute poisoning remains one of the commonest medical emergencies, accounting for 5–10% of hospital medical admissions. Although in the majority of cases the drug ingestion is intentional, the in-hospital mortality remains low (<0.5%).[1] There are specific antidotes available for a small number of poisons and drugs; however, in most intoxications, basic supportive care is the main requirement and recovery will follow. This chapter is a hands-on guide to the general management of acute poisoning and drug intoxication. For more detailed information than can be provided here, please refer to internet-based information services (e.g. Toxbase in the UK – http://www.spib.axl.co.uk) or a local/regional/national telephone poisons information service (e.g. National Poisons Information Service in the UK – 0844 8920111).

Clinical toxicology remains an experience-based specialty; consequently, many recommendations are based on a small literature of case reports, rather than controlled clinical studies. In recent years, toxicological experts have produced position statements and clinical guidelines on certain aspects of care, and these are referenced when possible.

GENERAL PRINCIPLES

The general principles of the management of poisoned patients are diagnosis based on history and clinical features, clinical examination, resuscitation, investigations and continued supportive care. Measures to reduce absorption or enhance elimination, and specific treatments, may be indicated in some cases. In the more acute situations, these actions often have to be carried out simultaneously.

ABC

In acutely poisoned patients who are unconscious, dentures should be removed and the oropharynx cleared of food and vomit. Tracheal intubation and airway protection is almost always necessary when a patient tolerates insertion of an oropharyngeal airway – perhaps the only exception to this rule is patients who have taken gamma hydroxybutyric acid (GHB) and gamma butyrolactone (GBL) (see later). Inadequate spontaneous ventilation, determined clinically or by arterial blood gas (ABG) analysis, obviously requires ventilatory support. Venous access should be established, and circulatory assessment must be made. Basic observations, including blood pressure, pulse rate, temperature, peripheral perfusion and urine output, should be recorded.

CLINICAL EXAMINATION

The clinical examination should include looking particularly for needle marks or evidence of previous self-harm. The Glasgow Coma Scale, designed for head-injured patients, is frequently used but descriptive documentation of the degree of impaired consciousness is much more valuable. In an unconscious patient with no history available, the diagnosis depends upon excluding other common causes of coma (**Box 88.1**) and circumstantial evidence. Specific attention should be paid to the temperature, pupil size, blood pressure, respiratory and heart rate, as these may help to restrict the list of potential toxins (**Box 88.2**). Patients should also have a detailed neurological examination, preferably before the administration of any muscle relaxants, documenting the presence/absence of abnormal tone and reflexes, spontaneous/inducible clonus and/or ocular clonus.

INVESTIGATIONS

Important initial investigations include the following:

- *Urinalysis*: keep a sample for later analysis if required. Although rapid reaction dipsticks are available to screen for common drugs of abuse/recreational drugs by immunoassay, their routine use is not recommended owing to false-positive results, detection of metabolites rather than parent drug and/or cross-reactivity with prescription and over-the-counter medicines.
- *Basic biochemistry*: many drugs are dependent on renal elimination. Significant renal insufficiency may alter management.
- *ABG analysis*: metabolic and/or respiratory acidosis is most common. Aspirin may initially cause a respiratory alkalosis, which in more significant ingestions can be followed by a metabolic acidosis or combined picture of a respiratory alkalosis/metabolic acidosis. Metabolic alkaloses are unusual.

Box 88.1 Common causes of coma other than acute poisoning

Intracranial bleeds
- Subarachnoid haemorrhage
- Subdural/extradural haematomas

Meningitis or encephalitis
Diabetic comas
Uraemic encephalopathy

Box 88.2 Clinical effects of the common poisons

Convulsions
Tricyclics, isoniazid, lithium, amfetamines, theophylline, carbon monoxide, phenothiazines, cocaine
Skin
Bullae: barbiturates, tricyclics
Sweating: salicylates, organophosphates, amfetamines, cocaine
Pupils
Constricted: opioids, organophosphates
Dilated: hypoxia, hypothermia, tricyclics, phenothiazines, anticholinergics
Temperature
Pyrexia: anticholinergics, tricyclics, salicylates, amfetamines, cocaine
Hypothermia: barbiturates, alcohol, opioids
Cardiac rhythm
Bradycardia: digoxin, beta blockers, organophosphates
Tachycardia: salicylates, theophylline, anticholinergics
Arrhythmias: digoxin, phenothiazines, tricyclics, anticholinergics

- *Anion gap*=$([Na^+]+[K^+])-([Cl^-]+[HCO_3^-])$: it is normally 10–14. Ethanol, methanol, ethylene glycol, metformin, cyanide, isoniazid or salicylates are the most frequent causes of a high anion gap metabolic acidosis in clinical toxicology.
- *Chest X-ray*: inhalation of gastric contents is not uncommon.
- *Drug levels*: these are rarely helpful except in specific poisonings. They include paracetamol, salicylates, iron, digoxin and lithium. It is important to note that, for most poisonings, drug concentrations guide rather than dictate treatment.

GUT DECONTAMINATION

EMESIS

Ipecacuanha-induced emesis is no longer recommended.[2] It is ineffective at removing significant quantities of poisons from the stomach, limits the use of activated charcoal and can increase the risk of aspiration in those patients who have a reduced level of consciousness.

Box 88.3 Drug intoxications where multiple-dose activated charcoal may be beneficial

Carbamazepine
Theophylline
Digoxin
Quinine
Phenobarbital
Dapsone
Sustained-release preparations

GASTRIC LAVAGE

The joint American and European toxicologists' statement suggests that gastric lavage removes an insignificant amount of poison, and may only propel unabsorbed poison into the small intestine; therefore it is no longer routinely recommended.[3] Additionally, it is important to note that gastric lavage often delays the use of activated charcoal, which is likely to have greater benefit with less unwanted effects or risks.

ACTIVATED CHARCOAL

Activated charcoal (AC) remains the first-line treatment for most acute poisonings.[4] Owing to its large surface area and porous structure it is highly effective at adsorbing many toxins with few exceptions. Exceptions include elemental metals, pesticides, alcohols including ethanol, strong acids and alkalis, and cyanide. It should be given to all patients who present within 1 hour of ingestion of a potentially toxic amount of a drug or drugs; it should not be given to those patients who are drowsy (unless they have a protected airway). International guidelines recommend administration of AC within 1 hour, so it is vital to identify rapidly those who present after a potentially serious overdose so that it can be given swiftly.[5] Longer than 1 hour it may still be effective if it follows an overdose of a substance that slows gastric emptying (e.g. opioids, anticholinergics, tricyclic antidepressants), but this depends on the clinical condition of the patient and amount ingested.

Repeated doses of AC can increase the elimination of some drugs by interrupting their entero-enteric and enterohepatic circulation.[6] Indications for repeated dose AC are shown in **Box 88.3**. It should be considered in patients who have ingested a modified or slow-release preparation or significant salicylate ingestions; in these situations multiple doses of AC are being administered to reduce absorption rather than enhance elimination. AC is given in 50 g doses for adults and 1 g/kg (max 50 g) for children. It commonly causes vomiting; therefore consider giving an antiemetic prior to administration. Multiple doses can be associated with constipation so patients should be given an appropriate laxative. Repeated doses are given at 4-hourly intervals until it is clinically indicated to stop.

WHOLE BOWEL IRRIGATION

This is a method of gut decontamination that is indicated for a limited number of poisons.[7] Whole bowel irrigation involves administration of non-absorbable polyethylene glycol solution to cause a liquid stool and reduce drug absorption by physically forcing contents rapidly through the gastrointestinal tract. Polyethylene glycol preparations are still occasionally used in surgical units for 'bowel preparation' prior to surgery. It may have a role in treating large ingestions of drugs that are not absorbed by AC. Indications include large ingestions of iron or lithium, ingestion of drug-filled packets/condoms ('body packers'), and large ingestions of sustained-release or enteric-coated drugs (e.g. theophylline or calcium channel blockers).

ENHANCING DRUG ELIMINATION

In the overwhelming majority of patients who present after an overdose, gut decontamination techniques and supportive care are all that is required. In a limited number of acute poisonings it may be necessary to consider methods to enhance elimination.

URINARY ALKALINISATION

Urinary alkalinisation (previously termed *forced alkaline diuresis*) may be useful for serious poisonings with:

- salicylates
- phenobarbital (with repeated dose AC)
- chlorpropamide
- methotrexate.

Intravenous 8.4% sodium bicarbonate is infused (the joint American and European toxicologists' statement recommends 225 mL over 1 hour in adults) to achieve a urine pH of approximately 7.5–8.5. The term 'urine alkalinisation' emphasises that urine pH manipulation is the prime objective of treatment; the terms 'forced alkaline diuresis' and 'alkaline diuresis' should be discontinued. According to international position statements it should be considered the treatment of choice for moderate to severe salicylate poisoning.[8] Care must be taken to ensure the potassium does not fall rapidly, and the urine pH should be measured every 30 minutes.

EXTRACORPOREAL TECHNIQUES

Numerous extracorporeal techniques are potentially available to aid drug removal in the poisoned patient, as well as correct metabolic and biochemical abnormalities as a result of the poisoning. These include plasmapheresis, haemodialysis, haemofiltration, haemodiafiltration and haemoperfusion. There are limited data on drug clearance by these techniques in the literature and it is not possible to extrapolate from one system to the other. At present, knowledge of the principles of the methods and the kinetics of the drug involved is relied upon.

Extracorporeal techniques should be considered only when there are clinical features or markers of severe toxicity, failure to respond to full supportive care coupled with poisoning by a drug that can potentially be removed. Impairment of the normal route of elimination of the compound may also influence the decision. Use of extracorporeal techniques is probably worthwhile only if total body clearance is increased by at least 30%. Haemoperfusion is rarely performed in most intensive care units and intermittent haemodialysis is often confined to renal units. Consequently, the use of continuous haemofiltration, with or without dialysis, using filtration rates of greater than 50–100 mL/kg per hour is likely to be as equally effective as when an extracorporeal technique is indicated.

An international multidisciplinary working party called EXTRIP (EXtracorporeal TReatments In Poisoning) is currently reviewing the role of extracorporeal elimination and will be issuing a number of guidelines for poisonings where extracorporeal elimination is used/considered shortly.[9]

LIPID EMULSION THERAPY

Intravenous lipid emulsion (ILE) is now recognised as an effective treatment for local-anaesthetic-induced cardiovascular collapse. The mechanism for benefit is not entirely clear, but is thought to relate either to the formation of an enlarged lipid sink, which may help to remove the offending drug from target tissues, or as an energy substrate for a shocked myocardium. Based on the lipid sink hypothesis, ILE has been considered a potential treatment for severe acute poisoning from a range of lipophilic drugs. There is good evidence from animal models and human cases/case series for its use in the management of local anaesthetic toxicity; there are an increasing number of case reports where ILE has been used in other poisonings, however, its use is not routinely recommended at this time. It is now frequently available in emergency rooms and other critical care settings. No optimal dosing regimen has yet been established, but it is clear that ILE has emerged as a possible powerful antidote in the last few years.[10] There have been reports of recurrence of toxicity after initial dosing with ILE, as well as complications such as pancreatitis.

CONTINUED SUPPORTIVE THERAPY

Self-poisoned patients do not always engender the empathy of the admitting medical team, but they are medical challenges, rather than merely instances of self-inflicted illness. Specific measures are described later, but good general supportive care of the unconscious unstable patient should be continued. This includes monitoring and provision of organ support when necessary, as well as fluid balance, correction of electrolytes, initiation of nutritional support, and prompt treatment of nosocomial infection.

Overall, in spite of the significant initial physiological disturbance, this group of patients usually has a good outcome.

SPECIFIC THERAPY OF SOME COMMON OR DIFFICULT OVERDOSES

This section emphasises only those features that may aid clinical diagnosis or prognosis. These are always intended to support those measures described under general principles. Some new and controversial therapies are mentioned.

AMFETAMINES (AMPHETAMINES) INCLUDING 'ECSTASY', MDMA

CLINICAL FEATURES

Symptoms of mild overdose include sweating, dry mouth and anxiety. Although the majority of ecstasy patients are dehydrated, a proportion have hyponatraemia from drinking water to excess; therefore it is important to measure serum sodium and electrolytes early in the patient's management. More severe features include tachycardia, hypertonia, hyperreflexia, hallucinations and hypertension. Supraventricular dysrhythmias may follow with coma, convulsions and the risk of haemorrhagic stroke. A hyperthermic syndrome may develop with hyperpyrexia leading to rhabdomyolysis, metabolic acidosis, acute renal failure, disseminated intravascular coagulation (DIC) and multiple organ failure. Where hyperthermia is suspected it is important that core body temperature (e.g. rectal) is measured to accurately record the degree of hyperthermia.[11]

TREATMENT

AC should be considered up to 1 hour post ingestion. Benzodiazepines are useful for agitated or psychotic patients and may have a central effect in reducing tachycardia, hypertension and hyperpyrexia. If benzodiazepines fail to control hypertension, other classes of antihypertensives should be started, such as alpha blockers or direct vasodilators. Beta blockers, even specific ones, should not be used due to the risk of unopposed alpha stimulation and subsequent hypertension developing. It should be noted that most patients are fluid-depleted rather than fluid-overloaded, and measurement of sodium concentrations should be undertaken early in fluid resuscitation. Hypertonic saline may rarely need to be considered in severe hyponatraemia. Hyperthermia should be treated in the standard manner, including administration of cold i.v. fluids, general cooling measures and benzodiazepines. For patients whose temperature remains elevated (particularly above 39°C), consider PO/NG cyproheptadine (a $5HT_{2A}$ antagonist) – the initial dose is 12 mg followed by 2 mg every 2 hours until temperature and other symptoms have settled. Additional methods for cooling, such as external and internal cooling devices or those used for therapeutic hypothermia post cardiac arrest, can be considered for rapidly reducing body temperature. Benzodiazepines and cyproheptadine should also be used in those patients with evidence of moderate/severe serotonin toxicity.[12]

BENZODIAZEPINES

CLINICAL FEATURES

Overdose is common, but clinical features are not usually severe unless complicated by other CNS depressant drugs (such as alcohol), pre-existing disease or the extremes of age. Toxicity commonly produces drowsiness, dysarthria, ataxia and nystagmus. Paradoxical agitation and confusion can occur less commonly.

TREATMENT

AC can be given if patients present within 1 hour of ingestion, yet supportive treatment is usually all that is required. Flumazenil is a specific antagonist (not licensed for use in poisoning) – there is the risk of significant cardiovascular (ventricular tachycardias) and neurological (status epilepticus) toxicity, as well as precipitating withdrawal in benzodiazepine-dependent patients.[13] Its use is therefore not recommended.

BETA BLOCKERS

CLINICAL FEATURES

There is a wide variation in the individual response to beta-blocker overdose. Those with cardiac disease are more at risk of complications. Hypotension and bradycardia predominate and are often refractory to standard resuscitation measures. The degree of heart block can range from a prolonged PR interval through to complete heart block and asystole. Cardiogenic shock and pulmonary oedema are not uncommon.[14]

TREATMENT

AC should be considered up to 1 hour post ingestion and multiple-dose charcoal in patients who have ingested sustained-release preparations. The role of atropine is not clear, although it is commonly used in patients who have bradycardia and hypotension. If symptomatic treatment with i.v. fluids for hypotension fails, glucagon (up to 10 mg i.v. as an initial bolus) is the next step. Further boluses and/or an infusion may be beneficial in addition to the initial bolus. Vomiting indicates that an 'adequate' dose of glucagon has been administered. Further options include hyperinsulinaemic–euglycaemic treatment, as described in the calcium channel blocker section is indicated. Inotropes and cardiac pacing (higher-voltage capture may be required) can be considered and based on the patient's clinical condition. Other measures such as intra-aortic balloon pumps and extracorporeal support (e.g. ECMO, bypass) may be locally available.

BUTYROPHENONES (INCLUDING HALOPERIDOL)

CLINICAL FEATURES

Drowsiness and extrapyramidal effects are most common. Rarely hypotension, QT prolongation, arrhythmias and convulsions develop. Serious toxicity is uncommon.

TREATMENT

AC should be considered up to 1 hour post ingestion, otherwise treatment is supportive. Extrapyramidal symptoms can be treated with procyclidine (5–10 mg i.v./i.m. in adults) or diazepam (10–20 mg in adults).

CALCIUM CHANNEL BLOCKERS

CLINICAL FEATURES

The cardiac effects of these drugs predominate in overdose, particularly hypotension and atrioventricular block, although reflex tachycardia occurs with nifedipine. Hypotension occurs owing to peripheral vasodilatation and negative inotropy. The therapeutic selectivity of actions is not typically seen in overdose. Severe toxicity may occur in patients who initially appear well, when sustained-release preparations have been ingested.

TREATMENT

AC should be considered up to 1 hour post ingestion and multiple-dose charcoal in patients who have ingested sustained-release preparations. Treatment remains supportive; however i.v. calcium chloride (10 mL of 10% solution) is often given in patients who remain hypotensive despite fluid administration. Further boluses and/or an infusion should be administered as guided by the clinical response. If calcium gluconate is used then administer 30 mL of 10% solution (it has one-third the ionised calcium compared with calcium chloride, and therefore doses should be increased by threefold where calcium gluconate is used). In those patients requiring multiple doses and/or an infusion, monitor the serum calcium concentration to ensure it remains below 3 mmol/L. Atropine is often used for bradycardia, and occasionally cardiac pacing may be necessary. In those with persistent hypotension not responding to i.v. fluids and calcium, the next step is hyperinsulinaemic–euglycaemic therapy is indicated.[15] An initial bolus of 1 unit/kg of short-acting insulin should be administered with 25–50 mL of 50% dextrose, followed by an infusion of 0.5–2 units/kg/h short-acting insulin; higher doses may be required in severely compromised patients. Careful monitoring of blood glucose and serum potassium should be undertaken, with replacement as necessary. There is anecdotal evidence that increasing glucose requirements suggest that the cardiovascular toxicity is starting to diminish.

CARBAMAZEPINE

Absorption is slow and unpredictable; moreover, maximum serum concentrations may not be achieved until 72 hours after ingestion. Carbamazepine undergoes enterohepatic recirculation leading to a prolonged overall half-life and is metabolised to an active metabolite.

CLINICAL FEATURES

Nystagmus, ataxia, tremor and fits are common but, in severe overdose, fluctuating coma and severe tachycardia or bradycardia may occur. Plasma concentrations of carbamazepine and the active metabolite can be measured, although they do not correlate well with toxicity. Life-threatening toxicity typically occurs with plasma concentrations greater than 40 mg/L (170 nmol/L).

TREATMENT

Multiple-dose AC is indicated in large ingestions or symptomatic patients, and may help elimination even if initiated several hours after the overdose. Further measures are based on the clinical course.

CARBON MONOXIDE (CO)

Haldane first described symptoms of CO toxicity in 1919 and the mechanisms of toxicity remain unclear. Smokers may have up to 10% of their haemoglobin bound to CO (i.e. carboxyhaemoglobin, COHb) without deleterious effects. Whereas coma and/or COHb levels >40% always indicate serious poisoning, delayed deterioration can occur in their absence. Affinity of CO for haemoglobin is approximately 240 times that of oxygen.

CLINICAL FEATURES

Neurological signs vary from mild confusion through to seizures and coma. A history of loss of consciousness should always be sought and may be the only indicator of significant poisoning. ST segment changes may be present on electrocardiogram (ECG). In the absence of respiratory depression or aspiration, Pa_{O_2} will be normal. It is essential that Sa_{O_2} is measured directly by a co-oximeter, and not calculated. Cherry-pink skin is seen only in textbooks; cyanosis is far more common.

TREATMENT

After basic resuscitative measures, high-flow oxygen (up to 100% if possible) should be administered and continued until the COHb level is less than 5%. This sometimes takes up to 24 hours. Hyperbaric oxygen (HBO), although often used, remains controversial. There have been eight randomised controlled trials of

HBO versus normobaric oxygen. Unfortunately, many of these are of poor quality and it is not possible to show any statistical benefit of HBO in reducing neurological sequelae at 1 month.[16] Considering the frequently encountered logistical difficulties in transferring an unconscious patient to an HBO centre, it cannot be routinely recommended based on the data currently available.

CHLOROQUINE

CLINICAL FEATURES

Hypotension, hypokalaemia, convulsions, ventricular arrhythmias and sudden cardiac arrest may result from severe poisoning. As little as 2 g of chloroquine have been reported to be fatal in adults. Symptoms typically tend to occur very early following ingestion, and normally within 3 hours of ingestion.

TREATMENT

AC should be considered up to 1 hour post ingestion. In patients who have ingested potentially significant amounts of chloroquine or who have features of significant poisoning, then high-dose diazepam (2 mg/kg over 30 minutes) with inotropic and ventilator support should be considered.[17] Hypokalaemia is common and may be protective in the early stage. It is self-correcting and consequently aggressive potassium replacement is not recommended.

COCAINE

CLINICAL FEATURES

The clinical features of acute cocaine toxicity are similar to those seen in the amfetamine section above. There is the additional risk of cocaine-related vasospasm, which can lead to ischaemia in any vascular bed, but is of particular significance from a cardiac and cerebral perspective. Cocaine-related myocardial ischaemia is due primarily to coronary artery vasospasm; additional mechanisms included increased myocardial oxygen demand due to increased heart rate, decreased vasodilators (nitric oxide), increased vasoconstrictors (endothelin) and increased platelet aggregation.[18]

TREATMENT

The treatment of the common unwanted effects related to cocaine are the same as those seen with amfetamines as described above. In terms of myocardial ischaemia, there are some differences between the management of this compared with classical atherosclerotic-related ischaemia. Patients should be treated with oxygen and aspirin; low-molecular-weight heparin and glycoprotein IIb/IIIa inhibitors should not be routinely used – their use should be guided by the blood pressure (increased risk of cerebral haemorrhage in those with significant hypertension). Vasodilators (e.g. S/L, buccal or i.v. nitrates) should be given early in an attempt to reverse coronary artery vasospasm; they may be contraindicated if there is a significant tachycardia due to the risk of a reflex tachycardia leading to an increased heart rate. Benzodiazepines should be administered to reduce sympathetic nervous system stimulation, reducing myocardial oxygen demand by reducing heart rate, as well as potentially causing coronary artery vasodilatation through peripheral cardiac benzodiazepine receptors. Beta blockers are contraindicated as they can lead to unopposed alpha stimulation leading to worsening hypertension, and in addition they can worsen cocaine-related coronary artery vasospasm. Other measures in those who fail to respond include other vasodilators (e.g. calcium channel blockers, alpha blockers) and/or primary angiography and angioplasty/intraluminal drug treatment.

CYANIDE

CLINICAL FEATURES

Severe toxicity is rapidly fatal; however, features include coma, respiratory depression, hypotension and metabolic acidosis. More moderate features include brief loss of consciousness, convulsions and vomiting. Rescuers must ensure that they do not get contaminated themselves. Expert advice is usually required in the management of these patients owing to the risk of significant toxicity.

TREATMENT

Inhaled amyl nitrate and 100% oxygen may well have been given at the scene, since it is present in 'cyanide antidote kits'. Following this there are a number of options:

1. Patients with severe features need dicobalt edetate 300 mg i.v. over 1 minute, followed by 50 mL dextrose 50% i.v., with a further 300 mg if there is no response. Dicobalt edetate is potentially very toxic when administered to patients who do not have cyanide poisoning.
2. Patients with mild-moderate features should be given sodium thiosulphate 12.5 g i.v. over 10 minutes.
3. An alternative for moderate poisoning is hydroxocobalamin i.v. 5 g in adults given over 15 minutes. This can also be considered in patients with smoke inhalation where cyanide exposure is suspected clinically (as it has less risk of toxicity than other antidotes).
4. Patients with a metabolic acidosis should be given sodium bicarbonate.

DIGOXIN

CLINICAL FEATURES

Toxicity may result from ingestion of greater than 2–3 mg, or more commonly from taking too high a daily dose and/or a reduction in renal elimination. Any cardiac arrhythmia may occur and adverse effects may be delayed for some hours. Severe poisoning can produce hyperkalaemia and hypotension.

TREATMENT

AC should be considered up to 1 hour post ingestion and multiple-dose charcoal may be effective by interrupting enterohepatic recirculation of the drug. A digoxin serum level may be helpful although it does not equate to the total body burden. Patients with hyperkalaemia should not be administered calcium gluconate (increased risk of cardiac toxicity); initial management is insulin–dextrose therapy. Those patients with persistent hyperkalaemia (>6.0–6.5), along with brady- or tachyarrhythmias associated with hypotension, should be treated with digoxin-specific antibody fragments.[19] Other treatments, particularly where digoxin-specific antibody fragments are not available, may be indicated but expert advice should be sought in these situations.

GAMMA HYDROXYBUTYRIC ACID (GHB) AND GAMMA BUTYROLACTONE (GBL)

CLINICAL FEATURES

In moderate to high ingestion, coma, convulsions, bradycardia, hypotension and severe respiratory depression can be seen, and other CNS depressant drugs potentiate the effects. Most patients who present to hospital merely require supportive care, and even those who present in coma are often awake within 2–4 hours; very few require intensive care.[20]

TREATMENT

Management is largely supportive; intubation is often not indicated even in those with significantly reduced levels of consciousness as airways reflexes tend to be maintained.[20] CT scanning should be considered in those with evidence of head injury, focal neurological signs or failure to wake after 1–2 hours. It is important before discharging a patient to determine whether they are potentially dependent users (daily use) and therefore at risk of withdrawal – expert advice on the management of these patients should be sought.

IRON

CLINICAL FEATURES

Iron poisoning classically has four phases:

- *phase 1:* initial GI symptoms secondary to direct corrosive action on gastric mucosa
- *phase 2:* latent asymptomatic phase
- *phase 3:* systemic iron toxicity
- *phase 4:* GI strictures several weeks after initial ingestion due to the initial direct GI corrosive effects.

The duration of phases 1 and 2 is dependent on the dose of iron ingested; some patients in very large ingestions may progress straight to a combined phase 1/3 presentation. Serum iron concentration is helpful in patient management.

TREATMENT

In those patients who present with features of severe iron poisoning, deferoxamine should be commenced at an initial rate of 15 mg/kg/h. The maximum licensed dose is 80 mg/kg/day; however, these patients may require more prolonged treatment and appropriate advice should be sought. For those presenting within 6 hours without severe symptoms, the management can be guided by a serum iron concentration 4–6 hours after ingestion (<55 μmol/L does not require treatment, >90 μmol/L treatment is recommended, 55–90 μmol/L treatment may be required depending on whether the concentration is not falling and/or the clinical condition of the patient). For those presenting more than 6 hours after presentation without severe features, the serum iron concentration is not as helpful in determining the need for treatment; expert advice should be sought for these patients.

ISONIAZID

CLINICAL FEATURES

Severe toxicity is characterised by coma, respiratory depression, hypotension and convulsions resistant to conventional treatments, and may result from doses >80 mg/kg. Protracted convulsions can cause rhabdomyolysis and acute renal failure.

TREATMENT

AC should be considered for large ingestions seen within 1 hour. Management of convulsions is initially benzodiazepines (i.v. 10–20 mg diazepam, or i.v. 4 mg lorazepam); those who fail to respond should be treated with 1 g of pyridoxine per gram of isoniazid ingested to a maximum of 5 g. Phenytoin should not be administered as it is ineffective and isoniazid inhibits the metabolism of phenytoin.

LITHIUM

CLINICAL FEATURES

There are two types of overdose: acute in lithium in naïve individuals/those on treatment, and chronic in those on long-term lithium treatment. For the latter this may be secondary to an intentional overdose or due to other factors such as dehydration or use of interacting drugs (e.g. NSAIDs, ACE-inhibitors, thiazide diuretics). Symptoms of toxicity can be divided as follows:

- *mild:* nausea, vomiting, fine tremor, polyuria, weakness

- *moderate:* confusion, urinary and faecal incontinence, myoclonic twitches/jerks, hypernatraemia, hyperreflexia
- *severe:* coma, renal failure, convulsions, cardiac arrhythmias.

TREATMENT

Lithium concentrations should be measured on arrival in chronic cases and then repeated every 4–6 hours; for acute overdoses, lithium concentrations should be measured 6 hours after ingestion and then every 4–6 hours. Patients should be adequately rehydrated, which may help with any renal impairment. Whole bowel irrigation (see above) should be considered in those who have ingested a potentially toxic amount of lithium. Extracorporeal elimination should be considered in those who have either severe features of lithium toxicity, or a serum lithium concentration of >7.5 mmol/L in acute overdoses or >4 mmol/L in chronic-related toxicity.

METHANOL AND ETHYLENE GLYCOL

CLINICAL FEATURES

Methanol and ethylene glycol are relatively non-toxic themselves, but their ingestion is a medical emergency because of their metabolism (following a latent period of 12–18 hours) to formic acid and glycolic acid respectively. These toxic metabolites account for the metabolic acidosis, ocular toxicity, renal failure and mortality that are occasionally seen. Mild features include dizziness, drowsiness and abdominal pain. When treatment is delayed, metabolic acidosis develops with drowsiness, coma and convulsions. The osmolal gap initially is elevated but then falls as the methanol or ethylene glycol is metabolised; the anion gap increases as the toxic metabolites build up.

TREATMENT

AC does not adsorb either methanol or ethylene glycol. The metabolic acidosis should be treated with sodium bicarbonate and the serum electrolytes measured. Ethanol prevents formation of the toxic metabolites and previously has been the most established treatment; its dosing is complex and it requires 1–2-hourly blood ethanol measurement and adjustment of the treatment. Additionally, it can cause significant CNS depression, necessitating critical care admission. Fomepizole (4-methypyrazole) has now become the antidote of choice – it is a twice-daily weight-based infusion without the need for specific monitoring and is not associated with neurological depression.[21] The initial dose is 15 mg/kg over 30 minutes, followed by a twice-daily infusion of 10 mg/kg for the next four doses and then increased to 15 mg/kg per treatment dose until treatment is no longer required. Ongoing management after initial loading dose often requires the involvement of clinical/medical toxicology services to facilitate ethylene glycol/methanol concentration measurement and interpretation of the results. It is important to remember with both ethanol and fomepizole that, should extracorporeal treatment be required, not only will the toxic alcohol be removed, but so too will the antidote; modifications to treatment regimens will be required.

NON-STEROIDAL ANTI-INFLAMMATORY DRUGS (NSAIDs)

CLINICAL FEATURES

NSAIDs are commonly ingested in overdose; symptoms tend to be mild and consist of gastrointestinal symptoms. GI haemorrhage is not commonly reported in acute overdose of NSAIDs (apart from secondary to Mallory–Weiss tears). Convulsions can occur, but are usually associated with mefenamic acid (up to 10–15% of patients). Large ingestions of NSAIDs can be associated with metabolic acidosis and/or renal impairment.[22] Patients who do not develop symptoms within 4 hours are unlikely to experience delayed toxicity.

TREATMENT

AC can be given for large ingestions that are seen within 1 hour of the overdose. Convulsions should be treated with a benzodiazepine. Although there is no indication for routine use, those patients with symptoms of GI irritation can be treated with a short course of oral proton pump inhibitor. Metabolic acidosis should be treated with sodium bicarbonate and other measures as indicated. Supportive care and appropriate investigation are required for patients with renal impairment.

OPIOIDS

CLINICAL FEATURES

Overdose is characterised by pinpoint pupils, drowsiness, shallow breathing and ultimately respiratory failure.

TREATMENT

AC may be effective for oral ingestions; otherwise treatment is supportive. Naloxone 100–200 microgram boluses should be given i.v. and increased as titrated to clinical response. In patients who fail to respond to 2 mg, alternative diagnoses should be considered. Those who respond may require repeat doses, particularly where a long-acting or sustained/modified release preparation has been ingested; an infusion of naloxone may be required in these patients. Intubation and mechanical ventilation are required if respiratory failure is not rapidly reversed by naloxone.

PARACETAMOL

There is increased metabolism of paracetamol to its toxic metabolite, *N*-acetyl-*p*-benzoquinonimine (NAPQI) as normal conjugation pathways are exceeded. This toxic metabolite irreversibly binds to hepatocytes leading to cell death and release of inflammatory and cytotoxic mediators and further hepatocyte death. There have been recent changes to the management of paracetamol management in the UK, which have not yet been finalised. The antidote for paracetamol poisoning is *N*-acetylcysteine. Although i.v. acetylcysteine administered more than 16 hours after ingestion may not prevent severe liver damage, it should still be given since outcome from paracetamol-induced fulminant hepatic failure is improved. Although severe hepatic injury has a 10% mortality, the majority of patients recover within 1–2 weeks.[23]

CLINICAL FEATURES

Paracetamol poisoning is often asymptomatic in early stages (first 24–48 hours); later presentations may be associated with evidence of acute liver injury/failure. Patients with very significant ingestions (initial 4-hour paracetamol concentrations of >800 mg/L) may present in coma with a lactic metabolic acidosis – this is a direct effect of the paracetamol.

TREATMENT

- Those patients who present within an hour – consider activated charcoal in significant ingestions.
- Current UK treatment guidelines for single known time point ingestions are based on a single treatment line starting at 100 mg/L at 4 hours post ingestion. Risk stratification is no longer required to determine the need for treatment.
- For those with staggered, supratherapeutic or unknown time of ingestions, treatment is not required for those who have ingested <75 mg/kg in the last 24 hours but is required for those who have ingested >150 mg/kg (these are based on actual body weight to a maximum of 110 kg). For those who have ingested between 75 and 150 mg/kg, advice should be sought on whether or not treatment is required.
- *N*-acetylcysteine 150 mg/kg in 200 mL 5% dextrose is infused over 1 hour, followed by 50 mg/kg in 500 mL 5% dextrose over 4 hours and 100 mg/kg in 1 L 5% dextrose over 16 hours (total dose 300 mg/kg in 20 hours). Maximum protective effect is time-dependent. An ingestion–treatment interval of less than 10 hours gives the best results.
- In those patients with evidence of liver injury, the last dose (100 mg/kg in 1 L 5% dextrose over 16 hours) is repeated until the patient's condition and biochemical and haematological results are improving.
- Although there is limited evidence, many recommend the use of prolonged *N*-acetylcysteine in patients with acute kidney injury.
- Expert opinion should be sought early on from a regional centre if liver failure is progressive since liver transplantation may become necessary.

PARAQUAT

In adult humans the lethal dose is 3–6 g (i.e. 15–30 mL of 20% w/v liquid concentrate). The mortality rate in patients ingesting the liquid concentrate is about 45%.[24] The lung is the primary target organ, with the injury being enhanced by oxygen. Peak concentrations are achieved between 0.5 and 2 hours.

CLINICAL FEATURES

Initial symptoms are gastrointestinal pain and vomiting with corrosive effects on the mouth, pharynx and oesophagus. Dyspnoea and pulmonary oedema follow within 24 hours, progressing to irreversible fibrosis and death. Cardiac, renal and hepatic dysfunctions are common.

TREATMENT

Those treating suspected paraquat-poisoned patients should wear appropriate personal protective equipment to prevent secondary exposure. An urgent qualitative urine test (dithionite spot test) should be undertaken to confirm exposure; a confirmatory plasma concentration should be measured in those where positive as this may guide prognosis. Management is largely supportive: analgesia for oropharyngeal burns and other measures as indicated by the patient's clinical condition. Oxygen therapy can increase the degree and severity of pulmonary fibrosis. Palliative care may be required in those with high paraquat concentrations who fail to respond to treatment. Expert advice should be sought in these patients, to determine whether other treatment options may be appropriate.

PHENYTOIN

CLINICAL FEATURES

Absorption is slow and unpredictable; moreover, maximum serum concentrations may not be achieved until 72 hours after ingestion. After initial nausea and vomiting, neurological symptoms develop including drowsiness, dysarthria and ataxia, and may ultimately progress to seizures. Cardiovascular toxicity is rare unless the overdose has been given i.v.

TREATMENT

Most patients require nothing more than supportive measures. There is some evidence from volunteer studies that multi-dose activated charcoal can increase the elimination of phenytoin; it is not clear whether this alters the outcome.

SALICYLATES (ASPIRIN)

Moderate toxicity occurs with serum concentrations 500–750 mg/L (3600–5500 μmol/L) and severe toxicity with concentrations >750 mg/L. Serum concentrations alone do not determine prognosis. The elimination half-life increases significantly with increasing concentrations. Small reductions in pH produce large increases in non-ionised salicylate, which then penetrates tissues.

CLINICAL FEATURES

Tinnitus, deafness, diaphoresis, pyrexia, hypoglycaemia, haematemesis, hyperventilation and hypokalaemia may all occur. Coma, hyperpyrexia, pulmonary oedema and acidaemia are reported as more common in fatal cases, which present late.

TREATMENT

Although multiple-dose AC is not recommended by some experts, most medical toxicologists would recommend its use in large ingestions since concretions of salicylates in the stomach can occur with delayed ongoing absorption. Urinary alkalinisation (see above) decreases the amount of non-ionised drug available to enter tissues and should be considered in those with moderate/severe toxicity. Extracorporeal techniques are very effective in removing salicylates and correcting acid–base disturbance.[25]

SELECTIVE SEROTONIN REUPTAKE INHIBITORS (SSRIS) OR 5-HT DRUGS

SSRIs include citalopram, fluoxetine, fluvoxamine, paroxetine and sertraline. These drugs have increasingly replaced the tricyclic antidepressants and generally appear to be much safer in overdose.

CLINICAL FEATURES

Drowsiness, tachycardia and mild hypertension are the commonest features. Seizures and coma can occur, as well as a serotonin syndrome in 14% of cases.[26]

TREATMENT

AC should be considered up to 1 hour post ingestion, otherwise treatment is supportive. Benzodiazepines should be used to treat agitated or hyperthermic patients. There are case reports of cyproheptadine being used to treat severe toxicity with SSRIs.[27] In those with hyperthermia, the advice as above for amfetamines should be followed in terms of assessment of the hyperthermia and appropriate management interventions.

THEOPHYLLINE

CLINICAL FEATURES

Acute theophylline poisoning is potentially very serious and severe poisoning carries a high mortality. Toxic effects such as agitation, tremor, nausea, vomiting and sinus tachycardia become evident at <30 mg/L (167 μmol/L). Concentrations >60 mg/L (333 μmol/L) in acute poisoning or >40 mg/L (222 μmol/L) in chronic usage frequently result in seizures, malignant ventricular arrhythmias, severe hypotension and death.[28] A key feature is hypokalaemia, which predisposes to arrhythmias and rhabdomyolysis. Measuring plasma theophylline levels confirms the ingestion and may help in deciding elimination methods; in the majority of poisoned patients they do not aid management. Sustained-release preparations may result in delayed onset and prolonged toxicity.

TREATMENT

Multi-dose AC should be considered, particularly in those with serum concentrations of greater than 40 mg/L. Although hypokalaemia does occur, there is not a total body depletion of potassium; therefore only potassium concentrations of less than 3 mmol/L should be cautiously replaced; monitor for a rebound hyperkalaemia. Convulsions should be treated with benzodiazepines and cardiac arrhythmias with beta blockers in non-asthmatic patients. Vomiting is often severe, and requires appropriate antiemetic administration.

TRICYCLIC ANTIDEPRESSANTS (TCAs)

CLINICAL FEATURES

These drugs remain the leading cause of death from overdose in patients arriving at the emergency department alive and account for up to one-half of all overdose-related adult intensive care admissions.[29] Features include anticholinergic effects such as warm dry skin, tachycardia, blurred vision, dilated pupils and urinary retention. Severe features include respiratory depression, reduced conscious level, cardiac arrhythmias, fits and hypotension. Arrhythmias may be predicted by a QRS duration >100 ms on the ECG; a QRS duration of >160 ms increases risk of seizures. All forms of rhythm and conduction disturbance have been described, and are not necessarily predicted by the ECG.[30] Amoxapine typically causes features of severe poisoning in the absence of QRS widening. Cardiac toxicity is due mainly to quinidine-like actions, slowing phase 0 depolarisation of the action potential. Other mechanisms include impaired automaticity, cholinergic blockade and inhibition of neuronal catecholamine uptake. Toxicity is worsened by acidaemia, hypotension and hyperthermia.

TREATMENT

After supportive care as outlined above, including multiple-dose AC, continuous cardiac monitoring is essential. Increasing arterial pH to ≥7.45 significantly reduces the available free drug and this may be the best way to avoid TCA toxicity. Mild hyperventilation and 8.4% sodium bicarbonate in 50 mmol aliquots achieves this strategy and may improve outcome.[31] Bicarbonate should probably be given in all cases of QRS prolongation (even in the absence of metabolic acidosis), arrhythmias with associated hypotension or metabolic acidosis; it should also be considered in those with convulsions. If arrhythmias occur, avoid class 1a agents; lidocaine may be best. Benzodiazepines are the drug of choice for sedation, treatment of seizures and may prevent emergence delirium.

VALPROATE

CLINICAL FEATURES

Most overdoses follow a benign course, with nausea, mild drowsiness and confusion. Coma can occur in large ingestions with cerebral oedema. There is the potential for metabolic derangement, including metabolic acidosis, hypernatraemia, hypoglycaemia and hyperammonaemia.

TREATMENT

Valproate levels are of little value, except to confirm the ingestion. There is poor correlation between depth of coma and free or total valproate levels. Supportive management is all that is usually required. Although in therapeutic use valproate is extensively protein-bound, with increasing plasma concentrations there is saturation of this binding leading to increased free drug; in these situations consider haemodialysis. Additionally, in those patients with significant overdoses and associated hepatic dysfunction and hyperammonaemia, consider the use of L-carnitine.

Access the complete references list online at http://www.expertconsult.com

1. Gunnell D, Ho D, Murray V. Medical management of deliberate drug overdose: a neglected area for suicide prevention? Emerg Med J 2004;21:35–8.
9. Lavergne V, Nolin TD, Hoffman RS, et al. The EXTRIP (EXtracorporeal TReatments In Poisoning) workgroup: guideline methodology. Clin Toxicol 2012;50:403–13.
10. Ozcan MS, Weinberg G. Intravenous lipid emulsion for the treatment of drug toxicity. J Intensive Care Med 2012;Jun 24 [Epub ahead of print].
15. Engebretsen KM, Kaczmarek KM, Morgan J, et al. High-dose insulin therapy in beta-blocker and calcium channel-blocker poisoning. Clin Toxicol 2011;49:277–83.
21. Hovda KE, Jacobsen D. Expert opinion: fomepizole may ameliorate the need for hemodialysis in methanol poisoning. Hum Exp Toxicol 2008;27:539–46.
23. Chun LJ, Tong MJ, Busuttil RW, et al. Acetaminophen hepatotoxicity and acute liver failure. J Clin Gastroenterol 2009;43:342–9.
25. Pearlman BL, Gambhir R. Salicylate intoxication: a clinical review. Postgrad Med 2009;121:162–8.

89

Sedation and pain management in intensive care

Luke E Torre

Despite the widespread use of sedative and analgesic agents in the intensive care unit (ICU), the goals of sedation and analgesia are not well established.[1] Having its roots in anaesthesia, ICUs would historically manage patients with full general anaesthesia including skeletal muscle paralysis and controlled ventilation modes and this was maintained until the disease process remitted. Sedation and analgesia were considered a necessary adjunct to the management of critically ill patients.

Combinations of opioids and benzodiazepines are commonly used to provide 'sedation' in the ICU. As high doses of opioids analgesics may result in significant sedation in their own right and are synergistic with sedative agents, the distinction between sedation and analgesia is blurred. This makes the definition and attainment of clear sedation goals elusive.

SEDATION

There has been a paradigm shift in thinking towards sedation practice in ICUs over the past 30 years. A combination of factors have led to this change, notably:

- improved ventilator technology and modes of ventilation allowing synchronised and spontaneous respiration
- improved drug development for sedation and analgesia with pharmacokinetic profiles that allow prompt titration, and pharmacodynamic profiles with fewer side-effects
- the development and implementation of sedation scoring systems in the ICU[2]
- the increasing use of percutaneous tracheostomy and/or non-invasive ventilation (NIV) for patients requiring prolonged ventilation
- the recognition of critical illness polyneuropathy and myopathy and the risk factors associated with it
- the separation and specialisation of intensive care physicians from other domains
- the emerging high-quality evidence in the field of sedation and analgesia in intensive care
- economic pressures and increased demand for finite intensive care resources.

Today, sedative use in the critically ill should be for one or more of the following purposes:

- a treatment for disease processes such as: seizures, raised intracranial pressure, serotonin syndrome and alcohol withdrawal
- to facilitate tolerance of intensive care therapies such as intubation, mechanical ventilation and active cooling
- to reduce oxygen consumption by reducing patient arousal, activity and anxiety
- to maintain the safety of patient and carers when dealing with the hyperactive delirious patient
- palliation
- procedural sedation.

Sedation of patients in the ICU is an integral part of what health care workers perceive to be care and compassion for the critically ill patient. Presumed benefits of sedative agents include:

- reducing patient anxiety over their illness, the welfare of relatives or the risk of death
- providing adequate rest
- reducing the distress of unpleasant sensations, invasive treatments and monitoring
- blunting awareness of the environment over which the patient has very little control and in which he/she may be unable to communicate.

Non-pharmacological methods should preferentially be used to help manage these issues. Avoiding potentially distressing situations, allowing adequate access to caring visitors, maintenance of good communication with the patient and a positive outlook by carers will satisfy many of these goals. Small comforts, such as ice chips by mouth, a comfortable mattress, relaxation music and maintaining a daytime/night-time environment all help this process.

LEVEL AND ASSESSMENT OF SEDATION

Critical to delivery of sedation is an accurate sedation assessment tool. Sedation scoring systems were first introduced in the 1970s.[2] Since that time, several validated scoring systems for critically ill patients have become available. The Ramsay Sedation Scale (RSS) and Richmond Agitation Sedation Scale are two of the most popular used worldwide (**Tables 89.1** and **89.2**). Despite their availability, validation and evidence base, their

Table 89.1 Ramsay Sedation Scale

LEVEL	RESPONSE
AWAKE LEVELS	
1	Patient anxious and agitated or restless or both
2	Patient cooperative, orientated and tranquil
3	Patient responds to commands only
ASLEEP LEVELS	
4	Brisk response to a light glabellar tap or loud auditory stimulus
5	Sluggish response to a light glabellar tap or loud auditory stimulus
6	No response to a light glabellar tap or loud auditory stimulus

Table 89.2 The Richmond Agitation Sedation Scale[56]

POINT	PATIENT RESPONSE TO VERBAL AND PHYSICAL STIMULI
+4	Combative – combative, violent, immediate danger to staff
+3	Very agitated – pulls or removes tubes or catheters; aggressive
+2	Agitated – frequent non-purposeful movement, fights ventilator
+1	Restless – anxious, apprehensive but movements not aggressive or vigorous
0	Alert and calm
–1	Drowsy – not fully alert, but has sustained (>10 seconds) awakening (eye opening/contact) to voice
–2	Light sedation – drowsy, briefly (<10 seconds) awakens to voice or physical stimulation
–3	Moderate sedation – movement or eye opening (but not eye contact) to voice
–4	Deep sedation – no response to voice, but movement or eye opening to physical stimulation
–5	Unarousable – no response to voice or physical stimulation

incorporation into routine management of intensive care patients remains low.[3]

Electroencephalography (EEG), which may be either 'raw' or 'processed', is able to provide a measure of cerebral activity. This monitor is more suitable for assessing depth of anaesthesia and may be difficult to interpret in the encephalopathic patient. Newer, easy to use devices using integrated EEG (e.g. Bi-spectral Index (BIS)) are now available. Evidence of their efficacy is appearing, but their role in the ICU is not well established.[4] Their use is also limited by practical considerations, such as interference due to movement artefact. To date these monitors have not enjoyed widespread use in the ICU, but may be useful for specific indications such as ensuring an isoelectric EEG in patients being treated for very high intracranial pressure.

SEDATION STRATEGIES

Although the choice of sedative agent(s) must be a conscientious decision based on pharmacokinetic and pharmacodynamic factors relevant to the critically ill patient, it is perhaps of greater importance to decide on the sedation strategy employed.

A variety of strategies have been described, some more novel than others:

- goal-directed sedation
- patient-targeted sedation protocols
- daily interruption of sedation
- intermittent sedation
- 'analgosedation' or analgesia-based sedation
- patient-controlled sedation.

The purpose of these strategies should be to achieve a controlled and predetermined level of sedation in the patient. The chosen level of sedation will be intimately linked to the underlying disease process, patients' characteristics and the treatments and interventions they are receiving. The aim of sedation should be documented by the team and conveyed to the bedside nurse, who will have the largest impact on achieving and maintaining the chosen level. Once instituted, the level of sedation should be regularly assessed.

Goal-directed sedation was the first method described where sedatives are freely adjusted (usually by the bedside nurse) to attain a prescribed level of sedation from a sedation scoring system.[2]

Patient-targeted sedation protocols implement two main features: a structured approach to the assessment of patient pain and distress, coupled with an algorithm that directs drug escalation and de-escalation based on the assessments.[5]

Daily interruption of sedation: this strategy employs a similar goal of sedative and analgesic titration to a desired depth of sedation. In contrast to 'patient-targeted sedation protocols', no formal algorithm has been established for drug escalation. However, the risk of excessive sedation is minimised by a daily interruption of both sedative and analgesic infusions until the patient awakens or exhibits distress that mandates resumed drug administration, usually with an initial bolus followed by a reduced infusion rate.[5]

Intermittent sedation administration involves use of longer-acting sedative agents, typically lorazepam, given by intermittent bolus titrated via a sedation scoring system.

'Analgosedation' is a more modern approach gaining favour in selected patients where sedation is not required as a treatment of their disease process. In these patients, opioid analgesia is instituted first, and once pain is adequately controlled, verbal measures are used to calm the patient to a targeted sedation level (e.g. Ramsay score 3–4). Major tranquillisers (e.g. haloperidol) are given for delirium and only then are sedative agents (e.g. propofol) used for short-term infusion and promptly ceased.[6]

Proposed benefits of the above sedation strategies include:[5–9]

- shorter duration of mechanical ventilation
- shorter length of ICU and hospital stay
- economic benefit
- less need for diagnostic studies (e.g. computed axial tomography (CT) scans) to assess impaired conscious state
- less ventilator-associated pneumonia
- a possible mortality benefit.

Criticisms of these strategies include:

- high self-extubation rates
- promotion of myocardial ischaemia
- triggering of a withdrawal syndrome.

Concerns over increased long-term neuropsychological effects (e.g. post-traumatic stress disorder) have been unfounded. Instead, evidence suggests a reduced incidence of these complications using such strategies.[10,11]

SEDATIVE AGENTS

GABA-A RECEPTOR AGONISTS

Gamma amino butyric acid (GABA) is a major neurotransmitter in the central nervous system, and one that is involved in the complex process of sedation. It binds to the alpha subunit of the GABA-A receptor and, by activation, causes a conformational change that opens the ligand-gated channel, allowing chloride ion influx into the neuron. This hyperpolarises the neuronal membrane and reduces neuronal activity leading to sedation.[12]

The GABA-A receptor agonists used in intensive care are benzodiazepines, propofol and barbiturates. They all share amnesic, hypnotic, anxiolytic and anticonvulsant effects, but have no analgesic properties.

Benzodiazepines

Benzodiazepines (BZAs), as a class, are probably the most widely used sedatives in ICUs. BZAs are good anticonvulsant drugs and also provide some muscle relaxation. They bind to the gamma subunit of the GABA-A receptor, resulting in a conformational change causing increased opening frequency of the channel.[13] The commonest agents used worldwide are midazolam, lorazepam and diazepam.

These drugs may be given by many routes, but most commonly intravenously (i.v.) or orally (p.o.) in critically ill patients. Intravenous administration is by either continuous or intermittent i.v. infusion (e.g. midazolam in 1 mg/mL dilution, titrated to effect).

Dosage of these agents may vary widely depending on various pharmacokinetic and pharmacodynamic factors such as:

- prior exposure to BZA (increased tolerance)
- age and physiological reserve
- volume status (hypovolaemic patients are more sensitive)
- renal and hepatic dysfunction
- co-administered drugs (e.g. combined with an opioid)
- history of alcohol consumption (increased tolerance).

Although some BZAs (e.g. midazolam) are short-acting, water-soluble agents, there is potential for accumulation of both parent compound and active metabolites in patients with hepatic and/or renal dysfunction. This is especially pertinent in the critically ill, where there may be extensive derangement of BZA pharmacokinetic profiles.[14,15] This may result in prolonged sedation and increased length of mechanical ventilation and ICU stay. There is, therefore, some difficulty in predetermining suitable dosages of these agents. Midazolam, in doses of 0.02–0.2 mg/kg/h may be suitable, with the level titrated to individual response. Longer-acting agents, such as diazepam, may be given by intermittent i.v. injection (e.g. diazepam 5–10 mg) as necessary.

BZAs are often combined with opioids in a compound 'sedative' infusion. This allows lower doses of BZA to be used, while capitalising on the opioid effects of respiratory and cough suppression, to facilitate mechanical ventilation and tube tolerance.

Flumazenil (flumazepil), the specific BZA antagonist, may be used to reverse the effect of BZAs to reduce unwanted acute side-effects, such as severe hypotension or respiratory depression, or to allow acute neurological assessment of the sedated patient.

Propofol

The i.v. anaesthetic agent propofol (2,6-di-isopropylphenol) is frequently used for sedation in the ICU. It binds to the beta subunit on the receptor and causes a conformational change to the chloride channel.[13] It gives more profound hypnosis than BZAs, which have a ceiling effect. It is given by continuous i.v. infusion.

It has a favourable pharmacokinetic profile compared with BZAs due to rapid hepatic and extrahepatic conjugation reactions to inactive metabolites. Indeed, clearance of propofol exceeds hepatic blood flow. This gives it a relatively short context-sensitive half-time, resulting in rapid offset, particularly after prolonged infusion.

Although propofol has been shown to reduce time on mechanical ventilation compared with BZA (specifically midazolam) sedation, it has not been shown to reduce time in the ICU.[16,17] Its combination with remifentanil, however, may result in a shorter ICU length of stay compared with the combination of midazolam with either fentanyl or morphine.[18,19]

Caution is required in hypovolaemic patients or those with impaired myocardial function as severe hypotension may result.[20] Doses for ICU sedation are generally much lower than those required for anaesthesia. The diluent in which propofol is delivered is lipid-rich and may have to be taken into account as a source of nutrition and indeed cause of hyperlipidaemia, depending on dosage and duration of therapy. Disodium edetate, present in the propofol solution, does not appear to be harmful in patients receiving long-term infusions of propofol.[21]

There continues to be concern about 'propofol infusion syndrome' particularly in paediatric patients who have developed severe heart failure (preceded by metabolic acidaemia, fatty infiltration of the liver and striated muscle damage) after prolonged, high-dose infusions of propofol.[22] The pathophysiology of this condition remains elusive but may relate to uncoupling of oxidative phosphorylation in mitochondria. There may also be a genetic susceptibility.[23] Caution should therefore be exercised when using propofol for prolonged periods and infusion rates should be limited to 4 mg/kg/h. Hyperlipidaemia may be a warning sign for development of the syndrome and serum triglyceride monitoring should be considered in patients at risk.[24] Management requires immediate cessation of propofol and cardiovascular supports, which may necessitate ECMO.[25] The condition, although rare, has a high mortality.

Barbiturates

Thiopentone is reserved for specific indications, such as management of intractable intracranial hypertension, or for the treatment of status epilepticus. It is not commonly used as a general sedative agent due to a long context-sensitive half-time when given by continuous infusion.

VOLATILE ANAESTHETIC AGENTS

The use of volatile anaesthetic agents for sedation in the ICU has been limited by:

- the cost of prolonged administration
- the more complex set-up required for the administration of these agents (vaporiser, scavenging apparatus, etc.)
- specific side-effects such as; 'halothane' hepatitis; accumulation of fluoride ions and consequent renal dysfunction (sevoflurane (fluoromethyl hexafluoroisopropyl ether) and isoflurane), compound A accumulation and possible renal dysfunction (sevoflurane and absorbent interaction)
- occupational health and safety concerns (e.g. spontaneous miscarriage).

Isoflurane and sevoflurane provide hypnosis, amnesia and, at higher concentrations, immobility of the patient. They have no analgesic properties. Their mechanism of action remains hotly debated. Desflurane, due to its low boiling point, has not yet been successfully incorporated into intensive care ventilator systems.

Volatile agents are useful for short periods of anaesthesia during invasive procedures in the ICU. They have classically been used for longer periods of sedation in acute severe asthma, due to their bronchodilator effect.

Newer vaporiser systems, such as the AnaConDa® (Anaesthetic Conserving Device), allow safe administration and recirculation of volatile agent through a standard ICU ventilator. Approximately 90% of the volatile agent is recirculated, greatly reducing cost.[26]

Studies generally show reduced time to awakening and extubation with short-term volatile administration compared with BZAs. Although fluoride levels are higher in patients receiving volatile agents, no significant adverse renal events have been attributed to it.[26] A recent study in ICU patients receiving prolonged sedation showed that sevoflurane reduced time to extubation and post-extubation opioid requirements compared with GABA-A agonists.[27] Other potential advantages include:

- lack of a withdrawal syndrome
- predictable offset independent of renal or hepatic dysfunction
- cardioprotective effects
- no tachyphylaxis
- lower incidence of delirium
- ability to measure and titrate end-tidal volatile concentration.

NMDA RECEPTOR ANTAGONIST

Ketamine acts by blocking NMDA receptors. It produces a sedative state known as 'dissociative anaesthesia', with the following characteristics:

- mild sedation
- amnesia
- analgesia
- reduced motor activity.

The lack of respiratory and cardiovascular depression at lower doses makes this a relatively safe drug for use in the ICU. Limitations to its use include hallucinations, and delirium during the recovery/withdrawal phase. These may be ameliorated by BZA administration. Ketamine may be used specifically for sedation in severe asthmatics (for its bronchodilator effect), in patients following head injury (for its effect at the NMDA receptor) or in patients where analgesia is difficult (e.g. extensive burns).[28,29]

MAJOR TRANQUILLISERS

Butyrophenones (e.g. haloperidol) and phenothiazines (e.g. chlorpromazine) are very useful agents for the sedation of delirious patients in the ICU. They act via a range of receptors including dopaminergic (D1 and D2), alpha-adrenergic, histamine, serotonin and cholinergic receptors. Main actions include:

- reduced motor activity
- apathy and reduced initiative
- sedation and drowsiness
- reduced aggression
- antiemetic.

Unwanted effects with these drugs are common and include:

- extrapyramidal effects (dystonia, akathisia and parkinsonism)
- endocrine effects (e.g. lactation)
- anticholinergic effects (e.g. blurred vision, dry mouth, urinary retention, constipation)
- hypotension
- neuroleptic malignant syndrome.

The advantage of major tranquillisers is that they can be used to gain control in difficult situations (e.g. when delirious patients may be a risk to themselves or their carers), without major risk of respiratory depression. They should not be used for long-term sedation, except for the specific treatment of psychosis. Typically haloperidol, diluted to a 1 mg/mL solution, may be given by repeated i.v. injection in doses of 2–20 mg/h until the delirious patient is approachable. Repeat dosages would then be titrated to allow easy arousal of the patient. Haloperidol may also be given p.o. or by i.m. injection. Recent interest has emerged with haloperidol use in elderly surgical patients in intensive care as prophylaxis against delirium.[30]

Atypical antipsychotic agents, such as olanzapine and quetiapine, are also efficacious agents for the management of delirious patients.[31] They have a lower side-effect profile than the 'typical' antipsychotics, especially with respect to extrapyramidal side-effects. They are usually given orally, although olanzapine may be given as sublingual wafers, a particularly useful route of administration in these patients.

α_2-AGONISTS

Dexmedetomidine is a highly selective α_2-agonist with a half-life of 2 hours. It provides safe analgesia and sedation in the ICU when given as a single agent by i.v. infusion.[32–35] Although originally licensed in Australia for 24-hour use, longer-duration infusions have been safely administered.[36,37] Compared with benzodiazepines, dexmedetomidine results in less delirium and shorter time to extubation.[38] This may impact on ICU length of stay and provide a significant cost benefit. Furthermore dexmedetomidine is showing promise as an effective treatment of agitated delirium in critically ill patients.[39]

Dexmedetomidine aims to deliver a cooperative, calm and tube-tolerant patient, without respiratory depression.[33] Extubation is usually performed with the agent still infusing to maintain the tranquil cooperative state. Opioid analgesic requirements are less compared with GABA agonist sedation.[36]

A loading dose of 1 µg/kg over 10 minutes is recommended in healthy patients, but this should be avoided or attenuated in the critically ill. Infusion rates of 0.2–1.0 µg/kg/h are recommended. Higher rates have been reported, but bradycardia is more frequently seen.[32,37,40] Side-effects may be predicted from the mechanism of action and include hypotension and bradycardia.

Clonidine, an established long-acting α_2-agonist, may be used to enhance sedation and analgesia when GABA-A agonists and opioids are used as the mainstay of sedation in the ICU. The usual i.v. dose range is 50–150 µg, 4–6 hourly.

ANALGESIA

Pain management is a priority in the care of critically ill patients. Skilled use of analgesics in the modern ICU aims to ensure that critically ill patients no longer suffer pain. Pain management relies largely on the use of opioid analgesics together with regional anaesthetic techniques and other adjuncts.

Many patients present to the ICU with painful conditions or undergo painful procedures during their stay. Patients commonly report pain from routine ICU procedures like arterial and central venous cannulation, endotracheal suctioning, insertion of an indwelling urinary catheter or nasogastric tubes and even turning in bed.[41] In addition, other adverse symptoms commonly reported include: unsatisfied thirst, difficult sleeping, anxiety, unsatisfied hunger, depression and shortness of breath.[41]

Pain has a number of adverse consequences, such as:

- provoking anxiety
- contributing to lack of sleep
- worsening delirium
- increasing the stress response
- causing respiratory embarrassment due to atelectasis and sputum retention
- causing immobility with venous and gut stasis.

Pain management comprises a number of modalities in addition to pharmacological methods, including:

- a caring and supportive ICU team, whom the patient can trust
- warm and comfortable surroundings
- attention to pressure areas
- bowel and bladder care
- adequate hydration and amelioration of thirst (e.g. moistening the mouth)

- early tracheostomy where indicated to reduce the discomfort of endotracheal intubation
- supplemental treatments such as acupuncture, acupressure, massage and transcutaneous electrical nerve stimulation (TENS).

OPIOIDS

Opioids remain the mainstay of analgesia in the ICU. The most commonly used agents in the ICU used worldwide include:

- morphine and its analogues (e.g. diamorphine, codeine)
- semisynthetic and synthetic agents:
  - phenylpiperidine derivatives (e.g. pethidine, fentanyl, sufentanil, remifentanil)
  - methadone
  - thebaine derivatives (e.g. buprenorphine, oxycodone).

The effects of opioids are mediated via the four opioid receptor subtypes; mu, kappa, delta and nociceptin/orphanin FQ. These are G-protein-coupled receptors that inhibit adenyl cyclase to reduce cAMP. This results in analgesia mediated at supraspinal, spinal and peripheral nerve endings.[42] The side-effects of opioids are well described.

Opioids are titrated to effect by intermittent i.v. injection, or by continuous infusion. This may be controlled by the nurse (nurse-controlled analgesia or NCA) or by the patient (patient-controlled analgesia or PCA). Suitable regimens are 1 mg/mL of morphine, or 20 μg/mL of fentanyl titrated to effect.

NCA is often combined with a BZA such as midazolam to produce a 'sedative/analgesic' infusion for patients on mechanical ventilation (see sedation section). Opioids can also be administered via the subarachnoid, epidural, transdermal, oral, sublingual and intranasal routes.

The effect of analgesia in the clinical setting is judged by:

- patient response, if they are conscious, either verbally by describing the level of pain subjectively or by using a visual analogue score (**Fig. 89.1**) or other assessment, such as behavioural pain scales[43,44]
- physiological markers of distress (e.g. tachycardia, hypertension, diaphoresis, restlessness).

These indicators should be assessed in the clinical context – that is, to what degree is the pathophysiological process contributing to pain? In the critically ill, the use of opioids may be complicated by:

- wide inter-individual response to similar dosages, especially in debilitated and elderly patients. Partial opioid agonists (such as buprenorphine) may be advantageous in these scenarios. They may be administered transdermally or sublingually
- severe hypotension following rapid administration, particularly in hypovolaemic patients

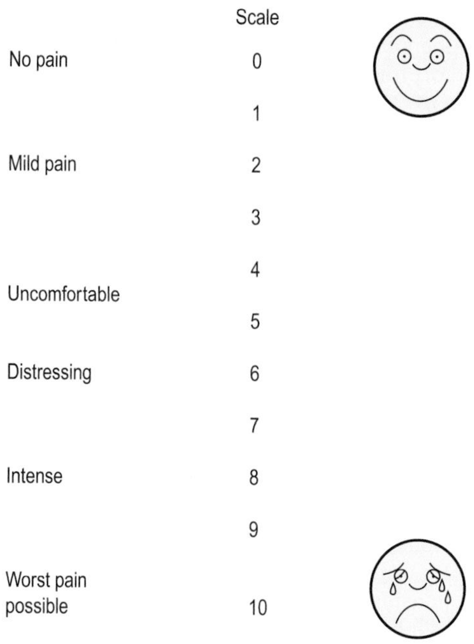

	Scale
No pain	0
	1
Mild pain	2
	3
	4
Uncomfortable	5
Distressing	6
	7
Intense	8
	9
Worst pain possible	10

Figure 89.1 Visual analogue score for the assessment of pain.

- prolonged duration of action, due to accumulation of parent compound and metabolites (e.g. morphine and its major metabolites morphine-3-glucuronide and morphine-6-glucuronide) in the elderly and in patients with renal and hepatic dysfunction. Use of drugs with shorter half-lives (e.g. fentanyl or sufentanil) or those with organ-independent metabolism (e.g. remifentanil) can reduce this problem
- constipation, often requiring concomitant administration of aperients to promote regular evacuation and prokinetics to prevent gastrostasis and allow enteral feeding
- the development of tolerance
- withdrawal symptoms on cessation or reduction of opioid medication.

Recognition of withdrawal symptoms is not always simple in ICU patients as they may mimic sepsis or delirium. Treatment is by reinstitution of and then slow withdrawal of the opioid. Alternatively, symptoms may be controlled by substitution for a long-acting opioid (e.g. methadone), BZAs or α_2-agonists.

The specific opioid antagonist naloxone has little role to play in the ICU, except for the treatment of severe hypotension, unwanted sedation or respiratory depression following opioid usage or overdose. Rapid reversal of opioid effect for the purpose of neurological assessment may be another valid use.

REMIFENTANIL

This is a synthetic, selective mu receptor agonist. It undergoes organ-independent hydrolysis by plasma, red blood cell and tissue esterases. It has a reliable context-sensitive half-time of 4 minutes, which makes it particularly attractive for critically ill patients.

Although an analgesic, it is gaining favour as a sedative agent in intensive care as it causes sedation, tube tolerance and a slowed respiratory rate. In addition, its pharmacokinetic profile makes it ideal for rapid neurological assessment. Studies show reduced extubation times and ICU length of stay when compared with traditional opioids.[18,19]

The loading dose is usually 1 μg/kg, however this should be avoided or attenuated in critically ill patients. Continuous infusion rates of 0.05–0.5 μg/kg/min are usually required and a starting rate of 0.1 μg/kg/min is recommended. Dosage alterations are usually in increments of 0.025–0.1 μg/kg/min. Due to the short half-life, adequacy of response can be assessed within 20 minutes.

Weaning should also be done by incremental dose reductions due to the risks of rebound hyperalgesia. Adding ketamine during the weaning process may modulate this risk.[45]

SIMPLE ANALGESICS

Paracetamol and other simple analgesics (e.g. salicylates) are particularly effective for:

- musculoskeletal pain
- perioperative pain
- inflammatory conditions
- multimodal analgesia, to reduce opioid requirements.

These drugs are given p.o., per rectum (p.r.) or i.v. to supplement analgesia in the critically ill (e.g. paracetamol 1–2 g 4–6-hourly). Paracetamol use is limited by the risk of hepatic dysfunction if used in high dose or for prolonged periods.

NSAIDs

The commonly used NSAIDs are carboxylic acids (e.g. indometacin (indomethacin), ibuprofen, mefenamic acid) or enolic acids (e.g. piroxicam). NSAIDs are useful for supplemental/multimodal analgesia in the ICU for the conditions listed for simple analgesics above. They are given p.o., p.r. or by intramuscular (i.m.) injection (e.g. indometacin 100 mg twice daily p.r.). Patient selection is paramount in the critically ill due to their serious side-effects, including:

- renal dysfunction
- gastrointestinal haemorrhage
- increased bleeding tendency due to platelet inhibition.

The newer cyclo-oxygenase-2 specific inhibitors (COX-2), such as valdecoxib and its injectable precursor parecoxib, have a much lower side-effect profile than traditional NSAIDs. This group of drugs should be used for only short periods, due to an increased cardiovascular morbidity associated with long-term use.[46] COX-2 inhibitors should be avoided in postoperative cardiac surgical patients due to an increased incidence of thromboembolic complications and sternal wound infection.[47,48]

TRAMADOL

Tramadol is a synthetic, racemic preparation with multiple analgesic actions. The (+) enantiomer is a mu receptor agonist and serotonin reuptake inhibitor, whereas the (–) enantiomer is a norepinephrine reuptake inhibitor.[49] In addition to mu receptor action, which accounts for approximately 30% of its analgesic effect, it also enhances the descending inhibitory pathways involved in pain modulation.[50] It is useful for moderate to severe pain in the postoperative patient in doses of 50–100 mg i.v., p.o. or i.m. 4-hourly to a maximum of 600 mg/day. Patients are at risk of developing serotonin syndrome whilst taking tramadol in combination with other pro-serotonergic agents.[51]

KETAMINE

(See 'NMDA receptor antagonist' above.) Ketamine is commonly used as part of multimodal analgesic regimens in surgical patients with severe pain, or if tolerant to opioids. Continuous infusion in a dosage range of 0.1–0.2 mg/kg/h is recommended.

NITROUS OXIDE

Short-term administration of Entonox (50% nitrous oxide in oxygen) is still useful for analgesia during painful procedures (e.g. burns dressings). This may be given by demand valve (controlled by the patient) or be administered by the medical staff.

LOCAL ANAESTHETICS – REGIONAL ANALGESIA

The use of local anaesthetic techniques in the critically ill patient is limited by:

- pain often emanating from multiple sources and therefore not amenable to a single regional technique
- the requirement for i.v. sedation/analgesia (for reasons previously outlined), making a regional technique for a source of pain superfluous
- the need to treat pain over a prolonged period, mandating either repetition of the regional block or the placement of an indwelling catheter (e.g. epidural catheter). Indwelling catheters have a defined duration of insertion (usually 3–4 days) before needing to be removed due to increasing infection risk

- coagulopathy and thrombocytopenia, frequently seen in this group of patients, making procedures such as epidural injection less safe.

When a regional technique is considered viable, then the following need to be considered:

- the procedure should be carried out by adequately trained personnel
- regional techniques may be time-consuming and require additional staff to properly position the patient and assist the proceduralist
- regional techniques carry serious complications (e.g. subarachnoid injection of local anaesthetic or epidural haematoma during placement of epidural catheters) as well as the risk of local anaesthetic toxicity
- good preparation is paramount:
  - informed consent from patient or legal surrogate
  - recent normal coagulation profile or correction of abnormal profile. Platelet counts above 75 000/µL are recommended and antiplatelet agents (other than aspirin) should be ceased at an appropriate time interval beforehand
  - the knowledge of and ability to deal with complications
  - experience and knowledge of the drugs being used. Typically ropivacaine 0.2% is used for regional infusions and can be combined with an opioid, such as fentanyl 2 µg/mL or 4 µg/mL, for epidural infusion. Recommended maximum bolus doses and continuous infusion rates must be known. For ropivacaine; a single bolus of up to 3 mg/kg is allowed (to a maximum of 300 mg), while continuous infusion rates should not exceed 400 µg/kg/h
- adequate training of nursing staff to monitor the level of block in neuraxial techniques, haemodynamic parameters and for possible complications.

Within the context above, the following blocks may be useful in patients:

- femoral nerve block for hip and femur injuries; 20–40 mL of 0.2% ropivacaine injected intermittently 8–12-hourly into the region of the femoral nerve immediately inferior to the inguinal ligament
- intercostal or paravertebral nerve blocks or catheters for thoracic and upper abdominal injuries or wounds; 20 mL of 0.2% ropivacaine injected into the region of appropriate intercostal nerve – a single injection site has been shown to cover multiple nerve root levels[52]
- brachial plexus or intravenous regional anaesthesia for isolated upper limb injuries or procedures (e.g. fracture manipulation)
- epidural analgesia for thoracic and abdominal pain (e.g. flail chest, pancreatitis)
- intrapleural analgesia/anaesthesia, applied either via a catheter placed for this purpose or via intercostal drains previously placed for treatment of pneumothorax.

SLEEP

Although, outwardly, sedated patients resemble the sleep state, there are notable neurophysiological differences. Typically, critically ill patients have shorter periods of sleep, with a distinct reduction of slow-wave ‘deep’ sleep and rapid eye movement (REM) sleep.[53] Critically ill patients have poor sleep patterns due not only to their primary illness, but also to a host of other factors including:

- loss of the sleep–wake cycle after prolonged sedation
- pain
- invasive devices and monitoring
- the ICU environment
- nursing duties.

The importance of sleep disturbance in the critically ill on outcome is unknown, but there is concern over its contribution to delirium.[54]

Much of the focus on improving sleep in critically ill patients relies on non-pharmacological measures, addressing the sleep environment and sleep hygiene of the patient. Pharmacological agents such as BZAs may help patients get to sleep quicker and wake less often, but do not seem to improve the quality of physiological sleep.[54]

THE FUTURE

Research into sedation and analgesia in critically ill patients is intensifying. Areas where future study is focusing include:

- patient-controlled sedation
- target-controlled infusions (TCI) in intensive care
- automated/semiautomated sedation delivery systems[55]
- melatonergic agents for nocturnal sleep (e.g. ramelteon, valdoxane).

Access the complete references list online at http://www.expertconsult.com

5. Schweickert WD, Kress JP. Strategies to optimize analgesia and sedation. Crit Care 2008;12(Suppl 3): S6.
6. Strom T, Martinussen T, Toft P. A protocol of no sedation for critically ill patients receiving mechanical ventilation: a randomised trial. Lancet 2010; 375(9713):475–80.
7. Kress JP, Pohlman AS, O'Connor MF, et al. Daily interruption of sedative infusions in critically ill patients undergoing mechanical ventilation. N Engl J Med 2000;342(20):1471–7.
8. Girard TD, Kress JP, Fuchs BD, et al. Efficacy and safety of a paired sedation and ventilator weaning protocol for mechanically ventilated patients in intensive care (Awakening and Breathing Controlled trial): a randomised controlled trial. Lancet 2008; 371(9607):126–13.
9. Bucknall TK, Manias E, Presneill JJ. A randomized trial of protocol-directed sedation management for mechanical ventilation in an Australian intensive care unit. Crit Care Med 2008;36(5):1444–50.
26. Soukup J, Schärff K, Kubosch K, et al. State of the art: sedation concepts with volatile anesthetics in critically ill patients. J Crit Care 2009;24(4):535–44.
39. Reade MC, O'Sullivan K, Bates S, et al. Dexmedetomidine vs. haloperidol in delirious, agitated, intubated patients: a randomised open-label trial. Crit Care 2009;13(3):R75.

90

Inotropes and vasopressors

John A Myburgh

The pharmacological support of the failing circulation is a fundamental part of critical care. The principal aim of these drugs is to restore inadequate systemic and regional perfusion to physiological levels.

DEFINITIONS

Inotropic agents are defined as drugs that act on the heart by increasing the velocity and force of myocardial fibre shortening. The consequent increase in contractility results in increased cardiac output and blood pressure. Characteristics of the ideal inotrope are shown in **Box 90.1**.

Vasopressors are drugs that have a predominantly vasoconstrictive action on the peripheral vasculature, both arterial and venous. These drugs are used primarily to increase mean arterial pressure.

The distinction between these two groups of drugs is often confusing. Many of the commonly used agents such as the catecholamines have both inotropic and variable effects on the peripheral vasculature that include venoconstriction, arteriolar vasodilatation and constriction.

Vasoregulatory agents may modulate the responsiveness of the peripheral vasculature to vasoactive drugs in pathological states such as sepsis. These agents include vasopressin and corticosteroids.

Given the overlap of pharmacodynamic effects of these drugs, the term 'vasoactive therapy' is a more appropriate description.

THE FAILING CIRCULATION

PHYSIOLOGY

Traditionally, cardiac output is discussed in terms of factors that govern cardiac function. These include preload, afterload, heart rate and rhythm, and contractility. Although this perspective is helpful in managing patients whose circulatory function is limited by cardiac disease, it is incomplete.

Cardiac output is controlled by venous return to the heart from the peripheral vasculature at an equal rate to that ejected during each cardiac cycle[1] (**Fig. 90.1**).

Blood is pumped down a pressure gradient that is determined by the force of myocardial ejection (contractility) and impedance to ventricular ejection (afterload). The resultant mean arterial pressure is the major 'afferent' determinant of regional perfusion pressure. Twenty per cent of the blood volume is contained in the arterial ('conducting') vessels. There is a marked drop in perfusion pressure and flow across the capillary beds to allow diffusion of substrates and oxygen. The difference between mean arterial pressure and the pressure in end capillaries ('efferent' perfusion pressure) determines regional, or organ-specific, perfusion pressure.

Blood enters the venous system and is returned to the heart via a pressure gradient determined by mean systemic pressure and right atrial pressure. The amount of blood returned to the heart determines the degree of ventricular filling prior to systole (preload), which subsequently determines stroke volume and cardiac output.

Under physiological conditions, the venous ('capacitance') system contains approximately 70% of the total blood volume, which acts as a physiological reservoir ('unstressed' volume). Under conditions where circulatory demands increase, increased sympathetic tone will cause contraction of this reservoir.[2] The resultant autotransfusion ('stressed' volume) may increase venous return by approximately 30% and subsequently cardiac output.[3]

Both the arterial and venous systems are integrated under complex neurohormonal influences. These include the adrenergic, renin–angiotensin–aldosterone, vasopressinergic and glucocorticoid systems in addition to local mediators such as nitric oxide, endothelin, endorphins and the eicosanoids.[4]

PATHOPHYSIOLOGY

Circulatory dysfunction or failure may be considered in terms of the major determinants of cardiac output, although there is marked interdependence between these factors.

HEART RATE FAILURE

Profound bradycardia will reduce both cardiac output and mean arterial pressure if sympathetic tone is compromised. Inotropes will increase both rate and speed of conduction, in addition to augmenting peripheral venous return, thereby restoring cardiac output and mean arterial pressure.

Tachycardia is associated with decreased left coronary artery perfusion, due to reduction of diastolic time, during which coronary perfusion occurs. This may exacerbate myocardial ischaemia in patients with coronary artery disease, particularly if mean arterial pressure, specifically diastolic blood pressure, is compromised. Therefore drugs that shorten diastolic time or compromise coronary perfusion should be used with caution in susceptible patients.

Box 90.1 The ideal inotrope

- Increases contractility
  - Increases mean arterial pressure
  - Increases cardiac output
  - Improves regional perfusion
- No increase in myocardial oxygen consumption
  - Avoidance of tachycardia
  - Non-arrhythmogenic
  - Maintenance of diastolic blood pressure
- Does not develop tolerance
- Titratable
  - Rapid onset
  - Rapid termination of action
- Compatible with other drugs
- Non-toxic
- Cost effective

PRELOAD FAILURE

Loss of intravascular blood volume or extracellular fluid is the most common cause of inadequate ventricular preload. This is corrected with fluids to maintain and restore a euvolaemia. Hypovolaemia must be recognised and treated as soon as possible, preferably before vasoactive therapy is used, although the early use of vasoactive therapy is increasingly being recommended.

There are other determinants of ventricular preload and venous return. Factors such as loss of muscle tone, positive intrathoracic pressure, loss of atrial contraction (atrial fibrillation) and ablation of sympathetic tone will compromise preload by reducing venous return. Under these circumstances, volume replacement alone may be insufficient to maintain adequate preload and vasoactive therapy may be required to increase venous return.

MYOCARDIAL FAILURE

Myocardial or 'pump' failure may be divided into disorders of systolic ejection (systolic dysfunction) and diastolic filling (diastolic dysfunction).

Systolic dysfunction occurs as a result of reduced effective myocardial contractility. This may be due to primary myocardial factors such as ischaemia,

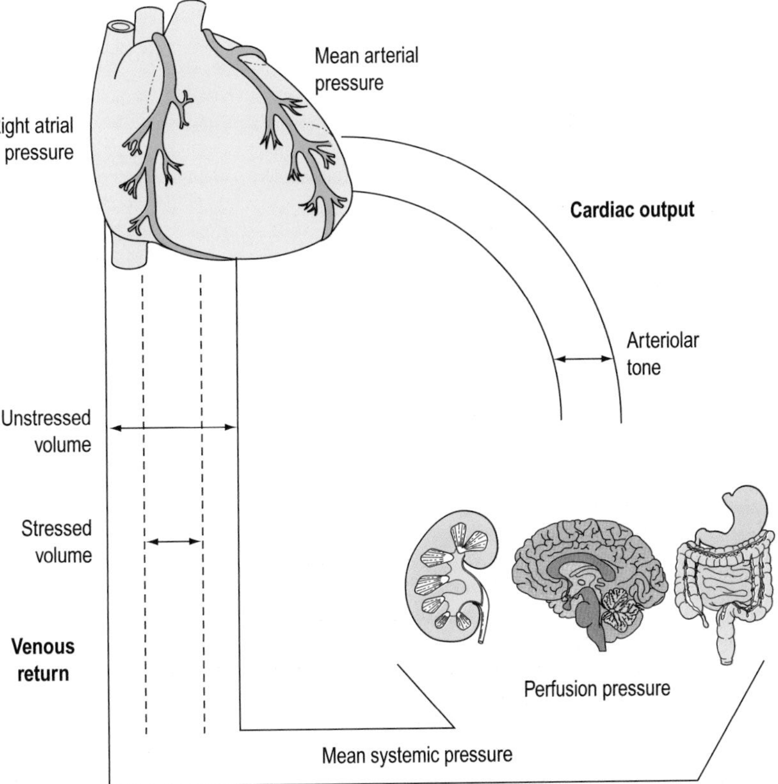

Figure 90.1 Schematic relationship of the determinants of cardiac output and venous return.

infarction or cardiomyopathy. Myocardial depression of both right and left ventricular function may occur in severe sepsis or following prolonged infusions of catecholamines. Increased impedance to ventricular ejection (e.g. hypertensive states) or structural abnormalities (e.g. aortic stenosis or hypertrophic obstructive cardiomyopathy) may cause systolic dysfunction.

Diastolic dysfunction is characterised by reduced ventricular compliance or increased resistance to ventricular filling during diastole. It may be due to mechanical factors such as structural abnormalities of the ventricle (e.g. restrictive cardiomyopathy) or to impaired diastolic relaxation that occurs with myocardial ischaemia or severe sepsis. This results in elevated end-diastolic pressure and pulmonary venous congestion. Episodic or 'flash' pulmonary oedema is a common clinical sign of diastolic dysfunction. Tachycardia that shortens diastolic time may exacerbate diastolic failure. Diastolic dysfunction frequently accompanies systolic failure, in both acute and chronic cardiac failure, particularly in elderly patients.

In the presence of systolic dysfunction, adequate stroke volume may be maintained by an increase in left ventricular end-diastolic volume (the Frank–Starling relationship), provided diastolic function is optimal. However, if the loss of effective myocardial mass is critical, the ventricle will be unable to maintain an adequate stroke volume and cardiac output will fall. In this situation, systolic dysfunction usually requires treatment with inotropic agents in order to augment stroke volume, thereby increasing cardiac output and mean arterial pressure.

VASOREGULATORY FAILURE

Disruption or impairment of regulation of the peripheral vasculature may result in circulatory failure. This includes acute sympathetic denervation, such as high quadriplegia, epidural or total spinal anaesthesia ('spinal' shock); distributive failure such as anaphylaxis; or pathological 'vasoplegia' that occurs in severe sepsis.

These syndromes are characterised by reduced responsiveness of the peripheral circulation to endogenous or exogenous sympathetic stimulation. This results in pooling in the venous circulation due to the inability to provide a 'stressed' volume.[5]

Management of these conditions has traditionally focused on the arterial circulation with attempts to increase systemic vascular resistance. However, the problem is predominantly impaired venous return, compounded to a lesser extent by pathological arteriolar vasodilatation.

Vasoactive agents may have a role in restoring vasoregulatory tone once adequate volume has been established.

CLASSIFICATION

The common ultimate cellular mechanism of action of these agents involves an influence on the release, utilisation or sequestration of intracellular calcium (**Fig. 90.2**). These agents are divided into two main groups based on whether or not their actions depend upon increases in intracellular cyclic adenosine 3,5-monophosphate (cAMP) and are outlined in **Table 90.1**.

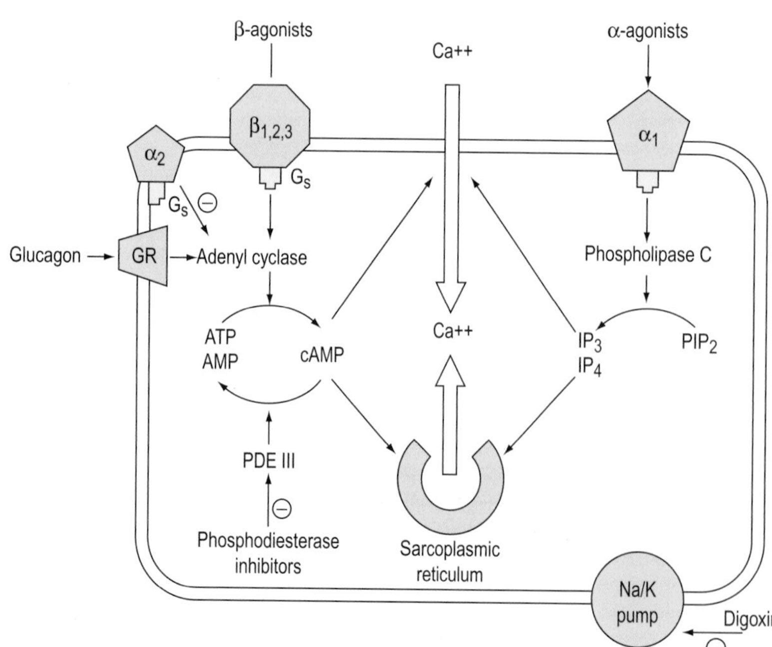

Figure 90.2 Schematic representation of the action of inotropic drugs on intracellular calcium in myocytes. GR=glucagon receptor; Gs=G protein complex; ATP=adenosine triphosphate, AMP=adenosine monophosphate; cAMP=cyclic AMP; PDE III=phosphodiesterase III; IP3=inositol phosphate 3, PIP2=phosphoinositol diphosphate.

Table 90.1 Classification of inotropes

cAMP DEPENDENT	cAMP INDEPENDENT
Catecholamines (beta-adrenergic agonists) Epinephrine (adrenaline) Norepinephrine (noradrenaline) Dopamine Dobutamine Dopexamine Isoprenaline Phosphodiesterase inhibitors Amrinone Milrinone Enoximone Levosimendan Calcium sensitisers Levosimendan Glucagon	Catecholamines (alpha-adrenergic agonists) Epinephrine (adrenaline) Norepinephrine (noradrenaline) Dopamine Digoxin Thyroid hormone

CATECHOLAMINES

Sympathomimetic amines are the most frequently used vasoactive agents in the intensive care unit (ICU) and include the naturally occurring catecholamines dopamine, norepinephrine (noradrenaline) and epinephrine (adrenaline), and the synthetic substances dobutamine, isoprenaline and dopexamine.

RECEPTOR BIOLOGY

Agonists bind to populations of adrenergic receptors, largely divided into α and β subgroups. Further subgroups of α- (α_{1A}, α_{1B}, α_{2A}, α_{2B}, α_{2C}) and β-receptors (β_1, β_2, β_3) have been identified.[4]

Signal transduction from agonist–receptor occupation to the effector cell is modulated by conformational changes in G proteins associated with these receptors. Under the additional influence of second messengers such as nitric oxide, endothelin and eicosanoids, these conformational changes promote the release of calcium from intracellular stores and increase membrane calcium permeability. Subsequent phosphorylation of substrate proteins via protein kinases act as third messengers to trigger a cascade of events that lead to specific cardiovascular effects.

β-Receptor occupancy predominantly activates adenyl cyclase to increase the conversion of adenosine triphosphate to cAMP. α-Receptor occupancy acts independently of cAMP by activation of phospholipase C, which increases inositol phosphates (IP_3 and IP_4) and diacyl glycerol.

This complex agonist–receptor–effector relationship is responsible for homeostatic mechanisms such as physiological responses to stress and autoregulation.

The activity and function of this system is dynamic and may be markedly influenced by pathological states. This may result in qualitative changes in the agonist–receptor–effector organ relationship (desensitisation) where receptors no longer respond to physiological or pharmacological sympathetic stimulation to the same extent. Quantitative changes such as reduced receptor density, receptor sequestration and enzymatic uncoupling (down-regulation) may also result in impaired responses.[6]

BIOSYNTHESIS

The biosynthesis and chemical structures of the naturally occurring catecholamines are shown in **Figure 90.3a**.

Catecholamines consist of an aromatic ring attached to a terminal amine by a carbon chain. The configuration of each drug is important for determining affinity to respective receptors.

Dopamine is hydroxylated to form norepinephrine, which is the predominant peripheral sympathetic chemotransmitter in humans, acting at all adrenergic receptors. The release of norepinephrine from sympathetic terminals is controlled by reuptake mechanisms mediated via α_2-receptors and augmented by epinephrine released from the adrenal gland at times of stress. Norepinephrine is converted to form epinephrine, which is subsequently metabolised in liver and lung.

All catecholamines have very short biological half-lives (1–2 minutes) and a steady state plasma concentration is achieved within 5–10 minutes after the start of a constant infusion. This allows rapid titration of drug to a clinical end-point such as mean arterial pressure.

Epinephrine and norepinephrine infusions produce blood concentrations similar to those produced endogenously in shock states, whereas dopamine infusions produce much higher concentrations than those naturally encountered. Dopamine may exert much of its effect by being converted to norepinephrine, thus bypassing the rate-limiting (tyrosine hydroxylase) step in catecholamine synthesis.

The synthetic catecholamines are derivatives of dopamine (Fig. 90.3b). These agents are characterised by increased length of the carbon chain, which confers affinity for β-receptors. Dobutamine is a synthetic derivative of isoprenaline. These agents have relatively little affinity for α-receptors due to the configuration of the terminal amine, which differs from the endogenous catecholamines.

Epinephrine, norepinephrine and isoprenaline all have hydroxyl groups on the β-carbon atom of the side chain, and this is associated with 100-fold greater potency than dopamine or dobutamine.

SYSTEMIC EFFECTS

The systemic effects of any of these agents will vary greatly between patients and within individuals at

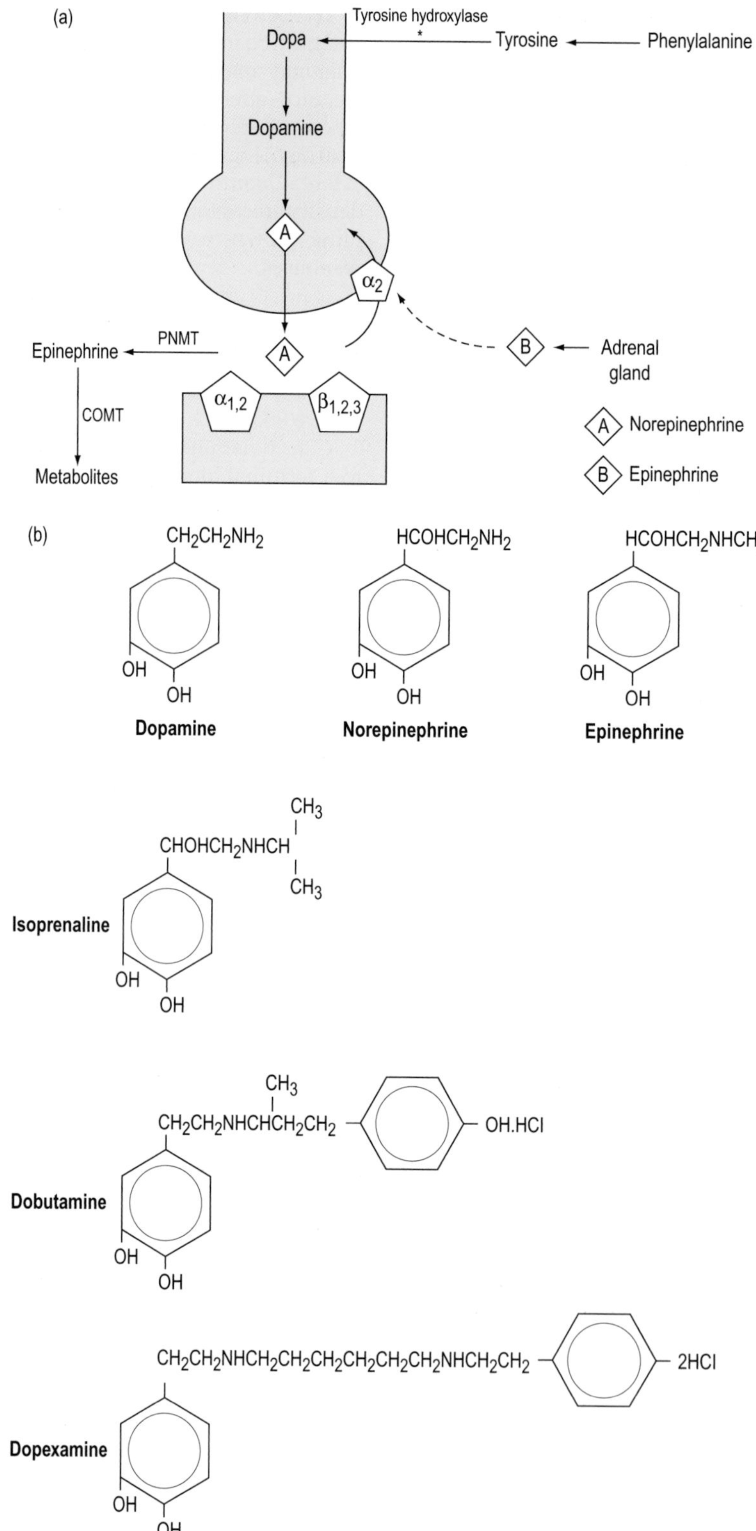

Figure 90.3 **(a)** Biosynthesis of catecholamines in sympathetic terminals. * = rate-limiting step by tyrosine hydroxylase; PNMT = phenethanolamine-*N*-methyltransferase, COMT = catechol-*o*-methyl-transferase. **(b)** Chemical structure of endogenous and synthetic catecholamines.

different times. Adequacy of response is often unpredictable and depends on the aetiology of circulatory failure and systemic co-morbidities. In some patients, dramatic responses to small doses may occur, whereas in others large doses of inotropes may be required to support the failing circulation.

The classification of sympathomimetic agents into alpha and beta agonists, based on the above structure–function relationships, is only a crude predictor of systemic effects.

Epinephrine, norepinephrine and dopamine are all predominantly beta agonists at low doses, with increasing α-effects becoming evident as the dose is increased.

The synthetic catecholamines are all predominantly beta agonists.

CARDIOVASCULAR

The cardiovascular effects of the catecholamines under physiological conditions are shown in **Table 90.2**.

Norepinephrine, epinephrine and dopamine all tend to increase stroke volume, cardiac output and mean arterial pressure, with little change in heart rate. Dopamine is associated with an increased incidence of dysrhythmias.[7] The effects on the peripheral vasculature are similar, with all agents increasing venous return without significant changes in calculated systemic vascular resistance.

Isoprenaline increases cardiac output predominantly by increasing heart rate and by moderate inotropy. This occurs without a significant change in blood pressure due to predominant β_2-receptor-induced veno- and vasodilatation.

The profile of dobutamine is similar to isoprenaline, although increases in heart rate are not as pronounced. Both of these agents may decrease mean arterial pressure, particularly in hypovolaemic patients, due to reduced venous return caused by venodilatation. The adverse effects of dobutamine and isoprenaline on heart rate and mean arterial pressure may compromise patients with ischaemic heart disease.

In the failing myocardium, particularly in patients with cardiac failure following cardiopulmonary bypass or septic shock, endogenous stores of norepinephrine are markedly reduced.[8] Furthermore, there may be significant desensitisation and down-regulation of cardiac β-receptors. In these situations, α_1- and α_2-receptors have an important role in maintaining inotropy and peripheral vasoresponsiveness.[9] This may be expressed clinically as 'tolerance' or tachyphylaxis to catecholamines, particularly with predominantly beta agonists such as dobutamine. This phenomenon may explain the requirement for high doses of catecholamines in refractory shock states. Consequently, the role of beta agonists in patients with severe myocardial failure has been questioned.

Catecholamines have a significant effect on the venous circulation. These drugs primarily restore or maintain 'stressed volumes' of the capacitance vessels under pathological conditions, thereby maintaining or increasing cardiac output and mean arterial pressure. This is important in 'vasoplegic' states such as septic shock.[5]

In clinically used doses, intravenously administered catecholamines have minimal direct vasoconstrictive effects on conducting arterial vessels.

The development of peripheral gangrene in refractory septic shock has been attributed to catecholamine-induced vasoconstriction. There is little evidence to support this as the development of tissue gangrene in these situations primarily occurs as a consequence of intravascular thrombosis caused by sepsis-mediated coagulopathy.

CEREBRAL

Under physiological conditions, catecholamines do not normally cross the blood–brain barrier. Cerebral blood flow is maintained at a constant rate over a range of perfusion pressure by cerebral autoregulation. Under conditions where the integrity of the blood–brain barrier is altered, such as following traumatic brain

Table 90.2 Cardiovascular effect of catecholamines

AGENT	β_1 EFFECTS	β_2 EFFECTS	α_1 EFFECTS	α_2 EFFECTS
	+ chronotropy + dromotropy + inotropy	+ inotropy vasodilatation bronchodilatation	+ inotropy vasoconstriction	+ inotropy vasoconstriction
Norepinephrine Epinephrine Dopamine	β effects predominate at low dose; α effects predominate at high dose			
Dobutamine	+	+	(+)	–
Isoprenaline	+	(+)	–	–
Dopexamine	+	+	–	–

+ = stimulation; (+) = mild effect; – = no effect.

injury and aneurysmal subarachnoid haemorrhage, exogenous catecholamines may directly enter the cerebral circulation.

The degree by which these agents directly affect the cerebral circulation following head injury is unknown, although there is some evidence suggesting that dopamine has a direct effect causing increased cerebral blood flow and intracranial pressure.[10]

RENAL

The kidney is an efficient autoregulator, maintaining constant glomerular filtration and renal blood flow by neurohumoral mechanisms such as the renin–angiotensin–aldosterone system.[11] All catecholamines will increase renal blood flow to a similar extent because of increased cardiac output and mean arterial pressure with a resultant natriuresis. Catecholamine-mediated increases in renal blood flow do not affect glomerular filtration rate.

A direct natriuresis may also result from inhibition of cAMP in the renal tubules. This effect has been attributed primarily to low doses of dopamine (2 μg/kg per min), although this occurs to a similar extent with epinephrine, norepinephrine and dobutamine. The use of low-dose 'renal' dopamine has been shown to be ineffective in preventing renal dysfunction in susceptible patients.[12]

SPLANCHNIC

Splanchnic autoregulation is not as robust as the brain and kidney. Perfusion is more dependent on mean arterial pressure and the duality of the mesenteric and portal systems. Concerns about catecholamine-induced splanchnic vasoconstriction with mesenteric and hepatic ischaemia have not been substantiated.[13]

Dopamine and dopexamine have been promoted as selective splanchnic vasodilators, but there are no conclusive studies indicating a significant benefit over norepinephrine or epinephrine. Many studies have used gastric intramucosal pH (pHi), a surrogate measurement of splanchnic blood flow, as the primary endpoint. However, as pHi remains an unvalidated measurement, the results of many of the comparative trials of the different sympathomimetics are inconclusive. All catecholamines are equally effective in increasing splanchnic perfusion by improving cardiac output and mean arterial pressure.

METABOLIC

Catecholamine-mediated β-stimulation may result in hyperglycaemia, hypokalaemia and hypophosphataemia, which may need monitoring and correcting.

Epinephrine is associated with the development of hyperlactataemia and acidaemia, due to activation of pyruvate dehydrogenase. Although pH may fall to levels around 7.2, the acidosis is not associated with impaired tissue perfusion or cellular dysoxia. In most patients who are haemodynamically stable, this is a self-limiting phenomenon and is not associated with adverse outcomes.[14,15]

NON-CATECHOLAMINES

PHOSPHODIESTERASE INHIBITORS

Phosphodiesterase inhibitors are compounds that cause non-receptor-mediated competitive inhibition of phosphodiesterase isoenzymes (PDE), resulting in increased levels of cAMP (see Fig. 90.2). Importantly, cAMP also affects diastolic heart function through the regulation of phospholamban, the regulatory subunit of the calcium pump of the sarcoplasmic reticulum. This enhances the rate of calcium resequestration and thereby diastolic relaxation.

For cardiovascular tissue, inhibition of isoenzyme PDE III is responsible for the therapeutic effects. Cardiac effects are characterised by positive inotropy and improved diastolic relaxation. The latter is termed lusitropy and may be beneficial in patients with reduced ventricular compliance or predominant diastolic failure.[16]

These agents also cause potent vasodilatation with reductions in preload, venous return and afterload as well as a reduction in pulmonary vascular resistance. The term 'inodilation' has been used to describe this dual haemodynamic effect.

Tolerance is not a feature. These agents may have a place in the management of patients with β-receptor down-regulation by causing intrinsic inotropic stimulation and by sensitising the myocardium to beta agonists. Other actions include inhibition of platelet aggregation and reduction of post-ischaemic reperfusion injury.

The pharmacokinetics of phosphodiesterase inhibitors are markedly different from catecholamines. Drug half-lives may be prolonged and excretion is predominantly renal. Hypotension may result from vasodilatation and combined use with catecholamines (e.g. norepinephrine or epinephrine) may be necessary to maintain mean arterial pressure.

Phosphodiesterase inhibitors that have been used in clinical practice include the bipyridine derivatives amrinone and milrinone, the imidazolones enoximone and piroximone, and the calcium sensitiser levosimendan. The cardiovascular effects are similar.

Milrinone is the most commonly used drug in clinical practice, with the latter exhibiting more inotropic effects than vasodilatation. Enoximone is more rapidly metabolised, but the metabolite is active and its cardiovascular effects persist for some hours.

Levosimendan is a dose-dependent selective phosphodiesterase inhibitor with a unique action on myocardial calcium metabolism.[17] By increasing myofilament calcium sensitivity throughout the cardiac cycle by binding to cardiac troponin C, associated conformational changes induce improved inotropic and lusitropic function. Vasodilatation is also induced through ATP-sensitive potassium channels. Calcium-sensitive actions predominate at low doses, whereas PDE-inhibition effects predominate at higher doses. The half-life of levosimendan is shorter than that of older PDE III inhibitors (approximately 1 hour) and it may be given by infusion.

HISTORICAL DRUGS

DIGOXIN

Digitalis glycosides have been used for the treatment of heart failure for 200 years and the vagotonic effects used to control the ventricular response in selected supraventricular tachyarrhythmias. Its use in the ICU has been superseded by catecholamines and antiarrhythmics such as amiodarone, although the role of digoxin in chronic heart failure is well established.

The role of digoxin in acute cardiac failure is limited. It has minimal effects as an inotrope and evaluation of its efficacy is difficult. The potential for toxicity in the critically ill patient is increased by hypokalaemia, hypomagnesaemia, hypercalcaemia, hypoxia and acidosis. Toxicity is manifested by dysrhythmias that may assume any form including supraventricular tachyarrhythmias, bradycardia, ventricular ectopy and conduction block at any level.

GLUCAGON

Glucagon is a naturally occurring polypeptide that directly stimulates adenyl cyclase via specific receptors to increase cAMP concentration in myocardial cells resulting in positive inotropy without producing myocardial excitability. No definitive cardiovascular role for this agent has been established apart from anecdotal reports of its use in severe beta-blocker and tricyclic poisoning.

THYROID HORMONE

Thyroid hormone is required for synthesis of contractile proteins and normal myocardial contraction. It is also a regulator of the synthesis of adrenergic receptors. Its use is limited in critically ill patients, but may have a limited, although unproven, role in haemodynamic support of brain-dead organ donors as a catecholamine-sparing agent.

SELECTIVE VASOPRESSORS

Vascular responsiveness is mediated via adrenergic receptors: α-mechanisms predominantly cause vasoconstriction; β-mechanisms, specifically β_2-receptors, mediate vasodilatation (see Table 90.2).

Norepinephrine, epinephrine and dopamine have variable effects on the peripheral vasculature and should not be regarded principally as vasoconstrictors or vasopressors.

There are few selective 'vasoconstrictors' that predominantly have a role in vasodilated states such as regional (epidural) anaesthesia or selected patients with acute spinal injury. Their utility in critically ill patients remains limited and they have an unproven role in patients with catecholamine-resistant septic shock and cardiopulmonary resuscitation.

PHENYLEPHRINE AND METARAMINOL

These agents are direct-acting alpha-2 agonists that are selective vasoconstrictors, both venous and arterial, with minimal beta activity. They have similar pharmacokinetics to catecholamines and may be given by infusion. In patients with normal sympathetic tone, these drugs may cause reflex bradycardia, particularly following bolus administration.

EPHEDRINE

Ephedrine is a synthetic, direct- and indirect-acting, non-catecholamine sympathomimetic that acts on both α- and β-receptors. Duration of action is longer than equivalent doses of epinephrine and it is generally unsuitable as an infusion.

VASOREGULATORY AGENTS

In addition to adrenergic regulation, neurohumoral influences have a 'permissive' or regulatory role in maintaining vasomotor tone. These are mediated through the renin–aldosterone–angiotensin axis and local mediators such as vasopressin, corticosteroids, nitric oxide and endothelin.

The response of the whole neurohumoral system may become blunted in conditions such as severe sepsis, where qualitative and quantitative changes may occur. In this context, failure of vasomotor responsiveness may be considered as part of the multiple organ failure.

VASOPRESSIN

Specific vasopressinergic receptors (V_1, V_2) have been identified in association with sympathetic terminals. Vasopressin is a naturally occurring peptide secreted by the posterior pituitary gland. Reduced serum levels of vasopressin have been demonstrated in septic shock and following cardiopulmonary bypass, suggesting an inflammatory-mediated mechanism. Levels are maintained during cardiogenic shock.

A proportion of patients with severe septic shock requiring high levels of catecholamines to support the circulation may respond to low doses of infused vasopressin (0.04 U/h). However, although vasopressin may improve catecholamine responsiveness in patients with less-severe shock, no benefit in mortality has been demonstrated and there is uncertainty about its use in shock states.[18]

STEROIDS

The role of steroid supplementation in circulatory failure has been studied for many years. Although immunosuppressive or anti-inflammatory doses have been shown to be ineffective, particularly in septic shock, replacement of 'stress response' doses (approximately 100–200 mg hydrocortisone per day) have been shown to improve catecholamine vasoresponsiveness in selected patients with septic shock.[19] However, the role of steroids in shock states remains uncertain, despite two large trials, and they are not routinely recommended.[20,21]

CLINICAL USES

Currently, there are no definitive studies comparing the efficacy of one inotrope (or combination of inotropes) over another in terms of improving survival.[22]

DRUG SELECTION

In most instances, individual experience and preference determine selection of inotrope(s).

On a pathobiological basis, exogenous catecholamines are essentially used to augment endogenous mechanisms that may be failing at a number of levels. In this context, vasoactive therapy should be regarded as 'cardiovascular neuroendocrine augmentation therapy'.

Norepinephrine or epinephrine may be considered as the first-line drug in most causes of circulatory failure. An emerging body of evidence confirms this statement.[7,14,15]

Dopamine predominantly acts as a precursor of norepinephrine and may be used as an alternative to norepinephrine, although it is associated with an increased incidence of arrhythmias.[7]

Prediction of the response of an individual to a catecholamine is problematic as marked inter- and intra-individual variability to the response of inotropic agents may occur.

The haemodynamic and metabolic response of an agent must be carefully monitored and evaluated. If there is not a satisfactory response, or if undesirable effects are obtained, the dose or agent should be changed.

MONITORING

Accurate monitoring of the circulation is essential in patients with circulatory failure to assess baseline parameters and the response of vasoactive drugs.

Clinical assessment of the circulation remains the cornerstone of monitoring these patients and includes frequent assessment and recording of pulse rate and rhythm, blood pressure, adequacy of peripheral perfusion, skin turgor, level of consciousness and urine output.

The majority of patients with circulatory failure managed in the ICU require haemodynamic monitoring as clinical signs may be masked or influenced by sedation, ventilation or organ failure. As a minimum, all patients receiving vasoactive drugs in all but trivial doses should have accurate monitoring of mean arterial pressure, ideally with an intra-arterial catheter referenced to the aortic root and an assessment of volume status such as central venous pressure.

In selected patients with primary myocardial failure, an assessment of cardiac output may be useful to quantify baseline function and to assess the response of the heart to drug therapy. Measurement of cardiac output may be done non-invasively using transthoracic or transoesophageal echocardiography or invasively using a pulmonary catheter, ideally using a continuous cardiac output display system, although the use of these catheters has decreased substantially.

Systemic vascular resistance is frequently calculated and used as a surrogate index of afterload. However, the clinical utility of systemic vascular resistance is limited to providing a crude estimate of global vascular tone, as it does not reflect afterload, arteriolar tone or venous return. Consequently, systemic vascular resistance should not be used as a criterion for selection of vasoactive drug or as a titratable end-point.

Restoration of reduced tissue perfusion is a primary aim of vasoactive therapy. This may be assessed clinically by improvements in urine output, serum urea and creatinine, reversal of metabolic acidosis and reduction in serum lactate.

DOSAGES AND DRUG ADMINISTRATION

Vasoactive drugs, such as catecholamines or vasopressors, are administered by continuous infusion through a dedicated central venous catheter using drug delivery systems such as infusion pumps or syringe drivers.

Infusion lines should be free of injection portals and clearly marked with identifying labels.

Concentrations of infusions should be standardised in accordance with individual unit protocols. Suggested infusion concentrations are shown in **Table 90.3**.

These infusions in mL/hour approximate μg/min. Absolute doses with regard to body weight are not relevant; rather it is the titrated clinical effect. Vasoactive drugs are usually prescribed as a titration against a desired mean arterial pressure.

CARDIOPULMONARY RESUSCITATION

Epinephrine has been used for circulatory collapse at least since 1907. The International Liaison Committee on Resuscitation guidelines recommends epinephrine as first-line vasoactive drug in cardiopulmonary

Table 90.3 Infusion concentrations of commonly used vasoactive drugs

AGENT	INFUSION CONCENTRATION	DOSE
Epinephrine	6 mg/100 mL 5% dextrose	Titrate mL/h (=μg/min)
Norepinephrine	6 mg/100 mL 5% dextrose	Titrate mL/h (=μg/min)
Dopamine	400 mg/100mL 5% dextrose	Titrate mL/h (approx μg/kg/min)
Dobutamine	500 mg/100 mL 5% dextrose	Titrate mL/h (approx μg/kg/min)
Isoprenaline	6 mg/100 mL 5% dextrose	Titrate mL/h (=μg/min)
Milrinone	10 mg/100 mL 5% dextrose	Loading dose: 50 μg/kg over 20 min Infusion: 0.5 μg/kg/min
Levosimendan	25 mg/100 mL 5% dextrose	Loading dose: 24 μg/kg over 10 min Infusion: 0.1 μg/kg/min
Phenylephrine	10 mg/100 mL 5% dextrose	Titrate mL/h (=100 μg/h)
Metaraminol	100 mg/100 mL 5% dextrose	Titrate mL/h (=mg/h)
Ephedrine	300 mg/100 mL 5% dextrose	Titrate mL/h (=3 mg/h)
Vasopressin	20 units/20 mL 5%dextrose	2.4 mL/h (0.04 u/min)
Hydrocortisone	100 mg/100 mL 5% dextrose	Loading dose: 100 mg Infusion: 0.18 mg/kg/h

resuscitation. Doses are 1 mg intravenously every 3 minutes.[23]

Epinephrine is recommended as first-line therapy for 'medical pacing' for severe bradyarrhythmias that do not respond to atropine. Isoprenaline has traditionally been used for this purpose; however, its use has been superseded by epinephrine due to concerns about efficacy and lack of alpha-adrenergic activity.

CARDIOGENIC SHOCK

Theoretically, catecholamine infusions may confer some advantages in cardiogenic shock, particularly in association with acute myocardial infarction. In patients with systolic heart failure, epinephrine, norepinephrine, dopamine and dobutamine have been shown to cause satisfactory short-term effects. This may allow the myocardium time to recover from post-ischaemic 'stunning', particularly after revascularisation. However, no increased long-term survival due to their use has been demonstrated.[24]

The role of phosphodiesterase inhibitors (e.g. milrinone) and calcium sensitisers (e.g. levosimendan) in acute heart failure has yet to be determined, but they may have a potential role in patients with diastolic heart failure, particularly those with associated high impedance states such as aortic stenosis and pulmonary hypertension. Due to their non-adrenergic mechanism of action, these agents may be useful in patients who are 'resistant' to catecholamines.

SEPARATION FROM CARDIOPULMONARY BYPASS

Numerous combinations of catecholamines have been used successfully to wean patients from cardiopulmonary bypass. However, there are no definitive studies demonstrating significant benefits of one catecholamine over another. Similarly, the question whether mechanical support devices, such as intra-aortic counterpulsation, offer a significant advantage over inotropes following cardiac surgery remains unanswered.

Epinephrine and norepinephrine have been found to increase cardiac output with little increase in heart rate or afterload and are often regarded as first-line drugs. Dobutamine may be associated with vasodilatation and hypotension.

There is no conclusive evidence that the catecholamines, including norepinephrine, cause vasospasm of arterial conduits in clinically used doses.

Phosphodiesterase inhibitors, such as milrinone and levosimendan, either as sole agents or in conjunction with epinephrine or norepinephrine, have been used with success. These may have a role following mitral valve replacement in patients with pulmonary hypertension or preoperative diastolic failure.[25]

Cardiopulmonary bypass may be associated with a systemic inflammatory response syndrome characterised by a hyperdynamic, vasodilated 'low systemic vascular resistance' state. Norepinephrine is frequently advocated as a 'vasopressor' agent in this context to restore mean arterial pressure, which may be reduced as a consequence. Although catecholamines may be required to achieve appropriate target mean arterial pressure and cardiac output, caution should be applied if high doses (e.g. >30 μg/min norepinephrine) are required. This may be associated with tachyphylaxis and potentiation of catecholamine dependency.[26]

RIGHT VENTRICULAR FAILURE

Right ventricular infarction and major pulmonary embolism may be associated with acute right ventricular failure. Right ventricular depression may also occur in severe sepsis. Restoration of preload is critical in these conditions, as the failing right ventricle is particularly susceptible to reductions in preload.[27]

Inotropes such as norepinephrine and epinephrine are regarded as first-line drugs in these situations in order to maintain adequate mean arterial pressure so that right coronary artery perfusion, which occurs throughout the cardiac cycle, is maintained.

SEPTIC SHOCK

The cardiovascular effects of the sepsis syndrome and septic shock are complex and range from a hyperdynamic, vasodilated state to one of increasing myocardial failure and paralysis of the peripheral v asculature (vasoplegia). The latter represents inability of the venous circulation to respond to endogenous or exogenous catecholamines with resultant venous pooling.

An increasing body of literature now recommends the use of catecholamines as first-line agents in the treatment of septic shock. The Surviving Sepsis Campaign guidelines recommend either norepinephrine or epinephrine be used as the first-line choice vasopressor.[28] However, the basis for this recommendation is limited as there is no high-quality evidence to recommend one catecholamine over another.[22] Concerns about adverse metabolic and splanchnic side-effects of epinephrine are unsubstantiated, and there is an emerging body of evidence that norepinephrine and epinephrine are equally effective in treating septic shock.[14,15] There is evidence that dopamine may be associated with adverse outcomes[7] and its use is being questioned in the absence of superiority to norepinephrine or epinephrine.

The efficacy of dobutamine as a sole agent or in combination with norepinephrine in septic shock is questionable and appears to add little to the efficacy of norepinephrine or epinephrine in terms of resolution of shock or mortality.

Doses required to achieve adequate mean arterial pressure in septic shock may vary: norepinephrine or epinephrine infusions (up to 40 μg/min) may be necessary. Patients who develop marked catecholamine dependency, in the absence of other acute remediable causes such as active infection, may respond to low doses of vasopressin or 'stress response' doses of hydrocortisone, although there is marked interindividual variation in response to these drugs.

ANAPHYLAXIS

Epinephrine is the drug of choice for anaphylactic reactions and for life-threatening bronchospasm, as it blocks mediator release and specifically reverses end-organ effects (see Ch. 66).

A dose of 0.1 mg, as 1 mL of 1:10000 solution, may be injected subcutaneously, intramuscularly or intravenously. Repeated doses or infusions of up to 100 μg/min may be required. A strong slowing pulse indicates a pressor effect and provides a useful clinical end-point for the rate of infusion. This alpha-agonist effect is probably also of considerable importance in anaphylaxis, as deaths are frequently due to prolonged refractory hypotension caused by acute biventricular failure. Early intravenous fluid therapy is also important.

RENAL PROTECTION

'Renal' dose dopamine (2 μg/kg per min) had been advocated for many years as a renal protective agent by causing renal vasodilatation. However, this has not been substantiated in controlled clinical trials in susceptible patients or as an adjunctive agent with other inotropes in septic shock.[12] Consequently low-dose dopamine is no longer recommended.

CEREBRAL PERFUSION PRESSURE

Augmentation of cerebral perfusion pressure is an important strategy in patients with pathological reductions in cerebral blood flow, such as traumatic brain injury and subarachnoid haemorrhage. Norepinephrine and epinephrine have been used to augment cerebral perfusion pressure, although there is no conclusive evidence to recommend one drug over another.[10]

Access the complete references list online at http://www.expertconsult.com

7. De Backer D, Biston P, Devriendt J, et al. Comparison of dopamine and norepinephrine in the treatment of shock. N Engl J Med 2010;362:779–89.
14. Myburgh JA, Higgins A, Jovanovska A, et al. A comparison of epinephrine and norepinephrine in critically ill patients. Intensive Care Med 2008;34:2226–34.
15. Annane D, Vignon P, Renault A, et al. Norepinephrine plus dobutamine versus epinephrine alone for management of septic shock: a randomised trial. Lancet 2007;370:676–84.
18. Russell JA, Walley KR, Singer J, et al. Vasopressin versus norepinephrine infusion in patients with septic shock. N Engl J Med 2008;358:877–87.
19. Annane D, Bellissant E, Bollaert PE, et al. Corticosteroids in the treatment of severe sepsis and septic shock in adults: a systematic review. JAMA 2009;301: 2362–75.
22. Havel C, Arrich J, Losert H, et al. Vasopressors for hypotensive shock. Cochrane Database Syst Rev 2011; 5:CD003709.
28. Dellinger RP, Levy MM, Rhodes A, et al. Surviving Sepsis Campaign: international guidelines for the management of severe sepsis and septic shock: 2012. Intensive Care Med 2013;39:165–228.

91

Vasodilators and antihypertensives

Anthony C Gordon and John A Myburgh

Vasodilators are a generic group of drugs that are primarily used in the intensive care unit (ICU) for the management of acute hypertensive states and emergencies. In addition, they have an important role in the management of myocardial ischaemia, systemic and pulmonary hypertension and cardiac failure.[1]

PHYSIOLOGY

Blood pressure is controlled by a complex physiological neurohormonal system involving all components of the cardiovascular system.[2,3] Traditionally, clinical practice has focused on the arterial circulation as the major regulator of systemic pressure. The importance of venous circulation in determining mean arterial pressure and cardiac output is discussed in Chapter 90.

The role of the peripheral vasculature, including both arteriolar and venous systems, in the regulation of blood pressure may be conceptually regarded as a balance between vasodilatation and vasoconstriction[3] (**Fig. 91.1**).

CALCIUM FLUX

The concentration of intracellular ionised calcium is the primary determinant of vascular smooth muscle tone: increases lead to smooth muscle contraction; decreases cause relaxation. Control of calcium influx and efflux is determined by adrenergic receptor occupation and changes in membrane potential, mediated through voltage-gated channels (see Ch. 90, Fig. 90.2).

ENDOTHELIAL SYSTEM

The endothelium plays a central role in blood pressure homeostasis by secreting substances such as nitric oxide, prostacyclin and endothelin.[3] These substances are continuously released by the endothelium and are integral in regional autoregulation.[4]

Nitric oxide is synthesised from L-arginine by nitric oxide synthases and diffuses into underlying smooth muscle where it activates guanylate cyclase to increase cyclic guanosine monophosphate (cGMP) resulting in relaxation of underlying smooth muscle and vasodilatation.

Prostacyclin is synthesised via the arachidonic pathway and has a minor role in the control of vascular tone.

Endothelins are endothelium-derived vasoconstrictor peptides that are associated with increases in vascular smooth muscle intracellular calcium. They bind to endothelin receptors within the vascular smooth muscle and lead to vasoconstriction, usually in response to shear stresses, tissue hypoxia, angiotensin II and inflammatory mediators (e.g. interleukin-6 and nuclear factor-κB (NF-κB)).

RENIN–ANGIOTENSIN–ALDOSTERONE SYSTEM

Angiotensinogen is converted by renin to form angiotensin I, which is subsequently converted to angiotensin II by angiotensin-converting enzyme (ACE). Angiotensin II has a number of effects that are responsible for blood pressure homeostasis. These include release of aldosterone, direct activation of alpha-adrenergic (α-adrenergic) receptors on vascular smooth muscle and a direct effect in the endothelium. These effects are directed at maintaining blood pressure and are integral in the stress response. Angiotensin-converting enzyme is also responsible for the inactivation of bradykinins that have predominantly vasodilatory effects, coupled to arachidonic acid synthesis and generation of prostacyclin.

ADRENERGIC SYSTEM

The sympathetic nervous system is integrally involved with all of the above systems, regulating vascular tone at central, ganglionic and local neural levels. Adrenergic stimulation of β-receptors is associated with vasodilatation; α-receptor stimulation results in vasoconstriction. The vascular effects of the catecholamines and vasopressors are discussed in Chapter 90.

Adrenergic stimulation is the predominant system in regulating venous tone.[5] This is due to endothelial differences in veins resulting in less production of nitric oxide and reduced responsiveness to angiotensin II.

PATHOPHYSIOLOGY

Hypertensive states develop as a result of impaired or abnormal homeostatic processes, causing an imbalance between vasoconstrictive and vasodilatory effects.

Essential hypertension is the most common cause of hypertension and is due to abnormal neurohormonal

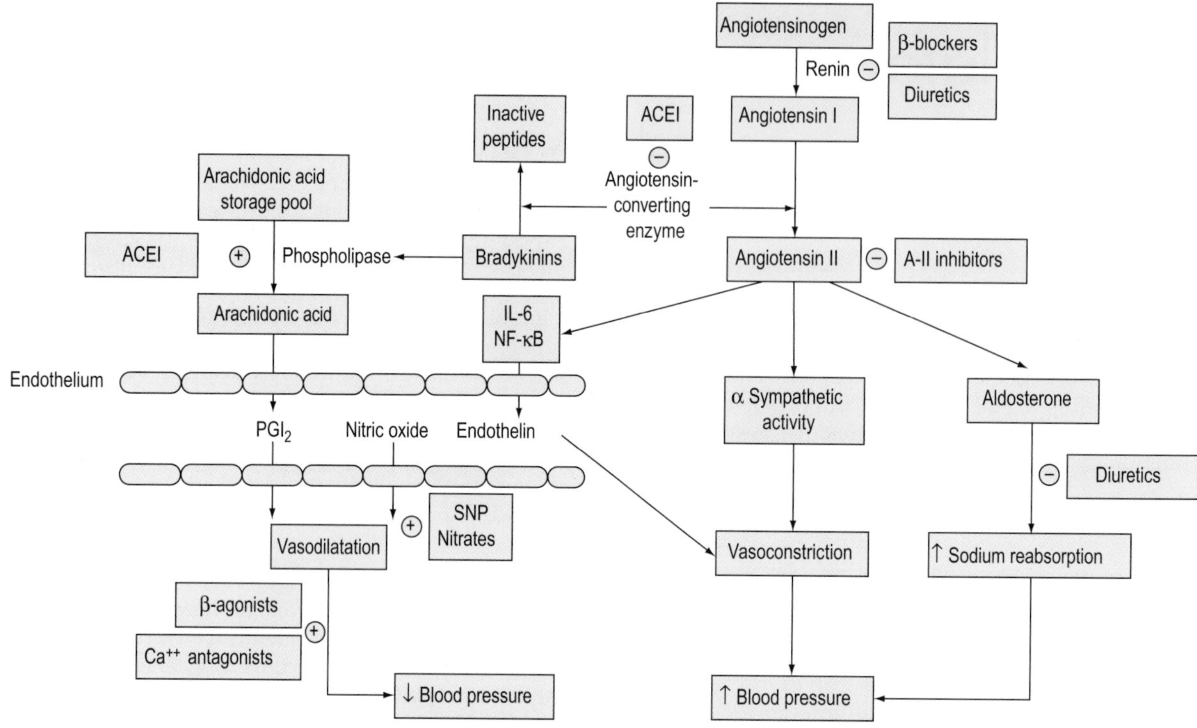

Figure 91.1 Schematic diagram of the neurohormonal factors determining vasomotor tone. Mechanism of action of vasodilators is shown by (–) for inhibition, (+) for stimulation. ACEI=angiotensin-converting enzyme inhibitors; A-II=angiotensin II; IL=interleukin; NF=nuclear factor; PGI_2=prostacyclin; SNP=sodium nitroprusside.

regulation, particularly exaggerated effects of renin-angiotensin activity.

Secondary causes of hypertension include structural abnormalities such as aortic stenosis or renal artery stenosis; endocrine conditions such as phaeochromocytoma, Cushing's syndrome and pregnancy-induced hypertension; and central causes such as hypertensive encephalopathy or raised intracranial pressure.

CALCIUM CHANNEL BLOCKERS

Calcium channel blockers have numerous effects on the cardiovascular system, influencing heart rate conduction, myocardial contractility and vasomotor tone. Entry of calcium through voltage-gated calcium channels is a major determinant of arteriolar, but not venous, tone.[6] Calcium channel blockers are recommended as first-step treatment for hypertension in Caucasian patients >55 years and Afro-Caribbean patients of any age.[7]

There are three major groups of calcium channel blockers that have different sites of action and thus different therapeutic effects: dihydropyridines (e.g. nifedipine, nimodipine, nicardipine, amlodipine, felodipine and clevidipine), phenylalkylamines (e.g. verapamil) and benzothiazepines (e.g. diltiazem).

Magnesium is a physiological calcium antagonist, and is used therapeutically as magnesium sulphate.

NIFEDIPINE

Nifedipine is a predominant arteriolar vasodilator, with minimal effect on venous capacitance vessels and no direct depressant effect on heart rate conduction.

It may be administered intravenously, orally or sublingually, and has a rapid onset of action (2–5 minutes) and duration of action of 20–30 minutes.

Nifedipine can be used to treat angina pectoris, especially that due to coronary artery vasospasm. Peripheral vasodilatation results in decreased systemic blood pressure, often associated with sympathetic stimulation resulting in increased cardiac output and heart rate, which may counter the negative inotropic, chronotropic and dromotropic effects of nifedipine. Nevertheless, nifedipine may be associated with profound hypotension in patients with ventricular dysfunction, aortic stenosis and/or concomitant beta blockade. For this reason, the use of sublingual nifedipine as a method of treating hypertensive emergencies is no longer recommended.[8]

Nifedipine and related drugs may cause diuretic-resistant peripheral oedema that is due to redistribution of extracellular fluid rather than sodium and water retention.

NIMODIPINE

Nimodipine is a highly lipid-soluble analogue of nifedipine. High lipid solubility facilitates entrance into the central nervous system where it causes selective cerebral arterial vasodilatation.

It may be used to attenuate cerebral arterial vasospasm following aneurysmal subarachnoid haemorrhage. Improved outcomes have been demonstrated in patients with Grade 1 and 2 subarachnoid haemorrhage.[9] Systemic hypotension may result from peripheral vasodilatation that may compromise cerebral blood flow in susceptible patients. Similarly, cerebral vasodilatation may increase intracranial pressure in patients with reduced intracranial elastance.

The recommended dose following aneurysmal subarachnoid haemorrhage is 60 mg orally 4-hourly, but it can be given at 30 mg 2-hourly to reduce variation in blood pressure. The use of intravenous nimodipine is not recommended owing to its profound effect on blood pressure.

AMLODIPINE

Amlodipine is an oral preparation that has a similar pharmacodynamic profile to nifedipine. In addition to arteriolar vasodilatory and cardiac effects, amlodipine has been shown to exert specific anti-inflammatory effects in hypertension, diabetic nephropathy and in modulating high-density lipoprotein (HDL) in patients with hypercholesterolaemia.[10] These effects have seen amlodipine increasingly being used for treatment of hypertension in high-risk patients, and may have a role in stable critically ill patients with associated comorbidities.

VERAPAMIL

The primary effect of verapamil is on the atrioventricular node and this drug is principally used as an antiarrhythmic for the treatment of supraventricular tachyarrhythmias. For this reason, concomitant therapy with beta blockers or digoxin is not recommended.

Verapamil is not as active as nifedipine in its effects on smooth muscle and it therefore causes less pronounced decrease in systemic blood pressure and is also negatively inotropic. It has a limited role as a vasodilator.[11]

DILTIAZEM

Diltiazem has a similar cardiovascular profile to verapamil, although its vasodilatory properties are intermediate between nifedipine and verapamil. Diltiazem exerts minimal cardiodepressant effects and is less likely to potentiate beta blockers.

MAGNESIUM SULPHATE

Magnesium regulates intracellular calcium and potassium levels by activation of membrane pumps and competition with calcium for transmembrane channels. Physiological effects are widespread, affecting cardiovascular, central and peripheral nervous systems and the musculoskeletal junction.[12]

It acts as a direct arteriolar and venous vasodilator causing reductions in blood pressure. Modulation of centrally mediated and peripheral sympathetic tone results in variable effects on cardiac output and heart rate.

Consequently, it has an established role in the treatment of pre-eclampsia and eclampsia,[13] perioperative management of phaeochromocytoma[14] and treatment of autonomic dysfunction in tetanus.[15] It has been proposed as a possible agent for the prevention of secondary ischaemia after aneurysmal subarachnoid haemorrhage; however, evidence of a benefit on outcome is still lacking.[16]

DIRECT-ACTING VASODILATORS

These drugs act directly on vascular smooth muscle and exert their effects predominantly by increasing the concentration of endothelial nitric oxide. These drugs are also known as nitrovasodilators.[17]

SODIUM NITROPRUSSIDE

Sodium nitroprusside is a non-selective vasodilator that causes relaxation of arterial and venous smooth muscle. It is compromised of a ferrous ion centre associated with five cyanide moieties and a nitrosyl group. The molecule is 44% cyanide by weight.

It is reconstituted from a powdered form. The solution is light sensitive so it requires protection from exposure to light (e.g. by wrapping administration sets in aluminium foil). Prolonged exposure to light may be associated with an increase in release of hydrogen cyanide, although this is seldom clinically significant.

When infused intravenously, sodium nitroprusside interacts with oxyhaemoglobin, dissociating immediately to form methaemoglobin while releasing free cyanide and nitric oxide. The latter is responsible for the vasodilatory effect of sodium nitroprusside.

Dosage is from 0.5 μg/kg/min to 8 μg/kg/min, but should always start at a low infusion rate and build up slowly.

Onset of action is almost immediate with a transient duration, requiring continuous intravenous infusion to maintain a therapeutic effect. Tachyphylaxis can occur and large doses should not be used if the desired therapeutic effect is not attained, as this may be associated with toxicity.

Sodium nitroprusside produces direct venous and arterial vasodilatation, resulting in a prompt decrease in systemic blood pressure. The effect on cardiac output is variable. Decreases in right atrial pressure reflect pooling of blood in the venous system, which may decrease cardiac output. This may result in reflex tachycardia that may oppose the overall reduction in blood pressure. In patients with left ventricular failure, the effect on cardiac output will depend on initial left ventricular end-diastolic pressure.

Sodium nitroprusside may potentially increase myocardial ischaemia in patients with coronary artery disease by causing an intracoronary steal of blood flow away from ischaemic areas by arteriolar vasodilatation. Secondary tachycardia may also exacerbate myocardial ischaemia.

Due to its non-selectivity, sodium nitroprusside has direct effects on most vascular beds. In the cerebral circulation, sodium nitroprusside is a cerebral vasodilator, leading to increases in cerebral blood flow and blood volume. This may be critical in patients with increased intracranial pressure. Rapid and profound reductions in mean arterial pressure produced by sodium nitroprusside may exceed the autoregulatory capacity of the brain to maintain adequate cerebral blood flow.

Sodium nitroprusside is a pulmonary vasodilator and may attenuate hypoxic pulmonary vasoconstriction, resulting in increased intrapulmonary shunting and decreased arterial oxygen tension. This phenomenon may be exacerbated by associated hypotension.

The prolonged use of large doses of sodium nitroprusside may be associated with toxicity related to the production and cyanide and, to a lesser extent, methaemoglobin.[18]

Free cyanide produced by the dissociation of sodium nitroprusside reacts with methaemoglobin to form cyanmethaemoglobin, or is metabolised by rhodenase in the liver and kidneys to form thiocyanate. A healthy adult can eliminate cyanide at a rate equivalent to a sodium nitroprusside infusion of 2 μg/kg per min or up to 10 μg/kg per min for 10 minutes, although there is marked inter-individual variability.

Toxicity should be of concern in patients who become resistant to sodium nitroprusside despite maximum infusion rates and who develop an unexplained lactic acidosis. In high doses, cyanide may cause seizures.

Treatment of suspected cyanide toxicity is cessation of the infusion and administration of 100% oxygen. Sodium thiosulphate (150 mg/kg) converts cyanide to thiocyanate, which is excreted renally. For severe cyanide toxicity, sodium nitrite may be infused (5 mg/kg) to produce methaemoglobin and subsequently cyanmethaemoglobin. Hydroxycobalamin, which binds cyanide to produce cyanocobalamin, may also be administered (5 g over 15 minutes, which may be repeated in severe cases).

GLYCERYL TRINITRATE

Glyceryl trinitrate is an organic nitrate that generates nitric oxide through a different mechanism from sodium nitroprusside.

The pharmacokinetics allows glyceryl trinitrate to be given by infusion, with a longer onset and duration of action than sodium nitroprusside. The intravenous dosage can start at 5 μg/min and increase incrementally to 200 μg/min (max dose 400 μg /min). Glyceryl trinitrate may also be administered sublingually, orally or transdermally.

Tachyphylaxis is common with glyceryl trinitrate; doses should not be increased if patients no longer respond to standard doses. Glass bottles or polyethylene administration sets are required as glyceryl trinitrate is absorbed into standard polyvinylchloride sets.

The effects on the peripheral vasculature are dose-dependent, acting principally on venous capacitance vessels to produce venous pooling and decreased ventricular preload. Together with furosemide, glyceryl trinitrate is particularly useful in treating acute cardiac failure and pulmonary oedema.

Glyceryl trinitrate primarily dilates larger conductance vessels of the coronary circulation, resulting in increased coronary blood flow to ischaemic subendocardial areas, thereby relieving angina pectoris. This is in contrast to sodium nitroprusside, which may cause a coronary steal phenomenon.

Reductions in blood pressure are more dependent on blood volume than with sodium nitroprusside. Precipitous falls in blood pressure may occur in hypovolaemic patients with small doses of glyceryl trinitrate. In euvolaemic patients, reflex tachycardia is not as pronounced as with sodium nitroprusside. At higher doses, arteriolar vasodilatation occurs without significant changes in calculated systemic vascular resistance. More recently glyceryl trinitrate has been suggested as one approach to improve microcirculatory flow in septic shock, but only after adequate fluid resuscitation.[19]

Glyceryl trinitrate is a cerebral vasodilator and should be used with caution in patients with known or suspected raised intracranial pressure. Headache due to this mechanism is a common side-effect in conscious patients.

ISOSORBIDE DINITRATE

Isosorbide dinitrate is the most commonly administered oral nitrate for the prophylaxis of angina pectoris. It has a physiological effect that lasts up to 6 hours in doses of 60–120 mg. The mechanism of action is the same as glyceryl trinitrate. Hypotension may follow acute administration, but tolerance to this develops with chronic therapy.[20]

HYDRALAZINE

Hydralazine is a potent, arterioselective, direct-acting vasodilator that acts via stimulation of cGMP and inhibition of smooth muscle myosin light chain kinase.

Following intravenous administration, 5–10 mg intravenously, hydralazine has a rapid onset of action, usually within 5–10 minutes. It can alternatively be given by continuous intravenous infusion, initially 200–300 μg/min and maintenance usually 50–150 μg/min, and may also be administered orally. The drug is partially metabolised by acetylation, for which there is marked inter-individual variability (35% of the population are slow acetylators). Although this does not have much clinical significance regarding the antihypertensive effects, it is important with respect to toxicity.[20]

Hydralazine causes predominantly arteriolar vasodilatation that is widespread but not uniform. It is associated with direct and reflex sympathetic activity, so that cardiac output and heart rate are increased. Prolonged use of hydralazine stimulates renin release and is associated with sodium and water retention. Consequently, hydralazine is frequently administered with beta blockers and/or diuretics.

Chronic use of hydralazine may be associated with immunological side-effects including lupus syndrome, vasculitis, haemolytic anaemia and rapidly progressive glomerulonephritis.

ALPHA-ADRENERGIC ANTAGONISTS

Several groups of compounds act as alpha-adrenergic blockers with variable affinity for populations of α-receptors. Physiology and pathophysiology may influence the responsiveness of the drug receptor–effector relationship. Receptor pathobiology is discussed in Chapter 90. Consequently, there may be marked inter- and intra-individual variability in the patient's response to these drugs.

There are six main groups of α-receptor antagonists: imidazolines (e.g. phentolamine), haloalkylamines (e.g. phenoxybenzamine), prazosin, beta-adrenergic antagonists with a receptor antagonism (labetalol, carvedilol), phenothiazines (chlorpromazine) and butyrophenones (haloperidol).

PHENTOLAMINE

Phentolamine is a non-selective, competitive antagonist at α_1- and α_2-receptors. At low doses, phentolamine causes prejunctional inhibition of norepinephrine (noradrenaline) release (via α_2-receptor inhibition). At higher doses, more complete α-receptor blockade is achieved, with enhancement of effects of beta agonists due to increased local concentration of norepinephrine produced by α_2-blockade (see Ch. 90, Fig. 90.3a).

Phentolamine is administered intravenously and may be given intermittently or by infusion. Onset is rapid (within 2 minutes), with a duration of action of 10–15 minutes.

Arteriolar and venous vasodilatation reduces systemic blood pressure. Effects on cardiac output are variable, and there is modest reflex sympathetic stimulation without significant increases in heart rate.

PHENOXYBENZAMINE

Phenoxybenzamine is a non-selective, non-competitive, α_1- and α_2-receptor antagonist. Blockade is also produced on histamine, serotonin and acetylcholine muscarinic receptors. Reuptake of norepinephrine is blocked, thereby potentiating the effects of beta agonists.

Phenoxybenzamine is usually administered orally, but may also be given intravenously (taking care to avoid extravasation as it is irritant to tissues). It has a long onset of action and prolonged duration of action (3–4 days). It causes a gradual reduction in systemic blood pressure, without rapid reflex sympathetic activity.

Prolonged use is associated with increased beta-adrenergic effects, predominantly increased heart rate, for which combination therapy with beta blockade is used. Phenoxybenzamine is primarily used in the management of phaeochromocytoma, either preoperatively or long term in inoperable patients. It may also be used to control autonomic hyperreflexia in patients with spinal cord transection.[21]

PRAZOSIN

Prazosin is a relatively arterioselective, competitive, α_1-receptor antagonist. It acts postjunctionally and therefore does not inhibit reuptake of norepinephrine. Consequently, it produces less tachycardia for a given reduction in systemic blood pressure.

It is administered orally and usually used for essential or renovascular (hyperreninaemia) hypertension. It is frequently used in combination with beta blockers and diuretics, particularly in patients with renal dysfunction.

LABETALOL

Labetalol is specific competitive antagonist at α_1-, β_1- and β_2-adrenergic receptors. Beta blockade effects predominate, with a approximate ratio of α_1:β-receptor blockade of 1:4–7. Labetalol has partial agonist effects on β_2-receptors.

It is administered intravenously (typically 10–50 mg), has a rapid onset of action (5–10 minutes) with a duration of 2–6 hours. It may be given by infusion (usually 15–180 mg/h).

Systemic blood pressure and cardiac output are reduced by a combination of negative inotropy, arterial and venous vasodilatation. Reflex tachycardia is attenuated by beta blockade. These properties make labetalol particularly useful in controlled hypotension during anaesthesia and surgery to reduce bleeding.

Side-effects such as bronchospasm and hyperkalaemia relate predominantly to beta blockade.

CARVEDILOL

Carvedilol is a non-selective beta blocker with α_1-antagonist activity. Most of the vasodilator activity relates to α_1-antagonism, although at high concentrations it also blocks calcium entry. The ratio of α_1:β-receptor blockade is 1:10.

It is administered orally; no intravenous preparation is available.

Recent studies have demonstrated slowing of progression of congestive cardiac failure and improved mortality, particularly when used in conjunction with ACE inhibitors in patients with mild to moderate cardiac failure.[22,23] It may also be used in patients who cannot be treated with ACE inhibitors.

HALOPERIDOL AND CHLORPROMAZINE

These drugs act as competitive α-receptor antagonists causing non-selective vasodilatation and blockade of norepinephrine reuptake.

These drugs are primarily used as major tranquillisers or antipsychotics; their effect on the peripheral vasculature should be regarded as a side-effect, rather than a specific therapeutic action.

Reduction of systemic blood pressure is variable and may be precipitous, particularly in hypovolaemic patients with high sympathetic drive. These drugs may be useful in neurogenic hypertension, and are not regarded as first-line vasodilators.

INODILATORS

Many inotropic drugs have peripheral vascular effects and these are discussed in more detail in Chapter 90.

At low doses, epinephrine, norepinephrine and dopamine are predominantly beta agonists and cause both arterial and venous vasodilatation, which may cause reductions in mean arterial pressure.

Dobutamine and isoprenaline are predominantly beta agonists and may cause decreases in mean arterial pressure, particularly in hypovolaemic patients or those with increased sympathetic drive. These agents may have a role in reducing left ventricular afterload in patients with systolic heart failure.

Milrinone is a selective type III phosphodiesterase inhibitor that prevents the breakdown of cAMP within cardiac and vascular tissues. The increased cAMP levels lead to increased levels of intracellular calcium and thus increased contraction of cardiac muscle. Within vascular smooth muscle the cAMP inhibits myosin light chain kinase producing less contraction and thus vascular relaxation.

Levosimendan is a newer calcium sensitiser that leads to a greater ventricular contraction for the same intracellular calcium concentration. It also leads to vasodilatation, mediated by activation of ATP-sensitive sarcolemmal and mitochondrial potassium channels. The drug itself has a relatively short half-life, but it has a long-acting active metabolite so that haemodynamic effects may be maintained for up to 7 days.

Both milrinone and levosimendan can lead to marked hypotension, particularly if a bolus dose is given. Therefore in critically ill patients a loading dose is best avoided and any excessive vasodilation may need to be balanced by a low dose of a vasoconstrictor. Usual infusion rates of milrinone are 0.375–0.75 μg/kg/min and levosimendan 0.05–0.2 μg/kg/min.

ANGIOTENSIN-CONVERTING ENZYME INHIBITORS

Angiotensin-converting enzyme (ACE) inhibition has become a cornerstone in the management of patients with hypertension, cardiac failure and ischaemic heart disease.[24,25] They are now recommended as first-stage treatment for hypertension in Caucasian patients <55 years and patients with diabetic nephropathy.[7] These drugs act by non-selective, competitive, irreversible inhibition to the angiotensin I binding site thus reducing conversion to angiotensin II.

There are a very large number of ACE inhibitors on the market with very high penetration into the ambulant patient population. These drugs are administered orally; there are no routinely used parenteral preparations. Consequently, many critically ill patients admitted to the ICU may be taking ACE inhibitors. As a general rule, ACE inhibitors are stopped in most critically ill patients until vital organ (specifically renal) function is stabilised and the patient can take them enterally. Thereafter, doses are gradually increased over time with close monitoring of renal function.

PREPARATIONS

Captopril has a short half-life and therefore may be useful for initiating treatment within the ICU. It is administered orally in increasing doses and intervals to a maximum dose of 50 mg 8-hourly. It may be administered sublingually in acute hypertension (5–25 mg), with an onset of action in 20–30 minutes, and duration of 4 hours. There are no significant differences in the cardiovascular effects between captopril and other preparations.

Enalapril is a prodrug, effective by hepatic metabolism to enalaprilat, producing a slower and more controlled action. It is administered orally in 5 mg increments to a total of 20 mg twice daily.

Lisinopril has the advantage of single daily dosing and may be useful in stable critically ill patients.

CARDIOVASCULAR EFFECTS

The cardiovascular effects of ACE inhibition are widespread, with effects that influence the peripheral vasculature, cardiac performance, and salt and water homeostasis. Consequently, ACE inhibitors are not principally regarded as vasodilators, although they have both direct and indirect effects on the peripheral vasculature.

Increased production of endothelial vasodilators such as prostacyclin and decreased production of endothelin by angiotensin result in generalised venous and arteriolar vasodilatation. This occurs in the absence of reflex sympathetic activity or changes in heart rate, due to the modulation of adrenergic stimulation. Systemic blood pressure is reduced without changes in cardiac output or heart rate.

ACE inhibition is associated with improved myocardial performance following acute myocardial infarction due to left ventricular remodelling and improvement in neurohumoral activation. These drugs have been shown to improve survival following myocardial infarction in patients with left ventricular dysfunction.[26]

'First-dose hypotension' is described in patients receiving ACE inhibitors for the first time. This may occur particularly in patients who are salt- and water-depleted, or those who develop sensitivity to the drug. Drug sensitivity may also present as a sudden decrease in renal function following commencement of the drug (see below).

RENOVASCULAR EFFECTS

ACE inhibitors may cause renal failure, particularly in patients with renovascular disease, hyperreninaemic hypertension and acute kidney injury. The renal effects of ACE inhibitors may be potentiated by diuretics, non-steroidal anti-inflammatory drugs and beta blockers. ACE inhibitors are contraindicated in patients with bilateral renal artery stenosis.

As a rule in intensive care patients, ACE inhibitors are started in suitable patients once renal function has stabilised and the patient no longer requires inotropic support. Initial doses should be low and increased as tolerated.

SIDE-EFFECTS AND TOXICITY

In addition to renal dysfunction, ACE inhibitors may be associated with a number of side-effects. The most common of these is cough, which is due to the increased production of kinins.[27]

Severe angioneurotic oedema causing upper-airway obstruction may occur with all ACE inhibitors, although this is less common with enalapril and lisinopril. This is due to increased activation of bradykinins. ACE inhibitors are contraindicated in patients with a history of hereditary or idiopathic angioneurotic oedema[28] and should be avoided in pregnancy.

Neutropenia and agranulocytosis are uncommon but potentially lethal side-effects in susceptible patients.

ANGIOTENSIN RECEPTOR BLOCKERS

These are a newer class of antihypertensive drugs that cause irreversible, selective blockade of angiotensin II at AT_1 receptors.[29,30]

Losartan is the prototype, which has been followed by newer compounds such as irbesartan, valsartan and telmisartan. These drugs are oral preparations; there is no parenteral form.

The cardiovascular profile of angiotensin receptor blockers is similar to the ACE inhibitors, but selective blockade of angiotensin II offers several possible advantages over ACE inhibitors. These drugs are long-acting and may be given once daily; onset of action is slow, thereby avoiding first-dose hypotension; side-effects such as cough and angioneurotic oedema are less common.[31] Angiotensin receptor blockers may be used as an alternative to ACE inhibitors but they should not be combined.[7]

CENTRALLY ACTING AGENTS

These agents modulate adrenergic stimulation at central nervous system and spinal cord level. The vasomotor centre of the medulla mainly controls sympathetic pressor influences, although other brainstem, midbrain and spinal centres have a role.

Most central responses are mediated through α_2-adrenergic receptors, which modulate the release and reuptake of norepinephrine, with subsequent effects on the peripheral vasculature and cardiac function.

CLONIDINE

Clonidine is a centrally acting α_2-agonist that stimulates inhibitory neurons in the vasomotor centre. This results in a reduction in sympathetic outflow from the central nervous system and is associated with negative inotropy and reduction in heart rate. Systemic blood pressure is reduced by this mechanism, with associated arteriolar and venous vasodilatation. Clonidine has centrally acting analgesic properties, which make it a suitable drug in patients with postoperative hypertension.

Peripherally, it stimulates prejunctional α_2-receptors, thereby decreasing norepinephrine release, but may also have an effect at postjunctional α_1-receptors, causing vasoconstriction. This may present as rebound hypertension following initial reduction of blood pressure, as there is variable duration of the central and peripheral effects.

Clonidine can be administered orally (50–100 μg 8-hourly) or by intravenous injection (25–150 μg) or by infusion (maximum 750 μg in 24 hours). It has a rapid onset of action (5–10 minutes) and duration of action of 20–30 minutes.

METHYLDOPA

Methyldopa acts as a centrally acting 'false' transmitter following metabolism to methylnorepinephrine and subsequent stimulation of α_2-receptors leading to reduced sympathetic outflow, although the precise mechanism is not clear.

It has a limited role in hypertensive emergencies, but is useful in accelerated essential, renovascular and pregnancy-induced hypertension.

It is administered orally in doses of 250 mg to 3 g per day although side-effects (abnormal function, depression) may be minimised if the daily dose is <1 g. It may lead to a positive direct Coombs test in 20% of patients.

OTHER ANTIHYPERTENSIVE AGENTS

BETA-ADRENERGIC ANTAGONISTS

Beta blockers have been used for the treatment of hypertension for over 30 years and have an increasingly important role in the management of cardiac failure.[32–34] Although no longer recommended as first-step treatment of hypertension they may be used if ACE inhibitors are poorly tolerated.[7]

In addition to decreasing heart rate and contractility, beta blockers have other neurohumoral effects that affect vascular tone. These relate to inhibition of renin release from juxtaglomerular cells (see Fig. 91.1) and prejunctional inhibition of norepinephrine that result in reduction in vascular tone and blood pressure. A central effect of beta blockers has also been proposed.

The mode of action has been described in terms of selectivity to blockade of beta-adrenergic receptors (β_1 and/or β_2). While this is an appropriate pharmacological distinction, the clinical activity of these drugs is not as predictable due to mixed populations of β_1- and β_2-receptors in most organs and variable receptor responsiveness in physiological and pathophysiological conditions. Consequently, there is marked inter-individual variability in the response to these drugs. In high-enough doses, whether intentionally or due to toxicity, all beta blockers will cause generalised antagonism with resultant therapeutic and toxic effects.

Lipid-soluble beta blockers include propranolol and metoprolol, which are predominantly excreted by the liver; atenolol and sotalol are water-soluble and predominantly renally excreted, warranting caution with these drugs in patients with renal dysfunction.

Beta blockers may be given orally or intravenously. As there is significant first-pass metabolism, doses for oral and intravenous administration are markedly different.

Esmolol is an intravenous beta blocker that is rapidly metabolised by red cell esterases and is therefore not dependent on renal or hepatic function. Its rapid onset of action and short duration allow infusion of drug, making it a useful drug in patients with acute hypertensive states associated with tachycardia. Labetalol and carvedilol are discussed above.

Beta blockers are frequently used as adjuncts to vasodilators in the treatment of hypertensive emergencies and states, particularly where reflex tachycardia and sympathetic stimulation occur (e.g. hydralazine, nifedipine and prazosin).

Side-effects and toxicity of beta blockers include bradycardia (which may be profound), hypotension, bronchoconstriction (caution in patients who have asthma), aggravation of peripheral vascular ischaemia, hyperkalaemia and masking of the sympathetic response to hypoglycaemia.

DIURETICS

As with beta blockers, diuretics have an established place in the management of hypertension. In addition to their effects on salt and water excretion and inhibition of aldosterone, direct vasodilatory effects are associated with diuretics such as furosemide and the thiazides.

These drugs have a rapid venodilatory action, which may be due to inhibition of norepinephrine-activated chloride channels on veins. Reductions of blood pressure and right atrial pressure may occur following low doses, and may present before an associated diuresis.

All diuretics should be used with caution in patients with renal dysfunction and avoided if hypovolaemia is present or suspected.

PULMONARY VASODILATORS

Pulmonary vasodilators may be used in the ICU mainly to treat acute right-sided heart failure commonly after cardiac surgery/transplantation. Many of the systemic vasodilators detailed above (namely calcium channel blockers, sodium nitroprusside and nitrates) will also have vasodilatory effects within the pulmonary circulation. Specific pulmonary vasodilators may be inhaled or administered intravenously.

NITRIC OXIDE

As detailed above, nitric oxide (NO) is an endogenous vasodilator. When inhaled it leads to vasodilation in only the ventilated areas of the lung, and rapid combination with haemoglobin prevents systemic vasodilation. This may improve ventilation–perfusion mismatch resulting in an improved oxygenation but controlled trials have not demonstrated any beneficial effect on outcomes in severe acute lung injury and it may have an adverse effect on kidney function.[35] Its use is now mainly confined to treatment of acute pulmonary hypertension post cardiac surgery.

NO is oxidated to NO_2 particularly in a high-oxygen environment and therefore NO_2 levels should be carefully monitored. Similarly appropriate scavenging systems must be employed.

Rebound pulmonary hypertension may occur and so NO therapy should be slowly weaned rather than abruptly stopped.

PROSTACYCLIN

Inhaled epoprostenol or iloprost (a prostacyclin derivative) can be used as alternatives to NO. Care should be taken to avoid systemic hypotension.

SILDENAFIL

Sildenafil is a phosphodiesterase type 5 inhibitor used in the management of chronic pulmonary hypertension, as well as erectile dysfunction. There are reports of its use for acute pulmonary hypertension within the ICU and that it can improve haemodynamics, however, by increasing shunt fraction it might worsen oxygenation when used in acute lung injury.[36]

DRUG SELECTION

The clinical use of vasodilators in intensive care is different from their use in ambulatory patients. In the critically ill patient, these drugs are primarily used to control acute rises in mean arterial pressure associated with sympathetic stimulation, or as specific treatment of hypertensive emergencies.[37]

The ideal vasodilator is therefore one that has a rapid and predictable onset of action, allows titration to achieve a desired systemic blood pressure, does not compromise cardiac output, does not cause significant reflex tachycardia and is non-toxic.

The selection of drug to treat hypertensive states will depend on the predominant cause of hypertension and the mechanism of action in the homeostatic pathway (outlined in Fig. 91.1).

There are no large studies investigating optimum therapy in patients presenting with hypertensive emergencies. These conditions occur in a heterogeneous group of patients and drug selection is essentially determined by the underlying pathophysiology, personal preference and experience.[37]

MONITORING

The principles of haemodynamic monitoring in patients receiving vasoactive drugs are outlined in Chapter 90.

Patients with severe hypertension or those receiving infusions or doses of potent vasodilators such as sodium nitroprusside and glyceryl trinitrate must be monitored via an intra-arterial catheter. Non-invasive measurement devices are not rapid or accurate enough and are not recommended in patients with hypertensive emergencies.

As peripheral vasodilators have significant effects on both the arterial and venous systems, assessment of volume status is important. In the majority of patients, establishing a euvolaemic state is essential before commencing a vasodilator.

DOSAGES AND DRUG ADMINISTRATION

Vasodilators administered via infusion are delivered through a dedicated central venous catheter using infusion pumps or syringe drivers and titrated to achieve a target mean arterial pressure. Infusion lines should be free of injection portals and clearly marked with identifying labels. Common drug doses are shown in **Table 91.1**.

SPECIFIC SITUATIONS

The following is a summary of the clinical uses of the above drugs in hypertensive states commonly encountered in the ICU. Specific pharmacology and physiological effects are discussed above.

ACUTE HYPERTENSION

The most common cause of hypertension in intensive care patients is pain or agitation, particularly in postoperative patients. It is important that patients have adequate analgesia and sedation before antihypertensives or vasodilators are used. Other common causes of hypertension include hypothermia, urinary retention, positional discomfort and omission of pre-admission antihypertensives, particularly beta blockers. The majority of instances of acute hypertension in the ICU will respond to simple measures addressing the above.[38]

Sustained hypertension may be treated acutely with incremental doses or infusions of short-acting drugs such as glyceryl trinitrate, sodium nitroprusside, labetalol, hydralazine, nifedipine or clonidine. Infusions of vasodilators may be required if hypertension persists, or if the patient in unable to take longer-acting oral agents such as prazosin or amlodipine. Hypertension associated with tachycardia may be treated with beta blockers.

HYPERTENSIVE ENCEPHALOPATHY

Hypertensive encephalopathy is defined as an acute organic brain syndrome occurring as a result of failure of cerebrovascular autoregulation. There may be differences in the degree of hypertension that cause encephalopathy and it may be the rate of increase of blood pressure that is more important than the absolute value. It may present as confusion, visual disturbances, blindness, seizures or stroke. Uncontrolled hypertension is

Table 91.1 Dose and infusion concentrations of commonly used vasodilators and antihypertensives in intensive care

AGENT	INFUSION/DOSE	CAUTION
Sodium nitroprusside	Diluted in 5% dextrose; range 0.5–8 μg/kg/min	Cyanide toxicity (> total dose 0.5 mg/kg per 24 hours) Photodegradation Raised intracranial pressure Rebound hypotension Shunt and oxygen desaturation
Glyceryl trinitrate	Diluted in 5% dextrose; range 5–200 μg/min	Drug binding to polyvinylchloride Tachyphylaxis Raised intracranial pressure
Hydralazine	10–20 mg i.v. bolus 20–50 mg 6–8-hourly	Tachycardia Myocardial ischaemia
Phentolamine	1–10 mg i.v. boluses 5–30 mg/h infusion	Tachycardia
Phenoxybenzamine	Oral: 10 mg/day until postural hypotension i.v.: 1 mg/kg per day	Idiosyncratic hypotension
Prazosin	2–10 mg/day, 8-hourly	
Nifedipine	5–10 mg oral/sublingual	Precipitous hypotension
Amlodipine	5–10 mg oral/day	Caution in renal impairment
Captopril	6.25–50 mg orally, 8-hourly Acute hypertension: 6.5–25 mg sublingually p.r.n.	Caution in renovascular hypertension and renal failure Pregnancy Angioneurotic oedema
Enalapril	5–20 mg/day	
Enalaprilat	0.625–5 mg bolus	Caution in renal failure and hypovolaemia
Losartan	25–100 mg/day	Caution in renal failure
Clonidine	25–150 μg i.v. bolus	Acute, perioperative centrally mediated hypertension May cause rebound hypertension with chronic use
Atenolol	1–10 mg i.v. boluses 25–100 mg oral b.d.	Caution in poor left ventricular function, asthma Hyperkalaemia Potentiated in renal failure
Metoprolol	50–100 mg 12-hourly; 5 mg i.v. bolus	As for atenolol, safe in renal failure
Esmolol	Loading dose 0.5 mg/kg 50–200 μg/kg/min infusion	
Labetalol	10–50 mg i.v. boluses 0.5–4 mg/min infusion	
Magnesium sulphate	40–60 mg/kg loading (or 6 g) 2–4 g/h infusion	Maintain serum magnesium >1.5–2 mmol/L

one of the causes of the posterior reversible encephalopathy syndrome (PRES), along with pre-eclampsia, immunosuppressant drugs and sepsis. If not adequately treated, hypertensive encephalopathy may result in intracerebral haemorrhage, coma or death.[39]

Hypertensive encephalopathy may occur in patients with untreated or undertreated hypertension or in association with other diseases such as renal disease (e.g. glomerulonephritis, renovascular disease), thrombotic thrombocytopenic purpura, immunosuppressive therapy, collagen vascular diseases or eclampsia. Consequently, drug treatment will depend on the context in which it occurs. It is also important to rule out other causes of neurological deterioration that may also present with hypertension (e.g. stroke, intracranial haemorrhage or space-occupying lesion).

There is no evidence from randomised controlled trials to conclude one therapy is superior to another at improving outcomes. The aim of drug therapy in these patients is to reduce blood pressure in a controlled, predictable and safe way. Acutely, short-acting, titratable parenteral drugs are suitable in emergency situations. Assuming there are no absolute contraindications to beta blockers, labetalol and esmolol are ideal drugs to use. Sodium nitroprusside can be used although it may increase intracranial pressure and reduce cerebral blood flow. Phentolamine may be equally effective.[8,36]

Other agents that are useful in controlling severe hypertension include hydralazine, clonidine and ACE inhibitors (although these must be used cautiously in patients with associated renal dysfunction). Severe drops in blood pressure that might compromise end-organ perfusion have been reported after the use of nifedipine and therefore its use in the emergency setting is not recommended.[8] Combination therapy is often required, although this should be done with caution to minimise additive effects with resultant hypotension.

Patients with hypertensive emergencies are frequently hypovolaemic due to excessive sympathetic stimulation. In the absence of left ventricular failure, judicious fluid replacement may reduce blood pressure and improve renal function, thereby minimising precipitous hypotension that may result following administration of some drugs. Diuretics are generally avoided in these conditions unless there is evidence of left ventricular failure.[40]

ACUTE STROKE

Acute stroke syndromes frequently occur in the setting of severe hypertension. The reduction of mean arterial pressure must be balanced by the maintenance of adequate cerebral perfusion pressure and cerebral blood flow. Ischaemic brain is vulnerable to critical reductions in cerebral blood flow, while excessive mean arterial pressure may increase the risk of cerebral haemorrhage.[41]

Acutely, blood pressure should be maintained in a normal range until intracranial pathology has been identified by CT scan. Aggressive reduction in blood pressure is not recommended in patients with ischaemic stroke, whilst hypertension in patients with aneurysmal subarachnoid haemorrhage or intracranial haemorrhage may be managed by drugs outlined above.

AORTIC DISSECTION

Aortic dissection is the most dramatic and most rapidly fatal complication of severe hypertension. The aim of medical treatment is to control blood pressure and left ventricular ejection velocity to minimise propagation of the dissection. Blood pressure should be decreased as rapidly as possible to a normal or slightly hypotensive level. Titrations are usually made to achieve systolic blood pressures of 100–110 mmHg or mean arterial pressure of 55–65 mmHg. This will depend on the patient's premorbid blood pressure and the accuracy of blood pressure measurement. It is important to maintain blood pressure at levels compatible with adequate cerebral and renal perfusion.[42]

This is best achieved initially by use of opioid analgesia, intravenous beta blockers (e.g. esmolol, labetalol or atenolol), and possibly adding a vasodilator such as sodium nitroprusside or glyceryl trinitrate. Tachycardia must be avoided as this is a significant determinant of aortic shear force that may exacerbate the dissection. Verapamil or diltiazem are suitable alternatives for patients who have a contraindication to beta blockade.

Aortic dissection distal to the left subclavian artery is managed conservatively with antihypertensive therapy. Proximal dissections are managed surgically after acute control of blood pressure.

ACUTE MYOCARDIAL ISCHAEMIA

Myocardial ischaemia in the absence of obstructive coronary atherosclerosis may be precipitated by severe hypertension. This occurs by increased left ventricular wall stress, reduced preload, tachycardia and increased myocardial metabolic demand. Severe ischaemia may result in acute left ventricular failure.

Intravenous glyceryl trinitrate is useful in this situation and may be used in combination with beta blockers such as esmolol, labetalol or carvedilol.

ACE inhibitors may be used in the acute situation and may be required for longer-term treatment.

PHAEOCHROMOCYTOMA

Tumours of the adrenal medulla secrete catecholamines that result in initial paroxysmal, then sustained, severe hypertension. They may present to the ICU as a hypertensive emergency or perioperatively for surgical ablation.[43]

Acute hypertensive crises associated with phaeochromocytoma are managed with incremental doses or infusions of phentolamine. Untreated patients may be significantly hypovolaemic and may require judicious volume replacement. Beta blockers should not be used in the acute setting as these will potentiate unopposed alpha-adrenergic stimulation.

Phenoxybenzamine forms the mainstay of treatment and preparation for surgery. This is commenced in 20–30 mg increments and continued until blood pressure is controlled. Excessive beta-adrenergic effects are treated with beta blockers only after sufficient alpha blockade with phenoxybenzamine.[21]

Magnesium sulphate is useful in the perioperative management of phaeochromocytoma. It is given by infusion at 2–4 g/hour.[14]

RENAL FAILURE

Renal insufficiency may be a cause or consequence of a hypertensive emergency. Patients on haemodialysis (particularly those receiving erythropoietin therapy) and renal transplant patients (especially those receiving ciclosporin or corticosteroids) commonly present with severe hypertension. In patients with new-onset renal failure accompanying severe hypertension, blood pressure must be controlled without potentiating renal dysfunction. Drugs such as calcium channel blockers, phentolamine or prazosin may preserve renal blood flow and are appropriate in these patients. ACE inhibitors and diuretics should be used with caution until renal function has stabilised or improved.

Patients in the recovery phase of acute renal failure are usually hypertensive. This is a normal physiological response and should not be treated unless there is associated myocardial or cerebral ischaemia.[44]

PRE-ECLAMPSIA AND ECLAMPSIA

In addition to delivery of the baby and placenta, parenteral magnesium sulphate is the treatment of choice to prevent the evolution of pre-eclampsia to eclampsia (seizures and deteriorating encephalopathy[13]). The recommended drugs for the treatment of severe hypertension in critically ill women during pregnancy or soon after birth include labetalol, hydralazine and nifedipine.[45]

ACE inhibitors and angiotensin receptor blockers are contraindicated in pregnancy. This is discussed in Chapter 63.

DRUG INTERACTIONS

Severe rebound hypertension may result following abrupt cessation of antihypertensive treatment. Drugs associated with this discontinuation syndrome include clonidine, methyldopa, beta blockers, guanethidine and diuretics. The degree of rebound depends on the rapidity of drug withdrawal, dosage, renovascular and cardiac function. Antihypertensives should be reintroduced according to the status of the patient and the degree of hypertension managed accordingly.

Interaction with monoamine oxidase inhibitors and drugs such as indirect sympathomimetics, narcotics and tyramine-containing foods may result in a hypertensive emergency. This is best managed acutely with alpha and/or beta blockers.

Access the complete references list online at http://www.expertconsult.com

7. National Institute for Health and Clinical Excellence. Hypertension – The Clinical Management of Primary Hypertension. 2011. Online. Available: http://guidance.nice.org.uk/CG127.
8. Marik PE, Varon J. Hypertensive crises: challenges and management. Chest 2007;131:1949–62.
40. Vaughan CJ, Delanty N. Hypertensive emergencies. Lancet 2000;356:411–17.
41. Sokol SI, Kapoor JR, Foody JM. Blood pressure reduction in the primary and secondary prevention of stroke. Curr Vasc Pharmacol 2006;4:155–60.
42. Ahmad F, Cheshire N, Hamady M. Acute aortic syndrome: pathology and therapeutic strategies. Postgrad Med J 2006;82:305–12.
45. National Collaborating Centre for Women's and Children's Health. Hypertension in pregnancy – the management of hypertensive disorders in pregnancy. 2011. Online. Available: http://guidance.nice.org.uk/CG107.

Part Fourteen

Metabolic Homeostasis

92

Acid–base balance and disorders

Thomas J Morgan

THEORETICAL CONSIDERATIONS

Optimal enzyme action in the cell cytosol and organelles requires tight control of proton activity. Although intracellular acid–base status can be tracked using magnetic resonance imaging, this is impractical. Physicians must therefore interpret extracellular data, usually via tests on arterial blood, knowing that plasma pH exceeds intracellular pH by an average of 0.6 pH units.

WATER DISSOCIATION AND ACID–BASE

Mammals are approximately 60% water. Stewart reminded us of the central role of water in aqueous acid–base equilibria.[1,2] In simple terms, water dissociates as follows:

$$H_2O \leftrightarrow H^+ + OH^-$$

By the Law of Mass Action, at any equilibrium $[H^+][OH^-] = Kw\ [H_2O]$, where Kw is the temperature-dependent dissociation constant. The concentration of water ($[H_2O] = 55.5$ M) exceeds that of its two dissociation products by several orders of magnitude ($[H^+] = 160$ nM at 37°C). Thus water acts as a vast reservoir for protons and hydroxyl ions. Because of its numeric predominance, $[H_2O]$ can be combined with Kw to form a new constant, K'w. The equilibrium equation then simplifies to:

$$[H^+][OH^-] = K'w \qquad (92.1)$$

pH AND ACID–BASE NEUTRALITY

The negative logarithm of the proton concentration, or more exactly proton 'activity', is termed 'pH'. In aqueous solutions, neutrality occurs when $[H^+] = [OH^-]$, so that $([H^+])^2 = K'w$. Thus neutral pH = 0.5 pK'w. At 37°C, neutral pH is 6.8. Of note, this is the normal mean intracellular pH, whereas the pH of the surrounding extracellular fluid is usually >7.3, which is relatively alkaline.

THE Pa_{CO_2}/pH RELATIONSHIP IS THE ACID–BASE 'WINDOW' FOR CLINICIANS

About 15 moles of CO_2 are generated daily by aerobic metabolism. CO_2 travels from its intracellular source (P_{CO_2} >50 mmHg (6.65 kPa)) down a series of partial pressure gradients to the atmosphere (P_{CO_2} = 0.3 mmHg (0.04 kPa)). The primary exit point is the lungs, where transit is facilitated by a large, perpetually refreshed blood–air interface. En route CO_2 equilibrates with all aqueous environments, in which the P_{CO_2} is an equilibrium value determined by regional CO_2 production, regional blood flow, alveolar perfusion and alveolar ventilation.

Clinicians use the relationship between arterial P_{CO_2} (Pa_{CO_2}) and arterial pH as their primary acid–base assessment platform. This is appropriate, because the acute Pa_{CO_2}/pH curve is a fundamental physiological property (**Fig. 92.1**). Several factors determine the shape and position of this curve.

THE Pa_{CO_2}/pH RELATIONSHIP IS DEFINED BY SEVERAL SIMULTANEOUS EQUATIONS

In all body fluids pH is a function of water dissociation modified by CO_2, other weak acids and certain electrolytes. Final equilibria obey the Laws of Mass Action, Mass Conservation, and Electrical Neutrality. In addition, non-diffusible (impermeant) ions trigger electrochemical forces known as Gibbs Donnan forces across semipermeable membranes. These influence the acid–base result.

Therefore several equations in addition to equation 92.1 must be satisfied at any equilibrium. They relate to:

1. *The interaction of carbon dioxide and water:*

   $$CO_2 + H_2O \leftrightarrow H_2CO_3 \leftrightarrow H^+ + HCO_3^-$$

   By applying the Law of Mass Action and substituting [dissolved CO_2] for $[H_2CO_3]$, the following expression is derived:

   $$pH = 6.1 + \log_{10}([HCO_3^-] / \alpha P_{CO_2}) \qquad (92.2)$$

   This is the Henderson–Hasselbalch equation, where α is the plasma CO_2 solubility coefficient (0.03), and 6.1 is the pKa, the negative logarithm of the dissociation constant.
2. *Bicarbonate dissociation:* carbonate is present in micromolar concentrations only:

   $$[H^+][CO_3^{2-}] = Keq\,[HCO_3^-] \qquad (92.3)$$

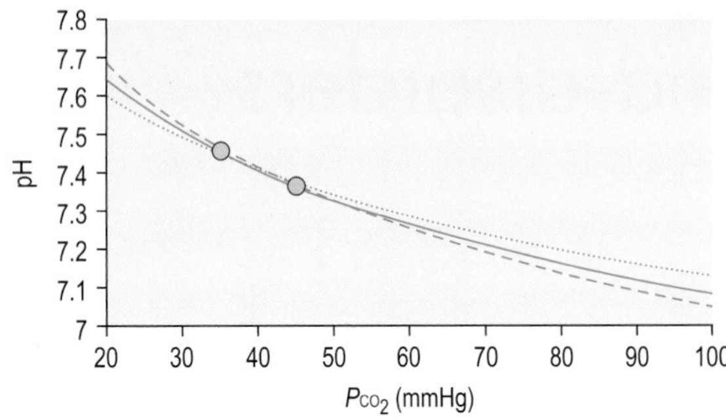

Figure 92.1 P_{CO_2}/pH relationships. The solid line shows the normal in vivo Pa_{CO_2}/pH relationship. The normal Pa_{CO_2} range is between the filled circles. To the left of the circles there is an increasing acute respiratory alkalosis, and to the right an increasing acute respiratory acidosis. The interrupted curve represents the normal in vitro whole-blood relationship, and the dotted curve is the same relationship for separated plasma. A point of commonality exists at P_{CO_2} = 40 mmHg (5.32 kPa).

3. *Non-volatile weak acid dissociation:* fluid compartments have varying concentrations of non-volatile (non-CO_2-generating) molecules possessing weak acid properties. Like all weak acids the overall negative charge of these molecules alters with pH. In plasma, they consist mainly of albumin and inorganic phosphate. In red cells haemoglobin predominates. Interstitial fluid contains much smaller concentrations, primarily phosphate. For convenience Stewart modelled all non-volatile weak acids as having a single anionic form (A^-) and a single conjugate base form (HA).

$$HA \leftrightarrow H^+ + A^-$$

By applying the Law of Mass Action:

$$[H^+][A^-] = KeqHA \quad (92.4)$$

4. *The Law of Mass Conservation:* Stewart termed the total concentration of non-volatile weak acids in any compartment 'A_{tot}', where:

$$A_{tot} = [HA] + [A^-] \quad (92.5)$$

A_{tot} is an imposed mass constant. It does not vary with pH. A pH change merely shifts the balance between HA and A^-.

5. *The Law of Electrical Neutrality:* linked to Stewart's concept of strong ion difference.[1,2] Certain elements in body fluids such as Na^+, K^+, Ca^{2+}, Mg^{2+} and Cl^- exist as completely ionised entities. At physiological pH they include anions with pKa values ≤4, for example sulphate, lactate and beta-hydroxybutyrate. Stewart described these compounds as 'strong ions'. In body fluids there is a surfeit of strong cations, which he referred to as the 'strong ion difference' (SID). In other words, SID = [strong cations] − [strong anions]. Being a 'charge' space, SID is expressed in mEq/L. SID calculated from measured strong ions in normal plasma is 42 mEq/L.

Hence, by the Law of Electrical Neutrality:

$$SID + [H^+] - [HCO_3^-] - [CO_3^{2-}] - [A^-] - [OH^-] = 0 \quad (92.6)$$

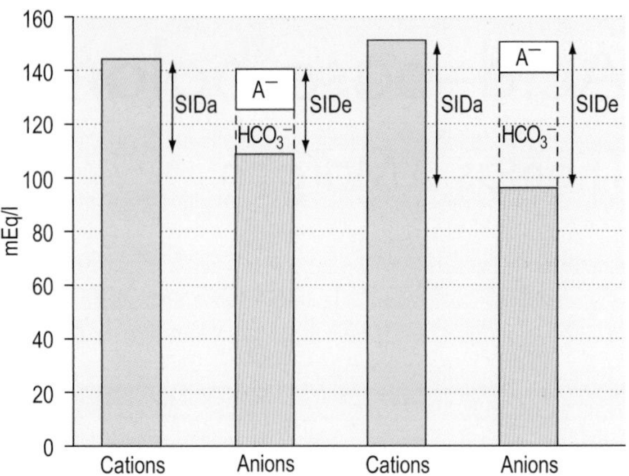

Figure 92.2 Gamblegrams of plasma strong and weak ions (in vitro data from CO_2 equilibrated normal blood). On the left, P_{CO_2} < 20 mmHg (2.66 kPa). On the right, the same blood with P_{CO_2} > 200 mmHg (26.6 kPa). The transition from hypocapnia to hypercapnia increases SIDa, with ionic redistribution between red cells and plasma due to altered Gibbs Donnan forces. There are almost identical increases in SIDe ($[A^-] + [HCO_3^-]$), also known as 'buffer base', although $[A^-]$ actually falls. Note that the SIG, which is SIDa − SIDe, remains close to zero.

6. *Gibbs Donnan forces:* impermeant ions influence equilibria across semipermeable membranes, causing redistribution of permeant ions to balance electrical and concentration gradients. The plasma compartment (volume 3 L), erythrocyte compartment (volume 2 L) and interstitial space (volume 13.5 L) contain different concentrations of impermeant anions, mainly albumin or haemoglobin. The highest concentration occurs within erythrocytes, in which negatively charged haemoglobin molecules attract diffusible cations (such as Na^+, K^+) from the adjacent plasma compartment while repelling diffusible anions (primarily Cl^-). To prevent cell swelling and haemolysis sodium, potassium and other cations are continually redistributed against the Donnan forces by energy-dependent transmembrane pumps. Importantly chloride, the major anion, remains susceptible to Donnan effects.

Because there are differing compartmental concentrations of impermeant weak acids a pH change causes differential charge alterations driving further redistributions, mainly chloride, between compartments. The net effect is that plasma SID goes up and down with Pa_{CO_2} (**Fig. 92.2**), the origin of the so-called Hamburger effect. Ionic shifts appear largely confined within the contiguous space occupied by the interstitial fluid (I), plasma (P) and erythrocytes (E) (the IPE space).[3] In other words SID_{IPE} does not alter with P_{CO_2}, a phenomenon underpinning the CO_2 - invariance of standard base excess - see below.

At equilibrium, equations 92.1 to 92.6 plus the Donnan equilibria must be satisfied. In the Stewart physical chemical model,[2] direct manipulation of pH, HCO_3^-, CO_3^{2-}, A^- and OH^- is impossible. Their values can be altered only indirectly via three independent variables imposed on but not controlled by the system. These are Pa_{CO_2}, which is externally regulated by alveolar ventilation, SID (more precisely SID_{IPE}, immune to Gibbs Donnan forces) and A_{totIPE}.

Thus for any individual the Pa_{CO_2}/pH relationship is a unique acid–base 'signature' (see Fig. 92.1), and ultimately a complex function of SID_{IPE} and A_{totIPE}. This aspect of the Stewart approach and its implications are disputed.[4]

WEAK IONS AND BUFFER BASE

SID is a charge space occupied by weak ions including H^+, OH^-, HCO_3^-, CO_3^{2-} and A^- arising from variably dissociating conjugate bases. Their total net charge must equal the inverse of SID. However, HCO_3^- and A^- numerically occupy the entire space (see Fig. 92.2). Other ions are in minute concentrations, either micromoles/L or with protons, nanomoles/L. SID therefore dictates the buffer base concentration and is numerically identical to it, so that $SID=[HCO_3^-]+[A^-]$. With Figge's linear approximations for A^-.[5] this allows us to reduce Stewart's equations from six to three without sacrificing accuracy.[6]

$$[A^-] \quad [Alb]\times(0.123\times pH-0.631)+[Pi]\times(0.309\times pH-0.469)$$

$$[HCO_3^-] \quad 0.0301\times P_{CO_2}\times 10^{(pH-6.1)}$$

$$SIDe \quad [HCO_3^-]+[A^-]$$

[Alb] is albumin concentration (g/L). [Pi] is phosphate concentration (mmol/L). P_{CO_2} is in mmHg. SIDe is effective plasma SID, also known as the 'buffer base' (see Fig. 92.2).

SID calculated from measured plasma concentrations of strong ions is termed the 'apparent' SID, or SIDa (see Fig. 92.2). Disparities between SIDe and SIDa imply the presence of unmeasured ions in plasma (see below).

ISOLATED CHANGES IN SID AND A_{tot}

At any given Pa_{CO_2}, a falling SID or a rising A_{tot} reduce pH, forcing the equilibrium towards metabolic acidosis. Conversely, a rising SID or a falling A_{tot} favour a metabolic alkalosis. Some argue that SID and A_{tot} act individually. We could thus have a strong ion acidosis or alkalosis combined with either a hyperalbuminaemic (high A_{tot}) acidosis or a hypoalbuminaemic (low A_{tot}) alkalosis.[7] However, SID and A_{tot} may be linked, with the SID set point adjusting to A_{tot}, presumably by renal chloride adjustment.[8,9]

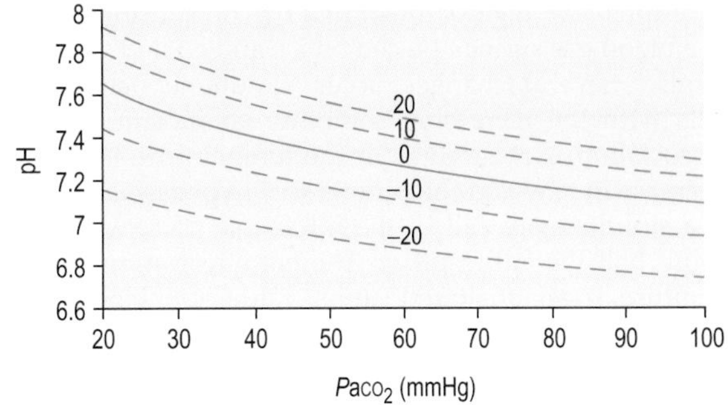

Figure 92.3 Pa_{CO_2}/pH curve shifts and associated SBE values (mEq/L). Alterations in metabolic acid–base status shift the curve down in metabolic acidosis (SBE increasingly negative) or up in metabolic alkalosis (SBE increasingly positive).

HOW ACID–BASE DISTURBANCES AFFECT THE Pa_{CO_2}/pH RELATIONSHIP

Acute respiratory disturbances move data points along the Pa_{CO_2}/pH curve, to the left in respiratory alkalosis, and to the right in respiratory acidosis (see Fig. 92.1). In contrast, metabolic disturbances (altered extracellular SID and/or A_{tot}) shift the entire curve up or down (**Fig. 92.3**). A down-shifted curve means the pH at any given Pa_{CO_2} is lower than normal, which depending on the Pa_{CO_2} represents either a primary metabolic acidosis or else metabolic compensation for a respiratory alkalosis. With an up-shifted curve, the pH at any given Pa_{CO_2} is higher than normal, signifying a primary metabolic alkalosis or else compensation for a respiratory acidosis.

TEMPERATURE CORRECTION OF BLOOD GAS DATA – 'ALPHA-STAT' VERSUS 'pH-STAT' APPROACHES

Blood gas analysers operate at 37°C. Their software can convert pH and gas tensions to values corresponding to the patient core temperature for interpretation. This is the 'pH-stat' approach. The alternative is to act on values as measured at 37°C: the 'alpha-stat' approach. Neither approach is clearly superior.[10]

'Alpha' is the ratio of protonated to total imidazole on histidine moieties in protein molecules. At 37°C with a normal mean intracellular pH of 6.8 (neutral pH for that temperature), alpha is approximately 0.55. Maintaining alpha close to 0.55 optimises enzyme structure and function and is a fundamental goal of the alpha-stat approach.

'Alpha-stat' logic is illustrated by considering blood in a blood gas syringe placed on ice and cooled anaerobically. Several changes occur simultaneously. P_{CO_2} falls with the increasing solubility coefficient. Water dissociation is reduced with the temperature-induced decrease in K'w and the progressive hypocarbia. There is a simultaneous fall in the imidazole pKa, which is about half the fall in pK'w. The net effect at any temperature is an unaltered alpha value. On blood gas analysis the specimen is rewarmed anaerobically to 37°C. The hypocarbia resolves while K'w and the imidazole pKa regain their original values. Again there is no change in alpha.

Hence, alpha is kept at 0.55 at any patient core temperature by maintaining uncorrected Pa_{CO_2} and pH measurements in their 37°C reference ranges,[11,12] a practice that mimics the physiology of ectothermic (cold-blooded) animals. With this approach cerebral autoregulation may be better preserved.[11] Similar arguments apply in fever, the more common ICU scenario. Many intensivists follow the alpha-stat approach.

Others argue that the pH stat approach is consistent with the physiology of hibernating endothermic mammals, and that it maintains superior cerebral oxygenation and greater cerebral perfusion in induced hypothermia.[13] This was the approach during an influential trial of mild hypothermia following out-of-hospital ventricular fibrillation (VF) arrest.[14]

RENAL PARTICIPATION IN ACID–BASE

In renal failure there is a progressive metabolic acidosis. About 60 mEq of strong anions including sulphate, hippurate and others accumulate daily as metabolic end-products, reducing extracellular SID. Free water is retained, again reducing SID. Hyperphosphataemia increases A_{tot}, commonly offset in acute renal failure by coexistent hypoalbuminaemia.[15]

Traditionally, renal acid–base homeostasis is described in terms of proton excretion, filtered HCO_3^- resorption and new HCO_3^- generation. Proton excretion is facilitated by titration of urinary buffers at low urinary pH, especially the $HPO_4^{2-}/H_2PO_4^-$ system (titratable acidity), and by up-regulation of distal tubular NH_3 production to facilitate luminal proton 'trapping' as NH_4^+.[16]

From the physical chemical perspective, any analysis based on H^+ or HCO_3^- 'balances' is misleading. In the Stewart model, $[H^+]$ and $[HCO_3^-]$ balance sheets cannot apply since these are dependent variables, responsive exclusively to P_{CO_2}, SID and A_{tot}. The physical chemical explanation is simple. The kidneys regulate extracellular SID via urinary SID,[17] the principle tool being tubular NH_4^+ acting as an adjustable cationic partner for tubular Cl^- and other urinary strong anions.[18] The kidneys modify A_{tot} via phosphate excretion, which is a different concept from that of 'titratable acidity'.

ACID–BASE ASSESSMENT – THE TWO 'SCHOOLS'

By convention acid–base disorders are divided into respiratory (Pa_{CO_2}) and metabolic (non-Pa_{CO_2}). Pa_{CO_2} is the undisputed index of respiratory acid-base status. Two 'schools', Boston and Copenhagen,[19] have formed around the identification and quantification of metabolic acid–base disturbances. Both succeed as navigation systems if used correctly.

Stewart's concepts neither invalidate nor supplant the traditional approaches,[20,21] but rather help us understand their physiological basis and extend their utility.[22] SID by itself is unreliable as a measure of metabolic acid–base status. Plasma SID, the only SID directly measurable by clinicians, is subject to Donnan effects, and thus varies with Pa_{CO_2} (the only CO_2-invariant SID being SID_{IPE}).

For a pure metabolic index to succeed, it must integrate the effects of SID and A_{tot}, irrespective of the Pa_{CO_2}. The best of these is standard base excess, the flagship of the Copenhagen school. However, Boston school devotees can navigate successfully using empirical plasma bicarbonate-based 'rules of thumb' (**Table 92.1**).

BASE EXCESS AND STANDARD BASE EXCESS

In 1960 Siggaard-Andersen introduced 'base excess' (BE),[23] defined as zero when pH=7.4 and P_{CO_2}=40 mmHg (5.32 kPa) (both at 37°C). If pH≠7.4 or P_{CO_2}≠40 mmHg, BE was defined as the concentration of titratable hydrogen ion required to return the pH of ex vivo blood to 7.4 while maintaining P_{CO_2} at 40 mmHg.

In the lead-up, Astrup, Siggaard-Andersen, Engel and others equilibrated the blood of Danish volunteers with known CO_2 tensions at varying haemoglobin concentrations after adding known amounts of acid or base. The data were used to create an 'alignment nomogram' that allowed the determination of BE from simultaneous measurements of pH, P_{CO_2} and haemoglobin concentration.

Seventeen years later, Siggaard-Andersen published the Van Slyke equation.[24] It was derived from known physical chemical relationships, and superseded the empirical nomogram. The equation computes BE as $(\Delta[HCO_3^-]+\Delta[A^-])$, in other words as the deviation from normal of the buffer base concentration in whole blood (P+E). From the Stewart perspective, buffer base and SID are interchangeable terms. Hence Stewart would describe BE as the abnormality in SID_{PE} at the prevailing A_{tot}.

It became clear that BE loses CO_2 invariance in vivo, where Gibbs Donnan forces drive ionic shifts between intravascular and interstitial compartments. A change in Pa_{CO_2} forces SID_{PE} and thus BE in the opposite direction. The solution was to model the total IPE space more closely by calculating BE at a haemoglobin concentration of approximately 50 g/L.[25,26] This is standard base excess (SBE).

Table 92.1 Compensation – mechanisms and rules

DISORDER	COMPENSATION	SIMPLE RULES	BOSTON RULES
Uncompensated respiratory acidosis and alkalosis	Nil	SBE −3.0 to +3.0	Resp acidosis: $HCO_3^-=24+0.1\times(Pa_{CO_2}-40)$ Resp alkalosis: $HCO_3^-=24+0.2\times(Pa_{CO_2}-40)$
Compensated respiratory acidosis and alkalosis	Resp acidosis: Extracellular SID increased by decreasing urinary SID Resp alkalosis: Extracellular SID decreased by increasing urinary SID	pH is normal or $SBE=0.4\times(Pa_{CO_2}-40)$	Resp acidosis: $HCO_3^-=24+0.35\times(Pa_{CO_2}-40)$ Resp alkalosis: $HCO_3^-=24+0.5\times(Pa_{CO_2}-40)$
Metabolic acidosis	Hyperventilation reduces Pa_{CO_2}	Pa_{CO_2}=2 digits after decimal point of pH or $Pa_{CO_2}=40+SBE$ (Pa_{CO_2} rarely <10 mmHg (1.33 kPa))	$Pa_{CO_2}=1.5\times(HCO_3^-)+8$
Metabolic alkalosis	Hypoventilation increases Pa_{CO_2}	Pa_{CO_2}=2 digits after decimal point of pH or $Pa_{CO_2}=40+SBE$ (Pa_{CO_2} rarely >60 mmHg (7.98 kPa))	$Pa_{CO_2}=0.9\times(HCO_3^-)+9$

As a metabolic acid–base index SBE is close to ideal, being both a quantitative therapeutic target and demonstrably independent of Pa_{CO_2}.[27] A useful formula is:

$$SBE \quad 0.93\times([HCO_3^-]+14.84\times(pH-7.4)-24.4)$$

with SBE and $[HCO_3^-]$ values in mEq/L. The formula can be refined to allow for variations in albumin and phosphate,[26] although the end-result is similar because haemoglobin is the predominant non-volatile weak acid in the IPE space.

A typical SBE reference range (in mEq/L) is −3.0 to +3.0. If SBE<−3.0 mEq/L, there is a down-shifted Pa_{CO_2}/pH curve. This could represent either a primary metabolic acidosis or else compensation for a primary respiratory alkalosis, depending on the Pa_{CO_2} (see below). SBE quantifies the increase in SID_{IPE} (in mEq/L) needed to return the curve to the normal position at the prevailing A_{tot} (see Fig. 92.3). In terms of the original BE definition, this is roughly the required dose of sodium bicarbonate in mmol per litre of extracellular fluid (more exactly per litre of I+P+E fluid). Similarly, if SBE>3.0 mEq/L, there is an up-shifted curve, either a metabolic alkalosis or compensation for a respiratory acidosis. The SBE value is the decrease in SID_{IPE} needed to return the curve to the normal position at the prevailing A_{tot}. Conceptually, it approximates the dose of HCl required per litre of 'extracellular' (I+P+E) fluid. In the past SBE has been termed 'extracellular SID excess' or 'SIDex' although a more correct term would be 'SID_{IPE} excess'. A complex formalism is required to express SBE in terms of SID_P and A_{totP}.[28,29]

THE BICARBONATE-BASED APPROACH TO METABOLIC ACID–BASE – THE BOSTON 'RULES OF THUMB'

Boston 'school' devotees match the plasma $[HCO_3^-]$ against the $[HCO_3^-]$ deemed appropriate for the measured Pa_{CO_2}, using empirical 'rules of thumb' derived from clinical and experimental data (see Table 92.1).[30] An offset denotes a metabolic acid–base disturbance.

The Boston method is largely qualitative. By focusing on plasma $[HCO_3^-]$ it ignores the A^- component of the buffer base (SIDe) (see Fig. 92.2). The rules of thumb reveal whether the Pa_{CO_2}/pH curve is shifted up or down but not by how much, unlike SBE, which functions as a therapeutic target.

ACID–BASE DISORDERS – CLASSIFICATION

PRIMARY ACID–BASE DISORDERS

Primary acid–base disorders dictate the direction of the pH disturbance. They are designated by the suffix 'osis', and can be either respiratory (Pa_{CO_2}) or metabolic. Hence we can have a respiratory or metabolic acidosis or alkalosis. The final pH abnormality (if any) is designated by the suffix 'aemia'. In acidaemia, plasma pH<7.35. In alkalaemia, plasma pH>7.45. In opposing primary acid–base disturbances the pH can be normal.

COMPENSATION AND ITS EFFECT ON pH

Compensation is a counter-response to a primary disorder, reducing the severity of the pH disturbance. When the primary disturbance is respiratory (Pa_{CO_2}), compensation is metabolic (renal alteration of SID and thus SBE). If the primary disturbance is metabolic (abnormal SBE), the compensation is respiratory (Pa_{CO_2}).

Metabolic compensation

In respiratory acid–base disturbances, the kidneys adjust SID_{IPE} by regulating urinary SID, primarily via urinary chloride. Sustained hypocarbia increases urinary SID causing a compensatory fall in SID_{IPE} and thus SBE. Sustained hypercarbia decreases urinary SID, increasing SID_{IPE} and thus SBE. Compensation for chronic respiratory disturbances takes time, but is ultimately effective. Over the Pa_{CO_2} range 25–80 mmHg (3.33–10.64 kPa), which encompasses most chronic respiratory disturbances, full compensation normalises the arterial pH.[27,31,32] However, this can take 5 days.

Respiratory compensation

By contrast, respiratory compensation for metabolic disturbances is faster, but less effective. A normal pH is *never* regained. Metabolic acid–base disturbances activate feedback loops linked to alveolar ventilation, forcing Pa_{CO_2} in the direction that reduces the pH perturbation. The loops are driven by CSF and plasma pH acting on the central and peripheral chemoreceptors respectively. In severe metabolic acidosis, minute ventilation can increase more than eightfold. The full response evolves over 12–24 hours, at first driven entirely by the peripheral chemoreceptors. Paradoxically the central chemoreceptors dampen the initial response, since SID equilibration between plasma and CSF is gradual, whereas P_{CO_2} equilibration is immediate.

ACID–BASE 'SCANNING TOOLS'

ELECTRICAL GAPS (Table 92.2)[33]

Accumulating strong anions reduce SID, causing metabolic acidosis. Other than chloride and L-lactate, strong anions are not measured routinely. However, they can be especially injurious for example in certain poisonings. Critical care practitioners use electrical 'gaps' as early warning systems.

Anion gap (AG)

The plasma AG is calculated (in mEq/L) as $[Na^+]+[K^+]-[Cl^-]-HCO_3^-]$. $[K^+]$ is omitted in many laboratories, which reduces the typical reference range to 5–15 mEq/L. The AG quantifies [unmeasured anions]–[unmeasured cations], both strong and weak. It is increased by unmeasured anions, and reduced by unmeasured cations. In health most of the AG consists of A^-, the negative charge on albumin and phosphate. The AG is altered by A_{tot} fluctuations and pH disturbances, both of which affect A^- (see Table 92.2). When used to scan for unmeasured strong anions, sensitivity and specificity are low.

Albumin-corrected anion gap (AGc)[7]

The AGc was devised to correct for variations in plasma [albumin], allocating a negative charge to

Table 92.2 Factors affecting the anion gap (AG), the albumin-corrected anion gap (AGc) and the strong ion gap (SIG)

FACTOR	AG	AGC	SIG
[Pi] ⇑	⇑	⇑	No effect
[Pi] ⇓	⇓	⇓	No effect
pH ⇑	⇑	⇑	No effect
pH ⇓	⇓	⇓	No effect
$[Ca^{2+}]$ and $[Mg^{2+}]$ ⇑	⇓	⇓	No effect
$[Ca^{2+}]$ and $[Mg^{2+}]$ ⇓	⇑	⇑	No effect
[Alb] ⇑	⇑	No effect	No effect
[Alb] ⇓	⇓	No effect	No effect
L-Lactate	⇑	⇑	No effect
Unmeasured strong anions (e.g. D-lactate, keto-acids, salicylate)	⇑	⇑	⇑
Unmeasured weak anions (polygelinate, myeloma IgA bands)	⇑	⇑	⇑
Unmeasured strong cations (lithium)	⇓	⇓	⇓
Unmeasured weak cations (THAMH+, myeloma IgG bands)	⇓	⇓	⇓
Chloride overestimation (bromism, hyperlipidaemia, high bicarbonate)	⇓	⇓	⇓
Sodium underestimation (hypernatraemia)	⇓	⇓	⇓

albumin appropriate for acidaemic conditions. The calculation is AG+0.25×(40−[albumin]), assuming a normal plasma [albumin] of 40 g/L. Severe alkalaemia reduces accuracy.

Strong ion gap (SIG)[33]

SIG is calculated as SIDa−SIDe, where SIDa=$[Na^+]$+$[K^+]$+$[Ca^{2+}]$+$[Mg^{2+}]$−$[Cl^-]$−[L-lactate], and SIDe=$[A^-]$+$[HCO_3^-]$. The unmeasured ions creating the 'gap' can be either strong or weak, but the term 'strong ion gap' has persisted. Its signal is subject to the summated variability of multiple analytes. Theoretically the SIG should be zero unless there are unmeasured ions, the list of which is smaller than with AG and AGc (Table 92.2). In many centres the normal SIG is 4 mEq/L or more, the positive bias presumably due to local variations in measurement technologies and analytic reference standards.

Other scanning tools

One refinement of the SIG, 'net unmeasured anions' (NUI), has been successfully incorporated into an acid-base diagnostic module and linked to a laboratory information system.[34] Two newer scanning tools are the 'BEua' parameter of Wolf & DeLand[25] and Anstey's 'UIX' index.[35] Both are referenced to the IPE space to quantify the unmeasured ionic component of SBE in the same dimension.[36]

THE OSMOLAL GAP

The osmolal gap scans for unmeasured osmotically active molecules. It is calculated as follows:

osmolal gap (mOsmol/kg)
measured osmolality − calculated osmolality

The formula for calculated osmolality of Bhagat and colleagues[37] is often preferred:

calculated osmolality (mOsmol/kg)
1.89 [Na] + 1.38 [K] + 1.03 [urea] + 1.08 [glucose] + 7.45 (all electrolyte concentrations in mmol/L)

The normal osmolal gap is <10 mosmol/kg. With an unexplained high AGc, a simultaneously raised osmolal gap suggests poisoning by methanol or ethylene glycol. However, a number of other molecules elevate the osmolal gap. These include other alcohols, mannitol and glycine, acetone and glycerol in ketoacidosis, and unknown solutes in lactic acidosis and renal failure.

PRACTICAL CONSIDERATIONS

THE DIAGNOSTIC SEQUENCE

After taking a history and examining the patient, a set of arterial blood gases should be evaluated focusing on the measured variables Pa_{CO_2} and pH. A sequence of questions can then be addressed:

Table 92.3 Acid–base status – primary survey

pH	Pa_{CO_2} (mmHg)	PRIMARY PROCESS(ES)
7.35–7.45	35–45	None
7.35–7.45	>45	1. Chronic respiratory acidosis or 2. Respiratory acidosis, metabolic alkalosis
7.35–7.45	<35	1. Chronic respiratory alkalosis 2. Respiratory alkalosis, metabolic acidosis
<7.35	<35	Metabolic acidosis
<7.35	>45	Respiratory acidosis
<7.35	35–45	Respiratory acidosis, metabolic acidosis
>7.45	>45	Metabolic alkalosis
>7.45	<35	Respiratory alkalosis
>7.45	35–45	Respiratory alkalosis, Metabolic alkalosis

WHAT IS THE PRIMARY PROCESS?

1. The primary process determines the direction of pH change.
2. Scan for primary disorders by matching the Pa_{CO_2} with the pH generated. If the direction of pH change is appropriate for the Pa_{CO_2} direction of change, there is a primary respiratory disturbance. If not, there is a primary metabolic disturbance.
3. There are nine possible combinations of Pa_{CO_2} and pH (**Table 92.3**).
4. A normal pH combined with an abnormal Pa_{CO_2} means one of two things. Either there are two opposing primary acid-base disorders, one respiratory and one metabolic, or else there is a primary respiratory acid-base disturbance with metabolic compensation. A 'normal' Pa_{CO_2} combined with an abnormal pH always represents two primary acid-base disturbances (see Tables 92.1 and 92.3).

IS THERE COMPENSATION?

1. In primary metabolic acid-base disturbances, respiratory compensation alters Pa_{CO_2} to reduce the pH disturbance. Hence there should be compensatory hypocarbia in metabolic acidosis and hypercarbia in metabolic alkalosis.
2. In primary respiratory acid-base disorders, compensation is present if the pH change is offset by an altered metabolic acid-base status. Hence in a compensated primary respiratory acidosis there should be a metabolic alkalosis (SBE>3 mEq/L), and in a compensated primary respiratory alkalosis there should be a metabolic acidosis (SBE<−3 mEq/L).

IS COMPENSATION APPROPRIATE?

1. Apply 'rules of thumb' (see Table 92.1) where applicable.
2. Remember that the pH is usually normal in fully compensated respiratory acid–base disturbances (although this can take days), whereas the pH is never normal in appropriately compensated metabolic acid–base disturbances.
3. In primary metabolic acid–base disorders, identify absent or inappropriate respiratory compensation as a separate acid–base disturbance. For example, in diabetic ketoacidosis, if the arterial pH=7.20 and the Pa_{CO_2}=20 mmHg (2.66 kPa), the patient has a metabolic acidosis with normal respiratory compensation (see Table 92.1). If, however, the pH=7.20 with a Pa_{CO_2}=32 mmHg (4.26 kPa), there is an accompanying respiratory acidosis (despite the hypocarbia). Conversely, if Pa_{CO_2}=12 mmHg (1.6 kPa) at the same pH, there is an added respiratory alkalosis.

IF METABOLIC ACIDOSIS IS PRESENT, HOW SEVERE IS IT?

1. The SBE is a quantitative index of metabolic acid–base status.
2. SBE=–4 mEq/L to –9 mEq/L indicates a mild metabolic acidosis (either primary or compensatory).
3. SBE=–10 mEq/L to –14 mEq/L indicates a moderate metabolic acidosis (either primary or compensatory).
4. SBE<–14 mEq/L indicates a severe metabolic acidosis.

IF METABOLIC ALKALOSIS IS PRESENT, HOW SEVERE IS IT?

1. SBE=+4 mEq/L to +9 mEq/L indicates a mild metabolic alkalosis (either primary or compensatory).
2. SBE=+10 mEq/L to +14 mEq/L indicates a moderate metabolic alkalosis (either primary or compensatory).
3. SBE>+14 mEq/L indicates a severe metabolic alkalosis.

WHAT IS THE AG OR PREFERABLY THE AGc?

1. If either is elevated, unmeasured anions are likely.
2. If the AGc is low or negative, suspect laboratory error, but consider lithium intoxication, IgG myeloma and others (see Table 92.2).

IS THE AGc INCREASE (IF ANY) ACCOMPANIED BY A SIMILAR REDUCTION IN SBE OR [HCO_3^-]?

1. An elevated AGc should be accompanied by a similar reduction in SBE or [HCO_3^-]. If not, there are dual disorders.
2. For example, if AGc=20 mEq/L and SBE=–15 mEq/L, there is a mixed normal AGc and raised AGc metabolic acidosis. If AGc=20 mEq/L and the SBE=0 mEq/L, there is a mixed metabolic alkalosis and raised AGc metabolic acidosis.

Box 92.1 Causes of metabolic acidosis

Normal AGc	Raised AGc
Saline infusions	L-lactate acidosis
Organic anion excretion	Ketoacidosis
Ketoacidosis	β-hydroxybutyrate, acetoacetate
Glue sniffing (hippurate, benzoate)	Renal failure
Loss high SID enteric fluid	Sulphate, hippurate, other organic anions
Small intestinal, pancreatic, biliary	Phosphate accumulation increases A_{tot}
Urinary/enteric diversions	Ethylene glycol poisoning
High urinary SID	Glycolate, oxalate
Renal tubular acidosis	Methanol poisoning
High urinary SID	Formate
Post hypocapnia	Salicylate overdose
High urinary SID	Salicylate, L-lactate, keto-anions
TPN and NH_4Cl administration	Pyroglutamic acidosis
	Pyroglutamate
	Toluene (glue sniffing)
	Hippurate, benzoate
	Short bowel syndrome
	D-lactate

IF THE AGc IS INCREASED, WHAT IS THE CAUSE?

1. There are several potential causes of a raised AGc (**Box 92.1**). Common causes include L-lactate and the ketoanions (beta-hydroxybutyrate and acetoacetate).
2. If there is no obvious cause, perform other specific assays (e.g. D-lactate, salicylate). A concurrently raised osmolal gap suggests methanol (unmeasured anion formate) or ethylene glycol toxicity (unmeasured anions glycolate and oxalate), but can also be present in ketoacidosis and hyperlactaemia. Urinary organic anions may reveal pyroglutamate.

CLINICAL ACID–BASE DISORDERS

METABOLIC ACIDOSIS

In metabolic acidosis, the SID_{IPE} is low relative to the corresponding A_{tot}. This can represent a narrowed difference between [Na^+] and [Cl^-] (normal AGc, Box 92.1), or an accumulation of other anions (elevated AGc, Box 92.1). Although a normal AGc acidosis is often hyperchloraemic, the absolute [Cl^-] is not important, but just its value relative to [Na^+].

Clinical features

Clinical features are those of acidaemia itself (Box 92.1), combined with toxicities of individual anions. These include blindness and cerebral oedema (formate), crystalluria, renal failure and hypocalcaemia (oxalate), and tinnitus, hyperventilation and fever due to uncoupling of oxidative phosphorylation (salicylate).

The adverse effects of acidaemia (**Box 92.2**) are more evident at low pH (<7.2). Acidaemia also has potential benefits. For example, the Bohr effect increases tissue oxygen availability, although rapidly counteracted by reduced 2,3-diphosphoglycerate concentrations. Lowering pH is protective in certain hypoxic stress models. During mild acidaemia therefore, the net result of harm versus benefit can be debated.

Infusion-related acidosis[38]

Large volumes of intravenous 0.9% sodium chloride cause a normal AGc metabolic acidosis. This may cause harm.[39] The SBE rarely falls below −10 mEq/L, so that with appropriate respiratory compensation the pH remains above 7.3. Cell culture and animal experiments plus low-level human evidence point to pro-inflammatory effects and other adverse consequences including hypotension, reduced renal perfusion, splanchnic dysfunction and coagulation disturbances. However, it is unclear whether hyperchloraemia rather than acidaemia is the culprit.[40]

Box 92.2 Adverse effects of metabolic acidosis

- Reduced myocardial contractility, tachy- and brady-dysrhythmias, systemic arteriolar dilatation, venoconstriction, centralisation of blood volume
- Pulmonary vasoconstriction, hyperventilation, respiratory muscle failure
- Reduced splanchnic and renal blood flow
- Increased metabolic rate, catabolism, reduced ATP synthesis, reduced 2,3-DPG synthesis
- Confusion, drowsiness
- Increased iNOS expression, pro-inflammatory cytokine release
- Hyperglycemia, hyperkalaemia
- Cell membrane pump dysfunction
- Bone loss, muscle wasting

Infusion-related acidosis is driven by the 'effective' SID of the administered crystalloid, since rapid infusion forces SID_{IPE} towards this value. The SID of administered fluid is zero whenever there are equal concentrations of the strong cation Na^+ and the strong anion Cl^-, for example in 0.9% sodium chloride, 0.45% sodium chloride and in dextrose and dextrose saline preparations. With these fluids rapid infusion will reduce extracellular SID at a rate outstripping the metabolic alkalosis of A_{tot} dilution, resulting in a metabolic acidosis.

To balance saline preparations, some Cl^- must be replaced with HCO_3^-, or else with strong anions that undergo metabolic 'disappearance' such as lactate, gluconate, or acetate. Sufficient chloride must be replaced to ensure that the fall in extracellular SID balances the A_{tot} dilution effect. In animal and human studies, this value is 24 mEq/L.[41,42]

Renal tubular acidosis (RTA)[16]

In RTA, urinary SID is high relative to the SID_{IPE}, with an inadequate nadir following an acid load. The disturbance is in renal tubular Cl^- handling, from either reduced ammonia production (Types 1 and 4), or increased chloride resorption (Type 2). Causes are legion (**Table 92.4**).

Apart from treating underlying causes and preventing hypercalcuria, management in Types 1 and 2 RTA is based on administering sodium bicarbonate or citrate to correct extracellular SID, and preventing and treating hypokalaemia using potassium citrate (not chloride). In

Table 92.4 Types of renal tubular acidosis

	TYPE 1	TYPE 2	TYPE 4
MECHANISM	Impaired distal NH_4^+ secretion	Increased proximal chloride resorption	Hyperkalaemic suppression of proximal tubular NH_4^+ production
SOME CAUSES	Idiopathic, hypercalcuric, amphotericin B, lithium carbonate, rheumatoid arthritis, Sjögren's disease, SLE, cirrhosis, renal transplant rejection, obstructive uropathy, primary hyperparathyroidism, hyperglobulinaemia	*With other proximal tubular defects (Fanconi syndrome)*: genetic, light chain nephropathy, acetazolamide, heavy metals, aminoglycosides, valproate, chemotherapy, renal transplantation, amyloidosis, paroxysmal nocturnal haemoglobinuria	*Reduced aldosterone secretion or sensitivity*: hyporeninaemia, adrenal insufficiency, ACE inhibitors, NSAIDS, cyclosporine, heparin, amiloride, spironolactone, triamterene, pentamidine, diabetes, obstructive uropathy, interstitial nephropathies, renal transplant rejection, analgesic nephropathy
SBE	Can be <−15 mEq/L	−6 to −15 mEq/L	−6 to −8 mEq/L
PLASMA [K^+]	Usually low	Low	High
URINE pH POST FUROSEMIDE	>5.5	<5.5 (bicarbonaturia with $NaHCO_3^-$ infusion)	Usually <5.5
URINARY AG	Positive	Negative	Usually positive
URINARY NH_4^+	Reduced	Normal or high	Usually reduced

Type 4 RTA, inciting agents are ceased, and adrenal insufficiency treated with mineralocorticoid replacement. Alkali supplements and furosemide are occasionally necessary.

Lactic acidosis

See Chapter 19.

Management of metabolic acidosis

Management is directed at the underlying cause. Care must be taken when instituting mechanical ventilation, since a sudden reduction in minute volume can be lethal. For example, an arterial pH of 6.9 and Pa_{CO_2} of 10 mmHg (1.33 kPa) implies maximal hyperventilation. If the Pa_{CO_2} suddenly returns to 'normal' (40 mmHg (5.32 kPa)), the arterial pH will fall to 6.7. If the Pa_{CO_2} rises further to 60 mmHg (7.98 kPa), the pH will be 6.6.

Administration of alkalinising agents – sodium bicarbonate, 'Carbicarb®', sodium lactate and tham[43] The term 'alkalinising agent' is preferred to 'buffer'. True chemical buffering implies resistance to pH change on addition of an acid or base, whereas an alkalinising agent increases the pH at any given P_{CO_2}.

In lactic acidosis and organic acidoses in general, it is difficult to justify the administration of alkalinising agents (see Ch. 19). However, it can be appropriate to infuse $NaHCO_3$ to correct a severe normal AGc acidosis. Other conditions where $NaHCO_3$ administration is often indicated include severe hyperkalaemia, methanol and ethylene glycol poisoning, and tricyclic and salicylate overdose. A $NaHCO_3$ dose of 1 mmol/kg increases SBE approximately 3 mEq/L.

Administering $NaHCO_3$ increases SID. The active agent is therefore sodium, not bicarbonate. NaOH is not used because of its alkalinity (pH 14). However, two problems arise from the high CO_2 content (CO_{2tot}) of $NaHCO_3$ (approximately 1028 mmol/L in a 1M solution). One is the need for expensive CO_2-impermeable containers during autoclaving and storage. The other is the possibility of paradoxical intracellular respiratory acidosis on administration. Although demonstrable in vitro,[44] this is unlikely to be a problem in clinical practice provided $NaHCO_3$ administration is slow (over 30–60 minutes) to prevent a surge in $\dot{V}CO_2$ and intravascular P_{CO_2}. This precaution should be effective except when pulmonary perfusion is massively reduced, such as in cardiac arrest.

Nevertheless the CO_{2tot} of bicarbonate preparations can be reduced, the trade-off being a rise in pH. For example in Carbicarb® (CO_{2tot}=750 mmol/L, P_{CO_2}= 2 mmHg (0.266 kPa), pH=9.8), half the monovalent bicarbonate becomes divalent carbonate. In Europe, sodium lactate (0.167M, pH 6.9) is an alternative. Note that lactate does not 'generate' bicarbonate. It is replaced by bicarbonate on metabolism to glucose by gluconeogenesis or CO_2 via the Krebs pathway.

Infusing a weak base (B_{TOT}) will also shift the Pa_{CO_2}/pH curve upward. THAM is tromethamine or tris buffer, a weak base with a pKa of 7.7 at 37°C. On addition of $THAMH^+$, buffer base charge becomes more negative to maintain electrical neutrality. SBE increases without changing SID_{IPE} or A_{tot}. THAM is CO_2-consuming, with good cell penetration, and causes an immediate intracellular metabolic and respiratory alkalosis. Presumably this phenomenon in CSF explains its propensity to cause sudden apnoea. THAM accumulates in renal impairment, and can cause hypoglycaemia, hyperosmolality, and coagulation and potassium disturbances.

Potential adverse effects of all alkalinising agents include a sudden increase in haemoglobin–oxygen affinity, the production of a hyperosmolar state, reduced $[Ca^{2+}]$ and $[Mg^{2+}]$, and rebound alkalosis on resolution of an organic acidosis.

METABOLIC ALKALOSIS

In metabolic alkalosis, SID_{IPE} is high relative to A_{tot}. Metabolic alkalosis has been described as the most common acid–base disturbance in hospital patients, but with modern definitions is more often part of a 'mixed' disorder.

Causes (**Box 92.3**)

Metabolic alkalosis can be precipitated by:

1. Low urinary SID (e.g. diuretics)
2. Loss of low SID enteric fluid (e.g. small gut fistulae)
3. Gain of high SID fluid (e.g. $NaHCO_3$ administration).

Clinical features

A high plasma pH (>7.55) has a number of adverse effects (**Box 92.4**). Mortality in critical illness escalates as the pH rises above 7.55, although how much is causation versus association is unclear.

Treatment

The first step is to remove the cause. Measures can then be instituted to accelerate the reduction in extracellular SID. They include:

1. Correcting effective volume depletion (reduced skin turgor, postural hypotension, high urea:creatinine ratio, urinary $[Cl^-]$<20 mmol/L). The term 'saline-responsive metabolic alkalosis' implies that saline overcomes the alkalinising renal response to hypovolaemia (low urinary SID). In fact, all metabolic alkaloses will respond if sufficient saline can be administered safely, since saline induces a 'counter' metabolic acidosis. Common colloid preparations have similar in vitro acid–base effects and could be infused as alternatives.[45]
2. Administering KCl to correct potassium depletion. The vital component is the chloride. Simplistically, potassium (strong cation) enters the depleted intracellular compartment in excess of administered chloride (strong anion), increasing SID_{IPE}. This explanation ignores associated Gibbs Donnan phenomena.
3. Acetazolamide therapy to increase urinary SID (requires adequate renal function).

Box 92.3 Metabolic alkalosis – causes

Low urinary SID	Enteric losses of low SID fluid	Gain of high SID fluid
Loop or thiazide diuretics	Pyloric stenosis, vomiting/gastric outlet obstruction, nasogastric suction	$NaHCO_3$ administration
Post-hypercapnia	Villous adenoma	Sodium citrate (plasma exchange, >8 units stored blood)
Corticosteroids	Laxative abuse	Renal replacement fluids with high SID (>35 mEq/L)
Cushing's syndrome		Milk alkali syndrome
Primary mineralocorticoid excess		
Carbenoxolone, glycyrrhetinic acid (licorice)		
Hypercalcaemia		
Milk alkali syndrome		
Magnesium deficiency		
Bartter's and Gitelman's syndromes		

Box 92.4 Severe metabolic alkalosis – multi-system effects

Central nervous system
- Vasospasm
- Seizures
- Confusion, drowsiness

Neuromuscular
- Weakness, tetany, muscle cramps

Cardiovascular
- Arrhythmias – supraventricular and ventricular
- Decreased contractility

Respiratory
- Decreased alveolar ventilation
- Atelectasis, hypoxaemia

Metabolic
- Hyperlactaemia
- Low [Pi], $[Ca^{2+}]$, $[Mg^{2+}]$ and $[K^+]$

Hemoglobin-oxygen affinity
- Initially increased (until counteracted by increased 2,3-DPG)

Box 92.5 Conditions predisposing to respiratory alkalosis

Acute	Chronic
Hypoxaemia	Pregnancy
Hepatic failure	High altitude
Sepsis	Chronic lung disease
Asthma	Neurotrauma
Pulmonary embolism	Chronic liver dysfunction
Pneumonia, acute lung injury	
CNS disorders – stroke, infection, trauma	
Drugs – salicylates, SSRI	
Opiate and benzodiazepine withdrawal	
Mechanical hyperventilation – intentional or inadvertent	
Pain, anxiety, psychosis	

4. Administration of HCl, which has a negative SID, through a central venous catheter. Minute ventilation, hypercarbia and oxygenation will usually improve. HCl can also be given indirectly, as NH_4Cl, or as arginine or lysine hydrochloride. All require hepatic deamination.
5. Renal replacement therapy.

As with metabolic acidosis, care is required when instituting mechanical ventilation. Minute volume settings should be reduced to avoid precipitating extreme alkalaemia.

RESPIRATORY ACIDOSIS

Causes (Table 92.5)

The risk is increased when CO_2 production is high and when ventilation is inefficient (large alveolar or apparatus dead space, respiratory muscle disadvantage due to hyperinflation).

Clinical features

These include the effects of acidaemia (see Box 92.2). However, acute hypercarbia has important central nervous effects, including asterixis, confusion, drowsiness, fitting and raised intracranial pressure. Hypercarbia also activates the sympatho-adrenal and renin–angiotensin systems, reducing renal perfusion, glomerular filtration rate and urine output.

Treatment

Management is directed at the underlying cause. Mechanical ventilation, either non-invasive or invasive, may be required.

RESPIRATORY ALKALOSIS

Causes

Respiratory alkalosis arises in a number of clinical scenarios (**Box 92.5**).

Clinical features

With the exception of the complications of hypoventilation, all the multisystem effects of alkalaemia apply.

Treatment

Management should be directed towards the underlying cause.

Table 92.5 Some causes of respiratory acidosis

MECHANISM/AFFECTED SITE	ACUTE	CHRONIC
Respiratory centre suppression	Sedative and narcotic drugs, CNS injury, CNS infection, brainstem vasculitis or infarction	Obesity, hypoventilation syndrome
Airway obstruction	Inhalational injury, Ludwig's angina, laryngeal trauma	Obstructive sleep apnoea, vocal cord paresis, subglottic and tracheal stenosis
Mechanical ventilation	Permissive hypercarbia	
Neural/neuromuscular	Spinal cord injury, Guillain–Barré syndrome, myasthenia gravis, muscle relaxants, envenomation, acute poliomyelitis, critical illness myoneuropathy	Phrenic nerve damage, paraneoplastic syndromes, post-polio syndrome
Muscle	Myopathy, low [K^+], high [Mg^{2+}], low [Pi], diaphragmatic injury, shock	Muscular dystrophies, motor neuron disease
Decreased chest wall compliance	Abdominal distension, burns, pneumothorax, large pleural effusions	Obesity, kyphoscoliosis, ankylosing spondylitis
Loss of chest wall integrity/geometry	Flail segment	Thoracoplasty
Increased small airways resistance	Asthma, bronchiolitis	Chronic obstructive pulmonary disease
Deceased lung compliance	Acute lung injury, pneumonia, pulmonary oedema, vasculitis, and haemorrhage	Pulmonary fibrosis

Access the complete references list online at http://www.expertconsult.com

1. Stewart PA. How to Understand Acid-Base. A Quantitative Acid-Base Primer for Biology and Medicine. New York: Elsevier; 1981.
2. Morgan TJ. The Stewart approach - one clinician's perspective. Clin Biochem Rev 2009;30(2):41–54. Epub 2009/07/01.
4. Kurtz I, Kraut J, Ornekian V, et al. Acid-base analysis: a critique of the Stewart and bicarbonate-centered approaches. Am J Physiol Renal Physiol 2008;294(5): F1009-1031. Epub 2008/01/11.
7. Fencl V, Jabor A, Kazda A, et al. Diagnosis of metabolic acid-base disturbances in critically ill patients. Am J Respir Crit Care Med 2000;162(6):2246–51. Epub 2000/12/09.
16. Soriano JR. Renal tubular acidosis; The clinical entity. J Am Soc Nephrol 2002;13:2160–70.
22. Kellum JA. Clinical review: reunification of acid-base physiology. Crit Care 2005;9(5):500–7. Epub 2005/11/10.
24. Siggaard-Andersen O. The Van Slyke equation. Scand J Clin Lab Invest Suppl 1977;37(146):15–20. Epub 1977/01/01.
33. Morgan TJ. Unmeasured ions and the strong ion gap. In: Kellum JA, Elbers PWG, editors. Stewart's Textbook of Acid Base. Amsterdam: AcidBase.org; 2009. p. 323–37.
38. Morgan TJ. The meaning of acid-base abnormalities in the intensive care unit: part III - effects of fluid administration. Crit Care 2005;9(2):204–11. Epub 2005/03/19.
43. Morgan TJ, Buffers. In: Kellum JA, Elbers PWG, editors. Stewart's Textbook of Acid Base. Amsterdam: AcidBase.org; 2009. p. 281–91.

93

Fluid and electrolyte therapy

Anthony Delaney and Simon Finfer

The management of patients' fluid and electrolyte status requires an understanding of body fluid compartments as well as an understanding of water and electrolyte metabolism. These principles will be considered along with the commonly encountered fluid and electrolyte disturbances. Recent evidence for the use of fluid therapy in a number of common clinical scenarios will also be presented.

FLUID COMPARTMENTS (TABLE 93.1, FIG. 93.1)

TOTAL BODY WATER

In humans, water contributes approximately 60% of body weight, with organs varying in water content (**Table 93.2**). The variation of the percentage of total body weight as water, between individuals, is largely governed by the amount of adipose tissue. The average water content as a percentage of total body weight is 60% for males and 50% for females. Total body water as a percentage of total body weight decreases with age, due to a progressive loss of muscle mass, causing bone and connective tissue to assume a greater percentage of total body weight[1–3] (**Table 93.3**).

Total body water is commonly divided into two volumes: the extracellular fluid (ECF) volume and the intracellular fluid (ICF) volume.[2] Sodium balance regulates the ECF volume, whereas water balance regulates the ICF volume. Sodium excretion is normally regulated by various hormonal and physical ECF volume sensors, whereas water balance is normally regulated by hypothalamic osmolar sensors.[4]

EXTRACELLULAR FLUID

ECF is defined as all body water external to the cell, and is commonly subdivided into plasma and interstitial fluid volumes. The ECF is normally 40% of total body water and 25% of total body weight. With acute or chronic illness, ICF volume is reduced, and ECF volume is increased and may even exceed the ICF volume. The ECF volume can be divided into the plasma volume, the extracellular fluid volume, and the interstitial volume.

INTRACELLULAR FLUID

ICF is defined as all the body water within cells and, unlike the ECF compartment, is an inhomogeneous, multicompartmental entity, with different pH and ionic compositions depending upon the organ or tissue being considered. The ICF volume is often determined by inference from the difference in measurements of the total body water and ECF spaces. This estimation suffers from the inaccuracies inherent in both ECF and total body water measurements. In general, the ICF is considered to be 60% of total body water and 35% of total body weight.

TRANSCELLULAR FLUID

Fluids in this compartment have a common characteristic of being formed by transport activity of cells. The fluid is extracellular in nature and will be considered as part of the interstitial volume. It may vary from 1 to 10 L, with larger volumes occurring in diseased states (e.g. bowel obstruction or cirrhosis with ascites), and is formed at the expense of the remaining interstitial and plasma volumes.

WATER METABOLISM

Water balance is maintained by altering the intake and excretion of water. Intake is controlled by thirst, whereas excretion is controlled by the renal action of antidiuretic hormone (ADH). In health, plasma osmolalities of about 280 mOsm/kg suppress plasma ADH to concentrations low enough to permit maximum urinary dilution.[5] Above this value, an increase in ECF tonicity of about 1–2% or a decrease in total body water of 1–2 litres causes the posterior pituitary to release ADH, which acts upon the distal nephron to increase water reabsorption. Maximum plasma ADH concentrations are reached at an osmolality of 295 mOsm/kg.[5] The osmotic stimulation also changes thirst sensation and, in the conscious ambulant individual, initiates water repletion (drinking), which is more important in preventing dehydration than ADH secretion and action. Thus, in health, the upper limit of the body osmolality (and therefore serum sodium) is determined by the

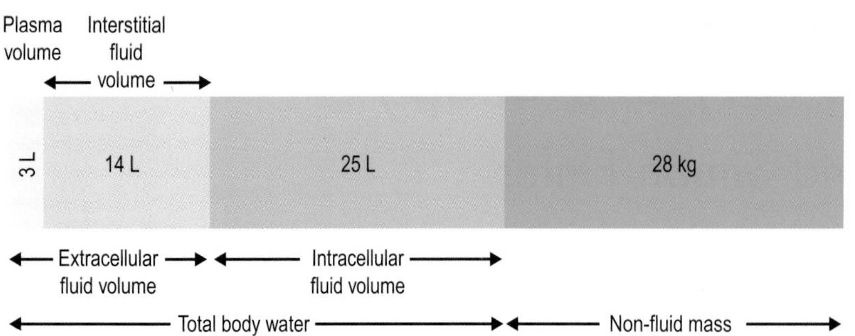

Figure 93.1 Body fluid compartments.

Table 93.1 Body fluid compartments

FLUID COMPARTMENT	VOLUME (ML/KG)	% TOTAL BODY WEIGHT
Plasma volume	45	4.5
Blood volume	75	7.5
Interstitial volume	200	20
Extracellular fluid volume	250	25
Intracellular fluid volume	350	35
Total body fluid volume	600	60

Table 93.2 Water content of various tissues

TISSUE	% WATER CONTENT
Brain	84
Kidney	83
Skeletal muscle	76
Skin	72
Liver	68
Bone	22
Adipose tissue	10

Table 93.3 Water content as a percentage of total body weight

AGE (YEARS)	MALES (%)	FEMALES (%)
10–15	60	57
15–40	60	50
40–60	55	47
>60	50	45

osmotic threshold for thirst, whereas the lower limit is determined by the osmotic threshold for ADH release.[6]

Increase in osmolality caused by permeant solutes (e.g. urea) does not stimulate ADH release. ADH may also be released in response to hypovolaemia and hypotension, via stimulation of low- and high-pressure baroreceptors. ADH release is extremely marked when more than 30% of the intravascular volume is lost. ADH may also be stimulated by pain and nausea, which are thought to act through the baroreceptor pathways.[4] ADH release may also be stimulated by a variety of pharmacological agents (**Table 93.4**). Renal response to ADH depends upon an intact distal nephron and collecting duct, and a hypertonic medullary interstitium. The capacity to conserve or excrete water also depends upon the osmolar load presented to the distal nephron.[4]

Table 93.4 Drugs affecting ADH secretion

STIMULATE	INHIBIT
Nicotine	Ethanol
Narcotics	Narcotic antagonists
Vincristine	Phenytoin
Barbiturates	
Cyclophosphamide	
Chlorpropamide	
Clofibrate	
Carbamazepine	
Amitriptyline	

WATER REQUIREMENTS

Water is needed to eliminate the daily solute load, and to replace daily insensible fluid loss (**Table 93.5**). With a normal daily excretion of 600 mOsm solute, maximal and minimal secretions of ADH will cause urine osmolality to vary from 1200 to 30 mOsm/kg respectively, and the urine output to vary from 500 mL to 20 L/day respectively. Skin and lung water losses vary, and may range from 500 mL to 8 L/day depending on physical activity, ambient temperature and humidity.

DISORDERS OF OSMOLALITY

TONICITY

Osmolality is a measure of the number of osmoles per kilogram (Osm/kg) of water. The osmolality of the ECF

Table 93.5 Daily fluid balance (for a 70-kg man at rest in a temperate climate)

	INPUT (ML)			OUTPUT (ML)	
	SEEN	UNSEEN		SEEN	UNSEEN
Drink	1000	–	Urine	1000	–
Food	–	650	Skin	–	500
Water of oxidation	–	350	Lungs	–	400
			Faeces	–	100
Total	1000	1000	Total	1000	1000

is due largely to sodium salts. Clinical effects of hyperosmolality, due to excess solute, depend upon whether the solute distributes evenly throughout the total body water (e.g. permeant solutes of alcohol or urea) or distributes in the ECF only (e.g. impermeant solutes of mannitol or glucose). With impermeant solutes, hyperosmolality is associated with a shift of fluid from the ICF to the ECF compartment. Hyperosmolality due to increased impermeant solutes is known as hypertonicity. This condition may also be associated with a reduction in the serum sodium concentration (see below).

WATER EXCESS

In a 70-kg man, for every 1 litre of excess water, ECF increases by 400 mL and ICF increases by 600 mL, on average. The osmolality also decreases by 6–7 mOsm/kg and the serum sodium falls by 3.0–3.5 mmol/L.

WATER DEFICIENCY

In a 70-kg man, for every 1 litre of water loss, 600 mL is lost from the ICF and 400 mL from the ECF. The osmolality also increases by 7–8 mOsm/kg and the serum sodium rises by 3.5–4.0 mmol/L.

ELECTROLYTES

Chemical compounds in solution may either:

- Remain intact (i.e. undissociated), in which case they are called non-electrolytes (e.g. glucose, urea)
- Dissociate to form ions, in which case they are called electrolytes. Ions carry an electrical charge (e.g. Na^+, Cl^-). Ions with a positive charge are attracted to a negative electrode or cathode, and hence are called 'cations'. Conversely, ions with a negative charge travel towards a positive electrode or anode and are called 'anions'. Each body water compartment contains electrolytes with different composition and concentration (**Table 93.6**).

Table 93.6 Electrolyte composition of body fluid compartments

	ICF (MMOL/L)	ECF (MMOL/L)	
		PLASMA	INTERSTITIAL
Sodium	10	140	145
Potassium	155	3.7	3.8
Chloride	3	102	115
Bicarbonate	10	28	30
Calcium (ionised)	<0.01	1.2	1.2
Magnesium	10	0.8	0.8
Phosphate	105	1.1	1

SODIUM

Sodium is the principal cation of the ECF and accounts for 86% of the ECF osmolality. In a 70-kg man, total body sodium content is 4000 mmol (58 mmol/kg) and is divided into a number of compartments (**Table 93.7**).

Table 93.7 The sodium compartments in a 70-kg man

	TOTAL (MMOL)	(MMOL/KG)
Total body sodium	4000	58
Non-exchangeable bone sodium	1200	17
Exchangeable sodium	2800	40
Intracellular sodium	250	3
Extracellular sodium	2400	35
Exchangeable bone sodium	150	2

ECF concentration of sodium varies between 134 and 146 mmol/L. The intracellular sodium concentration varies between different tissues, and ranges from 3 to 20 mmol/L.

The standard Western society dietary sodium intake is about 150 mmol/day, but the daily intake of sodium varies widely, with urinary losses ranging from <1 to >240 mmol/day.[7] Sodium balance is influenced by renal hormonal and ECF physical characteristics. The complete renal adjustment to an altered sodium load usually requires 3–4 days before balance is restored.

Box 93.1 Common causes of hyponatraemia

1. **Spurious result**
   - Isotonic
     - Hyperlipidaemia
     - Hyperproteinaemia
   - Hypertonic
     - Hyperglycaemia
     - Mannitol, glycerol, glycine or sorbitol excess
2. **Water retention**
   - Renal failure
   - Hepatic failure
   - Cardiac failure
   - Syndrome of inappropriate ADH secretion
   - Drugs
   - Psychogenic polydipsia
3. **Water retention and salt depletion**
   - Postoperative, post trauma or patients with excess fluid losses given inappropriate fluid replacement
   - Adrenocortical failure
   - Diuretic excess

HYPONATRAEMIA

Hyponatraemia is defined as serum sodium less than 135 mmol/L and may be classified as isotonic, hypertonic or hypotonic, depending upon the measured serum osmolality (**Box 93.1**).

Isotonic hyponatraemia

Plasma normally contains 93% water and 7% solids (5.5% proteins, 1% salts and 0.5% lipids). If the solid phase is elevated significantly (e.g. in hyperlipidaemia or hyperproteinaemia), any device that dilutes a specific amount of plasma for analysis will give falsely lower values for all measured compounds. This effect produces 'factitious hyponatraemia' and is associated with a normal measured serum osmolality.[8] Measurement of plasma sodium by an ion-selective electrode is not affected by the volume of plasma 'solids' and therefore 'pseudohyponatraemia' will not occur with this method.[8]

Hypertonic hyponatraemia

In patients who have hypertonicity due to increased amounts of impermeant solutes (e.g. glucose, mannitol, glycerol or sorbitol), a shift of water from the ICF to the ECF occurs to provide osmotic equilibration, thus diluting the ECF sodium. Such resultant hyponatraemia is often associated with an increased measured osmolality. For example, in the presence of hyperglycaemia, for every 3 mmol/L rise in glucose the serum sodium decreases by 1 mmol/L.[9]

Hypotonic hyponatraemia

Hyponatraemia is almost always caused by an excess of total body water, due to excessive hypotonic or water-generating i.v. fluids (e.g. 1.5% glycine, 0.45% saline or 5% glucose) or to excessive ingestion of water, particularly in the presence of high circulating ADH concentrations. It may rarely be caused by loss of exchangeable sodium or potassium. In the latter circumstances, a loss of approximately 40 mmol of sodium or potassium, without a change in total body water content, is required to lower the serum sodium by 1 mmol/L. As hyponatraemia may be associated with an alteration in both total body water and total body sodium, the ECF may be increased (hypervolaemia), decreased (hypovolaemia) or exhibit no change (isovolaemia).[5]

In health, a fluid intake up to 15–20 litres may be tolerated before water is retained and hyponatraemia occurs. In psychogenic polydipsia, if the water intake exceeds the renal capacity to form dilute urine, water retention and hyponatraemia will occur. With this disorder, the plasma osmolality exceeds urine osmolality. In circumstances where ADH is increased (e.g. hypovolaemia, hypotension, pain or nausea), or where renal response to ADH is altered (i.e. in renal, hepatic, pituitary, adrenal or thyroid failure), water retention occurs with lower intakes of fluid.

SPECIFIC CAUSES OF HYPONATRAEMIA

Transurethral resection of prostate (TURP) syndrome

Clinical features The TURP syndrome consists of hyponatraemia, cardiovascular disturbances (hypertension, hypotension, bradycardia), an altered state of consciousness (agitation, confusion, nausea, vomiting, myoclonic and generalised seizures) and, when using glycine solutions, transient visual disturbances of blurred vision, blindness and fixed dilated pupils, following TURP. It has also been described following endometrial ablation.[10] It may occur within 15 minutes or be delayed for up to 24 hours postoperatively,[11] and is usually caused by an excess absorption of the irrigating fluid, which contains 1.5% glycine with an osmolality of 200 mOsm/kg. Hyponatraemic syndromes have also been described when irrigating solutions containing 3% mannitol or 3% sorbitol have been used. Symptomatology usually occurs when >1 litre of 1.5% glycine or >2–3 litres of 3% mannitol or sorbitol are absorbed.[12]

The excess absorption of irrigating fluid causes an increase in total body water (which is often associated with only a small decrease in plasma osmolality), hyponatraemia (as glycine, sorbitol or mannitol reduces the sodium component of ECF osmolality) and an increase in the osmolar gap.[12,13] When glycine is used, other features include hyperglycinaemia (up to 20 mmol/L; normal plasma glycine concentrations range from 0.15 to 0.3 mmol/L), hyperserinaemia (as serine is a major metabolite of glycine), hyperammonaemia (following deamination of glycine and serine), metabolic acidosis and hypocalcaemia (due to the glycine metabolites glyoxylic acid and oxalate). Because glycine is an inhibitory neurotransmitter, and as it passes freely into the intracellular compartment when glycine solutions are used, hyperglycinaemia may be more important in the pathophysiology of this disorder than a reduction in body fluid osmolality and cerebral oedema.[14]

Treatment Treatment is largely supportive with the management of any reduction in plasma osmolality being based on the measured plasma osmolality and not the plasma sodium. If the measured osmolality is >260 mOsm/kg and mild neurological abnormalities exist, and if the patient is haemodynamically stable with normal renal function, close observation and reassurance (e.g. the visual disturbances are reversible and will last for less than 24 hours) are usually all that is needed. If the patient is hypotensive and bradycardic with severe and unresolving neurological abnormalities, haemodialysis may be warranted. Hypertonic saline is used only if the measured osmolality is <260 mOsm/kg and severe non-visual neurological abnormalities exist.[15]

Syndrome of inappropriate ADH secretion (SIADH)

This syndrome is a form of hyponatraemia in which there is an increased concentration of ADH inappropriate to any osmotic or volume stimuli that normally affect ADH secretion.[16] Diagnostic criteria and common causes are listed in **Boxes 93.2** and **93.3** respectively.

Clinical features Whereas cerebral manifestations are usually absent when the sodium concentration exceeds 125 mmol/L, progressive symptomatology of headache, nausea, confusion, disorientation, coma and seizures are often observed when plasma sodium is below 120 mmol/L.[17]

Treatment Initial treatment should be fluid restriction with close monitoring of serum sodium. If serum sodium concentration is not increasing with fluid restriction, judicious administration of sodium as intravenous normal or hypertonic saline may be required. As the true duration and rapidity of onset of hyponatraemia are often unclear, the presence and severity of symptoms may be used as the trigger for active correction of hyponatraemia.[17] The evidence base available to guide therapy is limited and there is consequently no consensus on the optimum rate at which to correct the serum sodium concentration. The major concern is to avoid neurological damage from untreated seizures, cerebral oedema, or myelinolysis.[17] In the absence of good evidence, recommended rates at which to increase the sodium concentration vary from 0.5 to 2 mmol/L per hour. Unless the treating clinician feels that more rapid correction is indicated, it seems prudent to correct the serum sodium concentration at a slower rather than a faster rate.

Box 93.2 Criteria for the diagnosis of syndrome of inappropriate antidiuretic hormone (SIADH)

- Hypotonic hyponatraemia
- Urine osmolality greater than plasma osmolality
- Urine sodium excretion greater than 20 mmol/L
- Normal renal, hepatic, cardiac, pituitary, adrenal and thyroid function
- Absence of hypotension, hypovolaemia, oedema and drugs affecting ADH secretion
- Correction by water restriction

Cerebral salt wasting

Cerebral salt wasting (CSW) is a syndrome occurring in patients with a cerebral lesion and an excess renal loss of sodium and chloride.[18] The exact aetiology of the syndrome remains unclear. Although hyponatraemia is not necessary for the diagnosis, the syndrome is commonly associated with hyponatraemia.[19] The diagnosis of CSW is suspected in patients with a cerebral lesion, such as subarachnoid haemorrhage, traumatic brain injury or a cerebral tumour, when there is an elevated urine output, with elevated urinary sodium in the absence of a physiological cause for increased sodium excretion.[19] The syndrome can be differentiated from the SIADH, as patients with CSW will have evidence of ECF depletion (e.g. negative fluid balance, tachycardia, increased haematocrit, increased urea, low central venous pressure) as opposed to the SIADH where ECF volume will be normal or slightly expanded.[20] Treatment of patients involves exclusion of other causes of hyponatraemia and increased urine output, replacement of sodium and fluid losses, and possibly fludrocortisone.[21]

SPECIFIC TREATMENTS USED FOR HYPONATRAEMIA

Hypertonic saline

Hypertonic saline, most commonly as 3% saline, is used as a therapy for patients with symptomatic

Box 93.3 Aetiologies of syndrome of inappropriate antidiuretic hormone (SIADH)

Ectopic ADH production by tumours
- Small cell bronchogenic carcinoma
- Adenocarcinoma of the pancreas or duodenum
- Leukaemia
- Lymphoma
- Thymoma

Central nervous system disorders
- Cerebral trauma
- Brain tumour (primary or secondary)
- Meningitis or encephalitis
- Brain abscess
- Subarachnoid haemorrhage
- Acute intermittent porphyria
- Guillain–Barré syndrome
- Systemic lupus erythematosus

Pulmonary diseases
- Viral, fungal and bacterial pneumonias
- Tuberculosis
- Lung abscess

hyponatraemia. Due to the osmolarity (1000 mOsm/L) of 3% saline, it must be given through a central line, and care must be taken to avoid the known complications of its use, including chronic heart failure and central pontine and extrapontine myelinolysis (osmotic demyelination syndrome).[22,23] Careful haemodynamic and electrolyte monitoring throughout saline administration is required. There is still no uniform agreement that osmotic demyelination is produced by a rapid correction of hyponatraemia.

Although hypertonic saline has been proposed as a therapy for raised intracranial pressure in a number of clinical settings,[24] its use remains controversial.[25] In a recent methodologically sound (adequate allocation concealment, blinded and using intention-to-treat analysis) randomised clinical trial, which included 229 patients with severe traumatic brain injury, resuscitation with 250 mL of 7.5% saline was not associated with improved mortality or functional outcomes compared with Hartmann's solution.[26]

Vasopressin receptor antagonists

V_2 receptor antagonists, such as lixivaptan, tolvaptan and OPC-31260, have recently been developed. These agents come from a novel class of non-peptide agents that bind to V_2 receptors in the distal tubule of the kidney and prevent vasopressin-mediated aquaporin mobilisation, and thus promote aquaresis.[27] These agents have been trialled as therapeutic options for the treatment of hyponatraemia in a number of clinical settings including hyponatraemia associated with heart failure, cirrhosis and SIADH.[27,28] At present the role of V_2 receptor antagonists in the management of hyponatraemia in the critically ill remains uncertain.

HYPERNATRAEMIA

Hypernatraemia, defined as a serum sodium greater than 145 mmol/L, is always associated with hyperosmolality and may be caused by excessive administration of sodium salts (bicarbonate or chloride), water depletion or excess sodium and loss of water (**Box 93.4**).

Excessive ingestion of sodium salts is rare, but intravenous infusion of large volumes of sodium-containing fluids is common in the management of hospitalised patients. Hypernatraemia often occurs in the recovery phase of acute illness when spontaneous diuresis or diuretic therapy results in more rapid clearance of free water than sodium. Pure water depletion is uncommon, unless water restriction is applied to a patient who is unconscious or unable to obtain or ingest water, as the thirst response normally corrects water depletion. If it occurs, the serum sodium concentration increases, in association with loss of both ECF and ICF.

Box 93.4 Causes of hypernatraemia

Water depletion
- Extrarenal loss
  - Exposure
  - GIT losses (often with excess saline replacement)
- Renal loss
  - Osmotic diuresis – urea, mannitol, glycosuria
  - Diabetes insipidus
    - Neurogenic
      - Post-traumatic, fat embolism
      - Metastatic tumours, craniopharyngioma, pinealoma, cysts
      - Meningitis, encephalitis
      - Granulomas (TB, sarcoid)
      - Guillain–Barré syndrome
      - Idiopathic
    - Nephrogenic
      - Congenital
      - Hypercalcaemia, hypokalaemia
      - Lithium
      - Pyelonephritis
      - Medullary sponge kidney
      - Polycystic kidney
      - Post-obstructive uropathy
      - Multiple myeloma, amyloid, sarcoid

Salt gain
- Hypertonic, saline or sodium bicarbonate

Clinical features

Hypernatraemia usually produces symptoms if the serum sodium exceeds 155–160 mmol/L (i.e. osmolality >330 mOsm/kg). The clinical features include increased temperature, restlessness, irritability, drowsiness, lethargy, confusion and coma.[29] Convulsions are uncommon. The diminished ECF volume may reduce cardiac output, thereby reducing renal perfusion, leading to prerenal renal failure.

Treatment

For pure water depletion, this consists of water administration. If i.v. fluid is required, 5% glucose or hypotonic saline solution (0.45% saline) is often used, as sterile water infusion causes haemolysis. In rare cases, i.v. sterile water may be used by administering through a central venous catheter.[30] Since rapid rehydration may give rise to cerebral oedema, the change in serum sodium should be no greater than 0.5 mmol/L per hour.[29]

POTASSIUM

Potassium is the principal intracellular cation and accordingly (along with its anion) fulfils the role of the ICF osmotic provider. It also plays a major role in the functioning of excitable tissues (e.g. muscle and nerve). As the cell membrane is 20-fold more permeable to potassium than to sodium ions, potassium is largely responsible for the resting membrane potential. Potassium also influences carbohydrate metabolism and glycogen and protein synthesis.

Total body potassium is 45–50 mmol/kg in the male (3500 mmol/70 kg) and 35–40 mmol/kg (2500 mmol/65 kg) in the female; 95% of the total body potassium is exchangeable. As ECF potassium ranges from 3.1 to 4.2 mmol/L, the total ECF potassium ranges from 55 to 70 mmol. About 90% of the total body potassium is intracellular: 8% resides in bone, 2% in ECF water and 70% in skeletal muscle. With increasing age (and decreasing muscle mass), total body potassium decreases.

FACTORS AFFECTING POTASSIUM METABOLISM

The potassium content of cells is regulated by a cell wall pump-leak mechanism. Cellular uptake is by the Na^+/K^+ pump, which is driven by Na^+/K^+ ATPase. Movement of potassium out of the cell is governed by passive forces (i.e. cell membrane permeability and chemical and electrical gradients to the potassium ion).

Acidosis promotes a shift of potassium from the ICF to the ECF, whereas alkalosis promotes the reverse shift. Hyperkalaemia stimulates insulin release, which promotes a shift of potassium from the ECF to the ICF, an effect independent of the movement of glucose. Beta$_2$-adrenergic agonists promote cellular uptake of potassium by a cyclic AMP-dependent activation of the Na^+/K^+ pump, whereas alpha-adrenergic agonists cause a shift of potassium from the ICF to the ECF.[31] Aldosterone increases the renal excretion of potassium; glucocorticoids are also kaliuretic, an effect that may be independent of the mineralocorticoid receptor.

Normally, mechanisms to reduce the ECF potassium concentration (by increasing renal excretion and shifting potassium from the ECF to the ICF) are very effective. However, mechanisms to retain potassium in the presence of potassium depletion are less efficient, particularly when compared with those of sodium conservation. Even with severe potassium depletion, urinary loss of potassium continues at a rate of 10–20 mmol/day. Metabolic alkalosis also enhances renal potassium loss, by encouraging distal nephron Na^+/K^+, rather than Na^+/K^+ exchange.

HYPOKALAEMIA

Hypokalaemia is defined as a serum potassium of less than 3.5 mmol/L (or plasma potassium less than 3.0 mmol/L). It may be due to decreased oral intake, increased renal or gastrointestinal loss, or movement of potassium from the ECF to the ICF (**Box 93.5**).

Clinical features

These include weakness, hypotonicity, depression, constipation, ileus, ventilatory failure, ventricular tachycardias (characteristically torsades de pointes), atrial tachycardias and even coma.[32] With prolonged and severe potassium deficiency, rhabdomyolysis and thirst and polyuria, due to the development of renal diabetes insipidus, may occur. The ECG changes are relatively non-specific, and include prolongation of the PR interval, T-wave inversion and prominent U-waves.

Box 93.5 Causes of hypokalaemia

- Inadequate dietary intake (urine K^+ <20 mmol/L)
- Abnormal body losses
  - Gastrointestinal (urine K^+ <20 mmol/L)
    - Vomiting, nasogastric aspiration
    - Diarrhoea, fistula loss
    - Villous adenoma of the colon
    - Laxative abuse
  - Renal (urine K^+ >20 mmol/L)
    - Conn's syndrome
    - Cushing's syndrome
    - Bartter's syndrome
    - Ectopic ACTH syndrome
      - Small-cell carcinoma of the lung
      - Pancreatic carcinoma
      - Carcinoma of the thymus
  - Drugs
    - Diuretics
    - Corticosteroids
    - Carbapenems, amphotericin B, gentamicin
    - Cisplatin
  - Renal tubular acidosis
  - Magnesium deficiency
- Compartmental shift
  - Alkalosis
  - Insulin
  - Na^+/K^+ ATPase stimulation
    - Sympathomimetic agents with β_2 effect
    - Methylxanthines
  - Barium poisoning
  - Hypothermia
  - Toluene intoxication
  - Hypokalaemic periodic paralysis
  - Delayed following blood transfusion (see Ch. 95)

Treatment

Intravenous or oral potassium chloride will correct hypokalaemia, particularly if it is associated with metabolic alkalosis. If the patient has renal tubular acidosis and hypokalaemia, potassium acetate or citrate may be preferred to potassium chloride. Intravenous administration of potassium should normally not exceed 40 mmol/h, and plasma potassium should be monitored at 1–4-hourly intervals.[33] In patients with acute myocardial infarction and hypokalaemia, traditional recommendations were to maintain the serum potassium at 4.0 mmol/L,[34] but more recently the need to administer supplemental potassium when the serum potassium is >3.5mmol/L has been questioned.[35]

HYPERKALAEMIA

Hyperkalaemia is defined as a serum potassium greater than 5.0 mmol/L or plasma potassium greater than 4.5 mmol/L. It may be artefactual (from sampling errors

Box 93.6 Causes of hyperkalaemia

Collection abnormalities
- Delay in separating RBC
- Specimen haemolysis
- Thrombocythaemia

Excessive intake
- Transiently following blood transfusion (see Ch. 95)
- Exogenous (i.e. i.v. or oral KCl, massive blood transfusion)
- Endogenous (i.e. tissue damage)
  - Burns, trauma
  - Rhabdomyolysis
  - Tumour lysis

Decrease in renal excretion
- Drugs
  - Spironolactone, triamterene, amiloride
  - Indometacin
  - Captopril, enalapril
- Renal failure
- Addison's disease
- Hyporeninaemic hypoaldosteronism

Compartmental shift
- Acidosis
- Insulin deficiency
- Digoxin overdosage
- Succinylcholine
- Arginine hydrochloride
- Hyperkalaemic periodic paralysis
- Fluoride poisoning

such as in vitro haemolysis); true hyperkalaemia may be due to excessive intake, severe tissue damage, decreased excretion or body fluid compartment shift (**Box 93.6**).

Clinical features

These include tingling, paraesthesia, weakness, flaccid paralysis, hypotension and bradycardia. The characteristic ECG effects include peaking of the T-waves, flattening of the P-wave, prolongation of the PR interval (until sinus arrest with nodal rhythm occurs), widening of the QRS complex, and the development of a deep S-wave. Finally, a sine wave ECG pattern that deteriorates to asystole may occur at serum potassium levels of 7 mmol/L or greater.

Treatment

This is directed at the underlying cause, and may include dialysis. Rapid management of life-threatening hyperkalaemia may be achieved by:[36]

- Calcium chloride 5–10 mL i.v. of 10% (3.4–6.8 mmol, which is used to reduce the cardiac effects of hyperkalaemia)
- Sodium bicarbonate, 50–100 mmol i.v.
- Glucose, 50 g i.v. with 10 units of soluble insulin
- Oral and rectal resonium A, 50 g
- Diuresis with furosemide, 40–80 mg i.v.
- Beta agonists e.g. salbutamol 5–10 mg nebulised.

CALCIUM

Almost all (99%) of the body calcium (30 mmol or 1000 g or 1.5% body weight) is present in bone. A small but significant quantity of ionised calcium exists in the ECF, and is important for many cellular activities including secretion, neuromuscular impulse formation, contractile functions and clotting. Normal daily intake of calcium is 15–20 mmol, although only 40% is absorbed. The average daily urinary loss is 2.5–7.5 mmol. The total ECF calcium of 40 mmol (2.20–2.55 mmol/L) exists in three forms: 40% (1.0 mmol/L) is bound to protein (largely albumin), 47% is ionised (1.15 mmol/L) and 13% is complexed (0.3 mmol/L) with citrate, sulphate and phosphate. The ionised form is the physiologically important form, and may be acutely reduced in alkalosis, which causes a greater amount of the serum calcium to be bound to protein.[37] Although the serum ionised calcium can be measured, the total serum calcium is usually measured, and this can vary with the serum albumin concentrations. A correction factor can be used to offset the effect of serum albumin on serum calcium: this is 0.02 mmol/L for every 1 g/L increase in serum albumin (up to a value of 40 g/L), added to the measured calcium concentration. For example, if measured serum calcium is 1.82 mmol/L, and serum albumin is 25 g/L, corrected serum calcium $=1.82+[(40-25)\times0.02]$ mmol/L $=2.12$ mmol/L. It has been suggested that ionised calcium, where available, is a better indicator of calcium status in the critically ill.[38]

HYPOCALCAEMIA

Common causes of hypocalcaemia include hypoparathyroidism and pseudohypoparathyroidism, septic shock, acute pancreatitis and rhabdomyolysis.[39] Clinical features of reduced serum ionised calcium include tetany, cramps, mental changes and decrease in cardiac output. Symptomatic hypocalcaemia should be treated with i.v. calcium, as either calcium chloride or calcium gluconate. It should be remembered that 1 mL of calcium chloride has three times as much elemental calcium as 1 mL of calcium gluconate, and so the former is the preferred formulation in acute situations. Calcium should be administered via a central vein when practical, owing to the risk of tissue damage if extravasated.[39]

HYPERCALCAEMIA

The clinical features of hypercalcaemia include nausea, vomiting, pancreatitis, polyuria, polydipsia, muscular weakness, mental disturbance and ectopic calcification. Some of the common causes of hypercalcaemia include endocrine diseases such as hyperparathyroidism and thyrotoxicosis, renal failure, malignancy, thiazide diuretics and prolonged immobilisation.[39]

Severe hypercalcaemia (>3.3 mmol/L) or more moderate symptomatic hypercalcaemia will require specific therapy. A cause for the elevated calcium concentration should be sought, and specific treatment may be warranted. General measures include restoration of intravascular volume with normal saline, followed by the use of a loop diuretic such as furosemide to promote calcium excretion. The use of bisphosphonates, such as pamidronate, is recommended for severe cases.[40] Other therapies to consider include steroids, calcitonin and mithramycin.

MAGNESIUM

Magnesium is primarily an intracellular ion that acts as a metallo-coenzyme in numerous phosphate transfer reactions. It has a critical role in the transfer, storage and utilisation of energy.

In humans, the total body magnesium content is 1000 mmol, and the plasma concentrations range from 0.70 to 0.95 mmol/L. The daily oral intake is 8–20 mmol (40% of which is absorbed) and the urinary loss, which is the major source of excretion of magnesium, varies from 2.5 to 8 mmol/day.[41]

HYPOMAGNESAEMIA

Hypomagnesaemia is caused by decreased intake or increased loss (**Box 93.7**). Clinical features include neurological signs of confusion, irritability, delirium tremors, convulsions and tachyarrhythmias. Hypomagnesaemia is often associated with resistant hypokalaemia and hypocalcaemia. Treatment consists of i.v. magnesium sulphate as a bolus of 10 mmol, administered over 5 minutes, followed by 20–60 mmol/day.

Box 93.7 Causes of magnesium deficiency

- Gastrointestinal disorders
  - Malabsorption syndromes
  - GIT fistulas
  - Short-bowel syndrome
  - Prolonged nasogastric suction
  - Diarrhoea
  - Pancreatitis
  - Parenteral nutrition
- Alcoholism
- Endocrine disorders
  - Hyperparathyroidism
  - Hyperthyroidism
  - Conn's syndrome
  - Diabetes mellitus
  - Hyperaldosteronism
- Renal diseases
  - Renal tubular acidosis
  - Diuretic phase of acute tubular necrosis
- Drugs
  - Aminoglycosides
  - Carbenicillin, ticarcillin
  - Amphotericin B
  - Diuretics
  - Cis-platinum
  - Ciclosporin

HYPERMAGNESAEMIA

Hypermagnesaemia is often caused by excessive administration of magnesium salts or conventional doses of magnesium in the presence of renal failure. Clinical features include drowsiness, hyporeflexia and coma, vasodilatation and hypotension, and conduction defects of sinoatrial and atrioventricular nodal block and asystole may occur. Treatment is directed towards increasing excretion of the ion, which may require dialysis. Intravenous calcium chloride may be used for rapidly treating the cardiac conduction defects.[41]

MAGNESIUM THERAPY

There are increasing reports of the use of magnesium as a therapy for a variety of conditions. A randomised control trial of over 10 000 women with pre-eclampsia demonstrated the efficacy of magnesium in the prevention of eclampsia,[42] and it is also a recommended treatment for established eclampsia. It has been used to treat atrial fibrillation, to achieve both rate control and reversion to sinus rhythm in a number of settings, including post cardiac surgery, and in the emergency department.[43,44] Magnesium, given either intravenously or nebulised, may be beneficial for patients with acute severe asthma.[45,46] There are also preliminary trials to suggest that magnesium may prevent delayed cerebral ischaemia due to vasospasm in patients with subarachnoid haemorrhage.[47]

PHOSPHATE

While most of the body phosphate exists in bone, 15% is found in the soft tissues as ATP, red blood cell 2,3-DPG, and other cellular structural proteins, including phospholipids, nucleic acids and phosphoproteins. Phosphate also acts as a cellular and urinary buffer.[41]

HYPOPHOSPHATAEMIA

Hypophosphataemia may be caused by a decreased intake, increased excretion or intracellular redistribution (**Box 93.8**). Although hypophosphataemia may be symptom-free, clinical features have been described that include paraesthesia, muscle weakness, seizures,

Box 93.8 Causes of hypophosphataemia

- Hyperparathyroidism
- Vitamin D deficiency
- Vitamin-D-resistant rickets
- Renal tubular acidosis
- Alkalosis
- Parenteral nutrition
- Alcoholism
- Refeeding syndrome

coma, rhabdomyolysis and cardiac failure. Hypophosphataemia may be a prominent feature of the refeeding syndrome when it may be accompanied by other electrolyte disturbances such as hypokalaemia and hypomagnesaemia. Treatment consists of close monitoring and replacement as oral or i.v. sodium or potassium phosphate, 50–100 mmol/24 h.

HYPERPHOSPHATAEMIA

Hyperphosphataemia is usually caused by an increased intake or decreased excretion (**Box 93.9**). Clinical features include ectopic calcification of nephrocalcinosis, nephrolithiasis and band keratopathy. Treatment may require haemodialysis; otherwise oral aluminium hydroxide and even hypertonic glucose solutions to shift ECF phosphate into the ICF can be used.

Box 93.9 Causes of hyperphosphataemia

- Rhabdomyolysis
- Renal failure (acute or chronic)
- Vitamin D toxicity
- Acidosis
- Tumour lysis
- Hypoparathyroidism
- Pseudohypoparathyroidism
- Diphosphonate (bisphosphonate) therapy
- Excess i.v. administration

FLUID AND ELECTROLYTE REPLACEMENT THERAPY

GENERAL PRINCIPLES

In critical illness many of the body's normal homeostatic mechanisms are deranged and basic life-preserving senses such as hunger and thirst may be abolished by disease processes or by treatments such as the use of sedation. As a result, the survival of critically ill patients depends on the administration of appropriate volumes of fluids, and appropriate quantities of electrolytes and nutrition by their medical and nursing attendants. Basal requirements for water, electrolytes and nutrients are discussed in Chapter 94. In addition to basal requirements, many critically ill patients have abnormal fluid and electrolyte losses that must be replaced; examples are discussed below.

GASTROINTESTINAL LOSSES

The daily volumes and composition of gastrointestinal tract (GIT) secretions in mmol/L are shown in **Table 93.8**. Clinical effects of fluid loss from the GIT are largely determined by the volume and composition of the fluid, and therapy is usually directed at replacing the losses. Gastric fluid loss (e.g. from vomiting and nasogastric suction) results in water, sodium, hydrogen ion, potassium and chloride depletion. Hence metabolic alkalosis, hypokalaemia, hypotension and dehydration develop if the saline and potassium chloride losses are not correctly replaced.

Pancreatic and biliary fluid losses (e.g. pancreatic or biliary fistula)

These may result in hyperchloraemic acidosis with hypokalaemia, hypotension and dehydration if the losses of bicarbonate, potassium and saline are not correctly replaced.

Intestinal losses (e.g. fistula or ileostomy losses, diarrhoea and ileus)

These result in hypokalaemia, hypotension and dehydration if the saline and potassium losses are not replaced.

RESUSCITATION FLUIDS

Systemic hypotension is a common feature of acute critical illness and first-line treatment is usually the administration of intravenous resuscitation fluid. The fluids available to clinicians to maintain or expand intravascular volume include crystalloids, colloids and blood products; the properties of colloid solutions and blood products are discussed in Chapters 95 and 96.

Whether the choice of resuscitation fluid influences patients' outcomes has been the subject of long-running debate. This debate, which was been fuelled by the conflicting and inconclusive results of a number of meta-analyses[48–49] may now be nearing resolution. Recent data from clinical trials may help guide clinicians with the choice of resuscitation fluids. The first adequately powered trial, the Saline versus Albumin Fluid

Table 93.8 Daily volume and electrolyte composition of GIT secretions

ELECTROLYTES (MMOL/L)	VOL. (L)	H^+	Na^+	K^-	CL^-	HCO_3^-
Saliva	0.5–1.0	0	30	20	10–35	0–15
Stomach	1.0–2.5	0–120	60	10	100–120	0
Bile	0.5	0	140	5–10	100	40–70
Pancreatic	0.75	0	140	5–10	70	40–70
Small and large gut	2.0–4.0	0	110	5–10	100	25

Evaluation (SAFE) Study, found that saline and albumin produced comparable outcomes in a heterogeneous population of adult patients,[50] but in patients with traumatic brain injury resuscitation with albumin was associated with a significant increase in mortality[51] Choice of fluid for resuscitation may also be important in patients with severe sepsis. In a trial led by the Scandinavian Critical Care Trials Group[52] patients with severe sepsis who were resuscitated with hydroxylethyl starch 130/0.42 in Ringer's acetate had an increased risk of death compared with resuscitated only with Ringer's acetate. Although rapid fluid resuscitation remains a strongly recommended treatment for adults with severe sepsis in the developed world, a trial in African children with severe infections has challenged the assumption that this is the correct strategy in all situations. In the FEAST study, children with severe infections who received 20–40 mL/kg of either normal saline or 5% albumin as fluid boluses had an increased risk of death compared with those who received only maintenance fluids.[53] The relevance of these findings for adult and developed world medicine is unclear. Further investigator-initiated trials are currently under way (such as the CHEST study, NCT00935168) and their results may further assist clinicians to develop evidence-based fluid resuscitation strategies.

Access the complete references list online at http://www.expertconsult.com

51. Myburgh J, Cooper DJ, Finfer S, et al. Saline or albumin for fluid resuscitation in patients with traumatic brain injury. N Engl J Med 2007;357(9): 874–84.
52. Perner A, Haase N, Guttormsen AB, et al. Hydroxyethyl starch 130/0.42 versus Ringer's acetate in severe sepsis. New Engl J Med 2012;367(2): 124–34.
53. Maitland K, Kiguli S, Opoka RO, et al. Mortality after fluid bolus in African children with severe infection. New Engl J Med 2011;364(26):2483–95.

94

Enteral and parenteral nutrition

Richard Leonard

It is standard practice to provide nutritional support to critically ill patients in order to treat existing malnutrition and minimise wasting of lean body mass. However, despite the universality of this practice, the evidence underlying it is often conflicting and of disappointingly poor quality.[1] The failings in the evidence seem to extend to some of the resulting debates, in which extreme positions are defended.[2,3] Inevitably these difficulties have led many to seek clarity in meta-analyses; perhaps equally inevitably,[4,5] these have usually disappointed. On so basic a question as the relative merits of enteral and parenteral routes of feeding, the two most recent meta-analyses have produced conflicting results.[6,7]

The problem persists with the publication of numerous clinical practice guidelines,[8–14] which differ radically in important areas.[15] Three studies have examined the effect of introducing such guidelines into ICUs using a cluster-randomisation design; whereas the first – the ACCEPT study – found a 10% reduction in mortality, which narrowly failed to reach statistical significance,[8] the other two detected no outcome benefit.[16,17]

NUTRITIONAL ASSESSMENT

Objective assessment of nutritional status is difficult in ICU, because disease processes confound methods used in the general population. Anthropometric measures such as triceps skin-fold thickness and mid-arm circumference may be obscured by oedema. Voluntary handgrip strength is impractical in unconscious patients. Laboratory measures, including transferrin, pre-albumin and albumin levels, lymphocyte counts, and skin-prick test reactivity, are abnormal in critical illness. Clinical evaluation – the so-called subjective global assessment – is better than objective measurement at predicting morbidity.[18] Historical features of malnutrition include weight loss, poor diet, gastrointestinal symptoms, reduced functional capacity and a diagnosis associated with poor intake. Physical signs include loss of subcutaneous fat, muscle wasting, peripheral oedema and ascites.

Although laboratory measures are of little value in assessing nutritional status in critically ill patients, they may be useful before elective major surgery. Serum albumin and operative site are closely associated with the risk of postoperative complications.[19] This raises the possibility that outcomes may be improved by treating preoperative malnutrition identified by a simple screening test.

PATIENT SELECTION AND TIMING OF SUPPORT

There are reasonable grounds to believe that it is better to provide nutritional support to critically ill patients than not to do so. This belief is based on the close association between malnutrition, negative nitrogen and calorie balance and poor outcome, and the inevitability of death if starvation continues for long enough. In otherwise healthy humans this takes several weeks to occur. There is also some direct evidence from one study of jejunal feeding in patients operated on for severe pancreatitis,[20] in which the control group received only intravenous fluids until normal diet resumed. Mortality markedly decreased in the group receiving nutritional support.

Two questions arise from this, relating to the important problem of when nutritional support should start:

- How long is it safe to leave a critically ill patient without nutrition? In other words, which patients need to be fed artificially because they would otherwise be starved for too long, and who can safely wait until they are able to eat?
- If the patient will clearly exceed whatever period is deemed reasonable, is it better to begin feeding immediately? In other words, when should we start to feed?

Quite good evidence now supports the early institution of nutritional support, and the trend is both to tolerate much shorter periods without nutrition and to begin feeding more rapidly after initial resuscitation.

In 1997, recommendations from a conference sponsored by the US National Institutes of Health, the American Society for Parenteral and Enteral Nutrition and the American Society for Clinical Nutrition suggested that nutritional support be started in any critically ill patient unlikely to regain oral intake within 7–10 days.[21] The basis for this was that, at a typical nitrogen loss of 20–40 g/day, dangerous depletion of lean tissue may occur after 14 days of starvation. Others have suggested a maximum acceptable delay of 3–7 days. Small studies comparing earlier with delayed institution of nutritional support have had conflicting results. A meta-analysis comparing early (first 48 hours after admission to ICU) with late enteral feeding revealed a reduction in infectious complications.[22] Two subsequent meta-analyses comparing early and delayed enteral feeding both found a reduction in mortality with early support,[23,24] although the authors commented that the total number of patients and the methodological quality of the studies included were both low. Early institution of enteral feeding within 24 hours of ICU admission in patients unlikely to feed orally in that time was an important component of the ACCEPT study guideline (**Fig. 94.1**).[8] The weight of evidence is presently in favour of this more aggressive approach, but it can hardly be regarded as conclusively proven.[25]

NUTRITIONAL REQUIREMENTS OF THE CRITICALLY ILL

ENERGY

Some muscle wasting and nitrogen loss are unavoidable in critical illness, despite adequate energy and protein provision.[26] This fact, coupled with the realisation that caloric requirements had previously been overestimated, has led to downward revision of intake, a process which may be continuing. In 1997, the American College of Chest Physicians (ACCP) published guidelines recommending a daily energy intake of 25 kcal/kg,[11] and this has remained the standard target energy intake for critically ill patients.

More recently, concerns have been raised that this standard intake may be excessive. An observational study found lower mortality in those patients who received 9–18 kcal/kg/day than in those with higher

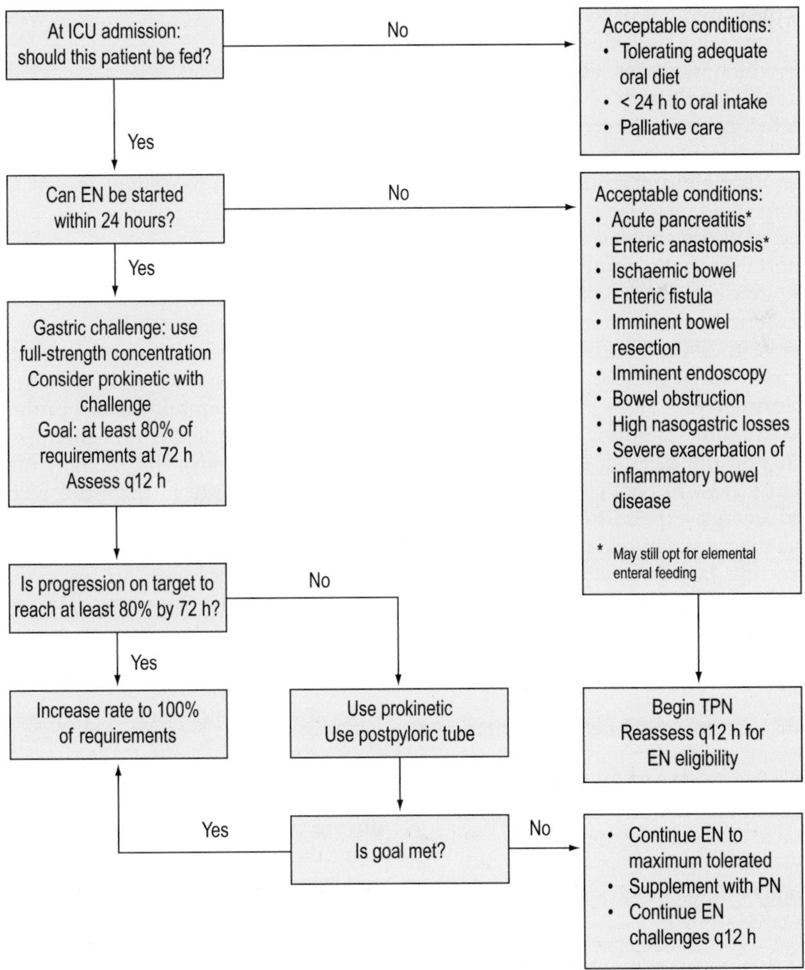

Figure 94.1 Algorithm for nutritional support used in the ACCEPT trial.[8] EN=enteral nutrition; PN=parenteral nutrition.

and lower intakes.[27] One small study showed no change in ICU or 28-day mortality, but a reduction in hospital and 180-day mortality, in patients fed with a target of 60–70% of their calculated requirement compared with those fed at 90–100% of required energy intake. However, the difference in delivered intakes was small.[28] In contrast, a much larger study comparing full enteral feeding with 'trophic' low-dose feeding for the first week after patients were admitted with acute lung injury could not identify any effect.[29] At present, unequivocal benefits of hypocaloric feeding have yet to be demonstrated in large prospective trials. It remains extremely important to realise that enterally fed patients frequently fail to achieve their target intake, and that significant under-feeding is certainly associated with worse outcomes.[27,30,31]

Attempts have also been made to tailor the energy provided to critically ill patients to their individual needs. Two methods are commonly used: indirect calorimetry and predictive equations. Indirect calorimetry is the gold standard, and its use is becoming easier with the availability of devices designed for ICU patients. It permits measurement of the resting energy expenditure (REE). This value excludes the energy cost of physical activity, which increases later in the course of an ICU admission.[32] Calorimetry reveals deviations from values predicted by equations, such that two-thirds of patients in one study were being either under- or overfed.[33] On the other hand, it could not be shown that outcomes are improved by the use of calorimetry,[34] although a more recent study showed a trend towards reduced hospital mortality in the group whose feeding was calorimetrically guided (and who received in consequence a higher caloric intake).[35] Moreover, there are no clear data to relate measured REE to total energy expenditure in the individual patient. Presently most ICUs do not use calorimetry.

There are several equations claiming to predict basal metabolic rate (BMR) on the basis of weight, sex and age. Correction factors exist to convert predictions of BMR into estimated energy expenditure by adjusting for such variables as diagnosis, pyrexia and activity. In the past these correction factors have been excessive and may have contributed to overfeeding; a more conservative approach is now advocated. The recommendations of the British Association for Parenteral and Enteral Nutrition are:[36]

1. Determine BMR from Schofield's equations (**Table 94.1**).
2. Adjust BMR for stress (**Table 94.2**).
3. Add a combined factor for activity- and diet-induced thermogenesis:
   bed-bound, immobile: +10%
   bed-bound, mobile/sitting: +20%
   mobile around ward: +25%.

Despite the popularity of measurements or estimates of energy expenditure it is not clear that their routine use improves outcome. Many clinicians dispense with both and simply aim to deliver the ACCP's recommended target of 25 kcal/kg/day.

Table 94.1 Basal metabolic rate in kcal/day by age and gender[37]

AGE	FEMALE	MALE
15–18	13.3 W+690	17.6 W+656
18–30	14.8 W+485	15.0 W+690
30–60	8.1 W+842	11.4 W+870
>60	9.0 W+656	11.7 W+585

W=weight in kg.

Table 94.2 Stress adjustment in the calculation of basal metabolic rate[36]

Partial starvation (>10% weight loss)	Subtract 0–15%
Mild infection, inflammatory bowel disease, postoperative	Add 0–13%
Moderate infection, multiple long bone fractures	Add 10–30%
Severe sepsis, multiple trauma (ventilated)	Add 25–50%
Burns 10–90%	Add 10–70%

PROTEIN

Assessment of nitrogen balance by measuring urinary urea nitrogen is too variable to be useful in estimating protein requirements in ICU.[38] As there is an upper limit to the amount of dietary protein that can be used for synthesis,[39] there is no benefit from replacing nitrogen lost in excess of this. A daily nitrogen provision of 0.15–0.2 g/kg/day is therefore recommended for the ICU population; this is equivalent to 1–1.25 g protein/kg/day. Severely hypercatabolic individuals, such as those with major burns, are given up to 0.3 g nitrogen/kg/day, or nearly 2 g protein/kg/day.[36]

MICRONUTRIENTS

Critical illness increases the requirements for vitamins A, E, K, thiamine (B1), B3, B6, vitamin C and pantothenic and folic acids.[40] Thiamine, folic acid and vitamin K are particularly vulnerable to deficiency during total parenteral nutrition (TPN). Renal replacement therapy can cause loss of water-soluble vitamins and trace elements. Deficiencies of selenium, zinc, manganese and copper have been described in critical illness, in addition to the more familiar iron-deficient state. Subclinical deficiencies in critically ill patients are thought to cause immune deficiency and reduced

Table 94.3 Vitamin requirements in critical illness[40]

VITAMIN	FUNCTION	DOSE
Vitamin A	Cell growth, night vision	10 000–25 000 IU
Vitamin D	Calcium metabolism	400–1000 IU
Vitamin E	Membrane antioxidant	400–1000 IU
Beta carotene*	Antioxidant	50 mg
Vitamin K	Activation of clotting factors	1.5 µg/kg/day
Thiamine (vitamin B1)	Oxidative decarboxylation	10 mg
Riboflavin (vitamin B2)	Oxidative phosphorylation	10 mg
Niacin (vitamin B3)	Part of NAD, redox reactions	200 mg
Pantothenic acid	Part of coenzyme A	100 mg
Biotin	Carboxylase activity	5 mg
Pyridoxine (vitamin B6)	Decarboxylase activity	20 mg
Folic acid	Haematopoiesis	2 mg
Vitamin B12	Haematopoiesis	20 µg
Vitamin C	Antioxidant, collagen synthesis	2000 mg

*Not strictly a vitamin.

Table 94.4 Trace element requirements in critical illness[40]

ELEMENT	FUNCTION	DOSE
Selenium	Antioxidant, fat metabolism	100 µg
Zinc	Energy metabolism, protein synthesis, epithelial growth	50 mg
Copper	Collagen cross-linking, ceruloplasmin	2–3 mg
Manganese	Neural function, fatty acid synthesis	25–50 mg
Chromium	Insulin activity	200 mg
Cobalt	B12 synthesis	
Iodine	Thyroid hormones	
Iron	Haematopoiesis, oxidative phosphorylation	10 mg
Molybdenum	Purine and pyridine metabolism	0.2–0.5 mg

Table 94.5 Water and electrolyte requirements per kilogram per day

Water	30 ml
Sodium	1–2 mmol
Potassium	0.7–1 mmol
Magnesium	0.1 mmol
Calcium	0.1 mmol
Phosphorus	0.4 mmol

resistance to oxidative stress. Suggested requirements for micronutrients in critically ill patients vary between authors and depending on route of administration; the most comprehensive guidance[40] is reproduced in **Tables 94.3** and **94.4**. More recent but broadly similar recommendations for some compounds are also available.[41,42]

Commercial preparations of both enteral and parenteral feeding solutions contain standard amounts of micronutrients. Supplementation of intake of certain antioxidant vitamins and trace elements above these levels is discussed below.

WATER AND ELECTROLYTES

Water and electrolyte requirements vary widely depending on the patient's condition; typical basal intakes are shown in **Table 94.5**.

ROUTE OF NUTRITION

When possible patients should be fed enterally. The advantages over the parenteral route are the lower cost, greater simplicity and possibly fewer infective complications. These appear to be the only advantages of the enteral route. Despite the fervour with which some pursue the debate,[2,3] there is little basis for the widespread belief that the enteral route provides a clear benefit in terms of outcome.

Two hypotheses are commonly advanced in support of the putative superiority of enteral feeding. First, it appears that the lipid contained within TPN is immunosuppressive. Intravenous lipid is known to suppress neutrophil and reticulo-endothelial system function, and a comparison of TPN with and without lipid in critically ill trauma patients showed a lower complication rate in those not receiving lipid.[43] Secondly, enteral feeding may protect against infective complications. Absence of complex nutrients from the intestinal lumen is followed in rats by villus atrophy and reduced cell mass of the gut-associated lymphoid tissue (GALT). Starved humans show these changes to a much lesser extent. Lymphocytes produced in the GALT are redistributed to the respiratory tract, and contribute heavily to mucosal immunity. In mice, this contribution is lost during TPN. The possibility that multiple organ failure may be driven by translocation of bacteria or endotoxin across an impaired mucosal barrier has been extensively investigated in animals. Although it is known that TPN is associated with increased gut permeability to macromolecules in humans, this does not seem to result in translocation.[44] Although translocation does occur following surgery, and seems to be associated with sepsis,[45] a causal relation with multiple organ failure is unproven.

In fact, a reduction in septic morbidity has been found only in certain groups, primarily abdominal trauma victims,[46,47] in whom parenteral nutrition was associated with a higher incidence of abdominal abscess and pneumonia. A third study found no difference.[48] In head-injured patients there is one trial showing no effect and one each supporting either route; however, in the study favouring TPN the enteral nutrition group were significantly underfed.[49–51] None of these studies is less than 20 years old, and the techniques of both enteral and parenteral feeding have changed a great deal in that time. Reductions in infective complications have also been found using enteral feeding in pancreatitis.[52] In contrast, no benefit was found in sepsis, though enteral feeding was instituted late.[53]

More recent systematic analyses have, as mentioned earlier, produced conflicting results. One found a reduction in infectious complications with enteral feeding, but no difference in mortality.[7] The most recent meta-analysis considered only high-quality trials using an intention-to-treat principle. It showed a clear reduction in mortality in patients fed parenterally.[6]

This mortality difference disappeared when early enteral and parenteral feeding were compared. On this basis, as in the ACCEPT study, the authors recommended early use of the enteral route, with recourse to parenteral nutrition if this was not possible. A well-powered randomised study comparing early parenteral with early enteral feeding is presently recruiting.[54] However, in view of the practical and financial advantages of enteral feeding, it will probably need to find a significant mortality difference in favour of the parenteral route if it is to change the present pragmatic preference for enteral feeding.

One related area of controversy remains the practice - advocated in the European guidelines, deprecated in the two North American ones - of supplementing partially successful but inadequate enteral intake with intravenous feeding relatively early in the course of an ICU admission.[9,13,14] One large multicentre study compared early parenteral supplementation of inadequate enteral intake (within 48 hours of ICU admission) with supplementation delayed until day 8.[55] There was no mortality difference, but patients in the delayed-supplementation group left ICU earlier and suffered fewer infective complications. However, interpretation of this study is complicated by the fact that the early-supplementation group received 25–30 kcal/kg/day, raising the possibility that high intake, rather than the route of feeding, was responsible for the increase in infections. The study also used tight glycaemic control. These differences from common practice make it difficult to generalise the findings. It is presently uncertain whether, when and at what dose parenteral feeding should be used to supplement inadequate enteral intake, but very early, aggressive intravenous supplementation does not seem warranted.

ENTERAL NUTRITION

ACCESS

Nasal tubes are preferred to oral, except in patients with a basal skull fracture, in whom there is a risk of cranial penetration. A large-bore (12–14 Fr) nasogastric tube is usually used at first. Once feeding is established and gastric residual volumes (see below) no longer need to be checked this can be replaced with a more comfortable fine-bore tube. A stylet is needed to assist in passage of fine-bore tubes. The position of all tubes must be checked on X-ray before feeding is started, as misplacement is not uncommon and intrapulmonary delivery of feed is potentially fatal.

Nasojejunal tubes may be beneficial if impaired gastric emptying is refractory to prokinetic agents[8] (see below); their unselective use is not indicated even in patients with mildly elevated gastric residual volumes.[56,57] Spontaneous passage through the pylorus following blind placement is not reliable, but may be increased by the administration of single doses of 200 mg erythromycin or 20 mg metoclopramide.[58] Endoscopic or fluoroscopic assistance is needed for truly reliable transpyloric tube placement, although use of electromagnetic guidance systems may obviate the logistic difficulties these traditional methods entail.[59] There are conflicting data on the question of whether nasojejunal feeding reduces the risk of aspiration or ventilator-associated pneumonia.[57,60,61] The lack of evidence of a clear benefit, coupled with the cost and logistic difficulty of placing them, precludes the routine use of nasojejunal tubes for all patients.

An alternative method of access in those needing long-term enteral feeding is percutaneous gastrostomy, which can be performed endoscopically or radiologically. Percutaneous jejunal access can be obtained either via a gastrostomy or by direct placement during incidental laparotomy.

REGIMEN

Slowly building up the rate of feeding is not proven to avoid diarrhoea or high gastric residual volumes. Head-injured patients fed with target intake from the outset have fewer infective complications,[62] and the practice has subsequently been shown to be safe in unselected ICU patients.[63] Nevertheless, it is presently common practice to start delivering around 30 mL/h and build up to the target intake depending on tolerance, as judged by gastric residual volumes. These are assessed by aspiration of the tube every 4 hours. Gastric residual volumes over 150 mL on two successive occasions have been associated with an increased incidence of ventilator-associated pneumonia in one study;[64] in contrast others have found no link between high residual volumes and the risk of aspiration.[65] Nevertheless, if the residual volume is consistently greater than 200 mL, treatment with prokinetic agents (metoclopramide 10 mg q. 8 h or erythromycin 250 mg q. 12 h intravenously) appears to increase tolerance of feeding, though there is no discernible effect on mortality or morbidity.[58] This is unsurprising in light of two recent studies showing that it is safe to tolerate gastric residual volumes up to 500 mL[66] or even not to check the volume at all.[67] An interesting report that acupuncture is more effective than a combination of metoclopramide, cisapride and erythromycin requires confirmation.[68] In refractory cases a nasojejunal tube often permits successful enteral feeding, because small bowel function is resumed quicker than gastric emptying. A nasogastric tube is still needed to drain the stomach. Diarrhoea, abdominal distension, nausea and vomiting may suggest intolerance, despite low gastric volumes. Absence of bowel sounds is common in ventilated patients and should not be taken to indicate ileus.

Fine-bore tubes should not be aspirated as this causes them to block. Various folk remedies have been tried for unblocking tubes, including instillation of Coca-Cola™, fruit juice and pancreatic enzyme supplements. The instillates should be left in situ for an hour or more.

COMPOSITION

Commercially available enteral feeding solutions vary widely in composition. Polymeric feeds contain intact proteins (derived from whey, meat, soy isolates and caseinates) and carbohydrates in the form of oligo- and polysaccharides. These require pancreatic enzymes for absorption.

Elemental feeds with defined nitrogen sources (amino acids or peptides) are not of benefit when used routinely, but may enable feeding when small bowel absorption is impaired, for instance in pancreatic insufficiency or following prolonged starvation. Lipids are usually provided by vegetable oils consisting mostly of long-chain triglycerides, but some also contain more easily absorbed medium-chain triglycerides. The proportion of non-protein calories provided as carbohydrate is usually two-thirds.

Electrolyte composition varies widely, with sodium- and potassium-restricted formulations available. Vitamins and trace elements are usually added by the manufacturers so that daily requirements are present in a volume containing roughly 2000 kcal. The possible benefits of providing additional doses of some of these substances to critically ill patients are considered below.

COMPLICATIONS

Enteral feeding is an independent risk factor for ventilator-associated pneumonia.[69] Sinusitis due to nasogastric intubation may necessitate changing to an orogastric tube. Fine-bore tubes are vulnerable to misplacement in the trachea or to perforation of the pharynx, oesophagus, stomach or bowel. Percutaneous endoscopic gastrostomy is associated with a high 30-day all-cause mortality in acutely ill patients, in whom it may be best avoided.[70] Other complications include insertion site infection, serious abdominal wall infection and peritonitis. Surgically placed jejunostomies can cause similar problems, and may also obstruct the bowel.

Diarrhoea is common in ICU patients, particularly those being fed enterally. It is often multifactorial and causes considerable distress and morbidity, particularly when the patient is repeatedly soiled with watery stool. Common causes include antibiotic therapy, *Clostridium difficile* infection, faecal impaction and a non-specific effect of critical illness. Malabsorption, lactose intolerance, prokinetic agents, magnesium, aminophylline, quinidine and medications containing sorbitol (for instance, paracetamol syrup and cimetidine) are occasional culprits. Rate of administration of enteral feed also plays a role. Faecal impaction, medication-induced diarrhoea and *Clostridium difficile* infection must be excluded or treated, while malabsorption may respond to elemental diet. Slowing the rate of feeding sometimes helps; diluting the formula does not. It is unclear whether addition of probiotics to enteral feed is of benefit; one small study has suggested they may reduce the incidence of diarrhoea, whereas another showed no benefit to patients with established feed-related diarrhoea.[71,72]

Metabolic complications include electrolyte abnormalities and hyperglycaemia. Severely malnourished patients are at risk of refeeding syndrome (see below) if nutritional support is begun too rapidly.

PARENTERAL NUTRITION

Parenteral nutritional support is indicated when adequate enteral intake cannot be established within an acceptable time. In some cases absolute gastrointestinal failure is obvious, whereas in others it becomes apparent only after considerable efforts to feed enterally have failed. As discussed above, there is increasing evidence that if enteral feeding cannot be established early then the parenteral route should be used until it can. Nevertheless, the aim in all patients fed intravenously should be to revert to enteral feeding as this becomes possible.

Box 94.1 Minimum monitoring during TPN – less stable patients may require more intensive surveillance

Nursing	Weekly (at least)
Temperature	Full blood picture
Pulse	Coagulation screen
Blood pressure	Liver function tests
Respiratory rate	Magnesium, calcium and phosphate
Fluid balance	Weight
Blood sugar (4-hourly when commencing feed)	**As indicated**
Daily (at least)	Zinc
Review of fluid balance	Uric acid
Review of nutrient intake	
Blood sugar	
Urea, electrolytes and creatinine	

The question of whether to supplement inadequate enteral feeding with intravenous support has also been discussed earlier.

Parenteral feeding solutions may be prepared from their component parts under sterile conditions. Ready-made solutions also exist, but any necessary additions must be made in the same way.

In ICU patients the daily requirements are infused continuously over 24 hours. Careful biochemical and clinical monitoring is important, particularly at the outset (**Box 94.1**).

ACCESS

The major concern with central venous access for TPN is prevention of infection. The following considerations apply.[73]

- *Insertion site:* subclavian lines have lower infection rates than internal jugular or femoral lines.
- *Tunnelling* may reduce infection rates in internal jugular lines but apparently not in short-term subclavian lines. It is not recommended for routine use.
- *Expertise* of operator and adequacy of ICU *nurse staffing levels* affect infection rate.
- *Skin preparation:* 2% chlorhexidine in alcohol is the most effective.
- *Sterile technique:* maximal sterile barrier procedures (mask, cap, gown, gloves, and large drape) are known to reduce catheter-related bacteraemia rates sixfold. There is a bewildering resistance to use of these precautions outside ICUs.
- *Dressings:* permeable polyurethane transparent dressings are superior to impermeable.
- *Antimicrobial catheters:* catheters coated with either chlorhexidine and silver sulfadiazine or rifampicin and minocycline are several times less likely to cause bacteraemia than standard polyurethane catheters. The duration of the anti-infective effect appears to be longer with the antibiotic-coated catheters (2 weeks versus 1).
- *Scheduled exchange* has not been proven to reduce catheter-related sepsis.
- *Guide-wire exchange* is associated with increased bacteraemia rates, which in routine use outweigh the reduced mechanical complications.

In practice pre-existing central access is used in the first instance. If a multi-lumen catheter is used, one lumen should be dedicated to administration of TPN and not used for any other purpose. Three-way taps should be avoided and infusion set changes carried out daily under sterile conditions. For long-term TPN (more than 2 months) specialised catheters with a tunnelled cuff or a subcutaneous port are recommended.

COMPOSITION

ENERGY

Energy is provided by a combination of carbohydrate and lipid. The optimal balance between the two is unknown; often 30–40% of non-protein energy is given as lipid. Alternatively, glucose may be relied upon for almost all the energy, with lipid being infused once or twice a week to provide essential fatty acids.

Glucose is the preferred carbohydrate and is infused as a concentrated solution. Exceeding the body's capacity to metabolise glucose (4 mg/kg/min in the septic patient) can lead to hyperglycaemia, lipogenesis and excess CO_2 production. Endogenous insulin secretion increases to control blood sugar levels. However, many patients require additional insulin, particularly diabetics. This may be infused separately, but when requirements are stable it is more safely added to the TPN solution. Persistent hyperglycaemia is better addressed by reducing the glucose infusion rate than by large doses of insulin.

Lipid provides essential fatty acids (linoleic and linolenic acids) and is a more concentrated energy source than glucose. It may thus avoid the complications of excess glucose administration. However, there are concerns of immunosuppression from lipid infusion, as discussed above. Current lipid preparations consist of soybean oil emulsified with glycerol and egg phosphatides. Replacement of some or all of the soybean oil with olive-oil- or fish-oil-based lipids or with medium-chain triglycerides has been proposed to offer immunological benefits; however, clear evidence of this has so far been elusive.[74]

NITROGEN

Nitrogen is supplied as crystalline solutions of L-amino acids. Commercially available preparations vary in their provision of conditionally essential amino acids. Glutamine, tyrosine and cysteine are absent from many because of instability.

MICRONUTRIENTS

Vitamin and trace element preparations are added to TPN solutions in appropriate amounts. Thiamine, folic acid and vitamin K are particularly vulnerable to depletion and additional doses may be necessary.

ELECTROLYTES

Amino acid preparations contain varying quantities of electrolytes; additional amounts may need to be added to the solution.

COMPLICATIONS

Parenteral nutrition has the potential for severe complications.

- *Catheter-related sepsis* is addressed above. Other complications of central venous cannulation are discussed elsewhere.
- *Electrolyte abnormalities* include hypophosphataemia, hypokalaemia and hypomagnesaemia, especially in the first 24–48 hours.
- *Hyperchloraemic metabolic acidosis* may result from amino acid solutions with a high chloride content. Replacing some chloride with acetate in the TPN solution will resolve this where necessary.
- *Rebound hypoglycaemia* may occur when TPN is discontinued suddenly. TPN should be weaned over a minimum of 12 hours. If it cannot be continued, an infusion of 10% dextrose should be started and blood sugars closely monitored.
- *Refeeding syndrome* may occur when normal intake is resumed after a period of starvation. It is associated with profound hypophosphataemia, and possibly hypokalaemia and hypomagnesaemia. With the restoration of glucose as a substrate, insulin levels rise and cause cellular uptake of these ions. Depletion of adenosine triphosphate (ATP) and 2,3-diphosphoglyceric acid (2,3-DPG) results in tissue hypoxia and failure of cellular energy metabolism. This may manifest as cardiac and respiratory failure, with paraesthesiae and seizures also reported. Thiamine deficiency may also play a part.
- *Liver dysfunction* is common during TPN. Causes include hepatic steatosis, intrahepatic cholestasis and biliary sludging from gallbladder inactivity. The problems necessitating TPN in the first place may also cause liver dysfunction.
- *Deficiencies* of trace elements and vitamins (especially thiamine, folic acid and vitamin K) may occur.

NUTRITION AND SPECIFIC DISEASES

ACUTE RENAL FAILURE

The advent of continuous renal replacement therapy means that dietary fluid and protein restriction is rarely necessary in ICU. Use of specialised lipid or amino acid formulations in TPN is not supported by evidence, and in general normal nutritional support is appropriate in acute renal failure.

LIVER DISEASE[21,75]

Energy requirements in ICU patients are not altered by the presence of chronic liver disease. Lipolysis is increased, so lipid must be used with caution to avoid hypertriglyceridaemia (not more than 1 g/kg/day). Protein restriction may be required in chronic hepatic encephalopathy; starting with 0.5 g/kg/day the dose may be cautiously increased towards a normal intake. Hepatic encephalopathy may in part be due to depletion of branched-chain amino acids (BCAAs) permitting increased cerebral uptake of aromatic amino acids, which produce inhibitory neurotransmitters. In protein-intolerant patients the use of feeds enriched with BCAAs may permit greater protein intake without worsening encephalopathy. Their routine use is not indicated.[76] Thiamine and fat-soluble vitamin deficiencies are common in patients with chronic liver disease. Fulminant hepatic failure reduces gluconeogenesis; hypoglycaemia is a common problem necessitating glucose infusion. Lipid is well tolerated. Energy and protein requirements are similar to those above. BCAAs have not been shown to be superior to standard amino-acid solutions.

RESPIRATORY FAILURE

Oxidation of fat produces less carbon dioxide than glucose. There have been attempts to use this to assist in weaning from mechanical ventilation by providing 50% of energy intake as lipid, with mixed results. Avoidance of overfeeding is much more important. The supplementation of omega-3 fatty acids in patients with acute lung injury (ALI) or acute respiratory distress syndrome (ARDS) is discussed below.

ACUTE PANCREATITIS

Formerly, TPN was a cornerstone of the management of severe acute pancreatitis to minimise pancreatic stimulation. This has changed with the publication of studies showing both gastric and jejunal feeding to be safe, effective and associated with reductions in infective complications compared with TPN.[51,77] Elemental feeds and pancreatic enzyme supplements are logical if malabsorption is a problem. Despite the shift towards enteral feeding of patients with pancreatitis, some can be fed only intravenously.

OBESITY

Although both the US clinical practice guideline and a subsequent consensus workshop recommend hypocaloric, high-protein feeding for obese patients, the strength of the recommendation is low and the evidence for it weak.[14,78] Their suggested caloric requirement is 22–25 kcal/kg ideal body weight/day or 11–14 kcal/kg actual body weight/day, of which 60–70% should actually be provided, together with 2 g/kg/day protein. No other guideline makes such a recommendation. At present there is insufficient evidence to justify feeding obese patients differently from others.

ADJUNCTIVE NUTRITION

Certain substances have been used as adjuncts to feeding solutions, in attempts to modulate the metabolic and immune responses to critical illness. In general no conclusive benefit has yet been shown in unselected critically ill patients. The situation has been complicated by a tendency to study several compounds simultaneously, at arbitrary doses and in heterogeneous populations, then to perform retrospective subgroup analysis in order to demonstrate an effect. The evidence would be a great deal clearer if supplements with an established therapeutic window were evaluated individually. Such interventions are at least as much matters of pharmacology as of nutrition, and should be investigated as such.

GLUTAMINE

Glutamine serves as an oxidative fuel and nucleotide precursor for enterocytes and immune cells, mainly lymphocytes, neutrophils and macrophages. It also appears to regulate the expression of many genes related to signal transduction and to cellular metabolism and repair. During catabolic illness glutamine is released in large quantities from skeletal muscle in order to supply this need. In these circumstances it may become 'conditionally essential' and is vulnerable to depletion, with potentially adverse effects on gut barrier and immune function, which may in turn impair the ability to survive a sustained period of critical illness once glutamine stores are depleted.

The evidence on glutamine supplementation in critical illness remains somewhat contradictory. Reductions in infectious complications and length of ICU stay were shown in small early studies of enterally fed trauma and burns patients, but a much larger study in unselected ICU patients found no effect on any outcome.[79] Intravenous supplementation with glutamine in patients fed by either route (but mostly enterally) showed a reduction in ICU mortality in the treatment arm on a per protocol analysis. However, this was not accompanied by any improvement in illness severity scoring, was not detectable at 6 months, and was not present on an intention-to-treat analysis.[80] Routine glutamine supplementation in enterally fed ICU patients is at present not supported by evidence.

TPN solutions have historically contained no glutamine because of problems with stability and solubility. These have now been overcome by use of dipeptides, but clinical studies of intravenous glutamine supplementation during TPN have also been conflicting. One early trial in ICU patients requiring TPN showed a reduction in late mortality that became apparent only after 20 days, and persisted at 6 months.[81] A similar finding of reduction in late mortality was confined to those requiring TPN for more than 9 days.[82] These studies are often cited as supporting the concept of glutamine as a conditionally essential amino acid that becomes depleted during prolonged intravenous feeding. In contrast, the SIGNET study was unable to find a benefit from providing glutamine for 7 days to parenterally fed ICU patients.[83] It has been argued that this simply reflected an inadequate period either to produce or to correct glutamine depletion. In the absence of evidence of harm, some ICUs now supplement all TPN with glutamine; other more selective units reserve it for those likely to require intravenous feeding for more than 9 days.

SELENIUM

Selenium is necessary in the regulation of glutathione peroxidase, the major scavenging system for oxygen free radicals. Low plasma selenium levels are common in ICU patients, and a number of small studies have shown potential benefits, but these could not be reproduced in two recent larger trials.[83,84]

ANTIOXIDANT VITAMINS

Vitamins A, C and E are also involved in systemic defence against oxidant stress, and have been studied in various combinations and doses, with and without selenium or omega-3 fatty acids. Of the trials not using other adjuncts, only one has shown a reduction in deaths using large enteral doses of vitamins C and E; the control group, however, had a very high mortality rate.[85] It is hard to recommend routine supplementation with antioxidant vitamins on present evidence.

ARGININE AND IMMUNONUTRITION

Arginine is a non-essential amino acid that acts as a precursor of nitric oxide, polyamines (important in lymphocyte maturation) and nucleotides. Animal studies suggest enhanced cell-mediated immunity and survival when arginine is supplemented. Several commercially available enteral feeding solutions combine omega-3 fatty acids, arginine, nucleotides and in one case glutamine to produce so-called immune-enhancing diets. There is some evidence for their use following burn injury or major surgery, but little in general ICU patients. Subsequent meta-analysis suggested an increase in mortality when arginine supplementation was given to septic patients,[86] and interim safety assessment of a trial led to its early cessation when this finding was replicated in the subgroup of patients with sepsis.[87]

There has been continued interest in using feeds enhanced with omega-3 fatty acids, often in combination with antioxidant vitamins. Some studies have found benefits in patients with ALI, ARDS or sepsis, leading some guideline-emitting bodies to support this practice. However, these results could not be repeated by other more recent studies in which individual components were evaluated separately,[88,89] and current knowledge does not warrant supplementation with omega-3 fatty acids.

Access the complete references list online at http://www.expertconsult.com

6. Simpson F, Doig GS. Parenteral vs. enteral nutrition in the critically ill patient: a meta-analysis of trials using the intention to treat principle. Intensive Care Medicine 2005;31:12–23.
8. Martin CM, Doig GS, Heyland DK, et al. Multicentre, cluster-randomized clinical trial of algorithms for critical-care enteral and parenteral therapy (ACCEPT). CMAJ 2004;170:197–204.
18. Baker JP, Detsky AS, Wesson DE, et al. Nutritional assessment: a comparison of clinical judgement and objective measurements. N Engl J Med 1982;306: 969–72.
24. Doig GS, Heighes PT, Simpson F, et al. Early enteral nutrition, provided within 24 h of injury or intensive care unit admission, significantly reduces mortality in critically ill patients: a meta-analysis of randomised controlled trials. Intensive Care Med 2009; 35:2018–27.
26. Streat SJ, Beddoe AH, Hill GL. Aggressive nutritional support does not prevent protein loss despite fat gain in septic intensive care patients. J Trauma 1987;27: 262–6.
39. Larsson J, Lennmarken C, Martensson J, et al. Nitrogen requirements in severely injured patients. Br J Surg 1990;77:413–16.
57. Davies AR, Morrison SS, Bailey MJ, et al. A multicenter, randomized controlled trial comparing early nasojejunal with nasogastric nutrition in critical illness. Crit Care Med 2012;40:2342–8.
66. Montejo JC, Minambres E, Bordeje L, et al. Gastric residual volume during enteral nutrition in ICU patients: the REGANE study. Intensive Care Med 2010;36:1386–93.
69. Drakulovic MB, Torres A, Bauer TT, et al. Supine body position as a risk factor for nosocomial pneumonia in mechanically ventilated patients: a randomised trial. Lancet 1999;354:1851–8.
83. Andrews PJ, Avenell A, Noble DW, et al. Randomised trial of glutamine, selenium, or both, to supplement parenteral nutrition for critically ill patients. BMJ 2011;342:d1542.

Part Fifteen

Haematological Management

95

Blood transfusion

James P Isbister

Blood component therapy has a central therapeutic role in clinical medicine, but blood banking and transfusion medicine have tended to focus on the blood component supply rather than the demand/patient perspective. The clinical focus should naturally be on 'what is best for the patient?' and not, 'what is best for the blood supply?' This shift from blood product focus to problem-based focus is now referred to as patient blood management.[1–3]

Demand for blood components continues to increase owing to the greater burden of chronic disease due to ageing of the population, increasing severity of illness of intensive care unit (ICU) patients and both a widening range of clinical indications for blood components and newer blood-intensive surgical procedures. This is being tempered by greater focus on appropriate use.

When prescribing blood component therapy, the clinical problem and patient's needs must be accurately identified and clearly understood. Often therapy is required for haematological deficiencies until the basic disease process can be corrected (e.g. surgical control for acute haemorrhage, or support for bone marrow suppression until the marrow recovers). Therapy may be aimed at controlling the effects of a deficiency or preventing secondary problems. Alternatively, the indication is passive immunotherapy (e.g. Rhesus prophylaxis) or high-dosage intravenous immunoglobulin as immunomodulatory therapy.

In recent years the role of blood transfusion in a wide range of clinical settings is being critically reassessed, especially in relationship to the labile blood components (red cell and platelet concentrates and fresh frozen plasma). Careful risk assessment and the use of blood conservation techniques have made 'bloodless' surgery possible in most uncomplicated elective surgical settings. Added to the uncertainty about the indications and benefits of allogeneic blood transfusion is the accumulating evidence that blood transfusion is an independent risk factor for poorer clinical outcomes. Clearly many transfusions are both indicated and life-saving, but it is appropriate that there is greater focus on techniques to minimise exposure, transfusion alternatives and closer attention to the quality and immediate efficacy of blood components.

There is a dearth of evidence supporting a role for red cell concentrates in improving clinical outcomes for haemodynamically stable patients, indeed the contrary appears to be the case.[4,5]

Traditionally, transfusion has been regarded as the 'default' decision when there is clinical uncertainty. The benefits of transfusion have been assumed with little or no evidence to support this assumption and patients are thereby unnecessarily exposed to potential morbidity or even mortality. Given that the decision-making process for using blood component therapy can be difficult, that indications may be controversial or when there is no evidence for potential benefit, there are good common sense and scientifically evidence-based reasons to adopt a non-transfusion default position.[6,7] If allogeneic blood component therapy can be avoided, the potential hazards cease to be an issue.

Both evidence-based transfusion medicine and the fact that blood is altruistically donated should ensure that blood is seen as a valuable and unique natural resource that should be conserved and managed appropriately. It should be used as therapy only when there is evidence for potential benefit, when alternatives have been considered and potential for harm has been minimised. Potential hazards must be balanced against benefits and wherever possible the benefits and risks should be explained to the patient/relatives.

In considering the use of allogeneic blood transfusion the following questions need to be addressed:

- What is the timeframe of the decision-making process?
- Is it an elective decision?
- What is the haemopoietic defect?
- What is the most appropriate therapy for the patient?
- Are there alternatives to allogeneic transfusion?
- What component is indicated and where should it be obtained?
- Except for serological compatibility are there any other patient-specific requirements (e.g. irradiated, CMV-negative)
- How should the component be administered and monitored?
- What are the potential hazards of the blood component therapy?
- Can the risk of adverse effects be avoided or minimised?
- What is the cost of the haemotherapy?

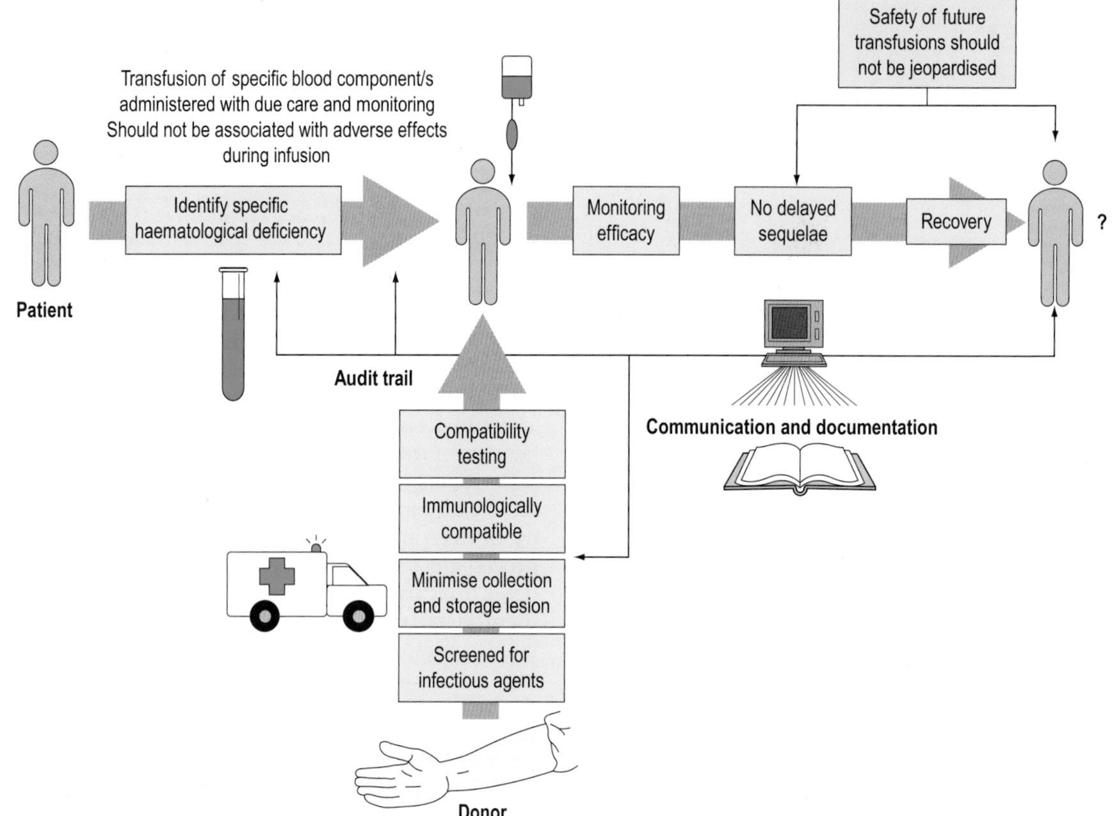

Figure 95.1 What is a safe transfusion?

- Is the patient fully informed of the medical decisions?

Safe and effective transfusion requires attention to the following details (**Fig. 95.1**):

- clearly defined indication and benefits of blood components
- accurate patient identification for blood group compatibility
- identification and careful management of high-risk patients
- appropriate handling, administration and monitoring
- provision of adequate amounts and quality of component(s)
- communication of benefits and risk to the patient/relatives
- the infusion should not be associated with preventable ill effects
- awareness of possible transfusion-related complications
- early diagnosis and prompt action in relation to adverse events of transfusion
- accurate documentation
- input into quality-assurance programmes.

BLOOD STORAGE AND THE STORAGE LESIONS

Blood is altered from the moment of collection and the 'lesions' of collection – anticoagulation, separation, cooling, preservation and storage – compound and progressively increase until the date of expiry.[8] The extent of these changes is determined by collection technique, the specific blood component, the preservative medium, the container, storage time and storage conditions. The threshold storage time for blood components has generally been arbitrarily determined by in vitro studies and assessment of in vivo survival. In the case of red cell concentrates, greater than 75% of transfused cells should survive post transfusion.

Storage results in quantitative and/or qualitative deficiencies in blood components, which may reduce the immediate efficacy of a transfusion. In parallel with these storage changes is an accumulation of degenerate material (e.g. microaggregates and procoagulant material), release of vasoactive agents, cytokine generation and haemolysis.[4] Many of the changes occurring during storage are related to the presence of leucocytes and can be minimised by pre-storage leucoreduction.[9] Red cells undergo a change from their biconcave disc shape to spiky spherocytes (echinocytes) and in so doing lose their flexibility. There are also changes in the red cell membrane resulting in an increased tendency to adhere to endothelial cell surfaces in the microcirculation, especially if there is activation of endothelial cells, for example in the presence of the systemic inflammatory response (e.g. with shock or sepsis).[10] There is evidence that the immediate post-transfusion function of stored red cells and haemoglobin in delivering oxygen to the microcirculation and unloading is questionable, and several hours are required for red cell oxygen carriage and delivery to return to normal.[11–13] It is important to differentiate between the storage lesion being responsible for failure to achieve clinical/laboratory end-points due to reduced survival and/or qualitative defects in cellular function and the 'toxic' effects of blood storage (**Fig. 95.2**).

The use of blood filters has been an acknowledgement of the existence of the blood storage lesion and its possible clinical significance. The 170 μm blood-giving filters were first introduced into transfusion medicine to stop the occlusion of blood-giving sets. Ironically, there was little concern that the fibrin clots may harm the patient, but fortunately the lung is one of nature's remarkable filters. Adult respiratory distress syndrome (ARDS) and the Vietnam War increased interest in unfiltered microaggregates accumulating during storage. Both logic and animal data suggested their implication in ARDS and that microfilters to remove microparticles 20–40 μm in size may be protective. This proved difficult to confirm, but microaggregate filters do not adequately address the problem of the storage lesion and its clinical significance. Use of pre-storage leucoreduction filters, and prevention of the development of the storage lesion in both blood and platelets from its inception, is more logical and scientific. Universal pre-storage leucoreduction is now standard practice in many countries, although it was primarily introduced as a precautionary measure against the possible transmission of variant Creutzfeldt–Jakob disease (vCJD) and not to address the numerous other indications for the removal of leucocytes.[14]

The clinical significance of blood storage lesions is still controversial. Further studies are needed to assess their relevance in conditions such as ARDS, multi-organ failure (MOF), vasoactive reactions and alterations in laboratory parameters.[15–21] It is assumed that blood components have been appropriately collected, processed, stored, transported and transfused but, despite much greater attention to standard operating procedures and regulation generally, the quality of the final product cannot be guaranteed.[22] The 'assumed' quality of labile cellular blood products is based on research data and monitoring of standard operating procedures. There is rarely detailed individual product assessment prior to transfusion. It is accepted that the adverse effects of storage increase with time and an arbitrary 'cut-off' is mandated on the basis of research studies.

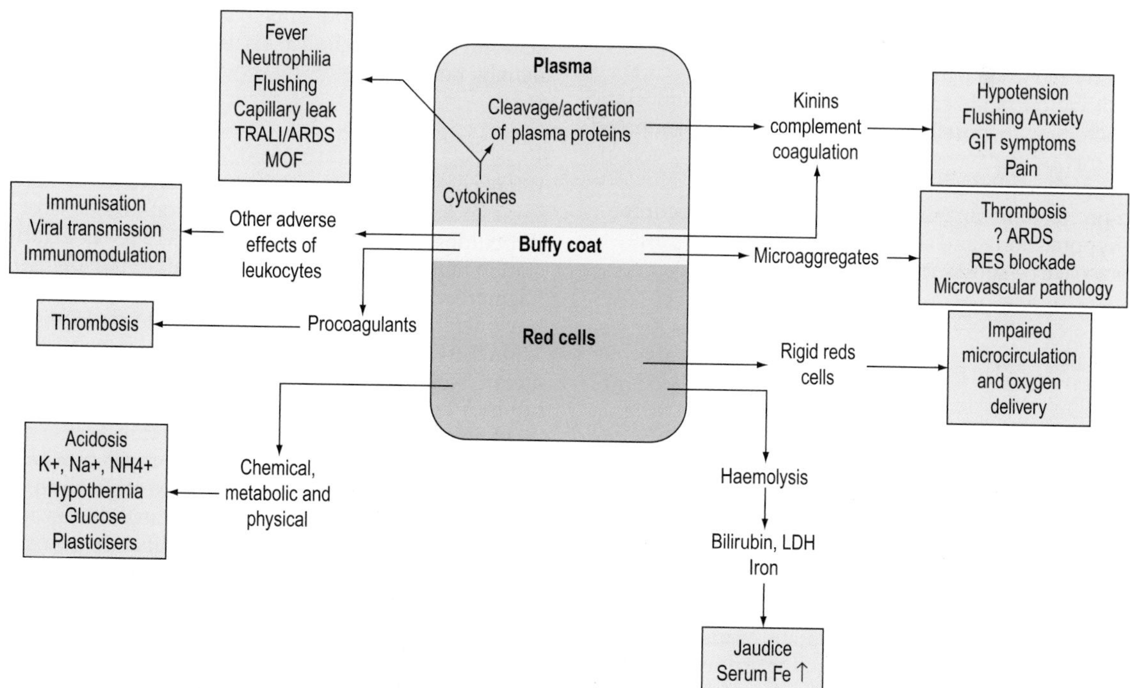

Figure 95.2 The storage lesions. ARDS=adult respiratory distress syndrome; GIT=gastrointestinal tract; MOF=multi-organ failure; RES=reticulo-endothelial system; TRALI=transfusion-related acute lung injury, LDH =lactic dehydrogenase.

In relation to the possible clinical significance of the storage lesion, the following should be considered:

- quantitative and qualitative deficiency of blood component
  - failure to achieve anticipated end-points due to reduced quantity and/or quality of the blood product
  - exposure to excessive numbers of donors in achieving efficacy
- physical characteristics
  - hypothermia
  - chemical characteristics
  - citrate toxicity
  - acid–base imbalance
  - glucose
- contamination
  - bacterial resulting in endotoxaemia or septicaemia
  - plasticisers
- accumulation of 'toxic' or degenerate products
  - role of the storage lesion in transfusion-related immunomodulation
  - role of cytokines
  - role of reticuloendothelial system blockade
  - accentuation of free radical pathophysiology due to free iron
- effects of transfusion on laboratory parameters (e.g. elevations in bilirubin, neutrophils, serum iron and lactic dehydrogenase), which may lead to incorrect interpretation
- large-volume transfusions (proportional to storage age) as a risk factor for MOF and ARDS
- early hyperkalaemia, late hypokalaemia
- activation and consumption of the haemostatic factors with possible contribution to disseminated intravascular coagulation (DIC) and venous thromboembolism
- non-haemolytic, non-febrile transfusion reactions
- hypotension and circulatory instability due to vasoactive substance (kinins, histamine).

THE ROLE OF LEUCOCYTES AS A 'CONTAMINANT' IN LABILE STORED BLOOD AND THE ROLE OF PRE-STORAGE LEUCOREDUCTION

Leucocytes may be responsible for a wide range of blood component quality and safety issues, but there are difficulties in assessing potential adverse effects.[14] Specific adverse outcomes in some patients have been shown to be due to the presence of leucocytes (e.g. non-haemolytic febrile transfusion reaction, platelet refractoriness and transfusion-associated graft-versus-host disease (TAGVHD)), but this is the minority. In the broader context the overall available evidence, in the absence of adequate large randomised clinical trials, suggests that universal pre-storage leucoreduction may reduce transfusion-related morbidity and mortality as well as generating cost savings.[23] Leucoreduction of red cell and platelet concentrates minimises the clinical consequences of the immunomodulatory effects of allogeneic transfusion. Hence it may decrease the incidence of recurrence of some cancers, of postoperative infections and of bloodstream infections and reduce ICU and hospital length of stay. In many patients transfusion-related acute lung injury (TRALI) is a multifactorial disorder and in 'at-risk' patients non-leucoreduced blood may be a risk factor. Patients in whom there is activation of the systemic inflammatory response syndrome (SIRS) are at risk of developing the multi-organ failure syndrome.[24,25] Patients at particular risk include those with trauma, burns, critical bleeding, shock, sepsis and those undergoing cardiopulmonary bypass.[26–29] The quality and function of pre-storage leucoreduced red cell concentrates is better maintained on storage, ensuring better post-transfusion efficacy and survival.[30]

CLINICAL GUIDELINES FOR BLOOD COMPONENT THERAPY

The following is a brief summary of the clinical guidelines for the use of commonly used blood components. The use of specific concentrates or recombinant products is beyond the scope of this book. As alluded to, there is a shift in the current development of clinical practice guidelines from focusing on specific indications for blood components to problem-oriented understanding of the clinical issues (i.e. patient blood management).[31]

RED CELL TRANSFUSIONS

What constitutes appropriate use of red cell transfusions in acute medicine is contentious because of the difficulties in identifying the benefits of red cell transfusion in many circumstances.[32] Pursuit of the lowest safe haematocrit continues to receive considerable attention, but pushing any aspect of a system to its limits risks 'sailing too close to the wind', which may be appropriate in some situations but potentially hazardous in others.[33,34]

In an otherwise stable patient, the transfusion of red cell concentrates is likely to be inappropriate when the haemoglobin level is >100 g/L. On the other hand, their use may be appropriate when haemoglobin is in the range 70–100 g/L if there are other defects in the oxygen transport system, such as cardiorespiratory dysfunction. The decision to transfuse should be supported by the need to relieve clinical signs and symptoms of impaired oxygen transport and prevent morbidity and mortality. The transfusion of red cell concentrates is likely to be appropriate when hemoglobin is <70 g/L and the anaemia is not reversible with specific therapy in the short term, but lower levels may be acceptable in patients who are asymptomatic, especially in the younger age group.[5]

PLATELET TRANSFUSIONS

Platelet transfusion therapy may benefit patients with platelet deficiency or dysfunction. The following are the indications for platelet transfusions:[35]

PROPHYLAXIS

- Bone marrow failure when the platelet count is $<10\times10^9$/L without associated risk factors for bleeding or $<20\times10^9$/L in the presence of additional risk factors
- To maintain the platelet count at $>50\times10^9$/L in patients undergoing surgery or invasive procedures
- In qualitative platelet function disorders, depending on clinical features and setting (platelet count is not a reliable indicator for transfusion).

BLEEDING PATIENT

- In any haemorrhaging patient in whom thrombocytopenia secondary to marrow failure is considered a contributory factor
- When the platelet count is $<50\times10^9$/L in the context of massive haemorrhage/transfusion and $<100\times10^9$/L in the presence of diffuse microvascular bleeding.

The transfusion of platelet concentrates is not generally considered appropriate:

- when thrombocytopenia is due to immune-mediated destruction
- in thrombotic thrombocytopenic purpura and haemolytic uraemic syndrome
- in uncomplicated cardiac bypass surgery.

FRESH FROZEN PLASMA

There are few specific indications for fresh frozen plasma, but its use may be appropriate:[36]

- for replacement of single-factor deficiencies where a specific or combined factor concentrate is not available
- for treatment of the multiple coagulation deficiencies associated with acute systemic coagulopathies:
  - DIC
  - massive blood transfusion
  - trauma-induced coagulopathy
  - cardiac bypass surgery
  - liver disease
  - peripartum coagulopathies
  - venom-induced coagulopathies
- for treatment of inherited deficiencies of coagulation inhibitors in patients undergoing high-risk procedures where a specific factor concentrate is unavailable
- for immediate reversal of warfarin-induced anticoagulation in the presence of potentially life-threatening bleeding when prothrombin concentrates (PCC) are not available[37] (see Ch. 98).

The use of fresh frozen plasma is generally not considered appropriate in cases of:

- hypovolaemia
- plasma exchange procedures unless post-exchange invasive procedures are planned
- treatment of immunodeficiency states.

CRYOPRECIPITATE

Cryoprecipitate is prepared from freshly collected plasma and contains factor VIII, fibrinogen, von Willebrand factor, factor XIII and fibronectin. Cryoprecipitate was originally developed for treatment of haemophilia due to factor VIII deficiency, but is now prescribed to treat congenital or acquired hypofibrinogenaemia, usually in the context of liver disease, trauma, DIC, hyperfibrinolysis or massive transfusion. Increasingly fibrinogen concentrates are recommended in these clinical settings.

IMMUNOGLOBULIN

Normal human immunoglobulin is available in intramuscular and intravenous forms for the treatment or prevention of infection in patients with proven hypogammaglobulinaemia.[38,39] Intravenous immunoglobulin G has been recommended as adjunctive therapy in patients with fulminant sepsis syndrome, especially those with toxic shock syndrome caused by group A streptococci.[40]

Intravenous immunoglobulin therapy also has a role in therapy of some autoimmune disorders, such as idiopathic thrombocytopenic purpura, autoimmune polyneuropathy and others (see Ch. 97).

FACTOR CONCENTRATES

There is an increasing number of plasma protein concentrates available for clinical use. Some are prepared from donor plasma and some by recombinant technology. Factor VIII and factor IX concentrates have an established role in the management of haemophilia, but others are in the process of establishing their clinical efficacy and indications. Antithrombin III (ATIII) concentrates are available for thrombophilia due to ATIII deficiency and have been recommended in other disorders where ATIII may be depleted (e.g. DIC, MOF) but evidence for efficacy is sparse.[41] Recombinant human activated protein C has antithrombotic, anti-inflammatory and profibrinolytic properties, but its role in the treatment of patients with severe sepsis remains controversial and it is generally not recommended.[42,43]

Of recent interest is the use of the recombinant activated haemostatic proteins and inhibitors. Recombinant activated factor VII (rFVIIa) was developed for the management of haemophilic patients with coagulation factor inhibitors; rFVIIa is commonly used 'off label' for controlling haemorrhage in the non-haemophilic setting and there is considerable controversy as to its benefits and risks.[44,45] There are an increasing number of case reports and series reporting on the use of rFVIIa in critical life-threatening haemorrhage. Patients with uncontrolled critical bleeding and coagulopathy, despite large transfusions and surgical intervention, have significant mortality rates and rFVIIa in these clinical situations is used as salvage therapy. Its use has been studied in controlled trials where there is critical bleeding in various clinical settings, but evidence for efficacy has been disappointing and thrombotic complications are a potential problem; rFVIIa initiates the extrinsic coagulation pathway when complexed to tissue factors at sites of injury and on activated platelet surfaces.

POTENTIAL ADVERSE EFFECTS OF ALLOGENEIC TRANSFUSION

The pathophysiology of blood transfusion reactions can broadly be divided into five categories (**Fig. 95.3**):

- Reactions may occur due to *immunological differences* between the donor and recipient, resulting in varying degrees of blood component incompatibility. In general, in order for a reaction to occur, the recipient needs to have been previously immunised to a cellular or plasma antigen.[46]
- A wide range of *infectious agents* may be transmitted by allogeneic blood component therapy.
- *Alterations in blood products due to preservation and storage* may result in quantitative and/or qualitative deficiencies in the blood components, which will reduce transfusion efficacy and expose the patient to potentially adverse consequences from storage accumulants in the component.
- *Technical or clerical errors* may result in adverse events in all the above categories.
- *Psychological* – this includes informed consent issues and patient anxiety about compatibility and infectivity.

In terms of causation of an adverse clinical event, the possible role of blood transfusion can be classified into three categories on the basis of probability[47] (**Fig. 95.4**):

- *Definite – unifactorial – transfusion caused*: the well-understood and reported hazards of transfusion (i.e. immunological, technical, infectious) are generally unifactorial with a 1:1 causal relationship between the blood component transfused (usually a specific individual unit) and the adverse consequence for the patient. ABO blood group incompatibility, transfusion-related infection transmission, TAGVHD and TRALI due to donor leucoagglutinins are examples in this category.
- *Probable – oligofactorial – transfusion related*: some adverse consequences of transfusion result from interaction with other insults, pathophysiology or host factors, but the contribution of the transfusion can usually be specifically identified. Fever, allergic reactions, hypotensive reactions, pulmonary oedema,

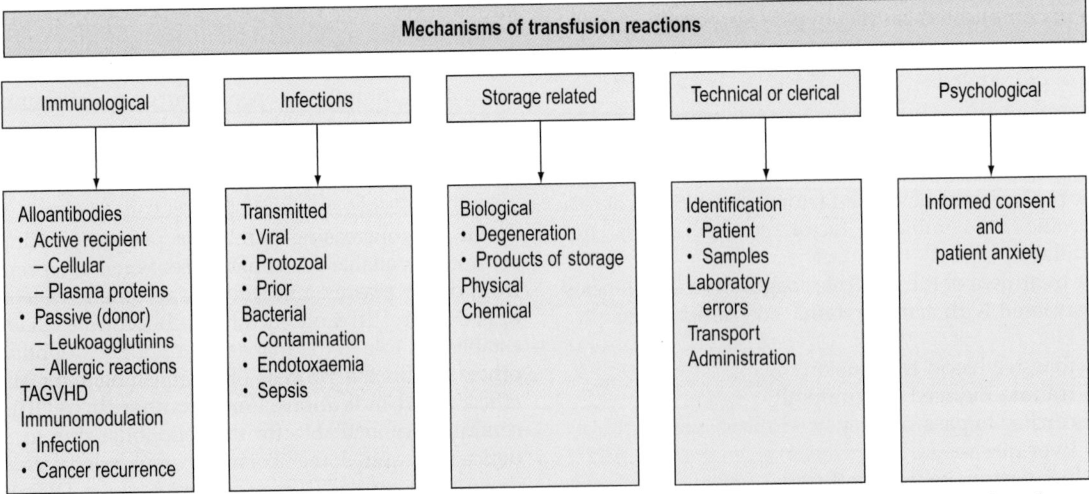

Figure 95.3 Possible mechanisms of adverse effects to blood transfusion. TAGVHD=transfusion-associated graft-versus-host disease.

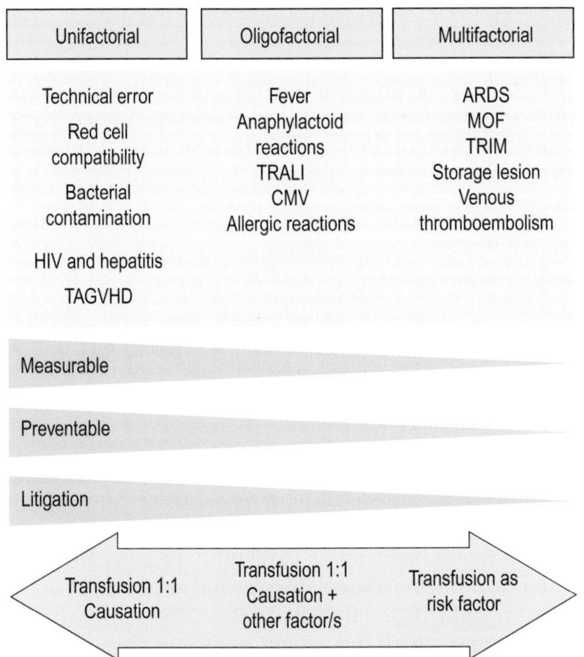

Figure 95.4 Algorithm for analysis for the possibility of a transfusion reaction. ARDS=adult respiratory distress syndrome; CMV=cytomegalovirus; MOF=multi-organ failure; TAGVHD=transfusion-associated graft-versus-host disease; TRIM=transfusion-induced immunomodulation; TRALI=transfusion-related acute lung injury.

some cases of TRALI, hyperbilirubinaemia and cytomegalovirus (CMV) transmission are examples in this category.

- *Possible – multifactorial – transfusion associated*: transfusion may be a contributor to a complication or poor clinical outcome. In these circumstances it may be difficult to implicate transfusion directly in an individual case, nor is it necessarily the major factor. Transfusion-induced immunomodulation (TRIM) and the clinical consequences of storage lesions fall into this category. The role of transfusion being associated with adverse consequences has been established in observational studies, but causation cannot be confidently concluded. Accumulating evidence, in the absence of randomised clinical trials, supports causation, thus demanding a more precautionary approach to allogeneic blood transfusion, examination of alternatives to transfusion and implementation of methods to improve the quality of transfused blood components (especially red cell and platelet concentrates). Universal pre-storage leucoreduction is currently the most important and effective strategy for minimising the clinical impact of TRIM and the blood storage lesions.

Adverse reactions to blood component therapy may present in a wide range of 'guises' and transfusion must always be considered in the differential diagnosis of any unexpected clinical presentation or indeed as a contributory factor to a clinical picture that may have several contributory factors[48] (**Fig. 95.5**).

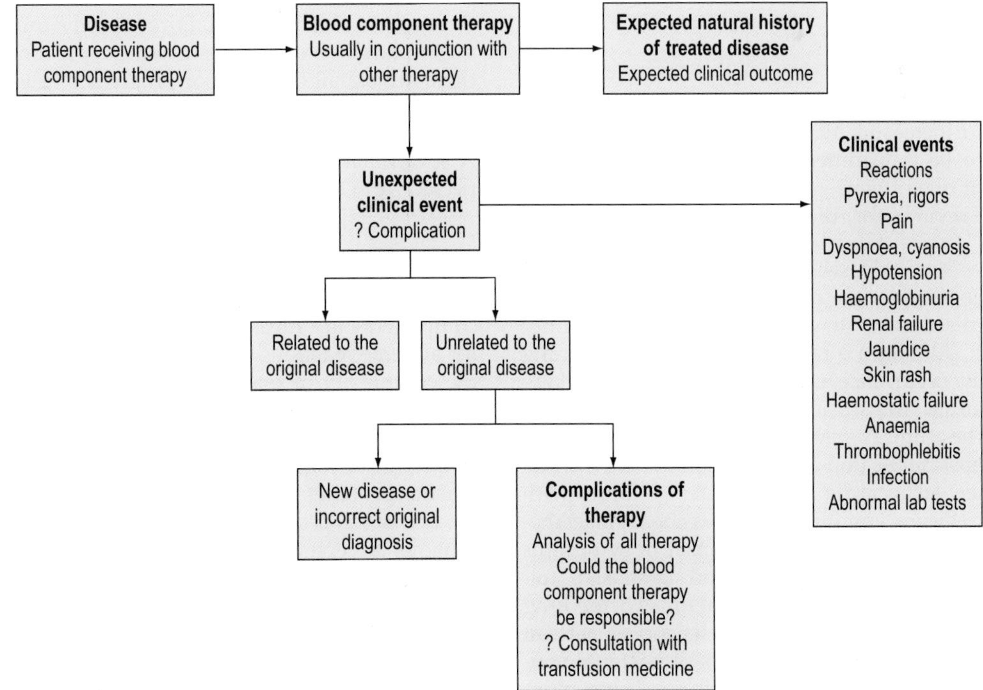

Figure 95.5 Adverse reactions to blood component therapy may just be one of the contributory factors in the differential diagnosis of any unexpected clinical presentation.

PYREXIA

Mild febrile reactions are not usually a matter of concern, but rigors and temperatures above 38°C should not be ignored. The majority of febrile reactions are now considered to be an immunological reaction against one or more of the transfused cellular or plasma components, usually leucocytes.

TRANSFUSION-RELATED INFECTIONS

HEPATITIS

Post-transfusion hepatitis is a potential complication of allogeneic transfusion; donor selection, serological and nucleic acid tests ensure exclusion of infective donors. Hepatitis B and C are now almost totally preventable transfusion-transmitted diseases.

HUMAN IMMUNODEFICIENCY VIRUS

Donor selection, antibody screening and nucleic acid testing of blood donors have almost eliminated transfusion-associated HIV infection.

MONONUCLEOSIS SYNDROMES

The development of swinging pyrexia with varying degrees of peripheral blood atypical mononucleosis, 7–10 days following transfusion, can cause diagnostic confusion. Abnormalities in liver function are common. CMV infection is the commonest cause of this syndrome. When correctly diagnosed CMV is not a serious infection assuming the patient does not have immune compromise.

OTHER TRANSFUSION-TRANSMISSIBLE INFECTIONS

There is an increasing range of agents that have the potential to be transmitted by blood transfusion, the most recent one of concern being vCJD. The reader is referred to reviews for further information.[49]

BACTERIAL CONTAMINATION

Bacterial contamination of stored blood has always been recognised as a potential cause of fulminant endotoxic shock. Although a rare complication, continuing reports of its occurrence, especially in relation to platelet concentrate transfusion, have increased awareness.[50,51] The clinical features of transfusion-related bacterial sepsis in the non-anaesthetised patient include rigors, fever, tachycardia and vascular collapse, with prominent nausea, vomiting and diarrhoea. Anaesthetised patients may have a delayed onset of symptoms (fever, tachycardia, hypotension and cyanosis), followed by DIC, renal failure and sometimes acute lung injury. The requirement to store platelet concentrates at room temperature increases the risks of bacterial contamination. Pre-release bacterial testing is being more widely advocated as a measure to minimise the problem.

HAEMOLYTIC TRANSFUSION REACTIONS

Most severe acute haemolytic transfusion reactions are due to ABO incompatibility, have an identifiable cause and are avoidable, in contrast to delayed haemolytic reactions that are immune in nature and are difficult to prevent.

INITIAL SYMPTOMS AND SIGNS

The classic symptoms and signs of an acute haemolytic transfusion reaction, typical of ABO incompatibility, include apprehension, flushing, pain (e.g. at infusion site, headache, chest, lumbosacral and abdominal), nausea, vomiting, rigors, hypotension and circulatory collapse.

HAEMOSTATIC FAILURE

Haemorrhagic diathesis due to DIC may be a feature, resulting in severe generalised haemostatic failure, with haemorrhage and oozing from multiple sites.[52] As the responsible transfusion is likely to have been administered for haemorrhage, increasing severity of local bleeding may be the first clue to an incompatible transfusion, especially if the patient is unconscious or anaesthetised in the operating room.

OLIGURIA AND RENAL IMPAIRMENT

Renal impairment may complicate a haemolytic transfusion reaction and its prevention or the appropriate management of established renal failure is important. If circulating volume and urinary output are rapidly restored, established renal failure is unlikely to occur. Death from acute renal failure directly caused by an incompatible blood transfusion is preventable, and there are usually other poor prognostic factors.

ANAEMIA AND JAUNDICE

A severe haemolytic transfusion reaction may be suspected from the development of jaundice or anaemia.

ALLERGIC AND ANAPHYLACTOID REACTIONS

Non-cellular blood (plasma and plasma derivatives) components are rarely considered to be a major cause for adverse reactions to transfusion therapy. However, the complexity of plasma and its various components and the effects from component processing results in a broader spectrum of potential adverse effects than is frequently recognised. The antigenic heterogeneity of plasma proteins and the presence of antibodies make the non-cellular components of blood responsible for a range of adverse effects, many of which remain poorly understood and commonly pass unrecognised in clinical practice.[53]

There has been debate over the years as to the classification of allergic reactions to blood components. Clinical severity may range from minor urticarial reactions or flushing through to fulminant cardiorespiratory collapse and death. Some of these reactions are probably true anaphylaxis, but in others the mechanisms have been less clear and the term 'anaphylactoid' has been used. To avoid implying the mechanism of the reaction, the term 'immediate generalised reaction' has also been used.

The clinical syndromes of immediate reactions have been classified as follows:

- *Grade I:*
  - skin manifestations
- *Grade II:*
  - mild to moderate hypotension
  - gastrointestinal disturbances (nausea)
  - respiratory distress
- *Grade III:*
  - severe hypotension, shock
  - bronchospasm
- *Grade IV:*
  - cardiac and/or respiratory arrest.

PLASMA AND PLASMA COMPONENTS MAY CAUSE ADVERSE EFFECTS BY SEVERAL PATHOPHYSIOLOGICAL MECHANISMS

Immunological reactions to normal components of plasma may occur in two ways:

- plasma proteins being antigenic to the recipient; they may contain epitopes on their molecules different from those on the recipient's functionally identical plasma proteins (e.g. anti-IgA antibodies)
- antibodies in the donor plasma reacting with cellular components of the recipient's blood cells or plasma proteins.

Physicochemical characteristics and contaminants of donor plasma, such as temperature, chemical additives, medications and micro-organisms, may be responsible for recipient reactions.

The preparation techniques and storage conditions of blood and blood products may potentially cause adverse reaction through:

- *accumulation of metabolites* or cellular release products
- *plasma activation* (i.e. activation of some of the proteolytic systems). Importantly, the complement and kinin/kininogen systems may generate vasoactive substances and anaphylatoxins which may be responsible for reactions. Some apparently allergic reactions to blood products may be due to vasoactive substances in the infusion. Subjective sensations may be missed in an unconscious patient. Hypotension occurring during rapid infusion of a hypovolaemic patient is likely to be interpreted as further volume loss, particularly with some plasma protein fractions that have been reported as consistently producing a transient fall in blood pressure, and a situation fraught with risk of overload can be produced
- *histamine generation*: histamine levels increase in some stored blood components and levels may be correlated with non-febrile, non-haemolytic transfusion reactions. Histamine release may be stimulated in the patient by plasma components, synthetic colloids and various medications
- *generation of cytokines* during storage may be responsible for non-haemolytic transfusion reactions
- *chemical additives*: there are various chemical additives (ethylene oxide, formaldehyde, drugs, latex) that may be responsible for immunological or non-immunological recipient reactions.

TRANSFUSION-ASSOCIATED GRAFT-VERSUS-HOST DISEASE (TAGVHD)

Graft-versus-host disease, classically observed in relationship to allogeneic bone marrow transplantation, may occur following a blood transfusion owing to the infusion of immunocompetent lymphocytes precipitating an immunological reaction against the host tissues of the recipient.[54] It is most commonly observed in immunocompromised patients, but may also be seen in recipients of directed blood donation from first-degree relatives, and occasionally where donor and recipient are not related, owing to homozygosity for HLA haplotypes for which the recipient is heterozygous. The syndrome usually occurs 3–30 days post allogeneic transfusion with fever, liver function test abnormalities, profuse watery diarrhoea, erythematous skin rash and progressive pancytopenia. Gamma irradiation of blood products is currently the standard of care for the prevention of TAGVHD.[55]

TRANSFUSION-RELATED ACUTE LUNG INJURY (TRALI)

TRALI is receiving a great deal of attention as a potentially serious complication of blood transfusion.[56] In the classic plasma neutrophil antibody-mediated form of the disease, symptoms usually arise within hours of a blood transfusion.[57] In contrast to most patients with ARDS, recovery usually occurs within 48 hours. The underlying pathophysiology of 'classic' TRALI is due to the presence of leucoagglutinins in donor plasma. When complement is activated, C5a promotes neutrophil aggregation and sequestration in the microcirculation of the lung, causing endothelial damage leading to an interstitial oedema and acute respiratory failure. This classic form of transfusion-related acute lung injury has been recognised for over five decades, but was thought to be a rare complication of allogeneic plasma transfusion. As leucoagglutinins occur typically in plasma from multiparous females there is a move to using male-donor-only fresh frozen plasma.

It is now accepted that there has been under-recognition and underdiagnosis of TRALI, due partly to a lack of clinical awareness, but also to a broader understanding of mechanisms by which blood transfusion may cause or be a contributory factor to lung injury.[58,59] The term 'TRALI' is now being expanded to include cases in which transfusion is identified as an independent risk factor predisposing patients to lung injury. The reader is referred to recent reviews addressing the expanding area of concern in which transfusion, per se, is being identified as an independent risk factor for poor clinical outcomes, of which TRALI is only one.[47] There is also recent experimental evidence supporting a 'two-hit' hypothesis in which patients may be 'primed' by shock, sepsis or extracorporeal circulation making them more susceptible to acute lung injury from blood transfusion.[60]

TRANSFUSION-RELATED IMMUNOMODULATION (TRIM)

Allogeneic blood transfusion is immunosuppressive having implications in relation to resistance to infection and the likelihood of cancer recurrence.[61-63] Donor leucocytes probably play the most important role in this immunomodulation. TRIM, along with the clinical effects of the blood storage lesion, is probably the mechanism by which allogeneic blood transfusion is responsible for poorer clinical outcomes discussed in the next section.

ALLOGENEIC TRANSFUSION AS AN INDEPENDENT RISK FACTOR FOR POORER CLINICAL OUTCOMES

Over the last decade experimental and clinical studies have identified blood transfusion as an independent risk factor for morbidity and mortality as well as increased admission rates to ICUs, assisted ventilation, increased length of hospital stay and additional costs.[64,47,65,66] Blood transfusion being implicated as part of the problem rather than optimal therapy has been a surprise to many clinicians, health administrators and patients, as it has always been assumed that blood transfusion can only be of benefit to the bleeding or anaemic patient. This long-standing belief is now being effectively challenged and currently the debate on the management of the acutely haemorrhaging or anaemic patient has moved significantly from a paradigm with a focus on transfusion to one in which the urgent control of critical bleeding is the paramount priority, with avoidance and/or minimisation of blood transfusion. There is thus increasing evidence that transfusion-related immunomodulation (TRIM) and the transfusion effects of storage lesions, especially with older stored blood, are responsible for poorer clinical outcomes in a range of clinical settings.[67-72]

However, it is not possible to categorically conclude causation and that pre-storage leucoreduction will eliminate or minimise the risk. Although the case for causation is strengthening, it is important to be aware that there is minimal evidence for the efficacy or appropriateness of many transfusions, and there is evidence that restrictive red cell transfusion policies do not jeopardise clinical outcomes in haemodynamically stable patients; indeed, the reverse may be the case.[73-75] Thus, until these issues are resolved, a precautionary approach should be adopted, with the modus operandi being to avoid or minimise allogeneic transfusion and use appropriate patient blood management techniques.[2,34,76] Additionally there is an association with transfusion and a higher incidence of venous thromboembolism.[77,78]

CRITICAL HAEMORRHAGE AND MASSIVE BLOOD TRANSFUSION

There is a reappraisal of clinical practice guidelines for the use of blood components in the bleeding patient.[79-81] The guidelines are no longer for the management of massive blood transfusion, but rather for the management of critical bleeding and avoiding getting into the massive transfusion coagulopathy quagmire in which the patient can spiral down into the 'triad of death'– coagulopathy, acidosis and hypothermia.

This reappraisal of management of patients with acute haemorrhage is resulting in the challenging of long-standing dogmas. There is greater tolerance of hypotension until haemorrhage is controlled, and lower haemoglobin levels are tolerated with closer attention to the clinical context of the anaemia and its impact on systemic and local oxygen delivery, especially if there are any compromises in cardiorespiratory function. More attention and research are being directed toward the role of clear fluids and the importance of plasma viscosity, colloid oncotic pressure and functional capillary density.[69] The search for safe and more effective plasma substitutes and haemoglobin-based oxygen carriers continues.[82]

If blood loss has been massive or there are defects in the haemostatic system, specific component therapy may be indicated. Advances in patient retrieval, resuscitation protocols, techniques for rapid and real-time diagnosis, trauma teams and early 'damage control' surgery have improved the management of acutely haemorrhaging patients. Patients are now surviving with larger volumes of blood transfusion, but sepsis, acute lung injury and multi-organ failure remain major challenges, and blood transfusion is increasingly being recognised as a two-edged sword and probably a contributory factor to these complications in which microcirculatory dysfunction and impaired tissue cellular metabolism are recognised as important in the pathophysiology. As already discussed, the evidence that the immediate post-transfusion ability of stored red cells and haemoglobin to deliver and unload oxygen to the microcirculation may be impaired is resulting in stored red cell concentrates not being automatically the first therapy for acutely enhancing oxygen delivery. Indeed, recent animal data indicate that the immediate clinical benefit of transfused red cells in treating hypovolaemic shock relates to reconstitution of the macrocirculation, with adverse effects on the functional capillary density in the microcirculation.[83] Concerns around the storage age of blood at the time of transfusion are now receiving considerable attention with impressive observational and mechanistic evidence pointing towards the likelihood that blood less than 2 weeks old will be optimal. If results of RCTs confirm this to be so then there will be significant challenges for the blood sector in supply chain management.

In previously healthy patients who have suffered an acute blood loss of less than 25% of their blood volume, restoring that volume is more important than replacing oxygen-carrying capacity. Plasma volume expanders may preclude the necessity for allogeneic transfusion, especially if bleeding can be controlled. Clear fluids also allow time for transfusion compatibility testing. In the context of acute bleeding and hypovolaemic shock, the haemoglobin level is not the primary indicator for determining the need for allogeneic red cell transfusion. A normal human may survive a 30% deficit in blood volume without fluid replacement, in contrast to an 80% loss of red cell mass if normovolaemia is maintained. Minimisation of allogeneic blood transfusion is important and haemodilution with tolerance of anaemia is now accepted clinical practice. However, there are limits to haemodilution, not only from the perspective of oxygen-carrying capacity. Marked reduction in blood viscosity is counterproductive as reactive peripheral vasoconstriction to maintain total peripheral resistance results in reduction in functional capillary density in the microcirculation. The role of clear fluids and the importance of plasma viscosity, colloid oncotic pressure, electrolyte composition and functional capillary density are the subject of current research.[84]

A protocol approach to blood component therapy is generally not recommended, as each patient should be treated individually. However, this remains a controversial issue with advocates for 'blind', up-front component therapy with red cell and haemostatic components, especially fresh frozen plasma and cryoprecipitate or fibrinogen concentrates. There are also enthusiastic advocates for 1:1:1 (red cells, platelets, plasma) replacement protocols based on recent military experience and this is recommended in some critical-bleeding protocols.

Many hospitals now have massive transfusion protocols that are activated on the basis of specific criteria. With better understanding of coagulopathy in the critical haemorrhage setting and the importance of hypofibrinogenaemia and hyperfibrinolysis, there is a reanalysis of the approach to blood component therapy.[85–87] In an elective situation in which normovolaemia is generally maintained from the outset, defects can be predicted and appropriate blood components prescribed, a protocol approach may be justified. This should be done in close consultation with the haematologist and hospital transfusion service.

Failure of haemostasis is common in critically bleeding patients and may be complex and multifactorial in pathogenesis.[85] The importance of avoiding acidosis and hypothermia cannot be overemphasised as the triad of coagulopathy, acidosis and hypothermia has an extremely poor prognosis. Coagulopathy associated with critical haemorrhage is related to other aspects of the pathophysiology of the clinical setting. The assumption that there is a 'generic coagulopathy' vaguely referred to as DIC is incorrect and can result in inappropriate therapeutic decisions. The reader is referred to an expanding literature on this topic where it will be seen that there can be no standard approach to therapy.[77] This author is increasingly convinced that the pathophysiology of coagulopathy, when occurring in the context of critical haemorrhage, should be viewed as related to the primary insult/initiating event, and that a 'secondary' coagulopathy (e.g. massive stored blood transfusion, haemodilution, hypothermia, continuing tissue hypoxia, etc.) may compound the problem in the resuscitated patient. The primary mechanisms of coagulopathy relating to the initiating event may relate to trauma, hypoxia, pregnancy, microbial infection, envenomation or iatrogenic (antithrombotic) agents. In all circumstances there is activation or inhibition of some aspect of the haemostatic system, and therapy is better informed if the varied mechanisms are understood. Frequently, complex tests are required for definitive diagnosis, but the urgency of the situation cannot always await the results, and therapy may be initiated on clinical evidence with minimal laboratory information.

Many trauma patients have coagulopathy at presentation that is related more to hypovolaemic shock and not to consumption or dilution. Excessive activation of the protein C system and hypofibrinogenaemia secondary to secondary hyperfibrinolysis are important.[86,87] Except for severe abnormalities, haemostatic laboratory parameters correlate poorly with clinical evidence of haemostatic failure. In the massively transfused patient, thrombocytopenia and impaired platelet function are the most consistent significant haematological abnormalities, correction of which may be associated with control of microvascular bleeding. Coagulation deficiency from massive blood loss is initially confined to factors V and VIII. Activated partial thromboplastin time (APTT), prothrombin time (PT) and fibrinogen assay should be performed, but the urgency of the situation does not usually allow for other specific factor assays. Fibrinogen, the bulk protein of the haemostatic system and essential for effective fibrin clot formation, is receiving greater attention with wider recommendations for replacement using concentrates or cryoprecipitate.

A problem with the standard screening tests of coagulation function is that they do not give information about the actual formation of the haemostatic plug, its size, structure or stability. For this reason there is increasing interest in global tests of haemostatic plug formation and stability such as thromboelastography, thrombin generation tests and clot waveform analysis in which changes in light transmission in routine APTT are measured. Fresh frozen plasma should be infused if the test results are abnormal, including cryoprecipitate or fibrinogen concentrates in the presence of hypofibrinogenaemia. Fibrinogen levels <1 g/L have generally been the trigger for replacement, but this is being reassessed, especially in the peripartum setting.[88,89]

With ongoing bleeding with associated microvascular oozing, various approaches may be taken. Having ensured that all identifiable haemostatic defects have been corrected, questions arise as to the role of fresh blood and, more recently, recombinant activated factor VII (rFVIIa).[45,90] The use of freshly collected whole blood remains controversial and is an 'emotive' subject needing some comment, but is advocated in the military setting. The provision of fresh whole blood can present logistic, ethical and safety problems needing consideration. Many transfusion medicine specialists categorically state that there is never an indication for fresh whole blood. Such dogma can be difficult to defend in the clinical setting of the massive haemorrhage and transfusion syndrome where pathophysiology remains poorly understood and specific blood component therapy may be ineffective.

The following statements reasonably summarise the current status of fresh blood transfusion:

- fresh blood provides immediately functioning oxygen-carrying capacity, volume and haemostatic factors in the one product
- the number of allogeneic donors to whom a patient is exposed is reduced
- problems associated with infusion of massive volumes of stored blood can be minimised/avoided
- the risk of transfusion-related viral infections is possibly higher than fully tested and stored blood.

SPECIFIC HAZARDS OF MASSIVE BLOOD TRANSFUSION

Massive blood transfusion may be defined in several ways:

- replacement of the circulating volume in 24 hours
- >4 units of blood in 1 hour with continuing blood loss
- loss of 50% of circulating blood volume within 3–4 hours.

Any patient receiving massive blood component therapy is likely to be seriously ill and have multiple problems. Many adverse effects must be considered in conjunction with the injuries and multi-organ dysfunction. It is not always possible to define the complications caused or aggravated by massive blood transfusion.

CITRATE TOXICITY

A patient responds to citrate infusion by the removal of citrate and mobilisation of ionised calcium. Citrate is metabolised by the Krebs cycle in all nucleated cells, especially the liver. A marked elevation in the citrate concentration is seen with transfusion exceeding 500 mL in 5 minutes; the level rapidly falls when the infusion is slowed. Citrate metabolism is impaired by hypotension, hypovolaemia, hypothermia and liver disease. Toxicity may also be potentiated by alkalosis, hyperkalaemia, hypothermia and cardiac disease. The clinical significance of a minor depression of ionised calcium remains ill defined, and it is accepted that a warm, well-perfused adult patient with normal liver function can tolerate a unit of blood each 5 minutes without requiring calcium. The rate of transfusion is more significant than the total volume transfused. Common practice is to administer 10% calcium gluconate 1.0 g i.v. following each 5 units of blood or fresh frozen plasma. Such a practice remains controversial as there is concern regarding calcium homeostasis and cell function in acutely ill patients.

ACID–BASE AND ELECTROLYTE DISTURBANCES

Acid–base

Stored bank blood contains an appreciable acid load and is often used in a situation of pre-existing or continuing metabolic acidosis. The acidity of stored blood is mainly due to the citric acid of the anticoagulant and the lactic acid generated during storage. Their intermediary metabolites are rapidly metabolised with adequate tissue perfusion, resulting in a metabolic alkalosis. Hence the routine use of sodium bicarbonate is usually unnecessary and is generally contraindicated. Alkali further shifts the oxygen dissociation curve to the left, provides a large additional sodium load and depresses the return of ionised calcium to normal following citrate infusion. Acid–base estimations should be performed and corrected in the context of the clinical situation. With continuing hypoperfusion, however, metabolism of citrate and lactate will be depressed, lactic acid production will continue and there may be an indication for i.v. bicarbonate and calcium to correct acidosis and low ionised calcium.

Serum potassium

Although controversial, it is unlikely that the high serum potassium levels in stored blood have pathological effects in adults, except in the presence of acute renal failure. However, hypokalaemia may be a problem 24 hours after transfusion as the transfused cells correct their electrolyte composition and potassium returns into the cells. Thus, although initial acidosis and hyperkalaemia may be an immediate problem with massive blood transfusion, the net result of successful resuscitation is likely to be delayed hypokalaemia and alkalosis. With CPD (citrate–phosphate–dextrose) blood, the acid load and red cell storage lesion are less. Constant monitoring of the acid–base and electrolyte status is essential in such fluctuating clinical situations.

Serum sodium

The sodium content of whole blood and fresh frozen plasma is higher than the normal blood level due to the sodium citrate. This should be remembered when large volumes of plasma are being infused into patients who have disordered salt and water handling (e.g. in renal, liver or cardiac disease).

HYPOTHERMIA

Blood warmed from 4°C to 37°C requires 1255 kJ (300 kcal) – the equivalent heat produced by 1 hour of muscular work – with an oxygen requirement of 62 L. Hypothermia impairs the metabolism of citrate and lactate, shifts the oxygen dissociation curve to the left, increases intracellular potassium release, impairs red cell deformability, delays drug metabolism, masks clinical signs, increases the incidence of arrhythmias, reduces cardiac output and impairs haemostatic function. Thus a thermostatically controlled blood-warming device should be routinely used when any transfusion episode requires the rapid infusion of more than 2 units of blood.

HYPERBILIRUBINAEMIA

Jaundice is common following massive blood transfusion as a significant amount of transfused stored blood may not survive, resulting in varying degrees of hyperbilirubinaemia. During hypovolaemia and shock, liver function may be impaired, particularly in the presence of sepsis or multi-organ failure. An important rate-limiting step in bilirubin transport is the energy-requiring process of transporting conjugated bilirubin from the hepatocyte to the biliary canaliculus. Thus, although an increased load of bilirubin from destroyed transfused red cells may be conjugated, there may be delayed excretion leading to a conjugated hyperbilirubinaemia. This 'paradoxical' conjugated hyperbilirubinaemia may be misinterpreted, leading to unnecessary investigations. The effect of resorbing haematoma and the possibility of an occult haemolytic transfusion reaction should also be considered.

BASIC IMMUNOHAEMATOLOGY

Red cell serology is a highly specialised area of knowledge and it is not possible to expect clinicians to have more than a basic working knowledge essential for patient safety. The following is a summary of core knowledge for the clinician.

SALINE AGGLUTINATION

Safe red cell transfusion has revolved around this traditional serological technique. A saline suspension of red cells is mixed with serum and observed for agglutination. Saline agglutination is used for ABO blood grouping and is one of the techniques for compatibility testing of donor blood.

THE DIRECT AND INDIRECT ANTIGLOBULIN TEST

In red cell serology, the antiglobulin test (Coombs test) is used to detect IgG immunoglobulins or complement components. The direct antiglobulin test (DAT) detects immunoglobulin or complement components present on the surface of the red cells circulating in the patient. The result is positive in autoimmune haemolytic anaemia and haemolytic disease of the newborn and during a haemolytic transfusion reaction. The indirect antiglobulin test (IAT) detects the presence of non-agglutinating antibodies in the patient's plasma, usually IgG type. Antibody screening for atypical antibodies and pre-transfusion compatibility testing are the main applications of the IAT.

REGULAR AND IRREGULAR (ATYPICAL) ANTIBODIES

The regular alloantibodies (isoagglutinins) of the ABO system are naturally occurring agglutinins present in all ABO types (except AB), depending on the ABO group. Group O people have anti-A and anti-B isoagglutinins, group A have anti-B and Group B have anti-A. Group A cells are the cause of the commonest and most dangerous ABO-incompatible haemolytic reactions. Atypical antibodies are not normally present in the plasma, but may be found in some people as naturally occurring antibodies or as immune antibodies. Immune antibodies result from previous exposure due to blood transfusion or pregnancy. Naturally occurring antibodies more frequently react by saline agglutination and, although they may be stimulated by transfusion, are usually of minimal clinical significance. In contrast, many of the immune atypical antibodies are of major clinical significance and their recognition is the raison d'étre for pre-transfusion compatibility testing and antenatal antibody screening. Most of the clinically significant immune atypical antibodies are detected by the IAT.

Blood group antigens vary widely in their frequency and immunogenicity. The D antigen of the Rhesus blood group system is common and highly immunogenic. Thus, when a Rh-negative (i.e. D-negative) patient is exposed to D-positive blood there is a high likelihood of forming an anti-D antibody. It is for this reason that the D antigen is taken into account when providing blood for transfusion, in contrast to the numerous other red cell antigens that are less common or less immunogenic. Beyond the Rh (D), and sometimes the Kell (K) blood group antigens, it is not practical, or necessary, to take notice of other blood group antigens unless an atypical antibody is detected during antibody-screening procedures.

THE ANTIBODY SCREEN

On receipt of a blood sample by the transfusion service, the red cells are ABO and Rh D typed and the serum is screened for atypical antibodies. This screen consists of testing the patient's serum with group O screening cells. The screening panel consists of red cells obtained usually from two group O donors containing all common red cell antigens occurring with a frequency of greater than approximately 2% in the community. If an atypical antibody is detected on the antibody screen, further serological investigations are carried out to identify the specificity of the antibody. These investigations are time-consuming and when possible should be carried out electively.

THE CROSSMATCH (COMPATIBILITY TEST)

The crossmatch is the final compatibility test between the donor cells and the patient's serum. The crossmatch test tends to be overemphasised, to the detriment of the antibody screen. With sophisticated knowledge of serology the emphasis in the supply of compatible blood is now concentrated on the steps prior to the final compatibility crossmatch.

THE TYPE AND SCREEN SYSTEM

As pre-compatibility testing has assumed the major role in the selection of blood for transfusion, there has been a rethinking of policies relating to the supply of blood for elective transfusions. Whenever elective surgery is planned for a patient who is likely to require blood transfusion, the transfusion service must receive a clotted blood sample well before the anticipated time of surgery. The pre-compatibility testing should be carried out during the routine working hours when facilities are geared for large workloads and enough staff is available to handle all contingencies.

THE PROVISION OF BLOOD IN EMERGENCIES

When quick clinical and laboratory decisions are made under conditions of stress it is frequently difficult for all involved personnel to appreciate the difficulties of others. The decision to give uncrossmatched, partially crossmatched or wait for crossmatched compatible blood is not easy, and certain basic serological considerations may clarify for the clinician some of the problems faced by the serologist. Depending upon the degree of urgency and the extent of previous knowledge about the patient's red cell serology, blood can be provided with varying degrees of safety. However, it should be emphasised that when a patient is exsanguinating and likely to die, the giving of ABO-compatible uncrossmatched blood, especially if the antibody screen is negative, is safe and appropriate therapy.

UNIVERSAL DONOR GROUP O BLOOD

Group O blood under normal circumstances will be ABO compatible with all recipients. The transfusions should be given as red cell concentrates screened for high-titre A or B haemolysins and used only in extreme emergencies. If the recipient is of childbearing age, every attempt should be made to give Rh-D-negative blood until the patient's blood group is known.

ABO-GROUP-SPECIFIC BLOOD

Transfusion of blood of the correct ABO type circumvents the isoagglutinin problems alluded to above. Simple as this approach may seem, its safety is dependent on meticulous attention to grouping. Previous blood group information, such as a 'bracelet' group or 'unofficial' group written in the patient's records, may be incorrect and there may be considerable risk if blood is administered on the basis of this information.

SALINE-COMPATIBLE BLOOD

The administration of saline-compatible blood is, for practical purposes, the administration of ABO-group-specific blood.

Access the complete references list online at http://www.expertconsult.com

4. Marik PE, Corwin HL. Efficacy of red blood cell transfusion in the critically ill: A systematic review of the literature. Crit Care Med 2008;36(9):1–8.
31. NH&MRC/ANZSBT. National Patient Blood Management Guidelines. National Blood Authority. Online. Available: http://www.nba.gov.au/guidelines/review.html (Accessed 31 August 2012).
34. Shander A, Javidroozi M, Ozawa S, et al. What is really dangerous: anaemia or transfusion? Br J Anaesthesiol 2011;107(Suppl 1):i41–59.
47. Isbister JP, Shander A, Spahn DR, et al. Adverse blood transfusion outcomes: establishing causation. Transfus Med Rev 2011;25(2):89–101.
60. Silliman CC, Fung YL, Ball JB, et al. Transfusion-related acute lung injury (TRALI): current concepts and misconceptions. Blood Rev 2009;23(6):245–55.
80. Neal MD, Marsh A, Marino R, et al. Massive transfusion: an evidence-based review of recent developments. Arch Surg 2012;147(6):563–71.

96

Colloids and blood products

Michael MG Mythen and Matthias Jacob

Colloids are used to maintain or restore deficits in blood volume. Hydrostatic and osmotic forces dictate movement of fluid between the different compartments of the body across semipermeable membranes, a phenomenon that is traditionally called Starling's principle within the circulatory system. Recently, the glycocalyx, an additional structure, is now thought to be crucial for a properly working vascular barrier.[1] It consists of membrane-bound proteoglycans and glycosaminoglycans with negatively charged side chains binding plasma proteins. Only an intact endothelial surface layer (ESL) guarantees a physiological vascular barrier, generating an inwardly directed oncotic gradient only across the protein-loaded ESL layer and a small, protein-free space directly beneath, completely at the luminal side of the endothelial cell line (**Fig. 96.1**). The traditionally presumed gradient across the anatomical vessel wall appears to be of minor importance. The ESL, and therefore vascular barrier competence, is endangered by many noxas common in critical illness and major surgery (e.g. inflammation, trauma, ischaemia/reperfusion injury and hypervolaemia). If the barrier is working, the intravascular osmotic pressure is an important determinant of the amount of intravascularly bound extracellular fluid and, therefore, of the quantitative component of cardiac preload, the target of colloidal infusion measures.

The osmotic pressure generated by a solute is proportional to the number of molecules or ions and independent of molecular size.

Colloid osmotic pressure (COP) is that exerted by macromolecules (proteins and colloids).[2,3] It can be measured using a membrane transducer system in which the membrane is freely permeable to small ions and water but largely impermeable to the colloid molecules.[4] The membrane pore size and the molecular size distribution of the colloid being studied will dictate the measured value (**Figs 96.2** and **96.3**).[3,4] The intact vascular barrier is freely permeable to electrolytes and other small osmolytes (glucose, mannitol), but relatively impermeable to macromolecules (see Fig. 96.3). An iso-oncotic colloid or protein preparation is a noncrystalline substance consisting of those macromolecules, the oncotic pressure being equal to that of the human plasma.

These types of fluid should theoretically, when infused into the intravascular space, expand the preexisting blood volume by the volume infused – that is, the so-called volume effect should be around 100%.[4,5] Meanwhile, it has become evident that this is not inevitably true for all situations in vivo; colloidal volume effects are context sensitive.[6] It could be demonstrated in human patients that close to 100% of an iso-oncotic preparation of human albumin or hydroxyethylstarch remains within the circulatory compartment when infused to maintain normovolaemia during acute blood loss. When infused into a normovolaemic circulatory compartment, the volume effect comes down towards 40%, the rest directly shifting towards the interstitial space causing a marked alteration of the ESL.[7] The mechanism behind this might be the release of atrial natriuretic peptide-activating metalloproteases, which digest the endothelial glycocalyx. Accordingly, avoiding hypervolaemia might be an advantage in patients undergoing major surgery.

Crystalloids have larger volumes of distribution depending on their composition[8] (**Fig. 96.4** and **Table 96.1**). Whereas isotonic solutions target the whole extracellular compartment, hypotonic preparations additionally load the intracellular space. Colloids or plasma substitutes initially target the intravascular compartment. Ideal properties include:

- stable with a long shelf life
- pyrogen, antigen and toxin free
- free from risk of disease transmission
- intravascular volume effect lasts for several hours
- metabolism and excretion do not adversely effect the recipient
- no tissue storage
- no direct adverse effects (e.g. causing a coagulopathy).

COLLOID SOLUTIONS

There are two major groups of colloids: plasma derivatives and semisynthetics.[1] Plasma derivatives include human albumin, plasma protein fraction, fresh frozen plasma and immunoglobulin solutions. Three principal types of semisynthetic colloids are commonly used in

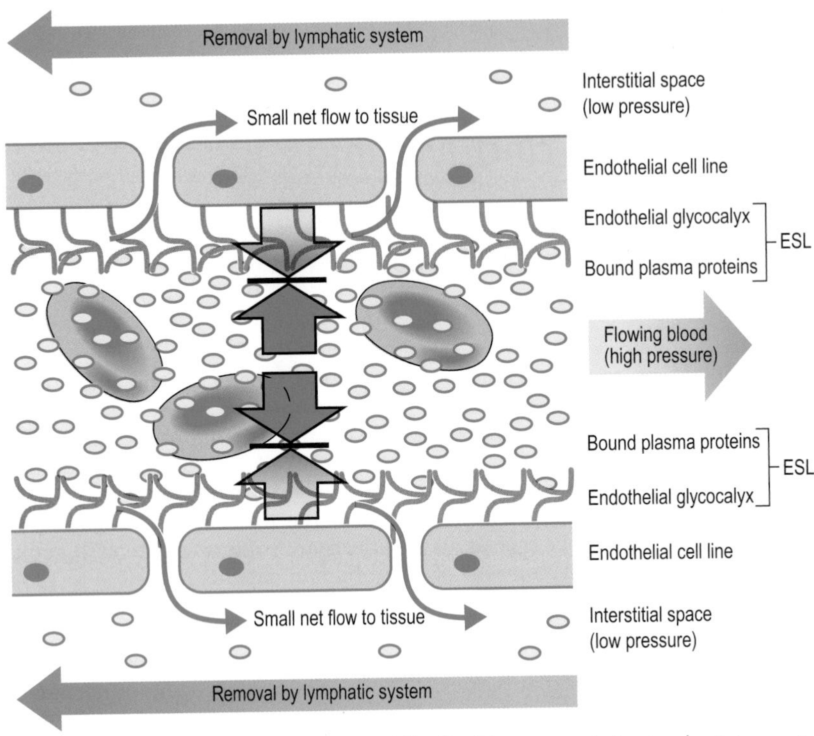

Figure 96.1 The role of the endothelial surface layer (ESL) for fluid homeostasis in steady state: an inwardly directed oncotic gradient across the ESL (orange arrows) opposes the hydrostatic force towards the interstitial space (thick black arrows). The net result is only a small fluid flux (thin black arrows), which is removed by the lymphatic system.

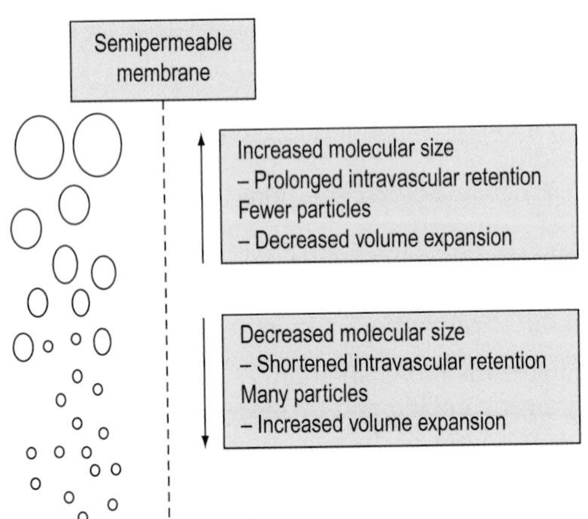

Figure 96.2 Polydispersity of colloid molecular size. *(Reproduced with permission from Grocott MPW, Mythen MG. Fluid therapy. In: Goldhill DR, Strunin L, editors.* Clinical Anaesthesiology. *London: Baillière Tindall; 1999. p. 363–81.)*

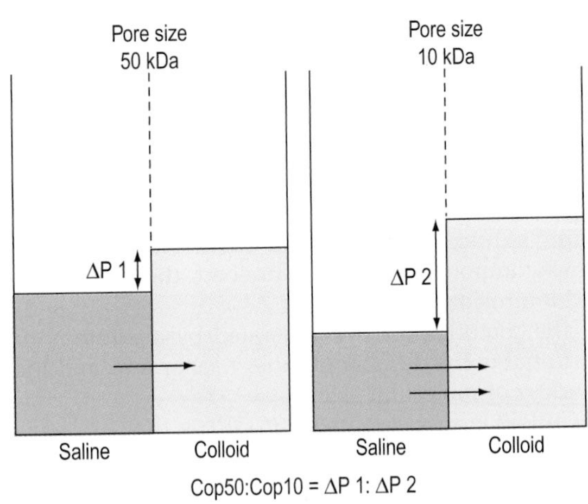

Figure 96.3 Schematic of technique for measurement of the COP50 : COP10 ratio. *(Reproduced with permission from Grocott MPW, Mythen MG. Fluid therapy. In: Goldhill DR, Strunin L, editors.* Clinical Anaesthesiology. *London: Baillière Tindall; 1999. p. 363–81.)*

intravenous solutions: gelatins, dextrans and hydroxyethyl starches. All colloids are presented dissolved in a crystalloid solution, isotonic saline still being the most common one, but isotonic glucose, hypertonic saline and isotonic balanced electrolyte solutions are also used.

Whereas human albumin solution contains more than 95% albumin with a uniform molecular size (monodispersity), all the semisynthetic colloids have a distribution of molecular sizes (polydispersity).[3,4] The size-weight relationship is relatively constant although some colloids can have equivalent molecular weight

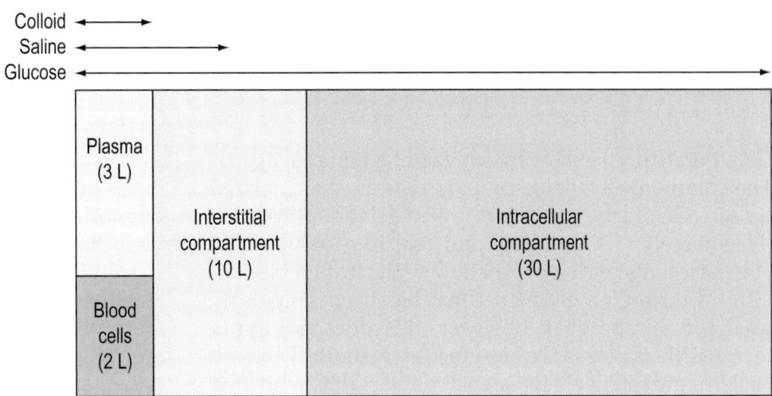

Figure 96.4 Simplified theoretical volumes of distribution of infused isotonic solutions of an ideal colloid, saline and glucose. *(Reproduced with permission from Grocott MPW, Mythen MG. Fluid therapy. In: Goldhill DR, Strunin L, editors.* Clinical Anaesthesiology. *London: Baillière Tindall; 1999. 363–81.)*

Table 96.1 Comparison of contents, osmolarity and pH of crystalloid solutions for intravenous administration

SOLUTION	OSMOLAR (MOSMOL/L)	PH	NA^+ (MMOL/L)	CL^- (MMOL/L)	K^+ (MMOL/L)	CA^{2+} (MMOL/L)	GLUCOSE (MG/L)	HCO_3^- (MOL/L)	LACTATE (MMOL/L)
Glucose 5%	252	3.5–6.5	–	–	–	–	50	–	–
Glucose 25%	1260	3.5–6.5	–	–	–	–	250	–	–
Glucose 50%	2520	3.5–6.5	–	–	–	–	500	–	–
Saline 0.9%	300	5.0	154	154	–	–	–	–	–
Glucose–saline	282	3.5–6.5	30	30	–	–	40	–	–
Ringer's	309	5.0–7.5	147	156	4	2.2	–	–	–
C. Na lactate*	278	5.0–7.0	131	111	5	2	–	–	29
Plasmalyte B	298.5	5.5	140	98	5	–	–	50	–

*Compound sodium lactate: Hartmann's solution or Ringer's lactate solution.
Reproduced with permission from Grocott MPW, Mythen MG. Fluid therapy. In: Goldhill DR, Strunin L, editors. Clinical Anaesthesiology. London: Baillière Tindall; 1999. p. 363–81.

(MW) with different molecular size – succinylated and urea-linked gelatins have almost identical molecular weights but the succinylated product undergoes conformational change due to an increase in negative charge and is physically larger.[4,5]

HUMAN ALBUMIN SOLUTION

Naturally occurring human albumin is thought of as an ideal colloid and is commonly the reference solution against which other colloids are judged; solutions are prepared from human plasma and heat treated to ensure that neither hepatitis nor HIV can be transmitted. It has a relatively short (~1 year) shelf life at room temperature, but a 5-year shelf life at 2–8°C. Human albumin 5% (the 4% version is a cost-free by-product of the production of packed red cells, exclusively used in Australia) is used for the treatment of hypovolaemia in a wide variety of clinical conditions. Concentrated salt-poor 20% human albumin is used for the treatment of hypoalbuminaemia in the presence of salt and water overload (e.g. hepatic failure with ascites). Albumin has putative advantages that include limiting free radical-mediated damage but the importance of a normal serum albumin level remains uncertain.[9–11]

Human-derived colloid has a number of disadvantages. It is an expensive product and concerns have been raised about transmission of infectious agents – such as new-variant Creutzfeldt–Jakob disease (nvCJD) associated with bovine spongiform encephalopathy (BSE) – that are not removed by currently available techniques. Concerns have also been raised by the conclusions of a highly controversial meta-analysis suggesting that the use of human albumin solution may be associated with increased mortality in the critically ill.[11–13] These conclusions were probably unjustified for most collectives except for traumatic brain injury,[14] but there is currently no evidence that the use of human albumin has any advantages over less expensive semisynthetic alternatives[15,16] or indeed crystalloids. However, the latter still applies to all colloids.[14,17,18] The volume effect of 5% human albumin is approximately

90% when used to maintain blood volume during acute blood loss.[16]

GELATINS

Gelatins are prepared by hydrolysis of bovine collagen.[19] The commonly available preparations are succinylated gelatin (Gelofusine) and urea-linked gelatin–polygeline (Haemaccel).[2,3] The significant calcium content of Haemaccel makes it incompatible with citrated blood if infused through a giving set that has been previously used for this product; however, this does not apply to SAGM (saline–adenine–glucose–mannitol) blood. Gelatins are relatively inexpensive and stable, with long shelf lives. The gelatins' plasma-volume-expanding effect lasts only about 90–120 minutes.[5] They are mainly eliminated by renal excretion.

Incidences of reactions to gelatins are acceptable (<0.5%) and range from mild skin rash and pyrexia to life-threatening anaphylaxis. The gelatins appear to have the least impact on haemostasis and it is not clear whether they have any impact over and above simple haemodilution of clotting factors. A theoretical specific safety issue has arisen with bovine-derived gelatin products since the advent of sporadic cases of nvCJD associated with exposure to tissue infected with BSE. The gelatin used in the commercially available products in the UK, for example, is sourced from the US (which is regarded as BSE-free) or from certified BSE-free herds in France. The UK Spongiform Encephalopathy Advisory Committee concluded that gelatin was safe to use in this context.

The intravascular volume effect of older gelatin preparations appears to be inferior to that of human albumin or hydroxyethylstarch.[20] Reliable data on the newer generation are rare.

DEXTRANS

Dextrans are polysaccharides biosynthesised commercially from sucrose by the bacterium *Leuconostoc mesenteroides* using the enzyme dextran sucrase.[2,3] This produces a high-molecular-weight dextran that is then cleaved by acid hydrolysis and separated by repeated ethanol fractionation to produce a final product with a relatively narrow molecular weight range. The products are described by their MW - Dextran 40 and Dextran 70 having MWs of 40000 and 70000 Da respectively.

Dextran preparations are stable at room temperature and have long shelf lives. Dextran 70 is used as a plasma substitute for the treatment of hypovolaemia and has an intravascular volume-expanding effect that lasts at least 6 hours. Dextran 40 is used for its effects on microcirculatory flow and blood coagulation in some types of surgery (e.g. vascular, neuro and plastic surgery). The beneficial effects on outcome when Dextran 40 is used as an 'anti-sludging agent' remain controversial. Dextran 40 should not be used as a plasma substitute for the treatment of hypovolaemia as, although it produces an immediate plasma volume expansion as a result of its low molecular weight, it may obstruct renal tubules and produce renal failure.

Dextrans can precipitate true anaphylactic reactions, as anti-dextran antibodies may be present due to synthesis of dextrans by lactobacilli that occur naturally as gut commensals. Dextran infusion, particularly of the high-molecular-weight products, can also precipitate anaphylactoid reactions. The risk of true anaphylactic reactions can be decreased about 10-fold by pretreatment with monovalent hapten–dextran. The dextrans are also associated with significant haemostatic derangements. These include:

- haemodilution of clotting factors
- reduction in factor VIII activity
- increase in plasminogen activation
- increase in fibrinolysis
- reduction in clot strength
- impairment of platelet function.

Red cell aggregation is also reduced with the lower-molecular-weight dextrans. In patients whose haemostatic function is normal prior to infusion, a maximum dose of 1.5 g/kg is often recommended to avoid risk of bleeding complications. The anticoagulant effects of dextrans can be utilised perioperatively as a prophylaxis against thromboembolism.[2,3]

Due to the relevant side-effect profile and the requirement to pretreat with the hapten, dextrans are, in 2012, of minor relevance in Europe.

HYDROXYETHYL STARCHES

Hydroxyethyl starches (HES) are produced by hydroxyethyl substitution of amylopectin, a D-glucose polymer obtained from potato or waxy maize.[2,3] The pattern of hydroxyethyl substitution on glucose moieties influences the susceptibility to hydrolysis by non-specific amylases in the blood. A high C2 to C6 substitution ratio and a high overall degree of substitution (the proportion of glucose moieties that have been substituted) both protect against enzymatic breakdown and prolong the effective activity of HES. The different products are commonly described by their weight-averaged molecular weight (MWw: the number of molecules at each weight times the particle weight divided by the total weight of all the molecules) and their degree of substitution,[1–5] distinguishing hetastarches (0.6–0.7), pentastarches (≈0.5) and tetrastarches (≈0.4). Starch usage varies between countries.

There is a move towards the use of the non-saline-based starch as there is an association between the administration of high volumes of normal saline and a hyperchloraemic metabolic acidosis; the clinical significance of this phenomenon remains controversial.[21–27] Colloids presented in balanced electrolyte solutions are becoming available outside the USA. In Europe, the trend over the past 5 years has been towards the use of lower-molecular-weight (130 kDa) tetrastarches presented in saline and more recently in balanced electrolyte solutions.[21] Starch preparations are stable at room temperature and have long shelf lives. The duration of intravascular retention is proportional to molecular weight[3,4,28,29] but is >6 hours even for the 130 kDa tetrastarches.

The initial volume effect of isooncotic HES preparations (6%) when infused to substitute actual intravascular deficits is close to 100%, irrespective of the generation.[28–30] HES products are associated with an acceptable incidence of adverse events including anaphylactoid reactions. Tissue deposition may result in intractable itching if large volumes of HES are infused over several days.[31] Whether the administration of large volumes of HES may cause some renal dysfunction or affect mortality in septic patients remains controversial.[32] The VISEP trial suggested hyperoncotic preparations of older generations in high dosage should be avoided in haemodynamically stable septic patients.[33] The 6S study, which found a significantly increased 90-day mortality after HES use, included 800 septic patients only *after* initial stabilisation,[34] as did the CHEST study, which found no difference in mortality and an unaltered renal state (RIFLE) after HES in 7000 ICU patients despite an increase in the use of renal replacement therapy.[35] Overall, no data currently prohibit the use of HES for use as a preload in the ICU patient. The perioperative use of modern HES preparations is currently not seriously questioned by available data, but neither safety nor efficacy has been demonstrated in large RCTs with long-term follow-up.[36]

HES products can cause a coagulopathy.[37] In particular, factor VIII (FVIII) levels are reduced and platelet function is impaired, causing a von Willebrand-like syndrome. These effects are greater with high-molecular-weight HES molecules infused at larger volumes and less in the reformulated balanced electrolyte alternative.[21] It is likely that in new-generation HES products some of the side-effects are attenuated.[38] However, their safety still needs to be proven.[33–36]

THE ROLE OF HYPERTONIC SOLUTIONS

In recent years hypertonic (600–1800 mosmol) crystalloid and colloid solutions have been introduced for certain clinical indications.[39–43] The theoretical advantage is that a small volume of administered fluid will provide a significant plasma volume expansion. The high osmolarity should draw tissue fluid into the intravascular space and thus should minimise tissue oedema for a given plasma volume increment. Colloids presented in a hypertonic saline carrier have been shown to achieve adequate resuscitation in a number of clinical settings. However, whether in fact a smaller volume of hypertonic solution really leads to a similar plasma volume expansion, in comparison to solutions with isotonicity, has never reliably been shown by direct blood volume assessment. From a physiological standpoint the idea that hypertonic crystalloid will drag water from the interstitial compartment may be optimistic, as electrolytes and other small osmolytes are not retained by the intact vascular barrier, in clear contrast to the blood–brain barrier. These solutions might result in reduced cerebral oedema in those patients at risk of this complication and these solutions may have a place in treating refractory cerebral oedema.[41–43] Outside the perioperative arena they are finding use in the management of burns patients and in prehospital resuscitation of trauma victim, being limited at present to single-dose administrations.

BLOOD SUBSTITUTES – PERFLUOROCARBON AND HAEMOGLOBIN THERAPEUTICS

In future, the use of artificial or semisynthetic oxygen-carrying solutions might become increasingly common.[44] A number of products have been and are currently under evaluation: perfluorocarbon, modified human haemoglobin (Hb), modified bovine Hb and recombinant Hb solutions. These products not only function as oxygen carriers but also are capable of sustained plasma volume expansion. Unlike Hb present in intact red cells, they often have a linear O_2-Hb dissociation profile and the effects on O_2 uptake in the lungs and release in the tissues are not yet clearly defined. Additionally, they may have specific pharmacological effects like nitric oxide scavenging, resulting in vasoconstriction. Nevertheless, a real artificial alternative to red cells as an oxygen carrier applicable in clinical routine will not be available in the near future.

PLASMA DERIVATIVES

FRESH FROZEN PLASMA

Fresh frozen plasma (FFP) contains normal plasma levels of all the clotting factors, albumin and immunoglobulin. A unit is typically 200–250 mL and has a FVIII level of at least 0.7 IU/mL (i.e. 70% of normal levels) and about 0.5 g of fibrinogen. It is kept at a temperature of –18°C or less in order to preserve coagulant levels. FFP is used for the replacement of multiple clotting factor deficiencies (e.g. liver disease, coumarin anticoagulant overdose and coagulopathy associated with massive blood transfusion).[45–47] An initial dose of at least 15 mL/kg (four packs for a 70-kg adult) is considered to be appropriate. Physiologically, in a normovolaemic patient, it might be better to correct any clotting factor deficit using a concentrate and then maintain the appropriate level using FFP instead of colloids in the face of ongoing bleeding or other volume deficit. This might decrease the risk of intravascular hypervolaemia, but currently there are no data to support using FFP in this way. FFP should not be used as a plasma volume expander, solely for the treatment of hypovolaemia.

CRYOPRECIPITATE

Cryoprecipitate is prepared by freeze-thaw of FFP, collection of the precipitate and then its resuspension in human plasma. It is a concentrate of FVIII, von Willebrand factor and fibrinogen and contains about 50% of the coagulant factor activity of the original unit (e.g. fibrinogen 250 mg, FVIII 100 IU). Cryoprecipitate is stored at −18°C and remains stable for up to a year.[45] It is indicated in the treatment of coagulation defects, including massive haemorrhage and DIC, if there is microvascular bleeding associated with a fibrinogen level <0.5 g/L. Also, it is, in principle, an alternative to the preferable FVIII or von Willebrand factor concentrates in the treatment of inherited deficiencies of those proteins.[46,47]

FACTOR VIII

Recombinant factor VIII is available but concentrates are also still prepared from pools of donor plasma and heat or chemically treated to inactivate HIV-1. It has a shelf life of 2–3 years. Chromatographic concentration results in high-purity FVIII, and the relative merits of high- and intermediate-purity products are being investigated.

Indications are the treatment of haemophilia A.[48] The dosage should carefully follow the recommendations of the respective manufacturers, targeting at plasma activities between 30 and 100%, depending on the clinical situation. Preferably, the strategy should be planned together with a specialist and will usually lead to a bolus of 25–50 U/kg, which can be repeated, for example, 12-hourly.

FACTOR IX COMPLEX

Factor IX complex (prothrombin complex concentrate, also called 'PPSB') contains the vitamin-K-dependent factors II, VII, IX and X in varying amounts, and is prepared from pools of plasma.[45] It is a freeze-dried preparation reconstituted with water immediately before use. Factor IX complex is mainly used to correct bleeding disorders due to an overdose of the vitamin K antagonistic coumarin anticoagulants in patients who cannot tolerate large volumes of FFP.[45] Purified factor IX concentrates are now available and appear preferable in haemophilia B.

OTHER PLASMA CONCENTRATES

Activated factor VII concentrate can be used in the very rare deficiency of FVII, but also, in principle, in patients with inhibitors to factor VIII or IX, as it bypasses the requirement for these factors.[45] The use of the specific factor concentrations is preferable. The use of activated factor VII in the management of severe life-threatening haemorrhage remains controversial.[49] Other concentrates, such as antithrombin III, C1 esterase inhibitor and proteins C and S, have been used experimentally with varying success for the treatment of DIC and septic shock. Recombinant activated protein C preparation (Drocegogin alfa, Xigris™, Eli Lilly, Indianapolis, USA) for the treatment of septic shock[50] (see Ch. 15) was withdrawn in 2011 owing to its unclear benefit and an increased risk of bleeding.

IMMUNOGLOBULINS (GAMMA GLOBULINS)

Human immunoglobulin preparations are pooled from plasma from normal blood donors. It contains antibodies to hepatitis A, measles, mumps, varicella, polio and prevalent bacteria, reflecting the plasma of the donors.[45] Immunoglobulins are indicated in the prevention or treatment of patients with hypogammaglobulinaemia, and may have a role in the treatment of autoimmune diseases, such as thrombocytopenic purpura and myasthenia gravis. Specific immunoglobulins are available for a range of infectious agents including tetanus, hepatitis B, rubella, measles, rabies and varicella zoster. They are made from donor plasma known to contain high levels of the specific IgG antibodies and are used for prophylaxis and treatment in patients who have not been actively immunised. Rhesus-D immunoglobulin is prepared from plasma containing high levels of anti Rh-D antibodies and it prevents sensitisation of Rh-negative mothers to Rh-D positive cells that may enter their circulation. The principal use of Rh-D immunoglobulin is in the prevention of haemolytic disease of the newborn.[51]

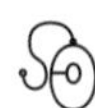

Access the complete references list online at http://www.expertconsult.com

3. Vercueil A, Grocott MP, Mythen MG. Physiology, pharmacology, and rationale for colloid administration for the maintenance of effective hemodynamic stability in critically ill patients. Transfus Med Rev 2005;19:93–109.
7. Chappell D, Jacob M, Hofmann-Kiefer K, et al. A rational approach to perioperative fluid management. Anesthesiology 2008;109:723–40.
8. Jacob M, Chappell D, Hofmann-Kiefer K, et al. The intravascular volume effect of Ringer's lactate is below 20%: a prospective study in humans. Crit Care 2012;16:R86.
28. James MF, Latoo MY, Mythen MG, et al. Plasma volume changes associated with two hydroxyethyl starch colloids following acute hypovolaemia in volunteers. Anaesthesia 2004;59:738–42.
37. Roche AM, James MF, Bennett-Guerrero E, et al. A head-to-head comparison of the in vitro coagulation effects of saline-based and balanced electrolyte crystalloid and colloid intravenous fluids. Anesth Analg 2006;102:1274–9.

97

Therapeutic plasma exchange and intravenous immunoglobulin therapy

Ian Kerridge, David Collins and James P Isbister

Blood letting to remove 'evil humours' has been practiced for over 2000 years. But although the restoration of 'balance' and the removal of 'noxious' agents from the blood remains the rationale for apheresis, contemporary practice is now based upon an extensive scientific understanding of the pathophysiology of the diseases treated by plasma exchange.[1] Exchange transfusions revolutionised the management of haemolytic disease in the newborn, and paved the way for therapeutic plasmapheresis and plasma exchange – the removal of plasma, with replacement by albumin-electrolyte solutions or fresh frozen plasma. Initially used in the management of hyperviscosity associated with malignant paraproteinaemia, it is now also used in the treatment of more than 100 autoimmune disorders but is expensive, not risk-free and debate continues on its therapeutic role in many diseases.

Intravenous immunoglobulin (IVIG) – once used purely as replacement therapy for patients with primary humoral immune deficiency – has also become increasingly used as an immunomodulatory agent. Its relevance in this chapter is that it is now being used in many disorders in which plasma exchange is effective, but the convenience and safety of IVIG therapy is preferred as an alternative. The underlying principles in managing autoimmune diseases with IVIG are similar to those of therapeutic plasma exchange. The immunomodulatory mechanism of action of IVIG remains controversial and it is likely, as with plasma exchange, that there is more than one mechanism in play. Therapeutic efficacy of IVIG has been established in controlled trials for a range of diseases including idiopathic thrombocytopenic purpura, Kawasaki disease, Guillain–Barré syndrome, dermatomyositis and others. There is compelling evidence that IVIG can modulate immune reactions of T cells, B cells and macrophages, thus interfering with antibody production and degradation, but also modulating the complement cascade and cytokine networks.

RATIONALE FOR PLASMA EXCHANGE

Theoretically, plasma exchange should be effective to treat any disorder in which there is a pathogenic circulating factor responsible for disease. However, it is increasingly clear that this premise is too simplistic as many other mechanisms have been found to contribute to its beneficial effects (**Box 97.1**). Plasma exchange brings about numerous alterations in the plasma's *milieu interieur* – which may be clinically beneficial or detrimental.

PATHOPHYSIOLOGY OF AUTOIMMUNE DISEASE

Autoimmune disease originates from the breakdown of immunoregulation (i.e. immune tolerance), allowing the immune system to become autoaggressive. Autoimmune diseases with underlying humoral mechanisms result from either a circulating autoantibody against a self-antigen (alone or in combination with an environmental antigen), or circulating immune complexes (which may be deposited in the microcirculation of various organs, resulting in end-organ damage). Cellular and tissue damage are effected by the autoantibody or immune complexes activating the cellular and humoral components of the inflammatory response. The circulating proteolytic systems involved include the complement, coagulation, fibrinolytic and kinin systems. On the cellular side, neutrophils and macrophages are involved, with eosinophils and basophils also playing a part.

The varied clinical manifestations of autoimmune disorders relate more to the cell, tissue or organ involved, rather than the pathophysiological process. However, basic pathophysiological mechanisms by which autoimmune diseases occur need to be understood in order to standardise treatment. Although some cells of the host defence system, in particular the macrophages and lymphocytes, may have special differentiation appropriate to individual organs, their basic functional processes are not all that dissimilar between different organs.

In general, autoimmune disease can be an acute, self-limiting ('one-hit') disorder, intermittent or a chronic perpetuating disorder. Acute autoimmune disease may have an identifiable trigger, such as an infection, followed by a 10-day to 3-week gap until the pathogenic humoral or cellular factors appear in the circulating blood. At this point, end-organ damage commences, and clinical features of the disease appear.

Box 97.1 Rationale for plasma exchange

Removal of circulating toxic factor antibodies
- Monoclonal antobodies
- Autoantibodies
- Alloantibodies

Immune complexes
Chemical drugs
Depletion of mediators of inflammation
Replacement of deficient plasma factor(s)
Potentiation of drug action
Enhanced reticuloendothelial function
Altered immunoregulation
Potentiating effect of plasma exchange on other modes of therapy (e.g. glucocorticoids)

The course of the disease will be determined by several factors:

- biological function and importance of the system involved
- extent of damage
- replaceability or otherwise of the cells under attack
- time course of the damaging insult.

The extent of damage, in turn, is a product of the:

- characteristics of the antibodies or lymphocytes involved (e.g. antibody affinity, complement fixing capabilities and titre)
- function of other components of the host defence system (e.g. neutrophils, platelets, proteolytic systems and reticuloendothelial system)
- presence of other aggravating factors (e.g. infection, hormonal responses and circulatory responses).

The kinetics of the end-cell involved in the immunological damage is relevant in determining the final outcome of the disease. Ultimate recovery of organ function after 'burn-out' of a self-limiting autoimmune disease, or control of a chronic autoimmune disease, is determined by the ability of the cell to replace and restore function to normal.

Cells are broadly divided into three kinetic characteristics:

- *Continuous replicators:* these cells are continuously replaced in the normal state, are readily replaced when damaged, and if the immunological insult is removed or controlled then full replacement of the end-cells occurs. Typically seen with the haemopoietic system, the cells lining the gut and skin cells.
- *Discontinuous replicators:* these are cells that are not being constantly replaced in the normal state, but when damaged, cell division is initiated and replacement occurs. This is seen with hepatocytes, renal tubular cells and the neuronal Schwann cell.
- *Non-replicating cells:* these cells when damaged are irreplaceably destroyed with permanent loss of function. This is seen with neuronal cells, muscle cells and renal glomeruli.

The clinical features and final outcome of any autoimmune disease are determined by many different factors, including the ability of the end-organ to repair following removal or control of the immunological insult. In many self-limiting autoimmune diseases, if the end-cell is a continuous or intermittent replicator then full recovery can be expected, after recovery from the acute phase of the illness. Examples are acute tubular necrosis, acute demyelination, acute hepatic failure and some forms of marrow aplasia. In contrast, in disorders involving non-replicating cells such as acute glomerulonephritis, therapy must be aimed at removing the immunological insult or dampening its damaging affects as soon as possible so as to minimise irreparable damage to the end-cells and thus long-term organ function. Immunological mediators may also produce disease without direct destruction of end-cells. This occurs when autoantibodies develop against cell receptors with blocking or destruction of the receptor, as may typically be seen in myasthenia gravis and thyrotoxicosis.

Therapy in acute and chronic autoimmune disease aims to minimise irreparable end-organ damage and support patients during the acute illness. This therapy may include:

- non-specific therapy to suppress the effector mechanisms (e.g. corticosteroids, antiplatelet therapy, nonsteroidal anti-inflammatory drugs, anticoagulation and depletion of humoral effector mechanisms by plasma exchange or defibrination)
- therapy to reduce the circulating levels of a humoral factor, which is achieved with plasma exchange or immunoabsorption technique
- specific or broad-spectrum immunosuppressive agents to suppress or block the immune response (e.g. corticosteroids, cytotoxic agents, anti-lymphocyte globulin, high-dose intravenous gamma-globulin therapy)
- therapy directed at altering reticuloendothelial function, which may then have effects on autoantibody and immune complex clearance, or clearance of circulating damaged cells
- intravenous immunoglobulin (IVIG) immunomodulatory therapy.

As most disorders are multifactorial, it is unlikely that a single form of therapy will be successful, so a multipronged approach to therapy needs to be based upon analysis of the underlying pathophysiology. The stage of the disease is also important (**Fig. 97.1**). Clearly, plasma exchange will have a different response when autoantibody production is rising rapidly, compared with a stage when autoantibody has ceased production. Also, immunoregulation is a complex process and therapies may interfere at different points in the immune mechanisms.

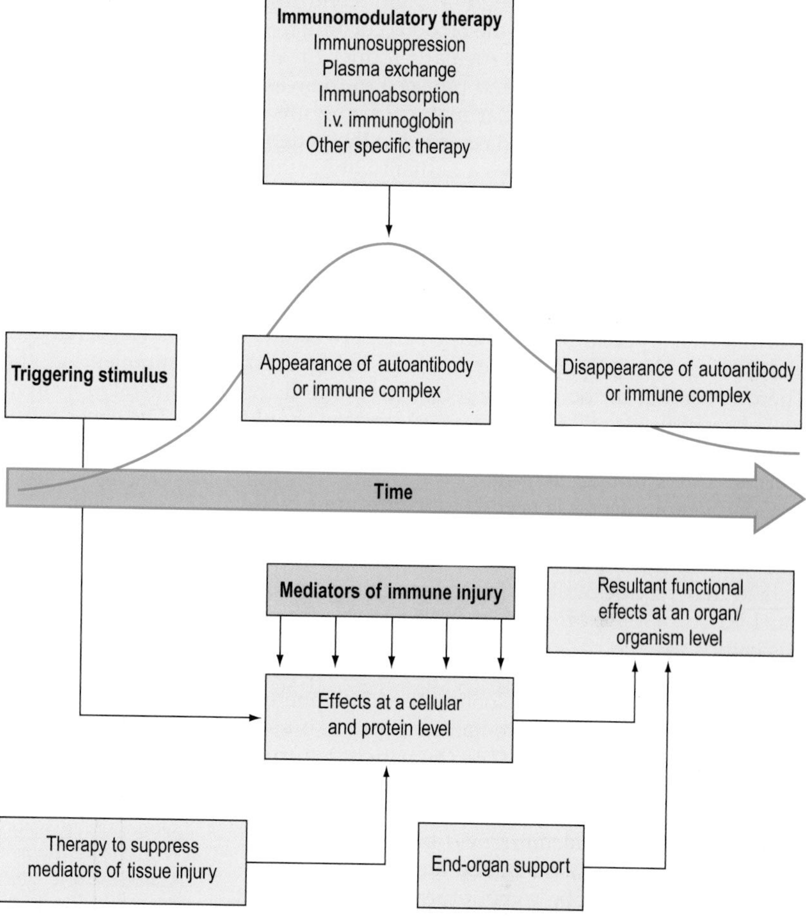

Figure 97.1 The therapy of 'one-hit' autoimmune disease.

In some circumstances, specific and directed therapy may attack the most relevant link in the pathophysiological chain, but overall multiple approaches to therapy may be required. In general, plasma exchange is a temporising procedure and concomitant immunosuppressive therapy is required to maintain control. Plasma exchange should generally be regarded as a first step in immunomodulatory therapy, and restricted to acute or fulminant situations in which autoantibodies or immune complexes are responsible for life-threatening or end-organ-damaging complications. If the humoral factor is only transient (' a one antigen hit' disorder), then no follow-up immunosuppression is required (e.g. acute post-infectious polyneuritis). Increasingly, monoclonal antibody therapy with rituximab (an anti-CD20 antibody) is finding a role in the longer-term management of autoimmune diseases.[2,3]

The recognition of the immunomodulatory effects of IVIG has resulted in an exponential increase in its use in immune and inflammatory disorders – with availability being one of the main drivers of the supply of human-derived plasma products. Indeed, in most of the immune and inflammatory disorders in which plasma exchange has been used, IVIG has been used – often with equal efficacy.[4]

TECHNICAL CONSIDERATIONS

Plasma exchange can be by filtration, centrifugation, or a combination of both, depending on the equipment available. There are a number of apheresis machines on the market. Filtration plasma exchange is found on a number of dialysis machines and uses a semipermeable membrane with small holes or pores up to 0.2 μm in diameter; this is approximately 30 times the diameter of the pores found in conventional high-flux haemofilter membranes.[5] Blood is pumped into this chamber and the plasma passes through the membrane; this membrane will allow the passage of substances up to 3×10^6 Da, separating substances such as immunoglobulins, immune complexes and complement factors from the cellular part of the blood.[5] The plasma is then diverted to a waste bag and the remaining cellular product mixed with replacement fluid and returned to the patient.

Apheresis machines using centrifugation use continuous or intermittent blood flow. The continuous flow machines pump blood through a band centrifuge; applied G-force separates out the blood according to its molecular weight, and the particular product (in this case the plasma) is removed and pumped to the waste bag, with the remaining cellular material being mixed with the replacement fluid and returned to the patient.[6] Intermittent centrifugation uses a Latham bowl, which fills with blood, is centrifuged, the plasma separated to a waste bag and the cellular products returned to the patient with replacement fluid. This procedure can be carried out through one vein; however, it is a longer procedure than the continuous-flow machines.[6]

The extracorporeal blood is anywhere between 150 and 250 mL depending on the machine being used. There is cooling in the extracorporeal circuit, and the replacement fluids will be cool so consideration should be given to maintain body temperature, with a blood warmer and warming blankets.[7]

Good venous access is needed for continuous blood flow, at between 30 and 100 mL/min depending on the replacement fluid and the patient's condition. As the patient may require multiple procedures, consideration must be given for appropriate venous access such as a vas-cath.

Most apheresis machines use regional anticoagulation, with citrate added as blood enters the apheresis circuit. Pooled plasma also contains citrate so, if used, the amount of citrate returned to the patient is further increased. It should be noted, however, that citrate toxicity can also occur when albumin is used, as this is a calcium-free and calcium avid-binding solution.[7] Although citrate is plasma-bound and relatively short-acting there will still be some returned to the patient where it is metabolised. Patients with abnormal liver functions will take longer to metabolise the citrate and therefore have an increased risk of citrate toxicity. Citrate toxicity produces hypocalcaemia with symptoms including acral or oral paraesthesia, light-headedness, tetany, nausea, vomiting and cardiac arrhythmias.[8] The drop in calcium levels occurs within the first 15 minutes of the procedure,[7] therefore attention should be paid to the patient's serum calcium and if required supplementation commenced prior to the start of the procedure. Calcium gluconate 10% at a dose of 2 mL per 250 mL of replacement fluid has been recommended; this can be added to the albumin or run as a concurrent infusion.[9,10] Other electrolytes can also become depleted, and should therefore be monitored and replaced as required.[7] Magnesium also binds to citrate and there can be up to a 60% fall in the blood levels of patients; however, concurrent supplementation is not recommended as routine.[7]

Occasionally the apheresis circuit is secondary to heart bypass, extracorporeal membrane oxygenation (ECMO) or renal dialysis. The literature is limited but it has been reported as safe.[7] For ECMO and heart bypass, the apheresis practitioner must work closely with the medical staff and perfusionist to ensure the patient's safety. Where renal dialysis is involved there should be negotiation as to the timing of the procedures. In most cases it is preferable for plasma exchange to be performed prior to dialysis so that any extra fluid given during the procedure can be removed by dialysis.

INDICATIONS (BOX 97.2)

Plasma exchange is most beneficial for immunoproliferative and autoimmune diseases. In some conditions with unclear pathophysiology, the beneficial effects of plasma exchange may be due to infusion of a deficient component in the replacement plasma, rather than removal of a circulating factor.

The American Society for Apheresis (ASFA) has published comprehensive 'Guidelines on the Use of Therapeutic Apheresis in Clinical Practice: Evidence-based

Box 97.2 Acute diseases in which plasma exchange may be beneficial*

Immunoproliferative diseases with monoclonal immunoglobulins
Hyperviscosity syndrome
Cryoglobulinaemia
Renal failure in multiple myeloma

Autoimmune diseases due to autoantibodies or immune complexes
Goodpasture syndrome
Myasthenia gravis
Guillain–Barré syndrome
Chronic inflammatory demyelinating polyneuropathy (CIDP)
Stiff-man syndrome
Systemic lupus erythematosus
Fulminant antiphospholipid syndrome
Thrombotic thrombocytopenic purpura
Haemolytic uraemic syndrome
Rapidly progressive glomerulonephritis
Coagulation inhibitors
Autoimmune haemolytic anaemia
Pemphigus
Paraneoplastic syndromes

Conditions in which replacement of plasma may be beneficial +/− removal of toxins
Disseminated intravascular coagulation
Multi-organ dysfunction syndrome
Overwhelming sepsis syndromes (e.g. meningococcaemia)

Conditions in which the mechanisms are unknown
Reye's syndrome

Removal of protein-bound or large-molecular-weight toxins
Paraquat poisoning
Envenomation

*This is an incomplete list and includes only disorders that are relatively common or in which plasma exchange has a definitive role to play.

approach from the Apheresis Applications Committee of the American Society for Apheresis'.[11] The ASFA guidelines describe four categories of disorder on the basis of a review of the available literature on the efficacy of TPE. These are as follows:

- *Category I*: 'Disorder for which apheresis is accepted as first-line therapy, either as a standalone treatment or in conjunction with other modes of treatment.'
- *Category II*: 'Disorders for which apheresis is accepted as second-line therapy, either as a standalone treatment or in conjunction with other modes of treatment.'
- *Category III*: 'Optimum role of apheresis therapy is not established. Decision-making should be individualised.'
- *Category IV*: 'Disorders in which published evidence demonstrates or suggests apheresis to be ineffective or harmful. Internal Review Board approval is desirable if apheresis treatment is undertaken in these circumstances.'

Category I disorders include: myasthenia gravis, Guillain–Barré syndrome, Goodpasture syndrome (anti-GBM antibody disease), cryoglobulinaemia, chronic inflammatory demyelinating polyradiculoneuropathy (CIDP), sickle cell disease (acute stroke) and Wegener's granulomatosis.

Category II disorders include: multiple sclerosis, neuromyelitis optica, acute disseminated encephalomyelitis, ABO-incompatible solid organ transplantation and catastrophic antiphospholipid syndrome.

Category III disorders include: aplastic anaemia, autoimmune haemolytic anaemia, paraneoplastic neurologic syndromes, erythrocytosis, acute liver failure, immune complex rapidly progressive glomerulonephritis and sepsis and multi-organ failure.

Category IV disorders include: dermatomyositis or polymyositis, ITP, rheumatoid arthritis, chronic progressive multiple sclerosis, scleroderma, amyloidosis and inflammatory bowel disease.

MONOCLONAL ANTIBODIES ASSOCIATED WITH IMMUNOPROLIFERATIVE DISEASES

Monoclonal immunoglobulins are a classical feature of multiple myeloma and Waldenström's macroglobulinaemia, but may also be associated with other lymphoproliferative disorders. These monoclonal proteins may be associated with numerous clinical effects, many of which may be reversed by plasma exchange:

- *Hyperviscosity syndrome:* characteristic clinical features of hyperviscosity in association with monoclonal proteins include visual disturbance, neurological dysfunction and hypervolaemia. All are rapidly relieved by plasma exchange.[12]
- *Haemostatic disturbances:* monoclonal proteins may impair haemostasis by adversely affecting platelet function or by inhibitory effects on coagulation factors. Plasma exchange is usually effective in controlling haemorrhage and may also be helpful in preparing patients for surgery.
- *Renal failure*: the development of renal failure in the course of multiple myeloma is generally regarded as a sign of poor prognosis. The renal failure is often multifactorial in origin, but some of these factors may be reversible by plasma exchange. Patients presenting acutely with hyperviscosity, dehydration and hypercalcaemia may show recovery of renal function following adequate hydration, alkaline diuresis and plasma exchange.

IMMUNOLOGICAL DISEASES

DISEASES MEDIATED BY SPECIFIC AUTOANTIBODIES

Goodpasture syndrome

In Goodpasture syndrome circulating antiglomerular basement membrane antibodies can often be demonstrated. The disease classically has a fulminant presentation with rapidly progressive renal failure and life-threatening pulmonary haemorrhage. Early diagnosis and intensive plasma exchange may be necessary to preserve renal function and control pulmonary haemorrhage. Patients who are already in anuric renal failure rarely show improvement in renal function.[13]

Myasthenia gravis

Removal of the acetylcholine receptor autoantibody is often associated with clinical improvement, but the beneficial effects of plasma exchange are usually transient, so the procedure should be used in conjunction with other forms of therapy (see Ch. 57, Myasthenia gravis). The major role of plasma exchange is in myasthenic crisis, in patients whose condition is resistant to other forms of therapy, and prior to surgery. Therapy can be monitored by acetylcholine receptor autoantibody assays and respiratory function tests. During the procedure patients may transiently deteriorate, owing to a combination of the physical exertion and removal of medication from the circulation. Adequate ventilatory support should be available. IVIG may also be use in myasthenia gravis.[14–16]

Stiff-man syndrome

Stiff-man syndrome is a rare neurological disorder characterised by involuntary axial and proximal limb rigidity and continuous motor unit activity on electromyography. Autoantibodies to glutamic acid decarboxylase are usually demonstrable and plasma exchange is often successful in those in whom autoantibody can be demonstrated, but if negative they are less likely to respond.[17,18]

Autoimmune haematological disorders

Haemostatic failure due to autoantibodies directed against coagulation factors may present a major management problem. Antibodies directed against factor VIII are the commonest, occurring spontaneously or in association with replacement therapy in haemophiliacs. First-line therapy in patients with coagulation factor inhibitors usually requires activated factor VII therapy with recombinant VIIa or appropriate prothrombin concentrates.[19]

IMMUNE COMPLEX DISEASE

Rapidly progressive glomerulonephritis

Immune-complex-induced rapidly progressive glomerulonephritis may occur by itself or be associated with several systemic disorders (e.g. systemic lupus erythematosus, polyarteritis nodosa, IgA nephropathy, post-streptococcal infection and Wagener's granulomatosis).[20–22] Plasma exchange may result in improvement in renal function even in patients who present with anuria. The decomplementing and defibrinating effects of plasma exchange may be partly responsible for clinical improvement. The therapeutic role of plasma exchange in rapidly progressive glomerulonephritis is difficult to assess, but most experienced physicians feel that the procedure leads to a more rapid and complete recovery of renal function in fulminant, rapidly deteriorating cases. However, the ultimate prognosis of the disease depends on adequate immunosuppression to inhibit immune complex formation, or spontaneous disappearance of the inciting antigen.

Systemic lupus erythematosus (SLE)

In acute life-threatening or organ-damaging relapses of SLE, plasma exchange should be considered if there is rapid deterioration in renal function, cerebritis, or acute fulminant lupus pneumonitis.[23]

Cryoglobulinaemia

The various forms of cryoglobulinaemia may be associated with vasculitis or hyperviscosity. If there is an acute fulminant presentation with cutaneous vasculitis, renal failure, and neurological impairment then plasma exchange should be considered an urgent definitive form of therapy.

OTHER IMMUNE-MEDIATED DISEASES

Renal transplant rejection

Humoral mechanisms appear to play a part in hyperacute renal allograft rejection. Plasma exchange +/− IVIG may be useful in tiding patients over episodes of acute graft rejection. However, results of clinical trials have been conflicting.[24,25] General opinion is that plasma exchange helps in a limited number of patients who cannot be currently preselected by any clinical or laboratory criteria.

Thrombotic microangiopathies

The thrombotic microangiopathies describe a number of syndromes characterised by disseminated microvascular thrombosis, thrombocytopenia and (often) anaemia. They include thrombotic thrombocytopenic purpura (TTP), haemolytic uraemic syndrome (HUS), disseminated intravascular coagulation (DIC), catastrophic antiphospholipid syndrome (CAPS) and paediatric thrombocytopenia-associated multiorgan failure (TAMOF).

Thrombotic thrombocytopenic purpura

TTP is a potentially fulminant and life-threatening disorder characterised by platelet microthrombi in small vessels, resulting in microangiopathy. The clinical syndrome is manifest by the pentad of thrombocytopenia, microangiopathic haemolytic anaemia, fever, renal dysfunction and neurological abnormalities. Abdominal symptoms, hepatic dysfunction and pulmonary abnormalities may also occur. With the appropriate clinical features, thrombocytopenia and a microangiopathic blood film, diagnosis is established.

TTP has been linked to a severe deficiency in ADAMTS13 with metalloprotease activity with its target cleavage sequence in von Willebrand factor (VWF). The presence of an autoantibody inhibitor to this vWF-reducing metalloproteinase has been documented in patients with both acute TTP and those with chronic relapsing forms. In normal plasma vWF undergoes proteolysis by a specific protease and deficiency of this cleaving protease reduces or abolishes the plasma clearance of ultralarge vWF multimers, resulting in intravascular aggregation of platelets particularly at sites of intravascular shear stress. The inhibitor to the metalloproteinase has been demonstrated to be an IgG autoantibody.

There is a primary idiopathic form of the disease that usually has an acute presentation and probably has an underlying autoimmune mechanism. This form may be associated with a variety of prodromal infections (viral or bacterial). Bacterial cytotoxins, produced by *Shigella dysenteriae* 1 and certain *E. coli* serotypes, have been related to TTP and HUS, probably by initiating damage to vascular endothelial cells possibly via cytokine mechanisms. TTP may be associated with various drugs (cytotoxic agents), toxins and bites. CMV, HIV and herpes viruses have also been implicated. Chemotherapy-associated thrombotic thrombocytopenic purpura/haemolytic uraemic syndrome is being increasingly recognised and may be associated with a range of cytotoxic medications. Severe microangiopathy resembling TTP has also been reported as a complication of acute graft-versus-host disease in patients receiving ciclosporin prophylaxis following allogeneic BMT.

TTP used to be fatal disease in 90% of patients, but dramatic improvement in its outcome has occurred over the past two decades. Plasma exchange has become the cornerstone of the treatment with cryoprecipitate-poor plasma (depleted in VWF).[26,27] It is now possible to achieve remissions in the majority of patients and cures are now common, although unfortunately relapse may occur. The clinical course at relapse is usually milder than the disease at presentation and less-aggressive therapy may be needed.

Haemolytic uraemic syndrome (HUS)

This syndrome has many similarities to TTP, but in contrast to cerebral TTP, renal involvement is the hallmark of microangiopathy and thrombocytopenia.[28] HUS is commonly categorised into 'typical' and 'atypical' HUS.

Typical HUS, the majority of cases, is commonly associated with infection and diarrhoea – most commonly caused by the Shiga-toxin producing *Escherichia coli* 0157:H7, which induces release of ultra-large vWF from the endothelium and inhibits ADAMS-13. Less often, HUS may present insidiously and the cause, which may include chemotherapy, radiotherapy or other medications, may be unclear. Therapeutic plasma exchange is generally not recommended for typical HUS associated with infection – which is often self-limiting and has a mortality of less than 5%. Although it is often tried in adult patients with HUS and in patients with typical HUS of more indeterminate cause – the results are often disappointing.

Atypical HUS is thought to result from genetic mutations in the complement pathway or from acquired autoantibodies against factor H, which result in uncontrolled activation of the alternative complement pathway and direct injury to the microvasculature. Plasma exchange is recommended for atypical HUS – which has a mortality rate of approximately 25%.

It is often difficult to distinguish atypical HUS from typical HUS and HUS from TTP, particularly in the acute setting – so plasma exchange is often initiated until the results of genetic studies and biomarkers can assist in clarifying the diagnosis.

Inflammatory demyelinating neuropathies and Guillain–Barré syndrome

This acute self-limiting disease in which an acute demyelinating neuropathy occurs (usually following a viral infection) commonly results in admission to the ICU (see Ch. 57, Guillain–Barré syndrome). The demyelination is due to post-infectious autoimmunity, with both cellular and humoral arms of the immune system attacking myelin. There is now wide experience in the use of plasma exchange and IVIG therapy in Guillain–Barré syndrome, with controlled trials substantiating its benefits of shortening of the illness, and complications. Therapy should be instituted early.[16,29] As Guillain–Barré syndrome also responds to high-dose IVIG, there is debate as to which should be the first line of therapy; as the therapies have comparable efficacy and safety, decisions are usually made on the basis of local logistics and economics.[30] In some cases the onset of recovery after therapy may be delayed, probably due to time for remyelination to occur. Some patients show rapid improvement after plasma exchange, suggesting the presence of neuronal blocking factors. Chronic inflammatory demyelinating peripheral neuropathy (CIPD) is related to the GBS and plasma exchange and/or IVIG have important roles in treatment, in many cases requiring long-term therapy.

COMPLICATIONS

Plasma exchange is a relatively safe procedure, with a case–fatality rate of 3–5 per 10 000 procedures – mainly as a consequence of cardiac arrest, cardiac failure and transfusion-associated acute lung injury (TRALI). Minor complications due to fluid shifts, electrolyte abnormalities and exposure to blood products are common and for these reasons close supervision by experienced physicians and apheresis operators with a sound understanding of the haemodynamic, biochemical, haematological and immunological effects of plasma exchange is of paramount importance.[31,32]

Assessment prior to commencing the procedure should include vascular access, haemodynamic stability, transfusion history, relevant co-morbidities and concomitant medications. Any medication that is highly plasma-bound or has a low volume of distribution is likely to be removed.[33,34] If there is any concern that a drug may be removed during the procedure then it should be withheld until completion, or the effects monitored during the procedure and additional doses given as required.[35] Where possible, ACE inhibitors and angiotensin receptor blockers should be stopped 24 hours prior to plasma exchange.[36] This is because these drugs will decrease the patient's ability to activate bradykinin, which in turn can lead to flushing, hypotension, and respiratory distress.[34]

Potential complications of plasma exchange include: fluid imbalance, reactions to replacement fluids, vasovagal reactions, pyrogenic reactions, hypothermia, embolism (air or microaggregates), hypocalcaemia, anaemia, thrombocytopenia, haemostatic disturbances, hepatitis, hypogammaglobulinaemia, and altered pharmacokinetics of drugs. Specific note should be made of the following effects.

CIRCULATORY EFFECTS

Any extracorporeal procedure is likely to lead to problems of circulatory instability. Intravascular volume changes, vasovagal reactions, medications and infusion fluids may alone, or in combination, be responsible for circulatory problems. Often the patient will be able to compensate but if there are pre-existing issues (e.g. altered blood volume, vascular disease, or renal failure) then close monitoring is essential. A strict fluid and electrolyte balance should be kept at all times, both during the plasma exchange and also as a daily tally.

PLASMA ONCOTIC PRESSURE (COP)

Most patients compensate for minor fluctuations in COP. Patients who have oedema or local factors predisposing to interstitial fluid accumulation (e.g. raised intracranial pressure, interstitial pulmonary oedema, deep venous thrombosis, and renal impairment) need close attention.

INFECTION

Many patients who are undergoing plasma exchange are already immunosuppressed, either due to their disease or secondary to drug therapy. In patients requiring recurrent and frequent plasma exchange, attempts should be made to maintain serum immunoglobulin levels. When fresh frozen plasma is not used as replacement fluid, the bacteriocidal and opsonic activities of blood are probably impaired, and it is probably advantageous to infuse at least two units of fresh frozen plasma at the conclusion of the procedure. At the completion of a course of plasma exchange, consideration may need to be given to a dose of intravenous gammaglobulin.

HAEMOSTASIS

Plasma exchange, particularly where albumin is used as the replacement fluid, causes perturbations in the haemostatic system, which may result in either bleeding or thrombosis. The significance of these alterations will depend largely on the volume and frequency of exchange, pre-existing defects in the system, anticoagulation, other risk factors for thrombosis, replacement fluids and invasive procedures.[31]

REACTIONS TO REPLACEMENT FLUIDS

The rapid infusion of any blood component may be associated with allergic or vasomotor reactions. Plasma exchange is a rather unique situation as blood or blood products and plasma substitutes are being infused at resuscitation rates into normovolaemic, normotensive patients.

Hypotension can occur at any point in the procedure and although plasma exchange will maintain the patient as normovolaemic, there is always the risk of reaction to the exchange fluid or fluid shifts within the patient. Fluid shifts will normally respond to slowing down or halting the procedure and giving a bolus of fluids until there is recovery of the blood pressure.[37] It is helpful to ensure adequate hydration of the patient prior to commencing the procedure as this will also help reduce the risk. It should be noted that many patients have a small drop in their systolic blood pressure within minutes of commencing the procedure. Patients with neurological disorders may also benefit from running the procedure in a positive fluid balance to help counteract a lack of peripheral venous resistance.

Reactions to plasma can be seen as the development of pruritis or urticaria and necessitate the administration of an antihistamine. If there is chest tightness, acute dyspnoea, or hypoxia and the patient is receiving plasma as the replacement fluid then consideration should be given to transfusion-related lung injury (TRALI) (caused by infusion of Class I or II HLA or anti-neutrophil antibodies from donor plasma which react with recipient leucocytes and cause leucoagglutination in pulmonary circulation) and appropriate treatment commenced.[9]

Where albumin is the replacement fluid on consecutive days, attention should be paid to coagulation parameters as there may be dilution of clotting factors. In patients with normal liver function, it would be expected that these would return to normal within a few days of ceasing plasma exchange; however, if the patient has had a recent haemorrhage or is pre or post surgery then the use of donor plasma may be justified.[7]

EFFECTS OF INTRAVASCULAR PROTEINS

If plasma protein fractions or albumin are being used for replacement fluids, not only will coagulation and complement components be depleted, but various transport and binding proteins in the circulation are significantly reduced. These may have significant effects on drug activity and elimination (e.g. antithrombin III levels may have effects on heparin activity). The effects of corticosteroids may be potentiated after plasma exchange owing to a reduction in binding proteins.

INTRAVENOUS IMMUNOGLOBULIN

Intravenous immunoglobulin (IVIG) products were originally developed in the 1950s for the treatment of immunodeficiency states. Since then, the immunomodulatory properties of IVIG have led to much broader usage in autoimmune and inflammatory disorders – usually in much higher doses.[38] In many cases the use of IVIG is based upon very limited evidence and much of the IVIG used is prescribed for 'off-label' indications.[39] Consequent shortages of IVIG and concerns regarding the costs of IVIG have led governments worldwide to attempt to restrict its use to only those conditions in which it has an established or emerging role.

IVIG is a sterile fractionated blood product consisting of concentrated immunoglobulin derived from pooled human plasma from thousands of healthy blood donors. IVIG typically contains more than 95% unmodified IgG (which has intact Fc-dependent effector functions) and trace amounts of IgA and IgM, cytokines, soluble CD4, CD8 and HLA molecules. Because IVIG is derived from large numbers of donors this provides a rich diversity of antibody repertoires and specificities.

A range of IVIG products are available. Although all contain IgG molecules, they may differ in regards to their pH, osmolality, excipient compounds (sucrose/sodium) and consequently in their adverse effects. In recent years IVIG preparations have been progressively improved – with the elimination of sugars and normalisation of salt content and pH – which has significantly reduced the incidence of adverse reactions.[40] At present there is a lack of good comparative data to suggest that one IVIG preparation is superior to another.

IVIG has multiple immunomodulatory and anti-inflammatory activities including: modulation of complement activation with inhibition of generation of membrane attack complex (C5b-9) and subsequent complement-mediated tissue damage, suppression of idiotype antibodies, neutralisation of 'super-antigens', saturation of Fc receptors on macrophages and suppression of various inflammatory mediators including cytokines (TNF-α, IL-1α, IL-6), chemokines, adhesion molecules and metalloproteinases.[42] Importantly, many of these effects extend beyond the half-life of IVIG (IVIG lasts 6–22 days in circulation), suggesting that the immunomodulatory effects of IVIG are not simply due to enhanced passive clearance of autoantibodies or interference with pathogenic autoantibodies.

INDICATIONS FOR IVIG (BOX 97.3)

IVIG has an established role in the treatment of primary immune deficiency and in acquired humoral immunodeficiency states due to haematological malignancies (particularly chronic lymphocytic leukaemia and multiple myeloma) and organ transplantation.[41] It also has an established role in many other conditions associated with autoimmune dysregulation as an immunomodulatory therapy including Guillain–Barré syndrome (GBS), idiopathic thrombocytopenic purpura, myasthenia gravis, chronic inflammatory demyelinating polyneuropathies (CIDP) and Kawasaki disease. IVIG is often as efficacious as plasmapheresis and so is often recommended as first-line therapy with therapeutic plasma exchange used for patients who are unresponsive to IVIG and immunosuppressive therapy (generally corticosteroids).[42,43] IVIG is considered as second- or third-line therapy in a number of other conditions in which standard therapies have been ineffective or are contraindicated and/or where the available evidence is inconclusive. Opinion remains divided as to whether IVIG has any role in sepsis. Despite a biological rationale for its use (based largely on preclinical work demonstrating enhanced bacterial clearance, inhibitory effects on mediators of inflammation and attenuated lymphocyte apoptosis) there is inconsistent evidence regarding its therapeutic efficacy.[44–46]

Box 97.3 Diseases in which IVIG has an established benefit

Acquired hypogammaglobulinaemia secondary to haematological malignancies
Chronic inflammatory demyelinating polyneuropathy
Guillain–Barré syndrome
Idiopathic (autoimmune) thrombocytopenia purpura (ITP) in adults
Inflammatory myopathies
Kawasaki disease
Lambert–Eaton myasthenic syndrome
Multifocal motor neuropathy
Myasthenia gravis
Neonatal haemochromatosis
Primary immunodeficiency diseases
Stiff-person syndrome
Graft-versus-host disease
Acute disseminated encephalomyelitis
ANCA-positive systemic necrotising vasculitis
Autoimmune haemolytic anaemia
Pemphigoid and pemphigus
Evans syndrome – autoimmune haemolytic anaemia with ITP
Fetomaternal/neonatal alloimmune thrombocytopenia
Haemophagocytic syndrome
Idiopathic (autoimmune) thrombocytopenia purpura (ITP) in children
IgM paraproteinaemic neuropathy
Kidney transplantation
Multiple sclerosis
Opsoclonus myoclonus ataxia
Post-transfusion purpura
Secondary hypogammaglobulinaemia (including iatrogenic immunodeficiency)
Specific antibody deficiency (including IgG subclasses)
Toxic epidermal necrolysis/Stevens–Johnson syndrome
Toxic shock syndrome

ADVERSE EFFECTS OF IVIG

Adverse effects occur in 3–8% of patients. Most are mild and transient, including flushing, fever, headache, fever, chills, fatigue, nausea, diarrhoea, malaise, myalgia, dyspnoea, back pain, tachycardia and hypotension. Immediate adverse effects can be effectively treated by slowing or temporary discontinuation of the infusion and symptomatic therapy with analgesics, antihistamines, and glucocorticoids in more severe reactions. IgA deficiency-related anaphylactic reactions are rare and largely preventable by identification of patients with IgA deficiency and use of IgA-depleted immune globulin.

Late adverse effects, including acute renal failure, venous thromboembolism, neutropenia, haemolytic anaemia, arthritis and aseptic meningitis, are also rare. Acute renal failure is generally transient and generally occurs in dehydrated patients and following the use of sucrose-stabilised products owing to osmotic injury. Thromboembolic complications occur as a result of hyperviscosity, especially in patients who have received a rapid infusion of high-dose IVIG and in those with risk factors including: advanced age, immobilisation, previous venous thromboembolism, hypertension, diabetes mellitus and dyslipidaemia.[47] The blood group antibodies present in IVIG may act as haemolysins and coat red cells with immunoglobulins – resulting in a positive direct antiglobulin test (DAT) and, occasionally, haemolytic anaemia.

Access the complete references list online at http://www.expertconsult.com

4. Negi VS, Elluru S, Siberil S, et al. Intravenous immunoglobulin: an update on the clinical use and mechanisms of action. J Clin Immunol 2007;27(3): 233–45.
7. Balogun RA, Ogunniyi A, Sanford K, et al. Therepeutic apheresis in special populations. J Clin Apher 2010;25:265–74.
11. Szczepiorkowski ZM, Winters JL, Bandarenko N, et al. Guidelines on the use of therapeutic apheresis in clinical practice: Evidence-based approach from the apheresis applications committee of the American Society for Apheresis. J Clin Apher 2010;25: 83–177.
32. Nguyen TC, Kiss JE, Goldman JR, et al. The role of plasmapheresis in critical illness. Crit Care Clin 2012;28:453–68.
34. Winters JL editor. Theraputic Apheresis: A Physician's Handbook, 2nd ed. Bethesda, Maryland: AABB; 2008.
39. Foster R, Suri A, Filate W, et al. Use of intravenous immune globulin in the ICU: a retrospective review of prescribing practices and patient outcomes. Transfus Med 2010;20(6):403–8.
40. Gelfand EW. Intravenous immune globulin in autoimmune and inflammatory diseases. N Engl J Med 2012;367:2015–25.

98

Haemostatic failure

Chee W Tan, Christopher M Ward and James P Isbister

Haemostasis is the process whereby blood fluidity and vascular integrity are maintained in the event of vascular injury. Failure of haemostasis is common in critically ill patients and may be complex and multifactorial in pathogenesis. As haemostatic failure may complicate a wide range of medical, surgical and obstetric disorders definitive diagnosis and specific therapy can significantly impact on outcome. Therapy may need to be initiated on clinical evidence with minimal laboratory information. Consultation with a clinical haematologist is strongly recommended.

NORMAL HAEMOSTASIS

The haemostatic system is a delicately controlled component of the host defence system, the role of which is to initiate haemostasis where and when required and in adequate, but not excessive, amounts. There has been a paradigm shift in our understanding of the haemostatic system from one of interacting humoral factors to an integrated cell-based system (**Fig. 98.1a**).[1,2] As an increasing range of focused therapies become available that modulate the activity of the haemostatic process, it is important that core aspects of the structure and function of the system are summarised.

The triad of vascular constriction, platelet plugging and fibrin clot formation to produce haemostatic plugs provides the framework for haemostasis (see Fig. 98.1a). Fibrinogen is the bulk protein of the coagulation system and fibrin is the end-product of a cascade of proteolytic activity. Thrombin is the potent proteolytic enzyme of the coagulation sequence converting fibrinogen to fibrin soluble monomers, which subsequently polymerise to form the fibrin clot. The cascade involves precursor coagulation proteins activated to become potent proteolytic enzymes, which with the aid of cofactors produce further activated precursors downstream. The polymerised fibrin is acted on by factor XIII to form a stable fibrin clot. The process of thrombin generation in small amounts initially occurs in relationship to tissue-factor-bearing cells and the process is subsequently transferred to the activated platelet surface where amplification occurs, as highlighted by the cellular model of coagulation.[2]

Following injury, vascular constriction reduces bleeding, and allows time to initiate haemostasis. With large-volume haemorrhage, the consequent systemic hypotension is an important physiological mechanism to minimise blood loss and facilitate stabilisation of the haemostatic plug. Controlled or 'tolerated' hypotension is now accepted as an important aspect of managing critical haemorrhage.[3,4] Vascular constriction is accentuated by vasoconstrictors released in association with platelet plug formation. Vascular endothelial cells play an active part by synthesising substances that act at the membrane surface and/or interact with platelets and the coagulation system (e.g. prostacyclin, antithrombin III, plasminogen activator, von Willebrand factor, thrombomodulin, heparin cofactor II and nitric oxide).[5] Following the initial vascular reactions, successful haemostasis depends on adequate numbers of functioning platelets and coagulation cascade function.

The coagulation system is now thought to be triggered predominantly via the extrinsic pathway in vivo. Damaged tissues expose tissue factor (TF), a membrane-bound protein present in cells surrounding the vascular bed. Factor (F) VII and VIIa (a small amount circulates normally in the blood) are bound to TF, activating factor X. FXa interacts with the cofactor Va to form prothrombinase complexes, with the generation of a small amount of thrombin on the cell surface. FIX is also activated by the TF/VIIa complex; it does not play a significant role in the initiation phase of coagulation, but diffuses across to platelets in the vicinity that have adhered in proximity to the site of the TF-bearing cells. FIXa binds to a specific platelet surface receptor and interacts with cofactor VIIIa, leading to activation of factor X directly on the platelet surface. This results in the amplification and propagation of coagulation. The traditional concept of the intrinsic and extrinsic systems is clearly artificial, but the concept still has value in performing and assessing haemostatic laboratory tests.

Von Willebrand factor (VWF) is a multimeric glycoprotein that mediates adhesion of platelets to the exposed subendothelium and links the primary vascular/platelet phase with coagulation by being the carrier protein for coagulant factor VIII. Factor VIII dissociates from VWF to form a complex on the activated platelet surface with IXa (tenase complex) to activate factor X to Xa. Further VWF is released from Weibel–Palade bodies in nearby endothelial cells and platelet α-granules. Platelets interact with VWF via their surface

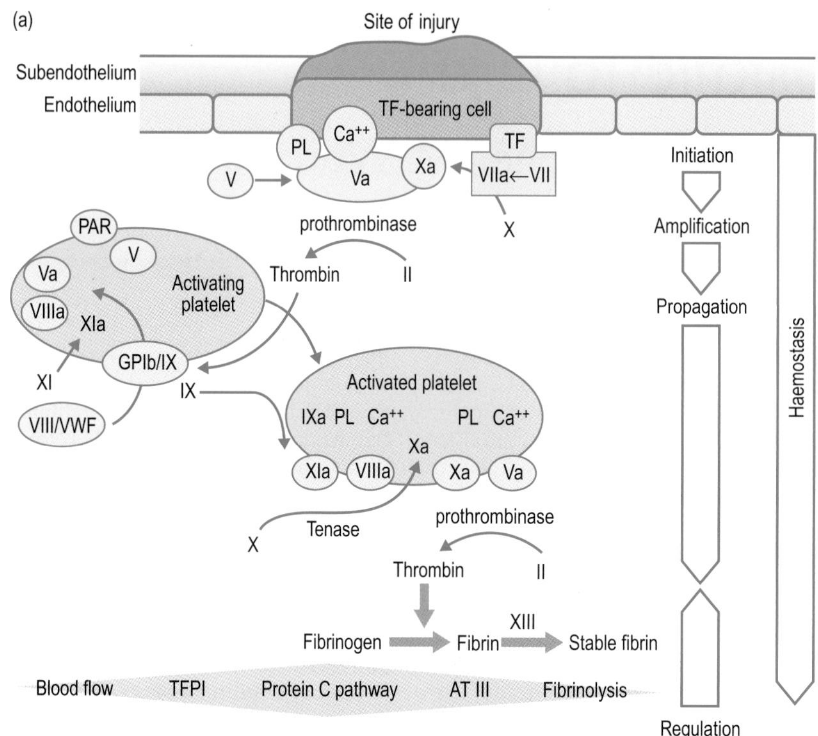

Figure 98.1 (a) The cellular model of coagulation emphasises the interplay between the endothelium, platelets and coagulation factors in the formation of a stable fibrin clot. TF=tissue factor; PL=phospholipids; PAR=protease activated receptors; TFPI=tissue factor pathway inhibitor; AT=antithrombin.

glycoprotein (GP) Ib–IX–V complexes. This results in platelet deceleration along the subendothelium, allowing platelet receptors to contact and bind collagen. Adhesion to collagen and subsequent platelet activation is now thought to be critical in haemostasis and is primarily facilitated by platelet glycoprotein VI (GPVI) and the GPIa–IIa receptor.[6,7] Recent literature suggests that GPIb–IX–V and GPVI may work in concert to mediate platelet activation, culminating in platelet aggregation via the activation of GPIIb–IIIa.[8,9]

Platelet adhesion, initiated by GPIb–IX–V binding to VWF and GPVI binding to collagen, produces a platelet monolayer over the injured subendothelium, and hence a procoagulant surface. Activation of the coagulation cascade results in local generation of thrombin, which binds to platelet protease-activated receptors (PARs), enhancing intracellular calcium mobilisation and platelet aggregation, resulting in production of a haemostatic plug and further facilitating coagulation. Further extension occurs due to platelet recruitment by platelet agonists, such as thrombin and other mediators, adenosine 5-diphosphate (ADP) and thromboxane A_2 released directly from platelets. P-selectin is expressed during activation and also plays a role in platelet-to-platelet cohesion.

Parallel to and within the coagulation system are complex feedback mechanisms to guard against inappropriate and excessive activation.[10–12] Several inhibitory proteins, including antithrombin III, thrombomodulin, protein C and S, tissue factor pathway inhibitor and in company with the fibrinolytic system, are important in controlling the degree and site of fibrin formation. Thrombin itself acts as either a procoagulant or anticoagulant depending on the context. Perturbations in this complex system can produce a wide range of clinical disorders from excessive arterial or venous thrombosis, microvascular obstruction and atheroma to haemostatic failure.

SYSTEMIC HAEMOSTATIC ASSESSMENT

There may be clinical features suggesting local or generalised failure of the haemostatic system (see **Fig. 98.1b**). Clinical history is important, especially with respect to previous bleeding, family history, co-morbid medical conditions and medications. The nature of surgery/invasive intervention may have haemostatic issues that need specific consideration.

Haemostatic system assessment can be broadly divided into laboratory tests of primary haemostasis, specifically platelet number and function, and tests of secondary haemostasis, which assess the integrity of the coagulation cascade (see Fig. 98.1b). Point-of-care haemostatic testing is increasing, particularly in the

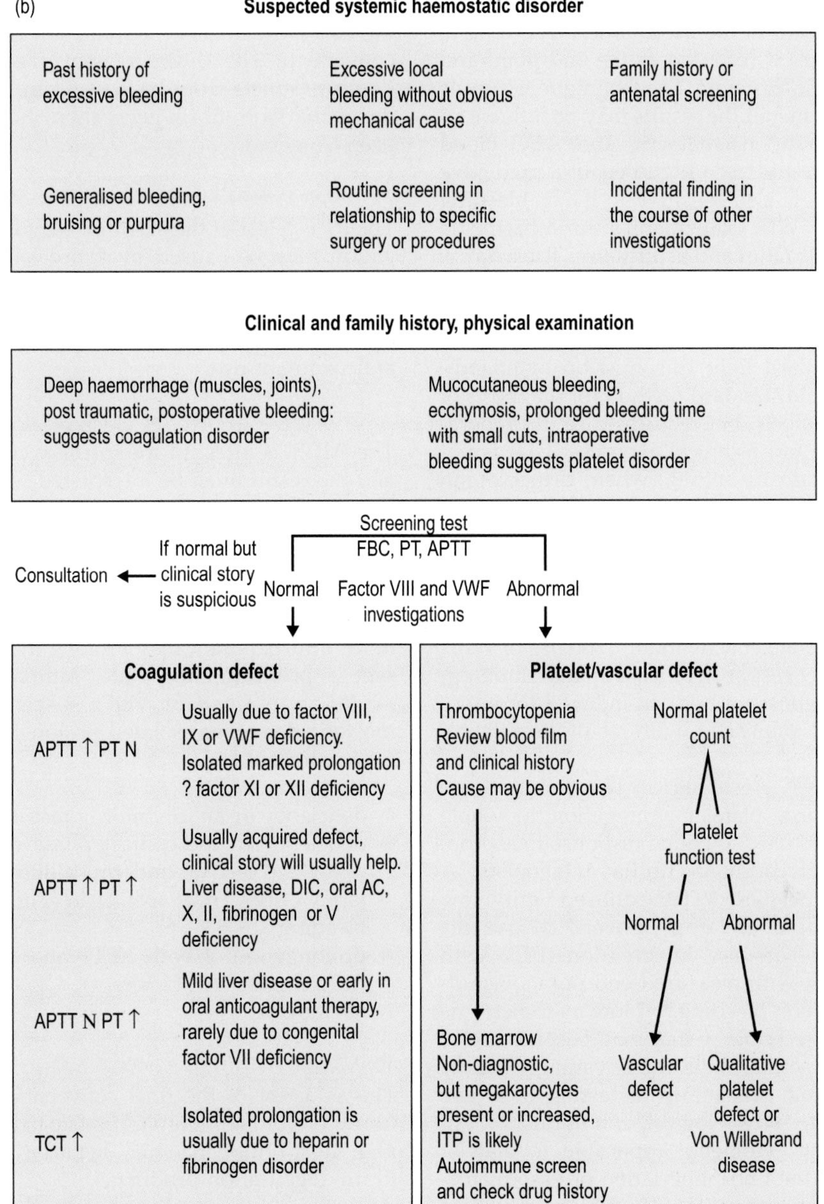

Figure 98.1, cont'd (b) Key features of history, examination and laboratory testing involved in the work-up of a patient suspected of a systemic haemostatic disorder. DIC=disseminated intravascular coagulation; AC=anticoagulants.

perioperative assessment of bleeding risk, in critical bleeding and massive blood transfusion, as well as in the assessment of bleeding risk attributable to new anticoagulant and antiplatelet therapy.

TESTS OF PRIMARY HAEMOSTASIS

A full blood count may reveal a depressed platelet count (thrombocytopenia). While a low count (less than 50×10^9/L) can contribute to haemostatic failure, a normal platelet count does not exclude platelet dysfunction as a cause of bleeding. Platelet function tests can be used both for the diagnosis of platelet disorders, and to monitor antiplatelet therapy at point of care.[13,14]

The platelet function analyser (PFA-100™) has replaced the bleeding time as a commonly used screening test for primary haemostatic defects. In the PFA-100™, citrated whole blood is subjected to high shear through a membrane coated with platelet agonists, collagen/epinephrine (adrenaline) or collagen/ADP, resulting in platelet adhesion, aggregation and closure of an aperture present in the membrane.[15] The time to occlude the aperture is recorded as the end-point and referred to as the closure time. The technique is simple and rapid to perform, but the results may be influenced by the platelet count, haematocrit, and ABO blood group. A normal result has a high negative predictive value, and the test is also sensitive to major bleeding disorders such as VWD, Glanzmann's thrombasthenia (deficiency in GP IIb/IIIa) and aspirin use. The assay is less sensitive to milder bleeding defects such as platelet storage pool disease, variably prolonged by platelet glycoprotein IIbIIIa antagonists and not affected by clopidogrel.[16] Standard light transmission aggregometry (LTA) is the gold standard method for diagnosis of platelet function defects, but requires careful preparation of the patient and technical expertise. LTA is not useful in the critical care setting, where drugs, organ failure and other stressors are likely to affect platelet responses. The recent development of whole blood multiple electrode platelet aggregometry (WBA) such as the Multiplate (Roche) to measure platelet function is promising, as it is a simple and rapid assay with less risk of artefactual platelet activation.[17] The use of WBA in assessing platelet response to aspirin and clopidogrel, and in the diagnosis of heparin-induced thrombocytopenia has been published, with results correlating well with LTA.[18,19]

The VerifyNow™ (Accumetrics) is a point-of-care test, which measures platelet aggregation in whole blood, and has been used to gauge response to aspirin, clopidogrel and glycoprotein IIbIIIa antagonists. A large randomised trial (GRAVITAS) utilised VerifyNow to individualise clopidogrel dose in over 2000 patients post percutaneous coronary intervention (PCI) with drug-eluting stents, with measured end-points including moderate/severe bleeding.[20] Flow cytometry is another emerging technology that may become useful in the critical care setting, with the advantages of low sample volume, and availability of testing of whole blood, representing physiological conditions.[21,22] An application of flow cytometry applicable to platelet function testing is the phosphorylation of vasodilator-stimulated phosphoprotein (VASP), which is used to assess the response to P_2Y_{12} antagonists such as clopidogrel.[23]

TESTS OF SECONDARY HAEMOSTASIS

In most clinical settings, a full blood count, prothrombin time (PT), activated partial thromboplastin time (APTT), fibrinogen level, D-dimer ± thrombin clotting time (TCT) provide a broad screen for most clinically significant haemostatic disorders (see Fig. 98.1b).[24–26] Based on these results, further specific tests of haemostasis may be performed (e.g. mixing studies, factor assays, platelet function tests and test of fibrinolytic function).

Broadly speaking, the PT tests the extrinsic system, the APTT the intrinsic system, and the TCT fibrinogen conversion. The D-dimer assay measures the breakdown products from lysis of fibrin, and serve as evidence that both fibrin generation and fibrinolysis have been triggered.

PROTHROMBIN TIME (PT)

The PT is a test of the extrinsic coagulation and prolongation may be caused by factor VII deficiency, liver disease, vitamin K deficiency or oral anticoagulant therapy. The PT is also expressed as the international normalised ratio (INR), specifically used to monitor anticoagulant use.

ACTIVATED PARTIAL THROMBOPLASTIN TIME (APTT)

The APTT is a test of the intrinsic coagulation system and the result must be interpreted with caution. There may be significant variation in test sensitivity and specificity between laboratories. In unselected patients there is poor correlation between the APTT prolongation and either the presence of haemostatic failure or the likelihood of a patient bleeding. Uncommonly a lupus anticoagulant may prolong the APTT and represent a prothrombotic state, rather than a bleeding tendency. In a patient with a suspected systemic haemostatic defect, an isolated prolongation of the APTT may represent:

- deficiency or an inhibitor of factor VIII, IX or XI
- deficiency in the contact phase of the coagulation cascade (i.e. FXII and prekallikrein, which importantly does not result in clinically significant bleeding)
- prolongation of both APTT and PT may be due to deficiencies of factors X, V, prothrombin or fibrinogen.

THROMBIN CLOTTING TIME (TCT)

This is a test of the final conversion of fibrinogen to fibrin. Prolongation of TCT is due to hypofibrinogenaemia, dysfibrinogenaemia, heparin, or generation of fibrin degradation products.

D-DIMER

The D-dimer assay measures cleavage fragments resulting from the proteolytic action of plasmin on fibrin, so is specific for fibrinolysis and not primary fibrinogenolysis. Elevation of D-dimer may be seen in the postoperative state, trauma, renal impairment, sepsis and venous thrombosis. High levels of D-dimer can occur with excessive fibrinolysis, as seen in disseminated intravascular coagulation.

SPECIFIC COAGULATION FACTOR ASSAYS

Fibrinogen is commonly measured in patients suspected of systemic haemostatic failure, using clottable protein methods, end-point detection techniques, or immunochemical tests. The Clauss method is the most common fibrinogen assay used.

Specific factor assays can be performed as secondary tests, after initial screening tests such as the APTT reveal abnormalities. With an isolated prolonged APTT, a mixing test, in which plasma from normal donors is added to patient sample plasma, can be performed. It will correct APTT prolongation secondary to factor deficiencies, but not if the prolongation is due to coagulation inhibitors. Non-specific inhibitors include drugs such as heparin and lupus anticoagulants; specific inhibitors such as acquired antibodies to FVIII are rare. An APTT corrected by a mixing test is further investigated with specific assays for FVIII, FIX and FXI. An isolated PT is investigated in a similar fashion, with FVII deficiency/inhibitor a possible cause.

EUGLOBULIN LYSIS TIME (ELT)

This test mainly reflects the presence of plasminogen activators and if shortened is indicative of system fibrinolytic activation.

GLOBAL COAGULATION ASSAYS

The PT and APTT, although useful in detecting coagulation factor deficiencies, have drawbacks and the APTT in particular does not accurately reflect haemostasis in vivo. Haemostasis does not just involve coagulation factors, but also cellular components including platelets and endothelial cells that play integral roles, so there is inevitably a limited assessment of coagulation profile via these tests. Global coagulation assays hence offer the advantage of assessing the haemostatic system as a whole, involving both coagulation factors and cellular components, and, as results are individualised, offer the potential of individualised treatment depending on the result.[27] Point-of-care testing with global coagulation assays offers significant advantages in the critical care setting. Global coagulation testing includes thrombin generation assays and whole blood thromboelastography.

Thrombin generation assays measure the final step of the coagulation pathway. They inform on both the bleeding risk and hypercoagulability of a patient, as thrombin has both prothrombotic and fibrinolytic roles. The calibrated automated thrombogram (CAT) assesses thrombin generation by using fluorogenic substrates.

Several studies have shown attenuated thrombin generation in patients with haemophilia and FXI deficiency with a severe clinical bleeding phenotype, independently of FVIII/FIX levels.[28,29] Thrombin generation was also reported to correlate with clinical response to bypassing agents such as recombinant factor VIIa (rFVIIa) in patients with severe haemophilia with high-titre inhibitors in the perioperative setting.[30] These assays appear promising for clinical use, but require specialised equipment and are still largely restricted to research settings at present.

TEG® and ROTEM® are both methods of whole blood thromboelastography used to assess haemostasis, particularly in the perioperative period as a point-of-care test. Both TEG and ROTEM enable ongoing evaluation of a clot as it forms. In both methods, a sample is placed in a cup, with a pin present in the centre of the cup as the device is operating. In the TEG the cup is spinning, whereas in the ROTEM it is the pin that rotates. The formation of a clot results in reduced movement of the pin, with the information translated into computer tracings such as that depicted in **Figure 98.2**.

Figure 98.2 illustrates the utility of the TEG and ROTEM to provide information on all stages of haemostasis, including fibrinolysis and clot stability, via challenge with tissue plasminogen activator. Both TEG and ROTEM have been widely used in liver transplantation and in cardiac bypass surgery in particular. It can also be utilised in clinical settings where changes in haemostasis can occur rapidly, with high bleeding risk, likely concomitant use of anticoagulants, frequent use of blood transfusion and likelihood of multi-organ failure and disseminated intravascular coagulation. Serial monitoring with thromboelastography has been used for haemostatic assessment of critically ill patients and has guided clinical management, including use of tranexamic acid and FXIII.[31,32] Thromboelastography results have also correlated with both clinical bleeding phenotype and response to bypassing agents, such as rFVIIa, in patients with haemophilia and inhibitors.[33,34] As they provide a more comprehensive clinically relevant assessment of the haemostatic status at point of care, it is likely that the use of global coagulation assays will increase.

CONGENITAL HAEMOSTATIC DEFECTS

Congenital bleeding disorders are rare, but should be suspected in the clinical setting with discrepant or unexpected major bleeding or with abnormal laboratory results (i.e. an isolated prolonged APTT). It is important to identify the defect so that specific replacement therapy can be administered, with dosage guided by regular coagulation factor level monitoring. Congenital bleeding disorders include haemophilia A (FVIII deficiency), haemophilia B (FIX deficiency) and von Willebrand disease. Haemophilia A and B are characterised by musculoskeletal and soft-tissue bleeding. Apart from specific factor concentrates, antifibrinolytics such as tranexamic acid are useful adjunctive therapy (discussed later in this chapter), with desmopressin also effective therapy in mild haemophilia A and certain types of vWD by stimulating endogenous release of FVIII and VWF.

Congenital platelet disorders are also rare, the commonest severe disorder being Glanzmann's thrombasthenia, which is a deficiency or dysfunction of GPIIbIIIa.[35] A history of repeated mucocutaneous bleeding

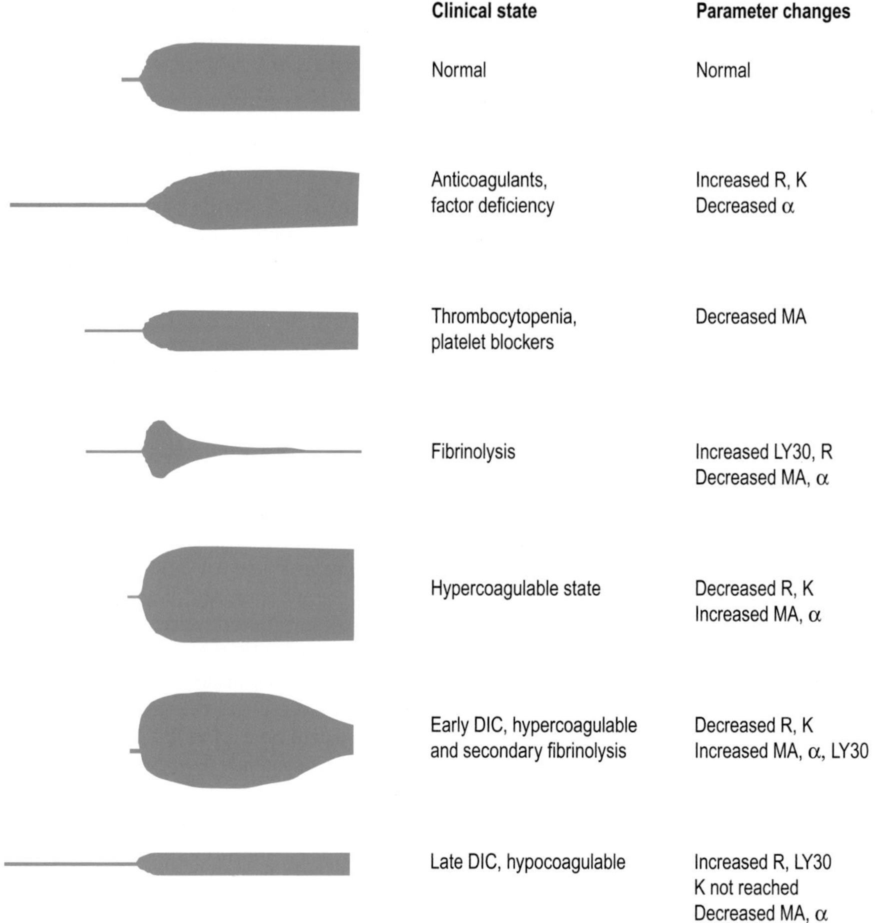

Figure 98.2 Comparative thromboelastograph tracings in normal and pathological states, with measured parameters assessing different aspects of haemostasis. These include: R time, which is the time elapsed until initial fibrin formation; K time gauges the dynamics of clot formation, α-angle assesses the kinetics of fibrin accumulation and cross-linkage, MA (maximum amplitude) assesses the effectiveness of platelet–fibrin interactions, while lysis time assesses fibrinolysis. *(Modified from Srinivasa et al.[65])*

with an abnormal PFA-100 test result may be suggestive of such disorders. Platelet transfusions may be required for acute bleeds or in relation to elective surgery; desmopressin acetate (DDAVP) ± antifibrinolytic therapy and rFVIIa may all have a role in management.

ACQUIRED HAEMOSTATIC DISORDERS

The acquired disorders of coagulation are usually more complex and multifactorial than the hereditary disorders. A unified approach is essential for the successful management of these potentially life-threatening situations, and transfusion therapy cannot be isolated from other treatment. Acquired haemostatic defects are commonly seen in extracorporeal circulation cardiac surgery and, like congenital abnormalities, can also be broadly divided into platelet defects and abnormalities involving coagulation factors.

EXTRACORPOREAL CIRCULATION CARDIAC SURGERY

Extracorporeal circulation, especially cardiopulmonary bypass, is associated with a range of haemostatic disturbances and the risks of bleeding versus thrombosis must be constantly balanced.[36] Time on bypass and multiple-valve replacements or reoperations impact on this risk. Haemostatic failure usually becomes apparent in the operating room or soon after and appropriate laboratory investigations should be performed. Plasma products or platelets will be less effective if anticoagulants such as heparin have not been adequately reversed. Increased fibrinolytic activity may in some cases also contribute to bleeding.

QUANTITATIVE PLATELET DEFECTS

DRUG-INDUCED THROMBOCYTOPENIA

The clinical presentation of drug-induced thrombocytopenia ranges from dramatic and fulminant with marked haemostatic failure to minor abnormalities. Drugs with a predilection for inducing thrombocytopenia include quinine (also in bitter drinks), quinidine, antituberculous drugs, heparin, thiazide diuretics, penicillins, sulfonamides, rifampicin and anticonvulsants.

Heparin-induced thrombocytopenia (HIT) is an important and potentially life-threatening complication of heparin therapy.[37-39] An immune reaction to heparin typically occurs after 7–10 days of therapy, leading to platelet aggregation and thrombocytopenia. The thrombocytopenia seen in HIT is often only moderate, and platelet numbers may remain within the normal range. In contrast to other causes of drug-induced thrombocytopenia, this condition is not associated with bleeding, but rather represents a prothrombotic state, with potentially devastating arterial, microvascular or venous thrombosis associated with the resultant platelet aggregation. Medical staff must be vigilant to the possibility of HIT occurring, and to keep heparin therapy as brief as possible. The incidence is less with the use of low-molecular-weight heparin (LMWH), but a strong clinical suspicion of HIT (probability of HIT based on four criteria of the 4T score: timing and nadir of the thrombocytopenia, the presence of thrombosis, and the possibility of other causes accounting for the thrombocytopenia – see **Table 98.1**) should result in the cessation of unfractionated heparin (UFH)/LMWH, and commencement of an alternate anticoagulant, such as danaparoid or thrombin inhibitors such as argatroban and lepirudin, while awaiting laboratory results.[40]

HIT can be challenging to diagnose in the critical setting, particularly with many potential causes of thrombocytopenia coexisting in the same clinical scenario. New scoring systems for HIT have emerged to address this issue.[41] Several screening tests for heparin–platelet factor 4 antibodies are available, but these also detect non-pathogenic antibodies, which can occur commonly in the setting of cardiac surgery. 'Functional' HIT assays, such as the serotonin release assay or whole blood aggregometry,[18] which show platelet activation in the presence of heparin and patient serum/plasma can confirm a diagnosis of HIT but are performed only in reference laboratories.

THROMBOTIC THROMBOCYTOPENIC PURPURA/HAEMOLYTIC URAEMIC SYNDROME

Thrombotic thrombocytopenic purpura/haemolytic uraemic syndrome (TTP/HUS) comprises disorders characterised by haemolytic anaemia and thrombocytopenia, with evidence of microangiopathy as suggested by the presence of red cell fragments on the blood film. While TTP and HUS can be difficult to distinguish from each other clinically, reduced activity of the vWF-cleaving protease ADAMTS13 is diagnostic of TTP, due to either an autoantibody or a congenital deficiency. Importantly, TTP/HUS can be distinguished from DIC by the absence of abnormal coagulation testing. TTP can also be associated with use of medications such as clopidogrel and quinine, and in settings such as pregnancy and bone marrow transplantation. This condition and its management are discussed in more detail in Chapter 97.

IDIOPATHIC THROMBOCYTOPENIC PURPURA (ITP)

ITP is an autoimmune disorder where autoantibodies (IgG) are directed against platelets, which are subsequently destroyed by the monocyte–macrophage system, predominantly in the spleen. ITP remains a diagnosis of exclusion, and is typically a disease of children and young adults. Corticosteroids should generally be regarded as short-term therapy in acute flares of this condition, particularly if the platelet count were to

Table 98.1 4T score to assess clinical probability of HIT; a score of 0–3 represents low probability, 4–5 intermediate and 6–8 high clinical probability of HIT

CATEGORY	2 POINTS	1 POINT	0 POINT
Thrombocytopenia	>50% fall, or nadir ≥20 × 10^9/L	30–50% fall, or nadir 10–19 × 10^9/L	<30% fall, or nadir <10 × 10^9/L
Timing of the decrease in platelet count	Days 5 to 10, or ≤day 1 with recent heparin (past 30 days)	>Day 10 or timing unclear, or <day 1 if heparin exposure within past 30–100 days	<Day 4 (no recent heparin)
Thrombosis or other sequelae	Proven thrombosis, skin necrosis, or acute systemic reaction after heparin bolus	Progressive, recurrent, or silent thrombosis; erythematous skin lesions	None
Other causes of thrombocytopenia	Non evident	Possible	Definite

Modified from Lo et al.[40]

fall to <10 000/μL +/− bleeding. In adults, the majority of patients respond with a rise in the platelet count. An initial high dose (1 mg/kg) of prednisolone a day is given until response occurs, after which the dose is gradually reduced. High-dose intravenous immunoglobulin is effective in most patients and is specifically indicated in fulminant acute disease resulting in major bleeding and/or not responding to corticosteroids, and is particularly useful preoperatively and in pregnancy. Platelet transfusions should be reserved for major, life-threatening bleeding.

Options for management of chronic ITP have increased recently with the availability of medications such as romiplostim that stimulate platelet production via binding to receptors for thrombopoietin, which is the primary regulator of both megakaryopoiesis and platelet production. Targeting pathogenic antibodies with rituximab has also shown some efficacy in ITP.

THROMBOCYTOPENIA IN CRITICAL CARE SETTINGS

Platelets play an important role in the inflammatory response and a reactive thrombocytosis is usually seen in infection. However, if there is overwhelming sepsis, associated disseminated intravascular coagulation (DIC) or marrow suppressive influences, thrombocytopenia can be seen. Sepsis, shock, DIC, alcoholism and nutritional deficiency are common factors contributing to thrombocytopenia in critically ill patients. Thrombocytopenia also often occurs in cardiothoracic surgery after extracorporeal blood circulation.

QUALITITATIVE PLATELET DEFECTS

The most common cause of acquired platelet dysfunction seen in the critical care setting is the use of antiplatelet therapy, which is discussed later in the chapter. Other causes of platelet dysfunction include uraemia, hepatic cirrhosis, multiple myeloma and myeloproliferative disorders. Platelet dysfunction can also occur post cardiac-bypass surgery, and can result in bleeding in the presence of a normal or near-normal platelet count. In this setting, platelet transfusions are administered, and antifibrinolytics are useful as adjunctive therapy.

CRITICAL HAEMORRHAGE AND MASSIVE BLOOD TRANSFUSION

The nature and management of haemostatic defects secondary to acute and/or massive blood loss are explained in greater detail in a preceding chapter. There has been increasing interest in the role of fibrinogen and the use of specific fibrinogen in trauma as part of a massive transfusion protocol. More recent guidelines have suggested that fibrinogen concentrations exceed 1.5 g/L to maintain haemostasis, compared with 1 g/L, with higher levels targeted in specific populations, such as cardiac surgery (3.9 g/L).[42]

Fresh frozen plasma (FFP) and platelet concentrates are often infused to correct significant coagulopathy in massive bleeding. However, the efficacy of FFP has not been established in such settings, including cardiac surgery.[43] FFP also carries the risk of bacterial and viral infections, incompatibility reactions, transfusion-related acute lung injury (TRALI) and fluid overload. Concerns over variant Creutzfeldt–Jakob disease have led to recommendations to cease FFP derived from the UK. Cryoprecipitate use, which is a source of fibrinogen, has been withdrawn in many countries of the European Union. Fibrinogen concentrates, on the other hand, are virally inactivated and carry a lower risk of transmitting infection, are not blood group specific, and can be stored at room temperature and given without delay owing to thawing. The use of fibrinogen concentrates in a wide variety of clinical settings in which bleeding risk is high, including aortic aneurysm graft surgery and coronary bypass graft surgery, has resulted in a significant reduction in blood product support (FFP, platelets, RBCs), correction of laboratory abnormalities in coagulation and significant reduction in perioperative bleeding.[42–44] In these studies, fibrinogen dose was guided by thromboelastography, emphasising the utility of global coagulation assays in guiding clinical management of patients with massive blood loss. ROTEM and TEG provide real-time assessment of the viscoelastic properties of clot formation whereas fibrinogen levels, although they can be used to guide administration of fibrinogen concentrates, are not known immediately hence do not reflect current haemostatic status. Larger prospective trials are required before the role of fibrinogen concentrates in the treatment of massive bleeding can be clearly defined, but results so far have been promising.

HAEMOSTATIC FAILURE ASSOCIATED WITH LIVER DISEASE

The liver is the production site of nearly all the coagulation factors involved, apart from FVIII and VWF. Bleeding is challenging to evaluate in patients with liver impairment, with prohaemostatic changes (including reduced levels of natural anticoagulants and plasminogen) and antihaemostatic changes (thrombocytopenia, platelet dysfunction, impaired synthesis of clotting factors, excessive fibrinolysis) likely to coexist. Mild to moderate prolongation of PT does not correlate with bleeding risk. Recent guidelines have advised assessing FFP use prior to invasive procedures, based on individual patient characteristics.[45,46] FFP also carries the theoretical risk of increasing portal pressure and aggravating bleeding. Prothrombin complex concentrates (PCCs) are a viable alternative, particularly in patients with fluid overload.[47] Haemostatic defects due to deficient vitamin-K-dependent coagulation factors (in patients with predominantly cholestatic liver disease) may be rapidly reversed with vitamin K therapy, and plasma transfusion may not be required.

Hypofibrinogenaemia and dysfibrinogenaemia are common in patients with liver impairment. As discussed previously, cryoprecipitate, and more recently, specific fibrinogen concentrates, can be administered in patients with chronic liver disease and bleeding with fibrinogen levels <1.5 g/L, or in patients not responding to plasma transfusion, as dysfibrinogenaemia is likely to be present in this setting.

DISSEMINATED INTRAVASCULAR COAGULATION (DIC)

Disseminated intravascular coagulation is a pathophysiological process characterised by an inappropriate, excessive and uncontrolled activation of the haemostatic process. The perpetuation of the process may be due to continuation of the stimulus and/or consumption of the natural inhibitors of haemostasis. Initially adequate compensation results in defects being demonstrable only in the laboratory tests, but if the initiating disorder is severe the clinical syndrome of uncontrolled acute DIC can result in significant bleeding, usually associated with end organ failure. A compensatory secondary fibrinolysis occurs, which in some cases may accentuate the bleeding.

PATHOPHYSIOLOGY

DIC is characterised by the initial consumption of clotting factors and platelets within the circulation, resulting in varying degrees of microvascular obstruction due to fibrin deposition (see **Fig. 98.3**). When significant platelet and coagulation factor consumption occurs, bleeding may become a major feature.

Mechanisms that may inappropriately activate the haemostatic system include:

- activation of the coagulation sequence by release of tissue thromboplastins into the systemic circulation (e.g. following extensive tissue trauma, during surgery, malignancy and during acute intravascular haemolysis)
- vessel wall endothelial injury causing platelet activation followed by activation of the haemostatic system (e.g. Gram-negative sepsis from endotoxin release, viral infections, extensive burns, prolonged hypotension, hypoxia or acidosis, see **Box 98.1**)
- induction of platelet activation (e.g. septicaemia, viraemia, antigen–antibody complexes).

CLINICAL FEATURES

The clinical presentation of DIC varies, with patients showing thrombotic, haemorrhagic, or mixed manifestations in various organ systems. The major clinical problem and presenting feature of acute DIC is bleeding. This may manifest as generalised bruising, or bleeding at sites of therapeutic or traumatic invasion (venepuncture sites and surgical wounds). DIC may occur in association with a wide range of clinical disorders (see Box 98.1). When DIC occurs in acutely ill patients with multisystem organ failure the prognosis is poor.

Box 98.1 Conditions associated with disseminated intravascular coagulation

Infection	Severe allergic reaction
Bacterial sepsis	Drug reactions
Viral haemorrhagic fevers	Extracorporeal circulations
Protozoal (malaria)	Snake bite envenomation
Trauma	Vascular disorders
Extensive tissue injury	Giant haemangioma
Head injury	Aortic aneurysm
Fat embolism	Pregnancy associated:
Malignancy	Septic abortion
Carcinoma	Abruptio placentae
Leukaemia (especially promyelocytic)	Eclampsia
	Amniotic fluid embolism
Immunological disorders	Placenta praevia
Transplantation rejection	Burns
Incompatible haemolytic blood transfusion reactions	Hyperthermia
	Liver disease and acute hepatic necrosis

LABORATORY FINDINGS

Results of tests may be variable and difficult to interpret. Significant DIC can be present despite normal standard coagulation tests (i.e. PT, APTT and TCT). The key tests in diagnosis are those that provide evidence for excessive conversion of fibrinogen to fibrin within the circulation and its subsequent lysis. Platelet–fibrin clots create a mesh in the microcirculation in which passing red cells may be traumatised, resulting in red cell fragmentation and haemolysis. The blood film may demonstrate fragmentation of the red cells (microangiopathic haemolytic anaemia), but this is more commonly seen in chronic DIC, especially in association with malignancy.

The diagnosis is usually based on a combination of the appropriate clinical picture with a supportive pattern of laboratory tests of the haemostatic system (**Table 98.2**).[48] Thrombocytopenia, hypofibrinogenaemia, with prolongation of the APTT, PT and TCT in conjunction with an elevation of fibrin degradation products (D-dimer test), is supportive evidence for the diagnosis. More specialised tests such as elevation of fibrinopeptide A and reduced levels of antithrombin III add further weight to the diagnosis. To assist in the accurate diagnosis of DIC, the International Society on Thrombosis and Haemostasis (ISTH) has developed a scoring algorithm based on laboratory results (**Table 98.3**).

In chronic DIC the laboratory findings are different from acute DIC. Many of the usual tests of haemostasis are normal or near normal. However, this is a

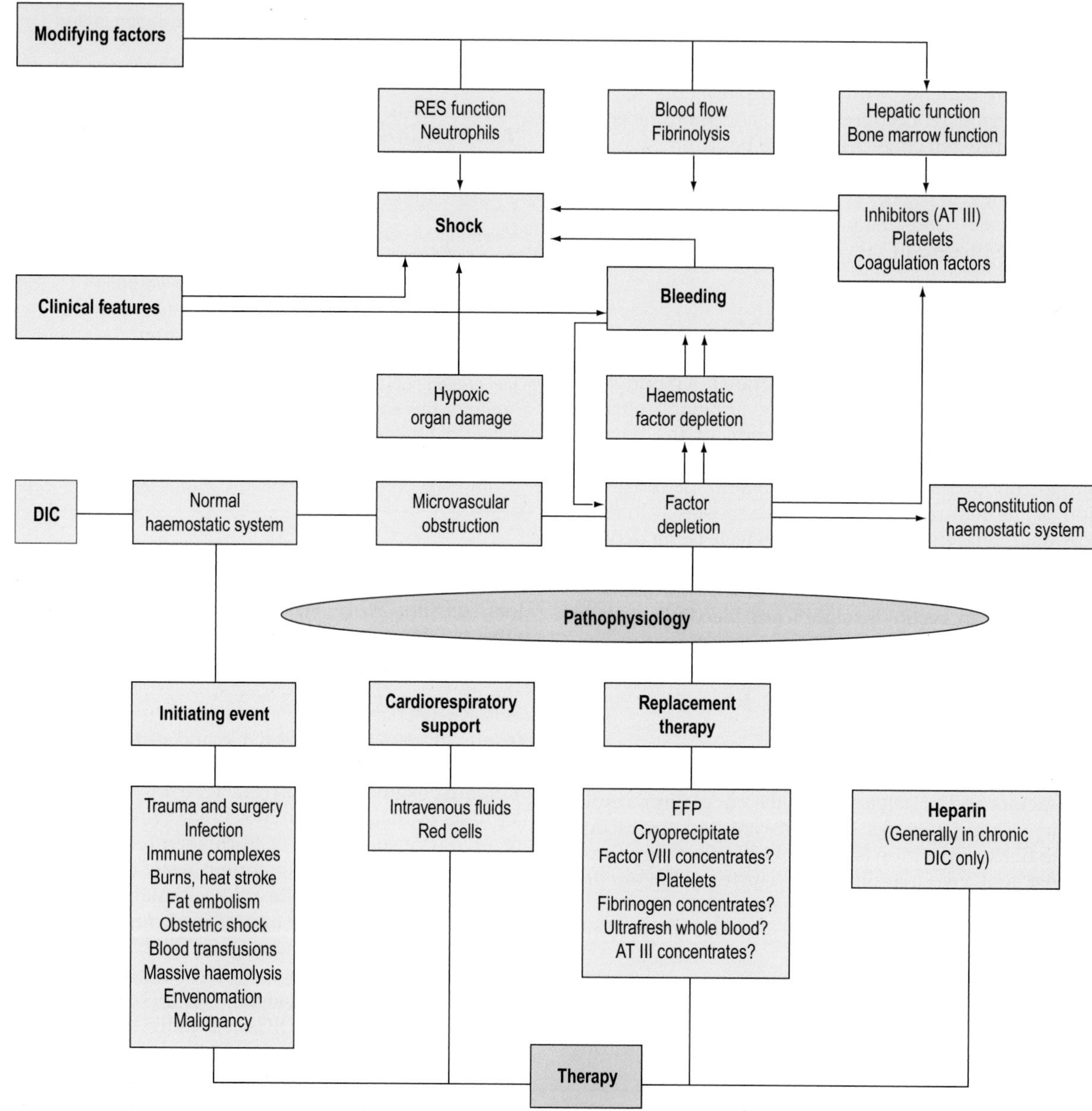

Figure 98.3 The pathophysiology and management of disseminated intravascular coagulation (DIC). RES=reticulo-endothelial system; AT=antithrombin.

compensated state in which there is increased turnover of each of the haemostatic components. D-dimer is elevated in this setting and a microangiopathic red cell picture is often seen on the peripheral blood film.

THERAPY

The most important measure in the management of DIC is treatment of the initiating cause in conjunction with general resuscitation. Blood component therapy should be given only in patients with bleeding or prior to major invasive procedures. Local institutions routinely establish laboratory parameters to guide transfusion therapy, usually aiming to maintain fibrinogen levels >1–1.5 g/L and platelet counts >20-30×10^9/L, maintaining around 50×10^9/L and PT below 1.5 times normal. Transfusion of blood products has the theoretical risk of 'feeding the fire', providing substrates for microthrombi formation, potentially leading to multi-organ failure. Heparin should be used judiciously in the setting of DIC, and can be beneficial in settings where major thrombotic complications have occurred, rather than bleeding. Small doses of UFH should be used initially. Therapeutic exchange can be considered in severe DIC, in which fluid overload has

Table 98.2 Laboratory test for the diagnosis of disseminated intravascular coagulation

ANALYSIS	EARLY	LATE
Platelet count	↓	↓↓
Activated partial thromboplastin time (APTT)	↑	↑↑
Prothrombin time (PT)	↑	↑
Thrombin clotting time (TCT)	↑	↑
Fibrin degradation products (D-dimer assay)	↑	↑↑
Hypofibrinogen	↓	↓↓
Other coagulation factors II, VII, VIII, X	↓	↓↓
Coagulation inhibitors: antithrombin III, protein C	↓	↓↓↓
Blood film	Usually normal in early stages	Fragmented red cells can be seen in subacute/ chronic cases
Supplementary and research tests – prothrombin fragment 1+2, thrombin–antithrombin complex (TAT complex), procalcitonin (PCT), plasmin–antiplasmin complexes (PAP complex)	↑	↑

Table 98.3 The ISTH scoring system; a score of ≥5 is indicative of overt DIC

	0 POINTS	1 POINT	2 POINTS
Platelet count ($\times10^9$/L)	>100	<100	<50
Elevated fibrin-degradation products	No increase	Moderate increase	Strong increase
Prolonged PT (s)	<3	<6	>6
Fibrinogen (g/L)	>1.0	<1.0	

From Toh & Hoots, with permission.[66]

occurred, as activated coagulation factors and pro-inflammatory cytokines are removed in the process. There have also been reports in the literature regarding the use of antithrombin in the setting of DIC, with varying impact on patient mortality.[49] There are currently no randomised controlled trials regarding the efficacy of rFVIIa in the setting of DIC.

ANTITHROMBOTIC THERAPY

There are an increasing number of antithrombotic agents available and associated with wider clinical use there has been a resultant increase in iatrogenic bleeding in patients presenting with other co-morbidities (e.g. trauma, surgery and invasive procedures). Intensivists must be aware of the methods for rapid reversal of therapy.[50,51] Bleeding problems in patients on well-controlled anticoagulation are usually due to surgery, trauma or a local lesion (e.g. peptic ulceration). Otherwise, bleeding can be due to over-anticoagulation, sometimes as a result of drug interactions. Elective surgery in this group of patients needs careful planning if haemorrhagic and thrombotic complications are to be avoided. Patients on antithrombotic therapy involved in traumatic events are a challenge in whom there is the risk of progression of the original insult, increased risk of post-traumatic complications, and mortality.

VITAMIN K ANTAGONISTS

These agents, including warfarin, induce a functional deficiency of the vitamin-K-dependent clotting factors (II, VII, IX and X), the anticoagulant action being measured by prolongation of PT (INR). The indications for reversing vitamin K antagonists depends on the clinical indication for therapy. Warfarin is now used increasingly in stroke prevention in the setting of atrial fibrillation. Reversal of over-anticoagulation should occur in most patients with an INR over 5, in bleeding patients, or in those at high risk of bleeding. In most cases oral anticoagulation can be ceased temporarily without further intervention. Vitamin K will reverse the warfarin effect as new factors are synthesised – for more rapid reversal, prothrombin complex concentrates (PCCs) should be used. PCCs have emerged as an effective alternative to FFP, to rapidly reverse the anticoagulant effects of warfarin, including protein C correction. Recent publications in the literature have advocated PCCs for urgent reversal of vitamin K antagonists, and several studies recommend PCCs, instead of FFP, for reversal in neurological emergencies.[52,53] PCCs provide important advantages over FFP, including viral inactivation, reduced risk of fluid overload, lack of a need for a cross-match, and also no risk of TRALI (transfusion-associated acute lung injury). There is as yet no definite consensus on optimal dosing of PCCs. They may carry an increased risk of thromboembolic events.

Vitamin K_1 is essential for sustained reversal, but care must be taken not to give an excessive dose if the patient needs to return to oral anticoagulation in the long term. For most surgical interventions or invasive procedures an INR of 1.5 or less is acceptable. This can usually be achieved by temporarily ceasing warfarin. If urgent reversal with vitamin K is required, the injectable form is preferred to oral administration in view of its more rapid onset of action. Doses of up to 5 mg of vitamin K can reverse the INR prolongation without causing significant warfarin resistance when the drug is resumed.

HEPARINS

Heparins act by potentiating the action of antithrombin III, a natural coagulation inhibitor. Unfractionated heparin (UFH) neutralises both thrombin and FXa, in contrast to the LMWHs, which predominantly neutralise FXa. The anticoagulant effect of UFH is usually measured by prolongation of the APTT. LMWHs do not prolong the APTT and are generally administered on weight basis and are not routinely monitored by a laboratory test. When monitoring is required, a drug-specific anti-Xa assay can be used.

Similar to over-anticoagulation with warfarin, cessation of heparins may be sufficient if bleeding occurs. If major bleeding has occurred, immediate reversal of UFH activity can be achieved with protamine sulphate. Protamine itself can paradoxically act as an anticoagulant in excess doses, hence doses of protamine required to neutralise 80% of estimated circulating UFH (e.g. 1 mg protamine sulphate will neutralise 100 units of heparin given in the previous 2–3 hours) have been suggested.[47] Protamine sulphate should be injected slowly by the intravenous route. Bleeding on LMWH is more difficult to manage than UFH, owing to the longer effective half-life - protamine also only partially reverses the LMWH effect (1 mg for each 1 mg enoxaparin in previous 8 hours).

ANTIPLATELET AGENTS

Antiplatelet agents are used widely for the treatment of arterial disease, and many of the non-steroidal anti-inflammatory agents are also platelet-inhibitory drugs. Aspirin has an irreversible effect on platelet function and platelet function tests may show abnormalities for up to 10 days after medication. Most of the other non-steroidal anti-inflammatory drugs have a reversible effect lasting a matter of hours or occasionally days. Perioperative bleeding is usually mild, but occasionally may be serious, depending on the surgery, and in some situations a platelet transfusion may be necessary.

Agents such as clopidogrel act as inhibitors of platelet aggregation by inhibiting the binding of ADP to its platelet receptor P2Y12, thus suppressing ADP-mediated activation of the GPIIb/IIIa complex. Prasugrel, another ADP antagonist, has emerged as effective therapy for ACS in the setting of PCI when combined with aspirin. Ticagrelor, which antagonises ADP via a different binding site to clopidogrel and prasugrel, is another treatment option. As with aspirin, platelets exposed to ADP antagonists are affected for their lifespan and recovery of normal platelet function occurs as new platelets are produced. ADP antagonists are thought to be more potent than aspirin in antiplatelet effect and hence associated with higher bleeding risk.[54] Prasugrel achieves more predictable antagonism of ADP compared with clopidogrel, at the expense of increased bleeding.[55] The bleeding risk is also high with ticagrelor.[56] The bleeding risk associated with antiplatelet agents has also increased with more frequent use of dual antiplatelet therapy, particularly with the advent of drug-eluting coronary stents and the risk of late in-stent thrombosis.

Antiplatelet agents have a central role in preventing arterial thrombosis. Clinicians are now regularly confronted by balancing the haemorrhagic risks associated with these agents, especially in the perioperative setting, against the thrombotic risks associated with their discontinuation. Platelet transfusions are the mainstay of treatment to reverse the effects of antiplatelet therapy when major bleeding occurs. Aspirin is considered less potent than ADP antagonists in terms of bleeding risk. Hence, it is generally agreed that continuing acetylsalicylic acid during vascular surgery procedures and in most other settings in which the bleeding risk is likely to be low is acceptable, with platelet transfusions administered only in high-risk settings, such as neurosurgery or eye surgery. There should be a lower clinical threshold to administer platelets for reversal of the more potent ADP antagonists, particularly prasugrel. It is generally recommended that ADP antagonists, such as clopidogrel, be ceased 5 days before surgery to allow regeneration of the platelet pool. Although withdrawal of the competitive GPIIb/IIIa inhibitors at the beginning of surgery will decrease the risk of bleeding, it should be emphasised that thrombotic events in patients waiting for urgent myocardial revascularisation are a significant risk and acceptance of perioperative bleeding risk may take priority in certain scenarios. The antiplatelet effect of abciximab lasts for days, whereas normal platelet function is restored within 4–6 hours with tirofiban. Hence withdrawal of tirofiban may be sufficient in bleeding episodes in the absence of thrombocytopenia. Apart from platelet transfusion, desmopressin and rFVIIa are suitable considerations in the management of major bleeding attributable to antiplatelet therapy.

NOVEL ORAL ANTICOAGULANTS (NOACs)

Newer anticoagulants specifically targeting thrombin (dabigatran, bivalirudin, lepirudin, argatroban) or factor Xa (rivaroxaban, fondaparinux, apixaban) have emerged in the management of both arterial and venous thromboembolism and have been shown to be

Table 98.4 Pharmacological properties of new anticoagulants and antiplatelet medications

	DABIGATRAN	RIVAROXABAN	APIXABAN	PRASUGREL	TIGACRELOR
Target	Thrombin	Factor Xa	Factor Xa	Platelet P2Y12 receptor	Platelet P2Y12, different binding site to ADP
Prodrug	Yes	No	No	Yes	No
Elimination half-life	12–14 h	7–13 h	8–13 h	~7 h (active metabolite)	7 h (tigacrelor), 9 h (active metabolite)
Clearance	80–85% renal	66% renal clearance	~60% hepatobiliary, ~25% renal	~70% renal, ~30% hepato-biliary	~60% renal, ~30% hepato-biliary
Cytochrome pathway involvement	—	CYP3A4	CYP3A4	CYP3A4, CYP2B6 (weak)	CYP3A4, CYP3A5 (less)
Direct antidote	No	No	No	No	No

efficacious and safe in these settings.[57,58] They offer significant advantages over vitamin K antagonist therapy, with fixed dosing, fewer drug and dietary interactions, and do not require routine laboratory monitoring (**Table 98.4**).

However, like all antithrombotic therapies, these agents have the potential to cause bleeding complications but, unlike warfarin, few have antidotes or reversal agents. Currently, there is little peer-reviewed literature regarding emergent reversal of the new anticoagulants, of which dabigatran and rivaroxaban are the most widely used. While experience grows, consensus and expert opinion emphasise the importance of risk stratification and general supportive measures depending on the degree of bleeding of patients on these anticoagulants.[59–61] Minor bleeding can be managed with withdrawal of the medication. Identification of a bleeding source and local measures to control the bleeding (which may be achieved via surgical or radiological means) are important, as are regular clinical monitoring, fluid resuscitation and red blood cell transfusions in major or life-threatening bleeding. Fluid replacement and maintenance of good urine output are particularly relevant with dabigatran, which is primarily renally excreted.

Laboratory monitoring with APTT and PT cannot provide precise information on drug levels of these agents on which to make clinical decisions. More research is required to confirm their utility in bleeding attributable to rivaroxaban or dabigatran, but a normal APTT (dabigatran) or PT (rivaroxaban) in this setting would suggest that haemostatic function is preserved, and that the NOAC is unlikely to be contributing significantly to major bleeding. Drug-specific assays for the NOACs are emerging, and will become more widely available in the near future.

It has been suggested that oral activated charcoal ingestion may be useful within 2 hours of dabigatran administration.[62] In extreme cases, acute haemodialysis or haemoperfusion can be considered in patients suspected of dabigatran overdose, especially if there is coexistent renal failure. There are currently no data on the use of oral activated charcoal in human studies with rivaroxaban, and haemodialysis would likely be ineffective in the setting of rivaroxaban overdose as it is a highly protein-bound drug.

There is no consensus on the use of FFP or PCCs in bleeding attributable to the newer anticoagulants. Abnormal laboratory parameters as a result of rivaroxaban (e.g. PT) were reversed by the administration of 4-factor PCCs in a cohort of healthy volunteers (4-factor PCCs contain similar amounts of non-activated thrombin, FVII, FIX and FX; 3-factor PCCs contain similar amounts of non-activated thrombin, FIX, and FX, but contain less FVII).[63] Such a finding was not reproduced in healthy individuals taking dabigatran. It is not known whether such findings can also be related to reversing bleeding in patients on these new anticoagulants. Furthermore, 4-factor PCCs are not routinely available in many countries including the USA and Australia.

Currently, the effectiveness of rFVIIa in reversing bleeding complications attributable to the new anticoagulants in humans is unclear and data from animal models are conflicting.[59] It has been postulated that rFVIIa acts proximally to FXa and thrombin, and hence may not alleviate the coagulopathy attributable to these new agents. rFVIIa is also prothrombotic and hence it must be used cautiously in all patients with an indication for anticoagulants.

The effectiveness of PCCs and rFVIIa for bleeding attributable to rivaroxaban and dabigatran will become clearer as familiarity with the use of both drugs increases. Currently, supportive care and local measures are the mainstays of management, with PCCs and rFVIIa a reasonable consideration in dire clinical situations, particularly if the last dose of newer anticoagulants is less than 12 hours.

ANTIFIBRINOLYTICS

Antifibrinolytic drugs such as tranexamic acid (TXA) and epsilon aminocaproic acid (EACA) are useful adjunctive drugs in the setting of major bleeding. TXA and EACA are lysine analogues, and work by competitive binding of lysine binding sites on plasminogen molecules, hence inhibiting fibrinolysis via its effects on plasmin formation. In a recent large review, the use of TXA and EACA has been found to be effective in reducing blood loss before and after surgery, without serious adverse effects.[64] Hence the use of these agents, as for PCCs, appears to be reasonable in major bleeding, including bleeding attributable to rivaroxaban and dabigatran. Aprotinin, another antifibrinolytic drug, was withdrawn from world markets after serious concerns relating to end-organ damage, including renal failure, myocardial infarction and encephalopathy, but such associations have not been observed with TXA or EACA.

The key pharmacological properties of the new anticoagulants and new antiplatelet agents are briefly described in Table 98.4.

ACQUIRED INHIBITORS OF COAGULATION

Major bleeding can be seen with rare inhibitors of coagulation factors. Autoantibodies against factors VIII (commonest), IX, X, V, and VWF have been reported. Bypassing agents such as rFVIIa and activated prothrombin complex concentrates such as FEIBA (factor VIII inhibitor bypassing activity) have been shown to be efficacious in arresting bleeding in this setting, particularly high-titre inhibitors. The other main aim of treatment is eradication of the offending antibodies. Previously, steroids and cyclophosphamide have been used to achieve this aim. Effectiveness of other treatment approaches, such as immune tolerance regimens and rituximab, has recently emerged. In acute emergencies, particularly in patients with high-titre inhibitors in whom bleeding has not responded to bypass agents, plasmapheresis and immunoadsorption with staphylococcal protein A can be used.

Access the complete references list online at http://www.expertconsult.com

1. Hoffman M, Monroe DM. Coagulation 2006: a modern view of hemostasis. Hematol Oncol Clin North Am 2007;21(1):1–11.
13. Favaloro EJ, Lippi G, Franchini M. Contemporary platelet function testing. Clin Chem Lab Med 2010;48(5):579–98.
30. Dargaud Y, Lienhart A, Negrier C. Prospective assessment of thrombin generation test for dose monitoring of bypassing therapy in hemophilia patients with inhibitors undergoing elective surgery. Blood 2010;116(25):5734–47.
49. Hook KM, Abrams CS. The loss of homeostasis in hemostasis: new approaches in treating and understanding acute disseminated intravascular coagulation in critically ill patients. Clin Transl Sci 2012;5(1):85–92.
59. Kaatz S, Kouides PA, Garcia DA, et al. Guidance on the emergent reversal of oral thrombin and factor Xa inhibitors. Am J Hematol 2012;87(Suppl 1):S141–5.

99

Haematological malignancy

Pascale Gruber and Timothy Wigmore

Haematological malignancies are tumours that involve the bone marrow, blood and lymphoid tissue. They account for 9% of all cancers. The overall prevalence of haematological malignancies is rising, with the greatest increase in non-Hodgkin's lymphoma and multiple myeloma.[1]

Patients with haematological malignancy account for approximately 1.5% of intensive care admissions.[2] They may develop critical illness due to either their underlying cancer or cancer-related treatments such as chemotherapy, radiotherapy or haematopoietic stem cell transplant (HSCT). Some clinical presentations are unique, for example only seen post HSCT, whereas others are more general.

CLASSIFICATION OF HAEMATOLOGICAL MALIGNANCIES

Over the last 30 years, many different classifications have been proposed. Traditional descriptive epidemiology divides haematological malignancies into four broad categories: leukaemia, Hodgkin lymphoma, non-Hodgkin lymphoma and myeloma, with national and international organisations publishing data in this format.[3-5] The revised World Health Organization (WHO) classifies haematological malignancies according to morphology, immunophenotype, genetic and clinical features.[6,7] Myeloid malignancies are categorised into the following groups: myeloproliferative neoplasms, myelodysplastic/myeloproliferative neoplasms, myelodysplastic syndromes, acute myeloid leukaemias, acute leukaemias of ambiguous lineage, precursor lymphoid neoplasms. Lymphoid malignancies are categorised into mature B cell neoplasms, mature T and NK cell neoplasms, Hodgkins lymphoma, histiocytic and dendritic cell neoplasms and post transplantation lymphoproliferative disorders.[8]

LEUKAEMIA

Over 350 000 people are diagnosed with leukaemia each year, worldwide accounting for 2.8% of all cancers.[3] Presenting features include fatigue, lymphadenopathy, hepatosplenomegaly and general symptoms of bone marrow failure such as anaemia, bleeding and reduced resistance to infection. Diagnosis is based on peripheral blood and bone marrow demonstrating blast cells, immunophenotyping, cytogenetic and molecular genetic analysis. The severity of disease, rate of progression and treatment varies greatly between leukaemias, so precise identification of the specific form of leukaemia is crucial to optimum management.

ACUTE MYELOID LEUKAEMIA (AML)

AML is characterised by uncontrolled proliferation of immature myeloid precursor cells. AML rises sharply in middle age and peaks at age 70. The WHO classifies AML into the following subtypes:

- AML with recurrent genetic abnormalities
- AML with myelodysplasia-related features
- Therapy-related myeloid neoplasms
- AML not otherwise specified
- Myeloid proliferations related to Down syndrome
- Blastic plasmacytic dendritic cell neoplasms.

Acute promyelocytic leukaemia (APML) falls within the first subtype. In APML the promyelocytes have dense cytoplasmic granules and Auer rods. The promyelocytes release thromboplastins commonly resulting in disseminated intravascular coagulation. APML responds well to all-trans-retinoic acid (ATRA) treatment.[9,10]

ACUTE LYMPHOBLASTIC LEUKAEMIA (ALL)

ALL is a malignant disorder of lymphoid precursor cells, commonly seen in childhood, with a good overall prognosis. ALL induction chemotherapy typically consists of a 4- or 5-drug regimen of prednisolone, vincristine, anthracycline, L-asparginase and/or cyclophosphamide.[11,12] Patients with ALL frequently have central nervous system involvement, therefore intrathecal chemotherapy or craniospinal irradiation is additionally required. Remission is consolidated with further chemotherapy or HSCT.[10] Prolonged maintenance therapy is often required to eradicate any residual leukaemic cells. A combination of daily methotrexate and 6-mercaptopurine constitutes the basis of most maintenance regimens. Five-year survival is 85–90% for children and less in adults.[13]

CHRONIC LYMPHOCYTIC LEUKAEMIA (CLL)

CLL may be classified as a form of leukaemia or low-grade lymphoma. It is most commonly found in elderly people. Clinical presentation includes fatigue, bone marrow failure, night sweats, lymphadenopathy, painful splenomegaly and autoimmune haemolytic anaemia. The natural history of CLL is variable with a median survival of 8–12 years.[10] Richter's transformation to diffuse large B-cell lymphoma is associated with a poor prognosis (median survival <1 year).[14] First-line treatment is fludarabine, cyclophosphamide and/or rituximab (monoclonal anti-CD20 agent).[15] Alemtuzumab (a monoclonal anti-CD52 agent) is useful in refractory CLL.[16]

CHRONIC MYELOID LEUKAEMIA (CML)

CML is linked to a translocation of chromosomes 22 and 9 (Philadelphia chromosome) leading to formation of BCR-ABL (a tyrosine protein kinase) causing uncontrolled proliferation in mature and immature white cells.[17] CML typically begins in the *chronic phase*, over several years progresses to an *accelerated phase* and eventually results in *blast crisis*. Patients present with weight loss, splenomegaly, fevers and night sweats. Imatinib (a tyrosine kinase inhibitor), a new form of treatment for CML, results in complete remission in approximately 80% of patients avoiding the need for HSCT, which was previously the only curative option for CML.[18]

LYMPHOMA

Lymphomas are tumours of B, T or NK lymphoid cells. Over 420 000 people are diagnosed with lymphoma each year, worldwide accounting for 3.3% of all cancers.[3] Traditionally, lymphomas are divided into Hodgkin's lymphoma and non-Hodgkin's lymphoma (NHL). Lymphomas are staged 1–4 according to lymph node spread and designated A or B depending on the absence or presence of 'B' symptoms: night sweats, fever and weight loss.

HODGKIN'S LYMPHOMA

Hodgkin's lymphoma is common in young people aged between 20 and 30 years. Classic presentation is of cervical lymphadenopathy, fever, night sweats, weight loss and pruritus. Reed–Sternberg cells are characteristic on histology. Choice of combination chemotherapy for Hodgkin's lymphoma depends on the patient's age, sex, tumour size and the histological subtype. Radiotherapy may be given for localised or bulky disease.[19] Combination chemotherapy with or without radiotherapy is curative in 75% of newly diagnosed patients with Hodgkin's disease.[10]

NON-HODGKIN'S LYMPHOMAS (NHL)

NHL is a heterogeneous group of conditions with over 30 subtypes. NHL are broadly divided into high and low grade. High-grade lymphomas tend to be aggressive but chemosensitive, whereas low-grade lymphomas are typically slow-growing, indolent and incurable.[10]

Low-grade lymphomas

Low-grade lymphomas encompass follicular lymphoma (most common), mantle cell lymphoma, marginal zone lymphomas and Waldenstrom macroglobinaemia. The clinical presentation, rate of disease progression and treatment modalities vary widely. The disease may continue for years and treatment is not always indicated.

High-grade lymphomas

The most common high-grade lymphoma is diffuse large B-cell lymphoma (DLBCL), accounting for about 30% of new cases of NHL. It typically affects elderly or middle-aged adults. First-line treatment of early-stage DLBCL includes CHOP chemotherapy (cyclophosphamide, doxorubicin, vincristine and prednisolone) with or without involved field radiotherapy.[20] Early-stage DLBCL is potentially curable with a 5-year survival of 70–80%.[21] Burkitt's lymphoma produces fast-growing tumours. There are three distinct variants of Burkitt's lymphoma: (1) endemic (African), (2) sporadic and (3) immunodeficiency associated. These forms differ in their clinical presentation and epidemiology but share the same aggressive nature. Childhood Burkitt's lymphoma is highly responsive to combination chemotherapy with a 5-year survival >90%. Risk of tumour lysis syndrome with Burkitt's lymphoma is high.[22]

MULTIPLE MYELOMA

Multiple myeloma is a plasma cell malignancy that accounts for 0.8% of all cancers and 10% of the haematological malignancies.[3] Patients present with bone pain, fractures and bone marrow failure with associated cytopenias. Renal failure is common due to light chain deposition in renal tubules, amyloidosis and hypercalaemia from bone destruction. Multiple myeloma is not curable but chemotherapy induces temporary remission. Typically, patients experience repeated episodes of relapse, treatment and remission over several years until the disease can no longer be controlled. Overall 5-year survival for multiple myeloma is around 35%. High-dose chemotherapy with HSCT is increasingly being used to reduce symptoms and increase survival.[23]

TREATMENT OF HAEMATOLOGICAL MALIGNANCIES

Haematological malignancies are treated using chemotherapy, radiotherapy or a combination of both with the intent of inducing remission or cure. HSCT offers the only hope of cure in some conditions, but is not without risks.

CHEMOTHERAPY

Chemotherapeutic agents, either individually or in combination, are used to induce cure or remission. Chemotherapeutic agents and regimens commonly used for treatment of haematological malignancies are outlined in **Table 99.1**. The goal of *induction therapy* is to achieve remission by reducing the number of leukaemic cells to an undetectable level; the goal of *consolidation therapy*, which follows induction therapy, is to eliminate any residual undetectable disease and achieve cure. *Maintenance therapy* is frequently used in ALL and APML to prolong remission. Chemotherapy may also be used as part of a conditioning regimen with or without total body irradiation prior to HSCT. Recent advances in the understanding of haematological cancers have led to an increase in the variety of chemotherapy and targeted therapies now available. Administration of some chemotherapeutic agents may result in life-threatening side-effects.

IFSOFAMIDE NEUROTOXICITY

Ifosfamide may be used in the treatment of lymphomas. It causes reversible neuropsychiatric disorders in 10–30% of patients including visual or auditory hallucinations, confusion, personality disorders, anxiety, extrapyramidal symptoms, seizures and coma. Symptoms occur from 2 to 48 hours after infusion and improve 48 hours after discontinuation of the drug. Risk factors include serum albumin <35 mg/dL, hyponatraemia, elevated serum creatinine, previous cisplatin use and bulky abdominal disease. Treatment involves normalisation of serum electrolytes and albumin, benzodiazepines (for seizures) and methylene blue.

RETINOIC ACID SYNDROME

Patients with APML treated with ATRA are at risk of retinoic acid syndrome. The condition is potentially life threatening and the diagnosis is based on the presence of dyspnoea, fever, weight gain, peripheral oedema, shock, acute kidney injury, heart failure, pericardial and pleural effusions. Management involves discontinuation of ATRA and administration of steroids.[9]

RADIOTHERAPY

Radiotherapy can be used alone or in combination with chemotherapy for lymphoma and myeloma. Total body irradiation (TBI) may be instituted as part of the myeloablative regimen in HSCT. Side-effects include gastrointestinal dysfunction, mucositis, pneumonitis, alopecia and skin irritation.

HAEMATOPOIETIC STEM CELL TRANSPLANTATION (HSCT)

HSCT has now become the standard treatment for many haematological malignancies because it is potentially curative. Approximately 50 000 to 60 000 patients undergo HSCT per year.[24] Reported rates of ICU admission range from 11 to 20% with higher rates of ICU admission after allogeneic transplant.[25–27] HSCT are divided according to the source of the stem cells (peripheral, bone marrow or umbilical cord) and donor of the cells (autologous or allogeneic). Autologous transplant involves re-infusing harvested peripheral blood taken from the patient during periods of remission after myeloablative conditioning. With autologous transplant patients risk the possibility of re-infusion of the patient's tumour cells and future disease relapse however treatment related mortality is less than 5%.[28,29] Allogeneic transplants involve the infusion of donor cells (sibling or mixed unrelated donor). Immunosuppression is required to reduce the risks of graft-versus-host-disease (GvHD) and graft failure. Treatment related mortality for allogeneic transplants are higher due to the intensive myeloablative regimens and immunosuppression required.

Prior to HSCT patients undergo myeloablative conditioning to destroy endogenous bone marrow cells using radiotherapy and/or chemotherapy. Typical myeloablative regimens include a combination of busulfan, cyclophosphamide and TBI. Reduced-intensity conditioning regimens such as fludarabine and low-dose TBI or fludarabine and busulfan are used for patients who are older, have multiple co-morbidities, or are undergoing repeat transplants. They are less toxic to the bone marrow but are sufficiently immunosuppressive to permit engraftment of donor cells.

CONDITIONS SPECIFIC TO HSCT PATIENTS

Infection

Following HSCT, the immune system takes several weeks to recover; the rapidity of recovery is dependent on the type of transplant, source of stem cells, age of the recipient and donor, conditioning regimen, presence of GvHD and degree of immunosuppression.[30] Most ICU admissions are during the early phase. The period of engraftment is divided into three phases subjecting the transplant recipient to risks of different infections:[31]

1. *Pre-engraftment (<30 days):* the recipient is at risk of bacterial infections due to neutropenia.
2. *Early post-engraftment (30–100 days):* cell-mediated immunity is impaired and the recipient is at risk of viral and fungal infections (cytomegalovirus (CMV), *Pneumocystis jirovecii* and *Aspergillus* spp.).
3. *Late post-engraftment (>100 days):* impaired reticulo-endothelial, cell-mediated and humoral functions mean recipients are at risk of *Mycobacteria* and viruses.

The use of novel broad-spectrum antibiotics with excellent Gram-negative coverage has resulted in Gram-positive organisms (*Staphylococcus* spp., *Streptococcus, Enterococcus*) being responsible for the majority of bacteraemias following HSCT.

Table 99.1 Common chemotherapeutic agents used in haematological malignancies[10]

CATEGORY	MODE OF ACTION	CHEMOTHERAPEUTIC AGENTS	SIDE-EFFECTS
Alkylating agents	Cells directly damage DNA by forming covalent bonds	Alkyl sulfonates Busulfan	Pulmonary fibrosis Seizures Thromboembolism
		Mustard gas derivatives Chlorambucil Cyclophosphamide Ifosfamide Melphalan	Haemorrhagic cystitis Neurotoxicity Myelosuppression GI disturbance Hepatotoxicity
		Triazines Dacarbazine Procarbazine	Myelosuppression GI disturbance
Anti-metabolites	Interferes with DNA and RNA growth by acting as inhibitors of enzymes processing purine and pyrimidines	Folic acid antagonist Methotrexate	Pneumonitis Myelosuppression Hepatotoxicity
		Purine antagonist 6-mercaptopurine	Myelosuppression GI disturbance
		Pyrimidine antagonists Capecitabine Cytarabine Gemcitabine	Myelosuppression Pneumonitis Cardiac arrhythmias GI disturbance
		Adenosine deaminase inhibitor Fludarabine	Myelosuppression Autoimmune haemolytic anaemia
Anti-tumour antibiotics	Interfere with enzymes necessary for DNA replication	Anthracyclines Doxorubicin Daunorubicin	Cardiomyopathy
		Miscellaneous Bleomycin	Pulmonary fibrosis
Plant alkaloids	Inhibit mitosis by interfering with the assembly of microtubule structure	Vinca alkaloids Vinblastine Vincristine	Peripheral neuropathy Hyponatraemia Myelosuppression
Topoisomerase II inhibitors	Interferes with enzymes involved in regulating DNA coiling	Etoposide	Myelosuppression GI disturbance Rash
Tyrosine kinase inhibitors	Binds to the site of tyrosine kinase activity, preventing its activity and causing tumour cell apoptosis	Imatinib	Cardiac failure Pneumonitis Rash Fluid retention
Miscellaneous	Ribonucleotide reductase inhibitor	Hydroxyurea	Myelosuppression Hepatotoxic Nephrotoxic Mucositis
	Binds to retinoid-dependent receptors (RAR) involved in cellular growth, proliferation and differentiation	All-trans retinoic acid (ATRA)	Retinoic acid syndrome Headache Hypertriglyceridaemia
	Depletion of cellular asparagine	Asparaginase	Pancreatitis Thromboembolism Myelosuppression

Table 99.1 Common chemotherapeutic agents used in haematological malignancies—cont'd

CATEGORY	MODE OF ACTION	CHEMOTHERAPEUTIC AGENTS	SIDE-EFFECTS
Immunotherapy	Monoclonal antibodies to CD20	Rituximab	Fever Muscle and joint pain Cardiotoxicity Hepatotoxicity Nephrotoxicity
	Monoclonal antibodies to CD52	Alemtuzumab	
	Non-specific immunotherapy	Interferon alpha	
	Immunomodulatory agents	Thalidomide Lenalidomide	Thromboembolism Peripheral neuropathy Thrombocytopenia

NOMENCLATURE OF COMMONLY USED COMBINATION CHEMOTHERAPEUTIC REGIMENS

	CHEMOTHERAPY	HAEMATOLOGICAL MALIGNANCY
FCR	Fludarabine+cyclophosphamide+rituximab	CLL
ABVD	Doxorubicin+bleomycin+vinblastine+dacarbazine	HL
BEACOPP	Bleomycin+etoposide+doxorubicin+cyclophosphamide+vincristine+procarbazine+prednisone	HL
R-CVP	Rituximab+cyclophosphamide+vincristine+prednisone	NHL
R-CHOP	Rituximab+cyclophosphamide+doxorubicin+vincristine+prednisone	NHL
R-FCM	Rituximab+fludarabine+cyclophosphamide+mitoxantrone	NHL
ProMACE-CytaBOM	Prednisone+doxorubicin (Adriamycin)+cyclophosphamide+etoposide+cytarabine+bleomycin+vincristine (Oncovin)+methotrexate+leucovorin	NHL
m-BACOD	Methotrexate+leucovorin+bleomycin+doxorubicin (Adriamycin)+cyclophosphamide+vincristine (Oncovin)+dexamethasone	NHL
MACOP-B	Methotrexate+leucovorin+doxorubicin (Adriamycin)+cyclophosphamide+vincristine (Oncovin)+prednisone+bleomycin	NHL
VAD	Vincristine+doxorubicin (Adriamycin)+dexamethasone	Multiple myeloma

Please note the table above highlights only some of the commonly used regimens. GI disturbance=gastrointestinal disturbance; CLL=chronic lymphocytic leukaemia; HL=Hodgkin's lymphoma; NHL=non-Hodgkin's lymphoma.

CMV infection is a major cause of morbidity and mortality after HSCT. CMV infection may present as a meningitis, colitis, uveitis and pneumonitis. The reported mortality in HSCT patients with CMV pneumonia is 85%.[32] CMV antigen surveillance and use of prophylactic ganciclovir in HSCT recipients who are CMV positive or have received transplants from CMV donors have led to a decrease in CMV infections.[31] Similarly, *P. jirovecii* pneumonia is less common with the effective use of trimethoprim–sulfamethoxazole prophylaxis. Fungal infections continue to be problematic with *Aspergillus* spp. and *Candida* spp. predominating. The routine use of azole prophylaxis has reduced the number of *C. albicans* infections but resulted in the emergence of azole-resistant species.

Graft-versus-host disease (GvHD)

GvHD occurs when the donor marrow recognises the host tissue as foreign and generates an immune response. The incidence of GvHD is 30–50% post-allogeneic transplant and increases with HLA mismatch, advanced age of the donor and recipient, inadequate immunosuppression, intensive myeloablative conditioning and the use of peripheral blood as the stem cell source. Acute GVHD presents with a maculopapular skin rash (especially affecting palms and soles), diarrhoea and intrahepatic cholestasis 7–28 days post-transplant. Acute GVHD is staged and graded according to the number and extent of organ involvement[33] (**Tables 99.2** and **99.3**).

The diagnosis of acute GvHD may be confirmed with a skin, rectal, or liver biopsy. Prophylaxis involves the use of immunosuppressants such as prednisolone, ciclosporin (cyclosporine) and mycophenolate mofetil. Treatment of severe acute GvHD involves high-dose pulsed methylprednisolone and/or additional immunosuppressive agents. Gastrointestinal involvement with secretory diarrhoea may necessitate the need for parenteral nutrition and octreotide. The degree

Table 99.2 Clinical staging of acute GvHD

STAGE	SKIN RASH	LIVER (BILIRUBIN μMOL/L)	GASTROINTESTINAL TRACT (DIARRHOEA IN L/DAY)
1	Maculopapular rash <25% of BSA	35–50	0.5–1
2	Maculopapular rash 25–50% of BSA	51–102	1–1.5
3	Maculopapular rash >50% of BSA	102–225	>1.5
4	Generalised eythroderma with bullae	>225	Severe abdominal pain with or without ileus

BSA=body surface area.

of acute GVHD is predictive of 100-day survival.[34] Chronic GvHD is a multi-organ syndrome which occurs >100 days post-transplant. It can be limited or extensive with skin (itchy dry skin, scleroderma), pulmonary (bronchiolitis obliterans), eye (sicca, keratitis), salivary glands (xerostomia) and neuromuscular (polyneuropathy, polymyositis, myasthenia gravis) involvement and liver dysfunction (hepatitis, cirrhosis). Treatment is often difficult and progression can be limited by increasing the dose of immunosuppression (with a consequent risk of infection).

Table 99.3 Grading of acute GvHD

GRADE	CLINICAL MANIFESTATIONS
I	Stage 1–2 skin, no gut or liver involvement
II	Stage 3 skin, stage 1 gut or stage 1 liver
III	Stage 3 skin, stage 2–4 gut or stage 2–3 liver
IV	Stage 4 skin, stage 4 gut or liver

Graft failure

Graft failure occurs when there is a failure to establish haematological engraftment after HSCT. It occurs in less than 5% of patients following allogeneic HSCT. Causes of graft failure include inadequate stem cell infusion, infection and GvHD. Graft failure is associated with an increased transplant mortality and risk of infection. Management consists of augmentation by granulocyte-colony stimulating factor (G-CSF), infusion of stem cells without additional chemotherapy or a repeat HSCT.

Diffuse alveolar haemorrhage (DAH)

DAH occurs in 5% of HSCT patients. It occurs within 30 days of transplant and is caused by injury to the pulmonary endothelial lining from chemo- and radiotherapy. Age, acute GvHD, intensive pre-transplantation chemotherapy, TBI and allogeneic transplant are important risk factors. Patients typically present with pyrexia, dyspnoea, cough, anaemia and diffuse infiltrates on chest radiographs in the absence of infection. Haemoptysis is rare. Bronchoalveolar lavage (BAL) is bloody and cytology shows haemosiderin-laden macrophages. Treatment is with high-dose steroids and the response is variable.

Idiopathic pneumonia syndrome (IPS)

The incidence of IPS is approximately 7% and it is commonly seen 3 weeks after HSCT. Typical presentation is of diffuse infiltrates on chest radiography or CT scan in the absence of an infective aetiology. Risk factors include allogeneic transplant, GvHD and CMV-positive donor status, pre-transplant radiation, and chemotherapy (busulfan, cyclophosphamide). Treatment is mainly supportive and, even with aggressive care, the mortality is over 70%.

Engraftment syndrome

Engraftment syndrome (also known as capillary leak syndrome) typically presents 4–5 days after autologous HSCT with fever, erythematous rash and non-cardiogenic pulmonary oedema. Other features include abnormal liver function tests, transient encephalopathy and multi-organ failure. The underlying pathophysiology is related to the release of pro-inflammatory cytokines and neutrophils. Use of G-CSF increases the prevalence of this syndrome and, should it occur, G-CSF must be discontinued. CT scan of the chest typically demonstrates bilateral ground-glass opacification. Management is supportive and steroids may be useful.

Cryptogenic organising pneumonia (COP)

COP, also known as bronchiolitis obliterans organising pneumonia, occurs in 1% of recipients 1–3 months following HSCT and presents with dyspnoea, fever and cough. CT scan of the chest typically demonstrates a ground-glass appearance and lung biopsy shows granulation tissue and fibroblasts in the small airways. Treatment response to steroids is usually good.

Veno-occlusive disease (VOD)

VOD, also known as sinusoidal obstruction syndrome, presents as a triad of painful hepatomegaly, jaundice and ascites 3 weeks following HSCT. Other features include weight gain, encephalopathy, bleeding, and hepato-renal syndrome. The disease spectrum ranges from a mild reversible condition to multi-organ failure.

Risk factors for VOD include myeloablative conditioning (busulphan, cyclophosphamide), pre-existing abnormal liver tests, intra-abdominal radiotherapy and repeat HSCT. The diagnosis is made by hepatic dopplers showing reversed or reduced portal flow of the hepatic vessels. A transjugular liver biopsy may also help establish the diagnosis. Management and prophylaxis in high-risk patients involve the use of defibrotide, a polydeoxyribonucleotide with anti-thrombotic, anti-inflammatory and fibrinolytic effects.[35] Severe VOD has a mortality of 85%.

Posterior reversible encephalopathy syndrome (PRES)

PRES is a syndrome characterised by confusion, headache, visual loss, and seizures commonly associated with HSCT and immunosuppressive agents (e.g. ciclosporin). T_2-weighted MRI characteristically shows diffuse hyperintensity involving the parieto-occipital white matter (**Fig. 99.1**).

The treatment is targeted at the underlying cause.

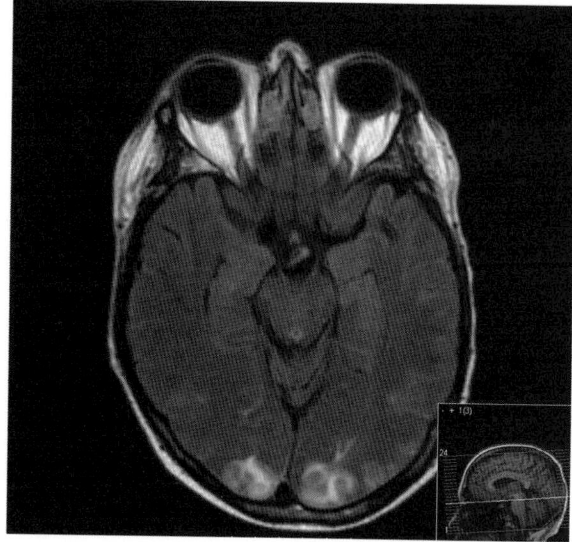

Figure 99.1 MRI scan of posterior reversible encephalopathy syndrome, showing the characteristic diffuse hyperintensity.

Post-transplant lymphoproliferative disorder (PTLD)

PTLD is a well-recognised but uncommon complication of allogeneic transplant. It is characterised by uncontrolled proliferation of EBV-infected B cells and results in impairment of T-cell immunity. Risks factors include previous EBV donor or recipient exposure, aggressive immunosuppression and T-cell-depleted transplants. EBV viral load should be monitored regularly on serial blood samples. Treatment involves reduction or withdrawal of immunosuppression with the potential risk of GvHD. Intravenous immunoglobulin, anti-B-cell monoclonal antibodies, rituximab and infusion of donor T cells have all been used with variable success.

Thrombotic thrombocytopenic purpura (TTP)

Secondary TTP following HSCT is thought to be due to chemotherapy-induced endothelial damage. Classic presentation is of renal failure, fever, thrombocytopenia, fluctuating neurological signs (confusion, mood changes, seizures and drowsiness) and microangiopathic haemolytic anaemia. The blood film typically shows red cell fragments and the haemolysis screen is positive. Treatment is supportive and involves plasmapheresis, broad-spectrum antibiotics and high-dose steroids. Haemolytic uraemic syndrome is a similar entity and may be distinguished from TTP by the lack of neurological signs and fever.

ACUTE ONCOLOGICAL EMERGENCIES

ACUTE ONCOLOGICAL EMERGENCIES REQUIRING URGENT CHEMOTHERAPY OR RADIOTHERAPY

A small number of patients are admitted directly to ICU with complications of their haematological malignancy requiring urgent chemotherapy and/or radiotherapy. These include:

1. *CNS involvement:* CNS involvement resulting in focal deficits, seizures, alteration of consciousness or high spinal cord compression is an indication for urgent chemotherapy and/or radiotherapy.
2. *Mediastinal masses and pericardial disease:* bulky mediastinal masses with compression of trachea, main bronchi or major vessels are often due to NHLs and require urgent chemotherapy and/or radiotherapy to relieve the compression (**Fig. 99.2**).
3. *Disseminated intravascular coagulation (DIC):* DIC may be a presenting feature of APML. Specific chemotherapy such as ATRA and supportive measures such as regular platelet transfusions and fresh frozen plasma reduce the risk of bleeding. Use of low-dose unfractionated heparin is not recommended as routine practice.
4. *Hyperviscosity syndromes:* hyperviscosity syndromes occur with multiple myeloma, leukaemia and Waldenstrom's macroglobinaemia. Clinical manifestations include headaches, coma, seizures, visual impairment, retinal haemorrhages, and bleeding. Emergency management is directed at decreasing blood viscosity by plasmapheresis followed by urgent chemotherapy aimed at reducing monoclonal immunoglobulins.
5. *Macrophage activation syndrome (MAS):* MAS, also known as haemophagocytic lymphohistiocytosis, is a recognised presentation of NHL and HD. Typical manifestations of MAS are fever, hepatosplenomegaly and thrombocytopenia. Vasodilatory shock, acute respiratory distress syndrome and acute kidney injury may also occur. Laboratory findings include low erythrocyte and leucocyte counts,

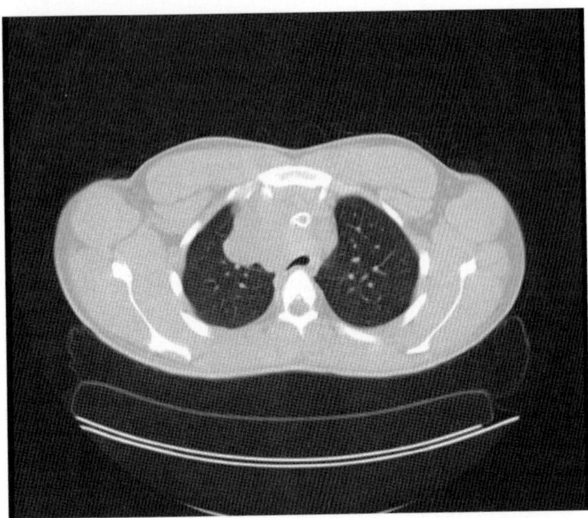

Figure 99.2 A mediastinal mass.

hypoalbuminaemia, hypertriglyceridaemia, hypofibrinogenaemia, hyperferritinaemia (>500 μg/L). Bone marrow findings show activated macrophages phagocytosing platelets, erythrocytes and leucocytes. Steroids and etoposide are the mainstays of treatment.

6. *Leukostasis:* Leukostasis is defined as a total leucocyte count of $>100 \times 10^9$/L. It is seen in patients with AML or AML in blast crisis. White cell plugs in the vasculature cause decrease tissue perfusion and result in neurological dysfunction and respiratory failure.[36] Leukostasis is associated with a high mortality and prompt treatment with chemotherapy and leukapheresis is indicated.

In some circumstances starting chemotherapy in the ICU, even when infection or organ failure is present, may be appropriate to limit disease progression that may result in death. Modification of chemotherapeutic regimens may be required to limit organ toxicity and the duration of neutropenia. In carefully selected cases of patients given chemotherapy in the ICU, published outcomes have been reasonable with an in-hospital mortality of 43%.[37] In fact, the administration of chemotherapy, in the ICU setting or within the last 3 weeks prior to ICU admission, does not appear to be associated with an increased risk of death.[38]

NEUTROPENIA AND NEUTROPENIC SEPSIS

Neutropenia is defined as an absolute neutrophil count (ANC) of $\leq 0.5 \times 10^9$/L. Fever is common in patients with haematological malignancies and differentiating infectious from non-infectious causes of fever is notoriously difficult. Assessment relies on the early identification of a likely source, microbiological surveillance and surrogate information from biomarkers. Severe sepsis and septic shock in patients with haematological malignancies has a reported mortality of 36–45%.[39,40] High-risk patients are those with significant co-morbidities and prolonged (>7 days) and profound neutropenia. Neutropenic sepsis is potentially fatal if left untreated.[41] Patients with neutropenic sepsis and evidence of organ failure must have antibiotics administered within 1 hour of presentation. A minimum of two sets of blood cultures should be collected: with a set collected from each lumen of a vascular access device, if present, and from a peripheral vein site; 2 blood culture sets from separate venepunctures should be sent if no central venous catheter is present. A chest radiograph and culture specimens from other sites of suspected infection (sputum, stool, urine) should also be taken. The Infectious Diseases Society of America recommends first-line antimicrobial treatment with an anti-pseudomonal beta-lactam agent, such as cefepime, a carbapenem (meropenem or imipenem–cilastatin), or piperacillin–tazobactam. Aminoglycosides, fluoroquinolones, and/or vancomycin should be added to the initial regimen in the event of septic shock or if antimicrobial resistance is suspected.[42] Vancomycin (or another agent active against Gram-positive cocci) should also be added if there is a suspected catheter-related infection, skin or soft-tissue infection or pneumonia. In intensive care units where there is a high incidence of multiresistant organisms, it may be necessary to use a second-line agent such as linezolid. Empirical antifungal therapy should be considered for patients with persistent or recurrent fever after 4–7 days of antibiotics. The need for antiviral agents or trimethoprim–sulfamethoxazole should be evaluated on an individual patient basis. G-CSF is often used to promote neutrophil recovery in patients with profound neutropenia. Blood cell counts should be obtained daily, and the G-CSF should be discontinued when the neutrophil count is $\geq 1.0 \times 10^9$/L. Side-effects of G-CSF include rash, injection site reactions, bone pain, flu-like symptoms and rarely splenic rupture. Finally, environmental precautions should be taken when managing febrile neutropenic patients with meticulous hand hygiene, full barrier precautions (gloves, gowns, and in some cases overshoes and masks) and patients should be kept in protective isolation. In the United Kingdom, the National Institute for Health and Clinical Excellence (NICE) has provided comprehensive guidance on the management of neutropenic sepsis following the National Confidential Enquiry into Patient Outcome and Death (NCEPOD) report (Systemic Anti-Cancer Therapy: For better, for worse? 2008).[43,44]

NEUTROPENIC ENTEROCOLITIS

Neutropenic enterocolitis is also known as typhlitis. Patients typically present with abdominal pain, fever, and diarrhoea after chemotherapy (especially cytosine arabinoside, vinca alkaloids, and doxorubicin). It is caused by a combination of chemotherapy-induced colonic mucosal wall damage, thrombocytopenia-related gastrointestinal bleeding, and colonisation of the bowel by pathogenic bacteria. Complications include bacteraemia, gastrointestinal bleeding, and perforation (5–10%). Abdominal CT scanning may demonstrate pneumoperitoneum or colonic pneumatosis indicating colonic damage with imminent perforation. Bowel-wall thickening on ultrasound scanning may also help confirm the diagnosis. Management is conservative with bowel rest, parenteral nutrition and antimicrobial therapy that target enteric Gram-negative and anaerobic organisms, including *Clostridium difficile*. Surgery may be required in patients with uncontrolled sepsis, bowel perforation or life-threatening gastrointestinal bleeding.

RESPIRATORY FAILURE

Acute respiratory failure is the most common cause of ICU admission in patients with haematological malignancies. The reason for respiratory failure is often infection, although other non-infectious causes including non-cardiogenic pulmonary oedema, acute respiratory distress syndrome, GvHD, diffuse alveolar haemorrhage, idiopathic pneumonia syndrome, chemotherapy (methotrexate, bleomycin, fludarabine, gemcitabine), cryptogenic organising pneumonia, and tumour infiltration of the lung should be considered (**Table 99.4**). Invasive mechanical ventilation is a poor prognostic indicator.[25,45] Reported mortality for patients who are invasively ventilated following HSCT is 52–96%.[46] Lung-protective ventilation strategies, use of non-invasive ventilation and use of bronchoalveolar lavage (BAL) to aid diagnosis have all contributed to improvements in outcome.[47,48] The diagnostic yield of BAL is 45% and leads to modification in treatment in up to two-thirds of patients but the procedure may precipitate the need for invasive mechanical ventilation. Routine transbronchial biopsy is not recommended as it rarely provides additional useful information but increases the risk of complications.

ACUTE KIDNEY INJURY

Acute kidney injury may be a result of the underlying cancer (monoclonal light chain deposition in multiple myeloma), tumour lysis syndrome, administration of nephrotoxic agents (amphotericin B, foscarnet, aminoglycosides, methotrexate, platin derivatives, cyclophosphamide, ciclosporin), hepato-renal syndrome from veno-occlusive disease, or sepsis. In some cases renal replacement therapy may be required. Studies have shown that the need for renal replacement therapy is an independent predictor of mortality in patients with haematological malignancy.[49,50]

TUMOUR LYSIS SYNDROME

Tumour lysis syndrome is caused by rapid lysis of tumour cells following chemotherapy leading to release of excessive quantities of intracellular contents into the systemic circulation. The metabolic disturbance is characterised by hyperkalaemia, hyperphosphataemia, hypocalcaemia and hyperuricaemia, which may lead to acute kidney injury and cardiac arrhythmias. It is commonly associated with the acute leukaemias and high-grade lymphomas (e.g., Burkitt's lymphoma). Close monitoring of renal function, potassium, calcium, phosphate, and urate levels is required in patients with high tumour burden after starting chemotherapy. Allopurinol or rasburicase (a recombinant urate oxidase enzyme) are used as prophylaxis.[51] Treatment includes aggressive fluid hydration, rasburicase and occasionally renal replacement therapy.

NEUROLOGICAL DYSFUNCTION

Neurological dysfunction may have a number of aetiologies including infection (bacterial, viral or fungal), bleeding, tumour infiltration, hyperviscosity syndromes (multiple myeloma, Waldenstrom haemoglobinaemia), cerebral infarcts, and cerebral venous thrombosis. Some chemotherapy and immunosuppressive agents (methotrexate, cytarabine, 5-fluorouracil, ciclosporin) may present with CNS toxicity and cerebellar syndromes. High-dose cisplatin can cause encephalopathy and optic nerve damage.

GASTROINTESTINAL AND LIVER DYSFUNCTION

Gastrointestinal and liver dysfunction may be associated with chemotherapy (ciclosporin, methotrexate, platinum derivatives), acute GvHD, infection (CMV, EBV, hepatitis, adenovirus, rotavirus, *Clostridium difficile*), veno-occlusive disease and tumour infiltration.

CARDIAC COMPLICATIONS

Cardiac complications such as cardiac failure, arrhythmias, pericardial effusion, myocarditis or endocarditis may be the result of the underlying cancer, chemotherapy (anthracyclines, cyclophosphamide, cisplatin) or infections (EBV, CMV, *Staphylococcus aureus*, *Aspergillus* spp., *Candida* spp.).

PREDICTORS OF MORTALITY IN PATIENTS WITH HAEMATOLOGICAL CANCER

Several studies have looked at predictors of mortality to help identify those patients with haematological malignancy most likely to benefit from ICU care. Some predictors have changed with time such as neutropenia, autologous transplant and underlying haematological diagnosis which are no longer indicative of poor outcome.[52–54] Advanced age, multi-organ failure, mechanical ventilation, vasopressor use, GvHD, elevated serum lactate on admission, allogeneic transplants continue to be associated with poor outcomes.[2,27,45,25,55] Acute Physiology and Chronic Health Evaluation (APACHE) II scores and Simplified Acute Physiology Score (SAPS) II scores often underestimate mortality.[26,56]

Table 99.4 Causes of respiratory failure in a patient with haematological malignancy

CAUSES	EXAMPLES	
Non-infectious	General	Acute respiratory distress syndrome Aspiration pneumonia Cryptogenic organising pneumonia Pulmonary leukaemic infiltration Tumour causing upper or lower airway obstruction Non-cardiogenic pulmonary oedema Chemotherapy-induced pulmonary toxicity Pulmonary interstitial fibrosis
	Specific to HSCT	Diffuse alveolar haemorrhage syndrome Idiopathic pneumonia syndrome Engraftment syndrome
Infectious	Bacterial	*Pseudomonas, Klebsiella, Acinetobacter, Staphylococcus, Enterococcus, Streptococcus, Legionella, Mycoplasma*
	Viral	Influenza, parainfluenza, adenovirus, respiratory syncytial virus, cytomegalovirus, herpes simplex virus, varicella zoster virus
	Fungal	*Candida* spp., *Aspergillus* spp., *Pneumocystis jirovecii*
	Mycobacteria	*Mycobacterium* tuberculosis

HSCT=haematopoietic stem cell transplant.

OUTCOMES OF PATIENTS WITH HAEMATOLOGICAL MALIGNANCY ADMITTED TO THE ICU

Previous studies have reported that patients with haematological malignancies who require intensive care often face a poor prognosis with in-hospital mortality rates of >80% reported in the mid-1990s. However, more recent reports have demonstrated better survival. The largest case series to date has demonstrated an in-hospital mortality of 59%.[2] This reduction in mortality is attributed to improvements in chemotherapeutic regimens, better patient selection, targeted therapies with less organ toxicity, appropriately tailored reduced intensity conditioning regimens for HSCT patients and improved ICU care.[57] This trend towards lower mortality also provides a strong argument against the traditionally held negative perception of patients with haematological malignancy admitted to the ICU.

Access the complete references list online at http://www.expertconsult.com

2. Hampshire PA, Welch CA, McCrossan LA, et al. Admission factors associated with hospital mortality in patients with haematological malignancy admitted to UK adult, general critical care units: a secondary analysis of the ICNARC Case Mix Programme Database. Crit Care 2009;13:R137.
3. Ferlay J, Shin HR, Bray F, et al. GLOBOCAN 2008, Cancer Incidence and Mortality Worldwide: IARC Cancer Base No. 10 [Internet]. Lyon, France: International Agency for Research on Cancer; 2010. Available from: http://globocan.iarc.fr
6. Jaffe ES, Harris LN, Stein H, Vardiman JW. World Health Organization Classification of Tumours: Pathology and Genetics of Tumours of Haematopoietic and Lymphoid Tissues. Lyon, France: IARC Press; 2001.
10. National Cancer Institute. Health professional version. Available from: http://www.cancer.gov/cancertopics
31. Center for International Blood and Marrow Transplant Research (CIBMTR); National Marrow Donor Program (NMDP); European Blood and Marrow Transplant Group (EBMT); American Society of Blood and Marrow Transplantation (ASBMT); Canadian Blood and Marrow Transplant Group (CBMTG); Infectious Diseases Society of America (IDSA); Society for Healthcare Epidemiology of America (SHEA); Association of Medical Microbiology and Infectious Diseases Canada (AMMI); Centers for Disease Control and Prevention (CDC). Guidelines for preventing infectious complications among hematopoietic cell transplant recipients: a global perspective. Bone Marrow Transplant 2009;44(8):453–558.
37. Benoit DD, Depuydt PO, Vandewoude KH, et al. Outcome in severely ill patients with hematological malignancies who received intravenous chemotherapy in the intensive care unit. Intensive Care Med 2006;32:93–9.

46. Afessa B, Azoulay E. Critical care of the hematopoietic stem cell transplant recipient. Critical Care Clin 2010;26(1):133–50.
47. Azoulay E, Schlemmer B. Diagnostic strategy in cancer patients with acute respiratory failure. Intensive Care Med 2006;32:808–22.
55. Benoit DD, Vandewoude KH, Decruyenaere JM, et al. Outcome and early prognostic indicators in patients with a hematologic malignancy admitted to the intensive care unit for a life-threatening complication. Crit Care Med 2003;31:104–12.
57. Azoulay E, Soares M, Darmon M, et al. Intensive care of the cancer patient: recent achievements and remaining challenges. Ann Intensive Care 2011; 1(1):5.

Part Sixteen

Transplantation

Organ donation

Stephen J Streat

Transplantation of organs and tissues is an established effective treatment for end-stage organ failure and other conditions.[1,2] Demand for transplantation is increasing as recipient outcomes continue to improve. However, organ donation from deceased donors has not correspondingly increased, leading to strident calls for 'solutions to the organ shortage crisis'.[3] Transplant numbers have been maintained or modestly increased by a number of strategies[3] including donation after cardiac death (DCD, formerly called non-heart-beating donation), live donors and varieties of chains of kidney exchange (including altruistic donors, paired and more complex kidney exchange[4]), the use of split livers for two recipients,[3] accepting more organs at higher risk of failure[1] and transplanting two such kidneys into one recipient.[5] Despite professional condemnation of the practice[6] desperate recipients from wealthy countries continue to take part in 'transplant tourism'[7–9] in poorer countries. Concerns have been expressed about internet-facilitated altruistic but directed live donation being potentially vulnerable to commercial exploitation.[10,11] Slow progress continues in alternative approaches to end-stage organ failure, including artificial organs, xenotransplantation and the engineering of organs (and tissues) from stem cells, but no such organ replacement is yet available for clinical use.

Over the last decade in particular there have been marked demographic changes in deceased donors, with no change or a fall in (younger) donors after traumatic brain injury and an increase in (older) donors following cerebrovascular accident, hypoxic–ischaemic encephalopathy and other non-traumatic conditions. Underlying these demographic changes are the combined effects of primary prevention of traumatic brain injury, better treatment of this and other intracranial catastrophes (subarachnoid and intracerebral haemorrhage in particular), changes in intensive care practice and changes in donor acceptability to transplant services. The true incidence of brain death in intensive care settings is largely unreported, in part owing to inconsistent clinical practice with respect to the determination of brain death in patients with apparent loss of brainstem function.[12] In many countries the number of organ donors after brain death is not rising and increases in the number of organ donors have come from DCD.[13,14]

Decompressive craniectomy does not improve long-term outcome after (at least diffuse[15]) traumatic brain injury, but it does control refractory intracranial hypertension,[15] and may thereby reduce the incidence of brain death. Institution of mechanical ventilatory support in poor-prognosis patients with apparent stroke (to facilitate CT scanning) has probably led to more such patients being admitted to ICU, sometimes after family discussion about possible future organ donation. The effectiveness of induced hypothermia for hypoxic–ischaemic encephalopathy after 'shockable' cardiac arrest[16] has led some to suggest its use after resuscitation from 'non-shockable' rhythms[17] where robust evidence of efficacy is absent.[18] Nevertheless this may have led to an increase in the number of poor-prognosis patients admitted to ICU (and cooled) with hypoxic–ischaemic encephalopathy.

RESPONSIBILITIES OF THE INTENSIVIST

Most intensivists support deceased-donor organ donation.[19,20] Those few who do not should make arrangements with other intensivist colleagues for the care of potential organ donors and discussions with their families.[21] Intensivists' responsibilities include the care of dying patients and of their families in the intensive care unit (ICU) – where donation occurs. Increasingly other agencies are defining best organ donation practice (and its language and metrics) in utilitarian ways[22] – e.g. 'transforming the greatest possible number of existing cadavers, in any centre, region or country, into real donors'[23] perhaps because intensive care organisations have largely failed to define what constitutes best practice in organ donation and to take responsibility for ensuring that it takes place. Increasingly, the family discussion of organ donation is being strategically planned, including the involvement of 'trained or designated requestors', and framed in ways which encourage, expect or 'nudge' the family to donate while seeking to overcome what are described as 'barriers or objections' to donation.

Regardless of the personnel involved in organ donation processes, intensivists should surely ensure that the processes involved in deceased-donor organ donation, including DCD, are of the highest standard and continue to be seen as such.[21] These processes include the care of the dying patient and their family, determination of death, identification of the potential for organ donation to occur, discussing organ donation with the family, maintenance of physiological stability after brain death throughout the time until organ retrieval, withdrawal of treatment and determination of death in DCD, and aftercare for the family of the deceased irrespective of whether organ donation took place.[21]

CARE OF THE DYING PATIENT AND THEIR FAMILY

Intensivists are familiar with the care of the dying patient, including the need to avoid suffering and maintain patient dignity. The respect of the ICU staff for the humanity of the dying person is expressed in the 'patient comfort care' provided by the nursing staff, the continued involvement and attentiveness of the medical staff, and in evident compassion of all staff for the family.[24]

On behalf of all the treating team, an intensivist should establish rapport during an early meeting (e.g. the morning after admission) with the family of every intensive care patient. This is particularly important for families of patients at high risk of death or disability with whom there will often need to be several 'bad news' meetings over several days. Family meetings should be attended by whomsoever the family defines itself to include, by the intensivist, and by a member of the nursing staff supporting the family (preferably the 'bedside nurse' looking after the patient). If the family wishes, the meeting might include a chaplain, social worker or cultural health worker. The 'support' role should be kept separate from the 'bearer of bad news' role. Family meetings should be held in a separate private room large enough to accommodate all the participants, away from the bedside and protected from interruption. The intensivist should convey an accurate account of the sequence of events, a realistic prognosis (in as much as this is possible) and the immediate treatment plan. There must be enough time for family members to speak[25] for discussion and to ensure that any questions that the family may have are answered. At the end of the meeting the intensivist should ascertain that the family understands what has been said[24] and agrees with the immediate plan. Ensuring that all team members give the family congruent messages is an essential part of maintaining the trust of the family in the ICU team. Ideally, one intensivist should speak with the family but where this is impractical it is vital that there be detailed and explicit discussions between one intensivist and another before the next family meeting. A relationship of mutual understanding and trust will enable the ICU team and the family to work together through difficult and painful issues, including withdrawal of intensive therapies,[26] death of the patient and consideration of organ donation.

Many patients who develop apparent loss of brainstem function do so during a period of active surgical and medical treatment. In these circumstances, brain-oriented intensive therapies (including sedatives, opioids, neuromuscular blockers, hypothermia and osmotherapy) should be withheld pending formal assessment of brain death. In order to meet the preconditions for brain death assessment,[21] extracranial physiological stability must be maintained, and these conditions also preserve the future possibility of organ donation.

Withdrawal of intensive therapies is common practice in ICUs worldwide.[26-28] Before recommending withdrawal of therapy in the setting of severe brain damage it is essential to establish prognosis, to the best extent that this is possible. An unconfounded clinical assessment of CNS function, imaging (usually CT but increasingly supplemented by MRI in some conditions – e.g. diffuse axonal injury) and neurophysiology (in particular short-latency somatosensory evoked potentials) all provide important information. During the period of sedative-free CNS assessment, some patients lose apparent brainstem function. If brain death does not occur but devastating brain damage has clearly occurred, those treating the patient (e.g. intensivists, neurosurgeons and others) should achieve a consensus view of prognosis and a recommended treatment plan, which might include withdrawal of intensive treatments (e.g. artificial airway, ventilatory or inotropic support, further neurosurgery). The intensivist should then discuss the prognosis and a recommended plan with the family and facilitate a consensus. Withdrawal of treatment may subsequently occur, either because death is seen to be imminent and inevitable or because the likely survival outcome would not be in accord with the patient's previously expressed wishes or inferred best interests. It is appropriate to withdraw all intensive therapies from such patients, while continuing to provide 'comfort care' to the patient and support to the family.[29] The possibility of future organ donation must have no influence on a decision to limit or withdraw specific brain-oriented therapies. Some patients having intensive treatments withdrawn will die within a timeframe (e.g. 1–2 hours) that makes DCD a possibility. Prediction of early death after withdrawal of therapy (including extubation) is imprecise but such patients usually have deep coma and impaired brainstem function.[30,31] In these situations it is appropriate to discuss DCD with the patient's family. However, the possibility of DCD must not be raised by the treating team before the family and the treating team have reached a consensus that treatment will be withdrawn.

Increasingly families of dying patients volunteer that they (or the patient) would wish for organ donation to take place, if possible. These views are commonly expressed before the determination of brain death in patients who seem very likely to become or may already be brain dead, but sometimes when the patient still has brainstem function and even prior to a decision that intensive treatments will be withdrawn. The intensivist should sensitively acknowledge these statements and assure the family that this issue will be addressed, without further family prompting, if and when clinical circumstances are appropriate.[21]

IDENTIFICATION OF THE POTENTIAL FOR ORGAN DONATION TO OCCUR

Most ICUs admit ventilated patients with very severe brain damage whose probability of recovery is low. The rationale for this practice is to identify any (small) subgroup of patients with reversible conditions and provide them with the necessary treatment to facilitate their recovery. There are, however, more extreme situations when the chance of recovery is thought so remote that either investigation (CT scanning, usually following intubation and ventilation), active treatment (osmotherapy and emergency surgery) or admission of the patient to ICU[32] would not usually occur.

Some ICUs now routinely admit these patients, either with the rationale that providing them (and their family) with good end-of-life care in an emergency department is not readily achievable, or solely for the possibility that organ donation might subsequently occur. Routinely admitting these patients to ICU has been called for[33] and could probably be expected to increase the number of organs available for transplant,[34] but various ethical, legal and clinical concerns have been raised about such practice.[35–38] Some have suggested that ICU admission should be 'automatic' (without prior family discussion) for these patients while some intensivists admit these patients subject to the informed consent of the family – including an understanding that possible future organ donation is the only reason to admit the patient to ICU, that organ donation might not be possible, and that they are prepared to consider organ donation in the near future should clinical circumstances permit it.

Organ donation is possible in most situations where brain death has been confirmed or when death occurs soon after withdrawal of treatment. The rare absolute contraindications to organ donation are when there is an unacceptably high risk of transmission of disease (usually malignancy or infection) to the recipient, or when the long-term function of all possible donor organs is likely to be unacceptably poor.

Tissue donation (including eyes for corneas and sclera, heart valves and vascular tissue, skin and bone) is also frequently possible in most patients dying in ICUs, including from those who cannot donate organs. Because of the relative benefits and risks to recipients of donated organs and tissues, tissue donation may not be possible in some circumstances where organ donation is acceptable (e.g. low-risk possible food exposure to variant CJD).

Advanced age, most treated bacterial sepsis, treated HSV encephalitis, positive HCV or HBV serology, and some 'apparently cured' malignancies are no longer absolute contraindications. Most extracerebral malignancies and certain infections (e.g. HIV) are likely to remain so, although organs from HIV-positive donors have recently been transplanted into HIV-positive recipients with acceptable outcomes.[39] Similarly, organ-specific relative contraindications to organ donation have reduced as the outcomes of recipients transplanted with donor organs formerly rejected have been found to be acceptable. Finally, all contraindications vary somewhat between transplant centres and continue to change in a more permissive direction. Intensivists should discuss possible absolute and organ-specific contraindications to donation and subsequent transplantation with the appropriate organ donation or procurement agency (who will liaise with transplant services as required) and not decide independently that donation in general or donation of any particular organ is contraindicated on medical grounds. The intensivist should ensure that the information necessary for these decisions is provided (**Box 100.1**).

In most jurisdictions an appropriate authority (e.g. a coroner or medical examiner) may legally interdict organ donation under certain circumstances (e.g. homicide) and this issue must also be clarified before donation proceeds.

DETERMINATION OF BRAIN DEATH

This is a clinical responsibility of the intensivist and must be carried out according to appropriate codes of practice. Although there are no universal criteria for the determination of brain death, codes of practice around

Box 100.1 Information likely to be required by transplant teams

- Age, sex, weight, approximate height
- Medical and social history (including co-morbidity, surgery, medication, alcohol, smoking, illicit drug use, tattoos, body piercing, sexual history and allergies)
- Detailed clinical history of fatal illness (including cause of death, history of cardiac arrest, periods of hypotension or hypoxia, evidence of aspiration or sepsis)
- Current clinical status (including physiological parameters and the extent of ventilatory and inotropic support)
- Current investigations (including blood group, arterial blood gases, chest X-ray, ECG, serum urea, creatinine, electrolytes, glucose, bilirubin, transaminases, alkaline phosphatase and γ-glutamyl transpeptidase, prothrombin ratio, activated partial thromboplastin time, haemoglobin, white cell count, platelets and all microbiology results)
- Other investigations may sometimes be required (e.g. echocardiogram, coronary arteriogram, bronchoscopy)

the world are very similar and all require[21,40,41] (at least) these three elements:

1. Establishing the presence of a condition known to produce severe and irreversible structural brain damage
2. Exclusion of possible confounding factors
3. Determination by clinical examinations (usually by two independent doctors) that there is profound unresponsive coma and persistent absence of brainstem function.

The clinical examination for the determination of brain death is facilitated by a proforma (e.g. the ANZICS protocol[42]), which should be included in the medical record. When clinical examination is not possible (e.g. when it is confounded by medications or when brainstem reflexes cannot be examined), then the absence of cerebral blood flow must instead be demonstrated by reliable imaging.[21]

The intensivist should convey the fact of brain death and its medical and legal implications to the family. It can be difficult to accept brain death as death, given the life-like appearance of the skin, the rise and fall of the chest and the warmth of the hands that are preserved by ventilatory and circulatory support. Some family members will accept an offer to view the clinical examination for brain death (with prior careful explanation of the possibility of spinal reflexes), or the cerebral blood flow study when clinical examination is confounded. This may help some to understand and accept the final awful implication of this diagnosis. Intensivists should be open to offering these options. In the absence of organ donation, it is appropriate to remove ventilatory support after brain death when family needs have been met.

DONATION AFTER CARDIAC DEATH

Donation after cardiac death (DCD), previously known as non-heart-beating donation, is increasing around the world but is not yet worldwide practice. Kootstra and colleagues from Maastricht[43] described four categories of 'non-heart-beating' donors and this classification remains in common use.

- *category I:* those who are dead on arrival
- *category II:* those in whom cardiopulmonary resuscitation is ceased
- *category III:* those in whom cardiac arrest is expect to soon occur
- *category IV:* those who have cardiac arrest while brain dead.

In all but Category III the situation is 'uncontrolled'.[43] DCD practice varies considerably worldwide. Category II donors are most common in the Dutch experience but donation does occur from all categories. Almost all DCD donors in the UK, USA, Canada and Australasia are Category III (and a small number are Category IV). By contrast, in Spain, although withdrawal of treatment in ICU is far less common than in Holland or the UK[44] and Category III donors are rare, most DCD donors are Categories I and II.[45] Recently DCD after euthanasia has been reported, so far only from Belgium.[46]

It is at times asserted about DCD that 'all organ donation occurred this way' before brain death was legally accepted as death, but this assertion ignores real differences between DCD in the modern era and historical organ removal after brain death in the past. The syndrome of brain death had been recognised many years before deceased donation; for example, absent cerebral blood flow was reported in 1956[47] and the clinical syndrome in 1959.[48,49] The final awful meaning of the brain death syndrome ('apnoea, fixed dilated pupils, polyuria, hyperglycaemia and spontaneous hypothermia')[50] was understood by intensivists and nephrologists in the 1960s and 1970s and conveyed to families at that time, before there was a discussion of organ donation (PB Doak, RV Trubuhovich, personal communications). Organ donation was not discussed with the family if some brainstem function (usually only a tracheal reflex) was known to be present. Apnoea despite hypercarbia was not specifically tested for but the shared expectation of the family and the treating team was that the patient would not breathe after withdrawal of ventilatory support (although in fact a few did, for a short time and inadequately). Cardiac arrest usually occurred in 15–20 minutes, at which point the patient was determined to be dead and the kidneys were removed.

There are differences between organ donation after brain death (DBD) and (Category III) DCD that have ethical and clinical consequences. These include that in DCD the patient is known to be alive, and not to be (brain) dead, at the time that organ donation is discussed, may well breathe after extubation and may not die within the timeframe in which organ donation is possible.

The legal, ethical and medical issues raised by DCD have been widely explored.[21,43,51–55] These include ensuring that there has been a consensus decision to withdraw treatment before organ donation is discussed with the family, estimating the likelihood of death soon after withdrawal of treatment, use of agents (e.g. heparin) and procedures (e.g. instrumentation) prior to death that are for 'organ benefit only', the location of withdrawal of treatment (ICU, operating room or other location), presence of family members after withdrawal of treatment, use of opioids and sedatives after withdrawal of treatment, separation of clinical responsibility for end-of-life care (including opioids, sedatives and determination of death) from responsibility for organ procurement, the exact method used for determination of death, the timing of organ removal after death, the procedure to be followed if the patient does not die within a timeframe where donation is possible, ensuring that the family are fully informed and supported throughout the process, ensuring that all participating personnel are familiar with, and accepting of, DCD procedures and ensuring that agreed protocols that explicitly address all of these issues are in place. Several national guidelines or recommendations have been produced that address these issues.[21,54-56] DCD should take place only after broad clinical, ethical and societal consensus has been achieved and expressed in such a document. Where such a measured process has been followed, DCD has been viewed favourably by both families and hospital staff and has modestly increased the number of organs available for transplant.

Delayed graft function is more common in recipients of DCD kidney grafts, but long-term recipient outcomes are equivalent to those who receive a graft from a brain-dead donor.[57] Lower graft and patient survival with DCD liver grafts, compared with DBD grafts, is commonly reported (e.g. 5-year graft survival 52% vs 66%, 5-year patient survival 65% vs 72%),[58] but equivalent outcomes (e.g. 5-year graft survival 83% vs 81%, 5-year patient survival 88% vs 85%)[13] have been achieved where DCD grafts have been used more cautiously. Recipient and graft outcomes after pancreas[59] and lung transplantation[60] from DCD donors are similar to those after DBD. Although successful heart transplantation from DCD donors has been reported, experience is insufficient so far to characterise the long-term recipient outcomes.

DISCUSSION OF ORGAN DONATION WITH THE FAMILY

Organ donation (from deceased donors) is an activity that takes place at the end of life, usually in an ICU. Organ donation is quite separate from transplantation, which is concerned with the care of patients with end-stage organ failure who may receive organ transplants. Appreciating this distinction enables an understanding of important issues that are not often discussed in transplant-oriented publications. Organ donation fundamentally modifies human rituals at the time of death, even of death in the ICU. Organ removal is an invasive procedure carried out in the operating room. Although done respectfully and with identical surgical processes to those used on living people, it is nevertheless viewed by some as 'mutilating'. Discussion of organ donation is an emotionally intense activity involving a newly bereaved family and a health professional, and requires very clear and sensitive communication. This discussion takes place in the midst of grief – when family members are experiencing the death of a family member. Awareness of transplantation varies widely in the community and there is even less knowledge of organ donation processes. Some families may not previously have known that organ donation and transplantation occur! Similarly, discussion of and support for organ donation vary widely in the community. There is greater support of 'organ donation in principle' than either individual willingness to donate or willingness to agree to donation on behalf of a family member. Discussion of organ donation among families is promoted as a way of increasing organ donation rates and it may do so. However, some family members hold strong views against organ donation based on spiritual, religious or cultural beliefs.[61] There are utilitarian views about organ donation including the notion that organ donation is the only possible positive outcome that can occur in the setting of brain death,[62] that it is appropriate to refer to dead or dying persons in a utilitarian way as sources of organs for transplant,[63] that organ donation can 'help the next of kin cope with grief',[64] and that fulfilling the previously expressed wishes of the donor should be the primary or indeed the only[65] consideration. In some jurisdictions these wishes have been deemed legally sufficient for organs to be retrieved, and are often assumed to be a means of increasing the organ donation rate[66] by excluding the family from the opportunity to prohibit organ donation and 'returning control to the individual'. This assumption may well be erroneous.[67,68] Many countries have defined the status of an individual's wishes about organ donation after their death as constituting legally sufficient 'consent'. However, the validity of the concept of 'consent' can be questioned as the person is dead at the time that the issue is real and because it is unlikely that current 'register-based' records of such wishes meet accepted standards for informed consent[69] in a personal healthcare context.[70] Implicit in a 'transplant-oriented' value system is the view that for a family to agree to organ donation is both desirable and of greater moral value ('the right thing to do') than the contrary decision, particularly if organ donation was the previously expressed wish of the dead person. This view, in which close family relationships[71] give no legitimacy to the family to determine what should happen to their loved one after death, is now explicitly acknowledged, practised and advocated by many USA organ procurement organisations (e.g. S Gunderson, personal communication). Similar views are increasingly expressed in the UK and Australia. Even in countries that legally allow the previously expressed wishes of the deceased to determine whether organ donation may take place, usual practice continues to both involve the family and not to proceed against family objection – accepting that the impact on the deceased's family is the most important factor determining consent practice.[72] However, in many countries this has resulted in the evolution, exposition and advocacy of strategies to overcome 'refusal to donate'[73] and to thereby achieve 'target conversion rates'. Possible adverse effects of such strategies on family bereavement[74] are not reported by those who advocate for them and whose sole measure of 'quality' or 'success' in organ donation practice is the proportion of situations in which donation occurs. Intensivists should reflect on their own views on these matters, and be aware of the views of others who might discuss organ donation with family members.

Although intensivists most often initiate discussion of organ donation with families in Australasia, this is increasingly unusual elsewhere. Whoever undertakes this discussion should be skilled in communication with grieving people. In Australasian clinical practice, the intensivist has already established a relationship with the family, involving mutual trust and respect, in prior family meetings during the patient's final illness. This relationship naturally allows the intensivist to initiate and facilitate discussion of organ donation. Describing this encounter as 'discussing organ donation' rather than 'obtaining consent' (or 'seeking consent' or even 'persuasion'[75]) is not 'organ focused' or coercive in language and enables the intensivist to provide complete and unbiased information, support the family in their decision making and thank them for their consideration, whatever they might decide about donation.

The intensivist must ensure that the fact of death (in the situation of brain death) is understood. When (Category III) DCD is a possibility, there must be prior consensus agreement by the family and the treating team that treatment must be withdrawn before the option of possible organ donation is raised by the intensivist. The patient is clearly not dead at this time, although death is certainly anticipated to be imminent. This imminent death should also be understood by the family before the option of DCD is offered. In either situation there must be sufficient time for the intensivist to inform the family about what organ donation entails (including the subsequent benefits to transplant recipients of those organs), to answer any questions and if necessary to facilitate decision making by the family. The discussion may take into account previously expressed wishes, previous family discussions, values and beliefs of the patient and of family members. Some language is particularly insensitive from the perspective of grieving families and should be avoided[21] (e.g. the use of the term 'harvest' rather than 'organ retrieval' to describe the process of organ retrieval, or 'the body' rather than the person's name to describe the brain-dead person).

Increasingly, intensivists are being expected to facilitate the involvement of other people in this discussion – including members of organ procurement agencies and others with specific training about this discussion – with the implicit or explicit aim of 'increasing the consent rate' – most commonly to a 'target' of ~75%.[76] Various models are advocated including 'collaborative requesting', where both ICU staff and others are involved and the 'designated or trained requestor' model wherein ICU staff introduce the 'requestor' and take no part in the discussion of donation. Highly explicit strategic plans have been developed, most notably in the US, to achieve 'target consent rates'. Although such an approach has been reported to 'increase organ donation' in non-randomised time series and other observational studies,[77,78] this was not found in the only randomised study of 'collaborative requesting' so far conducted.[79] 'Repeated requesting' has been reported to increase the number of families who agree to donate and language that is variously persuasive or coercive (e.g. 'fulfilling the deceased's wishes', 'doing what he would have wanted', 'something good may come of this', 'many families take comfort in donation', 'there are many people dying on waiting lists, including in your community') might also achieve that utilitarian objective. Despite the moral distress of many intensivists, including this author, arising in response to strategic plans that, for example, 'help staff overcome obstacles, plan re-approaches, address family needs and concerns, and ensure consistency and quality in their vigorous pursuit of donation',[80] it is increasingly evident that 'conversion-rate'-focused approaches are coming to dominate the discussion of donation with families.

The intensivist should facilitate the family spending time at the bedside prior to organ removal if they wish. Some investigations (e.g. echocardiography or bronchoscopy) may be performed during this time and the family should be informed about these. The intensivist should ensure that the family is offered the opportunity to spend time with the deceased after organ removal.

MAINTENANCE OF EXTRACEREBRAL PHYSIOLOGICAL STABILITY IN BRAIN DEATH

Immediately prior to brain death there is often a limited period of hypertension, tachycardia and occasionally dysrhythmia, mediated by both autonomic activity and catecholamine secretion. Pulmonary oedema, cardiac dysfunction and myocardial injury may develop and may have implications for subsequent heart and lung graft function.[81] Treatment of this temporary sympathetic phenomenon should preferably be with short-acting beta blocker (esmolol). Cardiac arrest can rarely occur during this phase, usually due to tachydysrhythmia, but is often reversible. Hypertension is soon followed by hypotension (which may be profound in the presence of hypovolaemia or cardiac dysfunction) and can lead to cardiac arrest or loss of donor organ viability. Blood pressure should be maintained (e.g. MAP ~70 mmHg (9.31 kPa)) with inotropic support and volume expansion. Diabetes insipidus soon occurs in most but not all brain-dead persons, manifest by brisk hypo-osmolar polyuria, leading quickly to hyperosmolality and later to hypovolaemia if untreated. Other hormone abnormalities do not have therapeutic implications.[82]

After loss of cerebral metabolism there is a fall of around 25% in oxygen consumption and carbon dioxide production[83] so that less ventilatory minute volume is necessary for normocarbia. The fall in energy expenditure (heat production) together with the loss of vasomotor tone and loss of possible thermogenesis from shivering exacerbate the risk of hypothermia.

Spontaneous movements and spinal motor reflexes commonly persist in brain death.[21] These rarely include bizarre movements,[21] which are often reproducible. Family members may be offered the opportunity to view the (perhaps second) clinical examination for brain death and should be warned about the possibility of these responses (which may not have occurred at the first examination) and given a prior explanation of them. These movements and sympathetic circulatory responses can also occur during organ retrieval in the operating room. The use of neuromuscular blockade and opioids is recommended in the operating room.[21]

STRATEGIES FOR MAINTAINING PHYSIOLOGICAL STABILITY

The onset of brain death is usually heralded by rises in intracranial pressure (if measured), hypertension and tachycardia, and progressive loss of brainstem function (coma, pupillary dilatation). These features should initiate preparation for specific support strategies, which include ensuring that central venous access, inotropic support, intravenous access for rapid volume expansion, DDAVP and a source of external heat (e.g. a warming blanket) are all available.

VENTILATORY MANAGEMENT

The aims of ventilatory management are to maintain good oxygenation and normocarbia, minimise circulatory depression and maintain, if possible, sufficiently good lung function to allow for future lung donation to occur. Usual pulmonary care including changes of position and sterile endotracheal suctioning must continue. When pulmonary dysfunction is severe, high levels of PEEP may be required to prevent airway frothing or provide adequate oxygenation. Establishing that there is apnoea at hypercarbia in such patients may require mechanical hypoventilation prior to apnoea and CPAP during it. Compared with a conventional ventilatory strategy, the use of a lung-protective strategy (including tidal volumes of 6–8 mL/kg of predicted body weight, PEEP of 8–10 cm H_2O, testing for apnoea on CPAP rather than at zero end-expiratory pressure, and closed-circuit airway suction) has been shown in a randomised controlled trial to increase the number of potential lung donors meeting suitability criteria at 6 hours (32/59 conventional vs 56/59 protective, $p<0.001$) and the number of actual lung donors (16/59 conventional vs 32/59 protective, $p=0.004$) with similar 6-month recipient survival (11/16 conventional vs 24/32 protective, not significant (NS)).[84] In a matched cohort study, oxygenation impairment remained 2 hours after an apnoea test at zero end-expiratory pressure but a recruitment manoeuvre immediately after the apnoea test was associated with no such impairment.[85] Although a Pa_{O_2} of more than 300–350 mmHg (40–46.5 kPa) on 100% oxygen and 5 cmH_2O PEEP was once thought essential for lung donation, lower Pa_{O_2}/Fi_{O_2} ratios (and higher PEEP) have been found acceptable[86] and some transplant centres have used ECMO to support (including electively) recipients of lungs with more serious but reversible impairment with acceptable outcomes.[87]

CIRCULATORY AND METABOLIC MANAGEMENT

The aims of circulatory management are to maintain adequate organ perfusion and arterial pressure without fluid overload or harmful vasoconstriction, and without prejudicing cardiac donation where this might be possible. Reasonable initial haemodynamic goals include normotension (e.g. MAP >70 mmHg (9.31 kPa)), heart rate of <100 beats per minute, and central venous pressure of ~8 mmHg (1.06 kPa). Some inotropic support is usually required. Having established normotension with an inotrope infusion, the haemodynamic response to a volume challenge should be assessed. The choice of inotrope is the subject of more controversy than evidence. Dobutamine is not recommended. Norepinephrine (noradrenaline), usually less than 500 µg/h, is preferred in Australasia (e.g. 85% of the 375 donors in 2011 in Australia and New Zealand received norepinephrine)[13] without apparent harm to organ function in recipients. Dopamine is not commonly used in Australasia (3% of 375 donors in 2011).[13] Low-dose dopamine infusion (4 µg/kg/min) has been shown in a randomised controlled trial to slightly increase urine volume (208±140 mL/h vs 178±106 mL/h, $p=0.009$) but without any effect on serum creatinine (0.82±0.29 vs 0.84±0.27 mg/dL).[88] Dopamine infusion (for ~6 hours in the donor) was associated with a slight reduction in the number of recipients receiving multiple dialyses before renal function recovered (56/227 [24.7%; 95% CI, 19.0–30.3%] vs 92/260 [35.4%; 95% CI, 29.5–41.2%]; $p=0.01$).[88] Epinephrine (adrenaline) may have specific benefit on renal blood flow in brain death,[89] but may also increase glycaemia and thereby osmotic diuresis. Catecholamine infusion may reduce the up-regulation of organ immunogenicity that occurs in brain death and lower the incidence of acute rejection in subsequent recipients of kidney grafts.[90] Although levels of thyroid hormones fall after brain death, this is probably the 'sick euthyroid syndrome' and replacement of thyroid hormone does not improve the circulation after brain death.[82] Importantly, and with more general cautionary value, this recent systematic review of the use of thyroid hormones found that benefit was shown in all 16 separate case series or retrospective audits but in none of the seven randomised controlled trials.[82] Corticosteroids are often given just prior to organ removal from brain-dead donors and commonly recommended (on the basis of retrospective analyses) to increase the number of organs, particularly thoracic organs, retrieved and transplanted. Although steroids improve haemodynamics in an experimental model,[91] an early randomised human study[92] did not show any benefit in kidney graft outcomes. A more recent study showed that treatment of brain dead liver donors with methylprednisolone (~1.6 g over ~14 hours) did not alter the use of fluids and catecholamines compared with a no-steroid group, but was associated with lower serum levels of inflammatory cytokines in the donors, lower recipient transaminase levels in the early post-transplant period and a somewhat reduced incidence of acute rejection within 6 months (11/50 vs 19/50, $p<0.05$).[93] Two trials of the combination of steroid and tri-iodothyronine (T_3) similarly did not show beneficial circulatory effects.[94,95] Vasopressin infusion can eliminate or substantially reduce the amount of catecholamine required to support arterial pressure[95,96] without apparent detriment to subsequently transplanted organs. Control of excessive polyuria will minimise the risks of developing hyperosmolality, hypovolaemia or hyperglycaemia secondary to infusion of large amounts of dextrose-containing fluids. Synthetic desmopressin (1-D amino-8 D arginine vasopressin) is commonly given to control diabetes insipidus and appears safe and effective.[13,97] Control of diabetes insipidus is an essential aspect of rational fluid therapy, and hypovolaemia should be corrected with resuscitation fluids. Advocacy continues for use of so-called 'hormonal resuscitation'[98] (combined use of T_3, steroid and vasopressin) on the basis of reports using retrospective analysis with multiple logistic regression,[99,100] despite the negative findings of a randomised controlled trial in 80 potential cardiac donors.[95] This study did show that haemodynamic improvement occurs with time after brain death and that 14/40 hearts initially considered unsuitable for transplant were suitable 6 hours later, suggesting that a determination of unsuitability for heart donation should not be made early after brain death.

Haemoconcentration occurs early after experimental brain death. Crystalloid infusion has been reported to worsen pulmonary function in brain death and somewhat larger volumes will be required than if colloid is used.[101] At least moderate anaemia is well tolerated in brain death, but red cells may be given if needed to maintain packed cell volume at around 0.25 pending organ retrieval. Free water should be given as necessary (1–2 mL/kg per hour as 5% dextrose) to maintain serum osmolality in the range of 280–310 mOsm/kg, corresponding to serum sodium below 155 mmol/L. Severe hyperosmolality (probably a marker of inadequate donor care) is associated with poor graft function in subsequent liver recipients.[102] Low-dose insulin infusion is commonly required (e.g. 41% of 375 donors in Australia and New Zealand in 2011)[13] to prevent hyperglycaemia. Failure to control diabetes insipidus will lead to increased requirements of free water to control serum osmolality and if large amounts of 5% dextrose are used for this then hyperglycaemia and osmotic diuresis may result. Serum potassium should be kept above 3.5 mmol/L, but correction of hypophosphataemia does not improve haemodynamics in brain death.[103]

Oxygen consumption, carbon dioxide production, heat production and glucose oxidation all fall in brain death owing to the loss of cerebral metabolic activity.[83] Hypothermia may readily develop in association with vasoparesis, loss of shivering, exposure to room temperature, warm polyuria and infusion of room temperature intravenous fluids. Core temperature should be kept above the 35–36.5°C required to confirm brain death.[21] Keeping the ambient temperature high (24°C) and using infusion fluid warmers, heated humidifiers and external warming systems may be required.

AFTERCARE OF THE DONOR FAMILY

Routine aftercare is increasingly recommended[104] for all families of patients who die in ICUs. Aftercare programmes are well received[24] and have the potential to improve the care of subsequent families by revealing areas of inadequate or inappropriate communication. There may be issues specific to organ donation that need to be addressed, sometimes by way of a family meeting with an intensivist at some later stage. Most organ donation agencies provide donor families with ongoing emotional support (which may extend over many years), provide them with limited anonymous information about recipients, and accept and facilitate limited anonymous communication (i.e. by letter) between recipients and donor families by mutual consent; direct contact is not recommended.[21]

Access the complete references list online at http://www.expertconsult.com

1. Sayegh MH, Carpenter CB. Transplantation 50 years later – progress, challenges, and promises. N Engl J Med 2004;351(26):2761–6.
6. International Summit on Transplant Tourism and Organ Trafficking. The Declaration of Istanbul on Organ Trafficking and Transplant Tourism. Clin J Am Soc Nephrol 2008;3(5):1227–31.
19. Pearson IY, Zurynski Y. A survey of personal and professional attitudes of intensivists to organ donation and transplantation. Anaesth Intensive Care 1995;23:68–74.
21. Australian and New Zealand Intensive Care Society. The ANZICS Statement on Death and Organ Donation. 3.1 ed. Melbourne: ANZICS; 2010. Online. Available: http://www.anzics.com.au/downloads/doc_download/399-anzics-statement-on-death-and-organ-donation-edition-31 (Accessed December 6th 2012).

31. Rabinstein AA, Yee AH, Mandrekar J, et al. Prediction of potential for organ donation after cardiac death in patients in neurocritical state: a prospective observational study. Lancet Neurol 2012;11(5):414–19.
55. Shemie SD, Baker AJ, Knoll G, et al. National recommendations for donation after cardiocirculatory death in Canada: donation after cardiocirculatory death in Canada. CMAJ 2006;175:S1.
56. Bernat JL, D'Alessandro AM, Port FK, et al. Report of a national conference on donation after cardiac death. Am J Transplant 2006;6:281–91.
69. Woien S, Rady MY, Verheijde JL, et al. Organ procurement organizations Internet enrolment for organ donation: abandoning informed consent. BMC Med Ethics 2006;7:E14.
79. ACRE Trial Collaborators. Effect of 'collaborative requesting' on consent rate for organ donation: randomised controlled trial (ACRE trial). BMJ 2009;339:b3911.
82. Macdonald PS, Aneman A, Bhonagiri D, et al. A systematic review and meta-analysis of clinical trials of thyroid hormone administration to brain dead potential organ donors. Crit Care Med 2012;40(5):1635–44.

101

Liver transplantation

Anish Gupta, Simon Cottam and Julia Wendon

Liver transplantation has revolutionised the care of patients, with both acute and chronic end-stage liver disease. It has become an almost routine procedure, with the majority of patients having a short postoperative intensive care unit (ICU) stay and 1-year survival >90%.[1–4] Indications have widened, and contraindications decreased. As a consequence, the number of patients awaiting transplantation continues to outstrip cadaveric donor rates; waiting times lengthen, hence patients become critically ill before receiving a transplant, increasing risk and perioperative complications, and impairing long-term outcome.[5] Innovative strategies have evolved as possible solutions to the lack of cadaveric donor organs, including widening the donor pool to include previously unsuitable donors (so-called marginal donors), paediatric and adult living-related donation, reduced size and splitting techniques and the use of 'non-heart-beating donation'.

PATIENT SELECTION

There are currently relatively few absolute contraindications to liver transplantation and no specific age limitation. Listing requires a multidisciplinary consensus of a 50% chance of 5-year survival once all risks are considered. Donor organs are preciously scarce, and allocation principles must therefore take into account the severity of the recipient's condition and the perioperative risk profile. Portopulmonary and hepatopulmonary syndromes are now an active indication for transplantation as opposed to a contraindication.[6] Such patients are likely to have a more complex postoperative course, especially if graft function is borderline or they develop sepsis. Patients must have the required cardiorespiratory reserve to tolerate the procedure. Guidelines are available in regard to hepatocellular carcinoma and liver transplantation.[7,8] Such patients increasingly, if not inevitably, require disease-modifying treatments (transarterial chemoembolisation and radio-frequency ablation). Periodic imaging of the liver is mandatory to monitor disease progression whilst waiting for a suitable cadaveric donor.

Much work has gone into the development of prognostic tools to allow accurate prediction of the need and timing for transplantation, and increasingly the system used is the model for end-stage liver disease (MELD). This was initially developed for predicting survival following transjugular intrahepatic portosystemic shunt (TIPS), but has been shown to be equally useful in predicting survival in those awaiting liver transplantation. Survival depends on the physiological reserve of the recipient and the quality of the donor organ. Cardiovascular 'fitness' should remain the key determinant for receiving high-risk donor organs, which are increasingly used in order to match demand. Perioperative outcome scoring systems are becoming more robust (survival outcomes following liver transplantation (SOFT) and balance of risk score (BAR)), but are still limited to specific types of donor organs and are often disease-non-specific.[9,10] Once multi-organ failure has developed in a debilitated patient awaiting transplantation, survival rates decrease to 20–30% and these patients often require weeks to months of postoperative hospitalisation.[2,11]

Cardiorespiratory function requires detailed assessment prior to listing. There is not one specific test that will determine fitness for transplantation; however, a combination of routine blood tests, CT imaging, ECG, echocardiography, cardiopulmonary exercise testing and brain imaging if encephalopathy is a feature serves as a minimum. CT imaging may uncover underlying pulmonary pathology as well as any coronary calcification (a weak predictor of critical ischaemia). Cardiopulmonary exercise testing promulgates invaluable information of the cardiac, pulmonary and skeletal muscle-mitochondrial unit. In addition to providing dynamic information on these systems, we are able to gauge the β-adrenoceptor response and the peak oxygen consumption, which has some proven prognostic value.[12] The anaerobic threshold is frequently discussed, but is subject to major limitations – anaemia, smoking, beta-blocker therapy, exercise tolerance prior to illness, cirrhotic cardiomyopathy and hepatorenal disease. This test is not validated as a discriminator for accurately determining success in the perioperative period, but forms an integral part of each assessment. Cardiovascular disease is the third commonest cause of death following liver transplantation, after disease recurrence/chronic rejection and malignancy. The risk factors for coronary artery disease require scrupulous investigation prior to listing, particularly as obesity and diabetes may develop post-transplantation, further increasing cardiac risk. Angiography and carotid Doppler studies must form part of the additional work-up in those patients with multiple risk factors.

Obesity is an increasingly common feature in patients listed for transplantation, and non-alcoholic steatohepatitis is the only indication for transplantation that is rising in frequency, soon to be the leading indication. The associated co-morbidities need to be quantified, and the overall risk profile cautiously considered prior to listing. Postoperative complications including infection, wound dehiscence, and ventilator dependency are more prevalent, with cardiovascular complications the main cause for mortality. Obese patients with diabetes or coronary artery disease are 40% less likely to reach 5-year survival.[13] However, even transplanted obese patients show a survival benefit over those on the waiting list despite their higher complication rate, and this provides a difficult ethical debate over resource allocation.[14] There are no thresholds in body mass index for listing. Optimisation prior to surgery should focus on controlling medical co-morbidities as well as weight loss and dietary changes.[15]

HEPATIC SYNDROMES

Changes in the cardiovascular system associated with chronic liver disease may contribute to the spectrum of cardiopulmonary disease associated with chronic liver disease and portal hypertension. A hyperdynamic state with high cardiac output, long-standing portal hypertension with the development of collateral flows, together with an imbalance of vasoactive mediators either synthesised or metabolised by the liver, may lead to characteristic changes in both flow and pressure through the pulmonary vasculature. This may be associated with hypoxia and orthodeoxia. Two ends of the spectrum are hepatopulmonary syndrome (HPS) and portopulmonary hypertension (PPH). The two conditions are uncommon but important, as they have vastly different impacts on risk associated with liver transplantation and long-term outcome (**Table 101.1**). The role of agents used in the management of primary pulmonary hypertension is yet to be examined in a controlled manner in liver disease, but data thus far suggest benefit.

HEPATOPULMONARY SYNDROME

HPS is present in approximately 20% of cirrhotic patients. It can be seen from Table 101.1 that hypoxia is a characteristic finding in this condition. It results from intrapulmonary vascular dilatation at the pre- and post-capillary level, leading to decreased ventilation/perfusion ratios; more uncommonly, anatomical shunt is present with arteriovenous communication. One of the postulated mechanisms of this vasodilatation is overactivity of pulmonary vasculature nitric oxide synthetase; pre-transplant patients have raised levels of exhaled nitric oxide that decrease post transplant with resolution of the syndrome. Diagnosis is confirmed by contrast-enhanced echocardiography or radionuclide lung perfusion scanning. Medical treatment of the syndrome has been disappointing; indeed, most transplant centres agree that the syndrome is an indication for transplantation in itself, as resolution is reported in up to 85% after transplantation.[16] Risk stratification based on severity is important, as vastly increased peri-transplant mortality is associated with severe hypoxia and high levels of vascular shunt. Severe hypoxia qualifies for MELD exception prioritisation. Mortality overall is 16% at 90 days and 38% at 1 year. Predictors of mortality in this group are severe hypoxia (Pa_{O_2}<6.5 kPa (<50 mmHg)) and shunt fraction >20%.[16] Refractory hypoxia is the indirect cause of death, which may be due to multi-organ failure, intracerebral haemorrhage and sepsis due to bile leaks. Whilst it is true that the recipient's organs are conditioned to function in the chronic pre-operative hypoxic state, the liver graft must be protected from hypoxia immediately following transplantation, with a gradual weaning of oxygen levels. Resolution of the syndrome is variable and can take up to 1 year, lending support to the theory that it is vascular remodelling rather than just acute reversal of vasodilatation that reverses hypoxia.[17,18]

Table 101.1 Diagnostic criteria for hepatopulmonary syndrome and portopulmonary hypertension

HEPATOPULMONARY SYNDROME	PORTOPULMONARY HYPERTENSION
Chronic liver disease (±cirrhosis)	Portal hypertension
Arterial hypoxaemia	Mean pulmonary artery pressure >25 mmHg (3.33 kPa)
PaO_2<75 mmHg (10 kPa) or A–a O_2 gradient >20 mmHg (2.66 kPa)	Pulmonary artery occlusion pressure <15 mmHg (2 kPa)
Intrapulmonary vascular dilatation	Pulmonary vascular resistance >120 dynes/s per cm^{-5}

PORTOPULMONARY HYPERTENSION

Up to 20% of pre-transplant patients have pulmonary hypertension; this probably constitutes increased flow through the pulmonary vasculature and is not associated with increased resistance. These patients do well after transplantation. A much more ominous syndrome is the presence of pulmonary hypertension with high pulmonary vascular resistance (seen in <4%). The aetiology of this syndrome is complex but it is characterised by a hyperdynamic high flow state with excess central volume and non-embolic pulmonary vasoconstriction. The pathological changes associated with this syndrome match those associated with primary pulmonary hypertension except that cardiac output is high in this group.

In comparison with HPS, there are several differences in terms of response to medical treatment and outcome after transplantation. The response to epoprostenol, a PGI_2 analogue, is encouraging. Decreases in pulmonary artery pressure but more importantly transpulmonary gradient (TPG) have been noted, although at least 3 months' treatment seems necessary, suggesting remodelling rather than vasodilatation is the important mechanism. A limiting factor in the treatment may also be progressive thrombocytopenia and splenomegaly. Endothelin receptor antagonists (bosentan, ambrisentan) have been shown to almost normalise PVR in selected patients by blocking the vascular reactivity of the pulmonary vascular bed. Phosphodiesterase inhibitors (e.g. sildenafil) increase the availability of nitric oxide within the pulmonary vasculature. These oral agents hold some advantage for outpatient management; however, intravenous prostacyclin remains the treatment of choice in severe cases.[19]

Another difference is the perioperative risk and post-transplant prognosis. Resolution is not associated with transplantation and progression can be a feature. Perioperatively, the higher the mean pulmonary artery pressure (MPAP), pulmonary vascular resistance (PVR) and TPG the greater is the risk of death, which is usually due to acute right ventricular decompensation. Right heart pressures need to be closely monitored with pulmonary artery catheterisation preferably commenced preoperatively to establish prostacyclin infusion. Milrinone may be added to gain further control of pulmonary pressures in the perioperative process. TOE monitoring provides invaluable assessment of right heart function, and enables more accurate volume replacement during reperfusion. If the MPAP is >35 mmHg (4.66 kPa) or the PVR is >250 dyne/s per cm (250 mN/m), mortality reaches 40%. If MPAP is >50 mmHg (6.66 kPa) some have even suggested delisting or even intraoperative cancellation as the mortality may be as high as 100%.[20] Intravenous pulmonary vasodilators are usually weaned to oral medications, which about half will require long term. Resolution in the remaining half occurs over several months.[19]

HEPATORENAL SYNDROME

Hepatorenal syndrome (HRS) is a potentially reversible cause of renal dysfunction in a small proportion of acute kidney injury (AKI) cases with cirrhosis. Two subtypes exist: type 1 results in acute renal deterioration following a precipitating event (sepsis, post-paracentesis syndrome), whereas type 2 is a progressive form occurring over weeks. It represents an advanced stage of haemodynamic dysfunction, characterised by splanchnic vasodilatation, reduced systemic vascular resistance and reduced effective arterial blood volume. This contraction in central blood volume stimulates a powerful neuroendocrine response mimicking volume depletion and predisposing to prerenal failure (hepatorenal syndrome).[21] The diagnosis is essentially one of exclusion in a patient with cirrhosis (**Box 101.1**).[22] The prognosis of HRS is poor with the worst survival rates out of all the causes of AKI (3-month survival for type 1 is 20%, and type 2 is 40%). Vasoconstrictor agents, albumin, transjugular intrahepatic portosystemic shunts and improved antimicrobial therapy have all proven benefits in serving as a bridge to transplantation.

Box 101.1 Diagnostic criteria for hepatorenal syndrome[22]

- Cirrhosis with ascites
- Serum creatinine >133 µmol/L (1.5 mg/L)
- No improvement in serum creatinine (to <133 µmol/L) after 2 days of diuretic withdrawal and albumin replacement (1 g/kg per day or maximum 100 g/day)
- Absence of shock
- Absence of nephrotoxic drugs
- Absence of renal parenchymal disease

Transplantation is the only treatment for HRS, with normalisation of sodium excretion, serum creatinine and neurohormonal levels occurring within 1 month. The renal vasoconstrictive indices require 12 months before recovering. HRS does increase the complication rate and reduce survival following transplantation, with renal function never recovering in up to 25%. Those on renal replacement therapy for more than 8 weeks prior to transplantation should be offered combined liver–kidney transplantation. Interestingly, the risk of acute rejection for combined liver–kidney grafts is the same as for liver transplantation, as compared with the higher rate of rejection that is seen for renal transplant alone.[22-24]

EXTRACORPOREAL HEPATIC SUPPORT

The liver has metabolic, excretory and synthetic functions, all of which need to be maintained in a patient who has liver failure until either an organ becomes available or regeneration takes place. Two groups of devices are available; purely mechanical devices provide detoxification whereas bioartificial devices, which require an abundant source of hepatocytes, also provide synthetic and biotransformation activities. Artificial devices include plasma exchange and albumin dialysis, which may incorporate extracorporeal albumin dialysis (MARS (molecular adsorbents recirculating system, Gambro)) or fractionated plasma separation and absorption (Prometheus). Clinical trials are in progress to evaluate the place for these devices. To date, none of these artificial devices has conferred a survival benefit in liver failure in prospective randomised trials, though there has been some success with improvements in neurological status and reduced cerebral oedema.[25-27] Bioartificial devices suffer from limited hepatocyte supply and prospective clinical trials conveying survival benefits, though some early results may prove promising. In addition to efficacy, still to be elucidated is the timescale over which these devices can be used and whether they can bridge the gap to regeneration, thus sparing the patient from transplantation.

PERIOPERATIVE ASPECTS

OPERATIVE TECHNIQUE

Orthotopic liver transplantation (OLT) involves recipient hepatectomy, revascularisation of the donor graft and biliary reconstruction. Two main techniques are used in adult liver transplantation: those with vena cava preservation ('piggyback technique') and those using portal bypass (either internal, temporary portocaval shunt or external, veno-venous bypass). The advantages of the piggyback technique include haemodynamic stability during the anhepatic phase, without large-volume fluid administration, and the negation of the need for veno-venous bypass with its associated risks and complications. Decreased transfusion requirements, shorter anhepatic time and shorter total operating time are also observed. There is no observed difference in renal function between the two techniques.[28-30] The donor hepatic artery is directly anastomosed, utilising an 'end-to-end' technique, or a conduit is constructed. Portal venous anastomosis must also be undertaken; in most patients this is an end-to-end anastomosis. Portal venous thrombosis is no longer a contraindication to transplantation and these patients may undergo a recannulisation procedure or require a jump graft technique. Such conduits and grafts are normally fashioned from donor vessels.

It is imperative that all those caring for the patients are aware of the surgical technique undertaken, as complications may vary. The radiologist must be aware of the technique used to allow appropriate interpretation of subsequent investigations and vascular imaging. This applies not just to the vascular anastomosis but also to the presence of a full graft, reduced size graft, right or left split graft or indeed an auxiliary graft. The biliary anastomosis is normally also undertaken as an end-to-end procedure, the donor bile duct being directly joined to the recipient duct. It is no longer standard for this to be undertaken over a T-tube, but this may be required where there is marked discrepancy between donor and recipient duct size. Some conditions (e.g. extrahepatic biliary atresia, primary sclerosing cholangitis) may preclude end-to-end anastomosis and formation of choledochojejunostomy may be required.

Split-liver grafts allow one liver to provide an organ for two recipients. Initially comprised of a child receiving the left lateral segment and an adult the remaining liver, nowadays two adults may receive grafts from one liver if the anatomy and size match allow. Such splits may be less than ideal when the recipient has a high MELD score, as is increasingly the case with the prioritisation of sick patients awaiting liver grafts. Such grafts are at increased risk of postoperative complications such as bile leaks and haematoma/collections at the cut surface.[3,31]

Auxiliary liver transplantation is a technique that involves subtotal recipient hepatectomy and implantation of a reduced size graft. It is a technically difficult procedure, as both portal and arterial supplies have to be constructed de novo. In addition, a duplicate biliary drainage system needs to be constructed. Hepatic venous outflow is anastomosed as usual. In acute liver failure, it has significant potential, since regeneration of the native liver may obviate the need for donor function, potentially allowing withdrawal of immunosuppression. It also has application in the treatment of some hereditary metabolic disorders where adequate metabolic function may be achieved with an auxiliary graft. The major advantage is withdrawal of immunosuppressive therapy if the patient develops severe complications, or when applicable gene therapy becomes available. The disadvantage of auxiliary transplantation in the face of acute liver failure is that the postoperative course is frequently more complicated; reasons are multifactorial, and failure can be due to the continued presence of a regenerating native liver or due to a smaller donor graft attempting to cope with a critical illness.

Non-heart beating transplantation (NHBD) has emerged in recent times as a potential way of increasing organs for transplantation.[32,33] The success in renal transplantation has led to exploration of its application in the fields of liver, pancreas and lung retrieval. Most retrievals are undertaken in the context of controlled NHBD (i.e. in the context of planned withdrawal of care). Warm ischaemia can be accurately assessed and cold ischaemia minimised. Early experience with NHBD was associated with inferior survival for patients and grafts but recent experience suggests that survival is approaching that for heart-beating donation. There are, however, continuing concerns over biliary and vascular complications. Prolonged cold ischaemia is associated with poor graft function and biliary complications, as are warm ischaemia times of greater than 30 minutes.[34] With regard to postoperative care, an understanding of the pre- and perioperative factors is essential in anticipating potential complications, initiation of monitoring and proactive management.

Living donor-related transplantation (LDRT) is now a routine undertaking in paediatric liver transplantation. It is becoming increasingly utilised in adult liver transplantation although its application in countries with good cadaveric donor pools is less established. Adult LDRT using right lobe grafts is an effective procedure with good survival outcomes, but is associated with significant complications. From a postoperative perspective the intensive care team may be responsible for the management of both the donor and the recipient. Morbidity rates for donors are significantly higher with use of a right lobe donation compared with a left lobe graft. Mortality for donors has been reported. Survival rates now reported for living related recipients are good, with rates of 80% at 12 months.[35,36]

Adequate function of undersized transplanted liver grafts is essential to successful outcome. Primary graft non-function is relatively rare and one of the main areas of concern is that of the so-called 'small for size syndrome'.[35,37] This was first recognised in the post-transplant setting but also occurs following liver resection. It is still an area under discussion but the clinical entity is that of hyperbilirubinaemia, graft dysfunction, ascites and portal hypertension with associated end-organ dysfunction/failure. The clinical picture is that of portal hyperaemia, with portal flow passing into a small liver remnant/graft with associated pathophysiological consequences, and at a histological level there is evidence of arteriolar constriction. In some patients consideration should also be given to the potential compounder of hepatic venous outflow limitation.[38,39] Other factors that predispose to the syndrome are an inappropriate graft weight to recipient and steatotic grafts. In regard of management of this syndrome most trials have focused on optimising venous outflow and limiting/preventing portal hyperaemia and limiting portal hypertension.[35,40] Animal studies have also examined the role of intrahepatic vasodilators with good effect. Management of the syndrome remains controversial but its early consideration allows the clinical team time to consider therapeutic options and interventions.

INTRAOPERATIVE MONITORING

In addition to routine monitors, invasive arterial blood pressure and central venous pressure measurements are invaluable. With modern advances in technology, it has now become routine practice to use some method of cardiac output monitoring. The trends in stroke volume variation and cardiac index can be used as a guide to fluid delivery, and to help gauge requirements for vasopressors and inotropes. The use of transoesophageal echocardiography (TOE) is often reserved for patients with known pulmonary hypertension, though this is gradually being used more frequently to assess fluid status, regional wall motion abnormalities, the presence of intracardiac thrombi, and even to locate the position and patency of transjugular intrahepatic portosystemic shunts (TIPS).[41,42]

FLUIDS, HAEMORRHAGE AND COAGULATION

There is no consensus on the amount or type of fluid that should be used during liver transplantation. The centrally deplete fluid compartment, if aggressively filled, will rapidly redistribute to the peripheral and portal circulation, exacerbating haemorrhage.[43] Incremental volume replacement is the key, ideally guided by some form of flow monitoring. Large volumes of crystalloids must be avoided to prevent excessive interstitial oedema. The choice of colloid remains an important topic of debate and ongoing research. The following points should be remembered when deciding which colloid to infuse. Starches with a molecular weight above 200 kDa may predispose to acute kidney injury and result in pruritus. Starches may remain within the intravascular compartment for longer than gelatines; however, this effect is questionable with modern, lower-molecular-weight starches.[44]

Orthotopic liver transplantation may be associated with massive blood loss. The causes are multifactorial and include preoperative coagulopathy secondary to end-stage liver disease, portal hypertension, surgical technique, adhesions related to previous surgery and intraoperative changes in haemostasis. The degree of clinical coagulopathy is impossible to predict, and relies on the imbalance in antihaemostatic and prohaemostatic drivers.[45] The low-grade fibrinolytic process in advanced cirrhotics may be exacerbated during surgery, particularly during the anhepatic and reperfusion stages. Platelet dysfunction, both quantitative and qualitative, is also common though the impact on haemostasis is variable.[46] The consequences of massive bleeding and replacement are significant, not only in terms of postoperative morbidity and mortality, but also intraoperatively when issues such as acute hypovolaemia, reduced ionised calcium due to elevated citrate levels, hyperkalaemia, acidosis and hypothermia become important. Transfusion-related acute lung injury (TRALI) is a potentially devastating complication. It is believed to result from neutrophil antibodies preformed in donor serum. The immunosuppressive effects of large-volume blood transfusions are well recognised and pertinent in a group of patients who are already functionally immunosuppressed. In addition to these immediate problems is the risk of transmission of, as yet, unidentified viral infection.

Much effort has gone into reducing the amount of exogenous blood products required intraoperatively. This includes the use of cell salvage techniques with autologous transfusion and frequent testing of haemostasis, utilising both laboratory-based tests and thromboelastography or rotational thromboelastometry. The prophylactic use of tranexamic acid may attenuate the degree of fibrinolysis during the early stages of transplantation. The severe post-reperfusion fibrinolysis often resolves once the donor liver begins to function and seldom requires immediate correction. Optimisation of clot stability with fibrinogen prior to coagulation factor and platelet replacement has led to reduced transfusion requirements in major haemorrhage. Fibrinogen and prothrombin complex concentrates are gaining popularity due to the reduced volume load and superior efficacy, though these products are not universally licensed or readily available. They are purified and virally inactivated by nature of the manufacture process, reducing the risks of viral transmission and TRALI.[47] There is a paucity of evidence-based thresholds for platelet transfusion, and the benefits in reducing haemorrhage and improving liver regeneration must be balanced with the adverse risks of ischaemia-reperfusion injury, TRALI and reduced survival.[46] These therapies must be judiciously employed in order to control bleeding at the potential expense of thromboembolic complications which may be as high as 4%.[41]

Although it is assumed that all patients with liver disease are subject to an increased risk of bleeding there are subgroups that are prothrombotic, as evidenced clinically and with thromboelastography. Patients with preoperative portal or hepatic venous thrombosis appear to carry a higher incidence of prothrombotic mutations than the general population, and patients with primary biliary cirrhosis and primary sclerosing cholangitis are frequently prothrombotic. Such patients may require anticoagulation in the early postoperative period. Other patient groups such as those with Budd–Chiari syndrome may have a recognised prothrombotic condition with a resultant early requirement for anticoagulation.

Electrolyte disorders are common in advanced liver disease, and careful monitoring of sodium, potassium and calcium levels is paramount. Hyponatraemia is associated with increased mortality in the pre-transplanted patient, and rapid changes in the perioperative period may lead to further morbidity (although mortality appears comparable).[48] Rapid changes in sodium concentration have been linked to rare cases of central pontine myelinosis. Calcium is required for haemostasis, and requires supplementation especially if citrated products have been administered. Life-threatening hyperkalaemia may develop on reperfusion, and must be anticipated and managed immediately. Cell-salvage apparatus can be used to wash the packed red cells to eliminate excess citrate and potassium administration.

POST-REPERFUSION SYNDROME

The post-reperfusion syndrome is a poorly understood phenomenon that occurs after reperfusion of the portal vein through the donor graft. It is characterised by hypotension, bradycardia, vasodilatation, pulmonary hypertension, hyperkalaemia and in some cases cardiac arrest. The aetiology is unclear, but a sudden increase in venous return, release of vasoactive substances, and cold potassium-rich preservation fluids are potentially implicated. The syndrome usually resolves within the first 5 minutes of reperfusion with appropriate fluid loading and electrolyte management. However, in approximately 30% of patients it lasts for significantly longer, necessitating the use of inotropes and/or vasopressors. The post-reperfusion syndrome seems more common in organs with longer preservation times and may well be associated with initial poor graft function.

POSTOPERATIVE CARE

The postoperative care of the recipient depends to some extent on preoperative co-morbidity, the presence of any of the immediate complications listed above, recipient stability during the procedure and lastly the pre-transplant cause of liver failure. Straightforward recipients who return to the ICU in a stable condition with good graft function may be woken up and weaned immediately. The tracheal tube and some of the invasive monitoring lines should be removed as soon as no longer required to reduce the risk of infection and encourage mobility. Close monitoring of all physiological systems is important in the early postoperative period (**Tables 101.2** and **101.3**).

EARLY COMPLICATIONS

As with all postoperative surgical intensive care admissions, some complications are applicable to all patients. These include haemorrhagic and pulmonary complications of any prolonged procedure in addition to specific complications pertinent to liver transplantation. These can be subdivided into technical complications, conditions and complications associated with pre-existing liver disease, and complications associated with immunosuppressive agents, graft function and massive transfusion.

CARDIOVASCULAR

End-stage liver disease is characterised by a hyperdynamic circulation, with low systemic vascular resistance, high cardiac index and a proportionately reduced central circulating volume. The majority of patients can be managed with judicious volume loading with or without vasopressors to maintain adequate perfusion

Table 101.2 Routine investigation of post-transplant patient in the ICU

	FBC	LFTS	COAGULATION	DRUG LEVELS	CULTURES	ULTRASOUND
Day 1	√	√	√		As indicated	Routine ultrasound including hepatic artery, hepatic and portal venous flow D1 and D5, and if clinically indicated at other times
Day 2	√	√	√	√	As indicated	
Day 3	√	√	√	√	As indicated	

Table 101.3 Monitoring of graft function in ICU

PARAMETER		COMMENT
GENERAL	Liver perfusion	Characteristics at surgery
	Bile production	Quality±volume if T-tube in situ
	Haemodynamics	Stabilisation, with cessation of vasopressor requirements
COAGULATION	INR/prothrombin time	8-hourly for first 24 hours, thereafter daily unless indicated. Fall in PT is more important than the actual value. FFP should be withheld to assess graft function although platelets given as indicated
BIOCHEMISTRY	Glucose	Hypoglycaemia is an ominous sign. 4-hourly for first 24 hours. Euglycaemia/hyperglycaemia requiring insulin infusion is normal
	Arterial blood gases and lactate	4–6-hourly depending on ventilatory requirement. Hyperlactataemia and acid–base disturbance should rapidly resolve. Other causes of base deficit such as renal tubular acidosis and hyperchloraemia should be excluded and managed appropriately
	AST	Should fall steadily (50% fall each day). The first measurement may reflect washout and thus the next may be higher. Daily measurements. The initial measurement reflects the degree of preservation injury
	Bilirubin	Early increases may reflect absorption of haematoma and do not reflect graft function. Haemolysis should be considered if the graft is not blood group matched, termed passenger lymphocyte syndrome
	ALP/GGT	Usually normal; increases may reflect biliary complications or cholestasis of sepsis

pressures. However, in some patients this state may compensate for degrees of cirrhotic cardiomyopathy, characterised by systolic and diastolic dysfunction, electrophysiological abnormalities and a blunted β-adrenoceptor response.[49–51] The massive increase in the volume of liver transplants performed in the last decade has revealed cardiac failure as an important cause of morbidity and mortality in the transplant recipient.[52] OLT can impose severe stresses on the cardiovascular system; haemorrhage, third-space loss, impaired venous return due to caval clamping, hypocalcaemia and acidosis impair myocardial contractility. Reperfusion can also be a time of profound circulatory instability. Rapid fluctuations in filling pressures place the compromised and stressed myocardium at risk of failure. In addition, the impaired exercise tolerance of the pre-transplant recipient may have limited the clinical importance of coronary ischaemia, which becomes pertinent in the post-transplant period.

Haemodynamic changes after OLT are also common; hypertension with an increased systemic vascular resistance is frequent and may be due to the restoration of normal liver function and portal pressure, as well as the hypertensive effect of the calcineurin immunosuppressants. The increased afterload in the early post-transplant period may unmask cardiac dysfunction. Management of myocardial failure post OLT is largely empirical; diuretics, afterload reduction and positive-pressure ventilation may all be required. In the longer term, control of cardiovascular risk factors is required and many of these patients may over the years return to the intensive care environs with other system failures and considerable burdens of hypertension, coronary ischaemia, diabetes, hyperlipidaemia and renal dysfunction.

PULMONARY

Pulmonary complications are common and occur in 40–80% of recipients. The presence of preoperative impairment (e.g. pleural effusions, hypoxaemia, pulmonary hypertension or the hepatopulmonary syndrome) is strongly associated with postoperative complications. Specific conditions related to liver transplantation include right hemidiaphragm palsy as a result of phrenic nerve damage, which can occur if suprahepatic caval clamping is used intraoperatively. The commonest postoperative problems are pleural effusions, ongoing shunting secondary to the hepatopulmonary syndrome, atelectasis and, over subsequent days, infection. De novo acute respiratory distress syndrome is relatively uncommon at this stage. Other complications such as TRALI and pulmonary oedema are almost certainly under-recognised and underreported.

Specific management of portopulmonary syndrome may be required in the postoperative period if right-sided pressures are elevated, to ensure that liver congestion and graft dysfunction do not ensue.[6,50,51] Control of pulmonary pressures may require a variety of therapeutic options, with the treatment options being similar to those utilised in primary pulmonary hypertension. Concern about potential hepatotoxicity needs to be balanced against the need to control right-sided pressures and provide optimal graft function. Similarly, hepatopulmonary syndrome may take a variable time to resolve and hypoxia during this period will require management and recognition. Respiratory complications are also seen in patients with poor muscle bulk and subsequent weakness. Similarly, the presence of osteoporosis in the pre-transplant patient is frequently associated with postoperative pain and poor cough.

The role of adequate analgesia is important, as in all patients, in promoting mobilisation and adequate respiratory function. In general, the management of a protracted respiratory wean follows conventional lines.

NEUROLOGICAL

The quoted incidence of central nervous system (CNS) complications varies widely from 10 to 40% in the published series. Most neurological complications occur within the first month of transplant. The commonest causes relate to persistence of pre-existing encephalopathy.[53,54] The causes are multiple, including hepatic, metabolic, infectious, vascular and pharmacological. A patient with acute liver failure will remain encephalopathic in the immediate post-transplant period, and is at risk of intracranial hypertension for 48 hours following transplantation, or longer in the face of graft dysfunction. De novo hepatic encephalopathy may develop in patients with severe graft dysfunction and/or primary graft non-function; again the patient is at risk of cerebral oedema. The effects of sepsis, rejection (and its treatment with high-dose steroids), drug therapy (especially the sedatives and analgesics used in the ICU setting) and the presence of renal failure may all contribute to the presence of altered conscious level. The calcineurin inhibitors are particularly associated with seizures and altered conscious level. All such patients will require brain imaging to further define the aetiology of their impaired neurology.

Other possible neurological complications are those of intracerebral haemorrhage. Such bleeds may relate to arteriovenous malformations, may be spontaneous or may be a complication of intracranial pressure monitoring, particularly in patients with acute liver failure. CNS infection normally presents later than the immediate postoperative period but should always be considered, especially in those patients with a prolonged and complicated postoperative course. All possible infecting agents, including bacterial, viral, fungal and opportunistic, should be considered. Central pontine myelinosis is a rare but potentially devastating complication associated with rapid sodium shifts. Modern technology and the use of haemofiltration techniques allow tight control of sodium shifts in the majority of patients, and this has become a rare neurological complication.

RENAL

Despite intraoperative efforts, renal dysfunction often progresses and acute renal failure is a relatively common complication, with an incidence of between 12 and 50% and a multifactorial aetiology.[55–57] Risk factors include the presence of pre-transplant co-morbidity (e.g. hypertension, diabetes mellitus, hepatorenal syndrome), severity of underlying liver disease, intraoperative instability, blood product requirement, drug toxicity and graft dysfunction. Mortality in those who require renal replacement is high, and graft survival is lower. To avoid exacerbation of existing renal impairment, agents with inherent nephrotoxicity, such as the calcineurin inhibitors, may be omitted or their dose significantly reduced in the early pre-transplant period. There must be a balance between the risk of rejection and that of side-effects of drug therapies. Mycophenolate mofetil, a cytotoxic immunosuppressant, may be substituted in the post-transplant course to limit or protect against renal dysfunction, and increasingly agents such as interleukin-2 (IL-2) blockers are utilised to decrease renal dysfunction.[58]

Intra-abdominal hypertension should always be considered in the post-transplant setting as a potential contributor to not only renal dysfunction but also cardiorespiratory embarrassment. Early consideration should be given to laparostomy in patients with elevated intra-abdominal pressures and associated organ dysfunction.[59,60]

PRIMARY NON-FUNCTION

This is a spectrum occurring in 2–23% of cases, which at worst requires urgent retransplantation. It is characterised by poor graft function from the time of reperfusion, with hyperlactataemia, coagulopathy, metabolic acidosis, hypoglycaemia, hyperkalaemia and a rapid elevation in aminotransferase concentrations, accompanied by a systemic inflammatory response. A major reason for the initial graft dysfunction is ischaemic injury to the graft, which depends on the type of preservation fluid used, and the duration of cold and warm ischaemia time. The aetiology of primary non-function remains unclear.[61] Vasodilator prostaglandins and antioxidants may have a role in 'rescue therapy', but controlled data are lacking.

SURGICAL PROBLEMS

Anastomotic thromboses are uncommon complications of liver transplantation, but can cause significant morbidity, which may require further invasive procedures and even urgent retransplantation. Hepatic artery thrombosis occurring in the early postoperative period is associated with a similar picture to PNF. Small vessel calibre is a risk factor, and is more prevalent in the paediatric recipient where it has also been associated with prothrombotic states such as protein C deficiency. Ultrasound is the first-line screening test and is undertaken both routinely in the immediate postoperative period and if there is a sudden rise in transaminase measurements. If the vessel is not visualised, the patient should proceed to CT angiography. If diagnosed quickly, emergency intervention can be undertaken to re-establish arterial flow; however, emergency retransplantation may be required.

Venous complications such as portal thrombosis are even less common, and are usually associated with intraoperative technical difficulty, recurrence of preoperative disease or undiagnosed thrombophilia. Portal thrombosis is normally associated with portal hypertension and massive ascites, but may also be associated with graft dysfunction, especially in the paediatric population. CT scanning will interrogate the vessels and also provide information on graft perfusion; regional ischaemia may be identified that may have presented as a transaminitis. Treatment is dependent on the severity of the injury but ranges from diuretics to angioplasty, surgical reconstruction or ultimately retransplantation. Regional ischaemia and areas of poor perfusion should be actively sought in patients with a transaminitis and especially in those who had received a reduced size or split-liver graft.

Biliary complications after liver-transplant are relatively common. The bile duct normally receives two-thirds of its arterial supply from the gastroduodenal artery and one-third from the hepatic artery. Post-transplant the only supply is from the hepatic artery, making it vulnerable to ischaemic injury whether that be at the time of retrieval, reperfusion or postoperatively. The resulting complication depends on the type of biliary anastomosis and the timing of the insult. Strictures are more commonly observed than leaks. Management of biliary complications is in the first instance endoscopic, with stent placement and/or balloon dilatation. In patients with a T-tube in situ, cholangiography may be undertaken by that route. Open reconstruction in the early postoperative period is uncommon (**Tables 101.4** and **101.5**, **Box 101.2**). Bile leaks may also be seen in the postoperative period from the cut surface of a split graft; they are associated with an increased risk of infection and potentially of pseudoaneurysm formation.

ACUTE REJECTION

Acute cellular rejection becomes a risk from approximately 5–7 days post transplant; the clinical signs of rejection are non-specific and include fever, deterioration in graft function and a rapid rise in serum aminotransferase concentration. Liver biopsy is the only

Box 101.2 Differential diagnosis of graft dysfunction in ICU

- Primary non-function
- Preservation injury
- Rejection – hyperacute/acute
- Vascular complications
- Biliary complications
- Drug-induced liver dysfunction
- Infection – viral, bacterial, fungal
- Recurrent disease (normally late)

Table 101.4 Technical complications of OLT

COMPLICATION	COMMENT
ABDOMINAL BLEEDING	
Anastomosis	Immediate
Graft surface (if cut down)	Immediate
General ooze secondary to coagulopathy	Immediate
Pseudo-aneurysm formation	Can present early or late and is usually associated with intra-abdominal sepsis and biliary leaks
VASCULAR COMPLICATIONS	
Hepatic artery thrombosis	Early and late
Portal vein thrombosis	Early and late; there may also be a stenosis of the portal vein rather than thrombosis
Inferior vena cava obstruction	May be infra-, supra- or retrohepatic in site
BILIARY COMPLICATIONS	
Biliary leak	Usually early
Biliary stricture	Usually late
Papillary dysfunction	Late
Roux-en-Y dysfunction	Usually late

Table 101.5 Biochemical and clinical features of technical problems

COMPLICATION	FEATURES	INVESTIGATION	MANAGEMENT
HEPATIC ARTERY THROMBOSIS	Early: rapid rise in transaminase, coagulopathy, graft failure Differential diagnosis: hyperacute rejection, primary non-/dysfunction	Ultrasound, angiogram	Thrombectomy, retransplantation
	Late: biliary complications, strictures, sepsis, liver abscess	Ultrasound, angiogram	Angioplasty
PORTAL VEIN THROMBOSIS	Early: rapid deterioration in graft function, acute liver failure, ascites, variceal bleeding	Ultrasound, CT, angiography, MRA	Thrombectomy, retransplantation, conservative management
	Late: mildly abnormal LFTs, portal hypertension, varices	Ultrasound, CT, angiography, MRA	

Table 101.6 Management of rejection in intensive care

	COMMENT	CHARACTERISTICS	LIVER BIOPSY	DIFFERENTIAL DIAGNOSIS	TREATMENT OPTIONS
HYPERACUTE REJECTION	Rare in OLT 1–10 days post-transplant	Rapid deterioration in graft function: AST > 1000 Coagulopathy, acidosis	Haemorrhagic necrosis	Primary non-function/ delayed function Hepatic artery thrombosis	Retransplantation Rarely: OKT3, cyclophosphamide, plasmaphoresis (unproven)
ACUTE REJECTION	30–70% Occurs at mean of 7–9 days	Often clinically silent apart from fever and RUQ pain High AST and bilirubin Coagulation and acid–base undisturbed	Portal inflammation Endotheliitis Bile duct damage	Sepsis Vascular Viral	Methylprednisolone 1 g daily for 3 days

In those who do not respond: Consider diagnosis; if correct, consider tacrolimus if induction agent is ciclosporin A, OKT3 or MMF/ sirolimus (rapamycin) if other new agents.

reliable diagnostic tool; however, biopsy may be relatively contraindicated owing to coagulopathy. In some circumstances transjugular biopsy offers a solution to this problem. The normal management regimen for an episode of acute rejection is that of pulsed methylprednisolone, 1 g for 3 days. The differential diagnosis may be that of sepsis, or problems with vascular integrity; there are some data to suggest that procalcitonin may be of use in the differentiation (**Table 101.6**).

INFECTIOUS COMPLICATIONS

Transplant recipients are uniquely vulnerable to bacterial infection: preoperative colonisation, prolonged and technically difficult surgery, large wounds, urinary catheterisation and the frequent need for central venous access postoperatively all combine to make them at vastly increased risk. However, compared with a decade ago, the overall incidence is reduced, probably owing to improved and patient-tailored immunosuppressive regimens. Sepsis remains an important and lifelong complication of liver transplantation, which may require readmission to intensive care.[62,63]

The epidemiology of pathogens is evolving; the incidence of Gram-positive bacterial infection (enterococci and staphylococci) is now more common than Gram-negative sepsis. More concerning is the emergence of multiple antibiotic-resistant bacteria, in particular meticillin-resistant *Staphylococcus aureus* (MRSA), vancomycin-resistant enterococci (VRE) and extended-spectrum beta-lactamase (ESBL)-producing Gram-negative organisms. Mortality and graft failure associated with infection caused by these multiply resistant organisms is significantly greater compared with other organisms.[64] A decline in the incidence of both *Pneumocystis jiroveci* (formerly *P. carinii*) and cytomegalovirus infection is probably a result of both modulating immunosuppressive regimens and more effective prophylaxis. Patients should be screened for viral infections, including herpes simplex virus (HSV) and cytomegalovirus (CMV) utilising polymerase chain reaction (PCR) techniques. Opportunistic fungal infection still remains problematic, especially in the context of environmental risk factors (**Table 101.7**).[65,66]

FEVER

In transplant recipients, 76% of febrile episodes have a documented infectious aetiology, but acute rejection needs to be considered in the differential diagnosis. In the ICU transplant recipient the aetiology is even more likely to be infectious – often nosocomial and bacterial. In one study, pneumonia, catheter-related bacteraemia and the biliary tree were the three most common sources in the ICU population (41%). Viral infections accounted for 9% of febrile episodes, fungal infections 3% and endocarditis 3%. As mentioned above, the epidemiology of pathogens is changing and it is important to have thorough knowledge of local problem pathogens on which to base meaningful antibiotic policy. These data have implications for the threshold to investigate febrile episodes, suspect bacterial infection and commence appropriate empirical antibiotic therapy. However, it should also be appreciated that immunosuppressed recipients do not always produce a febrile response to infection.

MANAGEMENT OF CMV INFECTION AFTER LIVER TRANSPLANTATION

CMV infection is rarely associated with symptomatic illness in healthy hosts, but is a major cause of morbidity and mortality in transplant recipients; it is the single most common opportunistic infection after solid organ transplantation. In the absence of antiviral prophylaxis

Table 101.7 Infection in the intensive care unit

	BACTERIAL	VIRAL	FUNGAL	PROTOZOAL
AETIOLOGY	Wound Nosocomial pneumonia Line sepsis UTI Liver Biliary	HSV CMV EBV Varicella	*Candida* *Aspergillus* PCP *Cryptococcus*	Toxoplasmosis *Strongyloides*
TIMING	Any time	HSV in first few weeks CMV 3–10 weeks EBV from 4 weeks Varicella later All may be earlier in ALF or retransplantation	Usually after 4 weeks	After 3 weeks

the overall incidence of CMV infection after OLT ranges from 23 to 85%, with approximately 50% of those developing clinical disease. CMV infection most commonly occurs in the first 3 months after OLT, with a peak incidence in the third and fourth week. Infection may be asymptomatic or it may cause a spectrum of illness including fever, thrombocytopenia, neutropenia, pneumonia and hepatitis. The indirect effects of infection probably contribute more to the adverse effects on graft function than direct effects. CMV infection further immunosuppresses the recipient, leading to increased opportunistic fungal infection and also increased risk of Epstein–Barr virus (EBV) infection, which can go on to be associated with post-transplant lymphoproliferative disease (PTLD). CMV infection is also implicated in increased rejection. In those patients who proceed to transplant who are already receiving immunosuppressive agents, or in those with acute liver failure, CMV disease may present earlier in the clinical course.

The risk of CMV infection post-transplant is dependent on the serological status of both the donor and recipient; the highest risk is associated with donor positive/recipient negative. Proven prophylactic strategies in the high-risk groups include valganciclovir or ganciclovir for 3 months. Currently, intravenous ganciclovir remains the gold standard in the treatment of CMV disease. Therapy will be converted to oral ganciclovir to facilitate discharge from hospital and rehabilitation. There is no evidence to support specific immunoglobulin in addition, but it is frequently added in the management of CMV pneumonitis.[64]

MANAGEMENT OF VIRAL HEPATITIS

Hepatitis C (HCV)-related cirrhosis is the commonest indication for transplantation in both Europe and the USA. Post-transplant HCV viraemia is universal. Recurrent liver disease, with a more accelerated and aggressive course, is often observed; indeed, 20% are cirrhotic at 5 years.[67] Those with histological evidence of recurrence also have a greater incidence of acute rejection. Immunosuppression, especially with steroids, directly increases the HCV RNA serum load. Most post-transplant programmes therefore convert to single- or double-agent immunosuppression regimens as soon as possible.[68] Still to be fully elucidated is the role of antiviral therapy (interferon and ribavirin) in both the pre- and post-transplant period. Provisional data are optimistic, although it requires considerable workload and supportive drug therapy. It would not normally be undertaken in the intensive care setting. Theoretically, early antiviral therapy is attractive as viral load is low, immunosuppressive therapy has just started and acute rejection necessitating pulsed steroids is relatively common. However, risk of infection and thrombocytopenia often contraindicates antiviral therapy in the early postoperative period. Retransplantation for HCV recurrence has been shown to be a successful possibility should the transplanted liver begin to fail.[69]

Initial results of transplantation for hepatitis B infection (HBV) were discouraging, largely owing to recurrent disease with rapid and fatal progression. Passive immunoprophylaxis with hepatitis B immune globulin (HBIG) during and after transplant and the use of antiviral agents pre-transplant to suppress viral replication dramatically reduce re-infection rate. However, such therapy must be continued indefinitely following transplant to prevent disease recurrence. In respect of modulation of immunosuppression regimens, the comments made with respect to HCV are similarly applicable.

IMMUNOSUPPRESSION

As the field of transplantation evolves, new immunosuppressive regimens and drugs become available. For all combinations, however, there is a balance to be struck between the optimal prevention of rejection and the toxicity and unwanted effects of the drugs. These agents affect T-cell-dependent B-cell activation, targeting different sites in the T-cell activation cascade by inhibiting T-cell activation or causing T-cell depletion. The incidence of acute rejection rises at about 1 week after OLT; it resembles a delayed-type hypersensitivity reaction, and immunosuppressive agents are highly effective at treating it. Chronic rejection occurs over months to years and is characterised by the 'vanishing bile-duct' syndrome; pathological mechanisms are poorly understood and immunosuppressant agents are largely ineffective.[58]

Currently, calcineurin inhibitors such as ciclosporin and tacrolimus, along with steroids, form the mainstay drugs after liver transplantation, certainly in the early stages. They have revolutionised the outcome of solid-organ transplantation, but both drugs are limited by their side-effects, predominantly nephro- and neurotoxicity, necessitating drug level monitoring. These manifestations of toxicity can be difficult in the management of post-transplant immunosuppression in patients who exhibited encephalopathy or renal dysfunction pre-transplant; the use of agents without nephrotoxic profiles may be considered in this context. It is usual to have an induction regimen beginning in the perioperative period; this usually involves a calcineurin inhibitor and steroids, which are administered in a high-dose taper regimen. With time after transplantation, the level of immunosuppression required decreases and drug doses may be reduced further. Cytotoxic drugs such as azathioprine or mycophenolate mofetil (MMF) may also allow further reduction of steroids and calcineurin inhibitors. The long-term effects of immunosuppression have to be considered but are less pertinent in the immediate postoperative period.

Another variation in the regimen is the introduction of antilymphocyte antibodies (ALA) for 10–14 days in order to delay the introduction of calcineurin inhibitors: this may be desirable in patients with impaired renal function. ALA interferes with lymphocyte function in several ways: enhanced removal of activated lymphocytes by the reticuloendothelial system, down-regulation of lymphocyte-binding cell surface receptors, with decreased lymphocyte activation and proliferation. Recently, monoclonal antibodies have been introduced (basiliximab). They bind to IL-2 receptors, which are only present on activated T-cells, and hence they have a more specific mode of action and favourable toxicity profile. The role of such agents, especially in those with renal dysfunction, is gaining greater recognition.

Sirolimus is a novel immunosuppressant that has been used extensively in renal transplantation and more recently in liver transplant recipients in whom the calcineurin inhibitors are contraindicated.[58] It resembles tacrolimus structurally, and binds to the same protein, but whereas ciclosporin and tacrolimus act by inhibiting *IL-2* gene transcription, sirolimus acts by blocking post-receptor signal transduction and IL-2-dependent proliferation. In addition to its immunosuppressive actions, sirolimus is also an antifungal and antiproliferative agent. Sirolimus lacks neuro- and nephrotoxicity. However, it can raise the intracellular concentrations of ciclosporin A and tacrolimus, indirectly potentiating their toxicity. Hyperlipidaemia has also been noted, although this may be a reflection of the often-higher-dose steroid regimens used in combination with sirolimus. Because of its antiproliferative effects, sirolimus can also cause thrombocytopenia, neutropenia and anaemia; there have also been concerns about its effects on wound healing. Sirolimus also requires therapeutic drug level monitoring, not only because serum concentrations have a high level of intra- and inter-individual variability, but also because there are significant interactions with drugs that use the cytochrome P-450 3A system. All immunosuppressive regimens should be tailored to individual patient needs and a balance struck between side-effects (short and long term) and risk of rejection.

RE-ADMISSION TO ICU/LATE COMPLICATIONS

The cause of re-admission to ICU after liver transplantation varies in relation to time after transplantation. Approximately 20% of recipients require re-admission, and this correlates with actuarial reduced patient and graft survival. In the period immediately after transplantation, cardiorespiratory failure is the commonest reason for re-admission, due to both fluid overload and infection. Indeed, an abnormal pre-discharge chest X-ray is predictive of re-admission, as is high central venous pressure and tachypnoea. Other predictors of re-admission are age, pre-transplant synthetic function, bilirubin, amount of intraoperative blood products and renal dysfunction. Graft dysfunction, severe sepsis and postoperative care of surgical complications are other important causes of readmission. Bleeding and biliary anastomotic leaks represent the commonest surgical causes for readmission.

LIVER TRANSPLANTATION FOR ACUTE LIVER FAILURE

Acute liver failure is a syndrome associated with an acute-onset coagulopathy, jaundice and encephalopathy; the causes are many and the syndrome is notable for its high morbidity and mortality. The acceptance of emergency liver transplantation in selected cases has revolutionised the clinical course, but outcome is sometimes disappointingly poor, often resulting from the rapid development of uncontrollable cerebral oedema, sepsis and multiorgan failure. There is also a short window of opportunity in listing these patients; despite highest priority listing they may receive 'marginal' organs or even ABO blood group incompatible organs. Early determination of prognosis and appropriate listing for transplant are clearly important. The King's College Hospital prognostic criteria for non-survival among patients with acute liver failure is a tool used to identify those at high risk while sparing those in whom

Table 101.8 King's College Hospital prognostic criteria for non-survival among patients with acute liver failure

PARACETAMOL INDUCED	NON-PARACETAMOL INDUCED
pH<7.3 (irrespective of grade of encephalopathy), following volume resuscitation and >24 hours post ingestion, *or*	PT>100 seconds (INR>6.5) irrespective of grade of encephalopathy, *or* pH<7.3 following volume resuscitation, *or*
PT>100 seconds (INR>6.5) *and* creatinine >300 µmol/L in patients with grade III–IV encephalopathy, occurring within a 24-hour timeframe	Any three of the following variables (in association with encephalopathy): Age <10 years or >40 years Aetiology: non-A, non-B or drug induced Jaundice to encephalopathy >7 days PT>50 seconds (INR>3.5) Serum bilirubin >300 µmol/L

spontaneous recovery will otherwise occur. It has been validated in both Europe and the USA (**Table 101.8**). Several advances in the supportive management of these patients have occurred since the original criteria were developed, but their prognostic value holds true.

PAEDIATRIC LIVER TRANSPLANTATION

OLT is the treatment of choice for children with end-stage liver disease. Cholestatic disorders make up the largest indication for transplantation, with extrahepatic biliary atresia plus or minus previous Kasai porto-enterostomy accounting for over 50% of paediatric transplants. Metabolic diseases and primary hepatic tumours are also common indications. As in adult recipients, multisystem effects of end-stage liver disease are common, and the occurrence of liver disease as part of a congenital syndrome (e.g. Alagille's) may warrant invasive preoperative evaluation of extrahepatic manifestation. Scarce availability of paediatric donors has driven innovations such as reduced size grafts, split-liver techniques and living donor programmes, which have all contributed to expand the pool of available donors and reduce the mortality for those children waiting for suitable organs.

One of the biggest problems associated with paediatric transplantation is the relatively high incidence of vascular complications such as hepatic artery thrombosis, portal vein thrombosis and venous outflow obstruction. Risk factors for these conditions include fulminant hepatic failure, long operation time, donor/recipient age and weight discrepancies, young recipient age, low recipient weight and arterial reconstruction techniques. In order to minimise these often devastating complications, strategies to minimise the risk include delayed primary closure of the abdominal wall, maintaining the haematocrit at 22–25% to ensure laminar flow, and avoidance of platelets and blood components combined with considered use of anticoagulants. Associated cardiac, pulmonary or renal abnormalities observed in some paediatric syndromes with liver disease may require particular attention and management such as the pulmonary stenosis seen in association with Alagille's.

Ten-year survival rates of 74 (age 12–17 years) – 84% (age 1–5 years) has brought about a new set of challenges relating to complications and management of long-term immunosuppression. The concept of tolerance-inducing immunosuppressive regimens has spurned a number of studies investigating this phenomenon.[70]

Access the complete references list online at http://www.expertconsult.com

6. Krowka MJ. Hepatopulmonary syndrome and portopulmonary hypertension: implications for liver transplantation. Clin Chest Med 2005;26:587–97.
16. Machicao VI, Fallon M. Hepatopulmonary syndrome. Semin Respir Crit Care Med 2012;33:11–16.
19. Krowka MJ. Portopulmonary hypertension. Semin Respir Crit Care Med 2012;33:17–25.
43. Moller S, Bendtsen F, Henrikson JH. Effect of volume expansion on systemic hemodynamics and central and arterial blood volume in cirrhosis. Gastroenterology 1995;109:1917–25.
64. Patel G, Huprikar S. Infectious complications after orthotopic liver transplantation. Semin Respir Crit Care Med 2012;33:111–24.

102

Heart and lung transplantation

Peter S Macdonald and Paul C Jansz

The first human-to-human heart transplant was performed in 1967 by Christiaan Barnard at Groote Schuur Hospital in South Africa. The donor heart functioned well immediately post-transplant and the patient survived for 18 days before dying from pneumonia complicating his immunosuppressive therapy. There followed an initial wave of surgical enthusiasm with multiple centres around the world commencing heart transplant programmes. Initial results were poor, however, with high early mortality rates and few long-term survivors. Many institutions abandoned the procedure and only a handful of heart transplant programmes persisted throughout the 1970s. The discovery of ciclosporin as an effective immunosuppressive agent and its introduction into clinical transplantation in the late 1970s led to renewed interest in heart transplantation with a rapid growth in transplant activity throughout the 1980s. Since then more than 100 000 heart transplants have been reported to the Registry of the International Society for Heart & Lung Transplantation (ISHLT).[1] Currently, it is estimated that more than 5000 transplants are performed each year in over 300 countries.[1] The survival rate after heart transplantation has improved steadily over the last two decades and currently approaches 90% at 1 year, 80% at 5 years and 60% at 10 years. Median survival is 11 years. Heart transplantation is now well established as the most effective treatment available for end-stage heart failure.

Human lung transplantation also commenced in the 1960s but as with heart transplantation early results were dismal and the procedure was largely abandoned until the 1980s. The first successful heart–lung transplant was performed at Stanford University Medical Center in 1981. During the next decade single-lung and bilateral-lung transplantation emerged as viable procedures for patients with end-stage lung disease. More than 40 000 lung transplants have been reported to the ISHLT registry and currently more than 3000 lung transplants are performed annually around the world.[2] Post-transplant survival although not as good as for other organs has improved steadily. In the most recent publication of the ISHLT registry median post-transplant survival was 5.5 years with 80% survival at 1 year, 53% at 5 years and 30% at 10 years.[2] Whereas heart transplant activity has plateaued in the last decade, lung transplant activity has been increasing steadily.[2]

Heart and lung transplantation are limited by donor organ availability. With rare exceptions, hearts and lungs donated for transplantation come from deceased persons. Historically, the vast majority of deceased donors for both heart and lung transplantation had undergone brain death (DBD). More recently, donation after circulatory death (DCD) has re-emerged as an important source of donor lungs as well as abdominal organs and in some cardiopulmonary transplant programmes up to one-third of lung transplants are performed from DCD donors.[3]

Virtually all of the improvement in heart and lung transplant survival over the last 20 years has been during the first few months after transplantation.[1,2] The improvement in survival can be explained by a number of factors including advances in immunosuppressive therapy with fewer deaths due to uncontrollable rejection or infection and better patient selection by excluding patients who are too sick to recover from the stresses of transplant surgery. Nevertheless, the first few days and weeks after transplantation is still a period of high mortality risk for transplant recipients, owing mainly to the complications of primary graft failure (PGF) or overwhelming infection.

THE POTENTIAL HEART DONOR

Of all organs retrieved from deceased donors for transplantation, the heart is the one most susceptible to the multiple insults that occur during brain death and the subsequent events that occur during donor organ retrieval and transplantation. Studies involving repeated echocardiographic examination of the brain-dead donor have revealed that left ventricular systolic dysfunction is common after brain death and that it often improves together with haemodynamic status after a period of aggressive donor management.[4]

In addition to its susceptibility to the adverse consequences of brain death, the heart is the donor organ with the least tolerability to the obligatory ischaemia reperfusion injury (IRI) that occurs during organ retrieval and implantation. Data from the ISHLT Registry indicates that, as the donor heart ischaemic time (the time from cross-clamp of the aorta in the donor to release of the aortic cross-clamp in the recipient) increases beyond 3 hours, there is a progressive increase in the mortality rate at 1 year post-transplant.[1] Donor heart ischaemic times in excess of 6 hours are associated with a 70% increase in the risk of death at 1 year post-heart transplantation.[1] Consequently, when coordinating the retrieval of donor organs, every effort is made to minimise the ischaemic time for the donor heart. In addition there is substantial evidence from large observational studies that hearts from older donors are more susceptible to IRI.[1,5] For this reason, the upper age limit for donor hearts in many programmes is restricted to a donor age less than 60 years. Even with this donor age restriction, hearts are still retrieved from only a minority of brain dead donors. In most jurisdictions hearts are retrieved from only about 30% of deceased donors.

DONOR ELIGIBILITY CRITERIA

Donor eligibility criteria vary between jurisdictions. Those that are currently utilised in Australia and New Zealand are summarised in **Table 102.1**.[6] As shown in the table, donors are subdivided into standard criteria and extended criteria donors based on a range of donor characteristics that if present are associated with an increased risk of graft failure and lower survival after transplantation. With rare exceptions, donor hearts are retrieved from brain-dead donors. There have been isolated case reports and small series of successful heart transplantation from DCD donors.[7] Given the rapid increase in organ donation from DCD donors in the last few years, there has been renewed interest in the utilisation of hearts from DCD donors for heart transplantation, but at present this remains an experimental activity. Echocardiographic assessment of the donor heart is recommended in all cases. Donor heart dysfunction does not necessarily imply pre-existing disease, but is associated with an increased risk of primary graft failure.[8] In donors with suspected coronary artery disease, coronary angiography is recommended if available.

DONOR MANAGEMENT

Although there has been considerable interest in donor management strategies aimed at optimising the quality of the donor heart, the most effective management strategy for the brain-dead potential organ donor in the period between determination of brain death and organ procurement for transplantation has not been established. Routine management of the potential cardiac donor after determination of brain death includes maintenance of ventilation, fluid and electrolyte balance. Central venous, arterial blood pressure and urinary catheters are recommended to monitor haemodynamic stability and ongoing fluid loss. Loss of autonomic tone and the onset of diabetes insipidus may result in severe haemodynamic instability and potentially large urinary volume losses. The majority of potential cardiac donors require a vasopressor agent to maintain arterial blood pressure and either intravenous vasopressin or subcutaneous DDAVP to correct diabetes insipidus. If donors fail to respond to these measures then more aggressive resuscitation including the use of a Swan–Ganz catheterisation to monitor central haemodynamics and combined hormonal administration have been recommended.[9]

Registry studies indicate that inotropic/vasopressor agents are administered to more than 90% of donors with norepinephrine (noradrenaline) being the most commonly administered agent.[10] Observational studies have suggested that the use of catecholamines may have divergent effects on different donor organs. For example, in one large retrospective analysis, Schnuelle and colleagues reported that the administration of

Table 102.1 Standard versus extended criteria for donor hearts

DONOR PARAMETER	STANDARD CRITERIA	EXTENDED CRITERIA (MARGINAL)
Age	<50 years	>50 years
Donor cardiac history	Nil	Pre-existing disease
Donor co-morbidities	Absent	Hepatitis B, C
Echocardiography*	Normal	Global dysfunction (LVEF<50%) Major regional wall motion abnormality Left ventricular hypertrophy (LV wall >13 mm)
Coronary angiography*	Normal or non-occlusive disease	Occlusive coronary artery disease
Haemodynamic status	Stable	Unstable with high CVP (and/or PAWP) and low BP
Inotropic support	Low	High (>0.2 µg/kg/min of norepinephrine or equivalent)
Ischaemic time	<6 hours	>6 hours

*Severe abnormalities will generally result in non-use of the organ.

catecholamines to multi-organ donors was associated with improved post-transplant outcomes for recipients of renal transplants, but worse outcomes for recipients of cardiac transplants.[11] In a subsequent large prospective randomised placebo-controlled trial of low-dose dopamine (4 μg/kg/min) in potential multi-organ donors, the same investigators found that dopamine administration to donors (who were already receiving norepinephrine in doses of less than 0.4 μg/kg/min) resulted in a reduced requirement for post-transplant dialysis in both renal transplant recipients and heart transplant recipients from the same donor.[12] Moreover, overall survival was improved in the heart transplant recipients.[13]

Vasopressin is another vasopressor agent that has been administered to the brain-dead donor often as part of a multihormonal cocktail usually with high-dose steroids and thyroid hormone.[14] Use of other hormonal therapies, particularly thyroid hormone administration, is controversial. In a recent systematic review, Macdonald and co-authors identified 16 separate case series and 7 prospective randomised controlled trials of thyroid hormone administration to brain-dead potential organ donors.[15] Whereas all case series reported a beneficial effect of thyroid hormone administration on a range of outcomes, including donor haemodynamic stability and donor heart utilisation, none of the randomised controlled trials reported any benefit from thyroid hormone administration. Despite this controversy, thyroid hormone administration in conjunction with other hormonal therapies has been recommended as part of an aggressive management protocol for the potential cardiothoracic donor and has been incorporated into the UNOS Critical Pathway for the organ donor.[9]

DONOR HEART PRESERVATION

The most common method of donor heart preservation involves cardioplegia with a cold hyperkalaemic crystalloid solution then cold static storage in a preservation solution in an ice chest during transport between donor and recipient hospitals. There are multiple preservation solutions that are in use, reflecting a lack of consensus regarding the optimal composition of these solutions.[16] All provide good preservation for up to 3 hours, but beyond this time there is a steady increase in the rate of PGF and mortality after heart transplantation. This has led to a renewed interest in the use of ex vivo machine perfusion devices to transport hearts between donor and recipient hospitals. These devices provide oxygen to the donor heart and restore aerobic metabolism during transport, thereby minimising the ischaemic insult to the donor heart. Small clinical trials have been conducted with these devices to date and it remains to be seen whether they improve the quality of the donor heart and broaden the pool of potential heart donors.

THE POTENTIAL LUNG DONOR

Experience has demonstrated that the donor lung has a greater tolerability to the adverse sequelae of brain death and subsequent insults associated with lung retrieval and transplantation than was initially thought to be the case. In particular, the tolerability of the donor lung to ischaemia reperfusion injury during retrieval and transplantation is better than that of the heart. Donor lung function appears to be less adversely affected by age than does donor heart function and in some jurisdictions donors up to age 70 are considered for lung donation.[6] In addition, the lungs of DCD donors have been found to be relatively resistant, compared with all other donor organs, to the warm ischaemia associated with withdrawal of life support. DCD donors have now become a major source of donor lungs contributing up to 30% of lung donors in some programmes.[3] For all these reasons, the numbers of lung transplants has been increasing both in absolute terms and as a proportion of all deceased donors.

DONOR ELIGIBILITY CRITERIA

As with heart transplantation, donor eligibility criteria for lungs vary between jurisdictions and there are separate categories for standard criteria and extended criteria donors (**Table 102.2**).[17,18] Although there have been concerns that the use of extended-criteria lung donors will lead to increased rates of early graft failure and death after lung transplantation, for some donor characteristics such as donor age, donor Pa_{O_2} or mode of death (DCD versus DBD) this has been found not to be the case.[17,19] Moreover, the increased risk associated with the use of lungs from donors with characteristics

Table 102.2 Standard versus extended criteria for donor lungs

DONOR PARAMETER	STANDARD CRITERIA	EXTENDED CRITERIA (MARGINAL)
Age	<55 years	>55 years
Smoking history	<20 pack years	>20 pack years
Chest trauma	Absent	Present
Aspiration	Absent	Present
Chest X-ray	Clear	Abnormal
Arterial blood gases	Pa_{O_2}>300 mmHg (40 kPa) on Fi_{O_2} of 100%	Pa_{O_2}<300 mmHg (40 kPa) on Fi_{O_2} of 100%
Sputum	Nil or minimal	Purulent, documented infection
Bronchoscopy	Clear or minimal secretions	Purulent secretions

associated with increased post-transplant mortality (e.g. donor smoking history) needs to be balanced against the risk of death on the waiting list.[20]

DONOR MANAGEMENT

A major challenge for the intensive care specialist caring for a potential multi-organ donor is balancing the haemodynamic goals that are optimal for one organ versus those of another. Whereas aggressive diuresis and fluid restriction may help to optimise lung gas exchange, the resultant volume depletion is likely to reduce perfusion to intra-abdominal organs. The main goals of haemodynamic management are to maintain normal central filling pressures and to use the lowest doses of vasopressor agents needed to maintain a mean arterial pressure above 70 mmHg (9.31 kPa).

In recent years there has been a significant shift in the ventilation strategy for brain-dead potential lung donors from a conventional (tidal volume 10–12 mL/kg and 3–5 cm H_2O PEEP) to a lung-protective strategy (6–8 mL/kg tidal volume and 8–10 cm H_2O PEEP). Other features of the lung-protective ventilation strategy are apnoea tests performed during continuous positive airway pressure and maintenance of a closed circuit during airway suction.[21] Use of a lung-protective ventilation strategy compared with a conventional ventilation strategy led to a doubling of the number of suitable lung donors in one large multicentre randomised trial.[21] There has also been interest in the administration of inhaled β_2-agonists to potential lung donors based on experimental evidence of improved donor lung quality and reduced primary graft dysfunction,[22] although preliminary results of a large study of over 500 potential lung donors were discouraging.

The other important aspect of management of the potential lung donor is donor bronchoscopy, particularly in donors with abnormal CXR findings. This is often performed by the lung retrieval team on arrival at the donor hospital. Bronchoscopy facilitates identification of any pathology that would contraindicate transplantation, clearance of inspissated secretions causing atelectasis and lavage sampling of the lower respiratory tract for potential pathogens that might precipitate infection in the recipient.

The very first human lung transplant like the very first human heart transplant was performed from a DCD donor. Interest in the use of lungs from DCD donors was reignited by Steen and colleagues in 2001 who also used an ex vivo lung perfusion system to assess donor lung quality.[23] Since then DCD lung donation has emerged as a major source of donor lungs for transplantation.[24] Indeed, the lung appears to demonstrate greater tolerability to ischaemia in this setting than any other organ so that warm ischaemic times of up to 90 minutes after withdrawal of life support have been tolerated prior to lung retrieval and successful lung transplantation.

DONOR LUNG PRESERVATION

As with heart preservation, the major method of donor lung preservation has been administration of a cold pneumoplegic solution followed by static storage in a lung preservation solution. Perfadex, a normokalaemic colloid solution based on dextran 40, has emerged as the favoured lung storage solution in most lung transplant programmes. It has been found to provide effective donor lung preservation from both DBD and DCD donors.

A major advance in donor lung preservation has been the use of ex vivo lung preservation (EVLP) devices. This concept was first advanced by Steen and colleagues[23,25] and later developed by Cypel and co-workers, who reported that EVLP could be used not only to prevent deterioration in lung function but also to restore function in lungs from extended criteria donors.[26]

HEART TRANSPLANTATION

SELECTION OF PATIENTS FOR HEART TRANSPLANTATION

Eligibility criteria for heart transplantation have been extensively reviewed elsewhere and will be discussed only briefly.[27,28] Heart transplantation is restricted to patients with end-stage heart disease who have exhausted all alternative therapies. Most patients have long-standing and intractable heart failure due to either ischaemic heart disease or some form of cardiomyopathy.[1] A substantial proportion of these patients require long-term mechanical circulatory support (so-called bridge to transplant) and in most jurisdictions between 30% and 50% of waiting-list patients are on mechanical circulatory support.[1] There has been a dramatic evolution in the design of mechanical devices to support the circulation – from large pulsatile pumps to small continuous flow devices that can be implanted in much smaller recipients and have proven to be far more durable.[29] Two-year survival rates for persons supported on continuous flow devices are now better than 80%.[30] Patients on long-term ventricular assist device (VAD) support can generally be managed as outpatients and undergo cardiac rehabilitation to optimise their physical condition prior to transplant surgery. VAD support has also been used in patients who are otherwise marginal candidates for heart transplantation owing to factors such as renal impairment and pulmonary hypertension (so-called bridge to decision). Long-term VAD support has been associated with reversal of these co-morbidities in several case series.[31,32]

A small proportion of patients who require consideration for heart transplantation present acutely in cardiogenic shock following acute myocardial infarction, cardiac surgery (post-cardiotomy syndrome) or in association with myocarditis. Short-term survival of these critically ill patients is usually dependent on acute mechanical circulatory support (e.g. with veno-arterial extracorporeal membrane oxygenation (VA ECMO)). Following stabilisation of vital organ function and establishment that the heart will not recover, these patients will usually be transitioned to a VAD designed for long-term support. There has been considerable interest in the use of mechanical circulatory support as a 'bridge to recovery'. This is most commonly observed when the indication for support is acute fulminant myocarditis. Spontaneous recovery of cardiomyopathic hearts following long-term mechanical support has also been reported, although this appears to be the exception rather than the rule.

HEART TRANSPLANT SURGERY

Heart transplantation can be performed either as an orthotopic or heterotopic procedure. The vast majority of heart transplants are performed orthotopically by excising the native heart and implanting the donor heart in its place. The original surgical technique described by Shumway and Lower[33] is still widely performed. This technique involves anastomosis of the left and right donor atria to the back walls of the corresponding recipient atria containing the central connections of the vena cava and pulmonary veins. An alternative surgical technique for orthotopic heart transplantation involves bicaval anastomosis. The right atrial bicaval anastamosis can be performed alone or in conjunction with anastomosis at the level of the pulmonary veins rather than at the level of the left atrium. The proposed advantages of this technique include better preservation of atrial anatomy and function with reduced risk of atrial thrombosis, atrial arrhythmias and atrioventricular valve regurgitation during long-term follow-up. Surgical series comparing these two approaches, however, suggest that long-term clinical outcomes are similar.

Heterotopic heart transplantation refers to the technique in which the native heart is retained and the donor heart is implanted 'in parallel'. First described by Barnard and colleagues,[34,35] the operation is achieved by anastomosing the left and right atria 'back to back' and then connecting the donor pulmonary artery and aorta to the recipient pulmonary artery and aorta with end-to-side anastomoses. A synthetic pulmonary artery graft is usually required to enable anastomosis between donor and recipient pulmonary arteries. Heterotopic transplantation is now rarely performed. The most common indication is for recipients with fixed pulmonary hypertension. In this setting an allograft that is used to operating against normal pulmonary pressures would fail once transplanted into an environment of pulmonary hypertension; however, in a heterotopic transplant the trained right ventricle of the recipient continues to maintain flow through the pulmonary vascular bed while the heterotopic heart functions primarily as a left ventricular assist. Permanent pacing wires, defibrillator wires and the corresponding systems are removed at the time of the transplant. During the implant the heart is no longer afforded the protection of hypothermia. This critical period of warm ischaemia must be kept to a minimum. To assist in the protection and resuscitation if the heart during this period a dose of blood cardioplegia is administered after the atrial anastomoses are completed.

Once the atrial, pulmonary artery and aortic connections are completed vents are placed in the left ventricle and the aorta, the heart is de-aired and the cross-clamp released. Temporary pacing wires are placed onto the heart and the heart is allowed a period of reperfusion whilst on cardiopulmonary bypass. The duration of the unloaded reperfusion varies and is related to the ischaemic time. A heart that has endured an ischaemic time (from cross-clamp in the donor to reperfusion in the recipient) of 4 hours may be given up to 1 hour of reperfusion before commencing separation from cardiopulmonary bypass and allowing the heart to work. Separation from cardiopulmonary bypass and the completion of the procedure needs to proceed carefully as the transplanted heart, in particular the right ventricle, is prone to acute failure.

POST-TRANSPLANT MANAGEMENT

IMMEDIATE POST-TRANSPLANT CARE AND MONITORING

As with routine cardiac surgical cases, heart transplant recipients are transferred from the operating room to the ICU bed still anaesthetised, intubated and ventilated. In the stable uncomplicated case after transfer to the ICU, sedation will be weaned and the patient extubated when sufficiently conscious, usually after 6–8 hours. Routine monitoring includes an ECG, arterial line, Swan–Ganz catheter and urinary catheter. In some centres, separate left atrial and CVP lines have been used instead of the Swan–Ganz catheter; however, the latter has the advantage of providing a direct measure of the pulmonary vascular resistance, which if elevated may cause acute right heart failure of the 'untrained' donor heart. Pericardial, mediastinal and one or more pleural drains (depending on the complexity of the transplant surgery) will be in place.

PHYSIOLOGY OF THE TRANSPLANTED HEART

The cardiac rhythm of the transplanted heart in the immediate post-transplant period is highly variable. Although there may be early establishment of sinus rhythm at a rate commensurate with the denervated state of the heart, usually the heart is profoundly bradycardic during the first few days after transplantation. Typically the sinus rate increases steadily over the first 1–2 weeks post-transplant and eventually stabilises at a resting rate between 90 and 100 per minute. Drugs that act by augmenting or inhibiting vagal efferent activity (e.g. digoxin, atropine) will have no effect on the heart rate of the transplanted heart. The transplanted heart is often 'stunned' by the reperfusion injury that occurs in the first 24 hours after transplantation. During this period the heart often demonstrates diastolic dysfunction with a restrictive filling pattern, which may persist for days after transplant surgery. Persistence of diastolic dysfunction beyond the first week post-transplant suggests the development of acute rejection.

CARDIAC RHYTHM AND PACING

A–V sequential pacing with temporary pacing wires is routine in the immediate post-transplant period. Filling pressures of 10–15 mmHg (1.33–2 kPa) may be required to ensure adequate diastolic filling and AV sequential pacing at rates up to 110 per minute may be required to maintain a normal cardiac output and stable arterial pressure. Pacing is gradually weaned over the first week post-transplant. During this period the sinus rhythm of the transplanted heart usually increases steadily. Temporary pacing is suspended when a stable sinus rhythm above 60 per minute is established, usually within the first week after transplantation when the heart has also recovered from its initial 'stunning'. Administration of amiodarone to the recipient *prior to* transplantation may delay sinus node recovery. Between 5 and 10% of transplanted hearts remain profoundly bradycardic or develop tachy–brady syndrome (possibly due to sinus node injury during recovery of the donor heart) and require implantation of a permanent pacemaker. Usually 3 weeks are allowed for recovery of sinus rhythm. Oral beta agonists have been used to accelerate sinus node recovery, but it is unclear whether they are effective or reduce the need for permanent pacing.

Tachyarrhythmias are uncommon after transplantation. Atrial fibrillation is probably less common than after other forms of cardiac surgery possibly owing to better preservation of atrial myocardium. Atrial flutter occurring beyond the first week post-transplant is suggestive of acute rejection and should prompt endomyocardial biopsy. If pacing wires are still present they can be used to attempt atrial overdrive pacing (AOD). Alternatively AOD pacing can be performed at the completion of the biopsy procedure. Ventricular tachyarrhythmias are very uncommon and usually observed in the setting of severe acute graft dysfunction and primary graft failure.

INOTROPIC AGENTS

Isoproterenol (isoprenaline) has been used traditionally in the immediate post-transplant ICU phase based on its chronotropic, inotropic and pulmonary vasodilator properties. There have been no large-scale controlled trials comparing different inotropic and chronotropic drugs in the immediate post-transplant period, however, so it is unclear whether these properties of isoproterenol make it any more effective than alternative i.v. inotropic agents such as dobutamine and epinephrine (adrenaline). Epinephrine is often co-administered if the patient is hypotensive with mean arterial pressures below 70 mmHg (9.31 kPa). Thyroid hormone administration to the heart transplant recipient has been advocated by some authors but, as with its use in the donor, its administration to the recipient after heart transplantation is controversial. In the routine case, inotropic and vasopressor support can usually be weaned within the first 48–72 hours as the donor heart recovers.

ARTERIAL BLOOD PRESSURE CONTROL

Prior to heart transplant, the recipient's arterial circulation in many cases has adapted to chronic systemic hypotension with systolic blood pressures in the range 80–90 mmHg (10.64–11.97 kPa). Replacement of an end-stage failing heart with a healthy donor heart often leads to a rapid increase in arterial blood pressure in the recipient as the donor heart regains normal function over the first few days post-transplant. This may be further exacerbated by the introduction of ciclosporin, which causes both renal and systemic vasoconstriction. Systolic blood pressures in excess of 140 mmHg (18.62 kPa) in the first weeks after heart transplantation may result in hypertensive encephalopathy, which may manifest as headache, drowsiness and seizures. Strict control of blood pressure, initially with intravenous vasodilators such as glyceryl trinitrate then with oral agents, may be required to prevent dangerous increases in arterial blood pressure during this early postoperative phase.

IMMUNOSUPPRESSION

Maintenance immunosuppression initially involves the administration of three drugs in combination: high-dose corticosteroids, an antimetabolite (mycophenolate mofetil (MMF) or azathioprine) and a calcineurin inhibitor (CNI, ciclosporin or tacrolimus). Approximately 50% of transplant units also use *induction* therapy, either a T-cell cytolytic agent (e.g. antithymocyte globulin) or an antibody that specifically blocks the activated IL-2 receptor (e.g. basiliximab).[1] The T-cell cytolytic agents are more potent immunosuppressive agents but are also associated with more side-effects related to the acute destruction of large numbers of T cells in the circulation – so-called cytokine release syndrome. Their use is associated with an increased risk of viral and fungal infections as well as later development of post-transplant lymphoproliferative disease (PTLD). They may be administered as a fixed daily dose or adjusted according to the daily T-cell count. The IL-2R inhibitors have a much better side-effect profile and their use is not associated with any increased risk of infection or PTLD. Some transplant units use induction agents routinely, whereas others restrict their use to specific situations (e.g. where there is a delay in commencement of the calcineurin inhibitor, usually because of persistent renal dysfunction in the recipient). Other transplant units use induction agents rarely if at all. Induction agents are usually commenced intraoperatively prior to reperfusion of the transplanted heart. Postoperative administration varies according to the agent used.

Dosing schedules of maintenance immunosuppressive drugs vary considerably between transplant units, although there is little evidence to support one approach over another. Steroids are initially administered intravenously in high doses, typically methylprednisolone 500 mg i.v. in the anaesthetic bay and again prior to reperfusion. A further 3 doses of 125 mg methylprednisolone are administered over the first 24 hours post-transplant, after which the recipient will commence a tapering dose of oral prednisolone starting at 1 mg/kg/day tapering to approximately 0.2 mg/kg/day by the 3rd week post-transplantation. MMF (or azathioprine) is administered with the premed then continued at 1.5 g b.d. either i.v. or orally. Ciclosporin or tacrolimus dosing is more variable. Some units administer the CNI preoperatively provided the recipient has normal renal function. Other units delay administration until after surgery when any acute perioperative renal dysfunction has resolved. Units also vary in their approach to CNI dosing and MMF dosing. Some use fixed dosing whereas others use therapeutic drug monitoring, adjusting the dose to meet target blood levels.

INFECTION PROPHYLAXIS

With currently used immunosuppressive drug protocols, the risk of infection is relatively low. Routine precautions including hand washing are applied as for standard ICU patients; however, patient isolation and barrier nursing are generally not required unless the patient is already colonised with multiresistant organisms.

Prophylactic antibiotic therapy is routine. A cephalosporin administered intravenously over the first 24 hours is routine; however, the choice of antibiotic may vary if the recipient is known to be colonised with one or more multiresistant organisms. *Pneumocystis* prophylaxis in the form of oral co-trimoxazole is commenced in the first week post-transplantation and continued indefinitely. Nystatin oral solution to prevent oropharyngeal candidiasis is also administered for the first 2 weeks post-transplant. Prophylaxis against other fungi particularly *Aspergillus* varies between units and may depend on local resistance patterns. Inhaled amphotericin for the first week followed by oral itraconazole for 3 months is one approach. In the event of a CMV mismatch (CMV-positive donor with CMV-negative recipient) oral valganciclovir is administered for the first 3 months post-transplant. Some units also administer valganciclovir to CMV-positive recipients.

Other routine drugs administered in the immediate post-transplant period include an insulin infusion as required to control hyperglycaemia, which is common following administration of high-dose steroids, proton pump inhibitors to prevent peptic ulceration and a statin. A typical post-transplant drug treatment protocol is shown in **Table 102.3**.

COMPLICATIONS

PRIMARY GRAFT FAILURE (PGF)

PGF is a syndrome in which the transplanted heart fails to meet the circulatory requirements of the recipient in the immediate post-transplant period as a consequence of either single or biventricular dysfunction. It is manifested as hypotension and low cardiac output in the presence of adequate filling pressures.[36] In most instances, it is likely to result from a multifactorial process with contributing elements from the donor, recipient and the transplant process.[8] Primary graft failure is the most feared early complication after heart transplantation and accounts for approximately 40% of all deaths within the first month.[1] The reported incidence of PGF after heart transplantation varies widely between studies with estimates ranging between 2.3 and 26%.[8] Most of the variability can be attributed to inconsistent definitions of PGF used by different authors. When PGF has been defined as the need for high-dose inotropes or mechanical assist devices in the immediate post-transplant period, most investigators have reported incidence rates of 10–20% or higher. Suggested diagnostic criteria for primary graft failure are listed in **Table 102.4**. Recognised risk factors for PGF are listed in **Table 102.5**.

Management of PGF depends on the severity and the mechanism of graft failure. In cases of selective or predominant right ventricular (RV) failure, pre-existing pulmonary hypertension (with or without acute exacerbation following cardiopulmonary bypass) is usually the cause. Selective pulmonary vasodilators such as inhaled nitric oxide or inhaled prostacyclin may provide sufficient RV unloading to restore cardiac output: however, the impact of these therapies on overall outcome is uncertain.[38–40] In severe cases implantation of an acute right ventricular assist device (RVAD) may be required. Longer-acting agents such as oral sildenafil may be required to allow weaning of nitric oxide and RVAD support in such cases.[41] In severe cases of left or bi-ventricular failure, early institution of total mechanical circulatory support is essential to avoid multi-organ failure.[42,43] A number of acute mechanical support options are available but the most widely used device is VA ECMO, which can be deployed by either peripheral or central cannulation.[42,43] Total circulatory support may be required for 7 days or longer.

INFECTIONS

Infections encountered in heart transplant recipients during the ICU phase of management are similar to those affecting routine cardiac surgical cases. Risk

Table 102.3 Perioperative heart and lung transplant drug treatment protocols currently utilised in the Heart and Lung Transplant Unit at St Vincent's Hospital, Sydney

AREA	HEART	LUNG
Preoperative on ward	Mycophenolate mofetil 1.5 g p.o.	Azathioprine 3 mg/kg p.o. Ciclosporin capsules p.o. 2 mg/kg if creatinine≤120 µmol/L 1 mg/kg if creatinine=130 µmol/L Omit if creatinine>130 µmol/L (CF patients must take pancreatic enzymes as for 'snack' with oral ciclosporin capsules)
In anaesthetic bay	Basiliximab 20 mg i.v.: if creatinine >120 µmol/L on night of transplant, or previously recorded creatinine >120 µmol/L, or LVAD, BiVAD or TAH (Give second dose of 20 mg i.v. on day 4) Vitamin K 10 mg i.v.: if on warfarin Methylprednisolone 500 mg i.v. Ganciclovir 5 mg/kg i.v.: if CMV mismatch (D+/R–). Cefazolin 500 mg	Methylprednisolone 500 mg i.v. Ganciclovir 5 mg/kg i.v.: if CMV mismatch Cefotaxime 1g i.v.; however, antibiotics based on donor and recipient micro, consult respiratory physician
In theatre off bypass	Methylprednisolone 500 mg i.v. Cefazolin 500 mg i.v.	Methylprednisolone 500 mg i.v. Cefotaxime 1 g i.v.; however, antibiotics often based on donor and recipient micro, consult respiratory physician
ICU or ward	IMMUNOSUPPRESSION	IMMUNOSUPPRESSION
	DAY 1	
	Tacrolimus 0.5 mg p.o. or via nasogastric tube: if Cr<140 µmol/L: give test dose or, if unable to commence oral therapy, commence infusion at 0.015 mg/kg/day i.v. given as continuous infusion over 24 h If Cr>140 µmol/L: hold tacrolimus until creatinine <140 µmol/L Methylprednisolone 125 mg i.v. q. 8 h×3 doses Myocphenolate mofetil 1 g i.v./p.o. b.d.	Ciclosporin 1 mg/kg i.v. as continuous infusion while intubated, increasing to 2 mg/kg depending on first steady state level (within 24–48 hours post-transplant). Initial target steady-state level=400–450 µg/L Ciclosporin p.o. b.d. once extubated (NB: p.o. dose is approximately 3 times the i.v. dose) CF patients: ciclosporin p.o. t.d.s. given with pancreatic enzymes, dose as for 'snack' Azathioprine 2 mg/kg i.v./p.o. nocte Methylprednisolone 125 mg i.v. q. 8 h x 3 doses, *then*
	DAY 2 ONWARDS	
	Methylprednisolone 40 mg i.v. b.d.×2 doses, *then* Prednisolone 0.6 mg/kg/day p.o. in 2 divided doses until 2 weeks post-transplant then wean by 0.1 mg/kg/day each week until complete withdrawal Mycophenolate mofetil 1 g i.v./p.o. b.d. Tacrolimus capsules p.o. b.d. as charted (titrate to target trough level of 8–12 µg/L by day 7) Basiliximab 20 mg i.v. on day 4 – *if given as induction.*	Prednisolone 1 mg/kg/day p.o. in 2 divided doses, tapering by 5 mg every second day to a single daily dose of 0.2 mg/kg (until first transbronchial biopsy)
	BACTERIAL PROPHYLAXIS	BACTERIAL PROPHYLAXIS
	Cefazolin 1 g i.v. q. 8 h×3 doses	Cefotaxime 1 g i.v. t.d.s. for 5 days – (may vary according to cultures) Roxithromycin 300 mg p.o. nocte – *Chlamydia* management Co-trimoxazole 800 mg/160 mg p.o. (Bactrim DS®), 1 tablet mane on Mondays and Fridays only

Table 102.3 Perioperative heart and lung transplant drug treatment protocols currently utilised in the Heart and Lung Transplant Unit at St Vincent's Hospital, Sydney—cont'd

AREA	HEART	LUNG
	FUNGAL PROPHYLAXIS	FUNGAL PROPHYLAXIS
	Nystatin drops 1 mL p.o. q.i.d. Sulfamethoxazole 800 mg p.o. *and* Trimethoprim 160 mg (Bactrim DS), one daily on Mondays and Fridays. Itraconazole 200 mg p.o. b.d. to be given until 12 weeks post-transplant Measure itraconazole trough level on day 14 (target >500 µg/L) Tacrolimus level must be rechecked when itraconazole ceased	Nystatin oral drops 1 mL p.o. q.i.d. Sulfamethoxazole 800 mg p.o. *and* Trimethoprim 160 mg (Bactrim DS), one daily on Mondays and Fridays (If *sulphur allergy*, check with consultant: give dapsone 100 mg daily on Mon/Wed/Fri) Nebulised salbutamol 5 mg b.d. 30 minutes before Nebulised amphotericin (Fungizone®) 10 mg b.d. until discharge from hospital
	VIRAL PROPHYLAXIS	VIRAL PROPHYLAXIS
	If CMV mismatch: ganciclovir 5 mg/kg/day i.v. on Monday, Wednesday and Friday until i.v. line is removed Then continue with valganciclovir 450 mg p.o. b.d. (adjusted to renal function) to be given until 12 weeks post-transplant	*CMV MISMATCH* Ganciclovir 5 mg/kg i.v. daily Mon/Wed/Fri until i.v. removed, then p.o. valganciclovir 450 mg b.d. (dose adjusted according to renal function) indefinitely CMV hyperimmune globulin i.v.: 2 vials days 1, 2, 3, 7, 14, 21 *CMV-POSITIVE RECIPIENT* Ganciclovir 5 mg/kg i.v. daily Mon/Wed/Fri until i.v. removed, then valganciclovir 450 mg p.o. b.d. (dose adjusted according to renal function) for 12 months *EBV-NEGATIVE PATIENTS (IF NOT ALREADY ON VALGANCICLOVIR)* VALACICLOVIR 500 MG P.O. B.D. (DEPENDING ON RENAL FUNCTION) INDEFINITELY
	PAIN MANAGEMENT	PAIN MANAGEMENT
	Morphine 1–2.5 mg i.v. p.r.n. Morphine 5–10 mg i.v. p.r.n. Paracetamol 1 g p.o./i.v. q.i.d.	Epidural anaesthesia (max. 5 days), if appropriate. Morphine 1–2.5 mg i.v. p.r.n. Morphine 5–10 mg i.m./s.c. p.r.n. Paracetamol 1 g p.o. q. 6 h Oxycodone 5 mg p.o. q. 6 h p.r.n.
	BOWEL MANAGEMENT	BOWEL MANAGEMENT
	Docusate with sennosides (50 mg, 8 mg) p.o. 2 b.d. Movicol p.o. 1 sachet daily	Docusate with sennosides (50 mg, 8 mg) p.o. 2 b.d. Movicol p.o. 1 sachet daily For CF patients check with consultant if diatrizoic acid (Gastrografin) 25–50 mL p.o. p.r.n. to be given
	GIT PROTECTION	GIT PROTECTION/REFLUX MANAGEMENT
	Ranitidine 50 mg i.v. t.d.s., followed by Ranitidine 150 mg p.o. b.d. on ward LIPID MANAGEMENT Pravastatin 40 mg p.o. nocte	Pantoprazole 40 mg i.v. daily or Ranitidine 50 mg i.v. t.d.s., then Rabeprazole 20 mg p.o. daily when on ward. If reflux symptoms persist, consider addition of: Domperidone 10–20 mg p.o. q.i.d. Sucralfate 1 g p.o. q.i.d.

Continued

Table 102.3 Perioperative heart and lung transplant drug treatment protocols currently utilised in the Heart and Lung Transplant Unit at St Vincent's Hospital, Sydney—cont'd

AREA	HEART	LUNG
	BONE PROTECTION	BONE PROTECTION
	Cholecalciferol 1000 U p.o. daily	Cholecalciferol 1000 U p.o. daily
	CALCIUM CITRATE 2 TABLETS P.O. NOCTE	CALCIUM CITRATE 2 TABLETS P.O. NOCTE, *PLUS* IF BMD <–1: CONSULT ENDOCRINE TEAM – ZOLEDRONIC ACID 4 MG I.V. EVERY 12 MONTHS

Table 102.4 Suggested diagnostic criteria for primary graft failure after heart transplantation

PRESENCE OF	EVIDENCED BY
Ventricular systolic dysfunction – left, right or biventricular dysfunction	Echocardiographic evidence of dysfunction
Cardiogenic shock lasting more than 1 hour	Low systolic blood pressure <90 mmHg (11.97 kPa) *and/or* Low cardiac output – <2 L/min/m² despite adequate intracardiac filling pressures – CVP>15 mmHg (2 kPa) and/or PAWP>20 mmHg (2.66 kPa)
Circulatory support	Use of ≥2 inotropic agents/vasopressors including high-dose epinephrine or norepinephrine *and/or* Use of a mechanical assist device – IABP, ECMO, VAD
Appropriate time frame	Onset <24 hours post-transplantation
Exclusion of secondary causes of PGF	e.g. cardiac tamponade, hyperacute rejection

Table 102.5 Recognised risk factors for primary graft failure after heart transplantation

DONOR FACTORS	RECIPIENT FACTORS	PROCEDURAL FACTORS
Age >30 years	Age >60 years	Ischaemic time >180 minutes
Cardiac dysfunction on Echo	Ventilator support	Donor recipient weight mismatching
High-dose inotropic support	Intravenous inotropic support, mechanical support	Female donor to male recipient
Cause of brain death	Pulmonary hypertension	Concomitant lung retrieval
Primary graft dysfunction of other organs	Overweight, diabetes mellitus	

factors for bacterial sepsis that are of particular importance for the heart transplant recipient include pretransplant mechanical or ventilator support and the need for high-dose perioperative immunosuppression. Other factors associated with an increased risk of sepsis in the ICU patient such as previous colonisation with multiresistant bacteria, large-volume blood loss and transfusion, acute renal failure and prolonged ventilation or placement of intravenous lines also apply to the heart transplant recipient. Classic signs of sepsis such as high fever may be masked or blunted by immunosuppressive therapy so a high index of suspicion is required. Infections usually respond to conventional antibiotic therapy but choice will depend on local sensitivities. Herpes simplex is common in the early post-transplant period but usually responds to oral aciclovir (acyclovir). Clinical infections with other viruses (e.g. herpes zoster and cytomegalovirus) usually have a more delayed onset after the ICU phase of treatment. Oropharyngeal candidiasis is probably the most common fungal infection and is usually preventable with oral nystatin. Occasionally, patients may present with early candidaemia, which is an important differential in the acutely septic patient. Other fungal infections such as *Aspergillus* may also occur during the immediate postoperative period but more typically occur at a later time point.

ACUTE REJECTION

Acute rejection is an adaptive immune response mounted by the recipient against the transplanted donor organ. Classical acute rejection is predominantly a T-lymphocyte-mediated inflammatory response directed against the grafted organ. As the rejection response progresses, graft injury in the form of myocyte necrosis and myocardial oedema develop. In more severe rejection, other inflammatory cells such as eosinophils and neutrophils are recruited into the myocardium and myocardial haemorrhage may occur. Acute cellular rejection can occur at any time post-transplantation but is unusual during the first week postoperatively. Acute rejection may be suspected on clinical grounds but is often completely asymptomatic. Symptoms are often non-specific and include fatigue, dyspnoea and fever.

Diagnosis is based on the pathological finding of a lymphocytic inflammatory infiltrate on endomyocardial biopsy and the grading of severity is based on the extent of the inflammatory infiltrate and the presence or absence of myocyte necrosis.[44] Most transplant programmes perform regular surveillance endomyocardial biopsies commencing at about 1 week post-transplant. Biopsies are repeated weekly for the first month post-transplant, fortnightly between months 1 and 3, monthly between months 4 and 6 then less commonly thereafter. Endomyocardial biopsy may be performed at any time between scheduled biopsies if there is clinical suspicion of rejection. The preferred vascular access for endomyocardial biopsy is the right internal jugular vein and this should be considered when placing central venous lines for critical care purposes.

The overall rate of biopsy proven acute rejection has been declining in recent years probably as a result of more effective maintenance immunosuppressive therapy.[1] Historically, most patients experienced one or more episodes of acute rejection requiring 'pulsed' steroid therapy (e.g. i.v. methylprednisolone 0.5–1.0 g daily for three doses) during the first 3 months after transplantation; however, recent registry reports indicate that only one in three heart transplant recipients will experience an acute rejection episode requiring pulsed immunosuppressive treatment during the first 12 months.[1]

Antibody-mediated rejection is also now recognised as a major cause of graft injury and loss.[45] It occurs as a result of the formation of donor-specific antibodies (DSA) in the recipient that are directed usually against donor HLA antigens. These may be present pre-transplant as a result of previous transfusions, organ transplants, viral infections or pregnancies. Hyperacute rejection (HAR) occurring during the first hours or days post-transplant is usually triggered by the presence of preformed DSA in high circulating titres. Fortunately, this is now a rare event as DSAs are normally detected by prospective or virtual cross-matching between the donor and recipient.[46] HAR often presents with rapid onset of severe graft dysfunction and may be difficult to distinguish from primary graft failure. Apart from acute circulatory support, treatment involves high-dose intravenous steroids, plasmapheresis and intravenous immunoglobulin (IVIG). In more severe cases, monoclonal antibody treatments have been used including rituximab, bortezomib and eculizumab.

LUNG TRANSPLANTATION

SELECTION OF PATIENTS FOR LUNG TRANSPLANTATION

As with heart transplantation, the primary indication for lung transplantation is the presence of advanced lung disease for which there is no alternative therapy. Guidelines for eligibility and selection criteria for lung transplantation have been extensively reviewed elsewhere.[47,48] The major disease categories are COPD/emphysema including α_1-antitrypsin deficiency, pulmonary fibrosis, cystic fibrosis, bronchiectasis and pulmonary vascular disease.[2] Collectively these diseases account for more than 90% of cases. Transplant procedures for pulmonary fibrosis have increased steadily during the last decade from 16% of all procedures in 2000 to 28% in 2009.[2] Bilateral lung transplantation has become the most commonly performed lung transplant procedure for all major lung diseases and in the most recent report of the ISHLT Registry accounted for 72% of all transplants.[2] Single lung is still occasionally performed for non-AAT-deficiency-associated COPD/emphysema and pulmonary fibrosis but rarely for other lung diseases. Combined heart–lung transplantation is now a relatively rare procedure and is largely restricted to patients with pulmonary vascular disease in association with complex congenital heart disease or coincidental severe end-stage heart and lung disease.

A critical aspect of the decision making regarding suitability for lung transplantation is the capacity of the patient to survive the stresses of lung transplant surgery. For this reason, patients who are too unwell either acutely or chronically have been considered unsuitable for lung transplantation. Objective criteria for defining these characteristics have been lacking, however, and decisions regarding capacity to survive the stress of surgery have to a large extent been based on clinical judgement.[46] Among the former are those with terminal respiratory failure requiring prolonged ventilator support with or without other organ failure. Among the latter are those who are malnourished, weak and cachectic due to chronic illness. Quantitative measures of frailty may provide a more objective measure on which to base decisions regarding suitability for transplantation; however, considerable further research is required.[49] The problem has been further compounded by the lack of a safe and effective 'artificial lung' to enable patients with advanced respiratory failure to be weaned from acute ventilator support and to participate in some form of rehabilitation programme prior to transplant surgery. ECMO support in awake patients or the use of pumpless carbon dioxide removal devices (e.g. Novalung) may go some way towards addressing this limitation.[50,51]

LUNG TRANSPLANT SURGERY

Bilateral lung transplantation was initially developed as an en bloc technique with a single tracheal anastomosis; however, the high incidence of tracheal anastomotic complications has led to this procedure largely being replaced by the technically simpler bilateral sequential single-lung transplant (BSSLT) procedure. BSSLT is most commonly performed with the larger right lung transplanted first followed by the left lung. The surgical approach may be via a midline sternotomy, horizontal bilateral thoracosternotomy (clam shell incision), or two smaller anterolateral thoracotomies (where the sternum is not divided). The operation may be performed with or without cardiopulmonary bypass, depending on the ability of the native lung to sustain the cardiac output and ventilation during implantation of the first lung and then the ability of the transplanted lung to sustain the cardiac output and ventilation during implantation of the second lung. Although cardiopulmonary bypass ensures the maintenance of adequate ventilation and vital organ perfusion, it requires anticoagulation and its use is associated with an increased risk of perioperative bleeding. Cardiopulmonary bypass does, however, offer the advantage of better operating conditions and importantly it allows control of donor lung reperfusion conditions. In the absence of cardiopulmonary bypass, the newly transplanted right lung must take over ventilation in order for the left lung to be implanted. At this time the transplanted right lung will receive the entire cardiac output and this can be detrimental. Cardiopulmonary bypass appears to have no deleterious effect on early lung function or clinical outcome.[52] A cuff of donor left atrial tissue containing the confluence of the two pulmonary veins is anastomosed to the recipient left atrium followed by the anastomosis of the donor to recipient pulmonary artery and finally the donor to recipient main bronchus.

Single-lung transplantation is performed via a thoracotomy on the corresponding side with the order of anastomoses being bronchus, left atrium and pulmonary artery. Combined heart–lung transplantation is the most extensive cardiothoracic transplant and is now restricted almost exclusively to patients with complex congenital heart disease complicated by irreversible pulmonary vascular disease. The operation is performed on cardiopulmonary bypass as an en bloc procedure with sequential anastomosis of the trachea, right atrium and aorta. Uncontrollable bleeding from adhesions formed during previous thoracic operations or from systemic to pulmonary arterial collaterals is a major cause of operative death in these patients. Surgical damage to major nerves (e.g. vagus, phrenic and recurrent laryngeal) is a potential complication of heart–lung transplantation and may contribute to postoperative morbidity.

POST-TRANSPLANT MANAGEMENT

IMMEDIATE POST-TRANSPLANT CARE AND MONITORING

Lung transplant recipients, like heart transplant recipients, are transferred from the operating room to the ICU bed still anaesthetised, intubated and ventilated. Bronchoscopy is performed in the operating room and later in the ICU. This is to check the bronchial anastomosis and to suction any secretions. In the uncomplicated case after transfer to the ICU, sedation will be weaned and the patient extubated when sufficiently conscious, usually within 24 hours of surgery. Routine monitoring includes an ECG, arterial line, Swan–Ganz catheter and urinary catheter. Upper and basal pleural drains will be in place and are placed on continuous suction. Air leaks can occur in the first few days post-transplant but are usually of small volume and self-limiting.

PHYSIOLOGY OF THE TRANSPLANTED LUNG

Transplantation of the lungs results in denervation below the level of the bronchial anastomosis (or below the tracheal anastomosis in the case of heart–lung transplantation). The main functional consequence is loss of the normal cough reflex and markedly impaired mucociliary clearance distal to the anastomosis, so patients are at high risk of sputum retention during the early postoperative phase. Respiration both at rest and in response to exercise is unaffected by lung denervation. Pulmonary vascular resistance, airway resistance and reactivity also appear to be unaffected by lung denervation.

VENTILATORY AND INOTROPIC SUPPORT

Postoperative ventilatory support varies according to the type of transplant. A normal endotracheal tube can be placed for double-lung and heart–lung transplant recipients. Occasionally, single lung transplant recipients may require placement of a double-lumen endotracheal tube to allow differential ventilation of the native and transplanted lungs. Chronotropic and inotropic support are routine for heart–lung transplantation but are not routinely required after single and BSSL transplantation.

Ventilator settings are similar to those used for patients undergoing major lung surgery with the aim being to minimise the risk of ventilator-induced lung injury. The Fi_{O_2} is rapidly reduced to the lowest level sufficient to maintain a Pa_{O_2} in the range 80–120 mmHg (10.64–15.96 kPa). Where possible, the tidal volume is kept below 6–8 mL per kg and the ventilator frequency is adjusted to maintain a peak inspiratory pressures below 30 cm H_2O. Positive end-expiratory pressure

(PEEP) will be set at 5–10 cm H_2O but may be increased depending on requirements. If arterial blood gasses are adequate the patient is woken and progressed towards extubation. This will involve a gradual withdrawal of ventilatory support.

IMMUNOSUPPRESSION

Induction therapy is used in approximately half of all lung transplant programmes. There has been an increase in the use of induction therapy in the most recent era, with a move away from polyclonal antithymocyte preparations to IL-2R antagonists or alemtuzumab.[2] ISHLT Registry data suggest a small improvement in survival in patients receiving induction therapy; however, this is based on a retrospective, non-randomised comparison.

As with heart transplantation, maintenance immunosuppression in lung transplant recipients initially involves the administration of three drugs in combination: high-dose corticosteroids, an antimetabolite (mycophenolate mofetil (MMF) or azathioprine) and a calcineurin inhibitor (CNI, ciclosporin or tacrolimus). Tacrolimus and MMF are the preferred CNI and antimetabolite in the majority of lung transplant programmes.[2] Recipients with cystic fibrosis are administered their calcineurin inhibitor with a pancreatic enzyme supplement on a t.d.s. schedule.

INFECTION PROPHYLAXIS

Lung transplant recipients are at high risk of infection, more so than other organ transplant recipients. In addition to being transplanted into a heavily immunosuppressed recipient, the transplanted lung uniquely is in direct contact with the external environment and any potential airborne pathogens. Often the donor has evidence of lower airway colonisation or even infection prior to lung retrieval. There is impaired ciliary function and loss of the cough reflex below the bronchial/tracheal anastomosis resulting in retained secretions below the anastomosis. In addition, a substantial proportion of lung transplant recipients - those with cystic fibrosis or bronchiectasis - are invariably colonised with multiresistant bacteria in the upper respiratory tract at the time of transplantation. These organisms can rapidly spread to the lower respiratory tract.

Bacterial prophylaxis

Donor sputum or bronchoscopy samples are taken prior to or at the time of lung retrieval and are used to guide antibiotic therapy in the recipient. For recipients with chronic suppurative lung disease prior to transplant, antibiotic prophylaxis will depend on sensitivities determined from pre-transplant surveillance. For other lung transplant recipients a third-generation cephalosporin with broad spectrum against Gram-positive and -negative organisms (e.g. cefotaxime) is administered.

Fungal prophylaxis

As with heart transplantation, *Pneumocystis jiroveci* prophylaxis usually in the form of oral co-trimoxazole is commenced in the first week post-transplantation and continued indefinitely. For patients who are allergic to sulfonamides, oral dapsone or monthly inhaled pentamidine is a suitable alternative. Nystatin oral solution to prevent oropharyngeal candidiasis is also administered for the first few weeks post-transplant. *Aspergillus* infections are less common but potentially catastrophic. Inhaled amphotericin (preceded by inhaled bronchodilators) has been shown to significantly reduce the incidence of *Aspergillus* and other fungal infections and is administered routinely as a b.d. or t.d.s. dose until hospital discharge.[53]

Viral prophylaxis

CMV may cause life-threatening pneumonitis in the lung transplant recipient and has been associated with increased risk of later development of bronchiolitis obliterans syndrome. Risk is highest in recipients of lungs from CMV-seropositive donors, particularly when the recipient is CMV negative (D+/R–). Although clinical infection is extremely uncommon in the first month post-transplant, it is essential to commence prophylaxis immediately post-transplant. Intravenous ganciclovir is administered initially followed by oral valganciclovir (dose adjusted for renal function) once the recipient is able start oral medications. Valganciclovir is continued indefinitely in D+/R– patients and for 6 months in D+/R+ and D–/R+ recipients. CMV hyperimmune globulin is also administered for up to 1 month to D+/R– recipients in some institutions. Recipients who are Epstein–Barr Virus (EBV) naïve who receive lungs from EBV-seropositive donors (D+/R–) are at high risk of developing post-transplant lymphoproliferative disease (PTLD), which carries a very high mortality. If not already receiving oral valganciclovir, EBV D+/R– recipients are maintained on valaciclovir indefinitely.

Other routine drugs administered in the immediate post-transplant period include an insulin infusion as required to control hyperglycaemia, which is common following administration of high-dose steroids, proton pump inhibitors to prevent peptic ulceration, domperidone and sucrulfate to prevent gastro-oesophageal reflux and calcium and vitamin D supplements to prevent osteoporosis. A typical post-transplant drug treatment protocol is shown in Table 102.3.

COMPLICATIONS

PRIMARY GRAFT DYSFUNCTION AND FAILURE

Primary graft dysfunction (PGD) is defined as an acute non-immune-mediated injury to the transplanted lung occurring within the first 72 hours postoperatively. PGD has been reported in up to 25% of lung transplant

Table 102.6 ISHLT Grading system for primary graft dysfunction after lung transplantation

PGD GRADE	Pa_{O_2}/Fi_{O_2}	RADIOGRAPHIC INFILTRATES CONSISTENT WITH PULMONARY OEDEMA
0	>300	Absent
1	>300	Present
2	200–300	Present
3	<200	Present

Table 102.7 Recognised risk factors for primary graft dysfunction after lung transplantation

DONOR FACTORS	RECIPIENT FACTORS	PROCEDURAL FACTORS
Age >50 years	Age >60 years	Prolonged ischaemic time
Smoking >10 pack years	Ventilator or ECMO support	
Pneumonia on CXR or purulent secretions on bronchoscopy	Pulmonary fibrosis	
Primary graft dysfunction of other organs	Pulmonary hypertension	
	Obesity	

recipients. The syndrome is manifested as impaired oxygenation and the presence of pulmonary alveolar opacities on CXR. The extent of the abnormalities in these two parameters has been used to grade the severity of the syndrome from absent (Grade 0) to severe (Grade 3) (**Table 102.6**).[51] In its most severe form, PGD3 results in a fulminant adult respiratory distress syndrome (ARDS). In this instance, there is rapid deterioration in gas exchange associated with increased pulmonary vascular resistance, reduced lung compliance and diffuse bilateral alveolar infiltrates on CXR. The major underlying cause is thought to be ischaemia reperfusion injury to the transplanted lungs, but other factors such as acid aspiration, pneumonia and ventilator-induced barotrauma may contribute (**Table 102.7**). Risk factors include prolonged graft ischaemia, increasing donor age and recipient diagnosis of pulmonary hypertension.[7]

Severe PGD is the major cause of early mortality after lung transplantation with a reported mortality of up to 50%. It is also associated with increased acute morbidity related to the need for prolonged ventilation and ICU stay, prolonged hospital stay and delayed recovery of lung function. For recipients who survive an episode of severe primary graft dysfunction, there are data suggesting that long-term outcomes are adversely affected.

Treatment is supportive and aimed at maintaining adequate gas exchange until the syndrome resolves. Inhaled nitric oxide has been shown to improve gas exchange and lower pulmonary vascular resistance acutely in PGD but has not been found to affect overall survival. In the most severe cases, ECMO support may be required to maintain oxygenation and remove carbon dioxide.

INFECTIONS

The infectious agents of most concern during the immediate post-transplant period are multiresistant bacterial pathogens, particularly in those undergoing transplantation for chronic suppurative lung disease. Pneumonia is the most common infectious complication and the risk is further increased by the need for prolonged ventilation (in the case of primary graft dysfunction) and airway complications (discussed below). Choice of antibiotic is based on in vitro sensitivities. As mentioned, fungal infections are less common but may be catastrophic. Angioinvasive *Aspergillus* infection may result in rapidly progressive necrotising pneumonia, bronchial anastomotic dehiscence or even pulmonary arterial or venous anastomotic dehiscence leading to exsanguinating haemoptysis. An aggressive diagnostic approach including bronchoscopy with bronchial washings or CT-guided fine needle aspiration of focal pneumonic lesions is essential to facilitate early diagnosis and initiation of appropriate antibiotic or antifungal treatment.

ACUTE REJECTION

The incidence of acute rejection after lung transplantation has been declining as it has for heart transplantation. Based on the most recent report from the ISHLT Registry, approximately one-third of lung transplant recipients develop acute rejection during the first 12 months after transplantation. Symptoms and signs of rejection are non-specific and include dyspnoea, cough, sputum production, fever, declining FEV_1 on spirometry and the appearance of alveolar infiltrates on CXR. The major differential diagnosis is lower respiratory tract infection. If unrecognised and untreated, acute rejection can lead to rapid onset of severe graft dysfunction and a clinical picture of ARDS. It is important to remember that rejection and infection can occur simultaneously. Transbronchial lung biopsy performed at the time of bronchoscopy and bronchial washing is required to confirm the diagnosis pathologically. As with heart transplantation, the severity of acute lung rejection is graded histologically.[54] Treatment for biopsy proven acute rejection in the first instance involves pulsed intravenous or oral steroid therapy.

Graft dysfunction occurring during the first 72 hours after transplantation is usually due to primary graft dysfunction; however, graft dysfunction occurring at any time after this suggests another cause – usually either infection or rejection. Acute cellular rejection is very uncommon in the first week post-transplant but acute antibody-mediated rejection (AMR) may occur if there are preformed donor-specific antibodies. AMR may result in severe graft dysfunction and be difficult to distinguish from PGD. Treatment of acute AMR is intensive and involves a combination of plasmapheresis, administration of high dose intravenous immunoglobulin (IVIG) and rituximab.

AIRWAY COMPLICATIONS

In most lung transplant operations, the surgeon does not attempt to restore the bronchial blood flow to the transplanted lung. Establishment of bronchial blood flow to the transplanted lung does occur over the first month post-transplant via ingrowth of collaterals from the recipient, but until then the transplanted lung is reliant on low-pressure retrograde collateral bronchial flow of (deoxygenated) blood from the pulmonary artery.[55] For these reasons the donor bronchus is relatively ischaemic during the first few weeks after transplantation and this predisposes to a number of airway complications including bronchial stenosis at or beyond the anastomosis, bronchomalacia, endobronchial infections and bronchial anastomotic dehiscence. The latter is often associated with persistent large air leaks from pleural or mediastinal drains and development of fatal mediastinitis. Repeated bronchoscopic assessment of the anastomosis is undertaken during the first 4–6 weeks until healing is complete. A variety of bronchoscopic interventional procedures have been developed to treat the different airway complications.[55]

CONCLUSIONS

Heart and lung transplantation have emerged as the most effective treatments available for patients with end-stage heart or lung disease. Transplantation of both organ transplants is limited by donor numbers so that only a small percentage of patients who might benefit are able to undergo the procedure. The severe shortage of donor organs has resulted in an increased utilisation of marginal donors with an associated risk of primary graft dysfunction or failure, which poses significant challenges during the initial ICU management of these patients. Nevertheless, the large majority of heart and lung transplant recipients make an excellent recovery following transplant surgery and return to a quality of life that is close to that of normal people of the same age. Almost two-thirds of heart transplant recipients live for more than 10 years and one-third live for more than 20 years after transplantation. Long-term survival of lung transplant recipients is less than that of heart transplant recipients but has been improving steadily. Improvements in donor management and organ preservation should increase the number of cardiothoracic organs available for transplantation, while ongoing refinements to post-transplant management are likely to result in further improvements in the long-term survival of these patients.

Access the complete references list online at http://www.expertconsult.com

1. Stehlik J, Edwards LB, Kucheryavaya AY, et al. The Registry of the International Society for Heart and Lung Transplantation: Twenty-eighth Adult Heart Transplant Report – 2011. J Heart Lung Transplant 2011;30(10):1078–94.
2. Christie JD, Edwards LB, Kucheryavaya AY, et al. The Registry of the International Society for Heart and Lung Transplantation: Twenty-eighth Adult Lung and Heart-Lung Transplant Report – 2011. J Heart Lung Transplant 2011;30(10):1104–22.
8. Iyer A, Kumarasinghe G, Hicks M, et al. Primary graft failure after heart transplantation. J Transplant 2011;2011:175768.
9. Zaroff JG, Rosengard BR, Armstrong WF, et al. Consensus conference report: maximizing use of organs recovered from the cadaver donor: cardiac recommendations, March 28–29, 2001, Crystal City, Va. Circulation 2002;106(7):836–41.
15. Macdonald PS, Aneman A, Bhonagiri D, et al. A systematic review and meta-analysis of clinical trials of thyroid hormone administration to brain dead potential organ donors. Crit Care Med 2012;40(5): 1635–44.
26. Cypel M, Yeung JC, Liu M, et al. Normothermic ex vivo lung perfusion in clinical lung transplantation. N Engl J Med 2011;364(15):1431–40.
28. Mehra MR, Kobashigawa J, Starling R, et al. Listing criteria for heart transplantation: International Society for Heart and Lung Transplantation guidelines for the care of cardiac transplant candidates 30 2006. J Heart Lung Transplant 2006;25(9): 1024–42.
30. Slaughter MS, Rogers JG, Milano CA, et al; HeartMate II Investigators. Advanced heart failure treated with continuous-flow left ventricular assist device. N Engl J Med 2009;361(23):2241–51.
48. Orens JB, Estenne M, Arcasoy S, et al; Pulmonary Scientific Council of the International Society for Heart and Lung Transplantation. International guidelines for the selection of lung transplant candidates: 2006 update – a consensus report from the Pulmonary Scientific Council of the International Society for Heart and Lung Transplantation. J Heart Lung Transplant 2006;25(7):745–55.

Part Seventeen

Paediatric Intensive Care

103

The critically ill child

Shelley D Riphagen

The chapters on paediatric intensive care are intended to help intensivists outside specialist paediatric centres manage common paediatric emergencies. They should be read in conjunction with relevant adult chapters, as there are many areas of commonality.

Compared with adults, there are a number of differences in neonates, infants and young children that render them more susceptible to disease and the progression to critical illness.

Very importantly, young children are unable to verbalise their complaints and the concerned responsible care-giver/parent must be listened to and taken seriously. Parents are usually very knowledgeable about their child's normal behaviour, and a non-specific change in behaviour, especially a change in the level of activity, alertness or feeding, may be the young child's only sign of developing critical illness. This difference from adults makes children more at risk of being 'ignored' or parents of being falsely reassured until the child is quite evidently critically ill with organ dysfunction.

There are, however, many similarities with adults in terms of organ support and monitoring, and the provision of intensive care for children is in many respects a scaled-down version of available adult technology.

Some of the important differences between adults and children are described below.

CARDIORESPIRATORY ADAPTATION AT BIRTH

Dramatic physiological adaptation takes place at birth. Intracardiac pressure relationships in the fetal circulation undergo significant changes associated with clamping of the umbilical cord and disconnection of the placenta, with its supply of vasodilating hormones. At the same time, the newborn takes the first breath of air, resulting in a sudden fall in pulmonary vascular resistance, increase in pulmonary blood flow and left atrial return with increase in left-sided pressures and subsequent physiological closure of both the foramen ovale and the ductus arteriosus. All blood, which previously short-circuited the right side of the fetal heart and lungs via the foramen ovale is forced to follow the postnatal/adult pattern of circulation.

Although there is a dramatic fall in pulmonary vascular resistance at birth, changes initiated at the time of birth are incomplete and progressive, with further reduction in pulmonary vascular resistance associated with regression in arteriolar muscularisation.

Reversion to fetal physiology, however, may occur during the first days to weeks of life in the case of respiratory pathology, or other causes of hypoxia and acidosis. Reversion to fetal pattern circulation means that desaturated blood short-circuits the lungs through the foramen ovale, resulting in further profound desaturation and hypoxaemia, with consequent increases in pulmonary vascular resistance and the development of a vicious cycle. Urgent reversal of the hypoxaemia must be instituted to prevent progression to death.

Pulmonary circulation pathophysiology is probably related to abnormalities of endogenous nitric oxide production and manipulation of this agent has proven useful in therapy.[1]

CAUSES OF TRANSITIONAL (POST-NATAL REVERSION TO FETAL) CIRCULATION

A 'fetal' pattern may persist due to:

- low lung volume states (e.g. hyaline membrane disease and perinatal asphyxia)
- pulmonary hypoplasia (e.g. diaphragmatic hernia and Potter's syndrome)
- meconium aspiration syndrome
- chronic placental insufficiency
- perinatal hypoxia and acidosis from any cause
- sepsis (e.g. group B streptococcal infection)
- hyperviscosity syndrome.

Return to fetal circulation may need to be medically or surgically induced in the case of 'duct dependent' congenital cardiac defects associated with either obstructive lesions on the right or left side of the heart, and as a temporising measure in the case of transposition of the great arteries. This may be achieved by infusion of prostaglandin E_2 (a placental-derived dilating hormone) and/or re-opening of the foramen ovale by balloon atrial septostomy via the femoral or umbilical vein/or open septectomy.

Some intracardiac or vascular shunt lesions result in high pulmonary blood flow and increasing pulmonary pressure states. Left untreated this elevated pulmonary vascular resistance may become fixed, and make subsequent surgical repair unfeasible.

GROWTH AND DEVELOPMENT

There is progressive growth and maturational development of all organ systems throughout childhood. This necessitates knowledge of normal/expected parameters and organ function at different ages in childhood. Drug and equipment calculations are age or weight based, and there is less room for error. Small miscalculations, depending on the size of the child, may have significant implications. Physiologically, organs in children are still undergoing maturation, and have not reached full potential to deal with superadded stresses and drug metabolism in some instances. Incomplete maturation of renal and liver function, specifically in neonates needs to be considered. Similarly, the ability to recover from injury in children is better than in adults because of the ongoing growth and development occurring in early childhood. Premature infants with significant 'chronic lung disease' may still have potential to recover near-normal lung function in adulthood. The brain in children undergoes significant continued maturation and development in early childhood and neural plasticity may allow for seemingly remarkable recovery from certain types of brain injury.

MATURATION

The immaturity of systems and biochemical processes at birth alters the physiological response to stress and drugs. Thermoregulation, immune function, respiratory, renal, hepatic and neurological function are all immature at birth, even in the full-term infant. This immaturity is magnified in the preterm infant with associated surfactant deficiency causing respiratory distress, liver glucuronyl transferase deficiency causing jaundice, and the necessity to be nursed in a thermo-controlled environment. Human body temperature is maintained within narrow limits. This is achieved most easily in the thermoneutral zone – the range of ambient temperature within which the metabolic rate is at a minimum. Once ambient temperature is outside the thermoneutral zone, heat production (shivering or non-shivering thermogenesis) or evaporative heat loss processes are required to maintain body temperature within normal limits. Regulatory mechanisms are less effective in the neonate (there is no shivering or sweating), who is otherwise disadvantaged by a high surface area to body weight ratio and lack of subcutaneous insulation.

The thermoneutral zone is higher in premature infants and falls with increasing postnatal age. Oxygen consumption is minimal, with an environmental or abdominal skin temperature of 36.5°C. Oxidation of brown fat found in the interscapular and perirenal areas (non-shivering thermogenesis) is the major source of heat production when 'cold stressed'.

Alteration of body temperature above or below normal leads to increased or decreased metabolism respectively. Attempts by the body to maintain body temperature within normal limits are associated with increased metabolism and cardiorespiratory demands. Radiation is a major source of heat loss in the neonate and is effectively minimised by double-walled incubators or by servo-controlled radiant heaters. The latter allow better access to critically ill babies for monitoring and procedures. Cold stress per se, increases neonatal mortality. In the presence of respiratory or cardiac disease, it may lead to decompensation.

SPECTRUM OF DISEASE

Congenital structural abnormalities of major systems including the heart, lung, brain and skeleton, among others, are usually evident at birth, however some may become exposed in early childhood.

Inborn errors of metabolism, although present from birth, may become evident only during an intercurrent period of stress, something as seemingly insignificant as weaning onto solids or a mild respiratory tract infection.

The immature immune system puts children at higher risk than adults for the development of serious bacterial and viral illnesses. The inflammatory response of the newborn is attenuated. Febrile response to infection may be lacking and both cellular (chemotaxis and phagocytosis) and humoral (complement activity and opsonisation) responses may be impaired. Cell-mediated immunity is significantly compromised in infants born without thymic function (DiGeorge syndrome) but in the normal newborn, T-cell function appears to be quite well developed. Rejection of skin allografts is slower in the newborn but this seems to be related mainly to the attenuated inflammatory response. The B-cell system, responsible for antibody production, is immature at birth, however the neonate has passive immunity against some infections because of transplacental transfer of maternal antibodies. Additional natural immunity is acquired as a result of immunoglobulin A (IgA) in breast milk, which protects against some acquired gastrointestinal infections. Overall, the immaturity and inexperience of the immune system result in a markedly increased susceptibility to infection in the first 6 months of life. Congenital abnormalities of the immune system usually present in childhood with recurrent or overwhelming infection.

The response to any illness may be physiologically immature and the mode of presentation much less well defined than in adults. For the most part, however, children are the scaled-down version of adults and, after the neonatal period, physiological principles that apply in adults generally apply also in children.

MANAGEMENT OF THE CRITICALLY ILL CHILD

Of paramount importance in the management of critically ill children are early recognition, appropriate resuscitation and adequate stabilisation prior to transfer to a tertiary institution with paediatric intensive care facilities.[2]

RECOGNITION

Recognition of critically ill children is slightly more difficult than in adults for a number of reasons. Children of various ages have different normal physiological parameters and it is important for those dealing with children to be familiar with these norms. For those unfamiliar or infrequently involved in the care of critically ill children, it is important to have a readily available information source of normal values for the specific aged child they are dealing with at the time. Resources are available on the internet and as hand-held applications to provide ready access to this information.

Non-verbal and younger children lack the communication skills to express their malaise in a specific manner. Generically as children become more unwell they will become lethargic, go off their meals and eventually may start vomiting. Older children respond in the same ways as adults with appropriate pyrexia to an infective trigger, whereas very young children, and especially neonates, may become hypothermic. Tachycardia is one of the most important signs in the deteriorating child, and an unexplained tachycardia or one that does not respond to antipyresis and analgesia must be regarded very seriously. As a child's condition deteriorates, the child may progress from being cool peripherally with a palpable peripheral to central temperature difference, to peripheral mottling and eventually a prolonged central capillary refill time. Pulses in the deteriorating child may be noticeably different peripherally from those taken centrally, even in those with a preserved blood pressure. Disinterest in eating and then drinking, which may progress to vomiting, suggests the development of ileus and gastric stasis as perfusion to the gut is reduced. Visceral perfusion abnormality may also be noticed by the parents, as they report abdominal distension or reduction in wet nappies or passing urine. During all this time, the deteriorating child may still have perfectly normal saturations and remain lucid, though with increasing drowsiness. Increasing tachypnoea may not necessarily identify a respiratory focus of decompensation, but may represent the attempt to compensate for the metabolic acidosis associated with shock.[3,4]

In summary, the skill involved in recognising the deteriorating child early, relies on careful history-taking with acknowledgement that the parents know what is normal for their child. Alteration from normal must not be ignored or dismissed until the child has been thoroughly and thoughtfully examined. Physiological and biochemical parameters that are not normal must be critically evaluated to ensure that the early signs of decompensation are not missed. Attempt must be made to treat what is presumed wrong, with the intention that the response to treatment results in normalisation of the physiological disturbance. If this is not the case, the child should remain under vigilant review, with a senior or specialist opinion sought to ensure that a diagnosis has not been missed.

RESUSCITATION

Identification and treatment of the most likely diagnosis, awareness of the potential differential diagnosis and repeated evaluation of response to treatment are all key to the successful management of a critically ill or injured child. Successful treatment should return physiological parameters to normal. If this does not occur, escalation of resuscitation may require more invasive organ support in the form of ventilation, infusion of inotropes, provision of renal, hepatic and haematological support. In extreme cases, extracorporeal life support may be required.[2]

STABILISATION AND TRANSFER

Stabilisation of a critically ill child at a referral hospital prior to transfer infers resuscitation has begun, physiological parameters are stable or returning towards normal and the appropriate level of all organ support required is in place. In some situations, the organ support required (for example haemofiltration) may not be available during the retrieval process, and it is important to minimise delay of the transfer to a place where equipment and staffing levels are present to optimise the eventual outcome of the child.[5]

Good stabilisation implies that the child has had all resuscitation procedures completed at the referral hospital and the child has appropriate airway and vascular access contingency plans to deal with destabilisation during the transfer. Ventilated children, for example, should have the appropriate-sized endotracheal tube confirmed in ideal position, a gastric tube to decompress the stomach and facilitate ventilation and the adequacy of ventilation monitored with continuous oxygen saturations and end-tidal carbon dioxide monitoring.

Children who have required volume resuscitation, are on inotropes or who are potentially cardiovascularly unstable should have enough vascular access to allow commencement or escalation of inotropes during transfer. Adequate cardiovascular monitoring, in the form of continuous cardiac trace and regular intermittent non-invasive or continuous invasive blood pressure monitoring, should be in place.

Arterial access in children is indicated in those who are cardiovascularly unstable and/or on inotropes, those who need targeted blood pressure (e.g. for intracranial perfusion pressure) and those who require frequent blood gas monitoring. Peripheral arteries including radial, dorsalis pedis and posterior tibial are preferable. Central arterial access attempts should completely avoid the brachial artery, as it is an end artery, and thrombosis may lead to limb loss. Attempt should be made to minimise blood gas monitoring by correlation of end-tidal CO_2 with Pa_{CO_2}. Excessive blood gas monitoring and the performance of blood tests that do not result in changes of treatment eventually result in the need for red cell transfusion. The risk–benefit of this practice must be considered.

Vascular access may be extremely challenging in critically ill children and familiarity with intraosseous needle insertion[6,7] and the use of the external jugular vein, may provide rapid access for the early commencement of resuscitation fluids. Intraosseous access is technically easy and provides 'central' access to a non-collapsible venous system, into which almost all resuscitation drugs can be rapidly infused. The limb accessed must be carefully monitored.[8] Placement of central venous lines (femoral and jugular) in children is technically more difficult than in adults, because of the diminutive size of the vessels, short neck in small children and bleeding problems that may be present in critical illness. Central venous cannulation should be attempted only by those skilled in this procedure.[9] Femoral central venous access is preferable to jugular access in children who have a coagulopathy or any suggestion of raised intracranial pressure. Catheters utilising the Seldinger technique have greatly increased successful placement. Ultrasonography is useful to determine the exact location of veins. Multilumen catheters are recommended when infusing multiple drugs and for parenteral nutrition. Complications including catheter-related sepsis are the same as in adults. This risk can be reduced by adherence to a bundle of measures.[10] The need for prolonged venous access may warrant regular catheter changes, or surgical implantation of a central venous device (e.g. Infusaport, Broviac or Hickman catheter).

In children undergoing resuscitation, a urinary catheter with hourly fluid balance allows a more complete assessment of adequacy of resuscitation. It is not expected that the child will immediately recover during the resuscitation and stabilisation process and so the delay in transferring the child to a definitive place of care should be minimised and be specific to the requirements of each patient.

PAEDIATRIC INTENSIVE CARE TRANSFER

Transfer by a team skilled in the retrieval of critically ill children is associated with reduced morbidity, critical incidents and mortality.[11] There are, however, some circumstances where the disease process is time critical, and the time delay in awaiting a paediatric retrieval team imposes an unacceptable risk.[12] In these cases it is important to use the most competent and skilled team available at the time, usually an anaesthetist, paediatrician and adult intensive care nurse. Advice and remote telephonic assistance should be available from the paediatric retrieval team or accepting PICU. For those performing time critical retrievals, it is essential that delay is minimised and only life-saving procedures are allowed to delay the transfer. In these cases it is helpful to have a discussion with the accepting team, in terms of their expectations for transfer and also of what to expect about the patient's condition. A checklist for retrieval is helpful to ensure that all eventualities have been considered.

PAEDIATRIC INTENSIVE CARE

The development of paediatric intensive care units (PICU) separate from adults, recognised the unique diseases, problems and requirements of critically ill children. Centralisation and modernisation of paediatric intensive care, along with dedicated paediatric retrieval teams, have dramatically improved outcomes in children. Critical illness or injury in children is not common, and the reduced incidence of disease means that centres that see more of a specific illness become more skilled at dealing with it, and children have better outcomes. Super-specialisation of paediatric intensive care is evolving, for example in the care of children with highly complex congenital cardiac lesions.[13]

The paediatric intensive care unit does not function in isolation and the intensive care team needs support from all other paediatric sub-specialties in providing the highest level of comprehensive care for this group of children. The PICU is only one part of the delivery of tertiary paediatric hospital care to children, which starts with the provision of excellent pre-hospital care; advice and support for level I and 2 hospitals in the resuscitation and stabilisation of critically ill children; and the subsequent safe transfer by specialised paediatric intensive care retrieval teams to the appropriate paediatric intensive care unit.

The adult intensive care unit, with its technically skilled nursing and medical team, may be an appropriate and safe place for a critically ill child to await retrieval, as long as the adult ICU team is appropriately supported by local paediatric consultants, and the paediatric retrieval team or accepting PICU continue to provide management advice on the critically ill child.

MINIMUM STANDARDS

Suggested minimum standards for a PICU should be adopted. In general a PICU should provide:

- a specialist trained in paediatric intensive care available at short notice, and available 24/7 for ongoing management advice
- a comprehensive range of paediatric sub-specialty support
- immediately available junior medical staff with advanced life support skills including advanced airway and vascular access competence
- nursing staff with experience in paediatric intensive care, and a nurse : patient ratio to facilitate the appropriate level of care

- allied health professionals with specific training in paediatrics including ready access to physiotherapists, dieticians, pharmacists, speech and language therapists, occupational therapists and child psychologists as well as ancillary support staff including clerical and portering staff
- specialised advanced life support equipment for children ranging in age from neonates to adolescents
- 24-hour laboratory, radiological and pharmacy services
- purpose-built PICU, recognising the special physical and emotional needs of critically ill children and their families
- a programme for teaching, continuing education, research and quality assurance
- the skills and expertise to transfer critically ill children within the hospital for investigations and treatment
- an in-house paediatric intensive care retrieval team, or at least an arrangement with an external retrieval team to provide critical care transfer of children into the PICU.

Neonatal intensive care units have many similar, but also additional other requirements.

PAEDIATRIC MONITORING

Technology has allowed most aspects of adult monitoring to be applied to neonatal and paediatric practice. The ideal paediatric haemodynamic and respiratory monitoring system should:[14,15]

- be non-invasive, painless and readily interfaced with the child
- constitute minimal risk to the child
- provide specific data relevant to the child's status that are reproducible and readily understood
- respond rapidly to changes in status
- provide continuous visual and/or auditory display of data
- have appropriate alarms
- have facilities for recording data
- be inexpensive and require low maintenance.

PULSE OXIMETRY

Pulse oximetry provides continuous non-invasive measurement of arteriolar saturation (Sa_{O_2}) and provides a rapid indication of hypoxaemia. Accurate information is given:

- when the oxyhaemoglobin dissociation curve is shifted to the left (e.g. fetal haemoglobin and alkalosis) or to the right (e.g. sickle-cell disease and acidosis)
- in the presence of carboxyhaemoglobin (functional saturation is accurate)
- with moderately severe desaturation (e.g. cyanotic heart disease)
- with anaemia (haemoglobin concentrations above 5 g/dL)
- when skin is pigmented.

Errors occur with extreme hypoperfusion, excessive movement and rapidly changing ambient light. A range of sensors are now available to monitor children of all ages.

TRANSCUTANEOUS P_{O_2} AND P_{CO_2} MONITORING

Oxygen and carbon dioxide diffuse through well-perfused skin from the superficial capillary network and can be measured using modified polarographic and glass electrodes respectively. The electrodes are heated to 43–45°C to arterialise the capillary blood and maximise capillary blood flow. Under optimal conditions, there is good correlation between arterial and transcutaneous gas tensions. Hence continuous monitoring of blood gas tensions is possible in a non-invasive way. The Ptc O_2 (transcutaneous)–Pa_{O_2} gradient and the output of the heating element have been used as indices of microcirculation. The accuracy of these devices is mainly confined to the neonatal period.

DRUG INFUSIONS

All drugs used in the care of critically ill children, including those used for cardiovascular support, should be administered according to body weight; accurate delivery is crucial. Accurate drug infusions require accurate devices, of which syringe pumps are the most useful. Potentially lethal errors in calculating drug dilutions are minimised by the use of dose/dilution/infusion rate guidelines that should be agreed upon within an institution by pharmacy and paediatric intensive care collaboration.[16] It is safer, with fewer drug errors and communication errors, time saving and potentially cost saving to have infusions made up in the same way by all referring institutions within the PICU network. These should be disseminated to referral institutions by the PICU and agreed at a clinical, clinical governance and management level.

PAIN RELIEF AND SEDATION IN CHILDREN

Management of pain and agitation in children has received inadequate attention and has tended to be underestimated and under-rated. Infants and children are often unable or unwilling to complain of pain. In the past, some believed that the neonate could not perceive pain.[17] It is now clear that neonates possess all the anatomical and neurochemical systems necessary for pain perception and exhibit physiological and behavioural responses to pain. Stress responses associated with pain and agitation may increase morbidity and mortality in critically ill patients. Analgesia can be provided by narcotic infusions, local blocks and regional techniques in children of all ages. Painful procedures in the PICU must always be accompanied by appropriate analgesia. Sedative agents can reduce agitation and minimise harmful stress responses; however, all opiates and benzodiazepines may result in withdrawal reaction after discontinuation and attempt should be made to wean agents to a minimum once noxious procedures have been completed. Agents like oral or intravenous cloinidine[18] are useful as opiate-sparing and benzodiazepine-avoiding adjuncts, with minimal withdrawal effects on discontinuation. Having parents at the bedside for most of the child's waking day, distraction with play therapy, reading and videos, and appropriate surroundings including noise and light levels all help to alleviate children's anxiety, and do not come at the cost of withdrawal.

OUTCOME OF PAEDIATRIC INTENSIVE CARE

Depending on admission criteria, mortality in paediatric ICUs ranges from 5 to 15%.[19] If patients with pre-existing severe disabilities are excluded, the majority of survivors have a normal or near-normal life expectancy. A number of scoring systems have been developed or modified for paediatric application to predict ICU mortality. These scoring systems allow comparison between different ICUs, internal audits, stratification of patients for research purposes and analysis of cost–benefit. The Paediatric RISk of Mortality (PRISM) score[20, 21] and the Paediatric Index of Mortality (PIM) score[22] are applicable to a wide range of critically ill infants and children. Although PRISM performs marginally better, PIM is easier to collect and hence less prone to errors in data collection. PIM also has the advantage that it predicts mortality based on admission parameters whereas PRISM is based on the worst variables in the first 24 hours. In many paediatric ICUs, deaths occur within the first 24 hours. PRISM is often recording the dying process rather than predicting it. Specialised scores have been developed for specific problems, e.g. the Modified Injury Severity Scale (MISS) and Paediatric Trauma Score (PTS) for paediatric trauma, and the modified Glasgow Coma Scale (GCS) for neurological insults. Numerous scoring systems have been developed for meningococcaemia, the best validated being the Glasgow Meningococcal Septicaemia Prognostic Score (GMSPS).[23]

Compared with adult intensive care, children with equivalent Therapeutic Intervention Scoring System (TISS) scores have a lower in-hospital and 1-month mortality.[16] Although multiple organ failure increases mortality, the prognosis is considerably better than for adults.[24] There is evidence that mortality is lower in specialist paediatric ICUs[25] and that paediatric ICUs with a larger workload have better outcomes than those looking after fewer children.[26] General hospitals should therefore have facilities for urgent resuscitation of children prior to early transport to a specialised paediatric ICU. Unless unavoidable, critically ill children, particularly those requiring mechanical intervention, should not be cared for in an adult ICU for longer than 24 hours. The American Academy of Pediatrics, the Society of Critical Care Medicine, the British Paediatric Association and the Australian National Health and Medical Research Council have all stated that children should receive intensive care in specialist paediatric units.

Access the complete references list online at http://www.expertconsult.com

3. Carcillo JA, Fields AI. Clinical practice parameters for haemodynamic support of pediatric and neonatal patients in septic shock. Crit Care Med 2002;30:1365–78.
11. Orr RA, Felmet KA, Han Y, et al. Pediatric specialised transport teams are associated with improved outcomes. Pediatrics 2009;124(1):40–8.
18. Arenas-Lopez S, Riphagen S, Tibby SM, et al. Use of oral clonidine for sedation in ventilated paediatric intensive care patients. Intensive Care Med 2004;30:1625–9.
19. Wilkinson JD, Pollack MM, Ruttimann UE, et al. Outcome of pediatric patients with multiple organ system failure. Crit Care Med 1986;14:271–4.
25. Pollack MM, Alexander SR, Clarke N, et al. Improved outcomes from tertiary center pediatric intensive care: a statewide comparison of tertiary and non-tertiary care facilities. Crit Care Med 1991;19:150–9.

104

Upper airway obstruction in children

Paul James and Sara Hanna

Upper airway obstruction is a particular clinical challenge in the paediatric population. The physics of air flow, the relative narrowness of the paediatric airway combined with the high rate of oxygen consumption in the child can produce rapid and unexpected deterioration in the clinical condition of a child. Moreover, severe airway obstruction occurs infrequently in non-specialist centres, but will require immediate intervention by the team present to secure a safe airway and maintain oxygenation. Successful management relies on an understanding of the paediatric airway, knowledge of the symptoms and signs that suggest unusual diagnoses or life-threatening obstruction, a realisation of what can and cannot be diagnosed without endoscopy and meticulous attention to basic anaesthetic principles.

ANATOMICAL AND DEVELOPMENTAL CONSIDERATIONS

The upper airway technically extends from the nares to the junction of the larynx with the trachea. It includes the nose, the paranasal sinuses, the pharynx and the larynx. It changes in size, shape and position from the neonatal period through infancy and childhood to resemble the adult airway by the age of 8 years.[1]

Children have a proportionally larger head and occiput relative to body size. The large head forces the neck into flexion when supine, which is a potential cause of airway obstruction.

NOSE

The nose is made up of nasal bones, nasal part of the frontal bones and frontal processes of the maxillae. The septum divides the cavity into two with the exterior opening at the nares and the opening into the nasopharynx at the choanae.

If the membrane that separates the palatal processes during development does not rupture the neonate will have choanal atresia and will present with airway obstruction.

Infants are obligate nasal breathers and secretions, oedema and blood easily block the small nasal apertures.

Similarly cellulitis, oedema or abscess formation in the paranasal sinuses will lead to airway obstruction.

PHARYNX

The pharynx forms the common upper pathway of the respiratory and alimentary tracts. It is divided into three regions: the nasopharynx, oropharynx and laryngopharynx, which open into the nasal cavity, mouth and larynx respectively.

The pharyngeal isthmus separates the nasopharynx and oropharynx. It closes off during swallowing.

The adenoids lie on the roof and posterior wall of the nasopharynx. These atrophy with age, but enlargement in early childhood may obstruct breathing. They may also be dislodged during instrumentation of the nose.

The oropharynx extends from the soft palate to the tip of the epiglottis. It is attached anteriorly to the base of the tongue via the glossoepiglottic folds, between which lies the valleculae.

At the entrance to the oropharynx is a collection of lymphoid tissue known as Waldeyer's ring. This consists of the lingual tonsil at the base of the tongue and bilateral palatine tonsils as well as the adenoids and tubal tonsils. Inflammation, infection or invasion of this tissue may obstruct breathing. The shape and dimension of the oropharynx affect airway function particularly during sleep.

The relatively large tongue decreases the size of the oral cavity and more easily obstructs the airway. Decreased muscle tone also contributes to passive obstruction of the airway by the tongue.

The laryngopharynx extends from the tip of the epiglottis to the lower border of the cricoid cartilage. The larynx bulges back into the centre of the laryngopharynx leaving a recess on either side known as the piriform fossa. This is a common site for impaction of swallowed foreign bodies.

LARYNX

The larynx is situated between the pharynx and trachea, extending from the base of the tongue to the cricoid cartilage.

The larynx consists of the thyroid cartilage, the cricoid cartilage, the paired arytenoids and the epiglottis, together with the small corniculate and cuneiform cartilages.

The laryngotracheal tube forms from the ventral wall of the foregut. The primitive glottis is formed at 10 weeks' gestation when the true vocal cords split. Failure of this process results in a congenital laryngeal web or atresia of the larynx. Incomplete division of the embryonic foregut results in a tracheo-oesophageal fistula.

The cricoid cartilage is shaped like a signet ring with the widest portion lying posterior. This is the only complete cartilage ring in the respiratory tract and is the narrowest portion of the larynx. Any oedema, infection or inflammation at this level results in airway compromise. Acquired subglottic stenosis as a result of prolonged or repeated tracheal intubation also occurs at this level. The larynx lies more anteriorly and higher, being at the level of the 4th cervical vertebra at birth, the 5th cervical vertebra at 6 years and the 6th cervical vertebra in the adult.

The epiglottis is a leaf-shaped structure attached to the posterior border of the thyroid cartilage by the thyroepiglottic ligament. The infant epiglottis is narrower, softer and more horizontally positioned than in the adult.

The more superior location of the larynx in children may create difficulty in visualising the laryngeal structures because of the acute angulation between the base of the tongue and the laryngeal opening.

The vocal cords are innervated by the recurrent laryngeal nerve, which if damaged results in paralysis of the corresponding vocal cord, causing it to lie motionless in the midline and at a lower level than the opposite side. Bilateral paralysis results in complete loss of voice and the two vocal cords may then flap together causing a valve-like obstruction during inspiration.

The highly compliant and poorly developed cartilage leads to increased susceptibility to dynamic airway collapse in the presence of obstruction. Loss of muscle tone in the pharynx leads to airway obstruction at the level of the soft palate and epiglottis. Laryngomalacia is a congenital abnormality of the larynx and results from the laryngeal structure being more pliable and less rigid than in the adult.[2]

PATHOPHYSIOLOGY

Resistance to laminar air flow increases in inverse proportion to the fourth power of the radius (Poiseuille's law) resulting in a marked increase in resistance to air flow with airway narrowing. The perpendicular cartilaginous ribs, which reduce the effect of the 'bucket handle' movement of the rib cage, and the immature intercostal muscles result in a mechanical 'disadvantage' and children are more reliant on the diaphragm for inspiration. Signs of increased respiratory effort to overcome airway obstruction include head bobbing (use of neck muscles), subcostal and sternal recession, tracheal tug and forced expiration (abdominal muscle contraction in expiration). Chronic airway obstruction may lead to chest wall deformity.

A higher metabolic rate and oxygen consumption, together with a smaller functional residual capacity and fewer fatigue-resistant fibres in the diaphragm, means there is little respiratory reserve and children with airway compromise can deteriorate very quickly.

However, children with chronic obstruction may manage surprisingly well with 'tolerable' airway noises and increased levels of respiratory work. Acute changes in airway calibre in these children may cause precipitous deterioration with accompanying hypoxia.

CLINICAL PRESENTATION

Stridor is a harsh, vibratory sound produced by turbulent air flow and is the cardinal feature of upper airway obstruction. Symptoms and signs vary with the level of obstruction, the aetiology and age of the child.

When faced with a child with possible airway obstruction the clinician must decide whether investigation and intervention are necessary and, if so, in what time scale. Very few diagnoses are truly clinical as it is only on direct endoscopy that the true cause of the problem can be confirmed. However, a careful history and examination are key to the decision-making process. Features that suggest obstruction needing urgent evaluation include episodes of colour change (pallor, cyanosis), apnoea, biphasic stridor, stridor when asleep and stridor from birth.

Extrathoracic obstruction is more pronounced during inspiration as the negative intraluminal pressure causes further airway narrowing. Obstruction is characterised by stridor and prolongation of inspiration. Intrathoracic airway diameter increases on inspiration and signs and symptoms occur mainly on expiration. There is prolonged expiration, wheeze and air trapping as seen in asthma, a common misdiagnosis.

Biphasic stridor is characteristic of mid-tracheal lesions or impending complete obstruction at any level (**Fig. 104.1**).

AETIOLOGY

The aetiology may be classified in a number of ways including according to the site of obstruction (i.e.

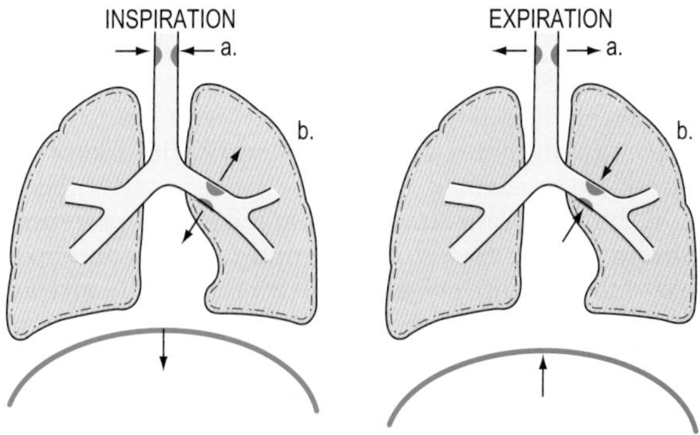

Figure 104.1 Dynamics of (a) extrathoracic and (b) intrathoracic airways obstruction.

Box 104.1 Common causes of upper airway obstruction in neonates/infants

Nose
- Choanal atresia

Oral cavity
- Encroachment of tongue on airway
- Macroglossia: Beckwith–Wiedeman, hypothyroidism
- Micrognathia: Pierre–Robin syndrome
- Haemangioma or venous/lymphatic malformation of tongue

Laryngeal abnormalities
- Laryngeal atresia
- Laryngomalacia
- Vocal cord paralysis
- Laryngeal cleft

Subglottic abnormalities
- Subglottic stenosis – congenital or acquired
- Subglottic haemangioma

Extrinsic lesions
- Mediastinal masses
- Cystic hygroma
- Foregut malformations
- Vascular abnormalities including rings and slings

nose, pharynx or larynx), whether it is congenital or acquired, or whether it is due to infection, malignancy, trauma, etc.

Boxes 104.1 and **104.2** list the more common causes according to the age of the child.

Box 104.2 Common causes of upper airway obstruction in children

Oral cavity

Encroachment of tongue on airway
- Macroglossia: Beckwith–Wiedeman, hypothyroidism
- Micrognathia: Pierre–Robin syndrome
- Haemangioma or venous/lymphatic malformation of tongue

Other oral mass lesions
- Ectopic–lingual thyroid/thyroglossal duct cyst/dermoid cyst/ranula

Nasopharynx/oropharynx/retropharyngeal space
- Adenoid/tonsillar inflammation and abscess
- Lymphatic malformation
- Supraglottitis
- Foreign bodies
- Trauma/burns
- Neoplasms

Larynx/cervical trachea

Supraglottic
- Laryngomalacia
- Epiglottitis

Glottic abnormalities
- Vocal cord paralysis
- Laryngeal cleft
- Recurrent respiratory papillomatosis

Subglottic abnormalities
- Croup
- Subglottic stenosis
- Congenital
- Acquired (prolonged or traumatic intubation)
- Subglottic haemangioma

INFECTIONS OF THE UPPER AIRWAY

Viral and bacterial infections causing upper airway obstruction present in a very similar way and are often concurrent. A logical and useful approach to diagnosis is to identify the site of infection and consider the nature of the condition.[3]

PHARYNGEAL INFECTIONS

In the pharynx the site of infection is the peritonsillar bed in 49% of cases, the retropharyngeal space in 22% of cases and the parapharyngeal spaces resulting in abscess formation in 2%.[4]

Bacterial tonsillitis and peritonsillar abscess (quinsy)

Tonsillitis is caused by the aerobes *Streptococcus pyogenes*, *Streptococcus pnemoniae* and *Staphylococcus aureus* and the anaerobes *Fusobacterium* spp., *Prevotella* spp., *Porphyromonas* spp. and *Actinomyces* spp. Aerobes predominate in the acute primary infection, whereas anaerobes are associated with abscess formation or extension across tissues. Treatment is with third-generation cephalosporins or co-amoxyclav as there is a high incidence of penicillin resistance.[5]

Metronidazole or carbapenems should be added if there is extension or abscess formation. Clindamycin or linezolid should be added to reduce bacterial exotoxin release if toxic shock is suspected.

Surgical removal in the acute setting is controversial as there is potentially an increased risk of bleeding, but if there is pus then drainage is indicated to prevent spontaneous rupture.[6]

Infectious mononucleosis

Infectious mononucleosis is caused by the Epstein–Barr virus.

Airway obstruction can occur and, despite steroids, 40–88% of patients with airway obstruction require tonsillectomy.[7]

The use of steroids does reduce duration of fever, pharyngitis and abnormal haematological findings.[8]

Retro- and parapharyngeal abscess

Retropharyngeal abscesses are more common in boys (ratio 2:1) and occur at a median age of 3 years. The incidence appears to be rising.[9]

The principal symptoms are fever, sore throat, trismus, torticollis, neck swelling and pain. Airway obstruction is rare.[10]

Staphylococci and streptococci are the usual causal agents but growth is often polymicrobial and treatment is with broad-spectrum antibiotics. Surgical drainage is indicated if there are symptoms persisting for 2 days or more, prior administration of antibiotics, and fluid on computed tomography scan with a cross-sectional area of >2 cm^2. Complications include mediastinitis and Lemierre's syndrome.

Lemierre's syndrome

Described in 1936, Lemierre's syndrome occurs when a pharyngeal/tonsillar infection is complicated by thrombophlebitis and septic emboli. The organism is usually *Fusobacterium necrophorum*. Local effects classically include thrombosis in the ipsilateral internal jugular vein and more distant spread with suppuration most commonly affecting the lungs, but also causing septic arthritis, osteomyelitis, meningitis and liver, renal and skin abscesses.[11]

Ludwig's angina

Ludwig's angina is a diffuse infection of the submandibular and sublingual spaces. Severe pain, fever, malaise and dysphagia occur with swelling that can be large enough to cause airway compromise. Antibiotic choice is as for tonsillar abscess and surgical drainage is indicated if there is pus formation.[12]

LARYNX/TRACHEAL INFECTIONS

Croup

Croup (laryngotracheobronchitis) is common and usually caused by the virus parainfluenza, influenza type A or B, respiratory syncytial virus or rhinovirus. It is the commonest cause of acquired acute stridor in children and is a clinical diagnosis. There is a sudden onset of a seal-like barking cough usually accompanied by stridor, hoarse voice and respiratory distress. Symptoms are usually worse at night. It commonly affects children age 6 months to 3 years with a peak incidence at 2 years. Only 2% of cases are admitted to hospital each year, of which only 0.5–1.5% will require intubation.[13]

A Cochrane review investigated the use and effectiveness of steroids in the treatment of children with croup and recommended all children should receive either dexamethasone 0.15 mg/kg or prednisolone 1–2 mg/kg orally.[14]

Nebulised epinephrine (adrenaline) 1/1000, 0.5 mL/kg to a maximum of 5 mL may be used to reduce airway swelling acutely in severe croup. This is a short-term measure and may allow time for the steroids to work or experienced personnel to be called to the child. It may be repeated if necessary after 30–60 minutes, but further doses should be used with caution as repeated need suggests an extremely narrow airway.

If intubation is indicated visualisation of the larynx should not be a problem; however, a smaller tracheal tube than normal for the age is usually required because of subglottic oedema. Once the obstruction is bypassed most children can be managed on a Swedish nose with minimal sedation and arm splinting. Extubation may be attempted after 72 hours (or earlier if a large leak develops). Around 10% will require re-intubation.

Epiglottitis

Very few clinicians have seen epiglottitis since the introduction of *Haemophilus influenzae* type B vaccination in 1992. In children, it is still almost always due to infection with *H. influenzae* type b (Hib), although it can be caused by beta-haemolytic streptococci, staphylococci or pneumococci. In a recent retrospective study, 10% of children presenting with epiglottitis were found to have Hib infection, despite having being vaccinated.[15]

It occurs usually in children aged 2–6 years, with a peak incidence at 3 years.

Epiglottitis is painful. There is an abrupt onset of high fever, sore throat, dysphagia, soft stridor and drooling. The child may prefer to sit leaning forwards with mouth open.

The key to management is to secure the airway under inhalation anaesthesia with an ENT surgeon standing by if a tracheostomy becomes necessary. Visualisation of the laryngeal inlet may be difficult. A bacterial swab of the epiglottis should be taken once the airway is secure. Antibiotic treatment with an extended-spectrum cephalosporin (e.g. ceftriaxone) is indicated. Recovery usually occurs about 48 hours after the institution of antibiotic therapy and confirmed by visualisation of a normal epiglottis on laryngoscopy.

Bacterial tracheitis

Bacterial tracheitis is uncommon. The condition may occur at any age. The usual pathogens are *S. aureus*, *H. influenzae*, streptococci, and *Neisseria* species.[16]

The signs and symptoms of bacterial tracheitis are frequently intermediate between those of viral croup and epiglottitis. Coughing produces copious tracheal secretions and retrosternal pain. The voice may be hoarse and stridor prominent. The larynx, trachea and bronchi can become acutely obstructed with purulent debris and inflammation with adherent pseudomembranes overlying friable tracheal mucosa.

Most patients with bacterial tracheitis will require tracheal intubation.

At laryngoscopy, the epiglottis and supraglottic structures will appear normal, although slough and pus may be visible beyond the vocal cords. Significant pneumonia and systemic symptoms of bacterial septicaemia are not unusual. Ceftriaxone is a reasonable first-line antibiotic therapy. The average duration of tracheal intubation is 6–7 days and antibiotic therapy and hospitalisation may be required for up to 14 days.

Diphtheria

Diphtheria is caused by *Cornyebacterium diphtheriae* and *Cornyebacterium ulcerans*. It begins with a croup-like illness, cough and sore throat, but often progressing to death through sepsis, suffocation by the 'pseudomembranes' of serocellular exudate and direct effects of the powerful exotoxin, which has an affinity for neural endings (paralysis), cardiac muscle (heart block and myocardial failure) and the adrenal glands (hypotension with endocrine failure). Unless there is a high index of suspicion, it is a diagnosis easily missed. Treatment includes administration of specific antitoxin and appropriate antibiotics.

Respiratory papillomatosis

Respiratory papillomatosis is characterised by recurrent proliferations of squamous papillomata within the airway, anywhere from lips to lungs. The viral pathogen is most commonly human papilloma virus types 6 and 11. The recurrent nature of this condition often necessitates multiple surgical procedures. The current management philosophy is toward a more conservative approach, aimed at ameliorating airway symptoms while limiting subsequent scarring of the larynx. Surgical debulking is the treatment of choice and several modalities have been used, including 'cold steel', microdebrider, CO_2 laser and radiofrequency ablation.

The use of adjuvant medical treatments, such as intralesional cidofovir remains controversial.[17]

TRAUMA

INHALATIONAL BURNS

Inhalational injury should be suspected with burns occurring in a closed space, and when facial burns, singed nasal hairs and oropharyngeal carbonaceous material are present. Respiratory complications are the major cause of mortality in children who are burnt. Direct airway burns or inhalation of products of combustion may lead to rapidly progressive oedema. The situation may be compounded by small airway and lung injury and by the need to provide adequate analgesia. Early intubation is strongly recommended prior to an emergency situation developing. Tracheal tube fixation is critical and may be problematic with extensive facial burns; it may require suturing of the tube to the nasal septum or securing the tube to the teeth.

FOREIGN BODY ASPIRATION

Foreign body aspiration is one of the leading causes of death in children. It is most common in those under 3 years, but can occur at any age.[18] Most deaths occur at the time of aspiration due to complete upper airway obstruction. Of those children who reach hospital, the mortality is low.[19] The most common aspirated object is 'food', usually nuts. Peanuts account for one-third of all foreign body aspirations.

Often the inhalation event is not witnessed, and the history may be less clear than expected. Presentation varies from severe acute upper airway obstruction through to a well, pink child with a persistent cough.

More than 90% of foreign bodies lodge below the upper airway in a main bronchus, slightly more commonly on the right side in children.[20]

As the majority of inhaled material is organic in origin a plain radiograph may fail to demonstrate an abnormality – especially in the first 24 hours, although X-rays in inspiration and expiration may show evidence of gas trapping.[18]

Management is as per the 'choking child' basic life support algorithm. Children with effective cough should be closely observed and encouraged to cough by themselves. If the cough is not effective and the child is conscious, the rescuer may intervene with five back blows followed by five chest thrusts (or abdominal thrusts in older children).

If the child is not conscious, the child should have airway, breathing and circulation assessed and managed as per the basic life support guidelines, with assisted ventilation and chest compressions.

Most children who reach hospital with an inhaled foreign body, or possibility of such, should have a rigid bronchoscopy under general anaesthesia.[21]

Most anaesthetists will use an inhalational induction with sevoflurane in order to maintain spontaneous ventilation.

N_2O is avoided particularly if there is radiological evidence of gas trapping. The cords and upper trachea are sprayed under direct laryngoscopy with 4 mg/kg lidocaine. Maintenance of ventilation and oxygenation during rigid bronchoscopy in children is controversial. The options are a spontaneously breathing technique (reduces the chance of distal movement or dislodgement of the foreign body) or muscle relaxation and use of positive-pressure ventilation (reduces atelectasis and desaturation episodes). It is difficult to demonstrate the superiority of one technique over another.[19]

SUBGLOTTIC STENOSIS

Subglottic stenosis may be congenital or acquired (usually due to post-intubation laryngeal injury).

The main feature is chronic, inspiratory stridor often made worse by intercurrent viral respiratory tract infection. When a child presents acutely the management is as for croup. However, ENT referral is necessary for diagnosis and management. The surgeon will grade the severity of the stenosis according to the size of endotracheal tube that can pass relative to that expected for age. This assessment and clinical condition will inform the decision to intervene.[22]

Treatment is laryngotracheal reconstruction (LTR) whereby a cartilage graft, from either the costal cartilages or the thyroid cartilage, is inserted into a vertical laryngotracheal fissure in order to expand the stenotic segment. Some stenoses will also require a posterior graft inserted into a posterior cricoid chondrotomy. In a double-stage LTR a tracheostomy is inserted to safeguard the airway postoperatively and the grafted area is stented for approximately 6 weeks. A further procedure is then performed to remove the stent and assess the airway. A tracheostomy is not used in a single-stage LTR and the child is left intubated with an age-appropriate endotracheal tube for 5–7 days postoperatively, both stenting and safeguarding the airway. All patients receive anti-reflux medication postoperatively to negate the negative impact of gastric contents on mucosal healing.

CONGENITAL

PIERRE ROBIN SEQUENCE

Pierre Robin sequence is a congenital anomaly presenting with micrognathia, glossoptosis and a cleft palate. Although there is a spectrum of airway obstruction most children can be managed by conservative measures or with a nasopharyngeal airway (NPA) for a few months. The natural history shows that, with normal growth, airway compromise resolves without immediate surgical intervention as previously advocated. However, a few children do require tracheostomy.[23]

CYSTIC HYGROMA

Conspicuous at birth, cystic hygroma or lymphangioma is a relatively rare cause of upper airway obstruction in infancy. The tumours consist of masses of dilated lymphatic channels. They usually occur in the neck but may involve tissues of the tongue and larynx and occasionally extend into the mediastinum. Airway obstruction may be due to infection or haemorrhage into the lesion. Surgical excision has been the mainstay of treatment, although complete removal is difficult and recurrence is common. Although some authors have reported watchful waiting of cystic hygroma, it should be considered only in patients who are asymptomatic. The medical treatment consists of the administration of sclerosing agents.

LARYNGOMALACIA

Laryngomalacia is the commonest cause of congenital stridor and usually presents within the first 2 weeks of life. Clinicians should not give this diagnosis without full airway assessment to any baby with life-threatening symptoms or stridor that is obvious at birth. Airway obstruction results from collapse of supraglottic structures on inspiration, and expiratory symptoms are not a feature. Stridor often gets worse initially for 6–9 months before gradually improving, with most children being free of symptoms by 18–24 months.[24]

It is a dynamic condition and the supraglottic collapse is most obvious during the 'waking phase' of anaesthesia if a formal airway assessment is done.

The majority of children will not require surgical intervention, but the remaining 5–10% require some form of surgical treatment. Surgical options include division of the aryepiglottic folds to 'open' the constricted supraglottis, resection of the redundant mucosa and suspension of the prolapsing epiglottis to uncover the laryngeal introitus. A degree of gastro-oesophageal reflux disease (GORD) is often associated with laryngomalacia and all children should therefore receive anti-reflux medication. This possibly reflects changes in airway and intrathoracic pressures in response to the airway obstruction, as opposed to being a causal factor. A neurological form of the condition exists and may be seen in children with neurological or neuromuscular conditions, such as cerebral palsy. In such cases, surgical intervention should be approached with caution and it may be most appropriate to manage severe airway collapse with a tracheostomy.[25]

OTHER

INFANTILE HAEMANGIOMA

Infantile haemangiomas are the most common tumours of infancy, affecting approximately 1 in 10 children.[26] These are highly proliferative vascular tumours that may grow very quickly, causing obstruction when the airway is involved; if these are left untreated there is a 50% mortality rate. Most airway haemangiomas will coexist with cutaneous lesions (but not vice versa).[27] The PHACES syndrome comprises airway haemangiomas with associated deep or diffuse cutaneous, segmental haemangiomas as well as posterior fossa malformations, arterial anomalies, cardiac/aortic defects, eye anomalies and sternal defect.[28]

Medical and surgical interventions have included steroids, chemotherapeutic agents (vincristine, interferon-α), laser treatment, surgical excision, tracheostomy, or a combination of these, but the spectacular effect of propranolol on cutaneous haemangiomas of infancy was described for the first time in 2008[29] and confirmed by a meta-analysis as being the best treatment available for infantile haemangiomas.[30] The mean dose of propranolol was 2 mg/kg/day (range 0.5–3 mg/kg/day). The mean treatment duration was 6 months (range 1.5–10 months). Clinical improvement was seen in a range of 24 hours–3 weeks (mean 3.8 days). Complications related to propranolol usage were found in one child (2.94%) who developed bronchoconstriction during the first week of treatment.

Because of the possible side-effects of propranolol, current infantile haemangioma treatment centres recommend that a full cardiovascular and respiratory review be performed prior to initiation of therapy.

VOCAL CORD PALSY

Vocal cord palsy may be idiopathic, a result of a neurological abnormality, or traumatic (birth or iatrogenic).[31] It may be uni- or bilateral.

Unilateral palsy presents with stridor and dysphonia, which often resolves with time as the contralateral vocal cord compensates.

Bilateral vocal cord palsy is potentially life threatening and a tracheostomy may be necessary in approximately half of cases. Magnetic resonance imaging of the brain is mandatory in order to exclude an Arnold–Chiari malformation with hydrocephalus.[32] Spontaneous recovery rates of up to 70% are reported.[31]

ANAESTHESIA FOR RELIEF OF UPPER AIRWAY OBSTRUCTION

The principle behind safe induction of anaesthesia in the obstructed airway is the maintenance of spontaneous ventilation. Muscle relaxants should be avoided before the airway is secure in order to avoid the potentially disastrous 'can't intubate, can't ventilate' scenario.

A gaseous induction using 100% oxygen with either sevoflurane or halothane is the technique of choice. The aim is to attain a plane of anaesthesia that is deep enough to allow laryngoscopy, but this is a slow process. If the airway becomes obstructed following loss of consciousness, it can be improved by applying CPAP, changing the patient's position (lateral or semiprone position), using simple airway manoeuvres or simple airway adjuncts such as a nasal airway.

Sufficient depth of anaesthesia for laryngoscopy may not be achieved because of the obstructed airway. A laryngeal mask airway may help. If it is impossible to secure the airway then direct access to the trachea via a cricothyroidotomy or tracheostomy should be gained.

Important points are:

- A prepared induction should be undertaken with efficient suction apparatus, a range of tracheal tubes, suitable stylets, bougies, trained staff, full monitoring, etc.
- Induction in the adopted position, for example sitting in epiglottitis, is advocated. The child is laid flat after induction and prior to intubation.
- Care must be taken not to distend the stomach as this will compound difficult ventilation.
- Orotracheal intubation is quickest and safest, and should be performed initially. After adequate tracheal suction, the tube is changed to a nasotracheal one. Muscle relaxants may be used at this point if the operator is confident of the ability to intubate and/or ventilate.[33]

CARE OF THE SECURED AIRWAY

Successful management of upper airway obstruction in children requires optimal care of the nasotracheal tube. Such children must always be nursed in an ICU with adequate nursing ratios. The nasotracheal tube must be positioned at the level of the clavicular heads (T_2) on chest X-ray. A meticulous technique of fixation must be employed to prevent accidental extubation. Adequate humidification is important to prevent obstruction of narrow tubes by secretions.

Repeated suctioning of secretions is required. Instillation of saline (0.5–1.0 mL) prior to suction may be necessary to encourage removal of secretions. Light sedation is used to improve tolerance of the tracheal tube and to reduce the risk of self-extubation. Arm restraints may also be advisable, particularly in very young children.

In the event of clinical deterioration after intubation, a simple mnemonic may aid successful management; DOPES represents *d*isplacement of the tube, *o*bstruction of the tube, *p*neumothorax, *e*quipment failure and stomach distension.

A true 'can't intubate or ventilate' scenario is rare in children. More often the situation has arisen due to 'operator error' for example suboptimal positioning of the child, inadequate anaesthesia, a distended stomach, a blocked endotracheal tube or understandable panic. However, the only objective in this situation is to maintain oxygenation and if none of the basic manoeuvres resolves the situation the options are to perform a needle cricothyrotomy or a formal tracheostomy.

TRACHEOSTOMY

Tracheostomy remains a life-saving procedure and must be undertaken if tracheal intubation is impossible. It is best performed under general anaesthesia with the neck extended. The airway can be maintained by facemask or laryngeal mask airway. Tracheostomies have been formed under local anaesthesia.

Care of a newly created tracheostomy is similar to that of an endotracheal tube, with the additional problem of some discomfort and the likelihood of fresh blood in the airway. Stay sutures in the tracheal wall lateral to the incision aid recannulation if accidental dislodgement occurs prior to formation of a well-defined tract.

The first tracheostomy tube change is undertaken once a tract has been established, usually between 5 and 7 days.

NEEDLE CRICOTHYROIDOTOMY

Cricothyroidotomy is the creation of an opening in the space between the anterior inferior border of the thyroid cartilage and the anterior superior border of the cricoid cartilage, to gain access to the airway below the glottis. It is difficult and risky in a small child. There are purpose-made paediatric kits available and these should be immediately available in every paediatric anaesthetic room.

Newer cannulae have both a 15 mm and a Luer-lock connector. It is not possible to ventilate a patient with a self-inflating bag via a needle cricothyrotomy and the cannula should be connected via the Luer-lock connection to an oxygen flowmeter via a Y-connector. The oxygen flow rate is initially set at the child's age in years. Ventilation occurs by occluding the open end of the Y-connector with a thumb for 1 second. If this does not cause the chest to rise, the flow should be increased by increments of 1 L/min.

Expiration must occur via the upper airway, even in situations of partial upper airway obstruction. If upper airway obstruction is complete, the gas flow must be reduced to 1–2 L/min. This will provide some oxygenation but little ventilation. Insufflation will buy a little time in which to secure a surgical airway. Complications include bleeding, pneumothorax, pneumomediastinum, subcutaneous emphysema, tracheo-oesophageal fistula, infection, haematoma and catheter dislodgement.

The recent national audit of major complications of airway management in the UK showed that the 'can't intubate, can't ventilate' scenario is rare in paediatric practice. Cricothyroidotomy and jet ventilation is difficult and risky, with the only reported attempt being unsuccessful. Tracheostomy by an ENT surgeon was used successfully more frequently.[34]

Access the complete references list online at http://www.expertconsult.com

2. Adewale L. Anatomy and assessment of the pediatric airway. Pediatr Anesth 2009;19(S1):3–10.
5. Brook I. Current management of upper respiratory tract and head and neck infections. Eur Arch Otorhinolaryngol 2009;266:315–23.
14. Russell KF, Liang Y, O'Gorman K, et al. Glucocorticoids for croup. Cochrane Database of Systematic Reviews 2011;(1):CD001955. Online. Available: http://onlinelibrary.wiley.com/doi/10.1002/14651858.CD001955.pub3/full.
17. Bruce I, Rothera M. Upper airway obstruction in children. Pediatr Anesth 2009;19(S1):90–101.
19. Farrell PT. Rigid bronchoscopy for foreign body removal: anaesthesia and ventilation. Paediatr Anaesth 2004;14:84–9.
25. Bruce I, Rothera M. Upper airway obstruction in children. Pediatr Anesth 2009;19(S1):90–101.
30. Stamatios P, Gemma P, Ioannis A, et al. A meta-analysis on the effectiveness of propranolol for the treatment of infantile airway haemangiomas. Int J Pediatr Otorhinolaryngol 2011;75:455–60.
34. Cook TM, Woodall N, Frerk C. Fourth National Audit Project. Major complications of airway management in the UK: results of the Fourth National Audit Project of the Royal College of Anaesthetists and the Difficult Airway Society. Part 1: anaesthesia. Br J Anaesth 2011;106:617–31.

105

Acute respiratory failure in children

Tavey Dorofaeff and Kevin Plumpton

Acute respiratory failure in children, as in adults, is a failure of gas exchange – inadequate oxygenation and/or carbon dioxide clearance. Respiratory distress refers to both the sensation of breathlessness and the signs of increasing effort to breathe as a consequence of deteriorating gas exchange (**Box 105.1**).[1,2]

EPIDEMIOLOGY[3,4]

Established or imminent respiratory failure is the commonest reason for admission to a neonatal intensive care unit (NICU) or paediatric intensive care unit (PICU). There were approximately 9200 paediatric admissions to Australian and New Zealand intensive care units in 2011 (adult ICUs and PICUs). Of these, approximately 53% had invasive ventilation. Respiratory disease as the lead diagnosis was the single commonest reason for admission (2661 patients ~29%). Infants between 1 and 12 months of age make up the largest majority with just over 1000 admissions per annum. There is a peak of admissions for respiratory diagnoses during the winter months that is predominantly due to acute viral bronchiolitis. Bronchiolitis makes up 12.9% of all non-elective ICU admissions in children. Mortality due to respiratory disease occurs in 1.9% of all paediatric admissions to ICU, representing 17.1% of paediatric deaths in ICUs around Australasia (ANZPIC unpublished data 2010/2011).

VENTILATORY DISADVANTAGES OF CHILDREN[5–7]

Neonates and small infants have a higher resting metabolic requirement for oxygen – estimated to be 7 mL/kg/min compared with 4 mL/kg/min for a school-age child or adult. Small infants are primarily diaphragmatic breathers with a compliant rib cage that makes for less efficient mechanics of breathing. The resultant reduced intrapleural pressure of –1 to –2 cm means there is less distending pressure applied to the lung. At end-expiration infant lung volumes approximate their functional residual capacity. This means less reserve and a tendency to collapse airways and lung parenchyma. The respiratory musculature also has proportionately more fatigable muscle fibres than in older children.

In sickness, infants can increase their respiratory rate only to increase minute ventilation. Without the ability to increase tidal volume, which is commonly reduced in illness, infants and small children get into a downward spiral of decreased distended lung, further hypoventilation and further lung derecruitment.

The airways of a young child are also disproportionately smaller than an adult's. Any obstruction of the lumen of the airways with increased mucous production or bronchoconstriction also increases airways resistance to the fourth power of the radius (Hagen–Poiseuille equation: $\Delta P = 8\ \mu LQ/\pi r^4$). Hence, anatomically small airways are a distinct disadvantage.

This lack of lung reserve and tendency to hypoxia is vitally important when intubating a sick infant. Infants need to be artificially (manually) ventilated until intubation is attempted. A true 'rapid sequence' induction with no assisted ventilation post sedation and muscle relaxant is not achievable and will usually result in further deterioration so that assisted ventilation prior to intubation is almost always required.

SIGNS AND SYMPTOMS OF ACUTE RESPIRATORY FAILURE

Signs and symptoms of respiratory failure in children that indicate the need for an increasing level of respiratory support are not subtle and are usually apparent from a brief focused clinical exam of the respiratory system. They relate to the developmental changes that influence the ways in which children compensate for, or decompensate from, respiratory failure. Due to pulmonary mechanics neonates and small infants tend to become tachypnoeic, but can also develop apnoeas from early in an illness. They exhibit signs of intercostal, subcostal and tracheal tug when distressed. Mild cyanosis is generally well tolerated but extreme tachypnoea, deep cyanosis, relative bradypnoea or apnoea and bradycardia are all signs of serious compromise where respiratory support needs to be instituted immediately. It may or may not be possible to determine focal clinical signs on examination of the chest.

Infants and toddlers also compensate with tachypnoea to increase minute ventilation but do not tend to exhibit apnoea unless severely decompensated. Focal signs are easier to elucidate. As children become more

Box 105.1 Causes of respiratory failure in children

Common causes of respiratory failure in the neonate

Congenital

Respiratory distress syndrome of prematurity

Congenital heart disease

Laryngo/tracheo/bronchomalacia

Vascular rings and slings

Diaphragmatic hernia

Pulmonary hypoplasia

Gastroschisis and omphalocele

Neuromuscular and skeletal disorders

Acquired

Transient tachypnoea of newborn

Meconium aspiration syndrome

Neonatal pneumonia

Pulmonary haemorrhage

Diaphragmatic palsy

Common causes of respiratory failure beyond the neonatal period

Bronchiolitis

Pneumonia

Asthma

Croup

Tumours

Trauma

Acute-on-chronic respiratory failure with chronic neuromuscular conditions

Acute respiratory failure with acute neuromuscular conditions

ARDS

Respiratory failure related to immunocompromised host

upright and mobile they develop more of an adult body habitus. Signs and symptoms are similar to adult respiratory failure. By the time a child is a teenager the signs and symptoms parallel those in adult respiratory medicine.

PREMATURITY AND NEONATAL CHRONIC LUNG DISEASE[8,9]

The lungs develop throughout the fetal period until late childhood. Lung development is divided into five stages; embryonic, pseudoglandular, canalicular, saccular and alveolar. The embryonic and pseudoglandular phases have very little gas exchange ability. At 28 weeks of gestation, the middle of the canalicular stage is where a significant amount of the ventilation can occur within the respiratory bronchioles; 28–32 weeks corresponds to the saccular stage. Alveoli are developing and surfactant production begins around 32 weeks and continues into childhood with increasing maturity of alveoli, replication and increasing numbers. Consequently children born at increasingly premature gestations and those of smaller size have increasing risk of severe lung disease. Factors such as infection, stress and exogenous steroids may influence the development of gas exchange tissues and of the production of surfactant. Underdevelopment of the lungs of the premature infant is only one of the issues that affect these infants. As a result they require a complex system of intensive care and aftercare as they are medically delicate for the first few years of life.

There is some relationship between prematurity and body weight. They are described as follows: a term newborn is delivered from 37 weeks after the mother's last menstrual period; prematurity occurs when a newborn is <37 weeks of completed gestation; extremely low birth weight is <1000 g, very low birth weight <1500 g and low birth weight is <2500 g.

Chronic neonatal lung disease (CNLD) is defined as either: oxygen requirement at 28 days post delivery (irrespective of premature gestation), or oxygen requirement at 36 weeks of gestational age. However, all premature infants will have some degree of abnormal lung development. Bronchopulmonary dysplasia and hyaline membrane disease are pathological findings on biopsy or autopsy of premature infants who have respiratory failure. They are often used synonymously to describe CNLD and respiratory distress syndrome. The pathological features of CNLD include alveolar septal fibrosis with alternating collapse and hyperinflation of acini. Smooth muscle hypertrophy/hyperplasia may also be present. Chest X-ray (CXR) may reveal generalised hyperinflation, multiple cystic areas and opacities. A novel type of CNLD exists (Wilson Mikity syndrome) where babies may not have an initial oxygen requirement but go on to develop an oxygen requirement towards term or beyond.

Complications of prematurity would be the most common reason for admission to a PICU for severe respiratory failure. This is frequently in the context of an acute viral chest infection. CNLD, airway reactivity and pulmonary hypertension exacerbate any symptoms the infant may have otherwise suffered, increasing the need for invasive and non-invasive respiratory support.

Apnoea is a feature of prematurity and is a common symptom of illness in premature infants from birth until about 3 months of corrected age. Important differentials include sepsis (bacterial and viral), intraventricular haemorrhage and pain. Respiratory stimulants such as caffeine can be used to treat apnoea. This is not always effective. Not infrequently, the infant may need non-invasive support such as continuous positive-airway pressure (CPAP) or bi-level positive-airway pressure (BiPAP) or ultimately invasive ventilation to manage the underlying condition and the apnoea. Central hypoventilation due to a *PHOX2B* mutation is increasingly recognised as a congenital form of depressed ventilatory drive beyond the neonatal period. It manifests as hypoventilation during sleep. These children usually need non-invasive or invasive support. If undiagnosed these children can present as sudden infant deaths.

Maternal tobacco use in pregnancy is a significant cause of prematurity and impairs lung development. Environmental tobacco smoke exposure exacerbates chronic lung disease, asthma and recurrent bronchiolitis in older infants.

LARYNGOMALACIA/TRACHEOMALACIA/BRONCHOMALACIA[10]

This results from cartilaginous weakness of the larynx, trachea, main bronchi or any combination of these. This causes a 'floppy' airway that tends to collapse during inspiration and/or expiration. Minor respiratory illnesses can result in increased turbulent flow due to increased respiratory rate and significant dynamic airway obstruction. What might be a mild illness for a normal infant becomes one that may require ventilation for a child with malacia. Ventilator weaning is often troublesome in these infants. Severe long-segment malacia can be an indication for long-term non-invasive home ventilation or tracheostomy and invasive ventilation. Over the first 18–24 months of life there is growth of the cartilage and improvement in the airway rigidity.

Although malacia in the trachea may occur de novo, intrathoracic anomalies (congenital heart disease, tracheoesophageal fistula, etc.) or space-occupying lesions can affect the development and rigidity of the airways.

CONGENITAL HEART DISEASE

Many of the congenital cardiac lesions present with respiratory features. Close examination may or may not reveal congenital heart disease as a cause for the patient's illness. Although antenatal ultrasound scanning detects a significant number of lesions, early discharge or home birth means that symptoms can develop and not be appreciated until acute decompensation occurs.

Congenital heart lesions producing acute respiratory failure fall into four main groups:

- *Left heart obstruction (e.g. critical aortic stenosis, interrupted aortic arch and coarctation of aorta):* this leads to pulmonary oedema, reduced pulmonary compliance and respiratory failure.
- *Large left-to-right shunts (e.g. ventricular septal defect and patent ductus arteriosus):* excessive pulmonary blood flow can cause pulmonary oedema, airway compression and obstruction. Minor intercurrent infection results in decompensation. Correction of the defect improves lung mechanics.
- *Cyanotic lesions:*
  - there is obstruction to pulmonary blood flow (e.g. tetralogy of Fallot and critical pulmonary stenosis)
  - the pulmonary and systemic circuits are in parallel (e.g. transposition of the great arteries)
  - there is complete mixing of systemic and pulmonary blood (e.g. single ventricle and truncus arteriosus).

In lesions with reduced pulmonary blood flow, lung compliance is high. High-pressure ventilation may further impede pulmonary blood flow, leading to increased hypoxaemia. Lesions associated with increased pulmonary blood flow have problems of reduced lung compliance and air trapping (due to small airways and bronchial compression) in addition to hypoxaemia (due to mixing).

- *Vascular lesions:* these are associated with compression or stenosis of large airways (see below).

Early institution of intravenous prostaglandins in company with other supportive measures such as intubation, ventilation, judicious fluid therapy and inotropes will be life saving in these infants. There are no contraindications to the commencement of prostaglandins in a collapsed infant where a paediatric cardiologist is not available to make an immediate assessment. An exception is that, in total anomalous pulmonary venous drainage, prostaglandin use could make the cyanosis worse, but most likely will be ineffectual and can be stopped if cyanosis worsens. This diagnosis requires expert assessment not immediately available to many collapsed infants at their initial presentation.

VASCULAR RINGS AND SLINGS[11]

Vascular rings and slings may be considered complete or incomplete and result from aberrant vessels and the ductus arteriosis (or ligamentum arteriosis, if the duct is closed) leading to a constricting lesion of the trachea or bronchi. Obstruction requires surgical correction and tracheobronchomalacia often remains once the obstruction is relieved. The commonest type of sling is the pulmonary artery sling: an anomalous left pulmonary artery and the ductus encircling the trachea posteriorly. Vascular rings most commonly result from a right-sided aortic arch or a double aortic arch. There are a number of combinations: double aortic arch and derivatives causing complete ring, right-sided aortic arch and anomalous right subclavian artery, right-sided aortic arch, mirror image vessel branching and left ductus arteriosis, and an anomalous innominate artery.

CONGENITAL DIAPHRAGMATIC HERNIA (CDH)[12,13]

There are two types:

BOCHDALEK HERNIA

A Bochdalek hernia involves a deficiency in the posterolateral part of the diaphragm. Most occur on the left side. A variable amount of the abdominal viscera herniates through into the chest. Presentation is dependent upon whether the hernia is diagnosed antenatally or not and whether pulmonary hypoplasia and pulmonary hypertension are present. Antenatal diagnosis may allow for use of fetal intrauterine therapy; however, this is still experimental. The spectrum of clinical course ranges from profound, non-survivable hypoxia and pulmonary hypertension in the newborn to mild tachypnoea in infancy or an incidental finding diagnosed when a child comes to medical attention. Therapy involves respiratory support as appropriate and surgical closure of the defect. Children with severe respiratory failure may need extensive medical stabilisation with high-frequency oscillator ventilation (HFOV), nitric oxide therapy and extracorporeal life support (ECLS). Partial liquid ventilation has also been used in some centres. About 10% of children with CDH have a chromosomal abnormality.

MORGAGNI'S HERNIA

A Morgagni hernia is in the anterior diaphragm. Typically only bowel will herniate through the defect. It is extremely uncommon for this hernia to cause respiratory embarrassment. It is often an incidental finding or associated with mild respiratory disease. Clinically insignificant hernias are repaired electively.

PULMONARY HYPOPLASIA[14]

This is usually secondary to a space-occupying lesion within the chest, which limits room for lung development and also results in abnormal pulmonary vasculature and pulmonary hypertension. Congenital diaphragmatic hernia, cystic adenomatous malformation, congenital neuroblastoma and great vessel abnormalities are common causes. Pulmonary hypoplasia can be idiopathic.

OMPHALOCELE AND GASTROSCHISIS[15,16]

An omphalocele results from failed development of the abdominal wall musculature. The abdominal organs are contained within a protruding thin-walled peritoneal sac. There is a high incidence of associated abnormalities (50–70%) and chromosomal defects (30%). Gastroschisis is herniation of the small bowel (usually) through an ischaemic defect in the abdominal wall. Approximately 15% of these children have associated defects or chromosomal abnormalities. Neither abnormality causes respiratory failure. However, surgical reduction may lead to increased intra-abdominal pressure, which limits excursion of the diaphragm and ventilation of the lungs. This is more likely with an omphalocele as more abdominal viscera are exteriorised.

NEUROMUSCULAR AND SKELETAL DISORDERS[5,17]

Any disorder that affects the ability of the muscles to 'drive' the ventilatory pump, or that causes a chest wall deformity, can compromise the effectiveness of ventilation. In the neonatal period these present with hypoventilation, desaturation and apnoea. Ventilator dependence as a neonate with these disorders indicates that the child is unlikely to survive without intensive support and, most likely, mechanical ventilation. Parents should be counselled appropriately. Spinal muscular atrophy (SMA) type 1 is the commonest example of this. Less severe neuromuscular disorders may survive the neonatal period but go on to develop respiratory failure later (e.g. Duchene's muscular dystrophy, SMA types 2 and 3). The amount of support offered needs to take into consideration ethical treatment, rational expenditure of resources and the wishes of the family and child (if appropriate).

ACQUIRED NEONATAL DISEASES

TRANSIENT TACHYPNOEA OF THE NEW BORN (TTN)

TTN is transient delayed clearance of fetal lung fluid. In transition from intrauterine life the infant has to aerate the majority of its alveoli within a few minutes. It is truly an amazing feat. Not surprisingly some infants may be slow to progress through this process. It is often an issue in infants that have little exposure to catecholamines due to a rapid operative delivery. Although these infants may require oxygen or CPAP, it is seldom that they need invasive ventilation.

MECONIUM ASPIRATION SYNDROME[18]

Meconium is the faecal material of an infant prior to and in the first days of life. Passage of meconium is normal after birth. Passage of meconium prior to or during birth is an indicator of fetal stress. If inhaled or aspirated by the infant during delivery it induces a chemical pneumonitis and obstructive lung disease. If there is meconium present and if the neonate is apnoeic, it is recommended that he/she is suctioned below the vocal cords before bag mask ventilation. Either intubation and suction via the endotracheal tube (ETT) or the use of a specialised meconium aspirator is recommended.

Once an infant develops meconium aspiration syndrome (MAS) the infant will need some degree of respiratory support. Non-invasive respiratory support and invasive ventilation are standard treatment options. Antibiotics are commonly administered as there is concern that sepsis might be an additional cause of fetal distress. Surfactant is deactivated by meconium and so surfactant therapy is used in severe cases. Surfactant lavage may also be employed as a rescue measure to facilitate the 'wash-out' of the lungs and replace surfactant deficiency. ECLS (extracorporeal life support) is indicated for severe MAS. Of all disease entities treated with ECLS (including all neonatal, paediatric and adult causes) it has the greatest survival. ELSO database figures show that survival from severe respiratory failure due to MAS is upward of 90% with some units boasting near-100% survival.

NEONATAL PNEUMONIA[19]

Neonates are at constant risk from pneumonia. Due to the relative immaturity of their immune system they are particularly sensitive to encapsulated bacteria and to Gram-negative bacteria such as *Escherichia coli*, *Klebsiella* and *Serratia*. Group B *Streptococcus* is carried as a vaginal commensal by up to 50% of women so is a common neonatal pathogen. These organisms also cause sepsis and meningitis in infants and newborns. Early infections <14 days are likely to have come from the mother at birth, either prior to birth (chorioamnionitis, prolonged rupture of membranes) or by transplacental infection (*Listeria monocytogenies*).

Viruses such as cytomegalovirus, varicella and other herpesviruses tend to cause a generalised viraemia rather than an isolated pneumonia. Fungal and protozoan infections are virtually unheard of in causing a neonatal pneumonia and tend to cause a systemic infection.

PULMONARY HAEMORRHAGE[14]

Prematurity, surfactant deficiency and persistent fetal circulation with pulmonary hypertension all predispose an infant to risk of pulmonary haemorrhage. Vitamin K deficiency can also present with pulmonary haemorrhage, but gastrointestinal bleeding and intracerebral bleeding are far more common. Children with abnormal pulmonary vascularity of the bronchial arteries can present with catastrophic pulmonary haemorrhage; however, this tends to present later in life. Disseminated intravascular coagulation can result in pulmonary haemorrhage in the setting of severe sepsis.

DIAPHRAGMATIC PALSY[14]

Palsy of the diaphragm is almost exclusively a complication of cardiothoracic surgery. These infants are difficult to wean from ventilation. If there is paradoxical upward movement of the affected diaphragm during inspiration, surgery to plicate the diaphragm is required. This stabilises the affected hemidiaphragm so that the normal hemidiaphragm can still create a negative pleural pressure for inspiration. The palsy will often improve with time.

COMMON ACQUIRED DISEASES BEYOND THE NEONATAL PERIOD

BRONCHIOLITIS[20–24]

Bronchiolitis is the commonest cause of respiratory failure beyond the neonatal period in children. Bronchiolitis is caused by infection and inflammation in the bronchioles resulting in obstructive lung disease leading to hypoxia, tachypnoea and air trapping. CXR shows hyperinflation (and collapse) of lung segments and often right upper lobe collapse and /or consolidation. Respiratory syncytial virus (RSV), human metapneumovirus (hMPV), human bocavirus, adenovirus, parainfluenzae, influenza virus and rhinovirus are all implicated in the hospitalisation of children. Data from the Australasian ANZPIC registry shows that in 2011 RSV virus continues to make up the majority of acute viral bronchiolitis – 60% of children admitted to an ICU had RSV identified.

Treatment is largely supportive. The majority of infants can be supported with non-invasive respiratory support. About 65% of the children (mentioned above) were supported with non-invasive ventilation (NIV) techniques and high-flow nasal cannula oxygen (HFNC). Similar proportions are seen in the non-RSV bronchiolitis group. Only a few infants require invasive ventilation. These tend to be the very young infants in whom apnoea is a feature of the disease and infants with underlying medical conditions such as chronic lung disease, cardiovascular disease and neuromuscular disease.

Up to 20% of infants who require invasive ventilation for bronchiolitis have a concurrent bacterial infection so antibiotics are often started empirically until haematology and inflammatory markers become reassuring and cultures are negative. A number of infants with bronchiolitis who need respiratory support must be transferred from their regional hospital to the nearest PICU. Although transfer with non-invasive support can be done safely for short road transfers, aeromedical transfer often necessitates intubation to secure the airway for the limitations of the aeromedical environment.

Steroids, epinephrine (adrenaline), bronchodilators and hypertonic saline have been investigated for the treatment of bronchiolitis. None has consistently shown significant benefit in hospitalised children. Specific antiviral therapy is not indicated in the immunocompetent. Recombinant RSV antibody provides passive prophylaxis against RSV and is indicated in infants with chronic lung disease or congenital heart disease.

Bronchiolitis by definition is limited to the under-12-months age group. A number of other definitions apply to children of older ages such as viral pneumonia, reactive airways disease (if there is bronchodilator responsiveness) or wheezy bronchitis. These definitions change every few years reflecting the poor understanding we have of this very common disease.

PNEUMONIA[5,25]

ANZPIC data show about 16% of respiratory admissions were for pneumonia. About half of these patients required invasive ventilation. Community-acquired pneumonia is caused predominantly by viruses followed by staphylococcal and streptococcal bacteria.

Atypicals such as *Mycoplasma pneumoniae* and *Chlamydia* also feature. Respiratory support is escalated as required to support the work of breathing and provide acceptable gas exchange. Tidal volumes kept at between 5 and 8 mL/kg and permissive hypercarbia and hypoxia are the usual goals. Treatment with empirical antimicrobials based on local sensitivity patterns should commence as soon as possible. Antibiotics should be changed to narrow-spectrum agents once organism sensitivities are known. The exception to this rule is in the treatment of cystic fibrosis where broad-spectrum cover may be needed to mitigate against the development of antimicrobial resistance. Bronchoscopy for samples is often not possible owing to the small calibre of the endotracheal tube. Blind bronchoalveolar lavage is almost routine for intubated patients. Endotracheal suction samples are also used; however, poor sensitivity and specificity limit their value.

ASTHMA[26–28]

Asthma is frequently diagnosed in childhood but not all wheezy exacerbations are asthma. They may be manifestations of an acute viral illness that presents with a constellation of symptoms including wheezing and tachypnoea but do not respond to bronchodilators. As an intensive care physician it is important to make an assessment of these patients as to the underlying aetiology. The management of a wheezy lower respiratory infection is purely supportive but may often require some mechanical respiratory support.

Acute severe asthma requires specific treatments for the inflammation and bronchoconstriction that are the pathophysiological basis of asthma. For all but the most severe, metered dose inhalers and spacers have been shown to have superior drug deposition. If there is significant hypoxia, oxygen-driven nebulisers are necessary. Nebulisers of salbutamol and ipratropium bromide should be given as a matter of urgency. Salbutamol nebulisers may need to be given continuously. Once the oxygen and nebulised bronchodilators have commenced then steroids are the next most important part of the asthma management. Gastric stasis is common in acute severe asthma so oral steroids should not be relied upon. Anti-inflammatory doses of intravenous steroid should be given urgently to all patients who do not significantly improve with the initial burst of bronchodilators. Frequently, patients are also mildly dehydrated due to poor oral intake and increased insensible losses so a small fluid bolus can be helpful along with commencement of maintenance intravenous fluids.

Intravenous salbutamol is sometimes necessary but can lead to side-effects of tachycardia, tremor, lactic acidosis and resultant compensatory increase in respiratory drive. An intravenous bolus of magnesium sulphate and/or aminophylline will often improve bronchoconstriction in severe refractory asthma but can have adverse effects. These last three medications are contentious and have protagonists and antagonists. However, the side-effects of medical therapy are less than the risks of invasive ventilation.

NIV with CPAP or BiPAP is increasingly used in asthma. Asthma was thought to be a contraindication but NIV is now thought to have a place in acute severe asthma. It should not replace invasive ventilation if this is deemed to be necessary. Invasive ventilation should be approached with caution and with preparations made for managing cardiac arrest and pneumothorax should these occur. The approach taken for the ventilation of severe paediatric asthma is the same as for an adult patient. The reader is referred to Chapter 35 on asthma for the salient issues regarding ventilation of patients with asthma. Volume ventilation is preferred as this will adapt to the changing compliance of the lungs as the bronchi relax. High pressures may be needed. The alveoli are protected from these pressures by the airway obstruction. The combination of steroid therapy and muscle relaxants puts the child at risk for critical illness neuropathy/myopathy. Fortunately most children do not require more than 48 hours of ventilation. General anaesthesia and ECLS have been used on rare occasions.

Acute asphyxial asthma can present as a community cardiorespiratory arrest in children. The profound bronchoconstriction may have resolved by the time the child presents in the emergency department. These children have usually suffered a severe hypoxic ischaemic brain injury. It is exceptionally rare for a child who presents with severe asthma to have a respiratory arrest once therapy has begun but aggressive up-front therapy is mandatory.

Twelve per cent of respiratory admissions to Australasian PICUs in 2011 were for asthma and approximately 70% required no supportive ventilation; 10% were ventilated and the remaining 20% were treated with high-flow nasal cannula oxygen or NIV.

CROUP[5]

Croup or laryngotracheobronchitis is infection and inflammation of the upper and lower airways. Children are more prone to croup owing to the smaller airway radius. Further narrowing leads to marked increase in resistance (Poiseuille's law) and turbulent flow. In the past intubation was frequently required. Use of steroids and epinephrine (adrenaline) nebulisers now means very few children require intubation. If required, intubation for severe croup is best done in the operating theatre with a gaseous induction and preservation of spontaneous breathing. If there is no significant lower airway or lung parenchymal inflammation these children are often able to be supported with a nasal endotracheal tube and awake, sometimes ambulant. Parainfluenza virus is the commonest cause of this condition. Important differentials to consider with severe stridor are: foreign body, bacterial tracheitis and epiglottis. Epiglottitis has become very uncommon with effective *Haemophilus influenzae* B vaccination.

TUMOURS

Neuroblastoma and lymphomas are the commonest tumours that develop in children and cause respiratory compromise. Lymphomas tend to arise centrally from mediastinal nodes. A rapidly growing mediastinal T-cell lymphoma is a true oncological emergency. Mediastinal compression results in life-threatening respiratory and cardiovascular compromise. Maintenance of spontaneous breathing and positioning the patient in a forward-sitting position are simple measures that may improve ventilation. Children will often find their own preferred position. Intravenous steroids may need to be commenced prior to diagnosis if the respiratory compromise is severe. Intubation of these patients is risky and best done in theatre with a gas induction and ENT surgeons on standby.

ACUTE NEUROMUSCULAR DISEASE

For the most part, the acute neuromuscular conditions that children succumb to are similar to those for adults. The reader is referred to the relevant chapters. Guillain–Barré, tetanus, botulism, acute demyelinating encephalomyelitis and acute spinal injury are supported and treated with supportive ventilation whilst expectantly awaiting return of neurological function. In Australia, tick bite paralysis can cause a severe paralysis in children. The toxin binds covalently with the acetylcholine receptor complex. The cholinergic block lasts long after the source of the toxin is removed. Not uncommonly, children require prolonged courses of supportive ventilation and intensive care. This is in contrast to the North American tick.

CHRONIC NEUROMUSCULAR CONDITIONS

Chronic neuromuscular disorders that are not diagnosed at birth are often diagnosed in infancy and early childhood. These children often require intermittent respiratory support with intercurrent illnesses. Many of these diseases are life-limiting and eventually children with severe neuromuscular or progressive conditions will suffer severe respiratory infections that need ventilation for prolonged periods. Cerebral palsy, Duchenne muscular dystrophy and spinomuscular atrophy are examples. Intubation can be difficult owing to scoliosis, limited jaw opening or facial dysmorphism. Ventilation is often troublesome due to chest wall deformity and underlying chronic lung disease. Weaning from ventilation is slow and laborious and may involve a protracted stay in the PICU on invasive ventilation and NIV. Some children cannot be weaned from invasive ventilator support after a severe infection so there is an increasing risk for these children that they will die a very medicalised death. End-of-life care and limitation of interventions are important issues to discuss with parents and care givers. Ideally these issues should be discussed prior to an acute illness so that parents and the child, if old enough, have time to consider the options without the stress of an imminent deterioration. Hopefully, some agreement can be reached and potential conflict between parents and PICU staff minimised at the time when the child is most unwell.

TRAUMA

The reader is referred to the chapters on head, chest and paediatric trauma. Pulmonary contusions and rib fractures are less common in small children. Head injury is common. As children grow, their bones ossify and they become involved in more risky activities so pulmonary contusions and rib fractures become more common. Infants tend to cope better with rib fractures, but older children have issues with pain and lung expansion, as experienced by adult patients.

Management of severe chest trauma in children is not different to that in adults: maintain distension of as much of the lung as possible, ensuring adequate ventilation with conventional or high-frequency oscillation and drainage of pneumothorax and haemothorax. Bronchoscopy can be useful for pulmonary toilet and removal of blood casts from the bronchial tree. Lung isolation and independent ventilation are difficult in children and seldom necessary.

ACUTE RESPIRATORY DISTRESS SYNDROME[3,4,29–31]

Acute respiratory distress syndrome (ARDS) may occur in children of all ages from a variety of direct and indirect lung insults, as it does in adults. In children, common causes of ARDS include shock, pneumonia, sepsis, near-drowning, aspiration and pulmonary contusion. ARDS is characterised by respiratory distress or failure, diffuse pulmonary infiltrates, reduced pulmonary compliance and hypoxia in the presence of a known precipitating cause and in the absence of left ventricular failure. ARDS is diagnosed when the ratio of the partial pressure of oxygen in arterial blood (Pa_{O_2}) to the fraction of inspired oxygen (Fi_{O_2}) is less than 200. This is the P/F ratio. Acute lung injury is diagnosed when the P/F ratio is less than 300. The P/F ratio in a healthy individual is approximately 500. Clinically P/F ratios are of little use. They define a degree of impaired gas exchange that makes some homogeneity of a heterogeneous situation, primarily for research purposes. Neonatal respiratory distress syndrome refers to respiratory distress that occurs in prematurely born infants as a result of inadequate surfactant production by their immature lungs. Treatment modalities for paediatric ARDS are very similar to those for adults with the open-lung/low-tidal-volume strategy, and acceptance of permissive hypoxia and hypercarbia. High-frequency oscillatory ventilation is commonly employed and ECLS is considered if there is a reversible or treatable cause. The reader is referred to Chapter 33 on ARDS.

FOREIGN BODIES

Laryngeal, tracheal and bronchial foreign bodies are commonplace in children. Most commonly foreign bodies that enter the airway (as opposed to oesophagus) become lodged, if they traverse the cords, at the level of the cricoid membrane (the narrowest part of the paediatric airway). The shape of the foreign body is of crucial importance as to its final resting place. Sharp and slender foreign bodies (such as needles) and particulate food material (i.e. pieces of nuts) travel further down the bronchial tree. Nut fragments and food particles are an important cause of morbidity. In particular, peanuts release arachidonic acid, which causes local inflammation. The resultant inflammation causes stenosis of the airway and pneumonia beyond the level of the obstruction. Bronchoscopy (flexible and rigid) should be performed if there is any concern of a foreign body.

IMMUNOCOMPROMISED PATIENTS[29,32]

A PICU within a hospital with an active oncology service and importantly a bone marrow transplant service will see a significant number of immunocompromised children. Not uncommonly, they present with generalised sepsis, localised pulmonary sepsis, or with pulmonary complications of conditioning regimens for transplant. Similarly if there is a solid organ transplant service (heart, liver, kidneys, lungs and small bowel) they all require degrees of systemic immunosuppression.

The amount of HIV that is seen in a paediatrics unit mirrors that seen in the heterosexual community as the majority is from maternal transmission. Developing and Third-World countries where HIV rates are extremely high in the adult population will see a lot more HIV in their critically unwell patients.

Undiagnosed leukaemia and lymphomas can present with respiratory failure due to: immunosuppression and sepsis, extremely high peripheral white cell counts causing sludging in the pulmonary circulation, or local compression of respiratory structures (see above). Some malignancies present with respiratory sequelae of disseminated intravascular coagulation (acute myeloid leukaemia) or with multisystem failure (haemophagocytic lymphohistiocytosis).

Genetic immunodeficiency states are rare. Severe combined immunodeficiency (SCID), combined variable immunodeficiency (CVID) and chronic granulomatous disease can all present with severe respiratory failure in undiagnosed patients. T-cell defects present with opportunistic infections such as *Pneumocystis*, *Nocardia* and fungal infections. B-cell deficiencies generally present with severe viral or encapsulated bacterial infection. Chronic granulomatous disease presents with recurrent bacterial infections that need an effective oxidative burst to destroy them (e.g. *Staphylococcus aureus*). Infection with an unexpected organism or severe respiratory failure in an infant that cannot be explained warrants a thorough investigation and assessment of the patient's immunocompetence.

Treatment of respiratory failure in the immunocompromised is directed toward the primary problem along with the respiratory support and antimicrobial therapy as appropriate. In some cases the immunosuppression, with steroids for example, may need to be decreased. In many chemotherapy and bone marrow transplant regimens, bone marrow stimulation or autologous stem cell rescue is used to minimise the period of neutropenia and minimise the risk of sepsis in the face of aggressive chemotherapy.

INVESTIGATIONS

RADIOLOGY[33,34]

Although chest X-ray is often mandatory in patients with respiratory disease to delineate the extent of lung involvement, the presence of pneumothorax or effusion or to check the position of the ETT and central venous lines, routine radiology investigations can expose children to unnecessary ionising radiation. Investigations that use ionising radiation should be done only if they will answer questions important to diagnosis or management of the patient. Exposure to medical radiation as a percentage of total lifetime radiation has been estimated to have risen from 15% to 50% in the USA over the last 30 years: CXRs are a significant contributor to this radiation. Children are most at risk. A chest computed tomography scan (CT) has a 1:1000 chance of inducing malignancy. Lateral CXR in children only rarely provides additional information over the anterioposterior view so is a waste of medical radiation if used routinely.

Standard CT and high-resolution spiral CT with thin cuts can provide better diagnostic detail than a plain CXR; however, their use should be justified in light of the increasing lifelong radiation exposure and the risk of transporting a critically ill patient to the scanner.

Magnetic resonance imaging (MRI), though not a good modality for the lung parenchyma, does not use ionising radiation and is safe with cumulative dosing.

Ultrasound is becoming routine in emergency departments and ICUs. Focused chest ultrasound can assist in the diagnosis of pneumonia, pleural effusions and pneumothorax with only a small amount of training. Ultrasound should be used routinely for the placement of central venous lines and is able to assist with the insertion of chest drains, placement of intra-arterial lines and peripheral intravenous lines (where veins are not visible on the skin surface).

MICROBIOLOGY[19,22,24,35,36]

Appropriate microbiological samples have a crucial role in diagnosis and therapy. It is important to sample blood and respiratory secretions prior to administering antimicrobial therapy if possible.

Nasopharyngeal aspirate or nasal brushings for immunofluoresence and viral DNA/RNA polymerase chain reaction (PCR) can detect a significant number of viral infections of the respiratory system. RSV and hMPV are by far the most common.

Bronchoscopy is used in the PICU but to a lesser extent than in the adult ICU. It is used to inspect the airways, clear secretions and obtain samples. The need to use very small bronchoscopes for infants, limited experience and reduced availability of equipment limit the utility of this modality in the PICU. When required it is undertaken by respiratory physicians or intensivists with a keen interest.

THERAPY FOR CHILDREN WITH SEVERE RESPIRATORY FAILURE

SUPPORTIVE CARE/FAMILY-CENTRED CARE

Even in the most critically ill children, parents are encouraged to be involved with the care of the child as much as is practical. The calming influence of a parent or grandparent cannot be understated, and is an important adjunct to sedation regimens in PICU and NICU. By inviting parents to participate in the care of their critically ill child, a partnership is forged that promotes trust and compliance with necessary medical interventions. In the event that the child does not survive, the benefit for the parents in the subsequent grieving process should not be underestimated. Siblings may also benefit. Occasionally, the sickest children are very sensitive to stimuli so deep sedation, muscle relaxation and minimal handling are required.

NORMOTHERMIA, FLUID BALANCE AND NUTRITION[37]

Maintenance and promotion of homeostasis is the hallmark of good intensive care. This includes adequate nutrition, euvolaemic fluid balance and normothermia (unless therapeutic hypothermia is undertaken). Small infants have a large body surface to weight ratio so maintenance of normothermia can be challenging, particularly during procedures and transportation around and between hospitals. Clinicians and nursing staff need to pay particular attention at these times. Adequate nutrition promotes recovery from critical illness so nutritional goals should be set early in the course and all attempts made to reach these goals, including the use of transpyloric feeding tubes and intravenous nutrition if required. Usually it is a struggle to achieve required goals but avoidance of overfeeding is also important. Impaired carbon dioxide clearance in severe respiratory failure makes this vital. Minimisation of fluid overload and increased lung water are crucial and can lead to prolonged ventilator weaning if not addressed. Diuretics are commonly used to treat generalised oedema but have side-effects of electrolyte imbalance and metabolic alkalosis. If fluid overload can be avoided then this is recommended.

ANTIMICROBIAL USE

Antimicrobial use should always be with consideration of the local pattern of pathogen sensitivities and promote good antimicrobial stewardship to minimise the impact of resistance patterns. Patients on antimicrobial therapy often benefit from specific input by infectious diseases specialists and routine consultation is an important part of antimicrobial stewardship.

GOOD HOUSE-KEEPING/ NOSOCOMIAL ISSUES

Children suffer complications of critical-illness-related therapies and immobilisation. Ventilator-associated pneumonias and other nosocomial infections can complicate the PICU course. Patients are at risk for dependent skin pressure areas and at contact points with medical devices. Thromboprophylaxis is important but it is less clear exactly who to treat. Protocolised care and the use of 'bundles' help to minimise the impact of these hospital-related morbidities. Local quality audit, assessment and focusing on improving areas peculiar to the specific unit are important. Good 'house keeping' in NICU and PICU is as important as the treatment of the underlying condition causing respiratory failure.

NON-INVASIVE RESPIRATORY SUPPORT

HIGH-FLOW NASAL CANNULA (HFNC) OXYGEN THERAPY[38–45]

HFNC oxygen therapy has made its way rapidly into the PICU armament of support. Its introduction has preceded the supportive research relating to its use. None the less, it appears to be a very useful tool at the lower end of respiratory support. HFNC oxygen therapy consists of a simple circuit comprising of a gas flow regulator, an oxygen mixer, a humidifier, a gas warmer, large-calibre tubing and a patient interface. The patient interface is most commonly a soft plastic or silicone nasal cannula. The cannula may be semiocclusive of the nares or non-occlusive. The idea is that gas inspired by the patient is preferentially derived by the flow through the circuit. Hence the flow must be at least the instantaneous peak inspiratory flow of the patient to avoid entrainment of environmental gas. HFNC is also thought to provide a small amount of positive airway pressure. This therapy is used increasingly in NICUs and PICUs for patients who need mild respiratory support. HFNC is safe, cheap and provides the support that a number of patients need beyond standard low-flow oxygen therapy.

Data from the ANZPIC registry 2011 reveal the impact HFNC therapy is having. HFNC accounts for almost 20% of the sole support given to patients with a respiratory diagnosis. Approximately 24% were supported with invasive ventilation and 35% with NIV. The remainder of patients were managed with a combination of the three therapies.

NASAL AND FACE MASK NON-INVASIVE VENTILATION[32,46–48]

The benefit that neonates derive from NIV is matched by the number of different systems to provide this type of support. Supporting premature neonates in this way is effective and beneficial and avoids many risks associated with long-term invasive ventilation. Even very premature infants can have a brief period of invasive ventilation, surfactant instillation and then the majority of their time they are supported on bubble CPAP for the weeks and months they are in the NICU. Neonatologists as a rule use a nasal prong patient interface. This is due to its simplicity, lack of bulk, ease of securing and effectiveness. As patients grow the use of masks becomes easier and the NIV devices are more able to synchronise and provide BiPAP effectively. Soft malleable facial structure, general uncooperativeness of patients and difficulties with adequate seal make patient interfaces difficult to match with individual patients. Newer plastics, manufacturing of devices and improved cushioning help to decrease these problems. Older children, like adults are most suited to mask ventilation support. However, with persistence and a range of masks younger children can be supported with NIV.

Triggering and delivery of support can be limited in some devices. Despite the advertising and salesmanship of ventilator companies, very few devices are suitable for small children. This is likely to change in the future.

The single most important resource, other than equipment, is experienced personnel who are able to persevere, use alternative interfaces and understand the equipment. In the acute setting it is very common to require sedation to augment patient compliance with the NIV. This should be used only where suitable staff members are present and emergency equipment is available for intubation.

INVASIVE VENTILATION[6,7,25,48]

CUFFED VERSUS UNCUFFED ETT/NASAL VERSUS ORAL[49,50]

The debate regarding cuffed versus uncuffed ETT is not likely to be resolved. Both types are reasonable to use and each type has its advantages and disadvantages. For short-term use, security and reliable ventilation most paediatric anaesthetists would prefer a cuffed ETT. In PICU when ventilation is expected to be difficult or when changing the ETT is likely to cause significant deterioration, cuffed ETTs are preferred. For longer-term PICU management the issue is less clear. Cuffed ETTs need to be the appropriate size and care taken to monitor inflation pressure and positioning of the cuff. With either cuffed or uncuffed ETT, a leak of inspired gas around the ETT (cuff deflated if present) is a desirable finding when considering extubation and risk of post-extubation stridor. Presence of a leak does not guarantee the patient will not suffer this complication. Usually it is local policy that directs the use of one or the other.

Nasal verses oral positioning for long-term ETTs is another contentious issue. Either route is used up to the age of around 8 years when maxillary and ethmoid sinuses become aerated. Oral intubation is used first when intubating a critically unwell child due to lack of reserve and the need to expedite positive-pressure ventilation. If the intubation is uncomplicated and the patient tolerates the procedure then the ETT may be changed to a nasal ETT. However, this is dependent on local PICU policy and preference rather than clear evidence. Arguably, a nasal ETT is more comfortable for the patient and easier to secure but can cause pressure areas. The risk of changing the ETT should override any decision to match the culture of the PICU with respect to positioning of the ETT.

CONVENTIONAL VENTILATION[51,52]

The debate as to volume- or pressure-regulated ventilation is ongoing although it appears that volume control may be more lung protective. Pressure control ventilation has historically been used in children owing to early ventilators not being able to guarantee delivery of the small tidal volumes that babies and infants require. With newer, more sophisticated ventilators the volume control can be adjusted up the nearest millilitre. Accurate volume measurement also requires the use of cuffed ETT in a majority of cases.

Triggered modes are used in patients who are spontaneously breathing. The aim is to have the patient lightly sedated, exercising the respiratory muscles and synchronising well with the ventilator. Appropriate triggering, inspiratory time and cycling to expiration are all important to synchrony.

Positive end-expiratory pressure (PEEP) of at least 5 cmH_2O (0.66 kPa) is routinely used in all paediatric and neonatal patients, albeit empirically. Children expire to near their functional residual capacity so that any loss of muscle tone will lead to greater likelihood of pulmonary atelectasis – hence a small amount of distending pressure is desirable. As in adults, PEEP is increased and recruitment manoeuvres are used to promote open lung ventilation. PEEP is unlikely to be increased beyond 15 cmH_2O (2 kPa). Adult strategies advocate higher PEEP but neonatal and paediatric preference is usually to change to high-frequency oscillator ventilation (HFOV) if adequate gas exchange cannot be maintained.

HIGH-FREQUENCY OSCILLATOR VENTILATION[30,53,54]

HFOV has been instrumental in the care of infants with severe respiratory failure from any number of causes. In essence it is a set pressure – the mean airway pressure (MAP), with oscillation of 6–12 Hertz around this. Oscillations are sinusoidal with negative and positive deflections. MAP, frequency and amplitude of the ventilator waveform influence oxygen and carbon dioxide clearance in discrete but not entirely independent ways. MAP and inspired oxygen are the primary determinants of oxygenation. Frequency and amplitude are the primary determinants of carbon dioxide clearance. Alveolar ventilation is said to occur by convective and diffusional mechanisms. These include bulk gas movement, laminar and turbulent flow, Pendeluft ventilation (between alveoli), collateral ventilation by alveolar channels and Taylor dispersion.

Children ventilated with HFOV are often heavily sedated and have neuromuscular-blocking agents administered. However, depending on pathology and stability, they may be allowed to breath on top of the oscillations of the ventilator. These spontaneous breaths are not supported so the clinician must ensure that the bias flow through the circuit is sufficient to maintain the MAP and allow for this tidal ventilation by the patient. For neonates and small infants this tidal volume is negligible compared with the bias flow. For older children this can be challenging and unachievable. Secretion clearance and humidification of gases can be challenging. High bias flow results in inadequate humidification while rain-out within circuits is frequently an issue. Weaning can be achieved while on HFOV, but most units convert to conventional ventilation for weaning, especially in older children who need larger tidal volumes.

VENTILATOR STRATEGIES[6,30,54]

Many ventilation concepts such as permissive hypercarbia, permissive hypoxia and open-lung ventilation came from the NICU and the management of respiratory distress syndrome in premature infants and the management of pulmonary hypoplasia in CDH. The single-organ disease and the desire of clinicians to improve outcomes and minimise morbidity drove the development in this area and credit must be given to the large number of clinicians and researchers who advanced this area.

ARDSNET has taken these concepts and demonstrated they can be translated to adult practice. Further studies followed. Although there are many criticisms of the studies they have taught us a lot about ventilation and iatrogenic morbidity that is potentially avoidable.

The best ventilation strategy gives a reasonable amount of gas exchange to meet metabolic tissue demands whilst minimising trauma (barotrauma, volutrauma, sheer stress, bio-trauma, etc.) on the lungs. Debate will rage for generations as to the best way to ventilate a critically unwell patient.

ICUs are dangerous places for patients. The modality keeping most patients in ICU is mechanical ventilation. Ventilation is hazardous and it is important to liberate the patient from dependence on mechanical support of any type as expeditiously as possible. Physicians, nurses and allied health staff must be proactive and creative to achieve this.

EXTRACORPOREAL LIFE SUPPORT (ECLS)[18,55,56]

Historically, adult ICUs had abandoned ECLS in the face of poorly constructed studies while NICUs and PICUs fostered and nurtured its development. Dramatic improvements in ECLS were promoted by improvements in cardiopulmonary bypass technology, developments in congenital heart surgery and the need to support neonates with severe respiratory failure such as meconium aspiration. Neonates across the spectrum of the ELSO registry have the greatest survival rates.

ECLS for neonates, infants and small children is typically achieved by surgical cannulation in the neck with the right common carotid and right internal jugular vein being accessed. Femoral vessels may also be used in older children but are unable to provide adequate flows in babies and infants. Veno-arterial ECLS is common, but veno-venous ECLS via a double-lumen catheter or two-vein cannulation is becoming more common for pure respiratory support.

Access the complete references list online at http://www.expertconsult.com

2. Duncan AW. The burden of paediatric intensive care: an Australian and New Zealand perspective. Paediatr Respir Rev 2005;6(3):166–73.
10. Masters IB, Chang AB. Tracheobronchomalacia in children. Expert Rev Respir Med 2009;3(4):425–39.
18. Singh BS, Clark RH, Powers RJ, et al. Meconium aspiration syndrome remains a significant problem in the NICU: outcomes and treatment patterns in term neonates admitted for intensive care during a ten-year period. J Perinatol 2009;29(7):497–503.
19. Nissen MD. Congenital and neonatal pneumonia. Paediatr Respir Rev 2007;8(3):195–203.
25. Turner D, Cheifetz IM. Pediatric acute respiratory failure: areas of debate in the pediatric critical care setting. Expert Rev Resp Med 2011;5(1):65–73.
51. Farias JA, Alía I, Esteban A, et al. Weaning from mechanical ventilation in pediatric intensive care patients. Intensive Care Med 1998;24(10):1070–5.

106

Paediatric fluid and electrolyte therapy

Frank Shann

Children need a much higher intake of water and electrolytes per kilogram of body weight than adults; this makes children more susceptible to dehydration if they have abnormal losses of water or a reduced intake. On the other hand, an inability to excrete a water load, due to immature kidneys (in neonates) or high levels of antidiuretic hormone (ADH), means that children can easily be given too much water intravenously. There are good reviews of fluid and electrolyte therapy in paediatric and neonatal intensive care[1–5] (see **Box 106.1**).

WATER

The full-term neonate is 80% water; this figure falls to about 60% by 12 months of age, and then remains almost constant throughout childhood. The intravenous (i.v.) fluid requirements for children in hospital are shown in **Tables 106.1** and **106.2**. The widely used formula for an active child shown in Table 106.2 was published in 1957,[6] and some of the measurements of energy expenditure were made almost a hundred years ago. The formula is a compromise between the requirements of a fully active child and the much lower requirements at basal metabolic rate – for example, the estimate of 100 mL/kg/day for an active 10-kg child in hospital is double the 50 mL/kg/day needed for a sick child at basal state (Table 106.2).[6,7]

Table 106.3 shows that very ill children in intensive care often need much less water than the 'standard' amounts that are often given.[1,6,8–13] For example, if a 15-kg child ('standard' maintenance fluid of 50 mL/h,[6] Table 106.1) sustains a head injury and has evidence of high levels of ADH (maintenance fluid×0.7),[9] is ventilated with humidified gas (maintenance×0.75),[8] is paralysed (basal state, maintenance×0.7),[6] and is maintained at a rectal temperature of 36°C (maintenance−12%),[1] then his actual full maintenance fluid requirement is (50×0.7×0.75×0.7) − 12%=16 mL/h. Even less water should be given initially if the child is overhydrated.

In very small children, all fluid administered has to be taken into account – including the volume of drugs (bicarbonate, dextrose and antibiotics) and 'flushes' used to clear i.v. lines (after blood sampling or administration of drugs).

The estimates of water requirements in Tables 106.1–3 are only approximate, and water balance must be monitored closely in any child in intensive care. Unfortunately, regular, accurate weighing of very sick children is often impractical, and hydration has to be assessed using the serum sodium concentration, skin turgor, urine output (minimum 0.5–1.0 mL/kg/h) and central venous pressure.

In a child with oliguria following a severe ischaemic or hypoxic insult (such as birth asphyxia, drowning or cardiac arrest), it may be helpful to measure the urine sodium concentration.[14] In oliguria due to acute tubular necrosis, where restriction of fluid intake may be necessary, the urine sodium is usually more than 40 mmol/L. In oliguria due to hypovolaemia, the urine sodium is usually less than 20 mmol/L.

SODIUM[15,16]

Sodium is predominantly an extracellular ion, so total body sodium is well represented by the serum concentration; it must be interpreted in the context of both total hydration and the relative amounts of water and sodium. Acute changes in serum sodium are usually due to changes in body water rather than changes in body sodium.

In the first 1 or 2 days of life, small preterm babies often have poor urine output and high transcutaneous fluid losses. They are therefore prone to hypernatraemia and hyperkalaemia, and such infants should usually be given 5% or 10% dextrose without sodium or potassium. From 2 days of age, 2–4 mmol/kg/day of sodium and potassium will usually be sufficient, but much higher intakes of sodium are needed in some preterm neonates owing to their impaired renal conservation of sodium.

Hyponatraemia may be due to:[16]

- increased body water due to excessive water intake, especially in the presence of high levels of ADH (CNS disease, intermittent positive-pressure ventilation (IPPV), lung disease, vomiting, stress)
- low body sodium due to diuretic therapy, poor renal conservation of sodium, or a low sodium intake (e.g. breast milk).

Acute hyponatraemia causes cerebral oedema, with a grave risk of cerebral herniation and death or severe brain damage.[17] Hyponatraemia due to sodium deficit

Table 106.1 Approximate intravenous fluid requirements for children (mL per hour)

	WEIGHT IN KG											
	3	5	7	10	15	20	25	30	40	50	60	70
Active	12	20	30	40	50	60	65	70	80	90	95	100
Sick	6	10	14	20	25	30	35	40	45	55	60	70
Intubated	4	7	10	14	17	21	25	28	32	40	45	50

Box 106.1 Key points

- Children in intensive care usually need much less water than the 'standard' maintenance amounts (see Table 106.1)
- Hypovolaemia should be corrected with 10 mL/kg boluses of 0.9% saline
- Isotonic 0.9% saline should be used as the maintenance fluid in ill children, with careful monitoring of the serum sodium
- Hypoglycaemia is very dangerous in infants, and hyperglycaemia is less dangerous than in adults
- In hyponatraemia, the serum sodium should rise no faster than 8 mmol/L per 24 hours
- In hypernatraemia, the serum sodium should fall no faster than 0.5 mmol/L per hour
- Potassium should be given intravenously no faster than 0.3 mmol/kg per hour
- Oedema with low serum osmolality and high urine osmolality is often due to excess water administration to a child with high levels of antidiuretic hormone – the main treatment is fluid restriction
- Oedema caused by capillary leak will not respond to diuretic therapy or dialysis – large amounts of fluids may be needed to preserve the intravascular volume
- In adults resuscitated with 4% albumin rather than 0.9% saline, mortality tended to be lower in sepsis and higher in trauma, but the differences were not statistically significant – saline is much less expensive

should be corrected by careful administration of sodium (**Table 106.4**). However, hyponatraemia is usually due to water excess rather than sodium deficiency, and this should be treated with restriction of water intake; if symptomatic, it can be corrected by careful administration of 3% sodium at 0.5 mL/kg/h (Table 106.4), and furosemide 0.5 mg/kg intravenously if there are high ADH levels. Hyponatraemia must be corrected slowly: the serum sodium should increase by no more than 8 mmol/L each 24 hours, and even less in patients with long-standing hyponatraemia.[16]

Hypernatraemia may be due to:[15]

- reduced body water (dehydration) from a large insensible fluid loss (caused by radiant heaters or phototherapy), diarrhoea, osmotic diuresis (caused by glycosuria) or inadequate fluid intake

Table 106.2 Approximate intravenous fluid requirements for children (mL/kg/day)

ACTIVE CHILD IN HOSPITAL	
<10 kg	100 mL/kg/day
10–20 kg	1000 mL+(50 mL/kg/day for each kg over 10 kg)
>20 kg	1500 mL + (20 mL/kg/day for each kg over 20 kg)
SICK, BUT NOT INTUBATED	
<10 kg	50 mL/kg/day
10–20 kg	500 mL+(30 mL/kg/day for each kg over 10 kg)
>20 kg	800 mL+(20 mL/kg/day for each kg over 20 kg)
INTUBATED, WITH HUMIDIFIED INSPIRED GASES	
<10 kg	35 mL/kg/day
10–20 kg	350 mL+(20 mL/kg/day for each kg over 10 kg)
>20 kg	550 mL + (12.5 mL/kg/day for each kg over 20 kg)

Table 106.3 Modifications to the fluid intakes for active children shown in Table 106.2

	ADJUSTMENT
DECREASE	
Humidified inspired air[8]	×0.75
Basal state (e.g. paralysed)[6]	×0.7
High ADH (IPPV, brain injury)[9]	×0.7
Hypothermia[1]	12% per °C
High room humidity[1]	×0.7
Renal failure[1]	×0.3 (+urine output)
INCREASE	
Full activity + oral feeds[6]	×1.5
Fever[1]	+ 12% per °C
Room temperature >31°C[1]	+ 30% per °C
Hyperventilation[10]	×1.2
Neonate – preterm (1–1.5 kg)[11]	×1.2
– radiant heater[12]	×1.5
– phototherapy[13]	×1.25
Burns – first day[1]	+4% per 1% area burnt
– subsequently[1]	+2% per 1% area burnt

ADH=antidiuretic hormone; IPPV=intermittent positive-pressure ventilation.

Table 106.4 Doses and formulae in paediatric fluid and electrolyte therapy

Albumin 20%	Undiluted: 2–4 mL/kg
5%	5% in 5% dextrose or saline:
Bicarbonate (number of mmol of deficit):	Under 5 kg: base excess×wt (kg)×0.5 (give half of this) Over 5 kg: base excess×wt (kg)×0.3 (give half of this)
Blood volume	85 mL/kg in neonate 70 mL/kg in older child
Calcium	Chloride 10% (0.7 mmol/mL Ca^{2+}): maximum 0.2 mL/kg i.v. stat, requirement 1.5 mL/kg/day Gluconate 10% (0.22 mmol/mL Ca^{2+}): maximum 0.5 mL/kg i.v. stat, requirement 5 mL/kg/day
Dextrose	For hypoglycaemia: 1 mL/kg 50% dextrose i.v. in neonate: 4 mg/kg/min (2.4 mL/ kg/h 10% dextrose) day 1, increasing to 8 mg/kg/min (up to 12 mg/kg/min with hypoglycaemia) For hyperkalaemia: 0.1 u/kg insulin and 2 mL/kg 50% dextrose i.v. stat
Magnesium	Chloride 0.48 g/5 mL (1 mmol/mL Mg^{2+}): 0.4 mmol (0.4 mL)/kg/dose slow i.v. 12-hrly Sulphate 50% (2 mmol/mL Mg^{2+}): 0.4 mmol (0.2 mL)/kg/dose slow i.v. 12-hrly
Mannitol	0.25–0.5 g/kg/dose i.v. (1–2 mL/kg of 25%) 2-hrly, provided serum osmolality <330 mosm/kg
Packed cells	10 mL/kg raises Hb 3 g%; 1 mL/kg raises PVC 1%
Potassium	Maximum 0.3 mmol/kg/h, requirement 2–4 mmol/kg/day, 1 g KCl = 13.3 mmol K^+. Hyperkalaemia: see dextrose
Sodium	Depletion: 3% saline at 0.5 mL/kg/h (maximum Na rise 8 mmol/L in 24 h); requirement 2–6 mmol/kg/day, 1 g NaCl =17.1 mmol/Na^+
Urine	Minimum acceptable is 0.5–1.0 mL/kg/h

- increased body sodium from administration of large amounts of sodium (e.g. sodium bicarbonate) or salt poisoning.

With hypernatraemic dehydration, shock should be treated with boluses of 10 mL/kg of 0.9% saline. The water deficit should then be corrected very slowly using 0.9% saline so that the serum sodium falls no faster than 0.5 mmol/L/h, to prevent cerebral oedema.[15] If salt ingestion causes severe acute hypernatraemia without dehydration, peritoneal dialysis or haemofiltration may be indicated.

POTASSIUM[18]

Potassium is predominantly an intracellular ion, so total body potassium is poorly represented by the serum concentration. The concentration of potassium in the serum depends on pH as well as the total body potassium (which is usually about 50 mmol/kg). A child may have hypokalaemia without a deficit of total body potassium in the presence of alkalosis and, conversely, there may be a large deficit of potassium without hypokalaemia in the presence of acidosis. Potassium should rarely be infused at more than 0.3 mmol/kg/h, and it should not normally be given to a patient with severe oliguria or anuria.

CALCIUM, MAGNESIUM AND PHOSPHATE

Hypocalcaemia in children occurs in:

- sick neonates in the first 2 days of life
- infants of diabetic mothers
- exchange transfusion with citrated blood (a temporary effect)
- magnesium deficiency
- infants fed cows' milk (which has a high phosphate content).

Hypocalcaemia and hypomagnesaemia cause jitters, tetany, cardiac arrhythmias and convulsions. The doses of calcium and magnesium are given in Table 106.4. The normal intravenous maintenance requirements in infants are 1 mmol/kg/day of calcium and 0.3 mmol/kg/day of magnesium.

STANDARD PAEDIATRIC MAINTENANCE FLUIDS

'Maintenance solution' is an unfortunate term, since these solutions do not provide maintenance calorie or protein requirements (see Parenteral nutrition, below). Until recently, it was common practice to give children a hypotonic maintenance solution of approximately 0.2% saline in 4% dextrose in generous amounts - based on the water requirements of an active child.[6] This policy resulted in a high incidence of hyponatraemia - and far too many children developed cerebral oedema that resulted in death or severe brain damage.[17,19–22]

Several factors have contributed to the high incidence of hyponatraemia in children. First, the amount of dehydration present is often overestimated,[23] and rapid administration of an excessive amount of fluid will cause hyponatraemia even if 0.9% saline is given - because the increase in intravascular volume will cause the production of urine containing more than 154 mmol/L of sodium (the amount present in 0.9% saline).[24] Secondly, the formula that is widely used to calculate maintenance water requirements is based on the needs of active children, and prescribes too much fluid for a sick child (Table 106.2).[17] Thirdly, many sick children have increased secretion of antidiuretic hormone even in the absence of hypovolaemia,[25,26] so they are unable to excrete the excess water when they are given large amounts of fluid. Fourthly, some sick children lose substantial amounts of sodium in their urine, perhaps due in part to the excretion of ketones as sodium salts.[22]

There is general agreement that an isotonic fluid such as 0.9% saline should be used to correct hypovolaemia, but there has been spirited debate about whether hypotonic 0.2% saline or isotonic 0.9% saline should be used for maintenance.[5,27,28] The supporters of using 0.2% saline argue that it is logical and safe provided the volume of fluid given is never in excess of actual requirements,[29–31] but there is limited empirical evidence to support this theory.[31] The supporters of using 0.9% saline for initial maintenance therapy in sick children (with careful monitoring of the serum sodium) argue that, in practice, this has been preferable,[17,19–22] because it is difficult to ensure that no excess fluid is administered, and there is a lower risk of hyponatraemia and cerebral oedema if any excess fluid that is given is isotonic. It is especially important to use isotonic fluid during and after surgery, and whenever there is a high risk of cerebral oedema (for example, amongst children with diabetic ketoacidosis or brain injury).[5,19–22,27,28]

Ill children with clear signs of hypovolaemia should be treated with 5–10 mL/kg boluses of 0.9% saline until the intravascular volume has been restored, and then given 0.9% saline (with potassium and dextrose as required) in the volumes shown in Tables 106.1 and 106.2 (or calculated from Table 106.3). The serum sodium concentration should be monitored carefully. If it is less than 138 mmol/L and falling, then less 0.9% saline should be infused. If the serum sodium is more than 142 mmol/L and rising, then 0.45% or 0.2% saline should be infused with a cautious increase in the rate.

Great care should be taken to avoid hypoglycaemia in children. Hypoglycaemia is particularly dangerous in young infants,[32] whereas hyperglycaemia is probably less dangerous in children than it is in adults in intensive care.[33]

The key messages are:

- correct hypovolaemia using 10 mL/kg boluses of 0.9% saline
- most sick children need far less maintenance fluid than previously thought (Table 106.1)
- use isotonic maintenance fluid for the first few days of treatment with careful monitoring of the serum sodium
- avoid hypoglycaemia.

DEHYDRATION AND SHOCK

Weight loss is the best guide to the degree of dehydration, if a recent weight is known. Many of the commonly used clinical signs of dehydration in children are inaccurate, and this leads to dehydration being diagnosed when it is not present, and to overestimation of the degree of dehydration.[23] The clinical signs of mild to moderate dehydration become apparent with only 3–4% dehydration in children.[23] The most reliable signs are:[34]

- decreased peripheral perfusion (as shown by pallor or reduced capillary return)
- deep breathing
- decreased skin turgor.

In children with shock, intravenous access may be difficult. In these circumstances, parenteral fluid can be given rapidly into the bone marrow, which is an intravascular compartment.[35] The usual sites chosen are the junction of the upper and middle third of the tibia (0–12 months of age), the medial malleolus (1–5 years) and the iliac crest (over 5 years). A 0.9 mm (20 gauge) lumbar puncture needle or an intraosseous needle can be used; the needle is held perpendicular to the bone and pushed in *gently* with a rotary motion about its long axis - a slight decrease in resistance will be felt as the needle enters the medulla. In infants with a patent anterior fontanelle, the superior sagittal sinus is an excellent way to gain intravenous access in an emergency.[36]

Shock should be treated with an initial bolus of 10 mL/kg of 0.9% saline, followed by further boluses of 10 mL/kg until the intravascular volume has been restored.[37] After shock has been corrected with a rapid infusion of fluid, the remainder of the deficit is

Table 106.5 Composition of some body fluids in children

FLUID	NA$^+$ (MMOL/L)	K$^+$ (MMOL/L)	CL$^-$ (MMOL/L)	HCO_3^- (MMOL/L)	OTHER
Gastric fluid	20–80	10–20	100–150	0	H$^+$ 30–120
Bile	140–160	3–15	80–120	15–30	
Pancreatic fluid	120–160	5–15	75–135	10–45	Basal state
Jejunal fluid	130–150	5–10	100–130	10–20	
Ileal fluid	50–150	3–15	20–120	30–50	
Diarrhoeal fluid	10–90	10–80	10–110	20–70	
Sweat					
Normal	10–30	3–10	10–35	0	
Cystic fibrosis	50–130	5–25	50–110	0	
Burn exudate	140	5	110	20	Protein 30–50 g/l
Saliva	10–25	20–35	10–30	2–10	Unstimulated

replaced over the next 48–72 hours, while giving maintenance requirements using 0.9% saline with dextrose and potassium chloride. Thus, a 5-kg child with 10% dehydration from diarrhoea (500 mL deficit) might receive 100 mL (20 mL/kg) of isotonic saline rapidly to restore the circulation, leaving a 400 mL deficit to be replaced over 48 hours. If the maintenance requirement is 250 mL/day (Table 106.2), then the child should be given a further 450 mL of 0.9% saline per day for the next 2 days (approximately 20 mL/h) in addition to the initial 100 mL. Further abnormal fluid losses should be replaced with an appropriate fluid (see **Table 106.5**).

In a randomised study of 3141 East African children with severe febrile illness and signs of poor peripheral perfusion, children given 20–40 mL/kg boluses of 5% albumin or 0.9% saline had a significantly *higher* mortality at 48 hours and 4 weeks than children not given a fluid bolus.[38] However, only 2.1% of the children satisfied WHO's criteria for shock, and many of the 3141 children had severe anaemia, pneumonia, meningitis or encephalopathy and were at risk of overhydration.[39] The study therefore does not show that fluid boluses are dangerous in hypovolaemic shock.

With hypernatraemic dehydration, shock should be treated as above, with rapid infusion of 10–20 mL/kg of isotonic saline. The remaining deficit should then be replaced *slowly* with 0.9% saline so the serum sodium falls no faster than 0.5 mmol/L/h, to prevent cerebral oedema.[15]

In dehydration due to pyloric stenosis there is a deficit of water, hydrogen ion, chloride and potassium. Hypovolaemia should be treated by rapid infusion of 10–20 mL/kg of 0.9% saline, then 0.9% saline in 5% dextrose with 40 mmol/L of potassium chloride should be given at 50 mL/kg/day with careful monitoring of the serum electrolytes and blood glucose.

OEDEMA

Oedema is common in children in intensive care units. It may be due to:

- excess water intake, often with high levels of ADH (from CNS disease, IPPV, or lung disease)
- capillary leak (due to the effects of hypoxia, ischaemia, acidosis or sepsis)
- hypoalbuminaemia
- heart failure or renal failure.

Several possible causes are often present in one child, and it can be difficult to decide which is the most important. Children with oedema and high levels of ADH will have a serum osmolality less than 270 mmol/kg (with hyponatraemia) and a urine osmolality greater than 270 mmol/kg; the appropriate treatment is fluid restriction. On the other hand, in children with oedema due to capillary leak, fluid restriction and attempts to remove water (diuretics, dialysis) are unlikely to cure the oedema, and often cause hypovolaemia; in fact, large amounts of fluid (e.g. blood and normal saline) may be needed to preserve the intravascular volume in these children – the oedema will disappear only when the capillary damage resolves.

CRYSTALLOID OR COLLOID FLUIDS

There have been many reviews of the contentious issue of the relative merits of crystalloid or colloid fluids in critically ill patients. A widely quoted review concluded that, compared with crystalloids, albumin increased mortality by 6% (95% CI, 3–9%).[40] However, a subsequent large study in 6997 adults in Australia found no significant difference in overall mortality between normal saline and 4% albumin[41] – the mortality with albumin tended to be lower in sepsis and higher in trauma, but the differences just failed to reach statistical significance in both subgroups. The Cochrane analysis is heavily influenced by the large Australian study, and it concluded that there is no evidence that albumin reduces mortality when compared with cheaper alternatives such as saline.[42]

There have been very few studies comparing crystalloid to colloid fluids in children, so most of the evidence comes from studies in adults. The use of albumin in paediatric and neonatal intensive care has been reviewed.[43,44] The meta-analyses do not suggest that colloid is better than crystalloid, and colloid is more expensive and carries a small risk of transmitting infection. Until more evidence is available, it seems sensible to use crystalloid as a routine, but give concentrated albumin to children with severe hypoalbuminaemia (perhaps if their serum albumin is less than 25 g/L) – unless the low albumin is caused by chronic malnutrition, when albumin should *not* be given.[45]

PARENTERAL NUTRITION[46–49]

'Maintenance solution' is an unfortunate medical term, particularly when small children are concerned – a solution of 5% dextrose with sodium and potassium chloride provides maintenance amounts of water, sodium, potassium and chloride, but little or no calories, protein, trace elements or vitamins. For example, 100 mL/kg/day of 5% dextrose provides 20 Cal/kg/day (84 kJ/kg/day), which is only 20% of the requirement of a normal infant (let alone a child with increased calorie requirements). It has been estimated that, although an adult has the energy reserve to survive for about a year on 3 litres of 10% dextrose a day, a small preterm infant will survive only 11 days on 75 mL/kg/day of 10% dextrose.[50]

Many children in intensive care units are unable to absorb adequate amounts of food from the gut, and their nutritional reserves are small so they often need parenteral nutrition. However, parenteral nutrition is difficult to administer and dangerous in small children – such patients should be referred to a specialist paediatric unit as soon as possible.

The usual requirements for amino acids, dextrose and fat in parenteral nutrition in children are shown in **Table 106.6**. The amino acid solution can be mixed with dextrose in the pharmacy department to make a 'nutrient solution'. A standard nutrient solution might provide 4 mmol/kg/day of sodium, 3 mmol/kg/day of potassium, and 7.5 mmol/day of calcium and phosphate (with up to 12 mmol/L for neonates). The standard solution should also contain 4 mmol/L of magnesium, 0.2 µmol/kg/day of manganese, 3 µmol/kg/day of zinc, 0.5 µmol/kg/day of copper, 0.04 µmol/kg/day of iodide, 0.005 µmol/kg/day of chromium, 20 µg/L of hydroxycobalamin, 2 mg/L of phytomenadione, 1 mg/L of folic acid, and a multivitamin preparation. For short-term nutrition, the solution need not provide fluoride, iron or vitamins A, D and E, but a paediatric multivitamin preparation should be given to children on long-term parenteral nutrition. Fat can be given as a 20% emulsion, either through a separate i.v.

Table 106.6 Approximate requirements in paediatric parenteral nutrition

	TOTAL FLUID (ML/KG PER DAY)*	AMINO ACIDS (G/KG PER DAY) DAY 1	2	3+	DEXTROSE (G/KG PER DAY) DAY 1	2	3+	LIPID (G/KG PER DAY) DAY 1	2	3	4+	TOTAL CALORIES (KCAL) NEEDED (1 KCAL=4.2 KJ)†
Neonates	100	1.5	2	2	10	10–15	15–20	1	2	2	2–3	100/kg
Under 10 kg	100	1.5	2	2	10	10	15–20	1	2	2	2–3	100/kg
10–15 kg	90	1	1.5	2	5	10	15	1	1.5	2	2–3	1000+(50/kg over 10 kg)
15–20 kg	80	1	1.5	1.5–2	5	10	10–15	1	1	1.5	2–3	1000+(50/kg over 10 kg)
20–30 kg	65	1	1	1–2	5	10	10–15	1	1	1	1–2	1500+(20/kg over 20 kg)
30–50 kg	50	1	1	1–2	5	5–10	10	1	1	1	1–2	1500+(20/kg over 20 kg)

*One mL/kg per day of fluid is needed for each kcal/kg per day; for adjustments to requirements, see Table 106.3 [Total kcal/kg per day equals g/kg per day of (amino acids×4)+(dextrose×4)+(fat×10). To calculate calories please note %=g/100 mL.]
†Calorie requirement of an active child in hospital.

line or alternating with the nutrient solution. Nutrient solutions for paediatric use contain high concentrations of calcium, magnesium and phosphorus and they should not be mixed with the fat emulsion, even in a Y-connection placed just before the cannula.

In a child on parenteral nutrition, it is important that abnormal fluid losses (Table 106.5) be replaced with an appropriate solution (in addition to the nutrient solution), and that parenteral nutrition always be introduced and withdrawn slowly. A dislodged i.v. cannula should be replaced immediately in a child on parenteral nutrition, to prevent rebound hypoglycaemia. If nutrient solution is not available at any time, it should be replaced with an infusion of a similar amount of dextrose (e.g. 20% dextrose with 40 mmol/L of sodium chloride and 20 mmol/L of potassium chloride).

Children receiving parenteral nutrition are liable to develop:

- hyperglycaemia (with glycosuria and dehydration)
- hypoglycaemia
- sepsis
- extravasation of solutions with necrosis of tissue
- thrombocytopenia
- hypoproteinaemia
- electrolyte imbalance
- acidosis
- anaemia
- hyperlipaemia
- uraemia
- cholestatic jaundice.

Box 106.2 Monitoring in paediatric parenteral nutrition

- Daily: inspect i.v. site, electrolytes, acid/base, serum triglyceride (reduce lipid infusion rate if triglyceride is greater than 2–2.5 mmol/L)
- Twice weekly: haemoglobin (transfuse if anaemia develops), platelets, proteins
- Weekly: creatinine, magnesium, calcium, phosphate, bilirubin, aspartate aminotransferase
- Blood glucose 8-hourly until the dextrose intake is stable
- Test urine for glucose 8-hourly (reduce dextrose intake if more than trace)
- Weigh frequently (daily if possible)

Frequent, careful monitoring is essential (**Box 106.2**). Initially, monitoring may need to be more frequent than suggested in Box 106.2, particularly in preterm babies. Monitoring can be less frequent once a child is stabilised on parenteral nutrition.

Access the complete references list online at http://www.expertconsult.com

1. Winters RW, editor. The Body Fluids in Pediatrics. 1st ed. New York: Little, Brown & Company; 1973.
2. Finberg L, Kravath R. Water and Electrolytes in Pediatrics: Physiology, Pathology, and Treatment. 2nd ed. Philadelphia: Saunders; 1993.
3. Greenbaum L. The pathophysiology of body fluids and fluid therapy. In: Kliegman R, Behrman R, Jenson H, et al, editors. Nelson Textbook of Pediatrics. 19th ed. Philadelphia: Saunders; 2011:212–49.
4. Dell K, Davis I. Fluid and electrolyte management. In: Martin R, Fanaroff A, Walsh M, editors. Fanaroff and Martin's Neonatal-Perinatal Medicine. 8th ed. Philadelphia: Mosby; 2005:695–712.
5. Paut O, Lacroix F. Recent developments in the perioperative fluid management for the paediatric patient. Curr Opin Anaesthesiol 2006;19(3):268–77.
6. Holliday MA, Segar WE. The maintenance need for water in parenteral fluid therapy. Pediatrics 1957;19(5):823–32.
7. Talbot F. Basal metabolism standards for children. Am J Dis Child 1938;55:455–9.
8. Sosulski R, Polin RA, Baumgart S. Respiratory water loss and heat balance in intubated infants receiving humidified air. J Pediatr 1983;103(2):307–10.
9. Bouzarth WF, Shenkin HA. Is 'cerebral hyponatraemia' iatrogenic? Lancet 1982;1(8280):1061–2.

107

Sedation and analgesia in children

Geoff Knight

All children, including preterm infants, feel and remember pain and discomfort.[1] The provision of optimal levels of analgesia sedation should therefore be a priority in the management of all critically ill children.

Pain in the paediatric intensive care unit (PICU) may be surgical or procedural in origin (e.g. central venous catheterisation, lumbar puncture, removal of drains) or due to the patient's underlying illness. Sedation is frequently necessary to allow a child to tolerate an endotracheal tube and mechanical ventilation. It may also be needed to allow sleep in a brightly lit, noisy environment. As young children are unlikely to cooperate during investigations such as an echocardiogram or computed tomographic (CT) scan, sedation is often necessary to prevent excessive movement.

In addition to its humane benefits, sedation and analgesia can suppress non-advantageous physiological responses to noxious stimuli. Analgesic suppression of the marked post-surgery stress response has been associated with significant improvements in postoperative morbidity and mortality.[2–4]

ASSESSMENT

Adequacy of pain relief and sedation is dependent on the accuracy of the assessment of the degree of discomfort. This assessment is often difficult in the critically ill child who may be preverbal, developmentally delayed, intubated and/or paralysed, or simply uncooperative. Thorough assessment requires careful and frequent consideration of a number of factors. These include the nature of the noxious stimulus, variations in physiological parameters (e.g. heart rate and blood pressure) and interpretation of subjective clues (e.g. facial expressions and posture). Parental interpretations are a reliable adjunct and should be incorporated into the overall assessment.

Particular challenges in both pain and sedation assessments arise in a number of patient groups and validated assessment tools should be utilised whenever possible. Neonates and infants are particularly difficult to assess. The Premature Infant Pain Profile (PIPP) and CRIES scales are objective measures of pain in this group of patients.[5] For the equally problematic preverbal child the Multidimensional Assessment of Pain Scale (MAPS) is a useful validated tool for assessing postoperative pain.[6] Established assessment tools such as the Face, Legs, Activity, Cry and Consolability (FLACC) scale have been modified to enhance the pain assessment of children with cognitive impairment.[7] The COMFORT and the modified COMFORT 'Behavior' are validated observer-reported sedation scales for children 1–3 years.[8] In older children, self-reporting measurement scales can be used but these require a degree of patient cooperation.

The most challenging patients to manage optimally are those receiving muscle paralysis. Attempts to enhance the limited clinical parameters available for interpretation with an objective measure have centred on the bispectral index (BIS). Validation studies in the paediatric intensive care environment are, however, limited and highlight the probable inaccuracy of current methods of assessing sedation in this group.[9] In general it is preferable to err on the side of over- rather than undersedation in the paralysed patient.

MANAGEMENT

The management of discomfort, anxiety and pain should be multifaceted. Consensus guidelines from the United Kingdom Paediatric Intensive Care Society incorporate a detailed analysis of the evidence for various assessment and management strategies.[10]

Management should, whenever possible, begin prior to the child's admission to the intensive care unit. Orientation to the unit should be accompanied by a clear, age-appropriate explanation of the planned procedure or operation and the expected postoperative course. Parental presence during this phase and at other critical times is also important to help allay anxiety and fear. Close attention should also be paid throughout a child's admission to potentially distressing physiological factors, such as hunger and urinary retention. In addition to these supportive measures, many paediatric patients require a pharmacological form of analgesia or sedation.

Delivery of sedation and analgesia should be tailored to the patient's particular requirements. It is therefore essential that there be continuous assessment and frequent adjustment of therapy to ensure that optimal levels of sedation and adequate analgesia are delivered at all times. Nurse-titrated sedative and

Table 107.1 Single-dose and infusion rates of sedative and analgesic drugs*

DRUG	SINGLE DOSE	INTRAVENOUS INFUSION
Midazolam	0.1–0.2 mg/kg i.v. 0.5 mg/kg oral	50–200 μg/kg per hour
Ketamine	1–2 mg/kg i.v.	10–20 μg/kg per min (sedation) 4 μg/kg per min (analgesia)
Propofol	1–3 mg/kg i.v.	<4 mg/kg per hour (short term)
Clonidine	1–2 μg/kg i.v.	0.1–2 μg/kg per hour
Dexmedetomidine	0.5–1 μg/kg	0.2–1 μg/kg per hour (<24 hours)
Morphine	0.1–0.2 mg/kg i.v.	10–40 μg/kg per hour
Fentanyl	1–2 μg/kg i.v.	1–10 μg/kg per hour
Remifentanil	0.1–0.5 μg/kg i.v.	0.1–0.5 μg/kg per min

*Infusion rates are per hour except for fentanyl, remifentanil and ketamine (per minute).

analgesia regimens can optimise outcomes by allowing timely adjustments. This approach requires clear communication by medical staff of the aims of management, including the targeted level of sedation and clear understanding by nursing staff of the pharmacology of the agents being administered. Relief of pain should be achieved with analgesic agents and care must be taken to avoid excessive doses of sedative agents when the patient's primary need is for pain relief (**Table 107.1**). Although emphasis should be on achieving optimal comfort, consideration should also be given to minimising side-effects. A single drug may be effective but often a combination of medications and delivery methods (e.g. i.v./oral, i.v./epidural) will be useful and may avoid the side-effects of high doses of a single agent.

The differences in drug handling between children and adults should be considered when planning analgesia and sedation regimens. Drug distribution, rates of drug metabolism and relative organ blood flows differ in children, particularly in young infants. These differences may result in greater concentrations of free drug and differing volumes of distribution. Neonates have relatively larger total body water, extracellular fluid volume, blood volume and cardiac output and significantly less body fat than adults. Their blood–brain barrier is less efficient and allows more ready entry of some drugs to the brain. Mixed-function oxidases mature quickly to adult levels by 6 months of age, and acetylation and glucuronidation mechanisms mature by about 3 months. Renal blood flow and glomerular filtration rate are low in the immediate neonatal period. However, both increase significantly in the first 2–3 days and reach adult values by around 5 months. Tubular secretory capacity reaches adult levels by 6 months of age. In general, therefore, drug metabolism and clearance are relatively mature by 6 months of age, but great care is required when dealing with the neonate and young infant.

DRUGS

MIDAZOLAM

Midazolam is water-soluble, and has a rapid onset of action. Metabolism occurs in the liver and by 6 months of age is comparable to that of an adult. The standard i.v. sedative dose is 0.1–0.2 mg/kg and this is effective for uncomfortable procedures such as echocardiography and cardioversion. The oral route (0.5 mg/kg) may also be useful although there is a 15-minute delay to onset of sedation. Nasal administration (0.2 mg/kg) can be useful in children who do not have established i.v. access and in whom oral agents are not appropriate. Although midazolam may be effective as the sole sedative agent for ventilated patients, higher doses or additional agents are commonly required in young children (1–4 years)[11] – 50–200 μg/kg per hour, in combination with an opioid (morphine 10–40 μg/kg per hour), is generally effective in facilitating mechanical ventilation. Dose-related respiratory depression occurs and hypotension can be significant in hypovolaemic patients and in those with depressed myocardial function. During continuous infusion, accumulation can occur, particularly in young infants (under 6 months) and in patients with liver dysfunction.

Midazolam has been shown to induce neuronal apoptosis in animal models.[12] Alternatives, such as dexmedetomidine or fentanyl, should therefore be considered particularly in the neonate. Midazolam's use in neonatal intensive care is controversial because of concerns regarding both safety and effectiveness in the newborn.[13]

KETAMINE

Ketamine is a dissociative anaesthetic agent with sedative, analgesic and amnesic properties. Biotransformation occurs via the microsomal enzyme system. Thus, there is little metabolism in the newborn and clearance is less and elimination half-life greater in infants than in older children and adults.[14]

An i.v. dose of 1–2 mg/kg is usually adequate to induce deep sedation. Cardiovascular disturbance is minimal and ketamine is therefore particularly useful as the induction agent in status asthmaticus and in patients with a compromised haemodynamic state, such as cardiac tamponade. Prolonged sedation for ventilated children can be achieved with a continuous infusion of 10–15 μg/kg per minute and analgesia can be provided by an infusion of 4 μg/kg per min. Concomitant use of an antisialogogue, such as glycopyrrolate, may help control the often seen increase in respiratory tract secretions. The unpleasant emergent phenomena seen frequently in adults probably occur less often in children. The traditional practice of concurrently administering a benzodiazepine with the aim of minimising these effects has minimal demonstrable benefit.[15] As with midazolam, ketamine has been shown to be neurotoxic in animal models and prolonged use in young infants should be minimised.[16]

PROPOFOL

Propofol is a rapidly acting hypnotic agent that is widely used in paediatric anaesthesia and in paediatric intensive care for short- and longer-term sedation.[17] Although it has no analgesic properties its short half-life makes it an attractive agent for sedation. The half-life decreases with age, probably owing to development of metabolising capacity and increasing hepatic flow.[18] Sedation can be achieved in the spontaneously breathing patient, with an induction dose of 1 mg/kg, followed by intermittent smaller doses; 2–3 mg/kg per hour has delivered uncomplicated satisfactory sedation to ventilated children.[19] Propofol should, however, be used with caution for sedation in the PICU because of the reported association between high-dose (>4 mg/kg per hour), prolonged (>29 hours) infusions and a clinical syndrome (propofol infusion syndrome) consisting of metabolic acidosis, lipaemia, cardiac failure, arrhythmias and death.[20] (It should be noted that the manufacturers advise against the use of propofol for sedation of children during intensive care.) The pathogenesis of this syndrome remains unclear, although it has been postulated that a disturbance of mitochondrial function leads to disordered hepatic lipid regulation.[21] Lipaemia may be an early indicator of developing problems and haemodialysis in the early phase is the only treatment described to date.[22]

There are sufficient concerns to limit the use of propofol in the PICU to short-term sedation in the stable ventilated child. A recent survey in Germany identified widespread use in paediatric intensive care with a time limitation of <24 hours in most cases and a median dose limit of 4 mg/kg/hour.[17] Limiting the duration of infusion to 6 hours at <4 mg/kg per hour is recommended. Use of propofol should also be avoided in the presence of shock, hypoxaemia or acute liver dysfunction.

CHLORAL HYDRATE

Chloral is an effective oral hypnotic and sedative agent with no analgesic effect. The hypnotic dose is 50 mg/kg and appropriate sedation may be achieved with lower doses. Gastric irritation can be a problem in some children. Toxic doses produce depression of respiration and cardiac contractility. Despite the disadvantage of delayed onset, chloral can be useful given prior to procedures, or as a supplemental sedative agent in the ventilated child, and it can effectively induce nocturnal sleep. On a cautionary note, there is some evidence that it may not be suitable in acutely wheezing infants.[23]

CLONIDINE AND DEXMEDETOMIDINE

Clonidine is an α_2-adrenoreceptor agonist with significant neurological, neuroendocrine and cardiovascular effects that result in sedation, analgesia and reduced sympathetic outflow. It is rapidly absorbed after oral administration and has a half-life of 9–12 hours. Metabolism is via the liver and kidney and approximately 50% is excreted unchanged in the urine. A single oral dose (4 μg/kg) can provide both preoperative sedation and postoperative analgesia following moderately painful surgery.[24] An i.v. infusion (0.1–2 μg/kg per hour) in combination with midazolam (50 μg/kg per hour) has been shown to produce effective sedation in ventilated children without haemodynamic disturbance.[25] Clonidine in similar doses can also have a role in the management of opioid withdrawal and in controlling the autonomic 'storms' seen following severe traumatic brain injury.

Dexmedetomidine is a selective α_2-agonist that has many of the properties of clonidine and may produce less respiratory depression. It is metabolised in the liver and the elimination half-life of 2 hours is similar in adults and older children and marginally longer in infants.[26] Retained respiratory drive during continuous infusion is particularly valuable and has allowed successful extubation of patients who had previously failed because of agitation.[27] The addition of dexmedetomidine to a sedative regimen has allowed a reduction in the required dose of benzodiazepines and opioids while delivering satisfactory levels of sedation with preserved respiratory drive.[28] Current licensing restrictions are for <24 hours' use in adults. The MIDEX and PRODEX trials assessed the efficacy of dexmedetomidine as an alternative to midazolam or propofol in adult intensive care patients.[29] Dexmedetomidine was comparable to both alternatives, and was associated with reduced ventilation time compared with midazolam. Studies in children are awaited, but dexmedetomidine is becoming accepted in the PICU as an adjunctive sedative agent (0.2–1 μg/kg per hour) and as an alternative to benzodiazepines.

Bradycardia and hypotension are seen with both clonidine and dexmedetomidine during continuous infusion and a risk–benefit assessment must be made prior to their use.

MORPHINE

Morphine is frequently used to provide analgesia and as part of a sedative regimen for children on mechanical ventilation. Marked variation in pharmacokinetics in the neonatal period has been demonstrated, but infants over 1 month of age eliminate morphine efficiently and should not be more sensitive to respiratory depression than adults. Clearance and half-life (2 hours) are at adult values by 6 months of age.[30] The active metabolite is renally excreted and can therefore accumulate with renal impairment.

The standard i.v. dose is 0.1–0.2 mg/kg, and an infusion rate of 10–40 μg/kg per hour should be titrated to effect for postoperative pain relief in spontaneously breathing patients. With careful titration of dose to effect, higher rates can be administered, particularly to the child on mechanical ventilation. Patient-controlled analgesia devices delivering fixed doses of opioid, with or without a background infusion, can be used successfully by the majority of school-aged children and may occasionally be appropriate in intensive care. Histamine-related side-effects, in particular nasal itch, may warrant a change of opioid, and fentanyl is an alternative.

FENTANYL AND ALFENTANIL

Fentanyl has theoretical advantages over morphine in certain situations because of its rapid onset and its systemic and pulmonary haemodynamic stability. Termination of the effects of a single dose is by redistribution. Clearance is more rapid in neonates and infants compared with adults and does not change with time during continuous infusion. However, after prolonged infusion, unchanged fentanyl is returned to the circulation from peripheral compartments, resulting in a prolonged terminal elimination half-life of approximately 21 hours.[31]

The effective dose for painful procedures is 1–2 μg/kg. Fentanyl is useful as an anaesthetic agent in patients with labile pulmonary vasculature, as it can blunt changes in pulmonary vascular resistance seen with stimulation.[4] It does not, however, prevent the increase in pulmonary vascular pressure caused by hypoxia.[32] Infusions of 1–5 μg/kg per hour produce effective sedation in neonates on mechanical ventilation; 1–10 μg/kg per hour is required for analgesia in older children. Tolerance can develop rapidly in both neonates and older children.[33]

Alfentanil, because of its shorter duration of action, may have advantages for analgesia or sedation for very short procedures.

REMIFENTANIL

Remifentanil is a synthetic opioid with potent analgesic properties, rapid onset of action and, following initial redistribution, a short half-life of around 8 minutes. Metabolism occurs via non-specific esterases and is therefore relatively independent of renal and hepatic mechanisms. The short duration of action allows rapid emergence from general anaesthesia, thereby facilitating extubation or assessment of the patient's neurological state.[34] Postoperative pain needs to be managed with an alternative analgesic regimen and a longer-acting opioid (morphine) should be administered prior to discontinuing remifentanil.

Infusions of 0.1–0.5 μg/kg per minute have produced satisfactory analgesia and sedation in ventilated adult patients and there is evidence that ventilation times are shorter and weaning from ventilation more rapid in comparison to standard sedation regimens.[35] Although remifentanil is widely used in paediatric anaesthesia there are few data available on its use in children in intensive care. Uncomplicated and successful use in the induction and sedation of a ventilated preterm neonate has been described.[36] As metabolism is relatively independent of renal and hepatic mechanisms, remifentanil could be considered for use in patients with liver and/or renal impairment who would not have continuing pain and in whom rapid termination of sedation is required.

THIOPENTAL

Thiopental is useful as an anaesthetic induction agent in critically ill children, although its hypotensive effects limit its use in shocked patients. The standard dose is 5 mg/kg, and this should be reduced to 2–3 mg/kg when there is a risk of hypotension. Thiopental is useful in the management of refractory status epilepticus and may have a role in difficult cases of raised intracranial pressure. In such cases, it is administered by continuous infusion (1–5 mg/kg per hour). Accumulation can lead to prolonged sedation.

PARACETAMOL AND NON-STEROIDAL ANTI-INFLAMMATORY DRUGS

The addition to an analgesic regimen of either paracetamol or a non-steroidal anti-inflammatory drug (NSAID) should be considered provided there are no contraindications.

Paracetamol is useful for mild to moderate pain and is an effective supplement to opioids for more severe pain. Enteral preparations, though useful, are prone to erratic absorption. The intravenous preparation is more useful in the intensive care setting and has been shown to reduce opioid requirements in adults with few side-effects following orthopaedic surgery.[37] The recommended initial i.v. dose in children is 15 mg/kg and the total daily i.v. dose should be limited to 60 mg/kg. Lower i.v. doses (7.5 mg/kg 6-hourly) are recommended for infants <10 kg. Contraindications to paracetamol include liver dysfunction, and care must be taken with dosage to avoid liver injury in all children.

NSAIDs should also be considered as supplemental analgesics. Care should be taken, however, regarding the risk of bleeding, particularly in the postoperative period and in the highly stressed patient in whom gastric bleeding is more likely. Ketorolac (0.6 mg/kg) can be given i.v. and therefore has the potential to reduce the dose of opioid required in the immediate postoperative period when enteral medications are not appropriate.

NITROUS OXIDE

Nitrous oxide is a potent analgesic agent. It is useful in intensive care during short painful procedures such as removal of surgical drains. A mixture of 50% nitrous oxide with oxygen provides analgesia in awake and cooperative patients. It is unsuitable for repeated or continuous use because of toxicity, and administration to younger children may cause distress because of the need for application of a mask.

ISOFLURANE

Isoflurane has been used for long-term sedation in intensive care in adults. As elimination is independent of hepatic and renal mechanisms, there are theoretical advantages in many critically ill patients. However, an association between isoflurane sedation and neurological abnormalities has been reported in children.[38] These abnormalities, including ataxia, agitation, hallucination and confusion, although all reversible by 72 hours, were a considerable clinical problem. They make this technique unsuitable in the PICU.

WITHDRAWAL SYNDROMES

Opioid withdrawal is a well-recognised problem and symptoms include poor feeding, tremors, agitation, poor sleeping, tachycardia, diarrhoea, sweating, increased muscle tone, dystonic posturing and seizures. Withdrawal occurs particularly following prolonged high-dose infusions. The risk of withdrawal following a fentanyl infusion is associated with the duration of infusion and the total dose. Infusion for >5 days or a total dose >1.5 mg/kg is associated with a greater than 50% incidence of withdrawal.[39] Benzodiazepine withdrawal (agitation, anxiety, sweating, tremor) is also seen and the risk following a midazolam infusion is associated with a total dose >60 mg/kg.[40]

Careful attention to weaning an infusion in high-risk patients can minimise withdrawal symptoms. Longer-term pharmacological management is occasionally required and is best managed by administering the agent from which the patient is withdrawing. Tapered infusions can be substituted for by enteral morphine, methadone or diazepam and clonidine has also been utilised.[41] The weaning programme can be as short as 5 days.[42]

Assessment is difficult but is assisted by the use of a validated assessment tool; the Withdrawal Assessment Tool-1 (WAT-1) is a promising assessment instrument.[43] Although withdrawal can be a significant problem, adequate sedation or analgesia should not be withheld because of fears of the development of drug dependence.

LOCAL ANAESTHESIA

Local anaesthesia can produce effective analgesia without systemic effects and therefore has significant advantages in many patients, particularly the postoperative group. In the intensive care setting, it can be used as the sole method of providing analgesia or in combination with i.v. agents. The risk of toxicity is related both to the dose and to the rapidity of absorption, which is dependent on local blood flow. Metabolism of the amide local anaesthetics (lidocaine, bupivacaine) is via the cytochrome P-450 system and their half-life is longer in infants less than 6 months of age. Unbound drug does not produce analgesia but is potentially toxic as infants have lower levels of the binding protein α-glycoprotein. The use of local anaesthesia in infancy therefore requires careful assessment and close monitoring.

TOPICAL

Analgesia for some painful procedures is possible with minimal sedation using topical preparations or careful local infiltration. The total dose of local anaesthetic agent infiltrated must be monitored to ensure that maximum doses are not exceeded. The total dose of lidocaine should not exceed 4 mg/kg (7 mg/kg if combined with epinephrine (adrenaline)). Systemic absorption of the prilocaine component in topical preparations occurs and neonates, because of their relative deficiency of methaemoglobin reductase, are at particular risk of methaemoglobinaemia. Topical preparations should be used with caution in this group.

NERVE BLOCK

Femoral nerve blockade is a simple technique that produces effective analgesia in cases of femoral shaft fracture. A single injection is effective for approximately 3 hours and longer-term analgesia can be provided by a continuous infusion of bupivacaine (0.125%) at 0.2–0.3 mL/kg per hour through a fine catheter placed adjacent to the femoral nerve.[44] As this technique can decrease opioid requirements, it is particularly useful in trauma patients who have suffered a coexistent head injury.

Intercostal nerve blocks may be useful after thoracotomies and liver transplants in children.[45] A single dose of 0.125% bupivacaine (maximum single dose 2 mg/kg) can produce up to 8 hours of analgesia. The dose must be carefully monitored, because the relatively high blood flow to the area increases the risk of toxicity. Continuous infusions via an intercostal catheter can provide ongoing pain relief. There is a risk of pneumothorax with this technique and it should therefore be avoided when there is significant coexistent lung disease.

EPIDURAL

Caudal, lumbar and thoracic epidural anaesthesia can provide effective control of postoperative pain in children.[46,47] The procedures must be performed by skilled experienced staff who clearly understand the risks and benefits. A complication rate of 1.5 per 1000 has been reported, with dural puncture and intravascular injection seen most commonly.[48] Other risks include cord injury, epidural infection and excessive motor blockade. Infants under 6 months are at highest risk because of their size and immature metabolism of local anaesthetic agents.

Many epidural catheter insertions are performed in the operating theatre as general anaesthesia is a prerequisite in most paediatric patients. PICU care may subsequently be required because of the nature of the surgery (e.g. thoracotomy, liver transplant) or because of underlying patient factors (e.g. neurological disorders, morbid obesity, age). Epidurals have been used in paediatric cardiac surgery without a clear benefit over conventional postoperative analgesia.[49] Particular indications for commencing epidural analgesia in the PICU include burns in a suitable distribution (e.g. abdomen and lower limbs) and blunt chest trauma with rib fractures. Contraindications include shock, hypovolaemia, meningitis, coagulopathy and local skin infection.

Bupivacaine is the most commonly used local anaesthetic. A single dose should not exceed 2.5 mg/kg and the maximum infusion rate is 0.4 mg/kg per hour (0.2 mg/kg per hour in infants). Opioids (morphine and fentanyl) may be added and have a synergistic effect, thereby allowing less local anaesthetic agent to be used. However, epidural opioids can cause sedation and respiratory depression.

SUMMARY

Delivering optimal levels of analgesia and sedation in the paediatric intensive care unit is challenging and requires careful assessment and a management approach incorporating both pharmacological and non-pharmacological aspects. Use of age-appropriate validated assessment tools combined with continuous adjustment of drug delivery is required. Withdrawal is common in children but the risk should not impact on the delivery of effective sedation or analgesia. Alternatives to the conventional approaches are required at times and the PICU team should be open to novel drug therapies or methods of drug delivery.

Access the complete references list online at http://www.expertconsult.com

1. Anand KJS, Hickey PR. Pain in the foetus and neonate. N Engl J Med 1987;317:1321–9.
6. Ramelet AS, Rees N, McDonald S, et al. Development and preliminary psychometric testing of the Multidimensional Assessment of Pain Scale: MAPS. Paediatr Anaesth 2007;17:333–40.
10. Playfor S, Jenkins I, Boyles C, et al. Consensus guidelines on sedation and analgesia in critically ill children. Intensive Care Med 2006;32:1125–36.
13. Ng E, Taddio A, Ohisson A. Intravenous midazolam infusion for sedation of infants in the neonatal intensive care unit. Cochrane Database Syst Rev 2003;1:CD002052.
29. Jakob SM, Ruokenen E, Grounds RM, et al. Dexmedetomidine vs midazolam or propofol for sedation during prolonged mechanical ventilation: two randomised trials. JAMA 2012;307(11):1151–60.
41. Tobias JD. Tolerance, withdrawal and physical dependency after long-term sedation and analgesia of children in the paediatric intensive care unit. Crit Care Med 2000;28:2122–32.
43. Franck LS, Harris SK, Soetanga DJ, et al. The Withdrawal Asssessment Tool-1 (WAT-1): an assessment instrument for monitoring opioid and benzodiazepine withdrawal symptoms in pediatric patients. Pediatr Crit Care Med 2008;9(6):573–80.
44. Johnson CM. Continuous femoral nerve blockade for analgesia in children with femoral nerve fractures. Anaesth Intensive Care 1994;22:281–3.

108

Shock and cardiac disease

Johnny Millar

SHOCK

Shock is the clinical state resulting from insufficient oxygen delivery to meet oxygen demand, described in detail in Chapter 15. Shock in children is most commonly due to hypovolaemia or sepsis and remains an important cause of global infant and child mortality. The cellular effects of tissue hypoxia in shock are the same in children and adults, but there are important developmental changes in anatomy, physiology and immunity during childhood that influence the incidence, presentation and natural history of shock.

DEVELOPMENTAL DIFFERENCES

BODY FLUID COMPARTMENTS[1]

Although the extracellular fluid volume in children is greater than in adults when indexed to body weight, the small absolute volumes involved are critical when blood or fluid loss causes shock; 100 mL blood loss is inconsequential for an adult, but represents one-third of the blood volume for a neonate (**Table 108.1**).[1]

CARDIAC[2–4]

There are many differences between the newborn and the mature heart that have important effects on function, particularly under stress. The newborn heart has a relatively small left ventricular muscle mass that must cope with the newly imposed demands of the systemic circulation. In response to increased afterload, the neonatal myocardium increases in mass by both hypertrophy and hyperplasia, with the capacity for the latter of these mechanisms being lost after the first 6 months of life. Neonatal cardiac myocytes appear small and blunted with a higher proportion of non-contractile elements than mature myocytes. The fewer myofibrils are poorly aligned and there are sparser, disorganised-looking mitochondria. Less efficient handling of calcium by the myocyte membrane and sarcoplasmic reticulum make the neonatal myocyte more dependent on extracellular fluid calcium concentration, which may contribute to limited cardiac reserve.

The physiological consequence is a stiffer, less compliant ventricle that is less able to generate contractile force. Physiological changes at birth (see below) increase both volume and pressure load to the left ventricle. The ability of the ventricle to increase output in response to further volume or pressure loading is limited. The neonatal heart functions at a high state of beta-adrenergic stimulation and therefore has a restricted capacity to increase contractility and rate. Following birth there is a steady increase in stroke volume index and cardiac index over the first 3 years of life.

VASCULAR

Antenatal pulmonary blood flow is low (<10% of combined ventricular output) through a relatively muscularised high-resistance circulation. Blood ejected by the right ventricle is mostly diverted through the ductus arteriosus to the systemic circulation. Pulmonary vascular resistance (PVR) falls abruptly at birth with a concomitant increase in pulmonary blood flow. The PVR then falls more slowly, reaching adult levels over the next 6 weeks as a result of pulmonary vascular remodelling. The increase in pulmonary blood flow immediately following birth results in increased preload to the left ventricle. Coincident with this the systemic vascular resistance rises acutely. Following the transition from fetal to neonatal circulation, systemic vascular resistance index remains relatively constant throughout early childhood.[5]

MICROCIRCULATION

There are animal and human data to support the notion of maturation of the microcirculation.[6,7] The infant and young child's microcirculation is leakier at baseline and functions at a higher turnover of fluid and protein than the adult. This state of higher turnover may predispose the child to greater capillary leak in response to inflammatory and traumatic stimuli resulting in hypovolaemic shock.

IMMUNITY AND THE INFLAMMATORY RESPONSE[8]

The newborn has had little prior exposure to pathogens and has limited capacity to respond to infection, so is at increased risk of invasive infection. This risk persists beyond the newborn period as the immune system

Table 108.1 Body fluid compartments during childhood (mL/kg)[1]

AGE	TOTAL BODY WATER	EXTRACELLULAR FLUID	INTRACELLULAR FLUID	BLOOD
Pre-term newborn	800	550	300	95
Birth	750	450	300	85
1 year	700	350	350	80
5 years	650	250	400	75
Adult	600	200	400	70

remains immature through infancy and early childhood, with deficits in both innate and adaptive immunity. In addition to immature barriers to infection, infants have lower levels of circulating complement components and defective natural killer cell function. A mature pattern of cytokine and chemokine production is not attained until later in childhood. B cells are geared toward producing IgM rather than IgG or IgA and there are multiple distinct deficiencies in T-cell function. The inflammatory response to sepsis also appears to undergo complex developmental changes, the implications of which are hard to define. Aspects of the pro- and anti-inflammatory response are qualitatively and quantitatively different in children compared with adults, including a relative exaggeration of the anti-inflammatory response.

Like adults, children are placed at risk of infection by therapeutic immunosuppression but there are also a large number of congenital diseases that are characterised by generalised or specific defects in immune function.

RECOGNITION OF SHOCK

Recognition of early shock is very important as children compensate well initially, but their capacity to do so is rapidly exhausted and decompensation can then be sudden; during the early stages of compensated shock in infants, signs may be limited to tachycardia and tachypnoea (**Table 108.2**). Hypotension is a late finding and demands urgent attention.

INITIAL ASSESSMENT AND INVESTIGATION

HISTORY

- Fever, feeding, urine output, diarrhoea, vomiting
- Rapid breathing, sweating, tiring while feeding
- Irritability, lethargy
- Trauma
- Potential for trauma in infants
- Potential for ingestion
- Vaccination history.

EXAMINATION

- Temperature
- Conscious level

Table 108.2 95% ranges for heart rate, blood pressure and respiratory rate in childhood[48]

AGE	HEART RATE (BEATS PER MINUTE)	MEAN BLOOD PRESSURE (mmHg)	RESPIRATORY RATE (BREATHS PER MINUTE)
Birth	95–145	40–60	30–66
6 months	110–175	50–90	28–57
1 year	105–170	50–100	25–55
4 years	81–131	50–100	20–26
7 years	66–111	60–90	20–24
14 years	56–106	65–95	15–20

- Peripheral perfusion, capillary refill
- Rash
- Skin turgor
- Mucous membranes
- Pulses
- Heart rate, rhythm
- Blood pressure
- Respiratory rate.

INITIAL INVESTIGATIONS

- Chest X-ray
- Arterial blood gas, lactate
- Full blood count and film examination
- Blood glucose
- Plasma electrolytes, urea, creatinine, liver function tests.

If there is evidence of sepsis or if there is no obvious cause for shock take cultures and start antibiotic therapy (**Table 108.3**).[9–11]

- Blood cultures – peripheral blood and from any lines already in place
- Urine cultures (suprapubic aspirate or in-out urinary catheter in young infants)
- Throat swab
- Urine, stool and nasopharyngeal aspirate for virology
- Do not do a lumbar puncture in a shocked child. Commence antibiotics following other cultures. CSF for bacterial and viral culture and PCR can be obtained later.

Table 108.3 Initial antibiotic treatment of septic shock in children

FIRST FEW DAYS OF LIFE	
Benzylpenicillin	60 mg/kg 12-hourly
Gentamicin	5 mg/kg 36-hourly
BEYOND FIRST FEW DAYS OF LIFE	
Flucloxacillin	50 mg/kg 6-hourly
Cefotaxime	50 mg/kg 6-hourly
Gentamicin	6 mg/kg 24-hourly
IF HOSPITAL ACQUIRED, REPLACE FLUCLOXACILLIN WITH	
Vancomycin	25 mg/kg load then 15–20 mg/kg 8-hourly

TYPES OF SHOCK

The traditional classification of shock (Ch. 15) is valid in children, but a combination of these is likely to be present in any given clinical situation. In particular it is best to think of septic shock as a clinical entity that incorporates features of several shock types.

HYPOVOLAEMIC SHOCK

This is a common presentation in childhood, particularly secondary to water and electrolyte losses with diarrhoea and vomiting.

The initial compensatory response to hypovolaemia is an increase in catecholamine secretion, leading to poor peripheral perfusion, tachycardia and a normal blood pressure with diminished pulse pressure. Lethargy and tachypnoea secondary to increasing metabolic acidosis are variably present. Up to 15–20% of the circulating blood volume may be lost before hypotension occurs. With further volume loss end-organ perfusion and oxygen delivery are compromised leading to worsening acidosis, coma, oligo/anuria and ultimately myocardial dysfunction.

The cause of hypovolaemia is usually evident from the history and examination, but hidden blood loss must be considered, particularly in infants where unreported head or abdominal trauma may have occurred with few external signs.

TREATMENT

Ensure adequate airway protection and breathing and administer oxygen. After establishment of intravenous (or intraosseous) access, early and aggressive intravenous fluid resuscitation is vital to restore the circulating blood volume. Give fluid (10–20 mL/kg 0.9% NaCl) rapidly with frequent clinical reassessment to verify signs of reversal of shock. Give blood if shock is due to ongoing blood loss.

CARDIOGENIC SHOCK

See section on Cardiac disease below.

DISTRIBUTIVE SHOCK

CAUSES

These include anaphylaxis, spinal cord injury or administration of vasodilators. Septic shock in children may have a distributive component, but this is not as common a finding as in adults (see below).

PRESENTATION

In distributive shock tissue perfusion is inadequate despite an initially normal circulating blood volume and normal (or high) cardiac output. Abnormal vasomotor tone with profound vasodilatation leads to a reflex tachycardia (in spinal cord injury absence of sympathetic activity may result in bradycardia). Examination reveals warm peripheries, tachycardia and hypotension with a wide pulse pressure. The cause of distributive shock is likely to be clear from clinical examination.

TREATMENT

Attend to airway and breathing, obtain intravenous access and give rapid fluid boluses (20 mL/kg 0.9% NaCl). If there is inadequate reversal of shock then vasopressors may be necessary to restore blood pressure (or counteract the effects of vasodilator drugs).

Anaphylaxis must be treated specifically and urgently. **Table 108.4** gives paediatric epinephrine (adrenaline) doses.

OBSTRUCTIVE SHOCK

CAUSES

These include pericardial tamponade, tension pneumothorax and mediastinal mass.

PRESENTATION

In obstructive shock extracardiac restriction of cardiac output prevents adequate oxygen delivery. There may be obstruction to the pulmonary or systemic outflow tract or circulation, or compression by pericardial tamponade or tension pneumothorax.

TREATMENT

Treatment is aimed at ensuring adequate circulating volume and identifying and remedying the cause of the obstruction. Tamponade and tension pneumothorax require urgent drainage.

SEPTIC SHOCK[8,12–14]

The clinical presentation of septic shock in young children is different to adults, who reliably present with peripheral vasodilation, hypotension and a relatively high cardiac output ('warm shock'). In children the

Table 108.4 Paediatric cardiac drug doses[48]

DRUG	DOSE
Adenosine	0.1 mg/kg (max 3 mg); increase by 0.1 mg/kg/dose to 0.3 mg/kg (max 12 mg)
Alprostadil (PGE_1)	10–50 ng/kg/min
Amiodarone	25 µg/kg/min for 4 h, then 5–15 µg/kg/min
Atropine	0.02 mg/kg (max 0.6 mg)
Bicarbonate (10%$NaHCO_3$)	1–2 mL/kg
Digoxin	15 µg/kg, then 5 µg/kg after 4 hours, then 3–5 µg/kg 12-hourly
Dobutamine	2–10 µg/kg/min
Epinephrine	
bolus	10 µg/kg (0.1 mL/kg 1 : 10000)
infusion	0.05–0.5 µg/kg/min
anaphylaxis	10 µg/kg (0.01 mL/kg 1 : 1000) by deep i.m. injection
Esmolol	500 µg/kg over 1 min, then 25–250 µg/kg/min
Isoproterenol	0.05–0.5 µg/kg/min
Levosimendan	12.5 µg/kg over 10 min, then 0.2 µg/kg/min for 24 h
Metaraminol	
bolus	0.01 mg/kg
infusion	0.05–0.5 µg/kg/min
Metoprolol	0.1 mg/kg over 5 min (max 5 mg)
Midazolam	
bolus	0.1 mg/kg
infusion	1–4 µg/kg/min
Milrinone	0.25–0.75 µg/kg/min
Morphine	
bolus	0.1 mg/kg
infusion	10–60 µg/kg/hour
Nitric oxide (inhaled)	10–20 parts per million
Norepinephrine	0.05–0.5 µg/kg/min
Sodium nitroprusside	0.5–3 µg/kg/min
Vasopressin	0.0005–0.002 U/kg/min

picture is usually dominated by myocardial suppression and peripheral vasoconstriction ('cold shock'). Hypovolaemia occurs rapidly due to capillary leak secondary to the sepsis-induced inflammatory response. Septic shock in children may be difficult to distinguish from cardiogenic shock or hypovolaemic shock. Neonatal sepsis often presents with features of persistent pulmonary hypertension, with right heart failure and a degree of cyanosis depending on patency of the ductus arteriosus and foramen ovale.

TREATMENT[13,15]

Recent guidelines emphasise the importance of prompt and aggressive fluid resuscitation and early institution of inotropic therapy.[13]

Airway

Administer supplemental oxygen to all children with shock. Intubate patients who are unable to protect their airway or have impending respiratory failure.

Circulation and access (see Ch. 105)

If peripheral access is difficult and the child is obtunded or severely shocked consider intraosseous access early. Give fluid boluses (20 mL/kg 0.9% NaCl) to restore circulating blood volume. Children with septic shock often require large amounts of fluid resuscitation – occasionally more than 100 mL/kg. In patients who do not have reversal of signs following 60 mL/kg of fluid, gain central venous access. This allows measurement of central venous pressure, administration of inotropes or vasoconstrictors and measurement of central venous saturation (see below). Insert an arterial line for frequent sampling and invasive monitoring of blood pressure.

Echocardiography is an important means of guiding inotrope and vasopressor management, allowing assessment of cardiac filling, contractility and PVR. Invasive measurement of cardiac output is rarely performed in children; pulmonary artery catheter insertion is technically difficult and although several non-invasive methods are available to estimate cardiac output in children none are widely used.

Inotrope/vasodilator/vasoconstrictor therapy (see Table 108.4 for drug doses)

Do not delay starting vasoactive drugs if there is difficulty gaining central venous access. Dilute infusions of inotropes and vasoconstrictors may be administered through a peripheral line, with care taken to avoid and check for extravasation.

Decreased contractility on echo or clinical suspicion

Dobutamine is a useful first-line inotrope in children and is relatively safe to administer through a peripheral intravenous line. Although dopamine is still widely used, it inhibits anterior pituitary release of thyrotropin, growth hormone and prolactin[16] and may be relatively ineffective in young infants. Epinephrine should be started as a second-line drug if cardiac function remains inadequate despite dobutamine.

Hypotension and warm peripheries

A vasoconstrictor may be used alone if myocardial function is adequate or is added to an inotrope if contractility is poor. Norepinephrine is the drug of choice, but an inadequate response to it may be due to downregulation of catecholamine receptor numbers or function. Apparent norepinephrine resistance warrants a trial of vasopressin, but a randomised controlled trial in paediatric shock failed to demonstrate any outcome benefit with vasopressin treatment (and showed a trend towards increased mortality).[17]

Hypotension and cool peripheries

Treat decreased contractility as above. As discussed earlier, peripheral vasoconstriction is a compensatory mechanism to maintain adequate perfusion pressure. Do not add a vasodilator to an already hypotensive patient. A vasoconstrictor may be needed in addition to an inotrope if hypotension persists.

Normotension and cool peripheries

If blood pressure is normal or high, addition of a vasodilator may reduce afterload and improve cardiac output. Sodium nitroprusside (SNP) has a short half-life and can be discontinued rapidly if the blood pressure falls. In addition to being a powerful vasodilator, milrinone has inotropic effects but should be used with care because of its relatively long half-life.

Pulmonary hypertension

If there is evidence of pulmonary hypertension during shock start an inotrope (dobutamine or epinephrine) to support the right ventricle. Intubate (if not already done), ventilate using a high Fi_{O_2} to a normal Pa_{CO_2} and correct acidosis. Inhaled nitric oxide should be added to reduce PVR.

Antibiotics

Early and appropriate antibiotic therapy is associated with improved survival.[18] Administer antibiotics to patients in whom the cause of shock is not immediately apparent. After appropriate cultures, selection of antimicrobials is guided by the clinical picture including any available results from prior cultures. In the absence of specific information, a suggested first-line treatment schedule is shown in Table 108.3. A search for the source or site of infection should be undertaken and it may be necessary to drain collections or remove infected tissue.

Blood transfusion

Transfusion of packed red cells to replace blood loss is essential. In a patient with ongoing evidence of inadequate oxygen delivery there is some evidence to support transfusion to maintain a haemoglobin of >10 g/L, particularly in septic shock.[13]

Corticosteroids

Give hydrocortisone to shocked patients who are at risk of absolute adrenal insufficiency (recent or ongoing treatment with corticosteroids, known hypothalamic/pituitary/adrenal disease or purpura fulminans). The routine use of hydrocortisone in septic shock does not reduce mortality in adults, although there may be some benefit to a prolonged low-dose course.[19] In children there is less evidence on which to base a recommendation and this remains a controversial area.[13,15]

Intravenous immunoglobulin

Intravenous pooled immunoglobulin (IVIG) has been used in both children and adults with septic shock, but evidence for an effect on mortality is poor.[20] IVIG has the potential to neutralise superantigens in toxic shock syndrome and its use is often recommended in this setting, but again clear evidence regarding clinical efficacy is lacking.[21] Anticytokine and antiendotoxin monoclonal immunoglobulin therapies remain experimental.

Extracorporeal membrane oxygenation (ECMO)

Current guidelines recommend ECMO for refractory septic shock.[13,15] There is emerging evidence that central ECMO cannulation via sternotomy is superior to peripheral or neck cannulation paediatric sepsis, allowing insertion of larger cannulae and consequently higher ECMO flows.[22]

Insulin

Hyperglycaemia is common in shock and may be exacerbated by epinephrine and corticosteroid treatment. Treat sustained hyperglycaemia with insulin infusion, but critically ill children are relatively sensitive to insulin[23] and have limited metabolic reserve, increasing the risk of hypoglycaemia. There is conflicting evidence regarding the benefits of tight glycaemic control in children and neonates, and hypoglycaemia has been a significant problem in many of these studies.[24–27]

GOALS OF TREATMENT

The goals of treatment are to reverse the shock state and ensure ongoing adequate tissue oxygen delivery. Frequent clinical reassessment is aided by laboratory investigations including:

- *heart rate:* normal for age (see Table 108.2)
- *blood pressure:* normal for age (see Table 108.2)
- *central venous pressure:* 10–12 mmHg (1.33–1.96 kPa)
- *central capillary refill:* <3 seconds
- *mental state:* normal
- *urine output:* >0.5 mL/kg/h
- *serum lactate:* <2.0 mmol/L
- *central venous saturation:* >70%.

Plasma lactate concentrations are indicative of inadequate tissue oxygenation and therefore a useful marker of shock. Hyperlactaemia can also be due to dead gut, liver dysfunction or epinephrine infusion.[28]

Measurement of central venous saturation (Scv_{O_2}) can be used to assess adequacy of oxygen delivery in the absence of a pulmonary artery catheter.[29] A sample taken from the superior vena cava (SVC) or SVC/RA (right atrium) junction is best; sampling from within the right atrium may be polluted by poorly saturated blood from the coronary sinus or by interatrial shunting. Goal-directed treatment of septic shock in children with a target Scv_{O_2}>70% is associated with improved survival.[30] In children with structural heart disease and intracardiac mixing, aim for an Sa_{O_2} – Scv_{O_2} difference of ≤30%.

CARDIAC DISEASE

Appropriate drug doses for this section are given in Table 108.4.

CARDIOGENIC SHOCK

Cardiogenic shock can be difficult to distinguish from septic shock. Causes of cardiogenic shock are listed in **Box 108.1**.

Patients present with tachycardia, low pulse volume and poor peripheral perfusion as vasoconstriction maintains blood pressure in the initial stages. Tachypnoea, obtundation and decreased urine output are present early. Examination may reveal a gallop rhythm, hepatomegaly, sweating and peripheral oedema. The presence or absence of a cardiac murmur is unlikely to be helpful in acute diagnosis. Ongoing shock leads to progressive hypoperfusion of end organs.

INVESTIGATION

Initial investigations include chest X-ray, ECG and echocardiogram, with further tests prompted by individual findings. Take blood cultures and start antibiotics if there is no known cause for cardiogenic shock.

TREATMENT

Treat as described for septic shock in the preceding section (see Table 108.4).

Consider ECMO early if the patient is deteriorating or unresponsive to therapy.

Box 108.1 Causes of cardiogenic shock

- Primary cardiac disease
  - Congenital heart disease
  - Post cardiac surgery
  - Cardiac trauma
  - Myocarditis
  - Cardiomyopathy
  - Arrhythmias and conduction defects
  - Endocarditis
- Local disease with cardiac effects
  - Constrictive pericarditis
  - Pericardial tamponade
  - Compression of heart by tumour, tension pneumothorax
- Systemic disease with cardiac effects
  - Sepsis
  - Hypoxic ischaemic injury
  - Autoimmune disease
  - Kawasaki disease
  - Drug ingestion

CARDIAC FAILURE[31–33]

Children with heart failure are a diverse group of patients with a heterogeneous group of diseases leading to worsening heart function. Cardiac failure can be due to primary or secondary myocardial disease, or the effects of congenital heart disease or its treatment (**Table 108.5**).

INVESTIGATIONS

- Chest X-ray
- Electrocardiogram
- Echocardiogram
- Further imaging with CT, MRI and catheter may be warranted
- Blood gas
- Electrolytes, renal and liver function
- Coagulation
- BNP, troponin I
- Viral cultures – urine, stool and nasopharyngeal aspirate
- Serum amino acids
- Urine amino and organic acids
- Serum carnitine.

TREATMENT

Treat any identified underlying cause for heart failure (sepsis, correctable congenital heart disease, arrhythmias, anaemia). Further treatment is in the following sections on cardiomyopathy, congenital heart disease and disorders of cardiac rhythm.

CARDIOMYOPATHY[34,35]

Primary cardiomyopathy is rare in childhood (1.13–1.24 per 100 000 children per year) with the highest incidence in the first year of life. Dilated and hypertrophic cardiomyopathies account for the majority (~80%) of cases and most do not have an identifiable cause. There is considerable phenotypic overlap between the different types of cardiomyopathy, and the clinical presentation is usually congestive cardiac failure. The 5-year mortality or transplant rate for children with dilated cardiomyopathy is 46%, with younger children and those who are sickest at presentation being at highest risk.

Infants present with poor feeding and failure to thrive, along with tachycardia, tachypnoea and sweating. There may be a hyperdynamic precordium and a gallop rhythm. In older children a careful history will often elicit decreased physical activity in comparison to their peers for many months. The clinical

Table 108.5 Causes of heart failure in children

CAUSE	EXAMPLES
BIRTH–2 WEEKS	
Sepsis	Neonatal sepsis, group B *Streptococcus*
Hypoxic ischaemic injury	Birth asphyxia
SVT	Congenital/neonatal
Congenital heart block	Isolated or with structural heart disease
Arteriovenous malformations	Vein of Galen malformation
Duct-dependent systemic circulation	Aortic coarctation or stenosis, HLHS
Persistent pulmonary hypertension of newborn	Secondary to sepsis, hypoxic ischaemic injury etc.
Anaemia	Twin-to-twin transfusion, Rhesus incompatibility
Cardiomyopathy	Infant of diabetic mother, congenital
Neonatal myocarditis	Enterovirus
Cardiac tumour	Rhabdomyoma
2 WEEKS–6 MONTHS	
Large volume left to right shunt lesions	VSD, AVSD, truncus arteriosus, AP window
Cardiomyopathy, myocarditis	
Coronary lesion	ALCAPA
Metabolic	Hypothyroidism
LATER CHILDHOOD	
Unrepaired congenital heart disease Left ventricular failure Right ventricular failure Systemic right ventricular failure	 Left to right shunt lesions Aortic or mitral valve disease Pulmonary or tricuspid valve disease Pulmonary hypertension Congenitally corrected transposition
Operated congenital heart disease Left ventricular failure Right ventricular failure Systemic right ventricular failure Single ventricular failure Arrhythmia	 Residual aortic or mitral valve disease Subaortic stenosis Pulmonary valve disease (repaired TOF) Pulmonary hypertension Post Senning or Mustard Post aortopulmonary shunt, Glenn or Fontan Post Fontan, Senning, Mustard
Cardiomyopathy, myocarditis	
Acquired cardiac disease	Rheumatic heart disease, endocarditis, Marfan syndrome, cor pulmonale
Transplant rejection	

HLHS=hypoplastic left heart syndrome; VSD=ventricular septal defect; AVSD=atrioventricular septal defect; AP=aorto-pulmonary; ALCAPA=anomalous origin of left coronary artery from pulmonary artery; TOF=tetralogy of Fallot.

presentation becomes more like that seen in adults, with hepatomegaly, ascites, oedema and poor peripheral perfusion.

TREATMENT (SEE TABLE 108.4 FOR DRUG DOSES)

There are few data on which to base treatment of heart failure in children. Mainstays of chronic treatment are diuretic therapy and ACE inhibitors, or beta blockers. The sicker child in the ICU will require further measures.

Oxygen

Treat decompensated heart failure with facemask oxygen.

Ventilation
Intubation and positive-pressure ventilation improve gas exchange and reduce work of breathing. Although positive pressure probably has no direct effect on left ventricular contractility, it improves output by reducing left ventricular afterload.[36] High pressures may impair cardiac output by reducing preload and increasing afterload to the right ventricle.

Afterload reduction
Vasodilator therapy is useful as long as an adequate blood pressure can be maintained. Sodium nitroprusside is a potent pure vasodilator. Milrinone has the additional advantage of some inotropic and lusitropic effects.

Inotropes
Dobutamine or milrinone (if vasodilatation is tolerated) can be used as first-line agents. Despite limited data in children, levosimendan is being used increasingly in paediatric heart failure. It appears capable of increasing cardiac output at minimal metabolic cost and is also a potent vasodilator.

Blood transfusion
Correct anaemia. Transfuse packed red blood cells to maintain Hb>10 g/dL.

Cardiac resynchronisation therapy[37,38]
Cardiac resynchronisation has become accepted therapy in subpopulations of adults with cardiomyopathy. In children there is evidence of benefit, but patient selection is made difficult by the heterogeneous nature of the underlying diseases. Dilated cardiomyopathy may respond less well than some types of congenital heart disease.

Mechanical support[39,40]
Veno-arterial ECMO (see Ch. 41) provides excellent short-term mechanical support, but is unsuitable for the longer periods necessary for bridging to transplantation. There are very few ventricular assist devices (VADs) available for support of the smaller child. The Excor Paediatric VAD ('Berlin Heart') is the most widely used of these, with a range of ventricular chambers down to 10 mL. Successful support to transplantation or recovery can be achieved in 70–90% of cases, but there is a high risk of infective, bleeding and thrombotic complications. Larger (>30 kg) children can be supported with smaller continuous flow implantable devices designed for adults, which may carry less risk of complications. Development of miniaturised versions of these devices for children is ongoing but as yet none is ready for clinical use.

AN APPROACH TO CONGENITAL HEART DISEASE

An in-depth discussion of congenital heart disease and its management is beyond the scope of this chapter. What follows is an overview of situations in which the intensivist or emergency physician may encounter congenital heart disease, based loosely on age and mode of presentation.

NEWBORN WITH CYANOSIS[41,42]

Most cyanosed newborns have respiratory disease and this needs to be treated appropriately. Cyanosis in the absence of respiratory distress is likely to be due to congenital heart disease. Cyanotic heart disease is likely if the Pa_{O_2} does not rise to 150 mmHg (≈20 kPa) after the baby has been breathing 100% oxygen for 10 minutes. Presence or absence of a murmur is not particularly helpful; many children with cyanotic heart disease do not have a murmur and murmurs can be heard in many newborn infants. There may be diagnostic clues on examination and chest X-ray, but all such infants need an urgent echocardiogram for definitive diagnosis.

SEVERE CYANOSIS (Sa_{O_2}<70%) (SEE TABLE 108.4 FOR DRUG DOSES)

Table 108.6 shows the features of congenital heart lesions presenting with severe cyanosis at birth. These infants must be treated urgently.

1. Intubate and ventilate to reduce oxygen consumption and treat any respiratory disease. Use a high Fi_{O_2} and avoid high pressures that might increase PVR.
2. Start alprostadil (prostaglandin E_1 (PGE_1), Prostin®) to keep the ductus arteriosus open. There is a risk of exacerbating pulmonary oedema in obstructed total anomalous pulmonary venous drainage (TAPVD), but unless this diagnosis has been made with certainty the ductus should be kept open.
3. Correct metabolic acidosis.
4. Use an inotrope if there is evidence of heart failure (see above).
5. Inhaled nitric oxide may be helpful in persistent pulmonary hypertension of the newborn and severe Ebstein anomaly.
6. Refer for advice and urgent transport to a specialist paediatric cardiac centre. Persistent severe cyanosis may require ECMO support prior to definitive treatment.

LESS SEVERE CYANOSIS (<90%)

Less-profound cyanosis is seen in neonates with transposition of the great arteries (TGA) and adequate mixing, milder forms of pulmonary stenosis (including tetralogy of Fallot) and Ebstein anomaly. There is a degree of cyanosis associated with all defects where there is mixing of pulmonary and systemic venous blood (e.g. unobstructed anomalous pulmonary venous drainage, single ventricle lesions). These infants are less sick and desaturation may be relatively difficult to detect without pulse oximetry. All such children require

Table 108.6 Differential diagnosis of severe cyanosis in the newborn

LESION	PATHOPHYSIOLOGY	CHEST X-RAY	MANAGEMENT
Transposition of great arteries	Pulmonary and systemic circulations in parallel, without mixing	Normal cardiac size Narrow pedicle ('egg on side' appearance) Normal/increased pulmonary vascularity	Alprostadil Balloon atrial septostomy
Pulmonary atresia/critical pulmonary stenosis	No forward flow from right ventricle Intracardiac right to left shunting Pulmonary blood flow via ductus arteriosus	Normal cardiac size Absent pulmonary artery silhouette Reduced pulmonary vascularity	Alprostadil Will need surgery or catheter procedure
Neonatal Ebstein anomaly	Severe tricuspid regurgitation Intracardiac right to left shunting +/− pulmonary valve disease	Massive atrial enlargement Lung fields difficult to see	Alprostadil Inhaled nitric oxide May need surgical procedure
Obstructed TAPVD	Severe pulmonary venous obstruction Pulmonary oedema	Normal cardiac size Diffuse pulmonary interstitial oedema	Cardiac surgical emergency
Persistent pulmonary Hypertension of the newborn	High PVR Right heart failure Right to left shunting through ductus arteriosus	Normal cardiac size and silhouette Reduced pulmonary vascularity	Alprostadil Inhaled nitric oxide Inotropes Look for and treat underlying cause

careful assessment and prompt referral to a paediatric cardiac centre.

NEWBORN WITH CARDIAC FAILURE

In lesions that cause obstruction to the left side of the heart (aortic stenosis, coarctation, hypoplastic left heart syndrome) systemic blood flow is provided by the right ventricle through the ductus arteriosus. Patients may not present until the ductus arteriosus begins to close when systemic blood flow diminishes and the left ventricle fails in the face of greatly increased afterload. There is a rapidly deteriorating clinical picture of pallor, cold peripheries and barely palpable pulses. Tachycardia and tachypnoea are universal and there is progressive hepatomegaly, cardiomegaly and pulmonary oedema. This is accompanied by profound metabolic acidosis and oliguria.

Other conditions presenting with cardiovascular collapse in the first 2 weeks of life are sepsis, inborn errors of metabolism, myocarditis/cardiomyopathy and sustained tachyarrhythmia. These can be difficult to differentiate initially and all neonates presenting in this fashion should be treated with appropriate antibiotics (see Table 108.3) until a definitive diagnosis is made.

TREATMENT (SEE TABLE 108.4 FOR DRUG DOSES)

1. Intubate and ventilate with resuscitation drugs to hand.
2. Sedate and ventilate to reduce oxygen consumption.
3. Start inotropes – dobutamine or epinephrine depending on severity of cardiac dysfunction.
4. Start alprostadil – a high dose (50 ng/kg/min) may be needed to reopen the ductus arteriosus.
5. Refer for advice and urgent transport to a paediatric cardiac centre.

INVESTIGATIONS

- Chest X-ray
- Echocardiogram
- ECG
- Arterial blood gas, electrolytes, renal and hepatic function
- Full blood count and film examination
- Coagulation
- Blood cultures
- Serum amino acids
- Urinary amino and organic acids.

CYANOSIS BEYOND THE NEWBORN PERIOD

Infants and young children with unoperated tetralogy of Fallot may present with episodic profound cyanosis associated with crying and agitation. These 'tet spells' are mostly due to dynamic obstruction of the right ventricular outflow tract with consequent right to left shunting through the VSD. Administration of oxygen and bringing the child's knees up tight to the chest will often terminate the spell (presumably by increasing systemic vascular resistance). Volume expansion may be helpful. If there is persisting cyanosis try sedation with morphine. In very resistant spells either a beta blocker (esmolol) or a peripheral vasoconstrictor (metaraminol) can be used. Inotropes and vasodilators will worsen the cyanosis.

Children with unrepaired or undiagnosed atrial or ventricular septal defects (or residual defects following repair) may become cyanosed under conditions of increased PVR, for example during acute respiratory illness. Cyanosis due to progressive pulmonary vascular disease with unrepaired long-standing left to right shunt (Eisenmenger's complex) is increasingly rare.

Certain operations for congenital heart disease leave patients with obligatory intracardiac mixing, producing cyanosis. Pulse oximetry in these patients will usually be in the range of 70–85% (parents will know their child's usual saturations). These children often have pulmonary blood flow supplied via an aorto-pulmonary shunt (e.g. modified Blalock Taussig ('BT') shunt or central shunt).

Two operations redirect systemic venous return directly to the pulmonary artery, bypassing the heart: the Glenn, or bidirectional cavopulmonary connection (SVC to pulmonary artery) and the Fontan (inferior vena cava (IVC) and SVC to pulmonary artery). Patients with a Glenn remain cyanosed, whereas patients with a Fontan have variable desaturation. In both cases pulmonary blood flow is extremely sensitive to PVR. If these patients require mechanical ventilation it is important to use low pressures and low rates if possible as positive intrathoracic pressure will impair pulmonary blood flow.

EMERGENCIES AND IMPORTANT PRESENTATIONS

Dehydration

Dehydration is particularly dangerous in cyanosed patients. These patients often have a high haematocrit and further haemoconcentration places them at risk of thrombosis. Intravenous rehydration should be aggressively pursued in dehydrated children with cyanotic heart disease.

Profound desaturation

Acute profound desaturation in a patient with shunt-dependent pulmonary blood flow suggests the possibility of shunt blockage and is a life-threatening emergency. Give volume (20 mL/kg 0.9% NaCl) and repeat if necessary. Discuss urgently with a paediatric cardiac centre and consider giving heparin (100 U/kg).

Intercurrent respiratory illness

Respiratory tract infections are common in childhood and these have important effects on children with limited or shunt-dependent pulmonary blood flow (see above). Increased work of breathing and increased PVR will worsen cyanosis. Respiratory failure must be treated on its merits, but the nature of pulmonary blood flow and the potential for increasing PVR must be borne in mind if mechanical ventilation is necessary.

HEART FAILURE BEYOND THE NEWBORN PERIOD[33]

Congenital-heart-disease-related heart failure beyond the newborn period is often due to the consequences of an unrepaired left to right shunt lesion. High pulmonary blood flow places a volume load on the left ventricle. Left ventricular enlargement and increased end-diastolic pressures ensue and the patient presents with tachycardia, tachypnoea, sweating, poor feeding and poor growth. There is often a gallop rhythm and a systolic murmur and peripheral vasoconstriction leads to cool peripheries. These children respond well to diuretics and ACE inhibitors, but may need inotropes and positive-pressure ventilation at presentation. Worsening cardiac failure in the first few months of life is often due to the normal fall in haematocrit at this age and will respond to blood transfusion.[43] These children will need repair of the underlying lesion, but this is rarely urgent.

An important lesion to consider in the infant with previously undiagnosed disease is anomalous origin of the left coronary artery from the pulmonary artery (ALCAPA). These children present with poor growth and episodic inconsolable crying in the first few months of life. There is cardiomegaly and evidence of anterolateral infarction on ECG. Echo confirms markedly diminished ventricular function, ventricular dilation and mitral regurgitation. This lesion warrants rapid surgical repair.

There may be ongoing ventricular dysfunction in repaired or unrepaired congenital heart disease owing to intrinsic ventricular systolic or diastolic function, or left- or right-sided valve disease. Ischaemic cardiomyopathy occurs rarely but can be seen following repair of coronary artery abnormalities or operations involving manipulation or reimplantation of the coronaries, most notably the arterial switch operation.[44]

EMERGENCIES AND IMPORTANT PRESENTATIONS

Intercurrent respiratory illness

Respiratory tract infections will cause an exacerbation of heart failure in children with congenital heart disease. Increased work of breathing and fever are poorly tolerated and often necessitate hospitalisation. This is most commonly seen in infants with unrepaired left to right shunt lesions and viral respiratory tract infections during the winter. It may be difficult to differentiate the effects of the respiratory disease from the heart failure, but initial attention to treatment of respiratory failure must be accompanied by careful assessment of the underlying disease.

DISORDERS OF CARDIAC RHYTHM[45–47] (SEE TABLE 108.4 FOR DRUG DOSES)

SINUS BRADYCARDIA

Sinus bradycardia (see Table 108.2) may appear more dramatic due to the frequent occurrence of sinus arrhythmia in children. Pathological causes of bradycardia include sinus node dysfunction, hypothermia, high intracranial pressure, cervical spinal cord injury, hypothyroidism, drug effects (beta blockers, digoxin, amiodarone, clonidine) and organophosphate poisoning. Sinus bradycardia very rarely needs treatment apart from addressing any underlying cause. Atropine or isoproterenol (isoprenaline) will increase the heart rate if necessary (Table 108.4).

SINUS NODE DYSFUNCTION

Sinus node dysfunction causes bradycardia, sinus pauses, and alternating bradycardia/tachycardia. It is most common following operations for congenital heart disease, particularly those involving extensive atrial surgery, and can occur many years later. Sinus node dysfunction is rare in children with structurally normal hearts and is well tolerated in this group. Emergency treatment involves treatment of bradycardia, if symptomatic, and consideration for pacemaker insertion.

COMPLETE HEART BLOCK

Complete heart block is usually congenital in children, with more than 90% being due to transplacental passage of maternal autoantibodies in autoimmune disease. In later childhood complete heart block is most likely to be associated with recent cardiac surgery or complex forms of congenital heart disease (congenitally corrected TGA, left atrial isomerism), but may also occur with myocarditis, cardiomyopathy, cardiac transplant rejection and some muscular dystrophies.

MANAGEMENT

Atropine will increase the ventricular rate and an infusion of isoproterenol will maintain it pending establishment of temporary or permanent cardiac pacing.

Inotropes should be used in patients with poor ventricular function due to long-standing bradycardia or underlying myocardial disease.

Transvenous temporary pacing is difficult in small children and external cardiac pacing may be necessary as a resuscitative measure.

Asymptomatic patients may still require insertion of a pacemaker, depending on cause, ventricular escape rate and myocardial function.

FIRST-DEGREE HEART BLOCK

A prolonged PR interval (see **Table 108.7**) can be seen in normal children during periods of increased vagal tone. Pathological causes of first-degree block include hypothermia, electrolyte abnormalities, acute rheumatic fever and any of the causes of complete heart block described above.

SECOND-DEGREE HEART BLOCK

Isolated Mobitz type I block (Wenckebach) is usually well tolerated. Mobitz type II is more likely to be symptomatic and require a pacemaker. Either form of second-degree AV block should be investigated for an underlying cause.

TACHYARRHYTHMIAS

Sinus tachycardia (see Table 108.2) is more common than tachyarrhythmia. Underlying causes (fever, pain or agitation, drugs) should be considered and treated.

SUPRAVENTRICULAR TACHYCARDIA (SVT) (SEE CH. 21)

Re-entrant SVT is common in childhood. Most cases occur in the first few months of life in the absence of congenital heart disease. Structural heart disease should be ruled out in all cases, however.

The re-entry circuit usually involves the atrioventricular (AV) node and an accessory conduction pathway. These tachycardias are abrupt in onset and have a relatively fixed rate. In neonates and infants the accessory pathway is discrete from the AV node and may conduct in either direction (accessory-pathway-mediated SVT). In older children and adults the alternative conduction route is often within the AV node itself, with two limbs of the node conducting at different frequencies and with different refractory periods (AV node re-entrant tachycardia).

Diagnosis

The ECG shows a narrow complex (see Table 108.7) tachycardia at greater than 200 beats per minute. P-waves are often difficult to discern, but occur with a 1:1 ratio to the QRS complexes. P-waves are usually inverted, but morphology and position will depend on the nature of the re-entry circuit.

Treatment

If shocked give:

- oxygen by mask, and sedation (midazolam)
- synchronised DC cardioversion (1 J/kg).

Table 108.7 Age-related approximate ECG intervals (and upper limits of normal)[49]

	NEWBORN	6–12 MONTHS	5–8 YEARS	12–16 YEARS
PR interval (ms)	100 (120)	110 (140)	130 (160)	135 (180)
QRS duration (ms)	65 (85)	65 (85)	80 (100)	90 (110)
QTc interval (ms)	420 (450)	410 (450)	410 (445)	410 (450)

All intervals in milliseconds. QTc= corrected QT interval=QT√(heart rate/60).

If stable:

1. *Vagal stimulation:* apply ice water to entire face for <30 seconds, gag, tracheal suction or held inspiration if ventilated. Give carotid sinus massage in older children. Do not apply eyeball pressure.
2. *Adenosine rapid i.v. bolus and flush:* give as centrally as possible. If unresponsive increase the dose (see Table 108.4). Adenosine is painful and causes vasodilatation.
3. *Atrial or transoesophageal overdrive pacing:* may terminate the arrhythmia.
4. *If unsuccessful or the tachycardia reverts after successful termination:* consider amiodarone or digoxin.
5. Do *not* use digoxin or verapamil if there is pre-excitation on the ECG (they both may enhance anterograde conduction in the accessory pathway).
6. Do *not* use verapamil in infants (it can cause shock and cardiac arrest).
7. *Following conversion to sinus rhythm:* check ECG for evidence of pre-excitation and look for structural disease.

Automatic SVTs are caused by an 'ectopic' rapidly firing focus within the atrium or AV conducting tissue. These are unusual in the absence of structural heart disease and are commonly seen following cardiac surgery. Typically there is variability of ventricular rate.

Ectopic atrial tachycardia (EAT) has an abnormal P-wave axis on the ECG with normal conduction to ventricles. Junctional ectopic tachycardia (JET) arises at the AV node or high in the bundle of His. There is complete AV dissociation on the ECG, the ventricular rate being greater than the atrial rate.

Treatment is aimed at reducing automaticity with adequate sedation and analgesia, and avoiding catecholamines and other chronotropes. Keep serum potassium, calcium and magnesium in the high normal range. Whole-body cooling is useful. Amiodarone can be used in resistant postoperative JET.

Atrial fibrillation

Atrial fibrillation is rare in children and is usually associated with cardiomyopathy or previous atrial surgery.

Box 108.2 Causes of ventricular arrhythmias in children

- Congenital heart disease (repaired tetralogy of Fallot, aortic stenosis)
- Cardiomyopathy
- Myocarditis
- Ischaemia (coronary abnormalities, Kawasaki disease)
- Transplant rejection
- Electrolyte abnormalities (hypo/hyperkalaemia, hypocalcaemia)
- Drugs (tricyclic antidepressants)
- Cardiac channelopathies (long QT syndrome, Brugada syndrome)
- Cardiac tumours
- Commotio cordis

Atrial flutter

Atrial flutter is an atrial re-entrant tachycardia. It can occur in newborns in the absence of structural heart disease but is more common in older patients with congenital heart disease, particularly those who have had surgery involving extensive atrial manipulation. Atrial flutter rates in children are faster than adults (>400 per minute in newborns). Diagnosis may be evident from the sawtooth baseline pattern of the ECG, but this may not be revealed until adenosine is given, blocking AV conduction.

Treat shocked patients as described above for SVT.

In the stable patient, atrial or transoesophageal overdrive pacing may terminate the arrhythmia.

VENTRICULAR ARRHYTHMIAS

Isolated premature ventricular contractions are common in infants and children with normal hearts. Ventricular arrhythmias are very rare in children (most cases of paediatric cardiac arrest present with severe bradycardia or asystole). Documented ventricular fibrillation or ventricular tachycardia must prompt an exhaustive search for an underlying cause (**Box 108.2**).

Emergency treatment of ventricular arrhythmias is described in Chapter 113.

Access the complete references list online at http://www.expertconsult.com

4. Price JF. Unique aspects of heart failure in the neonate. In: Shaddy RE, editor. Heart Failure in Congenital Heart Disease. London: Springer; 2011. p. 21–42.
8. Wynn J, Cornell TT, Wong HR, et al. The host response to sepsis and developmental impact. pediatrics 2010;125(5):1031–41.
13. Brierley J, Carcillo JA, Choong K, et al. Clinical practice parameters for hemodynamic support of pediatric and neonatal septic shock: 2007 update from the American College of Critical Care Medicine. Crit Care Med 2009;37(2):666–88.
31. Hsu DT, Pearson GD. Heart failure in children. Circulation: Heart Failure 2009;2(5):490–8.
32. Hsu DT, Pearson GD. Heart failure in children. Circulation: Heart Failure 2009;2(1):63–70.
41. Silberbach M, Hannon D. Presentation of congenital heart disease in the neonate and young infant. Pediatr Rev 2007;28(4):123–31.

109

Neurological emergencies in children

Anthony J Slater

Neurological emergencies are the most common life-threatening emergencies in children. In developed societies, after the first year of life, the leading cause of death in childhood is injury, particularly traumatic brain injury. There is a range of conditions affecting the brain, spinal cord and peripheral nervous system that require prompt recognition, resuscitation and definitive management. The pathophysiology, clinical features, treatment and outcome of these acute neurological emergencies are influenced by several important differences between adults and children. These differences include response to injury, developmental maturity and capacity for growth and recovery.

PATHOPHYSIOLOGY OF BRAIN INJURIES IN CHILDREN

Brain injuries are usually caused by a primary event (e.g. trauma, ischaemia, infection or metabolic disturbance) and are frequently accompanied by secondary injuries including oedema, altered cerebrovascular autoregulation, tissue hypoxia or other cytotoxic events. Therapy administered after the event will not influence the outcome of the primary injury, however, appropriate resuscitation, treatment and the avoidance of iatrogenic complications may prevent or reduce the impact of secondary injuries.

Features of brain injury particular to the paediatric patient are described below.

DIFFUSE CEREBRAL SWELLING

Diffuse brain swelling in the absence of oedema is a frequent early finding in paediatric brain injury, and is due to generalised cerebral vasodilation. It often resolves in 1–2 days if there is no other significant brain injury. With more severe primary traumatic injury diffuse cerebral swelling may be accompanied by areas of contusion, multifocal petechial haemorrhage, and vasogenic oedema that progress over several days.

CEREBRAL BLOOD FLOW AND METABOLISM

The cerebral perfusion pressure (CPP) represents the difference between mean arterial pressure (MAP) and intracranial pressure (ICP):

$$CPP = MAP - ICP$$

If autoregulation is disturbed as part of the illness, CPP becomes the major determinant of cerebral blood flow, particularly in areas with more severe damage. The ideal CPP in childhood is not known. The normal range of MAP varies with age from 40 mmHg (5.32 kPa) in a term neonate to 80 mmHg (10.64 kPa) in an adolescent. The target CPP is usually adjusted with age, taking into consideration the normal blood pressure for age. For example, for an adolescent patient the therapy may be directed at maintaining a CPP of 60 mmHg (7.98 kPa), whereas for a child aged 5 years the aim may be to maintain a CPP of 50 mmHg (6.65 kPa).

In conditions where vasogenic oedema occurs, arterial hypertension may increase vascular shift of fluid and worsen brain swelling. However, treatment aimed at lowering arterial pressure (e.g. with vasodilators) may interfere with homeostatic mechanisms and should be used cautiously.

The brain comprises 12% of body weight in infancy compared with 2–3% in adulthood. Cerebral oxygen and glucose consumption are therefore proportionately greater in childhood and glycogen stores are readily depleted. Hypoglycaemia occurs commonly in severe illnesses such as sepsis; therefore blood glucose should be monitored regularly.

HYPOVOLAEMIA

Children have small blood volumes and commonly develop hypovolaemia from scalp bleeding or intracranial haemorrhage. For example, hypovolaemia will develop in a 5 kg infant (blood volume 400 mL) following blood loss of less than 100 mL. Hypovolaemia should be treated aggressively with fluid boluses of 20 mL/kg to ensure adequate cerebral perfusion.

RELATIVE GROWTH

The child's short stature and proportionately large head confer a number of risks. The toddler's head is at the level of the front of a motor vehicle and isolated head injury is therefore common following pedestrian injury in this age group. The neck muscles are relatively weak in infancy and they support a large head. This renders the brain prone to deceleration injury in motor vehicle crashes and in cases of domestic violence. Injury inflicted by shaking an infant by the shoulders snaps the head to and fro leading to compression of brain tissue and rupture of delicate bridging veins.

BONE DEVELOPMENT

The skull bones in the first year of life are thin with open sutures and open fontanelles. Beyond 2 years, the skull sutures close and the cranial vault thickens. In young children there tends to be less bony protection from high-impact trauma, although the non-rigid skull may expand to partially decompress expanding lesions.[1]

UNDIAGNOSED COMA

An ordered approach to diagnosis and treatment is required for a child with depressed conscious state of unknown origin. This approach must consider common life-threatening and rare treatable diseases (**Box 109.1**).

INITIAL MANAGEMENT

Management should always begin with rapid assessment of the adequacy of airway, ventilation and circulation. If inadequacies are detected, interventions aimed at correcting them should occur immediately. Once venous access is obtained, blood should be collected for routine tests including immediate measurement of blood glucose. If hypoglycaemia is demonstrated 1–2 mL/kg of 25% glucose or 2.5–5 mL/kg of 10% glucose should be given intravenously as the neurological sequelae of unrecognised hypoglycaemia can be profound.

Box 109.1 Causes of trauma in children

Structural	Metabolic
Trauma	Post-ictal state
Accidental	Infection
Inflicted	Meningitis
Hydrocephalus	Encephalitis
Haemorrhage	Acute disseminated encephalomyelitis
AVM	Drugs and toxins
Aneurysm	Hypoxia–ischaemia
Tumour	Circulatory shock
Tumour	Biochemical
Cerebral abscess	Hypoglycaemia
	Sodium and/or water disorder
	Calcium disorder
	Acid–base disorder
	Hyperthermia
	Hepatic failure
	Haemolytic–uraemic syndrome
	Inborn errors of metabolism

Concurrent with the initial assessment and resuscitation, relevant details of the present and past history should be obtained. A detailed neurological and general physical examination should be performed. It is important to document accurately the conscious state so that changes over time, particularly deterioration, can be easily recognised. The Glasgow Coma Scale (GCS) is appropriate for this purpose; the responses of children change with development and therefore the GCS requires modification for paediatric use (**Table 109.1**). After completing the clinical assessment, the likely diagnosis is often apparent and appropriate investigation and treatment can commence. Multiple factors may compound to produce coma. For example, a child with severe gastroenteritis may have hyperthermia, hyponatraemic dehydration, metabolic acidosis and hypovolaemic shock.

CONTROLLED VENTILATION

Indications for ventilating a comatose child are:

- upper airway obstruction or loss of airway reflexes
- apnoea or respiratory failure
- rapidly worsening coma
- signs of progressive elevation of ICP (i.e. bradycardia, hypertension, abnormal pupillary light reflexes and localising signs).

Once ventilation is initiated the stomach should be drained with a gastric tube and blood pressure checked every 5 minutes. Raised ICP should be considered in any case of rapidly progressive coma. If critical intracranial hypertension is suspected clinically, management should include moderate hyperventilation and intravenous mannitol (0.25 g/kg). Hypertonic saline given as 3 mL/kg of 3% solution (0.5 mmol/mL) can also rapidly reduce ICP.[2] Once stability is achieved then adequate sedation and analgesia are required. Muscle relaxants may be necessary to facilitate ventilation and prevent straining; however, their use precludes further neurological assessment and therefore, if long-acting muscle relaxants are continued, ICP monitoring is advisable. Hyperventilation is a short-term manoeuvre and, if used during the early resuscitation phase, a gradual return to a low–normal Pa_{CO_2} should be the aim. This is best achieved with end-tidal CO_2 and ICP monitoring. Particular attention should be paid to restoring intravascular volume and maintaining an adequate CPP.

CRANIAL COMPUTERISED TOMOGRAPHY

A CT scan is required in comatose children with localising signs and in those in whom the diagnosis is not clear. A CT should also be performed if the conscious state is abnormal and there is history of trauma. Even if the general condition doesn't warrant controlled ventilation, a CT is often best performed under general

Table 109.1 Glasgow Coma Scale for children

GLASGOW COMA SCALE (4–15 YEARS)		CHILD'S GLASGOW COMA SCALE (<4 YEARS)	
RESPONSE	*SCORE*	*RESPONSE*	*SCORE*
EYE OPENING		EYE OPENING	
Spontaneously	4	Spontaneously	4
To verbal stimuli	3	To verbal stimuli	3
To pain	2	To pain	2
No response to pain	1	No response to pain	1
BEST MOTOR RESPONSE		BEST MOTOR RESPONSE	
Obeys verbal command	6	Spontaneous or obeys verbal command	6
Localises to pain	5	Localises to pain or withdraws to touch	5
Withdraws from pain	4	Withdraws from pain	4
Abnormal flexion to pain (decorticate)	3	Abnormal flexion to pain (decorticate)	3
Abnormal extension to pain (decerebrate)	2	Abnormal extension to pain (decerebrate)	2
No response to pain	1	No response to pain	1
BEST VERBAL RESPONSE		BEST VERBAL RESPONSE	
Orientated and converses	5	Alert, babbles, coos, words to usual ability	5
Disorientated and converses	4	Less than usual words, spontaneous irritable cry	4
Inappropriate words	3	Cries only to pain	3
Incomprehensible sounds	2	Moans to pain	2
No response to pain	1	No response to pain	1

anaesthesia. Unwanted movement will cause poor-quality images and sedation alone may place the child at risk of hypoventilation or aspiration.

LUMBAR PUNCTURE

Lumbar puncture (LP) should be performed when there is reasonable suspicion of meningitis or encephalitis. The risks and contraindications to LP are discussed under bacterial meningitis.

ADDITIONAL INVESTIGATIONS

Additional investigations include arterial blood gas analysis, serum electrolytes, glucose, urea and creatinine, liver function tests, serum ammonia, serum and CSF lactate and pyruvate and urine analysis. Appropriate screening of blood and urine will exclude common poisons and drug intoxications.

SPECIFIC TREATMENT

The clinical signs and results of investigations generally guide treatment. If hypoglycaemia occurs, it should be corrected rapidly and care should be taken to ensure that it does not recur by the administration of appropriate glucose-containing i.v. fluid and regular blood glucose monitoring. Herpes simplex encephalitis can present in many ways and is not excluded by the absence of CSF pleocytosis. Acyclovir therapy should therefore be considered in any patient in whom herpes cannot be confidently excluded.

STATUS EPILEPTICUS

Convulsive status epilepticus (CSE) is usually defined as a continuous convulsion lasting 30 minutes or longer or repeated convulsions lasting 30 minutes or longer without recovery of consciousness between convulsions.[3] As 30 minutes is generally considered too long to wait before starting treatment, an alternative 'operational definition' of a seizure lasting more than 5 minutes has been proposed for adults and older children (>5 years old). It is acknowledged that the biology and clinical features of CSE in young children differ from that in adults.[4] The common causes of CSE in children are:

- prolonged febrile convulsion
- epilepsy associated with the first presentation, anticonvulsant withdrawal or intercurrent illness
- central nervous system infection (e.g. meningitis or encephalitis)
- metabolic disturbance (e.g. hypoglycaemia, hyponatraemia, hypocalcaemia)
- trauma, including inflicted injury.

PATHOPHYSIOLOGY

Many physiological changes occur during prolonged seizures. There is an initial phase of compensation lasting less than 30 minutes. Following a period of transition there is a phase of decompensation commencing between 30 and 60 minutes and evolving over hours. Physiological changes during the compensated phase include tachycardia, hypertension, increased catecholamine release and increased cardiac output. Changes within the brain include increased cerebral blood flow and increased cerebral utilisation of glucose and oxygen. After 30–60 minutes the mechanisms for homeostatic compensation fail. During the decompensated phase there may be falling blood pressure and cardiac output, hypoglycaemia, hypoxia, acidosis, electrolyte disturbance, and rhabdomyolysis. The cerebral physiology is characterised by failing autoregulation and reduced cerebral blood flow and oxygen and glucose utilisation. Over hours a deficit in brain energy develops and this is associated with the development of brain damage.[5]

EXCITATORY AMINO ACIDS AND BRAIN INJURY

Mesial temporal sclerosis is the most common acquired brain lesion following CSE. There is evidence that the accumulation of a number of excitatory and inhibitory amino acids has a role in the pathophysiology of neuronal injury. In particular, glutamate accumulation and stimulation of NMDA receptors lead to an influx of intracellular calcium, which triggers a number of cytotoxic events and ultimately cell death.[6]

MANAGEMENT

The initial management is as for other neurological emergencies with attention to airway and oxygenation. Most seizures in childhood cease spontaneously in a short time, but if they persist after presentation to an emergency department they should be stopped to avoid metabolic and ischaemic neuronal damage. Hypoglycaemia should be excluded or detected early.

FIRST-LINE THERAPY

Benzodiazepines remain the first-line antiepileptic drug (AED) for stopping seizures and should be administered for seizures that do not stop spontaneously within 5 minutes. The efficacy of benzodiazepines is reduced if administration is delayed.[7] Therefore there is strong argument for first-line therapy to be administered prehospital either by the parents, care providers, or paramedics.[8] Intravenous access is unlikely in the community; however, midazolam can be administered via the buccal, intranasal, or intramuscular route. Buccal midazolam is more effective, easier and more socially acceptable to administer then rectal diazepam.[9-11] Once intravenous access is available lorazepam is usually considered the drug of choice as, compared with diazepam, it is at least as effective, safer and has a longer duration of action.[12-14] If a seizure has not responded to two doses of benzodiazepine, a second-line AED should be administered. If a benzodiazepine has been administered pre-hospital then only one further dose should be administered in the emergency department.

SECOND-LINE THERAPY

Phenytoin is the second-line AED of choice in most situations. It is given as 20 mg/kg i.v. over 30 minutes, which is followed by maintenance dosing (4–8 mg/kg/day in 2-3 doses). It causes minimal sedation or respiratory depression, but is not suitable in neonates and in patients who are already on maintenance doses. Fosphenytoin, a prodrug of phenytoin, can be administered intramuscularly and has less irritant effect when given i.v.[15] Its place in the management of CSE in children is not yet clear. When phenytoin is contraindicated, phenobarbitone (20 mg/kg i.v. over 30 minutes) should be given. Respiratory depression and hypotension occur, particularly after benzodiazepines. Further doses can be safely administered to ventilated children who have ongoing seizures.

THIRD-LINE THERAPY

Levetiracetam is effective against a broad range of seizure types and can be administered enterally or intravenously. Case series have described the use of intravenous levetiracetam (20–60 mg/kg over 5–15 minutes) in children with CSE. These reports suggest that the drug is safe and effective either as a single agent or in combination with other AEDs.[16] Valproate is commonly used for maintenance therapy in epilepsy. There are several reports of successfully using intravenous valproate to abort CSE in children. The doses reported range from 20 to 40 mg/kg. The rate of infusion reported also varies from 5 to 30 minutes.[17] Valproate can rarely cause encephalopathy or hepatotoxicity. Therefore levetiracetam may have a safety advantage over valproate as a third-line agent for CSE. In many centres rectal paraldehyde (0.3 mL/kg, max 5 mL, mixed with an equal quantity of olive oil) is frequently used in the management of CSE. One advantage of paraldehyde is that, like diazepam, it can be administered rectally if i.v. access is difficult to obtain.

FOURTH-LINE THERAPY

If CSE continues for longer than 30–60 minutes despite the administration of two or at most three different AEDs, induction of intravenous anaesthesia should occur followed by intubation and ventilation and admission to intensive care. Thiopentone 2–5 mg/kg slowly i.v. then 1–5 mg/kg per hour by continuous infusion into a central vein can be given. Thiopentone necessitates endotracheal intubation and mechanical ventilation, and possibly inotropic drugs to counter its myocardial depressant effects. Blood concentrations need to be monitored during prolonged use. Seizures are only controlled by anaesthetic doses of thiopentone. Midazolam infusion has been used as an alternative to thiopentone. After a bolus of 0.2 mg/kg (maximum 10 mg) an infusion is commenced at 0.1 mg/kg per hour. If seizures continue or recur the bolus dose is repeated and the infusion increased up to 1 mg/kg per hour if tolerated, although even higher doses have been reported.[18-20] When muscle relaxants are used to facilitate intubation, they should be short-acting to ensure ongoing seizure activity is not masked.

The patient must be protected from self-injury during seizures. Severe respiratory and metabolic acidosis are common and are best managed by rapid control of the seizure and maintenance of adequate ventilation and oxygenation. Once seizures are controlled, the cause should be sought. A detailed history is invaluable. A CT scan should reveal structural lesions. An LP should be deferred if the child is unconscious after a seizure. However, if the conscious state improves and there are no signs of raised intracranial pressure (see below) an LP will confirm or exclude meningitis. When the diagnosis remains unclear, viral encephalitis (e.g. herpes simplex or enterovirus), metabolic encephalopathy, poisoning and inflicted injury should be considered.

OUTCOME

The outcome of CSE is dependent on the aetiology. Neurologically normal children in whom CSE is precipitated by fever are considered to have a good prognosis with mortality reported between 0 and 2%.[21] The incidence of neurological deficits or cognitive impairment in this group is also very low. In acute symptomatic CSE (where CSE is a symptom of an acute neurological process such as infection, or trauma) mortality is 12–16% and the incidence of new neurological dysfunction is more than 20%.[21] In this setting, however, it is very difficult to tease out the extent to which prolonged seizures contribute to neurological sequelae.

BACTERIAL MENINGITIS

PATHOPHYSIOLOGY

Bacterial meningitis (BM) usually occurs following haematogenous spread of organisms carried in the nasopharynx. In childhood the common bacteria causing BM are *Streptococcus pneumoniae*, *Neisseria meningitidis* and *Haemophilus influenzae* type b (Hib). Group B *Streptococcus*, *Escherichia coli* and *Listeria monocytogenes* are the most common causative organisms of neonatal BM. Occasionally, meningitis occurs as a complication of other pathology such as base of skull fracture, chronic middle ear infection, or infection of a congenital dermoid sinus.

In the early stages of the disease cerebral hyperaemia occurs. This can be followed by cerebral ischaemia, which may occur by several different mechanisms. Local vasculitis of vessels traversing the subarachnoid space can progress to arterial thrombosis and focal infarction. Other vascular abnormalities including vasospasm and sagittal sinus thrombosis can also occur. Cerebral oedema is relatively common in meningitis and is caused by a combination of vasogenic, cytotoxic and hydrostatic factors. If cerebral oedema is severe then raised ICP and impaired cerebral perfusion can occur leading to global cerebral ischaemia.

CLINICAL FEATURES

In children the typical features of BM are fever, headache, photophobia, neck stiffness and vomiting. The history may extend over several days; however, in fulminant cases the time from first symptom to coma and death may only be a few hours. Neonates and young infants do not present with the typical localised symptoms and signs. Instead, they present with generalised signs of illness including lethargy, poor feeding and pallor. Generalised or focal convulsions or apnoea may be present at presentation. Tuberculous meningitis usually presents with a more insidious onset of symptoms and may be associated with focal neurological signs.

Complications occur commonly in BM. During the early phase, meningitis may be associated with septic shock and disseminated intravascular coagulation (DIC). Fluid and electrolyte abnormalities are relatively common, particularly hyponatraemia and hypoglycaemia. Focal and generalised convulsions are also relatively common and may progress to status epilepticus. During the recovery phase subdural effusions or hydrocephalus may occur.

INVESTIGATIONS

Lumbar puncture (LP) for CSF microscopy, culture and polymerase chain reaction (PCR) testing is required for definitive diagnosis of BM and to guide antibiotic therapy. Although a lumbar puncture can be performed safely in the majority of children with BM, LP may precipitate brainstem herniation if raised intracranial pressure (ICP) is present.[22] Identifying children at risk of this complication is difficult; however, it is generally recommended that empirical antibiotic therapy be commenced and LP deferred if any of the following clinical features are present: depressed conscious state, decorticate or decerebrate posturing, focal neurological signs or other signs of raised ICP. A normal CT scan does not exclude the possibility of elevated ICP.[22] Therefore the decision to defer an LP should be based on clinical rather than radiological signs. In addition to signs of increased intracranial pressure, other indications for deferring the LP include cardiorespiratory instability and severe coagulopathy.

If LP is deferred then alternative methods of establishing a bacterial diagnosis include blood culture and bacterial antigen testing in urine and PCR testing of blood.[23,24]

MANAGEMENT

RESUSCITATION

Severely ill patients require rapid resuscitation. Comatose patients require intubation and ventilation to prevent airway obstruction and hypoventilation. Hypovolaemia should be treated rapidly with boluses of fluid. Patients with septic shock will also require inotropic support.

Cerebral resuscitation

General principles of supporting brain injury apply to BM. These include optimising cerebral oxygen delivery, controlling intracranial pressure and preventing cerebral metabolic stress. The role of ICP monitoring is controversial. There is some anecdotal evidence to support the use of ICP monitoring in a small number of selected cases. Unfortunately, there are no large studies that assess the benefit or harm of ICP monitoring and ICP-targeted therapy in BM.

ANTIBIOTIC THERAPY

Empirical broad-spectrum antibiotics should be selected based on likely pathogens and local resistance patterns. A common protocol for BM is to use ampicillin plus cefotaxime for the 3 months of life and to use a third-generation cephalosporin (cefotaxime or ceftriaxone) after the first month.[25–26] In regions where penicillin- and cephalosporin-resistant *Pneumococcus* occurs, vancomycin should be added to the initial empirical antibiotics until the causative organism is identified and the antibiotic sensitivities are known. When cephalosporin-resistant *Pneumococcus* are found to be the causative organism in meningitis, both a third-generation cephalosporin and vancomycin should be continued as vancomycin penetrates into CSF poorly and therefore should not be used as a single agent. The addition of rifampicin should be considered.[27]

ADJUVANT THERAPY

If dexamethasone is used as adjuvant therapy it should be used only for children over 3 months of age and ideally be given before the first dose of antibiotics and continued for 48 hours (0.4 mg/kg 12-hourly).[28] There is evidence that dexamethasone reduces the incidence of neurological sequelae and sensorineural deafness; however, the beneficial effects are greatest in Hib meningitis (*Haemophilus influenzae*).[29,30] With immunisation, changing epidemiology and the emergence of antibiotic-resistant pneumococcal strains, it is possible that the relationship between risk and benefit of dexamethasone therapy has changed. However, current recommendations support the use of dexamethasone for children greater than 3 months of age with bacterial meningitis.[26,27,31] Oral glycerol also has promise as an adjuvant agent. One recent large randomised controlled trial demonstrated that oral glycerol administration, with or without dexamethasone, was associated with reduced neurological sequelae compared with placebo.[32]

FLUID THERAPY

There is consensus that hypovolaemia should be treated rapidly and aggressively; however, fluid therapy after the initial resuscitation is controversial. It is important to consider the tonicity of i.v. fluids as well as the rate of fluid administration. Hypotonic fluids should not be administered in BM owing to the risk of hyponatraemia and cerebral oedema.[33,34] Hyponatraemia is often attributed to the syndrome of inappropriate antidiuretic hormone secretion and therefore fluid restriction is logical. There is evidence, however, that ADH is *appropriately* elevated in response to hypovolaemia[35] and that hyponatraemic patients with BM tend to be more dehydrated than normonatraemic patients.[36] Compared with fluid restriction, fluid therapy aimed at providing maintenance plus correcting the fluid deficit has been reported to result in a more rapid correction of sodium and ADH[35,37] and has also been associated with reduced short-term morbidity and neurological sequelae at follow-up.[38] The trials of fluid therapy in BM have all been undertaken in low-income countries where delayed presentation is common. The effect of fluid therapy on the outcome of BM in populations where children present early and mortality is low is unknown.

OUTCOME

Bacterial meningitis is associated with significant mortality and morbidity. Overall mortality for BM in childhood is 5–10%; however, in children requiring mechanical ventilation, a mortality rate of 30% has been reported with major neurological sequelae occurring in 33% of survivors.[39]

ENCEPHALITIS

Common causes of encephalitis include enteroviruses, mycoplasma, cytomegalovirus, herpes, Epstein–Barr and respiratory viruses (adenovirus and parainfluenzae). The most significant causes worldwide are the insect-transmitted arbovirus encephalitides including Australian (Ross and Murray Valley), Japanese B and St Louis. These can cause profound coma and are associated with significant incidence of residual neurological deficit.

Presenting symptoms of encephalitis include seizures, focal neurological deficits in the setting of an acute febrile illness, confusion and coma. Meningeal irritation may not be obvious. CSF analysis may show a pleocytosis and in the early phase this can consist predominantly of neutrophils. As mentioned, herpes is the most important diagnosis to make, because it is treatable. Electroencephalography (EEG), CT and magnetic resonance imaging (MRI) are helpful in making the diagnosis. MRI is more sensitive than CT for detecting signs of encephalitis, particularly during the early stages of the illness. PCR on CSF may also aid rapid diagnosis.[40,41] Acyclovir if used early improves outcome and should be commenced when the diagnosis is suspected.

The enteroviruses are important causes of encephalitis in children. In addition they cause other acute neurological illnesses including acute flaccid paralysis due to transverse myelitis and Guillain–Barré syndrome.[42] Pleconaril is a promising new antiviral agent that appears to have clinical benefit in enteroviral infections, including CNS disease.[43] Outcome of viral encephalitis is worse in infancy than in older age groups.[44]

NON-TRAUMATIC INTRACRANIAL HAEMORRHAGE

Non-traumatic intracranial haemorrhage (ICH) is uncommon in children. Arteriovenous malformations (AVM) are a more common cause of haemorrhage in children than aneurysms[45] (**Box 109.2**). The presenting features are similar to those seen in adults, and include sudden severe headache, altered conscious state and seizures. Diagnosis can usually be made by CT scan. Raised ICP, if present, is managed in the usual manner. A mass lesion or acute obstructive hydrocephalus requires neurosurgical assessment. Following diagnosis of ICH, further investigations may be required to clarify the underlying cause. These include coagulation profile and platelet count. Angiographic images can be obtained with CT, magnetic resonance (MRA) or digital subtraction. In some cases definitive cerebral angiography may be required to define the underlying vascular malformation or tumour. Definitive surgery or endovascular treatment of an AVM can be planned once the underlying lesion has been defined. A period of close observation is required as children may be at greater risk of rebleeding from an AVM than adults. The efficacy of therapies (e.g. calcium channel blockers) used to prevent vasospasm in adults has not been studied in children with aneurysmal haemorrhage. Sequelae of ICH include hemiparesis, aphasia, seizures and hydrocephalus.

HYPOXIC–ISCHAEMIC ENCEPHALOPATHY

AETIOLOGY

The most common causes of hypoxic–ischaemic encephalopathy outside the neonatal period are:

- near-miss sudden infant death syndrome
- immersion
- accidents, including drug ingestion and strangulation
- inflicted injury.

Box 109.2 Aetiology of spontaneous intracranial haemorrhage in children

- Vascular malformations
  - Arteriovenous malformation
  - Capillary telangiectasia
  - Cavernous malformation
  - Venous malformation
- Aneurysm
  - 'Berry'
  - Mycotic
  - Post-traumatic
- Coagulopathy
  - Thrombocytopenia
  - Haemophilia
  - Anticoagulant therapy
- Tumours
  - Gliomas
- Hypertension

PATHOLOGY

The brain depends on an uninterrupted supply of oxygen and glucose to produce, via aerobic glycolysis, sufficient high-energy adenosine triphosphate (ATP) to maintain neuronal membrane and synthetic function. Under anoxic conditions anaerobic glycolysis occurs, which produces lactic acid but less ATP (by 18 times). As there are virtually no stores of ATP, rapid neuronal failure ensues. If ischaemia accompanies hypoxia, there is associated failure of both substrate delivery and metabolic waste removal, which amplifies the cellular insult. Ischaemia produces coma in less than 10 seconds and cerebral damage in as little as 2 minutes.

Following restoration of cerebral blood flow there is a period of relative hyperaemia followed by relative hypoperfusion. Cytotoxic cerebral oedema may subsequently develop, but significant elevation of ICP is unusual unless ischaemia and damage are profound.

MANAGEMENT

The principles of therapy are similar to those for other brain injuries. It is mandatory to provide rapid cardiopulmonary resuscitation and prevent secondary insults. In cases of out-of-hospital cardiac arrest, full resuscitation must be attempted while the history is sought. Post-resuscitation care is important for optimising outcome. Comatose patients with hyper- or hypotonia and a Glasgow Coma Scale (GCS) score <8 are probably best managed by mechanical ventilation and sedation for at least 1–2 days, although benefits are not proven. Ventilation should be targeted at normocapnoea, and hyperventilation avoided owing to the risk of further cerebral ischaemia.[46] Haemodynamic disturbance may develop because of primary cardiac dysfunction or hypovolaemia secondary to fluid loss from capillary leak syndrome. Circulating volume should be restored and inotropic agents considered so as to improve the state of the circulation. The dose and choice of vasoactive agent should be individualised based on haemodynamic monitoring.

Following cardiac arrest children are usually hypothermic. Fever commonly develops during the subsequent hours and is associated with worse outcome.[47] Therefore fever should be anticipated and prevented. Further to preventing fever, there is evidence that therapeutic hypothermia of 32–34°C improves outcome. There are trials in adults following cardiac arrest[48,49] and trials in newborns following birth asphyxia[50,51] demonstrating improved neurological outcome if hypothermia is used for between 12 and 72 hours. Although there are no paediatric trials, therapeutic hypothermia should be considered as a treatment option in children who are comatose following hypoxic ischaemic events. Hyperglycaemia has been associated with a worse prognosis and, although it may simply be a marker of injury severity, active treatment has been advocated. The role of ICP measurement is limited as intracranial hypertension usually occurs only in the setting of severe injury and poor outcome.[52]

PROGNOSIS

The major determinants of recovery are ischaemic time, cerebral metabolic rate and quality of resuscitation. In immersion injuries in young children, full recovery may be possible despite prolonged ischaemia if sufficient rapid cerebral cooling has occurred. In these cases the onset of ischaemia may be delayed by bradycardia with preferential cerebral flow (the 'diving reflex'). In general, survival from out-of-hospital cardiac arrest is unlikely, even with expert CPR, if asystole is present on arrival at hospital.[53] The rare exception is the hypothermic child who presents following immersion; prolonged CPR may be justified in selected cases when profound hypothermia was induced rapidly. If cardiac output is present on arrival at hospital, with either flexion or extension to pain, recovery is likely. Normothermic patients, who present apnoeic, flaccid and unresponsive to pain, are likely to die or have serious neurological deficits. This group is also prone to further deterioration several days after the insult, with progression of cerebral oedema. Coma persisting for more than 24 hours is a predictor of poor prognosis and minimal long-term improvement is likely in this group.[54] Residual neurological deficits present at the end of the first week are less likely to improve following ischaemic injury than following traumatic brain injury.

A number of ancillary tests have been investigated as predictors of neurological outcome. Somatosensory evoked potentials (SEPs) performed at the bedside are the most useful aid to prediction. One report of 109 children with severe brain injury concluded that, with appropriate patient selection, the positive predictive value for poor outcome of bilaterally absent SEPs is 100% (95% CI 92–100%).[55]

GUILLAIN–BARRÉ SYNDROME

CLINICAL FEATURES

Guillain–Barré syndrome (GBS) is characterised by acute areflexic paralysis with raised CSF protein and normal CSF cell counts. It is the most common cause of acute motor paralysis in children. There is strong evidence to support an autoimmune cause with many patients having raised anti-ganglioside antibodies. Many cases are preceded by symptoms of upper respiratory tract infection or diarrhoea. Infectious agents associated with subsequent development of GBS include *Campylobacter jejuni*, cytomegalovirus, Epstein–Barr virus, varicella zoster virus and *Mycoplasma pneumoniae*. The syndrome includes a number of peripheral nerve disorders that have been classified based on the distribution of weakness, antibody profiles and nerve conduction studies.[56]

Although most patients develop typical ascending, symmetrical areflexic weakness, GBS may present insidiously with apparent lethargy or loss of motor milestones in the young child. There may also be rapid progression and admission criteria to the ICU include respiratory failure, bulbar palsy, severe autonomic disturbance, or rapidly progressive weakness. Sensory loss is usually minimal and transient. Pain in the back and legs, possibly neurogenic in origin, is common and may be the presenting feature.[57] This pain may be severe and is often difficult to control. Papilloedema and encephalopathy occasionally occur.[58] The complications of deep-venous thrombosis and thromboembolism are not common problems in young children but may occur in adolescents.

INVESTIGATIONS

A lumbar puncture (LP) should be done ideally before treatment with intravenous immunoglobulin (IVIG) is commenced. CSF typically shows a WCC $<10\times10^6$, while CSF protein is usually raised but may be normal during the first week of illness. Nerve conduction studies may be normal if performed early. Neurophysiological criteria have been used to classify GBS subtypes according to either demyelinating or axonal neuropathies and whether or not both sensory and motor nerves are involved.[59] Anti-ganglioside antibodies are raised in some but not all patients.[60]

If there is uncertainty about the clinical diagnosis then brain and spinal cord imaging, as well as screening for infection, should be considered. Contrast-enhanced spinal MRI demonstrates contrast enhancement of spinal nerve roots and the cauda equina in most patients with GBS.[61,62]

MANAGEMENT

Adequate respiratory care is the basis of minimising morbidity and mortality in GBS. Up to one-third of patients require ventilatory support and, ideally, mechanical ventilation should be undertaken electively. Early indications are increased work of breathing, fatigue, poor cough, and progressive bulbar palsy. Hypercarbia is a late sign and should be avoided. In children who are old enough to cooperate, forced vital capacity (FVC) should be monitored during the progressive phase of the illness. Mechanical ventilation should be considered if FVC falls below 15–20 mL/kg. Careful frequent clinical assessment is necessary. Once mechanically ventilated, many patients require some degree of hyperventilation to prevent 'air hunger'. Although nasotracheal intubation is satisfactory initially, a tracheostomy should be performed if recovery is delayed. This will improve comfort and allow speech via the ventilator generating an air leak around the tracheostomy tube. Successful weaning is unlikely unless vital capacity exceeds 12 mL/kg and maximum negative inspiratory force is at least 20 cm H_2O (2 kPa).

Autonomic dysfunction is an important cause of morbidity and mortality in children with GBS. Airway manipulation or induction of anaesthesia, particularly in the presence of hypoxia, may provoke serious cardiac arrhythmias. Fluctuating blood pressure, urinary retention and gut dysfunction also occur.

Plasma exchange (PE) and intravenous immunoglobulin (IVIG) are effective therapies. The indications for either are rapid progression, respiratory insufficiency or weakness to the point of being unable to walk unassisted. The strongest evidence for these therapies is from adult trials.[63–65] Large trials adequately powered to separately test the efficacy of PE and IVIG in children have not been performed; however, a number of small retrospective studies have described local experiences with these immune therapies in children with mixed results.[66–70] As IVIG has significant potential technical advantages over PE, IVIG is generally the first-line therapy in children. Indications for IVIG are based on the degree of functional impairment and time from onset of symptoms. The indications are not influenced by the clinical or neurophysiological subtype or the results of antibody screening. There is no evidence to support sequential treatment using both PE and IVIG.[71,72]

Pain is a common feature of GBS and may have a neuropathic basis. Paracetamol, non-steroidal anti-inflammatory drugs are useful, while drugs to treat neuropathic pain including gabapentin, carbamazepine and amitriptyline may also be beneficial.

The problems of long-term ventilation in a conscious patient compounded by emotional immaturity, speech failure, fear of procedures and family disruption make the management of a child with GBS and their family particularly challenging. A sensitive team approach is essential.

PROGNOSIS

The prognosis in acute GBS may be better for children than for adults. Full recovery is likely if the time from maximal deficit to onset of recovery is less than 18 days. Complete recovery, despite a longer plateau phase, has been reported, however.[73] Good recovery can occur in patients who have required ventilation and the need for ventilation may not be a poor prognostic factor in children.[66] Those presenting with a subacute course are at risk of relapse and permanent motor deficits.

ACUTE DISSEMINATED ENCEPHALOMYELITIS

Acute disseminated encephalomyelitis (ADEM) is defined as an episode of inflammatory central nervous system demyelination with polyfocal neurological deficits accompanied by encephalopathy (behavioural change or altered consciousness). Clinical features include encephalopathy, which is required to make the diagnosis, ataxia, hemiparesis, seizures, upper airway respiratory obstruction and polyfocal neurological deficits.[74] The encephalopathy varies in severity from subtle signs of irritability and headache to life-threatening coma and decerebrate rigidity. Severe cases frequently require support with a period of mechanical ventilation.[75]

ADEM is often preceded by a viral infection or vaccination. The most common agents responsible for the prodromal phase include Epstein–Barr virus, cytomegalovirus, herpes simplex virus, and *Mycoplasma*; however, in the majority of cases a specific agent cannot be identified. The condition is thought to result from an autoimmune process with formation of antibodies against myelin.

INVESTIGATION

Lumbar puncture should be performed to exclude infectious encephalomyelitis. There may be a modest elevation of the CSF white cell and red cell count. CSF oligoclonal bands and raised CSF immunoglobulin levels occur more commonly in multiple sclerosis than in ADEM.[74] MRI with T2 and FLAIR show bilateral asymmetrical hyperintense demyelinating lesions. The lesions predominantly involve the white matter at the grey–white matter junction; however, the grey matter may also be involved. The size of lesions varies from punctate to large tumefactive (puffy/swollen) mass-like lesions.[76] Some patients with ADEM have normal MRI findings on initial presentation but develop features typical of ADEM if the study is repeated several weeks later. In some patients the MRI changes first appear at a time when clinical improvement is occurring.

MANAGEMENT

Although there are no randomised therapeutic trials in ADEM, high-dose corticosteroids are considered the treatment of choice. Intravenously methylprednisolone 20–30 mg/kg/day (maximum 1 g/day) for 3–5 days followed by oral prednisolone tapered over 2–3 weeks often results in rapid clinical improvement. Other treatment options include intravenous immunoglobulin (2 g/kg intravenously for 2–3 days) and plasmapheresis.[74]

OUTCOME

Most children with ADEM recover completely although a small percentage of children have significant neurological and neuropsychological sequelae. Rarely ADEM is fatal. Approximately 20% of children initially diagnosed with ADEM experience a recurrence of neurological symptoms and subsequently receive the diagnosis of multiple sclerosis.[77]

METABOLIC ENCEPHALOPATHY

Approximately 0.1% of babies have an inborn error of metabolism. Acute encephalopathy is one of the many ways neurometabolic diseases present in childhood.[78,79] In general, acute presentations occur in the neonatal period and early infancy. Symptoms are often vague and include lethargy, poor feeding and vomiting. Older infants and children more commonly present with a chronic encephalopathy, with features that may include seizures, long-tract signs, visual impairment and loss of milestones.

APPROACH TO DIAGNOSIS

A careful history and examination may elicit clues to a possible metabolic problem. Family history and history of drug exposure are extremely important. Valproate, in particular, has been associated with liver dysfunction and encephalopathy. The following readily available investigations are useful to allow a broad categorisation and direct further detailed investigations: blood gas analysis, blood sugar, serum ammonia, serum lactate, plasma amino acids, urine metabolic screen, and urine ketones. While lactic acidosis and hypoglycaemia can occur in a number of disease states including sepsis, persisting abnormalities require further investigation. Lactic acidosis can be further assessed with measurement of lactate/pyruvate ratio. **Figure 109.1** provides an algorithm proposed by Ellaway and colleagues to direct the investigation of metabolic disease presenting in the newborn period based on the metabolic abnormalities detected from baseline investigations.[80] This is best done in collaboration with a metabolic disease specialist or a clinical biochemist.

MANAGEMENT

Initial management includes elimination of toxic metabolites and administration of calories to switch

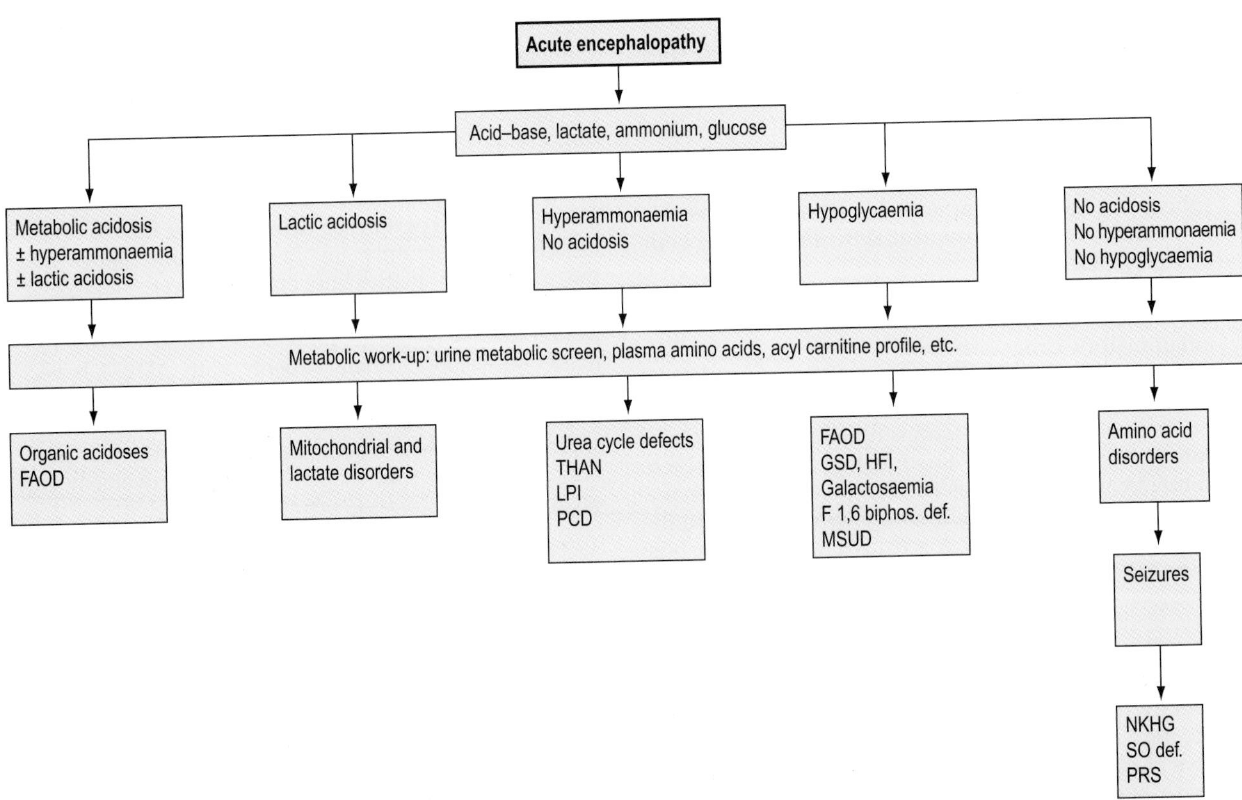

Figure 109.1 Flow diagram to guide investigation of inborn errors of metabolism presenting in the newborn period. FAOD=fatty acid oxidation disorder; F1,6 biphos. def., =fructose 1,6 biphosphatase deficiency; GSD=glycogen storage disorder; HFI=hereditary fructose intolerance; LPI=lysinuric protein intolerance; MSUD=maple syrup urine disease; NKHG=non-ketotic hyperglycinaemia; PCD=pyruvate carboxylase deficiency; PRS=pyridoxine-responsive seizures; SO def.=sulphite oxidase deficiency; THAN=transient hyperammonaemia of the newborn.

off catabolism. Metabolic derangements such as acidosis and hypoglycaemia should be corrected. The role of ICP monitoring for acute intracranial hypertension is controversial; however, patients with suspected raised ICP and unconscious patients should receive standard modalities of support including intubation and mechanical ventilation. Hyperammonaemia should be managed by stopping enteral feeds to limit protein intake. Agents such as arginine and sodium benzoate can be administered to increase ammonia metabolism. Providing calories intravenously in the form of glucose and fat limits the extent of catabolism and thereby helps to curtail the metabolic crisis. Dialysis is used to control severe hyperammonaemia and acidosis. Continuous venovenous haemodiafiltration is more effective than peritoneal dialysis.[81]

SPINAL INJURY

INCIDENCE

Paediatric spinal trauma is relatively rare, comprising <5% of all spinal injuries. Approximately 5% of children with severe head trauma will have a cervical spine injury. However, a high proportion of children who die following motor vehicle trauma, particularly those who suffer immediate cardiorespiratory arrest, or who die before arrival at hospital, have disruption of the spinal cord above C3, particularly at the cervico-medullary junction.[82,83]

AETIOLOGY

The most common causes of paediatric spinal trauma are motor vehicle crashes, as either a pedestrian or passenger, falls and diving injuries. Sports-related injuries are uncommon.

PATHOPHYSIOLOGY

The patterns of spinal injury in children differ from those seen in adults in many ways. Spinal cord injury without radiographic abnormality (SCIWORA) occurs almost exclusively in children (20–60% of spinal cord injuries). It is associated with a high incidence of complete neurological deficit. Spinal injury in the first decade of life occurs most commonly in the first two cervical segments, with atlanto-axial rotatory subluxation, bony or ligamentous injuries, or SCIWORA and severe cord injury. Although not as common as upper cervical injuries, lower cervical injuries (below C4) do occur in young children,[84] while injury may occur at more than one level. Atlanto-axial rotatory subluxation is rarely associated with neurological deficit while ligamentous injury is more likely to be associated with permanent neurological deficit than high cervical fractures.[85] As the bony spine matures, the pattern of injury becomes more adult-like, with lower cervical and thoracic injuries seen in the second decade.[86,87]

CLINICAL FEATURES

The immediate effects of spinal cord damage are similar at any age. Frequently an associated head injury can render clinical assessment extremely difficult; confirmation of cord injury is sometimes delayed. Clues to the diagnosis in the unconscious patient include:

- flaccidity, immobility and areflexia below the level of the lesion
- hypoventilation with paradoxical chest movement; this occurs in the absence of airway obstruction where the intercostal muscles are paralysed and the phrenic nerves are intact
- apnoea with rhythmic flaring of the alae nasi (Duncan's sign), seen when the lesion is above C3
- hypotension with inappropriate bradycardia and cutaneous vasodilatation below the level of injury, due to absent spinal sympathetic outflow
- priapism, which occurs frequently.

There may be visible or palpable evidence of trauma to the spine and surrounding soft tissues, including retropharyngeal or retrolaryngeal haematomas. Spinal shock is common with temporary complete loss of function. As this resolves after 3–5 days, reflexes progressively return, usually starting with bulbocavernosus and anal reflexes. Incomplete lesions, including the Brown-Sequard cord hemisection, and anterior and central cord syndromes may become apparent at this stage.

INVESTIGATIONS

Resuscitation, including emergency intubation, should not be delayed to perform X-rays. However, the entire spinal column should be X-rayed subsequently, to demonstrate the presence of subluxation, fractures, or dislocations. MRI is useful both in the acute setting and in assessment at later stages and is now accepted as the standard for identifying haemorrhage, contusion or compression of the cord. CT produces better definition of bony injuries, and may also show cord involvement by haematomas, bone fragments and foreign bodies. SCIWORA was defined in an era before MRI was routinely available. In the majority of children with SCIWORA, MRI will also be normal; however, if intramedullary lesions are demonstrated with MRI, permanent neurological deficits are more likely.[88,89] Somatosensory evoked potentials may be useful to evaluate the integrity of the spinal cord, particularly in the comatose patient.

MANAGEMENT

Achieving control of airway, ventilation and circulation is always of first priority. If tracheal intubation is indicated, and if stability of the neck is unknown, skilled assistance is necessary to immobilise the head and neck and prevent flexion or extension. Because of the sympathectomised state in high cord injuries, a relatively low blood pressure can be expected even after hypovolaemia is corrected. Significant hypotension becomes more likely the higher the lesion and the younger the patient. Haemodynamic support with a vasoconstrictor such as norepinephrine (noradrenaline) is useful if hypotension is problematic following restoration of intravascular volume. As up to 20% of patients will have multiple trauma, many will require major surgical procedures, during which the spinal cord must remain protected. If muscle relaxants are required 2–3 days following the injury, suxamethonium is contraindicated owing to the risk of fatal hyperkalaemia.

The use of steroids is controversial and there are no studies specific to children. Two randomised controlled trials in adults demonstrated that high-dose methylprednisolone administered soon after injury improved outcome.[90–91] These studies have significant limitations and the results have not been universally accepted.[92–94]

As with brain injuries, preventing secondary injury is vital. Adequate perfusion of the cord should be ensured, as autoregulation of blood flow is lost after trauma. Immobilisation can be maintained by skull tongs with axial traction or external bracing. Operative intervention is controversial with little evidence of neurological improvement from decompressive surgery. Laminectomy and decompression in children with complete cord injuries carry significant mortality.

The incidence of venous thromboembolism after spinal injury in adolescents approaches that in adults and therefore patients in this age group should receive standard prophylaxis. Venous thromboembolism is rare in prepubertal children (approximately 1%), and the risk–benefit ratio of routine prophylaxis in this age group is unknown.[95] There should be early consultation with a specialised spinal injuries unit. Optimal rehabilitation requires a team of orthopaedic and neurosurgeons, rehabilitation specialists, nurses, physiotherapists, occupational therapists, psychiatrists, social workers and schoolteachers.

PROGNOSIS

The prognosis of all spinal injuries in children may be better than in adults. In one series of 113 children with spinal column injuries, 55 (48%) had no neurological deficit, 38 (34%) had an incomplete deficit, and of these 23 (20%) made a complete recovery and 11 (10%) improved. The remaining 20 (18%) children had a complete cord injury and, of these, 4 improved and 3 died.[82] In a smaller series 44% had neurological deficits, SCIWORA was seen in 21% and 11% of injuries were immediate, complete and permanent. Of the 18 children with SCIWORA, 4 had a permanent, complete deficit.[85]

Access the complete references list online at http://www.expertconsult.com

18. Abend NS, Gutierrez-Colina AM, Dlugos DJ. Medical treatment of pediatric status epilepticus. Semin Pediatr Neurol 2010;17:169–75.
21. Raspall-Chaure M, Chin RF, Neville BG, et al. Outcome of paediatric convulsive status epilepticus: a systematic review. Lancet Neurol 2006;5:769–79.
32. Peltola H, Roine I, Fernández J, et al. Adjuvant glycerol and/or dexamethasone to improve the outcomes of childhood bacterial meningitis: a prospective, randomized, double-blind, placebo-controlled trial. Clin Infect Dis 2007;45:1277–86.
38. Maconochie IK, Baumer JH. Fluid therapy for acute bacterial meningitis. Cochrane Database Syst Rev 2008;1:CD004786. DOI: 10.1002/14651858.CD004786.pub3.
51. Gluckman PD, Wyatt JS, Azzopardi D, et al. Selective head cooling with mild systemic hypothermia after neonatal encephalopathy: multicentre randomised trial. Lancet 2005;365:663–70.
69. Ortiz-Corredor F, Pena-Preciado M. Use of immunoglobulin in severe childhood Guillain-Barré syndrome. Acta Neurol Scand 2007;115:289–93.
75. Absoud M, Parslow RC, Wassmer E, et al. Severe acute disseminated encephalomyelitis: a paediatric intensive care population-based study. Mult Scler 2011;17:1258–61.
80. Ellaway CJ, Wilcken B, Christodoulou J. Clinical approach to inborn errors of metabolism presenting in the newborn period. J Paediatr Child Health 2002;38:511–17.
87. McCall T, Fassett D, Brockmeyer D. Cervical spine trauma in children: a review. Neurosurg Focus 2006;20:E5.
89. Liao CC, Lui TN, Chen LR, et al. Spinal cord injury without radiological abnormality in preschool-aged children: correlation of magnetic resonance imaging findings with neurological outcomes. J Neurosurg 2005;103:17–23.

110

Paediatric trauma

Kevin McCaffery

In developed countries, trauma continues to be the leading cause of death in children over 1 year of age.[1] When the additional vast burden of morbidity is added, it is clear that this spectrum of pathologies deserve urgent, ongoing and proactive attention.

Paediatric trauma is *complex* – an easily overlooked concept, particularly for those who mostly care for traumatised adults, yet this understanding is crucial to the provision of an effective paediatric trauma service.

This chapter is written principally from the viewpoint of the intensive care specialist faced with a seriously injured child. As intensive care involvement frequently begins with a request to assist with pre-hospital care or retrieval, key management priorities for this phase are included in the wider intensive care discussion.

OPPORTUNITIES FOR INTERVENTION

Death following trauma has long been considered to have a trimodal distribution (immediate, early <4 hours, and delayed). Later publications challenge this pattern of distribution, though the concept remains philosophically useful. Pre-hospital health care practitioners focus on the pre-hospital phase of trauma management, whereas hospital-based acute practitioners are more cognisant of the immediate and intermediate phases of trauma care. Taking a bigger picture, however, it is clear that there are a number of definable phases in the journey of a severely traumatised patient requiring different types of intervention (**Fig. 110.1**). A mature 'trauma system' or 'trauma team' would be expected to be cognisant of and active in all phases of trauma management from injury to outcome.

Trauma

This phase is commonly unexpected and sudden, with little opportunity to mitigate harm. All useful interventions here are derived from those emplaced during the pre-trauma phase. The most important interventions in the management of trauma are those that prevent injury occurring in the first place.

Pre-trauma

In a number of areas, legislation and public safety campaigns have led to decreased morbidity and mortality. Notable successes lie in the areas of motor vehicle legislation (seatbelt laws, drink–driving legislation, speed restriction and vehicle design), bicycle legislation (cycle helmets and education), water safety (pool fencing, water safety and swimming lessons) and burn reduction (smoke detectors, limitation of hot water temperature).

By any measure, politicians and legislators rank amongst the most effective members of the expanded 'trauma team,' though it should be noted that they can be susceptible to influence by pressure groups, as exemplified by the turbulent (and ongoing) evolution of swimming-pool fencing regulations in Australia.[2]

Pre-hospital care

Two models for pre-hospital care predominate in the Western world.[3] In the United States, the prevailing concept is that of 'scoop and run' by paramedical staff to designated 'trauma centres'. The principal driver of this process was the decreased battlefield mortality seen between World War II (4.5%) and the Vietnam War (1.9%). A number of innovations contributed to this decrease, but increasing rapidity of casualty evacuation to well-equipped surgical hospitals was a key feature.

Conversely, the model adopted by several European and Scandinavian countries involves use of paramedic-crewed ambulances supported by a well-developed network of physician-manned ambulances, essentially mobile intensive care units.

No robust data currently exist to demonstrate the superiority of one system over the other, for it is likely that differences in such variables as geography and distance, prevalence of penetrating versus blunt trauma and cost and resource implications will favour different models in different areas.

Furthermore, in comparison with adults, seriously traumatised children are more likely to require secondary transfer to a paediatric trauma centre after initial stabilisation is undertaken, owing to concentration of paediatric expertise in a smaller number of centres.

THE DEVELOPMENT OF 'TRAUMA TEAMS, CENTRES AND SERVICES'

The concept of multidisciplinary teams and institutions with specific interest and expertise in trauma

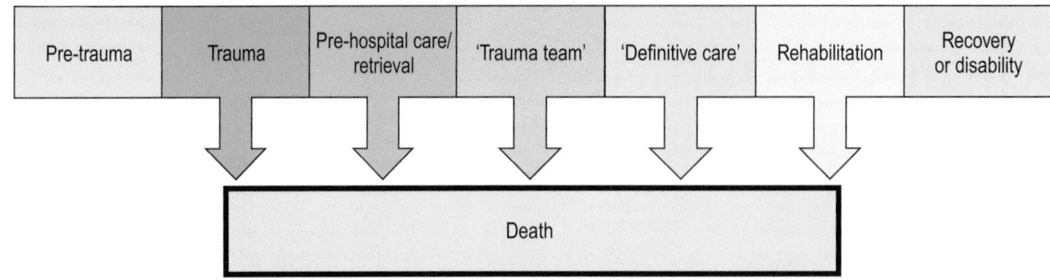

Figure 110.1 Phases of severe paediatric trauma.

management began to develop in the 1950s and 1960s. Currently, most developed countries have accreditation processes for trauma services and designate different centres by 'level' based on their capabilities.

In addition to doctors and nurses from acute specialties such as the emergency department, surgical subspecialties, anaesthesiology and critical care, the wider multidisciplinary team frequently includes trauma coordinators, research staff and rehabilitation specialists such as physiotherapists, psychologists and social workers. Similarly, the remit of trauma teams, centres and services has expanded beyond simple care of the traumatised patient, and now includes data collection and analysis, development of injury-prevention strategies and coordination of regional trauma services.

There is growing evidence that development of trauma teams, centres and services improves outcomes for injured adults[4] and children.[5] Opinion is more divided on whether or not outcomes for seriously traumatised children are improved when managed in designated paediatric trauma centres compared with adult trauma centres, however.[6,7]

SPECIFIC PAEDIATRIC TRAUMA PRESENTATIONS

Differing mechanisms of injury may be associated with specific patterns of injury in both children and adults, though anatomical and physiological differences between age groups will alter the pattern seen. Children requiring intensive care admission will have serious injury to one or more of the following.

TRAUMATIC BRAIN INJURY

Brain injury, resulting either directly from trauma or indirectly from hypoxic–ischaemic insult, accounts for the majority of deaths and long-term severe morbidity in paediatric trauma. Once the insult has occurred, management is entirely focused on prevention of secondary insults and further damage. Conventionally this involves control of intracranial hypertension, defence of cerebral perfusion pressure (CPP) and minimisation of injurious factors such as seizures, hypo- or hyperglycaemia and fever. An overview of this topic is provided below, but those wishing a comprehensive review of the current evidence base behind current management of paediatric traumatic brain injury (TBI) are directed to guideline documents published by the Brain Trauma Foundation.[8]

PAEDIATRIC TBI: ANATOMICAL AND PHYSIOLOGICAL CONSIDERATIONS

Adult brain volume is reached around 6 years of age, whereas skull growth continues until around 16 years of age. Children thus have less room for brain swelling within the rigid skull. This is compounded by differences between children and adults in adaptive mechanisms to defend against raised intracranial pressure, including smaller relative cerebrospinal fluid volumes, higher intracellular concentrations of sodium and impaired ability of neurons to extrude sodium. In addition to the propensity of smaller children to raised intracranial pressure (ICP), cerebral perfusion pressure may be further compromised by the similarities in autoregulation of cerebral blood flow between small and larger children, affording smaller patients less safety margin.[9]

NEUROLOGICAL ASSESSMENT AND MONITORING OF CHILDREN

Priorities of the assessment process are as follows:

- to benchmark neurological function over time
- to identify lesions and problems requiring treatment
- to identify prognostic markers.

Neurological assessment in childhood presents challenges in compliance with examination. An appreciation of child development and the use of age-appropriate tools (such as a modified Glasgow Coma Score) greatly facilitate this assessment. Assessment is best done as a process involving frequent clinical assessments over time, supplemented where indicated by targeted investigations such as computed tomography (CT) or magnetic resonance imaging (MRI).

Invasive monitoring of intracranial pressure and arterial blood pressure allows identification of deleterious intracranial pressure and permits calculation of cerebral perfusion pressure.

Intracranial pressure monitoring should be zero calibrated at the tragus of the ear with the patient inclined 30°. The target ICP threshold requiring management has not been defined in paediatrics, but current evidence would support an upper value of 20 mmHg (2.66 kPa). Lower values of 15–20 mmHg (2–2.66 kPa) may be more appropriate for small infants.

Cerebral perfusion pressure is defined as *mean arterial pressure (MAP) – mean intracranial pressure.* Mean arterial pressure should be zero calibrated at the level of the right atrium with the patient inclined 30°. It should be noted that the difference in zero level between ICP and MAP will not give a true CPP as stated and that the error will increase with increasing patient length. It does, however, allow for standardisation of measurement within routine clinical practice. Target CPP thresholds requiring management have not been defined in paediatrics, but current evidence would support a CPP target of between 40 and 50 mmHg (5.32 and 6.65 kPa).

MANAGEMENT PRIORITIES IN THE CHILD WITH HEAD INJURY

Management of paediatric neurotrauma is entirely focused on minimising secondary injury to neurons. Principles include the following:

Management of intracranial pressure

This involves manipulation of intracranial contents as described in the Monroe–Kellie hypothesis. Thus, the intracranial volume lying within the incompressible skull is composed of brain tissue, blood and cerebrospinal fluid (CSF), and any increase in the volume of one of the components must be compensated for by a reduction in volume of the others. Interventions manipulate the following volumes as follows:

- **Blood compartment:** decreasing intracranial blood volume may be tackled in three ways:
  - *Extravasated blood:* significant collections require surgical evacuation.
  - *Venous compartment:* venous drainage may be optimised by avoidance of venous obstruction (spinal collar, internal jugular lines, excessive PEEP) and patient positioning (30° head up, head midline). One small paediatric study demonstrated that increased head-up bed angle decreased ICP but not CPP.[10] Judicious sedation and muscle relaxation decrease the incidence of coughing, shivering and asynchrony with mechanical ventilation.
  - *Arterial compartment:* manipulation of this compartment requires brain tissue with preserved autoregulation to P_{CO_2}, pH, viscosity and metabolic demand. Thus, mild hyperventilation will vasoconstrict these areas, thereby decreasing the volume of the arterial bed. Prolonged or extreme hypocarbia should be avoided due to the potential for ischaemia, particularly to vulnerable penumbral areas of injured brain. Hypercarbia must also be avoided as it will increase ICP. Volume-controlled ventilation may permit more stable blood gases.

  Osmotic agents such as 3% (hypertonic) saline or mannitol exert a rheological effect by dehydrating red blood cells. The resultant decrease in blood viscosity permits a degree of cerebral vasoconstriction while still meeting metabolic demands. Use of hypertonic saline in preference to mannitol appears better supported in the literature to date.

  Decreasing neuronal metabolic demand can lower ICP. Seizures should be controlled and hyperthermia avoided. Second-tier therapies such as barbiturates and therapeutic hypothermia (32–33°C) have been demonstrated to decrease refractory raised ICP. However, both have potential serious side-effects and limited evidence to support routine use. Recent RCTs of therapeutic hypothermia versus normothermia in children have failed to demonstrate differences in functional outcome, and either no difference in mortality[11] or a trend towards increased morbidity and mortality in the cooled group.[12] A further study – Cool Kids – was stopped early on grounds of futility and has yet to publish its results.
- **CSF volume:** external ventricular drainage of the lateral ventricles allows decrease in CSF volumes in addition to ICP monitoring. This may not be practical if the ventricles have already been effaced, however.
- **Brain volume:** osmotherapy with hypertonic saline or mannitol may decrease intracranial volume by dehydrating neurons in areas with an intact blood–brain barrier.

A fourth mechanism for decreasing intracranial pressure is to undertake a decompressive craniectomy. Although recent randomised controlled trial data in adults demonstrated decreased ICPs in patients receiving this intervention, the operated group also experienced worse outcomes.[13] In paediatrics, although a number of small studies have demonstrated the utility of decompressive craniectomy in reducing raised ICP, evidence of effect on outcomes is lacking.[4,14]

Centres with limited experience in managing paediatric neurotrauma may benefit from structured guidelines, an example of which is the Scottish Intercollegiate Guideline Network (SIGN) guideline 110: Early management of patients with a head injury.[15]

A number of prognostic markers in head injury have been identified. These include the Glasgow Coma Scale, Injury Severity Score and initial hypotension.[16] Of note, the motor score component of the Glasgow Coma Scale may be as predictive as using the entire score.[17]

THORACIC TRAUMA

ANATOMICAL AND PHYSIOLOGICAL CONSIDERATIONS

The immature rib cage is largely cartilage, and ossifies through childhood. Compliant ribs allow transmission of greater impact energy to underlying viscera, allowing severe contusion without necessarily fracturing. Furthermore, the compliant infant chest and relatively transverse ribs impair tolerance of upper airway obstruction.

Increased basal metabolic rate and reduced functional residual capacity result in a more rapid onset of hypoxaemia in younger children, and this may be compounded in infancy by physiologically low haemoglobin.

ASSESSMENT AND MANAGEMENT OF THORACIC TRAUMA

Immediate assessment of a child with thoracic trauma is focused on identifying life-threatening injuries, which include:

- large airway disruption
- tension pneumothorax
- open pneumothorax
- massive haemothorax
- flail segment
- cardiac tamponade.

Management is guided by the specific findings from the primary survey, but severe thoracic trauma is likely to require intubation and ventilation, with pleural or pericardial drainage as indicated. Rare but severe injuries that may be difficult to detect during resuscitation and therefore require a high index of suspicion would include major vascular injuries, thoracic spinal injuries and traumatic diaphragmatic hernia.

A chest X-ray is a component of routine trauma assessment and may be supplemented as indicated by ultrasound assessment and computed tomography. Angiography of the great vessels may be undertaken formally or as part of the CT scan. Serial arterial gases guide requirements for ventilatory support.

ABDOMINAL TRAUMA

ANATOMICAL AND PHYSIOLOGICAL CONSIDERATIONS

The orientation of the compliant ribs in small children affords less protection to the disproportionately large liver and spleen when compared with older children or adults, while the shallow pelvis leaves the bladder at similar risk.

Small children are difficult to examine. They are also prone to aerophagia with distension of the stomach increasing emesis risk, and in some cases leading to diaphragmatic splinting.

Paediatric abdominal trauma is largely blunt in nature, and solid organ injury occurs far more commonly than hollow visceral injury. Certain mechanisms of injury should lead to the suspicion of characteristic injuries. These include handlebar into epigastrium associated with pancreatic or duodenal injury, lap-belt injuries in motor vehicle accidents leading to small bowel rupture, diaphragmatic injury or Chance fracture (flexion) of the lumbar spine. Given the difficulties in diagnosis, a high index of suspicion for abdominal injuries in trauma in children is essential.

When suspicion of abdominal injury exists, repeated clinical examination over time is supplemented by plain abdominal X-rays, ultrasonography, or CT scanning as indicated. In haemodynamically stable blunt paediatric trauma, focused abdominal sonography for trauma (FAST) currently lacks the sensitivity and positive predictive power for use as a definitive screening tool.[18] CT scanning of the abdomen is considered the 'gold standard'.

In most paediatric trauma involving the abdomen, management is expectant. Laparotomy is generally reserved for the following situations:

- penetrating injury
- hollow viscus perforation (bladder rupture/pneumoperitoneum)
- haemodynamic instability despite adequate fluid resuscitation (≥40 mL/kg)
- peritonism (later sign)
- diaphragmatic rupture.

Even high grades of splenic or hepatic laceration may be managed conservatively, provided assessment is frequent and the patient is managed in a facility with the ability to intervene surgically at short notice.

SPINAL INJURY

Spinal injury in children is rare, often difficult to diagnose and potentially devastating if missed. Challenges include the anatomical and physiological differences between adults and children, which change the types of injury commonly seen, and make radiological interpretation difficult and clinical examination challenging. Furthermore, as spinal injuries are rare, the benefits of managing injured children in a paediatric facility must be balanced against the expertise available in adult spinal injury centres.

ANATOMICAL AND PHYSIOLOGICAL CONSIDERATIONS

Differences in the immature spine and the proportionally more massive head change patterns of paediatric injury compared with adults. High lesions from the occipitoaxial junction to C3 are more common than the more typical C4–C5 lesions seen in older patients. In addition, the elasticity of paediatric ligaments may lead to the phenomenon of spinal cord injury without radiological abnormality (SCIWORA), present in 17–43% of paediatric cord injuries.[19, 20]

Mechanisms of injury change at different stages of development, with increasing incidence of sports injuries in older children.[19]

Pre-verbal children present challenges in assessment and even older children may regress and become uncompliant with clinical examination. Additionally, progressive ossification of the spine during childhood renders radiological interpretation problematic.

Spinal cord injury in children, particularly when very young, leads to an increased incidence of scoliosis, tracheostomy (due to the increased incidence of high lesions) and progressive pulmonary insufficiency.

ASSESSMENT AND MANAGEMENT

The possibility of spinal cord injury should be considered in all significant trauma, and particularly following motor vehicle accidents, rapid deceleration injuries or in the presence of multisystem trauma, head injuries, other injuries above the clavicle or abnormal neurological signs.

The first priority is spinal immobilisation, which should occur in the pre-hospital phase.

Clinical assessment is supplemented by plain radiography in the initial assessment. In severely traumatised patients, early neck clearance by clinical examination is not possible, and even plain radiography in three views - which has 94% sensitivity - may fail to detect SCIWORA. Computerised tomography and magnetic resonance imaging contribute additional information, but still will not detect all lesions even when motor signs are present.[21]

Spinal precautions must be maintained until either the neck is deemed to be uninjured or stable on clinical and radiological grounds, or until fixation has occurred.

Use of steroids or hypothermia in paediatric spinal injury is not supported by evidence at this time and is not regarded as mainstream therapy.

Early feeding, gastric protection with proton pump inhibitors, bowel care, care of skin and pressure points and prevention of contractures are important interventions if not precluded by other injuries. Similarly, early access to rehabilitation services may improve functional outcomes.

BURNS

Burns are a common cause of accidental death in childhood.[22] Younger children predominantly suffers scalds, whereas older children are more likely to present with flame burns. Burns are often included within the extended scope of trauma as many mechanisms leading to burns are also associated with traumatic injury (motor vehicle accidents, explosions, etc.). Additionally, when confronted by the prospect of burning, patients will frequently risk or incur traumatic injuries during attempted escape.

ANATOMICAL AND PHYSIOLOGICAL CONSIDERATIONS

The increased surface area/weight ratio of children compared with adults leads to a number of problems. Fluid loss from the burn may rapidly lead to dehydration, and any surface cooling undertaken increases the risk of iatrogenic hypothermia. Furthermore, alteration in body proportions from birth to adulthood mandates the use of specific methods for estimating paediatric burn surface area such as the modified Lund and Browder chart. Estimated burn surface area may be made using the area of the child's palm with outstretched fingers. Each such area corresponds to 1% of body surface area (areas of erythema should *not* be included in estimation of burn surface area).

Mechanisms of injury and patterns of burn are different to adults. Small, curious children below the level of kitchen work-surfaces are commonly scalded on the face, head and upper body when pulling pans and kettles down, an injury exacerbated by a disproportionately large head. Similarly, severe hand injuries may follow attempts to grasp hot objects or, in older children, fireworks.

The small paediatric airway is particularly vulnerable to upper airway obstruction following smoke inhalation.

Finally, paediatric burn injury may result in profound and progressive disability. Thick burn scarring may distort normal somatic growth, and psychological scarring may severely compromise social development.

INITIAL MANAGEMENT

First aid for burns involves cooling for no longer than 20 minutes, using tepid (not cold) water. As burns and trauma frequently coexist, a trauma primary survey (**a**irway+cervical spine control, **b**reathing, **c**irculation, **d**isability) should be rapidly carried out. The findings of particular relevance are listed in **Box 110.1**.

Box 110.1 Primary survey findings in burns

Airway: Is there actual or impending airway compromise?
- History of burn in enclosed space
- Facial burns/swelling
- Stridor or respiratory distress
- Carbonaceous sputum

Breathing: Is there respiratory compromise?
- Respiratory distress
- Cyanosis
- Thoracic or upper abdominal burns
- Circumferential thoracic burns

Circulation: Is there evidence of hypotension or hypovolaemia?
- Calculate burn surface area, ascertain time of injury to facilitate fluid management
- Shock from associated injuries?

Disability (neurology): Is there impairment of conscious level?
- Carboxyhaemoglobin level?
- Other toxins from smoke, e.g. cyanide?
- Associated head injury?

Once cooled, burns should be covered with sterile, non-occlusive dressings. Creams or ointments should not be applied unless advised by the local burns surgeon. Adequate hydration is required to optimise perfusion of injured areas. Fluid regimens such as the Parkland, Brooke or Galveston formulae (or modifications thereof – see **Box 110.2**: modified Parkland formula) are routinely initiated.

Pain relief with opioids and consideration of need for escharotomy where burns are circumferential should occur early, and be repeated frequently as required.

DEFINITIVE CARE

Major burns are best managed by burns centres. Burned patients in the intensive care unit are commonly ventilated for inhalational injury or to facilitate pain management. These patients require meticulous attention to fluid and electrolyte balance, nutrition, analgesia and wound care. Frequent trips to the operating room for dressing changes, wound debridement or skin grafting are expected. Routine antibiotics are not indicated, but patients require close monitoring for signs of evolving sepsis. Wound swabs and debrided tissue for culture assist in surveillance for sepsis.

NON-ACCIDENTAL INJURY

A significant proportion of children presenting with trauma will have been injured deliberately or through neglect, often by a parent or care giver. Although confrontational, this is an important diagnosis to consider as it has profound implications for the future safety of both the affected child and the family at large. In many countries there is an obligation on health care practitioners to report concerns to child protective services.

Although presentations are highly variable and may be covert, there are a number of risk factors that may increase the likelihood of an injury being factitious, as follows.

INJURY CHARACTERISTICS

- Delayed presentation of injury
- Injury inconsistent with history provided
- Injury inconsistent with child's developmental stage
- Injury with suspicious pattern as follows:

Bruising

- Specific patterns, e.g. belt buckle, handprints, loop marks from flex
- Multiple bruises of differing ages

Fractures

- Fractures of different ages
- Specific patterns, e.g. spiral humeral fracture

Burns

- Specific patterns, e.g. immersion (glove/stocking/thighs, sometimes sparing buttocks and backs of knees), cigarette or cooker-top
- Burns of different ages

Others

- Retinal haemorrhages
- Bite marks
- Bleeding from, or trauma to, anus or genitalia.

In addition to features of the injury, there are numerous patient and social factors increasing the risk of factitious injury, which include amongst others:

- *patient factors:* young age, congenital anomalies, physical or intellectual disability, adoption, etc.
- *social factors:* young or single parents, unstable family situations, substance abuse and parents who were themselves abused. Environmental stresses include divorce or financial/legal/professional difficulties.

SUMMARY

Paediatric trauma differs in important respects from trauma in adults, and is associated with a vast burden of morbidity and mortality. The development of dedicated paediatric trauma teams or services appears to be associated with improved outcomes, and represents a powerful mechanism for developing and disseminating regionally appropriate protocols, undertaking research and engaging legislators.

Box 110.2 Modified Parkland formula

Patients require resuscitation fluids+maintenance fluids.

Resuscitation fluids: 3–4 mL Hartmann's solution×weight (kg)×%total body surface area burned.

Half of this volume is given in the first 8 hours from time of injury, with the remainder given over the subsequent 16 hours.

Maintenance fluids (commonly Hartmann's+5% dextrose): 100 mL/kg/day for the first 10 kg, 50 mL/kg/day for the next 10 kg then 20 mL/kg/day for every kg thereafter.

- Formula is used in burns exceeding 15% total body surface area.
- Fluid boluses given during resuscitation may be subtracted *unless* pre-existing dehydration or associated injuries exist.
- Aim is for *adequate* urine output: 1–2 mL/kg/h<30 kg; 0.5–1 mL/kg/h>30 kg

Access the complete references list online at http://www.expertconsult.com

1. Deaths, final data for 2009. National Vital Statistics Reports 2012. Centers for Disease Control and Prevention. Online. Available: http://www.cdc.gov/nchs/data_access/Vitalstatsonline.htm.
3. Nathens AB, Brunet FP, Maier RV. Development of trauma systems and effect on outcomes after injury. Lancet 2004;363:1794–801.
5. Rupp RA, Megargel R, Reed III J, et al. Traumatic pediatric mortality based on Injury Severity Score (ISS): a retrospective study from the Delaware Trauma System 1998–2007. Ann Emerg Med 2011;58(4s):S241.
8. Kochanek PM, Carney N, Adelson PD, et al. Guidelines for the acute medical management of severe traumatic brain injury in infants, children, and adolescents - second edition. Pediatr Crit Care Med 2012;13(Suppl 1):S1–82.
12. Hutchison JS, Ward RE, Lacroix J, et al. Hypothermia therapy after traumatic brain injury in children. N Engl J Med 2008;358:2447–56.
13. Cooper DJ, Rosenfeld JV, Murray L, et al. Decompressive craniectomy in diffuse traumatic brain injury. N Engl J Med 2011;364(16):1493–502.

111

Withholding and withdrawing life-sustaining medical treatment in children

James Tibballs

Withholding and withdrawing life-sustaining medical treatment is common in hospitals, particularly in intensive care units. Usually, decisions regarding limitation of therapy are based on ethical considerations and derived by discussion and mutual agreement between parents and clinicians. However, disputes sometimes arise. When such disputes are settled in court, the judgements constitute common law.

All common law cases have been decided in the child's 'best interests', which is a nebulous term. Although each case has its own circumstances, a composite view reveals three legal and hence ethical criteria for 'best interests'. These are based on the present and future *'quality of life'*, *'futility'* of present treatment and a comparison of *'burdens versus benefits'* of present and future treatment and its discontinuance. These principles may facilitate difficult decisions. This chapter considers the principles in such legal cases, which serve as the ethical basis for withholding and withdrawing life-sustaining medical treatment.

BACKGROUND LEGALITIES

Although no legislation exists, judgements in common-law cases on withholding or withdrawing life-sustaining treatment establish the legal basis for limitation of medical treatment. Common-law cases often involve disputes between parents and doctors.

Palliative care cannot lawfully be withheld or withdrawn. Such care includes provision of reasonable medical procedures for relief of pain, suffering and discomfort, and the reasonable provision of food and water. However, artificial provision of food and water such as by nasogastric tube, gastrostomy or intravenous administration is medical, not palliative, care and may be legally withdrawn.

Withholding and withdrawing of life-sustaining medical treatment occurs in paediatric institutions, particularly in intensive care units.[1–7] When the parents and doctors agree to withhold or withdraw treatment, their decisions are usually made on ethical grounds. However, disagreements between parents and hospital staff, and indeed between hospital staff, sometimes arise because of differences in ethical opinions. This is not surprising since one's ethical position is derived from diverse social, cultural, religious, moral and familial influences.

The common ethical and legal mantra for withholding and withdrawing treatment is the so-called 'best interests' of the child. This term, somewhat nebulous, is enshrined in, but not clarified by, section 68F of the Family Law Act 1975 (Cth), in which courts are directed to determine a child's 'best interests'.

Although the 'best interests' considered by courts in each case are specific to the circumstances of the child, when all cases are considered together three recognisable circumstances permit lawful withholding or withdrawing treatment. Several 'withholding' cases have come before Australian courts but, as only one case of withdrawing treatment from children (Baby D) has been considered, it is necessary therefore to consider a few cases from other jurisdictions with similar systems of law.

Other legal requirements in this setting are presumed. These include:

- sanctity of life
- withholding and withdrawing of life-sustaining treatment are omissions not acts
- withholding and withdrawing treatment are legally equivalent
- any deliberate attempt to shorten life or cause death is a criminal act
- euthanasia either active or passive is unlawful
- competent persons, who may include teenagers, have the right of self-determination
- parents, as legal guardians, make decisions on behalf of their child, but they cannot demand a particular treatment, nor demand that a particular treatment be withdrawn or withheld, nor withhold consent for treatment if not in the child's 'best interests'
- a doctor cannot be ordered to provide treatment not in the child's 'best interests'
- sedation or analgesia may be administered with the purpose of relieving pain, suffering and distress, but which may also unintentionally shorten life
- death following lawful withholding or withdrawal of treatment is due to the underlying disease
- parents and doctors may together decide to withhold or withdraw treatment in a child's 'best interests', but neither should do so alone.

Although ethical standards and clinical guidelines are not legally enforceable, adherence to these may be scrutinised by courts in the context of meeting an appropriate standard of care according to the codes of practice of professional bodies or in relation to established medical practice.[8] It is obvious that ethical and legal principles are interdependent. It would be difficult, but not impossible, to imagine that legal judgements would be not be ethical and vice versa. Each espouses almost identical positions. Nevertheless, an occasional judgement may astound physicians, as for example the case of In the matter of baby K,[9] in which a judge ruled that mechanical ventilation could not be discontinued for an anencephalic infant.

QUALITY OF LIFE

That the future quality of life could be considered a factor in a decision to withhold or treatment was foreshadowed in Australia by the Victorian case of Baby M. Although the concept had already been accepted in Britain, it had been originally rejected in the Australian case of Re F; F v F.

RE F; F v F

This case,[10] concerning an infant with spina bifida, was brought hurriedly before the court in a father's affidavit, which (disputed by the mother) claimed that his infant was being denied sustenance and sedated for the apparent purpose of permitting or causing death. The judge stated that his concern was to deal only with the immediate and specific problem – that is, the administration of sustenance, which was ordered. However, he also said:

> *'... whatever may be the justification through some form of ethical assessment, for the adoption of a deliberate course of conduct designed to terminate the life of a child, the law in this community is clear and simple. It gives no warrant whatever for any such decision to be made. ... Difficult problems ... may be ... involved in the preservation or continuation of life, but no parent, no doctor, no court, has any power to determine that the life of any child, however disabled that child may be, will be deliberately taken from it. ... It does not permit decisions to be made concerning the quality of life, nor does it enable any assessment to be made as to the value of any human being'.*

Baby M

Although the Baby M case[11] was heard in the Victorian State Coroner's Court, whose findings did not at that time constitute law, nevertheless it suggested that a line of reasoning would be important in future cases before Australian courts. It concerned an infant born with a severe spina bifida with a large lumbar myelomeningocele, hydrocephalus, Arnold – Chiari malformation of the brain stem, vocal cord paresis and severe deformities of the lower limbs. She was relatively unresponsive, had little spontaneous movement and had difficulty swallowing, sucking and breathing. If surviving, she would unable to walk, be doubly incontinent, have no sexual function, probably require an artificial airway and would certainly require multiple operations on her spine and lower limbs. Her quality of future life was estimated extremely poor. Accordingly, the medical staff of the hospital and parents decided that no active treatment, including surgery to close the myelomeningocele, be undertaken. Feeding was restricted to that on demand and she was given paracetamol and phenobarbital. Subsequently, she developed respiratory difficulty, was treated with an infusion of morphine and died 12 days after birth. However, a member of the 'Right-to-Life' association complained to police about the infant's treatment. An autopsy was performed. The Deputy Coroner ruled that the infant had died of natural causes secondary to bronchopneumonia and hypoxia secondary to vocal cord paralysis obstructing the upper airway obstruction in the presence of toxic amounts of phenobarbital and morphine.

The case focused on the validity of withholding medical treatment in circumstances based on a *quality of life*. The Deputy Coroner, while noting that generally quality of life factors are not valid reasons to withhold treatment, the very serious disabilities of Baby M placed her in a group who would not be selected for surgery. Medical staff involved in the case was exonerated by the Deputy Coroner who stated that their decisions were legally, ethically and morally sound.

Baby D

This Victorian State case concerned Baby D,[12] who had been born at 27 weeks' gestation and required intubation and mechanical ventilation for apnoea of prematurity while a twin developed normally. Several extubation attempts were unsuccessful over several months due to development of tracheal stenosis. At one re-intubation, hypoxaemia caused cardiac arrest requiring external cardiac compression. A subsequent MRI scan revealed major hypoxic brain damage that was expected to result in severe cerebral palsy and blindness. However, she was conscious, had intact brainstem function and intact cardiorespiratory function except for life dependence on intubation. Her parents applied to the court to allow extubation (withdrawal of therapy) without re-intubation if airway obstruction re-occurred. The court sanctioned this withdrawal of therapy on the basis that continuation of life-maintaining treatment would result in a very poor quality of life, which was not in her best interests. The principle of 'double effect' of appropriate use of sedative agents to allay suffering but inevitably shortening life was also affirmed.

Re J

In this British case,[13] a 4-month-old infant was the subject of a medical recommendation to withhold mechanical ventilation. It was this case that introduced assessment of 'quality of life' as a touchstone.

The infant, asphyxiated and born prematurely at 27 weeks' gestation and weighing 1.1 kg, had required mechanical ventilation for 1 month initially and then recurrently over the course of the next 3 months. On one occasion he was resuscitated from pulselessness. At 3 months of age ultrasound studies revealed gross irreparable hypoxic brain damage. He was blind and neonatologists predicted that he would have spastic quadriplegia, deafness and be unlikely to develop even limited intellectual abilities. The judge ordered the hospital, in the infant's 'best interests', not to reventilate him.

On appeal it was argued that, as in Re C [1989] 2 All ER 782, court-sanctioned withholding of treatment applied to an infant who was dying or in whom death could only be postponed, whereas baby J was in no immediate danger. It was argued that a court is justified in withholding consent to such treatment only if it is certain that the quality of the child's subsequent life would be 'intolerable' to the child, 'bound to be full of pain and suffering' and 'demonstrably ... so awful that in effect the child must be condemned to die' as per Judges Dunn and Templeman in Re B [1990] 3 All ER 927.

The court baulked at the terms 'condemned to die' and 'the child must live'. Although 'Thou shalt not kill' is an absolute commandment in this context it is permissible to add 'but need'st not strive officiously to keep alive'. A court can never sanction steps to terminate life and as Judge Taylor stated, 'The court was concerned only with the circumstances in which steps should not be taken to prolong life'. Thus, 'What doctors and the court have to decide is whether, in the best interests of the child patient, a particular decision as to medical treatment should be taken which as a side effect will render death more or less likely'. There is a 'balancing exercise' to be performed in assessing the course to be adopted in the best interests of the child. Accordingly:

> *'account has to be taken of the pain and suffering and quality of life which the child will experience if life is prolonged. ... also ... of pain and suffering involved in the proposed treatment itself. ... I do not think that we are bound to, or should, treat (Judge) Templeman's use of the words 'demonstrably so awful' or Judge Dunn's use of the word 'intolerable' as providing a quasi-statutory yardstick. ... there will be cases in which it is not in the interests of the child to subject it to treatment which will cause increased suffering and produce no commensurate benefit'.*

The issue before Lord Donaldson was whether it would be in the 'best interests' of the child to restart mechanical ventilation and subject him to all the associated processes of intensive care if at some future time he could not continue breathing unaided. In dismissing the appeal, his judgement strongly speaks to the issue of quality of life, and introduces an unacknowledged concept of futility as a basis for withholding treatment in appropriate circumstances.

Judge Taylor, concurring, also introduced a concept observed in American judgements: that of 'a substituted judgement':

> *'the correct approach is ... to judge the quality of life the child would have to endure if given that treatment and decide whether in all circumstances such a life would be so afflicted as to be intolerable to that child. I say 'that child' because the test should not be whether the life would be tolerable to the decider. The test must be whether the child in question, if capable of exercising sound judgement, would consider the life intolerable'.*

The interpretation of the quality of life may be variable, depending on the circumstances of the patient, as illustrated by examples given by Judge Taylor in Re J. In a case of disability following an accident, as opposed to one of disability from birth, a perception by the child of what has been lost, rather than never known, may be relevant to judging the quality of life.

Re Wyatt

This is another English case[14] in which the parents of a severely disabled infant and doctors could not agree on treatment should the infant's condition deteriorate. It defined the role of a court order in subsequent medical management and re-examined the meaning of 'best interests'.

At the age of 1 year after birth at 26 weeks' gestation, this infant with microcephaly and profound brain damage was blind, deaf, incapable of voluntary movement or response and had severe spastic quadriplegia. In addition she had irreparable chronic lung damage necessitating permanent oxygen administration and had kidney dysfunction that would require dialysis. Following a dispute between the infant's parents and doctors, a court order was made that doctors could withhold mechanical ventilation otherwise necessary to prolong life, on the grounds that to do otherwise was not in the infant's best interests. Unexpectedly, mechanical ventilation was not needed. When the infant attained the age of 18 months, the parents applied to court to have the previous declaration discharged on the grounds that she was now not terminally ill. However, Judge Hedley declined to discharge the declaration after considering that her condition was unchanged. In doing so, he remarked on the utility of 'intolerability' as the test of best interests:

> *'it is in my view essential that the concept of "intolerable to that child" should not be seen as a gloss on, much less a supplementary test to, best interests. It is a valuable guide in the search for best interests in this kind of case'.*

The declaration was reviewed when the child was 2 years of age when again the concept of 'best interests' of the child was scrutinised. The court again de-emphasised 'intolerability' as the touchstone of 'best interests' and reaffirmed its meaning as enunciated in Re A, that ' "best interests" encompasses medical, emotional and all other welfare issues' and that 'The court must conduct a balancing exercise in which all the relevant factors are weighed'. Notwithstanding, since any case will be highly specific: 'any criteria which seek to circumscribe the best interests tests are … to be avoided'. On this occasion, as on the previous, the Court declined to discharge the initial declaration but added that the declaration was permissive, not mandatory and subject to discussion between parents and doctors before implementation. It was not the court's role to oversee the treatment plan for a gravely ill child, which was for the doctors in consultation with the child's parents.

FUTILITY

Futility is difficult to define and it may be quite different according to the perspectives of parent and physician – as illustrated in In the matter of baby K[9] when doctors, opposed by the mother, sought to discontinue mechanical ventilation for an anencephalic infant solely on the basis of futility. Nevertheless, the concept has been drawn upon in an Australian case involving an adult but no children, and it has appeared in American and British cases involving adults and children.

Airedale NHS Trust v Bland

Withdrawal of treatment from persons in persistent vegetative status (PVS) came to legal notice in Britain in 1993 with Airedale NHS Trust v Bland.[15] Physicians of Anthony Bland, a young man in PVS after being asphyxiated in a crowd stampede, proposed cessation of artificial feeding and withholding of antibiotic therapy in case of infection. These actions would culminate in his death by starvation and, although unpleasant for hospital staff, would not cause discomfort or stress to the patient. His 'best interests' lay in being able to lawfully discontinue all life-sustaining treatment and medical support.

Lord Hoffmann considered that it is not just the interests of the patient that are being considered and reminded us of the American substituted judgment when he opined:

> *'in the extraordinary case of Anthony Bland, we think it more likely that he would choose to put an end to the humiliation of his being and the distress of his family. Finally, Anthony Bland is a person to whom respect is owed and we think that it would show greater respect to allow him to die and be mourned by his family than to keep him grotesquely alive'.*

Moreover, 'the decision does not involve … a decision that he may die because the court thinks that "his life is not worth living". There is no question being worth living or not worth living because the stark reality is that Anthony Bland is not living a life at all.'

Lord Mustill delivered comprehensive and clear statements related to the benefits to be gained by different parties. It was in the best interests of the community that Anthony Bland be allowed die:

> *'it is the best interests of the community at large that Anthony Bland's life should now end. …. Nothing will be gained by going on and much will be lost. The stress of the family will get steadily worse. The strain on the devotion of a medical staff charged with the care of a patient whose condition will never improve, who may live for years and who does not even recognise that he is being cared for, will continue to mount. The large resources of skill, labour and money now being devoted to Anthony Bland might in the opinion of many be more fruitfully employed in improving the condition of other patients, who if treated may have useful, healthy and enjoyable lives for many years to come.'*

In addition, according to Lord Mustill, it would be in best interests of his family that he die, and therefore in his own best interest to die:

> *'He suffers no pain and feels no mental anguish … and (he experiences) the progressive erosion of the family's happy recollections by month after month of distressing and hopeless care'. 'By ending his life the doctors will not relieve him of a burden become intolerable, for others carry the burden and he has none … he has no interests of any kind'.*

The invasiveness of treatment, the indignity and its futility should be in the best interests of the family not to experience:

> *'account should be taken of the invasiveness of the treatment and the indignity to which, as the present case shows, a person has to be subjected if his life is prolonged by artificial means, which must cause considerable distress to the family – a distress which reflects not only their own feelings but their perception of the situation of their relative who is being kept alive. But in the end it is the futility of the treatment which justifies its termination' [emphasis added].*

Messiha v South East Health

This Australian case involved a 75-year-old man in deep coma with absent cortical activity several days after sustaining an hypoxic–ischaemic injury during asystolic cardiac arrest secondary to heart and lung disease.[16] Physicians proposed withdrawing mechanical ventilation, which would culminate in his death earlier than if treatment was continued. This was opposed by family members. A judge ruled that withdrawal of treatment was permitted on the grounds of futility:

> *'Apart from extending the patient's life for some relatively brief period, the current treatment is futile … burdensome and … intrusive. The withdrawal of treatment may put his life in jeopardy but only to the extent of bringing forward what I believe to be the inevitable*

in the short term. I am not satisfied that the withdrawal of his present treatment is not in the patient's best interests and welfare'.

Re L

Dame Elizabeth Butler-Sloss stressed that 'best interests' was the appropriate test and also clarified the role of futility and 'intolerability' in paediatric cases. The issue concerned a 9-month-old infant with trisomy 18 who had multiple heart defects, chronic respiratory failure, gastroesophageal reflux, severe developmental delay, epilepsy and hypotonia, and who had already suffered cardiac and respiratory arrests.[17] In supporting the judgement of Judge Hedley in Wyatt, she remarked:

> *'There is a strong presumption in favour of preserving life, but not where treatment would be futile, and there is no obligation on the medical profession to give treatment which would be futile. I agree with (Judge) Hedley that the court should be focusing on best interests rather than the concept of intolerability, although the latter may be encompassed within the former'.*

Re L.H.R.

Futility as noted above is sometimes difficult to define but it was done clearly in this American case in which the parents of a 4-month-old infant wanted unwilling doctors and a hospital to withdraw treatment.[18] The infant had suffered a 'medical catastrophe' 15 days after birth and had since been in a persistent vegetative state. A State Supreme Court, acknowledging that the infant never had an opportunity to develop and express ideas and was terminally and hopelessly ill with no reasonable possibility of ever attaining cognitive function, pronounced 'Under these circumstances, we find that the *life-support system was prolonging her death rather than her life*' (emphasis added). The author of this chapter has found this concept useful in explaining to relatives of patients the meaning of 'futility'.

BURDENS VERSUS BENEFITS

Sometimes determination of the 'best interests' is a matter of weighing the burdens and benefits.

This was described clearly by the judgement in In the matter of AB[19] in which an American court ruled that, upon a request from a mother, treatment could be withdrawn from her 3½-year-old child who had sustained hypoxic brain damage secondary to a cardiac arrhythmia. The decision hinged on the 'best interest' standard, which 'requires a weighing of the benefits and burdens of treatment options including non-treatment as objectively as possible. Factors that should be considered when making decisions about life-sustaining or life-saving treatments for a seriously ill newborn include: (1) the chance the therapy will succeed, (2) the risks involved with treatment and non-treatment, (3) the degree to which the therapy if successful will extend life, (4) the pain and discomfort associated with the therapy and (5) the anticipated quality of life with and without treatment'.

Benefit vs burden was also the issue in the British case of An NHS Trust v B[20] – a case in which doctors wanted to withdraw mechanical ventilation, against the wishes of parents, from an 18-month-old child who had spinal muscular atrophy type I. The child's illness had progressed to the point where the only spontaneous movement possible was that of eyebrows. The case is notable for three reasons. The first is that the court drew up an extensive list of burdens and benefits specific to the child that serve as a good illustration of factors needing consideration in an individual case. Secondly, although the burdens appeared to heavily outweigh the benefits and hence favour discontinuation of treatment, Judge Holman ruled in favour of continuing mechanical ventilation via endotracheal intubation. Thirdly, as the judge also ruled against the need for a tracheostomy, this created a difference between withdrawing treatment (cessation of mechanical ventilation) and withholding treatment (tracheostomy).

Mohammed's Case

This astounding decision attracted considerable media attention in Britain. The decision is not in agreement with a previous case of a 16-month-old ventilated child with SMA type I, Re C,[21] in which the judicial decision was to allow the withholding of mechanical ventilation against parental wishes in the event of a future respiratory arrest once the present mechanical ventilation had been successively weaned. The decision is also not in agreement with a subsequent case – Re K,[22] in which the court ruled that it was appropriate to cease parenteral nutrition and to allow die a 5½-month-old infant with congenital myotonic dystrophy who had required mechanical ventilation for intermittent episodes of septicaemia associated with central venous access. The judge distinguished the circumstances from those in An NHS Trust v B on the basis of age and development.

The recent Australian case of TS & DS v Sydney Children's Hospital Network ("Mohammed's case")[23] was adjudicated on the basis of a preponderance of burden over benefit in determining a child's best interests. Parents demanded invasive mechanical ventilation for their 9-month-old infant with a severe neurodevelopmental disorder due to pyruvate dehydrogenase deficiency. Their infant, after a prolonged period of hypoxaemia, was unresponsiveness, had seizures, blindness, deafness and cardiac failure requiring continuous positive airway pressure. Doctors advised against ventilation on the basis that the infant's condition was incurable. The court ruled that ventilation would cause pain and discomfort, would provide only temporary benefit and would not alleviate his underlying condition. Rather, his best interests were to receive pain relief and palliative care.

CLINICAL GUIDELINES ON WITHHOLDING AND WITHDRAWING TREATMENT

The withholding and withdrawal of life-sustaining treatment are the subjects of numerous guidelines.

Most relevant are those of the Royal College of Paediatrics and Child Health (RCPCH), those of the American Academy of Paediatrics and those of the General Medical Council (GMC).

RCPCH GUIDELINES

The RCPCH guidelines,[24] last published in 2004, claim to take into account recent changes in legislation and legal cases. They identify five situations where it is ethical and legal to withhold or withdraw life-sustaining treatment: the 'brain-dead' child, the 'permanent vegetative state', the 'no chance' situation, the 'no purpose situation' and the 'unbearable situation'. However, these divisions are somewhat confused. The state of 'brain death' requires no legal or ethical decision as it is, but not merely, a question of when to stop treatment depending upon the acceptance by and reasonable wishes of parents and any considerations of organ donation. Although both "no purpose" situation and the "unbearable" situations may be the basis for withholding or withdrawal of treatment, the "no purpose" situation is also described, confusingly, in terms of the child being unreasonably expected to "bear the situation". All categories are said to be determined by the 'child's best interests' yet heavy reliance is placed on the concept of 'intolerability', which has drawn strong judicial criticism in Re Wyatt,[14] R (Burke) v General Medical Council [2005] EWHC 1879 and in Re L.[17]

A guiding principle of the ethical framework is claimed to be adherence to legal duty, but which is curiously described as 'arguably inconsistent' – a term that is neither expounded nor justified. The legal basis is Re J (A Minor)(Wardship: Medical Treatment) [1990] 3 All ER 930: 'when the quality of life the child would have to endure if given the treatment would be so afflicted as to be *intolerable* to the child'. The guidelines declare that a number of legal judgements (but does not identify them) have established that there is no obligation to give treatment which is futile and burdensome, that feeding and other medical treatment may be withdrawn in patients in whom the vegetative state is thought to be permanent, and that treatment may be withdrawn from patients if continuation is not in their best interests. Although these statements may be true, the legal details are absent.

Nevertheless, these ethical principles have been lauded in common law cases such as An NHS Trust v B [2006] but, as expected, judges are always keen to point out that they do not constitute law.

AMERICAN ACADEMY OF PEDIATRICS GUIDELINES[25]

These are similar those of the RCPCH but use the term 'forgo' to refer to both stopping (withdrawing) treatment already begun and not starting (withholding) a treatment, and decisions turn on the 'best interests' standard. This involves balancing the benefits and burdens of treatment. Benefits may include prolongation of life (unless prolonged unconsciousness is not considered a benefit), improved quality of life after treatment (including reduction of pain or disability) and increased physical pleasure, emotional enjoyment and intellectual satisfaction. The burdens of treatment include intractable pain, irremediable disability or helplessness, emotional suffering, invasive or inhumane interventions designed to sustain life or other activities that detract from the patient's quality of life.

'Quality of life' refers to that perceived by the patient, not how others perceive it. Accordingly, a 'substituted judgement standard' should apply in which parents or surrogates must make inferences about the preferences of previously competent children. However, in states of prolonged unconsciousness, this standard cannot be applied easily.

Curiously, despite exhortation to regard quality of life only from the patient's perspective, 'Physicians and families should also consider whether continued treatment conforms with respect for the meaning of human life and accords with the interests of others, such as family members and other loved ones'.

GENERAL MEDICAL COUNCIL GUIDELINES[26]

These extensive ethical statements include references to common-law cases, legislation (limited) and to the European Convention on Human Rights.

The essential concepts are the doctor's ethical obligation to show respect for human life, to protect the patient's health and to make patient's best interests their first concern. This means offering those treatments where possible benefit outweighs any burdens and risks associated with the treatment, and avoiding those treatments where there is no net benefit to the patient.

Benefits and burdens are not limited to purely medical considerations. Doctors should not simply substitute, for the incompetent patient, their own values or those of people consulted. Prolonging life will usually be in the best interest of the patient, provided it is not excessively burdensome or disproportionate in relation to expected benefits. Not continuing or not starting a potentially life-prolonging treatment is in the best interests of the patient when it would provide no net benefit.

When death is drawing near, doctors should not strive to prolong the dying process with no regard to the patient's wishes, where known, or to current assessment of the benefits and burdens of treatment and non-treatment.

Where patients lack capacity, an assessment of the benefits, burdens and risks, and the acceptability of proposed treatment must be made on their behalf by the doctor, taking account of the patient's wishes, if known. Where these are unknown, it is the doctor's responsibility to decide what is in the patient's best interests after consulting those close to the patient.

The guideline contains a section of legal background including the following:

- Life-prolonging treatment may be lawfully withheld or withdrawn from incompetent patients when commencing or continuing treatment is not in their best interests (Airedale NHS Trust v Bland [1993] 1 All ER 821).
- There is no obligation to give treatment that is futile and burdensome (Re J (A Minor)(Wardship: Medical Treatment) [1990] 3 All ER 930).
- For children or adults who lack capacity, in reaching a view on whether a particular treatment would be more burdensome than beneficial, assessments of the likely quality of life for the patient with or without the particular treatment may be one of the appropriate considerations (Re B [1981] 1 WLR; Re C (A Minor) [1989] All ER 782; Re J (A Minor)(Wardship: Medical Treatment) [1990] 3 All ER 930; Re R (Adult: Medical Treatment) [1996] 2 FLR 99).
- In the case of patients in a permanent vegetative state, artificial nutrition and hydration constitute medical treatment and may be lawfully withdrawn (Airedale NHS Trust v Bland [1993] 1 All ER 821).
- Final responsibility rests with the doctor to decide what treatments are clinically indicated and should be provided to the patient, subject to a competent patient's consent or, in the case of an incompetent patient, any known views of that patient prior to becoming incapacitated and taking account of the views offered by those close to the patient (Re J (A Minor)(Child in Care: Medical Treatment) [1992] 2 All ER 614; Re G (Persistent Vegetative State) [1995] 2 FCR 46).
- The Human Rights Act 1998 has implications by incorporating into English law the European Convention on Human Rights. Relevant to withholding and withdrawing life-prolonging treatment are Article 2, which requires that life be protected, Article 3, which prohibits inhuman and degrading treatment, and Article 8, which requires respect for private and family life. It is noted that case law is consistent with the Convention.

These guidelines are arguably the best since recommendations are clearly based on legal decisions and, moreover, have been approved by the Court of Appeal (R v General Medical Council [2005] EWCA Civ 1003). However, prior to this judgement they had not escaped legal criticism (Burke v GMC [2004] 3 FCR 579), principally because they failed to acknowledge the incompetent person's wishes, stated when competent, for provision of treatment particularly of life-sustaining nutrition and hydration. Moreover, it was maintained that withdrawal of treatment contrary to advance direction was in breach of the European Convention on Human Rights and required judicial authorisation.

The GMC appealed the decision claiming that the judge had erred in relation to a patient's right to demand treatment, and in the use of an excessively narrow scope of 'intolerability' as the touchstone of the patient's best interests. The Appeal Court, reversing the lower court's ruling, held that a competent patient could not demand treatment that a doctor considered adverse to the patient's needs, and held that a doctor was not required to keep alive a patient who while competent had expressed a wish in an advance directive to be maintained alive when entering a persistent vegetative state. Furthermore, the test of 'best interests' of an incompetent patient was to be determined by the individual's circumstances, of which 'intolerability' was but one. The Appeal Court also held that, although there would be circumstances in which it would be advisable for a doctor to seek a court's approval before withdrawing artificial nutrition and hydration from a patient not in a persistent vegetative state, there was no legal duty to do so.

Far from being critical of the GMC's guidelines, the Appeal Court lent support to the guidelines and expressed its wish that the GMC promulgate, teach and implement their guidelines in every hospital.

CONCLUSIONS

In considering whether to withhold or withdraw life-sustaining treatment from a child, the appropriate test is that of 'best interests', which although a nebulous term essentially means

> *a determination of the quality of life, futility and a comparison of benefits and burdens.*

These three concepts are not independent as 'quality of life' with continuation of treatment may be derived by a 'comparison of benefits and burdens' flowing from treatment. 'Best interests' should also incorporate, but not exclusively, a notion of tolerability of continued treatment. The concept of futility was prominent in early cases and remains important but it is less easily defined unless related to prolongation of the dying process. These legal concepts may be helpful in the clinical situation when litigation is unlikely, but when parties nevertheless dispute courses of action each of which is considered correct under different ethical positions. It may be surprising to physicians that these principles are well described in law. Indeed, rather than consider withdrawal or withholding treatment under ethical principles, it perhaps more helpful to first ask 'Is it lawful?' and then ask 'Is it ethical?'. Whatever ethical position is adopted when contemplating withholding or withdrawing treatment from children, notwithstanding disputes, these principles should be observed because, in the end, the legal position is decisive.

Access the complete references list online at http://www.expertconsult.com

6. Isaacs D, Kilham H, Gordon A, et al. Withdrawal of neonatal mechanical ventilation against the parents' wishes. J Paediatr Child Health 2006;42:311–5.
12. Re: Baby D (NO.2). [2011] FamCA 176.
13. Re J [1990] 3 All ER 930.
14. Re Wyatt (a child) (medical treatment: continuation of order) [2005] EWCA Civ 1181.
15. Airedale NHS Trust v Bland [1993] 1 All ER 821.
16. Messiha v South East Health [2004] NSWSC 1061.
23. TS & DS v Sydney Children's Hospital Network ("Mohammed's case") [2012] NSWSC 1609.
24. Royal College of Paediatrics and Child Health. Withholding or withdrawing life sustaining treatment in children: A framework for practice. 2004. Online. Available: <http://www.rcpch.ac.uk>.
25. American Academy of Pediatrics. Guidelines on foregoing life-sustaining medical treatment. Pediatrics 1994;93:532–6.
26. General Medical Council. Withholding and Withdrawing Life-prolonging Treatments: Good Practice in Decision-making. 2002. Online. Available: <http://www.gmc-uk.org/standards/whwd.htm>.

112

Paediatric poisoning

James Tibballs

EPIDEMIOLOGY

The peak incidence of poisoning in childhood is among 1–4-year-olds. It usually occurs in the home when the child ingests a single prescribed or over-the-counter medication or a household product. Approximately 3500 young children are admitted to hospital each year in Australia.[1] This mode of poisoning is called 'accidental' - erroneously, because it is usually the result of inadequate supervision or unsafe storage of poisons. The mortality is very low and if hospitalisation is required, it is usually brief (1–3 days), so care must be taken to ensure that whatever treatment is applied, it does not cause additional illness.

Occasionally, poisoning in childhood is either truly accidental as in ingestion of a decanted chemical, or is part of a syndrome of child abuse, or is iatrogenic as when a parent mistakes medications at home or when medical or nursing staff make errors in drug administration in hospital. Unfortunately, medication errors occur with approximately 5% of paediatric inpatient medication.[2] Self-poisoning in older children is usually with the intention to manipulate their psychosocial environment or to commit suicide, or is the result of substance abuse. All such circumstances of poisoning require remedial action. Occasionally toxic gases are inhaled for example during fires.

PRINCIPLES OF MANAGEMENT

The four basic principles in management of poisoning are:

- support vital functions
- confirm the diagnosis
- remove the poison from the body
- administer an antidote[3,4] (**Table 112.1**).

Individual poisons may require specific measures. Consult current toxicology texts[5–7] for details and consult Chapter 88. Knowledge of important poisons is indispensable for paediatric practice. A number of poisons or classes of poison are potentially fatal to a small child if taken as a single tablet or a teaspoonful.[8] These include opiates (methadone, buprenorphine, lomotil), camphor, quinine derivatives, cyclic antidepressants, clonidine, sulfonylureas, salicylates, calcium channel blockers and colchicine. If a poison is unfamiliar, a poison information centre provides valuable information but clinical judgement rests with the physician.

The support of paediatric vital functions (life-support) is detailed in Chapters 103–105, 108–111 and 113 of this volume.

CONFIRMATION OF DIAGNOSIS

Commonly, the diagnosis of poisoning in paediatric practice is self-evident from a history detailed by parents or guardians. Although a single poison is usually involved, the possibility of several or multiple poisons should be considered. Occasionally the diagnosis is unknown on presentation. Any child who presents with unexplained obtundation, fitting, hypoventilation, hypotension or has a metabolic derangement must have the diagnosis excluded.

Recognition of a 'toxidrome', a constellation of symptoms and signs, may make the diagnosis.[5–7] Although numerous toxidromes exist, the four prominent types and their causative drugs or agents are shown in **Table 112.2**.

Laboratory analysis of body fluid specimens can assist in diagnosis and management of poisoning. For example, rapid routine analyses are widely available for glucose, potassium, calcium, pH, osmolarity, alcohols, paracetamol, phenytoin, digoxin, salicylate, theophylline, iron, lead, and methaemoglobin. If particular toxins are suspected, discussion with laboratory staff will optimize information to be gained.

REMOVAL OF THE POISON

Treatment should be determined by the poison, severity of poisoning as judged by the observed and expected effects of the poison, by the amount ingested, by the interval between ingestion and presentation and by the existence or otherwise of an antidote.

The range of treatment options is to: do nothing apart from advice and discharge home, observe for a short duration in the emergency department or ward, provide intensive nursing care, or treat medically. The modes of medical therapy include extracorporeal

Table 112.1 Antidotes to some poisons

POISON	ANTIDOTES	COMMENTS
Amphetamines	Esmolol i.v. 500 μg/kg over 1 min, then 25–200 μg/kg per min Labetalol i.v. 0.15–0.3 mg/kg or phentolamine i.v. 0.05–0.1 mg/kg every 10 minutes	Treatment for tachyarrhythmia Treatment for hypertension
Anticholinergic toxidrome (antimuscarinic)	Physostigmine 0.01–0.02 mg/kg i.v. slowly, repeatable but titrated to improve consciousness	Beware cholinergic effects including bradycardia, bronchospasm and weakness (treat with atropine)
Benzodiazepines	Flumazenil i.v. 3–10 μg/kg, repeat 1 minute, then 3–10 μg/kg per hour	Specific receptor antagonist. Beware convulsions
Beta blockers	Glucagon i.v. 50–150 μg/kg repeat after 3–5 min, then infusion of effective dose/h Isoproterenol i.v. 0.05–3 μg/kg per min Norepinephrine i.v. 0.05–1 μg/kg per min	Stimulates non-catecholamine cAMP (preferred antidote) Beware β_2 hypotension Antagonises toxin at receptors
Calcium channel blocker	Calcium chloride i.v. 10%, 0.2 mL/kg	Antagonises at receptors
Carbon monoxide	Oxygen 100%	Decreases carboxyhaemoglobin May need hyperbaric oxygen
Cyanide	Dicobalt edetate i.v. 4–7.5 mg/kg Hydroxocobalamin (vitamin B12) i.v. 70 mg/kg Amyl nitrite 0.2 mL perles by inhalation until sodium nitrite 3% i.v. 0.13–0.33 mL/kg over 4 min, then sodium thiosulphate 25% i.v. 1.65 mL/kg (max 50 mL) at 3–5 minutes	Give 50 mL 50% glucose after dose 'Cyanide antidote kit'; beware anaphylaxis, hypertension Beware hypotension; nitrites form methaemoglobin–cyanide (beware excess methaemoglobin >20%); thiosulphate forms non-toxic thiocyanate from methaemoglobin–cyanide
Digoxin	Magnesium sulphate i.v. 25–50 mg/kg (0.1–0.2 mmol/kg) Digoxin Fab i.v: acute – 10 vials per 25 tablets (0.25 mg each), 10 vials per 5 mg elixir; steady state: vials, serum digoxin (ng/mL) ×BW(kg)/100; empirical therapy: 10–20 vials acute poisoning, 1–2 vials chronic	Antagonises digoxin at sarcolemma Binds digoxin
Ergotamine	Sodium nitroprusside infusion 0.5–5.0 μg/kg per min Heparin i.v. 100 units/kg, then 10–30 units/kg per hour	Treats vasoconstriction; monitor BP continuously Monitor partial thromboplastin time
Lead	Dimercaprol (BAL) i.m. 75 mg/m^2 4-hourly, six doses, then i.v. $CaNa_2$ edetate (EDTA) 1500 mg/m^2 over 5 days or oral succimer (DMSA, dimercaptosuccinic acid) 350 mg/m^2 8-hourly (or 30 mg/kg/day) for 5 days, then 12-hourly 14 days if blood level >3.38 μmol/L; if asymptomatic and blood level 2.65–3.3 μmol/L, infuse $CaNa_2$EDTA 1000 mg/m^2 per day 5 days or oral succimer (DMSA, dimercaptosuccinic acid) 350 mg/m^2 8-hourly (or 30 mg/kg/day) for 5 days	Chelating agents

Continued

Table 112.1 Antidotes to some poisons—cont'd

POISON	ANTIDOTES	COMMENTS
Heparin	Protamine 1 mg/100 units heparin	Direct neutralisation
Hydrofluoric acid	Calcium chloride 10% i.v. 0.2 mL/kg Calcium gluconate gel, topically	For systemic toxicity For burns
Iron	Deferoxamine 15 mg/kg per hour 12–24 hours if serum iron >90 μmol/L (500 μg/dL) or >63 μmol/L (350 μg/dL) and symptomatic, give slowly	Beware anaphylaxis
Isoniazid (or hydrazine exposure)	Pyridoxine (vitamin B6) 70 mg/kg (max 5 g) i.v. 3–5 minutes if seizing, 30–60 minutes if not, *and* Diazepam	Metabolic acidosis may be mildly exacerbated
Local anaesthetic drug cardiovascular toxicity	Intralipid 20% i.v. 1.5 mL/kg over 1 min, repeat ×2 intervals 5 min then infusion 0.25–0.50 mL/kg/min as needed to maintain BP	Mechanism uncertain – may bind toxin; suitable for other lipophilic drugs including sertraline, bupropion, quetiapine and possibly clomipramine, propranolol, thiopentone, verapamil
Methanol, ethylene glycol, glycol ethers	Ethanol i.v. loading dose 10 mL/kg 10% diluted in glucose 5%, then 0.15 mL/kg per hour to maintain blood level 0.1% (100 mg/dL), *or* Fomepizole (4-methylpyrazole) 15 mg/kg over 30 minutes, then 10 mg/kg 12-hourly, four doses	Competes with poison for alcohol dehydrogenase Inhibits alcohol dehydrogenase (not available in Australia)
Methaemoglobinaemia	Methylene blue i.v. 1–2 mg/kg over several minutes	Reduces methaemoglobin to haemoglobin
Methotrexate	Leucovorin (folinic acid) i.v. 100–1000 mg/m^2 6-hourly until methotrexate 0.05–0.1μmol/L, *and* Glucarpidase 50 units/kg i.v.	Sustains folate cycle blocked by methotrexate Cleaves methotrexate to non-cytotoxic metabolites
Opiates	Naloxone i.v. 0.01–0.1 mg/kg, then 0.01 mg/kg per hour as needed	Direct receptor antagonist
Organophosphates and carbamates	Atropine i.v. 20–50 μg/kg every 15 minutes until secretions dry Pralidoxime i.v. 25 mg/kg over 15–30 minutes then 10–20 mg/kg per hour for 18 hours or more	Blocks muscarinic effects Reactivates cholinesterase; not for carbamates
Paracetamol	*N*-acetylcysteine i.v. 150 mg/kg in dextrose 5% over 1 hour, then 50 mg/kg per hour for 4 hours then 100 mg/kg for 16 hours (total 300 mg/kg over 20 hours), *or* oral 140 mg/kg, then 17 doses of 70 mg/kg 4-hourly (total 1330 mg/kg over 72 hours), if serum paracetamol exceeds 1500 μmol/L at 2 hours, 1000 at 4 hours, 500 at 8 hours, 200 at 12 hours, 80 at 16 hours, 40 at 20 hours	Restores glutathione-inhibiting metabolites; beware anaphylaxis
Phenothiazine (and other drug) dystonia	Benzatropine i.v or i.m. 0.01–0.03 mg/kg	Blocks dopamine reuptake

Table 112.1 Antidotes to some poisons—cont'd

POISON	ANTIDOTES	COMMENTS
Potassium	Calcium chloride 10% i.v. 0.2 mL/kg	Antagonises cardiac effects (immediate)
	Glucose i.v. 0.5 g/kg plus insulin i.v. 0.05 units/kg	Decreases serum potassium (rapid marked effect); monitor serum glucose
	Salbutamol aerosol 0.25 mg/kg	Decreases serum potassium (rapid marked effect)
	Sodium bicarbonate i.v. 1 mmol/kg	Decreases serum potassium (slight effect); beware hypocalcaemia
	Resonium oral or rectal 0.5–1 g/kg	Adsorbs potassium (slow effect)
Sulfonylureas and other drugs causing hypoglycaemia	Glucose 0.5–1.0 g/kg i.v. then infusion	Monitor serum glucose frequently
	Octreotide 1–2 μg/kg 8-hourly	Refractory hypoglycaemia from sulfonylureas and quinine; inhibits insulin release
Tricyclic antidepressants	Sodium bicarbonate i.v. 1–2 mmol/kg to maintain blood pH >7.45, aim for 7.55	Reduces cardiotoxicity
Valproic acid	L-carnitine i.v. if serum valproate ≥450 mg/L, no coma and ammonia and liver enzymes normal: 25 mg/kg 6-hourly (max 6 g/day); if coma with raised ammonia and hepatic enzymes 100 mg/kg load (max 6 g) over 30 min then 15 mg/kg 4-hourly over 10–30 min until improvement	Replaces depleted carnitine levels; measure valproate – if ≥1000 mg/L start haemodialysis or haemoperfusion

decontamination, diuresis or gastrointestinal decontamination, with the last-named of most importance. The task with all poisonings is to match the treatment and its intensity to the severity of the poisoning, thereby avoiding under- and overtreatment.

EXTRACORPOREAL DECONTAMINATION

Occasionally, removal from the circulation by an extracorporeal technique is needed by charcoal haemoperfusion, haemodialysis, plasma filtration or haemofiltration. Examples of toxins removable by these techniques are barbiturates, lithium, metformin, salicylates, theophylline, toxic alcohols, carbamazepine and valproic acid.[3,9] Such techniques, combined with extracorporeal circulatory support, should be applied when conventional therapy is failing or is anticipated to fail.

ALKALINE DIURESIS

Induce diuresis of 2–5 mL/kg/h with alkalinisation of the urine by 1–2 mmol/kg sodium bicarbonate i.v. then infuse 50–75 mmol/L in intravenous fluid titrated to maintain alkaline urinary pH without exceeding serum pH of 7.55. Monitor serum pH, sodium, potassium, calcium and avoid clinical problems of fluid overload. This reduces reabsorption in distal renal tubules of drugs including phenobarbitone, salicylate, methotrexate, and chlorpropamide.[3]

GASTROINTESTINAL DECONTAMINATION

Since the vast majority of poisoning in childhood is by ingestion, potential exists for removal from the gastrointestinal tract before absorption. However, the correct choice and timing of a gastrointestinal decontamination technique are crucial to uncomplicated recovery. The usual choices are activated charcoal, induced emesis, gastric lavage, whole bowel irrigation, or a combination of these techniques. Occasionally endoscopic removal may be needed. The efficacy, indications, contraindications and disadvantages and complications of these techniques are discussed below. A general plan of management is presented in **Figure 112.1**.

A crucial point in management is initial recognition that the patient is in a state of either 'full-consciousness' or 'less-than-full consciousness'. Traditionally, management has been dependent on a judgement of whether the gag reflex is present or absent, but in practice this is rarely tested. Since aspiration pneumonitis is a common feature of poisoning management, particularly among (but not confined to) obtunded patients, it is prudent to regard all obtunded patients as having incompetent pharyngeal reflexes.

The decision to attempt removal of a poison should always be made with due reference to two facts:

- The vast majority of childhood poisonings recover with merely supportive care or no treatment at all.
- Aspiration pneumonitis is more serious than most poisonings.

Table 112.2 Toxidromes

TOXIDROME	SIGNS AND SYMPTOMS			DRUGS/AGENTS (EXAMPLES)
Anticholinergic	Agitation Coma Delirium Mydriasis Dry mouth Hyperthermia Tachycardia (sinus) Hypertension Skin flushed and dry Urinary retention Ileus or decreased motility			Antihistamines Atropine and related drugs and substances (inc. plants) Carbamazepine Phenothiazines Tricyclic antidepressants Benzatropine
Cholinergic	MUSCARINIC	NICOTINIC	CENTRAL	
	Diarrhoea Urinary incontinence Miosis Bradycardia Bronchorrhoea Vomiting Lacrimation Salivation	Weakness/paralysis Fasciculation Tachycardia Hypertension	Obtundation/coma Agitation Seizures	Organophosphates Carbamates
Sympathomimetic	Agitation Delirium/coma Seizures Mydriasis Hyperthermia Sweating Hypertension Tachycardia Hyperpnoea			Amphetamines and derivatives Cocaine Caffeine Catecholamines Ketamine Phenylcyclidine Theophylline Lysergic acid diethylamide
Opioid/opiate	Obtundation/coma Hypoventilation Hypotension Miosis			Morphine Heroin Methadone Fentanyl Oxycodone Buprenorphine Propoxyphene

ACTIVATED CHARCOAL

Charcoal adsorbs many drugs and is regarded as a 'universal antidote'.[3,10] Although advocated as sole treatment in most poisonings, it is overused for minor poisonings and for many poisons no data exist regarding efficacy.

Treatment of charcoal with chemicals and heat increases its surface area to approximately 950 m^2/g in so-called low-surface-area activated charcoal and to 2000 m^2/g in superactivated charcoal. The latter adsorbs paracetamol better and is more palatable.[11,12] Activated charcoal is not pleasant to drink and is associated with vomiting in 20% of poisoned children.[13] It is superior to induced emesis and gastric lavage in treatment of symptomatic poisoned patients,[14–16] but its efficacy diminishes with time after ingestion. Activated charcoal reduces absorption of ingested experimental drugs in volunteers by 85–100% when administered 5 minutes after ingestion,[17–19] by 40–75% at 30 minutes[20] and by 30–50% at 60 minutes.[19,21] At mean times of 98 minutes[22] or more than 2 hours[23] after poisoning, it was not effective at all.

Activated charcoal alone is as effective as when combined with either emesis or with lavage,[24] but in combination with these methods has an 8.5% incidence of aspiration, compared with zero when used alone.[18]

Repeated doses of activated charcoal (multi-dose) enhance elimination of some drugs by increased adsorption and by post-absorption elimination by

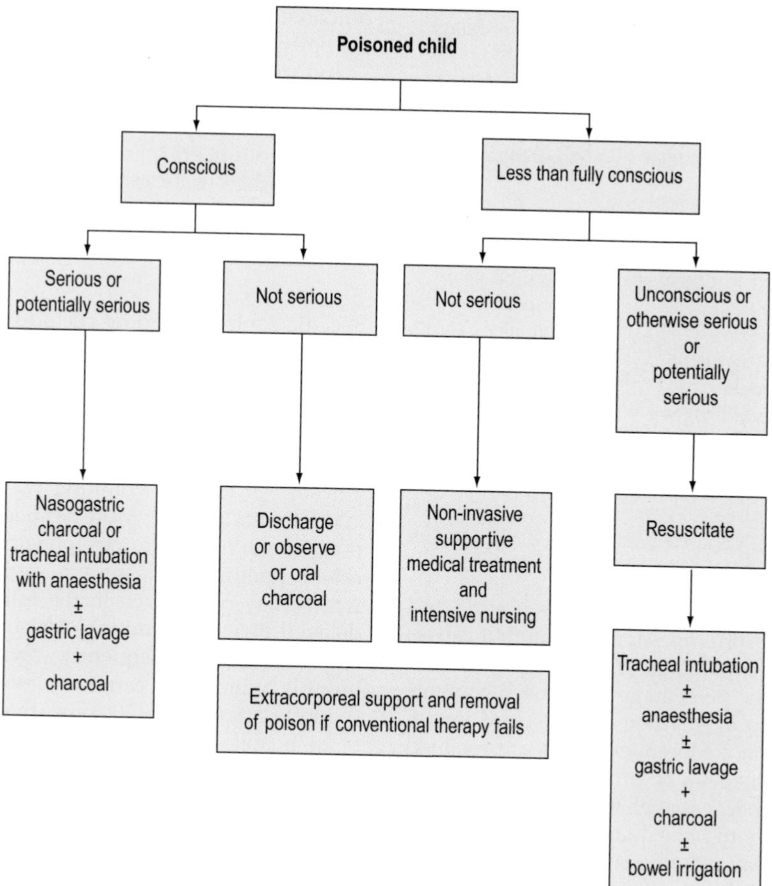

Figure 112.1 General management of the poisoned child.

interruption of an enterohepatic circulation and by removing drug from the gastrointestinal mucosa ('gastrointestinal dialysis'). Although multiple reports exist in experimental and clinical practice (**Box 112.1**),[25] there is no hard evidence to show that this therapy reduces mortality or morbidity. Only in life-threatening poisoning by carbamazepine, dapsone, phenobarbital, quinine or theophylline should multiple-dose activated charcoal be considered.[25]

A suitable single dose is 1–2 g/kg. A multiple-dose regimen for children is 1–2 g/kg stat followed by 0.25–0.5 g/kg 4–6-hourly. An alternative is 0.25–0.5 g/kg hourly for 12–24 hours.[26]

Contraindications

- Ileus
- A less-than-fully-conscious patient unless already intubated
- Substances not adsorbed – for example, strong corrosive acids and alkalis, cyanide, metals (iron, lithium, mercury, lead), alcohols, glycols, petroleum distillates (not all) and essential oils[5–7]

Complications

Aspiration of charcoal causes severe and often fatal pneumonitis, bronchiolitis obliterans and adult respiratory distress syndrome. Inadvertent intratracheal instillation of activated charcoal causes a significant increase in lung microvascular permeability and arterial blood gas derangements.[27]

Constipation is common after charcoal, but bowel obstruction is fortunately rare. The addition of a laxative (e.g. sorbitol or magnesium sulphate) is not recommended because, although transit time through the gut is decreased, efficacy of the charcoal is reduced and life-threatening fluid and electrolyte imbalance may occur.[28]

INDUCED EMESIS

For many reasons, induced emesis with ipecacuanha (ipecac) has disappeared from hospital practice and should not be performed routinely in this setting.[29] Ipecac contains alkaloids, mainly emetine and cephaeline, that induce emesis by stimulation of the chemoreceptor trigger zone of the medulla and by irritation of the gastric mucosa.

Box 112.1 Elimination and lack of elimination of drugs by multiple-dose activated charcoal[25]

Elimination increased in experimental and clinical studies	Elimination increased in volunteer studies	Elimination not increased in experimental or clinical studies
Carbamazepine	Amitriptyline	Astemizole
Dapsone	Dextropropoxyphene	Chlorpropamide
Phenobarbital	Digitoxin	Doxepin
Quinine	Digoxin	Imipramine
Theophylline	Disopyramide	Meprobamate
	Nadolol	Methotrexate
	Phenylbutazone	Phenytoin
	Phenytoin	Sodium valproate
	Piroxicam	Tobramycin
	Sotalol	Vancomycin

The efficacy of ipecacuanha (ipecac) is limited and decreases with time from ingestion. Although it causes vomiting in a high percentage (93–100%) of children within 25 minutes, the percentage of stomach contents ejected is small (28%) even when administered immediately after ingestion.[30] Moreover, solids are retained in the stomach or may even be propelled into the duodenum.[20] In adults, ipecac is even less useful and has to be given immediately to have quantifiable effects.[31]

It does not improve outcome and may reduce effectiveness of the alternative treatments of activated charcoal, oral antidotes and whole bowel irrigation. However, its use in the home is safe and is associated with fewer paediatric emergency department attendances,[32] and it is still recommended by authoritative paediatric health organisations in the USA.[33] Although ipecac was recommended inappropriately in 20% of cases reported to poisons information centres, it caused little morbidity.[34]

Experimentally, approximately 50–83% of ingested experimental drug is removed if ipecac is given after 5 minutes,[17] falling to 2–44% if given at 30 or 60 minutes.[21,35–38] In paediatric paracetamol poisoning, the 4-hour post-ingestion serum level was approximately 50% of controls if ipecac-induced vomiting occurred within 60 minutes of ingestion, but no benefit was derived if emesis occurred beyond 90 minutes after ingestion.[39] Similarly, serum levels of paracetamol were reduced approximately 50% if ipecac was administered at home, inducing emesis at a mean of 26 minutes after ingestion, compared with ipecac administered at a medical facility at a mean of 83 minutes.[40]

Critics claim that induced emesis merely creates work, delays discharge from the emergency department[41] increases complications[41] and does not benefit the patient who presents more than 1 hour after ingestion.[42] Importantly, ipecac did not alter the clinical outcome of patients who presented awake and alert to the emergency department.[15]

Induced emesis appears superior to gastric lavage but inferior to activated charcoal. In salicylate poisoning, emesis retrieved twice as much as gastric lavage.[43] In adult volunteers ipecac-induced vomiting, occurring at an average of 19 minutes after ingestion, removed 54% of a tracer compared with 30% with gastric lavage performed at the equivalent times after ingestion.[14,44,45]

Contraindications

Specific contraindications include actual or impending loss of full consciousness or ingestion of corrosives or hydrocarbons.[29]

Complications

Potential complications include time-related lack of efficacy, protracted vomiting (17%), diarrhoea (13%) and lethargy (12%).[46] More serious, but rare, complications include gastric, oesophageal or brain haemorrhage, pneumomediastinum, aspiration pneumonitis, which may occur even in the fully conscious patient, delayed onset of vomiting, which is a threat if loss of consciousness subsequently occurs, and abuse in bulimia, which may cause cardiotoxicity as well as the sequelae associated with repetitive vomiting.

In hospital, induced emesis has no practical role. Even when a child presents very early after significant poisoning, oral or nasogastric charcoal is preferred. Importantly, whenever induced emesis is used the child must be fully conscious on administration and is expected to be fully conscious when vomiting occurs.

GASTRIC LAVAGE

The place of this in the management of the poisoned victim is very limited.[47] It is invasive, ineffective and potentially harmful. It should be reserved for the child who presents very soon after a life-threatening ingestion such as iron.

It involves passage of a large-bore oro- or nasogastric tube into the stomach and the repeated instillation of fluid, usually water, but some authorities advocate normal or half-normal saline. The oral route is preferred because of less potential for traumatic injury but an oropharyngeal airway may be needed to prevent tube occlusion by chomping. A smaller tube may be used if the poison is a liquid. Traditionally, the child should be placed in the left lateral position to limit stomach emptying, but volume of intragastric contents rather than body position determines gastric emptying.[48]

Experimental studies on liquids indicate that gastric lavage retrieves 90% at 5 minutes,[49] 45% at 10 minutes[45] and 30% at 19 minutes[44] and reduces absorption or bioavailability by 20–32% at 1 hour after ingestion.[35,50] When performed 5 minutes after ingestion of tablet drugs, it failed to prevent absorption, presumably because the tablets had not disintegrated.[18] In true overdose situations, gastric lavage within 4 hours of admission reduced serum paracetamol levels by 39%.[51]

Efficacy of gastric lavage, even with large-bore tubes, is poor because tablets are not removed and lavage encourages propulsion into the duodenum.[30] In symptomatic patients, gastric lavage alone compared with gastric lavage and activated charcoal increased pneumonic aspiration and did not alter the duration of intubation or the stay in the emergency department or the intensive care unit (ICU),[16] and was not beneficial unless performed within 1 hour of ingestion.[15] An RCT of gastric lavage in acute overdose[24] (criticised methodologically),[24,52] suggested that it made no difference to outcome of obtunded patients when preceding activated charcoal.

Contraindications

- Less-than-fully conscious patient (unless already intubated) because of the risk of aspiration pneumonitis – which is not negligible even during full consciousness[16]
- After ingestion of corrosives because of the risk of perforation
- After ingestion of hydrocarbons or petrochemicals because of the risk of pneumonitis.

Complications

- Aspiration pneumonitis
- Water intoxication
- Minor trauma to oropharynx (gastro-oesophageal perforation occurs rarely)
- Intrabronchial instillation of lavage fluid.

As expected, infants and children never cooperate fully for gastric lavage, thus increasing risks of complications and the degree of psychological trauma.

If lavage is indicated (i.e. for life-threatening poisoning), rapid sequence induction of anaesthesia with intubation is mandatory. The largest possible lubricated tube of diameter similar to an appropriate-sized endotracheal tube should be used and correct placement in the stomach confirmed. Small volumes (1–2 mL/kg) of warm tap water or 0.9% saline may be used to lavage until clear. However, most fluids should be retrieved to avoid complications with fluid and electrolytes, particularly hyponatraemia if water is used.

WHOLE BOWEL IRRIGATION

Irrigation of the bowel with an iso-osmolar solution of polyethylene glycol and electrolytes is effective in reducing absorption of experimental drug by 24–67% at 1 hour after ingestion[53,54] and up to 73% at 4 hours after ingestion.[55] However, it is not conclusively proven to improve the outcome. The technique has limited applications to sustained-release or enteric-coated drugs and remains a theoretical option for ingestions of iron, lead, zinc (substances not adsorbed by activated charcoal), packets of illicit drugs[56] and for lithium.[57] Whole bowel irrigation may be useful in delayed presentations when poisons have progressed beyond the stomach.

Since irrigation solutions are adsorbed by activated charcoal and cause desorption of drug, this necessitates prior administration of charcoal if a combined technique is used.[58] However, whole bowel irrigation did not add to the benefits of activated charcoal in an experimental model of sustained-release theophylline poisoning.[59]

A suitable regimen is approximately 30 mL/kg per hour for 4–8 hours until rectal effluent is clear. A regimen of 25 mL/kg per hour has been used safely for 5 days (total 44.3 litres),[60] but a total of 3 litres was as effective as 8 litres in a simulated poisoning.[61]

Contraindications

Risk of aspiration during:

- less-than-full consciousness
- bowel obstruction or ileus.

PLAN OF MANAGEMENT

A general plan of management is suggested in Figure 112.1, but each case of poisoning mandates a specific management according to circumstances: consciousness and risk of aspiration, timing of presentation in relation to the severity of poisoning and the existence or otherwise of an effective antidote dictate if removal should be attempted, and by what means.

POISONING BY SPECIFIC SUBSTANCES

Like adults, children are poisoned regularly by therapeutic prescription or over-the-counter therapeutic drugs and substances (see Ch. 88). The poisons probably reflect their availability in the home. In a survey, the most common agents responsible for hospital admission of children were benzodiazepines, anticonvulsants, antiparkinsonism drugs, paracetamol, major tranquillisers, antidepressants and cardiovascular drugs.[62] The inquisitive nature of young children results in poisoning by substances not normally regarded as dangerous and not encountered in adults. A few of these are considered here briefly.

BUTTON OR DISC BATTERIES

Ingestion may cause electrolytic injury and potentially corrosive, toxic or pressure injury. There are many types of batteries that contain a variety of substances; the most important are lithium, mercury and potassium hydroxide.

Impaction in the oesophagus is the most significant situation; this can result in oesophageal perforation and tracheo-oesophageal fistula or aorto-oesophageal fistula. An impacted battery must be removed endoscopically as soon as possible. Lithium batteries are large and impact readily and they have higher voltages than other types. Electrolysis commences as soon as the battery surfaces are immersed in oesophageal fluid. The consequence is local and surrounding tissue destruction, including the trachea.[63] Strong alkali is produced at the cathode and strong acid is produced at the anode. Mercury batteries are more likely to fragment[64] but mercury poisoning is very uncommon.

Sufficient follow-up is necessary to exclude oesophageal and tracheal damage and to ensure that a battery in the stomach or distal bowel is eliminated.

PETROLEUM DISTILLATES

Numerous by-products of petroleum distillation are utilised for industrial and domestic purposes. Ingestion of these hydrocarbons may cause CNS toxicity (comprising obtundation and convulsion), gastrointestinal irritation, occasional hepatorenal toxicity, and pneumonitis.

Pneumonitis is the most significant and it may occur during ingestion or subsequent vomiting. Although variable, these substances have low surface tensions, which enables their rapid dispersement throughout contiguous mucosal surfaces including the respiratory tree. Prime examples are petrol, kerosene, lighter fluid, lamp oil and mineral spirits. Any child who ingests a distillate must be assessed for pneumonitis and this should include clinical examination, a chest X-ray and at least a non-invasive measurement of oxygenation such as pulse oximetry. Although most children who ingest petroleum distillates do not develop pneumonitis, the onset of this complication may be within 30 minutes[65] and progress rapidly to severe lung disease. An adequate period of observation (6 hours) is necessary to exclude this complication. There is a poor correlation between the amount ingested and the severity of pulmonary toxicity.

Deliberate inhalation of volatile hydrocarbons such as petrol or aerosolised paint has the additional toxicity on myocardial tissue, including fatal tachydysrhythmia, possibly due to sensitisation to endogenous catecholamines. The deliberate inhalation of paint fumes, usually via a plastic bag, is known as 'chroming'.

ESSENTIAL OILS

The oils from certain plants contain mixtures of terpenes, alcohols, aldehydes, ketones and esters, which are used domestically for various purposes. The well-known oils are eucalyptus, turpentine, citronella, cloves, tea tree, peppermint, wintergreen and lavender. In general, small amounts cause depression of conscious state, irritation of gastrointestinal tract, liver dysfunction and pneumonitis if inhaled. Each has different toxicity. For example, as little as 5 mL of eucalyptus oil[66] or 15 mL of turpentine may cause depression of conscious state.

Emesis should not be induced and gastric lavage performed only if airway protection is required.

LEAD

Children are more susceptible to lead poisoning after ingestion than are adults, possibly because of better absorption.

Acute poisoning usually occurs after ingestion of a lead salt or metallic foreign body or a lead-containing product, such as paint, traditional remedy or cosmetic. Acute poisoning by a salt may cause life-threatening cardiovascular collapse and encephalopathy.

Chronic poisoning can occur with ingestion of lead-contaminated water, or by inhalation of leaded petrol fumes or contaminated house dust. Chronic poisoning causes multi-organ dysfunction including neuromuscular dysfunction and encephalopathy.

Treatment consists of gastric decontamination in the case of recent ingestion of lead salts. The use of intravenous or oral chelating agents may be indicated.[67] In the case of ingestion of a lead foreign body, serial X-rays should be taken to ensure elimination, otherwise surgical removal is indicated. In the case of multiple embedded gunshot pellets and in all cases of chronic poisoning, serum lead levels should be measured to guide chelation therapy (see Table 112.1).

PARACETAMOL

This is the most common drug ingested by children in an accidental, iatrogenic or deliberate overdose situation. Overdose has the potential for hepatic failure and, less commonly, renal failure. The onset of toxicity is delayed – up to several days. Consequently, the need for acute gastric decontamination is uncommon, but would be justifiable for acute large-dose presentations. The toxicity in part is caused by the hepatic metabolite of the drug (*N*-acetyl-*p*-benzoquinoneimine), which accumulates when endogenous glutathione, which facilitates conversion of *N*-acetyl-*p*-benzoquinoneimine to non-toxic substances, becomes exhausted. Adequate supply of glutathione is ensured by administration of the antidote *N*-acetylcysteine, a glutathione precursor that can be administered intravenously or orally (see Table 112.1).

Time of presentation after ingestion, as well as dose, determines management. If presentation is within 1 hour of ingestion, effective gastric removal or administration of activated charcoal may be all that is required pending a serum paracetamol level. In contrast, if presentation is several hours after ingestion, administration of the antidote according to serum paracetamol level takes precedence and, although it may be administered orally or intravenously, the intravenous route is generally preferred.[68] In one study, hepatic toxicity was slightly less in patients treated with the intravenous regimen compared with the oral regimen in patients whose treatment was initiated within 12 hours of ingestion, but later than 18 hours hepatic toxicity was slightly less in patients treated with the oral regimen compared with the intravenous regimen, with no difference in toxicity in those treated with either regimen at presentations between 12 and 18 hours after ingestion.[69]

Near-simultaneous administration of activated charcoal and acetylcysteine may be of some benefit but it may also cause vomiting or desorption, thus decreasing the effectiveness of the oral antidote. If presentation is many hours after the poisoning, activated charcoal is not indicated, so the antidote could be administered orally if necessary according to serum paracetamol levels. In all cases, evidence of liver dysfunction mandates administration of the antidote.

The threshold single toxic dose of paracetamol indicating *N*-acetylcysteine administration is generally regarded as 150 mg/kg, although it has been suggested that a single dose less than 200 mg/kg in children less than 6 years of age may be safely managed at home.[70] However, in situations of repeated sub-150 mg/kg doses hepatotoxicity has a high mortality among children[71] and in adults.[72] Unfortunately, toxic overdosing by chronic administration is not uncommon even in paediatric institutions.[73]

No sufficient data exist on which to firmly base a decision when to administer *N*-acetylcysteine to children. In lieu of this, time-related serum levels of paracetamol should be measured and reference made to a guideline to administer the antidote (see Table 112.1) as derived from single toxic dose adult data.[74] The serum paracetamol level indicating antidote has been predicted as >225 mg/L (1500 µmol/L) at 2 hours after ingestion of a single overdose of elixir in children 1–5 years of age.[22] If serum levels of paracetamol cannot be obtained and >150 mg/kg has been ingested as a single dose, or liver dysfunction is present after chronic poisoning, the antidote should be given.

Adverse reactions to *N*-acetylcysteine (approximately 7–8%) respond to an antihistamine[75] and its temporary cessation.

IRON

Small quantities of elemental iron (>20 mg/kg) are toxic to children. This dose may be reached by ingestion of a few iron tablets. The initial effects are gastrointestinal, which may include gastric erosion, followed sometimes by an interval before cardiovascular failure occurs at 6–24 hours and then followed by multi-organ failure (including encephalopathy) and hepatic and renal failure up to some 48 hours after ingestion. In addition to general supportive measures, specific management should include abdominal X-ray to determine if unabsorbed tablets are present, in which case gastric lavage or whole bowel irrigation may be useful. Activated charcoal is useless. Chelation therapy with deferoxamine (see Table 112.1) should be guided by serum iron level and clinical status.

CAUSTIC SUBSTANCES

In a study of 743 children,[76] the incidence of oesophageal burns caused by ingestion of automatic machine dishwashing detergents was 59%, caustic soda 55% and drain cleaners 55%. All are strongly alkaline and are corrosive. Dishwasher detergents are presented as liquids, powders or tablet blocks and are commonly accessed in an open dishwasher.[77] Pharyngeal and oesophageal irritation, burns or corrosion may occur. There may be simultaneous ocular and dermal toxicity. Any child presenting with a history of ingestion of a caustic substance, irrespective of clinical signs, should be considered for oesophagoscopy and follow-up since the correlation between symptoms and signs and oesophageal burns is poor[76] and significant oesophageal damage may occur in the absence of more proximal injury.[78]

Access the complete references list online at http://www.expertconsult.com

3. Smith SW. Drugs and pharmaceuticals: management of intoxication and antidotes. Mol Clin Environ Toxicol 2010;2:397–460.
6. Erickson TB, Ahrens WR, Aks SE, et al, editors. Pediatric Toxicology. Diagnosis and Management of the Poisoned Child. New York: McGraw Hill; 2005.
8. Michael JB, Sztajnkrycer MD. Deadly pediatric poisons: nine common agents that kill at low doses. Emerg Med Clin North Am 2004;22:1019–50.
10. Lapus RM. Activated charcoal for pediatric poisonings: the universal antidote? Curr Opin Pediatr 2007;19:216–22.
29. Krenzelok EP, McGuigan M, Lheur P. Position statement: ipecac syrup. American Academy of Clinical Toxicology; European Associations of Poisons Centres and Clinical Toxicologists. J Toxicol Clin Toxicol 1997;35:699–709.
47. Academy of Clinical toxicology and European Association of Poisons Centres and Clinical Toxicologists. Position statement: gastric lavage. J Toxicol Clin Toxicol 2004;42:933–43.
56. Tenenbein M. Position statement: whole bowel irrigation. American Academy of Clinical Toxicology; European Association of Poisons Centres and Clinical Toxicologists. J Toxicol Clin Toxicol 1997;35:753–62.
64. Litovitz T, Schmitz BF. Ingestion of cylindrical and button batteries: an analysis of 2382 cases. Pediatrics 1992;89:747–57.
67. Bradberry S, Vale A. Dimercaptosuccinic acid (succimer; DMSA) in inorganic lead poisoning. Clin Toxicol 2009;47:617–31.
69. Yarema MC, Johnson DW, Berlin RJ, et al. Comparison of the 20-hour intravenous and 72-hour oral acetylcysteine protocols for the treatment of acute acetaminophen poisoning. Ann Emerg Med 2009;54:606–14.

113

Paediatric cardiopulmonary resuscitation

James Tibballs

Basic and advanced cardiopulmonary resuscitation (CPR) for infants and children are described. The essentials of resuscitation are presented in figures for the infant and child (**Fig. 113.1**) and for the newly born infant (**Fig. 113.2**). Recommendations are based on guidelines published by resuscitation organisations[1–3] that are derived from evaluation of the science of resuscitation by the International Liaison Committee on Resuscitation.[4]

This chapter is focused on medical and nursing personnel in hospital and complements Chapters 21 (Adult cardiopulmonary resuscitation) and 103 (The critically ill child). To add ability to knowledge, it is advisable to undertake a specialised paediatric cardiopulmonary resuscitation course, such as the Advanced Paediatric Life Support (APLS) or Paediatric Advanced Life Support (PALS) courses.

Distinctions within the term 'paediatric' are based on combinations of physiology, physical size and age. Some aspects of CPR are different for the 'newly born', infant, small (younger) child and large (older) child:

- *'newly born'* (newborn): the infant at birth or within several hours of birth
- *'infant'*: an infant outside the 'newly born' period and up to the age of 12 months
- *'small/young child'*: a child of preschool and early primary school from the age of 1–8 years
- *'large/older child'*: a child of late primary school from the age of 9 up to 14 years
- children older than 14 years may be treated as adults, but they do not have the same propensity for ventricular fibrillation as do adults.

EPIDEMIOLOGY

The causes of cardiopulmonary arrest (CPA) in infants and children are many and include any cause of hypoxaemia or hypotension, or both. Common causes are trauma (motor vehicle accidents, near-drowning, falls, burns, gunshot), drug overdose and poisoning, respiratory illness (asthma, upper-airway obstruction, parenchymal diseases), postoperative (especially cardiac), septicaemia and sudden infant death syndrome. As many as 10% of newly born infants require some form of resuscitation for varied conditions of which birth asphyxia is the most common.

PREVENTION

Cardiopulmonary arrest occurring in hospital may be preventable. Every institution which admits children should have a system to recognise deterioration, call for assistance and to provide rapid enhancement of the level of care, hence the use of medical emergency teams, rapid response teams and paediatric early warning scores.[5]

BASIC LIFE SUPPORT

ASSESSMENT OF AIRWAY AND BREATHING

If the child is not responsive to tactile and auditory stimulation, not breathing normally and not moving, the rescuer should assess the airway and breathing, which can be achieved in either the supine or lateral position. Obvious causes of airway obstruction in the pharynx should be removed. Fluids such as vomitus or blood should be aspirated with a Yankauer sucker. Solid or semi-solid objects such as food particles or foreign objects should be removed with an instrument (e.g. Magill's forceps). Since the most common cause of airway obstruction in an obtunded state is the tongue, first-aid manoeuvres to elevate it should be performed. These manoeuvres are backward head tilt, chin lift and jaw thrust. Head tilt and chin lift are often combined. If neck injury is present or suspected, neither the head tilt nor the chin lift manoeuvre should be used. Following establishment of an airway, the presence or absence of adequate breathing is assessed by inspection of movement of the chest and abdomen, and by listening and feeling for escape of exhaled air from the mouth and nose (look, listen and feel). If adequate breathing is occurring the patient should be placed on the side in a coma position.

RESCUE BREATHING (EXPIRED AIR RESUSCITATION)

If breathing is inadequate then expired air resuscitation or bag-(valve)-mask ventilation should be commenced

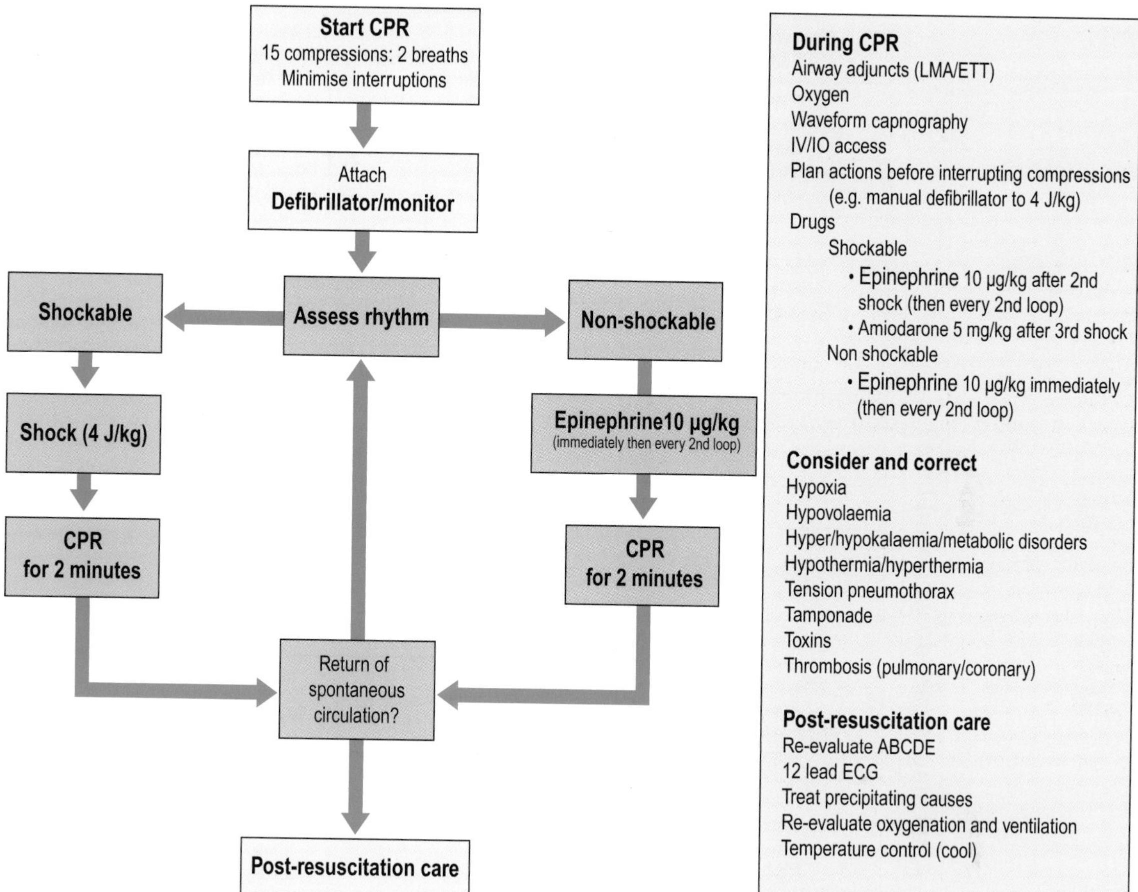

Figure 113.1 Advanced life support for infants and children. PEA=pulseless electrical activity; VF=ventricular fibrillation; VT=ventricular tachycardia. *(Reproduced with permission from the Australian Resuscitation Council, Melbourne.)*

immediately. Initially at least two breaths are recommended, but some guidelines suggest up to five. (There is no definitive evidence.) While maintaining the airway, administer slow breaths over 1–1.5 seconds to achieve adequate chest inflation. In children of all sizes, a mouth-to-mouth technique is possible by pinching the nostrils closed. In the newly born and infants, a mouth-to-mouth-and-nose technique is recommended, but if the rescuer has a small mouth then a mouth-to-nose technique is an alternative. Lack of chest rise may signify obstruction of the airway requiring repositioning of the head and neck.

ASSESSMENT OF CIRCULATION

If the child is unresponsive and not breathing, external cardiac compression (ECC) should be commenced immediately. Pulse by palpation may be performed, but the 'pulse check' has been removed from CPR guidelines for lay-persons because of their inability to reliably check the pulse, which may also be an issue for healthcare personnel. Palpation of any major pulse (carotid, brachial, femoral) is appropriate. If a pulse cannot be detected within 10 seconds or the rate is inadequate (<60 beats/min) then external cardiac compression (ECC) should be commenced.

EXTERNAL CARDIAC COMPRESSION (ECC)

Different techniques are used for infants and children of different sizes but in all patients the depth of compression is one-third the depth of their chest. For newly born infants and infants, two techniques are in common use. In the 'two-finger technique', the middle finger and forefinger are used. This technique is taught to lay-persons and is also the preferred technique for a single healthcare rescuer. With the better 'two-thumb technique', the hands encircle the thorax, approaching the

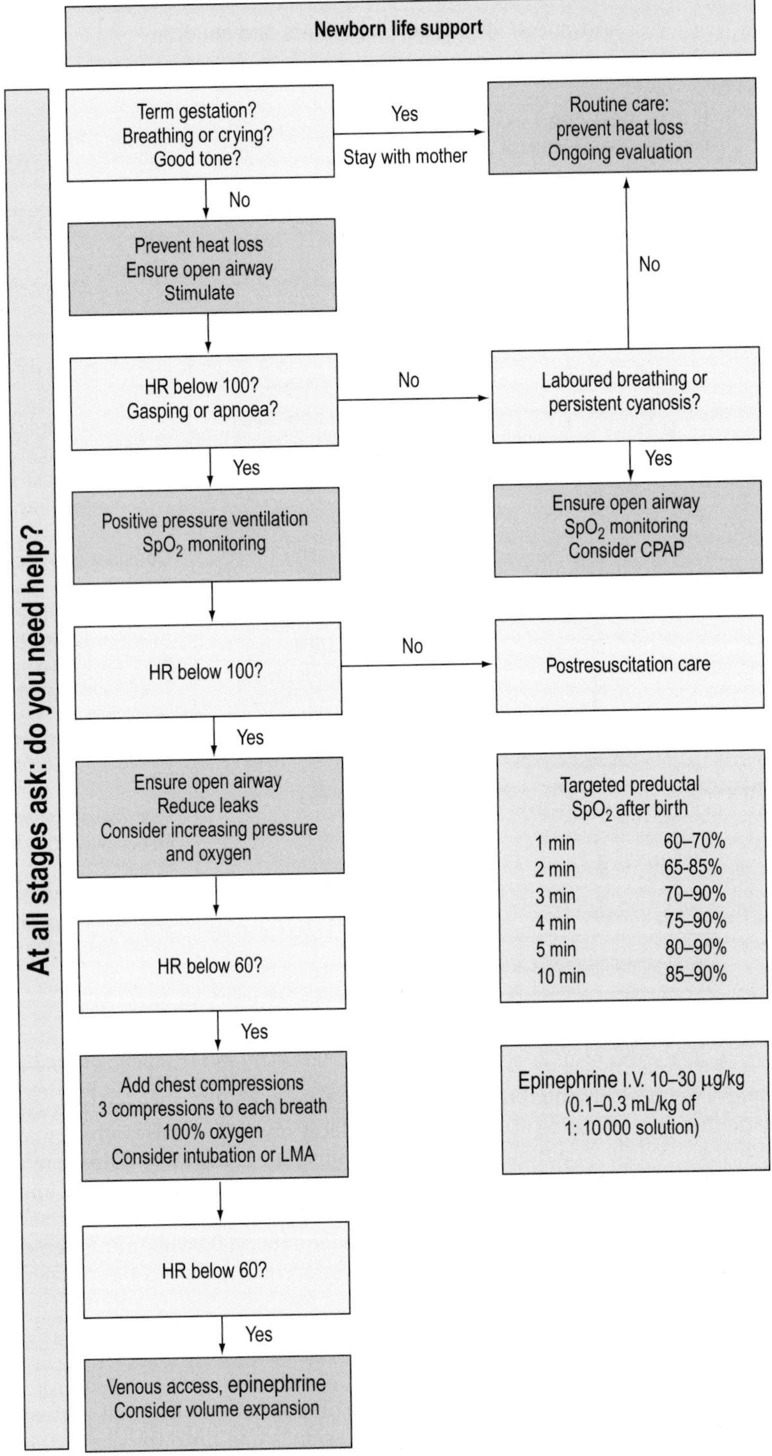

Figure 113.2 Newly born infant resuscitation. *(Reproduced with permission from the Australian Resuscitation Council, Melbourne.)*

chest from either above or below, and the thumbs are placed either opposite, alongside or atop one another. With this technique, the rescuer must take care to avoid restriction of the patient's chest during inflation. With premature newly born and small infants, the rescuer's encircling fingers may reach and stabilise the vertebral column without limiting chest inflation. With both techniques, the sternum is compressed above the xiphoid or about one fingerbreadth below the inter-nipple line.

Either a single hand or both hands may be used for infants and children as determined by the relationship between the size of the patient's chest and the hands of the rescuer. For young children, ECC can be performed with the heel of one hand. For older children, a bimanual technique as per adults may be used. In all ages, the 'centre of the chest' – which corresponds to the lower sternum – is compressed. Approximately 50% of each cycle should be compression. Every effort should be made to minimise 'hands-off' time (interruptions). This requires coordinated teamwork when, for example, ECC is paused to allow rhythm analysis or the application of DC shock.

RATES OF COMPRESSION AND RATIO OF COMPRESSION TO VENTILATION

In hospitals (two or more rescuers), the ratio of compression to ventilation for infants and children should be 15:2. Resuscitation may be commenced with either ventilations or compressions. After every 15 compressions, a pause should allow delivery of two ventilations whenever expired air resuscitation or any type of mask ventilation is given. ECC can be given during the second exhalation. The aim should be to achieve about 5 cycles per minute (i.e. about 75 compressions and 10 breaths per minute). If circulation returns, but respiration remains inadequate, the number of ventilations should be higher but care should be taken to avoid hypocarbia, which results in cerebral ischaemia. A sole healthcare rescuer may use the lay-person ratio of 30:2, aiming to achieve about 5 cycles in 2 minutes (i.e. about 75 compressions and 5 breaths per minute).

For infants and children, compressions should be delivered at a rate of 100/min (i.e. 1 compression every 0.6 seconds or approximately 2 per second). As ventilation is interposed between compressions, the actual compressions delivered will be less than 100 each minute. If the airway has been secured (e.g. by endotracheal intubation), strict coordination of compression and ventilation is not crucial; ventilation can be given against resistance imposed by chest compression. In this case about 100 compressions/minute will be achieved, but ventilation should be limited to about 10–12 per minute and wherever possible guided by arterial blood gas analysis. This low rate is all that is needed to match low cardiac output achieved during ECC. Excessive ventilation detracts from effectiveness of ECC and causes hypocarbia.

For newly born infants the total number of recommended 'events' per minute is 120, with the aim of achieving 90 compressions and 30 inflations each minute (i.e. in a ratio of 3:1). Beyond the newly born period (i.e. when the lungs have been inflated), the compression–ventilation ratio of 15:2 should be used.

ADVANCED LIFE SUPPORT

As soon as practicable, mechanical ventilation with added oxygen should be commenced with either a bag-mask or via endotracheal intubation. Although intubation is preferred (see below), valuable time should not be wasted in numerous unsuccessful attempts. Initial effective bag-mask ventilation is sufficient and necessary prerequisite for successful paediatric CPR. Bags of appropriate sizes should be available for infants, small children and large children. A bag of ~500 mL volume should be available for newly born infants. Insertion of an oropharyngeal (Guedel) airway may be necessary to facilitate bag-mask ventilation. Access to the circulation and display of the electrocardiograph and oximetry should also be achieved as soon as possible. Thereafter treatment should be guided by the cardiac rhythm. Underlying causes of CPA should be sought and treated.

AIRWAY MANAGEMENT

If attending personnel are skilled, the trachea should be intubated as soon as practicable. This establishes and maintains an airway, facilitates mechanical ventilation with 100% oxygen, minimises the risk of pulmonary aspiration, enables suctioning of the trachea and provides a route for the administration of selected drugs. If difficulty is experienced at initial intubation, oxygenation should be established with bag-mask ventilation before a re-attempt at intubation. Initial intubation should be via the oral route (not nasal), because oral intubation is invariably quicker than nasal, is less likely to cause trauma and haemorrhage, and enables the endotracheal tube to be more easily exchanged if the first choice is inappropriate. On the other hand, a tube placed nasally can be better affixed to the face and so is less likely to enter a bronchus or be subject to inadvertent extubation, and is preferred for transport and long-term management. A nasogastric tube should be inserted after intubation to relieve possible gaseous distension of the stomach sustained during bag-mask ventilation.

Correct placement of the endotracheal tube in the trachea must be confirmed. In the hurried conditions of emergency intubation at cardiopulmonary arrest, it is not difficult to mistakenly intubate the oesophagus or to intubate a bronchus. There is no substitute for:

- visualising the passage of the tip of the endotracheal tube through the vocal cords at intubation

- confirmation of bilateral pulmonary air entry by auscultation in the axillae
- continuous observation of bilateral rise and fall of the chest on ventilation
- observation of the patient becoming and remaining pink.

Immediately after intubation, tracheal placement of the tube should be confirmed by capnography or colorimetric CO_2 detection. The former is preferred because it also affords ongoing assessment of adequacy of ECC and ventilation as well as a continuous warning of accidental extubation. Excretion of CO_2 needs effective pulmonary blood flow and ventilation of the lungs. Failure to detect CO_2 while there is either spontaneous or ECC-generated cardiac output necessitates immediate exclusion of oesophageal intubation by direct laryngoscopic inspection. If the tube is correctly located in the trachea, and CO_2 is not detected or is low, ECC should be improved and hyperventilation, if occurring, limited. Oxygenation should be confirmed with use of a pulse oximeter or measurement of arterial gas tension.

Uncuffed tube sizes (internal diameter)

- 2.5 mm tube for a premature newborn <1 kg; 3.0 mm for infants 2.0–3.0 kg; 3.0 or 3.5 mm for infants >3.0 kg and up to age 6 months; 4 mm for infants 7 months to 1 year
- for children over 1 year, the size is approximately determined by the formula: size (mm)=age (years)/4+4.

Cuffed tube sizes (internal diameter)

- 3.0 mm for newborns ≥3 kg and ≤1 year; 3.5 mm for children 1–2 years
- for children over 2 years, the size is approximately determined by the formula: size (mm)=age (years)/4+3.5

Larger and smaller tubes should be available. The correct size should allow a small leak on application of moderate pressure but also ensure adequate pulmonary inflation. Cuffed tubes have the advantage of avoiding a change when deemed too small in a hazardous situation but occupy more volume in a small airway.

The tube is inserted a specific depth to avoid accidental extubation and endobronchial intubation, both of which may threaten oxygenation. Assessment of the depth of insertion at laryngoscopy is not reliable because this is performed with the neck extended and when the laryngoscope is removed the head assumes a position of neutrality or flexion with the depth of insertion increasing automatically. Whether oral or nasal intubation, on a chest X-ray taken with the head in neutral position, the tip of the tube should be at the interclavicular line. If not, its depth should be adjusted.

Appropriate initial depths of insertion measured from the centre of the lips for an oral tube are:

- 9.5 cm for a term newly born; 11.5 cm for a 6-month-old; 12 cm for a 1-year-old
- after 1 year of age the depth is given by the formula: depth (cm)=age (years)/2+12.

Appropriate initial depths of insertion measured at the nares for a nasal tube are:

- 11–11.5 cm for a term newly born; 13 cm for a 6-month-old; 14 cm for a 1-year-old
- after 1 year of age the depth is given by the formula: depth (cm)=age (years)/2+15.

Laryngeal mask airways (LMA) may be used to establish and maintain an airway in the spontaneously breathing patient and for emergency relief of upper airway obstruction, but they have a limited role during CPR. Their role in provision of mechanical ventilation remains uncertain. Like bag-mask ventilation, they do not protect the airway from aspiration. Although insertion of an LMA is easier to learn than endotracheal intubation, training should not replace mastery of bag-mask ventilation. An LMA is not suitable for long-term use or during transport when endotracheal intubation is preferred. Sizes are available to suit body weight (kg) of newborns, infants and children: <5 kg size 1, 5–10 kg size 1½, 10–20 kg size 2, 20–30 kg size 2½, 30–50 kg size 3, 50–70 kg size 4, 70–100 kg size 5, and >100 kg size 6.

ELECTROCARDIOGRAPH

The electrocardiograph (ECG) should be displayed with either leads or paddles. Drug therapy or immediate direct current (DC) shock is determined by the existing rhythm.

ACCESS TO THE CIRCULATION

Access to the circulation via a peripheral or central vein should be attempted immediately (depending on skill). Any site is acceptable. Visible or palpable peripheral veins are to be found on the dorsum of the hand, wrist, forearm, cubital fossa, chest wall, foot and ankle. In infants, scalp veins are accessible and the umbilical vein can be used up to about 1 week after birth. Although the external jugulars are usually distended and easily cannulated at CPR, this may be impeded by performance of intubation or bag-mask ventilation. Cannulation of femoral, subclavian or internal jugular veins is an option, but difficult and hazardous in this situation. Surgical cutdown onto a long saphenous, saphenofemoral junction or basilic vein is a valuable skill sometimes required in traumatic exsanguination. Any pre-existing functioning line can be used provided it does not contain any drug or electrolyte precipitating the CPA.

INTRAOSSEOUS INJECTION

If intravenous (i.v.) access cannot be achieved rapidly (within 60 seconds), intraosseous (i.o.) access should be obtained. This route has been used for patients of all ages and provides rapid, safe and reliable access to the circulation. It serves as an adequate route for any parenteral drug and fluid administration.

A metal needle with a trocar (e.g. disposable intraosseous needle; Cook, Illinois, USA) is preferable. Although many sites have been used for bone marrow injection, the easiest to identify is the anteromedial surface of the upper or lower tibia, especially in children less than 6 years. The site of the former is a few centimetres below the anterior tuberosity and the latter a few centimetres above the medial malleolus. The handle of the device needle is held in the palm of the hand while the fingers grip the shaft about a centimetre from the tip. It is inserted perpendicular to the bone surface and a rotary action is used to traverse the cortex. Sudden loss of resistance signifies entry to bone marrow. Correct positioning of the needle is confirmed by aspiration of bone marrow (which may be used for biochemical and haematological purposes) but that is not always possible. Bone injection guns (e.g. Wais Med Ltd), which propel a needle to a preset depth or drills (e.g. EZ-IO, Mayo Healthcare), enable easy intraosseous injection for infants, children and adults. The latter devices are preferred.

Volume expanders need to be given by syringe to achieve rapid restoration of circulating volume and rapid access of drugs to the central circulation. This is best achieved using a 10 mL syringe with a three-way tap in the i.v. tubing so that the i.o. needle does not become dislodged inadvertently.

Care should be exercised to avoid complications, particularly cutaneous extravasation, compartment syndrome of the leg and osteomyelitis. Contraindications include local trauma and infection.

ENDOTRACHEAL ADMINISTRATION OF DRUGS

Lipid-soluble drugs – epinephrine (adrenaline), atropine, lidocaine and naloxone – may be administered via the endotracheal tube if neither i.v. nor i.o. access is possible. Although the optimal doses of these drugs by this route are not known, work in animal models suggests doses should be 10 times the i.v. doses. The drugs should be diluted in normal saline up to 2 mL for infants, 5 mL for small children and 10 mL for large children. It is acceptable and simplest to squirt the drugs from the syringe (after removing the needle) directly into the endotracheal tube and disperse them throughout the respiratory tree with bagging. Neither sodium bicarbonate nor calcium salts should be administered via the tracheal route because they injure the airways.

DC SHOCK

Defibrillators should have paediatric paddles of cross-sectional area 12–20 cm^2 for use in children <10 kg body weight. For others, adult-sized paddles (50–80 cm^2) are satisfactory provided the paddles do not contact each other. Selectable energy levels should enable delivery of doses 0.5–4 J/kg. The closest level to the dose should be selected. One paddle is placed over the mid-axilla opposite the xiphoid or nipple, and the other to the right of the upper sternum below the clavicle. Conductive gel (confined to the area beneath the paddles) or gel pads and firm pressure are needed to deliver optimum energy to the heart without causing skin burns. The doses for monophasic and biphasic shock are the same.

In the treatment of refractory arrhythmias, equipment failure should be excluded. An anteroposterior position of the paddles (one over the cardiac apex, one over the left scapula) may be efficacious in refractory arrhythmia. Dextrocardia may be present with congenital heart disease and the position of the paddles should be altered accordingly.

Monophasic and biphasic automated external defibrillators (AEDs) with attenuated energy doses (approximately 50 J or less) may be used for children 1–8 years of age (approximately 10–25 kg). Adult energy doses of 150–200 J may be used in children older than 8 years of age or 25 kg body weight. Although AEDs are not recommended for use in infants as they may not reliably distinguish ventricular fibrillation from tachycardia and hence pose a risk of harmful DC shock, in the situation of a 'shockable' rhythm with poor or no cardiac output, an AED with dose attenuation may be used. If that is not available, an adult AED may be used.

Rescuers should be cognisant of the risk of inadvertent shock to themselves and colleagues during operation of defibrillators. They should ensure that they have no physical contact with the patient directly or indirectly at the time of electrical discharge. Surgical gloves provide minimal protection against shock. Paddles should be charged only when already placed on the chest of the patient. If the need to give DC shock abates while the paddles are charged, they should be disarmed before replacing them in their cradles.

TREATMENT OF SPECIFIC ARRHYTHMIAS

The following discussion of specific arrhythmias assumes that mechanical ventilation with oxygen and external cardiac compression has been commenced. The treatment of pulseless arrhythmias is summarised in **Figure 113.3**. Reversible causes of arrhythmias should be sought and treated during resuscitation. For example:

- *hypoxaemia or hypotension causing bradycardia:* may respond to ventilation
- *hypocalcaemia and toxicity caused by calcium channel blockade:* may be treated with calcium i.v. or i.o. (chloride 10% 0.2 mL/kg, gluconate 10% 0.7 mL/kg)

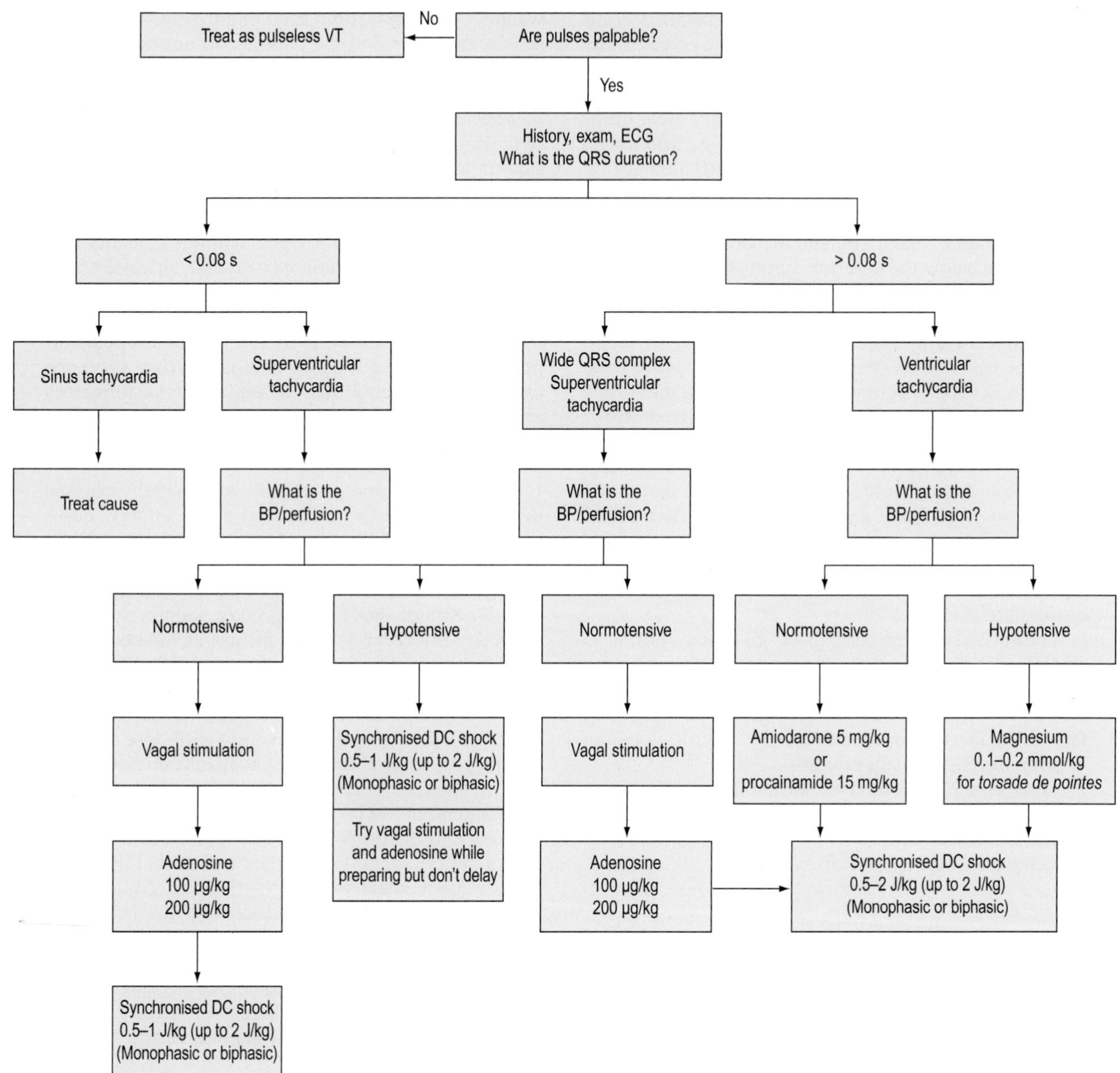

Figure 113.3 Treatment of tachyarrhythmias. *(Reproduced with permission from the Australian Resuscitation Council, Melbourne.)*

- *hyperkalaemia:* may be antagonised with a calcium salt then the serum level lowered with insulin (0.05 U/kg)+dextrose (0.5 g/kg), but beware of hypoglycaemia. Additional treatments of hyperkalaemia are salbutamol, sodium bicarbonate, hyperventilation or combinations.

All drugs should be flushed into the circulation with a small bolus of isotonic fluid. To prevent their inactivation, drugs should not be mixed together in the syringe or in infusion lines.

ASYSTOLE AND BRADYCARDIA

Asystole and hypotensive bradycardia (<60 beats/min) should be treated with epinephrine 10 μg/kg i.v. or i.o. If these routes are not available, epinephrine 100 μg/kg should be administered via endotracheal tube (ETT).

Unresponsive asystole should be treated with additional similar doses of epinephrine (10 μg/kg i.v., i.o.; 100 μg/kg ETT) every 3–5 minutes. Higher doses, up to 200 μg/kg i.v. or i.o., may be indicated in special circumstances (e.g. beta-blocker toxicity) but should not be used routinely as they have not altered outcome and predispose to complications (post-arrest myocardial dysfunction, hypertension, tachycardia). In newly born infants, the initial bolus dose is 100–300 μg/kg.

Recurrent bradycardia or asystole may require an infusion of epinephrine at 0.05–3 μg/kg per min: doses <0.3 μg/kg per min are predominantly beta adrenergic; doses >0.3 μg/kg per min are predominantly alpha adrenergic. Infuse into a secure large vein. If sinus rhythm cannot be restored, sodium bicarbonate 1 mmol/kg i.v. or i.o. may be helpful, but do not allow mixing with epinephrine since catecholamines are inactivated in alkaline solution.

Sinus bradycardia, sinus arrest with slow junctional or idioventricular rhythm, and atrioventricular block are the most common preterminal arrhythmias in paediatric practice. Untreated, bradycardia progresses to asystole. Bradycardia caused by vagal stimulation should be managed with cessation of the stimulus and/or atropine 20 μg/kg i.v. or i.o. (minimum dose 100 μg) but persistent vagal-mediated bradycardia should be treated with epinephrine 10 μg/kg i.v. or i.o.

If facilities are available, bradycardia may be treated with pacing (oesophageal, transcutaneous, transvenous, epicardial) if sinus node dysfunction or heart block exists, but it is not helpful in asystole.

VENTRICULAR FIBRILLATION AND PULSELESS VENTRICULAR TACHYCARDIA

The initial dose for ventricular fibrillation (VF) or pulseless ventricular tachycardia (VT) is a single unsynchronised DC shock of 4 J/kg followed by immediate resumption of ECC without pausing to analyse the rhythm. If VF or pulseless VT persists, subsequent single shocks of 4 J/kg are given, each followed by 2 minutes of ECC. Higher doses may be given in refractory VF.

Failure of VF to revert to sinus rhythm after the first shock should also be treated with epinephrine 10 μg/kg i.v. or i.o. or 100 μg/kg ETT every 3–5 minutes. Persistent (refractory) or recurrent VF or VT may also be treated with the antiarrhythmic drug amiodarone interspersed with single DC shocks. The dose of amiodarone is 5 mg/kg i.v. or i.o. as a bolus, which may be repeated to a maximum of 15 mg/kg. If amiodarone is not available, lidocaine in a dose of 1 mg/kg i.v. or i.o. or 2–3 mg/kg via ETT may be used, but the evidence for its efficacy is poor. An infusion of lidocaine at 20–50 μg/kg per min may be used to suppress excitability. Alternatives to epinephrine as a vasopressor, such as other catecholamines or vasopressin, have not been adequately investigated for use during CPR for children.

The witnessed (monitored) onset of VF or pulseless VT, such as in the cardiac catheter laboratory or intensive care unit setting, should be treated with successive (if needed) unsynchronised DC shocks up to a stack (salvo) of three shocks all of 4 J/kg. Rescuers should maintain the paddles on the chest and be prepared to deliver the series of the three shocks in quick succession, pausing only to verify the rhythm. Automatic external defibrillators are not suitable for this purpose because of time delays in their recognition of rhythms and charging. A precordial thump may be given before DC shock but its efficacy has not been proven.

Magnesium, 25–50 mg/kg (0.1–0.2 mmol/kg) i.v. or i.o., is indicated for polymorphic VT (*torsade de pointes*).

ELECTROMECHANICAL DISSOCIATION AND PULSELESS ELECTRICAL ACTIVITY

A normal ECG complex without pulse or circulation is called electromechanical dissociation (EMD). If untreated, the ECG initially deteriorates to an abnormal but still recognisable state when it is called pulseless electrical activity (PEA). Both conditions should be treated as for asystole and their causes ascertained and treated.

PULSATILE VENTRICULAR TACHYCARDIA

Haemodynamically stable VT may be treated with an antiarrhythmic agent such as amiodarone (5 mg/kg i.v. over 20–60 minutes) or procainamide (15 mg/kg i.v. over 30–60 minutes). Since both drugs prolong the QT interval, they should not be given together. If *torsade de pointes* is present, magnesium (25–50 mg/kg, 0.1–0.2 mmol/kg i.v. or i.o.) may be used. If cardioversion is needed, it should be synchronised at 0.5–2 J/kg under sedation/anaesthesia. Pulsatile VT may be difficult to distinguish from wide-complex supraventricular tachycardia (SVT) when its QRS duration is >0.08 seconds.

SUPRAVENTRICULAR TACHYCARDIA

Supraventricular tachycardia (SVT) is the most common spontaneous arrhythmia in childhood and infancy. It may cause life-threatening hypotension. It is usually re-entrant with a rate of 220–300/min in infants, less in children. The QRS complex is usually narrow (<0.08 seconds) making it difficult sometimes to discern from sinus tachycardia (ST). However, whereas ST is a part of other features of illness, SVT is a singular entity, and whereas the rate in ST is variable with activity or stimulation, it is uniform in SVT. In both rhythms, a P-wave may be discernible. SVT with aberrant conduction (QRS>0.08 seconds) may resemble VT. Relative treatment of these tachycardias is summarised in Figure 113.3.

If SVT is haemodynamically stable (adequate perfusion and blood pressure), initial treatment should be vagal stimulation. For infants and young children, application to the face of a plastic bag filled with iced water is often effective. Older children may be treated with carotid sinus massage or guided to perform a Valsalva (e.g. blowing through a narrow straw). If the patient is ventilated, apply vagal stimulation by tracheal or pharyngeal suction. If vagal stimulation is unsuccessful, give adenosine 100 μg/kg i.v. (maximum 6 mg) as a rapid bolus aided by an injection of 0.9% saline. If unsuccessful, double the dose to 200 μg/kg (maximum 12 mg) and again inject rapidly. An adenosine-induced pro-tachyarrhythmia (e.g. *torsade de pointes*) is rare.

An alternative drug treatment of haemodynamically stable SVT is amiodarone whose schedules are either infusions of 5 mg/kg over 1 hour followed by 5 μg/kg/min, or initially 25 μg/kg/min for 4 hours followed by 5–15 μg/kg/min. Amiodarone may cause hypotension, hypothyroidism and pulmonary toxicity. Other alternative drugs include procainamide in a dose of 15 mg/kg i.v. over 30–60 minutes, digoxin, a beta blocker or a calcium channel blocker. However, calcium channel blockers should not be used at all to treat SVT in infants and should be avoided or used with extreme caution in children because they may induce hypotension and cardiac depression. Haemodynamically stable SVT unresponsive to vagal stimulation and drug therapy may be treated with synchronised DC shock (cardioversion) in a dose of 0.5–1.0 J/kg.

SVT may cause severe hypotension or pulselessness, in which case synchronised DC shock (cardioversion) at 0.5–1.0 J/kg should be given immediately, progressing to 2 J/kg if necessary. While preparations are made to give DC shock, vagal stimulation and adenosine (i.v. or i.o.) may be tried provided they do not delay cardioversion.

POST-RESUSCITATION CARE

Supportive therapy should be provided until there is recovery of function of vital organs. This may require provision of oxygen therapy, mechanical ventilation, inotropic/vasopressor infusion, renal support, parenteral nutrition and other therapy for several days or longer. However, the percentage of inspired oxygen should be reduced as soon as possible after resuscitation to achieve only normal levels of Pa_{O_2}. Hyperoxaemia, like hypoxaemia, should be avoided. Recovery of infants and children is usually slow because cardiorespiratory arrest is often secondary to prolonged global ischaemia or hypoxaemia, which implies that other organs sustained damage before cardiorespiratory arrest. Particular care should be taken to ensure adequate cerebral perfusion with well-oxygenated blood. Hyperventilation is not useful for this purpose.

Therapeutic hypothermia post resuscitation (32–34°C) up to 3 days may improve neurological outcome, but is controversial and may predispose to infection and coagulopathy. However, an inadvertently hypothermic patient (e.g. one nearly drowned in icy water), provided the temperature is above 33°C, should not initially be actively warmed. During therapeutic hypothermia, shivering should be prevented with sedation and/or neuromuscular blockade, seizures should be actively sought and treated with anticonvulsant and the cause of the CPA should be investigated and treated appropriately (e.g. sepsis or drug overdose). Hyperthermia should be aggressively treated, in all instances.

Complications of CPR should be sought, especially if secondary deterioration occurs. A chest X-ray should be obtained to check the position of the endotracheal tube, to exclude pneumothorax, lung collapse, contusion or aspiration, and to check the cardiac silhouette – although an echocardiographic examination is preferable to specifically check contractility and to exclude a pericardial effusion. Measurements of haemoglobin, pH, gas tensions, electrolytes and glucose are important.

CESSATION OF CARDIOPULMONARY RESUSCITATION

Long-term outcome from paediatric CPR is mediocre, but better if arrest is respiratory alone or if CPA occurs in hospital. The decision to cease CPR should be based on a number of factors including the duration and quality of resuscitation, response to treatment, pre-arrest status, remediable factors, likely outcome if ultimately successful, opinions of personnel familiar with the patient and, whenever appropriate, the informed wishes of the parents. In general, unless hypothermia or drug toxicity exists, survival to normality is unlikely if there has been a failure to respond to full competent CPR after 30 minutes and several doses of epinephrine. In the newly born infant, discontinuation of treatment is appropriate if CPR does not establish a spontaneous circulation within 10–15 minutes. Family members should be kept informed, allowed to be present or asked if they want to be present during resuscitation.

POST-RESUSCITATION STAFF MANAGEMENT

Unfortunately, CPA occurring in hospital is often unexpected – for example, when a moribund patient arrives unannounced in the emergency department, a patient's condition deteriorates rapidly on the ward or when a mishap occurs under anaesthesia. These situations test the readiness, training, abilities and skills of individuals and the organisation of the institution. Performance should be audited with a view to improvement. These events have significant psychological impact on individuals and sensitive debriefing sessions should be encouraged.

Access the complete references list online at http://www.expertconsult.com

1. Australian Resuscitation Council and New Zealand Resuscitation Council. Guidelines 12.1-12.7. Online. Available: http://www.resus.org.au.
2. Kleinman ME, Chameides L, Schexnayder SM, et al. Part 14: pediatric advanced life support: 2010 American Heart Association Guidelines for Cardiopulmonary

Resuscitation and Emergency Cardiovascular Care. Circulation 2010;122:S876–908.
3. Biarent D, Bingham R, Eich C, et al. European Resuscitation Council Guidelines for Resuscitation 2010 Section 6. Paediatric Life Support. Resuscitation 2010; 81:1364–88.
4. Kleinman ME, de Caen AR, Chameides L, et al; Pediatric Basic and Advanced Life Support Chapter Collaborators. Part 10: Pediatric basic and advanced life support: 2010 International Consensus on Cardiopulmonary Resuscitation and Emergency Cardiovascular Care Science With Treatment Recommendations. Circulation 2010;122:S466–515.
5. Tibballs J. Systems to prevent in-hospital cardiac arrest. Paediatrics and Child Health 2011;21:322–8.

Appendix 1

Normal biochemical values

Refer to local reference range for site specific interpretation

I BLOOD CHEMISTRY

S=serum
P=plasma
HWB=heparin whole blood

α_1-Acid glycoprotein (S)		0.5–1.4 g/L
Aldosterone (S)	Supine:	140–530 pmol/L
	Erect:	220–970 pmol/L
Ammonia (P) to lab without delay		4–50 μmol/L
Amylase (S or P)		70–300 U/L
α_1-Antitrypsin (S or P)		2.1–4.0 g/L
Aspartate aminotransferase (AST) (P)		6–42 U/L
Bicarbonate (P)		22–32 mmol/L
Bilirubin (total) (S or P)		3–17 μmol/L
Bilirubin (direct) (S or P)		2–9 μmol/L
Caeruloplasmin (S or P)		0.20–0.60 g/L
Calcium (S or P)		2.25–2.65 mmol/L
Carotene (S or P)		1.0–4.8 μmol/L
Chloride (S or P)		98–108 mmol/L
Cholesterol (S or P)		3.1–6.5 mmol/L
Copper (S or P)		11–23 μmol/L
Cortisol (S or P)	8–9 a.m.	300–800 nmol/L
	4–5 p.m.	100–600 nmol/L
Creatinine (P)		50–120 μmol/L
Creatinine clearance		>1.3 mL/s
Creatinine kinase (P)		20–130 U/L
Creatinine kinase MB isoenzymes		<7 μg/L
Digoxin (S)	Toxic	>2 μg/L
Effective thyroxine ratio (ETR) (S)		0.90–1.09
FSH (S) Male		3–19 U/L
Female Follicular		5–20 U/L
Mid-cycle		15–30 U/L
Luteal		5–15 U/L
Postmenopausal		50–100 U/L
Glucose (fasting) (fluoride) (P)		3.9–6.2 mmol/L
γ-Glutamyl transferase (γ-GT) (P)	F	7–30 U/L
	M	10–50 U/L
Growth hormone (fasting, resting) (S)	M	<6 mU/L
	F	<16 mU/L
	Child	<10 mU/L
Insulin (fasting) (S)		3–28 mU/L
Iron (S or P) (1) Iron 8–10 a.m.	M	14–31 μmol/L
	F	11–29 μmol/L
(2) Iron-binding capacity	M	41–70 μmol/L
	F	37–77 μmol/L

Continued

Lactate (special collection)		0.3–1.3 mmol/L
LDH (S or P)		<80 U
Lead (HWB)		<2 μmol/L
Lithium (S) not plasma		0.8–1.2 mmol/L (therapeutic range)
Magnesium (S or P)		0.7–1.1 mmol/L
Oestriol (pregnancy) (S)		Depends on gestation
Osmolality (S or P)		275–295 mOsm/kg
Phosphatase		
A. Prostatic (S or P) (stabilise plasma with 5 mg/mL of $NaHSO_4$ or freeze)		0–4 U/L
B. Alkaline (S or P)		100–350 U/L
Phosphate (inorganic) (P)		0.8–1.4 mmol/L
Porphyrins (red cell) (HWB)		<1.2 μmol/L
Potassium (P)		3.4–5.0 mmol/L
Prolactin (S) (resting)		25 μg/L
Proteins		
A. (1) Total (S)		63–78 g/L
(2) Albumin (S)		35–45 g/L
B. Electrophoresis (S) not plasma:		
Albumin		35–45 g/L
α_1-Globulin		2–4 g/L
α_2-Globulin		5–9 g/L
β-Globulin		6–10 g/L
γ-Globulin		8–16 g/L
Pyruvate (special collection)		30–80 μmol/L
Renin (special tubes - keep blood cold)		
100–180 mmol Na intake:		
Supine (6 hours)		<0.58 ng/s/L
Upright (4 hours)		0.28–1.25 ng/s/L
Sodium (P)		134–146 mmol/L
Thyroxine (S)		60–150 nmol/L
Transferrin (S or P)		2.1–3.5 g/L
Triglyceride (fasting) (P)		1.80 mmol/L
Tri-iodothyronine (S)		1.3–2.9 nmol/L
Troponin T		<30 ng/L
TSH (S)		1–11 mU/L
Urea (P)		3.0–8.0 mmol/L
Uric acid (P)	M	0.18–0.48 mmol/L
	F	0.12–0.42 mmol/L
Zinc (P)		12–20 μmol/L

II URINE

AA=20 mL 50% acetate
d=24-hour collection
Sp= spot urine

Aldosterone (d, AA)		14–55 nmol/d
ALA (delta amino laevulinic acid) (Sp or d, AA)	Sp:	<50 μmol/L
	d:	10–50 μmol/d
Amylase (Sp or d, *no acid*)	Sp:	<900 U/L
	d:	100–1000 U/d
Calcium (d, AA)		<7.5 mmol/d

Continued

Catecholamines and derivatives (d, 20 mL 50% HCl):		
1. HMMA (VMA) Hydroxymethoxymandelic acid		<35 µmol/d
2. Metepinephrine		<5.6 µmol/d
3. Catecholamine		<1.6 µmol/d
Copper (d, AA)		<1.6 µmol/d
Coproporphyrin (collect 24-hour urine into 8 g sodium carbonate)		<245 nmol/d
Creatinine (d, AA)		10–20 mmol/d
5-Hydroxyindole-acetic acid (5-HIAA) (d, AA)		5–37 µmol/d
Hydroxyproline (d, AA)		<0.35 mmol/d (gelatin-free diet)
Indican (d, AA)		0.04–0.36 mmol/d
Lead (d, AA)		0.4 µmol/d
Magnesium (d, AA)		2.0–6.6 mmol/d
Melanin (fresh Sp)		Qualitative
Oestriol (in pregnancy) (d, AA)		50–160 µmol/d at 36 weeks' gestation
Osmolality (Sp)		300–1300 mOsm/kg
Oxalate (d, AA)		<300 µmol/d
Phosphorus (d, AA)		10–42 mmol/d
Porphobilinogen (fresh Sp)		Qualitative
Potassium (d or Sp, AA)		25–100 mmol/d
Protein (d or Sp, AA)		0.02–0.06 g/d
Sodium (d or Sp, AA)		40–210 mmol/d
Steroids (d, AA):		
1. 17-Oxosteroids	M	28–80 µmol/d
	F	14–60 µmol/d
2. 17-Hydroxy corticosteroids	M	14–70 µmol/d
	F	7–50 µmol/d
Urea (d or Sp, AA)		170–500 mmol/d
Uric acid (d, 8 g sodium carbonate)		<3.6 mmol/d (purine-free diet)
Urobilinogen (fresh Sp)		Qualitative
Uroporphyrin (collect as for coproporphyrin)		<50 nmol/d
Xylose absorption:		
Xylose excretion in 5 hours		>27 mmol
Plasma value at 2 hours		1.7–3.4 mmol/L

III FAECES

Fat (3-day collection)	<5 g/L
Porphyrins (single stool)	
Coproporphyrins	<30 nmol/g dry wt
Protoporphyrins	<135 nmol/g dry wt

IV CSF

Protein	0.15–0.45 g/L
Glucose	2.7–4.2 mmol/L
IgG	<0.05 g/L
IgG: total protein ratio	5–14%

Appendix 2

Système International (SI) units

BASIC SI UNITS / PREFIXES

Physical quantity	Name	Symbol	Factor	Name	Symbol	Factor	Name	Symbol
Length	Metre	m	10^{18}	Exa-	E	10^{-18}	Atto-	a
Mass	Kilogram	kg	10^{15}	Peta-	P	10^{-15}	Femto-	f
Time	Second*	s	10^{12}	Tera-	T	10^{-12}	Pico-	p
Electric current	Ampere	A	10^{9}	Giga-	G	10^{-9}	Nano-	n
Thermodynamic temperature	Kelvin	K	10^{6}	Mega-	M	10^{-6}	Micro-	µ
Luminous intensity	Candela	cd	10^{3}	Kilo-	k	10^{-3}	Milli-	m
Amount of substance	Mole	mol	10^{2}	Hecto-	h	10^{-2}	Centi-	c
			10^{1}	Deca-	da	10^{-1}	Deci-	d

*Minute (min), hour (h) and day (d) will remain in use although they are not official SI units.

DERIVED SI UNITS

Quantity	SI units	Symbol	Expression in terms of SI base units or derived units
Frequency	Hertz	Hz	1 Hz = 1 cycle/s (1 s^{-1})
Force	Newton	N	1 N = 1 kg.m/s^2 (1 kg.m.s^{-2})
Work, energy, quantity of heat	Joule	J	1 J = 1 N.m (1 kg.m^2.s^{-2})
Power	Watt	W	1 W = 1 J/s (1 J.s^{-1})
Quantity of electricity	Coulomb	C	1 C = 1 A.s
Electric potential, potential difference, tension, electromotive force	Volt	V	1 V = W/A (1 W.A^{-1})
Electric capacitance	Farad	F	1 F = 1 A.s/V (A.s.V^{-1})
Electric resistance	Ohm	W	1 W = 1 V/A (1 V.A^{-1})
Flux of magnetic induction, magnetic flux	Weber	Wb	1 Wb = 1 V.s
Magnetic flux density, magnetic induction	Tesla	T	1 T = 1 Wb/m^2 (1 Wb.m^{-2})
Inductance	Henry	H	1 H = 1 V.s/A (V.s.A^{-1})
Pressure	Pascal	Pa	1 Pa = 1 N/m^2 (1 N.m^{-2}) = 1 kg/m^2.s^2 (1 kg.m^{-2}.s^2)

The litre (L) (10^{-3} m^3 = dm^3), though not official, will remain in use as a unit of volume, as also will the dyne (dyn) as a unit for force (1 dyn = 10^{-5} N).

PRESSURE MEASUREMENTS

SI unit	Old unit	Conversion factors: Old to SI (exact)	Conversion factors: SI to old (approx.)
kPa	mmHg	0.133	7.5
kPa	1 standard atmosphere (approx. 1 Bar)	101.3	0.01
kPa	cmH_2O	0.0981	10
kPa	lb/sq in	6.894	0.145

HAEMATOLOGY

Measurement	SI unit	Old unit	Conversion factors: Old to SI	Conversion factors: SI to old
Haemoglobin (Hb)	g/dL	g/100 mL	Numerically	equivalent
Packed cell volume	No unit*	Per cent	0.01	100
Mean cell Hb concentration	g/dL	Per cent	Numerically	equivalent
Mean cell Hb	pg	µug	Numerically	equivalent
Red cell count	Cells/litre	Cells/mm^3	10^6	10^{-6}
White cell count	Cells/litre	Cells/mm^3	10^6	10^{-6}
Reticulocytes	Per cent	Per cent	Numerically	equivalent
Platelets	Cells/litre	Cells/mm^3	10^6	10^{-6}

*Expressed as decimal fraction.

PH	$[H^+]$
pH	nmol/litre
6.80	158
6.90	126
7.00	100
7.10	79
7.20	63
7.25	56
7.30	50
7.35	45
7.40	40
7.45	36
7.50	32
7.55	28
7.60	25
7.70	20

Appendix 3

Respiratory physiology symbols and normal values

SYMBOLS

Primary		Secondary symbols for gas phase	
C	Concentration of gas in blood	A	Alveolar
F	Fractional concentration in dry gas	B	Barometric
f	Frequency of respiration (breaths/min)	D	Dead space
P	Pressure or partial pressure	E	Expired
Q	Volume of blood	I	Inspired
$\dot{Q}$	Volume of blood per unit time	L	Lung
R	Respiratory exchange ratio	T	Tidal
S	Saturation of haemoglobin with O_2	*Secondary symbols for blood phase*	
$\dot{V}$	Volume of gas per unit time	a	arterial
		c	capillary
		ć	end-capillary
		i	ideal
		v	venous
		$\bar{v}$	mixed venous

– above any symbol denotes a mean value.
· above any symbol denotes a value per unit time.

NORMAL VALUES

1. **Blood**
   (a) *Arterial*

pH	:	7.36–7.44	(H^+=44–36 nmol/L)
PaO	:	85–100 mmHg	(11.3–13.3 kPa)
$PaCO_2$	:	36–44 mmHg	(4.8–5.9 kPa)
O_2 content	:	20–21 vols%	(8.9–9.4 nmol/L)
CO_2 content	:	48–50 vols%	(21.6–22.5 nmol/L)

   (b) *Venous*

pH	:	7.34–7.42	(H^+=38–46 nmol/L)
PO_2	:	37–42 mmHg	(5–5.6 kPa)
PCO_2	:	42–50 mmHg	(5.6–6.7 kPa)
O_2 content	:	15–16 vols%	(6.7–7.2 mmol/L)
CO_2 content	:	52–54 vols%	(23.3–24.2 mmol/L)

2. **Gases**
   (a) *Inspired air*

O_2	:	20.93%	
PI_{O_2}	:	149 mmHg	(19.9 kPa)
N_2	:	79.04%	
PI_{N_2}	:	563 mmHg	(75 kPa)
CO_2	:	0.03%	

   (b) *Expired air*

O_2	:	16–17%	
PE_{O_2}	:	113–121 mmHg	(15–16 kPa)
N_2	:	80%	
PE_{N_2}	:	579 mmHg	(77 kPa)
CO_2	:	3–4%	
PE_{CO_2}	:	21–28 mmHg	(2.8–3.7 kPa)

3. **Ventilation:perfusion**
   (a) *Alveolar–arterial oxygen gradient:*
   5–20 mmHg (0.7–2.7 kPa) breathing air
   25–65 mmHg (3.3–8.6 kPa) breathing 100% oxygen
   (b) *Venous admixture* ($\dot{Q}_S:\dot{Q}_T$): 5% of cardiac output
   (c) *Right to left physiological shunt*: 3% of cardiac output
   (d) *Anatomical dead space*: 2 mL/kg body weight
   (e) *Dead space:tidal volume ratio* $V_D:V_T$): 0.25–0.4 or 33+(Age/3) percent
4. **Lung volumes**
   Approximate values in adults are listed. Values are less in smaller subjects and in females.

Tidal volume	:	400 mL or 6 mL/kg
Inspiratory capacity	:	3.6 litres
Inspiratory reserve volume	:	3.1 litres
Expiratory reserve volume	:	1.2 litres
Functional residual capacity	:	2.4 litres
Residual volume	:	1.2 litres
Total lung capacity	:	6.0 litres
Vital capacity	:	4.8 litres

   or 2.5 L/sq m body surface *or* 2.5 L/m height in males
   2.0 L/sq m body surface *or* 2.0 L/m height in females
   or 65–75 mL/kg
5. **Lung mechanics**

(a) *Peak expiratory flow rate*	:	450–700 L/min (males)	
	:	300–500 L/min (females)	
(b) *Forced expiratory volume in 1 second* (FEV_1)	:	70–83% of vital capacity	
(c) *Compliance* (approximate values)			
(i) Lung compliance (CL)		*Static*	*Dynamic*
conscious (erect)	:	200 mL/cmH_2O	180 mL/cmH_2O
paralysed anaesthetised (supine)*	:	160 mL/cmH_2O	80 mL/cmH_2O
(ii) Chest wall compliance (CCW)	:	200 mL/cmH_2O	
(iii) Total compliance (CT):			
conscious (erect)	:	150 mL/cmH_2O	100 mL/cmH_2O
paralysed anaesthetised (supine)*	:	74 mL/cmH_2O	56 mL/cmH_2O
(d) *Airways resistance*:			
conscious	:	0.6–3.2 cmH_2O/L per second	
sedated, partially paralysed and ventilated (includes resistance of endotracheal tube and catheter mount)	:	5–10 H_2O/L per second	

   (e) *Work of breathing*: 0.3–0.5 kg m/min
   or oxygen consumption of 0.5–1 mL/L ventilation

*Compliance values would be lower for the sedated, partially paralysed, ventilated patient in the intensive care unit, i.e. effective dynamic compliance=40–50 mL/cmH_2O.

6. **Cardiovascular** – pressures in kPa are given within brackets
   (a) Cardiac index : 2.5–3.6 L/min per m^2
   (b) Stroke volume : 42–52 mL/m^2
   (c) Ejection fraction : 0.55–0.75
   (d) End-diastolic volume : 75±15 mL/m^2
   (e) End-systolic volume : 25±8 mL/m^2
   (f) Left ventricular stroke work index : 30–110 g-m/m^2
   (g) Left ventricular minute work index : 1.8–6.6 kg-m/min per m^2
   (h) Oxygen consumption index : 110–150 mL/L
   (i) Right atrial pressure : 1–7 mmHg (0.13–0.93)
   (j) Right ventricular systolic pressure : 15–25 mmHg (2.0–3.3)
   (k) Right ventricular diastolic pressure : 0–8 (0–1)
   (l) Pulmonary artery systolic pressure : 15–25 mmHg (2.0–3.3)
   (m) Pulmonary artery diastolic pressure : 8–15 mmHg (1–2)
   (n) Pulmonary artery mean pressure : 10–20 mmHg (1.3–2.7)
   (o) Pulmonary capillary wedge pressure : 6–15 mmHg (0.8–2.0)
   (p) Systemic vascular resistance : 770–1500 dyne-s/cm^5
   : 77–150 kPa-s/L
   (q) Pulmonary vascular resistance : 20–120 dyne-s/cm^5
   : 2–12 kPa-s/L

Appendix 4

Physiological equations

RESPIRATORY EQUATIONS

(a) *Oxygen consumption* (250 mL/min)
Oxygen consumption=amount of oxygen in inspired gas minus amount in expired gas

i.e. $\dot{V}O_2 = (\dot{V}I \times FI_{O_2}) - (\dot{V}E \times FE_{O_2})$

(b) *Carbon dioxide production* (200 mL/min)
Volume CO_2 eliminated in expired gas=expired gas volume×CO_2 concentration in mixed expired gas

i.e. $\dot{V}CO_2 = \dot{V} \times F\bar{E}_{CO_2}$

As expired volume is made up of alveolar and dead space gas,

$$\dot{V}CO_2 = (\dot{V}A \times FA_{CO_2})(\dot{V}D \times FI_{CO_2})$$

As Fi_{CO_2} is negligible, especially if there is no rebreathing,

$$\dot{V}CO_2 = \dot{V}A \times FA_{CO_2}$$

or

$$FA_{CO_2} = \frac{\dot{V}CO_2}{\dot{V}A}$$

or

$$PA_{CO_2}(\text{mmHg}) = \frac{\dot{V}_{CO_2}(\text{mL/min STPD})}{\dot{V}A(\text{L/min BTPS})} \times 0.863$$

or

$$PA_{CO_2}(\text{kPa}) = \frac{\dot{V}_{CO_2}(\text{mmol/min})}{\dot{V}A(\text{L/min BTPS})} \times 2.561$$

STPD: Standard temperature (0°C) and pressure (760 mmHg or 101.35 kPa) dry gas
BTPS: Body temperature and ambient pressure, saturated with water vapour

(c) *Physiological dead space*

Bohr's equation, $\frac{V_D}{V_T} = \frac{PA_{CO_2} - P\bar{E}_{CO_2}}{PA_{CO_2}}$

or

$$\frac{V_D}{V_T} = \frac{Pa_{CO_2} - P\bar{E}_{CO_2}}{Pa_{CO_2}}$$

(d) *Alveolar oxygenation*

$$PA_{O_2} = PI_O - \frac{Pa_{CO_2}}{R}$$

where R is the respiratory quotient (normally 0.8).

$$PA_{O_2} = PI_{O_2} - Pa_{CO_2}\left(\frac{PI_{O_2} - P\bar{E}_{O_2}}{P\bar{E}_{CO_2}}\right)$$

or $$PA_{O_2} = PI_{O_2} - PA_{CO_2}\left(\frac{FI_{O_2} + 1 - FI_{O_2}}{R}\right)$$

when $FI_{O_2} = 1.0$ (patient breathing 100% oxygen),

then $PA_{O_2} = (PB - \text{saturated water vapour pressure}) - PA_{CO_2}$

$= (PB - 47) - Pa_{CO_2}$

(e) *Venous admixture*

$$\frac{\dot{Q}_S}{\dot{Q}_T} = \frac{C\acute{c}_{O_2} - Ca_{O_2}}{Cc'_{O_2} - C\overline{v}_{O_2}}$$

$$= \frac{(PA_{O_2} - Pa_{O_2}) \times 0.0031}{CaO_2 + (PA_{O_2} - Pa_{O_2}) \times 0.0031 - C\overline{v}_{O_2}}$$

$$= \frac{(PA_{O_2} - Pa_{O_2}) \times 0.0031}{(PA_{O_2} - Pa_{O_2}) \times 0.0031 + 5} \text{ (simplified)}$$

(f) *Fractional inspired oxygen concentration*

$$Fi_{O_2} = \frac{O_2 \text{ flow in L/min} + (\text{air flow in L/min} \times 0.21)}{\text{Total } O_2 + \text{air flow in L/min}}$$

(g) *Henderson–Hasselbalch equation*

$$\text{pH} = \text{pKA} + \log\frac{(\text{HCO}_3^-)}{(\text{CO}_2)}$$

$$\text{pH} = 6.1 + \log\frac{(\text{HCO}_3^- \text{ in mmol/L})}{(PCO_2 \text{ in mmHg}) \times 0.03}$$

$$[\text{H}^+]\,\text{nmol/L} = 24 \times \frac{(PCO_2 \text{ in mmHg})}{(\text{HCO}_3^- \text{ in mmol/L})}$$

$$[\text{H}^+]\,\text{nmol/L} = 180 \times \frac{(PCO_2 \text{ in kPa})}{(\text{HCO}_3^- \text{ in mmol/L})}$$

CARDIOVASCULAR EQUATIONS

(a) *Mean blood pressure* (BP) = DBP + ⅓ (SBP − DBP)
(b) *Rate pressure product* (RPP) = P × SBP
(c) *Body surface area* (BSA) in $m^2 = (\text{Ht})^{0.725} \times (\text{Wt})^{0.425} \times 71.84 \times 10^{-4}$
(d) **Cardiac index* (CI) $= \frac{\text{CO}}{\text{BSA}}$ = mL/min per m^2
(e) *Stroke volume* (SV) $= \frac{\text{CO}}{P}$ = mL/beat
(f) **Stroke volume index* (SVI) $= \frac{\text{SV}}{\text{BSA}}$ = mL/beat per m^2
(g) **Left ventricular stroke work index* (LVSWI) = (BP − PCWP) (SVI) (0.0136) = g-m/m^2 per beat
(h) *Systemic vascular resistance* (SVR) $= \frac{\text{BP} - \text{RAP}}{\text{CO}}$ resistance units

(Multiply × 79.9 to convert to absolute resistance units, dynes-s cm^{-5})

(i) *Pulmonary vascular resistance* (PVR) $= \frac{\text{PAP} - \text{PCWP}}{\text{CO}}$ resistance units

(Multiply × 79.9 to convert to absolute resistance units, dynes-s cm^{-5})

(j) *Left ventricular pre-ejection period* (PEP) = QS_2 − LVET m s
(k) *Other systolic time index ratios* may easily be calculated:

$$\frac{1}{PEP^2} \text{ and } \frac{PEP}{LVET}$$

*For interpatient comparisons and reference standards, the 'index' term, output normalised to body surface, may be used when:

SBP = systolic blood pressure in mmHg
DBP = diastolic blood pressure in mmHg
P = heart rate in beats/min
Ht = height in cm
Wt = weight in kg
CO = cardiac output in mL/min
PCWP = pulmonary capillary wedge pressure in mmHg
RAP = right atrial pressure in mmHg
PAP = mean pulmonary artery pressure in mmHg
LVET = left ventricular ejection time in m s
QS_2 = total electromechanical systole in m s.

RENAL EQUATIONS

(a) *Standard creatinine clearance* (mL/min/1.73 m²)

$$= \frac{\text{urine creatinine (mmol/L)}}{\text{serum creatinine (mmol/L)}} \times \text{urine volume (mL/min)} \times \frac{1.73}{\text{body surface area (m}^2\text{)}}$$

(b) *Per cent filtered Na^+ excreted*

$$= \frac{\text{urine Na}^+ \text{ (mmol/L)}}{\text{serum Na}^+ \text{ (mmol/L)}} \times \frac{\text{serum creatinine (mmol/L)}}{\text{urine creatinine (mmol/L)}} \times 100$$

(c) *Free water clearance* (mL/min)

$$= \text{urine volume (mL/min)} - \frac{\text{urine osmolality (mOsm/kg)}}{\text{plasma osmolality (mOsm/kg)}} \times \text{urine volume (mL/min)}$$

(d) *Additional calculated parameters*:

(i) $\frac{\text{urine}}{\text{plasma}}$ osmolality ratio

(ii) $\frac{\text{urine}}{\text{serum}}$ creatinine ratio

(iii) $\frac{\text{blood urine}}{\text{serum creatinine}}$ ratio

(iv) $\frac{\text{urine}}{\text{plasma}}$ urea ratio

(v) urinary Na^+ and K^+ excretion (mmol)

(vi) $\frac{\text{urinary Na}^+}{\text{urinary K}^+}$ ratio

Appendix 5

Plasma drug concentrations and American nomenclature

Refer to local laboratory reference range for site specific values

PLASMA DRUG LEVELS

Drug	Normal or therapeutic concentration mg/L	Toxic concentration mg/L	Lethal or potentially lethal concentration mg/L
Acetazolamide	10–15	–	–
Acetohexamide	21–56	–	–
Acetone	–	200–300	550
Aluminium	0.13	–	–
Aminophylline (theophylline)	10–20	20	–
Amitriptyline	50–200 μg/L	400 μg/L	10–20
Amphetamine	20–30 μg/L	–	2
Arsenic	0.0–20 μg/L	1.0	15
Barbiturates			
Short-acting	1	7	10
Intermediate-acting	1–5	10–30	30
Phenobarbital	15	40–70	80–150
Benzene	–	Any measurable	0.94
Beryllium	Tissue levels generally used (lung and lymph)	–	–
Boric acid	0.8	40	50
Bromide	50	0.5–1.5 g/L	2 g/L
Brompheniramine	8–15 μg/L	–	–
Cadmium	0.1–0.2 μg/L	50 μg/L	–
Caffeine	–	–	100
Carbamazepine	6–12	12	–
Carbon monoxide	1% saturation of Hb	15–35% saturation of Hb	50% saturation of Hb
Carbon tetrachloride	–	20–50	–
Chloral hydrate	10	100	250
Chlordiazepoxide	1.0–2.0	6	20
Chloroform	–	70–250	390
Chlorpromazine	0.3	1–2	3–12
Chlorpropamide	30–140	–	–
Codeine	25 μg/L	–	–

Continued

Drug	Normal or therapeutic concentration mg/L	Toxic concentration mg/L	Lethal or potentially lethal concentration mg/L
Copper	1–1.5	5.4	—
Cyanide	0.15	—	5
DDT	13 µg/L	—	—
Desipramine	0.59–1.4	—	10–20
Dextropropoxyphene	50–200 µg/L	5–10	57
Diazepam	0.5–2.5	5–20	50
Dieldrin	1.5 µg/L	—	—
Digitoxin	20–35 µg/L	—	320 µg/L
Digoxin	1–2 µg/L	2–9 µg/L	—
Dinitro-*o*-cresol	—	30–40 µg/L	75
Diphenhydramine	5	10	—
Disopyramide	3–7	—	—
Ethosuximide	40–80	—	—
Ethyl chloride	—	—	400
Ethylene glycol	—	1.5 g/L	2–4 g/L
Fluoride	0.5	—	2
Gentamicin trough level	<2	>2	—
Glutethimide	1–5	10–30	30–100
Gold (sodium aurothiomalate)	3–6	—	—
Hydrogen sulphide	—	—	0.92
Hydromorphone (dihydromorphinone)	—	—	0.1–0.3
Imipramine	0.1–0.3	0.7	2
Iron	500 (erythrocytes)	6 (serum)	—
Lead	0.05–1.3	1.3	—
Lidocaine	2–4	6	—
Lithium	0.8–1.2 mmol/L	1.5 mmol/L	4 mmol/L
LSD (lysergic acid diethylamide)	—	1–4 µg/L	—
Magnesium	0.7–1.1 mmol/L	—	—
Manganese	0.15	4.6	—
Meprobamate	10	100	200
Mercury	60–120 µg/L	—	—
Mesuximide	2.5–7.5	—	—
Methadone	480–860 µg/L	2	4
Methanol	—	200	890
Methapyrilene	2 µg/L	30–50	50
Methaqualone	1–2	5–30	30
Methylamphetamine	—	5	40
Methyprylon	10	30–60	100
Mexiletine	0.6–2.5	—	—
Morphine	0.1	—	0.5–4
Nickel	0.41	—	—
Nicotine	—	10	5–52
Nitrofurantoin	1.8	—	—
Nortriptyline	50–200 µg/L	400 µg/L	10–20
Orphenadrine	—	2	4–8

Continued

Drug	Normal or therapeutic concentration mg/L	Toxic concentration mg/L	Lethal or potentially lethal concentration mg/L
Oxalate	2	–	10
Papaverine	1	–	–
Paracetamol (Refer to paracetamol nomogram for time-dependent interpretation and treatment)	5–25	30	250 at 4 hours, 50 at 12 hours
Paraldehyde	50	200–400	500
Paramethoxyamphetamine (PMA)	–	–	2–4
Pentazocine	0.1–1	2–5	10–20
Perphenazine	–	1	–
Pethidine	600–650 μg/L	5	30
Phenacetin	5–25	30	400
Phencyclidine	–	0.5	1
Phensuximide	10–19	–	–
Phenylbutazone	100	–	–
Phenytoin (Dilantin)	8–20	30	100
Phosphorus	Concentration in tissues usually used	–	–
Primidone	10	50–80	100
Probenecid	100–200	–	–
Procainamide	3–8	10	–
Prochlorperazine	–	1	–
Promazine	–	1	–
Propoxyphene	0.1–1	5–20	57
Propranolol	0.025–0.1	–	8–12
Propylhexedrine	–	–	2–3
Quinidine	3–6	10	30–50
Quinine	–	–	12
Salicylate (acetylsalicylic acid)	100–350	350–400	500
Strychnine	–	2	9–12
Sulfadiazine	80–150	–	–
Sulfaguanidine	30–50	–	–
Sulfafurazole	90–100	–	–
Sultiame	4–10	–	–
Theophylline	10–20	20	–
Thioridazine	1–1.5	10	20–80
Tin	0.12	–	–
Tobramycin trough level	<2	>2	–
Tolbutamide	53–96	–	–
Toluene	–	–	10
Tribromoethanol	–	–	90
Tricyclics	50–200 μg/L	400 μg/L	10–20
Trimethobenzamide	1.0–2.0	–	–
Valproate	50–100	–	–
Warfarin	0.8–2.4	–	–
Zinc	0.68–1.36	–	–
Zoxazolamine	3–13	–	–

AMERICAN NOMENCLATURE

INN (BAN)	USAN
Epinephrine (adrenaline)	Epinephrine
Cinchocaine	Dibucaine
Deferoxamine (sesferrioxamine)	Deferoxamine
Dextropropoxyphene	Propoxyphene
Dihydromorphinone	Hydromorphone
Ergometrine	Ergonovine
Hyoscine	Scopolamine
Isoproterenol (isoprenaline)	Isoproterenol
Meclozine	Meclizine
Mepivacaine	Carbocaine
Methylamphetamine	Methamphetamine
Norepinephrine (noradrenaline)	Norepinephrine, levarterenol
Orciprenaline	Metaproterenol
Oxybuprocaine	Benoxinate
Paracetamol	Acetaminophen
Pethidine	Meperidine
Salbutamol	Albuterol

FURTHER READING

Davies DS, Prichard BNC. Biological Effects of Drugs in Relation to their Plasma Concentrations. London: Macmillan; 1973.

Koch-Weser J. Serum drug concentrations as therapeutic guides. N Engl J Med 1972;287:227–31.

Koch-Weser J. The serum level approach to individualization of drug dosage. Eur J Clin Pharm 1975;9:1–8.

Richens A, Warrington S. When should plasma drug levels be monitored? Curr Ther 1979;20:167–85.

Winek CL. Tabulation of therapeutic, toxic and lethal concentrations of drugs and chemicals in blood. Clin Chem 1976;22:832–6.

Appendix 6

Confirmation of intubation

This is a frequently performed procedure in anaesthesia, in the ICU and in a wide range of emergency situations with very variable availability of sophisticated equipment. It is also the cause of significant morbidity and mortality.

This is a simple checklist that can be modified depending on the equipment available.

Always:

- *Visualise:* the passage of the tip of the endotracheal tube through the vocal cords at intubation, where possible (most reliable but not perfect)
- *Observe:* continuous observation of rise and fall of the chest on ventilation
- *Auscultate:* confirm air entry by auscultation in the axillae and also listen over the stomach. The axillae will confirm bilateral air entry (and indicate endobronchial intubation if air entry is unilateral). Auscultation over the stomach will allow differential breath sounds between axillae and stomach and may indicate oesophageal tube placement if the stomach sounds are louder
- *Observe the patient's colour:* it should remain pink.

Equipment should be available that will also assist includes:

- *Capnography:* CO_2 in the exhaled air is a reliable indicator of correct tube placement. Capnography should always be available for anaesthesia and certainly for transfer of critically ill patients. Ideally, it should be easily available in any ICU
- *Oximetry:* helps to confirm oxygenation.

Of these, visualisation and capnography are most reliable for intubation, but all have a part to play and anyone intubating a patient must have a checklist to confirm correct placement.

'If in doubt, take it out.' Sometimes some of the four basic signs are unconvincing, but if there is any doubt the tube should be replaced or mouth-to-mouth/mask ventilation should be used.

Appendix 7

Parameters monitored and measured by the PiCCO monitor

New non-invasive monitors have introduced some new 'measurements' into clinical practice.

Parameter normal value	Symbol
Pulse contour cardiac output/index CI 3.0–5.0 L/min per m^2 Pulse contour cardiac output is calibrated by means of a simple transcardiopulmonary thermodilution measurement	PCCO/PCCI
Global end-diastolic volume/index 680–800 mL/m^2 (indexed) The total end-diastolic volume of all four chambers of the heart	GEDV/I
Intrathoracic blood volume/index 850–1000 mL/m^2 (indexed) The global end-diastolic volume plus the pulmonary blood volume	ITBV/I
Extravascular lung water/index 3.0–7.0 mL/kg (indexed) Quantifies lung status in terms of pulmonary permeability	EVLW/I
Cardiac function index 4.5–6.5 L/min (indexed) CO/GEDV = preload independent variable of heart function	CFI
Stroke volume/index 40–60 mL/m^2	SV/I
Stroke volume variation <10% Percentage difference of biggest to smallest stroke volumes over the last 30 seconds	SVV
Left ventricular contractility 1200–2000 mmHg/s (159.6–266 kPa/s) Maximum velocity of blood pressure curve corresponds to maximum power or contractility of the left heart	dP/dt_{max}
Systemic vascular resistance/index 1200–2000 dyn/s/cm^{-5} per m^2 (indexed)	SVR/SVRI

EVLW: There are two mechanisms by which the EVLW may be raised: increased intravascular filtration pressure (left heart failure, volume overload), and increased pulmonary vascular permeability as in endotoxic shock and sepsis. There is a direct relationship between the mortality of intensive care patients with acute respiratory distress syndrome and high extravascular lung water.

SVV: Large variations in stroke volume are an indication of reduced intravascular volume (also atrial fibrillation, heart valve disease).

Appendix 8

Mortality/dysfunction risk scores and models

PAEDIATRIC RISK OF MORTALITY (PRISM) SCORE

Mortality risk assessment.

Parameter	Age limit	Ranges		Points
Systolic blood pressure		(mmHg)	(kPa)	
	Infants	130–160	17.3–21.3	2
		55–65	7.3–8.7	2
		>160	>21.3	6
		40–54	5.3–7.2	6
		<40	<5.3	7
	Children	150–200	20–26.7	2
		65–75	8.7–10	2
		>200	>26.7	6
		50–64	6.7–8.5	6
		<50	<6.7	7
Diastolic blood pressure		(mmHg)	(kPa)	
	All ages	>110	>14.6	6
Heart rate (beats/min)	Infants	>160		4
		<90		4
	Children	>150		4
		<80		4
Respiratory rate (breaths/min)	Infants	61–90		1
		>90		5
		Apnoea		5
	Children	51–70		1
		>70		5
		Apnoea		5
$Pa_{O_2} : Fi_{O_2}$ ratio		(mmHg)	(kPa)	
	All ages	200–300	26.6–39.9	2
		<200	<26.6	3
Pa_{CO_2}		(torr (mmHg))	(kPa)	
	All ages	51–65	6.8–8.7	1
		>65	>8.7	5
Pupillary reactions	All ages	Unequal or dilated		4
		Fixed and dilated		10
PT/PTT	All ages	1.5 times control		2
Total bilirubin (mg/dL)	>1 month	>3.5		6
Potassium (mEq/L)	All ages	3.0–3.5		1
		6.5–7.5		1
		<3.0		5
		>7.5		5
Calcium (mg/dL)	All ages	7.0–8.0		2
		12.0–15.0		2
		<7.0		6
		>15.0		6
Glucose (mg/dL)	All ages	40–60		4
		250–400		4
		<40		8
		>400		8
Bicarbonate (mEq/L)	All ages	<16		3
		>32		3

Infants: 0–1 year of age. PRISM score=(systolic blood pressure points)+(diastolic blood pressure points)+(heart rate points)+(respiratory rate points)+(oxygenation points)+(Glasgow Coma Score points)+(pupillary reaction points)+(coagulation points)+(bilirubin points)+(potassium points)+(calcium points)+(glucose points)+(bicarbonate points).

SEPSIS-RELATED ORGAN FAILURE ASSESSMENT (SOFA) SCORE

Easy to calculate, describes the sequence of complications in a critically ill patient rather than predicting outcome.

Organ system	Measure
Respiration	$Pa_{O_2} : Fi_{O_2}$ ratio
Coagulation	Platelet count
Liver	Serum bilirubin
Cardiovascular	Hypotension
Central nervous system	Glasgow Coma Score
Renal	Serum creatinine or urine output

Measure	Finding		Points
$Pa_{O_2} : Fi_{O_2}$ ratio	(mmHg)	(kPa)	
	≥400	≥53.2	0
	300–399	39.9– 53.1	1
	200–299	26.6–39.8	2
	100–199	13.3–26.5	3
	<100	<13.3	4
Platelet count	≥1500/μL		0
	1000–149 999/μL		1
	500–99 999/μL		2
	200–49 999/μL		3
	<200 per μL		4
Serum bilirubin	<1.2 mg/dL		0
	1.2–1.9 mg/dL		1
	2.0–5.9 mg/dL		2
	6.0–11.9 mg/dL		3
	≥12.0 mg/dL		4
Hypotension	(mmHg)	(kPa)	
	Mean arterial pressure ≥70	≥9.3	0
	Mean arterial pressure <70 then (no pressor agents used)	<9.3	1
	Dobutamine any dose		2
	Dopamine ≤5 μg/kg per min		2
	Dopamine >5–15 μg/kg per min		3
	Dopamine >15 μg/kg per min		4
	Epinephrine ≤0.1 μg/kg per min		3
	Epinephrine >0.1 μg/kg per min		4
	Norepinephrine ≤0.1 μg/kg per min		3
	Norepinephrine >0.1 μg/kg per min		4
Glasgow Coma Score	15		0
	13–14		1
	10–12		2
	6–9		3
	3–5		4
Serum creatinine or urine output	Serum creatinine <1.2 mg/dL		0
	Serum creatinine 1.2–1.9 mg/dL		1
	Serum creatinine 2.0–3.4 mg/dL		2
	Serum creatinine 3.5–4.9 mg/dL		3
	Urine output 200–499 mL/day		3
	Serum creatinine >5.0 mg/dL		4
	Urine output <200 mL/day		4

Pa_{O_2} is in mmHg/kPa and Fi_{O_2} in percentages, from 0.21 to 1.00. Adrenergic agents as administered for at least 1 hour with doses in μg/kg per min. A score of 0 indicates normal and a score of 4 indicates most abnormal. Data can be collected and the score calculated daily during the course of the admission. Interpretation: minimum total score: 0; maximum total score: 24. The higher the organ score, the greater is the organ dysfunction. The higher the total score, the greater is the multiorgan dysfunction.

MORTALITY RATE BY SOFA SCORE[1]

Organ system	0	1	2	3	4
Respiratory	20%	27%	32%	46%	64%
Cardiovascular	22%	32%	55%	55%	55%
Coagulation	35%	35%	35%	64%	64%
CNS	32%	34%	50%	53%	56%
Renal	25%	40%	46%	56%	64%

LOGISTIC ORGAN DYSFUNCTION SYSTEM (LODS)

Assess patients for severity of critical organ dysfunction. To predict the probability of death for the patient.

Data collection	During the first 24 hours in the ICU
Data point	If not measured then it is assumed to be normal for scoring purposes If several measurements, use the most severe value

LOD score=(neurological score)+(cardiovascular score)+(renal score)+(pulmonary score)+(haematological score)+(hepatic score).

NEUROLOGICAL SCORE

Glasgow coma score	Points
14–15	0
9–13	1
6–8	3
<6	5

Use lowest value. If sedated, estimate the score prior to sedation.

CARDIOVASCULAR SCORE

Heart rate (beats/min)		Systolic BP (mmHg)	Systolic BP (kPa)	Points
30–139	*and*	90–239	11.9–31.8	0
≥140	*or*	240–269	31.9–35.8	1
		70–89	9.3–11.8	1
		≥270	≥35.9	3
		40–69	5.3–9.2	3
<30	*or*	<40	<5.3	5

The most abnormal value for heart rate or systolic blood pressure, either minimum or maximum.

RENAL SCORE

Serum urea nitrogen (mg/dL)		Creatinine (mg/dL)		Urine output (L/d)	Points
<17	*and*	< 1.20	*and*	0.75–9.99	0
17–27.99	*or*	1.2–1.59			1
28–55.99	*or*	≥1.60	*or*	≥10	3
				0.5–0.74	3
≥56					5
				<0.5	5

Highest value for urea nitrogen and for creatinine; if the urine output data are for less than a 24-hour period, adjust that value to 24 hours, assuming the same rate of excretion. On haemodialysis, use the value of urine output prior to initiating haemodialysis

PULMONARY SCORE

On Ventilation or CPAP?		Ratio (Pa_{O_2} (mmHg) : Fi_{O_2})	Ratio (Pa_{O_2} (kPa) : Fi_{O_2})	Points
No				0
Yes	*and*	≥150	≥20	1
Yes	*and*	<150	<20	3

Respiratory support; use the lowest ratio of Pa_{O_2} to Fi_{O_2}.

HAEMATOLOGICAL SCORE

White blood cell count (10^9/L)		Platelet count (10^9/L)	Points
2.5–4.9/μL	*and*	≥50/μl	0
		≥50/μL	1
1–2.4/μL	*or*	<50/μL	1
<1/μL			3

Note: Most abnormal values for the white cell count are either minimum or maximum; minimum platelet count if several values are available.

HEPATIC SCORE[2]

Bilirubin		Prothrombin time	Points
<2.0 mg/dL (< 34.2 μmol/L)	*and*	≤3 seconds above standard (≥25% of standard)	0
≥2.0 mg/dL (≥34.2 μmol/L)	*or*	>3 seconds above standard (<25% of standard)	1

Highest value for bilirubin available. Highest value for prothrombin time in seconds.

MPM II, MORTALITY PROBABILITY MODELS[3,4]

Excluded
- Age <18 years
- Burn patients
- Coronary care patients
- Cardiac surgery patients
- (The scoring is either present or not present)

Definitions

Coma or deep stupor at time of ICU admission
- Not due to drug overdosage
- If patient is on paralysing muscle relaxant, awakening from anaesthesia or heavily sedated, use best judgement of the level of consciousness prior to sedation
- *Coma*: no response to any stimulation; no twitching, no movements in extremities, no response to pain or command; Glasgow Coma Score 3
- *Deep stupor*: decorticate or decerebrate posturing; posturing is spontaneous or in response to stimulation or deep pain; posturing is not in response to commands; Glasgow Coma Score 4 or 5

Heart rate at ICU admission
- Heart rate ≥150 beats/min within 1 hour before or after ICU admission

Systolic blood pressure at ICU admission
- Systolic blood pressure ≤90 mmHg (11.9 kPa) within 1 hour before or after ICU admission

Chronic renal compromise or insufficiency
- Elevation of serum creatinine >2 mg/dL and documented as chronic in the medical record
- If there is the acute diagnosis on chronic renal failure then record only yes for acute renal failure

Cirrhosis
- History of heavy alcohol use with portal hypertension and varices
- Other causes of liver disease with evidence of portal hypertension and varices
- Biopsy confirmation of cirrhosis

Metastatic malignant neoplasm
- Stage IV carcinomas with distant metastases
- Do not include involvement only of regional lymph nodes
- Include if metastases are obvious by clinical assessment or confirmed by a pathology report
- Do not include if metastases not obvious, or if pathology report is not available at the time of ICU admission
- Acute haematological malignancies are included
- Chronic leukaemias are not included unless there are findings attributable to the disease or the patient is under active treatment for the leukaemia. Findings include sepsis, anaemia, stroke caused by clumping of white blood cells, tumour lysis syndrome with elevated uric acid following chemotherapy, pulmonary oedema or the lymphangiectatic form of acute respiratory distress syndrome

Acute renal failure
- Acute tubular necrosis or acute diagnosis on chronic renal failure
- Prerenal azotaemia is not included

Cardiac dysrhythmia
- Cardiac arrhythmia, paroxysmal tachycardia, fibrillation with rapid ventricular response, second- or third-degree heart block
- Do not include chronic and stable arrhythmias

Cerebrovascular incident
- Cerebral embolism, occlusion, cerebrovascular accident, stroke, brainstem infarction, cerebrovascular arteriovenous malformation (acute stroke or cerebrovascular haemorrhage, not chronic arteriovenous malformation)

Gastrointestinal bleeding
- Haematemesis, melaena
- A perforated ulcer does not necessarily indicate GI bleeding; may be identified by obvious 'coffee grounds' in nasogastric tube
- A drop of haemoglobin by itself is not sufficient evidence of acute GI bleeding

Intracranial mass effect
- Intracranial mass (abscess, tumour, haemorrhage, subdural) as identified by CT scan associated with any of the following: (1) midline shift; (2) obliteration or distortion of cerebral ventricles; (3) gross haemorrhage in cerebral ventricles or subarachnoid space; (4) visible mass >4 cm; or (5) any mass that enhances with contrast media
- If the mass effect is known within 1 hour of ICU admission, it can be indicated as yes
- CT scanning is not mandated and is indicated only for patients with major neurological insult

Age in years
- Patient's age at last birthday

CPR within 24 hours prior to ICU admission
- CPR includes chest compression, defibrillation or cardiac massage
- Not affected by the location where the CPR was administered

Mechanical ventilation
- Patient is using a ventilator at the time of ICU admission or immediately thereafter

Medical or unscheduled surgery admission
- Do not include elective surgical patients (surgery scheduled at least 24 hours in advance) or preoperative Swan–Ganz catheter insertion in elective surgery patients

REFERENCES

1. Vincent JL, Moreno R, Takala J, et al. The SOFA (Sepsis-related Organ Failure Assessment) score to describe organ dysfunction/failure. Int Care Med 1996;22:707–10.
2. Le Gall J, Klar J, Lemeshow S, et al. The logistic organ dysfunction system. JAMA 1996;276:802–10.
3. Lemeshow S, Teres D, Klar J, et al. Mortality Probability Models (MPM II) based on an international cohort of intensive care patients. JAMA 1993;270:2478–86.
4. Lemeshow S, Le Gall J-R. Modeling the severity of illness of ICU patients. JAMA 1994;272:1049–55.

Index

Page numbers followed by 'f' indicate figures, 't' indicate tables, and 'b' indicate boxes.

A

B

C

D

H

I

M

O

P

Q

R

S

T

U

V

W

Y

Z